HANDBOOK OF PSYCHOPHYSIOLOGY

SECOND EDITION

This revised and expanded second edition of the *Handbook of Psychophysiology* replaces Professors Cacioppo and Tassinary's *Principles of Psychophysiology*. The revised second edition is an essential reference for students, researchers, and professionals in psychophysiology, psychology, psychiatry, neuroscience, and related biological and behavioral sciences.

This *Handbook* is divided into six sections covering topics such as the history of psychophysiology, systemic psychophysiology (ranging from the peripheral nervous system to the neuroendocrine and immune systems), principles of human behavior that have emerged from psychophysiological analyses, applications, and methodology. The final section of the *Handbook* provides detailed coverage of emerging topics in psychophysiology, including functional magnetic resonance imaging. With respect to fundamental psychological processes, this comprehensive reference discusses theoretical advances, empirical findings, and methodological developments and standards.

The scope and coverage of psychophysiology have expanded tremendously since the first edition of this book. This expanded second edition of the *Handbook of Psychophysiology* provides both a context for and coverage of the biological bases of cognition, emotion, and behavior. Psychophysiological methods, paradigms, and theories offer entry to a biological cosmos that does not stop at skin's edge, and this essential reference is designed as a road map for every explorer of this cosmos.

John T. Cacioppo is the Tiffany and Margaret Blake Distinguished Service Professor at the University of Chicago.

Louis G. Tassinary is Associate Professor of Architecture and Adjunct Professor of Psychology at Texas A & M University.

Gary G. Berntson is Professor of Psychology, Psychiatry, and Pediatrics at Ohio State University.

HANDBOOK OF PSYCHOPHYSIOLOGY

SECOND EDITION

Edited by

JOHN T. CACIOPPO
University of Chicago

LOUIS G. TASSINARY
Texas A & M University

GARY G. BERNTSON
Ohio State University

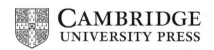

CAMBRIDGE
UNIVERSITY PRESS

PUBLISHED BY THE PRESS SYNDICATE OF THE UNIVERSITY OF CAMBRIDGE
The Pitt Building, Trumpington Street, Cambridge, United Kingdom

CAMBRIDGE UNIVERSITY PRESS
The Edinburgh Building, Cambridge CB2 2RU, UK   www.cup.cam.ac.uk
40 West 20th Street, New York, NY 10011-4211, USA   www.cup.org
10 Stamford Road, Oakleigh, Melbourne 3166, Australia
Ruiz de Alarcón 13, 28014 Madrid, Spain

First published 2000

Printed in the United States of America

Typefaces Sabon 9.75/12 and Univers   *System* AMS-TEX   [FH]

A catalog record for this book is available from the British Library

Library of Congress Cataloging in Publication Data
Handbook of psychophysiology / edited by John T. Cacioppo, Louis G.
Tassinary, Gary G. Berntson. – 2nd ed.
p. cm.
Rev. ed. of: Principles of psychophysiology.   1990.
Includes bibliographical references and index.
ISBN 0-521-62634-X (hardback)
1. Psychophysiology handbooks, manuals, etc.   I. Cacioppo, John
T.   II. Tassinary, Louis G.   III. Berntson, Gary G.   IV. Principles
of psychophysiology.
[DNLM: 1. Psychophysiology.   WL 103 H2363 2000]
QP360.P7515   2000
612.8 – dc21
DNLM/DLC
for Library of Congress   99-36718
                                                               CIP

ISBN 0 521 62634 X hardback

CONTENTS

PREFACE

Individuals are revered in Western societies for stolid independence, discerning perception, objective analyses, cultivated tastes, dispassionate analyses, and articulate disquisition. It is little surprise that those aspects of human discourse that can be articulated or timed have sometimes been accorded special status, set apart from millions of years of evolutionary forces, beyond the reach of the underlying biology. It is also a mistake. Equally mistaken are reductionistic approaches that anticipate the richness of the mind will be revealed comprehensively by peering through a membrane wall or while riding the human genome through behavioral terrain.

Even if evolution is too distant to inspect rigorously, its cousin, ontogeny, is not. During their early years, children demonstrate repeatedly that a great deal of human nature is shaped by biological forces, driven by bodily processes, and manifested in physiological events, only a subset of which are sometimes articulated verbally or behaviorally. From birth, reciprocal influences between social and physiological events are apparent and crucial to normal growth and development. In time, children acquire a keen faculty to comment on events, both internal and external, and to construe these events in terms of a coherent conceptualization. We are a species that ascribes meaning, so exploration, prediction, attribution, and control are not mere extravagances but rather heralds of a coherent state of being. However, like the organization and processes underlying the undeniable percept that the sun circles the earth, the organization and processes underlying human perception, reasoning, judgment, and behavior may be far subtler than apparent manifestations might lead one to suspect.

People routinely develop explanatory scenarios, but only the attentive and systematic observer tries also to disconfirm these accounts, to extend beyond common-sense observation and reasoning to do so, and to discover something about the governance of the world and of ourselves in doing so. This book is dedicated to the attentive and systematic observers who understand that, without contrivances to extend their faculties, the reach of their observations will fall short of their questions; that the Heisenberg principle is not limited to esoteric elements in physicists' laboratories or imaginations; that they cannot comprehend the full scope or processes of mental existence without delving into biological reality. We need instruments and intellectual tools to assist us in this endeavor. Psychophysiological methods, paradigms, and theories offer entry to a biological cosmos that does not stop at skin's edge. This book is designed as a road map for the explorer of this cosmos.

The most important instrument remains human genius, but psychophysiological methods, paradigms, and theories provide a gateway to a biological cosmos more fascinating and expansive than has been appreciated by most. This book is certainly not the first. The possibility that fundamental aspects of human nature might be discovered by focusing on the interaction between environmental stimuli and an information-processing organism was recognized more than 2,000 years ago. Only recently, however, have technological advances and scientific reasoning begun to enable investigators to use physiological principles and measures to address fundamental questions about the organization and governance of human nature and behavior.

Paralleling the growing interest in the concepts and methods of psychophysiology are technological developments in signal acquisition and analysis, as well as efforts in recent years to articulate standards for psychophysiological recording. As a result, psychophysiological analyses have never before been more powerful or accessible. Furthermore, decades of scientific research and debate on matters bridging the mind and brain have produced a wealth of knowledge that transcends techniques and measures. These developments have facilitated problem-oriented research in psychophysiology.

Despite important advances in and growing applications of psychophysiology, the last *Handbook of Psychophysiology* (Sternbach & Greenfield 1972) was published almost three decades ago, a stunning realization when one considers how active and vital the discipline is today. The scope and coverage of psychophysiology, as for most sciences over the same period, have expanded tremendously. No single book can cover completely all the diverse elements of psychophysiology, and we have not attempted to do so here. Instead, a major objective was to compile a technical sourcebook that would provide a broad context for and representative coverage of the basic and applied significance of contemporary research. We sought to cover materials at a level of scholarship that is informative to the specialist yet comprehensible to a thoughtful student of the discipline. In short, the book is designed to serve as a reference volume that we hope will be helpful to students and researchers for years to come. As such, it is perhaps most appropriate for a graduate course on psychophysiology, although various chapters could be used in conjunction with additional readings or texts in any number of topical graduate courses or seminars.

The book is divided into six parts: introduction, foundations, processes, applications, methodology, and appendices. Part One provides a brief introduction to the history, logic, and promise of the field of psychophysiology. The focus of Part Two is systemic psychophysiology, with chapters ranging from the activity or function of the human central (human electroencephalography, event-related brain potentials, brain imaging techniques, neuropsychology) and peripheral (electrodermal, cardiovascular, somatic, and gastrointestinal) nervous systems to the neuroendocrine (e.g., stress and sexual hormones) and immune (e.g., cellular, hormonal) systems. Each chapter is characterized by discussions of the physiological basis of the system and the responses of interest in psychophysiology, the technical issues involved in the recording and quantification of these physiological events, and the theory underlying psychological inferences based on these physiological events. Conceptual insights achieved in each area are also addressed.

The chapters in Part Three elaborate upon these foundations by highlighting principles of human behavior that have emerged from psychophysiological analyses. Included in this section are chapters on homeostasis and allostasis; visceral afference and interoception; attention, expectation, and learning; language processes; motivation and emotion; interpersonal and cultural processes; developmental states and processes; response selection, preparation, and execution; and altered states such as sleep and dreaming.

Coverage in Part Four complements the previous focus on basic processes in its emphasis on applications. Foremost among these in contemporary research are psychopathology, clinical health psychology, the detection of deception, human factors, and environmental design. A chapter on each topic is included.

Although the chapters in Part Two cover issues related to the extraction, analysis, and interpretation of physiological data, there are several important issues in psychophysiology that are sufficiently complex and general that they warrant tutorials of their own. Part Five is included for this purpose. It begins with a chapter on psychometric issues, which emphasizes the importance of a solid empirical foundation for the inferences that are to be drawn. Following are two chapters on statistical and design considerations; the first focuses on traditional psychophysiological measures and the second examines issues raised by imaging data. Part Five ends with a chapter on nonlinear analyses. Finally, the appendices in Part Six provide detailed coverage of two emerging topics in psychophysiology: laboratory safety and functional magnetic resonance imaging.

On a more personal note, we wish to thank the contributors to this book – all active researchers and scholars – who graciously consented to take time from their own research to prepare general and comprehensible reference chapters for other working scientists. We deeply appreciate the cooperation of these authors and offer our sincere thanks to all for the time and care expended in preparing their chapters. We would also like to thank our colleagues and students, from whom we have learned so much. And we thank our families and friends for their questions, suggestions, patience, support, and good humor.

CONTRIBUTORS

Peter A. Bandettini   *National Institute of Mental Health*
Jackson Beatty   *University of California – Los Angeles*
Gary G. Berntson   *Ohio State University*
Rasmus M. Birn   *Medical College of Wisconsin*
Margaret M. Bradley   *University of Florida*
K. A. Brownley   *University of North Carolina – Chapel Hill*
C. H. M. Brunia   *Tilburg University*
John T. Cacioppo   *University of Chicago*
Michael G. H. Coles   *University of Illinois*
Seana Coulson   *University of California – San Diego*
Antonio R. Damasio   *University of Iowa*
Richard J. Davidson   *University of Wisconsin – Madison*
Michael E. Dawson   *University of Southern California*
Amanda B. Diekman   *Northwestern University*
Kathleen M. Donahue   *Medical College of Wisconsin*
B. R. Dworkin   *Pennsylvania State University*
Monica Fabiani   *University of Missouri*
Kara D. Federmeier   *University of California – San Diego*
Diane L. Filion   *University of Kansas Medical Center*
Nathan A. Fox   *University of Maryland – College Park*
Shira Gabriel   *Northwestern University*
Wendi L. Gardner   *Northwestern University*
James H. Geer   *Louisiana State University*
Ronald Glaser   *Ohio State University*
Gabriele Gratton   *University of Missouri*
William A. Greene   *Eastern Washington University*
Robert A. M. Gregson   *Australian National University*
Alfons Hamm   *University of Greifswald*
Terry Hartig   *Uppsala University*
Andrew Harver   *University of North Carolina – Charlotte*
Heather A. Henderson   *University of Maryland – College Park*
Blair D. Hicks   *University of Illinois*
Kenneth Hugdahl   *University of Bergen*
B. E. Hurwitz   *University of Miami*
William G. Iacono   *University of Minnesota*
Laurie Iciek   *Loyola University Medical Center*
Daren C. Jackson   *University of Wisconsin – Madison*
Erick Janssen   *The Kinsey Institute*
J. Richard Jennings   *University of Pittsburgh*

Deborah J. Kasprowicz   *Loyola University Medical Center*
Jennifer Keller   *University of Illinois*
Janice K. Kiecolt-Glaser   *Ohio State University*
Jonathan W. King   *University of Missouri*
Kenneth L. Koch   *Milton S. Hershey Medical Center*
Christian Kohler   *University of Pennsylvania*
Arthur F. Kramer   *University of Illinois*
Marta Kutas   *University of California – San Diego*
Richard D. Lane   *University of Arizona*
Christine L. Larson   *University of Wisconsin – Madison*
Lisa Manzi Lentino   *Ohio State University*
Tyler S. Lorig   *Washington and Lee University*
William R. Lovallo   *University of Oklahoma*
Brennis Lucero-Wagoner   *California State University – Northridge*
Gregory A. Miller   *University of Illinois*
Tomas F. Münte   *University of California – San Diego*
Eric R. Muth   *Pennsylvania State University*
Arne Öhman   *Karolinska Institutet*
Russ Parsons   *University of Illinois*
R. T. Pivik   *Canadian Sleep Institute*
Jeffrey L. Pressing   *University of Melbourne*
Eric M. Reiman   *University of Arizona*
Virginia M. Sanders   *Loyola University Medical Center*
Anne M. Schell   *Occidental College*
Louis A. Schmidt   *McMaster University*
N. Schneiderman   *University of Miami*
Charles T. Snowdon   *University of Wisconsin – Madison*
Robert M. Stern   *Pennsylvania State University*
Lynn A. Stine   *University of Pittsburgh*
Catherine M. Stoney   *Ohio State University*
Michael J Strube   *Washington University*
Louis G. Tassinary   *Texas A & M University*
Terrie L. Thomas   *University of Oklahoma*
Daniel Tranel   *University of Iowa*
Bruce Turetsky   *University of Pennsylvania*
Bert N. Uchino   *University of Utah*
G. J. M. van Boxtel   *Tilburg University*
Cyma Van Petten   *University of Arizona*
Timothy Weber   *University of Illinois*
Toni E. Ziegler   *University of Wisconsin – Madison*

PART ONE

INTRODUCTION

CHAPTER ONE

PSYCHOPHYSIOLOGICAL SCIENCE

JOHN T. CACIOPPO, LOUIS G. TASSINARY, & GARY G. BERNTSON

What is the relationship between the mind and brain? Why is it that in intense fear and anger one's bodily processes feel as if they have a mind of their own? Do feelings and thoughts affect physiological processes and health? Can one learn to control physiological responses and, if so, does the control of these responses or the associated feedback from the responses modulate cognition and emotion? What is the basis of consciousness? How exactly does one person's mood spread to others? Psychophysiology is a field concerned with just such questions. In psychophysiology, the mind is viewed as having a physical substrate. Contrary to unidirectional reductionism, however, the mind is viewed as being more comprehensible if the structural and functional aspects of this physical substrate are considered in conjunction with broader aspects of the functional outputs of that substrate, including verbal, behavioral, and contextual data. As such, psychophysiology is an interdisciplinary field that emphasizes multiple levels of analysis.

It is an exciting time in the field of psychophysiology. Investigations of elementary physiological events in normal thinking, feeling, and interacting individuals are now feasible, and new techniques are providing windows through which psychological processes can be viewed unobtrusively. Instrumentation now makes it possible for investigators to explore the selective activation of discrete parts of the brain during particular psychological operations in normal individuals. Developments in ambulatory recording and computing equipment make it possible to measure peripheral physiological and endocrinological responses in naturalistic as well as laboratory settings. And the emergence of accepted recording standards, signal representation, and multivariate statistical analyses have facilitated study of the interrelationships among autonomic, somatic, brain, endocrinologic, and immunologic processes. However, the views from these windows are clear only because of the deliberate efforts of knowledgeable investigators.

Knowledge and principles of physiological mechanisms, biometric and psychometric properties of the measures, statistical representation and analysis of multivariate data, and the structure of psychophysiological inference are important if veridical information is to be extracted from psychophysiological data. These are among the topics covered in depth in this *Handbook*.

Objections have been raised to the notion that the mind can be understood any better by including investigation of its physiological manifestations. For instance, some have suggested that changes in consciousness are sufficient to explain social behavior, and that it is more important to study how people perceive and react to events than to reduce consciousness to physiological events (e.g. Allport 1947; Caldwell 1994). Consciousness has been classified in a variety of ways but is typically thought to include changes in awareness of emotions, needs, motives, cognitions, or expectations (cf. Kipnis 1997). However, concerns about the fragility of theoretical structures based on self-report data have been expressed for more than half a century (Cook & Selltiz 1964; Gutek 1978; Turner & Martin 1984). As Kipnis (1997) noted:

Unlike the physical and biological sciences, however, these classification systems describe dynamic mental processes that cannot be directly seen, touched, or measured.... Despite the splendor of these visions about how the mind works, these classifications are particularly vulnerable to challenge and replacement. This is because, as I said, there are no empirical procedures used to verify their independent existence. (p. 207)

Others have argued that we do not know, and are not soon to discover, the physical counterparts of psychological processes. Kipnis (1997), for instance, regarded the obstacles to discovering the physical counterparts to these dynamical processes as being overwhelming at present and therefore argued to explain "social behavior in relatively objective changes in technology, rather than in subjective changes in mental states" (p. 208).

There are undoubtedly psychological, social, and cultural phenomena whose secrets are not yet amenable to physiological analyses. Yet elementary cognitive and behavioral processes are being illuminated by psychophysiological methods, and more complex cognitive, affective, social, and clinical phenomena are increasingly succumbing to psychophysiological inquiries. Where most psychophysiologists differ from Kipnis (1997), therefore, is not in the importance placed on considering objective environmental factors and contexts, but rather in the value placed on pursuing the physical manifestations of psychological processes and of using biological data to inspire and constrain psychological research and theory.

Consider the range of human experiences that results from exposure to light. The human eye is a sensory receptor organ that is sensitive to only a narrow band of the electromagnetic spectrum. One could refer to this limited band of electromagnetic energy as the "psychological" domain, since electromagnetic phenomena falling within this band have clear and obvious effects on human experience. However, the visible light band is but a small part of a broader, coherent spectrum of electromagnetic energy that can also influence human experience and behavior and that can be revealed through the use of specialized equipment to extend the reaches of the human senses. Exposure to ultraviolet light, although imperceptible to the human eye, can alter visual perception by damaging receptors in the eye, or it can influence behavior indirectly by producing sunburn; exposure to infrared light, which is also imperceptible to the human eye, can affect thermal sensations as well as body temperature. Knowledge of the broader organization of the electromagnetic spectrum and its relationship to human vision also makes it possible to design specialized instruments that render ultraviolet and infrared light visible to the human eye. These developments, and our understanding of the effects of electromagnetic energy on various aspects of human behavior, would not be likely if methods were limited to verbal reports and observations limited to the band of visible light. An illustration is the "blindsight" of patients with visual cortical damage, who can accurately respond to light without conscious awareness (Weiskrantz 1986).

Recent studies further indicate that visual perception is not simply a faithful representation of the image cast by a stimulus on the retina; rather, it is a neural image formed by neural mechanisms over the entire visual pathway. When the visual features of an external stimulus produce the experience of a different external stimulus, we call it an illusion. This label does not explain the discrepancy between the external stimulus and the conscious experience of this stimulus, but recent psychophysiological investigations demonstrate how such a discrepancy may occur. Tootell et al. (1995), for instance, used functional magnetic resonance imaging (fMRI) to observe brain activity as individuals watched an expanding grid on a screen and again as individuals viewed the grid when it stopped expanding. When the grid stops expanding, individuals experience an illusion that makes it appear as if the grid is contracting rather than sitting motionless on the screen, an illusion known as the waterfall effect. Tootell et al. (1995) found that activity in the medial temporal (MT) region of the visual system continued during this illusion. These results, combined with animal studies in which stimulation of neurons in the MT region affected visual perception, are consistent with the notion that the pattern of neuronal activity in visual pathways (rather than the external stimulus per se) gives rise to the visual perception of movement.

Studies of the psychophysiology of cold provide another illustration of how consciousness can fit within a broader theoretical context, the nature of which would not be evident by an exclusive focus on verbal reports of feeling states. Physiological processes are temperature-sensitive, and various mechanisms have evolved to maintain core body temperature within the narrow ranges necessary for normal functioning. Most of these mechanisms (e.g., decreased eccrine gland activity to reduce cooling through evaporation, peripheral vasoconstriction to shunt heated blood away from the surface of the skin, shivering to produce additional body heat) are initiated and can operate entirely outside the range of consciousness. If automatic adjustments to raise body temperature prove insufficient, the individual becomes aware of the cold and of the need for willful action to raise body temperature. Mentation can also foster behavioral flexibility and creative adaptation. In this example an individual's actions could take any of a variety of forms, ranging from donning additional clothing to moving to a warmer environment. Thus, consciousness is not a divine endowment that orchestrates the organism's actions from a site on high but instead reflects brain processes that evolved because they confer adaptive advantage to the species. Consciousness may facilitate our ability to establish goals, engage in exploratory behavior, anticipate and predict rewards and punishments, contemplate the likely outcomes of behavioral options, learn vicariously, engage in counterfactual reasoning, and more. But rather than viewing consciousness as the ultimate achievement of the human species that can only be understood unto itself, most psychophysiologists view consciousness as an important but narrow band of influences, instantiated in brain processes and relevant to the governance of human experience and behavior. In this regard, the approach followed by contemporary psychophysiologists is reminiscent of that first adopted by seventeenth-century astronomers:

Nothing could be more obvious than that the earth is stable and unmoving, and that we are the center of the universe. Modern Western science takes its beginning from the denial of this commonsense axiom.... Common sense, the foundation of everyday life, could no longer serve for the governance of the world. When "scientific" knowledge, the sophisticated product of complicated instruments and subtle calculations, provided unimpeachable truths, things were no longer as they seemed. (Boorstin 1983, p. 294)

Accordingly, psychophysiological research has provided insights into almost every facet of human nature, from the attention and behavior of the neonate to memory and emotions in the elderly. This book is about these insights and advances – what they are, the methods by which they came about, and the conceptualizations that are guiding progress toward future advances in the discipline.

Historically, the study of psychophysiological phenomena has been susceptible to "easy generalizations, philosophical pitfalls, and influences from extrascientific quarters" (Harrington 1987, p. 5). Our objectives in this chapter are to define psychophysiology, review briefly major historical events in the evolution of psychophysiological inference, outline a taxonomy of logical relationships between psychological constructs and physiological events, and specify a scheme for strong inference within each of the specified classes of psychophysiological relationships.

The Conceptualization of Psychophysiology

"The body is the medium of experience and the instrument of action. Through its actions we shape and organise our experiences and distinguish our perceptions of the outside world from sensations that arise within the body itself" (Miller 1978, p. 14). Anatomy, physiology, and psychophysiology are all branches of science organized around bodily systems whose collective aim is to elucidate the structure and function of the parts of and interrelated systems in the human body in transactions with the environment. Anatomy is the science of body structure and the relationships among structures.

Physiology concerns the study of bodily function or how the parts of the body work. For both of these disciplines, what constitutes a "body part" varies with the level of bodily organization, ranging from the molecular to cellular to tissue to organ to body system to the organism. Thus, the anatomy and physiology of the body are intricately interrelated.

Psychophysiology is intimately related to anatomy and physiology but is also concerned with psychological phenomena – the experience and behavior of organisms in the physical and social environment. The complexity added when moving from physiology to psychophysiology includes both the capacity by symbolic systems of representation (e.g., language and mathematics) to communicate and to reflect upon history and experience as well as the social and cultural influences on physiological response and behavior. These factors contribute to plasticity,

adaptability, and variability in behavior. Psychology and psychophysiology share the goal of explaining human experience and behavior, and physiological constructs and processes are an explicit and integral component of theoretical thinking in psychophysiology.

The technical obstacles confronting early studies, the importance of understanding the physiological systems underlying observations, and the diverse goals and interests of the early investigators in the field fostered a partitioning of the discipline into areas of physiology and measurement. The organization of psychophysiology in terms of underlying physiological systems, or what can be called *systemic psychophysiology*, remains important today for theoretical and pedagogical reasons. Physiological systems provide the foundation for human processes and behavior and are often the target of systematic observation. An understanding of the physiological system(s) under study and the bioelectrical principles underlying the responses being measured contributes to plausible hypotheses, appropriate operationalizations, laboratory safety, discrimination of signal from artifact, acquisition and analysis of physiological events, legitimate inferences based on the data, and theoretical advancement.

Psychophysiology – like anatomy, physiology, and psychology – is a broad science organized in terms of a thematic as well as a systemic focus. The organization of psychophysiology in terms of topical areas of research can be called *thematic psychophysiology*. For instance, cognitive psychophysiology concerns the relationship between elements of human information processing and physiological events. Social psychophysiology concerns the study of the cognitive, emotional, and behavioral effects of human association as related to and revealed by physiological measures, including the reciprocal relationship between physiological and social systems. Developmental psychophysiology deals with ontological changes in psychophysiological relationships as well as the study of psychological development and aging through noninvasive physiological measurements. Clinical psychophysiology concerns the study of disorders in the organismic–environmental transactions and ranges from the assessment of disorders to interventions and treatments. Environmental psychophysiology elucidates the vagaries of organism–place interdependencies as well as the health consequences of design through unobtrusive physiological measurements. And applied psychophysiology deals with the implementation of psychophysiological principles in practice, such as operant training ("biofeedback"), desensitization, relaxation, and the detection of deception.

In each of these areas, the focus of study draws on but goes beyond the description of the structure or function of cells or organs in order to investigate the organism in transactions with the physical or sociocultural environment. Some of these areas, such as developmental psychophysiology, have counterparts in anatomy and physiology but refer to complementary empirical domains that focus on human experience and behavior. Others, such as social psychophysiology, have a less direct counterpart in anatomy or physiology because the focus begins beyond that of an organism in isolation. Yet the influence of social and cultural factors on physiological structures and functions, and their influence as moderators of the effects of physical stimuli on physiological structures and functions, leaves little doubt as to the relevance of these factors for anatomy and physiology as well as for psychophysiology (see e.g. Barchas 1976; Cacioppo & Petty 1983; Cacioppo, Petty, & Andersen 1988; Waid 1984). For instance, Meaney and colleagues (1996) provided evidence that rat pups who are ignored by their mothers develop a more reactive hypothalamic pituitary adrenocortical (HPA) axis than rat pups who are licked and groomed by their mothers.

Psychophysiology is intimately related to anatomy and physiology, and knowledge of the physiological systems and responses under study contribute to both theoretical and methodological aspects of psychophysiological research. However, as noted by Coles, Gratton, and Gehring (1987), knowledge of the physiological systems, though contributory, is logically neither necessary nor sufficient to ascribe psychological meaning to physiological responses. The ascription of psychological meaning to physiological responses ultimately resides in factors such as the quality of the experimental design, the psychometric properties of the measures, and the appropriateness of the data analysis and interpretation. For instance, although numerous aspects of the physiological basis of event-related brain potentials remain uncertain, functional relationships within specific paradigms have been established between elementary cognitive operations and components of these potentials by systematically varying one or more of the former while monitoring changes in the latter.

The point is not that either the physiological or the psychological perspective is preeminent, but rather that both are fundamental to psychophysiological inquiries; more specifically, that physiological and psychological perspectives are complementary. Inattention to the logic underlying psychophysiological inferences simply because one is dealing with observable physiological events is likely to lead either to simple and restricted descriptions of empirical relationships or to erroneous interpretations of these relationships. Similarly, "an aphysiological attitude, such as is evident in some psychophysiological research, is likely to lead to misinterpretation of the empirical relationships that are found between psychophysiological measures and psychological processes or states" (Coles, Donchin, & Porges 1986, pp. ix–x). Thus, whether organized in terms of a systemic or a thematic focus, psychophysiology can be conceptualized as a natural extension of anatomy and physiology in the scientific pursuit of understanding human processes and behavior. It is the joint consideration of physiological and functional perspectives, however, that is thought to improve operationalization, measurement, and

inference and therefore to enrich research and theory on cognition, emotion, and behavior.

There has been little consensus regarding the formal definition of psychophysiology. Some of the early definitions of the field were in operational terms such as research in which the polygraph was used, research published by workers in the field, and research on physiological responses to behavioral manipulations (Ax 1964b; Furedy 1983). Other early definitions were designed to differentiate psychophysiology from the older and more established field of physiological psychology or psychobiology. Initially, psychophysiology differed from physiological psychology in the use of humans in contrast to animals as participants, the manipulation of psychological or behavioral constructs rather than anatomical structures or physiological processes, and the measurement of physiological rather than behavioral responses (Stern 1964). Although this heritage is still in evidence, this distinction is often blurred by psychophysiologists who modify physiology with drugs or conditioning procedures and by psychobiologists who manipulate psychological or behavioral variables and measure physiological outcomes. Contemporary definitions are more likely to emphasize the mapping of the relationships between and mechanisms underlying psychological and physiological events (e.g. Ackles, Jennings, & Coles 1985; Hugdahl 1995).

A major problem in reaching a consensus has been the need to give the field direction and identity by distinguishing it from other scientific disciplines while not limiting its potential for growth. Operational definitions are unsatisfactory for they do not provide long-term direction for the field. Definitions of psychophysiology as studies in which psychological factors serve as independent variables and physiological responses serve as dependent variables distinguish it from fields such as psychobiology, but they have been criticized as being too restrictive (Coles 1988; Furedy 1983). For instance, such definitions exclude studies in which physiological events serve as the independent/blocking variable and human experience or behavior serve as the dependent variable (e.g., the sensorimotor behavior associated with manipulations of the physiology via drugs or operant conditioning, or with endogenous changes in cardiovascular or electroencephalographic activity), as well as studies comparing changes in physiological responses across known groups (e.g, the cardiovascular reactivity of offspring of hypertensive versus normotensive parents).

Moreover, psychophysiology and psychobiology – as well as behavioral, cognitive, and social neuroscience – share goals, assumptions, experimental paradigms, and sometimes databases, but they differ primarily in terms of analytic focus. In psychophysiology, the emphasis is on integrating data from multiple levels of analysis to illuminate psychological functions and mechanisms rather than physiological structures per se. All of these substantive areas have a great deal to contribute to one another, and ideally this complementarity should not be masked in their definition by the need to distinguish these fields. Indeed, the formulation of structure–function relationships is advanced to the extent that "top down" and "bottom up" information can be integrated.

At present, for instance, there are fundamental limitations in the ability of psychophysiological measures such as brain imaging to accurately reveal functional localization (Barinaga 1997; Sarter, Berntson, & Cacioppo 1996a). Even for functions that are in fact localized to specific neural circuits, these circuits may: be diffusely organized or widely distributed; overlap anatomically or even share common neuronal elements with circuits mediating different functions; or perform different functions (e.g., facilitate or inhibit a given operation) depending on the patterns of input and activation associated with different cognitive states or contexts. These possibilities would clearly complicate efforts to elucidate the cerebral localization of functions. Activation of diffusely organized circuits (or components of circuits), for example, may not yield a sufficiently intense signal to be differentiated from noise or from activity patterns of control tasks. This could lead to a failure to detect a localized function. Alternatively, a focal, detected region within a larger undetected area of activation could lead to an overestimate of the degree of functional localization. Similarly, the existence of functionally distinct but overlapping circuits could lead to an underestimate of the degree of functional localization, as the overlapping area would be activated during multiple cognitive or behavioral contexts.

Perhaps the more problematic possibility is that some central circuits may have differential and overlapping functions depending on the pattern of activation. A helpful example is provided by the research on the functions of "state-setting" systems (Mesulam 1990), particularly the attentional functions mediated via cortical cholinergic and noradrenergic afferents (Sarter et al. 1996b). Research in this area has resulted in fairly specific hypotheses about (i) the attentional processes that depend on the integrity of cortical cholinergic and noradrenergic afferents and (ii) the key role of attentional dysfunctions based on aberrations in activity of these systems in major neuropsychiatric disorders (Robbins & Everitt 1987; Sarter 1994; Sarter & Bruno 1994). Whereas imaging studies have pointed to cortical areas in frontal, temporal, and parietal lobes that may be involved in various types of attention (Cohen et al. 1992; Corbetta et al. 1990, 1991; Grossman et al. 1992; Pardo, Fox, & Raichle 1991; Posner et al. 1988; Posner & Petersen 1990), more "bottom up" approaches aim at the determination of the specific role of acetylcholine in different cortical areas in attentional functions (Metherate & Weinberger 1990).

An understanding of the role of the major afferent projections to cortical areas in attention is facilitated by a convergence of evidence from imaging studies in human patients and from animal studies on the cognitive effects of manipulations of the activity of cortical inputs (Sarter et al. 1996a). Imaging studies may continue to relate sustained attention to prefrontal and superior parietal areas (Pardo et al. 1991), for example, and decreases in the activity in these areas may indeed be associated with the cognitive decline in dementia (Mielke et al. 1994). In isolation, however, the imaging approach is unlikely to reveal the precise functional contribution of individual afferent systems of these areas and, more generally, cannot discriminate different neuronal activity patterns leading to identical signal levels. The point is not to contrast or even prioritize the heuristic power of psychophysiological (top-down) or psychobiological (bottom-up) approaches but rather to illustrate the significance of integrating relevant evidence from psychophysiology and the neurosciences.

The emergence of areas of research in psychoneuroendocrinology (Frankenhauser 1983; Grunberg & Singer 1990; Mason 1972), behavioral neurology (Lindsley 1951; Tranel & Damasio 1985), and psychoneuroimmunology (Ader 1981; Glaser & Kiecolt-Glaser 1994; Henry & Stephens 1977; Jermott & Locke 1984) raises additional questions about the scope of psychophysiology. It is important to note that anatomy and physiology encompass the fields of neurology, endocrinology, and immunology owing to their common goals and assumptions as well as to the embodiment, in a literal sense, of the nervous, endocrine, and immunologic systems within the organism.

Psychophysiology, therefore, is based on the assumptions that human perception, thought, emotion, and action are embodied phenomena, and that physical (e.g. neural and hormonal) responses can shed light on human nature. The level of analysis in psychophysiology is not on isolated components of the body but rather on organismic–environmental transactions. That is, psychophysiology represents a top-down approach within the neurosciences that complements the bottom-up approach of psychobiology. Thus, psychophysiology can be defined as the scientific study of social, psychological, and behavioral phenomena as related to and revealed through physiological principles and events in functional organisms.

In the following section, we review some of the major historical developments that have influenced contemporary thinking and research in psychophysiology. As might be expected from the discussion thus far, many of these early developments stemmed from studies of human anatomy and physiology.

Historical Developments

Psychophysiology is still quite young as a scientific field. Studies dating back to the turn of the century can be found involving the manipulation of a psychological factor and the measurement of one or more physiological responses (Berger 1929; Darrow 1929; Eng 1925; Jacobson 1930; Mosso 1896; Peterson & Jung 1907; Sechenov 1878;

Tarchanoff 1890; Wenger 1941; Wilder 1931; see also Wood-worth & Schlosberg 1954), and such studies would now be considered as falling squarely under the rubric of psychophysiology. Chester Darrow (1964), in the inaugural Presidential Address of the Society for Psychophysiological Research, identified Darwin (1873), Vigoroux (1879), James (1884), and Fere (1888) as among the field's earliest pioneers. Yet the first scientific periodical devoted exclusively to psychophysiological research, the *Psychophysiology Newsletter,* was not published until 1955 as an outgrowth of the *Polygraph Newsletter* (Ax 1964a). The Society for Psychophysiological Research was formed five years later, and the first issue of the scientific journal *Psychophysiology* was published but a quarter century ago. Precisely when psychophysiology emerged as a discipline is therefore difficult to specify, but it is usually identified with the formation of the Society for Psychophysiological Research in 1960 or with the publication in 1964 of the first issue of *Psychophysiology* (Fowles 1975; Greenfield & Sternbach 1972; Sternbach 1966).

Although psychophysiology as a formal discipline is less than 50 years old, interest in interrelationships between psychological and physiological events can be traced as far back as the early Egyptian and Greek philosopher–scientists. The Greek philosopher Heraclitus (c. 600 B.C.) referred to the mind as an overwhelming space whose boundaries could never be fully comprehended (Bloom, Lazerson, & Hofstadter 1985). Plato (c. 400 B.C.) suggested that rational faculties were located in the head; passions were located in the spinal marrow and, indirectly, the heart; and instincts were located below the diaphragm where they influenced the liver. Plato also believed the psyche and body to be fundamentally different; hence, observations of physiological responses provided no grounds for inference about the operation of psyche (Stern, Ray, & Davis 1980). Thus, despite the fact that the peripheral and central nervous system, brain, and viscera were known to exist as anatomical entities by the early Greek scientist–philosophers, human nature was dealt with as a noncorporeal entity not amenable to empirical study.

In the second century A.D., Galen (c. 130–200) formulated a theory of psychophysiological function that would dominate thought well into the eighteenth century (Brazier 1959, 1961; Wu 1984). Hydraulics and mechanics were the technology of the times, and aqueducts and sewer systems were the most notable technological achievements during this period. Bloom et al. (1985) suggested: "It is hardly by accident, then, that Galen believed the important parts of the brain to lie not in the brain's substance, but in its fluid-filled cavities" (p. 13). Based on his animal dissections and his observations of the variety of fluids that permeated the body, Galen postulated that humors (fluids) were responsible for all sensation, movement, thoughts, and emotion, and that pathologies – physiological or behavioral – were based on humoral disturbances. The role of bodily organs was to produce or process these humors, and the nerves, although recognized as instrumental in thought and action, were assumed to be part of a hydraulic system through which the humors traveled. Galen's views became so deeply entrenched in Western thought that they went practically unchallenged for almost 1,500 years.

In the sixteenth century, Jean Fernel (1497–1558) published the first textbook on physiology, *De Naturali Parte Medicinae* (1542). According to Brazier (1959), this book was well received, and Fernel revised and expanded the book across numerous editions. The ninth edition of the book was retitled *Medicina,* and the first section was entitled *Physiologia.* Although Fernel's categorization of empirical observations was strongly influenced by Galen's theory, the book "shows dawning recognition of some of the automatic movements which we now know to be reflexly initiated" (Brazier 1959, p. 2). This represented a marked departure from traditional views that segregated the control of human action and the affairs of the corporeal world.

Studies of human anatomy (e.g. Vesalius 1543/1947) during this period in history also began to uncover errors in Galen's descriptions, opening the way for questions of his methods and of his theory of physiological functioning and symptomatology. Within a century, two additional events occurred that had a profound impact on the nature of inference in psychophysiology. In 1600, William Gilberd (1544–1603) recognized a difference between electricity and magnetism and, more importantly, argued (in his book, *Magnete*) that empirical observations and experiments should replace "the probable guesses and opinions of the ordinary professors of philosophy."

In addition, the reign of authority as the source of answers to questions about the basis of human experience and behavior was challenged by the work of such scholars as Galileo, Bacon, and Newton. Galileo (1564–1642) challenged knowledge by authority in matters of science, by which Galileo meant physical sciences and mathematics. He argued that theologians and philosophers had no right to control scientific investigation or theories and that observation, experiment, and reason alone could establish physical truth (Drake 1967). Galileo was also aware of limitations of sense data. Concerned with the possibility of illusion and misinterpretation, Galileo believed that mathematics alone offered the kind of certainty that could be completely trusted. Galileo did not extend this reasoning beyond the physical sciences, but scientific investigations of the basis of human experience and behavior benefited from his rejection of authority as a source of knowledge about physical reality, his emphasis on the value of skepticism, and his insistence that more could be learned from results that suggested ignorance (disconfirmation) than from results that fit preconceptions (confirmation).

Francis Bacon (1561–1626) took the scientific method a step further in *Novum Organum* (1620/1855), adding induction to observation and adding verification to inference.

Bacon was not a scientist, yet he is regarded as a fore-runner of the hypothetico-deductive method (Brazier 1959; Caws 1967). Bacon's formulation and subsequent work on the logic of scientific inference (cf. Platt 1964; Popper 1959/1968) led to the now-familiar sequence underlying scientific inference: (1) devise alternative hypotheses; (2) devise a crucial experiment with alternative possible outcomes, each of which will disfavor if not exclude one or more of the hypotheses; (3) execute the experiment to obtain a clear result; and (4) recycle to refine the remaining possibilities. Such a scheme was accepted quickly in the physical sciences, but traditional philosophical and religious views segregating human existence from worldly events slowed its acceptance in the study of human physiology, experience, and behavior (Brazier 1977; Harrington 1987; Mecacci 1979).

William Harvey's (1578–1657) doctoral dissertation, "De Motu Cordis" (1628/1931), represented the first major work to use these principles to guide inferences about physiological functioning, and it also disconfirmed Galen's principle that the motion of the blood in the arterial and venous systems ebbed and flowed independently of one another (except for some leakage in the heart). Pumps were an important technological development during the seventeenth century, and Harvey perhaps drew on his observations of pumps in positing that blood circulated continuously through a circular system, pushed along by the pumping actions of the heart and directed through and out of the heart by the one-way valves in each chamber of the heart. Galen, in contrast, had posited that blood could flow in either direction in the veins. To test these competing hypotheses, Harvey tied a tourniquet above the elbow of his arm – just tight enough to prevent blood from returning to the heart through the veins, but not so tight as to prevent blood from entering the arm through the arteries. The veins swelled below but not above the tourniquet, implying that the blood could be entering only through the arteries and exiting only through the veins (Miller 1978). A variation on Harvey's procedure is used in contemporary psychophysiology to gauge blood flow to vascular beds.

During this period, which coincided with a world now burgeoning with machines, the human eye was conceived as functioning like an optical instrument. Images were conceived as projected onto the sensory nerves of the retina. Movement was thought to reflect the mechanical actions of passive ballonlike structures (muscles) that were inflated or deflated by the nervous fluids or gaseous spirits that traveled through canals in the nerves. And higher mental functions were still considered by many to fall outside the rubric of the physical or biological sciences (Bloom et al. 1985; Brazier 1959; Harrington 1987). The writings of René Descartes (1596–1650) reflect the presumed division between the mind and body. The actions of animals were viewed as reflexive and mechanistic in nature, as were most of the actions of humans. But humans alone, Descartes argued, also possess a consciousness of self and of events around them – a consciousness that (like the body) was a thing but (unlike the body) was not a thing governed by material principles or connections. This independent entity called "mind," Descartes proposed, presides over volition from the soul's control tower in the pineal gland located at the center of the head:

The soul or mind squeezed the pineal gland this way and that, nudging the animal fluids in the human brain into the pores or valves, "and according as they enter or even only as they tend to enter more or less into this or that nerve, they have the power of changing the form of the muscle into which the nerve is inserted, and by this means making the limbs move." (quoted in Jaynes 1973, p. 172)

Shortly following Descartes' publication of *Traite de l'Homme* (c. 1633), Steno (1638–1686) noted several discrepancies between Descartes' dualistic and largely mechanistic characterization of human processes and the extant evidence about animal and human physiology. For instance, Steno noted that the pineal gland (the purported bridge between the worlds of the human mind and body) existed in animals as well as humans, that the pineal gland did not have the rich nerve supply implied by Descartes' theory, and that the brain was unnecessary to many animal movements (cf. Jaynes 1973). Giovanni Borelli (1608–1679) disproved the notion that movement was motivated by the inflation of muscles by a gaseous substance. Borelli conducted experiments in which he submerged a struggling animal in water, slit its muscles, and looked for the release of bubbles (Brazier 1959). These observations were published posthumously in 1680, shortly after the suggestion by Francesco Redi that the shock of the electric ray fish was muscular in origin (Basmajian & DeLuca 1985, chap. 1; Wu 1984).

Despite the prevalent belief during this period that the scientific study of animal and human behavior could apply only to those structures they shared in common (Bloom et al. 1985; Harrington 1987), the foundations laid by the great seventeenth-century scientist–philosophers encouraged students of anatomy and physiology in the subsequent century to discount explanatory appeals to the human soul or mind (Brazier 1959). Consequently, experimental analyses of physiological events and psychological constructs (e.g., sensation, involuntary and voluntary action) expanded and inspired the application of technological advances to the study of psychophysiological questions. For instance, the microscope was employed (unsuccessfully) in the late seventeenth century to examine the prevalent belief that the nerves were small pipes through which nervous fluid flowed.

According to Brazier (1959, 1977), that electricity might be the transmitter of nervous action was initially seen as unlikely because, drawing upon the metaphor of electricity running down a wire, there was believed to be insufficient insulation around the nerves to prevent a dissipation of the electrical signal. Galvani and Volta's (c. 1800) experiments demonstrated that nerves and muscles were indeed electrically excitable, and research by Du Bois-Reymond (1849) established that nerves and muscles were electrically polarized as well as excitable. Based on reaction times, Helmholtz (c. 1850) correctly inferred that nerves and muscles were not like wires because they propagated electrical impulses too slowly. The work that followed ultimately verified that neural signals and muscular actions were electrical in nature, that these electrical signals were the result of biochemical reactions within specialized cells, and that there was indeed some dissipation of these electrical signals through the body fluids, dissipation that could be detected noninvasively at the surface of the skin. Specific advances during the nineteenth and twentieth centuries in psychophysiological theory and research are discussed in the remainder of this book. However, the stage had been set by these early investigators for the scientific study of psychophysiological relationships.

Psychophysiological Relationships and Psychophysiological Inference

We praise the "lifetime of study," but in dozens of cases, in every field, what was needed was not a lifetime but rather a few short months or weeks of analytical inductive inference.... We speak piously of taking measurements and making small studies that will "add another brick to the temple of science." Most such bricks just lie around the brickyard. (Platt 1964, p. 351)

The importance of the development of more advanced recording procedures to scientific progress in psychophysiology is clear, as previously unobservable phenomena are rendered observable. Less explicitly studied, but no less important, is the structure of scientific thought about psychophysiological phenomena. For instance, Galen's notions about psychophysiological processes persisted for 1,500 years – despite the availability for several centuries of procedures for disconfirming his theory – in part because the structure of scientific inquiry had not been developed sufficiently (Brazier 1959).

An important form of psychophysiological inference to evolve from the work of Francis Bacon (1620/1855) and Galileo (Drake 1967) is the hypothetico-deductive logic outlined previously (cf. Platt 1964; Popper 1959/1968). If the data are consistent with only one of the theoretical hypotheses, then the alternative hypotheses with which the investigator began become less plausible. With conceptual replications to ensure the construct validity, replicability, and generalizability of such a result, a subset of the original hypotheses can be discarded, and the investigator recycles through this sequence. One weakness of this procedure is the myriad sources of variance in psychophysiological investigations and the stochastic nature of physiological events, resulting in the sometimes poor replicability or

generalizability of the results. A second weakness is the intellectual invention and omniscience required to specify all relevant alternative hypotheses for the phenomenon of interest. Because neither of these shortcomings can be overcome with certitude, progress in the short term can be slow and uncertain. However, adherence to this sequence provides grounds for strong inference in the long term (Platt 1964).

SUBTRACTIVE METHOD IN PSYCHOPHYSIOLOGY

Physiological responses are often of interest only to the extent that they allow one to index a psychological process, state, or stage. A general analytic framework that has aided the design and interpretation of psychophysiological investigations is the "subtractive" method, which has been adapted from studies of mental chronometry (Donders 1868; cf. Cacioppo & Petty 1986; Coles 1989). At the simplest level, experimental design begins with an experimental and a control condition. The experimental condition represents the presence of some factor, and the control condition represents the absence of this factor. The experimental factor might be selected because it is theoretically believed to harbor n information processing stages, and the construction of the control condition is guided to incorporate $n - 1$ information processing stages. Differences between these conditions (e.g., on reaction time measures) are thought to reflect the impact (e.g. duration) of the nth information processing stage.

The principle underlying the inclusion of physiological measures in these designs is twofold: (a) physiological differences between experimental conditions thought to represent n and $n - 1$ processing stages support the theoretical differentiation of these stages; and (b) the nature of the physiological differentiation of experimental conditions (e.g., the physiological signature of a processing stage) may further support a particular psychological characterization of that information processing stage. According to the subtractive method, the systematic application of "stage deletion" makes it possible to deduce the physiological signature of each of the constituent stages underlying some psychological or behavioral response. For instance, if the experimental task ($n + 1$ stages) requires 50 msec longer to complete than the control task (n stages), this result is consistent with the theoretical conception of the experimental and control tasks differing in one (or more) processing stage(s) as well as with the differential processing stage(s) requiring approximately 50 msec to perform. Similarly, if the experimental task is characterized by greater activation of Broca's area than the control task, this is consistent with both the theoretical conception of the experimental and control tasks differing in one (or more) processing stage(s) and the differential processing stage(s) relating to language production.

When one of these stages is thought to be responsible for the differential impact of two conditions on behavior, analyses of concomitant physiological activity can again be informative in one of two ways. If the patterns of physiological activity resulting from the isolation of presumably identical stages are dissimilar, then the similarity of the stages is challenged even though there may be similarities between the subsequent behavioral outcomes. The greater the evidence from multiple operationalizations that a particular stage is accompanied by a specific physiological profile across the ranges of stimuli employed in the investigations, the more challenging is the dissimilarity in obtained physiological profiles (Cacioppo & Petty 1986).

If, on the other hand, similar patterns of physiological activity result from the isolation of stages that are hypothesized to be identical, convergent evidence is obtained that the same fundamental stage is operative. These data do not provide strong evidence that the stages are the same; still, the more peculiar the physiological profile is to a given stage within a particular experimental context, the greater the value of the convergent evidence (Cacioppo & Tassinary 1990).

There are two additional issues that should be considered when using a subtractive framework to investigate elementary stages of psychological processes. First, the subtractive method contains the implicit assumption that a stage can be inserted or deleted without changing the nature of the other constituent stages. But this method has long been criticized for ignoring the possibility that manipulating a factor to insert or delete a processing stage might introduce a completely different processing structure. Using multiple operationalizations to insert or delete a stage may be helpful but, as outlined in what follows, this does not ensure strong logical grounds for inference. If each operational insertion or deletion of a stage has the same effect, then investigators may have greater confidence that these effects are attributable to the conceptual processing stage of interest, or at least that the effects are not an artifact of an unintended confound. Parametric studies of each processing stage can also provide important information about the range over which a stage manifests as a particular physiological profile, thereby improving investigators' ability to generate appropriate comparison conditions. A failure to find the same physiological profile across a wide range of a stimulus believed to invoke a given processing stage does not itself indicate whether a new stage is invoked or whether the old stage manifests differently at various levels of stimulation; however, it does indicate an important limitation when one is interpreting the physiological profile in a subsequent study of this processing stage. As Donchin (1982) suggested, "each hypothesis so tested generates predictions for its own specific range of validity. The observed relations may or may not be universally applicable" (p. 460).

Second, in order to construct the set of comparison tasks using the subtractive method, one must already have a clearly articulated hypothesis about the sequence of events that transpires between stimulus and overt response. This assumption renders the subtractive method particularly useful in testing an existing theory about the stages constituting a psychological process and in determining whether a given stage is among the set constituting two separate processes. Note, however, that confirmatory evidence can still be questioned by the assertion that the addition or deletion of a particular stage results in an essentially different set of stages or substages. Again, the inclusion of several experimental and comparison tasks (i.e., multiple operationalizations) appears to be judicious.

Although there are important limitations on the assumption of simple additive models that make it more useful for studying some types of processes (see e.g. Sanders 1980), the subtractive method can also yield data that are helpful in deriving comprehensive, empirically based models of psychological processes. Again, assume that the comparison is between experimental conditions with different impacts on behavior. If the physiological profile that differentiates these conditions is similar to a distinctive physiological profile that has been found previously to characterize a particular processing stage, the possibility is raised that the same processing stage has been detected in another context. The stronger and more distinctive the link between a physiological profile and a processing stage within the ranges of stimuli used, the stronger is this possibility. Similarly, if the sequence of physiological activity differentiating two conditions can be modeled by concatenating the physiological responses found previously to characterize even more rudimentary processing types or stages, then a model of a set of stages distinguishing these two conditions would be suggested. Again, converging evidence for this empirically derived model could be marshalled from other (e.g., observational or verbal) measures obtained in the experiment and from subsequent experiments.

Whenever a physiological response (or profile) found previously to vary as a function of a psychological processing stage or state is observed, the possibility is raised that the same processing stage or state has been detected. Much of the research in psychophysiology is based on just such reasoning. A person might be thought to be anxious because they show physiological activation, inattentive because they show diminished activation, happy because they show an attenuated startle response, and so on. However, one cannot logically conclude that a processing stage or state has definitely been detected simply because a physiological response found previously to vary as a function of a psychological processing stage or state has been observed. (The logical flaw in this form of psychophysiological inference is termed "affirmation of the consequent.") In the next section, we present a general framework for thinking about relationships between psychological concepts and physiological events, and we discuss the rules of evidence

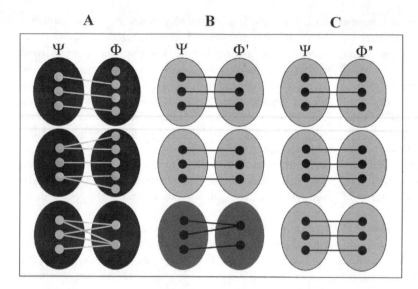

Figure 1. Depiction of logical relations between elements in the psychological (Ψ) and physiological (Φ) domains. Left panel: Links between the psychological elements and individual physiological responses. Middle panel: Links between the psychological elements and the physiological response pattern. Right panel: Links between the psychological elements and the profile of physiological responses across time.

for and the limitations to inference in each (see also Cacioppo & Tassinary 1990).

THE PSYCHOLOGICAL AND PHYSIOLOGICAL DOMAINS

A useful way to construe the potential relationships between psychological and physiological events is to consider these two types of events as representing independent sets (domains), where a *set* is defined as a collection of elements that together are considered a whole. Psychological events – by which we mean conceptual variables representing functional aspects of embodied processes – are conceived as constituting one set, which we shall call set Ψ. Physiological (e.g., brain, autonomic, endocrinological) events, by which we mean empirical physical variables, are conceived as constituting another, which we shall call set Φ.[1] Inspection of Figure 1 (upper left panel) reveals that all elements in the set of psychological events are assumed to have some physiological referent; that is, the mind is viewed as having a physical substrate.[2]

Focusing first on the top row of Figure 1, the existence of psychologically irrelevant physiological events (e.g., random physiological fluctuations; increased electrodermal activity due to minor variations in body temperature) is of importance in psychophysiology for purposes of artifact prevention or elimination. However, such elements within the physiological domain can be ignored if nonpsychological factors have been held constant, their influence on the physiological responses of interest has been identified and

removed, or they do not overlap with the physiological event of interest. These objectives are achieved through the application of proper psychophysiological recording techniques. The important point here is that the achievement of these objectives simplifies the task of specifying psychophysiological relationships, in the ideal case, by eliminating physiological events that have no direct relevance to psychological events (see Figure 1, top row of panel B).

We can now state five general relations that might be said to map the elements within the domain Ψ of psychological events to elements within the domain Φ of physiological events (see Figure 2); these may be listed as follows:

1. A one-to-one relation, such that an element in the psychological set is associated with one and only one element in the physiological set and vice versa.
2. A one-to-many relation, meaning that an element in the psychological domain is associated with a subset of elements in the physiological domain.
3. A many-to-one relation, meaning that two or more psychological elements are associated with the same physiological element.

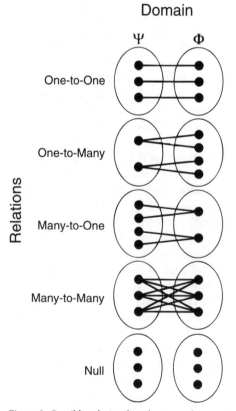

Figure 2. Possible relationships between elements in the psychological (Ψ) and physiological (Φ) domains.

4. A many-to-many relation, meaning that two or more psychological elements are associated with the same (or an overlapping) subset of elements in the physiological domain.

5. A null relation, meaning there is no association between an element in the psychological domain and that in the physiological domain.[3]

Of these possible relations, only the first and third allow a formal specification of psychological elements as a function of physiological elements (Coombs, Dawes, & Tversky 1970, pp. 351–71). This is important because, as we have noted, psychophysiological research typically involves the manipulation of (or blocking on) elements in the psychological domain and the measurement of elements in the physiological domain. The grounds for theoretical interpretations in psychophysiology can therefore be strengthened if a way can be found to specify the relationship between the elements within Ψ and Φ in terms of one-to-one or, at worst, many-to-one relationships.

PHYSIOLOGICAL ELEMENTS AS SPATIAL AND TEMPORAL RESPONSE PROFILES

If a one-to-one relation exists then an element in the psychological set is associated with one and only one element in the physiological set. Such relationships provide strong grounds for inference but are not common in psychophysiology (Cacioppo & Tassinary 1990; Coles et al. 1987; Donchin 1982). The functional opposite of the one-to-one relation is the null relation, which means that the element in the physiological domain is unrelated to (and hence harbors no information about) the element in the psychological domain.

Another form of relation between elements in the psychological and physiological domains is the one-to-many, meaning that an element in the psychological domain is associated with a subset of elements in the physiological domain. Note that one-to-many relations between sets of psychological and physiological elements can be greatly simplified by reducing them to one-to-one relations as follows. Define a second set Φ' of physiological elements such that any subset of physiological elements associated with the psychological element is replaced by a single element in Φ', which now represents a physiological syndrome or response pattern. Thus, one-to-one and one-to-many relations between elements in the psychological domain Ψ and elements in the physiological domain Φ both become one-to-one relations between Ψ and Φ' (see Figure 1, panel B).

The remaining relations that can exist between elements in these domains are the many-to-one, meaning that two or more psychological elements are associated with the same physiological element; and the many-to-many, meaning that two or more psychological elements in Ψ are associated with two or more of the same elements in Φ

(see Figure 1, lower row of panel A). These relations can also be simplified with a few changes in how one conceptualizes an element in the physiological domain.

As before, a new set Φ' of physiological elements is defined such that any subset of physiological elements associated with one or more psychological elements is replaced by a new element representing a profile of physiological responses. Thus, the elements in Φ' again represent a specific pattern or syndrome of physiological events, and many-to-many relations between elements in Ψ and Φ can be reduced to many-to-one (or, in some cases, one-to-one) relations by viewing elements within the physiological domain as representing singular physiological responses and physiological response syndromes.

However, such a reconceptualization may not be sufficient to cast all of the psychophysiological relations of interest in terms of one-to-one or many-to-one relations. This may still not be a problem, because the set Φ' of physiological elements can be redefined such that the forms of physiological events as they unfold over time are also considered to yield yet another set of physiological elements, Φ'' (Figure 1, panel C; cf. Cacioppo, Marshall-Goodell, & Dorfman 1983). By including both temporal and spatial information regarding the physiological events in the definition of the elements in Φ'', many complex psychophysiological relationships can be reduced to one-to-one or many-to-one relations.

ASYMMETRIES IN PSYCHOPHYSIOLOGICAL INFERENCE

Research in which psychological or behavioral factors serve as the independent (or blocking) variables and physiological structures or events serve as the dependent variable can be conceptualized as investigating the $P(\Phi \mid \Psi)$, the "probability of Φ given Ψ." Research in which physiological structures or events serve as the independent (or blocking) variables and psychological or behavioral factors serve as the dependent variable can, in contrast, be conceptualized as investigating the $P(\Psi \mid \Phi)$.

For example, when differences in brain images or physiological events (Φ) are found in contrasts of tasks that are thought to differ only in one or more cognitive functions (Ψ), the data are often interpreted prematurely as showing that brain structure (or event) Φ is associated with cognitive function Ψ. These data are also treated as revealing much the same information that would have been obtained had brain structure (or event) Φ been stimulated or ablated and a consequent change in cognitive function Ψ observed. This form of interpretation reflects the explicit assumption that there is a fundamental localizability of specific cognitive operations, as well as the implicit assumption that there is an isomorphism between Φ and Ψ (Sarter et al. 1996a). Causal hypotheses regarding a specific brain structure or process (Φ) underlying a cognitive operation (Ψ)

are of the form $\Psi = f(\Phi)$; they necessarily imply that Φ is always followed by Ψ but do not imply that Ψ is always preceded by Φ.[4] Furthermore, brain events (Φ) may be of interest to the extent that they index a cognitive operation or state, so that the inferences are of the form $\Psi = f(\Phi)$ rather than not-$\Psi = f(\text{not-}\Phi)$. Thus, an aim of psychophysiology can generally be specified by the conditional probability of Ψ, given Φ:

$$P(\Psi \mid \Phi) = 1.$$

The typical structure of the imaging study (and most psychophysiological studies) can be represented by the conditional probability of Φ, given Ψ:

$$P(\Phi \mid \Psi) = x.$$

That is, psychophysiological measures provide information about Φ as a function of Ψ, but the conditional probabilities are equivalent ($P(\Psi \mid \Phi) = P(\Phi \mid \Psi)$) if and only if there is a one-to-one relationship between physiological event Φ and cognitive function(s) or operation(s) Ψ (Cacioppo & Tassinary 1990). Interpreting psychophysiological studies of the form $P(\Phi \mid \Psi)$ as equivalent to psychophysiological studies of the form $P(\Psi \mid \Phi)$ is not misleading if one is dealing with one-to-one relationships. However, this is an assumption that must be tested. Assuming that brain areas become active during specific operations, for instance, reflects a one-to-one relationship and may hinder progress in psychophysiology unless this assumption is tested or its implications for inference recognized. These interpretations should be based on more than mere consistency with the imaging data; ideally, evidence would also be presented demonstrating that the $P(\text{not-}\Psi, \Phi) = 0$ in the assessment context (in which case Φ would be a marker of Ψ) or across contexts (in which case the relationship between Φ and Ψ would be invariant). Strong inferences would then be possible.

Approaches such as stimulation and ablation studies provide complementary rather than redundant information to traditional psychophysiological studies, in which physiological variables serve as dependent measures. This is because stimulation and ablation studies bear on the relationship $P(\Psi \mid \Phi)$, whereas studies in which physiological variables serve as dependent measures provide information about $P(\Phi \mid \Psi)$. Despite the formal parallelism between the expression $P(\Phi \mid \Psi)$ and $P(\Psi \mid \Phi)$, there is a fundamental asymmetry in the heuristic power of studies aimed at the demonstration of $P(\Psi \mid \Phi)$ versus $P(\Phi \mid \Psi)$. The causal role of Φ in process Ψ can be examined by direct experimental manipulation of the physiology. The loss of cognitive function by inactivation of neuronal processes (by mechanical, thermal, or neurochemical means) can serve to establish Φ as causal for function Ψ. Addressing a more complex avenue of research – facilitation of cognitive processes (e.g., attention or memory) by electrical or neurochemical brain

activation – can further establish that Φ is a sufficient condition for influencing process Ψ (Sarter et al. 1996a). Whether the observed relationships have import in normal, functioning humans is informed by studies in which Φ as a function of Ψ is examined.

Although both relationships $P(\Psi \mid \Phi)$ and $P(\Phi \mid \Psi)$ can be studied experimentally, the complexity implied in studies aimed at demonstrating $P(\Phi \mid \Psi)$ is based on the fact that experimental alteration of cognitive function Ψ necessarily alters brain activities $\Phi', \Phi, \ldots$ (including those, say Φ, that underlie Ψ). Thus, although a psychological context may yield concurrent manifestation in Ψ and Φ', the causal linkage remains in question because an alternate (even undetected) brain event Φ could be causally mediating both Ψ and Φ'. In this case, excluding Φ' as a necessary and/or sufficient condition for the observed Ψ may require a tedious and exhaustive evaluation of the alternative hypothesis not-$\Psi = f(\text{not-}\Phi')$. Note that this conclusion does not challenge the importance and utility of evidence generated by imaging methods, but it does point to fundamental limitations in the strength of the inference deduced from experimental approaches aimed solely at the demonstration of $P(\Phi \mid \Psi)$. The integration of methods and data from bottom-up and top-down approaches provides a means of circumventing some of the thornier interpretive problems of either approach alone, thereby permitting strong inferences in psychophysiology even in areas in which hypothesis-driven research is not yet possible (Sarter et al. 1996a).

AN ILLUSTRATION

As Gould (1985) noted:

We often think, naively, that missing data are the primary impediments to intellectual progress – just find the right facts and all problems will dissipate. But barriers are often deeper and more abstract in thought. We must have access to the right metaphor, not only the requisite information. Revolutionary thinkers are not, primarily, gatherers of facts, but weavers of new intellectual structures. (Essay 9)

It may be useful to illustrate some of these points using a simple physical metaphor in which the bases of a multiply determined outcome are known. Briefly, let Φ represent the heater and Ψ the temperature in a house. In the context of psychophysiology, the heater parallels a neural mechanism and the temperature represents the cognitive manifestation of the operation of this mechanism. Although the heater and the temperature are conceptually distinct, the operation of the heater represents a physical basis for the temperature in the house. Thus, $\Psi = f(\Phi)$. A bottom-up approach (i.e. $P(\Psi \mid \Phi)$) makes clear certain details about the relationship between Ψ and Φ, whereas a top-down approach (i.e. $P(\Phi \mid \Psi)$) clarifies others. For instance, when the activity of the heater is manipulated (Φ

is stimulated or lesioned), a change in the temperature in the house (Ψ) results. This represents a bottom-up approach to investigating the physical substrates of cognitive phenomena. That manipulating the activity of the heater produces a change in the temperature in the house can be expressed as $P(\Psi \mid \Phi) > 0$. Note that the $P(\Psi \mid \Phi)$ need not equal 1 for Φ to be a physical substrate of Ψ. This is because, in our illustration, there are other physical mechanisms that can affect the temperature in the house (Ψ), such as the outside temperature (Φ_1) and the amount of direct sunlight in the house (Φ_2). That is, there is a lack of complete isomorphism specifiable (at least initially) between the regulated variable (Ψ) and a physical basis (Φ).

In any given context, the temperature in the house may be influenced by any or all of these physical mechanisms. If the outside temperature or the amount of direct sunlight happens to vary when the heater is activated, then the temperature may not covary perfectly with the activation of the heater (i.e., $P(\Psi \mid \Phi) < 1$) even though the temperature is, at least in part, a function of the operation of the heater (i.e., $P(\Psi \mid \Phi) > 0$). If the outside temperature and amount of direct sunlight are constant or are perfectly correlated with the activation of the heater, then the temperature in the house and the activity of the heater may covary perfectly ($P(\Psi \mid \Phi) = 1$). In the context of psychophysiology, this is analogous to a brain lesion study accounting for some of the variance ($P(\Psi \mid \Phi) > 0$) or all of the variance ($P(\Psi \mid \Phi) = 1$) in the cognitive measure used in the study. The latter result does not imply that the lesioned brain region is a necessary component, just as temperature in the house covarying perfectly with heater activation does not mean that no other physical mechanisms could also influence the temperature. Thus, as long as $P(\Psi \mid \Phi) > 0$, Φ can be considered a predictor (or component) of Ψ; that $P(\Psi \mid \Phi) = 1$ does not imply that Φ is the only (or a necessary) cause of Ψ.

Also evident in this metaphor are the asymmetry between $P(\Psi \mid \Phi)$ and $P(\Phi \mid \Psi)$ and the interpretive problems that may result when simply assuming $P(\Psi \mid \Phi) = P(\Phi \mid \Psi)$. As outlined previously, the former term represents variations in temperature in the house given variations in the activity of the heater, whereas $P(\Phi \mid \Psi)$ represents the activity of the heater given variations in the temperature in the house. Although one would expect to find $P(\Phi \mid \Psi) > 0$ in some contexts, the fact that the temperature in the house increases reliably when the heater is activated does not necessarily imply that changes in the temperature in the house will be associated with variations in the activity of the heater. In the winter months, changes in the temperature in the house may be associated with corresponding changes in the activity of the heater. However, in another context (e.g., the summer months), the heater may be uniformly inactive yet housing temperature continues to vary owing to the operation of other physical factors (e.g., outside temperature Φ_1 or exposure Φ_2 to direct sunlight).

Thus, the finding that $P(\Phi \mid \Psi) = 0$ means not that Φ has no role in Ψ but only that Φ has no role in Ψ *in that context*. In the context of brain imaging studies, areas that are not found to become active as a function of a cognitive operation may nevertheless be part of a physical substrate for that cognitive operation (just as a heater may remain a part of the physical mechanism for the temperature in a house).

The preceding example illustrates why one would not want to exclude a brain area as potentially relevant to a cognitive operation based solely on the area not being illuminated in a brain image as a function of the cognitive operation. The converse also holds; that is, a brain area that is illuminated as a function of a cognitive operation may or may not contribute meaningfully to the production of the cognitive operation. Consider a light emitting diode (LED) on a thermostat (which we will call Φ') that illuminates when the heater (Φ) is operating. In this case, $P(\Phi \mid \Psi) = P(\Phi' \mid \Psi) > 0$. That is, the LED represents a physical element that would show the same covariation with the temperature in the house as would the operation of the heater – as long as a top-down approach were used. Were the complementary bottom-up approach to be used, it would become obvious that disconnecting (lesioning) the heater has effects on the temperature in the house whereas disconnecting (or directly activating) the LED has none.

The metaphor also illustrates the "categorical" error: the intuitively appealing notion that the organization of cognitive phenomena maps in a one-to-one fashion into the organization of the underlying neural substrates. The temperature of the house, for instance, does not map into a single "temperature center" in the house; rather, it is determined by several different physical mechanisms. One might argue that the problem is in how Ψ is being defined, that the temperature in the house is not the most useful way of conceptualizing the phenomenon. One solution may be to specify the heater-related contribution to temperature (reconceptualize the function dimension, Ψ as Ψ'), but this is not the only or even the best solution. Suppose, for instance, that the system is designed to maintain the temperature of the house within a narrow range. The problem in such a system may not be in the definition of Ψ but in the full delineation of its physical basis (Φ, Φ_1, Φ_2, and interactions) in order to achieve a closer approximation between functional concepts and models of mechanisms. Although we anticipate that some one-to-one mappings between Φ and Ψ may ultimately be achieved, reaching this ultimate aim requires a recognition of the preliminary state of our knowledge at present and the attendant implications for strong inference. Given the complementary nature of the data from brain imaging and from direct stimulation and lesion studies, progress in psychophysiology should be fostered by an integration rather than a progressive segregation of these approaches and literatures.

Four Categories of Psychophysiological Relationships

As illustrated in the preceding section, relations between elements in the psychological and physiological domains cannot be assumed to hold across situations or individuals. Indeed, elements in the psychological domain are delimited in the subtractive method in part by holding constant other processes that might differentiate the comparison tasks. Such a procedure is not unique to psychophysiology or to the subtractive method, since many psychological and medical tests involve constructing specific assessment contexts in order to achieve interpretable results. The interpretation of a blood glucose test, for instance, can rest on the assumption that the individual fasted prior to the onset of the test. Only under this circumstance can the amount of glucose measured in the blood across time be used to index the body's ability to regulate the level of blood sugar (Guyton 1971). Here, the relationship between the physiological data and theoretical construct is said to have a limited range of validity because the relationship is clear only in certain well-prescribed assessment contexts (Cacioppo & Petty 1986; Donchin 1982). The notion of limited ranges of validity thus raises the possibility that a wide range of complex relationships between psychological and physiological phenomena might be specifiable in simpler, more interpretable forms within specific assessment contexts.

In order to clarify these issues, it is useful to conceptualize psychophysiological relationships in terms of a 2 (one-to-one vs. many-to-one) by 2 (situation-specific vs. cross-situational) taxonomy. The specific families (i.e. categories) of psychophysiological relationships that can be derived from this taxonomy are depicted in Figure 3. The criterial attributes for, and theoretical utility in, establishing each of these categories are specified in the two dimensions illustrated in Figure 3; causal attributes of the relationships, and whether the relationships are naturally occurring or artificially induced, constitute yet other (orthogonal) dimensions and are explicitly excluded here for didactic purposes. For instance, the category in Figure 3 labeled "psychophysiological concomitants" refers only to the conditions and implications of covariation and is not intended to discriminate between instances in which the psychological factor is causal in the physiological response, vice versa, or a third variable causes both. In the sections that follow, each type of psychophysiological relationship and the nature of the inferences that each suggests are outlined.

PSYCHOPHYSIOLOGICAL OUTCOMES

In the idealized case, an *outcome* is defined as a many-to-one, situation-specific (context-dependent) relationship between Ψ and Φ. Establishing that a physiological response (i.e., an element in Φ) varies as a function of a psychological change (i.e., an element in Ψ) means that one is dealing at the very least with an outcome relationship between these elements. Note that this is often the first attribute of a psychophysiological relationship that is established in laboratory practice. Whether the physiological response follows changes in the psychological event across situations (i.e., is context-independent) or whether the response profile follows only changes in the event (i.e., is isomorphic) is not typically addressed initially. Hence, a given psychophysiological relationship may appear to be an outcome but subsequently be identified as being a marker as the question of isomorphy is examined; a relationship that appears to be an outcome may subsequently be reclassified as being a concomitant once the range of validity is examined; and a relationship that appears to be a marker (or concomitant) may emerge as an invariant upon studying the generalizability (or isomorphy) of the relationship. However, this progression is not problematic in terms of causing erroneous inferences; as we shall see, any logical inference based on the assumption that one is dealing with an outcome relationship holds as well for marker, concomitant, or invariant psychophysiological relationships.

Despite serving as the most elemental psychophysiological relationship, the outcome can provide the basis for strong inferences. Specifically, if two psychological models differ in predictions regarding one or more physiological outcomes, then the logic of the experimental design allows theoretical inferences to be drawn based on psychophysiological outcomes alone. That is, a psychophysiological outcome enables systematic inferences to be drawn about psychological constructs and relationships based on hypothetico-deductive logic. Of course, no single operationalization of the constructs in a crucial experiment is

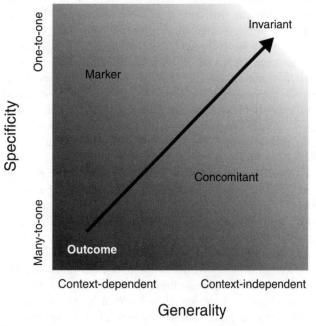

Figure 3. Taxonomy of psychophysiological relationships.

likely to convince the adherents of both theories. If multiple operationalizations of the theoretical constructs result in the same physiological outcome, however, then strong theoretical inferences can be justified.

The identification of a physiological response profile that differentiates the psychological element of interest is sufficient to infer the absence of one or more psychological elements, but it does not provide logical grounds to infer anything about the *presence* of a psychological element. Hence, the identification of psychophysiological outcomes can be valuable in disproving theoretical predictions, but they are problematic as indices of elements in the psychological domain. This caveat is often noted in discussions of the scientific method and is perhaps equally often violated in scientific practice (Platt 1964). Skin conductance, for instance, has been a major dependent measure in psychological research because emotional arousal is thought to lead to increased skin conductance (Prokasy & Raskin 1973). Similarly, EMG (electromyographic) activity over the forehead region has been a frequent target measure in relaxation biofeedback because tension has been found to increase EMG activity over this region (Stroebel & Glueck 1978). Yet as noted in the previous section, simply knowing that manipulating a particular element in the psychological domain leads to a particular response in the physiological domain does not logically enable one to infer anything about the former based on observations of the latter, because one does not know what other antecedents might have led to the observed physiological response. Procedures such as holding constant any variations in the elements in the psychological domain that are not of interest, measuring these elements in addition to those of immediate theoretical interest to determine which elements are likely to have caused the observed changes in physiological response, and excluding those physiological responses believed to covary with these irrelevant elements all represent attempts to reduce many-to-one relationships to one-to-one relationships (i.e., going from psychophysiological outcomes to psychophysiological markers; see Figure 3). Such procedures clearly strengthen the grounds for psychophysiological inference, but they neither assure that all relevant factors have been identified and controlled nor provide a means for quantifying the extent of other influences on psychophysiological responding.

For example, consider what can be expected if the probability of a physiological element, $P(\Phi)$, is greater than the probability of the psychological element of interest, $P(\Psi)$. Since this implies that $P(\Psi, \Phi) \mid P(\Psi) > P(\Psi, \Phi) \mid P(\Phi)$, it can be seen that $P(\Phi \mid \Psi) > P(\Psi \mid \Phi)$ and hence that research based only on outcome relationships would result in an overestimation of the presence of the psychological element.

We should emphasize that these probabilities are simply a way of thinking more rigorously about psychophysiological relations; one still needs to be cognizant that these relationships and probabilities may vary across situations. Indeed, comparisons of these probabilities across assessment contexts can provide a means of determining the individual or situational specificity of a psychophysiological relation. Before proceeding to this dimension of the taxonomy outlined in Figure 3, we elaborate further on psychophysiological relations within a specific assessment context when viewed within the framework of conditional probabilities. In particular, as $P(\Psi, \Phi)$ approaches 1 and $P(\text{not-}\Psi, \Phi)$ approaches 0, the element in the physiological domain can be described as being an ideal marker of the element in the psychological domain.

PSYCHOPHYSIOLOGICAL MARKERS

In its idealized form, a psychophysiological *marker* is defined as a one-to-one, situation-specific (context-dependent) relationship between abstract events Ψ and Φ (see Figure 3). The psychophysiological marker relation assumes only that the occurrence of one event (usually a physiological response, parameter of a response, or profile of responses) predicts the occurrence of the other (usually a psychological event) within a given context. Thus, markers are characterized by limited ranges of validity. Such a relationship may reflect a natural connection between psychological and physiological elements in a particular measurement situation, or it may reflect an artificially induced (e.g., classically conditioned) association between these elements. It is important to recognize that minimal violations of isomorphism between Ψ and Φ within a given assessment context can nevertheless yield a useful (although imperfect) marker when viewed in terms of conditional probabilities.

Markers can vary in their specificity and sensitivity. The more distinctive the form of the physiological response and/or the pattern of associated physiological responses, the greater is the likelihood of achieving a one-to-one relationship between the physiological events and the psychological construct – and the wider may be the range of validity of the relationship thereby established. This is because the utility of an element in Φ to index an element in Ψ is generally strengthened by defining the physiological element so as to minimize its occurrence in the absence of the element in the psychological domain.

In terms of sensitivity, a psychophysiological marker may simply signal the occurrence or nonoccurrence of a psychological process or event and possess no information about the temporal or amplitude properties of the event in a specific assessment context. At the other extreme, a psychophysiological marker may be related in a prescribed assessment context to the psychological event by some well-defined temporal function, so that the measure can be used to delineate the onset and offset of the episode of interest, and/or it may vary in amplitude and thus reflect the intensity of the psychological event.

In sum, markers represent a fundamental relationship between elements in the psychological and physiological domains that enables an inference to be drawn about the nature of the former given measurement of the latter. The major requirements in establishing a response as a marker are: (1) demonstrating that the presence of the target response reliably predicts the specific construct of interest; (2) demonstrating that the presence of the target response is insensitive to (e.g., uncorrelated with) the presence or absence of other constructs; and (3) specifying the boundary conditions for the validity for the relationship. The term "tracer" can be viewed as synonymous with "marker," for each refers to a measure so strictly associated with a particular organismic–environmental condition that its presence is indicative of the presence of this condition. On the other hand, the term "indicant" is more generic and includes invariants, markers, and concomitants, since each allows the prediction of Ψ given Φ. We turn next to a description of concomitants.

PSYCHOPHYSIOLOGICAL CONCOMITANTS

A psychophysiological *concomitant* (or correlate), in its idealized form, is defined as a many-to-one, cross-situational (context-independent) association between abstract events Ψ and Φ (see Figure 3). That is, the search for psychophysiological concomitants assumes there is a cross-situational covariation between specific elements in the psychological and physiological domains. The assumption of a psychophysiological concomitant is less restrictive than the assumption of invariance in that one-to-one correspondence is not required, although the relationship tends to be more informative given a stronger association between elements in the psychological and physiological domains.

Consider, for instance, the observation that pupillary responses vary as a function of individuals' attitudes toward visually presented stimuli – an observation followed by the conclusion that pupillary response is a "correlate" of people's attitudes (Hess 1965; Metalis & Hess 1982). However, evidence of variation in a target physiological response as a function of a manipulated (or naturally varying) psychological event establishes only an outcome relation, which is necessary but insufficient for the establishment of a psychophysiological concomitant or correlate.

First, the manipulation of the same psychological element (e.g., attitudes) in another context (e.g., using auditory rather than visual stimuli) may alter or eliminate the covariation between the psychological and physiological elements if the latter is evoked either by a stimulus that had been fortuitously or intentionally correlated with the psychological element in the initial measurement context or by a noncriterial attribute of the psychological element that does not generalize across situations. For instance, the attitude–pupil-size hypothesis has not been supported using nonpictorial (e.g., auditory, tactile) stimuli, where

it is possible to control the numerous light-reflex–related variables that can confound studies using pictorial stimuli (Goldwater 1972). It is possible, in several of the studies showing a statistical covariation between attitudes and pupillary response, that the mean luminance of individuals' selected fixations varied inversely with their attitudes toward the visual stimulus (Janisee 1977; Janisee & Peavler 1974; Woodmansee 1970).

Second, the manipulation of the same psychological element in another situation may alter or eliminate the covariation between the psychological and physiological elements if the latter is evoked not only by variations in the psychological element but also by variations in one or more additional factors that are introduced in (or are a fundamental constituent of) the new measurement context. Tranel, Fowles, and Damasio (1985), for instance, demonstrated that the presentation of familiar faces (e.g., famous politicians, actors) evoked larger skin conductance responses (SCRs) than did the presentation of unfamiliar faces. This finding, and the procedure and set of stimuli employed, were subsequently used in a study of patients with prosopagnosia (an inability to recognize visually the faces of persons previously known) to demonstrate that the patients can discriminate autonomically between the familiar and unfamiliar faces despite the absence of any awareness of this knowledge. Thus, the first study established a psychophysiological relationship in a specific measurement context, and the second study capitalized on this relationship. However, to conclude that a psychophysiological concomitant had been established between familiarity and SCRs would mean that the same relationship should hold across situations and stimuli (i.e., the relationship would be context-independent). Yet ample psychophysiological research has demonstrated a psychophysiological outcome opposite to that specified by Tranel et al. (1985) – namely, that novel or unusual stimuli can evoke larger SCRs than familiar stimuli (see e.g. Landis 1930; Lynn 1966; Sternbach 1966). Hence, it is safe to conclude that the relation between stimulus familiarity and skin conductance should not be thought of as a psychophysiological concomitant.[5]

Unfortunately, evidence of faulty reasoning based on the premature assumption of a true psychophysiological correlate (or invariant) is all too easy to find:

I find in going through the literature that the psychogalvanic reflex has been elicited by the following varieties of stimuli ... sensations and perceptions of any sense modality (sight, sounds, taste, etc.), associations (words, thoughts, etc.), mental work or effort, attentive movements or attitudes, imagination and ideas, tickling, painful or nocive stimuli, variations in respiratory movements or rate, suggestion and hypnosis, emotional behavior (fighting, crying, etc.), relating dreams, college examinations, and so forth.... Forty investigators hold that it is specific to, or a measure of, emotion of the affective qualities; ten others state that it is not necessarily of an emotional or affective nature; twelve men hold that it is somehow to be identified with conation, volition, or attention, while five hold very definitely that it is nonvoluntary; twenty-one authorities state that it goes with one or another of the mental processes; eight state that it is the concomitant of all sensation and perception; five have called it an indicator of conflict and suppression; while four others have used it as an index of character, personality, or temperament. (Landis 1930, p. 391)

The hindrances to scientific advances, it would seem, stem not so much from impenetrable psychophysiological relationships as from a failure to recognize the nature of these relationships and their limitations to induction.

As in the case of a psychophysiological marker, the empirical establishment of a psychophysiological concomitant logically allows an investigator to make a probability statement about the absence or presence (if not the timing and magnitude) of a particular element in the psychological domain when the target physiological element is observed. It is important to emphasize, however, that the estimate of the strength of the covariation used in such inferences should not come solely from evidence that manipulated or planned variations of an element in Ψ are associated with corresponding changes in an element in Φ. Measurements of the physiological response each time the psychological element is manipulated or changes can lead to an overestimate of the strength of this relationship and hence to erroneous inferences about the psychological element based on the physiological response. This overestimation occurs to the extent that there are changes in the physiological response not attributable to variations in the psychological element of interest. Hence, except when one is dealing with an invariant relationship, establishing that the manipulation of a psychological element leads cross-situationally to a particular physiological response or profile of responses is not logically sufficient to infer that the physiological event will be a strong predictor of the psychological element of interest; base-rate information about the occurrence of the physiological event across situations must also be considered. This is sometimes done in practice by quantifying the natural covariation between elements in the psychological and physiological domains and by examining the replicability of the observed covariation across situations.

PSYCHOPHYSIOLOGICAL INVARIANTS

The idealized *invariant* relationship refers to an isomorphic (one-to-one), context-independent (cross-situational) association (see Figure 3). To say that there is an invariant relationship therefore implies that: (1) a particular element in Φ is present if and only if a specific element in Ψ is present; (2) the specific element in Ψ is present if and only if the corresponding element in Φ is present; and (3) the relation between Ψ and Φ preserves all relevant arithmetical (algebraic) operations. Moreover, only in the case of invariants does $P(\Psi \mid \Phi) = P(\Phi \mid \Psi)$ and

$P(\text{not-}\Psi, \Phi) = P(\text{not-}\Phi, \Psi) = 0$. This means that the logical error of affirmation of the consequent is not a problem in psychophysiological inferences based on an invariant relation. Hence, the establishment of an invariant relationship between a pair of elements from the psychological and the physiological domains provides a strong basis for psychophysiological inference. Unfortunately, invariant relationships are often assumed rather than formally established; as we have argued, such an approach leads to erroneous psychophysiological inferences and vacuous theoretical advances.

It has been suggested occasionally that the psychophysiological enterprise is concerned with invariant relationships. As we have seen, the search to establish one-to-one psychophysiological relationships is important. Moreover, as noted by Stevens (1951):

The scientist is usually looking for invariance whether he knows it or not. Whenever he discovers a functional relation between two variables his next question follows naturally: under what conditions does it hold? In other words, under what transformation is the relation invariant? The quest for invariant relations is essentially the aspiration toward generality, and in psychology, as in physics, the principles that have wide application are those we prize. (p. 20)

It should be emphasized, however, that evidence for invariance should be gathered rather than assumed, and that the utility of psychophysiological analyses does not rest entirely with invariant relationships (Cacioppo & Petty 1985; Donchin 1982). Without this recognition, the establishment of any dissociation between the physiological measure and psychological element of interest invalidates not only the purported psychophysiological relationship but also the utility of a psychophysiological analysis. However, as outlined in the preceding sections of this chapter (and in the chapters to follow), psychophysiology need not be conceptualized as offering only mappings of context-independent, one-to-one relationships in order to advance our understanding of human processes and behavior.

In summary, the minimum assumption underlying the psychophysiological enterprise is that psychological and behavioral processes unfold as organismic–environmental transactions and hence have physiological manifestations, ramifications, or reflections (Cacioppo & Petty 1986). Although invariant psychophysiological relationships offer the greatest generality, physiological concomitants, markers, and outcomes also can provide important and sometimes otherwise unattainable information about elements in the psychological domain. These points hold for the neurosciences, as well. In laboratory practice, the initial step is often to establish that variations in a psychological element are associated with a physiological change, thereby establishing that the psychophysiological relationship is, at least, an outcome. Knowledge that changes in an element in the psychological domain are associated with changes in a physiological response or profile neither assures that the response will serve as a marker for the psychological state (since the converse of a statement does not follow logically from the statement) nor that the response is a concomitant or invariant of the psychological state (since the response may occur in only certain situations or individuals, or may occur for a large number of reasons besides changes in the particular psychological state). Nevertheless, both forms of reasoning outlined in this chapter can provide a strong foundation for psychophysiological inferences about behavioral processes.

Conclusion

Psychophysiology is based on the dual assumptions that (i) human perception, thought, emotion, and action are embodied and embedded phenomena and that (ii) the responses of the corporeal brain and body contain information that – in an appropriate experimental design – can shed light on human processes. The level of analysis in psychophysiology is not on isolated components of the body but rather on organismic–environmental transactions, with reference to both physical and sociocultural environments. Psychophysiology is therefore, like anatomy and physiology, a branch of science organized around bodily systems whose collective aim is to elucidate the structure and function of the parts of and interrelated systems in the human body in transactions with the environment. Like psychology, however, psychophysiology is concerned with a broader level of inquiry than anatomy and physiology and can be organized in terms of both a thematic and a systemic focus. For instance, the social and inferential elements as well as the physical elements of psychophysiology are discussed in the following chapters.

The importance of developing more advanced recording procedures to scientific progress in psychophysiology is clear, as previously unobservable phenomena are rendered tangible. However, advanced recording procedures alone are not sufficient for progress in the field. The theoretical specification of a psychophysiological relationship necessarily involves reaching into the unknown and hence requires intellectual invention and systematic efforts to minimize bias and error. Psychological theorizing based on known physiological and anatomical facts, exploratory research and pilot testing, and classic psychometric approaches can contribute in important ways by generating testable hypotheses about a psychophysiological relationship. It should be equally clear, however, that the scientific effectiveness of psychophysiological analyses does not derive logically from physiologizing or from the measurement of organismic rather than (or in addition to) verbal or chronometric responses. Its great value stems from the stimulation of interesting hypotheses and from the fact that, when an experiment agrees with a prediction about orchestrated actions of the organism, a great many alternative hypotheses

may be excluded. The study of physiological mechanisms and techniques can sharpen our thinking and reduce the error of our conceptualizations and measurements. Although necessary and important, one should bear in mind that such studies are means rather than ends in psychophysiology. Little is gained, for instance, by simply generating an increasingly lengthy list of correlates between specific psychological variables and additional psychophysiological measures.

A scientific theory is a description of causal interrelations. Psychophysiological correlations are not causal. Thus, in scientific theories, psychophysiological correlations are monstrosities. This does not mean that such correlations have no part in science. They are, in fact, the instruments by which the psychologist may test his or her theories (Gardiner, Metcalf, & Beebe-Center 1937, p. 385).

Thus, in order to further theoretical thinking, this chapter has outlined a taxonomy of psychophysiological relations and suggested a scheme for strong inference based on these relationships. This formulation can help address the following questions:

1. How does one select the appropriate variable(s) for study?
2. How detailed or refined should be the measurement of the selected variables?
3. How can situational and individual variability in psychophysiological relationships be integrated into theoretical thinking about psychophysiological relationships?
4. How can physiological measures be used in a rigorous fashion to index psychological factors?

However, the ultimate value of the proposed way of thinking about psychophysiological relationships rests on its effectiveness in guiding psychophysiological inference through the channels of judgmental fallacies. As Leonardo da Vinci (c. 1510) noted: "Experience does not ever err, it is only your judgment that errs in promising itself results which are not caused by your experiments."

NOTES

1. In our discussions here, the psychological domain is coextensive with the conceptual domain and the physiological domain is coextensive with the empirical domain (Cacioppo & Tassinary 1990).
2. The identity thesis states that there is a physical counterpart to every subjective or psychological event (Smart 1959). Importantly, the identity thesis does not imply that the relationship between physical and subjective events is one-to-one (i.e., invariant). Within the context of psychophysiology, for instance, the identity thesis does not necessarily imply that the physiological representation will be one-to-one in that: (a) there will be one and only one physiological mechanism able to produce a given psychological phenomenon; (b) a given psychological event will

be associated with, or reducible to, a single isolated physiological response rather than a syndrome or pattern of responses; (c) a given relationship between a psychological event and a physiological response is constant across time, situations, or individuals; (d) every physiological response has specific psychological significance or meaning; or (e) the organization and representation of psychological phenomena at a physiological level will mirror what subjectively appears to be elementary or unique psychological operations (e.g., beliefs, memories, images).

3. Both the many-to-many and the null relation may result in random scatter plots when measuring the natural covariation between elements in the psychological and physiological domains. However, these relations can be distinguished empirically by manipulating the psychological factors and quantifying the change in physiological response (and vice versa). The scatter plot between this psychological factor and physiological response should remain random in the case of a null relation between them, but not if they are part of a many-to-many relation.

4. See Cacioppo and Berntson (1992) for a discussion of the distinction between parallel and convergent multiple determinism.

5. Nevertheless, the application of the psychophysiological outcome and assessment context developed by Tranel et al. (1985) in the study of prosopagnosics by Tranel and Damasio (1985) illustrates the scientific value of psychophysiological investigations even when the relationship between elements in the psychological and physiological domains holds only within highly circumscribed assessment contexts.

REFERENCES

Ader, R. (1981). *Psychoneuroimmunology*. New York: Academic Press.

Ackles, P. K., Jennings, J. R., & Coles, M. G. H. (1985). *Advances in Psychophysiology*, vol. 1. Greenwich, CT: JAI.

Allport, G. (1947). Scientific models and human morals. *Psychological Review, 54,* 182–92.

Ax, A. F. (1964a). Editorial. *Psychophysiology, 1,* 1–3.

Ax, A. F. (1964b). Goals and methods of psychophysiology. *Psychophysiology, 1,* 8–25.

Bacon, F. (1620/1855). *Novum organum* (translated into English by T. Kitchin). Oxford University Press.

Barchas, P. R. (1976). Physiological sociology: Interface of sociological and biological processes. *Annual Review of Sociology,* 299–333.

Barinaga, M. (1997). What makes brain neurons run? *Science, 276,* 196–8.

Basmajian, J. V., & De Luca, C. J. (1985). *Muscles Alive: Their Functions Revealed by Electromyography,* 5th ed. Baltimore: Williams & Wilkins.

Berger, H. (1929). Uber das Elektrenkephalogramm des Menschen [On the electroencephalogram of man]. *Archiv für Psychiatrie und Nervenkrankheiten, 87,* 551–3. [Reprinted in English in Porges & Coles 1976.]

Bloom, F. E., Lazerson, A., & Hofstadter, L. (1985). *Brain, Mind, and Behavior*. New York: Freeman.

Boorstin, D. J. (1983). *The Discoverers: A History of Man's Search to Know His World and Himself*. London: Dent.

Brazier, M. A. (1959). The historical development of neurophysiology. In J. Field (Ed.), *Handbook of Physiology. Section I: Neurophysiology,* vol. I, pp. 1–58. Washington, DC: American Physiological Society.

Brazier, M. A. (1961). *A History of the Electrical Activity of the Brain*. London: Pitman.

Brazier, M. A. (1977). *Electrical Activity of the Nervous System,* 4th ed. Baltimore: Williams & Wilkins.

Cacioppo, J. T., & Berntson, G. G. (1992). Social psychological contributions to the decade of the brain: Doctrine of multilevel analysis. *American Psychologist, 47,* 1019–28.

Cacioppo, J. T., Marshall-Goodell, B., & Dorfman, D. D. (1983). Skeletal muscular patterning: Topographical analysis of the integrated electromyogram. *Psychophysiology, 20,* 269–83.

Cacioppo, J. T., & Petty, R. E. (1983). *Social Psychophysiology: A Sourcebook*. New York: Guilford.

Cacioppo, J. T., & Petty, R. E. (1985). Physiological responses and advertising effect: Is the cup half full or half empty? *Psychology and Marketing, 2,* 115–26.

Cacioppo, J. T., & Petty, R. E. (1986). Social processes. In M. G. H. Coles, E. Donchin, & S. Porges (Eds.), *Psychophysiology: Systems, Processes, and Applications,* pp. 646–79. New York: Guilford.

Cacioppo, J. T., Petty, R. E., & Andersen, B. L. (1988). Social psychophysiology as a paradigm. In H. L. Wagner (Ed.) *Social Psychophysiology and Emotion: Theory and Clinical Applications,* pp. 273–94. Chichester, U.K.: Wiley.

Cacioppo, J. T., & Tassinary, L. G. (1990). Inferring psychological significance from physiological signals. *American Psychologist, 45,* 16–28.

Caldwell, A. B. (1994). Simultaneous multilevel analysis. *American Psychologist, 49,* 144–5.

Caws, P. (1967). Scientific method. In P. Edwards (Ed.), *The Encyclopedia of Philosophy,* pp. 339–43. New York: Macmillan.

Cohen, R. M., Semple, W. E., Gross, M., King, A. C., & Nordahl, T. E. (1992). Metabolic brain pattern of sustained auditory discrimination. *Experimental Brain Research, 92,* 165–72.

Coles, M. G. H. (1988). Editorial. *Psychophysiology, 25,* 1–3.

Coles, M. G. H. (1989). Modern mind-brain reading: Psychophysiology, physiology, and cognition. *Psychophysiology, 26,* 251–69.

Coles, M. G. H., Donchin, E., & Porges, S. W. (1986). *Psychophysiology: Systems, Processes, and Applications*. New York: Guilford.

Coles, M. G. H., Gratton, G., & Gehring, W. J. (1987). Theory in cognitive psychophysiology. *Journal of Psychophysiology, 1,* 13–16.

Cook, S. W., & Selltiz, C. (1964). A multiple-indicator approach to attitude measurement. *Psychological Bulletin, 62,* 36–55.

Coombs, C. H., Dawes, R. M., & Tversky, A. (1970). *Mathematical Psychology: An Elementary Introduction*. Englewood Cliffs, NJ: Prentice-Hall.

Corbetta, M., Miezin, F., Dobmeyer, S., Shulman, G. L., et al. (1990). Attentional modulation of neural processing of shape, color, and velocity in humans. *Science, 248,* 1556–9.

Corbetta, M., Miezin, F. M., Dobmeyer, S., Shulman, G. L., & Petersen, S. E. (1991). Selective and divided attention during visual discriminations of shape, color, and speed: Functional anatomy by positron emission tomography. *Journal of Neuroscience, 11,* 2383–2402.

Darrow, C. W. (1929). Differences in the physiological reactions to sensory and ideational stimuli. *Psychological Bulletin, 26,* 185–201.

Darrow, C. W. (1964). Psychophysiology, yesterday, today and tomorrow. *Psychophysiology, 1,* 4–7.

Darwin, C. (1873). *The Expression of the Emotions in Man and Animals.* New York: Appleton. [Original work published in 1872.]

Donchin, E. (1982). The relevance of dissociations and the irrelevance of dissociationism: A reply to Schwartz and Pritchard. *Psychophysiology, 19,* 457–63.

Donders, F. C. (1868). Die schnelligkeit psychischer Prozesse. *Archive für Anatomie und Psychologie,* 657–81.

Drake, S. (1967). Galileo Galilei. In P. Edwards (Ed.), *The Encyclopedia of Philosophy,* p. 262. New York: Macmillan.

Eng, H. (1925). *Experimental Investigation into the Emotional Life of the Child Compared with That of the Adult.* London: Oxford University Press.

Fere, C. (1888). Notes on changes in electrical resistance under the effect of sensory stimulation and emotion. *Comptes Rendus des Seances de la Societe de Biologie, 5,* 217–19. [Reprinted in English in Porges & Coles 1976.]

Fernel, J. (1542). *De naturali parte medicinae.* Paris: Simon de Colies. [Cited in Brazier 1959.]

Fowles, D. C. (1975). *Clinical Applications of Psychophysiology.* New York: Columbia University Press.

Frankenhauser, M. (1983). The sympathetic-adrenal and pituitary-adrenal response to challenge: Comparison between sexes. In T. Dembroski, T. Schmidt, & G. Blumchen (Eds.), *Biobehavioral Bases of Coronary Heart Disease,* pp. 91–105. Basel: Karger.

Furedy, J. J. (1983). Operational, analogical and genuine definitions of psychophysiology. *International Journal of Psychophysiology, 1,* 13–19.

Gardiner, H. M., Metcalf, R. C., & Beebe-Center, J. G. (1937). *Feeling and Emotion: A History of Theories.* New York: American Book Company.

Glaser, R., & Kiecolt-Glaser, J. K. (1994). *Handbook of Human Stress and Immunity.* San Diego: Academic Press.

Goldwater, B. C. (1972). Psychological significance of pupillary movements. *Psychological Bulletin, 77,* 340–55.

Gould, S. J. (1985). *The Flamingo's Smile: Reflections in Natural History.* New York: Norton.

Greenfield, N. S., & Sternbach, R. A. (1972). *Handbook of Psychophysiology.* New York: Holt, Rinehart & Winston.

Grossman, M., Crino, P., Reivich, M., Stern, M. B., & Hurtig, H. I. (1992). Attention and sentence processing deficits in Parkinson's disease: The role of anterior cingulate cortex. *Cerebral Cortex, 2,* 513–25.

Grunberg, N. E., & Singer, J. E. (1990). Biochemical measurement. In J. T. Cacioppo & L. G. Tassinary (Eds.), *Principles of Psychophysiology,* pp. 149–76. Cambridge University Press.

Gutek, B. A. (1978). On the accuracy of retrospective attitudinal data. *Public Opinion Quarterly, 42,* 390–401.

Guyton, A. C. (1971). *Textbook of Medical Physiology,* 4th ed. Philadelphia: W. B. Saunders.

Harrington, A. (1987). *Medicine, Mind, and the Double Brain: Study in Nineteenth-Century Thought.* Princeton, NJ: Princeton University Press.

Harvey, W. (1628/1931). *Exercitatio anatomica de motu cordis et sanguinis in animalibus.* Frankfurt: Fitzeri. Translated into English by C. D. Leake. Springfield, IL: Thomas.

Henry, J. P., & Stephens, P. M. (1977). *Stress, Health, and the Social Environment.* New York: Springer-Verlag.

Hess, E. H. (1965). Attitude and pupil size. *Scientific American, 212,* 46–54.

Hugdahl, K. (1995). *Psychophysiology: The Mind–Body Perspective.* Cambridge, MA: Harvard University Press.

Jacobson, E. (1930). Electrical measurements of neuromuscular states during mental activities: III. Visual imagination and recollection. *American Journal of Physiology, 95,* 694–702.

James, W. (1884). What is an emotion? *Mind, 9,* 188–205.

Janisee, M. P. (1977). *Pupillometry: The Psychology of the Pupillary Response.* Washington, DC: Hemisphere.

Janisee, M. P. & Peavler, W. S. (1974). Pupillary research today: Emotion in the eye. *Psychology Today, 7,* 60–3.

Jaynes, J. (1973). The problem of animate motion in the seventeenth century. In M. Henle, J. Jaynes, & J. J. Sullivan (Eds.), *Historical Conceptions of Psychology,* pp. 166–79. New York: Springer.

Jermott, J. B. III, & Locke, S. E. (1984). Psychosocial factors, immunologic mediation, and human susceptibility to infectious diseases: How much do we know? *Psychological Bulletin, 95,* 78–108.

Kipnis, D. (1997). Ghosts, taxonomies, and social psychology. *American Psychologist, 52,* 205–11.

Landis, C. (1930). Psychology and the psychogalvanic reflex. *Psychological Review, 37,* 381–98.

Lindsley, D. B. (1951). Emotion. In S. S. Stevens (Ed.), *Handbook of Experimental Psychology,* pp. 473–516. New York: Wiley.

Lynn, R. (1966). *Attention, Arousal, and the Orientation Reaction.* Oxford, U.K.: Pergamon.

Mason, J. W. (1972). Organization of psychoendocrine mechanisms: A review and reconsideration of research. In N. S. Greenfield & R. A. Sternbach (Eds.), *Handbook of Psychophysiology,* pp. 3–124. New York: Holt, Rinehart & Winston.

Meaney, M. J., Bhatnagar, S., Larocque, S., McCormick, C. M., Shanks, N., Sharma, S., Smythe, J., Viau, V., & Plotsky, P. M. (1996). Early environment and the development of individual differences in the hypothalamic-pituitary-adrenal stress response. In C. R. Pfeffer (Ed.), *Severe Stress and Mental Disturbance in Children,* pp. 85–127. Washington, DC: American Psychiatric Press.

Mecacci, L. (1979). *Brain and History: The Relationship between Neurophysiology and Psychology in Soviet Research.* New York: Brunner/Mazel.

Mesulam, M. M. (1990). Large-scale neurocognitive networks and distributed processing for attention, language, and memory. *Annals of Neurology, 28,* 597–613.

Metalis, S. A., & Hess, E. H. (1982). Pupillary response/semantic differential scale relationships. *Journal of Research in Personality, 16,* 201–16.

Metherate, R., & Weinberger, N. M. (1990). Cholinergic modulation of responses to single tones reduces tone-specific receptive field alterations in cat auditory cortex. *Synapse, 6,* 133–45.

Mielke, R., Pietrzyk, U., Jacobs, A., Fink, G. R., Ichimiya, A., Kessler, J., Herholz, K., & Heiss, W. D. (1994). HMPAO SPET and FDG PET in Alzheimer's disease and vascular dementia: Comparison of perfusion and metabolic pattern. *European Journal of Nuclear Medicine, 21*, 1052–60.

Miller, J. (1978). *The Body in Question*. New York: Random House.

Mosso, A. (1896). *Fear* (translated by E. Lough & F. Riesow). New York: Longrans, Green.

Pardo, J. V., Fox, P. T., & Raichle, M. E. (1991). Localization of a human system for sustained attention by positron emission tomography. *Nature, 349*, 61–4.

Peterson, F., & Jung, C. G. (1907). Psychophysical investigations with the galvanometer and pneumograph in normal and insane individuals. *Brain, 30*, 153–218.

Platt, J. R. (1964). Strong inference. *Science, 146*, 347–53.

Popper, K. R. (1959/1968). *The Logic of Scientific Discovery*. New York: Harper & Row.

Porges, S. W., & Coles, M. G. H. (Eds.) (1976). *Psychophysiology*. Stroudsburg, PA: Dowden, Hutchinson & Ross.

Posner, M. I., & Petersen, S. E. (1990). The attention system of the human brain. *Annual Review of Neuroscience, 13*, 25–42.

Posner, M. I., Petersen, S. E., Fox, P. T., & Raichle, M. E. (1988). Localization of cognitive operations in the human brain. *Science, 240*, 1627–31.

Prokasy, W. F., & Raskin, D. C. (1973). *Electrodermal Activity in Psychological Research*. New York: Academic Press.

Robbins, T. W., & Everitt, B. J. (1987). Comparative functions of the central noradrenergic, dopaminergic and cholinergic systems. *Neuropharmacology, 26*, 893–901.

Sanders, A. F. (1980). Stage analysis of reaction processes. In G. E. Stelmach & J. Requin (Eds.), *Tutorials in Motor Behavior*. Amsterdam: North-Holland.

Sarter, M. F. (1994). Neuronal mechanisms of the attentional dysfunctions in senile dementia and schizophrenia: Two sides of the same coin? *Psychopharmacology, 114*, 539–50.

Sarter, M., Berntson, G. G., & Cacioppo, J. T. (1996a). Brain imaging and cognitive neuroscience: Towards strong inference in attributing function to structure. *American Psychologist, 51*, 13–21.

Sarter, M., & Bruno, J. P. (1994). Cognitive functions of cortical ACh: Lessons from studies on trans-synaptic modulation of activated efflux. *Trends in Neurosciences, 17*, 217–21.

Sarter, M., Bruno, J. P., Givens, B. S., Moore, H., McGaughy, J., & McMahon, K. (1996b). Neuronal mechanisms of drug effects on cognition: Cognitive activity as a necessary intervening variable. *Cognitive Brain Research 3*, 329–43.

Sechenov, I. M. (1878). *Elements of Thought*. Reprinted in R. J. Herrnstein & E. G. Boring (Eds.) (1965), *A Source Book in the History of Psychology*. Cambridge, MA: Harvard University Press.

Smart, J. J. C. (1959). Sensations and brain processes. *Philosophical Review, 68*, 141–56.

Stern, J. A. (1964). Toward a definition of psychophysiology. *Psychophysiology, 1*, 90–1.

Stern, R. M., Ray, W. J., & Davis, C. M. (1980). *Psychophysiological Recording*. New York: Oxford University Press.

Sternbach, R. A. (1966). *Principles of Psychophysiology*. New York: Academic Press.

Stevens, S. S. (1951). *Handbook of Experimental Psychology*. New York: Wiley.

Stroebel, C. F., & Glueck, B. C. (1978). Passive meditation: Subjective, clinical, and electrographic comparison with biofeedback. In G. E. Schwartz & D. Shapiro (Eds.), *Consciousness and Self-Regulation*, vol. 2, pp. 401–28. New York: Plenum.

Tarchanoff, J. (1890). Galvanic phenomena in the human skin during stimulation of the sensory organs and during various forms of mental activity. *Pflügers Archiv für die gesammte Physiologie des Menschen und der Tiere, 46*, 46–55. [Reprinted in English in Porges & Coles 1976.]

Tootell, R. B. H., et al. (1995). Visual motion after effect in human cortical area MT revealed by functional magnetic resonance imaging. *Nature, 375*, 139.

Tranel, D., & Damasio, A. R. (1985). Knowledge without awareness: An autonomic index of facial recognition by prosopagnosics. *Science, 228*, 1453–4.

Tranel, D., Fowles, D. C., & Damasio, A. R. (1985). Electrodermal discrimination of familiar and unfamiliar faces: A methodology. *Psychophysiology, 22*, 403–8.

Turner, C. F., & Martin, E. (1984). *Surveying Subjective Phenomena*. New York: Russell Sage Foundation.

Vesalius, A. (1543/1947). *De humani corporis fabrica*. Basle: Oporinus. Translated into English by J. B. de C. M. Saunders & C. D. O'Malley. New York: Schuman.

Vigoroux, R. (1879). Sur le role de la resistance electrique des tissues dans l'electro-diagnostic. *Comptes Rendes Societe de Biologie, 31*, 336–9. [Cited in Brazier 1959.]

Waid, W. M. (1984). *Sociophysiology*. New York: Springer-Verlag.

Weiskrantz, L. (1986). *Blindsight: A Case History and Implications*. Oxford University Press.

Wenger, M. A. (1941). The measurement of individual differences in autonomic balance. *Psychosomatic Medicine, 3*, 427–34.

Wilder, J. (1931). The "law of initial values," a neglected biological law and its significance for research and practice. *Zeitschrift für die gesammte Neurologie und Psychiatrie, 137*, 317–24. [Reprinted in English in Porges & Coles 1976.]

Woodmansee, J. J. (1970). The pupil response as a measure of social attitudes. In G. F. Summers (Ed.), *Attitude Measurement*. Chicago: Rand McNally.

Woodworth, R. S., & Schlosberg, H. (1954). *Experimental Psychology*. New York: Holt, Rinehart & Winston.

Wu, C. H. (1984). Electric fish and the discovery of animal electricity. *American Scientist, 72*, 598–607.

PART TWO

FOUNDATIONS

CHAPTER TWO

HUMAN ELECTROENCEPHALOGRAPHY

RICHARD J. DAVIDSON, DAREN C. JACKSON, & CHRISTINE L. LARSON

Introduction

The measurement of brain electrical activity using the electroencephalograph (EEG) provides a noninvasive and inexpensive method to directly measure brain function and make inferences about regional brain activity. It has many virtues as a direct measure of brain function that can be used in myriad applications in the biobehavioral sciences, ranging from studies of basic cognitive processes to emotional function, dysfunction, and development. It also has a number of limitations that the user must keep in mind as decisions about when and how to use such methods are made. The purpose of this chapter is to provide an overview of the major concepts and methods associated with use of EEG in biobehavioral research. In addition, some of the promising contemporary research efforts using EEG will be featured. Event-related potentials are not covered in this chapter, since they are addressed elsewhere in this volume.

HISTORICAL BACKGROUND

The measurement of human brain electrical activity is a recent development in the history of science. It was only about 70 years ago that the first demonstration of recording human brain electrical activity was published (Berger 1929). This first report was greeted with considerable skepticism in the scientific community. It wasn't until a live demonstration of scalp-recorded brain activity from the neuroscientist Adrian's head (at the 1935 meeting of the Physiological Society in London) that electroencephalographic measures became more widely accepted in the biomedical research community. In the ensuing years, rapid developments in data collection, data reduction, and data analysis have resulted in important progress in this area (Shagass 1972).

In his initial report, Berger used two large pad electrodes soaked in saline, one placed over the forehead and the other placed at the back of the head. Berger observed that there were regular rhythmic waves at about 10 Hz in relaxed adults and noticed that these waves were best seen when subjects had their eyes closed in the absence of stimulation or other mental activity such as imagining or problem solving. These waves subsequently became known as "alpha" waves. In later work, Berger had the opportunity to record directly from the cortical surface during neurosurgery and confirmed the important fact that scalp and direct recordings were essentially identical in form except that the amplitude at the scalp was attenuated.

A major event in the history of research on the EEG was the launching of the journal *Electroencephalography and Clinical Neurophysiology* in 1949. In the first volume of this journal, an article by Moruzzi and Magoun (1949) appeared that established the consequences of reticular stimulation on cortical EEG. Following stimulation of the brainstem reticular formation in cats, widespread increases in cortical arousal as reflected in EEG desynchronization were observed. This helped to launch the study of brain electrical activity as an integrated neurophysiological phenomenon and to establish a role for EEG measures in the assessment of arousal. While this and other similar experiments undoubtedly played an important role in highlighting the utility of these measures as indices of activation, the finding of global cortical activation as a consequence of brainstem stimulation also had the unwitting effect of reinforcing the view that EEG could not provide very useful information on cortical specificity (Davidson 1978). This notion was championed by some and led to the development of general arousal theory (e.g. Duffy 1962; see Thayer 1989 for modern version) in which the EEG is considered to be useful only for making inferences about global states of sleep and wakefulness.

John T. Cacioppo, Louis G. Tassinary, and Gary G. Berntson (Eds.), *Handbook of Psychophysiology*, 2nd ed. © Cambridge University Press 2000. Printed in the United States of America. ISBN 62634X. All rights reserved.

SPACE AND TIME IN MEASURES OF REGIONAL BRAIN FUNCTION

The use of EEG to make inferences about neural activation and other brain processes has a number of distinct advantages and disadvantages. In general, there is some trade-off between temporal and spatial resolution in measures of regional brain function. Measures derived from brain electrical activity have very good intrinsic temporal resolution. These indices are typically recorded in a way that permits resolution in the millisecond domain, which makes these measures ideal for linking with behavior that dynamically changes over short periods of time. Moreover, changes in neuronal activation can be instantaneously reflected in changes in EEG, whereas with hemodynamic measures such as functional magnetic resonance imaging (fMRI) there is always a delay between the time a neuronal change occurs and the onset of a detectable hemodynamic change (Cohen 1996). Measures derived from brain electrical activity are thus ideally suited for tracking the neural changes coincident with rapid phasic changes in behavioral state.

A particularly appropriate role for these measures is in examining the neural correlates of irregular, spontaneously occurring behavior. For example, EEG measures have been effectively utilized in the study of the neural substrates of emotion. By collecting continuous EEG and video-recorded facial behavior, brain electrical activity that was coincident with specific, objectively coded facial signs of emotion could be extracted off-line (Davidson et al. 1990b). The onset and offset times of the extracted activity are based upon the times at which the specific facial expressions occurred. Even very brief, fleeting expressions (shorter than one second in duration) could be studied using these techniques, owing to the method's time resolution. If the EEG is sampled 200 times per second then the resolution would be 5 msec, considerably better than the resolution of video. The video frame in which the onset of the expression was judged to begin can be used to identify the sample in the EEG that coincides with this time. In a subsequent section, we will consider issues concerning the reliability of brief epochs of EEG and the minimum duration of EEG needed to establish a reliable index of a particular behavioral state.

Whereas the temporal resolution of the EEG is clearly a major advantage of the method, the relatively poor spatial resolution is a major disadvantage. Even with high-density electrode arrays, the spatial resolution of this method will always be inferior to those based upon metabolic or hemodynamic imaging. There are several reasons for this state of affairs. The methodological issues associated with high-density EEG recording will be considered in more detail shortly. However, it is important to note here that, even with electrode arrays that include 128 channels, the average interelectrode distance on a typical adult head is approximately 2.25–2.50 cm, a full order of magnitude coarser than the spatial resolution achievable with modern functional MRI. Second, the spatial distribution of neuronal potentials is distorted by the highly resistive properties of the skull. The skull acts as a spatial low-pass filter and smears the electrical activity over a relatively large region of scalp. Third, there is no unique solution to the inverse problem. A particular distribution of scalp potentials can be produced by many different combinations of intracerebral generator sources. Thus, inferring the sources of observed voltage changes on the head is fraught with methodological complications and will rarely, if ever, be definitive. We therefore cannot assume that a particular scalp distribution isomorphically reflects an underlying neuroanatomical localization.

Despite these complexities, temporal and spatial changes in scalp-recorded brain electrical activity can provide useful information on brain–behavior relations, can help to confirm specific hypotheses about functional neuroanatomy when interpreted in light of the constraints and cautions just described, and can provide unique information on the time course of neural events associated with dynamically changing behavior. Moreover, these measures are relatively inexpensive to obtain and are completely noninvasive. This makes them ideally suited for use in studies with infants and children and in large studies where the use of hemodynamic neuroimaging methods would be prohibitively expensive. Examples of each of these will be provided in this chapter.

The Physiological Substrates of EEG

Most researchers now agree that the ongoing EEG is not a direct product of summated action potentials but rather derives from summated postsynaptic potentials. Because both neural tissue and the overlying skull act as low-pass filters, the fields created by the high-frequency transients associated with action potentials diminish sharply with distance from the source. Thus, it is very unlikely that action potentials – even summated action potentials – are represented at the scalp surface in the ongoing EEG. It is also generally agreed that while glial cells may contribute to slow, DC changes in brain electrical activity, they do not account for significant variance in the scalp-recorded EEG. Thus, the primary contributor appears to be summated postsynaptic potentials. In animal studies where intracellular recordings are compared with scalp-recorded EEG, there is a close correspondence between the overall shape of these waveforms (Elul 1968; Thatcher & John 1977) that is suggestive of the contributions of summated postsynaptic potentials to EEG generation. See Figure 1.

Although summated postsynaptic potentials are thought to be the proximal substrate of most of what we record as EEG on the scalp surface, uncertainty still remains regarding the mechanisms responsible for the pacing of the EEG.

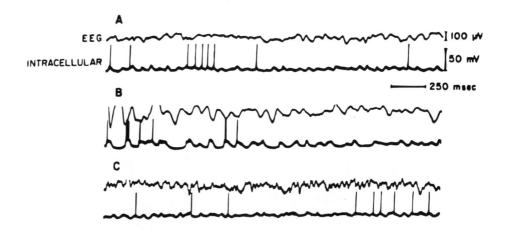

Figure 1. Neuronal activity recorded from the same cell in the posterior suprasylvian cortex, 750-μ depth; EEG taken from anterior suprasylvian cortex. Animal awake (A), sleeping (B), and intensely aroused (C), with EEG patterns characteristic of these states. Note corresponding changes in form of the neuronal waves. Reprinted with permission from Thatcher & John, *Foundations of Cognitive Processes.* Copyright 1977 Lawrence Erlbaum Associates, Inc.

Evidence from a variety of sources points toward the thalamus as a critical site for regulating the rhythmic activity of cortex.

In the early 1930s, a thalamocortical reverberating theory of rhythmicity was proposed. According to this model, rhythmic activity was not due to a particular pacemaker but rather arose as a consequence of the circular movement of impulses in a loop between cortical tissue and the thalamus. Several observations in animal studies performed within the next decade irreparably damaged the thalamocortical loop theory. First, Adrian (1941) recorded from thalamus and cortex directly and found that thalamic rhythmicity was not dependent upon an intact cortex. Morison and Bassett (1945) found that decortication did not prevent rhythmic activity in the thalamus. If rhythmic activity were dependent upon thalamocortical loops then these cortical manipulations should interfere with the expression of thalamic activity. These observations were, however, compatible with the view that the thalamus is a major pacemaker for rhythmic activity in the cortex.

The view that the thalamus is a major contributor to cortical rhythmic activity was championed in work by Andersen and colleagues (Andersen & Andersson 1968) in studies with anesthetized animals. They demonstrated that, in anesthetized cats, spontaneous barbiturate-induced cortical spindle activity was highly correlated with spindle activity in thalamus. The causal influence of thalamic activity on cortex was established in experiments that used selective cooling to produce reversible lesions. These studies demonstrated that if cortex is cooled, the amplitude of the cortical rhythms are attenuated but there is no change in frequency. However, if thalamus is cooled, dramatic changes in the frequency of cortical rhythmic activity are produced. Andersen and colleagues postulated that there were multiple thalamic pacemakers. According to this view, any thalamic nucleus was capable of exhibiting rhythmic oscillations that could then be imposed on relatively localized regions of cortex via thalamocortical cells.

More recently, Steriade and colleagues proposed an updated model of thalamic contributions to cortical rhythmic activity. In contrast to Andersen and Andersson's (1968) model, which suggests that any of the thalamic nuclei is capable of exhibiting rhythmic oscillations and imposing this rhythm on other nuclei, Steriade proposed that the nucleus reticularis in the thalamus is the true "pacemaker" (Steriade et al. 1985). Selective damage to this nucleus abolished rhythmic activity of the thalamus and cortex in rats (Buzsaki et al. 1988) and cats (Steriade et al. 1985). In addition, there are very few connections among most thalamic nuclei (Jones 1985). Only the nucleus reticularis projects to virtually all other thalamic nuclei (Scheibel & Scheibel 1966). Therefore, it was suggested that nucleus reticularis serves as the pacemaker and imposes its rhythmic oscillation on other thalamic nuclei and thalamocortical cells.

Few studies have examined the relation between thalamic activity and cortical EEG in humans. In a recent study (Larson et al. 1998), we measured regional glucose metabolism using positron emission tomography (PET) and EEG simultaneously. We extracted alpha-band activity from the EEG using standard spectral analysis methods (to be described shortly) and then averaged the EEG across sites to form a whole-head composite of alpha power. We then entered this whole-head average into a correlational analysis using statistical parametric mapping (see Friston 1994 for general overview) to determine the brain regions where metabolic activity was most strongly related to average whole-head alpha power. We found that the thalamus emerged as the site that was most strongly inversely correlated with alpha power. That is, those subjects who showed greater metabolic activity in the thalamus also showed less whole-head alpha power, indicative of greater cortical activity. In other words, activation of the thalamus

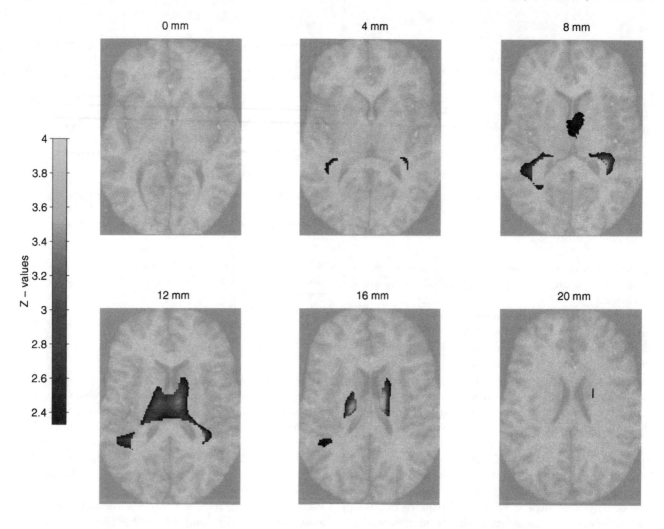

Figure 2. Negative correlation between regional glucose metabolism derived from PET from the entire brain volume and eyes-open 8–13-Hz alpha power averaged across 28 electrodes. The PET data display regions of significant negative correlations mapped onto axial MRI planes spanning the thalamus. The scale is in z-values. The lowest z-value displayed is 2.33, which is equivalent to an r-threshold of 0.43. Adapted from Larson et al. (1998).

was associated with desynchronization of the EEG (see Figures 2 and 3). Recently, using regions of interest drawn on co-registered structural MRI scans to specifically extract a thalamic region of interest (Lindgren et al. 1999), we replicated our previous finding and demonstrated that the association was present only in healthy control subjects, not in acutely depressed patients. Depressed and control subjects did not differ in absolute thalamic metabolism, nor did they differ in whole-head alpha power. Moreover, the variance of these measures within the depressed group was comparable to the control group. The fact that the depressed group failed to show a strong inverse relation between thalamic metabolism and alpha power – in the presence of normal EEG and thalamic metabolic means and variability – suggests an abnormality in thalamocortical interaction in the depressed patients. The

mechanisms that might account for such an abnormality are not currently known and must be studied in future research.

In two major, largely theoretical books, the physicist Paul Nunez (1981, 1995) challenged the view of the thalamus as primary contributor to the regulation of cortical rhythmicity. It is beyond the scope of this chapter to present his theory in detail, but Nunez underscored intrinsic properties of intracortical interaction in the production of cortical rhythmicity. Pyramidal cells account for between two thirds and three quarters of all cortical neurons. These cells occupy cylindrical columns and are situated so that their axons and dendrites are aligned perpendicular to the cortical surface. The two major forms of interconnection among cortical neurons are short-range (< 1 mm in humans) and cortico-cortical, extending up to several centimeters. In humans, the number of cortico-cortical connections is considerably larger than afferent connections to or efferent connections from cortex. The thalamus, which is the most extensive subcortical input to cortex of any structure, does not provide more than approximately 1% of the fibers entering any given region of cortex. Nunez (1981) argued that EEG frequencies are

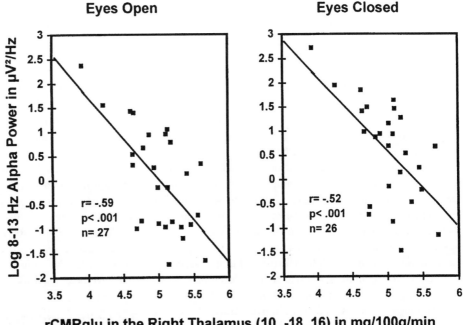

Figure 3. Scatter plot of the correlation between regional glucose metabolism (rCMR$_{glu}$) from one coordinate in the right thalamus and eyes-open and eyes-closed 8–13-Hz alpha power averaged across 28 electrodes. Adapted from Larson et al. (1998).

particularly sensitive to long-range cortico-cortical connections. He and his colleagues developed a model to predict EEG frequency based upon the following major variables: the circumference of the cortex, a long-range connection parameter (based upon cortico-cortical connections), the average velocity of action potential propagation in these long-range association fibers, and a threshold parameter that reflects the threshold for firing of pyramidal neurons. In support of this model, Nunez presented data illustrating that lesions made exclusively to white matter in cats altered EEG frequency. For now, however, scant data exist in support of this model. It is also possible that intrinsic cortical processes of the sort described by Nunez – as well as afferent influences from thalamus – both exert influence over cortical EEG frequency.

In his more recent book, Nunez (1995) speculated that the neocortex determines the resonant oscillatory activity of the brain while the thalamus adjusts its oscillatory frequencies to be synchronous with the neocortical resonant frequency. Nunez relied upon the experimental work of Steriade and colleagues (Steriade, Oakson, & Diallo 1976) to support his argument. In this latter study, Steriade et al. (1976) stimulated motor cortex electrically with a 10-Hz pulse delivered every 2 sec. After 28 passes, the thalamic nuclei began spontaneously to produce bursts of rhythmic activity near this 10-Hz driving frequency. Nunez (1995) also noted that thalamic oscillations coincident with neocortical rhythms will produce a larger cortical response than a thalamic rhythm that is unrelated to the neocortical resonant frequency. Nunez suggested that the combination of the larger neocortical response and the frequency plasticity of the thalamus causes the thalamic rhythms to become coincident with the neocortical rhythms.

Descriptive Characteristics of the EEG

In this section we describe the normal characteristics of the EEG that have been inferred from visual inspection and routine frequency analysis, and we delineate some of the major developmental changes that occur in these parameters. Normal EEG can be characterized with respect to many different parameters. However, the most common parameters used to characterize the EEG are frequency and amplitude. Methods used to extract these parameters will be described in the next section. It is primarily on the basis of frequency and amplitude that EEG differences among several major behavioral states have been described. In normal adults, deep sleep or slow-wave sleep is associated with large and very slow waves in the delta frequency range (1–4 Hz). Lighter sleep is associated with spindle bursts and some slow-wave activity. During drowsiness, amplitude is reduced to the low-amplitude theta range (5–7 Hz) and delta activity is common. "Relaxed wakefulness" is the term often used to characterize the state during which alpha activity is predominant (8–13 Hz). During alert attentiveness, the EEG is mainly characterized by low-amplitude fast activity (> 13 Hz) (see Pilgreen 1995). A commonly used strategy in EEG research is to quantify "activation" in alert waking subjects by examining the reduction in alpha power in a specific scalp location during an experimental condition compared with a control condition (see e.g. Pfurtscheller 1992; Steriade 1989). Inferences about activation asymmetry are often made by comparing the power in the alpha band from left and right homologous electrodes (Davidson 1988).

There are major developmental changes in the EEG that evolve from a disorganized, discontinuous pattern to one that is more organized and coherent (see Niedermeyer 1993 and Pilgreen 1995 for reviews). Very premature infants (less than 28 weeks conceptual age) have a burst-suppression EEG pattern that does not vary between wakefulness and sleep. The burst-suppression pattern consists of very low-amplitude periods lasting from one to several seconds interrupted by high-amplitude complex activity. Neonates (28 to 31 weeks conceptual age) continue to show no differentiation between states of wakefulness and sleep, but they do begin to show a pattern of fast activity superimposed upon a slow delta rhythm (less than 0.5 Hz). This pattern, referred to as a "delta brush" (Lombroso 1993), is one of the hallmarks of a normally developing EEG and usually persists until the fortieth week. Differentiation among states of wakefulness, active (REM) sleep, and quiet (non-REM) sleep begins between 32 and 35 weeks from conception. The EEG during wakefulness and active sleep is very similar, with waves consisting of diffuse delta activity and occasional bursts of faster frequencies that are superimposed on the delta. Eye movements during REM at this age are similar to those found in adults. Full-term neonates spend about 60% of their time in REM sleep. The percentage of REM sleep declines throughout life. The neonatal EEG patterns typically disappear by six weeks from birth in a full-term infant. Within the first three months of life, a posterior rhythm of about 4 Hz develops. This rhythm is believed to be the precursor of the adult posterior alpha rhythm, since it is accentuated with eye closure. Delta activity in the waking EEG gradually disappears as the child develops, and the frequency of the dominant rhythm increases until it reaches its maximum value of approximately 10 Hz at about 10 years of age. Activity at about 8 Hz is usually present by 2 years of age; this activity gradually declines until approximately 25–30 years of age, when the normal adult EEG pattern is established. Some authors have noted an association between the age at which the adult EEG pattern is fully established and the age at which the final state of myelination is complete (Pilgreen 1995). At the other end of the lifespan, episodic theta and delta activity is sometimes observed at particular (e.g. temporal) scalp regions, though the functional significance of these changes has not been systematically studied.

An electroencephalogram is often decomposed into bands defined on the basis of lower and upper frequency boundaries. The classic bands for the adult EEG include delta (0–4 Hz), theta (5–7 Hz), alpha (8–12 Hz), beta (13–20 or 30 Hz) and gamma (36–44 Hz) ranges. An important issue in research is the extent to which the band boundaries are arbitrary – whether they in fact cohere if

examined in a rigorous statistical fashion. Moreover, the extent to which they differ by scalp region is also of importance for making meaningful comparisons of band power among different scalp sites. In an effort to examine this question, we performed a principal component analysis of absolute power spectra from 26 scalp sites in a sample of 115 subjects (Goncharova & Davidson 1995). This analysis yielded five factors, with three corresponding to the traditional bands of delta, theta, and beta. We found support for two separate alpha bands: one at 9–10 Hz and the other at 11–13 Hz. Further analysis indicated that it was specifically the 10-Hz component that was most highly correlated with other, independent indices theoretically predicted to be associated with asymmetric anterior EEG.

There are many other important features of the EEG that have been extracted and described. These will be described after we consider the various analytic strategies that have been used for data reduction and analysis.

Recording and Measurement

INTRODUCTION

Despite the worldwide proliferation of EEG research laboratories, there are surprisingly varied data acquisition and reduction procedures used in the different labs. Few researchers agree on such basic methodological issues as choice of reference electrode, minimum number of electrodes needed, proper analysis techniques, and so forth. As turnkey high-density array EEG systems become commercially available (and increasingly more affordable), the need for a basic understanding of these issues becomes increasingly important. The following section presents a brief overview of EEG methodology, with a focus on state-of-the-art high-density recording technology. Its inclusion will help the interested researcher begin to answer this question: What is the most convenient and efficient way to collect, process, and analyze EEG data that will lead to the most useful inferences concerning underlying brain activity?

ELECTRODE LOCATIONS AND REFERENCE ISSUES; HIGH-DENSITY ARRAYS
Electrodes and Electrode Locations

Typical commercially available electrodes consist of hollow discs or cups (composed of chlorided silver, gold, or tin), which are filled with a conductive gel before application. It is essential that the metal used to construct the electrodes be the same for all electrodes that will be applied for EEG and that different metals not be mixed. This is particularly so when commercial caps are used for scalp recording yet different electrodes are applied for mastoids or ears. For example, the default metal for the Electro-Cap (Eaton, Ohio) system is tin. Investigators using this cap should use tin electrodes also for ear or mastoid placement, since the use of different metals will lead to electrical drift and slow DC artifact.

Electrodes may be applied singly using an adhesive material or as a group using a cap or net system. The primary goal of any electrode placement scheme should be to evenly sample the surface of the scalp. The original 10–20 system has been the traditional choice for most EEG researchers (Jasper 1958). Using the 10–20 system, electrodes may be placed in a pattern constrained by the position of several surface landmarks, including the nasion, inion, and left and right preauricular points. Electrodes are applied based upon the percentage of the distance between these various coordinates. For example, the vertex electrode is 50% of the distance between the inion and nasion on the midline. Individual electrodes are designated by a convenient nomenclature indicating brain hemisphere (odd numbers = left, even numbers = right) and general cortical zone (F = frontal, C = central, T = temporal, P = parietal, O = occipital). For example, T3 refers to the electrodes over the anterior temporal lobe on the left side of the head. It is the norm to report EEG findings by referencing standard 10–20 sites, enabling researchers to easily compare findings across studies and laboratories. It is thus crucial that electrode location be consistent across subjects and across studies. Although electrode placement is often the first task learned by EEG technicians and researchers, placement should be carefully checked across technicians to ensure compatible results across subjects. High-density arrays typically use different notation schemes to accommodate an increasing number of electrodes, but "translation" maps should be provided to enable quick interpretation of the data in terms of standard 10–20 sites.

Choice of Reference

Perhaps the most divisive issue among current EEG researchers is the choice of reference electrode. Happily, the popular fiction of a "monopolar" recording seems to be waning. All voltage recordings are in fact bipolar: they represent the difference in potential between the active site and the reference site (for a classic discussion of these issues, see Katznelson 1981). The choice of reference site has often been guided by a search for the most "inactive" available site (i.e., the site with the least EEG activity present). However, because of volume conduction, there is no site on the body that is electrically neutral with respect to brain activity; thus, the notion of an inactive site is a convenient myth. This is a particularly important issue for EEG studies that examine topographic differences, since the spatial distribution of the observed scalp voltage will depend upon the choice of reference electrode location. Many studies examine asymmetries in brain electrical activity to make inferences about hemispheric specialization and asymmetric hemispheric activation (e.g. Davidson et al. 1990a). In such studies, the choice of reference is crucial because dif-

ferent reference locations may provide a different pattern of results, depending upon the types of tasks that are used and the hypothesized underlying region of cortical activation involved. One strategy we have often used has been to present findings using multiple reference montages in order to establish the similarity of the basic pattern of results across reference (e.g. Davidson et al. 1990a; Henriques & Davidson 1991).

Despite the existence of theoretical and empirical justifications for the use of particular references, EEG researchers vary widely in their choice of reference electrode. At a recent professional meeting for psychophysiologists, endorsements were made for the average reference, linked-ears–linked-mastoids, sterno-vertebral, and nose reference, among others. Clearly there are differences of opinion as to which is the best reference location. The linked-ears and average reference are the most common, so these will be discussed in detail.

The linked-ears reference is perhaps the most commonly used in EEG research. The use of commercially available clip leads makes the use of an ears reference relatively easy to implement with no discomfort to the subject. One disadvantage of this reference scheme is that earlobe sensors have a tendency to pick up the ECG (electrocardiogram) signal. Physically linking the earlobe sensors may help solve this problem. Although some investigators unwittingly assume that the ears reference is particularly appropriate because it is relatively electrically neutral, this assumption is incorrect. Volume conducted brain activity can clearly be recorded at the ear (see Katznelson 1981). Moreover, in his influential chapter, Katznelson (1981) presented a theoretical argument asserting that physical linking of the ears could produce a low-resistive shunt between the two sides of the head, thus attenuating asymmetries that might be present in the brain electrical recordings (data from a single subject that appeared to support this assertion were presented). This claim provoked others to examine the issue more systematically, and a number of studies appeared that addressed whether physically linking the ears actually attenuated the magnitude of observed asymmetry. In Senulis and Davidson (1989) we examined this claim by electronically linking and unlinking the ears while recording EEG referenced to Cz (vertex). We then re-derived the EEG off-line, comparing the conditions of physically linked ears and computer-averaged ears (comparison data came from adjacent 1-min trials). We found no evidence for any impact of physically linking the ears on observed asymmetry. Averaged ears and physically linked ears yielded identical asymmetry estimates. This finding has been conceptually replicated in several other studies (Andino et al. 1990; Miller 1991). In retrospect, the idea that physically linking the ears might provide a low-resistive shunt capable of attenuating the magnitude of observed asymmetry was ill-conceived, since the electrode impedances, even when extremely low (e.g., 1 kΩ), would be higher than the internal resistance within the head. Thus, a physical link between electrodes on the two ears could not possibly provide a shunt that was lower in resistance than what is present under normal physiological conditions inside the body.

The evidence overwhelmingly demonstrates that physically linking the ears does not in any way influence the magnitude of observed asymmetry as a consequence of providing a low-resistive shunt between the two sides of the head. Still, it is prudent *not* to physically link the ears for a different reason. Generally, variations in electrode impedance among electrodes (and specifically between homologous electrodes) do not have any bearing on the observed voltage measurement. In fact, one can calculate the change in observed voltage measurement as a consequence of variations in electrode impedance. Because modern amplifiers have very high input impedance (typically in the range of 100 kΩ), variations in electrode impedance on the order of several thousand ohms will have a negligible effect on the observed voltage measurement.

When linking the ears or mastoids prior to input to the amplifier, different issues arise. Here, variations in the impedance of the left and right electrodes will change the effective spatial location of the reference and could potentially alter the magnitude and direction of observed asymmetry. For this reason, when physical linking of the ears or mastoids is performed, it is important to equate the impedances of the two ear or mastoid electrodes as closely as possible, particularly if questions regarding asymmetry are important. If the assessment of asymmetry is an important component of an EEG study that uses linked-ears or -mastoids reference, the investigators should ideally record their measurements of the impedance of each separate ear or mastoid. These values could then be used to examine the relation between impedance asymmetry and EEG asymmetry and so establish that any small variation in the former is not accounting for variance in the latter. This issue is particularly pertinent in studies that focus on individual differences in asymmetric activation, since such studies make comparisons of asymmetry across subjects. Complete within-subject studies would not be affected, since differences among tasks would be superimposed upon whatever bias might be introduced by variations in impedance asymmetry.

If an investigator wishes to use a linked-ears reference, for most purposes it is preferable to re-derive the data off-line using an averaged-ears reference. This is done by recording the data with an original reference of either a single ear or mastoid or some other location (e.g. vertex). If a single ear or mastoid is used for the original recording, the other ear or mastoid would be recorded as an active site. Off-line, the data can then be re-referenced to an average of the two ears (or mastoids). This referencing strategy avoids the pitfalls of using a physically linked ears or mastoids reference because variations in electrode impedance of the two ears would in this case have no effect on the data since they are each recorded as separate channels.

There are probably only two instances in which a linked-ears (-mastoids) reference might be preferred over an averaged-ears (-mastoids) reference. First, the linked reference can help to reduce artifact. For example, electrocardiogram artifact is typically reduced when using a linked-ears or -mastoids reference compared with a single ear or mastoid. In addition, there are special recording conditions during which specific types of artifact are prominent that might benefit from linked-ears recording. One such case is the simultaneous recording of EEG and impedance cardiography (ZCG); the latter involves the imposition of a high-frequency signal across the torso and often leads to prominent EEG artifact (Dalton & Davidson 1997). We have found that a physically linked ears reference, in conjunction with specific types of amplifiers, helps to attenuate the artifact and allows such simultaneous recordings to be made. The second instance in which an investigator might prefer a linked-ear or -mastoid reference is when there are a limited number of channels available. The averaged-ears or -mastoids reference requires one additional channel compared to the physically linked reference.

Some investigators (e.g. Tucker 1993) have argued that the average reference, although computationally intensive, is probably the best solution to the reference problem. The logic underlying the average reference solution is based on the following assumption: If a sufficient number of electrodes are sampled, then – given the variations in voltage and phase across the head – the average voltage across the entire braincase at any given moment should be zero. Of course, this assumption is predicated on the view that a sufficient number of electrodes are sampled and that these sampled electrodes are distributed fairly evenly across the entire head. Because of the geometry of the head, the ventral surface of the braincase is not adequately sampled, even in very high-density sensor applications. However, with a sufficiently large number of electrodes, this problem is minimized. Just how large a number of electrodes is acceptable for the computation of an average reference is not definitively known, but most investigators agree that a minimum of 20 electrodes (assuming they are evenly spaced on the scalp surface) is about the fewest number possible for an average reference computation. Of course, the more electrodes that comprise the average, the better. It is essential when using an average reference to ensure that the sampled electrodes are distributed relatively evenly across the scalp. With fewer than about 32 electrodes, the investigator must exercise caution in the construction of the average reference if significant artifact is present on several channels, necessitating that these channels not be included in the average. This scenario would result in different reference montages across subjects.

The average reference can be computed off-line and subsequently used as the reference for each "active" electrode. The on-line reference used makes no difference; the average reference can be re-derived using a recording made with any original reference (for a detailed explanation, see Lehman & Skrandies 1984; for a solution that takes into account the distance between electrodes, see Hjorth 1982).

It is worth reiterating that every recording is essentially a bipolar recording. Data should not be interpreted as reflecting scalp activity at the "active" site; rather, the voltage obtained reflects the potential difference between the target site and the reference site. This knowledge should lead to more cautious interpretation of topographic features of data derived from using any of the references described here. Oftentimes, the best solution is to report each data set using two or more reference schemes and so ascertain the extent to which similar findings emerge for each (see e.g. Davidson et al. 1990a; Henriques & Davidson 1991). Consistencies across reference in topographic patterning increase confidence in topographic interpretations.

High-Density Electrode Arrays

Recent advances in EEG technology have made high-density (up to 256-channel) recording systems commercially available. Such arrays provide more even coverage of the scalp than traditional 16- and 32-channel electrode arrays, with an average interelectrode distance of less than 3 cm (see Figure 4). Average reference derivations should be more accurate with an increasing number of electrodes (the average voltage across all electrodes should be closer to zero at any given time point). As EEG researchers use more sophisticated experimental designs, increase their knowledge of neural generators, and develop new analysis techniques, the use of high-density arrays will be important in identifying highly localized patterns of EEG activity. Using a paradigm of iterative subsampling of phantom ERP data, Srinivasan, Tucker, and Murias (1998) showed how focal "hot spots" can be washed out by 19- and 32-channel recording montages as a result of spatial aliasing.

However, important questions remain concerning the use of high-density recording arrays. The most important issue is a conceptual one and concerns the additional yield provided by these arrays. As we have noted, the skull acts as a spatial filter and smears brain electrical activity. The intercorrelations among closely spaced electrodes tend to be very high, typically in the range of 0.8 to 0.9. And most importantly, for certain types of questions, the likely size of the underlying aggregate generator might be quite large. For studies of simple sensory and motor function, where small discrete brain locations are

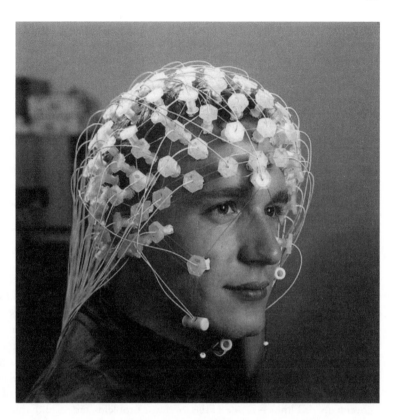

Figure 4. Photograph of the sensor net with 128 electrodes, manufactured by Electrical Geodesics, Inc. (EGI; www.egi.com). Photography by Greg Sutter.

likely, the increase in resolution afforded by high-density arrays is quite apparent (Srinivasan et al. 1998). However, with more complex cognitive and affective processes, it is not entirely clear at present how much additional information will be gained from these methods (using EEG frequency analysis methods and not event-related activity). It is critical, however, that studies be conducted with quantitative EEG using high-density sampling in order to examine the extent to which spatial aliasing is present in the lower-density recordings.

There are a number of important practical considerations in the use of high-density arrays. Application of electrodes must be fairly quick to avoid subject fatigue. Scalp abrasion must be kept to a minimum to avoid subject discomfort. Care must be taken to avoid any shunts between neighboring electrodes due to electrolyte leaking. (See Tucker 1993 for a practical discussion of these issues in high-density recording.) Price is obviously an important consideration for most researchers. A long-standing benefit of EEG recording has been its low cost as compared with other functional neuroimaging methodologies. High-density arrays must likewise be competitively priced if they are to become a realistic option for mainstream EEG researchers. Finally, analysis techniques must be developed that allow for the integration of the huge amount of data these arrays produce. The benefits of high-density recording are nullified if researchers examine data from a mere subset of electrodes. To the extent that these questions are answered and caveats resolved, the advent of high-density arrays promises to be a valuable new tool in EEG research.

ARTIFACT

Artifact can be a formidable problem for the investigator. In this context, it should be noted that EEG allows for considerable subject motion compared with other neuroimaging procedures. It is the only method available that can tolerate fairly substantial head movement, and it does not require the subject to be lying prone during experiments. If desired, the ambient noise in the environment can be almost completely eliminated. These features make the use of EEG particularly attractive in pediatric samples and other populations where it is not likely that head movement could be eliminated.

Biological Artifact

Muscle Artifact. "Noise" in the EEG data – including but not limited to electromyographic (EMG) activity near the recording sites, gross head/body movement, and eye movements or blinks – is one of the foremost problems facing EEG researchers. Standard procedures for recognizing and addressing various types of biological artifact (arising from cephalic or noncephalic sources) are an important component of preanalysis data processing. Reduction of artifact in the data is best dealt with in a prophylactic manner; subjects can be instructed to try to remain as still as possible during the recording trials, to try not to blink excessively, to try to relax as much as possible, and so forth. However, it is important to recognize that following these instructions becomes a de facto task that may divert attention away from the experiment itself. Moreover, certain types of experiments, such as those involving emotion induction, could be adversely affected by instructing subjects to remain still. In those experiments where the tasks under study do enable the experimenter to instruct subjects to keep motion to a minimum, muscle activity can often be reduced by careful observation during the recording session; subjects who appear tense should be encouraged to relax and possibly take a break from the experiment. If possible, trials can be re-presented if the experimenter judges the level of artifact to be excessive during a particular trial. However, in experiments where such flexibility is not possible or where it would be inappropriate to instruct the subject to refrain from movement, it is necessary to consider procedures other than simple instruction to reduce or eliminate artifact. Dealing with artifact on a post hoc basis is time-consuming but necessary to ensure the integrity of the data. Although some laboratories employ computer algorithms to detect and score out artifact (e.g., eliminating data epochs in which a predetermined amplitude criterion is surpassed), only visual scanning of the data will detect all artifact.

Electromyographic contamination by muscle activity is a common occurrence in EEG recording. High-frequency activity, particularly in the temporal and lateral-frontal sites, may represent tension or jaw movement and is commonly observed in certain task situations (see Figure 5). The EMG is a broadband signal that is most prominent in frequencies above the EEG frequencies (i.e., above 50 Hz). However, a simple low-pass filter cannot be used to remove all of the EMG contributions to the observed signal, since the EMG signal is typically very broad and includes frequencies all the way into the alpha-band range (10 Hz). In fact, the use of such a filter can be quite misleading, because it removes the visible muscle artifact but retains that component that is in the same frequency range as the EEG. Assuming that the amplifier filter settings are set to allow observation of the high-frequency EMG (the low-pass filter must be set to permit passage of signals up to about 100 Hz), the researcher may elect to score out such data epochs completely. If a sufficient quantity of data is available for a given condition, this strategy may be appropriate. However, it will bias the data toward the inclusion of epochs during which muscle activity is minimal and thus may skew the findings. For example, if an experiment compares the EEG during two emotion induction conditions, one of which results in more muscle activity than the other, and if the investigator excludes all epochs during which muscle artifact was present, then the comparison between the conditions may be biased because of the differential sampling of epochs in each of the two conditions. If such a bias is likely or if an insufficient amount of data exists to exclude data confounded by muscle activity, then other data analytic strategies are required.

An alternative strategy that we have advocated is to derive a measure of power in an EMG band from each of the EEG leads; then regress this value on power in the traditional EEG bands to derive measures of EEG power with the component accounted for by EMG removed. (See Pivik et al. 1993 for description of this technique and Ekman & Davidson 1993 for an example of its application.) This strategy is predicated on the assumption that power in different frequencies within the broad EMG band is linearly related, so that increases in power in higher-frequency EMG components are accompanied by increases in power in lower-frequency components (Pivik et al. 1993). In order to perform this analysis, brain electrical activity must be sampled at a sufficiently high sampling rate to derive a metric of power in an EMG band. We typically sample the EEG at 250 Hz; this puts the Nyquist frequency at 125 Hz, and one may then extract power in the 70–100-Hz band. To obtain a more reliable estimate of EMG band power, sampling of the EEG can be performed at a higher rate so that a broader EMG band can be extracted. Measures of EMG power are derived separately for each electrode site.

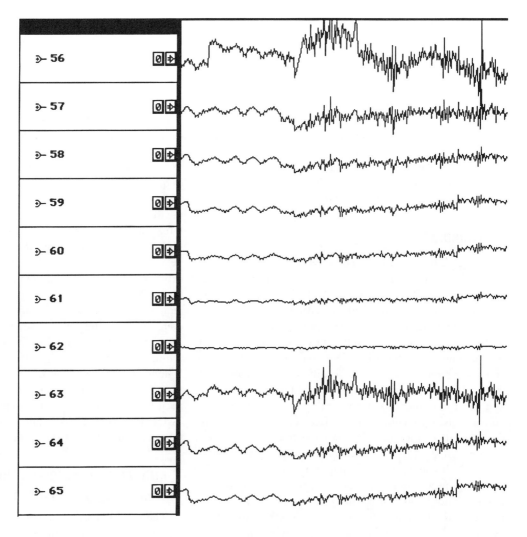

Figure 5. Example of muscle artifact in the EEG produced by jaw clenching. Note the high-frequency activity in channels 56, 57, and 63. These are the leftmost lateral temporal electrode sites on the EGI 128-channel net.

Assuming that a sufficient amount of data is available for each subject, the regression of the EMG on EEG power can be performed within subjects.

Special care must be taken to ensure the absence of EMG contamination when measuring power in the gamma band, typically defined as the 36–44-Hz range. Interest in the measurement of gamma activity has been generated by the observations in animals of gamma activity associated with the "binding" of perceptual features (Singer 1995). Although such observations have been from recordings directly in cortex, some investigators have suggested that scalp-recorded activity in the gamma frequency range may be observed and is associated with focused attention and perceptual binding (see e.g. Spydell & Sheer 1982). Unless adequate procedures are used to regress out EMG from the gamma band, measures of activity in this band should be suspected of being confounded with muscle activity.

Eye Movement Artifact. Eye movements and eye blinks are a problem in virtually all experimental paradigms. Large eye artifact can contaminate the EEG, especially in the frontal sites. Careful instructions to the subject to min-

imize these behaviors will help, but they seldom eradicate the problem. One strategy in dealing with eye artifact is to score out any contaminated EEG data, although this may lead to a dramatic loss of data in some paradigms. Another strategy is to use one of several computer algorithms designed to remove the effect of eye artifact from the EEG signal (Gasser, Ziegler, & Gattaz 1992; Gratton, Coles, & Donchin 1983). These programs generally rely on regression techniques to determine the magnitude of correlation between eye electrodes (vertical and horizontal leads) and each EEG signal. "Eye-corrected" EEG data may then be processed and analyzed as would any other data.

Nonbiological Artifact

Given the hardware involved in EEG research, it is inevitable that nonbiological sources of artifact will influence the data. For example, 60-Hz noise from nearby electrical devices is easy to identify but not so easy to eliminate. Initial suspects may be computer monitors, overhead lighting, power cables, and power strips. If the noise source cannot be located, 60-Hz notch filters may be used either off-line or during data collection in order to reduce the effect of the noise source on the data. High electrode impedances or a faulty ground connection can exacerbate 60-Hz noise problems. Another source of artifact comes from the recording electrodes themselves. Care must be taken to see that the electrodes are carefully washed after each use to prevent corrosion and the build-up of electrical potentials across the surface of the electrode.

RECORDING

The gain by which the EEG signal is amplified is generally chosen from a number of predetermined settings (generally from 5k to upwards of 30k). When choosing the gain, it is best to find the optimal setting: sufficiently high that the amplifier is sensitive enough to pick up small deflections in the signal, yet sufficiently low that saturation or "clipping" does not occur. In systems that allow differential selection of gain values for different EEG sensors, it is useful to set the gain for frontal and temporal channels at a lower level than that for central, posterior, and occipital channels, since contamination from eye artifact is more likely to affect the sites closer to the front of the head. Avoiding clipping in the eye channels and frontal-temporal EEG sites becomes especially important when eye artifact correction procedures are to be used, because clipped data points cannot be used when determining the EEG–eye lead correlations. It should be standard procedure to collect calibration values (gain and zero offset) by passing signals of known frequency and amplitude through each amplifier channel. Collection of calibration data both before and after each recording session provides a means to correct variable gain and offset in individual amplifier channels, and careful inspection of calibration data can often expose amplifier malfunction. In particular, if the recorded calibration data at the end of a session differ from that collected at the beginning of the session, there is some indication that a change of gain occurred during the session. This might signify amplifier malfunction or some other problem that would render the data questionable. Once the analog EEG signal has been digitized, amplitude is expressed as A-D (analog-to-digital) units. It is crucial that EEG data be reported in terms of microvolts; the calibration data are used to convert the raw A-D counts into real units.

Filters are used to selectively attenuate signals that are unwanted or not of interest. Filtering of the EEG signal may be accomplished by using analog filters during the recording or by using digital filters during or after the recording. Filter settings depend largely on the frequency bands of interest in the data. For example, if the experimenter is interested in examining alpha-band (8–13-Hz) activity, a bandpass filter – with a high-pass setting well below the lower boundary and a low-pass setting well above the upper boundary of the alpha band – is required, given the roll-off characteristics of analog filters. These characteristics (expressed in decibels per octave) will partially determine the appropriate filter setting. Care must be taken to attenuate as little as possible the frequency bands of interest, and investigators should be encouraged to examine a graph of the filter roll-off to ensure that the frequencies of interest are not attenuated.

Another methodological issue that depends largely on the frequency bands of interest is selection of sampling rate. When the EEG signal is sampled discretely, the Nyquist theorem states that the highest frequency that can be accurately resolved is half the sampling rate. If the experimenter were interested in examining frequencies of up to 90 Hz, a sampling rate of 200 Hz would prevent temporal aliasing in the digitized signal. In practice, however, the sampling rate is usually set at a level somewhat above twice the highest frequency of interest; in the preceding example, a sampling rate of 250 Hz would suffice. If high-frequency EMG is of interest, sampling rates of 500 Hz or even 1,000 Hz are sometimes used. However, the capacity for data storage increases along with sampling rate. Twice the disk space is required for data collected using a sampling rate of 1,000 Hz as for data sampled at 500 Hz.

ANALYTIC STRATEGIES AND ISSUES
Windowing, FFT, and FHT

The raw EEG signal may be thought of as being primarily composed of rhythmic sinusoidal patterns of activity. After the raw EEG signal has been recorded, saved to disk, and scored for artifact, the next step is to select epochs for the computation of the power spectrum. Epochs should be sufficiently short so that they meet the stationarity assumption, which holds that the data during the epoch do not change in their frequency composition. The frequency resolution of the analysis will be affected by the length of the epoch selected for analysis, with better frequency resolution associated with longer epochs. Epochs should be selected with a Hanning or Hamming window, essentially a cosine taper function. This type of window attenuates the contributions of the data from the ends of the epoch, thus minimizing spurious frequencies in the analysis that might arise from the abrupt transition to the analysis epoch. Most investigators use windows that overlap by 50% so that the data from the tails of each window are reflected in the adjacent window, thus providing maximal data yield.

The power spectrum provides information on the contributions of each frequency to the entire EEG spectrum. The fast Fourier transform (FFT) decomposes the complex EEG signal into its underlying sine wave constituents. (The fast Hartley transform, or FHT, is conceptually identical

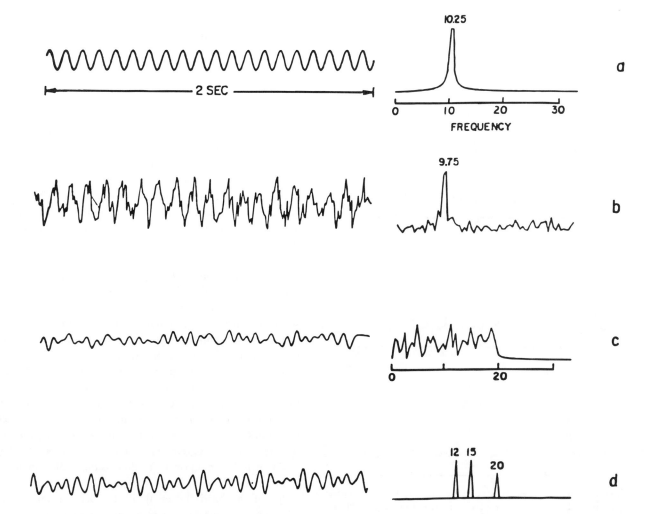

Figure 6. Raw signals (right) and corresponding power spectra (left) for various mathematical functions. (a) Sinusoidal oscillation of frequency 10.25 cps, sampled over an epoch length of 2 sec. (b) Oscillation at 9.75 cps with noise of equal power added. (c) Noise only, bandlimited to contain frequency components only below 20 cps. (d) Mixture of three sinusoidal oscillations having frequencies of 12, 15, and 20 cps. From *Electrical Fields of the Brain: The Neurophysics of EEG* by Paul Nunez. Copyright © 1981 by Oxford University Press, Inc. Used by permission of Oxford University Press, Inc.

but computationally less intensive; Bracewell 1984.) The results of the spectral decomposition are used to compute the amount of power at different frequencies. Figure 6 presents artificially generated EEG signals and their corresponding power spectra. The top portion of the figure displays the power spectra for a pure sine wave of 10.25 Hz. The second line of the figure displays the raw signal and power spectra for a 9.75-Hz signal, plus random noise of equal power added. In the third line of the figure, the power spectrum for random noise below 20 Hz is presented. Note the absence of any discernable peak in the power spectrum. In the bottom line of the figure, a mixture of three sinusoidal oscillations is depicted. Note how the spectral analysis neatly separates each of the frequencies in the complex raw signal.

Power is typically expressed in units of μV^2. Because distributions of power tend to be skewed, most investigators transform the data in order to normalize its distribution. The most common transform used is the natural log transformation (see Davidson et al. 1990a for a comparison of different transformations). Power is usually aggregated across frequency bins to form measures of band power. Also, different epochs of the same condition are averaged

to provide more reliable estimates of spectral power for a given condition. The effects of such averaging can be clearly seen in Figure 7. As the figure shows, noise that is random will become attenuated with additional epochs included in the average, so that the signal-to-noise ratio increases. We strongly advocate that all studies using spectral analysis of EEG report the average and minimum amounts of artifact-free data used to compute a within-subject average for each condition of an experiment.

Another decision faced by the EEG researcher is whether to express power in absolute or relative units. Typically, if power is expressed in relative units, then power in a particular band is expressed as a proportion of power in

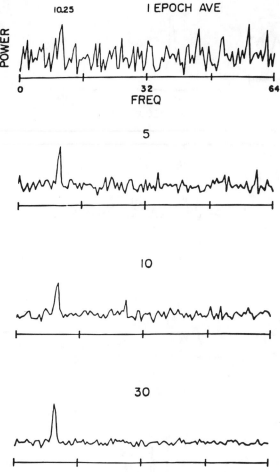

Figure 7. Average power spectra for a sinusoidal function (10.25 cps) plus noise having twice the power of the sine function. Plots are obtained by averaging the power spectra of various numbers of individual 2-sec epochs, as shown. From *Electrical Fields of the Brain: The Neurophysics of EEG* by Paul Nunez. Copyright © 1981 by Oxford University Press, Inc. Used by permission of Oxford University Press, Inc.

the entire spectrum. This computational strategy helps to minimize individual differences across subjects in absolute power magnitude. However, it has the disadvantage of obscuring just where in the power spectrum the differences among conditions or groups might reside. Other strategies are preferable for removing the influence of individual differences in absolute power, as we describe next. Also, the general issue of psychometric considerations in computing different EEG parameters will be addressed in a separate section.

Coherence Analysis

Examination of relations between pairs of EEG channels may be achieved using coherence analysis. The coherence between signals is a squared correlation coefficient expressed as a function of frequency that measures the phase consistency between two signals. Coherence measures will therefore always range between 0 and 1. Coherence is in-

dependent of amplitude, so it is possible to obtain high coherence over parts of the spectrum with low amplitude and low coherence in parts of the spectrum with high amplitudes. If two noise-free signals have a constant phase relation between them (regardless of what the actual phase is) at some frequency, then the coherence between them is always 1. Many factors can produce spuriously high coherence estimates; these are detailed in Nunez (1995, pp. 164–5). Some of the more important factors include statistical unreliability, volume conduction, and reference electrode effects. The first problem can be addressed by including a sufficient number of epochs and then averaging across epochs, just as was recommended for spectral analysis. If the phase is close to 0 degrees, it is likely that volume conduction and/or reference electrode effects are affecting the data. These effects can be reduced by either recording from closely spaced bipolar electrodes or by using the Laplacian. The Laplacian of the electrical potential results in a quantity that is proportional to either the source intensity or sink intensity, depending upon the sign. The Laplacian will highlight local sources and higher spatial frequencies in topographic data. Nunez (1981, p. 198–9) provided a computational method for deriving the Laplacian. It is computed as the second derivative in space of the potential field at each electrode. In practice, the computation of the Laplacian uses an array of closely spaced electrodes to derive a value for an electrode at the center of an array (see e.g. Hjorth 1975). A more accurate estimate is based upon three-dimensional (3D) spline interpolations for computing the Laplacian over the actual shape of the head (Le et al. 1994). Because the Laplacian amplifies high–spatial frequency noise, a spatial filter should be applied after the computation of the Laplacian (Le, Menon, & Gevins 1994). One drawback of all Laplacian methods is that it is not possible to estimate the Laplacian at peripheral electrodes, since there is an incomplete set of surrounding electrodes for these sites.

Coherence analysis has been suggested to reflect connections among different cortical generators (see e.g. Thatcher, Krause, & Hrybyk 1986). Thatcher and his colleagues (Thatcher, Walker, & Guidice 1987; Thatcher 1992) used such data to make inferences about developmental changes in the cortical connectivity. A particularly dramatic demonstration of the reflection of cortical connectivity in coherency can be found in data on interhemispheric coherence in normal subjects compared with split-brain individuals (i.e., patients who have undergone a surgical severing of the corpus callosum as a treatment for intractable epilepsy). Nunez (1981) reported on three split-brain subjects and three matched normal controls for resting eyes-closed data recorded from the left and parietal electrodes (P3 and P4) referenced to the ipsilateral mastoid. Among normal controls, average interhemispheric coherence for the peak in the alpha band was approximately 0.7. Among the split-brain patients, two individuals failed to show interhemispheric coherence above 0.4, while the third patient showed a maximum coherence between these sites of approximately 0.6. Thus, it appears that surgical severing of the corpus callosum resulted in a lowering of interhemispheric coherence, implying that the cortico-cortical connections provided by the corpus callosum are essential in the maintenance of normal coherence.

ASYMMETRY METRICS

One common use of EEG in psychophysiology is to make inferences about differential activation of regions of the two hemispheres. Various indices have been proposed to provide a convenient metric in which to express the magnitude and direction of asymmetry. Most commonly, the investigator will use power in the alpha band from two homologous electrodes in the derivation of the asymmetry index. For example, one of the most common asymmetry metrics is the log right minus log left ($\log R - \log L$) alpha power asymmetry index. In light of the fact that alpha tends to be inversely associated with activation in the waking EEG, positive numbers on this index denote left greater than right activation, whereas negative numbers denote right greater than left activation. As we shall explain in more detail, the $\log R - \log L$ alpha asymmetry index has been demonstrated to show moderate test–retest stability and excellent internal consistency reliability (Tomarken et al. 1992b). The validity of different asymmetry metrics can be established only by correlating values on the metric with independent variables that are predicted to be associated with the asymmetrical process in question. It is important when using an asymmetry metric to examine also the separate contributions of the two hemispheres to the effect in question. For example, in an experiment in which two conditions are compared on an asymmetry metric and condition A is found to have a significantly larger asymmetry index compared with condition B, we can only conclude that condition A produced greater *relative* left-sided activation compared with condition B. However, this difference could be a function of one of three different patterns:

1. condition A has greater left-sided activation than condition B and no difference in the right hemisphere;
2. condition A has less right-sided activation than condition B and no difference in the left hemisphere; and
3. condition A has *both* greater left-sided and less right-sided activation than condition B.

For certain theoretical models, the differentiation among these possibilities is crucial. In order to ascertain which of these alternatives might be accounting for a given asymmetry difference, the investigator must examine the separate activation levels from the left- and right-hemisphere electrodes. In the next section, we consider some of the methodological complications of such analyses.

WHOLE-HEAD RESIDUALIZED POWER

Some theoretical questions require an investigator to examine relations between power in a particular electrode or group of electrodes and some criterion variable. For example, we have investigated relations between asymmetric activation in anterior scalp regions and reactivity to emotional stimuli (Tomarken, Davidson, & Henriques 1990; Wheeler et al. 1993). In these studies, we used an asymmetry metric ($\log R - \log L$ alpha power) and correlated individual differences in baseline indices of this metric and measures of reactivity to short emotional film clips. In the Wheeler et al. (1993) study, once we observed a significant relation between the asymmetry metric and the affect variables, we wanted to determine which hemisphere was accounting for the effect in question. It would not be appropriate simply to take the power at a given electrode (e.g., the left medial frontal electrode, F3) and correlate alpha power at this site with the affect variable, because one of the major contributors to variations among individuals in absolute amount of alpha power is skull thickness (Leissner et al. 1970). When the asymmetry score is computed, it removes individual differences in skull thickness, since variation across subjects in skull thickness is far greater than variations among scalp locations within subjects. Thus, to determine which hemisphere was accounting for the effect in this example requires procedures other than simply using the raw (or log-transformed) power from an individual site. We have developed a straightforward procedure for this purpose.

Assuming that a sufficient number of sites are sampled, a measure of whole-head EEG power can be derived. We assume that the major contributor to individual differences in whole-head power is anatomical variability (primarily skull thickness) across individuals. By regressing the EEG from each site on whole-head power, we can then remove the contributions of this unwanted variable and determine the amount of variance in our outcome measure accounted for by the EEG measure following the removal of variance that is primarily produced by gross anatomical variability. We have suggested as a rule of thumb that at least 20 electrodes be used for the computation of the whole-head average. This will minimize the possibility of any single electrode or region dominating the whole-head average. The average whole-head power is computed by first obtaining the individual electrode site powers and then averaging these data across sites. We then use a hierarchical regression model, where our outcome measure is the variable to be predicted. First entered is the whole-head power average; next we enter the power from the site of interest and determine the percentage of variance accounted for by power at this site. We can directly compare the amount of variance accounted for by power at each of the homologous sites that constituted the original asymmetry metric.

SOURCE LOCALIZATION

It is important to emphasize that even high-density EEG, analyzed with various deblurring methods such as the Laplacian transform, do not provide direct information about the anatomical origins of the observed signals. When data from high-density EEG recordings are mapped onto a three-dimensional head surface, the data are not true 3D data but instead are 2D data displayed on a 3D surface. One of the hopes of high-density arrays is that they might be used with source localization techniques to provide information on just where in the brain the observed signals are generated. Source localization techniques involve methods to mathematically represent the location, orientation, and strength of a hypothetical dipolar point current source. This problem is a version of the inverse problem, the description from a surface distribution of the underlying sources that gave rise to such a distribution. There are differences of opinion regarding the utility of these techniques. Their major limitation is that there is no unique solution to the inverse problem. The solution to the problem must therefore be constrained by some a priori assumptions. In the case of simple sensory and motor processes, source localization techniques may be quite useful (Gevins 1996a,b). However, with more complex processes that likely involve several sources that partially overlap in time, source localization is more problematic. New developments on the horizon include testing the same subjects in the same paradigm using both fMRI and EEG methods and then using the fMRI data to constrain the source localization solution. The electrophysiological data can provide useful information on the temporal dynamics of the source that are unavailable with fMRI methods alone.

EVENT-RELATED DESYNCHRONIZATION

As we have noted, cortical activation is generally associated with an attenuation of alpha rhythms in the cortex. Phasic desynchronization of the alpha rhythm was first quantified and reported by Pfurtscheller (1977; Pfurtscheller & Aranibar 1977). Event-related desynchronization (ERD) is a measurement of the time-locked average power associated with desynchronization of alpha rhythms. This ERD is measured using an event-related potential (ERP) paradigm: an average is taken across multiple experimental events within the same condition in order to measure ERD in response to particular events. The ERD has been studied as a function of cortical activation (Van Winsum, Sergeant, & Geuze 1984) and arousal (Boiten, Sergeant, & Geuze 1992; Van Winsum et al. 1984) and has been shown to occur in paradigms using voluntary movement (Pfurtscheller & Aranibar 1979) and cognitive processing (Sergeant, Geuze, & Van Winsum 1987).

PSYCHOMETRIC ISSUES

When investigators use biological measures, they often unwittingly assume that such measures are reliable and therefore rarely bother to examine the psychometric characteristics of the data they generate. However, particularly in the EEG area, where many derived indices are obtained and where such indices are often used to reflect both instantaneous state as well as trait differences, the consideration of psychometric issues is important. There are several different parameters of reliability that can be computed. First, it is often useful to know whether the metric we extract displays *internal consistency* reliability. This form of reliability reflects the extent to which different trials or epochs of the same measure within a condition are reflecting the same process. It is typically used with paper-and-pencil measures, where individual items are entered to determine if they cohere as a unitary construct. We have applied measures of internal consistency reliability to metrics of activation asymmetry (Tomarken et al. 1992b) and have found these metrics to show excellent reliability, with reliability coefficients consistently exceeding 0.85. *Test–retest* reliability is another form of reliability. Often EEG metrics are used as traitlike indicators to differentiate among groups. When used in this way, it is imperative to establish that the metric in question shows adequate test–retest stability. The intraclass correlation is the preferred statistic to assess test–retest stability, since it is sensitive to both relative position within a group and to absolute value of the metric. Electroencephalogram measures of alpha-power asymmetry obtained during a resting state show moderate stability over a period of approximately one month, with stability estimates ranging between 0.65 and 0.75 (Tomarken et al. 1992b).

When computing measures of reliability, it is particularly important to use measures that are not strongly affected by individual differences in such anatomical variables as skull thickness. Thus, for example, the test–retest stability of absolute levels of power in the alpha band tends to be very high (above 0.85). However, it is likely that basic anatomical differences among subjects, which obviously do not change much over short periods of time, account for these high stability coefficients.

Research Applications

INTRODUCTION

In this section, we selectively highlight some applications of quantitative EEG methods to specific questions that have long occupied the attention of biobehavioral scientists. In light of space limitations, this review is meant to showcase examples of particular approaches and not to provide a comprehensive survey of the findings based on EEG methods in the study of psychological processes. The section is divided into four parts: cognition, affect, individual differences, and psychopathology; specific examples are provided in each of these areas. It is important to emphasize that we consider here only those studies that have used measures of the spontaneous EEG and not studies that examine event-related potentials. Moreover, there are topics (e.g. sleep) that we have omitted because they are covered elsewhere in this volume.

COGNITIVE PROCESSES

In EEG studies of task-induced changes in activity, it is important that tasks be matched on several basic characteristics. Two of the most important characteristics for matching include the difficulty level of the tasks being compared and the motor requirements of the tasks. If the tasks are not matched on these dimensions, it is difficult to conclude that the specific cognitive processes that may have been engaged by the task are responsible for the observed changes. Davidson et al. (1990a) performed a study comparing EEG changes elicited during psychometrically matched verbal and spatial cognitive tasks. These tasks were specifically chosen since we predicted that posterior activation asymmetry would differentiate between them, with the greater relative left-sided activation predicted for the verbal task compared with the spatial task and greater relative right-sided posterior activation during the spatial task compared with the verbal task. The verbal task was the word-finding task modeled after the Boston Naming Test (Kaplan, Goodglass, & Weintraub 1978). Subjects were presented with sentences that defined particular words such as "a box or house for bees to live in." Items varied in difficulty level. Following presentation of the sentence and after the subjects had arrived at their response, they pressed a button that terminated EEG data collection. At this point, they were instructed to write down their response.

The spatial task was the dot localization task, adapted from a measure developed by Hannay, Varney, and Benton (1976). The subject is shown a drawing of two open rectangles, one above the other. The top rectangle contains two dots and the bottom rectangle contains an array of numbers. The bottom rectangle is slightly offset to the right or left of the top rectangle. The subject is presented with the stimulus and is asked to indicate the numbers that the two dots would cover if the two rectangles were superimposed. Task difficulty was manipulated by varying the size of the number array, with larger arrays associated with more difficulty. The subject was instructed to press the response key when he or she arrived at the two numbers corresponding to the response. As in the word-finding task, this button press terminated data collection. The subjects then wrote the two numbers corresponding to the dot locations on their answer sheet.

The tasks that were used were carefully matched on basic psychometric properties including mean accuracy,

mean item difficulty, and coefficient alpha (based upon a behavioral-only study with 151 subjects). Because EEG was collected only during the presentation of the stimulus and since data collection was automatically terminated when subjects pressed their response key, there was no possibility that differential movement during each of the two tasks could have biased the results.

In this study, EEG was recorded from only a small number of anterior and posterior scalp locations – left and right medial frontal, central, and parietal electrodes. We compared two reference montages, vertex (Cz) and an averaged-ears reference. Band power was extracted in the delta, theta, alpha, and beta bands. Finally, relations between the EEG data and measures of performance were also examined. Several important findings emerged from this study. First, asymmetry of alpha power in the central and parietal regions differentiated between the verbal and spatial task, with greater relative left-sided activation associated with the verbal task. This finding was present for both the vertex and averaged-ears reference. The specific pattern of hemispheric activation in the central and parietal region differed. In the central region, greater activation in the left hemisphere (less alpha power) occurred during the verbal task compared with the spatial task. No difference was present in the right hemisphere. In the parietal region, it was the right hemisphere that differentiated between the two tasks, with greater activation (less alpha power) observed during the spatial compared with the verbal task. In the parietal region, there were no alpha power differences for the left hemisphere. This general pattern was present for both the averaged-ears and the vertex reference. That the specific individual hemispheric contributions to the overall laterality difference between tasks was different for the central and parietal regions underscores a point made earlier about the importance of decomposing asymmetry scores so that differential contributions by the left and right hemisphere can be identified.

When we examined differences in other frequency bands between the two tasks, we found that they were considerably less robust than the differences identified in the alpha band. However, when differences did occur in any of the other bands (delta, theta, and beta), they were in the same direction as those found for alpha: greater suppression of power in the hemisphere putatively activated and greater accentuation of power in the other hemisphere. Investigators sometimes assume that, when alpha power is attenuated during task performance, there is a "compensatory" increase in beta power. An alternative view holds that all synchronous activity in cortex is attenuated during states of cortical activation, and that – although most synchronous activity is in the alpha band – there is some activity in other bands and hence the power in these other bands should also decline. In this study, we examined correlations between alpha and beta power asymmetry to ascertain the extent to which these correlations would be positive or negative. One classical view would hold that they should be inversely correlated, since beta power would increase when alpha power is suppressed. However, on the view that activation should be associated with attenuation of power in all frequency bands, measures of alpha and beta asymmetry during task performance should actually be positively correlated. Most of the correlations we reported in this study were positive, challenging the older view that, when alpha power is suppressed, it is replaced by an increase in beta power. Our findings are consistent with the alternative notion that activation is associated with suppression of power across the entire spectrum.

When we examined correlations between measures of EEG asymmetry and task performance, we found that asymmetry in alpha power was most consistently and strongly correlated with task performance. For example, the correlation between parietal alpha asymmetry and performance on the word-finding task was 0.63. Correlations between alpha asymmetry and performance for dot localization were opposite in sign, though none failed to reach significance. In general, correlations were higher for the vertex-referenced than for the averaged-ears data. This likely reflects the fact that the vertex-referenced data involved recording between two more closely spaced electrodes and thus were likely to reflect more local sources. Clearly, the resolution of this issue would benefit from recording with high-density electrode arrays.

We compared the correlations between power asymmetry and measures of absolute power from a particular site or the average of left and right power for homologous sites. We consistently found that it was the difference in power between homologous sites – the asymmetry metric – that accounted for more variance in task performance than power in any individual site or region. This finding underscores the potential importance of asymmetry and suggests that the relative difference in activation between the hemispheres may, in certain cases, be far more important for behavior than the absolute amount of activation in a region.

In a study using high-density EEG recording methods, Gevins et al. (1997) examined the patterns of cortical activation associated with verbal or spatial working memory. The task studied was a version of the *n*-back task, requiring subjects to compare the current stimulus to one presented one or more trials previously. In the version used by Gevins et al. (1997), letter stimuli were presented on each trial and appeared in one of four quadrants of the visual field. Spatial matches required subjects to press a button if the spatial location of the stimulus on the current trial was the same as the spatial location of the stimulus that appeared three trials back. The identity of the letter was irrelevant on spatial match trials. For the verbal trials, the subjects' task was to press if the current stimulus was the same letter as was presented three trials back, independent of the spatial location of the stimulus. Verbal

and spatial control tasks consisted of the recognition of a particular letter or spatial position, respectively.

The EEG was recorded from a 115-channel array referenced to linked mastoids; EEG spatial topography was enhanced utilizing the "finite element deblurring" method (Le & Gevins 1993), which provides an estimate of the electrical fields as they would be recorded from the cortical surface. The method uses MRI-derived, anatomically realistic models of volume conduction to project the scalp-recorded signals downward onto the cortical surface. Local tissue thicknesses are derived for each subject from their individual MRI, and these data are then used to estimate the conductivity of each finite element on an individual subject basis. Fast Fourier transforms were computed on 2-sec samples of EEG, using a 50% overlapping Hanning window. Average power spectra were then averaged within condition for each subject.

Frontal midline theta power increased in magnitude with increasing memory load. Dipole modeling implicated the anterior cingulate region as the source of this signal. A low-frequency parietocentral alpha power signal (average of 9 Hz) decreased with increasing memory load. A faster occipitoparietal alpha power signal (average of 11 Hz) was relatively attenuated during the spatial version of the task, particularly over the right posterior hemisphere. The findings from this study suggest that decrements in alpha power during the difficult compared with the easy tasks indicates that this signal is inversely related to the amount of cortical resources devoted to the task. Results also demonstrated that the alpha signal increased with practice, implying that fewer cortical resources are required for task performance following skill development. The midline frontal theta signal was interpreted by these and other authors (e.g. Gundel & Wilson 1992; Inouye et al. 1994; Iramina, Ueno, & Matuoka 1996) to reflect attentive states that occur during complex task performance. Why such a process should be reflected in increases in theta activity is not clear from this or other reports.

In a complementary article based upon the same data set, Gevins et al. (1997) reported on the stimulus-locked ERP correlates associated with performance of these tasks. In discussing the different information provided by the spectral data versus the ERP data, the researchers suggested that "changes in EEG spectra are probably more closely related to changes in the state of the functional networks underlying task performance (cf. Lopes da Silva 1991), while the subsecond EP responses probably more closely index different operations being performed on internal representations (cf. Ritter et al. 1982)" (Gevins et al. 1997, p. 383). However, they do not offer any data on actual correlations between ERP and spectral measures. In a study that directly compared spectral to ERP measures, we found that the spectral measures were more sensitive to incentive variations compared with the ERP measures (Sobotka, Davidson, & Senulis 1992).

AFFECTIVE PROCESSES

One of the chief virtues of brain electrical activity measures is the excellent time resolution they afford. This is particularly advantageous when studying spontaneous emotion, since episodic bursts of emotion are often fleeting and so their occurrence cannot be predicted with certainty. We have performed a series of studies during which EEG measures were obtained while subjects were exposed to complex emotional stimuli (e.g., short film clips – see Davidson et al. 1990b; Ekman, Davidson, & Friesen 1990). In these studies, we unobtrusively videotaped subjects' facial behavior in response to the stimuli so that we could go back, objectively code facial behavior, and then extract portions of the EEG during which specific facial expressions were present. Used as such, the facial behavior provides a flag to index the occurrence of a specific emotion. In our first major article on this topic (Davidson et al. 1990b), we developed a set of methodological desiderata for the psychophysiological study of emotion:

1. adequate procedures must be used to independently verify the presence of the intended emotion;
2. epochs of different discrete emotions must be separable;
3. the physiological measures chosen for study must have a sufficiently fast time constant to reflect brief periods of emotion;
4. at least two emotions and a baseline condition must be compared;
5. the intensity of the elicited emotion must be matched across conditions; and
6. sufficient data for each condition must be collected to yield reliable estimates of the physiological parameters under study.

Comment on some of these desiderata is certainly warranted. The first desideratum refers to the use of some independent procedure – such as facial expression, emotion-modulated startle, facial EMG, or a similar measure – to verify that the intended emotional changes have been produced. Some of these procedures can also be used to isolate specific parts of the record during which a peak emotional response is present. The fourth desideratum is offered to establish that a particular profile of biological change that might be found for one emotion condition is unique to that specific emotion and is not something generically associated with emotion or states of arousal. The fifth desideratum on intensity matching is particularly important, because often two or more emotion conditions are compared that clearly differ in intensity or arousal. Any EEG difference observed in this case could be a function of intensity or arousal differences between conditions rather than differences in the specific emotional states that were produced. Lang developed a picture set specifically for this purpose from which appetitive and aversive pictures that are matched on arousal can be selected (Lang, Bradley, & Cuthbert 1995).

In the Davidson et al. (1990b) study, we compared EEG during film clips designed to elicit happiness and disgust. The intensity of amusement in response to the positive film clips and disgust in response to the negative film clips was matched. We found greater right-sided prefrontal activation (indexed by decrements in alpha power) during facial signs of disgust in response to the negative clips compared with facial signs of happiness in response to the positive clips. No differences between conditions were observed in posterior scalp regions for the same points in time. Anterior temporal alpha power asymmetry also differentiated between conditions (see Figures 8 and 9). It is important to note that these EEG differences were not present when data were aggregated over the entire film period, independent of the subjects' facial behavior. These findings highlight the utility of using the ongoing EEG in investigations of this kind, where the occurrence of discrete epochs of spontaneous emotion cannot be predicted in advance and are of short duration.

INDIVIDUAL DIFFERENCES

We have examined relations between individual differences in both anterior and posterior EEG asymmetry measures and measures of affect and cognitive function, respectively. In infants (Davidson & Fox 1989) as well as adults (Davidson & Tomarken 1989), we noticed that there were large individual differences in baseline electrophysiological measures of prefrontal activation and that such individual variation was associated with differences in aspects of affective reactivity. In infants, Davidson and Fox (1989) reported that 10-month-old babies who cried in response to maternal separation were more likely to have less left and greater right-sided prefrontal activation during a preceding resting baseline compared with those infants who did not cry in response to this challenge. In adults, we first noted that the phasic influence of positive and negative emotion elicitors (e.g., film clips) on measures of prefrontal activation asymmetry appeared to be superimposed upon more tonic individual differences in the direction and absolute magnitude of asymmetry (Davidson & Tomarken 1989).

During our initial explorations of this phenomenon, we needed to determine if baseline electrophysiological measures of prefrontal asymmetry were reliable and stable over time and thus could be used as a traitlike measure. Tomarken and colleagues (1992b) recorded baseline brain electrical activity from 90 normal subjects on two occasions separated by approximately three weeks. At each testing session, brain activity was recorded during eight 1-min trials, four eyes-open and four eyes-closed, presented in counterbalanced order. The data were visually scored to remove artifact and then Fourier transformed. Our focus was on power in the alpha band (8–13 Hz). We computed coefficient alpha as a measure of internal

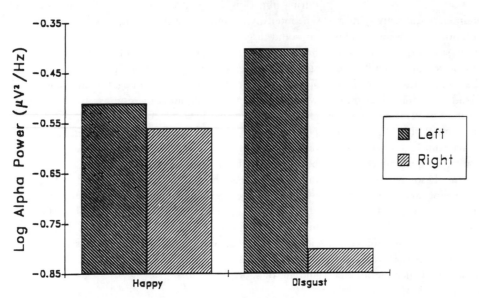

Figure 8. Mean log-transformed alpha power (in $\mu V^2/Hz$) for the left and right frontal regions (F3 and F4) during the happy and disgust facial expression conditions. Increasingly negative numbers indicate less alpha power; the negative numbers are a function of the log transformation, so lower (i.e., more negative) numbers are associated with increased activation. Reprinted with permission from Davidson, Ekman, Saron, Senulis, & Friesen, "Approach–withdrawal and cerebral asymmetry: Emotional expression and brain physiology 1," *Journal of Personality and Social Psychology,* vol. 58, pp. 330–41. Copyright © 1990 by the American Psychological Association.

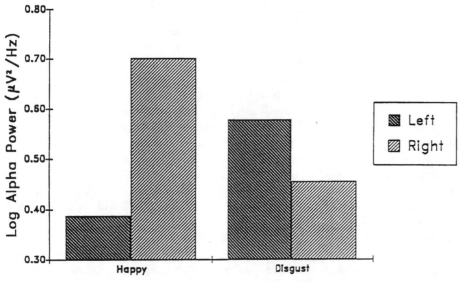

Figure 9. Mean log-transformed alpha power (in $\mu V^2/Hz$) for the left and right anterior temporal regions (T3 and T4) during the happy and disgust facial expression conditions (lower numbers are associated with increased activation). Reprinted with permission from Davidson, Ekman, Saron, Senulis, & Friesen, "Approach–withdrawal and cerebral asymmetry: Emotional expression and brain physiology 1," *Journal of Personality and Social Psychology,* vol. 58, pp. 330–41. Copyright © 1990 by the American Psychological Association.

consistency reliability from the data for each session. The coefficient alphas were quite high, with all values exceeding 0.85, indicating that the electrophysiological measures of asymmetric activation indeed showed excellent internal consistency reliability. The test–retest reliability was adequate, with intraclass correlations ranging from 0.65 to 0.75 depending upon the specific sites and methods of analysis. The major finding of import from this study was the demonstration that measures of activation asymmetry based upon power in the alpha band from prefrontal scalp electrodes showed both sufficiently high internal consistency reliability and acceptable test–retest reliability to be considered a traitlike index.

The large sample size in this reliability study enabled us to select a small group of extreme left and extreme right frontally activated subjects for MR scans to determine if there existed any gross morphometric differences in anatomical structure between these subgroups. None of our measures of regional volumetric asymmetry revealed any difference between the groups (unpublished observations). These findings suggest that whatever differences exist between subjects with extreme left versus right prefrontal activation are likely functional and not structural.

On the basis of our prior data and theory, we reasoned that extreme left and extreme right frontally activated subjects would show systematic differences in dispositional positive and negative affect. We administered the trait version of the Positive and Negative Affect Scales (PANAS; Watson, Clark, & Tellegen 1988) to examine this question and found that the left frontally activated subjects reported more positive and less negative affect than their right frontally activated counterparts (Tomarken et al. 1992a). More recently, Sutton and Davidson (1997) showed that scores on a self-report measure designed to operationalize Gray's concepts of Behavioral Inhibition and Behavioral Activation (the BIS/BAS scales; Carver & White 1994) were even more strongly predicted by electrophysiological measures of prefrontal asymmetry than were scores on the PANAS scales (see Figures 10 and 11). Subjects with greater left-sided prefrontal activation reported more relative BAS to BIS activity compared with subjects exhibiting more right-sided prefrontal activation.

We also hypothesized that our measures of prefrontal asymmetry would predict reactivity to experimental elicitors of emotion. The model that we have developed over the past several years (see Davidson 1992, 1994, 1995) features individual differences in prefrontal activation asymmetry as a reflection of a diathesis that modulates reactivity to emotionally significant events. According to this model, individuals who differ in prefrontal asymmetry should respond differently to an elicitor of positive or negative emotion, even when baseline mood is accounted for.

In order to examine this question, we performed the following experiment (Wheeler et al. 1993). We presented short film clips designed to elicit positive or negative emotion. Brain electrical activity was recorded prior to the presentation of the film clips. Just after the clips were presented, subjects were asked to rate their emotional experience during the preceding film clip. In addition, subjects completed scales that were designed to reflect their mood at baseline. We found that individual differences in prefrontal asymmetry predicted the emotional response to the films, even after measures of baseline mood were statistically removed. Those individuals with more left-sided prefrontal activation at baseline reported

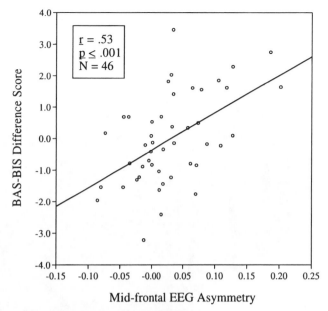

Figure 10. Scatter plot of the correlation between mid-frontal (F3 and F4) EEG asymmetry and BAS – BIS difference scores (score for Behavioral Approach System minus score for Behavioral Inhibition System). Higher EEG asymmetry scores reflect greater relative left-frontal activation. Higher BAS – BIS difference scores reflect greater relative BAS activity. Adapted from Sutton and Davidson (1997).

more positive affect to the positive film clips, and those with more right-sided prefrontal activation reported more negative affect to the negative film clips. These findings support the idea that individual differences in electrophysiological measures of prefrontal activation asymmetry mark some aspect of vulnerability to positive and negative emotion elicitors. That such relations were obtained following the statistical removal of baseline mood indicates that any differences in baseline mood between left and right frontally activated subjects cannot account for the prediction of film-elicited emotion effects that were observed.

In addition to studies using self-report and psychophysiological measures of emotion, we have also examined relations between individual differences in electrophysiological measures of prefrontal asymmetry and other biological indices, which in turn have been related to differential reactivity to stressful events. Two recent examples from our laboratory include measures of immune function and cortisol. In the case of the former, we examined differences between left and right prefrontally activated subjects in natural killer (NK) cell activity, since declines in NK activity have been reported in response to stressful, negative events (Kiecolt-Glaser & Glaser 1991). We predicted that subjects with right prefrontal activation would exhibit lower NK activity compared with their left-activated counterparts because the former type of subject has been found to report more dispositional negative affect, to show higher relative BIS activity, and to respond more intensely to negative emotional stimuli. We found that right frontally activated

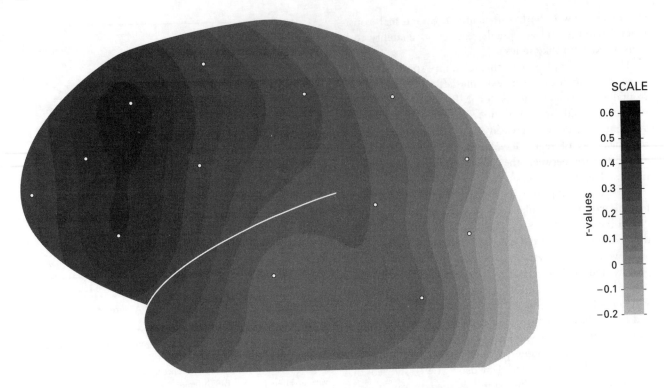

SCALE

Figure 11. Topographic map of the relation (Pearson correlation coefficient) between resting EEG asymmetry (log right minus log left alpha-band power density) and the BAS − BIS difference score (z-transformed score for BAS minus z-transformed score for BIS). The asymmetry score for each homologous electrode pair (represented by small circles) was correlated with the BAS−BIS difference score. These correlations were used to generate a spline-interpolated map across a lateral view of the head. This map is used for display purposes only; all inferential statistics are based on actual measured values at specific scalp electrode sites. Adapted from Sutton and Davidson (1997).

subjects indeed had lower levels of NK activity compared to their left frontally activated counterparts (Kang et al. 1991).

In collaboration with Kalin, our laboratory has studied similar individual differences in scalp-recorded measures of prefrontal activation asymmetry in rhesus monkeys (Davidson, Kalin, & Shelton 1992, 1993). In Kalin et al. (1998) we acquired measures of brain electrical activity from a large group of rhesus monkeys ($N = 50$); EEG measures were obtained during periods of manual restraint. A subsample of 15 of these monkeys was tested on two occasions, four months apart. We found that the test–retest correlation for measures of prefrontal asymmetry was 0.62, suggesting similar stability of this metric in monkey and man. In the group of 50 animals, we also obtained measures of plasma cortisol during the early morning. We hypothesized that if individual differences in prefrontal asymmetry were associated with dispositional affective style then such differences should be correlated with cortisol, since individual differences in baseline cortisol have been related to various aspects of trait-related

stressful behavior and psychopathology (see e.g. Gold, Goodwin, & Chrousos 1988). We found that animals with right-sided prefrontal activation had higher levels of baseline cortisol than their left frontally activated counterparts. Moreover, when blood samples were collected two years following our initial testing, animals classified as showing extreme right-sided prefrontal activation at age 1 had significantly higher baseline cortisol levels when they were 3 compared with animals who were classified at age 1 as displaying extreme left-sided prefrontal activation. These findings indicate that individual differences in prefrontal asymmetry are present in nonhuman primates and that such differences predict biological measures that are related to affective style.

PSYCHOPATHOLOGY

Electroencephalography has been extensively used to study brain dysfunction in psychopathology. Several reviews have appeared on EEG changes in schizophrenia (Kemali, Galderisi, & Maj 1988; Nunez 1995, pp. 616–19); these data will not be reviewed here. Brief mention will be made of the use of EEG to examine asymmetric activation hypothesized to characterize both affective and anxiety disorders. Readers interested in a review of EEG studies in depression may consult Davidson and Henriques (in press).

We have conducted several studies examining regional brain electrical activity in depression. We hypothesized that most depression is fundamentally associated with a deficit in the approach/appetitive motivation system and should therefore be specifically accompanied by decreased activation in the left prefrontal region as measured by scalp electrophysiology; see Davidson (1998) for a general review. Henriques and Davidson (1991) obtained support for this hypothesis. Moreover, in another study, these authors demonstrated that the decrease in left prefrontal activation found among depressives was also present in recovered depressives who were currently euthymic, compared with never-depressed controls who were screened for lifetime history of psychopathology in themselves and in their first-degree relatives (Henriques & Davidson 1990). The findings from patients with localized unilateral brain damage, together with neuroimaging and electrophysiology studies in psychiatric patients without frank lesions, converge on the notion that depression is associated with a deficit in at least the prefrontal component of the approach system. We view this pattern of left prefrontal hypoactivation as a neural reflection of the decreased capacity for pleasure, loss of interest, and generalized decline in goal-related motivation and behavior.

Based upon other evidence (Davidson 1998), it has been hypothesized that – in contrast to depression – anxiety disorders should be associated with an increase in right-sided rather than a decrease in left-sided prefrontal activation, particularly during an acute episode of anxiety. To test this hypothesis, we exposed social phobics who were particularly fearful of making public speeches to the threat of having to make a public speech (Davidson et al. in press). Brain electrical activity was recorded during an anticipation phase as subjects were presented with an audiotaped countdown that noted how much time remained before their speech. The tape-recorded message was presented every 30 sec for a total of 3 min. We found that the phobics showed a large and highly significant increase over baseline in right-sided prefrontal activation. During this anticipation period, the control subjects showed a very different pattern of regional changes. The only change to reach significance was in the left posterior temporal region. We interpret this latter change as likely a consequence of verbal rehearsal in anticipation of making the public speech. No region in the right hemisphere exceeded an even liberal statistical threshold for increased activation relative to a baseline condition. The change in prefrontal activation among the phobics is consistent with our hypothesis of increased right-sided activation associated with an increase in anxiety. A modest increase was also found in right parietal activation and is consistent with the hypothesis of increased right-sided activation associated with the arousal component of anxiety (Heller & Nitschke 1998). Indeed, simultaneous measures of heart rate in this study indicated that the phobics had higher heart rate compared with the controls, particularly during the anticipation phase.

Research using self-report measures of positive and negative affect as well as experienced increases in autonomic arousal indicate that decreased positive affect is uniquely associated with depression, whereas increased autonomic arousal is uniquely associated with anxiety. However, reported negative affect is something that has been found to be common to both anxiety and depression (Watson et al. 1995). We have hypothesized that the decrease in left prefrontal activation may be specific to depression and that the increase in right-sided prefrontal activation (as well as right parietal activation) may be specific to certain components of anxiety. Considerably more research is required to understand the contribution being made by the activated right prefrontal region to negative affect. Other work (see Posner & Petersen 1990 for a review) indicates that portions of the right prefrontal region are activated during certain types of vigilance and attention (Knight 1991). Anxiety-related negative affect is accompanied by heightened vigilance (McNally 1998), which may be reflected in the right prefrontal increase.

Conclusions

Although the human EEG provides a highly indirect measure of brain function, it has been used in a remarkably diverse array of applications and research paradigms. New developments in EEG recording and analysis methodology enable modern investigators to record from a large number of electrodes relatively inexpensively. Such measures provide an economical, noninvasive, and potentially informative window on certain aspects of brain function. The low cost of these measures, particularly in comparison with hemodynamic neuroimaging procedures, makes them ideally suited for studies requiring the testing of large samples of subjects. Among their other virtues (besides being noninvasive) is their fast time resolution. This makes these measures particularly well-suited for studying behavioral phenomena that occur with short duration. However, as noted in this chapter, the chief disadvantage of these methods is their relatively poor spatial resolution and the impossibility of making definitive conclusions about the sources that give rise to the scalp voltage distributions.

In the future, the combination of electrophysiological and hemodynamic measures may provide optimal complementary views of brain function. Recent research indicates that vascular and electrophysiological activity may be uncoupled (Cannestra et al. 1996) as a result of vascular "overspill," a phenomenon associated with the spreading of a vascular response outside the spatial boundaries of neuronal activity. Thus, although hemodynamic methods may provide better intrinsic spatial resolution, inaccuracies can arise owing to overspill. In addition, there is a hemodynamic delay following a local neuronal response, so that the time resolution of hemodynamic methods will always be inferior to those based upon electrophysiology.

It is our expectation that – when used with the appropriate methods and cautions – scalp-recorded EEG spectral activity will continue to provide noninvasive, useful information on integrative brain function for many years to come.

NOTE

The research reported in this chapter was supported by NIMH grants MH43454, MH40747, Research Scientist Award K05-MH00875 and P50-MH52354 to the Wisconsin Center for Affective Science (R. J. Davidson, Director), by a NARSAD Established Investigator Award, and by a grant from the John D. and Catherine T. MacArthur Foundation.

REFERENCES

Adrian, E. D. (1941). Afferent discharges to the cerebral cortex from peripheral organs. *Journal of Physiology, 100,* 159–91.

Andersen, P., & Andersson, S. A. (1968). *Physiological Basis of the Alpha Rhythm.* New York: Century-Crofts.

Andino, F. L. G., et al. (1990). Brain electrical field measurements are unaffected by linked earlobes reference. *Electroencephalography and Clinical Neurophysiology, 75,* 155–60.

Berger, H. (1929). Uber das Electrenkephalogramm des Menschen. Translated and reprinted in Pierre Gloor, Hans Berger on the electroencephalogram of man. *Electroencephalography and Clinical Neuropysiology (Supp. 28),* 1969. Amsterdam: Elsevier.

Boiten, F., Sergeant, J., & Geuze, R. (1992). Event-related desynchronization: The effects of energetic and computational demands. *Electroencephalography and Clinical Neurophysiology, 82,* 302–9.

Bracewell, R. N. (1984). The fast Hartley transform. *Proceedings of the Institute for Electrical and Electronics Engineers, 72,* 1010–18.

Buzsaki, G., Bickford, R. G., Ponomareff, G., Thal, L. J., Mandel, R., & Gage, F. H. (1988). Nucleus basalis and thalamic control of neocortical activity in the freely moving rat. *Journal of Neuroscience, 8,* 4007–26.

Cannestra, A. F., Blood, A. J., Black, K. L., & Toga, A. W. (1996). The evolution of optical signals in human and rodent cortex. *Neuroimage, 3,* 202–8.

Carver, C. S., & White, T. L. (1994). Behavioral inhibition, behavioral activation and affective responses to impending reward and punishment: The BIS/BAS scales. *Journal of Personality and Social Psychology, 67,* 319–33.

Cohen, M. S. (1996). Rapid MRI and functional applications. In A. W. Toga & J. C. Mazziota (Eds.), *Brain Mapping: The Methods,* pp. 223–55. New York: Academic Press.

Dalton, K. M., & Davidson, R. J. (1997). The concurrent recording of electroencephalography and impedance cardiography: Effects of EEG. *Psychophysiology, 34,* 488–93.

Davidson, R. J. (1978). Specificity and patterning in biobehavioral systems: Implications for behavior change. *American Psychologist, 33,* 430–6.

Davidson, R. J. (1988). EEG measures of cerebral asymmetry: Conceptual and methodological issues. *International Journal of Neuroscience, 39,* 71–89.

Davidson, R. J. (1992). Emotion and affective style: Hemispheric substrates. *Psychological Science, 3,* 39–43.

Davidson, R. J. (1994). Asymmetric brain function, affective style and psychopathology: The role of early experience and plasticity. *Development and Psychopathology, 6,* 741–58.

Davidson, R. J. (1995). Cerebral asymmetry, emotion and affective style. In R. J. Davidson & K. Hugdahl (Eds.), *Brain Asymmetry,* pp. 361–87. Cambridge, MA: MIT Press.

Davidson, R. J. (1998). Affective style and affective disorders: Perspectives from affective neuroscience. *Cognition and Emotion, 12,* 307–30.

Davidson, R. J., Chapman, J. P., Chapman, L. J., & Henriques, J. B. (1990a). Asymmetrical brain electrical activity discriminates between psychometrically-matched verbal and spatial cognitive tasks. *Psychophysiology, 27,* 528–43.

Davidson, R. J., Ekman, P., Saron, C., Senulis, J. A., & Friesen, W. V. (1990b). Approach–withdrawal and cerebral asymmetry: emotional expression and brain physiology 1. *Journal of Personality and Social Psychology, 58,* 330–41.

Davidson, R. J., & Fox, N. A. (1989). Frontal brain asymmetry predicts infants' response to maternal separation. *Journal of Abnormal Psychology, 98,* 127–31.

Davidson, R. J., & Henriques, J. B. (in press). Regional brain function in sadness and depression. In J. Borod (Ed.), *The Neuropsychology of Emotion.* New York: Oxford University Press.

Davidson, R. J., Kalin, N. H., & Shelton, S. E. (1992). Lateralized effects of diazepam on frontal brain electrical asymmetries in rhesus monkeys. *Biological Psychiatry, 32,* 438–51.

Davidson, R. J., Kalin, N. H., & Shelton, S. E. (1993). Lateralized response to diazepam predicts temperamental style in rhesus monkeys. *Behavioral Neuroscience, 107,* 1106–10.

Davidson, R. J., Marshall, J. R., Tomarken, A. J., & Henriques, J. B. (in press). While a phobic waits: Regional brain electrical and autonomic activity predict anxiety in social phobics during anticipation of public speaking. *Biological Psychiatry.*

Davidson, R. J., & Tomarken, A. J. (1989). Laterality and emotion: An electrophysiological approach. In F. Boller & J. Grafman (Eds.), *Handbook of Neuropsychology.* Amsterdam: Elsevier.

Duffy, E. (1962). *Activation and Behavior.* New York: Wiley.

Ekman, P., & Davidson, R. J. (1993). Voluntary smiling changes regional brain activity. *Psychological Science, 4,* 342–5.

Ekman, P., Davidson, R. J., & Friesen, W. V. (1990). Duchenne's smile: Emotional expression and brain physiology, II. *Journal of Personality and Social Psychology, 58,* 342–53.

Elul, R. (1968). Brain waves: Intracellular recording and statistical analysis help clarify their physiological significance. In R. Enslein (Ed.), *Data Acquisition and Processing in Biology and Medicine,* vol. 5. New York: Pergamon.

Friston, K. J. (1994). Statistic parametric mapping. In R. W. Thatcher et al. (Eds.), *Functional Neuroimaging: Technical Foundations,* pp. 79–93. San Diego: Academic Press.

Gasser, T., Ziegler, P., & Gattaz, W. F. (1992). The deleterious effect of ocular artefacts on the quantitative EEG, and a remedy. *European Archives of Psychiatry and Clinical Neuroscience, 241,* 352–6.

Gevins, A. (1996a). Electrophysiological imaging of brain function. In *Brain Mapping: The Methods,* pp. 259–72. San Diego: Academic Press.

Gevins, A. (1996b). High resolution evoked potentials of cognition. *Brain Topography, 8,* 189–99.

Gevins, A., Smith, M. E., McEvoy, L., & Yu, D. (1997). High-resolution EEG mapping of cortical activation related to working memory: Effects of task difficulty, type of processing, and practice. *Cerebral Cortex, 7,* 374–85.

Gold, P. W., Goodwin, F. K., & Chrousos, G. P. (1988). Clinical and biochemical manifestations of depression: Relation to the neurobiology of stress. *New England Journal of Medicine,* *314,* 348–53.

Goncharova, I. I., & Davidson, R. J. (1995). The factor structure of EEG: Differential validity of low and high alpha asymmetry in predicting affective style [Abstract]. *Psychophysiology,* *32,* S35.

Gratton, G., Coles, M. G., & Donchin, E. (1983). A new method for off-line removal of ocular artifact. *Electroencephalography and Clinical Neurophysiology, 55,* 468–84.

Gundel, A., & Wilson, G. F. (1992). Topographical changes in the ongoing EEG related to the difficulty of mental tasks. *Brain Topography, 5,* 17–25.

Hannay, H. J., Varney, N. R., & Benton, A. L. (1976). Visual localization in patients with unilateral brain disease. *Journal of Neurology, Neurosurgery and Psychiatry, 39,* 307–13.

Heller, W., & Nitschke, J. B. (1998). The puzzle of regional brain activity in depression and anxiety: The importance of subtypes and comorbidity. *Cognition and Emotion, 12,* 421–47.

Henriques, J. B., & Davidson, R. J. (1990). Regional brain electrical asymmetries discriminate between previously depressed subjects and healthy controls. *Journal of Abnormal Psychology, 99,* 22–31.

Henriques, J. B., & Davidson, R. J. (1991). Left frontal hypoactivation in depression. *Journal of Abnormal Psychology, 100,* 535–45.

Hjorth, B. (1975). An on-line transformation of EEG scalp potentials into orthogonal source derivations. *Electroencephalography and Clinical Neurophysiology, 39,* 526–30.

Hjorth, B. (1982). An adaptive EEG derivation technique. *Electroencephalography and Clinical Neurophysiology, 54,* 654–61.

Inouye, T., Shinosaki, K., Iyama, A., Matsumoto, Y., Toi, S., & Ishihara, T. (1994). Potential flow of frontal midline theta activity during a mental task in the human electroencephalogram. *Neuroscience Letters, 169,* 145–8.

Iramina, K., Ueno, S., & Matuoka, S. (1996). MEG and EEG topography of frontal midline theta rhythm and source localization. *Brain Topography, 8,* 329–31.

Jasper, H. H. (1958). The ten-twenty electrode system of the International Federation. *Electroencephalography and Clinical Neurophysiology, 10,* 371–5.

Jones, E. G. (1985). *The Thalamus.* New York: Plenum.

Kalin, N. H., Larson, C., Shelton, S. E., & Davidson, R. J. (1998). Asymmetric frontal brain activity, cortisol, and behavior associated with fearful temperament in Rhesus monkeys. *Behavioral Neuroscience, 112,* 286–92.

Kang, D. H., Davidson, R. J., Coe, C. L., Wheeler, R. W., Tomarken, A. J., & Ershler, W. B. (1991). Frontal brain asymmetry and immune function. *Behavioral Neuroscience, 105,* 860–9.

Kaplan, E. F., Goodglass, H., & Weintraub, S. (1978). *The Boston Naming Test.* Boston: E. Kaplan & H. Goodglass.

Katznelson, R. (1981). EEG recording, electrode placement, and aspects of generator localization. In P. L. Nunez (Ed.), *Electrical Fields of the Brain,* pp. 176–213. New York: Oxford University Press.

Kemali, D., Galderisi, S., & Maj, M. (1988). EEG correlates of clinical heterogeneity of schizophrenia. In D. Giannitrapani & L. Murri (Eds.), *The EEG of Mental Activities,* pp. 169–81. Basel, Switzerland: Karger.

Kiecolt-Glaser, J. K., & Glaser, R. (1991). Stress and immune function in humans. In R. Ader, D. L. Felten, & N. Cohen (Eds.), *Psychoneuroimmunology,* 2nd ed., pp. 849–67. San Diego: Academic Press.

Knight, R. T. (1991). Evoked potential studies of attention capacity in human frontal lobe lesions. In H. S. Levin, H. M. Eisenberg, & A. L. Benton (Eds.), *Frontal Lobe Function and Dysfunction,* pp. 139–53. New York: Oxford University Press.

Lang, P. J., Bradley, M. M., & Cuthbert, B. N. (1995). *International Affective Picture System (IAPS): Technical Manual and Affective Ratings.* Gainesville: University of Florida Center for Research in Psychophysiology.

Larson, C. L., Davidson, R. J., Abercrombie, H. C., Ward, R. T., Schaefer, S. M., Jackson, D. C., Holden, J. E., & Perlman, S. B. (1998). Relations between PET-derived measures of thalamic glucose metabolism and EEG alpha power. *Psychophysiology, 35,* 162–9.

Le, J., & Gevins, A. (1993). Method to reduce blur distortion from EEGs using a realistic head model. *IEEE Transactions on Biomedical Engineering, 40,* 517–28.

Le, J., Menon, V., & Gevins, A. (1994). Local estimate of surface Laplacian derivation on a realistically shaped scalp surface and its performance on noisy data. *Electroencephalography and Clinical Neurophysiology, 92,* 433–41.

Lehman, D., & Skrandies, W. (1984). Spatial analysis of evoked potentials in man – A review. *Progress in Neurobiology, 23,* 227–50.

Leissner, P., et al. (1970). Alpha amplitude dependence on skull thickness as measured by ultrasound technique. *Electroencephalography and Clinical Neurophysiology, 29,* 392–9.

Lindgren, K. A., Larson, C. L., Schaefer, S. M., Abercrombie, H. C., Ward, R. T., Oakes, T. R., Holden, J. E., Perlman, S. B., Benca, R. M., & Davidson, R. J. (1999). Thalamic metabolic rate predicts EEG alpha power in healthy controls but not in depressed patients. *Biological Psychiatry, 45,* 943–52.

Lombroso, C. (1993). Neonatal electroencephalograpy. In E. Niedermeyer & F. Lopes da Silva (Eds.), *Electroencephalography: Basic Principles, Clinical Applications and Related Fields.* Baltimore: Williams & Wilkins.

Lopes da Silva, F. (1991). Neural mechanisms underlying brain waves: From neural membranes to networks. *Electroencephalography and Clinical Neurophysiology, 79,* 81–93.

McNally, R. J. (1998). Information-processing abnormalities in anxiety disorders: Implications for cognitive neuroscience. *Cognition and Emotion, 12,* 479–95.

Miller, G. A. (1991). The linked-reference issue in EEG and ERP recording. *Journal of Psychophysiology, 5,* 273–6.

Morison, R. S., & Bassett, D. L. (1945). Electrical activity of the thalamus and basal ganglia in decorticate cats. *Journal of Neurophysiology, 8,* 309–14.

Moruzzi, G., & Magoun, H. W. (1949). Brain stem reticular formation and activation of the EEG. *Electroencephalography and Clinical Neurophysiology, 1,* 455–73.

Niedermeyer, E. (1993). Maturation and the EEG: Development of waking and sleep patterns. In E. Niedermeyer and F. Lopes de Silva (Eds.), *Electroencephalography: Basic Principles, Clinical Applications and Related Fields,* pp. 167–91. Baltimore: Williams & Wilkins.

Nunez, P. (1981). *Electrical Fields of the Brain: The Neurophysics of EEG.* New York: Oxford University Press.

Nunez, P. (1995). *Neocortical Dynamics and Human EEG Rhythms*. New York: Oxford University Press.

Pfurtscheller, G. (1977). Graphical display and statistical evaluation of event-related desynchronization (ERD). *Electroencephalography and Clinical Neurophysiology, 43*, 757–60.

Pfurtscheller, G. (1992). Event-related synchronization ERS: An electrophysiological correlate of cortical areas at rest. *Electroencephalography and Clinical Neurophsysiology, 83*, 62–70.

Pfurtscheller, G., & Aranibar, A. (1977). Event-related cortical desynchronization detected by power measurements of scalp EEG. *Electroencephalography and Clinical Neurophysiology, 42*, 817–26.

Pfurtscheller, G., & Aranibar, A. (1979). Evaluation of event-related desynchronization (ERD) preceding and following voluntary self-paced movement. *Electroencephalography and Clinical Neuropsychology, 46*, 138–46.

Pilgreen, K.L. (1995). Physiologic, medical and cognitive correlates of electroencephalography. In P. L. Nunez (Ed.), *Neocortical Dynamics and Human EEG Rhythms*, pp. 195–248. New York: Oxford University Press.

Pivik, R. T., Broughton, R. J., Coppola, R., Davidson, R. J., Fox, N., & Nuwer, M. R. (1993). Guidelines for the recording and quantitative analysis of electroencephalographic activity in research contexts. *Psychophysiology, 30*, 547–58.

Posner, M. I., & Petersen, S. E. (1990). The attention system of the human brain. In W. M. Cowan, E. M. Shooter, C. F. Stevens, & R. F. Thompson (Eds.), *Annual Review of Neuroscience*, pp. 25–42. Palo Alto, CA: Annual Reviews.

Ritter, W., Simson, R., Vaughan, H. G., Jr., & Macht, M. (1982). Manipulation of event-related potential manifestations of information processing stages. *Science, 218*, 909–11.

Scheibel, M. E., & Scheibel, A. B. (1966). The organization of the nucleus reticularis thalami: A Golgi study. *Brain Research, 1*, 43–62.

Senulis, J. A., & Davidson, R. J. (1989). The effect of linking the ears on the hemispheric asymmetry of EEG. *Psychophysiology, 26*, 555.

Sergeant, J., Geuze, R., & Van Winsum, W. (1987). Event-related desynchronization and P300. *Psychophysiology, 24*, 272–7.

Shagass, C. (1972). Electrical activity of the brain. In N. S. Greenfield & R. A. Sternbach (Eds.), *Handbook of Psychophysiology*, pp. 263–328. New York: Holt, Rinehart & Winston.

Singer, W. (1995). Development and plasticity of cortical processing architectures. *Science, 270*, 758–64.

Sobotka, S. S., Davidson, R. J., & Senulis, J. A. (1992). Anterior brain electrical asymmetries in response to reward and punishment. *Electroencephalography and Clinical Neurophysiology, 83*, 236–47.

Spydell, J. D., & Sheer, D. E. (1982). Effect of problem solving on right and left hemisphere 40 Hertz EEG activity. *Psychophysiology, 19*, 420–5.

Srinivasan, R., Tucker, D. M., & Murias, M. (1998). Estimating the spatial Nyquist of the human EEG. *Behavior Research Methods, Instruments, and Computers, 30*, 8–19.

Steriade, M. (1989). Brain electrical activity and sensory processing during waking and sleep states. In M. H. Kryger, T.

Roth, & W. C. Dement (Eds.), *Principles and Practice of Sleep Medicine*. Philadelphia: Saunders.

Steriade, M., Deschenes, M., Domich, L., & Mulle, C. (1985). Abolition of spindle oscillation in thalamic neurons disconnected from nucleus reticularis thalami. *Journal of Neurophysiology, 54*, 1473–97.

Steriade, M., Oakson, G., & Diallo, A. (1976). Cortically elicited spike-wave discharge in thalamic neurons. *Electroencephalography and Clinical Neurophysiology, 41*, 641–4.

Sutton, S. K., & Davidson, R. J. (1997). Prefrontal brain asymmetry: A biological substrate of the behavioral approach and inhibition systems. *Psychological Science, 8*, 204–10.

Thatcher, R. W. (1992). Cyclic cortical reorganization during early childhood. *Brain and Cognition, 20*, 24–50.

Thatcher, R. W., & John, E. R. (1977). *Functional Neuroscience, Vol. 1: Foundations of Cognitive Processes*. Hillsdale, NJ: Erlbaum.

Thatcher, R. W., Krause, P., & Hrybyk, M. (1986). Corticocortical association fibers and EEG coherence: A two compartmental model. *Electroencephalography and Clinical Neurophysiology, 64*, 123–43.

Thatcher, R. W., Walker, R. A., & Giudice, S. (1987). Human cerebral hemispheres develop at different rates and ages. *Science, 236*, 1110–13.

Thayer, R. E. (1989). *The Biopsychology of Mood and Arousal*. New York: Oxford University Press.

Tomarken, A. J., Davidson, R. J., & Henriques, J. B. (1990). Resting frontal brain asymmetry predicts affective responses to films. *Journal of Personality and Social Psychology, 59*, 791–801.

Tomarken, A. J., Davidson, R. J., Wheeler, R., & Doss, R. C. (1992a). Individual differences in anterior brain asymmetry and fundamental dimensions of emotion. *Journal of Personality and Social Psychology, 62*, 676–87.

Tomarken, A. J., Davidson, R. J., Wheeler, R., & Kinney, L. (1992b). Psychometric properties of resting anterior EEG asymmetry: Temporal stability and internal consistency. *Psychophysiology, 29*, 576–92.

Tucker, D. (1993). Spatial sampling of head electrical fields: the geodesic sensor net. *Electroencephalography and Clinical Neurophysiology, 87*, 154–63.

Van Winsum, W., Sergeant, J., & Geuze, R. (1984). The functional significance of event-related desynchronization of alpha rhythm in attentional and activating tasks. *Electroencephalography and Clinical Neurophysiology, 58*, 519–24.

Watson, D., Clark, L. A., & Tellegen, A. (1988). Development and validation of brief measures of positive and negative affect: The PANAS scales. *Journal of Personality and Social Psychology, 54*, 1063–70.

Watson, D., Clark, L. A., Weber, K., Assenheimer, J. S., Strauss, M. E., & McCormick, R. A. (1995). Testing a tripartite model: I. Evaluating the convergent and discriminant validity of anxiety and depression symptom scales. *Journal of Abnormal Psychology, 104*, 3–14.

Wheeler, R. E., Davidson, R. J., & Tomarken, A. J. (1993). Frontal brain asymmetry and emotional reactivity: A biological substrate of affective style. *Psychophysiology, 30*, 82–9.

CHAPTER THREE

EVENT-RELATED BRAIN POTENTIALS

Methods, Theory, and Applications

MONICA FABIANI, GABRIELE GRATTON, & MICHAEL G. H. COLES

Introduction and Historical Context

Ever since Berger (1929) demonstrated that it is possible to record the electrical activity of the brain by placing electrodes on the surface of the scalp, there has been considerable interest in the relationship between these recordings and psychological processes. Whereas Berger and his followers focused their attention on spontaneous rhythmic oscillations in voltage (i.e., on the electroencephalogram or EEG), more recent research has concentrated on those aspects of the electrical potential that are specifically time-locked to events (i.e., on event-related brain potentials or ERPs). The ERPs are regarded as manifestations of brain activities that occur in preparation for, or in response to, discrete events, be they internal or external to the subject. Conceptually, ERPs are regarded as manifestations of specific psychological processes.

The history of ERP research is closely linked with the development of technologies that allow the extraction of event-related brain activity from the background EEG oscillations, which are usually much larger in amplitude and therefore tend to obscure it (for an extended review see Donchin 1979). The first of these techniques was based on the photographic superimposition of several time-locked EEG traces (Ciganek 1964; Dawson 1947). This method, however, was very cumbersome, and it was soon replaced by the development of several analog signal averagers (see Donchin 1979). However, it was not until the 1960s and the advent of digital computers (and thus of digital signal averaging) that ERP research really took flight.

The last three decades have seen several paradigmatic shifts in the focus of this research. In the 1970s and early 1980s, the analysis and interpretation of ERPs was informed by the computer analogy of the human information processing system: ERP components (i.e., peaks and troughs in the waveforms that tend to covary in response

to experimental manipulations) could be viewed as subroutines within this system, each indexing some aspect of cognitive processing (Donchin 1979, 1981). Within this framework, the focus was mostly on the relationship between cognitive processes and ERP activity, without much reference to the possible underlying brain sources of the potentials. In the 1990s, however, the rapid expansion of noninvasive brain imaging methods (see e.g. Toga & Mazziotta 1996) and recent technological advances that allow simultaneous recordings from dense electrode arrays have brought forth two further changes (discussed more extensively in the next section): (i) several algorithms have been developed to derive the putative brain sources of surface-recorded electrical activity; and (ii) several attempts have been made at integrating the recording of ERPs with other brain imaging methods, such as positron emission tomography (PET), functional magnetic resonance imaging (fMRI), magneto-encephalography (MEG), and optical imaging (event-related optical signal, or EROS). At present, ERPs are one of the most established methods in cognitive neuroscience and are considered the "gold standard" in terms of temporal resolution among noninvasive imaging methods.

In the following section of this chapter we will review the procedures for ERP derivation, what is known about the underlying sources of ERPs and their relationship to physiological function, and the concept of component and some aspects of component quantification. Later in this chapter, we will focus on the relationship between ERPs and psychological function.

Physical Context

DERIVING EVENT-RELATED POTENTIALS

The procedures used to derive ERPs begin with the same amplifiers and filters used to obtain EEG (see Figure 1).

John T. Cacioppo, Louis G. Tassinary, and Gary G. Berntson (Eds.), *Handbook of Psychophysiology,* 2nd ed. © Cambridge University Press 2000. Printed in the United States of America. ISBN 62634X. All rights reserved.

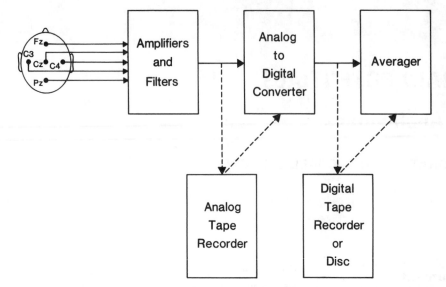

Figure 1. Schematic representation of the operations involved in the recording of event-related brain potentials. From left to right: (a) Top view of the head, indicating the placements of five electrodes (Fz, C3, Cz, C4, and Pz) from which EEG is recorded – note that other locations are also frequently used. (b) The EEG signal is then transferred to an amplifying and filtering system. (c) The amplified and filtered signal may be stored temporarily on an analog magnetic tape. (d) The analog signal is then converted into a digital signal by sampling the potential at a high frequency (usually at least 100 Hz) by an analog-to-digital converter. (e) The digitally transformed signal may be stored on a digital storage device (magnetic tape or disk). (f) Finally, ERPs are extracted from the digitized EEG signal via point-by-point averaging across a large sample of trials (more than 20).

signal-to-noise ratio. However, in all cases, the samples are selected so as to bear a constant temporal relationship to an event. Because all those aspects of the EEG that are not time-locked to the event are assumed to vary randomly from sample to sample, the averaging procedure should result in a reduction of these potentials, leaving the event-related potentials visible.[1] The resulting voltage × time function (see Figure 2) contains a number of positive and negative peaks, which are then subjected to a variety of measurement operations (see Chapters 32 and 33 of this volume).

Because ERP measures are always taken as differences in potential between two recording locations, they will vary as a function of (a) the electrode site at which they are recorded and (b) the reference electrode used. Spatial (topographic) distribution is regarded as an important discriminative characteristic of the ERP (Donchin 1978; Sutton & Ruchkin 1984). Therefore, positive and negative peaks in the ERP are generally described in terms of their characteristic scalp distribution, their polarity, and their latency.

Electrodes are attached to the scalp at various locations and connected to amplifiers. The recording locations are usually chosen according to the International 10–20 system (Jasper 1958) or expanded versions of this system (e.g. Nuwer 1987), so that between-laboratory and between-experiment comparisons are possible. The outputs of the amplifiers are converted to numbers by a device for measuring electrical potentials, an analog–digital converter. The potentials are sampled at a frequency ranging from 100 to 10,000 Hz (cycles per second) and are usually stored for subsequent analysis.

The ERP is small (a few microvolts) in comparison to the EEG (about 50 μV). Thus, the analysis generally begins with a procedure to increase the discrimination of the "signal" (the ERP) from the "noise" (background EEG). The most common procedure involves *averaging* samples of the EEG that are time-locked to repeated occurrences of a particular event. The number of samples used in the average is related to the

Figure 2. A schematic representation of ERP components elicited by auditory, infrequent target stimuli. The three panels represent three different voltage × time functions: the left bottom panel shows the very early sensory components (with a latency of less than 10 msec); the left top panel shows the middle latency sensory components (with a latency of between 10 and 50 msec); and the right panel shows late components (latency exceeding 50 msec). Note the different voltage and time scales used in the three panels, as well as the different nomenclatures used to label the peaks (components). Adapted from Donchin (1979) with permission from the author and Plenum Publishing.

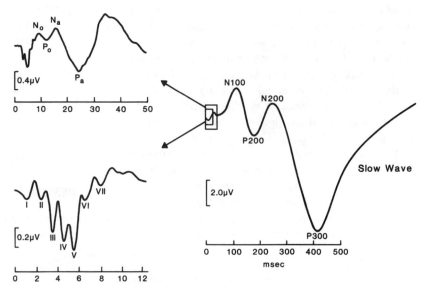

The labels given to the peaks of an ERP waveform usually include descriptors of polarity and latency. According to this logic, P300 refers to a positive peak with a modal latency of 300 msec. A similar labeling system involves a descriptor of polarity (P or N) followed by a number designating the ordinal latency of the component. Within this system, "P3" refers to the third positive peak in the waveform. Other descriptors that can be used in labeling peaks make reference to the scalp locations at which the potential is maximal (e.g., frontal P300), or to the psychological or experimental conditions that control the potential (e.g., novelty P3, readiness potential, mismatch negativity or MMN).

THE EXOGENOUS VERSUS ENDOGENOUS DISTINCTION

From a psychological point of view, it is convenient to distinguish between different types of ERPs. First we can identify those ERPs whose characteristics are mostly controlled by the physical properties of an external eliciting event. Such evoked potentials are considered to be obligatory and are referred to as "sensory" or "exogenous." Second, we can identify ERPs whose characteristics are determined more by the nature of the interaction between the subject and the event. For example, some ERPs vary as a function of the information processing activities required of the subject; others can be elicited in the absence of an external eliciting event. These potentials are referred to as "endogenous." (For a discussion of the distinction between exogenous and endogenous potentials, see Donchin, Ritter, & McCallum 1978.)

Although the exogenous–endogenous distinction is a useful method for classifying many ERP components, some potentials possess characteristics that are intermediate between these two groups and are therefore called "mesogenous." The N100 is such an example, for it is sensitive to both the physical properties of the stimulus as well as to the nature of the interaction between the subject and the event (e.g., whether the event is to be attended).

FROM THE BRAIN TO THE SCALP: THE GENERATION AND PHYSIOLOGICAL BASIS OF ERPs

In this section, we review evidence that relates the scalp-recorded electrical activity to its underlying anatomical and physiological basis (see also Allison, Wood, & McCarthy 1986; Nunez 1981). It is generally assumed that ERPs are distant manifestations of the activity of populations of neurons within the brain. This activity can be recorded on the surface of the scalp because the tissue that lies between the source and the scalp acts as a volume conductor. Because the electrical activity associated with any particular neuron is small, at the scalp it is only possible to record the integrated activity of a large number of neurons. Two requirements must be met for this integration to occur: (i) the neurons must be active synchronously, and (ii) the electric fields generated by each particular neuron must be oriented in such a way that their effects at the scalp cumulate. As a consequence, only a subset of the entire brain electrical activity can be recorded from scalp electrodes.

Two considerations further restrict the likely sources of the ERP. First, because the ERP represents the synchronous activity of a large number of neurons, it is probably not due to the summation of presynaptic potentials (spikes), since these potentials have a very high frequency and short duration. On the other hand, postsynaptic potentials, which have a relatively slower time course, are more likely to be synchronous and hence to summate and so produce scalp potentials. Thus, it is commonly believed that most scalp ERPs are the summation of the postsynaptic potentials of a large number of neurons that are activated (or inhibited) synchronously (Allison et al. 1986).

A second consideration concerns the orientation of neuronal fields. Because the electric fields associated with the activity of each individual neuron involved must be oriented in such a way as to cumulate at the scalp, only neural structures with a specific spatial organization may generate scalp ERPs. Lorente de Nò (1947) specified the spatial organizations that are required for the distant recording of the electrical activity of a neural structure. He distinguished between two types, "open fields" and "closed fields." A structure having an open-field organization is characterized by neurons that are ordered so that their dendritic trees are all oriented on one side of the structure while their axons all depart from the other side. In this case, the electric fields generated by the activity of each neuron will all be oriented in the same direction and summate. Only structures with some degree of open-field organization generate potentials that can be recorded at the scalp. Open fields are obtained whenever neurons are organized in layers – as in most of the cortex, parts of the thalamus, the cerebellum, and other structures.

A structure with a closed-field organization is characterized by neurons that are concentrically or randomly organized. In both cases, the electric fields generated by each neuron will be oriented in very different (sometimes opposite) directions and thus will cancel each other out. Examples of closed-field organization are given by some midbrain nuclei.

From this analysis it is clear that ERPs represent just a sample of the brain electrical activity associated with a given event. Thus, it is entirely possible that a sizeable portion of the information processing transactions that occur after (or before) the anchor event are silent as far as ERPs are concerned. For this reason, some caution should be used in the interpretation of ERP data. For instance, if an experimental manipulation has no effect on the ERP, we cannot conclude that it does not influence brain processes. By the same token, if two experimental manipulations have the same effect on the ERP, it cannot be concluded that they necessarily influence identical processes.

FROM THE SCALP TO THE BRAIN: INFERRING THE SOURCES OF ERPs

So far we have examined how particular properties of neuronal phenomena may determine whether they will be recorded at the scalp. We have approached the problem of ERP generation in a direct fashion, from properties of the generators to predictable scalp observations. In most cases, however, we have only limited information about the neural structure(s) responsible for a specific aspect of the ERP. Our database consists of observations of voltage differences between scalp electrodes or between scalp electrodes and a reference electrode. To determine which neural structures are responsible for the scalp potential (i.e., to identify the neural generators of ERPs), we must solve the "inverse problem"; that is, we have to infer the *unique* combination of neural generators whose activity results in the potential observed at the scalp.

In solving this problem, we are confronted with an indefinite number of unknown parameters. In fact, an indefinite number of neural generators may be active simultaneously, and each of them may vary in amplitude, orientation of the electric field, and location inside the head. Because a limited number of observations (the voltage values recorded at different scalp electrodes) is used to estimate an indefinite number of parameters, it is clear that the inverse problem does not have a unique solution (i.e., an infinite number of different combinations of neuronal generators could produce the same scalp distribution). A further complication is that the head is not a homogeneous medium. Therefore, the electric field generated by the activity of a given structure is difficult to compute. A particularly important distortion of the electric fields is caused by the skull – a very low-conductance medium that reduces and smears electric fields. For all these reasons, we cannot unequivocally determine which structures are responsible for the ERP observed at any given moment when the only information available is provided by the potentials recorded at scalp electrodes.

Notwithstanding these problems, investigators have tried to identify the neural sources of the scalp ERP using a variety of approaches, involving both noninvasive and invasive techniques. Noninvasive techniques include scalp recordings from dense electrode arrays combined with interpolated mapping and source analysis algorithms (which involve complex mathematical procedures and are based on a number of assumptions) as well as the combination of ERPs with other imaging methods that possess higher spatial resolution (e.g., PET, fMRI, MEG, EROS). Invasive techniques include recordings from indwelling macroelec-

trodes (in humans or in animals) and lesion data (also in humans or animals).

Dense Electrode Arrays and Source Modeling

During the last few years, several companies have marketed data acquisition systems for electrophysiology designed to record from a large number of channels (up to 256; see e.g. Tucker 1993). These systems allow investigators to derive detailed maps of brain electrical activity, which can (in principle) reveal differences that are of interest for the study of various experimental conditions and/or subject populations. Yet because the skull operates as a low-pass spatial filter, the question has arisen of what is the effective optimal spatial sampling for ERP recording. For instance, Srinivasan and colleagues (1996; see also Tucker 1993) have recently shown that 256 locations may accurately reproduce the most significant local variations in scalp electrical activity.

The increase in the number of recording locations has facilitated the study of the distribution of ERP activity across the scalp and, in particular, the construction of accurate maps of surface activity, which are usually based on interpolation procedures (Perrin et al. 1987). Another advantage of dense-array recording is the possibility of generating models of the three-dimensional locations of the brain generators involved in producing the surface ERP activity (i.e., equivalent dipole analysis). Computational approaches to dipole analysis involve generating several alternative hypotheses about the neural structures that may be active at a given moment and that may be responsible for an observed scalp ERP. The distribution of potentials across the scalp that would be generated by each of these structures can then be computed using a direct approach. Finally, the structure whose activity best accounts for the observed scalp distribution can be identified (Scherg, Vajsar, & Picton 1989; Scherg & Von Cramon 1986; see also Chapter 33).

ERPs and Other Imaging Methods

These computational approaches make a number of assumptions that cannot always be verified, and they also require the availability of specific neurophysiological knowledge about candidate underlying structures. In some cases, this knowledge can be based on data obtained with other imaging methods, such as the use of magnetic field recordings (MEG). Magnetic fields generated by brain activity are extremely small in relation to magnetic fields generated by environmental and other bodily sources. Therefore, their measurement is both difficult and expensive. The advantage of measuring the magnetic field is that it is practically insensitive to variations of the conductive media (such as those due to the presence of the skull). It is therefore easier to compute the source of a particular field. An in-depth discussion of the problems and characteristics of MEG is beyond the scope of this chapter and can be found elsewhere (Beatty et al. 1986). We will only note here that using MEG to determine the source of neural components still requires assumptions about the number of neural structures active at a particular moment in time.

In other cases, knowledge about candidate ERP sources can be based on the integration of data from a variety of different imaging methods applied to the same subjects in the same experimental conditions. In this way, one can exploit the differential spatial and temporal resolutions of the different methods. Some issues related to this approach are discussed by Gratton in Chapter 33 of this volume.

Invasive Methods

Invasive techniques can also be used for the identification of the sources of ERP components. One such technique involves implanting electrodes within the brain of humans or animals. Research on humans has been made possible by the need for recording EEG activity in deep regions of the brain for diagnostic purposes (Halgren et al. 1980; Wood et al. 1984). A problem with human research is that the indwelling electrodes are located according to clinical rather than scientific criteria and may therefore fail to map the regions involved in the generation of scalp ERPs. This issue may be partially addressed by research on animals (e.g., Buchwald & Squires 1983; Csepe, Karmos, & Molnar 1987; Javitt et al. 1992; Starr & Farley 1983). However, a problem with animal research is the difficulty of determining whether the ERP observed in animals corresponds to that observed in humans, since there are fundamental differences in the anatomy and physiology of animal and human brains. Finally, a general problem with depth recording is that it is difficult to know the extent to which the scalp-recorded ERP is due to the activity of the structures that have been identified by the indwelling electrodes. This problem can be addressed, at least in part, by lesion studies with animals and humans showing that lesions in the structure identified as the candidate generator result in the elimination of the scalp potential. Examples of animal lesion studies have been reported by Paller et al. (1988b) and by Javitt et al. (1992); studies of lesioned human patients have been made by Alho et al. (1994), Johnson (1988, 1989, 1993), and Knight (1984, 1997; see also Knight et al. 1981).

In summary, although solving the inverse problem does present difficulties, several techniques have been developed for identifying the source of ERP components. Although no single method may be able to give definitive answers in all cases, the convergence of several techniques may provide useful information about the neural structures whose activity is manifested at the scalp by the ERP.

THE CONCEPT OF COMPONENT AND ITS ALTERNATIVES

As we have noted, the ERP can be described as a voltage × time × location function. We assume that the various voltage fluctuations represented by this function reflect the summed activity of neuronal populations. This neurophysiological activity, in turn, is assumed to correspond to some psychological process. One concept that has evolved in the area of ERP research is that of *component*, which is commonly taken to reflect the tendency of segments of the ERP waveforms to covary in response to specific experimental manipulations. According to this logic, the total ERP is assumed to be an aggregate of a number of ERP components. Components can be defined in three different ways (Fabiani et al. 1987; Näätänen & Picton 1987). First, components can be defined in terms of the positive and negative peaks (maxima and minima) that are observed in the ERP waveform. Second, components can be defined as aspects of the ERP waveform that are functionally associated – in other words, that covary across subjects, conditions, and/or locations on the scalp. Third, components can be defined in terms of those neural structures that generate them. These definitions may converge in some circumstances. However, as Näätänen and Picton (1987) indicated, a peak in the ERP waveform (e.g., the N1) may represent the summation of several functionally and structurally distinct components. It can also be assumed that the same brain structure may contribute to more than one component and that different brain structures may produce activity that is functionally equivalent (e.g., homologous structures in the left and right hemispheres, such as the primary sensory and motor cortices). Thus, the adoption of one or another of these definitions will have important consequences for the interpretation of the component structure of the ERP waveform. A corollary of this is that different measurement procedures will be required depending on the type of component definition adopted. These procedures will be reviewed in subsequent sections after a brief discussion of general measurement issues.

Recently, other approaches to the interpretation of the ERP have been developed in which the "classic" concept of component is not required. For instance, investigators have used subtraction methods to isolate effects that may be riding over several different components. These include, among others, the repetition effect (i.e., the differential response observed for items that have been previously seen with respect to new items) and the attention effect (i.e., the differential response to items that are attended with respect to those that are not). Note that, by using this approach, the focus is shifted from an interest in describing the functional significance of the ERP component per se to an interest in what the observed ERP can tell us about the way stimuli are processed.

QUANTIFICATION OF ERP COMPONENTS

In this section, we describe some general measurement issues pertaining to the ERP as well as procedures that have been used to quantify ERP activity. As mentioned earlier, the precise choice of measurement operations will depend, at least in part, on the way in which ERP activity is interpreted. For further information about ERP measurement issues, see Chapter 33.

Artifacts

The potential recorded at the scalp can be influenced by sources of electrical activity that do not arise from the brain. Examples of these sources of artifact include the movement of eyeballs and eyelids, tension of the muscles in the head and neck, and the electrical activity generated by the heart. These artifacts can be dealt with in the following ways. First, one can set up the recording situation so that artifacts are minimized. This can be accomplished by suitable choice of electrode locations and of the subject's environment and task. Second, one can simply discard records that contain artifacts. Unfortunately, this procedure may lead to a bias in the selection of the observations and/or subjects. Third, one can use filters to attenuate artifactual activity. This procedure is useful when the frequency of the artifactual activity is outside the frequency range of the ERP signal of interest. For example, the frequency of electromyographic (EMG) activity is higher than that of most endogenous ERP components. Fourth, one can attempt to measure the extent of the artifact and then remove it from the data. This procedure has been used most frequently in the case of ocular artifacts, and a number of correction algorithms have been developed (for reviews see Brunia et al. 1989; Gratton 1998). The use of correction procedures is particularly useful whenever the number of trials that can be collected is limited or when participants have difficulty controlling their eye movements (e.g., children or patient populations).

Signal-to-Noise Ratio

Several procedures have been advocated to increase the signal-to-noise ratio, including filtering, averaging, and pattern recognition (Coles et al. 1986; see also Chapter 33). Filtering involves the attenuation of noise whose frequency differs from that of the signal. For example, most endogenous components have frequencies of between 0.5 Hz and 20 Hz. Thus, at the time of recording (or later, at the time of analysis), analog or digital filters can be used to attenuate activity outside this frequency range. Great care should be taken in the selection of filters. The amplitude and latency of an ERP component (as well as the general ERP waveform) will be distorted if the bandpass of the filter excludes frequencies of interest (see Figure 3).

Averaging involves the summation of a series of EEG epochs (or trials), each of which is time-locked to the event of interest. These EEG epochs are assumed to be the product of two sources: (i) the ERP, and (ii) other voltage fluctuations that are not time-locked to the event. Because, by definition, these other fluctuations are random with respect to the event, they should average to zero and so leave the time-locked ERP both visible and measurable. If

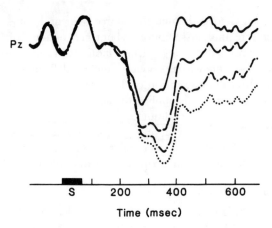

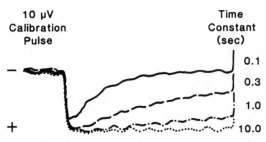

Figure 3. ERPs elicited by counted, rare tones (upper panel). The data recorded with four different high-pass filter settings ("time constant") are superimposed. Stimulus occurrence is indicated by an S on the time scale. Calibration pulses (lower panel) are plotted on the same voltage × time scale as the ERPs. Note the reduction in amplitude and deformation of the ERP waveshape produced by progressively shorter time constants, which reduce low-frequency activity. Reprinted from Duncan-Johnson & Donchin (1979) with permission from the authors and The Society for Psychophysiological Research.

(a) the ERP signals are constant over trials, (b) the noise is random across trials, and (c) the ERP signals are independent of the background noise, then the signal-to-noise ratio will be increased by the square root of the number of trials included in the average.

One of the problems with the averaging procedure is that the three assumptions described in the previous paragraph are typically not always satisfied. In particular, if the latency of the ERP varies from trial to trial (latency jitter), then the average ERP waveform will not be representative of the actual ERP of any individual trial. A related issue is that investigators may be interested in measures of the ERP on individual trials. Thus, a major thrust in ERP methodology has been to derive procedures for single-trial analysis.

Pattern recognition techniques allow the investigator to identify segments of the EEG epoch that contain specific features (e.g., a particular peak pattern that is characteristic of a given ERP component). Examples of pattern recognition techniques are cross-correlation, Woody filter (Woody 1967), and stepwise discriminant analysis (Donchin & Herning 1975; Horst & Donchin 1980; Squires

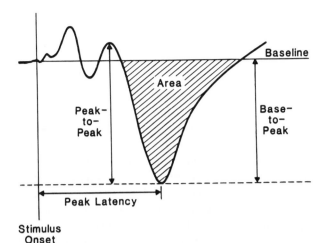

Figure 4. Schematic representation of an ERP waveform, indicating different procedures for component quantification. Three types of peak measures are indicated. The peak latency is obtained by measuring the interval (in msec) between the external triggering event and a positive or negative peak in the waveform. The base-to-peak amplitude measure is obtained by computing the voltage difference (in μV) between the voltage at the peak point and a baseline level (usually the average prestimulus level). The peak-to-peak amplitude measure is obtained by computing the voltage difference between the voltage at the peak point and the voltage at a previous peak of opposite polarity. The area measure is obtained by integrating the voltage between two timepoints.

& Donchin 1976). For more general discussions of pattern recognition techniques, see Fabiani et al. (1987), Glaser and Ruchkin (1976), and Chapter 33.

Peak Measurement

As we have indicated, ERP components can be defined in terms of peaks having characteristic polarities and latency ranges. Thus, a measurement operation that corresponds to this definition involves the assessment of peak amplitude (in microvolts) and/or peak latency (in milliseconds); see Figure 4. Amplitude is usually measured with reference either to the pre-event, or baseline, voltage level (base-to-peak amplitude) or to some other peak in the ERP waveform (peak-to-peak amplitude). Latency is measured with reference to the onset of the event. When the component under analysis does not have a definite peak, it is customary to measure the integrated activity (area measure) or the average activity (mean-amplitude measure) across a particular latency range.

Covariation Measures

Components can also be defined in terms of segments of the ERP waveform that exhibit covariation across subjects, conditions, and scalp locations. As a consequence, procedures are needed to identify and measure these segments. These procedures often entail measuring the extent to which a particular pattern of variation is represented in a waveform. This can be determined by measuring the covariation (or, sometimes, the correlation) of the waveform

(or a segment of it) with an idealized wave representing the component of interest. The "ideal" wave can be identified using statistical methods, such as principal components analysis (PCA; Donchin & Heffley 1978) or discriminant analysis (Donchin & Herning 1975). Alternatively, the ideal wave can be selected using arbitrary models, such as a cosinusoidal function (Fabiani et al. 1987; Gratton et al. 1989b). These types of analyses are advantageous in the presence of noise or when there is substantial component overlap; however, Fabiani et al. (1987) and Gratton et al. (1989b) showed that component recognition using peak procedures may actually be both reliable and valid, provided that data are adequately filtered.

Source Activity Measures

A third way of defining components is in terms of underlying sources. According to this definition, we should quantify the activity of these sources to provide latency and amplitude measures of the different components. As noted previously, the relationship between scalp electrical activity and source activity is difficult to describe and requires a number of assumptions. Recently, large strides have been made in this area with the development of algorithms for dipole (e.g., BESA – Scherg & Von Cramon 1986; Scherg et al. 1989) and distributed (EMSE – Greenblatt et al. 1997; LORETA – Baillet & Garnero 1997; Pascual-Marqui, Michel, & Lehmann 1994) source analyses. Both of these approaches are based on modeling efforts. Spatiotemporal dipole models fit a small number of individual point dipoles to data that vary over space and time. The location and orientation of the dipoles may be fixed, whereas amplitude and polarity are left free to vary over time. In this way it is possible to represent variations in surface activity in terms of variations of the activity of a few underlying brain structures.

In contrast to dipole models, distributed source models assume that extended segments of the cortex (or even the entire cortex) can be active simultaneously. To express local variations (and hence explain variations in surface distribution), these algorithms allow the relative contribution of individual areas of the cortex to vary over time. These models, although perhaps more realistic, are usually underdetermined from a statistical point of view (i.e., they include more free parameters than data points). Therefore, external criteria are necessary to constrain the number of possible solutions (e.g., minimum norm, correlation between adjacent data points). Note that both dipole and distributed modeling efforts can be guided and constrained by anatomical and functional data obtained with other methods (e.g., MRI, fMRI, PET).

Problems in Component Measurement

In this section we discuss two specific problems that arise during component measurement. The first problem concerns the commensurability of the measurements of different waveforms. Is a particular component, recorded under a particular set of circumstances, the same as that recorded in another situation? This is especially a problem when we define components as a peak observed at a given latency. For example, if the latency of the peak differs between two experimental conditions, we would be led to conclude that different components are present in the two sets of data. How can we be sure that the same component varies in latency between the two conditions, rather than that two different components are present in the two different conditions? A solution to this problem could be derived from a careful examination of the pattern of results obtained and from a comparison of these results with what we already know about different ERP components. Of course, this means that we are including a large number of empirical and theoretical arguments in the definition of each ERP component – definitions that may differ from one component to another and from time to time. For example, the definition of a component may include not only polarity and latency but also distribution across the scalp and sensitivity to experimental manipulations (see e.g. Fabiani et al. 1987). Thus, it is clear that a correct interpretation of the component structure of an ERP waveform requires some background information about the components themselves. In turn, this indicates that the concept of component is likely to evolve over time (as more knowledge is accumulated) and that revisions of traditional component classifications may sometime be necessary.

A second problem in component measurement is that of component overlap. Usually, ERP components do not appear in isolation, but several of them may be active at the same moment in time. This reflects the parallel nature of brain processes. When this occurs, it is difficult to attribute a particular portion of scalp activity to a particular component. Peak and area measures are particularly susceptible to this problem. Principal component analysis has been proposed as a tool to separate the contribution of overlapping components (Donchin & Heffley 1978), but in some cases even PCA can misallocate variance across different components (Wood & McCarthy 1984). As a result, we may attribute a difference obtained between two particular experimental conditions to the wrong component.

Several procedures have been proposed to solve the problem of component overlap, but none of them seems to have universal validity. In some cases, it can be assumed that only one component varies between two experimental conditions. In this case, the variation of this component can be isolated by subtracting two sets of waveforms and performing the measurement on the resulting "difference waveform." Unfortunately, we can not always assume that the effect of an experimental variable is so selective. Furthermore, the subtraction procedure implies that only amplitude – and not latency – varies across experimen-

tal conditions. This may not always be true, which may result in a particularly serious problem when subtracted waveforms are used and latency varies across conditions.

Another approach is based on using scalp distribution data to decompose overlapping components (vector filter – Gratton, Coles, & Donchin 1989a; Gratton et al. 1989b). A prerequisite for this procedure is that hypotheses about the scalp distributions of the components contributing to the data can be made in advance. Furthermore, if the scalp distributions of different components are correlated, then attribution of variance to one or another component may be arbitrary. Procedures such as discriminant analysis and PCA can be useful in deriving orthogonal sets of scalp distributions from the data. Note that distributional filters perform the same kind of operations in the spatial domain that frequency filters perform in the frequency domain. Whereas frequency filters apply different weights to activity in different frequency bands, distributional filters apply different weights to activity from different spatial locations.

Inferential Context

In this section, we review the procedures through which we come to make inferences about psychological and physiological processes and states from the measurement of ERPs. Previous work by Cacioppo and Tassinary (1990) describes different types of relationships between psychological and physiological variables, relations that limit the extent and generalizability of inferences that can be drawn from psychophysiological data. More recent papers (Kutas & Federmeier 1998; Miller 1996; Sarter, Berntson, & Cacioppo 1996) also discuss existing limitations in making inferences about brain function on the basis of brain imaging data. The general framework described in these papers is assumed in the approach presented here, which is more limited in scope and is intended as a description of the experimental logic that is often employed in ERP research.

EXPERIMENTAL LOGIC

If the ERP waveform is interpreted as an aggregate of several components, then some theory about the functional significance of each component would be useful for understanding the meaning of changes that this component will exhibit as a function of specific contexts. We should emphasize that by "functional significance" we mean a specification not of the neurophysiological significance of the component but rather of the information processing transactions that are manifested by it. In this sense, then, neurophysiological knowledge may be useful – but not necessarily critical – to the psychophysiological enterprise. Of course, neurophysiological knowledge is very important if we wish to use ERPs as a tool to make statements about brain function.

In the case of all ERP components, the initial phase in the process of establishing functional significance begins with the "discovery" of a component. A theory about the functional significance of a component is then developed, a complex process that involves the following.

1. Studies of the component's antecedents. Antecedent conditions refer to those experimental manipulations that will produce consistent variations – in amplitude, latency, and (in some cases) scalp distribution – in an ERP component.
2. Establishing the consequences of variation in the latency or amplitude of the component. An examination of the consequences can be used to test statements relating to functional significance.
3. Speculations about the psychological and/or neurophysiological function it manifests (Donchin 1981).

Examples of this logic applied to the P300 are reviewed in a later section. Here we consider the ways in which ERP measures are used to make inferences about psychological processes and, in some cases, to make inferences about brain activity. We shall review a series of inferential steps that depend to an increasing extent on assumptions about the functional significance of the ERP. For the purposes of elucidating the inferential process, we shall consider an experiment in which subjects are run in two different conditions.

USING ERP MEASURES: PSYCHOPHYSIOLOGICAL INFERENCE

Inference 1: Conditions Are Different

At the most fundamental level, we can ask whether or not the two conditions are associated with different ERP responses. Note that both this inference and the next do not depend on the classification of the ERP into components. Rather, they are based on the evaluation of the waveforms obtained in different conditions. The analytic procedure necessary to answer this question would involve a univariate or multivariate analysis of variance (with condition and peak, or data point, within a specified time window as factors). Given that such an analysis yields a significant effect of condition or a condition-by-peak or data-point interaction, we can infer that the conditions are different. If we assume that the ERP is a sign of brain activity and/or that it reflects some psychological process, then we can infer that the brain activity and associated psychological processing are different in the two conditions.

Inference 2: Conditions Differ at a Particular Time

The second level of inference concerns the time at which the two conditions differ. This inference could be made on the basis of post hoc tests of the significant condition-by-time interaction. It would take the form of "by at least msec X, processing of stimuli in condition A is different than processing of stimulus in condition B." This kind of inference is frequently made in studies of selective attention, where an important theoretical issue concerns the relative time at which an attended event receives preferential processing. As with the first, most primitive form of inference, we need only assume that the ERP is a reflection of some nonspecified aspect of psychological processing. Note that this same evidence can also be used to infer the time at which some (nonspecified) brain structure(s) shows differential processing for two events.

Inference 3: Conditions Differ with Respect to the Latency of Some Process

For this level of inference, additional assumptions and measurement operations must be made. Here we use ERPs to study the duration of processes preceding the occurrence of a particular physiological event (such as a component's peak). This requires that we can identify a particular physiological event (or component) across conditions and that this event varies in latency. Further, we usually assume that the ERP component can only occur *after* a particular psychological process is carried out. Note that, for this inferential level, we must first adopt a procedure to identify the component in question and measure its latency; we then use an analytic procedure (e.g., analysis of variance, *t*-test) to evaluate the difference between the conditions with respect to the component latency. As a result of this procedure, we make the inference that the conditions differ with respect to the timing of a given process.

Inference 4: Conditions Differ with Respect to the Degree to Which Some Process Occurs

The notion of component also allows us to use ERPs to infer that a particular process occurs to a greater extent under one condition than under another. In this case, we must assume that a particular ERP component is a manifestation of some process. We must further assume that changes in the magnitude of the component correspond directly to changes in the degree to which the process is invoked. Then, we must devise a suitable measurement procedure to identify and assess the magnitude of the component. Finally, we can proceed with the usual inferential test and determine whether or not the conditions differ with respect to the extent of the process. Of course, if precise knowledge were available about the underlying brain sources of a particular ERP activity, then statements made about the ERP could also apply to the brain structures in question.

Psychological Context: Selective Review of ERP Findings

In this section we review a number of findings in the ERP literature. We begin with a discussion of ERPs that are

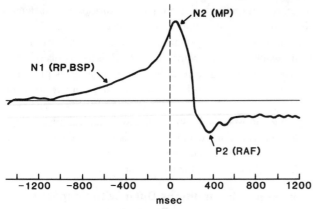

Figure 5. Typical movement-related potential (recorded from a central electrode, Cz) preceding a voluntary hand movement. Note that the potential begins about 1 sec before the movement (indicated by the dashed vertical line). The potential can be subdivided into different components as follows: N1 (RP = readiness potential, BSP = *Bereitschaftspotential*); N2 (MP = motor potential); P2 (RAF = reafferent potential). Adapted with permission from Kutas & Donchin, "Preparation to respond as manifested by movement-related brain potentials," *Brain Research*, vol. 202, pp. 95–115. Copyright 1980 Elsevier Science.

related to the preparation, execution, and evaluation of motor responses. This is followed by a brief overview of sensory and cognitive ERP components that occur after a marker event, with particular emphasis on ERP effects related to attention, memory, and language.

RESPONSE-RELATED POTENTIALS

In this section we review research on ERP activity that is typically observed in relationship to movement preparation and generation (readiness potential, lateralized readiness potential, contingent negative variation) or as a reaction to errors (error-related negativity).

Movement-Related Potentials

One class of event-preceding potentials includes those that are apparently related to the preparation for movement. These potentials were first described by Kornhuber and Deecke (1965), who found that – prior to voluntary movements – a negative potential develops slowly, beginning some 800 msec before initiation of the movement (see Figure 5). These "readiness potentials" (or *Bereitschaftspotentials*) were distinguished from those that followed the movement, the "reafferent" potentials. In similar conditions involving passive movement, only postmovement potentials were observed. Both readiness and reafferent potentials tend to be maximal at electrodes located over motor areas of the cortex. Furthermore, some components of the potentials are larger at electrode locations contralateral to the responding limb (at least for hand and finger movements). Indeed, this kind of lateralization has become an important criterion for movement-related potentials.

The investigation of movement-related potentials has developed along several different paths, including:

1. the discovery and classification of different components of the movement-related potential (for reviews see Brunia, Haagh, & Scheirs 1985; Deecke et al. 1984);
2. analysis of the neural origin using the scalp topography of ERPs (Vaughan, Costa, & Ritter 1972) or magnetic field recordings (Deecke, Weinberg, & Brickett 1982; Okada, Williamson, & Kaufman 1982);
3. analysis of the functional significance of different components (for reviews see Brunia et al. 1985; Deecke et al. 1984); and
4. recording of movement-related potentials in special populations (e.g., in mentally retarded children – Karrer & Ivins 1976; in Parkinson's patients – Deecke et al. 1977).

In general, these studies confirm that the potential described by Kornhuber and Deecke is generated, at least in part, by neuronal activity in motor areas of the cortex and is a reflection of processes related to the preparation and execution of movements.

The Lateralized Readiness Potential (LRP). Movement-related potentials have been applied to the investigation of human information processing. Studies reviewed in the previous section (Kornhuber & Deecke 1965) indicated that the readiness potential occurs prior to voluntary movements of the hand and is maximal at central sites, contralateral to the responding hand. In addition, the lateralized readiness potentials could also be observed in the foreperiods of warned reaction time tasks when subjects know in advance which hand to use in response to the imperative stimulus (Kutas & Donchin 1977).

Based on this evidence, researchers working independently at the Universities of Groningen (De Jong et al. 1988) and Illinois (Coles & Gratton 1986) concluded that one could exploit the lateralization of the readiness potential in choice reaction time tasks to infer whether and when subjects had preferentially prepared a response (see De Jong et al. 1988; Gehring et al. 1992; Gratton et al. 1988, 1990; Kutas & Donchin 1980).

The derivation of the LRP (Coles 1989) is based on the following steps, which are designed to ensure that any observed lateralization can be specifically attributed to motor-related asymmetries rather than to other kinds of asymmetrical brain activity. (1) Potentials recorded from electrodes placed over the left and right motor cortices are subtracted. This subtraction is performed separately for conditions where left-hand movements represent the correct response and for those where right-hand movements are correct. In each case, the potential ipsilateral to the side of the correct response is subtracted from the potential contralateral to the side of the correct response. (2) The asymmetry values for left- and right-hand movements are then averaged to yield a measure of the average lateralized activity as subjects prepare to move. This average measure is the LRP.

Measures of the LRP have been used to make three different kinds of inferences: (i) to infer whether a response has been preferentially activated or prepared (note that no LRP will be observed if both responses are equally activated); (ii) to infer the degree to which a response has been preferentially activated. This inference presupposes that the level of asymmetry as reflected by the LRP is related to the level of differential response activation. In fact, Gratton et al. (1988) observed that the level of the LRP at the time of an overt response was fixed: that is, there appeared to be a criterion level of the LRP which, when crossed, was associated with an overt response. Finally, LRP measures have also been used (iii) to infer when a response is preferentially activated. This inference has, perhaps, proved to be the most troublesome owing to the problems associated with the measurement of LRP onset (Smulders, Kenemans, & Kok 1996).

In order to use the LRP in the context of research in experimental and cognitive psychology, it is necessary to arrange the experimental design so that the question of interest can be phrased in terms of a question about the relative activation of the two responses, made with the left or right hands. To illustrate the LRP approach, we give two examples of work using the LRP.

The first experiment addressed a question about the nature of information transmission: Can partial information about a stimulus be transmitted to the response system before the stimulus is completely processed? (See e.g. Miller 1988; Sanders 1990.) The rationale is as follows. For a stimulus that contains two attributes, compare (a) conditions under which both attributes are mapped to the same (correct) response versus (b) conditions where the attributes are mapped to different (correct and incorrect) responses. If you observe incorrect response activation in the conflict condition, then partial information about the attribute must have been transmitted. Evidence in favor of partial transmission was reported by Gratton et al. (1988; see also Smid, Mulder, & Mulder 1990; Smid et al. 1991) using a noise compatibility paradigm (Eriksen & Eriksen 1974). They found that the incorrect response can be activated on the conflict trials even though the correct response is executed.

Similar findings were obtained in a Go–No-Go paradigm by Miller and Hackley (1992; see also Osman et al. 1992). In this case the trick is to map one stimulus attribute to response hand and the other attribute to response decision. If a response is activated when no response is required, then partial information about the attribute associated with response hand must have been transmitted.

In the experiment by Miller and Hackley, the stimuli were letters that had two attributes: size and identity, with size being deliberately made more difficult to determine than identity. Letter size was mapped to the Go–No-Go

decision, while letter identity was mapped to response hand. Miller and Hackley found that, on Go trials, there was the expected development of an LRP associated with the subject's response on these trials. For No-Go trials, there was also a (smaller) LRP even though the subject showed no sign of any response-related muscular activity. These data indicate that, on No-Go trials, a response was activated even though that response was never executed. Partial information about letter identity was being transmitted to the response system.

These two examples are illustrative of the kinds of inferences that can be made using the LRP. The LRP has also helped to identify the processing locus of particular experimental effects and individual differences. Furthermore, measures of the LRP have provided insights into the question of the level in the processing system at which inhibitory mechanisms act to stop a response (De Jong et al. 1990). For further information about these and other issues, the interested reader should consult the reviews by Coles, Gratton, and Donchin (1988) and Coles et al. (1991, 1995).

The Contingent Negative Variation (CNV). The CNV was first described by Walter and colleagues (1964) as a slow negative wave that occurs during the foreperiod of a reaction time task (see Figure 6). The wave tends to be largest over central (vertex) and frontal areas. Researchers investigating the functional significance of CNV have manipulated several aspects of the S1–S2 paradigm, including the subject's task, the discriminability of the imperative stimulus, foreperiod duration, stimulus probability, presence of distractors, and so forth. The component has been variously described as related to expectancy, mental priming,

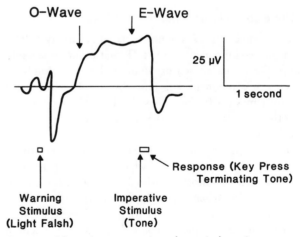

Figure 6. Schematic representation of a typical contingent negative variation (CNV) recorded from Cz. The CNV is the negative portion of the wave between the presentation of the warning and imperative stimuli. The early portion of the CNV is labeled "O-wave" (orienting wave); the late portion is labeled "E-wave" (expectancy wave). Adapted from Rohrbaugh & Gaillard (1983) with permission from the authors.

association, and attention (for a review see Donchin et al. 1978 or Rohrbaugh & Gaillard 1983).

A research controversy in this area concerns whether the CNV consists of one or rather several, functionally distinct, components. A further related question is whether the late portion of the CNV (just prior to the imperative stimulus) reflects more than the process of motor preparation as the subject anticipates making a response to the imperative stimulus. This controversy was raised by Loveless and his co-workers (e.g. Loveless & Sanford 1974; see also Connor & Lang 1969), who argued that the CNV consists of two components, an early orienting wave (the O-wave) and a later expectancy wave (the E-wave). Subsequent research by these investigators led them to argue that the E-wave is a readiness potential and reflects nothing more than motor preparation. Research by Rohrbaugh, Syndulko, and Lindsley (1976) and by Gaillard (1978; see also Rohrbaugh & Gaillard 1983) also supports this interpretation. However, the question of the functional significance of the latter component (the E-wave) remains controversial. Some investigators have claimed that, because a late E-wave is evident even in situations in which no overt motor response is required, the E-wave has a significance over and above that of motor preparation. However, it is clear that even though the overt motor response requirement may be removed from these situations, attention to a stimulus necessarily involves some motor activity associated with adjustment of the sensory apparatus. Perhaps the most persuasive arguments for a nonmotor role for the late CNV comes from a study of Damen and Brunia (1987), who found evidence for a motor-independent wave that precedes the delivery of feedback information in a time estimation task (see also van Boxtel & Brunia 1994).

The Error-Related Negativity (ERN)

As its name implies, the error-related negativity (ERN) is a negative component of the ERP that occurs when subjects make errors in sensorimotor and similar kinds of tasks. The component was first observed by Falkenstein and colleagues (1990), but it has also been observed in several other laboratories (Dehaene, Posner, & Tucker 1994; Gehring et al. 1993).

In the prototypical experiment, subjects perform a choice reaction time task in which they must respond to two different auditory (or visual) stimuli with their left or right hands. When they respond incorrectly – for example, by using the left hand to respond to a stimulus requiring the right-hand response – a negative potential is observed at the scalp. The negativity peaks at around 150 msec after response onset (defined in terms of EMG activity) and is maximal at fronto-central scalp sites. It is interesting that the negativity in the waveform for the incorrect trials begins to diverge from the waveform associated with correct trials at around the time of the response.

Several different studies have evaluated the functional significance of this component. For example, Gehring et al. (1993; see also Falkenstein et al. 1995) found that the amplitude of the ERN depends on the degree to which experimental instructions stress accuracy over speed (the amplitude is larger when accuracy is stressed). Bernstein, Scheffers, and Coles (1995) found that the amplitude also varies with the degree of error (defined in terms of movement parameters): it is larger when the incorrect response deviates from the correct response in terms of two rather than one parameter. Finally, although errors in these tasks are sometimes followed immediately by correct responses, error correction does not appear to be a necessary condition for the appearance of an ERN. An ERN is observed when subjects respond (incorrectly) to No-Go stimuli, a situation where the errors cannot be corrected by a second motor response (Scheffers et al. 1996).

The ERN is related to a variety of behaviors that together can be regarded as remedial actions taken to compensate for an error being made or having been made. These actions include attempts to inhibit the error, correct the error, or slow down so that the system does not make errors in the future (Gehring et al. 1993; Scheffers et al. 1996).

Evidence for the generality of the process manifested by the ERN was provided by Miltner, Braun, and Coles (1997). In this experiment, subjects were required to perform a time-interval production task. Shortly after subjects made a response indicating the end of a 1-sec interval, a feedback stimulus provided information about whether that interval was correct or incorrect. For incorrect feedback stimuli, an ERN-like negative potential was observed. These results suggest that the same error processing can be engaged by feedback stimuli as by incorrect actions themselves.

Finally, there is now evidence to suggest that the ERN is generated by frontal brain structures involving either the supplementary motor area or the anterior cingulate cortex. Equivalent dipole analyses for the ERN observed in choice reaction time tasks (Dehaene et al. 1994; Holroyd, Dien, & Coles 1998) and for the ERN-like negativity observed to feedback stimuli (Miltner et al. 1997) implicate activity in these neural structures as being responsible for the ERN signal recorded at the scalp.

Involvement of these structures is consistent with the picture that has begun to emerge from the functional studies of the ERN. That picture includes error monitoring and remedial action processes as essential aspects of the human cognitive system. Whenever humans perform tasks, they must set up not only their cognitive systems to execute the tasks but also a system to assure that performance on the tasks conforms to task goals. The ERN appears to be a manifestation of the activity of this system, although it is presently unclear whether it is more closely related to the error-detection process itself or to some consequence of error detection involving an aspect of remedial action (for reviews see Coles, Scheffers, & Holroyd 1998; Falkenstein et al. 1995; Gehring et al. 1995).

SENSORY COMPONENTS

The presentation of stimuli in the visual, auditory, or somatosensory modality elicits a series of voltage oscillations that can be recorded from scalp electrodes. In practice, sensory potentials can be elicited either by a train of relatively high-frequency stimuli or by transient stimuli. In the former case, the ERP responses to different stimuli overlap in time. The waveforms driven by the periodic stimulation have quite fixed periodic characteristics and are therefore referred to as "steady state" (Regan 1972). In the case of transient stimuli, the responses from different stimuli are separated in time.

Both steady-state and transient potentials appear to be obligatory responses of the nervous system to external stimulation. In fact, the earlier components of all sensory potentials (within, say, 100 msec) are invariably elicited whenever the sensory system of interest is intact. In this sense, they are described as exogenous potentials. They are thought to represent the activity of the sensory pathways that transmit the signal generated at peripheral receptors to central processing systems. Therefore, these components are "modality specific"; that is, they differ both in waveshape and scalp distribution as a function of the sensory modality in which the eliciting stimulus is presented. As would be expected of manifestations of primitive sensory processes, the sensory components are influenced primarily by such stimulus parameters as intensity and frequency. For a review of these components, see Hillyard, Picton, and Regan (1978).

For clinical purposes, sensory-evoked potentials are used in the diagnosis of neurological diseases (i.e., demyelinating diseases, cerebral tumors and infarctions, etc.). Of particular diagnostic importance are the auditory potentials (diseases involving the posterior fossa) and the steady-state visual potential (multiple sclerosis). Auditory potentials can also be used to diagnose hearing defects in uncooperative subjects (such as newborn infants). Because most sensory potentials appear to be insensitive to psychological factors, they have not been used extensively in the study of psychological processes.

THE EARLY NEGATIVITIES

Several negative components have been described in the period between 100 msec and 300 msec after the presentation of an external stimulus. In this section, we will examine two families of negative components that have been associated with selective attention, elementary feature analysis, and auditory sensory memory. Their scalp distribution and morphology vary as a function of the modality of the eliciting stimulus. These potentials may

be considered as mesogenous, since they lie at the interface between purely exogenous and purely endogenous components.

ERPs and the Locus of Selective Attention

"Selective attention" refers to the ability of the human information processing system to analyze selectively some stimuli and ignore others. The locus at which selective attention occurs within the information processing flow has long been an issue of contention in psychology (see e.g. Johnston & Dark 1986). Two metaphors have been associated with selective attention: filtering (Broadbent 1957) and resources (Kahnemann 1973; Norman & Bobrow 1975). Filtering theories have focused on the debate about the locus of the filter. Does filtering occur at an early, perceptual level (early selection theories – Broadbent 1957) or at later stages of processing (late selection theories – Deutsch & Deutsch 1963)? According to the resource metaphor, selective attention is a mechanism by which the system allocates more resources to process information coming through a particular attended channel than through other, unattended channels. Thus, research questions concern how many processing activities can be performed simultaneously, as well as what factors limit the availability of processing resources. These issues have been addressed mostly in the context of research on the P300 (briefly reviewed in a subsequent section).

Psychophysiologists in general and ERP researchers in particular have rephrased the question of the locus of selective attention to ask where – in the sequence of electrophysiological responses that follow stimulation – the effect of selective attention begins to emerge. The "attention effect" is usually defined as a larger response to stimuli when the subject's attention is directed to some of the stimulus features than when the subject's attention is directed elsewhere.

The first indications that ERPs could be used to investigate attentional processes came from studies in which the ERP response to attended stimuli was compared to that to unattended stimuli (Eason et al. 1964; Hillyard et al. 1973). These kinds of studies suggested that attended stimuli are associated with a more negative ERP between 100 and 200 msec. Subsequent research has been concerned with three issues: (i) the use of ERPs to test theories of selective attention; (ii) the nature of the attentional effect on ERPs; and (iii) the neurophysiological basis of selective attention effects.

In a typical paradigm (Hillyard et al. 1973), four types of stimuli are presented. The stimuli (e.g., tones) differ along two dimensions (e.g., location and pitch), each having two levels (left vs. right ear and standard vs. deviant pitch). The subject is instructed to attend to stimuli at a particular location and to detect target tones of a deviant pitch (e.g., left-ear tones of high pitch). In order to investigate attention effects, ERPs to standard tones occurring

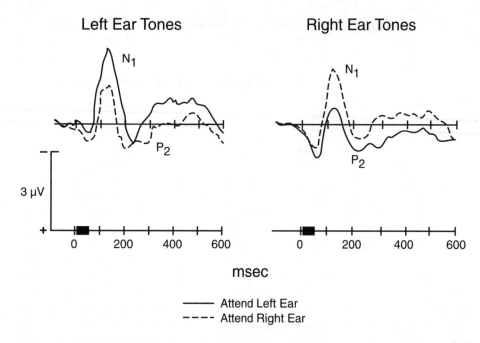

Figure 7. The effect of attention on early components of the auditory event-related potential recorded at the central electrode (Cz). The left panel shows ERPs for tones presented in the left ear. Note that the difference between the ERPs to attended tones (solid line) and those for unattended tones (dashed line) consists of a sustained negative potential. A similar difference can be seen for tones presented to the right ear (see right panel). Adapted with permission from Knight, Hillyard, Woods, & Neville, "The effects of frontal cortex lesions on event-related potentials during auditory selective attention," *Electroencephalography and Clinical Neurophysiology,* vol. 52, pp. 571–82. Copyright 1981 Elsevier Science.

in the attended location (channel) are compared to ERPs to standard tones in the unattended channel.

Using this paradigm, Hillyard and his colleagues have observed a larger negativity with a peak latency of about 100–150 msec for stimuli presented in the attended channel (see Figure 7, which shows data from a similar experiment by Knight et al. 1981). The moment in time at which the waveforms for attended and unattended stimuli diverge is considered as the time at which filtering begins to play a role.

Subsequent studies have shown that, by and large, ERP peaks are influenced by attention manipulations in one of three ways (see Hackley 1993).

1. They may be unaffected by the attention manipulation. In this case, the ERP activity is considered an automatic response to the stimulation. An ERP response with these properties is often referred to as an *exogenous* component.
2. They may be affected by the attention manipulation but occur even when attention is directed somewhere else. In this case, the ERP activity can be considered as a "semi-automatic" response in that it may occur even without attention, but it is larger (or smaller) when

attention is deployed to the stimulus. An ERP response with these properties is often labeled a *mesogenous* component.
3. They may require attention to occur. In this case, the ERP activity is "optional" in that it occurs only when the subject is actively engaged in processing the information provided by the stimulus. An ERP response with these properties is often labeled an *endogenous* component.

With respect to the locus of selective attention, the issue then arises of which are the earliest ERP responses (after stimulation) to be influenced by attention manipulation. A theory advanced by Hernandez-Peon, Scherrer, and Jouvet (1956), called the peripheral gating hypothesis, proposes that attention influences responses at a very initial level within the sensory pathway. In favor of this theory are anatomical observations of centrifugal fibers from the central nervous system directed toward sensory organs (such as the cochlea and the retina). Indeed, Lukas (1980, 1981) reported that the earliest brainstem auditory-evoked potentials (BAEPs) – with a latency of just a few milliseconds from stimulation and presumably generated in the cochlea itself or in the early portions of the auditory pathway – were already influenced by attention manipulations. Similar results were reported by Eason and colleagues (1964) in the visual modality (in this case, using the electroretinogram). However, numerous subsequent attempts to replicate these findings failed, and methodological concerns were raised (for a review, see Hackley 1993). For this reason, it is now accepted that the earliest auditory-evoked potentials that are affected by attention have a latency of approximately 20–25 msec (McCallum et al. 1983). These potentials are likely to be generated in primary auditory cortex (Romani, Williamson, & Kaufman 1982a; Romani et al. 1982b;

Woldorff et al. 1993) – in which case, selective attention effects will appear when the signal arrives at the cortex. Findings leading to similar conclusions have been obtained for the somatosensory modality (Michie et al. 1987).

In the visual modality, a different pattern of results emerges. In this case, the earliest responses that are usually attributed to cortical involvement (latency of approximately 50–70 msec) appear to be unaffected by selective attention manipulations (provided, of course, that eye movements are not involved – Hansen & Hillyard 1980, 1984; Mangun, Hillyard, & Luck 1993). Attention effects occur only later, leading several investigators to speculate that attention effects emerge when the signal is transferred from the primary visual cortex to surrounding cortical areas (Mangun et al. 1993). Source modeling efforts (Clark & Hillyard 1996) and a combination of ERPs and other imaging methods (Heinze et al. 1994) provided support for this hypothesis. Further support was offered by optical imaging data showing that early attention effects (latency around 100 msec) are visible in extrastriate (area 19) but not in striate (area 17) cortex (Gratton 1997).

The Middle Latency Cognitive Components

So far we have discussed early ERP activity that is influenced by attention manipulations. However, another set of ERP activities are influenced by the "history" (or sequence) of stimuli that precede the current eliciting event. Some of these activities appear to occur in an automatic fashion – that is, they occur in response to both attended and unattended events. The most studied of these ERP activities is the mismatch negativity or MMN (Näätänen 1982). Because the MMN occurs even in the absence of attention, it has been associated with some form of preattentive (or sensory) memory. Other ERP activities – such as the N200s and the P300 – are sensitive to changes in the stimulus sequence, but they occur only in response to attended stimuli. These latter components can therefore be considered optional responses and are associated with postattentive forms of memory (short-term or working memory). In the next two sections we will describe research on the MMN and on the N200s; research on the frontal (novelty) P3, parietal P300 (or P3b), and slow waves will be reviewed in the section on late positivities.

The MMN. The MMN was first described by Näätänen, Gaillard, and Mäntysalo (1978; for extended reviews see Näätänen 1992 and Ritter et al. 1995). The MMN is typically studied using a passive auditory "oddball" paradigm. In this paradigm, subjects are presented with two auditory stimuli (or classes of stimuli) that occur in a Bernoulli sequence. The probability of one stimulus is generally less than that for the other, but the subject's attention is not devoted to the series of tones but instead to another task, such as reading a book. To derive the MMN, the average waveform elicited by the standard (frequent) stimuli is subtracted from that of the deviant (rare) stimuli. This subtraction yields a negative component with an onset latency as short as 50 msec and a peak latency of 100–200 msec (see Figure 8). This component is usually largest at frontal and central electrode sites, and it inverts in polarity at the mastoids (when the reference electrode is on the nose tip; see e.g. Alho et al. 1986). This evidence of polarity inversion, as well as intracranial recordings in animals (Csepe et al. 1987; Javitt et al. 1992, 1994) and dipole modeling in humans (Scherg et al. 1989), suggests that the primary auditory cortex and/or the immediately adjacent areas may be the brain generators of the MMN.

An MMN is elicited whenever the standard and deviant stimuli are discriminable on any of a number of features (such as pitch, intensity, and duration; see Näätänen 1992 for a review). Its onset latency and amplitude are both dependent on the ease of discriminating the stimuli from one another (i.e., the more discriminable the stimuli, the larger the amplitude of the MMN and the shorter its onset latency – see Figure 8). However, it is usually necessary to present two or three standards in order for a deviant stimulus to elicit an MMN (Cowan et al. 1993). In addition, an MMN is elicited with an interstimulus interval (ISI) of up to 10 sec between a standard and a deviant stimulus (Böttcher-Gandor & Ullsperger 1992). Finally, the amplitude of the MMN is larger for stimuli that differ along more than one dimension than for those that differ on only one dimension (see Ritter et al. 1995).

Taken together, these characteristics suggest that:

1. the MMN may reflect the operation of a "mismatch detector" (hence the label "mismatch negativity");
2. because the MMN is obtained even when the subject is not attending the stimuli, it is likely to be related to the automatic and preattentive processing of deviant features (cf. Treisman & Gelade 1980);
3. the MMN may be based on a type of memory that is transient in nature, as an MMN is not recorded after long ISIs; and
4. because the presence of more that one deviant feature affects the amplitude of the MMN, the MMN may reflect the outcome of a comparison in which multiple features can be processed in parallel.

Thus, it has been suggested that the MMN may be used as an index of the operation of an early, preattentive sensory (echoic) memory (Näätänen 1992; cf. Cowan 1995 and Ritter et al. 1995).

However, additional evidence suggests that the memory underlying the MMN may be of longer duration than previously thought (Cowan et al. 1993) and that the sensory memory underlying the MMN and the sensory memory investigated in behavioral tasks may be different (Cowan 1995; Ritter et al. 1995). One final problem in using the MMN as an index of sensory memory is that, contrary to behavioral evidence, a visual analog of the MMN has been

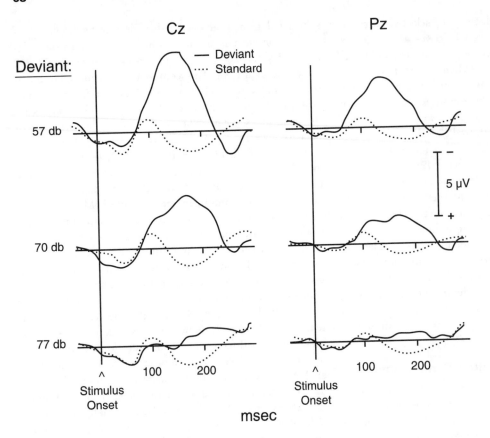

Figure 8. The effects of deviance on mismatch negativity (MMN). A standard (80-dB) tone was presented on 90% of the trials and a deviant tone (57, 70, or 77 dB, in different blocks) was presented on 10% of the trials. The ERP to the standard is indicated by the dotted line in each panel; the ERP to the deviant tone is indicated by the solid line. As the degree of mismatch between stimuli increases, the mismatch negativity also increases (i.e., the magnitude of the difference between standard and deviant ERPs increases). Redrawn from Näätänen & Picton (1987) with permission from the authors and The Society for Psychophysiological Research.

difficult to obtain. However, recent data obtained with optical imaging suggest that early memory effects (with a latency comparable to that of the MMN) can be observed in primary visual cortex and/or adjacent areas (Gratton 1997; Gratton et al. 1998).

The N200s. The label "N200" (or N2) is used to refer to a family of negative components that are similar in latency and whose scalp distribution and functional significance vary according to modality and experimental manipulations. For instance, different N200s can be observed for the visual modality (with maximum amplitude at occipital recording sites) and for the auditory modality (with maximum at the central or at frontal recording sites). In many experimental situations, the amplitude of the N200 appears to reflect the detection of some type of mismatch between stimulus features or between the stimulus and some previously formed template. The N200 differs from the MMN in that the subject's attention is usually engaged and the template for the comparison process may be actively generated by the subject.

Squires, Squires, and Hillyard (1975) first described the N200 using a paradigm in which they manipulated stimulus frequency and task relevance independently; they found that the N200 was larger for rare stimuli. Subsequent research has shown that several types of N200 can be described, even within the same modality. Specifically, Gehring et al. (1992) used a two-stimulus visual paradigm in which the first stimulus provided information about the most likely feature to be present in the second stimulus, thus creating expectations for specific stimulus features. They observed a larger N200 (with a frontal distribution) when the features in the second stimulus mismatched with the subject's expectancies (created by the first stimulus) than when the stimulus features were consistent with these expectancies. This paradigm differs from the typical MMN paradigm in that expectancy for particular features is dissociated from the physical presentation of the stimuli themselves. Therefore, the memory template to which the current stimulus is compared is generated internally and is not the result of previous presentations of the template itself. In the same paradigm, Gehring and colleagues also presented stimuli consisting of either homogenous or heterogenous features; they observed a larger N200 (with a central distribution) for the heterogenous than for the homogenous stimuli.

The N200 has also been used in the investigation of mental chronometry. In particular, Ritter et al. (1982) and Renault (1983) observed that the latency of this component covaries with reaction time. The high correlation between N200 latency and reaction time may reflect the importance of feature discrimination processes (signaled by the N200) in determining the latency of the overt response. However, the subtraction technique that Ritter et al. (1982) used to derive their measures of N200 must be interpreted with caution, because the latencies of components in the original waveforms differ. Furthermore, motor potentials, which are characterized by a large negativity, will also covary quite strictly with reaction times. Thus, it is important to disambiguate the N200 component from motor potentials when the former is used in the study of mental chronometry.

THE LATE COGNITIVE ERPs: MEMORY AND LANGUAGE EFFECTS

In this section we review a sample of the research dealing with two major families of endogenous components, the P300 (and similar late positivities) and the N400 (and other language-related components). For reasons of space we do not discuss in detail other late components, particularly a group of "slow waves." At the present time, the functional significance of these slow waves is largely unknown. However, for further information see Sutton and Ruchkin (1984) and the research on the O-wave (listed in earlier section on CNV).

The P300 and Other Late Positivities

In this section, we focus on studies of the relationship between memory and late positive components (including the P300, the frontal P3, and other positive components). These studies have focused on three types of effects: (1) effects that are associated with deviant, relevant items; (2) effects related to the memorability of items (in memory paradigms involving either direct or indirect memory tests); and (3) effects obtained during the retrieval of items (i.e., at the moment in which the direct or indirect memory test is administered).

Late Positivities Elicited by Deviant Stimuli: The "Classic" P300. As mentioned earlier, deviant items in an oddball paradigm elicit early and middle latency negative ERP activity. In addition, if the subject is attending the stimuli, deviant items also elicit various types of late positivities (with a typical latency exceeding 300 msec). The first of these positivities to be identified was the P300 (also labeled P3 or P3b; Sutton et al. 1965), which is elicited by task-relevant oddball stimuli and is maximum at posterior (parietal) scalp locations.

After more than 30 years of research on P300, there is still no conclusive indication of the brain sources underlying this scalp-recorded activity. The research conducted so far suggests that P300 may result from the summation of activity from multiple generators located in widespread cortical and possibly subcortical areas (Halgren et al. 1980; Johnson 1988, 1989, 1993; Knight et al. 1989; McCarthy et al. 1997). There has been some evidence that at least one of these sources may be located in the medial-temporal lobes (Halgren et al. 1980; Okada, Kaufman, & Williamson 1983). However, lesion data from animals (Paller et al. 1988b) and humans (Johnson 1988, 1989, 1993) indicate that it is unlikely that the scalp-recorded P300 is entirely generated in this area, as this component can still be recorded in the presence of medial-temporal lesions. In addition, Knight et al. (1989) reported that lesions of the temporo-parietal junction in certain conditions affected the amplitude of the scalp P300.

In contrast to the uncertainty about its neural origin, extensive information has been gathered on the factors that affect the amplitude and latency of the P300. For example, Duncan-Johnson and Donchin (1977) reported that P300 amplitude is sensitive to stimulus probability, provided that the stimuli are relevant to the subject's task. If the events occur while the subject is performing another task, then even rare events do not elicit the P300 (Figure 9; see also Gratton et al. 1990; Johnson & Donchin 1978). Further research has indicated that it is subjective, rather than objective, probability that controls the amplitude of P300 (Squires et al. 1976). In addition, P300 can be elicited by stimuli or stimulus classes in any modality, and the stimuli can be very diverse – as long as the subject is able to classify them unambiguously (Kutas, McCarthy, & Donchin 1977; Sutton et al. 1967; Towle, Heuer, & Donchin 1980). Finally, in another series of studies, Donchin, Kramer, and Wickens (1986; see also Sirevaag et al. 1989) demonstrated that the amplitude of P300 is related to the processing resources demanded by a particular task. In a dual-task situation, P300 amplitude to primary task events increases with the perceptual/cognitive resource demands while the P300 response to the concurrent secondary task decreases.

Research on P300 latency has focused on the identification of those processes that have elapsed prior to its elicitation. Donchin (1979) proposed that P300 latency may reflect stimulus evaluation or categorization time. This idea was supported by the observation that the correlation between P300 latency and reaction time is higher when subjects are given accuracy rather than speed instructions. Furthermore, as categorization becomes more difficult, P300 latency becomes longer (see Figure 10). Finally, it appears that the P300 latency is more dependent on the completion of processes of stimulus evaluation and categorization than on those related to the current overt response. Several studies (Magliero et al. 1984; McCarthy & Donchin 1981; Ragot 1984; Verleger 1997) demonstrate that manipulations that should affect the duration of response-related processes (i.e., stimulus–response compatibility) have relatively little effect on P300 latency (although a small effect is sometimes

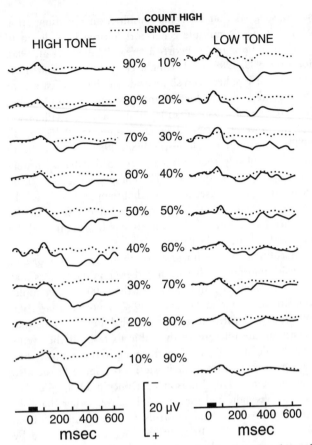

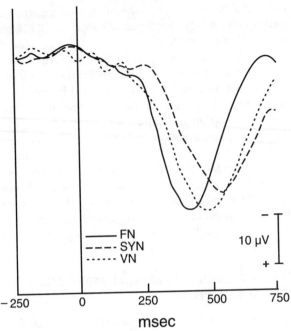

Figure 9. Grand-average ERP waveforms at Pz from 10 subjects for counted (high, left column) and uncounted (low, right column) stimuli (tones), with different a priori probabilities. The probability level is indicated by a percentage value beside each waveform. Waveforms from a condition in which the subjects were instructed to ignore the stimuli are also presented for a comparison. The occurrence of the stimulus is indicated by a black bar on the time scale. Positive voltages are indicated by downward deflections of the waveforms. Note that P300 amplitude is inversely proportional to the probability of the eliciting stimulus (probability effect) and, at the same probability level, P300 is larger for counted than uncounted stimuli (target effect). Redrawn from Duncan-Johnson & Donchin (1977) with permission from the authors and The Society for Psychophysiological Research.

Figure 10. ERP waveforms at Pz averaged across subjects for three different semantic categorization tasks. The solid line indicates ERPs obtained during a task in which the subjects had to distinguish between the word DAVID and the word NANCY (the FN condition). The dotted line indicates ERPs obtained during a task in which the subjects had to decide whether a word presented was a male or a female name (the VN condition). The dashed line indicates ERPs obtained during a task in which the subjects had to decide whether a word was or was not a synonym of the word PROD (SYN condition). These three tasks were considered to involve progressively more difficult discriminations. Note that the latency of P300 peak is progressively longer as the discrimination is made more difficult. Adapted with permission from Kutas, McCarthy, & Donchin, "Augmenting mental chronometry: The P300 as a measure of stimulus evaluation time," *Science,* vol. 197, pp. 792–5. Copyright 1977 American Association for the Advancement of Science.

observed; see Ragot 1984 or Verleger 1997), whereas manipulations of stimulus complexity have a large effect.

These observations led Donchin (1981; Donchin & Coles 1988a,b) to propose that the P300 may be a manifestation of a process related to the updating of models of the environment or context in working memory. Such an updating would depend on the processing of the current event but would also have implications for the processing of and the response to future events (including the subsequent memory for the event itself). Other theories of the functional significance of P300 have been offered by Desmedt (1980), Rösler (1983), and Verleger (1988). Both Desmedt and Verleger proposed that the P300 may be related to the termination or "closure" of processing periods, while Rösler

proposed that the P300 may reflect controlled processing. All of the theories provide a good account of the eliciting conditions for the parietal P300. Donchin's "context updating" hypothesis has also been used to generate predictions about the future consequences of the elicitation of a large (or small) P300 at a particular trial. Tests of these predictions have been taken as a validation benchmark for the context updating hypothesis. Because other theories did not generate competing hypotheses, it is difficult to determine whether or not they are confirmed by these data. One of the data sets used to validate the context updating hypothesis has been the research on the relationship between the amplitude of P300 elicited by an item and its subsequent memorability. This research will be reviewed in a subsequent section.

Statements relating to functional significance can be tested by an examination of the predicted consequences of variation in the latency or amplitude of the P300 for the outcome of the interaction between the subject and the

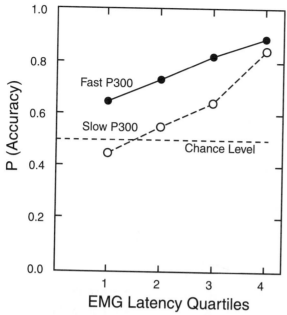

Figure 11. Accuracy of reaction time responses given at different latencies (speed–accuracy functions) for trials with fast and slow P300. Response latency (defined in terms of the onset of the EMG response) is plotted on the abscissa. The probability that a response would be correct is plotted on the ordinate. Note that the probability of giving a correct response increases as response latency increases. At very short response latencies, responses are at a chance level of accuracy (0.5). At long response latencies, responses are usually accurate. The speed–accuracy function for those trials with P300 latency shorter than the median latency ("fast P300" trials) are indicated by solid lines. The speed–accuracy function for those trials with P300 latency longer than the median latency ("slow P300" trials) are indicated by dashed lines. Note that, for each response latency, the probability of giving a correct response is higher when the P300 on that trial (reflecting the speed of stimulus processing on that trial) is fast than when it is slow. Redrawn with permission from Coles, Gratton, Bashore, Eriksen, & Donchin, "A psychophysiological investigation of the continuous flow model of human information processing," *Journal of Experimental Psychology: Human Perception and Performance*, vol. 11, pp. 529–53. Copyright © 1985 by The American Psychological Association.

environment. For example, if the P300 occurs after the stimulus has been evaluated, then the quality of the subject's response to that event should depend on the timing of that response relative to the occurrence of the P300. Thus, Coles and colleagues (1985; see also Donchin et al. 1988) showed that, for a given response latency, response accuracy is higher the shorter the P300 latency (see Figure 11).

The context updating hypothesis predicts further that, to the extent that the subject's future behavior depends on the degree to which an event leads to a change in their model of the environment, that behavior will be related to P300 amplitude. Several studies have demonstrated a relationship between the memorability of an event, assessed at some future time, and the amplitude of the P300 response to the event at the time of initial presentation (see three sections hence). As another example, it has been shown

that the subject's future strategy as revealed in overt behavior can be predicted from the P300 response to current events (Donchin et al. 1988; Gratton, Coles, & Donchin 1992). In particular, in a speeded choice reaction time task, the amplitude of the P300 following an error was related to the latency and accuracy of overt responses on subsequent trials.

Late Positivities Elicited by Novel Stimuli: The "Frontal" P3. Courchesne, Hillyard, and Galambos (1975) used a modified oddball task in which unrecognizable complex stimuli were unexpectedly interspersed within the oddball sequence. They found that the unexpected novel stimuli elicited a positivity with a latency similar to that of the classic P300 but with a more frontally oriented scalp distribution. Since this initial experiment, a number of additional studies (Friedman, Simpson, & Hamberger 1993; Knight 1987; Yamaguchi & Knight 1991) have confirmed that a frontally oriented P300 is elicited by deviant stimuli that are exceedingly rare and unexpected within the context and for which there is no previously formed memory template (novel stimuli). As a consequence, the frontal P300 elicited by these stimuli has also been labeled "novelty P3."

The relationship between the frontal and parietal P300 has been subject to debate, with some researchers considering the two as completely different components (Donchin & Coles 1988a) and others considering them as variations of the same component (Pritchard 1981). More recently, Fabiani and Friedman (1995) have shown that *all* attended deviant items elicit frontal P3s when the stimuli are first presented (i.e., during a practice block). However, with subsequent repetitions of the same stimuli, the scalp distribution of the P3 reverts to a parietal maximum, which is typical for the "classic" P300 in young adult subjects. Interestingly, older adult subjects do not show this scalp distribution change over time; rather, they produce a frontally focused P3 in response to all deviant and novel stimuli (see also Friedman & Simpson 1994).

Fabiani and Friedman (1995) proposed that the frontal P3 may be elicited by items for which no memory template is available (and "orienting" may be required) and that it diminishes when a template is formed (i.e., with repeated presentations of the same stimuli). Older subjects or subjects with frontal lobe dysfunction may have problems forming and/or maintaining the stimulus template and therefore exhibit a frontal P3 even in response to deviant stimuli that are repeated a number of times. Knight (1984, 1997) found that the frontal portion of the novelty P3 is suppressed in patients with frontal lobe lesions. This, in turn, suggests that the presence of a frontal P3 to subsequent repetitions of deviant items may be associated with frontal lobe dysfunction, as measured by neuropsychological tests (e.g., the Wisconsin Card Sorting Test; see Fabiani, Friedman, & Cheng 1998).

ERP Effects Associated with Subsequent Memory. The relationship between P300 and memory has been tested in various paradigms. For example, Karis, Fabiani, and Donchin (1984b) recorded ERPs to words presented in a series that contained a distinctive word (an "isolate" – cf. von Restorff 1933). The isolation was achieved by changing the size of the characters in which the word was displayed. As is well documented (von Restorff 1933; Wallace 1965), isolated items are better recalled than are comparable non-deviant items (the von Restorff effect). The isolated items, being rare and task-relevant, can be expected to produce large P300s. Thus, it was predicted that the recall variance would be related to the very factors that are known to elicit and control P300 amplitude. Karis et al. (1984b) found that the magnitude of the von Restorff effect depends on the mnemonic strategy employed by the subjects. Rote memorizers (i.e., subjects who rehearse the words by repeating them over and over) showed a large von Restorff effect – and poor recall performance – relative to elaborators (i.e., subjects who combine words into complex stories or images in order to improve their recall). For all subjects, isolates elicited larger P300s than nonisolates. For rote memorizers, isolates subsequently recalled elicited larger P300s on their initial presentation than did isolates that were not recalled. This relationship between recall and P300 amplitude was not observed in elaborators (see Figure 12). It is noteworthy that the amplitude of a frontal positive slow wave was correlated with subsequent recall in the elaborators, suggesting that this component may be related to the degree of elaborative processing.

Karis and colleagues (1984b) interpreted these data as evidence that all subjects "noticed" the isolated words and reacted by updating their memory representations and producing large P300s. However, differences among the subjects emerged when they tried to memorize the stimuli by using different types of rehearsal strategies. When subjects used rote strategies, changes in the stimulus representation – induced by the isolation and manifested by P300 – made it easier to recall the word. For the elaborators, whose recall depended on the networks of associations formed as the series were presented, the effects of the initial memory activation and updating manifested by P300 were not noticeable because they were overshadowed by the more powerful elaborative processing that occurred after the time frame of P300.

The hypothesis that the relationship between P300 amplitude and subsequent recall does depend on the mnemonic strategy used by the subject was supported by subsequent studies in which the effects of strategies were investigated by: (a) manipulating instruction on a within-subject basis (Fabiani, Karis, & Donchin 1990b); (b) demonstrating that, in children who do not spontaneously use elaborative strategies, the P300–memory relationship is evident in all subjects in the absence of strategy instructions (Fabiani et al. 1990a); and (c) showing that the

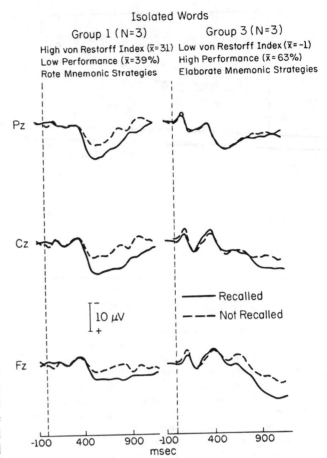

Figure 12. ERPs elicited by isolated words that were later recalled (solid line) or not recalled (dashed line). The left column shows ERPs for subjects who used rote mnemonic strategies; the right column shows ERPs for subjects who used elaborative strategies. Note that the amplitude of P300 is related to subsequent recall for the rote memorizers but not for elaborators. Reprinted with permission from Fabiani, Karis, & Donchin, "P300 and recall in an incidental memory paradigm," *Psychophysiology*, vol. 23, pp. 298–308. Copyright 1986 Elsevier Science.

P300–memory relationship is clearer in adults in incidental memory paradigms (i.e., when the memory test is unexpected and mnemonic strategies are unlikely to be used; Fabiani et al. 1986). Finally, Fabiani and Donchin (1995) investigated the P300–memory relationship for the case in which words are semantically isolated; they also studied the effects of the type of orienting task given during the von Restorff paradigm. They found that both semantic and physically isolated words that were subsequently recalled elicited larger P300s than those that were not, and that the type of orienting task given to the subjects had an effect on whether or not an isolation effect was obtained.

The memory effects that can be observed in the ERP during study are not limited to isolated or rare items. In several recent studies, memory paradigms have been used that do not capitalize on stimuli for which the P300 is expected to be enhanced, that is, paradigms in which neither the distinctiveness nor the probability of occurrence of the stimuli to be memorized are manipulated. A seminal study in this respect (Sanquist et al. 1980) found that, in a same–different judgment task, larger-amplitude P300s (or late positive components) were elicited by stimuli that were correctly recognized in a subsequent recognition test. Johnson, Pfefferbaum, and Kopell (1985) recorded ERPs in a study–test memory paradigm. They reported that the P300 associated with subsequently recognized words was slightly, but not significantly, larger than that elicited by nonrecognized words.

Paller, Kutas, and Mayes (1987a) recorded ERPs in an incidental memory paradigm. Subjects were asked to make either a semantic or a nonsemantic decision and were subsequently, and unexpectedly, tested for their recognition or recall of the stimuli. They found that ERPs elicited during the decision task were predictive of subsequent memory performance, being more positive for words subsequently recalled or recognized than to words not recalled or recognized. Similarly, Paller, McCarthy, and Wood (1988a) recorded ERPs in two semantic judgment tasks, which were followed by a free recall and a recognition test. The ERPs to words later remembered were again more positive than those to words later not remembered, even though the memory effect was smaller for recognition than for recall. Neville and colleagues (1986) recorded ERPs to words that were either congruous or incongruous with a preceding sentence; subjects were asked to judge whether or not the word was congruent with the sentence. They found that the amplitude of a late positive component (P650) predicted subsequent recognition.

Paller and colleagues (1987b) defined the larger positivity for items later memorized than for items not memorized as "Dm" (difference based on subsequent memory). They used this terminology to stress the possibility that this difference may not be associated with a parietal P300, in part because the scalp distribution of the effect does not correspond exactly to that of the P300. In subsequent studies, Paller and colleagues (1987b; Paller 1990) attempted to determine whether the Dm can be observed in indirect (priming) memory tasks as well as direct memory tasks or whether it is specific to one form of memory. The results were ambiguous: in the first study (Paller et al. 1987b) the Dm effect was evident for direct tasks as well as for the indirect test (stem completion), but in a subsequent study (Paller 1990) the effect was evident only for the direct memory tasks. Rugg (1995) summarized a large body of research investigating the relationship between ERPs and subsequent memory and concluded that there is an undisputed relationship between a late positivity in the ERPs and the subsequent memory for these items. However, whether or not this subsequent memory effect is in fact entirely due to an increased P300 is still subject to debate. It is possible that more than one memory effect may be observable in the ERP, and its nature and scalp distribution may depend on whether or not the memory task emphasizes explicit memory instructions and/or the distinctiveness/probability aspects of items. It is important to emphasize that memory is a complex phenomenon that can be influenced by a multitude of variables and that can be probed with a number of different tests. Thus, it is unlikely that a single component of the ERP can be identified as "the" memory component. It is much more likely, and indeed more interesting, that a series of ERP components will prove to be significant in different memory tasks.

Several investigators have recently focused on differences in the scalp distribution of effects as a function of stimulus dimension. For instance, Mecklinger and Muller (1996) presented subjects with a visual recognition paradigm in which stimuli varied in both position and shape. In different blocks, subjects compared the study and test stimuli on the basis of one of the two dimensions. The interest was in the differences between the potentials elicited by the same stimuli in the two tasks. These changes in the ERP were interpreted as being due to differential use of brain structures for memorization of the shape and position dimensions. The shape task was associated with a posterior (occipital) P200 component, which was not observed for the spatial memory task. In addition, Mecklinger and Muller replicated the P300 and frontal slow-wave effects first reported by Karis et al. (1984a), although the P300 had a different scalp distribution in the two tasks.

ERP Effects Associated with Repeated Presentations of a Stimulus. Since the 1970s, ERPs have been recorded in paradigms testing the recognition of a previously presented item. Some of these early studies employed the Sternberg memory search paradigm, in which the subject is first presented with a short list of items to be memorized (the memory set) and is then presented with test items (one at a time) and asked to indicate (using a speeded response) whether or not each item belongs to the memory set. Whereas most of this research focused on variations in the latency of P300 as a function of the number of items in the memory set (Ford et al. 1982), it was generally observed that positive (Yes) responses were associated with larger P300s (or more positive waveforms) than negative (No) responses. This phenomenon was later replicated in studies using a more traditional recognition paradigm (e.g., Karis et al. 1984b).

Several investigators have attempted to determine if the ERPs elicited by test items can be used to validate the so-called two-process model of recognition. According to this model, successful recognition may occur either because subjects experience the conscious recollection of having previously seen the test item or because the item was "familiar" (although the subject could not recollect explicitly the previous encounter with the test item). The distinction between "recollection" and "familiarity" (see Tulving 1985) has now become a central issue in the investigation of conscious (or explicit) and unconscious (or implicit) processes. A popular paradigm for this research involves using a recognition test that requires subjects to indicate whether they experienced recollection or familiarity when confronted with the test items (i.e., distinguish between Know and Remember judgments). Using this paradigm, Smith (1993) observed that a larger P300 (or positivity) was observed for items for which the subjects indicated explicit recollection than for items for which they only experienced familiarity. Items for which a negative response was given elicited the smallest P300s. Smith (1993) interpreted these findings as indicating that the larger positivity is associated with the conscious recollection experience. However, alternative interpretations are possible, including one which assumes that the memory trace is stronger for items that are recollected than for items that are judged familiar. The P300 would then be related to the "strength" of the memory trace rather than to conscious experience. Another explanation was advanced by Spencer, Vila, and Donchin (1994), who suggested (a) that different patterns of results were obtained by different subjects who performed the task in different ways and (b) that some of the amplitude differences obtained by Smith (1993) may also have been due to latency differences in the averaged waveforms.

Another body of research has focused on the effect of repeating task-relevant items in tasks in which memory is not directly tested. As with the recognition paradigm, the repeated items are associated with increased positivity with respect to nonrepeated items (Besson, Kutas, & Van Petten 1991; Hamberger & Friedman 1992; Rugg 1990; see Rugg 1995 for a review). The interpretation of this finding is unclear. Rugg (1995), summarizing a large body of research, suggested that the increased positivity reflects a reduction of the N400 that is obtained after repeated presentations of a particular item (see next section) rather than an increase in the amplitude of a positive component. He interpreted this reduction in N400 as a manifestation of a context integration process: the first presentation of an out-of-context item requires processing, which is not required at its subsequent presentations. However, direct tests of this hypothesis have yielded ambiguous results (for a discussion, see Rugg 1995).

Note that whereas repetitions of verbalizable items are usually associated with increased positivities, this does not appear to be the case for visual material that cannot be verbally categorized. For instance, Gratton, Corballis, and Jain (1997) reported a more negative ERP at parietal locations for old than for new test items in a recognition task using novel line patterns (see also Rugg, Soardi, & Doyle 1995; Van Petten & Senkfor 1996). In one experiment, Gratton et al. (1997) used lateral presentations during the study phase and foveal presentations during test. They showed an increased temporal negativity during the test phase (when the stimuli were presented centrally) that was systematically contralateral to the side at which the stimuli

were presented at study. They interpreted their findings as evidence of a hemispheric organization of visual memory.

Another example of negative activity (this time larger at right frontal locations) associated with recognition processes was reported by Friedman (1990). Although the significance of this activity is yet unclear, it is possible that it might be related to retrieval processes. Note that a negativity associated with retrieval processes was also described by Wijers and colleagues (1989) in a combined visual–memory search paradigm.

The N400 and Other Language-Related ERP Components

In this section we will review a number of ERP components that appear to index various linguistic processes (for a more extended review see Kutas 1997 or Chapter 21 of this volume). The first of these components to be described was the N400, originally recorded in a sentence reading task by Kutas and Hillyard (1980a). In this paradigm, words are presented serially and the subject is asked to read them silently in order to answer questions about the content of the sentence at the end of the experiment. In two studies reported by Kutas and Hillyard (1980a), 25% of the sentences ended with a semantically incongruous (but syntactically correct) word. These incongruous words elicited an N400 component that was larger than that elicited by words that were congruous with respect to the meaning of the sentence. Furthermore, the amplitude of the N400 appeared to be proportional to the degree of incongruity: moderately incongruous words ("he took a sip from the waterfall") had a smaller N400 than strongly incongruous words ("he took a sip from the transmitter"). Kutas and Hillyard (1982) reported that the N400 to incongruous endings was slightly larger and more prolonged over the right than the left hemisphere (see also Kutas, Van Petten, & Besson 1988b). More recent evidence from intracranial recordings suggests that the N400 may be generated in the parahippocampal anterior fusiform gyrus (McCarthy et al. 1995; Nobre, Allison, & McCarthy 1994; see also Kutas, Hillyard, & Gazzaniga 1988a for N400 in commissurotomy patients).

The basic incongruity effect reflected by the N400 has been replicated and extended repeatedly, using variations of the sentence reading paradigm just described. The aim of these studies has been to determine whether the N400 is a manifestation of a distinctively semantic process (i.e., a brain response to semantic violations) or whether it is elicited by other kinds of deviance. Kutas and Hillyard (1984) found that the amplitude of the N400 was inversely related to the subject's expectancy of the terminal word (cloze probability) but that it was insensitive to sentence constraints (i.e., to the number of possible alternative endings). Kutas and Hillyard (1980b) showed that an N400 followed semantic deviation, whereas a late positive complex (P300) followed physical deviation. In addition, Kutas

THE PIZZA WAS TOO HOT TO...

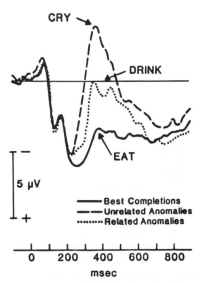

Figure 13. The effects of anomalous sentence endings on the N400. The ERPs (from Pz) depicted in the figure were recorded following visual presentation of words that varied in their relationship to the previous words in the sentence. For example, for sentences such as "The pizza was too hot to …", three endings were possible: *best completion* – "eat"; *related anomaly* – "drink"; *unrelated anomaly* – "cry". Note that the N400 component is present only for anomalies and is larger for unrelated than for related anomalies. Reproduced with permission from Kutas & Van Petten, "Event-related brain potential studies of language," *Advances in Psychophysiology*, vol. 3, pp. 139–87. Copyright 1988 Jessica Kingsley Publishers.

and Hillyard (1983) inserted a number of semantic and grammatical anomalies in prose passages. They found that large N400s were associated with the semantic anomalies embedded in the text but not with the grammatical errors. Kutas, Lindamood, and Hillyard (1984) found that anomalous words that were semantically related to the sentence's "best completion" (e.g., "the pizza was too hot to drink") elicited smaller N400s than anomalous words unrelated to the best completion (e.g., "the pizza was too hot to cry"). This suggests that the degree of semantic relatedness is an important determinant of the N400 (see Figure 13).

Work by Van Petten and colleagues (see Van Petten 1995) indicated that the N400 elicited by semantically congruent words is influenced by the interaction of word characteristics (such as frequency in the language) and the sentence context. For example, low-frequency words usually elicit larger N400s than high-frequency words, but this effect is only apparent early in the sentence, before the sentence context is established (Van Petten & Kutas 1990; see also Van Petten & Kutas 1991).

A large N400 component is also evoked by semantic anomalies presented in the auditory modality (Connolly et al. 1992; McCallum, Farmer, & Pocock 1984) and in anomalies embedded in American Sign Language (ASL) gestures (Neville 1985). However, Besson and colleagues did not find N400 responses to anomalies embedded in music, finding instead that these anomalies are associated with positivities (Besson, Faïta, & Requin 1994; Besson & Macar 1986; Macar & Besson 1987). Finally, N400-like components have also been recorded in paradigms other than sentence reading, such as the sentence verification paradigm (e.g. Fischler et al. 1983). In this paradigm, sentences are presented in segments ("a robin / is / a bird"), and two dimensions are orthogonally manipulated: whether the sentences are positive or negative ("is," "is not") and whether they are true or false. The subject is required to indicate whether the sentence is true or false. A large negativity was elicited by false affirmative ("a robin / is / a tree") and true negative ("a robin / is not / a tree") sentences – that is, by sentences in which the first and last elements were semantically unrelated (see also Fischler et al. 1985; Kounios & Holcomb 1992).

In general, research on the N400 suggests that this component is specifically sensitive to the violation of semantic expectancies. Measures of the N400 have proven useful in testing theories and models relating to semantic priming (Van Petten & Kutas 1987) and in understanding the time course of language processing. For example, Pynte and colleagues (1996) found that N400s were elicited by the last word in metaphors (such as "John is a lion") but not in literal sentences (such as "John is a courageous"). This suggests that the literal meaning of sentences is accessed early on in processing, even if a metaphorical meaning is ultimately understood.

Several other ERP components are recorded in response to language processing. For example, a positivity – labeled P600 or syntactic positive shift (SPS) – is elicited by syntactic anomalies (e.g., lack of subject–verb agreement; Kutas & Hillyard 1983). In addition, some slowly developing sentencewide effects are visible when low-pass filtering is applied to the ERP encompassing an entire sentence; these effects are reviewed in detail by Kutas (1997; see also Chapter 21).

Social and Applied Context

So far, we have discussed a number of experimental manipulations that affect various ERP components and allow investigators to make inferences about the cognitive significance of the electrical brain activity observed at the scalp. However, our brain is also processing emotions and attitudes and also plays a fundamental role in maintaining vital bodily functions (see Kutas & Federmeier 1998 for an extended discussion of an integrated view of brain function). Thus, it is not surprising that emotional and social factors may also influence the latency and amplitude of ERP components. For example, experimental instructions are an important determinant of endogenous components. In fact, strategy instructions (Fabiani et al. 1986), speed–accuracy instructions (Kutas et al. 1977), bargaining (Karis et al. 1984a), and payoff manipulations (Karis,

Chesney, & Donchin 1983) have all been shown to affect the ERP waveform.

As another example, Cacioppo and colleagues conducted a series of psychophysiological studies of social attitudes. They advocate the use of psychophysiological measures, especially for those cases in which subjects do not want (or are unable) to talk about their attitudes (Cacioppo et al. 1993, 1994a,b; Crites et al. 1995).

Several researchers have investigated the effects of emotional stimuli on the ERP. By and large, the data have been interpreted in terms of emotion effects on cognitive processing. For instance, Vanderploeg, Brown, and Marsh (1987) compared the ERP responses to faces and words that did or did not convey emotional meanings, finding that P3 was larger for neutral faces. Kestenbaum and Nelson (1992) compared the ERP elicited by angry and happy faces in 7-year-old children and adults, finding different effects of valence on P3 amplitude (see also Stormark, Nordby, & Hugdahl 1995). Naumann and colleagues (Diedrich et al. 1997; Naumann et al. 1992, 1997) have tried to identify ERP components specifically related to emotion rather than to cognitive processes. Their approach is based on an attempt to manipulate independently the emotional valence and the cognitive demands imposed by the stimuli. However, the results remain ambiguous, and the question of whether there are ERP components that are specifically related to emotional processes is still open.

There are now a considerable number of studies using ERPs in more applied areas. This includes work in human factors, for which we refer the reader to Chapter 29, as well as work on the use of ERPs in "lie detection" and on the effects of alcohol on the ERP. Studies of lie detection and ERP use a logic similar to that proposed by Cacioppo et al. (1994b) in that stimulus words or phrases relating to a crime may be categorized in one way if the information they represented were unknown to the individual but in another way if the information were known. The role of the ERPs, then, is to identify the categorization rule being used by the subject, who may otherwise be unwilling to reveal his or her "guilty knowledge." Both the P300 (Farwell & Donchin 1991) and the N400 (Boaz et al. 1991) have been used within this context.

As a final example of a more applied use of ERP research, investigators have been examining the effects of alcohol on P300 and other ERP components (such as the MMN and the O-wave) in the hope of identifying possible biological markers of high risk to developing alcoholism (Eckardt et al. 1996; Jaaskelainen et al. 1996b; see Jaaskelainen, Näätänen, & Sillanaukee 1996a and Porjesz & Begleiter 1996 for reviews).

Summary and Conclusions

Research conducted over the past four decades has established the ERP as one of the main tools available to cognitive neuroscientists. The advantages of ERPs include their exquisite temporal resolution, relatively low cost and portability, and their high level of sensitivity to cognitive processing. These qualities have allowed ERPs to be applied to the investigation of a number of theoretical issues that are relevant to cognitive psychology. Recently, several other neuroimaging techniques have joined ERPs as tools for investigating the function of the human brain. However, rather than replacing ERPs as a method of choice, it appears that a combination of different approaches (including not only imaging methods but also neuropsychological and neurophysiological data) may provide a more complete description than the use of one technique alone.

NOTES

Preparation of this chapter was supported in part by NIMH grant #5R01MH57125-01 to G. Gratton, McDonnell–Pew grant #97-32 to M. Fabiani, and NIMH grant #MH41445 to M. G. H. Coles.

1. Note that this assumption may not always be valid – as, for example, in the case of variability in the latency and other characteristics of the ERP from sample to sample. Furthermore, the ERP derived by averaging may include potentials that do not originate in the brain but are time-locked to the event.

REFERENCES

Alho, K., Paavilainen, P., Reinikainen, K., Sams, M., & Näätänen, R. (1986). Separability of different negative components of the event-related potential associated with auditory stimulus processing. *Psychophysiology, 23,* 613–23.

Alho, K., Woods, D. L., Algazi, A., Knight, R. T., & Näätänen, R. (1994). Lesions of frontal cortex diminish the auditory mismatch negativity. *Electroencephalography and Clinical Neurophysiology, 91,* 353–62.

Allison, T., Wood, C. C., & McCarthy, G. (1986). The central nervous system. In M. G. H. Coles, E. Donchin, & S. W. Porges (Eds.), *Psychophysiology: Systems, Processes, and Applications,* pp. 5–25. New York: Guilford.

Baillet, S., & Garnero, L. (1997). A Bayesian approach to introducing anatomo-functional priors in the EEG/MEG inverse problem. *IEEE Transactions on Biomedical Engineering, 44,* 374–85.

Beatty, J., Barth, D. S., Richer, F., & Johnson, R. A. (1986). Neuromagnetometry. In M. G. H. Coles, E. Donchin, & S. W. Porges (Eds.), *Psychophysiology: Systems, Processes, and Applications,* pp. 26–40. New York: Guilford.

Berger, H. (1929). Uber das Elektrenkephalogramm das Menschen. *Archiv für Psychiatrie, 87,* 527–70.

Bernstein, P. S., Scheffers, M. K., & Coles, M. G. H. (1995). "Where did I go wrong?" A psychophysiological analysis of error detection. *Journal of Experimental Psychology: Human Perception and Performance, 21,* 1312–22.

Besson, M., Faïta, F., & Requin, J. (1994). Brain waves associated with musical incongruities differ for musicians and non-musicians. *Neuroscience Letters, 168,* 101–5.

Besson, M., Kutas, M., & Van Petten, C. (1991). ERP signs of semantic congruity and word repetition in sentences. In C. H. M. Brunia, G. Mulder, & M. N. Verbaten (Eds.), *Event-Related Brain Research* (EEG Suppl. 42), pp. 259–62. Amsterdam: Elsevier.

Besson, M., & Macar, F. (1986). Visual and auditory event-related potentials elicited by linguistic and non-linguistic incongruities. *Neuroscience Letters, 63,* 109–14.

Boaz, T. L., Perry, N. W., Raney, G., Fischler, I. S., et al. (1991). Detection of guilty knowledge with event-related potentials. *Journal of Applied Psychology, 76,* 788–95.

Böttcher-Gandor, C., & Ullsperger, P. (1992). Mismatch negativity in event-related potentials to auditory stimuli as a function of varying interstimulus interval. *Psychophysiology, 29,* 546–50.

Broadbent, D. E. (1957). A mathematical model for human attention and immediate memory. *Psychological Review, 64,* 205–15.

Brunia, C. H. M., Haagh, S. A. V. M., & Scheirs, J. G. M. (1985). Waiting to respond: Electrophysiological measurements in man during preparation for a voluntary movement. In H. Heuer, U. Kleinbeck, & K. H. Schmidt (Eds.), *Motor Behavior. Programming, Control and Acquisition,* pp. 35–78. Berlin: Springer-Verlag.

Brunia, C. H. M., Mocks, J., Van Den Berg-Lenssen, M. M. C., Coelho, M., Coles, M. G. H., Elbert, T., Gasser, T., Gratton, G., Ifeachor, E. C., Jervis, B. W., Lutzenberger, W., Sroka, L., van Blokland-Vogelesang, A. W., van Driel, G., Woestenburg, J. C., Berg, P., McCallum, W. C., Tuan, P. D., Pocock, P. V., & Roth, W. T. (1989). Correcting ocular artifacts: A comparison of several methods. *Journal of Psychophysiology, 3,* 1–50.

Buchwald, J., & Squires, N. (1983). Endogenous auditory potentials in the cat: A P300 model. In C. Woody (Ed.), *Conditioning,* pp. 503–15. New York: Plenum.

Cacioppo, J. T., Crites, S. L., Berntson, G. G., & Coles, M. G. (1993). If attitudes affect how stimuli are processed, should they not affect the event-related brain potential? *Psychological Science, 4,* 108–12.

Cacioppo, J. T., Crites, S. L., Jr., Gardner, W. L., & Berntson, G. G. (1994a). Bioelectrical echoes from evaluative categorizations: I. A late positive brain potential that varies as a function of trait negativity and extremity. *Journal of Personality and Social Psychology, 67,* 115–25.

Cacioppo, J. T., Petty, R. E., Losch, M. E., & Crites, S. L. (1994b). Psychophysiological approaches to attitudes: Detecting affective dispositions when people won't say, can't say, or don't even know. In S. Shavitt & T. C. Brock (Eds.), *Persuasion: Psychological Insights and Perspectives,* pp. 43–69. Boston: Allyn & Bacon.

Cacioppo, J. T., & Tassinary, L. G. (1990). Inferring psychological significance from physiological signals. *American Psychologist, 45,* 16–28.

Ciganek, L. (1964). Excitability cycle of the visual cortex in man. *Annals of the New York Academy of Sciences, 112,* 241–53.

Clark, V. P., & Hillyard, S. A. (1996). Spatial selective attention affects early extrastriate but not striate components of the visual evoked potential. *Journal of Cognitive Neuroscience, 8,* 387–402.

Coles, M. G. H. (1989). Modern mind–brain reading: Psychophysiology, physiology and cognition. *Psychophysiology, 26,* 251–69.

Coles, M. G. H., De Jong, R., Gehring, W. J., & Gratton, G. (1991). Continuous versus discrete information processing: Evidence from movement-related potentials. In C. H. M. Brunia, G. Mulder, and M. N. Verbaten (Eds.), *Event-Related Brain Research* (EEG Suppl. 42), pp. 263–9. Amsterdam: Elsevier.

Coles, M. G. H. & Gratton, G. (1986). Cognitive psychophysiology and the study of states and processes. In G. R. J. Hockey, A. W. K. Gaillard, & M. G. H. Coles (Eds.), *Energetics and Human Information Processing,* pp. 409–24. Dordrecht: Martinus Nijhof.

Coles, M. G. H., Gratton, G., Bashore, T. R., Eriksen, C. W., & Donchin, E. (1985). A psychophysiological investigation of the continuous flow model of human information processing. *Journal of Experimental Psychology: Human Perception and Performance, 11,* 529–53.

Coles, M. G. H., Gratton, G., & Donchin, E. (1988). Detecting early communication: Using measures of movement-related potentials to illuminate human information processing. In B. Renault, M. Kutas, M. G. H. Coles, & A. W. K. Gaillard (Eds.), *Event-Related Potential Investigations of Cognition,* pp. 69–89. Amsterdam: North-Holland.

Coles, M. G. H., Gratton, G., Kramer, A. F., & Miller, G. A. (1986). Principles of signal acquisition and analysis. In M. G. H. Coles, E. Donchin, & S. W. Porges (Eds.), *Psychophysiology: Systems, Processes, and Applications,* pp. 183–221. New York: Guilford.

Coles, M. G. H., Scheffers, M. K., & Holroyd, C. (1998). Berger's dream? The error-related negativity and modern cognitive psychophysiology. In H. Witte, U. Zwiener, B. Schack, & A. Döring (Eds.), *Quantitative and Topological EEG and MEG Analysis,* pp. 96–102. Jena-Erlangen: Druckhaus Mayer Verlag.

Coles, M. G. H., Smid, H. G. O. M., Scheffers, M. K., & Otten, L. J. (1995). Mental chronometry and the study of human information processing. In M. D. Rugg and M. G. H. Coles (Eds.), *Electrophysiology of Mind: Event-Related Brain Potentials and Cognition,* pp. 86–131. Oxford University Press.

Connolly, J. F., Phillips, N. A., Stewart, S. H., & Brake, W. G. (1992). Event-related potential sensitivity to acoustic and semantic properties of terminal words in sentences. *Brain and Language, 43,* 1–18.

Connor, W. H., & Lang, P. J. (1969). Cortical slow-wave and cardiac rate responses in stimulus orientation and reaction time conditions. *Journal of Experimental Psychology, 82,* 310–20.

Courchesne, E., Hillyard, S. A., & Galambos, R. (1975). Stimulus novelty, task relevance and the visual evoked potential in man. *Electroencephalography and Clinical Neurophysiology, 39,* 131–43.

Cowan, N. (1995). Sensory memory and its role in information processing. In G. Karmos, M. Molnar, V. Csepe, I. Czigler, & J. E. Desmedt (Eds.), *Perspectives of Event-Related Potential Research* (EEG Suppl. 44), pp. 21–31. Amsterdam: Elsevier.

Cowan, N., Winkler, I., Teder, W., & Näätänen, R. (1993). Memory prerequisites of mismatch negativity in the auditory event-related potential (ERP). *Journal of Experimental Psychology: Learning, Memory, and Cognition, 19,* 909–21.

Crites, S. L., Cacioppo, J. T., Gardner, W. L., & Berntson, G. G. (1995). Bioelectrical echoes from evaluative categorization: II. A late positive brain potential that varies as a function of attitude registration rather than attitude report. *Journal of Personality and Social Psychology, 68*, 997–1013.

Csepe, V., Karmos, G., & Molnar, M. (1987). Effects of signal probability on sensory evoked potentials in cats. *International Journal of Neuroscience, 33*, 61–71.

Damen, E. J. P., & Brunia, C. H. M. (1987). Changes in heart rate and slow brain potentials related to motor preparation and stimulus anticipation in a time estimation task. *Psychophysiology, 24*, 700–13.

Dawson, G. D. (1947). Cerebral responses to electrical stimulation of the waking human brain. *Journal of Neurology, Neurosurgery, and Psychiatry, 10*, 134–40.

Deecke, L., Bashore, T., Brunia, C. H. M., Grunewald-Zuberbier, E., Grunewald, G., & Kristeva, R. (1984). Movement-associated potentials and motor control. In R. Karrer, J. Cohen, & P. Tueting (Eds.), *Brain and Information: Event-Related Potentials*, pp. 398–428. New York: New York Academy of Sciences.

Deecke, L., Englitz, H. G., Kornhuber, H. H., & Schmitt, G. (1977). Cerebral potentials preceding voluntary movement in patients with bilateral or unilateral Parkinson akinesia. In J. E. Desmedt (Ed.), *Attention, Voluntary Contraction, and Event-Related Cerebral Potentials* (Progress in Clinical Neurophysiology, vol. 1), pp. 151–63. Basel, Switzerland: Karger.

Deecke, L., Weinberg, H., & Brickett, P. (1982). Magnetic fields of the human brain accompanying voluntary movements. Bereitschaftsmagnetfeld. *Experimental Brain Research, 48*, 144–8.

Dehaene, S., Posner, M. I., & Tucker, D. M. (1994). Commentary: Localization of a neural system for error detection and compensation. *Psychological Science, 5*, 303–5.

De Jong, R., Coles, M. G. H., Gratton, G., & Logan, G. L. (1990). In search of the point of no return: The control of response processes. *Journal of Experimental Psychology: Human Perception and Performance, 16*, 164–82.

De Jong, R., Wierda, M., Mulder, G., & Mulder, L. J. M. (1988). Use of partial stimulus information in response processing. *Journal of Experimental Psychology: Human Perception and Performance, 14*, 682–92.

Desmedt, J. E. (1980). P300 in serial tasks: An essential post-decision closure mechanism. In H. H. Kornhuber & L. Deecke (Eds.), *Motivation, Motor, and Sensory Processes of the Brain* (Progress in Brain Research, vol. 54), pp. 682–6. Amsterdam: Elsevier.

Deutsch, J. A., & Deutsch, D. (1963). Attention: Some theoretical considerations. *Psychological Review, 70*, 80–90.

Diedrich, O., Naumann, E., Maier, S., & Becker, G. (1997). A frontal positive slow wave in the ERP associated with emotional slides. *Journal of Psychophysiology, 11*, 71–84.

Donchin, E. (1978). Use of scalp distribution as a dependent variable in event-related potential studies: Excerpts of preconference correspondence. In D. Otto (Ed.), *Multidisciplinary Perspectives in Event-Related Brain Potentials Research* (EPA-600/9–77–043), pp. 501–10. Washington, DC: U.S. Government Printing Office.

Donchin, E. (1979). Event-related brain potentials: A tool in the study of human information processing. In H. Begleiter (Ed.), *Evoked Potentials and Behavior*, pp. 13–75. New York: Plenum.

Donchin, E. (1981). Surprise!... Surprise? *Psychophysiology, 18*, 493–513.

Donchin, E., & Coles, M. G. H. (1988a). Is the P300 component a manifestation of context updating? *Behavioral and Brain Sciences, 11*, 354–6.

Donchin, E., & Coles, M. G. H. (1988b). On the conceptual foundations of cognitive psychophysiology: A reply to comments. *Behavioral and Brain Sciences, 11*, 406–17.

Donchin, E., Gratton, G., Dupree, D., & Coles, M. G. H. (1988). After a rash action: Latency and amplitude of the P300 following fast guesses. In G. Galbraith, M. Klietzman, & E. Donchin (Eds.), *Neurophysiology and Psychophysiology: Experimental and Clinical Applications*, pp. 173–88. Hillsdale, NJ: Erlbaum.

Donchin, E., & Heffley, E. (1978). Multivariate analysis of event-related potential data: A tutorial review. In D. Otto (Ed.), *Multidisciplinary Perspectives in Event-Related Brain Potential Research* (EPA-600/9–77–043), pp. 555–72. Washington, DC: U.S. Government Printing Office.

Donchin, E., & Herning, R. I. (1975). A simulation study of the efficacy of step-wise discriminant analysis in the detection and comparison of event-related potentials. *Electroencephalography and Clinical Neurophysiology, 38*, 51–68.

Donchin, E., Kramer, A. F., & Wickens, C. D. (1986). Applications of event-related brain potentials to problems in engineering psychology. In M. G. H. Coles, E. Donchin, & S. W. Porges (Eds.), *Psychophysiology: Systems, Processes, and Applications*, pp. 702–18. New York: Guilford.

Donchin, E., Ritter, W., & McCallum, C. (1978). Cognitive psychophysiology: The endogenous components of the ERP. In E. Callaway, P. Tueting, & S. H. Koslow (Eds.), *Event-Related Brain Potentials in Man*, pp. 349–411. New York: Academic Press.

Duncan-Johnson, C. C., & Donchin, E. (1977). On quantifying surprise: The variation of event-related potentials with subjective probability. *Psychophysiology, 14*, 456–67.

Duncan-Johnson, C. C., & Donchin, E. (1979). The time constant in P300 recording. *Psychophysiology, 16*, 53–5.

Eason, R. G., Aiken, L. R., Jr., White, C. T., & Lichtenstein, M. (1964). Activation and behavior: II. Visually evoked cortical potentials in man as indicants of activation level. *Perceptual and Motor Skills, 19*, 875–95.

Eckardt, M. J., Rohrbaugh, J. W., Stapleton, J. M., Davis, E. Z., et al. (1996). Attention-related brain potential and cognition in alcoholism-associated organic brain disorders. *Biological Psychiatry, 39*, 143–6.

Eriksen, B. A., & Eriksen, C. W. (1974). Effects of noise letters upon the identification of target letter in a non-search task. *Perception and Psychophysics, 16*, 143–9.

Fabiani, M., & Donchin, E. (1995). Encoding processes and memory organization: A model of the von Restorff effect. *Journal of Experimental Psychology: Learning, Memory and Cognition, 21*, 224–40.

Fabiani, M., & Friedman, D. (1995). Changes in brain activity patterns in aging: The novelty oddball. *Psychophysiology, 32*, 579–94.

Fabiani, M., Friedman, D., & Cheng, J. C. (1998). Individual differences in P3 scalp distribution in old subjects, and their relationship to frontal lobe function. *Psychophysiology, 35*, 698–708.

Fabiani, M., Gratton, G., Chiarenza, G. A., & Donchin, E. (1990a). A psychophysiological investigation of the von Restorff paradigm in children. *Journal of Psychophysiology, 4*, 15–24.

Fabiani, M., Gratton, G., Karis, D., & Donchin, E. (1987). The definition, identification, and reliability of measurement of the P300 component of the event-related brain potential. In P. K. Ackles, J. R. Jennings, & M. G. H. Coles (Eds.), *Advances in Psychophysiology*, vol. 1, pp. 1–78. Greenwich, CT: JAI.

Fabiani, M., Karis, D., & Donchin, E. (1986). P300 and recall in an incidental memory paradigm. *Psychophysiology, 23,* 298–308.

Fabiani, M., Karis, D., & Donchin, E. (1990b). Effects of mnemonic strategy manipulation in a von Restorff paradigm. *Electroencephalography and Clinical Neurophysiology, 75,* 22–35.

Falkenstein, M., Hohnsbein, J., & Hoormann, J. (1995). Event-related potential correlates of errors in reaction tasks. In G. Karmos, M. Molnar, V. Csepe, I. Czigler, & J. E. Desmedt (Eds.), *Perspectives of Event-Related Potentials Research* (EEG Suppl. 44), pp. 280–6. Amsterdam: Elsevier.

Falkenstein, M., Hohnsbein, J., Hoormann, J., & Blanke, L. (1990). Effects of errors in choice reaction tasks on the ERP under focused and divided attention. In C. H. M. Brunia, A. W. K. Gaillard, & A. Kok (Eds.), *Psychophysiological Brain Research*, pp. 192–5. Tilburg, The Netherlands: Tilburg University Press.

Farwell, L. A., & Donchin, E. (1991). The truth will out: Interrogative polygraphy ("lie detection") with event-related brain potentials. *Psychophysiology, 28,* 531–47.

Fischler, I., Bloom, P. A., Childers, D. G., Roucos, S. E., & Perry, N. W., Jr. (1983). Brain potentials related to stages of sentence verification. *Psychophysiology, 20,* 400–9.

Fischler, I., Childers, D. G., Achariyapaopan, T., & Perry, N. W., Jr. (1985). Brain potentials during sentence verification: Automatic aspects of comprehension. *Biological Psychology, 21,* 83–105.

Ford, J. M., Pfefferbaum, A., Tinklenberg, J. R., & Kopell, B. S. (1982). Effects of perceptual and cognitive difficulty on P3 and RT in young and old adults. *Electroencephalography and Clinical Neurophysiology, 54,* 311–21.

Friedman, D. (1990). ERPs during continuous recognition memory for words. *Biological Psychology, 30,* 61–87.

Friedman, D., & Simpson, G. V. (1994). ERP amplitude and scalp distribution to target and novel events: Effects of temporal order in young, middle-aged and older adults. *Brain Research. Cognitive Brain Research, 2,* 49–63.

Friedman, D., Simpson, G., & Hamberger, M. (1993). Age-related changes in scalp topography to novel and target stimuli. *Psychophysiology, 30,* 383–96.

Gaillard, A. (1978). Slow brain potentials preceding task performance. Dissertation, Institute for Perception (TNO), Soesterberg, The Netherlands.

Gehring, W. J., Coles, M. G. H., Donchin, E., & Meyer, D. E. (1995). A brain potential manifestation of error-related processing. In G. Karmos, M. Molnar, V. Csepe, I. Czigler, & J. E. Desmedt (Eds.), *Perspectives of Event-Related Potentials Research* (EEG Suppl. 44), pp. 287–96. Amsterdam: Elsevier.

Gehring, W. J., Goss, B., Coles, M. G. H., Meyer, D. E., and Donchin, E. (1993). A neural system for error-detection and compensation. *Psychological Science, 4,* 385–90.

Gehring, W. J., Gratton, G., Coles, M. G., & Donchin, E. (1992). Probability effects on stimulus evaluation and response processes. *Journal of Experimental Psychology: Human Perception and Performance, 18,* 198–216.

Glaser, E. M., & Ruchkin, D. S. (1976). *Principles of neurobiological signal analysis.* New York: Academic Press.

Gratton, G. (1997). Attention and probability effects in the human occipital cortex: An optical imaging study. *NeuroReport, 8,* 1749–53.

Gratton, G. (1998). Dealing with artifacts: The EOG contamination of event-related brain potential. *Behavior Research Methods, Instruments, and Computers, 30,* 44–53.

Gratton, G., Bosco, C. M., Kramer, A. F., Coles, M. G., Wickens, C. D., & Donchin, E. (1990). Event-related brain potentials as indices of information extraction and response priming. *Electroencephalography and Clinical Neurophysiology, 75,* 419–32.

Gratton, G., Coles, M. G., & Donchin, E. (1989a). A procedure for using multi-electrode information in the analysis of components of the event-related potential: Vector filter. *Psychophysiology, 26,* 222–32.

Gratton, G., Coles, M. G., & Donchin, E. (1992). Optimizing the use of information: Strategic control of activation of responses. *Journal of Experimental Psychology: General, 121,* 480–506.

Gratton, G., Coles, M. G. H., Sirevaag, E. J., Eriksen, C. W., & Donchin, E. (1988). Pre- and post-stimulus activation of response channels: A psychophysiological analysis. *Journal of Experimental Psychology: Human Perception and Performance, 14,* 331–44.

Gratton, G., Corballis, P. M., & Jain, S. (1997). Hemispheric organization of visual memories. *Journal of Cognitive Neuroscience, 9,* 92–104.

Gratton, G., Fabiani, M., Goodman-Wood, M. R., & DeSoto, M. C. (1998). Memory-driven processing in human medial occipital cortex: An event-related optical signal (EROS) study. *Psychophysiology, 35,* 348–51.

Gratton, G., Kramer, A. F., Coles, M. G., & Donchin, E. (1989b). Simulation studies of latency measures of components of the event-related brain potential. *Psychophysiology, 26,* 233–48.

Greenblatt, R. E., Nichols, J. D., Voreades, D., & Gao, L. (1997). Multimodal, integrated, PC-based functional imaging software [Abstract]. *NeuroImage, 5,* S631.

Hackley, S. A. (1993). An evaluation of the automaticity of sensory processing using event-related potentials and brain-stem reflexes. *Psychophysiology, 30,* 415–28.

Halgren, E., Squires, N. K., Wilson, C. L., Rohrbaugh, J. W., Babb, T. L., & Randall, P. H. (1980). Endogenous potentials generated in the human hippocampal formation and amygdala by infrequent events. *Science, 210,* 803–5.

Hamberger, M., & Friedman, D. (1992). Event-related potential correlates of repetition priming and stimulus classification in young, middle-aged and older adults. *Journal of Gerontology: Psychological Sciences, 47,* 395–405.

Hansen, J. C., & Hillyard, S. A. (1980). Endogenous brain potentials associated with selective auditory attention. *Electroencephalography and Clinical Neurophysiology, 49,* 277–90.

Hansen, J. C., & Hillyard, S. A. (1984). Effects of stimulation rate and attribute cueing on event-related potentials during selective auditory attention. *Psychophysiology, 21,* 394–405.

Heinze, H. J., Mangun, G. R., Burchert, W., Hinrichs, H., Scholz, M., Munte, T. F., Gos, A., Scherg, M., Johannes, S., Hundeshagen, H., et al. (1994). Combined spatial and temporal imaging of brain activity during visual selective attention in humans. *Nature, 372,* 543–6.

Hernandez-Peon, R., Scherrer, H., & Jouvet, M. (1956). Modification of electrical activity in cochlear nucleus during "attention" in unanesthetized cats. *Science, 123,* 331–2.

Hillyard, S. A., Hink, R. F., Schwent, V. L., & Picton, T. W. (1973). Electrical signs of selective attention in the human brain. *Science, 182,* 177–80.

Hillyard, S. A., Picton, T. W., & Regan, D. (1978). Sensation, perception, and attention: Analysis using ERPs. In E. Callaway, P. Tueting, & S. H. Koslow (Eds.), *Event-Related Brain Potentials in Man,* pp. 223–321. New York: Academic Press.

Holroyd, C. B., Dien, J., & Coles, M. G. H. (1998). Error-related scalp potentials elicited by hand and foot movements: Evidence for an output-independent error-processing system in humans. *Neuroscience Letters, 242,* 65–8.

Horst, R. L., & Donchin, E. (1980). Beyond averaging II: Single trial classification of exogenous event-related potentials using step-wise discriminant analysis. *Electroencephalography and Clinical Neurophysiology, 48,* 113–26.

Jaaskelainen, I. P., Näätänen, R., & Sillanaukee, P. (1996a). Effect of acute ethanol on auditory and visual event-related potentials: A review and reinterpretation. *Biological Psychiatry, 40,* 284–91.

Jaaskelainen, I. P., Pekkonen, E., Hirvonen, J., Sillanaukee, P., et al. (1996b). Mismatch negativity subcomponents and ethyl alcohol. *Biological Psychology, 43,* 13–25.

Jasper, H. H. (1958). The ten-twenty electrode system of the International Federation. *Electroencephalography and Clinical Neurophysiology, 10,* 371–5.

Javitt, D. C., Schroeder, C. E., Steinschneider, M., Arezzo, J. C., & Vaughan, H. G., Jr. (1992). Demonstration of mismatch negativity in the monkey. *Electroencephalography and Clinical Neurophysiology, 83,* 87–90.

Javitt, D. C., Steinschneider, M., Schroeder, C. E., Vaughan, H. G., & Arezzo, J. C. (1994). Detection of stimulus deviance within primate primary auditory cortex: Intracortical mechanisms of mismatch negativity (MMN) generation. *Brain Research, 667,* 192–200.

Johnson, R., Jr. (1988). Scalp-recorded P300 activity in patients following unilateral temporal lobectomy. *Brain, 111,* 1517–29.

Johnson, R., Jr. (1989). Auditory and visual P300s in temporal lobectomy patients: Evidence for modality-dependent generators. *Psychophysiology, 26,* 633–50.

Johnson, R., Jr. (1993). On the neural generators of the P300 component of the event-related potential. *Psychophysiology, 30,* 90–7.

Johnson, R., Jr., & Donchin, E. (1978). On how P300 amplitude varies with the utility of the eliciting stimuli. *Electroencephalography and Clinical Neurophysiology, 44,* 424–37.

Johnson, R., Jr., Pfefferbaum, A., & Kopell, B. S. (1985). P300 and long-term memory: Latency predicts recognition time. *Psychophysiology, 22,* 498–507.

Johnston, W. A., & Dark, V. J. (1986). Selective attention. *Annual Review of Psychology, 37,* 43–75.

Kahneman, D. (1973). *Attention and Effort.* Englewood Cliffs, NJ: Prentice-Hall.

Karis, D., Chesney, G. L., & Donchin, E. (1983). "... 'Twas ten to one; and yet we ventured ...": P300 and decision making. *Psychophysiology, 20,* 260–8.

Karis, D., Druckman, D., Lissak, R., & Donchin, E. (1984a). A psychophysiological analysis of bargaining: ERPs and fa-cial expressions. In R. Karrer, J. Cohen, & P. Tueting (Eds.), *Brain and Information: Event-Related Potentials,* pp. 230–5. New York: New York Academy of Sciences.

Karis, D., Fabiani, M., & Donchin, E. (1984b). P300 and memory: Individual differences in the von Restorff effect. *Cognitive Psychology, 16,* 177–216.

Karrer, R., & Ivins, J. (1976). Steady potentials accompanying perception and response in mentally retarded and normal children. In R. Karrer (Ed.), *Developmental Psychophysiology of Mental Retardation,* pp. 361–417. Springfield, IL: Thomas.

Kestenbaum, R., & Nelson, C. A. (1992). Neural and behavioral correlates of emotion recognition in children and adults. *Journal of Experimental Child Psychology, 54,* 1–18.

Knight, R. T. (1984). Decreased response to novel stimuli after prefrontal lesions in man. *Electroencephalography and Clinical Neurophysiology, 59,* 9–20.

Knight, R. T. (1987). Aging decreases auditory event-related potentials to unexpected stimuli in humans. *Neurobiology of Aging, 8,* 109–13.

Knight, R. T. (1997). Distributed cortical network for visual attention. *Journal of Cognitive Neuroscience, 9,* 75–91.

Knight, R. T., Hillyard, S. A., Woods, D. L., & Neville, H. J. (1981). The effects of frontal cortex lesions on event-related potentials during auditory selective attention. *Electroencephalography and Clinical Neurophysiology, 52,* 571–82.

Knight, R. T., Scabini, D., Woods, D. L., & Clayworth, C. C. (1989). Contributions of temporal-parietal junction to the human auditory P3. *Brain Research, 502,* 109–16.

Kornhuber, H. H., & Deecke, L. (1965). Hirnpotentialanderungen bei Wilkurbewegungen und passiven Bewegungen des Menschen: Bereitschaftpotential und reafferente Potentiale. *Pflügers Archiv für die gesammte Physiologie, 248,* 1–17.

Kounios, J., & Holcomb, P. J. (1992). Structure and process in semantic memory: Evidence from event-related brain potentials and reaction times. *Journal of Experimental Psychology: General, 121,* 459–79.

Kutas, M. (1997). Views on how the electrical activity that the brain generates reflects the functions of different language structures. *Psychophysiology, 34,* 383–98.

Kutas, M., & Donchin, E. (1977). The effect of handedness, of responding hand, and of response force on the contralateral dominance of the readiness potential. In J. Desmedt (Ed.), *Attention, Voluntary Contraction and Event-Related Cerebral Potentials* (Progress in Clinical Neurophysiology, vol. 1), pp. 189–210. Basel, Switzerland: Karger.

Kutas, M., & Donchin, E. (1980). Preparation to respond as manifested by movement-related brain potentials. *Brain Research, 202,* 95–115.

Kutas, M., & Federmeier, K. D. (1998). Minding the body. *Psychophysiology, 35,* 135–50.

Kutas, M., & Hillyard, S. A. (1980a). Reading senseless sentences: Brain potentials reflect semantic incongruity. *Science, 207,* 203–5.

Kutas, M., & Hillyard, S. A. (1980b). Event-related brain potentials to semantically inappropriate and surprisingly large words. *Biological Psychology, 11,* 99–116.

Kutas, M., & Hillyard, S. A. (1982). The lateral distribution of event-related potentials during sentence processing. *Neuropsychologia, 20,* 579–90.

Kutas, M., & Hillyard, S. A. (1983). Event-related brain potentials to grammatical errors and semantic anomalies. *Memory and Cognition, 11*, 539–50.

Kutas, M., & Hillyard, S. A. (1984). Brain potentials during reading reflect word expectancy and semantic association. *Nature, 307*, 161–3.

Kutas, M., Hillyard, S. A., & Gazzaniga, M. S. (1988a). Processing of semantic anomaly by right and left hemispheres of commissurotomy patients. Evidence from event-related brain potentials. *Brain, 111*, 553–76.

Kutas, M., Lindamood, T. E., & Hillyard, S. A. (1984). Word expectancy and event-related brain potentials during sentence processing. In S. Kornblum & J. Requin (Eds.), *Preparatory States and Processes*, pp. 217–37. Hillsdale, NJ: Erlbaum.

Kutas, M., McCarthy, G., & Donchin, E. (1977). Augmenting mental chronometry: The P300 as a measure of stimulus evaluation time. *Science, 197*, 792–5.

Kutas, M., & Van Petten, C. (1988). Event-related brain potential studies of language. In P. K. Ackles, J. R. Jennings, & M. G. H. Coles (Eds.), *Advances in Psychophysiology*, vol. 3, pp. 139–87. Greenwich, CT: JAI.

Kutas, M., Van Petten, C., & Besson, M. (1988b). Event-related potential asymmetries during the reading of sentences. *Electroencephalography and Clinical Neurophysiology, 69*, 218–33.

Lorente de Nò, R. (1947). Action potential of the motoneurons of the hypoglossus nucleus. *Journal of Cellular and Comparative Physiology, 29*, 207–87.

Loveless, N. E., & Sanford, A. J. (1974). Slow potential correlates of preparatory set. *Biological Psychology, 1*, 303–14.

Lukas, J. H. (1980). Human auditory attention: The olivocochlear bundle may function as a peripheral filter. *Psychophysiology, 17*, 444–52.

Lukas, J. H. (1981). The role of efferent inhibition in human auditory attention: An examination of the auditory brainstem potentials. *International Journal of Neuroscience, 12*, 137–45.

Macar, F., & Besson, M. (1987). An event-related potential analysis of incongruity in music and other non-linguistic contexts. *Psychophysiology, 24*, 14–25.

Magliero, A., Bashore, T. R., Coles, M. G. H., & Donchin, E. (1984). On the dependence of P300 latency on stimulus evaluation processes. *Psychophysiology, 21*, 171–86.

Mangun, G. R., Hillyard, S. A., & Luck, S. J. (1993). Electrocortical substrates of visual selective attention. In D. Meyer & S. Kornblum (Eds.), *Attention and Performance*, pp. 219–43. Cambridge, MA: MIT Press.

McCallum, W. C., Curry, S. H., Cooper, R., Pocock, P. V., & Papakostopoulos, D. (1983). Brain event-related potentials as indicators of early selective processes in auditory target localization. *Psychophysiology, 20*, 1–17.

McCallum, W. C., Farmer, S. F., & Pocock, P. V. (1984). The effects of physical and semantic incongruities on auditory event-related potentials. *Psychophysiology, 24*, 449–63.

McCarthy, G., & Donchin, E. (1981). A metric for thought: A comparison of P300 latency and reaction time. *Science, 211*, 77–80.

McCarthy, G., Luby, M., Gore, J., & Goldman-Rakic, P. (1997). Infrequent events transiently activate human prefrontal and parietal cortex as measured by functional MRI. *Journal of Neurophysiology, 77*, 1630–4.

McCarthy, G., Nobre, A. C., Bentin, S., & Spencer, D. D. (1995). Language-related field potentials in the anterior-medial temporal lobe: I. Intracranial distribution and neural generators. *Journal of Neuroscience, 15*, 1080–9.

Mecklinger, A., & Muller, N. (1996). Dissociations in the processing of "what" and "where" information in working memory: An event-related potential analysis. *Journal of Cognitive Neuroscience, 8*, 453–73.

Michie, P. T., Bearpark, H. M., Crawford, J. M., & Glue, L. C. T. (1987). The effects of spatial selective attention on the somatosensory event-related potential. *Psychophysiology, 24*, 449–63.

Miller, G. A. (1996). How we think about cognition, emotion, and biology in psychopathology. *Psychophysiology, 33*, 615–28.

Miller, J. (1988). Discrete and continuous models of human information processing: Theoretical distinctions and empirical results. *Acta Psychologica, 67*, 191–257.

Miller, J. O., & Hackley, S. A. (1992). Electrophysiological evidence for temporal overlap among contingent mental processes. *Journal of Experimental Psychology: General, 121*, 195–209.

Miltner, W. H. R., Braun, C. H., & Coles, M. G. H. (1997). Event-related brain potentials following incorrect feedback in a time-production task: Evidence for a "generic" neural system for error-detection. *Journal of Cognitive Neuroscience, 9*, 787–97.

Näätänen, R. (1982). Processing negativity: An evoked potential reflection of selective attention. *Psychological Bulletin, 92*, 605–40.

Näätänen, R. (1992). *Attention and Brain Function*. Hillsdale, NJ: Erlbaum.

Näätänen, R., Gaillard, A. W., & Mäntysalo, S. (1978). Early selective-attention effect on evoked potential reinterpreted. *Acta Psychologica, 42*, 313–29.

Näätänen, R., & Picton, T. (1987). The N1 wave of the human electric and magnetic response to sound: A review and an analysis of the component structure. *Psychophysiology, 24*, 375–425.

Naumann, E., Bartussek, D., Diedrich, O., & Laufer, M. E. (1992). Assessing cognitive and affective information processing functions of the brain by means of the late positive complex of the event-related potential. *Journal of Psychophysiology, 6*, 285–98.

Naumann, E., Maier, S., Diedrich, O., Becker, G., et al. (1997). Structural, semantic, and emotion-focused processing of neutral and negative nouns: Event-related potential correlates. *Journal of Psychophysiology, 11*, 158–72.

Neville, H. J. (1985). Biological constraints on semantic processing: A comparison of spoken and signed languages [Abstract]. *Psychophysiology, 22*, 576.

Neville, H. J., Kutas, M., Chesney, G., & Schmidt, A. L. (1986). Event-related brain potentials during initial encoding and recognition memory of congruous and incongruous words. *Journal of Memory and Language, 25*, 75–92.

Nobre, A. C., Allison, T., & McCarthy, G. (1994). Word recognition in the human inferior temporal lobe. *Nature, 372*, 260–3.

Norman, D. A., & Bobrow, D. G. (1975). On data-limited and resource-limited processes. *Cognitive Psychology, 7*, 44–64.

Nunez, P. L. (1981). *Electric Fields of the Brain: The Neurophysics of EEG.* Oxford University Press.

Nuwer, M. R. (1987). Recording electrode site nomenclature. *Journal of Clinical Neurophysiology, 4,* 121–33.

Okada, Y. C., Kaufman, L., & Williamson, S. J. (1983). The hippocampal formation as a source of the slow endogenous potentials. *Electroencephalography and Clinical Neurophysiology, 55,* 416–26.

Okada, Y. C., Williamson, S. J., & Kaufman, L. (1982). Magnetic fields of the human sensory-motor cortex. *International Journal of Neurophysiology, 17,* 33–8.

Osman, A., Bashore, T. R., Coles, M. G. H., Donchin, E., & Meyer, D. E. (1992). On the transmission of partial information: Inferences from movement related brain potentials. *Journal of Experimental Psychology: Human Perception and Performance, 18,* 217–32.

Paller, K. A. (1990). Recall and stem-completion priming have different electrophysiological correlates and are differentially modified by directed forgetting. *Journal of Experimental Psychology: Learning, Memory, and Cognition, 16,* 1021–32.

Paller, K. A., Kutas, M., & Mayes, A. R. (1987a). Neural correlates of encoding in an incidental learning paradigm. *Electroencephalography and Clinical Neurophysiology, 67,* 360–71.

Paller, K. A., Kutas, M., Shimamura, A. P., & Squire, L. R. (1987b). Brain responses to concrete and abstract words reflect processes that correlate with later performance on a test of stem-completion priming. *Electroencephalography and Clinical Neurophysiology (Suppl.), 40,* 360–5.

Paller, K. A., McCarthy, G., & Wood, C. C. (1988a). ERPs predictive of subsequent recall and recognition performance. *Biological Psychology, 26,* 269–76.

Paller, K. A., Zola-Morgan, S., Squire, L. R., & Hillyard, S. A. (1988b). P3-like brain waves in normal monkeys and in monkeys with medial temporal lesions. *Behavioral Neuroscience, 102,* 714–25.

Pascual-Marqui, R. D., Michel, C. M., & Lehmann, D. (1994). Low resolution electromagnetic tomography: A new method for localizing electrical activity in the brain. *International Journal of Psychophysiology, 18,* 49–65.

Perrin, F., Pernier, J., Bertrand, O., Giard, M. H., & Echallier, J. F. (1987). Mapping of scalp potentials by surface spline interpolation. *Electroencephalography and Clinical Neurophysiology, 66,* 75–81.

Porjesz, B., & Begleiter, H. (1996). Effects of alcohol on electrophysiological activity of the brain. In H. Begleiter & B. Kissin (Eds.), *The Pharmacology of Alcohol and Alcohol Dependence, Alcohol and Alcoholism,* no. 2, pp. 207–47. New York: Oxford University Press.

Pritchard, W. S. (1981). Psychophysiology of P300. *Psychological Bulletin, 89,* 506–40.

Pynte, J., Besson, M., Robichon, F. H., & Poli, J. (1996). The time-course of metaphor comprehension: An event-related potential study. *Brain and Language, 55,* 293–316.

Ragot, R. (1984). Perceptual and motor space representation: An event-related potential study. *Psychophysiology, 21,* 159–70.

Regan, D. (1972). *Evoked Potentials in Psychology, Sensory Physiology, and Clinical Medicine.* New York: Wiley.

Renault, B. (1983). The visual emitted potentials: Clues for information processing. In A. W. K. Gaillard & W. Ritter (Eds.), *Tutorials in Event-Related Potential Research: Endogenous Components,* pp. 159–76. Amsterdam: North-Holland.

Ritter, W., Deacon, D., Gomes, H., Javitt, D. C., & Vaughan, H. G., Jr. (1995). The mismatch negativity of event-related potentials as a probe of transient auditory memory: A review. *Ear and Hearing, 16,* 52–67.

Ritter, W., Simson, R., Vaughan, H. G., Jr., & Macht, M. (1982). Manipulation of event-related potential manifestations of information processing stages. *Science, 218,* 909–11.

Rohrbaugh, J. W., & Gaillard, A. W. K. (1983). Sensory and motor aspects of the contingent negative variation. In A. W. K. Gaillard & W. Ritter (Eds.), *Tutorials in Event-Related Potential Research: Endogenous Components,* pp. 269–310. Amsterdam: North-Holland.

Rohrbaugh, J. W., Syndulko, K., & Lindsley, D. B. (1976). Brain components of the contingent negative variation in humans. *Science, 191,* 1055–7.

Romani, G. L., Williamson, S. J., & Kaufman, L. (1982a). Tonotopic organization of the human auditory cortex. *Science, 216,* 1339–40.

Romani, G. L., Williamson, S. J., Kaufman, L., & Brenner, D. (1982b). Characterization of the human auditory cortex by the neuromagnetic method. *Experimental Brain Research, 47,* 381–93.

Rösler, F. (1983). Endogenous ERPs and cognition: Probes, prospects, and pitfalls in matching pieces of the mind–body problem. In A. W. K. Gaillard & W. Ritter (Eds.), *Tutorials in Event-Related Potential Research: Endogenous Components,* pp. 9–35. Amsterdam: Elsevier.

Rugg, M. D. (1990). Event-related brain potentials dissociate repetition effects of high- and low-frequency words. *Memory and Cognition, 18,* 367–79.

Rugg, M. D. (1995). ERP studies of memory. In M. D. Rugg & M. G. H. Coles (Eds.), *Electrophysiology of Mind: Event-Related Brain Potentials and Cognition,* vol. 25, pp. 133–70. Oxford University Press.

Rugg, M. D., Soardi, M., & Doyle, M. C. (1995). Modulation of event-related potentials by the repetition of drawings of novel objects. *Brain Research. Cognitive Brain Research, 3,* 17–24.

Sanders, A. F. (1990). Issues and trends in the debate on discrete vs. continuous processing of information. *Acta Psychologica, 74,* 123–67.

Sanquist, T. F., Rohrbaugh, J. W., Syndulko, K., & Lindsley, D. B. (1980). Electrocortical signs of levels of processing: Perceptual analysis and recognition memory. *Psychophysiology, 17,* 568–76.

Sarter, M., Berntson, G. G., & Cacioppo, J. T. (1996). Brain imaging and cognitive neuroscience: Toward strong inference in attributing function to structure. *American Psychologist, 51,* 13–21.

Scheffers, M. K., Coles, M. G. H., Bernstein, P., Gehring, W. J., & Donchin, E. (1996). Event-related brain potentials and error-related processing: An analysis of incorrect response to Go and No-go stimuli. *Psychophysiology, 33,* 42–53.

Scherg, M., Vajsar, J., & Picton, T. W. (1989). A source analysis of the late human auditory evoked potentials. *Journal of Cognitive Neuroscience, 1,* 336–55.

Scherg, M., & Von Cramon, D. (1986). Evoked dipole source potentials of the human auditory cortex. *Electroencephalography and Clinical Neurophysiology, 65,* 344–60.

Sirevaag, E. J., Kramer, A. F., Coles, M. G., & Donchin, E. (1989). Resource reciprocity: An event-related brain potentials analysis. *Acta Psychologica, 70*, 77–97.

Smid, H. G. O. M., Lamain, W., Hogeboom, M. M., Mulder, G., & Mulder, L. J. M. (1991). Psychophysiological evidence for continuous information transmission between visual search and response processes. *Journal of Experimental Psychology: Human Perception and Performance, 17*, 696–714.

Smid, H. G. O. M., Mulder, G., & Mulder, L. J. M. (1990). Selective response activation can begin before stimulus recognition is complete: A psychophysiological and error analysis of continuous flow. *Acta Psychologica, 74*, 169–201.

Smith, M. E. (1993). Neurophysiological manifestations of recollective experience during recognition memory judgments. *Journal of Cognitive Neuroscience, 5*, 1–13.

Smulders, F. T. Y., Kenemans, J. L., & Kok, A. (1996). Effects of task variables on measures of the mean onset latency of LRP depend on scoring method. *Psychophysiology, 33*, 194–205.

Spencer, K. M., Vila, E., & Donchin, E. (1994). ERPs and performance measures reveal individual differences in a recollection/familiarity task [Abstract]. *Psychophysiology, 31*, S93.

Squires, K. C., & Donchin, E. (1976). Beyond averaging: The use of discriminant functions to recognize event-related potentials elicited by single auditory stimuli. *Electroencephalography and Clinical Neurophysiology, 41*, 449–59.

Squires, K. C., Squires, N. K., & Hillyard, S. A. (1975). Decision-related cortical potentials during an auditory signal detection task with cued intervals. *Journal of Experimental Psychology: Human Perception and Performance, 1*, 268–79.

Squires, K. C., Wickens, C., Squires, N. K., & Donchin, E. (1976). The effect of stimulus sequence on the waveform of the cortical event-related potential. *Science, 193*, 1142–6.

Srinivasan, R., Nunez, P. L., Tucker, D. M., Silberstein, R. B., & Cadusch, P. J. (1996). Spatial sampling and filtering of EEG with spline Laplacians to estimate cortical potentials. *Brain Topography, 8*, 355–66.

Starr, A., & Farley, G. R. (1983). Middle and long latency auditory evoked potentials in cat: II. Component distribution and dependence on stimulus factors. *Hearing Research, 10*, 139–52.

Stormark, K. M., Nordby, H., & Hugdahl, K. (1995). Attentional shifts to emotionally charged cues: Behavioural and ERP data. *Cognition and Emotion, 9*, 507–23.

Sutton, S., Braren, M., Zubin, J., & John, E. R. (1965). Evoked potential correlates of stimulus uncertainty. *Science, 150*, 1187–8.

Sutton, S., & Ruchkin, D. S. (1984). The late positive complex. Advances and new problems. In R. Karrer, J. Cohen, & P. Tueting (Eds.), *Brain and Information: Event-Related Potentials* (Annals of the New York Academy of Sciences, vol. 425), pp. 1–23. New York: New York Academy of Sciences.

Sutton, S., Tueting, P., Zubin, J., & John, E. R. (1967). Information delivery and the sensory evoked potentials. *Science, 155*, 1436–9.

Toga, A. W., & Mazziotta, J. C. (Eds.) (1996). *Brain Mapping. The Methods*. San Diego: Academic Press.

Towle, V. L., Heuer, D., & Donchin, E. (1980). On indexing attention and learning with event-related potentials [Abstract]. *Psychophysiology, 17*, 291.

Treisman, A., & Gelade, G. (1980). A feature integration theory of attention. *Cognitive Psychology, 12*, 97–136.

Tucker, D. M. (1993). Spatial sampling of head electrical fields: The geodesic sensor net. *Electroencephalography and Clinical Neurophysiology, 87*, 154–63.

Tulving, E. (1985). Memory and consciousness. *Canadian Psychology, 26*, 1–12.

van Boxtel, G. J., & Brunia, C. H. (1994). Motor and non-motor components of the contingent negative variation. *International Journal of Psychophysiology, 17*, 269–79.

Vanderploeg, R. D., Brown, W. S., & Marsh, J. T. (1987). Judgments of emotion in words and faces: ERP correlates. *International Journal of Psychophysiology, 5*, 193–205.

Van Petten, C. (1995). Words and sentences: Event-related brain potential measures. *Psychophysiology, 32*, 511–25.

Van Petten, C., & Kutas, M. (1987). Ambiguous words in context: An event-related analysis of the time course of meaning activation. *Journal of Memory and Language, 26*, 188–208.

Van Petten, C., & Kutas, M. (1990). Interactions between sentence context and word frequency in event-related brain potentials. *Memory and Cognition, 18*, 380–93.

Van Petten, C., & Kutas, M. (1991). Influences of semantic and syntactic context on open- and closed-class words. *Memory and Cognition, 19*, 95–112.

Van Petten, C., & Senkfor, A. J. (1996). Memory for words and novel visual patterns: Repetition, recognition, and encoding effects in the event-related brain potential. *Psychophysiology, 33*, 491–506.

Vaughan, H. G., Costa, L. D., & Ritter, W. (1972). Topography of the human motor potential. *Electroencephalography and Clinical Neurophysiology, 25*, 1–10.

Verleger, R. (1988). Event-related potentials and memory: A critique of the context updating hypothesis and an alternative interpretation of P3. *Behavioral and Brain Sciences, 11*, 343–56.

Verleger, R. (1997). On the utility of P3 latency as an index of mental chronometry. *Psychophysiology, 34*, 131–56.

von Restorff, H. (1933). Uber die Wirkung von Bereichsbildungen im Spurenfeld. *Psychologische Forschung, 18*, 299–342.

Wallace, W. P. (1965). Review of the historical, empirical, and theoretical status of the von Restorff phenomenon. *Psychological Bulletin, 63*, 410–24.

Walter, W. G., Cooper, R., Aldridge, V. J., McCallum, W. C., & Winter, A. L. (1964). Contingent negative variation: An electrical sign of sensorimotor association and expectancy in the human brain. *Nature, 203*, 380–4.

Wijers, A. A., Mulder, G., Okita, T., & Mulder, L. J. (1989). Event-related potentials during memory search and selective attention to letter size and conjunctions of letter size and color. *Psychophysiology, 26*, 529–47.

Woldorff, M. G., Gallen, C. C., Hampson, S. A., Hillyard, S. A., Pantev, C., Sobel, D., & Bloom, F. E. (1993). Modulation of early sensory processing in human auditory cortex during auditory selective attention. *Proceedings of the National Academy of Sciences U.S.A., 90*, 8722–6.

Wood, C. C., & McCarthy, G. (1984). Principal component analysis of event-related potentials: Simulation studies demonstrate misallocation of variance across components. *Electroencephalography and Clinical Neurophysiology, 59*, 298–308.

Wood, C. C., McCarthy, G., Squires, N. K., Vaughan, H. G., Woods, D. L., & McCallum, W. C. (1984). Anatomical and physiological substrates of event-related potentials. In R. Karrer, J. Cohen, & P. Tueting (Eds.), *Brain and Information: Event-Related Potentials,* pp. 681–721. New York: New York Academy of Sciences.

Woody, C. D. (1967). Characterization of an adaptive filter for the analysis of variable latency neuroelectrical signals. *Medical and Biological Engineering, 5,* 539–53.

Yamaguchi, S., & Knight, R. T. (1991). P300 generation by novel somatosensory stimuli. *Electroencephalography and Clinical Neurophysiology, 78,* 50–5.

CHAPTER FOUR

POSITRON EMISSION TOMOGRAPHY AND FUNCTIONAL MAGNETIC RESONANCE IMAGING

ERIC M. REIMAN, RICHARD D. LANE, CYMA VAN PETTEN, & PETER A. BANDETTINI

Psychophysiology traditionally involves manipulations of psychological state in intact human beings coupled with examination of central and peripheral physiological changes using sensors on the *surface* of the body, face, or skull. Although the details of the associated brain functions have been of great interest, until relatively recently the methodology for examining brain function in intact human beings in an anatomically precise way was not available. In the past 30 years, however, there has been a revolution in the ability to visualize the three-dimensional structure and function of the brain, based in part on the advent of computer algorithms used to generate these images.

Computerized tomography (CT) and magnetic resonance imaging (MRI) scanning greatly advanced our ability to study brain structure noninvasively. Positron emission tomography (PET) was the first high-resolution technique to examine functional activity in the living human brain, beginning in the 1970s (Phelps et al. 1975). The advent of short half-life radiotracers, such as ^{15}O, transformed PET and brought it into the field of psychophysiology, enabling the examination of the neural substrates of brief mental events in intact people with far greater spatial resolution than was previously possible. Functional magnetic resonance imaging (fMRI), an extension and refinement of structural MRI, has – in the short time since its inception in 1991 (Belliveau et al. 1991) – become the leading functional neuroimaging technique and is likely to remain so in the future. However, many methodological challenges remain to be resolved with fMRI, and PET is a proven technique that is the method of choice in a number of applications.

In this chapter, we begin by presenting a review of PET methodology. Next we compare PET and fMRI along multiple dimensions of interest to psychophysiologists. (The reader is referred to Chapter 36 by Bandettini et al. for a detailed review of fMRI.) The goal of these methodological reviews is to enable researchers to understand and distinguish between these techniques in a thoughtful manner as they review published work or design research to address specific research questions. In the third and final section we illustrate these principles by presenting the application of PET and fMRI to the study of cognition. Because the ultimate goal of this chapter is to promote the use of PET and fMRI in the generation of new knowledge, we place particular emphasis in this final section on the advantages and disadvantages of PET and fMRI as they pertain to issues of experimental design.

Positron Emission Tomography

PET is an imaging technique that provides information about biochemical and physiological processes in the brain and other organs of the body (Raichle 1983). Neuroscientifically, PET is used to investigate the brain regions, pathways, and chemical processes that participate in normal human behaviors, those that are involved in normal development, aging, and the response to injury, and those that are involved in the pathophysiology and treatment of behavioral disorders. In order to understand the capabilities and limitations of this technique, it is helpful to understand the components of PET studies (see Table 1).

TABLE 1. Components of a PET Study

1. Positron emitting radiotracer
2. PET imaging system
3. Image processing
4. Tracer kinetic model
5. Experimental design
6. Image analysis
7. Data interpretation

John T. Cacioppo, Louis G. Tassinary, and Gary G. Berntson (Eds.), *Handbook of Psychophysiology*, 2nd ed. © Cambridge University Press 2000. Printed in the United States of America. ISBN 62634X. All rights reserved.

POSITRON EMITTING RADIOTRACER

PET studies require the synthesis and administration of a positron emitting radiotracer, a physiological or pharmacological compound that is labeled with a positron emitting radioisotope. Commonly used positron emitting radioisotopes include ^{15}O (half-life 2 min), ^{13}N (half-life 10 min), ^{11}C (half-life 20 min), and ^{18}F (half-life 110 min). Since oxygen, nitrogen, and carbon are normal constituents of the body and pharmaceutical compounds, these elements can be incorporated into physiological compounds, pharmacological compounds, and their analogs without affecting their behavior in the body. Since fluorine can serve as an analog of hydrogen, it can also be incorporated into some of these compounds without affecting their behavior in the body. For this reason, PET has the potential to study a wide variety of substrates, substrate analogs, and pharmacological compounds. For instance, ^{15}O-water is commonly used to measure cerebral blood flow (CBF) (Fox & Mintun 1989; Herscovitch, Markham, & Raichle 1983; Raichle et al. 1983); ^{18}F-fluorodeoxyglucose is commonly used to measure the cerebral metabolic rate for glucose (CMRgl) (Huang et al. 1980; Phelps et al. 1979; Reivich et al. 1979), and ^{11}C-raclopride can be used to estimate the density of available dopamine D2 receptors in the brain (Farde et al. 1985, 1986).

The commonly used positron emitting radiotracers have a radioactive half-life of 2–110 min, so these compounds must be produced in relatively close proximity to the imaging system. The synthesis of a positron emitting radiotracer typically involves a particle accelerator, most commonly a cyclotron, and sometimes complicated radiochemistry techniques (Nozaki & Hazue 1995; Saha, MacIntyre, & Go 1992). The cyclotron produces positron emitting radioisotopes by bombarding a target with rapidly accelerated protons or deuterons. Automated or manual techniques use these radioisotopes (generated in the form of a radiolabeled precursor) and other compounds to synthesize radiotracers. Quality adherence procedures are used to confirm that each batch of radiotracer material (e.g., ^{18}F-flourodeoxyglucose dissolved in normal saline) is radiochemically pure, chemically pure, and free of pyrogens. In order to reduce the cost and simplify the process involved in radiotracer synthesis, an ultracompact cyclotron is available for the production of ^{15}O-water (the cerebral blood flow tracer most commonly used in brain mapping studies) and other ^{15}O-labeled tracers (Cherry & Phelps 1996; Nozaki & Hazue 1995), and small linear accelerators are becoming available for the production of a variety of positron emitting radioisotopes. For clinical studies, replaceable generators are also available for the production of the myocardial perfusion tracers, such as ^{82}rubidium (^{82}Ru) and certain other radioisotopes (Knapp, Brihaye, & Callahan 1995). Most PET centers have a cyclotron and radiochemistry facility on-site, but some imaging centers receive the longer-lived radiotracers from a regional radiotracer distribution center that is less than a few minutes away (for both ^{11}C and ^{18}F) or a few hours away (for ^{18}F) by ground or air transportation. Although the short half-lives of positron emitting radioisotopes contribute to the high cost of PET studies, they make it possible to study subjects with relatively low radiation exposures, since radioactivity in the body is almost gone about five half-lives after radiotracer administration.

Once the tracer is synthesized, it is rapidly transported to the PET laboratory and administered to the subject intravenously or by inhalation. The administered radiotracer decays by the emission of a positron from the unstable nucleus of the radioisotope. A positron is a subatomic particle with the mass of an electron and a positive charge. Each positron travels a short distance (root mean square range 0.4–1.4 mm; Cherry & Phelps 1996) before it comes to rest and interacts with an electron in the surrounding tissue. This distance, which contributes to PET's theoretical limitation in spatial resolution, is directly related to the energy of the emitted positron; it is longest for ^{15}O and shortest for ^{18}F among the most commonly used radioisotopes (Cherry & Phelps 1996). The positron–electron pair undergoes annihilation, converting its combined mass into two high-energy (511-keV) photons, known as gamma rays, which travel in virtually opposite directions. These photons are detected by the PET imaging system. The principles of positron emission and annihilation are illustrated in Figure 1.

Brain Mapping Tracers

Since CBF and CMRgl are markers of local neuronal activity, CBF and CMRgl tracers are often used. The most commonly used CBF tracer is ^{15}O-water; other CBF tracers include ^{15}O-butanol and ^{15}O-carbon dioxide. The most commonly used CMRgl tracer is ^{18}F-fluorodeoxyglucose (FDG). Radiotracer techniques are also available for the measurement of cerebral blood volume (CBV) and the cerebral metabolic rate for oxygen (CMRO$_2$). Whereas increases in local neuronal activity are associated with increases in regional CBF, CBV, and CMRgl (Raichle 1987), they do not appear to be associated with increases in CMRO$_2$ (Fox & Raichle 1986). As discussed by Bandettini (Chapter 36 of this volume), the observation that local neuronal activity is associated with an increase in CBF in excess of oxygen demand appears to account for the ability of functional magnetic resonance imaging to detect regional increases in brain oxygenation in conjunction with increases in local neuronal activity using a technique known as "blood oxygenation level dependent" (BOLD) contrast.

Advantages of ^{15}O-water include the ability to acquire an image relatively quickly (typically, about 60 sec, but as quickly as 15–20 sec – Cherry et al. 1995; Volkow et al. 1991) and the ability to make multiple images in the same

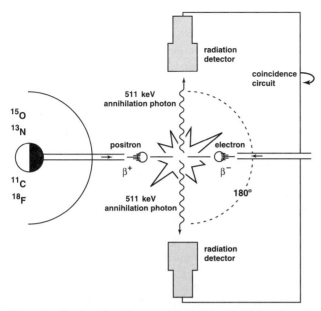

Figure 1. Physics of positron emission and coincidence detection. Radioisotopes employed in PET studies decay by the emission of positrons (+), particles that have the mass of an electron but a positive charge, from a nucleus that is unstable owing to a deficiency of neutrons. Positrons lose their kinetic energy after travelling about 0.4–1.4 mm, come to rest, and interact with local electrons (−). The two particles undergo annihilation, and their mass is converted into two high-energy (511-keV) photons that travel in opposite directions (approximately 180°). The two photons are detected by opposing detectors in the imaging system, which are connected by an electronic coincidence circuit that records an event only when the two photons reach the detectors at the same time. Redrawn with permission from Raichle, "Positron emission tomography," *Annual Review of Neuroscience,* vol. 6, pp. 249–67. Copyright 1983 Annual Reviews, Inc.

subject with an interval of only 10 min between scans. The ability to acquire images relatively quickly is attributable to the rapid transport of ^{15}O-water to the brain and its almost complete diffusibility across the blood–brain barrier during a single pass. During a single pass through the brain, the initial ^{15}O-water "uptake phase" is especially sensitive to the detection of increases in local neuronal activity (Cherry et al. 1995; Volkow et al. 1991); still, scans commonly continue through the radiotracer "washout phase" and beyond in order to accumulate more PET counts and thus reduce noise in the image. Since scans can be acquired relatively quickly, ^{15}O-water studies make it possible to study individuals during a relatively brief behavioral state (e.g., an experimentally induced emotion or a particular stage of sleep) and during a relatively uncomfortable behavioral state (e.g., experimentally induced anxiety or pain). The ability to acquire multiple sequential images is attributable to the 2-min half-life of ^{15}O and the resulting rapid decay of radioactivity from the preceding image.

^{15}O-water studies permit subjects to serve as their own control during a single scanning session. For this reason, this tracer is especially well suited for studies that benefit from the acquisition of multiple images during a single scanning session: investigating brain regions that participate in aspects of normal human behaviors, such as perception, motor control, attention, memory, language, emotion, the sleep–wake cycle, and consciousness (Frackowiak et al. 1997; Raichle 1987), as well as for investigating regions of the brain that are selectively affected by rapidly induced behavioral syndromes, such as biochemically induced panic attacks and behaviorally induced anxiety syndromes (Reiman 1997). Due to the brevity of scans, the main disadvantage of this brain mapping tracer is that the acquired images contain relatively few PET counts (on the order of 7–8 million counts per brain image). Because such images are relatively noisy, they are usually smoothed to a lower spatial resolution: about 10–20 mm full width at half-maximum (FWHM) in order to improve the signal-to-noise or S/N ratio (i.e., image quality). Furthermore, ^{15}O-water studies typically involve averaging conditions across subjects to further improve S/N. Nonetheless, the ability to compare images within subjects during experimental and baseline images – the ability to subtract the baseline image from the experimental image in order to generate a voxel-by-voxel "subtraction image" of state-dependent changes in regional CBF – usually outweighs concerns about poor spatial resolution.

Although ^{15}O-water is the radiotracer most commonly used in brain mapping studies, it does not completely diffuse across the blood–brain barrier in a single pass; this leads to a slight underestimation in CBF measurements, particularly at higher rates (Herscovitch, Markham, & Raichle 1987). In contrast, the radiotracer ^{15}O-butanol is completely diffusible; it thus provides a more accurate measure of blood flow and, at least theoretically, avoids underestimates of state-dependent increases in regional blood flow (Herscovitch et al. 1987). Since the underestimation of CBF with ^{15}O-water is small and the synthesis of this tracer is fully automated, most laboratories favor it over butanol in brain mapping studies.

Whereas CBF images are commonly acquired in the 1 min following the intravenous bolus injection of ^{15}O-water and its arrival to the brain, FDG images are commonly acquired over a 30–60-min period following the intravenous administration of FDG, its transport into brain cells, and its phosphorylation. As an analog of glucose, deoxyglucose undergoes phosphorylation (the initial step of glycolysis), leading to the accumulation of ^{18}F-fluorodeoxyglucose-6-phosphate (Huang et al. 1980; Phelps et al. 1979; Reivich et al. 1979; Sokoloff et al. 1977). Unlike glucose-6-phosphate, this metabolite cannot be further metabolized and is "trapped" in brain cells. The first 15–30-min interval following the intravenous administration of FDG is known as the *radiotracer uptake* period, during which the tracer is delivered to the brain and phosphorylated; radiotracer uptake during this period is reflected by changes in regional brain activity. The next 30–60-min interval is known as the *scanning* period (though scans can begin even earlier). During the scanning period, the image of brain activity is like a slowly degrading photograph and is relatively unaffected by the subjects' behavioral state. Advantages of FDG in brain mapping studies include the generation of relatively high-quality images (due to the relatively long scans and, when necessary, to completing the radiotracer uptake period outside the imaging system). The relatively long FDG scan leads to the acquisition of images with relatively high PET counts (on the order of 50–150 million counts per brain image), resulting in higher-quality images than those acquired using ^{15}O-water. It is thus easier to distinguish biological signals from noise in these images and so there is less need to smooth the images to a lower spatial resolution in order to improve the contrast between signal and noise. The ability to acquire images outside the imaging system is sometimes helpful in patients with unusually severe claustrophobia (a much less significant problem with PET than with MRI), in unusual circumstances that are not easy to replicate in the PET laboratory (e.g., an experimental provocation of an acrophobia), and in environments in which the clinical demand leads to restrictions in scanning time. Disadvantages of this radiotracer technique include the inability to repeat scans in the same subject during a single scanning session (it takes several hours for the residual brain activity to dissipate); the inability to study relatively brief or uncomfortable behavioral states (e.g., rapid-eye-movement or REM sleep; experimentally induced anxiety syndromes) or behavioral states that might be confounded by psychophysiological habituation during the radiotracer uptake period (although state-dependent changes in brain activity most strongly reflect the first few minutes of uptake); head movement during the scan; and the relatively small number of scans that one can acquire in a research subject due to the relatively longer half-life of ^{18}F, its accumulation in the bladder (the dose-limiting organ), and concerns about the safety of low-level radiation exposure. Nonetheless, the quality of FDG images makes them particularly well suited for comparing regional brain activity across scanning sessions in between-group comparisons (investigating alterations in regional brain activity in patients versus healthy control subjects, males versus females, older versus younger subjects, etc.) as well as between-session comparisons (studying the same subject on different days to investigate regions of the brain that are selectively affected by age, different stages of the menstrual cycle, the response to brain injury, medication and nonmedication treatments, the natural history of behavioral disorders, etc.).

Neurochemical Tracers

Researchers continue to develop, test, and apply positron emitting radiotracers with the potential for characterizing neurotransmitter and neuroreceptor processes. Radiotrac-

ers that bind to specific receptors, known as *radioligands,* have the potential to measure a variety of neuroreceptor processes, such as: the total receptor density (B_{max}); the unoccupied receptor density (B'_{max}), receptor affinity (using terms like $1/K_D$, k_{on}, k_{off}, k_3, and k_4, where K_D is the equilibrium receptor–ligand binding constant, k_{on} is the receptor–ligand association rate, k_{off} is the receptor–ligand dissociation rate, k_3 is the receptor–ligand association rate constant, k_4 is the receptor–ligand dissociation rate constant; $K_D = k_{off}/k_{on}$, $k_3 = k_{on}B'_{max}$, and $k_4 = k_{off}$); radioligand distribution volume (DV'', which tends to reflect the B'_{max}/K_D for some radioligands); and the receptor–ligand binding potential ($B'_{max}K_D$) (Huang, Barrio, & Phelps 1986; Koeppe et al. 1991; Mintun et al. 1984; Perlmutter et al. 1986). In order to measure these processes, radioligands must have several features:

1. they must be rapidly synthesized and purified;
2. they must have no pharmacological, clinical, or adverse effects in the radiotracer doses employed;
3. they must easily penetrate the blood–brain barrier;
4. they must bind to the receptor subtype of interest (e.g., dopamine D2 receptors) without binding to other receptors of the same type (e.g., other subtypes of dopamine receptors), a feature known as "receptor subtype selectivity";
5. they must bind the receptor of interest in much higher affinity than they bind to nonspecific, nonsaturable receptors (just about anything to which a radioligand might stick), a feature known as "receptor specificity";
6. they must not produce labeled or potentially confounding active metabolites during the scanning period; and
7. their kinetics must be compatible with the tracer kinetic model used to transform images of activity into neuroreceptor measurements (Huang et al. 1986; Sedvall et al. 1986).

When studies find an increased density of unoccupied receptors using many of the better-established radiotracer techniques, it could reflect an increase in total receptor density itself (e.g., an increase in dopamine D2 receptor density) or a decrease in the synaptic concentration of endogenous ligand (a decrease in the synaptic concentration of dopamine).

At this time, promising positron emitting radioligands have been developed for the characterization of dopamine D1, D2, D3, D4, and transporter receptors (although the concentrations of imaged D3 and D4 receptors are not very high), the serotonin 1A, 2A, and transporter receptors, acetylcholine muscarinic and nicotinic receptors, opiate mu and mu/delta receptors, the glutamate NMDA receptor, benzodiazepine 1 and 2 receptors, and estradiol receptors (Langstrom & Dannals 1995; Sedvall et al. 1996; Stocklin 1995). To the extent that these radiotracer techniques are validated, they can be used to investigate (i) the role of receptor subtype abnormalities in the pathophysiology of psychiatric disorders prior to the potentially confounding effect of prior medication exposure (Wong & Resnick 1995), (ii) the extent to which receptor occupancy is related to the beneficial or adverse effects of psychopharmacological treatments, and (iii) the extent to which receptor abnormalities could be used to characterize lesions – for example, abnormally increased benzodiazepine receptors in seizure foci (Frost & Mayberg 1995) and abnormally increased estradiol receptors in women with metastatic breast cancer (Mintun et al. 1991).

PET measurements of receptor density are affected in part by synaptic concentrations of neurotransmitters, endogenous ligands that compete with the radioligand for the receptor. Some studies suggest that a radioligand that rapidly and reversibly binds to its receptors, such as the selective D2 receptor ligand ^{11}C-raclopride, is more strongly affected by synaptic concentrations of neurotransmitter than a radioligand that binds less reversibly to its receptors, such as the D2/5HT2 receptor ligand ^{11}C-N-methyl-spiperone. Researchers have actually capitalized on this potential confound in order to estimate how synaptic concentrations of neurotransmitters (including synaptic concentrations of dopamine, serotonin, acetylcholine, and endorphins) are locally affected in response to pharmacological challenges (Dewey et al. 1990, 1992; Smith et al. 1997, 1998) and during behavioral tasks (Koepp et al. 1998). This technique can be used to investigate how synaptic neurotransmitter concentrations are regionally involved in the pathophysiology, medication treatment, and nonmedication treatment of psychiatric disorders, how they are regionally affected during different behavioral tasks or states (thus helping to characterize the chemical neuroanatomy of normal behaviors and experimentally induced behavioral syndromes), and potentially important neurotransmitter actions. Thus, PET can now be used to map the chemical processes that are involved in normal and abnormal human behaviors.

Finally, radiochemists have developed radiotracers for the characterization of other neurotransmitter processes, including estimates of DOPA decarboxylase activity (an enzyme involved in dopamine synthesis that provides a marker of intact dopaminergic neuronal terminals and is reduced in patients with Parkinson's disease), serotonin synthesis, and concentrations of monoamine oxidase A and B (enzymes involved in the degradation of norepinephrine, serotonin, and dopamine) (Langstrom & Dannals 1995; Stocklin 1995).

Other Tracers

In addition to the tracers just described, radiotracer techniques have been developed for other physiological processes. These include: amino acid uptake, which provides clinically useful information about the spatial extent of low-grade and high-grade tumors; CMRO$_2$, which has been used in conjunction with measures of CBF and CBV in the assessment of cerebrovascular disorders; the permeability–surface area product for water (PSw), a measure of blood–brain barrier permeability to water that is regulated by the central adrenergic system and increased by most antidepressants; and brain tissue pH, a reduction in which has been postulated to trigger anxiety attacks in patients with panic disorder (Conti 1995; Heiss & Podreka 1995; Herscovitch 1995; Reiman 1990). Radiochemists continue to develop and test positron emitting radiotracers with the potential for measuring biochemical and physiological processes of interest to researchers and clinicians. For this reason, the versatility of PET is limited only by the ingenuity and persistence of radiochemists and the interest (and patience) of researchers who wish to use the radiotracers to address interesting and important problems.

THE PET IMAGING SYSTEM

After the radiotracer is administered, an imaging system is employed to make regional measurements of PET counts in the brain. Available PET systems consist of concentric rings of detectors into which the head or body is placed (Cherry & Phelps 1996). Each detector consists of a scintillator crystal that transforms an incoming 511-keV photon (i.e., a gamma ray) into a flash of light and a photomultiplier tube that transforms the light into an electric current. Most commercial systems use the crystal bismuth germanate (BGO). Older commercial systems use the crystal cesium fluoride, which has the capacity to acquire counts with less dead time at higher rates and thus to acquire ^{15}O-water images with sufficient counts in a shorter period of time. Some commercial systems use the crystal sodium iodide, which is less expensive, less powerful, and less suitable for ^{15}O-water studies. Manufacturers have recently investigated the use of lutetium oxyorthosilicate (LSO), an expensive crystal with the potential to increase the detection of gamma rays by a factor of five (Cherry & Phelps 1996). Manufacturers have also considered the use of solid-state devices in place of, or in addition to, photomultiplier tubes to provide more accurate and less expensive imaging systems.

Each detector is connected to multiple opposing detectors by coincidence circuits. Coincidence circuits record those events in which the opposing detectors sense two annihilation photons simultaneously. Coincidence circuits thus record the number of annihilation events that have occurred somewhere along a straight line joining the two detectors. (These circuits also record a relatively small number of "random coincidence events" in which unrelated photons strike opposing detectors simultaneously and a small number of "scattered coincidence events" in which gamma rays have been deflected somewhere in the body to another detector, leading to inaccurate localization of the annihilation event.) Typically, PET systems record at least one million coincidence events per PET slice during a single scan. Measurements of regional PET counts in the head are reconstructed from the record of coincidence events by means of a computer-applied mathematical reconstruction algorithm (Cherry, Dahlbom, & Hoffman 1992; Cherry & Phelps 1996). The principle of coincidence detection was illustrated in Figure 1.

Until recently, most PET systems restricted the acquisition of coincidence events to those that struck opposing detectors in the same or adjacent horizontal planes by placing septa between adjacent rings that projected beyond the detectors into the field of view. While this two-dimensional (2D) mode of image acquisition greatly reduces the number of random and scattered events, it also decreases sensitivity to detect true coincident events to about 0.5%, because it misses the coincidence events that occur across sections (Cherry & Phelps 1996; Townsend 1991). The latest commercial systems enable the septa between adjacent rings to be retracted automatically, thus permitting the three-dimensional (3D) mode of image acquisition. By acquiring coincidence events using opposing detectors from any of the rings, the sensitivity to detect true coincidence is increased to about 3.0% (Townsend 1991). Three-dimensional imaging characteristically leads to higher-quality images (i.e., an increase in S/N), particularly at low counting rates (Cherry, Dahlbom, & Hoffman 1991). The 3D mode of image acquisition provides a particular benefit for neurotransmitter and neuroreceptor studies, increasing S/N by a factor of about five, since these processes occur in minute concentrations (Cherry & Phelps 1996; Townsend 1991). Although the 3D mode of image acquisition may be less useful for higher counting rates, it is now used in many ^{15}O-water studies (Cherry, Woods, & Hoffman 1993), since it is possible to acquire images at a lower radiotracer dose and so reduce the subject's radiation exposure. Because 3D imaging increases the number of scattered and random coincident events, involves a computationally intensive 3D-image reconstruction algorithm (Cherry et al. 1992), and involves unusually large data sets, some situations may be more appropriate for 2D imaging. In the future, different detector configurations (e.g., nearly spherical systems), shorter septa lengths, and more precise coincidence timing could provide images with unprecedented image quality (Townsend 1991).

Like other imaging techniques, PET systems can be described in terms of their spatial resolution (ability to image small objects), temporal resolution (ability to acquire data quickly), contrast resolution (ability to distinguish true signals from false signals and noise), and sensitivity (ability to acquire data from small amounts of radioactivity) (Daube-Witherspoon 1995). PET systems differ in other specifications, including: the size of the aperture into which the head or body is placed; the number of horizontal PET slices for which data are simultaneously acquired (an almost anachronistic concept with 3D imaging, but as many as 47 slices in commercially available systems); the distance between contiguous slices (about 3.5 mm in the latest systems); the thickness of each slice (about 5 mm); the axial field of view (about 15 cm in the latest systems, permitting researchers to acquire data in the entire brain); the ability to acquire images in only 2D versus either 2D or 3D mode; the external radiation source used to acquire transmission images before (or, possibly, at the same time as) the emission scan; and the electronics, computers, and software used in image processing (Daube-Witherspoon 1995).

The spatial resolution of an imaging system reflects the smallest distance between two point sources that permits a distinction between their respective images. When a point or line source is imaged, a count profile assumes the approximate shape of a Gaussian curve; the spatial resolution is most commonly defined as the width of the curve at half of its maximum value (i.e., the full width at half-maximum or FWHM). The latest generation of PET systems has a spatial resolution of about 3–5 mm FWHM in the plane of each slice, although the reconstructed images are typically smoothed further in order to improve contrast resolution (S/N). The theoretical limit of PET's spatial resolution is about 2–3 mm FWHM, owing to (i) the distance the positron must travel from the radionuclide before it interacts with an electron and (ii) the small extent to which the resulting gamma rays that arise from an annihilation event deviate from a 180° angle (Cherry & Phelps 1996). For this reason, PET is ultimately limited in its ability to detect and represent accurately data from very small structures (such as brainstem nuclei) and in the extent to which it can be used to study small animals. The extent of this limitation depends on: the resolution of the system; the radioisotope (best for ^{18}F owing to the lower energy and smaller distance travelled by the emitted positron; worst for ^{15}O); the size, shape, and orientation of the structure of interest; and the contrast in radioactivity between the structure of interest and its neighbors (Daube-Witherspoon 1995; Mazziotta et al. 1981).

Despite the PET system's limited spatial resolution, experimental studies can be designed to localize and discriminate regional changes in PET measurements that are as close as 1–2 mm apart (Fox et al. 1986; Mintun, Fox, & Raichle 1989). Thus, it has been possible to map the retinotopic organization of visual cortex and the somatotopic organization of supplementary motor cortex with remarkable precision (Fox et al. 1986; Fox, Burton, & Raichle 1987; Frackowiak et al. 1997).

PET's temporal resolution – the time it takes to acquire an image with adequate S/N – depends on the radiotracer technique (the time it takes for FDG uptake and phosphorylation, the time it takes to reach a state of equilibrium in most neuroreceptor studies, etc.); the time it takes to acquire sufficient PET counts (a factor that is influenced by the radiotracer dose and the sensitivity of the PET system for neurotransmitter, neuroreceptor, and other studies involving low count rates); and the ability to tolerate high count rates without significant dead time (the cumulative time interval during which the detectors are saturated and incoming photons are not detected, a factor in ^{15}O-water studies). The administered PET dose should be limited to that which produces dead time amounting to less than 20%–30% of the imaging period (Cherry & Phelps 1996).

PET is more sensitive than other imaging techniques, such as single photon emission tomography (SPECT), MRI, and magnetic resonance spectroscopy (MRS). For this reason (and the versatility of potential radiotracer techniques), PET continues to offer special promise in the study of neurotransmitters, neuroreceptors, and other processes that exist in minute concentrations.

PET's contrast resolution is directly related to the number of acquired counts. Thus, there is a trade-off between contrast resolution and the radiotracer dose employed (since higher doses are associated with more counts), temporal resolution (since more counts are acquired during longer scanning periods), spatial resolution (since counts from neighboring voxels contribute to data in each voxel), and the number of images acquired during the same state in one or more individuals that are averaged together. These factors can affect the radiotracer dose employed, the filters used to smooth the images, the number of scans acquired in a single subject, and the number of subjects that participate in a study.

IMAGE PROCESSING

PET images can be significantly affected by radiation attenuation (the extent to which gamma rays are absorbed by the tissue through which they pass, preventing them from reaching the detector), random coincidence events, scattered coincidence events, differences in detector efficiency, and the effects of dead time (especially at higher counting rates). Procedures are commonly used to correct for random events and dead time, normalize the detectors, correct for scatter and attenuation, and calibrate the images using a known radiation source. Images of PET counts can thus be converted into images of radioactivity in units of mCi/ml (Cherry & Phelps 1996; Daube-Witherspoon 1995).

Because of differences in tissue density and the distance a gamma ray must pass through the head or body to reach detectors, only a minority of gamma rays emitted ever reach opposing detectors. Two alternative methods are used to correct an emission image (an image that measures gamma rays that arise inside the head or body) for radiation attenuation. The *measured* attenuation correction method uses a transmission image (an image that measures radiation transmitted through the head from an external radiation source, in this case ^{68}Ge/^{68}Ga) to correct the emission images for attenuation on a voxel-by-voxel basis. The transmission image is typically acquired just prior to the emission images and assumes that there is minimal head movement between scans; efforts are now underway

to acquire transmission and emission images simultaneously, addressing the potential problem of misalignment (Daube-Witherspoon 1995). Alternatively, the *calculated* attenuation correction method uses the contours of the head and knowledge about the extent to which brain tissue and skull attenuate gamma radiation to correct emission images for attenuation. Although less precise, this procedure is commonly used in FDG studies if the subject is not in the scanner during the radiotracer uptake period (since radioactivity inside the head would confound the transmission image) and avoids the potentially confounding effect of movement between transmission and emission scans.

An image reconstruction algorithm is used to convert information about PET counts (originally represented as a sinogram) into horizontal images. The conventional algorithm used in the reconstruction of PET images is known as the filtered back-projection method (Cherry & Phelps 1996). A modification of this method, known as the back-projection–re-projection method, is used to reconstruct data collected in the 3D mode (Cherry et al. 1993; Cherry & Phelps 1996). The filter, which is applied to the data prior to image reconstruction, reduces noise in a manner that results in a reconstructed image with higher S/N but a lower spatial resolution. The filter one chooses to reduce noise and smooth the image depends on the number of acquired counts and a subjective assessment of image quality (Daube-Witherspoon 1995). Iterative algorithms, such as the maximum likelihood algorithm, repeatedly refine the image to achieve an optimal correspondence with the raw data. Although these techniques are quite labor-intensive, they have the potential not only to reduce noise and improve spatial resolution in the reconstructed image, particularly for images involving relatively few counts (e.g., neurotransmitter, neuroreceptor, and ^{15}O-water studies), but also to incorporate additional information (e.g., information from co-registered MRIs about the distribution of gray matter, white matter, and cerebrospinal fluid; Leahy & Yan 1991).

TRACER KINETIC MODELS

The imaging system provides an image of regional PET counts, corresponding to the local concentration of radionuclides (mCi/ml) in the brain. To convert this information into biochemical and physiological processes, a tracer kinetic model must be employed (see e.g. Chen et al. 1998, Huang et al. 1980, or Patlak, Blasberg, & Fenstermacher 1983 for CMRgl measurements; Herscovitch et al. 1983 for CBF; Farde et al. 1986, Huang et al. 1986, Mintun et al. 1984, Perlmutter et al. 1986, or Wong, Gjedde, & Wagner 1986 for dopamine D2 receptor measurements; and Koeppe et al. 1991 for benzodiazepine receptor measurements). A tracer kinetic model consists of mathematical equations that account for the behaviors of the radiotracer in the body, including its radioactive half-life, its rate of transport to the brain, its distribution into various tissue compartments (e.g., plasma, extracellular brain tissue, intracellular brain tissue, etc.), its active and labeled metabolites, and – in the case of neurotransmitter and neuroreceptor measurements – its specific and nonspecific binding. Models are commonly used to reduce these processes into different compartments (e.g., plasma FDG, brain FDG, brain FDG-6-phosphate, and four transport rate constants in a three-compartment model representing the kinetics of FDG) (Gjedde 1995). Some tracer kinetic models rely on data acquired after the radiotracer reaches a state of equilibrium; others rely on dynamically acquired data, capturing images in sequential frames each lasting a few seconds to a few minutes.

Tracer kinetic models often require the acquisition of peripheral measurements during the performance of PET scans. For instance, the tracer kinetic models used to measure CBF and CMRgl typically rely on multiple, sequential measurements of radioactivity through a radial artery catheter to estimate the rate of radiotracer delivery to the brain. By obtaining a series of samples, one can generate a time–activity curve; this permits the calculation of absolute radioactivity in the sample at any previous moment. Since the radiotracer is injected into a vein, passed through the heart, and distributed evenly into the arterial system, values in the radial artery (which is comparable in distance from the heart to the major cerebral arteries) provide an excellent estimate of the values in the cerebral arteries. The radioactivity detected in the PET scan is corrected for attenuation due to bone, muscle, and other tissue that the signal must pass through. When this information and that from the blood samples are combined, one can determine the absolute amount of radiactivity and thus blood flow (based on the tracer kinetic model) at any location in the brain.

A technique is now available to estimate the rate of FDG delivery to the brain using dynamically acquired images of the internal carotid arteries and a single measurement of venous activity after the scan is complete (Chen et al. 1998). This technique, which eliminates the discomfort (and, in seriously ill patients, the small risk) associated with arterial catheterization, has the potential to be applied to other radiotracer techniques, especially those involving radiosotopes other than ^{15}O.

In most cases, the accuracy of biochemical and physiological measurements with PET ultimately depends on the validity of the tracer kinetic model and its underlying assumptions. However, it is possible to conduct brain mapping studies without converting images of brain activity (in units of PET counts of mCi/ml) into quantitative measurements of CBF (in units of ml/min/100 g) or CMRgl (in units of mg/min/100 g) (Fox & Mintun 1989). With ^{15}O-water or FDG and conventional radiotracer techniques, there is a relatively linear relationship between the distribution of activity and CBF or CMRgl in the brain, respectively. In brain mapping studies, the regional data are typically normalized for the variation in absolute measurements using a linear scaling factor (e.g., a regional/whole-brain ratio) or the general linear model (e.g., analysis of covariance) (Fox & Mintun 1989; Frackowiak et al. 1997), resulting in a unitless term regardless of whether one uses nonquantitative information (PET counts) or quantitative information (in biochemical or physiological units). Thus, if one assumes that whole-brain CBF or CMRgl is not significantly different during experimental and baseline conditions, then it is not necessary to acquire quantitative measurements of CBF or CMRgl, perform an uncomfortable arterial catheterization, or make multiple measurements of arterial activity in order to investigate state-dependent changes in local neuronal activity. Still, it is important to recognize conditions associated with changes in whole-brain CBF (including decreases with sedation, non-REM sleep, and decreased PCO_2 levels) and to consider the use of quantitative measurements in these conditions.

EXPERIMENTAL DESIGN

In general, PET studies are designed to maximize the detection of potentially subtle alterations in CBF, CMRgl, and other PET measurements, to relate these alterations to specific traits and states, and to minimize the effects of possible confounds. In brain mapping studies, researchers commonly investigate regions of the brain that are preferentially involved in potentially dissectable behaviors. In within-group comparisons (i.e., studies involving multiple CBF studies acquired during experimental and control conditions in multiple subjects), researchers commonly study 6–12 subjects and acquire 6–12 images per scanning session. In considering sample size and the number of images in each condition, one considers the problem of statistical power; in considering maximal number of scans per imaging session, one considers subject tolerance (e.g., remaining in the same position during a 2-hr scanning session) and radiation dosimetry. Depending on the question being investigated, it is usually helpful to maximize the intensity of the task during the experimental condition (e.g., maximize the frequency of a visual stimulus, the number of previously seen items in a memory recognition task, or the intensity of an emotion), to choose a baseline condition that controls for aspects of the experimental condition (e.g., the visual stimulus, eye movements, motor response) that are thought to be unrelated to the behavior of interest, to measure other variables that could be related to alterations in local neuronal activity (e.g., reaction time, "hits" and "misses" in a memory recognition task, or psychophysiological expressions of emotion), and to consider the inclusion of an additional no-task baseline condition (e.g., eyes closed and directed forward) to provide an additional perspective about the CBF differences observed between experimental and baseline conditions.

Some experiments call for qualitative differences between experimental and baseline conditions (e.g., emotion versus emotionally neutral conditions), some call for quantitative differences between these conditions (e.g., high or low memory demand), and some call for an investigation of interactions (e.g., greater differences in film-generated than recall-generated emotion).

Because 20–60 seconds are typically required to acquire a ^{15}O-water PET image, behavioral conditions must be studied in blocks. Thus, if one were to conduct a PET study in subjects during an explicit memory task that has been previously studied (outside of a neuroimaging context) using randomly presented familiar and unfamiliar stimuli, it would be helpful to revise the experiment to address the needs of PET. For example, it would be useful to: (1) present as many familiar stimuli as possible during a recall condition without inducing a ceiling effect in the subject's recognition response and present as many unfamiliar stimuli as possible during a control condition; (2) conduct a "dress-rehearsal" study in representative subjects outside the PET laboratory to verify that the expected behavioral responses are observed in these blocked conditions; and then (3) repeat the procedure in a different group of subjects in the PET laboratory. To the extent that it is possible, scans should be randomized or counterbalanced to address the potentially confounding effects of scan order.

In the comparison of known groups, which is one type of between-group comparison (e.g., patients with a psychiatric disorder versus controls), it is helpful to:

1. identify homogeneous patient samples (e.g., only those who satisfy extremely rigorous criteria for a psychiatric disorder) who do not have comorbid psychiatric, neurologic, or serious medical disorders, centrally acting medications, or other possible confounds;
2. identify control subjects who have neither psychiatric, neurologic, or serious medical disorders nor centrally acting medications and who have no other confounds (e.g., age, gender, sociodemographic variables, intelligence, phase of the menstrual cycle);
3. consider the subjects' cognitive-emotional-behavioral state at the time of the scan (i.e., the extent to which a finding is related to the pathophysiology of the disorder or to differences in the subject's current state with regard to eye movement, task compliance, level of arousal, or anxiety);
4. consider the role, if any, of provocation and treatment studies (e.g., to investigate regions of the brain that participate in the predisposition to, elicitation of, and medication or nonmedication treatment of panic disorder); and
5. consider the possible role of specific cognitive activation conditions during the imaging study to help relate specific regions of the brain to dysfunctional mental operations.

At this time, some researchers prefer to acquire PET images in patients and controls during a resting baseline state (e.g., eyes closed and directed forward with no movement and minimal sensory stimulation) in order to avoid the potentially confounding effects of differential performance on a standardized task; some researchers prefer to acquire these images during a well-characterized task that is thought to be unaffected by the disorder (e.g., a relatively simple sensory stimulation or attentional task) in order to reduce possible variations in the subject's cognitive-emotional-behavioral state at the time of the scan; and some researchers prefer to acquire these images during a task that is differentially performed in patients and controls (e.g., a frontal lobe task or a masked facial emotion recognition task) in order to enhance postulated differences in specific brain regions. A potential problem with this last approach is the chicken-or-egg question of whether patients fail to perform the task as well because the investigated region is dysfunctional or, conversely, whether patients fail to activate the investigated region because (for other reasons) they are not complying with the task as well. Various approaches have been taken to deal with this issue, such as varying the difficulty of the task across groups so that performance is comparable in each group or examining whether performance and neural activity are correlated or otherwise systematically related.

Although the subtraction approach has yielded important new findings, its limitations are increasingly being recognized (Friston et al. 1996b; Price & Friston 1997; Sarter, Berntson, & Cacioppo 1996). The subtraction approach is based on the assumption of "pure insertion" – that the only difference between the experimental and control condition is the phenomenon of interest. This approach does not take into account any interaction between the cognitive context and the cognitive function in question. Thus, factorial designs have become increasingly popular since they are tailored to address exactly such interaction effects (Frackowiak et al. 1997). For example, in PET protocols involving 12 scans, 2 × 3 (with one repetition of each condition) or 2 × 6 factorial designs are common. Experimental designs that permit more detailed examination of differences also permit greater latitude in the examination of commonalities. Thus, statistical techniques for so-called conjunction analyses (Price et al. 1997) have been developed that permit the identification of regions of statistically significant overlap across conditions or methods.

Finally, experimental studies should attempt to address important questions; they should be designed to test specific hypotheses and generate additional hypotheses that can be tested in the future; they should capitalize on the capabilities of this technology and interpret findings in the context of its limitations; and they should complement other kinds of behavioral neuroscientific studies in human and nonhuman species.

IMAGE ANALYSIS

This section considers techniques used to analyze data from ^{15}O-water studies. Many of the principles (e.g., those involved in anatomical localization, image deformation and averaging, and statistical analysis) are applicable to other radiotracer techniques.

Although it is sometimes helpful to analyze data in pre-selected regions of interest (ROIs), automated algorithms are commonly used to detect state-dependent changes in regional brain activity. Currently used software packages have several components:

1. a smoothing procedure to increase S/N;
2. an interpolation procedure to provide data between slices and generate a three-dimensional image;
3. a method to normalize each PET image for the variation in whole-brain measurements;
4. an iterative procedure to align multiple, sequential PET images acquired in the same subject in case of subtle head movement;
5. an optional co-registration method to align each subject's PET image with a T1-weighted volumetric MRI;
6. an image deformation algorithm to transform each subject's PET images or co-registered PET and MRI images into the spatial dimensions of a standard brain atlas;
7. statistical procedures to compare spatially standardized images acquired during the same experimental and baseline states in different subjects (or, less commonly, multiple images acquired during the same experimental and baseline state in a single subject); and
8. statistical or experimental efforts to address the statistical problem of multiple comparisons (type-I error) (Fox et al. 1988; Frackowiak et al. 1997).

Let us consider some of these issues in more detail.

Smoothing

As previously noted (and illustrated in Figure 2), image smoothing reduces noise in an image, effectively increasing the number of counts that contribute to the measurement in each voxel (Daube-Witherspoon 1995). The extent to which an image is smoothed depends on the quality of the image and the size of certain regions of interest. Images consisting of fewer PET counts (e.g., CBF images that are acquired in a short period of time) require more smoothing than images of higher PET counts (e.g., FDG images). Note that if one analyzes data from a preselected ROI, then image smoothing is less important. By averaging the data from all voxels within the region, one decreases noise and thus increases the signal-to-noise ratio without increasing the contributions of measurements in neighboring voxels via partial volume averaging.

Interpolation

Although PET images are typically displayed in the form of two-dimensional horizontal slices, linear interpolation methods can be used to fill in data in the gaps between the slices, even when the image is acquired and reconstructed in two dimensions (Fox et al. 1988; Mintun et al. 1989). Once the data are represented in three dimensions, PET images can be reformatted in any plane, deformed into a standard size and shape, and compared in different subjects.

Normalization for the Variation in Absolute Brain Measurements

In order to characterize state-dependent alterations in local neuronal activity, one must normalize regional measurements of CBF, CMRgl, ^{15}O-water uptake, and FDG uptake for the variability in absolute brain measurements on a voxel-by-voxel or regional basis. For instance, unit recordings find a predictable relationship between increases in the frequency of a visual stimulus (an annular reversing checkerboard pattern) and increased neuronal activity in primary visual cortex; PET studies find the same relationship between the frequency of this stimulus and measurements of CBF and ^{15}O-water uptake in the same brain region after the PET data are normalized for the variation in whole-brain measurements (Fox & Raichle 1984). The *proportional scaling* method uses a simple ratio to normalize every PET image in a study to the same whole-brain value (Fox et al. 1988; Fox & Mintun 1989; Frackowiak et al. 1997). In many CBF studies, every voxel in the image is multiplied by 50 ml/min/g (a standard value for whole-brain blood flow) and divided by whole-brain measurements of CBF or ^{15}O-water activity in the particular image. The *general linear model* method normalizes regional PET measurements for the variation in absolute measurements using analysis of covariance (Frackowiak et al. 1997; Friston et al. 1990). The proportional scaling method may be preferable in experiments that involve a relatively small number of scans (since it is not adversely affected by fewer degrees of freedom) and those that involve substantial variations in whole-brain measurements (more likely in qualitative studies of whole-brain PET counts than in quantitative studies of whole-brain CBF or CMRgl; Frackowiak et al. 1997). The general linear model method is a more rigorous statistical method for normalizing the data in experiments that involve a relatively large number of scans and only minor variations in whole brain measurements (Frackowiak et al. 1997).

Whenever a normalization procedure is used, it is assumed that there are no significant differences in whole-brain activity during the experimental and control scans. For conditions in which such differences are apparent (e.g., a reduction in whole-brain CBF associated with hypocapnia, reductions in whole-brain CBF and CMRgl associated with sedative/hypnotic medication or sleep), it may be difficult to know whether an observed change in normalized measurements represents altered neuronal activity in this region, unchanged neuronal activity in this region in comparison to the rest of the brain, or some combination of these factors.

In some instances, there are significant reductions in regional CBF or CMRgl in many regions of the brain. In such cases (e.g., comparing measurements in patients with Alzheimer's dementia to normal control subjects, since this disorder is associated with reductions in whole-brain CMRgl during the latter stages of the illness), it may be preferable to normalize the data using a region of interest known to be relatively unaffected in the condition of interest (e.g., the pons in studies of Alzheimer's disease; Minoshima et al. 1995a) rather than the data from the whole brain.

Alignment of Sequential PET Images

In order to compare multiple PET images from the same subject, it is important to minimize the misalignment between scans. During the PET procedure, several procedures (e.g., thermoplastic facial masks and head molds) are commonly used to help minimize this problem, but they do not fully address it; although stereotactic devices that drill holes directly into the skull have a role in a small number of neurosurgery patients and experimental animals, they are too invasive for most research applications. Iterative algorithms are now available to characterize and correct for head movement (i.e., up to three translations and three rotations) between scans (Minoshima et al. 1992; Woods, Cherry, & Mazziotta 1992). The Woods algorithm is commonly used in brain mapping studies. Still, these techniques do not correct for misalignment between transmission and emission scans or head movements during a single-frame scan.

Localization, Co-registration, and Deformation

Since PET images consist of low-resolution physiological or biochemical images that lack precise anatomical landmarks, it is usually difficult to identify neuroanatomical ROIs in the PET image. Several strategies have been used to identify regions of interest, compare data from different subjects in these regions, and compare findings from different laboratories. These strategies include (1) visual inspection of the PET image, (2) visual comparison with a brain atlas, (3) definition of an ROI identification in a co-registered structural brain image, and (4) automated methods for the transformation of brain images into the coordinates of a standard brain atlas.

Although visual inspection is a simple method, it is a relatively inaccurate and unreliable way to identify ROIs in the PET image. Furthermore, the choice of a brain region relies on the inspection of the functional data (the dependent variable of interest), increasing the chance of observer bias. Some laboratories acquire PET images in horizontal planes that are parallel to identifiable craniofa-

cial landmarks, such as the orbitomeatal or canthomeatal line, and then attempt to compare these images visually to a tomographic atlas of the brain that uses the same landmarks. Unfortunately, this approach fails to account for the variable relationship between these craniofacial landmarks and the brain, including its angle and vertical extent (Fox, Perlmutter, & Raichle 1985). This strategy, too, relies on the inspection of the functional data and so increases the chance of observer bias.

A more sophisticated approach uses an automated algorithm to co-register each subject's PET image(s) with his or her own structural brain image (i.e., a computed tomography image or an MRI) (Collins et al. 1994a; Evans 1995; Evans et al. 1991; Pellizarri et al. 1989; Woods, Cherry, & Mazziotta 1993). Algorithms have sought to match homologous points (using anatomical or fiducial landmarks), brain surfaces, or voxel-by-voxel features in the PET and MRI brain images. PET–MRI co-registration can be used to identify precisely the structural correlates of PET images and PET subtraction images (when state-dependent CBF changes are distinguishable from noise) in an individual subject. For instance, this approach can be used in brain mapping studies designed to identify and avoid "eloquent" brain areas – regions that are critically involved in a clinically important behavior, such as articulation – in candidates for neurosurgery (Duncan et al. 1997; Fried et al. 1995; Leblanc & Meyer 1990; Leblanc et al. 1992; Pardo & Fox 1993); it can also be used to identify precisely preselected ROIs that have well-defined anatomical landmarks (e.g., a study that wishes to test the hypothesis that the amygdala is activated during a facial recognition task). Co-registration can be used in conjunction with other procedures to help "correct" PET images for the potentially confounding effects of atrophy and partial volume averaging (e.g., to determine the extent to which reductions in regional or whole-brain PET measurements are related to an increased contribution of cerebrospinal fluid; Evans 1995), and it can be incorporated into the procedure used to transform each person's PET images into the dimensions of a standard brain atlas. Limitations of this procedure include minor errors in co-registration accuracy (about 1–2 mm) and the problem of identifying ROIs where there are no precise anatomical landmarks (e.g., divisions of prefrontal cortex). In addition, there are problems associated with any procedure that relies exclusively on preselected ROIs: an inability to determine if the maximal alteration in brain function resides in the ROI or in a neighboring region (due to partial volume averaging), failure to detect differences in subregions (if the ROI is too large), an inability to determine the spatial extent of the alteration in brain function, and an inability to characterize alterations in explored regions. To the extent that this procedure localizes well-defined anatomical ROIs with greater accuracy than available image deformation algorithms, the analysis of preselected ROIs could complement voxel-by-voxel brain maps.

At this time, the most powerful brain mapping algorithms rely on procedures that automatically deform each person's PET images or coregistered PET and MRI images into the coordinates of a standard brain atlas (Collins, Peters, & Evans 1994b; Evans 1995; Fox et al. 1988; Frackowiak et al. 1997; Friston et al. 1991, 1995; Greitz et al. 1991; Kosugi et al. 1993; Miller et al. 1993; Minoshima et al. 1992, 1994; Seitz et al. 1990). By transforming every person's images into the same spatial coordinates, one can compare data from different subjects, use intersubject image averaging procedures that reduce noise and thus increase S/N in statistical brain maps, and compare findings generated in different laboratories. The standard coordinate system is that provided by the atlas of Talairach and Tournoux (1988); coordinates are reported as the distance in millimeters to the left or right of midline (the x-axis), the distance anterior or posterior to a coronal plane through the anterior commissure (the y-axis), and the distance superior or inferior to a horizontal plane through the anterior and posterior commissures (the z-axis). (Earlier studies used coordinates from Talairach et al. 1967, the previous version of this atlas; since the y-axis was computed as the distance anterior or posterior to a coronal plane midway between the anterior and posterior commissures, one needs to add 12 mm to a formerly published y-axis coordinate to translate it into the currently used coordinate system.) Some image deformation methods are trilinear – adjusting each person's brain image for its orientation and its size in the x, y, and z dimensions but making no adjustments for variations in shape or the position of individual structures. These methods work surprisingly well in brain mapping studies, for they provide a precision of about 5–8 mm depending on the structure's location in the brain (i.e., more accurate for voxels closer to the reference landmarks, less accurate for voxels at the periphery of the image) and permit substantial improvements in S/N when brain maps are superimposed from different subjects (because the imprecision in anatomical standardization is compensated in part by partial volume averaging in the relatively low-resolution PET images) (Fox et al. 1988). Other methods rely on relatively crude nonlinear image deformation algorithms to make additional adjustments for brain shape – an issue that is particularly important to studies that attempt to characterize between-group differences in regional PET measurements. Researchers continue to develop and test nonlinear image deformation algorithms with even greater accuracy (Bookstein 1989; Collins et al. 1994b; Friston et al. 1995; Miller et al. 1993; Minoshima et al. 1994, 1995b; Yun 1996).

Statistical Comparisons

As illustrated in Figure 2, statistical procedures can improve the ability to detect and localize regions of the brain that participate in normal and abnormal behaviors. This section considers image subtraction, intersubject and within-subject image averaging, statistical tests, and the problem of multiple comparisons.

Perhaps the simplest comparison involves the subtraction of an image acquired during a baseline control state (e.g., the resting state without movement) from an image acquired in the same subject during a behavioral state of interest (e.g., a fist-clenching and -unclenching task) on a voxel-by-voxel basis (after the data are normalized for the variation in whole-brain measurements). The resulting subtraction image (Figure 2) consists of a large number of changes in regional blood flow, some of which may be state-dependent but most of which are random (i.e. noise). An individual subtraction image makes it possible to localize a large state-dependent change in regional blood flow within 1–2 mm despite the limited resolution of PET (Fox et al. 1986; Mintun et al. 1989); it also improves the ability to detect these changes. In comparison to the original images, one can see that the subtraction image improves our ability to detect state-dependent increases in regional CBF (e.g., a large increase in left sensorimotor cortex and smaller increases in the supplementary motor area and right cerebellar vermis). However, it is still difficult to distinguish subtle state-dependent changes from noise in a single subtraction image. Additional steps are needed to reduce the noise.

Subtraction images derived from data repeatedly acquired during the same experimental and control states in one or more subjects can be averaged together on a voxel-by-voxel basis to produce an image of mean changes in regional CBF (see Figure 2). This procedure leads to predictable reductions in noise (since random changes cancel each other out in a predictable relationship to the total number of PET counts), preservation in state-dependent changes (assuming that regions are consistently activated during the behavioral state and that the voxels are in the same spatial coordinate system), and thus an increase in S/N (Fox et al. 1988). In brain mapping studies, *inter*subject image averaging is commonly performed by transforming subtraction images from 6–12 subjects into the coordinates of Talairach's brain atlas and computing an image of mean changes in regional CBF (Fox et al. 1988; Frackowiak et al. 1997). In some cases, *intra*subject image averaging can utilize two or more subtraction images from the same subject to generate an image of mean changes in regional CBF. Although this procedure assumes that there is little psychophysiological habituation during repeated performance of the experimental or baseline conditions in the same subject, the image of mean increases in regional CBF (or a statistical map representing the same data) can be superimposed onto the subject's co-registered MRI with or without any transformation into standard spatial coordinates.

One can generate images of the mean change in regional CBF, yet statistical tests can further characterize these changes. In order to contrast mean differences in

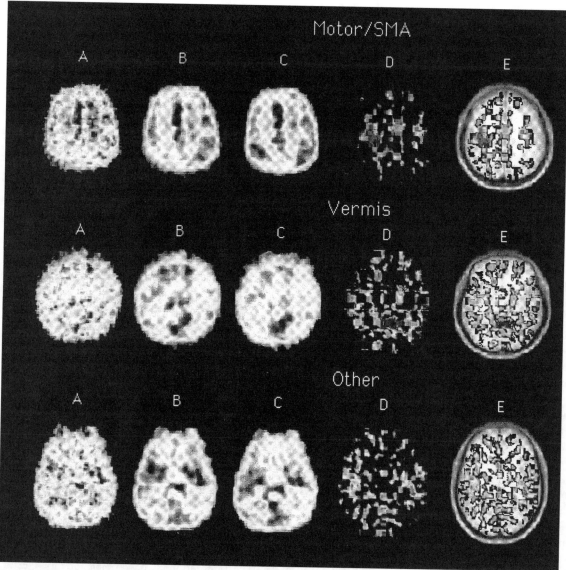

Figure 2. Image analysis techniques used to identify state-dependent changes in regional CBF. This figure illustrates how PET CBF images, image smoothing, image subtraction, PET–MRI co-registration, and intersubject image averaging improve the ability to detect and localize state-dependent changes in local neuronal activity. CBF images were normalized for the variation in whole brain measurements and warped into the same spatial coordinates. Each column shows three sections from a multislice, spatially standardized brain image. Top row: A section (Motor/SMA) containing (i) primary sensorimotor cortex (Motor), which participates in the execution of fist clenching, and (ii) the supplementary motor area (SMA), which participates in the planning and initiation of fist clenching. Middle row: A section containing the cerebellar vermis (Vermis), which participates in the coordination of fist clenching. Bottom row: A section containing none of the regions (Other) that actively participate in fist clenching. Column A: Sections from a high-resolution PET CBF image acquired in one subject during a baseline control state without fist clenching. The image is noisy and thus needs to be smoothed to improve image quality. Column B: Sections from the same baseline control CBF image smoothed to a lower spatial resolution. Noise in the image is greatly reduced. Column C: Sections from a smoothed CBF image acquired in the same subject as she repeatedly opened and closed her right hand. Note how difficult it is to detect and localize state-dependent changes in regional CBF in these blurry physiological images. Column D: A subtraction image, computed by subtracting the baseline image (column B) from the experimental image (column C) on a voxel-by-voxel basis. It is relatively easy to distinguish state-dependent CBF increases in the left sensorimotor cortex from noise. Indeed, it is possible to localize these large, discrete CBF changes within 1–2 mm. However, it is difficult to distinguish relatively subtle state-dependent CBF increases from noise, such as those in SMA and vermis. Column E: Subtraction image co-registered onto the subject's T1-weighted volumetric MRI. (The gray color scales were manually adjusted to help visualize the CBF increase in left motor cortex.) Co-registration makes it possible to localize anatomical regions of interest in the PET image and state-dependent changes in regional CBF (such as the cerebellar vermis) that are large enough to detect in a single subject. Column F: Statistical map of significant, state-dependent increases in regional CBF generated from CBF and co-registered MRI images in six subjects; $z > 2.58$, $P < 0.005$, uncorrected for multiple comparisons. Intersubject image averaging reduces noise (no longer visible in any of the sections) and improves the power to distinguish state-dependent changes in local neuronal activity (e.g., in SMA and vermis) from noise.

regional CBF on a voxel-by-voxel basis, researchers have commonly used *t*-score or *z*-score maps. Change distribution analysis, the original intersubject image averaging procedure, computes *z*-scores by characterizing the population of maximal mean changes in the image (i.e., the peaks and valleys) and comparing each mean change to the standard deviation of the population of mean changes (Fox et al. 1988). Another extensively used procedure computes *z*-scores using voxel-by-voxel information about the mean value in each set of images and a mean (or "pooled") variance computed from all of the voxels (Evans et al. 1992). Statistical parametric mapping (SPM), which is used in the largest number of laboratories, in its simplest application computes normalized *t*-score (i.e., *z*-score) maps using voxel-by-voxel information about the mean value and variance in each set of images (Frackowiak et al. 1997). It is important to recognize that not all *z*-score maps are alike: articles should specify the procedures used to normalize data for absolute measurements, the procedures used to deform data into standard spatial coordinates, and the procedures used to compute statistical maps.

The creators of SPM continue to update their methods; at the time of this writing, their latest version is SPM99. Statistical parametric mapping now permits a full application of the general linear model to the determinants of activity in each individual voxel. Thus, it readily permits the generation of maps of main effects and interactions (to examine the extent to which a CBF change in one comparison is significantly different from a CBF change in another comparison; Friston et al. 1996a) (Frackowiak et al. 1997), as well as the ability to examine or exclude the effects of covariates (e.g., age, a rating scale score, or a psychophysiological measurement). One can also use this approach to identify statistically significant asymmetries in activation (i.e., the extent to which a CBF change in one voxel is significantly different from a change in the homologous voxel in the opposite hemisphere).

In addition to parametric or nonparametric contrasts, it is possible to generate maps that relate PET measurements in one region to those in other regions. *Functional* connectivity refers to the simultaneous activation of two or more regions without specifying the cause or direction of this association, whereas *effective* connectivity examines the effect that a given region has on another given region using structural equation modeling and path analysis (Frackowiak et al. 1997; Friston et al. 1993a,b; McIntosh & Gonzalez-Lima 1994; McIntosh et al. 1994, 1996). This represents a considerable advance in the power of functional neuroimaging, as it begins to address the components and functional interactions within neural circuits that mediate specific functions.

Researchers like to test specific hypotheses, but they also like to explore findings throughout the brain. Since potentially significant findings could be identified in over 50,000 voxels, researchers must consider the statistical problem of multiple comparisons: as the number of comparisons increases, it becomes increasingly likely that one or more voxels will have statistical value greater than the critical value by chance alone (i.e., a type-I error). Before considering this issue, it is important to recognize that the multiple comparison problem is related to the number of independent comparisons. Owing to the smoothness (i.e., limited spatial resolution) of images, the analysis of a statistical map involves no more than several hundred independent resolution units or "resels" (Worsley et al. 1992), a concept now incorporated in some of the most sophisticated statistical methods used to address the problem of multiple comparisons (Frackowiak et al. 1997). But even this number overestimates the number of independent measurements owing to the extent to which data in different brain regions are functionally connected. For this reason, the optimal statistical approach for correcting multiple comparisons is not known – but it should maximize the trade-off between sensitivity to the detection of relatively subtle changes (a crucial issue, since brain mapping studies have limited statistical power) and the number of type-I errors (Frackowiak et al. 1997).

Procedures commonly used to correct for multiple comparisons include: those that depend on the magnitude (or intensity) of the maximal statistical value relative to the number of resels (or, less commonly, the number of identified "maxima") in the image (Evans et al. 1992; Fox et al. 1988; Worsley et al. 1992); those that depend on the spatial extent of voxels exceeding a particular statistical value (Friston et al. 1994); and those that depend on the combination of magnitude and spatial extent. See Frackowiak et al. (1997) for a detailed discussion of these issues and other image analysis strategies.

Another commonly used strategy is to use an empirically derived critical value (e.g., a *z*-score of 2.58 or 3.09; $p < 0.005$ or 0.001, uncorrected for multiple comparisons) to at least partially address the problem of type-I errors (Frackowiak et al. 1997; Reiman et al. 1997). In a study of relatively smooth PET images acquired in multiple subjects during well-characterized behavioral and control tasks, we found that a critical *z*-score of 2.58 yielded 0–1 type-I errors in the entire data set (much lower than expected if one does not consider the contribution of connectivity) and the best trade-off between type-I and type-II errors (Reiman et al. 1997). The extent to which this finding can be applied to higher-resolution PET or MRI data (in which one would expect more type-I errors), different sample sizes, and differences in the number of accumulated PET counts remains to be determined. Procedures less commonly used to address the problem of multiple comparisons include the gamma-2 statistic, an omnibus procedure empirically established to identify images that contain one or more significant changes in regional CBF in the population of local maxima (Fox et al. 1988) as well as a nonparametric procedure that uses permutation test theory to derive empirically a critical value in each data set (Holmes et al.

1996). The latter method might be especially well suited for studies involving a relatively small number of scans (e.g., those involving intrasubject image averaging) (Frackowiak et al. 1997). Perhaps the optimal way to address the multiple comparison problem is an independent replication of findings. Thus, an initial exploratory study could test hypotheses about alterations in specific brain regions and explore alterations in the rest of the brain. These additional alterations (i.e., the newly generated hypotheses) could be tested in a replication study.

When presenting data in a research article, one commonly includes a table listing the anatomical region, estimated Brodmann's areas, atlas coordinates, and statistical values for regions above a certain critical value. Figures commonly include entire brain maps together with: (a) multiple sections superimposed onto a single spatially standardized MRI, an average of spatially standardized MRIs acquired in all subjects, an average of spatially standardized MRIs from 305 subjects studied at the Montreal Neurological Institute (Evans et al. 1993), or a digitized brain atlas; (b) three-dimensional surface projection maps that project regional changes onto the medial and lateral surface of a spatially standardized brain MRI (Frackowiak et al. 1997; Minoshima et al. 1995b; Reiman et al. 1996); or (c) two-dimensional projection maps that project regional changes onto sagittal, coronal, and transverse sections (Frackowiak et al. 1997). Although brief reports commonly illustrate their findings using selected brain sections – and sometimes do so using their most convincing cases – these figures should not distract the reader from a careful inspection of the data. Since a failure to reject the null hypothesis does not prove that the alternative hypothesis is untrue, a "negative finding" does not rule out the possibility that the investigated region is not affected. For that reason, it is useful to report possibly significant findings even if one cannot rule out the possibility of type-I errors; the provisional nature of these exploratory findings should be emphasized in the discussion section.

DATA INTERPRETATION

When interpreting PET findings, it is important to consider the limitations of this imaging technique. Limitations in the spatial resolution of PET images, the contrast resolution of individual PET images, and the accuracy of the image deformation algorithm used to compute statistical maps all make it difficult to specify regions (e.g., specific thalamic nuclei) that are responsible for observed changes in regional brain measurements. Since increases in regional brain activity appear to reflect the activity of terminal neuronal fields (Schwartz et al. 1979) – including those from local interneuron and afferent projections arising in other sites – it is difficult to specify the neuronal projections that account for observed changes in regional activity. Although PET and other imaging techniques provide infor-

mation about the neuroanatomical correlates of emotion, lesion studies (including experimental lesions in laboratory animals, neurological patients with selective brain injuries, and perhaps the induction of temporary functional lesions in human subjects using transcranial magnetic stimulation) are required in order to determine whether the implicated regions are necessary or sufficient to produce the behavior of interest (e.g., an emotion) or its potentially dissectable components (e.g. experiential, expressive, and evaluative aspects of emotion). See Sarter et al. (1996) for a more extended discussion of this issue.

As previously noted, PET studies raise the possibility of type-I errors that merit confirmation in an independent data set. Even more problematic, failure to detect significant alterations in PET measurements (type-II errors) could reflect limitations in spatial resolution, statistical power, heterogeneity in the strategies used to perform a task, or a change in the pattern rather than the level of neuronal activity. It is also important not to overinterpret unilateral changes as being significantly lateralized, since a change in one hemisphere relative to that in the opposite hemisphere may not reach statistical significance; in order to identify lateralized changes, one needs to directly compare activity changes in one hemisphere to those in the other hemisphere on a regional or voxel-by-voxel basis. Similarly, one needs to directly compare voxel-by-voxel maps of state-dependent changes in regional brain activity to conclude that changes in one comparison are significantly greater than those in another comparison.

In studies that compare data from patients and controls, it is important to consider the possibility that observed differences are related to the pathophysiology of the disorder – for example, a genetic or learned predisposition to panic attacks in patients with panic disorder – or to differences in the subjects' behavioral state at the time of the study (e.g., anxiety, the attempt to refrain from compulsive rituals in patients with obsessive-compulsive disorder, eye movements, or differences in the performance of a behavioral task). One should also consider the possibility that observed differences in regional CBF or CMRgl are related to alterations in local neuronal activity, the density of glial cells or terminal neuronal fields that innervate a region, or the combined effects of atrophy and partial volume averaging. In some studies, additional procedures are required to address the combined and potentially confounding effects of partial volume averaging, carotid artery activity, and temporalis muscle activity on measurements in the anterior temporal lobe (Chen et al. 1996; Reiman 1997). Finally, it is important to consider other experimental confounds that could account for the observed findings.

RISKS TO HUMAN SUBJECTS

An important consideration in the performance of PET studies is the risk to human subjects. The usual risks to subjects who participate in PET studies can be attributed to radiation exposure and vascular catheterization.

Positron emitting radiotracers produce low-level, low–linear energy transfer (LET) radiation that consists of positrons and gamma rays. For appropriate diagnostic indications, the clinical benefit of PET studies typically exceeds the small risks of radiation exposure. For research studies, laboratories have relatively strict guidelines about the maximal radiation dose that a research volunteer can receive in a single scanning session or year. The dose depends on the radiation exposure of different radiotracers to individual organs and the whole body. The maximal radiation dose to a research subject must be lower than the limits established by the Food and Drug Administration (United States Code of Federal Regulations) and lower than an "effective dose equivalent" (computed from estimates of the radiation exposure to different organs and the susceptibility of each organ to radiation-induced cancer) of 50 millisieverts (5 rem). The limit for volunteers under 18 years of age is one tenth of this amount, severely restricting scientific PET studies of children unless the procedure has a clinical benefit. (Even if one could study children with a psychiatric disorder for strictly scientific purposes, it would be difficult to justify the study of control subjects.)

Exposure to very low-level, low-LET radiation exposure in PET studies and other radiological procedures may be associated with a small risk of leukemia and cancer of solid organs later in life. However, the risk is too small to measure directly, extrapolations from the study of Japanese atomic bomb survivors continue to be debated, and it remains unknown whether there is a threshold below which radiation is associated with no adverse effects (ICRP 1991; NRCC 1990). In our laboratory, we give research volunteers information about the risk of radiation-induced cancer and attempt to relate crude estimates of this risk to other everyday risks, such as smoking a carton of cigarettes in one's lifetime and exposure to the air pollution in a large city for one year (Brill et al. 1982). For a comparable number of scans, the risk of radiation exposure can be reduced by a factor of three using 3D imaging (Cherry et al. 1993).

Experts have studied additional risks of low-level LET radiation. The risk to the developing embryo (ICRP 1991; NRCC 1990) makes it necessary to exclude pregnant women from participating in PET studies. The risk of genetic abnormalities in subsequent generations due to irradiation of germ cells appears to be extremely small (ICRP 1991). Finally, the risks of infertility, aging, cataract formation, skin or blood changes, and radiation sickness require much higher levels of radiation exposure than is received in PET studies (NRCC 1990).

Most PET studies require venous catheterization for the purpose of radiotracer administration. This procedure is associated with only transient discomfort. Many quantitative PET studies also require arterial catheterization and blood sampling, typically through the radial artery, in an effort to estimate the rate of radiotracer transport to the brain. Arterial catheterization typically causes transient discomfort and sometimes causes an uncomfortable bruise. If an Allen's test is performed to assure collateral circulation to the hand through the ulnar artery, the risk of developing inadequate circulation to the hand almost never occurs in healthy subjects. Unless there is an interest in characterizing alterations in whole-brain CBF, arterial catheterization is usually not performed in ^{15}O-water studies.

EXPENSE AND AVAILABILITY

Another consideration in the performance of PET studies is their considerable expense. Installing a cyclotron, radiochemistry facility, and imaging system can cost from $3–$6 million (though the cost can be reduced using less expensive accelerators or centrally located radiotracer distribution facilities). In addition, the major PET centers rely on numerous personnel (e.g., radiochemists or radiopharmacists, physicists or engineers, nuclear medicine technologists, computer scientists, physiologists and biomathematicians, physicians, and researchers from related fields); the operating budget is commonly $1–$2 million per year. The break-even cost of each PET procedure is estimated to be between $615 and $2,780, depending on procedure volume (Evens et al. 1983); the typical procedural cost of a PET session is about $1,500 to $2,000.

A Comparison of Functional MRI and PET

In this section we compare fMRI and PET across a variety of domains. This comparison is based on the foregoing discussion of PET and a detailed review of fMRI methods in Chapter 36 of this volume. There are three types of fMRI imaging, which use blood flow, blood volume and blood oxygenation level–dependent (BOLD) signals. The BOLD signal has the highest functional contrast and is the most commonly used method for fMRI imaging. Therefore, the comparison of PET and fMRI will focus on BOLD imaging unless otherwise noted. This comparison addresses physical and technical issues, experimental design, artifact, ancillary measures during scanning, scanning environment, and accessibility issues; see Table 2 for a summary. Wherever possible, basic principles will be illustrated with examples drawn from the literature on functional neuroimaging of emotional states.

PHYSICAL AND TECHNICAL CONSIDERATIONS

Functional MRI has the distinct advantage of no radiation. There is no known limit to the number of times someone can be studied safely. By contrast, PET involves a significant amount of radiation that is a function of the

TABLE 2. Comparison of PET and BOLD fMRI

	BOLD fMRI	PET
Physical/Technical		
Radiation	None	++
Spatial resolution	3 mm	3 mm and 8–15 mm
Temporal resolution	From 4–8 sec to 200 msec	30 sec
Technical complexity	+	+
Whole-brain coverage	Some areas difficult to image	+
Origin of signal	Partially understood	Well understood
Quantifiability of signal	Percent change in signal	Relative and absolute CBF
Neurotransmitter release	Not possible	+
Experimental Design		
State-related	+	+
Event-related	+	Not possible
Repeat studies	++ (in theory)	Possible (dose limited)
Single-subject studies	+ (common)	Possible but rarely done
Artifact		
Motion sensitivity	Extreme	Readily controlled
Spatially dependent hemodynamic response fx	A problem with high spatial resolution	Not a problem
ECG	Can be removed	None
Respiration	Can be removed	None
Large vessel	Can be removed	Can be removed
Temporalis muscle	Not a problem	Can be removed
Other Measures during Scans		
EEG/ERP	Interleave between scans	+
EOG	Interleave between scans	+
EMG	Interleave between scans	+
ECG	+	+
Skin conductance	+	+
Startle	Any movement an issue	More feasible
Scan Environment		
Noise	Constant across conditions	No problem
Claustrophobia	5%–10% of subjects	No problem
Visual presentation	Some restrictions (size, resolution)	Fewer limitations
Accessibility of subject	Limited during scanning run	Readily accessible between scans
Verbal ratings	Any movement an issue	No problem between scans
Miscellaneous		
Number of centers (worldwide)	100–200 (1000s)	20–30 (300 cameras total)
Cost per subject	$500	$2,000
Amount of data to process	Major issue	Minor issue

Key: + denotes that this factor is present or feasible; ++ denotes that this factor is highly relevant or significant.

total dose of radiotracer and its nature. The risks associated with radiation exposure during PET imaging have just been described. Typically, subjects can participate in only one PET study per year.

Spatial resolution is superior with fMRI. Although spatial resolution of fMRI is a complex topic and varies as a function of imaging parameters, a useful estimate is that spatial resolution with conventional 1.5-Tesla systems is approximately 3 mm. Higher-strength magnets may increase spatial resolution down to 1 mm. As discussed previously, there is an inherent theoretical limit in the spatial resolution of PET, on the order of about 3 mm. In recent studies, the effective resolution of PET is on the order of 8–15 mm when standard image processing procedures (such as spatial normalization and a smoothing filter) are utilized.

Temporal resolution is also superior with fMRI. As indicated in Table 3, temporal resolution varies depending on how the functional neuroimaging data are being used. With any brain imaging technique, there is an inherent limit of temporal resolution that is a function of

TABLE 3. Time Resolution of fMRI

Maximum on–off switching rate	16 sec optional 4–8 sec possible
Minimum detectable stimulus duration	~30 msec
Minimum detectable difference in activation duration	100 msec
Minimum detectable stimulus interval in a single region	1 sec
Minimum detectable stimulus interval across separate brain regions	200 msec
Minimum time to create a functional (whole-brain) image	5 sec
Maximum image acquisition rate	20–40 frames/sec

hemodynamic response. Whereas the peak blood flow response occurs 6–9 sec after stimulus onset, the complete response and recovery lasts about 16 sec. It is possible to detect a "new" response 4–8 sec after the first stimulus. However, within that context there are several other time intervals of interest to researchers.

For example, a stimulus duration as brief as 30 msec can be detected with fMRI, and the minimum detectable difference in duration of regional brain activation is 100 msec. A stimulus interval as brief as 1 sec can be detected in a single region, but across two regions the minimum detectable stimulus interval is 200 msec. The minimum time to create a whole brain image is 5 sec, and the maximum image acquisition rate is 20–40 frames (or images) per second. By contrast, the temporal resolution of PET images in routine applications is about 30 sec (corresponding to the period of maximum signal acquisition). In theory, one could systematically vary stimulus duration across PET imaging conditions, thereby generating subtraction images corresponding to a stimulus duration difference. However, it is probably preferable to pursue research questions related to these temporal characteristics with fMRI because of its greater availability, lesser expense, and absence of radiation exposure.

PET and fMRI are comparable in technical complexity. Both require a physicist to design the image acquisition, an expert technologist to run the scanning system, and a statistical consultant to assist in the data analysis. Depending on the experimental design, technical assistance may be required for stimulus presentation or psychophysiological data collection in an fMRI context. PET may also require a radiochemist for radiotracer synthesis, although automated systems for generating radiotracers such as ^{15}O are now available.

There are no limits to the areas of the brain that can be imaged with PET. However, some of the older PET systems have an axial field of view of about 10 cm, which means that either the very top or very bottom of the brain is not included in the image. This typically does not

influence the outcome of the study. By contrast, specific regions are more difficult to image using fMRI owing to the differences in magnetic susceptibility across tissues or between tissue and air. Magnetic field inhomogeneities are created at these interfaces, causing signal dropout and/or image distortion. For example, orbitofrontal cortex can be difficult to image because of its proximity to the nasal sinuses. Specific solutions to these problems come with some expense in S/N, sensitivity, imaging time, or whole-volume imaging capability.

The signal measured with PET is a function of blood flow and is therefore very well understood. The area of blood flow increase is greater than the area of neural activation (the analogy of "watering the entire garden for the sake of one thirsty flower" is useful as a first approximation), but the lower spatial resolution of PET makes this irrelevant for all practical purposes.

By contrast, the BOLD signal results from a combination of blood flow changes, blood volume changes, and oxygen consumption (Boxerman et al. 1995; Buxton, Wong, & Frank 1997; Davis 1998; Frahm et al. 1996; Kim & Ugurbil 1997). The inherent physiological meaning of what is detected with BOLD fMRI is not fully understood (i.e., additional details regarding coupling between flow, volume, and metabolic rate during activation are still needed; see Mandeville 1998). Furthermore, it is not known whether the BOLD signal arises from venules or capillaries (Bandettini & Wong 1997), a distinction that can influence the interpretation of findings. Thus, the greater spatial resolution of fMRI raises questions not encountered in PET. These questions must be answered if the technical advantages of fMRI are to be fully exploited.

With PET one can obtain a resting image and compare resting images between subjects; the value obtained in the resting state is relative to a preset normalized mean for all subjects to which all blood flow values are statistically adjusted. In BOLD fMRI what is measured is a percentage change in signal in one condition relative to another. Such relative changes are very useful in a PET context as well, but with PET (as well as with arterial spin labeling–based or blood volume–based fMRI – Detre et al. 1992; Edelman, Siewert, & Darby 1994; Kim 1995; Kwong et al. 1995; Wong, Buxton, & Frank 1996, 1997) there is the option of comparing one condition across subjects. The reason for this difference between PET and BOLD fMRI is that the BOLD fMRI signal contains structural as well as functional information (more of the former than the latter), leading to greater variability between subjects. In contrast, PET provides purely functional information; when that information is placed in a standardized spatial template, the contribution of structural information is minimized and essentially eliminated when the smoothing filter is applied.

Another advantage of PET is that the signal can be absolutely quantified, as described previously. Absolute quantification is not possible with BOLD fMRI (but is possible with arterial spin labeling fMRI and with blood volume fMRI). It should be noted that several groups are now attempting to quantify BOLD contrast using the physiological stressor of hypercapnia.

This capacity for absolute quantification is particularly useful when using PET for neurochemical measurements. One can examine the binding of a radiotracer to a receptor in competition with an endogenous ligand. This provides an indirect measure of the binding of endogenous ligand. These methods can be used to quantify the number of receptors as well as the amount of released endogenous neurotransmitter. Such direct neurochemical measurements cannot be performed with fMRI. However, one can combine neurochemical manipulations – for example, fenfluramine injection versus placebo (Meyer et al. 1996) or apomorphine versus placebo (Dolan et al. 1995) – with indices of activation using ^{15}O or BOLD measurements to determine where changes in regional activation occur in association with such neurochemical changes.

EXPERIMENTAL DESIGN

It is customary in PET and fMRI studies to present stimuli in blocks (e.g., a series of pictures evoking emotional responses of a particular type), which can be compared with a baseline condition (Chertkow & Bub 1994). By contrast, a great advantage of fMRI for psychophysiological studies is the recently developed capacity to study event-related phenomena. The first studies of event-related fMRI have begun to appear in the literature (e.g. Büchel et al. 1998; see also Chapter 36 for a comprehensive list). For example, one could present a mixture of pleasant, unpleasant, and neutral pictures in a scanning block. With event-related analysis techniques it is possible to pick out the neural activation patterns associated with each individual stimulus and then average across events of a particular type. One could also examine whether the neural activation pattern differs as a function of whether it follows one particular valence condition as compared with another. This method also makes it possible to detect neural events whose time course may be too brief to be detected in the 30-sec scanning window associated with PET. For example, the activation pattern associated with a pinprick has been reported with fMRI but could not be detected with PET because of its lower temporal resolution (Tanaka et al. 1998).

In theory, another major advantage of fMRI is the capacity to perform repeat studies (Karni et al. 1993; Zarahn, Aguirre, & D'Esposito 1997). This option is not available in PET studies owing to annual limits in permissible radiation exposure – unless one modifies the number of scans and radiation dose so that the total exposure across repeat studies does not exceed that of a single study. In practice, it has been difficult to replicate results across or even

within fMRI sessions by comparing identical conditions at the beginning and the end. The reasons for such "session effects" are not fully understood. Most likely explanations involve motion artifact, problems in co-registration of images, changes in physiological state of the subject (e.g. fatigue), or habituation effects. Once this problem is solved it will significantly extend the range of questions that can be addressed with fMRI.

Single-subject studies are rarely performed with ^{15}O PET because the signal-to-noise ratio is relatively low, which is why intersubject image averaging is used to enhance it. One advantage of the latter is that it involves statistically analyzing the data from all of the subjects in the study, thus avoiding bias through the selective presentation of data. Single-case studies with FDG PET are common and are used clinically.

Single-case studies with fMRI are common and often yield results that are highly statistically significant. In fact, the reader of the fMRI literature should be aware that – when results are combined across subjects – spatial resolution is decreased because data are fit into normalized space and a smoothing filter is applied. Therefore, data will often be presented in the form of single cases with the statement that "similar results were obtained in other subjects." The reader should pay particular attention to whether the coordinates of the activations in other subjects are reported and, if so, whether they are consistent with the conclusion that the same region is activated in each subject. One way of ensuring that activity in the same location is being reported is to use a region-of-interest approach. In that case, the question becomes the degree to which the entire pattern of activity is similar across subjects.

ARTIFACTS

The PET signal (gamma rays) emanating from a point in the brain does not change when the head moves, but the scanner will falsely attribute that signal to another location in the image because the template used to create the image does not move. It is therefore important to place the head in exactly the same position prior to each scan as well as to control head movement during each scan. Just prior to each scan, the head can be positioned in the scanner in exactly the same location by precisely positioning landmarks on the subject's face with laser beams (located in the gantry of the scanner for this specific purpose). Various types of headholders are available to restrict movement during and between scans. After PET data are acquired, algorithms are applied to align the scans within each subject to one another. This typically leads to adjustments of only a few millimeters in any direction, particularly if care has been taken by the researcher to restrict motion during image acquisition. Application of attenuation correction algorithms is dependent upon adequate restriction of motion. In sum, motion can be adequately controlled with PET if properly attended to.

By contrast, motion artifact is a major issue in fMRI research. With the significantly greater spatial resolution of fMRI, moving the head less than 1 mm during the course of image acquisition heightens the need for precise co-registration of images. More importantly, the fMRI signal results from an interaction between exogenously applied magnetic gradients and the magnetic properties of the tissues in the head. In fMRI, head movement changes the signal emanating from any given locus in the brain and also (as with PET) creates a mismatch between the true locus of the altered signal and the location of that signal in the image. Therefore, considerable attention is given to minimizing head movement during fMRI image acquisition, including limiting the duration of scanning sessions. If one were content to adjust fMRI data through smoothing (or by other means, such as adjustment of voxel size to a spatial resolution comparable to that of PET) then motion artifact would be less of an issue.

Another source of movement artifact is physiological motion. Assuming the skull is stationary, the brain moves several millimeters with each cardiac and respiratory cycle, a source of motion artifact that can measured. Just as event-related changes can be quantified and positively identified, motion of the brain associated with the cardiac and respiratory cycles can be modeled in this context and removed during the data processing step.

It is typically assumed that neural activation in all areas of the brain leads to the same absolute blood flow response (i.e., that the hemodynamic response is spatially independent). This may or may not be the case; the area is currently under investigation. This is an issue with high–spatial resolution fMRI, as a given percentage change in signal could mean different things in different regions.

The aforementioned artifacts are issues for fMRI because of its high spatial resolution. There are sources of artifact that are relevant for PET because of its relative spatial imprecision – for example, large vessel artifact and temporalis muscle artifact. Both are correctable if properly attended to. The latter is not a problem with fMRI because of its high spatial resolution, but large vessel artifacts do exist with fMRI.

The internal carotid artery passes near to the midbrain and just medial to the medial temporal lobe. Under certain conditions (such as emotional arousal), cardiac output may increase in a state-dependent manner. This can lead to a greater concentration of radiotracer in the internal carotid arteries shortly after injection of the radiotracer (during the first 30 sec, when signal acquisition is at its maximum) relative to the control conditions. Because of partial volume averaging (adjacent voxels contribute to the blood flow value measured at any given voxel), greater blood flow may appear to be present in specific brain areas (e.g. hippocampus or amygdala) owing to greater activity in the internal carotid arteries. Although each PET image is typically corrected for global blood flow, this correction applies to the accumulated activity in the entire brain for the entire scan and may not eliminate this regionally specific increase. A procedure for eliminating large vessel artifact from PET images, developed by Chen and colleagues (1996), consists of identifying the pattern associated with activity in the internal carotid arteries in a separate study and subtracting this activity from the blood flow pattern of interest. Although conservative, if the medial temporal activation persists after this subtraction then it cannot be due to this artifact. In fMRI, special procedures are currently being evaluated and tested for restricting signal changes to capillary effects and for identifying and eliminating the contributions to signal change of large collecting veins or arteries.

During certain types of emotional arousal (e.g., anticipatory anxiety), subjects may clench their teeth, which leads to increased activity in the temporalis muscle. The latter lies only a few millimeters from the temporal pole, a structure that has been activated in several emotion studies. Since ^{15}O-water travels through the entire bloodstream, any structure that requires increased blood flow to meet its metabolic demands will receive an incremental increase in radiotracer delivery in proportion to the blood flow increase. Because of partial volume averaging, an increase in temporalis muscle activity could be misattributed to activity in the temporal pole. A procedure similar to that just described for internal carotid artery activity has been used to eliminate blood flow due to temporalis muscle activity (Reiman et al. 1997). Other procedures to correct this artifact include co-registration of PET and structural MRI data as well as measurement of temporalis EMG (electromyographic) activity and statistical elimination of this activity from the PET image in a covariance analysis.

OTHER MEASURES DURING SCANS

The psychophysiological measurements acquired during functional neuroimaging can add extremely useful information that can aid considerably in the interpretation of brain imaging data and add another dimension of physiological information. In the context of emotion research, for example, skin conductance and facial EMG data can be used to validate the success of the valence and arousal conditions being studied. When combined with quantitative EEG (electroencephalogram) data, PET or fMRI data can aid considerably in dipole localization.

An advantage of PET is that psychophysiological measures can be obtained without difficulty. In contrast, fMRI and psychophysiological data acquisition can interfere with one another. Special techniques are under development to deal with these issues, but it is important to emphasize that psychophysiological data collection in the context of fMRI is much more technically challenging.

Metal of any kind is dangerous in the MRI environment, since the strong magnetic fields can turn any metal object into a flying missile. Metal (e.g. electrodes) on the body surface can heat up and burn the subject. Furthermore, the presence of metal anywhere in the vicinity of the object being scanned can severely distort the MRI signal. This is particularly true for EEG or facial EMG electrodes. Thus, nonferromagnetic electrodes made of tin or graphite are being developed for psychophysiological data collection during fMRI scanning.

A magnetic field change will induce current in a wire. The rapidly changing magnetic gradients associated with fMRI induce currents in traditional copper wires that will appear as noise in the psychophysiological tracing. This source of noise can be filtered out of low-frequency signals such as ECG (electrocardiogram) or respiration. However, with EEG the frequency range of the signal overlaps with that of the changing magnetic gradients. Therefore, low- or high-pass filters will not eliminate the electrical artifacts. One solution is to record artifact-free EEG during the interval between each scan (typically about 1 sec, but this interval between scans can be extended if needed). Another option is to use a nonmetallic conducting medium for the electrical signals.

Recording skin conductance from the plantar surface of the foot has been explored to maximize the distance of the electrodes from the head coil. These skin conductance recordings were found to be inadequate because of the paucity of sweat glands in the foot. It has subsequently been observed in preliminary studies that electrodes on the palmar surface of the hand do not distort the functional neuroimaging signals and are the optimal location for skin conductance recordings (Margaret Bradley, personal communication).

The startle probe causes movement and is therefore to be avoided in the fMRI environment. However, the startle probe could be administered in the context of PET, which is relatively insensitive to tiny movements. To our knowledge, this has not yet been done.

SCAN ENVIRONMENT

The changing magnetic gradients create a loud noise, which requires that the subject use earplugs. The consistency of this auditory stimulus across all scanning conditions minimizes its effect on experimental results. New strategies are being developed that are based on image acquisition grouping and temporal spacing to minimize the interaction of the hemodynamics induced by scanner noise and the hemodynamics induced by the task. By contrast, auditory noise is not a significant consideration in PET experiments.

It is common in PET studies to converse with and obtain verbal ratings from the subject between scans, but manual rather than verbal responses *during* scans are preferred in order to avoid the head movement associated with speaking. During fMRI scanning, auditory noise interferes with (but does not prevent) verbal communication between subject and experimenter. Verbal communication by the subject during fMRI scanning is undesirable because the flow of air through the nose and mouth alters magnetic susceptibility of the nasopharynx and therefore the ability to image neighboring brain structures. Although a brief motion associated with speaking causes an immediate motion artifact, the induced hemodynamic change takes 5 sec or so. Therefore, one advantage of fMRI is its potential to decouple the motion artifact from the induced hemodynamic effect.

Approximately 5%–10% of subjects cannot undergo MRI scanning because of claustrophobia associated with being surrounded by the head coil and scanner. Although this could create a bias in the sample, it is typically not considered a significant issue.

Other aspects of the scanning environment are worth noting. With the head surrounded by the head coil, routine viewing of a computer or television monitor (as in PET) is not possible. Alternatives in fMRI include back-projection of images (onto a screen located at the foot of the scanning bed) that can be viewed with mirrors by the subject in the supine position. An alternative approach involves goggles through which the visual stimuli are presented. These systems are expensive but have resolution characteristics comparable to a computer monitor.

ACCESSIBILITY

A distinct advantage of fMRI is its greater accessibility relative to PET. At present there are only about 300 PET cameras in the world, and it is estimated that there are only about 20–30 PET centers publishing functional neuroimaging research. The number of PET centers could increase owing to the clinical utility of PET in detecting metastases (Silverman et al. 1998) and myocardial ischemia (Schwaiger 1995) and in differentiating brain tumors from radiation necrosis (Conti 1995), but the multimillion-dollar investment required means that this technology is likely to be available only in major medical or research centers. In addition to the capital investment required to establish a PET center, the cost per subject is approximately four times higher with PET than with fMRI ($2,000 vs. $500).

By contrast, there are probably thousands of MRI machines in medical centers around the world, and the cost of upgrading structural MRI systems for functional neuroimaging is "only" in the hundreds of thousands of dollars. At present there are about 100–200 U.S. centers conducting fMRI research. There are many more fMRI than PET investigators, which is likely to facilitate the development of solutions to the numerous technical challenges described here.

One factor that makes fMRI slightly less accessible is the computer resources needed to support it. The amount of data generated in scanning one fMRI subject is about one order of magnitude greater than with PET (gigabytes vs. hundreds of megabytes). The requirements for fMRI data transfer, data analysis, and data storage are considerable, whereas the quantity of data constitutes a relatively minor issue in PET research.

Functional Imaging Studies of Cognition

In this section we apply the principles discussed previously to research on cognition. The methodological issues that have been raised are carried a step further by illustrating how the advantages and disadvantages of PET and fMRI influence experimental design and thus the generation of new knowledge.

BETWEEN-SUBJECT VERSUS WITHIN-SUBJECT DESIGNS

Within-subject experimental designs compare among conditions, all of which are administered to a homogeneous group of participants. Between-subject designs include groups of participants that differ in the experimental conditions they partake of (e.g., different stimulus conditions, different pharmacological treatments) or in some stable pre-existing characteristic (e.g., age, gender). In functional imaging research, between-subject designs are most often used to investigate the brain regions and/or processes impaired in a clinically defined group relative to some control group. PET scans of regional cerebral glucose metabolism with the FDG tracer can reveal hypometabolism extending beyond the locus of a lesion visible in structural images or postmortem observations (Baron 1989; Szelies et al. 1991). Hypometabolism may arise because a lesion has deprived an area of some of its normal input or damaged one of its efferent targets, or because the disease process itself produces cellular damage or dysfunction short of cell death. Reduced function in these brain areas may contribute as much to an observed cognitive deficit as frank damage observable in structural images, so that correlations between regions of hypometabolism and cognitive performance are part of the neuropsychological strategy of understanding brain function by characterizing its dysfunctions.

Paller and colleagues (1997) exploited this capability to explore the similarity of the neural circuitry underlying two amnesic syndromes: (i) those following localized damage to the medial temporal lobe; and (ii) Korsakoff's syndrome, in which the primary structural damage appears to be localized to the diencephalon. Compared with alcoholic subjects without a memory impairment, the Korsakoff's subjects displayed reduced glucose metabolism in widespread areas of the frontal and parietal lobes. Surprisingly,

however, the Korsakoff's patients did not differ from controls in medial temporal glucose metabolism. These results thus failed to support the idea that the memory impairments of Korsakoff's and medial temporal lobe amnesia share a common anatomical locus; instead they suggest that disrupted thalamocortical interactions can also impair learning.

The Korsakoff's study of Paller and colleagues is fairly typical of PET studies in patient populations in its use of FDG as the radiotracer. Because FDG scans readily allow the quantification of single-subject data, they are well suited for detecting regional differences in resting metabolism between individuals. However, such differences may be accentuated by administering a "behavioral challenge" prior to the scan, during the uptake period for the radioisotope. For instance, most studies comparing Alzheimer's patients to normal controls have yielded good discrimination between groups when participants rested quietly prior to the scan yet perhaps even clearer separation when a cognitive task has been adminstered during the uptake period (Kessler et al. 1991; Miller et al. 1987; see also Duara et al. 1992).

The disadvantages of glucose metabolism measurements with FDG are that the maximum safe dosage of this isotope allows only one or two scans per subject and that its long half-life makes it most sensitive to brain activity that persists for some 45 min. These qualities make FDG scans a bad match for experimental designs that either require more than two conditions or involve cognitive activities that are difficult to sustain for long periods of time. Most studies of normal cognition have thus utilized the ^{15}O radioisotope, a measure of blood flow rather than glucose metabolism. Use of a ^{15}O tracer allows a larger number of shorter-duration scans within the same subject, up to twelve 40–60-sec scans. Even if an experimental design includes fewer than twelve distinct conditions, this larger number of scans allows each condition to reoccur at different times during the session so that one can avoid confounding experimental effects with practice or fatigue effects. The primary drawback of ^{15}O scans is a lower S/N, which precludes easy analysis of single-subject data. Instead, the most typical method of analysis collapses across subjects to discover regional differences between conditions. Anatomical variability between subjects will thus decrease the spatial precision of measurements and make it difficult to distinguish between adjacent brain structures. Another important difference between the two radioisotopes is in the timing of any experimental task that the subjects perform. For blood flow measures, the task and data collection are coincident; this constrains possible tasks to those that can be performed lying supine and without head movement. Measures of glucose metabolism impose fewer constraints on the selection of a behavioral challenge because the critical time frame occurs before the scanning.

The PET literature to date has been marked by a strong correlation between the choices of (1) radioisotope, (2) between- versus within-subject designs, and (3) normal versus disordered populations. For example, most comparisons between normal and clinically defined groups use long-duration FDG scans, whereas most studies of the normal population use within-subject designs and shorter-duration ^{15}O scans. But these are only the most typical cases; the procedures for any given experiment should be selected according to the goals of the study. Within-subject measures of glucose metabolism have been applied to questions about skill acquisition in normal subjects by comparing a scan conducted after initial performance to one conducted after well-practiced performance (Haier et al. 1992). Conversely, cerebral blood flow measurements have been used to compare normal and dyslexic readers (Rumsey et al. 1997); the multifaceted nature of reading calls for designs with more than two conditions and is thus more amenable to ^{15}O than FDG scans.

In contrast to ^{15}O PET, the signal-to-noise ratio in functional magnetic resonance imaging using the BOLD method is high enough that single-subject data can be examined and statistically analyzed. It is a strength of this methodology that the contribution of intersubject anatomical variability will not reduce the spatial resolution of data from individual subjects. Of course, the observation of a significant relationship between an experimental condition and a brain region in one subject does not guarantee that the relationship will generalize to the population. It may be useful to consider an analogy between fMRI and event-related potential (ERP) data, given that the impact of an experimental manipulation can also be easily visualized in ERP data from a single subject (see Chapter 3 of this volume). In theory, the voltage at each of the time points in two ERP waveforms obtained from the same subject could be compared with each other to indicate which time points are significantly influenced by the experimental manipulation, where the sample size is equal to the number of time points (N = [epoch length in seconds] × [sampling rate in Hertz]). In practice, however, ERP researchers typically measure voltage at the same time points in each subject and condition and use analyses in which sample size is equal to the number of subjects.[1] A statistically significant experimental effect is thus one that occurs in most of the subjects tested. In most cognitive ERP studies, variability in the timing of an experimental effect across subjects has not been a major stumbling block to a multisubject analysis or to comparisons between groups of subjects (see e.g. Iragui, Kutas, & Salmon 1996; Neville et al. 1993; Van Petten et al. 1997). Given that experimental effects in cognitive paradigms usually persist for at least 100 msec, voltage is typically measured not at a single time point but as an average across contiguous time points in a latency window based on prior results, or by inspection of a grand average of all the subjects. Although the latency window selected

for analysis may not correspond to the exact onset and offset of an experimental effect for any given subject, this measurement strategy evaluates the commonality across subjects by quantifying the same time frame in each individual. For fMRI data sets, it is less trivial to decide what counts as measuring the same thing across individual subjects. A cortical region can be defined by its (1) location relative to standard brain landmarks (e.g., the location of the anterior and posterior commissures in the coordinate system of Talairach & Tournoux 1988), (2) location relative to the gyral/sulcal patterns of an individual's cortex, (3) response to a standard stimulus that is not part of the experimental paradigm, or (4) response to the experimental stimuli.

The fMRI methods used for analyzing data from multiple subjects are still in a state of development, so that variants of each of these strategies can be found in the literature. Büchel, Turner, and Friston (1997) performed a spatial normalization on the structural MR images of each subject's brain to align them with the brain in Talairach's atlas, formed a grand average of the aligned functional images, and contrasted the activity of each voxel during visual stimulation versus rest. The spatial normalization procedure was successful in that activity of the lateral geniculate nucleus apparent in each individual subject was also apparent, and statistically significant, in the average across subjects. It will be of some interest to see if this procedure is equally successful in cognitive paradigms where the regions of greatest interest are in cortical association areas, which may show greater individual variability (Clark & Plante 1998). In a comparison of sentences to meaningless consonant strings, Bavelier and colleagues (1997, p. 668) report that "while the foci of activation fell within the same broad anatomical areas for all subjects, there was a large variability in the exact distribution of the activation within a given anatomical area across subjects." These investigators assessed the similarity of results across subjects by first dividing each brain into 62 regions (based on each individual's sulcal anatomy, apparent in structural MR images) and then measuring the percentage of voxels differentially active between conditions and the percentage of oxygenation change in those active voxels for each subject and region. This strategy for dealing with intersubject anatomical variability seems a reasonable one, but its effectiveness depends both on the extent to which cortical function follows sulcal boundaries and on the size of functionally specialized cortical areas, two parameters that are largely unknown for most of the human cortex.

For some parts of the human brain – most notably, visual cortex – functional neuroimaging data and prior knowledge of monkey neuroanatomy have converged to yield good descriptions of the location and function of single cortical areas (Tootel et al. 1996). Demb and colleagues applied this knowledge to the long-standing but controversial issue of whether or not developmental dyslexia involves a visual deficit. Given that the general location and stimulus preferences of primary visual cortex and area MT+ were known, these investigators used standard stimulus sequences to define the borders of both areas in each individual subject before proceeding to the main experimental paradigm (Demb, Boynton, & Heeger 1997). The central comparisons between the normal and dyslexic groups could thus be made with some degree of confidence that the same functionally defined cortical area had been measured in each subject. Because they had a strong a priori hypothesis about dyslexia and visual motion processing, Demb and colleagues were able to capitalize on existing anatomical data to produce a priori definitions of the regions of interest.

As the functional imaging database expands, more experiments should approach the ideal case of using prior results to make specific anatomical predictions about a new task or population. At present, a more typical situation is one in which the regions of interest are only weakly constrained by prior neuropsychological data or are essentially unknown. For example, neurologists and neuropsychologists over the last century have inconsistently defined "Wernicke's area" to include various parts of the left middle and superior temporal gyri, superior temporal sulcus, and even the angular and supramarginal gyri (Bogen & Bogen 1976), so that current investigators have some justification for making similar broad cuts when evaluating whether or not individual subjects show activations in the "same" region. We can hope, though, that the improvement in spatial localization offered by imaging over natural lesions will similarly sharpen our characterization of structure–function relationships.

TASK VERSUS ITEM MANIPULATIONS

Cognitive experimental designs can be broadly divided into (a) those that vary the task a subject performs on relatively similar subsets of stimuli versus (b) those that vary stimulus parameters within a single assigned task. Both experimental strategies have played important roles in the oldest method of cognitive neuroscience – neuropsychology. In studies of brain-damaged patients, dissociations between tasks have often played a pivotal role in the interpretation of structure–function relationships. For instance, the finding that anterior aphasics with "agrammatic" production and comprehension could nonetheless distinguish grammatical from ungrammatical sentences in a simple good–bad task forced a revision of the idea that these regions of frontal cortex *stored* grammatical knowledge and instead focused attention on their role in *deploying* grammatical knowledge (Bates & Goodman 1997; Linebarger, Schwartz, & Saffran 1983). Observations of intact versus impaired performance contingent on item type have been equally important for cognitive theories derived from neuropsychological data. For instance, the dual-route model

of reading aloud draws critical support from the existence of patients who can read words with irregular pronunciations but not nonwords (presumably because a lexical route from spelling to sound is intact but a rule-based route is impaired) and also from the existence of other patients with the opposite pattern of performance (Coltheart et al. 1993; Marshall & Newcombe 1980; Patterson & Morton 1985).

In studies of the normal population, the *item design* has been more prevalent than the *task design* for experiments using behavioral, ERP, or MEG (magnetoencephalographic) measures. In language processing experiments, subjects are typically asked to perform one task (e.g., pronounce words as rapidly as possible, make lexical decisions, read silently) while the experimenter compares reaction times, accuracies, or electrophysiological responses to semantically plausible versus implausible words, correctly versus incorrectly inflected verbs, rhyming versus nonrhyming words, regular versus irregular past tenses, high- versus low-frequency words, phonologically regular versus irregular words, words from dense versus sparse orthographic neighborhoods, and so forth. In memory experiments, the experimenter is likely to examine recall or recognition of previously studied versus unstudied items, items studied during "deep" versus "shallow" processing tasks, new items that are similar versus dissimilar to those previously studied, and so on.

Task manipulations have also played an important role in behavioral and ERP studies of cognition, but typically via their interactions with item type. In psycholinguistics, for example, it is generally assumed that lexical characteristics that are fundamentally important in word recognition will be evident across distinct tasks. Task-by-item interactions are often interpreted as an indication that a given factor may be relevant for a particular, arbitrary, artificial laboratory task but not for natural reading or listening. In memory research, interactions between stimulus type and test type (recall vs. recognition vs. various implicit tests, item vs. source recognition, etc.) have been a major tool for fractionating memory into subsystems and component processes (Paller 1990; Schacter & Tulving 1994; Senkfor & Van Petten 1999).

In contrast to the strong focus on item designs in behavioral and electrophysiological research, the first decade of functional imaging has relied heavily on pure task designs to activate the brain regions involved in a given cognitive process. A memory experiment may thus compare regional cerebral blood flow when subjects perform a yes–no recognition task to when they merely read previously studied and unstudied words (Cabeza et al. 1997). A language experiment may compare blood flow as subjects generate words related to the stimulus items with their blood flow while reading the stimulus items aloud (Petersen et al. 1989). Both examples are drawn from the PET literature, but the smaller cognitive fMRI literature to date has similarly focused on differences in blood oxygenation level between different tasks performed on similar subsets of stimuli.

The task design for functional imaging has at least two clear strengths. First, it is easy to ensure that the stimuli themselves do not trigger sensory or cognitive processes that differ between conditions, because very similar or identical stimuli can be used in each condition. Equating stimuli for characteristics that are not of interest in a particular experiment is a critical issue for all psychophysiological paradigms, more so than in behavioral experiments. Assessing performance in a particular task narrows the range of potentially influential variables in a way that brain activity measures do not. For accuracy and reaction time (RT) measures, the dependent measure is directly produced by the task – no task, no data. In behavioral studies, the choice of task can eliminate the influence of extraneous stimulus characteristics: lexical decision times will reflect lexical variables but not the fundamental frequency of the speaker's voice; judgments about the speaker's gender will be influenced by fundamental frequency but are unlikely to be influenced by lexical variables. For brain activity measures, the direct link between task and data is broken. Whether or not a subject is asked to do anything, some brain regions will respond to sound, light, or mechanical energy impinging on the sensory surfaces. Using the same stimuli across experimental conditions protects against confounds introduced by stimulus sets that differ in ways that are unknown to the experimenter.

The second strength of the task design for functional imaging is that explicitly instructing participants to engage different cognitive processes may maximize the likelihood that different brain regions will be active across tasks. Task manipulations are a straightforward means of encouraging qualitatively different processing across conditions. In contrast, pure task effects in behavioral measures are often difficult to interpret because accuracy and RT are simple scalars that do not reveal whether experimental effects are quantitative or qualitative in nature. Increased difficulty of a single cognitive process and addition of a second distinct process may yield similar behavioral effects. Similarly, electrophysiological experiments are typically designed to avoid direct comparisons between ERPs elicited in different tasks, because a qualitative change in the component structure of a voltage waveform across tasks may obscure quantitative differences in the amplitude or latency of components present in both tasks, and vice versa (Kutas & Van Petten 1994). Given that brain images are neither a unidimensional measure (like accuracy) nor subject to the problem of cancellation between temporally overlapping components (like ERPs), qualitative differences among conditions can be a desirable outcome of an experimental manipulation rather than an interpretative hazard.

One challenge in using a pure task design strategy is evaluation and control of task difficulty. In the most typical case, an experimenter will design two tasks that require different processes for successful performance. An additional difference in overall difficulty level will not alter the qualitative distinctions between tasks but may introduce additional brain activity that is not strictly necessary for task performance. A more difficult task may engender higher levels of internal accuracy monitoring, error detection, error correction, and – at the extreme – some level of frustration or irritation at one's poor performance. Conversely, an easier task may allow additional uncommitted time between stimuli to engage in anticipation of the next item or preparation of the next response; some of these metaprocesses are likely to have a common anatomical locus across tasks. It has been suggested that (among other functions) the anterior cingulate participates in error detection (Jueptner et al. 1997; Miltner, Braun, & Coles 1997), whereas the motor, premotor, and supplementary motor cortices are undoubtedly involved in response preparation (Miller, Riehle, & Requin 1992; Richter et al. 1997; Roland et al. 1980). But it is possible that other, as yet poorly characterized, brain areas are involved in domain-specific aspects of monitoring and preparation. Some advance knowledge about the relative difficulty of experimental tasks gathered via accuracy and RT measures will be beneficial in distinguishing specific from generic consequences of task difficulty. Finally, comparisons between regional activations in imaging experiments and the performance of patients with damage to those regions serve as the strongest test of whether a given region is merely active during a task or rather is actually critical for the successful performance of that task (Sarter et al. 1996; Swick & Knight 1996; Thompson-Schill et al. 1998).

There are also clear drawbacks to the pure task design for functional imaging. Perhaps the worst-case scenario is that differing instructional sets simply fail to influence the cognitive activity of interest, yielding no observable difference in brain regions that are indeed substrates for that cognitive process. This outcome is likely to arise not because the active task fails to engage the targeted process but rather because the baseline task does so as well. Presentation of similar stimuli across conditions may trigger similar cognitive operations, regardless of whether these are explicitly requested or required for performance of the assigned task. For example, the very first PET investigation of language processing yielded a suprising null effect in that a comparison designed to isolate semantic processes – production of a related verb versus reading aloud – failed to activate any portion of the cortical territory traditionally regarded as Wernicke's area (Petersen et al. 1989). In retrospect, this outcome was far from surprising given the robust behavioral evidence for semantic processing in reading aloud: faster RTs in the presence of semantic context make the pronunciation task a routine tool in psycholinguistic investigations of semantic processing. Mental operations above and beyond those strictly required during a baseline task are no less likely in the domain of memory research. Mere presentation of previously studied items is almost certain to trigger some level of spontaneous retrieval, as evidenced by the similarity of old–new differences in explicit recognition tasks and nonmemory tasks including incidentally repeated stimuli (Rugg & Doyle 1994; Van Petten & Senkfor 1996; but see Swick & Knight 1997). It can be argued that such incidental, uninstructed processing is ubiquitous across cognitive domains. After finding that electrical field potentials in large and widespread cortical and subcortical regions differentiated standard and rare tones in a simple auditory discrimination task, Halgren and colleagues (1995, p. 246) concluded that:

the brain seems to adopt the strategy of engaging all potentially useful areas, even though the probability that they will contribute to immediate task performance is very low. The potential benefit of engaging multiple structures is that incidental learning can occur, behavioral accuracy and consequences can be monitored and, more generally, stimulus information achieves a widespread integration with context and memory. While such "conscious" processing is intentionally rendered superfluous in many psychological tasks, it could be essential for survival and reproduction in the natural environment. In comparison to these benefits, the cost of such a strategy would seem to be minimal, given that in homeotherms all brain areas must be metabolically supported in any case, regardless of whether they are engaged by the task or not.... If areas tend to be engaged even if they have only a very slight probability of being needed, then it is likely that many of the essential areas in the "active" task will also be engaged in the "baseline" task, even though they are not essential. The subtraction may not reveal such areas and thus greatly underestimate the extent of the brain involved in a given cognitive process.

Although such underestimation may be the norm for experimental strategies that rely on contrasts between active and baseline tasks, steps can be taken to alleviate this problem. One is the inclusion of a "resting" baseline without stimulus presentation; although comparisons between rest and any task will not isolate any aspect of perception or cognition, comparisons between each experimental task and a common baseline will allow visualization of regional activations shared by all the tasks. A second strategy is to design baseline and active tasks that are fairly demanding, so that cognitive resources are diverted in the desired direction and a subject's ability to engage in extraneous cognitive activities is reduced. One simple way of increasing the demands of both tasks is by rapid stimulus presentation; correlational analyses have demonstrated that activity in at least some brain areas increases monotonically with stimulus presentation rate (Price et al. 1994; Wise et al. 1991).

The second major drawback to a pure task design strategy is that – even as tasks are designed to identify and

isolate brain regions involved in particular cognitive processes – we have an imperfect understanding of which cognitive processes are required or engaged by any particular task. In the short history of functional imaging research, investigators have largely relied on their intuitions when designing tasks; hence rhyme judgments on word pairs, generating a rhyming word, phoneme monitoring, and syllable counting have all been used as "phonological" tasks, and an even larger number of "semantic" tasks have been employed. The exact nature of the task requirements has been a focal point in a recent controversy surrounding a robust positive result in both PET and fMRI studies. Although activation of the left inferior frontal gyrus (IFG) has been observed in numerous comparisons between semantic and nonsemantic tasks (Gabrieli, Poldrack, & Desmond 1998), others have argued that it is difficult to separate the contribution of semantic analyses from spontaneous phonological processes in the word generation tasks that have been a mainstay of this research (Price et al. 1997) or from a more general cognitive process of selecting among competing sources of information (Thompson-Schill et al. 1997).

Controversies of this sort seem inevitable when one considers that neuropsychologists have been arguing about the proper description of the left IFG (Broca's area) in language processing for several decades. Rather than a sign of trouble, such arguments can be taken as reflecting a healthy research program that extends beyond the simple goal of mapping known functions onto locations. After all, characterizing the fundamental components of cognition is as much a part of functional imaging research as the other subdisciplines of cognitive science. We can hope that such arguments will both arise and be settled at a more rapid pace in functional imaging research than in neuropsychology, given that normal subjects are easier to find than patients with specific lesions. Explicit comparisons between nominally similar tasks (e.g., a set of phonological tasks each compared to a resting baseline) are likely to be more common as the capability of fMRI for repeated testing of the same subjects is more fully exploited, and such comparisons may be especially useful in identifying core cognitive processes.

Another powerful method for circumventing questions about the exact nature of a task contrast will be greater use of the item design in functional imaging research. Item manipulations within a single task can be used to create a gradient of difficulty; convergent results from easy-versus-difficult and active-versus-baseline comparisons will provide stronger support for structure–function conclusions than either experimental strategy alone. Moreover, it will be easier to forge links between functional imaging results and behavioral or electrophysiological studies using similar item-based designs. It is possible that conditions explicitly designed to vary along a unitary dimension will yield weaker hemodynamic contrasts than those designed to vary qualitatively, but several recent studies demonstrate the feasibility of the former approach. In a sentence comprehension task, Just and colleagues (1996) observed a graded influence of syntactic complexity in both Broca's and Wernicke's areas when three sentence types were each compared to a resting baseline. In a verb generation task, Thompson-Schill and colleagues (1997) compared nouns possessing a strongly associated verb (e.g. *scissors – cut*) to those with many possible answers (e.g. *rope – hang/tie/cut/stretch*). Greater activity in Broca's area for the "high selection" condition was paralleled in two other tasks using stimuli that varied in their demand for selecting among different sources of information (Thompson-Schill et al. 1997). In a task of detecting occasional animal names, we observed differential blood flow in the left superior temporal and angular gyri for lists of semantically related versus unrelated words (Van Petten, Reiman, & Senkfor 1995).

Item-based experimental designs need not start with the assumption that stimulus classes vary along some unitary dimension; they can also be used to explore the possibility that qualitatively different mechanisms are invoked by different stimulus types. For example, Fiez and Petersen (1998) reviewed PET studies comparing orthographically consistent and exception words (i.e., those like *lint* whose pronunciations follow regular grapheme-to-phoneme conversion rules versus those like *pint* with irregular pronunciations). Domains of partial regularity combined with exceptions abound in language (as in the past-tense system for English verbs), so that such contrasts between regular and irregular words have been at the heart of arguments pitting single-mechanism models against those that postulate a rule-based system for regular items and direct memory look-up for irregular items (Plaut et al. 1996; Plunkett & Marchman 1993). As Fiez and Petersen (1998) noted, the PET results to date can be accommodated by either single-mechanism or dual-route models, but these results suggest new critical comparisons that can be tested in neuropsychological studies. The relationship between orthography and phonology is only one circumscribed issue in cognition, but it has been an exemplary case where the use of similar paradigms has allowed psycholinguistic, computational, neuropsychological, and functional imaging methods to tackle the same problem.

Although item designs are now being used to good effect in language processing experiments, the picture has not been as bright in memory research. In recognition tasks, differential responses to studied versus unstudied items are mandatory for deriving a behavioral accuracy measure, and different brain responses for remembered old items (hits) versus new items have been a basic tool in electrophysiological studies of memory (Van Petten & Senkfor 1996). PET contrasts between studied and unstudied items have revealed less consistent results. The majority of experiments have found that blocks of old items elicit greater

blood flow in prefrontal cortex than new items, yet greater, lesser, and null changes in blood flow have been observed in the medial temporal lobe (Dolan & Fletcher 1997; Henke et al. 1997; Nyberg et al. 1995; Schacter et al. 1997; Tulving et al. 1996). A different strategy for localizing brain areas sensitive to successful retrieval of episodic memories has been to compare conditions with high recall or recognition rates (engendered by additional or deeper study prior to scanning) to those with lower accuracy rates. These contrasts have similarly revealed both positive and negative relationships between medial temporal blood flow and accuracy (Petersson, Elfgren, & Ingvar 1997; Rugg et al. 1997). One possible account of these discrepant findings is that the medial temporal lobe is involved in both the encoding of new (or poorly learned) stimuli and the retrieval of well-learned items. In an fMRI study comparing studied to unstudied items, Gabrieli and colleagues (1997) reported increased activity in one region of the medial temporal lobe but decreased activity in a neighboring region. It is possible that opposing activity changes in small adjacent brain structures are vulnerable to blurring and cancellation by PET methods of intrasubject averaging, so it will be of some interest to pursue old–new differences in fMRI experiments that allow examination of individual brains.

Item designs have been the minority of functional imaging studies because ^{15}O PET and the first generation of fMRI methods require averaging activity over 30–60 sec. Many of the item manipulations used to good effect in behavioral and electrophysiological studies are not amenable to blocked presentation of a given condition. Predictability as to what will come next undermines a good deal of the specific effort required to resolve a perceptual, linguistic, or memory challenge. The literature to date has included some methods for circumventing this problem of blocked presentation; for instance, contrasts between old and new items during recognition memory tests have been conducted by comparing blocks with *mostly* (~ 90%) old items to those containing mostly new items. Comparing stimulus blocks with different probabilities of stimulus types offers a compromise between the technical requirement of using long epochs and the cognitive requirement of avoiding complete predictability.

Some of the limitations on experimental design in functional imaging are eliminated by newer event-related analyses of fMRI data that selectively average responses from epochs corresponding to randomly intermixed stimuli (Rosen, Buckner, & Dale 1998). The most conservative use of this method is with slow presentation rates that allow the prolonged hemodynamic response to each item to begin and end before onset of the next item. Even in tasks for which a behavioral or electrophysiological response can be elicited within a second of stimulus onset, the BOLD signal may persist for close to 10 sec (Buckner et al. 1996; McCarthy et al. 1997). Using long stimulus–onset asynchronies (SOAs) affords a temporal separation between trial types but may also result in few trials and a low S/N. Very slow presentation rates may also alter cognitive processes in undesirable ways: most selective attention paradigms would be ruled out, and sentence comprehension at six words per minute would be a very different process than natural reading or listening. However, some recent studies have suggested that responses to sequential stimuli add in a nearly linear fashion, so that the contribution of one stimulus type can be distinguished from temporally adjacent stimuli with SOAs as short as 2 sec (Dale & Buckner 1997; Josephs, Turner, & Friston 1997; Kim, Richter, & Ugurbil 1997). As presentation rates approach or exceed two items per second, the BOLD signal is likely to saturate and the activity elicited by individual items will be unrecoverable (Friston et al. 1998; Rees et al. 1997). However, for many cognitive paradigms, this lower limit will not be problematic. More critical will be the analytic procedure used for isolating responses to one stimulus type from temporally overlapping responses. Preliminary studies have dealt with this problem by ensuring that each trial type is preceded and followed by each other trial type equally often, so that simple subtraction can be used to estimate and eliminate response overlap (Dale & Buckner 1997). Such perfect randomization of trial order is not possible for all cognitive questions. One may wish to compare trials accompanied by correct and incorrect behavioral responses (for instance, hits to false alarms in recognition memory), but these cannot be foreseen in advance of the subject's behavior. In sentence processing studies, grammar does not allow words of a particular class to be placed in any random order (in English, for example, articles are followed by nouns and never by verbs). Such cases of differential response overlap in different conditions pose the same analytical problem as that encountered in ERP research (Woldorff 1993), so that similar correction methods are under development (Buckner et al. 1998).

Full development of event-related fMRI methods will ease comparisons among hemodynamic, electrical, and magnetic measures of brain activity (George et al. 1995). These may or may not prove equally sensitive to the variety of mechanisms the brain uses to process information (see e.g. Riehle et al. 1997), but all will offer some view of the "enchanted loom where millions of flashing shuttles weave a dissolving pattern, always a meaningful pattern, though not ever an abiding one" (Sherrington 1940).

NOTE

1. This analytic strategy is the same as that used in most cognitive studies with reaction time measures. A single-subject analysis is possible with reaction times because each trial can be considered as a single data point and multiple trials from two conditions within one individual can be statistically compared. In practice, however, most researchers compute average reaction times from each subject in each condition and then compare these averages across a sample of subjects.

REFERENCES

Bandettini, P. A., & Wong, E. C. (1997). Magnetic resonance imaging of human brain function: Principles, practicalities, and possibilities. *Neurosurgery Clinics of North America, 8,* 345–71.

Baron, J. C. (1989). Depression of energy metabolism in distant brain structures: Studies with positron emission tomography in stroke patients. *Seminars in Neurology, 9,* 281–5.

Bates, E., & Goodman, J. C. (1997). On the inseparability of grammar and the lexicon: Evidence from acquisition, aphasia, and real-time processing. *Language and Cognitive Processes, 12,* 507–84.

Bavelier, D., Corina, D., Jezzard, P., Padmanabhan, S., Clark, V. P., Kami, A., Prinster, A., Braun, A., Lalwani, A., Rauschecker, J. P., Turner, R., & Neville, H. (1997). Sentence reading: A functional MRI study at 4 Tesla. *Journal of Cognitive Neuroscience, 9,* 664–86.

Belliveau, J. W., Kennedy, D. N., McKinstry, R. C., Buchbinder, B. R., Weisskoff, R. M., Cohen, M. S., Vevea, J. M., Brady, T. J., & Rosen, B. R. (1991). Functional mapping of the human visual cortex by magnetic resonance imaging. *Science, 254,* 716–19.

Bogen, J. E., & Bogen, G. M. (1976). Wernicke's region – Where is it? *Annals of the New York Academy of Sciences, 280,* 834–43.

Bookstein, F. L. (1989). Principal warps: Thin-plate splines and the decomposition of deformations. *IEEE Transactions on Pattern Analysis and Machine Intelligence, 11,* 567–85.

Boxerman, J. L., et al. (1995). MR contrast due to intravascular magnetic susceptibility perturbations. *Magnetic Resonance in Medicine, 34,* 555–66.

Brill, A. B., Adelstein, S. J., et al. (1982). *Low Level of Radiation Effects: A Fact Book.* New York: Society of Nuclear Medicine.

Büchel, C., Morris, J., Dolan, R. J., & Friston, K. J. (1998). Brain systems mediating aversive conditioning: An event-related fMRI study. *Neuron, 20,* 947–57.

Büchel, C., Turner, R., & Friston, K. (1997). Lateral geniculate activations can be detected using intersubject averaging and fMRI. *Magnetic Resonance in Medicine, 38,* 691–4.

Buckner, R. L., Bandettini, P. A., O'Craven, K. M., Savoy, R. L., Petersen, S. E., Raichle, M. E., & Rosen, B. R. (1996). Detection of cortical activation during averaged single trials of a cognitive task using functional magnetic resonance imaging. *Proceedings of the National Academy of Sciences U.S.A., 95,* 891–8.

Buckner, R. L., Goodman, J., Burock, M., Rotte, M., Koutstaal, W., Schacter, D., Rosen, B., & Dale, A. M. (1998). Functional-anatomic correlates of object priming in humans revealed by rapid presentation event-related fMRI. *Neuron, 20,* 285–96.

Buxton, R. B., Wong, E. C., & Frank, L. R. (1997). A biomechanical interpretation of the BOLD signal time course: The balloon model. *Proceedings of the ISMRM 5th Annual Meeting.* Vancouver.

Cabeza, R., Kapur, S., Craik, F. I. M., McIntosh, A. R., Houle, S., & Tulving, E. (1997). Functional neuroanatomy of recall and recognition: A PET study of episodic memory. *Journal of Cognitive Neuroscience, 9,* 254–65.

Chen, K., Bandy, D., Reiman, E. M., et al. (1998). Noninvasive quantification of the cerebral metabolic rate for glucose using positron emission tomography, 18F-fluorodeoxyglucose, the Patlak method, and an image-derived input function. *Journal of Cerebral Blood Flow and Metabolism, 18,* 716–23.

Chen, K., Reiman, E. M., Lawson, M., Yun, L.-S., Bandy, D., & Palant, A. (1996). Methods for the correction of vascular artifacts in PET O-15 water brain mapping studies. *IEEE Transactions on Nuclear Science, 43,* 3308–14.

Cherry, S. R., Dahlbom, M., & Hoffman, E.J. (1991). Three dimensional positron emission tomography using a conventional multislice tomograph without septa. *Journal of Computer Assisted Tomography, 15,* 655–68.

Cherry, S. R., Dahlbom, M., & Hoffman, E.J. (1992). Evaluation of a 3D reconstruction algorithm for multi-slice PET scanners. *Physics in Medicine and Biology, 37,* 779–90.

Cherry, S. R., & Phelps, M. E. (1996). Imaging brain function with positron emission tomography. In A. W. Toga & J. C. Mazziotta (Eds.), *Brain Mapping Methods,* pp. 191–221. San Diego: Academic Press.

Cherry, S. R., Woods, R. P., Doshi, N. K., et al. (1995). Improved signal-to-noise in PET activation studies using switched paradigms. *Journal of Nuclear Medicine, 36,* 307–14.

Cherry, S. R., Woods, R. P., & Hoffman, E. J. (1993). Improved detection of focal cerebral blood flow changes using three-dimensional positron emission tomography. *Journal of Cerebral Blood Flow and Metabolism, 13,* 630–8.

Chertkow, H., & Bub, D. (1994). Functional activation and cognition: The ^{15}O-water PET subtraction method. In A. Kertesz (Ed.), *Localization and Neuroimaging in Neuropsychology,* pp. 151–84. San Diego: Academic Press.

Clark, M. M., & Plante, E. (1998). Morphology of the inferior frontal gyrus in developmentally language-disordered adults. *Brain and Language, 61,* 288–303.

Collins, D. L., Neelin, P., Peters, T. M., & Evans, A. C. (1994a). Automatic 3D intersubject registration of MR volumetric data in standardized Talairach space. *Journal of Computer Assisted Tomography, 18,* 192–205.

Collins, D. L., Peters, T. M., & Evans, A. C. (1994b). An automatic 3D non-linear image deformation algorithm procedure for determination of gross morphometric variability in human brain. In *Proceedings of the 4th Conference on Biomedical Computing,* pp. 180–94. SPIE.

Coltheart, M., Curtis, B., Atkins, P., & Haller, M. (1993). Models of reading aloud: Dual route and parallel-distributed processing approaches. *Psychological Review, 100,* 589–608.

Conti, P. (1995). Oncology: Brain and spinal cord. In Wagner, Szabo, & Buchanan, pp. 1041–54.

Dale, A. M., & Buckner, R.L. (1997). Selective averaging of rapidly presented individual trials using fMRI. *Human Brain Mapping, 5,* 1–12.

Daube-Witherspoon, M. E. (1995). Positron emission tomography: Operational guidelines. In Wagner, Szabo, & Buchanan, pp. 346–62.

Davis, T. L. (1998). Calibrated functional MRI: Mapping the dynamics of oxidative metabolism. *Proceedings of the National Academy of Sciences U.S.A., 95,* 1834–9.

Demb, J. B., Boynton, G. M., & Heeger, D. J. (1997). Brain activity in visual cortex predicts individual differences in reading performance. *Proceedings of the National Academy of Sciences U.S.A., 94,* 13363–6.

Detre, J. A., et al. (1992). Perfusion imaging. *Magnetic Resonance in Medicine, 23,* 37–45.

Dewey, S. L., Brodie, J. D., Fowler, J. S., et al. (1990). Positron emission tomography (PET) studies of dopaminergic/cholinergic interactions in the baboon brain. *Synapse, 6,* 321–7.

Dewey, S. L., Smith, G. S., Logan, J., et al. (1992). GABAergic inhibition of endogenous dopamine release measured in vivo with 11C-raclopride and positron emission tomography. *Journal of Neuroscience, 12,* 3773–80.

Dolan, R. J., & Fletcher, P. C. (1997). Dissociating prefrontal and hippocampal function in episodic memory encoding. *Nature, 388,* 582–5.

Dolan, R. J., Fletcher, P., Frith, C. D., Friston, K. J., Frackowiak, R. S., & Grasby, P. M. (1995). Dopaminergic modulation of impaired cognitive activation in the anterior cingulate cortex in schizophrenia. *Nature, 378,* 180–2.

Duara, R., Barker, W. W., Chang, J., Yoshii, F., Loewenstein, D. A., & Pascal, S. (1992). Viability of neocortical function shown in behavioral activation state PET studies in Alzheimer disease. *Journal of Cerebral Blood Flow and Metabolism, 12,* 927–34.

Duncan, J. D., Moss, S. D., Bandy, D. J., Manwaring, K., Kaplan, A. M., Reiman, E. M., Chen, K., Lawson, M. A., & Wodrich, D. L. (1997). Use of positron emission tomography for presurgical localization of eloquent brain areas in children with seizures. *Pediatric Neurosurgery, 26,* 144–56.

Edelman, R., Siewert, B., & Darby, D. (1994). Qualitative mapping of cerebral blood flow and functional localization with echo planar MR imaging and signal targeting with alternating radiofrequency (EPISTAR). *Radiology, 192,* 1–8.

Evans, A. C. (1995). Correlative imaging. In Wagner, Szabo, & Buchanan, pp. 405–21.

Evans, A. C., Collins, D. L., Mills, S. R., et al. (1993). 3D statistical neuroanatomical models from 305 MRI volumes. *Proceedings of the IEEE Nuclear Science Symposium and Medical Imaging Conference.* Piscataway, NJ: IEEE.

Evans, A. C., Collins, L., Worsley, K., Dai, W., Milot, S., Meyer, E., & Bub, D. (1992). Anatomical mapping of functional activation in stereotactic coordinate space. *Neuroimage, 1,* 43–53.

Evans, A. C., Marrett, S., Torrescorzo, J., et al. (1991). MRI–PET correlative analysis using a volume of interest (VOI) atlas. *Journal of Cerebral Blood Flow and Metabolism, 11,* A69–A78.

Evens, R. G., Siegel, B. A., Welch, M. J., et al. (1983). Cost analyses of positron emission tomography for clinical use. *American Journal of Roentgenology, 141,* 1073–6.

Farde, L., Ehrin, E., Eriksson, L., et al. (1985). Substituted benzamides as ligands for visualization of dopamine receptor binding in the human brain by positron emission tomography. *Proceedings of the National Academy of Sciences U.S.A., 82,* 3863–7.

Farde, L., Hakan, H., Ehrin, E., et al. (1986). Quantitative analysis of D2 dopamine receptor binding in the living human brain by PET. *Science, 231,* 258–61.

Fiez, J. A., & Petersen, S. E. (1998). Neuroimaging studies of word reading. *Proceedings of the National Academy of Sciences U.S.A., 95,* 914–21.

Fox, P. T., Burton, H., & Raichle, M. E. (1987). Mapping human somatosensory cortex with positron emission tomography. *Journal of Neurosurgery, 65,* 34–63.

Fox, P.T., & Mintun, M.A. (1989). Noninvasive functional brain mapping by change-distribution analysis of averaged PET images of $H_2^{15}O$ tissue activity. *Journal of Nuclear Medicine, 30,* 141–9.

Fox, P. T., Mintun, M. A., Raichle, M. E., et al. (1986). Mapping human visual cortex with positron emission tomography. *Nature, 323,* 806–9.

Fox, P.T., Mintun, M. A., Reiman, E. M., & Raichle, M.E. (1988). Enhanced detection of focal brain responses using intersubject averaging and distribution analysis of subtracted PET images. *Journal of Cerebral Blood Flow and Metabolism, 8,* 642–53.

Fox, P. T., Perlmutter, J. S., & Raichle, M. E. (1985). A stereotactic method of anatomical localization for positron emission tomography. *Journal of Computer Assisted Tomography, 9,* 141–53.

Fox, P. T., & Raichle, M. E. (1984). Stimulus rate dependence of regional cerebral blood flow in human striate cortex, demonstrated with positron emission tomography. *Journal of Neurophysiology, 51,* 1109–21.

Fox, P. T., & Raichle, M. E. (1986). Focal physiological uncoupling of cerebral blood flow and oxidative metabolism during somatosensory stimulation in man. *Proceedings of the National Academy of Sciences U.S.A., 83,* 1140–4.

Frackowiak, R. S. J., Friston, K. J., Frith, C. D., Dolan, R. J., & Mazziotta, J. C. (1997). *Human Brain Function.* San Diego: Academic Press.

Frahm, J., et al. (1996). Dynamic uncoupling and recoupling of perfusion and oxidative metabolism during focal activation in man. *Magnetic Resonance in Medicine, 35,* 143–8.

Fried, I., Nenov, V. I., Ojemann, S. G., & Woods, R. P. (1995). Functional MR and PET imaging of rolandic and visual cortices for neurosurgical planning. *Journal of Neurosurgery, 83,* 854–61.

Friston, K. J., Ashburner, J., Frith, C. D., et al. (1995). Spatial registration and normalization of images. *Human Brain Mapping, 2,* 165–89.

Friston, K. J., Frith, C. D., & Frackowiak, R. S. J. (1993a). Time-dependent changes in effective connectivity measured with PET. *Human Brain Mapping, 1,* 69–80.

Friston, K., Frith, C., Liddle, P., Dolan, R., Lammertsma, A., & Frackowiak, R. (1990). The relationship between global and local changes in PET scans. *Journal of Cerebral Blood Flow and Metabolism, 10,* 458–66.

Friston, K. J., Frith, C. D., Liddle, P. F., & Frackowiak, R. S. J. (1991). Plastic transformation of PET images. *Journal of Computer Assisted Tomography, 15,* 634–9.

Friston, K. J., Frith, C. D., Liddle, P. F., & Frackowiak, R. S. J. (1993b). Functional connectivity: The principal component analysis of large (PET) data sets. *Journal of Cerebral Blood Flow and Metabolism, 13,* 5–14.

Friston, K. J., Josephs, O., Rees, G., & Turner, R. (1998). Nonlinear event-related responses in fMRI. *Magnetic Resonance in Medicine, 39,* 41–52.

Friston, K. J., Poline, J.-B., Holmes, A. P., Frith, C. D., & Frackowiak, R. S. J. (1996a). A multivariate analysis of PET activation studies. *Human Brain Mapping, 4,* 140–51.

Friston, K. J., Price, C. J., Fletcher, P., Moore, C., Frackowiak, R. S., & Dolan, R. J. (1996b). The trouble with cognitive subtraction. *Neuroimage, 4,* 97–104.

Friston, K. J., Worsley, K. J., Frackowiak, R. S. J., et al. (1994). Assessing the significance of focal activations using their spatial extent. *Human Brain Mapping, 1,* 214–20.

Frost, J. J., & Mayberg, H. S. (1995). Epilepsy. In Wagner, Szabo, & Buchanan, pp. 564–75.

Gabrieli, J. D. E., Brewer, J. B., Desmond, J. E., & Glover, G. (1997). Separate neural bases of two fundamental memory processes in the human medial temporal lobe. *Science, 276,* 264–6.

Gabrieli, J. D. E., Poldrack, R. A., & Desmond, J. E. (1998). The role of left prefrontal cortex in language and memory. *Proceedings of the National Academy of Sciences U.S.A., 95,* 906–13.

George, J. S., Aine, C. J., Mosher, J. C., Schmidt, D. M., Ranken, D. M., Schlitt, H. A., Wood, C. C., Lewine, J. D., Sanders, J. A., & Belliveau, J. W. (1995). Mapping function in the human brain with magnetoencephalography, anatomical magnetic resonance imaging, and functional magnetic resonance imaging. *Journal of Clinical Neurophysiology, 12,* 406–31.

Gjedde, A. (1995). Tracer kinetics: Compartment models. In Wagner, Szabo, & Buchanan, pp. 451–62.

Greitz, T., Bohm, C., Holte, S., & Eriksson, L. (1991). A computerized brain atlas: Construction, anatomical content and some applications. *Journal of Computer Assisted Tomography, 15,* 26–38.

Haier, R. J., Siegel, B. V., Jr., MacLachlan, A., Soderling, E., Lottenberg, S., & Buchsbaum, M. S. (1992). Regional glucose metabolic changes after learning a complex visuospatial/motor task: A positron emission tomographic study. *Brain Research, 570,* 134–43.

Halgren, E., Baudena, P., Clarke, J. M., Heit, G., Marinkovic, J., Devaux, B., Vignal, J.-P., & Biraben, A. (1995). Intracerebral potentials to rare target and distractor auditory and visual stimuli. II. Medial, lateral and posterior temporal lobe. *Electroencephalography and Clinical Neurophysiology, 94,* 229–50.

Heiss, W.-D., & Podreka, I. (1995). Cerebrovascular disease. In Wagner, Szabo, & Buchanan, pp. 531–48.

Henke, K., Buck, A., Weber, B., & Wieser, H.G. (1997). Human hippocampus establishes associations in memory. *Hippocampus, 7,* 249–56.

Herscovitch, P. (1995). Cerebral blood flow, volume, and oxygen metabolism. In Wagner, Szabo, & Buchanan, pp. 505–14.

Herscovitch, P., Markham, J., & Raichle, M. E. (1983). Brain blood flow measured with intravenous $H_2^{15}O$, I: Theory and error analysis. *Journal of Nuclear Medicine, 24,* 782–9.

Herscovitch, P., Markham, J., & Raichle, M. E. (1987). Positron emission tomographic measurement of cerebral blood flow and water permeability with O-15 water and C-11 butanol. *Journal of Cerebral Blood Flow and Metabolism, 7,* 527–42.

Holmes, A. P., Blair, R. C., Watson, J. D. G., & Ford, I. (1996). Non-parametric analysis of statistic images from functional mapping experiments. *Journal of Cerebral Blood Flow and Metabolism, 16,* 7–22.

Huang, S., Barrio, J. R., & Phelps, M. E. (1986). Neuroreceptor assay with positron emission tomography: Equilibrium versus dynamic approaches. *Journal of Cerebral Blood Flow and Metabolism, 6,* 515–21.

Huang, S., Phelps, M. E., Hoffman, E. J., et al. (1980). Noninvasive determination of local cerebral metabolic rate of glucose in man. *American Journal of Physiology, 238,* E69–E82.

ICRP [International Commission on Radiological Protection] (1991). *1990 Recommendations of the ICRP.* Oxford, U.K.: Pergamon.

Iragui, V., Kutas, M., & Salmon, D. P. (1996). Event-related brain potentials during semantic categorization in normal aging and senile dementia of the Alzheimer's type. *Electrophysiology and Clinical Neurophysiology: Evoked Potentials, 100,* 392–406.

Josephs, O., Turner, R., & Friston, K. (1997). Event-related fMRI. *Human Brain Mapping, 5,* 243–8.

Jueptner, M., Stephan, K. M., Frith, C. D., Brooks, D. J., Frackowiak, R. S. J., & Passingham, R. E. (1997). Anatomy of motor learning: Frontal cortex and attention to action. *Journal of Neurophysiology, 77,* 1313–24.

Just, M. A., Carpenter, P. A., Keller, T. A., Eddy, W. F., & Thulborn, K. R. (1996). Brain activation modulated by sentence comprehension. *Science, 274,* 114–16.

Karni, A., et al. (1993). Stimulus dependent MRI signals evoked by oriented line-element textures in human visual cortex. *Book of Abstracts, Society for Neuroscience 23rd Annual Meeting.* Washington, DC.

Kessler, J., Herholz, K., Grond, M., & Heiss, W. D. (1991). Impaired metabolic activation in Alzheimer's disease: A PET study during continuous visual recognition. *Neuropsychologia, 29,* 229–43.

Kim, S.-G. (1995). Quantification of relative cerebral blood flow change by flow-sensitive alternating inversion recovery (FAIR) technique: Application to functional mapping. *Magnetic Resonance in Medicine, 34,* 293–301.

Kim, S.-G., Richter, W., & Ugurbil, K. (1997). Limitations of temporal resolution in functional MRI. *Magnetic Resonance in Medicine, 37,* 631–6.

Kim, S.-G., & Ugurbil, K. (1997). Comparison of blood oxygenation and cerebral blood flow effects in fMRI: Estimation of relative oxygen consumption change. *Magnetic Resonance in Medicine, 38,* 59–65.

Knapp, F. F., Jr., Brihaye, C., & Callahan, A. P. (1995). Generators. In Wagner, Szabo, & Buchanan, pp. 150–65.

Koepp, M. J., Gunn, R. N., Lawrence, A. D., Cunningham, V. J., Dagher, A., Jones, T., Brooks, D. J., Bench, C. J., & Grasby, P. M. (1998). Evidence for striatal dopamine release during a video game. *Nature, 393,* 266–8.

Koeppe, R. A., Holthoff, V. A., Frey, K. A., et al. (1991). Compartmental analysis of [11C] flumazenil kinetics for the estimation of ligand transport rate and receptor distribution using positron emission tomography. *Journal of Cerebral Blood Flow and Metabolism, 11,* 735–44.

Kosugi, Y., Sase, M., Kuwatani, H., et al. (1993). Neural network mapping for nonlinear stereotactic normalization of brain MRI images. *Journal of Computer Assisted Tomography, 17,* 455–60.

Kutas, M., & Van Petten, C. (1994). Psycholinguistics electrified: Event-related brain potential investigations. In M. Gernsbacher (Ed.), *Handbook of Psycholinguistics,* pp. 83–143. New York: Academic Press.

Kwong, K. K., et al. (1995). MR perfusion studies with T1-weighted echo planar imaging. *Magnetic Resonance in Medicine, 34,* 878–87.

Langstrom, B., & Dannals, R. F. (1995). Carbon-11 compounds. In Wagner, Szabo, & Buchanan, pp. 166–78.

Leahy, R., & Yan, X. (1991). Incorporation of anatomical MR data for improved functional imaging with PET. In A. Colchester & D. Hawkes (Eds.), *Information Processing in Medical Imaging,* pp. 105–19. Wye, U.K.: Springer-Verlag.

Leblanc, R., & Meyer, E. (1990). Functional PET scanning in the assessment of cerebral arteriovenous malformations. *Journal of Neurosurgery, 73,* 615–19.

Leblanc, R., Meyer, E., Bub, D., et al. (1992). Language mapping with activation PET scanning. *Neurosurgery, 31,* 369–73.

Linebarger, M. C., Schwartz, M. F., & Saffran, E. M. (1983). Sensitivity to grammatical structure in so-called agrammatic aphasics. *Cognition, 13,* 361–92.

Mandeville, J. B. (1998). Dynamic functional imaging of relative cerebral blood volume during rat forepaw stimulation. *Magnetic Resonance in Medicine, 39,* 615–24.

Marshall, J. C., & Newcombe, F. (1980). The conceptual status of deep dyslexia: An historical perspective. In M. Coltheart, K. Patterson, & J. C. Marshall (Eds.), *Deep Dyslexia,* pp. 1–21. London: Routledge & Kegan Paul.

Mazziotta, J. C., Phelps, M. E., Plummer, D., & Kuhl, D. E. (1981). Quantitation in positron emission computed tomography: 5. Physical-anatomical effects. *Journal of Computer Assisted Tomography, 5,* 734–43.

McCarthy, G., Luby, M., Gore, J., & Goldman-Rakic, P. (1997). Infrequent events transiently activate human prefrontal and parietal cortex as measured by functional MRI. *Journal of Neurophysiology, 77,* 1630–4.

McIntosh, A. R., Bookstein, F. L., Haxby, J. V., & Grady, C. L. (1996). Spatial pattern analysis of functional brain images using partial least squares. *Neuroimage, 3,* 143–57.

McIntosh, A. R., & Gonzalez-Lima, F. (1994). Structural equation modelling and its application to network analysis in functional brain imaging. *Human Brain Mapping, 2,* 2–22.

McIntosh, A. R., Grady, C. L., Ungerleider, J. V., et al. (1994). Network analysis of cortical visual pathways mapped with PET. *Journal of Neuroscience, 14,* 655–66.

Meyer, J. H., Kapur, S., Wilson, A. A., DaSilva, J. N., Houle, S., & Brown, G. M. (1996). Neuromodulation of frontal and temporal cortex by intravenous d-fenfluramine: An [^{15}O]H$_2$O PET study in humans. *Neuroscience Letters, 207,* 25–8.

Miller, J. D., de Leon, M. J., Ferris, S. H., Kluger, A., George, A. E., Reisberg, B., Sachs, H. J., & Wolf, A. P. (1987). Abnormal temporal lobe response in Alzheimer's disease during cognitive processing as measured by 11C-2-deoxy-D-glucose and PET. *Journal of Cerebral Blood Flow and Metabolism, 7,* 248–51.

Miller, J., Riehle, A., & Requin, J. (1992). Effects of preliminary perceptual output on neuronal activity of the primary motor cortex. *Journal of Experimental Psychology: Human Perception and Performance, 18,* 1121–38.

Miller, M., Christensen, G., Amit, Y., & Grenander, U. (1993). Mathematical textbook of deformable neuroanatomies. *Proceedings of the National Academy of Sciences U.S.A., 90,* 433–4.

Miltner, W. H. R., Braun, C. H., & Coles, M. G. H. (1997). Event-related brain potentials following incorrect feedback in a time-estimation task: Evidence for a generic neural system for error detection. *Journal of Cognitive Neuroscience, 9,* 788–98.

Minoshima, S., Berger, K. L., Lee, K. S., & Mintun, M. A. (1992). An automated method for rotational correction and centering of three-dimensional functional brain images. *Journal of Nuclear Medicine, 33,* 1479–1585.

Minoshima, S., Frey, K. A., Foster, N. L., & Kuhl, D. E. (1995a). Preserved pontine glucose metabolism in Alzheimer's disease: A reference region for functional brain image (PET) analysis. *Journal of Computer Assisted Tomography, 19,* 541–7.

Minoshima, S., Frey, K. A., Koeppe, R. A., et al. (1995b). A diagnostic approach in Alzheimer's disease using three-dimensional stereotactic surface projections of fluorine-18-FDG PET. *Journal of Nuclear Medicine, 36,* 1238–48.

Minoshima, S., Koeppe, R. A., Frey, K. A., & Kuhl, D. E. (1994). Anatomic standardization: Linear scaling and nonlinear warping of functional brain images. *Journal of Nuclear Medicine, 35,* 1528–37.

Mintun, M. A., Fox, P. T., & Raichle, M. E. (1989). A highly accurate method of localizing regions of neuronal activation in the human brain using positron emission tomography. *Journal of Cerebral Blood Flow and Metabolism, 9,* 96–103.

Mintun, M. A., McGuire, A. H., Welch, M. J., Siegel, B. A., & Katzenellenbogen, J. A. (1991). PET imaging of estrogen receptors in breast cancer. In D. E. Kuhl (Ed.), *In Vivo Imaging of Neurotransmitter Functions in Brain, Heart, and Tumors,* pp. 277–92. Washington, DC: American College of Nuclear Physicians.

Mintun, M. A., Raichle, M. E., Kilbourn, M. R., et al. (1984). A quantitative model for the in vivo assessment of drug binding sites with positron emission tomography. *Annals of Neurology, 15,* 217–27.

Neville, H. J., Coffey, S. A., Holcomb, P. J., & Tallal, P. (1993). The neurobiology of sensory and language processing in language-impaired children. *Journal of Cognitive Neuroscience, 5,* 235–53.

Nozaki, T., & Hazue, M. (1995). Accelerators. In Wagner, Szabo, & Buchanan, pp. 144–50.

NRCC [National Research Council Committee on the Biological Effects of Ionizing Radiation] (1990). *BEIR V. Health Effects of Exposure to Low Levels of Ionizing Radiation.* Washington, DC: National Academy Press.

Nyberg, L., Tulving, E., Habib, R., Nilsson, L.-G., Kapur, S., Houle, S., Cabeza, R., & McIntosh, A.R. (1995). Functional brain maps of retrieval mode and recovery of episodic information. *Neuroreport, 7,* 249–52.

Paller, K. A. (1990). Recall and stem-completion priming have different electrophysiological correlates and are modified differentially by directed forgetting. *Journal of Experimental Psychology: Learning, Memory, and Cognition, 16,* 1021–32.

Paller, K. A., Acharya, A., Richardson, B. C., Plaisant, O., Shimamura, A. P., Reed, B. R., & Jagust, W. J. (1997). Functional neuroimaging of cortical dysfunction in alcoholic Korsakoff's syndrome. *Journal of Cognitive Neuroscience, 9,* 277–93.

Pardo, J. V., & Fox, P. T. (1993). Preoperative assessment of the cerebral hemispheric dominance for language with CBF PET. *Human Brain Mapping, 1,* 57–68.

Patlak, C., Blasberg, R. G., & Fenstermacher, J. D. (1983). Graphical evaluation of blood-to-brain transfer constants from multiple-time uptake data. *Journal of Cerebral Blood Flow and Metabolism, 3,* 1–7.

Patterson, K. E., & Morton, J. (1985). From orthography to phonology: An attempt at an old interpretation. In K. E. Patterson, J. C. Marshall, & M. Coltheart (Eds.), *Surface Dyslexia,* pp. 335–59. Hillsdale, NJ: Erlbaum.

Pellizzari, C. A., Chen, G. T. Y., Spelbring, D. R., et al. (1989). Accurate three-dimensional registration of CT, PET and/or MRI images of the brain. *Journal of Computer Assisted Tomography, 13,* 20–6.

Perlmutter, J. S., Larson, K. B., Raichle, M. E., Markham, K. J., Mintun, M. A., Kilbourn, M. R., & Welch, M. J. (1986). Strategies for in vivo measurement of receptor binding using positron emission tomography. *Journal of Cerebral Blood Flow and Metabolism, 6,* 154–69.

Petersen, S. E., Fox, P. T., Posner, M. I., Mintun, M., & Raichle, M. E. (1989). Positron emission tomographic studies of the processing of single words. *Journal of Cognitive Neuroscience, 1,* 153–70.

Petersson, J. M., Elfgren, C., & Ingvar, M. (1997). A dynamic role of the medial temporal lobe during retrieval of declarative memory in man. *Neuroimage, 6,* 1–11.

Phelps, M. E., Hoffman, E. J., Mullani, N. A., & Ter-Pogossian, M. M. (1975). Application of annihilation coincidence detection to transaxial reconstruction tomography. *Journal of Nuclear Medicine, 16,* 210–24.

Phelps, M. E., Huang, S. C., Hoffman, E. J., et al. (1979). Tomographic measurement of local cerebral metabolic rate in humans with [F-18] 2-fluoro-2-deoxy-D-glucose: Validation of method. *Annals of Neurology, 6,* 371–88.

Plaut, D. C., McClelland, J. L., Seidenberg, M. S., & Patterson, K. (1996). Understanding normal and impaired word reading: Computational principles in quasi-regular domains. *Psychological Review, 103,* 56–115.

Plunkett, K., & Marchman, V. A. (1993). From rote learning to system building: Acquiring verb morphology in children and connectionist nets. *Cognition, 48,* 21–69.

Price, C. J., & Friston, K. J. (1997). Cognitive conjunction: A new approach to brain activation experiments. *Neuroreport, 5,* 261–70.

Price, C. J., Moore, C. J., Humphreys, G. W., & Wise, R. J. S. (1997). Segregating semantic from phonological processes during reading. *Journal of Cognitive Neuroscience, 9,* 727–33.

Price, C. J., Wise, R. J. S., Watson, J. D. G., Patterson, K., Howard, D., & Frackowiak, R. S. J. (1994). Brain activity during reading. The effects of exposure duration and task. *Brain, 117,* 1255–69.

Raichle, M. E. (1983). Positron emission tomography. *Annual Review of Neuroscience, 6,* 249–67.

Raichle, M. E. (1987). Circulatory and metabolic correlates of brain function in normal humans. In B. V. Mountcastle, F. Plum, & S. R. Geiger (Eds.), *Handbook of Physiology, The Nervous System, V. Higher Functions of the Brain,* pp. 643–74. Bethesda, MD: American Physiological Society.

Raichle, M. E., Martin, M. R. W., Herscovitch, P., et al. (1983). Brain blood flow measured with intravenous $H_2{}^{15}O$, II: Implementation and validation. *Journal of Nuclear Medicine, 24,* 790–8.

Rees, G., Howseman, A., Josephs, O., Frith, C. D., Friston, K. J., Frackowiak, R. S. J., & Turner, R. (1997). Characterizing the relationship between BOLD contrast and regional cerebral blood flow measurements by varying the stimulus presentation rate. *Neuroimage, 6,* 270–8.

Reiman, E. M. (1990). PET, panic disorder, and the study of anxiety. In J. C. Ballenger (Ed.), *Neurobiology of Panic Disorder,* pp. 245–70. New York: Wiley-Liss.

Reiman, E. M. (1997). The application of positron emission tomography to the study of normal and pathological emotions. *Journal of Clinical Psychiatry, 58,* 4–12.

Reiman, E. M., Caselli, R. J., Lang, S. Y., Chen, K., Bandy, D., Minoshima, S., Thibodeau, S. N., & Osborne, D. (1996). Preclinical evidence of Alzheimer's disease in persons homozygous for the ε4 allele for apolipoprotein E. *New England Journal of Medicine, 334,* 752–8.

Reiman, E. M., Lane, R. D., Ahern, G. L., Schwartz, G. E., Davidson, R. J., Friston, K. J., Yun, L.-S., & Chen, K. (1997). Neuroanatomical correlates of externally and internally generated human emotion. *American Journal of Psychiatry, 154,* 918–25.

Reivich, M., Kuhl, D., Wolf, A., et al. (1979). The [18F] fluorodeoxyglucose method for the measurement of local cerebral glucose utilization in man. *Circulation Research, 44,* 127–37.

Richter, W., Andersen, P. M., Georgopoulos, A. P., & Kim, S. G. (1997). Sequential activity in human motor areas during a delayed cued finger movement task studied by time-resolved fMRI. *Neuroreport, 8,* 1257–61.

Riehle, A., Grun, S., Diesmann, M., & Aertsen, A. (1997). Spike synchronization and rate modulation differentially involved in motor cortical function. *Science, 278,* 1950–3.

Roland, R. E., Larsen, B., Lassen, N. A., & Skinhoj, E. (1980). Supplementary motor area and other cortical areas in organization of voluntary movements in man. *Journal of Neurophysiology, 43,* 118–36.

Rosen, B. R., Buckner, R. L., & Dale, A. M. (1998). Event-related MRI: Past, present, and future. *Proceedings of the National Academy of Sciences U.S.A., 95,* 773–80.

Rugg, M. D., & Doyle, M. C. (1994). Event-related potentials and stimulus repetition in direct and indirect tests of memory. In H.-J. Heinze, T. F. Munte, & G. R. Mangun (Eds.), *Cognitive Electrophysiology,* pp. 124–48. Boston: Birkhäuser.

Rugg, M. D., Fletcher, P. C., Frith, C. D., Frackowiak, R. S. J., & Dolan, R. J. (1997). Brain regions supporting intentional and incidental memory – A PET study. *Neuroreport, 8,* 1283–7.

Rumsey, J. M., Nace, K., Donohue, B., Wise, D., Maisog, J. M., & Andreason, P. (1997). A positron tomographic study of impaired word recognition and phonological processing in dyslexic men. *Archives of Neurology, 54,* 562–73.

Saha, G. B., MacIntyre, W. J., & Go, R. T. (1992). Cyclotron and positron emission tomography radiopharmaceuticals for clinical imaging. *Seminars in Nuclear Medicine, 22,* 150–61.

Sarter, M., Berntson, G. G., & Cacioppo, J. T. (1996). Brain imaging and cognitive neuroscience: Toward strong inference in attributing function to structure. *American Psychologist, 51,* 13–21.

Schacter, D. L., & Tulving, E. (1994). *Memory Systems 1994.* Cambridge, MA: MIT Press.

Schacter, D. L., Uecker, A., Reiman, E., Yun, L.-S., Bandy, D., Chen, K., Cooper, L. A., & Curran, T. (1997). Effects of size and orientation change on hippocampal activation during episodic recognition: A PET study. *Neuroreport, 8,* 3993–8.

Schwaiger, M. (1995). Left ventricular failure. In Wagner, Szabo, & Buchanan, pp. 826–37.

Schwartz, W. J., Smith, C. B., Davidsen, L., et al. (1979). Metabolic mapping of functional activity in the hypothalamoneurohypophysial system of the rat. *Science, 205,* 723–5.

Sedvall, G., Farde, L., Persson, A., et al. (1986). Imaging of neurotransmitter receptors in the living human brain. *Archives of General Psychiatry, 43,* 995–1005.

Seitz, R. J., Bohm, C., Greitz, T., et al. (1990). Accuracy and precision of the computerized brain atlas programme for localization and quantification in positron emission tomography. *Journal of Cerebral Blood Flow and Metabolism, 10,* 188–99.

Senkfor, A. J., & Van Petten, C. (1999). Who said what? Electrophysiological dissociations of source and item memory. *Journal of Experimental Psychology: Learning, Memory, and Cognition, 21,* 1005–25.

Sherrington, C. S. (1940). *On Man and His Nature.* Cambridge University Press.

Silverman, D. H., Hoh, C. K., Seltzer, M. A., Schiepers, C., Cuan, G. S., Gambhir, S. S., Zheng, L., Czernin, J., & Phelps, M. E. (1998). Evaluating tumor biology and oncological disease with positron-emission tomography. *Seminars in Radiation Oncology, 8,* 183–96.

Smith, G. S., Dewey, S. L., Brodie, J. D., et al. (1997). Serotonergic modulation of dopamine measured with [11C]raclopride and PET in normal human subjects. *American Journal of Psychiatry, 154,* 490–6.

Smith, G. S., Schloesser, R., Brodie, J. D., et al. (1998). Glutamate modulation of dopamine measured in vivo with positron emission tomography (PET) and 11C-raclopride in normal human subjects. *Neuropsychopharmacology, 18,* 18–25.

Sokoloff, L., Reivich, M., Kennedy, C., et al. (1977). The [14C]deoxyglucose method for the measurement of local cerebral glucose utilization: Theory, procedure and normal values in the conscious and anesthetized albino rat. *Journal of Neurochemistry, 28,* 897–916.

Stocklin, G. (1995). Fluorine-18 compounds. In Wagner, Szabo, & Buchanan, pp. 178–94.

Swick, D., & Knight, R. T. (1996). Is prefrontal cortex involved in cued recall? A neurophysiological test of PET findings. *Neuropsychologia, 34,* 1019–28.

Swick, D., & Knight, R. T. (1997). Event-related potentials differentiate the effects of aging on word and nonword repetition in explicit and implicit memory tasks. *Journal of Experimental Psychology: Learning, Memory, and Cognition, 23,* 123–42.

Szelies, B., Herhlz, K., Pawlik, G., Karbe, H., Hebold, I., & Heiss, W.-D. (1991). Widespread functional effects of discrete thalamic infarction. *Archives of Neurology, 48,* 178–82.

Talairach, J., Szikla, G., Tournoux, P., et al. (1967). *Atlas d'Anatomie Stereotaxique du Telencephale.* Paris: Masson.

Talairach, J., & Tournoux, P. (1988). *Co-Planar Stereotaxic Atlas of the Human Brain.* New York: Thieme Medical Publishers.

Tanaka, N., Josephs, O., Friston, K., & Frackowiak, R. S. J. (1998). Cortical responses to single episodes of mechanical pain: an event-related fMRI and PET study. *Neuroimage, 7,* S421.

Thompson-Schill, S. L., D'Esposito, M., Aguirre, G. K., & Farah, M. J. (1997). Role of left inferior prefrontal cortex in retrieval of semantic knowledge: A reevaluation. *Proceedings of the National Academy of Sciences U.S.A., 94,* 14792–7.

Thompson-Schill, S. L., Swick, D., Farah, M. J., D'Esposito, M., Kan, I. P., & Knight, R. T. (1998). Verb generation in patients with focal frontal lesions: A neuropsychological test of neuroimaging findings. *Proceedings of the National Academy of Sciences U.S.A., 95*, 15855–60.

Tootel, R. B. H., Dale, A. M., Sereno, M. I., & Malach, R. (1996). New images from human visual cortex. *Trends in Neurosciences, 19*, 481–9.

Townsend, D. W. (1991). Optimization of signal in positron emission tomography scans: Present and future developments. In D. J. Chadwick & J. Whelan (Eds.), *Exploring Brain Functional Anatomy with Positron Emission Tomography* (Ciba Foundation Symposium no. 163), pp. 57–75. West Sussex, U.K.: Wiley.

Tulving, E., Markowitsch, H. J., Craik, F. I. M., Habib, R., & Houle, S. (1996). Novelty and familiarity activations in PET studies of memory encoding and retrieval. *Cerebral Cortex, 6*, 71–9.

Van Petten, C., Reiman, E., & Senkfor, A. J. (1995). PET and ERP measures of semantic and repetition priming [Abstract]. *Psychophysiology, 32*, S81.

Van Petten, C., & Senkfor, A. J. (1996). Memory for words and novel visual patterns: Repetition, recognition, and encoding effects in the event-related brain potential. *Psychophysiology, 33*, 491–506.

Van Petten, C., Weckerly, J., McIsaac, H., & Kutas, M. (1997). Working memory capacity dissociates lexical and sentential context effects. *Psychological Science, 8*, 238–42.

Volkow, N. D., Mullani, N. A., Gould, L. K., et al. (1991). Sensitivity of measurements of regional brain activation with oxygen-15 water and PET to time of stimulation and period of image reconstruction. *Journal of Nuclear Medicine, 32*, 58–61.

Wagner, H. N., Szabo, Z., & Buchanan, J. W. (Eds.) (1995). *Principles of Nuclear Medicine*. Philadelphia: Saunders.

Wise, R., Chollet, F., Hadar, U., Friston, K., Hoffner, E., & Frackowiak, R. (1991). Distribution of cortical neural networks involved in word comprehension and word retrieval. *Brain, 114*, 1803–17.

Woldorff, M. G. (1993). Distortion of ERP averages due to overlap from temporally adjacent ERPs: Analysis and correction. *Psychophysiology, 30*, 98–119.

Wong, D. F., Gjedde, A., & Wagner, H. N., Jr. (1986). Quantification of neuroreceptors in the living human brain. I. Irreversible binding of ligands. *Journal of Cerebral Blood Flow and Metabolism, 6*, 137–46.

Wong, D. F., & Resnick, S. M. (1995). Mental illness: Neurotransmission. In Wagner, Szabo, & Buchanan, pp. 590–4.

Wong, E. C., Buxton, R. B., & Frank, L. R. (1996). Quantitative perfusion imaging using EPISTAR and FAIR. *Proceedings of the ISMRM 4th Annual Meeting*. New York.

Wong, E. C., Buxton, R. B., & Frank, L.R. (1997). Implementation of quantitative perfusion imaging techniques for functional brain mapping using pulsed arterial spin labeling. *NMR in Biomedicine, 10*, 237–49.

Woods, R. P., Cherry, S. R., & Mazziotta, J. C. (1992). Rapid automated algorithm for aligning and reslicing PET images. *Journal of Computer Assisted Tomography, 16*, 620–33.

Woods, R. P., Cherry, S. R., & Mazziotta, J. C. (1993). MRI–PET registration with automated algorithm. *Journal of Computer Assisted Tomography, 17*, 536–46.

Worsley, K. J., Evans, A. C., Marrett, S., & Neelin, P. (1992). A three-dimensional statistical analysis for CBF activation studies in the human brain. *Journal of Cerebral Blood Flow and Metabolism, 12*, 900–18.

Yun, L.-S. (1996). Scattered data modeling and deformation with transfinite constraints. Dissertation, Arizona State University, Tempe.

Zarahn, E., Aguirre, G., & D'Esposito, M. (1997). A trial-based experimental design for fMRI. *Neuroimage, 6*, 122–38.

CHAPTER FIVE

NEUROPSYCHOLOGY AND BEHAVIORAL NEUROLOGY

DANIEL TRANEL & ANTONIO R. DAMASIO

Introduction: Historical Context

Neuropsychology and *behavioral neurology* are terms designating related fields that have developed at the interface of clinical practice and scientific inquiry in the general domain of brain–behavior relationships. The principal objectives of these fields are to diagnose and manage brain disease and consequent neuropsychological dysfunction and to establish the neural basis of cognition and behavior.

For centuries, humans have evidenced a remarkable preoccupation with understanding their own brains – how they develop, how they are put together, how they work, what happens when they are damaged. Philosophers, anthropologists, and scientists from fields such as neurology and psychology (to name but two) have held a long-standing fascination with the relationship between the brain and behavior – in particular, with the enigmatic question of how brain and mind are related, or what is known classically as the "mind–body" problem. Answers have been presented and defended passionately, ranging from monism to dualism and including theories bizarre and absurd. Proponents have suffered persecution, castigation, expatriation and worse at the hands of politicians, religious zealots, and others who were outraged that human existence might be reduced to a fifteen hundred–gram mass of nerve fibers. Nonetheless, the curiosity has never waned entirely; now, in the fading twilight of the twentieth century, the study of brain–behavior relationships is very much a centerpiece of modern science.

Scientific consideration of brain–behavior relationships can be traced to a number of landmark observations beginning more than a century ago (see Benton 1988 for review). In the 1860s, Paul Broca (1865) reported on a patient, known as "Tan," who developed an inability to produce speech following damage to the left front part of the brain. The discovery led to the suggestion, at the time quite radical, that we humans speak with the left side of our brains. A few years later, Carl Wernicke reported a complementary finding: damage to the posterior part of the left hemisphere rendered patients unable to comprehend speech while leaving speech production relatively unaffected; this led to a remarkably prescient neurological model of language (Wernicke 1874), the essence of which is still a leading heuristic in clinical neurology and neuropsychology. About the same time, John Harlow (1868) reported on the case of Phineas Gage, who developed an unusual and seemingly unbelievable focal impairment in personality and social conduct following an accident in which an iron bar exploded through the front part of his brain, destroying prefrontal cortex bilaterally.

The study of brain–behavior relationships enjoyed another period of remarkable progress following World War II, due in some measure to the ravages of war, which provided a grim service to researchers by producing a large number of suitable subjects for careful experimentation – that is, persons who had sustained focal and stable brain wounds that could be correlated with performances on cognitive psychological tests (Newcombe 1969). In fact, this approach (which has come to be known as the "lesion method") has remained the methodological workhorse in systems-level cognitive neuroscience.

Other developments – centered around key case studies – can be cited. In 1957, Scoville and Milner reported for the first time on the patient known as HM, who developed severe and permanent anterograde amnesia (learning impairment) following bilateral resection of the mesial temporal lobes, which was done to control intractable epilepsy. Careful neuropsychological studies of HM yielded a number of key breakthroughs in our understanding of the neural basis of memory and, in particular, focused attention on the role of the mesial temporal region (especially the hippocampus and related structures in entorhinal, perirhinal,

John T. Cacioppo, Louis G. Tassinary, and Gary G. Berntson (Eds.), *Handbook of Psychophysiology*, 2nd ed. © Cambridge University Press 2000. Printed in the United States of America. ISBN 62634X.

and parahippocampal cortices) in memory. Studies by Roger Sperry, in collaboration with Joseph Bogen and Michael Gazzaniga (e.g. Gazzaniga 1987; Sperry 1968), sparked interest in the dramatic differences between the two hemispheres of the brain. These investigators showed that "split brain" patients, who had undergone surgical separation of the two hemispheres for control of seizures, retained two more or less separate modes of consciousness: one in the left hemisphere that was language-based and operated in sequential, analytical style; and one in the right hemisphere that was spatially based and operated in gestalt, holistic style. In the modern era, the trend has continued with prototypical cases such as EVR (Eslinger & Damasio 1985), NA (Squire & Moore 1979; Teuber, Milner, & Vaughan 1968), and Boswell (Damasio et al. 1985a).

Neuropsychology's emphasis on case studies prompted understandable concern that findings might not generalize or might not even prove repeatable. To a large extent, this criticism has been assuaged in modern-era studies, which have managed to assemble larger groups of brain-damaged patients and to put various hypotheses to rigorous empirical test. Nonetheless, the skeptics performed the important function of calling attention to the importance in neuropsychological research of factors such as overall intelligence, age, gender, and handedness. Other issues that have occupied the focus of contentious polemics in the field include the debate between localizationists and antilocalizationists, the notions of redundancy and equipotentiality, and the concepts of centers and networks (Geschwind 1965; Lashley 1950; for a review see Benton & Tranel in press). These debates have been constructive in focusing the field on key issues and in fueling theoretical refinements; on the practical side, they have facilitated the development of empirically driven rehabilitation programs.

It is worth highlighting some of the themes that have dominated the history of behavioral neurology and neuropsychology. Consider the age-old debate between localizationists and antilocalizationists, which was firmly joined more than a century ago. The localizationist side was exemplified – some might say caricatured – by the notion of *phrenology*, a system of brain–behavior relationships articulated by Franz Josef Gall and Johann Spurzheim in the late eighteenth and early nineteenth centuries. Gall and Spurzheim (Spurzheim 1815) outlined in detail how 27 different cognitive functions and personality traits were subserved by specific brain regions. Phrenology was based on skull saliencies, and bumps on the skull were used as clues about underlying brain specialization. For example, Gall noted that his classmates with superior memory had prominent eyes and reasoned that this was the result of overdevelopment of underlying brain regions that were important for memory. The notion of phrenology has been highly controversial since its inception. Not only did the phrenological maps contain a degree of detail about

cerebral localization that far outstripped the empirical evidence, but the evidence itself – correlations between skull bumps and mental capacities – bordered on the absurd. Another problem with phrenology was the inclusion of traits such as "God and religion" and "love for one's offspring." Not only was there poor consensus about the meaning of such constructs, their religious connotations attracted rancorous criticism, especially from those disturbed by the antidualistic nature of Gall's position.

The antilocalizationist position was exemplified by investigators such as Pierre Flourens, who argued that all parts of the brain subserved all perceptual, intellectual, and volitional functions equally (Flourens 1846). Flourens supported his claims with results from ablation experiments, which showed that the crucial factor determining how an organism was affected by brain damage was the extent of tissue removed (*size* of lesion) and not its location. Complete removal of brain lobes resulted in a complete loss of function; large but incomplete damage created a partial loss of function; but with smaller removals there was a complete recovery of function. The findings emphasized the notion of *redundancy* in brain–behavior relationships, a concept that was recapitulated several decades later in Karl Lashley's notion of equipotentiality (e.g. Lashley 1929).

In short, localizationists assigned specific functions to specific brain regions; the antilocalizationists insisted that the cerebral hemispheres operated as a unity, without specific specialization of function. This debate has been revisited at regular junctures throughout the twentieth century, often in ways that resembled the polemics of the nineteenth century. For example, discoveries such as those of Broca and Wernicke were countered by experiments such as those of Lashley demonstrating that all areas of the cerebral cortex were equally important for complex learning and memory. Echoing the ideas of Flourens, Lashley argued that the degree of behavioral impairment following a brain lesion was simply proportional to the amount of brain tissue that had been destroyed, with location being less important or perhaps entirely irrelevant. Lashley emphasized the key ideas of redundancy and equipotentiality.

A somewhat different form of redundancy was postulated by Hughlings Jackson (1870, 1873) in his hierarchical conception of the organization of the nervous system. In Jackson's scheme, sensory and motor functions were represented at each "level," with more complex aspects of function being represented at the highest level of nervous structure. However, the highest level also included nerve fibers from lower levels, making for "multiple representation" of a function at that level. As a consequence, a lesion at the highest level left many fibers intact and produced less (or no) impairment in some functions as compared to the same lesion placed at a lower level. "Hence large destroying lesions in the hemisphere will result in no palsy, whereas palsy will follow lesions equally large in the corpus striatum. No fact is better recognized than that a large part of one cerebral hemisphere may be destroyed when there are no obvious symptoms of any kind" (Jackson 1873). Thus, Jackson invoked a redundancy of neural elements to explain the sparing of certain elementary functions following brain injury. Still another form of redundancy was implied by Jackson's dictum that the behavioral capacities of a brain-lesioned patient were more an expression of the properties of the spared regions of the brain than of the lesioned area. The idea was applied primarily to account for differences in the extent of recovery from motor and speech impairments that were observed between younger and older patients, but in principle it could apply to all individual differences in brain capacity.

It is interesting to note that the fundamental idea popularized by Gall – that specific brain regions are specialized for specific mental functions – has probably turned out to be more right than wrong. In fact, a sort of "neophrenology" appears to be still very much alive and well. One would be hard-pressed to distinguish between some claims being made currently (e.g., that a religious "center" has been discovered in a particular region of the left temporal lobe; Ramachandran et al. 1997) and some of the ideas elaborated in Gall's phrenological system. We would caution against such extreme claims, but at the same time there is no question that, over the last couple of decades, systems neuroscience has yielded a cascade of breakthroughs supporting remarkably detailed brain–behavior relationships and has done so with a degree of precision that would have been virtually impossible to predict in the era prior to the advent of modern neuroimaging.

Physical Context: A Framework for Discussing the Neuroanatomical Basis of Higher Brain Functions

We turn now to a brief description of our framework of neural architecture subserving higher brain functions, which has been set forth in detail in previous publications (Damasio 1989a,b; Damasio & Damasio 1993, 1994); see Figure 1.

THE FRAMEWORK

The framework is governed by two sets of constraints: (i) neurobiological constraints, which correspond to basic neuroanatomical and structural features of the nervous system; and (ii) reality constraints, which correspond to characteristics of physical structure, operation, and frequency of various entities and events, as well as various combinations of entities and events.

When the brain interacts with the environment, these two sets of constraints lead to the following processes:

1. *domain formation,* which refers to a process whereby entities are categorized on the basis of properties such as physical structure, function, frequency, and value;

2. *recording of contextual complexity,* which refers to the formation of records of the temporal and spatial interactions of entities within sets of concurrent events; and

3. *functional regionalization,* which refers to the process whereby potentially fragmented, multimodal records of sensory–motor interactions, as well as the codes that bind the coincidence of such records in time and space, are assigned to relatively segregated brain systems.

The framework specifies a relative functional compartmentalization located in the human brain. One large set of systems, in early sensory cortices and motor cortices, explicitly represents "images" of varied modalities and potential movements. Another set of systems, located in higher-order cortices (e.g., of temporal, parietal, and frontal regions) and in subcortical nuclei such as the basal ganglia and amygdala, orchestrates the construction of those explicit representations in sensorimotor cortices. The latter set of systems promotes activity in separate sensory cortices and helps establish temporal correspondences among these cortices. Yet another set of neural systems ensures the attentional enhancement required for the concerted operation of the others. All of these systems operate under the influence of internal preferences and biases, which are expressed in brain core networks concerned with enacting survival-related biological drives and instincts (see Damasio & Damasio 1994).

The reconstruction of explicit representations of basic entities and actions – for example, an object or a regular sequence of movements – is accomplished in pertinent "early sensory" regions by means of long-range cortico-cortical feedback projections that mediate relatively synchronous excitatory activation. The time scale of the large-scale synchronization paced from higher-order cortices is on the order of several thousand milliseconds, the scale required for meaningful cognition. At more local levels, the scale is on the order of tens of milliseconds.

We have designated the neural device from which reconstructions are conducted as a *convergence zone* (Damasio 1989a,b). A convergence zone is an ensemble of neurons within which many feedforward/feedback loops make contact. A convergence zone: (i) receives forward projections from cortical regions located in the connectional level immediately below; (ii) sends reciprocal backward projections to the originating cortices; (iii) sends forward projections to cortical regions in the next connectional level; and (iv) receives projections from heterarchically placed cortices and from subcortical nuclei in thalamus, basal forebrain, and brainstem.

Knowledge retrieval is based on relatively simultaneous activity in many early cortical regions that is engendered over several recurrences. The result of such recurrences is an explicit representation, which is the basis for an image. In other words, concepts are represented dispositionally

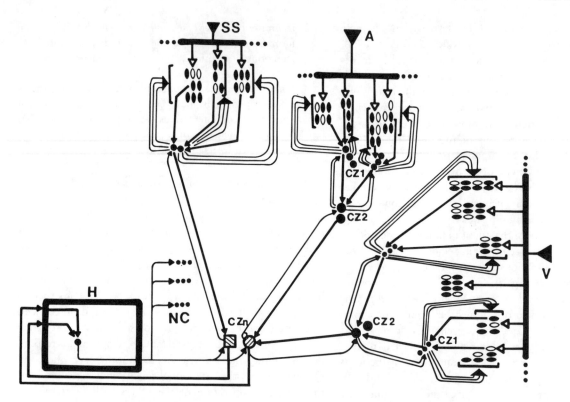

Figure 1. The diagram shows part of the systems architecture required for our framework of higher brain functions. Shown here are pathways directed towards the hippocampus (H), related to access of certain classes of concrete knowledge. Here, V, SS, and A denote early and intermediate sensory cortices in the visual, somatosensory, and auditory modalities, respectively. Separate functional regions within each sector (denoted by open and filled dots) send feedforward projections to various levels of convergence zones (CZ1, CZ2, ..., CZn). The convergence zones reciprocate these projections with feedback projections to the originating regions. Also, there are outputs from H to the last station of feedforward convergence zones (CZn) and to noncortical (NC) neural stations in basal forebrain and brainstem nuclei. Feedforward and feedback connections terminate in distributed fashion across neuron ensembles, not on specific single neurons, and these connections should not be viewed as rigid channels. Reprinted with permission from Damasio, "The brain binds entities and events by multiregional activation from convergence zones," *Neural Computation*, vol. 1, pp. 123–32. Copyright 1989 by MIT Press.

along a series of neural processing stations, and meaning is derived by multiple recurrences and iterations within such a system.

Knowledge can be retrieved at different levels of complexity, ranging from very specific (subordinate) to very broad (superordinate). Consider the following example. Knowledge about the unique dog "Tucker" is specific and unique and hence is considered to be at the subordinate level; less specific and unique knowledge about "dogs" (of which Tucker is an example) is classified at the level of a basic object; and still less specific knowledge concerning "living entities" (of which dogs and Tucker are examples) is classified as superordinate level.

The level at which knowledge is retrieved depends on the scope of multiregional activation, which in turn depends on the level of convergence zone activated. Low-level convergence zones bind signals relative to entity categories (e.g., shape, color, texture) and are placed in association cortices located immediately beyond ("downstream" from) the cortices whose activity defines featural representations. Higher-level convergence zones bind signals relative to more complex combinations and are placed at a higher level in the cortico-cortical hierarchy. The convergence zones capable of binding entities into events and describing their categorization are located at the top or front of the hierarchical streams in anterior temporal and frontal regions.

The *dispositional* representations embodied in convergence zones are the result of previous learning, during which forward projections and reciprocating backward projections were simultaneously active. During learning and retrieval both, the neurons in a convergence zone are under the control of a variety of cortical and noncortical projections. These include projections from thalamus, nonspecific neurotransmitter nuclei, and other cortical projections from convergence zones in prefrontal cortices; cortices located higher up in the feedforward hierarchy; homologous cortices of the opposite hemisphere; and heterarchical cortices of parallel hierarchical streams.

In short, the structures and processes required to store and access dispositional representations must be distinguished from the structures and processes needed for on-line explicit representations. In the framework used here, activation of neuron assemblies in the anterior temporal region does not produce, within the assembly itself, a topographically organized representation. As a consequence, we cannot be made conscious of the activity within anterior temporal cortex itself. Instead, when the neuron assemblies that hold dispositional representations are activated, they lead to the activation of early sensory cortices and cause topographically organized representations to be formed in those cortices. Eventually, we experience the latter as images, which may be less vivid than images produced during perception but not different in their essential nature.

According to our proposal, there is no single site for the integration of sensory and motor processes. Rather, the experience of spatial and temporal integration – that is, our subjective sense of seamless, integrated reality – is brought about by time-locked occurrences that are multiple, recursive, and iterative. There is no localizable single store for the meaning of a given entity or event within a cortical region. Rather, meaning is achieved by widespread multiregional activation of fragmentary records pertinent to a given stimulus and according to a combinatorial code specific or partially specific to the entity. Also, the meaning of an entity, in this sense, is not stored anywhere in the brain in permanent fashion; instead, it is re-created anew for every instantiation. Here, the instantiations may be highly similar (or not) from one occasion to the next, but they are never identical. The records pertinent to a given entity or event are inscribed over synaptic populations and over multiple loci of cerebral cortex and subcortical nuclei.

AN ILLUSTRATION

To illustrate some of the principal ideas of our framework, consider the process whereby we can look at various things and know what those things are. To put this in question form: How is it that we can look at a tool, or an animal, or a familiar person (or pictures of these things) and know what they are – that is, know their meaning (or what is often termed "semantics")? What neural processes support this cognitive operation? In a recent study, we addressed this issue by studying brain-damaged subjects who had lost the ability to recognize different subsets of such entities (Tranel et al. 1997a).

Our empirical observations were that:

1. subjects with damage to the right temporal polar region had defective recognition of familiar persons;
2. subjects with damage to the right mesial occipital/ventral temporal region, or to the left mesial occipital region, had defective recognition of animals; and
3. subjects with damage to the left occipital-temporal-parietal junction had defective recognition of tools.

We concluded that retrieval of knowledge for entities from different conceptual categories depends on partially segregated neural systems. As is typical of lesion experiments, damage to any of these sites did not preclude entirely the performance of a given task. Rather, performance was rendered defective relative to normal, indicating that the damaged areas are needed for optimal regular performance but leaving open the possibility (indeed, likelihood) that other mechanisms of task execution are available.

In the context of our theoretical framework, how does the circuitry at each of the identified sites (right temporal polar, left mesial occipital, etc.) contribute to the retrieval of conceptual knowledge – that is, to the recognition of concrete entities? First, it should be emphasized that we do not believe these neural sites to contain either facsimile representations of entities or lexicographic definitions of the concepts for those entities. Instead, we believe that each neural site is instrumental in generating the recall of separate pieces of knowledge whose collection describes sufficiently the concept of a given entity. The sites operate as catalysts for the retrieval of the multidimensional aspects of knowledge that are necessary and sufficient for the mental representation of a concept of a given entity. Although the retrieval of those separate aspects of knowledge occurs in a spatially segregated manner (as far as neural tissue is concerned), the retrieval is temporally correlated so that what we bring into mind is an integrated, seamless image or concept. Thus, we believe that the sites contain conceptual knowledge, in a dispositional sense, but that the explicit mental representation of the concept does *not* occur at the site. The sites are not "centers" containing conceptual knowledge of persons, animals, or tools. Rather, the sites are part of multicomponent systems, each containing circuitry necessary for the process of optimal concept retrieval.

In our view, conceptual knowledge is held in dispositional form (nonexplicit and nonmapped) in higher-order association cortices and subcortical nuclei within circuitry featuring convergence–divergence connectional properties. Dispositional knowledge coded in convergence/divergence zones can be made explicit (in mapped form) in early sensory cortices and in motor structures. The recall of knowledge pertinent to a particular concept requires the activation of multiple convergence/divergence sites; these sites direct the reconstruction, in pertinent early sensory cortices, of the explicit images that comprise the concept. Activation of early sensory cortices is essential for conscious processing of the concept to occur; however, activation of the primary cortices within the set of early sensory cortices is not essential.

Taking our illustration of conceptual knowledge retrieval one step further, we would suggest that the neural sites identified in our study play an *intermediary* role in concept retrieval. For example, when a stimulus depicting a given tool is shown to the subject and the visual properties of that stimulus are processed, an intermediary region becomes active and promotes the explicit sensorimotor representation of knowledge pertaining to that tool in the appropriate early sensory cortices and motor structures. Sensory images might represent the typical action of the tool in space, its typical relationship to the hand and to other objects, the typical somatosensory and motor patterns associated with the handling of the tool, and the possible sound characteristics associated with the tool's operation. The evocation of some part of the potentially large number of such images, over a brief lapse of time and in varied sensorimotor cortices, would constitute the conceptual evocation for a given tool. When a concept from another category is evoked – for example, that of an animal or a person – a different intermediary region is engaged. Again, note that we do not believe that the intermediary regions for conceptual knowledge contain in explicit form the concepts for concrete entities.

Also, we do not envision the intermediary regions as rigid "modules" or "centers"; rather, their structure and operation are seen as flexible and modifiable by learning. An individual's learning experience of concepts of a similar kind (e.g., concepts of animals) leads to the recruitment, within the available neural architecture, of a critical set of spatially proximate microcircuits. We presume that the anatomical placement of the region within which the microcircuits are recruited for a certain range of items is not random; rather, it is the one best suited to permit the most effective preferential interaction – by means of feedforward and feedback projections – between the regions of cerebral cortex that subtend visual perception and those required to represent explicitly the images that define the pertinent conceptual knowledge. The number of microcircuits recruited to operate as intermediaries for a certain range of concepts would vary with the learning experience. We would expect normal individuals to develop, under similar conditions, a similar type of large-scale architecture; however, we would also predict ample individual variation of microcircuitry within each key region, so that – at different times – the same individual would engage the same macroregions but not necessarily the same microcircuitry within them.

Finally, why is it that retrieval of concepts for different kinds of entities would be correlated with different neural sites? One reason is the overall physical characteristics of the entities in question, which would determine the sort of sensorimotor mapping generated during interactions between an organism and the entity as it was learned. Another reason involves the detailed physical characteristics and contextual linkages of entities, which would permit the mapping of certain unique items, such as familiar persons. Take for example a tool such as a saw. The multiple sensory channels (somatosensory, visual) and the hand motor patterns inherent in the conceptual description of the saw would lead to the preferential recruitment of a sector of cortex that is (i) capable of receiving such multiple sensory signals and (ii) close to regions involved in the processing of visual motion and hand motion.

Social and Psychological Context: Brain–Behavior Relationships

We turn now to a discussion of brain–behavior relationships. The discussion is not intended to be comprehensive; rather, we have chosen several topics that illustrate the key principles set forth in the foregoing section. Specifically, we focus on examples from the domains of executive functions and social conduct, emotion, memory, and perception and recognition.

EXECUTIVE FUNCTIONS AND SOCIAL CONDUCT

The term "executive functions" has been used to denote a set of loosely related cognitive and behavioral capacities that include judgment, planning, decision making, and social conduct. These capacities are linked intimately to the prefrontal region of the brain; in fact, it is not uncommon to see these abilities referred to as "frontal lobe" functions (Tranel, Anderson, & Benton 1994a). Executive functions are at the pinnacle of the cognitive hierarchy and draw upon virtually all other cognitive capacities, including perception, memory, and emotion. Social conduct can be considered an executive function that is a conflation of the other functions. In particular, social conduct depends critically on judgment and decision making, and (like other executive functions) social conduct is linked closely to the prefrontal lobes.

Acquired Sociopathy

As alluded to in our earlier mention of Harlow's seminal case of Phineas Gage, investigators throughout the history of neuropsychology have called attention to the dramatic changes in social behavior that occur subsequent to injuries to the prefrontal region of the brain (Brickner 1934; Eslinger & Damasio 1985; Harlow 1868; Hebb & Penfield 1940; Luria 1969; Stuss & Benson 1986). As case reports accrued over the past century, it became apparent that the affected patients have a number of features in common (see Damasio & Anderson 1993): inability to organize future activity and hold gainful employment, diminished capacity to respond to punishment, a tendency to present an unrealistically favorable view of themselves, a tendency to display inappropriate (or absent) emotional reactions, and normal intelligence. Several of these features are highly reminiscent of the personality profile associated with sociopathy, and we have actually gone so far as to dub this condition "acquired sociopathy" (Damasio, Tranel, & Damasio 1990c).

Others have called attention to such characteristics in patients with ventromedial prefrontal lobe damage. For example, Blumer and Benson (1975) noted a personality type characteristic of patients with orbital damage (which the authors termed "pseudo-psychopathic") in which salient features were puerility, a jocular attitude, sexually disinhibited humor, inappropriate and near-total self-indulgence, and complete lack of concern for others. Stuss and Benson (1986) emphasized that such patients demonstrate a remarkable lack of empathy and general lack of concern about others. The patients tend to show callous unconcern, boastfulness, and unrestrained and tactless behavior. Other descriptors include impulsiveness, facetiousness, and diminished anxiety and concern for the future.

Patients with ventromedial prefrontal lesions and acquired sociopathy demonstrate a proclivity to make decisions and engage in behaviors that have negative consequences for their own well-being. The patients are usually not destructive and harmful to others in society (a feature that distinguishes the "acquired" form of the disorder from the standard "developmental" form); however, they repeatedly opt for courses of action that are not in their best interest in the long run. They make poor decisions about interpersonal relationships, occupational endeavors, and finances. In short, they act as though they have lost the ability to ponder different courses of action and then select the option that promises the best blend of short- and long-term benefit. What makes this manifestation all the more striking – and what has defied simple explanation ever since the days of Harlow – is that most of the patients retain normal intelligence, conventional memory, language, perception, attention, and so on. In other words, there are no obvious neuropsychological impairments that might account parsimoniously for the erratic behavior.

The Somatic Marker Hypothesis

We have proposed a somatic marker hypothesis to account for the bizarre changes in social conduct, planning, and decision making that typify patients with ventromedial prefrontal damage (Damasio 1994, 1995, 1996; Damasio et al. 1990c). At the center of the hypothesis is the idea that what these patients have lost (as a consequence of their brain damage) – and what causes problems with planning and decision making – is the capacity to use emotions and feelings to help guide behavior. Emotional changes are termed "somatic states" in our account, following the ideas that (i) emotion is expressed most importantly through changes in the representation of body state and (ii) the results of emotion are primarily represented in the brain in the form of transient changes in the activity pattern of somatosensory structures. The somatic marker hypothesis provides a neurobiological explanation for this phenomenon, proposing that the patients do not have access to somatic guideposts that normally mark various behavioral alternatives as positive or negative and so facilitate advantageous decision making.

We see structures in ventromedial prefrontal cortex as providing the substrate for learning associations between complex situations and the types of bioregulatory states (including emotional states) usually associated with such situations in prior experience. Hence, the ventromedial region holds linkages between the facts that comprise a given situation and the emotion previously paired with that situation in an individual's experience. Following the general framework outlined previously, the linkages are "dispositional": they do not explicitly hold the representations of the facts or of the emotional state but instead hold the potential to reactivate an emotion by evoking activity in the pertinent cortical and subcortical structures. In short, the ventromedial sector performs a memory function: it establishes a linkage between the disposition for a certain aspect of a situation and the disposition for the type of emotion that (in the individual's experience) has been associated with the situation.

When a situation arises – say, a social scenario requiring certain decisions and courses of action (e.g., a holiday party at the boss's house) – dispositions are activated in higher-order association cortices, leading to the recall of pertinent facts and other related knowledge. The related ventromedial prefrontal linkages are activated concurrently, leading to the consequent activation of the emotional disposition apparatus (e.g., various limbic structures, such as the amygdala, cingulate, and insular cortex). The net result is a reconstruction of a previously learned factual–emotional set. We have proposed that the reactivation of the emotional disposition network can occur via either: (1) a *body loop,* in which somatic units (e.g., musculoskeletal, visceral, and other internal milieu components of the soma) actually change, with the changes being relayed to somatosensory cortices; or (2) an *"as if" loop,* in which the reactivation signals bypass the body and are relayed to the somatosensory cortices directly, with the latter adopting the appropriate pattern without bodily input. Finally, we have emphasized that the establishment of a somatosensory pattern, whether it be via the body loop or via the "as if" loop, can occur either overtly or covertly.

The somatosensory pattern evoked by a particular situation is co-displayed with factual knowledge pertinent to the situation. Insofar as decision making is concerned, here is the key idea: The somatosensory pattern operates to constrain the process of reasoning over multiple options and multiple future outcomes. Specifically, when the somatosensory image that defines a particular emotional response is juxtaposed to images that describe a particular scenario of a future outcome, the pattern *marks* the scenario as good or bad. In short, the images of the scenario are judged, and marked, by the juxtaposed images of the somatic state. Engaged in a complex decision-making space, this process greatly facilitates the operation of logical reasoning. The somatic markers allow certain option–outcome pairs to be rapidly endorsed or rejected. The decision-making space is made manageable for a logic-based cost–benefit analysis. Also, when there is a high degree of uncertainty regarding the future and regarding which course of action is optimal, the constraints imposed by somatic markers allow the individual to decide efficiently within reasonable time intervals. This would apply in particular to many complex social situations and the on-line navigation required in such situations.

In the characteristic absence of somatic markers in patients with ventromedial prefrontal injuries, response options and outcomes become somewhat equalized, and the process of deciding on an option will depend entirely on logic operations over many potential alternatives. This strategy can be extremely slow and laborious and may fail to take into account previous experience. As a consequence, decision making is neither timely, accurate, nor propitious; it may even be random or impulsive. The somatic marker hypothesis goes against popular and scientific lore that reasoning and decision making are optimal when a person is cool, calm, and calculated – in short, *un*emotional – and explains why too little emotion is no less deleterious for decision making than too much emotion.

The somatic marker hypothesis has received empirical support from recent studies of patients with ventromedial prefrontal damage. First, it was shown that – when playing a gambling game in which certain decisions were associated with short-term gain but long-term loss whilst others were associated with short-term loss but long-term gain – patients with ventromedial prefrontal damage opted for short-term gain even though this strategy was costly in the long run (Bechara et al. 1994). In contrast, normal subjects soon catch on to the game and begin pursuing a strategy that maximizes their long-term gains. A follow-up study showed that, unlike normal controls, ventromedial prefrontal patients fail to develop anticipatory skin conductance responses (SCRs) to decisions that turned out to be disadvantageous (Bechara et al. 1996). This absence of anticipatory SCRs was interpreted as a correlate of the patients' insensitivity to future outcomes and as compatible with the idea that patients fail to activate biasing signals that could function as value markers when distinguishing between choices with good versus bad outcomes. We suggested that such biasing signals derive from the bioregulatory machinery that sustains somatic homeostasis and can be expressed in emotion and feeling.

Also, we more recently explored the possibility that the overt reasoning used to decide advantageously in a complex situation would be *preceded* by a nonconscious biasing step that uses neural systems other than those that support declarative knowledge (Bechara et al. 1997; see Figure 2). In this study, normal subjects and patients with ventromedial prefrontal damage and decision-making defects performed the gambling task; behavioral, psychophysiological, and self-report measures were obtained in parallel. The self-report data were used to judge whether subjects had developed a conscious notion of how the game worked, and the behavioral and psychophysiological data were scored accordingly. The results showed that normal subjects began to play the game advantageously (i.e., to make good deci-

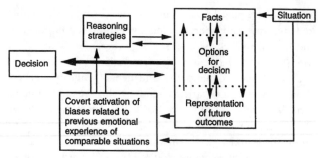

Figure 2. Diagram of our proposal for the steps involved in decision making. We have suggested that the sensory representation of a situation that requires a decision leads to two parallel, interacting chains of events. In one, the sensory representation of a particular situation, or a representation of the facts evoked by the situation, activates neural systems that hold nondeclarative dispositional knowledge related to the individual's previous emotional experience of similar situations. We believe the ventromedial prefrontal cortices are key structures holding such knowledge. Activation of these prefrontal cortices in turn activates autonomic and neurotransmitter nuclei, and the ensuing nonconscious signals act as covert biases influencing the circuits that support the processes of cognitive evaluation and reasoning. In the other chain, the representation of a particular situation generates: (1) overt recall of pertinent facts, especially those regarding various response options and future outcomes related to courses of action that might be taken in regard to the situation; and (2) the application of deliberate reasoning strategies to facts and options. Reprinted with permission from Bechara, Damasio, Tranel, & Damasio, "Deciding advantageously before knowing the advantageous strategy," *Science*, vol. 275, pp. 1293-5. Copyright 1997 American Association for the Advancement of Science.

sions) before they realized, in any sort of conscious fashion, which strategy worked best. The prefrontal patients, however, continued to play disadvantageously even after they knew the correct strategy. Also, normal subjects began to generate anticipatory SCRs whenever they pondered a decision that turned out to be risky *before* they knew explicitly (consciously) that it was, in fact, a risky decision. The prefrontal patients never developed anticipatory SCRs, although some of them did eventually realize which decisions were risky. We interpreted these results to suggest that (i) in normal individuals, nonconscious biases guide behavior before conscious knowledge does, and (ii) without the help of such biases, overt knowledge may be insufficient to ensure advantageous behavior (Bechara et al. 1997). Some interesting studies in social psychology have led to a similar notion – namely, that individuals can learn and make decisions with information that is not available to conscious awareness (see e.g. Lewicki, Hill, & Czyzewska 1992).

EMOTION AND AFFECT

Neuroscientific inquiry into the domain of emotion has enjoyed renewed popularity in the past several years (see Nadel & Lane in press). Empirical breakthroughs and theoretical developments alike have abounded and, after decades of neglect from the neuroscience community, the domain of emotion has become one of the most popular areas of study in the field.

Recognition of Emotion in Facial Expressions

Perhaps one of the most intriguing findings to emerge in recent years in the neuroscience of emotion is the curious but remarkably robust link between the amygdala and the processing of facial emotional expressions, particularly expressions with negative affective valence (e.g., fear or anger). This link has been established in lesion studies, which have shown that bilateral amygdala damage impairs the ability to recognize fear in faces (Adolphs et al. 1994, 1995; Calder et al. 1996; Young et al. 1995), and in functional imaging studies, which have shown that the amygdala is selectively activated in normal subjects by the perception of fear faces (Breiter et al. 1996; Morris et al. 1996). The link appears to be multimodal: one study has shown that bilateral amygdala damage impaired the ability to recognize fear in auditory stimuli (Scott et al. 1997), and another study showed activation of the amygdala by unpleasant olfactory stimuli (Zald & Pardo 1997).

Why should this be the case? We have presented a preliminary explanation, incorporating the known anatomical arrangements of the amygdala and following the general framework elaborated previously (see Adolphs et al. 1995 and Figure 3). From an anatomical viewpoint, the amygdala projects back to all visual cortices, including the striate cortex, and it is possible that high-level feedback from the amygdala can participate directly in the activity of those regions during perception and visual imagery. Hence, we envision the amygdala as a convergence zone for the social, homeostatic, and survival-related meaning of certain complex stimuli, including some facial expressions. When a fear face is encountered, for example, the amygdala activates a myriad of cortical and subcortical regions whose temporally coordinated activity would then constitute the concept of fear. Important components of this system would include limbic and somatic structures. Also, we see the amygdala as crucially important for processing stimuli that communicate emotional significance in social situations; specifically, the amygdala may orchestrate patterns of neural activation in disparate sectors of the brain that would encode the intrinsic, physical features of stimuli (e.g., shape and position in space) as well as the value that certain stimuli have to the organism, especially emotional significance (Adolphs et al. 1995). In this context, it is instructive to consider several findings from the animal literature. Neurons in the amygdala are active during social interactions (Kling, Steklis, & Deutsch 1979) and social communication (Jurgens 1982). Amygdalectomized monkeys develop social behavioral impairments that are so severe that the animals quickly die if left unattended in the wild (Kling & Brothers 1992). Our take on this is that the integration of complex sensory information (such as the recognition of facial expressions) with the motivational va-

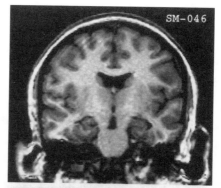
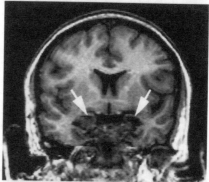
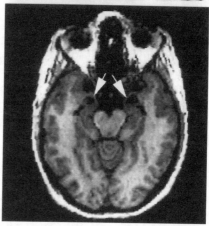

Figure 3. Magnetic resonance images of the brain of patient SM-046. Sections at the level of the amygdala are shown in coronal (middle) and horizontal (bottom) planes; the top panel shows a coronal section at the level of the hippocampus. SM-046 has selective, bilateral damage to the amygdala (arrows). The hippocampus (top) is not affected. The bilateral amygdala lesion resulted in a specific impairment in SM-046's ability to recognize fear in facial expressions. Reprinted with permission from Adolphs, Tranel, Damasio, & Damasio, "Fear and the human amygdala," *Journal of Neuroscience*, vol. 15, pp. 5879–91. Copyright 1995 Society for Neuroscience.

lence of a stimulus is especially important for recognizing social intentions and status and for guiding behavior on the basis of social cues (threats, warnings, submissive gestures).

The amygdala appears to be important for the processing of other information that has emotional significance (Cahill et al. 1995; Markowitsch et al. 1994). For instance, it has been shown that the amygdala is important for classical conditioning of autonomic responses and, in particular, for the acquisition of conditioned responses (behavioral and autonomic) to stimuli that have been paired with an aversive event (Bechara et al. 1995; Davis 1992; LaBar et al. 1995; LeDoux et al. 1990). Bechara and colleagues (1995) found that a patient with circumscribed bilateral amygdala damage (but with normal hippocampi) was able to acquire declarative knowledge normally but was impaired in acquiring conditioned autonomic responses to an aversive loud noise; a patient with circumscribed bilateral hippocampal damage (but with intact amygdalae) showed the opposite pattern, with normal acquisition of autonomic conditioning but impaired declarative knowledge. A more recent study by Adolphs et al. (1997) has extended these findings, showing that two subjects with bilateral amygdala damage had impairments in long-term declarative memory for emotionally arousing material. What the subjects lacked, specifically, was the ability to be influenced by the emotionally arousing nature of to-be-learned stimuli. Normally, such stimuli are learned better than neutral stimuli; however, neither subject with amygdala damage showed such an effect. These findings suggest that the amygdala serves to mediate between the evaluation and experience of emotional events and their acquisition and consolidation into long-term memory.

Anosognosia and Related Conditions

Anosognosia is a condition in which patients lose the ability to recognize disease states in themselves. In the most extreme cases, patients fail to recognize major disabilities such as a complete hemiplegia or hemianesthesia (Babinski 1914). Anosognosia can also occur in relation to cognitive and behavioral deficits (Anderson & Tranel 1989). Patients give no sign of understanding that their cognition and behavior are compromised and fail to appreciate the ramifications of their disabilities. Measurement of anosognosia can be difficult, but in general the term can be applied whenever there is a significant discrepancy between the patient's report of disability and the objective evidence regarding the patient's level of functioning.

Anosognosia is strongly associated with damage to the right somatosensory cortices in the parietal and insular regions. There appears to be a laterality effect for this condition that is of a magnitude comparable to that observed for language, although the results of some studies are probably skewed because aphasic patients are often excluded. Nonetheless, full-blown anosognosia is rarely observed in connection with left-hemisphere lesions, reflecting an arrangement that mirrors the situation regarding language (where there is an overwhelming dominance by the left hemisphere). The ventromedial prefrontal region, including the orbital and lower mesial frontal cortices, is another frequent neural correlate of anosognosia (Damasio et al. 1990c).

Anosodiaphoria, which is closely related to anosognosia, refers to the case where a patient acknowledges – but fails to appreciate the significance of – acquired impairments in physical or psychological function. In practice, there is a certain degree of overlap between anosodiaphoria and anosognosia. It is common to observe that pronounced anosognosia (e.g., complete denial of hemiplegia) tends to evolve over time, as the patient recovers, into anosodiaphoria.

Another related condition is a disorder of body schema (Benton & Sivan 1993) in which patients become unable to localize various parts of their bodies. The most common manifestations are autotopagnosia, finger agnosia, and right–left disorientation (the latter two being essentially partial forms of the former). Autotopagnosia refers to a condition in which the patient loses the ability to identify parts of the body, either to verbal command or by imitation. In its most severe form, the disorder affects virtually all body parts; however, this is quite rare, and it is far more common to observe partial forms of the condition, including deficits in finger localization (finger agnosia) and right–left discrimination.

Anosognosia and the related conditions just mentioned are associated most strongly with damage to right somatosensory cortices – notably, the very regions that are responsible for the external senses of touch, temperature, and pain as well as the internal senses of joint position, visceral state, and pain. These regions have been implicated as comprising the neural network that subserves the mapping of body states (Damasio 1994). Specifically, the somatosensory cortices receive a set of signals hailing from various parts of intra- and extrapersonal space, including signals from visceral and musculoskeletal systems (from both sides of the body) as well as extrapersonal signals pertinent to the current status of the body. These signals find a comprehensive meeting ground in right-hemisphere structures, which include the primary somatosensory region (areas 3, 1, and 2 in the parietal lobe), somatosensory association cortices in the insula, and a secondary somatosensory region known as S2 in the depth of the sylvian fissure. In anosognosia, such signals fail to trigger appropriate neural records. For example, the somatic signals that would denote the presence of a paralyzed leg do not activate the pertinent neural regions that would allow this perception to become conscious. Physiologically, then, anosognosia corresponds to the inability of somatosensory percepts to activate pertinently linked memories that would give them appropriate meaning. There is a disruption of the continually updated representation of normal somatic and psychological states and their placement in autobiographical context (Damasio 1994).

MEMORY

Memory refers to knowledge that is stored in the brain and to the processes of acquiring, storing, and retrieving such knowledge. Memory has a role in human mind and behavior that can hardly be overemphasized, as it contributes to nearly every aspect of higher nervous function, including perception, recognition, language, planning, problem solving, and decision making.

Amnesia refers specifically to an impairment in the ability to learn new information or to retrieve previously acquired knowledge. The impairment of learning is known as *anterograde* amnesia, whereas the impairment in retrieving previously acquired knowledge is known as *retrograde* amnesia, with the demarcation being the point in time at which neurological disease begins. Amnesia is one of the most frequent cognitive impairments suffered by brain-injured individuals (Squire & Shimamura 1996; Tranel & Damasio 1995) and one of the most debilitating. Studies of memory-disordered patients over the past four to five decades – dating back to the pathbreaking work of Scoville and Milner (1957) with patient HM – have yielded important insights into the neural basis of memory, and newer work using functional imaging techniques has also begun to make contributions (see e.g. Dolan & Fletcher 1997; Gabrieli et al. 1997).

Memory and the Mesial Temporal Lobe

The mesial temporal lobe contains several structures that are critical for memory, including the hippocampus, the amygdala, the entorhinal and perirhinal cortices, and part of the parahippocampal gyrus. Damage to some or all of these structures produces characteristic patterns of amnesia (Cohen & Eichenbaum 1993; Corkin 1984; Curran & Schacter 1997; Damasio et al. 1985a; Mishkin 1982; Squire 1992; Tranel & Damasio 1995; Zola 1997). First, there is a consistent (albeit imperfect) correspondence between the side of damage and the type of learning impairment; thus, unilateral lesions tend to produce material-specific amnesia. Specifically, left-sided lesions produce defects primarily in the learning of verbal information (e.g., words or written material) while nonverbal information is largely spared; conversely, right-sided lesions produce defects primarily in the learning of nonverbal material (e.g., complex visual and auditory patterns) while verbal information is largely spared (Milner 1972). Second, the mesial temporal region is critical for the acquisition of new information (anterograde memory), but its role in the retrieval of previously learned knowledge (retrograde memory) is minimal. That is, the ability to retrieve information that was acquired prior to the onset of the lesion is usually spared following damage to mesial temporal structures (Cohen & Eichenbaum 1993; Corkin 1984; Damasio et al. 1985a; O'Connor, Verfaellie, & Cermak 1995). Third, structures in the mesial temporal region are crucial for the acquisition of *declarative* information – knowledge that can be "declared" or brought to mind for conscious inspection (e.g., facts, words, names, faces). However, these structures do not appear to be necessary for the acquisition of *nondeclarative* information, such as sensorimotor skills

(e.g., skiing, dancing) that cannot be declared or brought to mind (Corkin 1965; Gabrieli et al. 1993; Thompson 1986; Tranel & Damasio 1993; Tranel et al. 1994b). In short, patients with damage confined to structures in the mesial temporal region will manifest an anterograde amnesia for declarative knowledge, with the material type (verbal vs. nonverbal) influenced by the side of lesion.

The precise roles of various mesial temporal structures in memory functioning have yet to be clarified, although there is considerable evidence suggesting that the hippocampal formation (defined as inclusive of cell fields of the hippocampus proper, the dentate gyrus, the subicular region, and the entorhinal cortex) is a key component of the mesial temporal system (see Zola 1997). In fact, specific cell fields within the hippocampus proper have been pinpointed as being particularly important, especially the CA1 field (Rempel-Clower et al. 1996; Zola 1997; Zola-Morgan, Squire, & Amaral 1986). Convergent evidence for this position comes from careful studies of the pathology of Alzheimer's disease, which have revealed that – in early stages of the disease – neurofibrillary tangles are present selectively in pivotal way stations for input to and output from the hippocampus (Hyman et al. 1984; Van Hoesen & Damasio 1987).

The role of the amygdala in memory has been controversial. Studies in nonhuman primates have yielded conflicting results, with some (e.g. Mishkin 1978) reporting that the amygdala is critical for normal learning and others indicating that the amygdala does not play a crucial role (Murray & Gaffan 1994; Zola-Morgan et al. 1989). Findings from the few human cases available are also somewhat equivocal (Nahm et al. 1993; Tranel & Hyman 1990). However, more recent studies have shed additional light on this issue, indicating that the amygdala has a role in the learning of information that has significant emotional valence (Bechara et al. 1995; Davis 1992; LaBar et al. 1995; LeDoux et al. 1990).

Memory and the "Nonmesial" Portions of the Temporal Lobe

Structures in the anterior, lateral, and inferior aspects of the temporal lobes, including the polar region and the anterior portion of the second, third, and fourth temporal gyri, can be referred to as "nonmesial" temporal structures, indicating that these structures are separable – functionally as well as anatomically – from those included in the "mesial temporal" designation. Damage to nonmesial portions of the temporal lobe is associated with a memory defect encompassing the retrograde compartment (Cermak & O'Connor 1983; Cohen & Squire 1981; Kapur 1993; Kapur et al. 1994; Kopelman 1992; Markowitsch et al. 1993; Squire & Alvarez 1995). In fact, if the damage spares the mesial temporal region then the memory defect may be confined to the retrograde compartment (Kapur 1993; Kapur et al. 1994; Markowitsch et al. 1993; see Hodges 1995 for a review).

Retrograde amnesia frequently affects retrieval of knowledge for unique material more than knowledge for nonunique material. For instance, a patient may have difficulty retrieving detailed information about such unique episodes as the birth of children, the purchase of a home, or facts about public events; however, the same patient will remain capable of retrieving nonunique knowledge – the meanings of words and the meaning of nonverbal stimuli such as common entities and actions. Structures in the right temporal region may play a predominant role in retrograde memory, with a lesser role for homologous left-sided structures, although this issue has not been extensively studied. However, one laterality effect that is well established regards the verbal specialization of the left side and the parallel nonverbal specialization of the right side. Hence, damage to the left anterior temporal region produces an impairment in the retrieval of words for unique entities (proper nouns) without affecting the capacity to retrieve nonverbal conceptual knowledge about those entities (Damasio et al. 1996), and damage to the homologous right temporal region will produce an impairment in the retrieval of conceptual knowledge for unique persons but not an impairment in the retrieval of unique names (Tranel et al. 1997a).

Memory and the Basal Forebrain

The basal forebrain, situated immediately behind the orbital prefrontal cortices, comprises a set of bilateral paramidline gray nuclei that include the septal nuclei, the diagonal band of Broca, the nucleus accumbens, and the substantia innominata. Damage to this region is frequently caused by ruptured aneurysms of the anterior communicating artery or of the anterior cerebral artery, leading to a characteristic amnesic syndrome (Alexander & Freedman 1984; Damasio et al. 1985b; Deluca & Diamond 1995). One problem in studying this condition, however, is that most of the affected patients have surgical clips that preclude magnetic resonance imaging, limiting the anatomical analysis that can be performed.

Patients with damage to the basal forebrain manifest difficulties in associating specific subcomponents of memory episodes with one another. A patient may recall a particular family event, for example, but place the event entirely out of context with respect to other events that occurred around the same time period. This errant binding of memory episode components affects new learning as well – for example, the patient may learn new faces but associate them with incorrect names. In a striking example of this type of impairment, one of our basal forebrain patients repeatedly set off each morning to a job that she had held some two decades earlier but from which she had long since retired. A related phenomenon is what has been termed "source amnesia" (Schacter, Harbluk, & McLachlan 1984). A patient may learn information (verbal and nonverbal) accurately yet be unable to recall the circumstances under which the learning took place. The patient recalls the content but not the source of the learning experience. One other characteristic of basal forebrain amnesia is that patients have a tendency to produce wild confabulations – for example, making up fantasy stories about various strange adventures that have no basis in fact.

Memory and the Diencephalon

Structures in the diencephalon, particularly the dorsomedial nucleus of the thalamus and the mammillary bodies, play an important role in memory. Damage to these structures produces a severe anterograde amnesia that resembles the amnesia associated with mesial temporal damage. Characteristically, there is a major defect in the acquisition of declarative knowledge while the learning of nondeclarative information is spared. However, more so than with the amnesia associated with mesial temporal lesions, diencephalic amnesia may involve the retrograde compartment as well. This retrograde amnesia tends to have a temporal gradient, so that retrieval of memories acquired closer in time to the onset of the lesion is more severely affected whereas retrieval of more remote memories is better preserved. Severe alcoholism and stroke are two frequent causes of damage to the diencephalon (Butters & Stuss 1989; Graff-Radford et al. 1990). The amnesia that develops after prolonged alcoholism is part of a distinctive condition known as Wernicke–Korsakoff syndrome, which has been extensively studied from both neuroanatomical and neuropsychological perspectives (see e.g. Victor, Adams, & Collins 1989).

Working Memory

Working memory is the short window of mental processing (on the order of minutes) during which information is held "on-line" while operations are performed on it – a sort of "mental scratch pad" (Baddeley 1992). This form of memory is distinguished from short-term memory largely on a conceptual basis: working memory is considered to have a somewhat longer processing frame and a larger capacity than short-term memory (although the two constructs probably overlap and may share neural substrates). Short-term memory covers only the very brief period (on the order of a minute or so) during which a limited amount – the classic seven (plus or minus two) chunks – of information can be held without rehearsal. Working memory is used to bridge temporal gaps, that is, to hold representations in a mental workspace long enough to make appropriate responses to stimulus configurations or contingencies in which some (or even all) of the basic constituents are no longer extant in perceptual space. In essence, working memory is a temporary storage and processing system used for problem solving and other cognitive operations that take place over a limited time frame.

The prefrontal cortex has been implicated in the mediation of working memory (Milner, Petrides, & Smith 1985;

Petrides et al. 1993), particularly in functional imaging studies (Cohen et al. 1997; Courtney et al. 1997; Jonides et al. 1993; McCarthy et al. 1994; Smith et al. 1995). Goldman-Rakic (1987; see also Wilson, O'Scalaidhe, & Goldman-Rakic 1993) has suggested that this may be more or less the exclusive memory function of the entire prefrontal cortex, with different subregions of the prefrontal cortex being connected to particular domains of operations (e.g., verbal working memory, spatial working memory). In fact, there is evidence for left- and right-sided specialization of the prefrontal regions in regard to working memory, following the typical left-verbal–right-spatial arrangement (Smith, Jonides, & Koeppe 1996).

One other intriguing formulation concerns psychological functions such as retrieval of information from semantic memory, encoding of information into episodic memory, and retrieving information from episodic memory, functions that have been associated with different parts of the frontal lobes in a model proposed by Tulving (Nyberg, Cabeza, & Tulving 1996; Tulving et al. 1996). Specifically, Tulving has suggested that the left frontal lobes are more involved in the retrieval of general knowledge (referred to as "semantic memory information") and are also more involved in the encoding of novel aspects of incoming information into episodic memory; the right frontal lobes are more involved with episodic memory retrieval and, in particular, with retrieval "attempts" that occur in episodic mode.

PERCEPTION AND RECOGNITION

Balint Syndrome

Balint syndrome is a disorder of perception and attention in the visual realm that consists of three distinct phenomena: (i) visual disorientation (also known as simultanagnosia); (ii) ocular apraxia (also known as psychic gaze paralysis); and (iii) optic ataxia (see Damasio 1985; Newcombe & Ratcliff 1989; Rizzo 1993; Rizzo & Hurtig 1987).

Visual disorientation is the key component of Balint syndrome. It entails an inability to attend to more than one limited sector of the visual panorama at any given time. The patient can home in on only one small portion of the visual field and is unable to monitor simultaneously what is happening in other parts of the field. The sector of clear vision may be unstable and can shift unpredictably, so that the patient suddenly loses a particular stimulus from view. Patients note that their visual focus appears to jump from one part of the field to another. This phenomenon precludes the ability to form a spatially coherent visual field, and the patients are unable to follow the trajectories of moving objects or place stimuli in their proper locations in space. Defective perception of motion is a frequent manifestation in patients with Balint syndrome (Schenk & Zihl 1997), and patients may fail to recognize the meaning of pantomime (e.g., wiggling a fin-

ger to signal "come here") or to recognize the identity of a familiar person based on gait. Defective depth perception (astereopsis) is another common correlate (Rizzo 1989).

Ocular apraxia is a defect in visual scanning – specifically, an inability to direct gaze voluntarily towards a particular target in the visual field. For example, patients may detect that something has entered the field on the left, but they miss the target when they try to shift their gaze so that it falls in central vision, making incorrectly calibrated saccades that fail to hit the target accurately.

Optic ataxia is a disturbance of visually guided reaching behavior, manifest by the patient's inability to point accurately and smoothly at a target or to reach out and deftly pick up an object. The reaching disturbance is confined to movements that are visually guided. Hence, if the patients try to point toward sound sources they will do so accurately, and they can also point accurately to targets on their own body using somatosensory information (proprioception).

The development of Balint syndrome is related to bilateral damage to occipitoparietal cortices in the superior sector of the visual association region. A lesion confined to the right occipitoparietal region may produce a less severe form of the condition, and lesions confined to the superior occipital region (without extension into the parietal region) usually cause visual disorientation but without ocular apraxia and optic ataxia. Balint syndrome is *not* caused by damage to the inferior sector of visual association cortices, illustrating the clear specialization of the inferior and superior visual systems for different types of processing (Ungerleider & Mishkin 1982).

Neglect

Neglect refers to a phenomenon in which a patient fails to attend normally to a portion of extrapersonal or intrapersonal space (or both) that cannot be explained by defective perception. Neglect can affect the visual, auditory, or tactile modalities or combinations thereof, but its manifestation is most striking and probably most common in the visual modality. The patient fails to attend to the left hemispace, ignoring objects, persons, and movements that occur on the left side (Bisiach & Luzzatti 1978; Heilman, Watson, & Valenstein 1993; Robertson & Marshall 1993; Weintraub & Mesulam 1989). Visual neglect is associated with lesions in the right parietal and occipitoparietal region. Neglect has also been associated with damage to other right hemisphere regions, including the anterior cingulate, the supplementary motor area, the dorsolateral prefrontal cortices, and the basal ganglia and other subcortical structures. There is a strong tendency for neglect to develop in relationship to the *left* hemispace of the patient, in connection with right hemisphere disease; this is true of all the sensory modalities. In fact, right-sided neglect is exceedingly rare. This tendency illustrates the dominant role of the right hemisphere in the mapping of extrapersonal and intrapersonal space (Damasio 1995), as discussed earlier in connection with anosognosia.

Agnosia

The term *agnosia* signifies lack of knowledge and is used to denote an impairment of recognition. Traditionally, two types of agnosia have been described (Lissauer 1890). One, termed *associative* agnosia, refers to a failure of recognition that results from defective activation of information pertinent to a given stimulus. The other, termed *apperceptive* agnosia, refers to a disturbance of the integration of otherwise normally perceived components of a stimulus.

Teuber (1968) gave a narrower definition of agnosia, noting that the phenomenon essentially involves "a normal percept that has somehow been stripped of its meaning" (p. 293). In this sense, agnosia was conceptualized more as a disorder of memory than as a disorder of perception, and only associative agnosia truly qualified as a disorder of memory. However, clinically and scientifically it has proved useful to retain the concept of apperceptive agnosia and to maintain a distinction between apperceptive and associative agnosia. Recognition is disturbed in both conditions, but in the apperceptive variety the problem can be traced (at least in part) to faulty perception.

Strictly speaking, agnosia encompasses cases where recognition impairments are confined to one sensory modality – for example, vision or audition or touch. If recognition defects extend across two or more modalities then the appropriate designation is amnesia (as discussed before). Also, agnosia is a term usually applied to conditions that develop suddenly and following the onset of acquired cerebral dysfunction, as opposed to developmental weaknesses or defects associated with psychiatric disease.

One other important distinction is between recognition and naming. Under normal circumstances, recognition of an entity is frequently indicated by naming (e.g., that's a "deer" or that's "Uncle Howard"). However, studies of brain-damaged subjects have shown that recognition and naming are dissociable capacities (Damasio et al. 1990a; Damasio et al. 1996). For example, patients may be able to recognize entities that they cannot name, as indicated by responses signifying that the patients understand the meaning of a particular stimulus. Conversely, patients may have a recognition impairment but not a naming impairment (see Tranel et al. 1997a for a fuller discussion of this issue). Hence, it is important to maintain a distinction between recognition and naming.

Pure forms of agnosia, especially the associative variety, are rare. Nonetheless, over the years quite a number of cases have been reported. The condition continues to attract considerable interest from cognitive scientists, owing in large measure to the window it provides into the manner in which the brain apprehends, records, and retrieves knowledge about various entities. Visual agnosia, especially agnosia for faces (prosopagnosia), is the most commonly encountered form of recognition disturbance affecting a primary sensory modality.

Category-Specific Visual Object Agnosia. Disorders of visual recognition rarely affect all categories of objects with equal magnitude; in fact, recognition impairments can be remarkably restricted to one category or another (see e.g. Sartori et al. 1993; Tranel et al. 1997a; Warrington & McCarthy 1994; Warrington & Shallice 1984). The most common profile is impaired recognition of living things (e.g. animals) together with normal recognition of artifactual objects (e.g. tools), but the reverse dissociation has also been reported (Tranel et al. 1997a; Warrington & McCarthy 1994). Such dissociations in visual recognition abilities have been interpreted as indicating that different types of stimuli are mapped by different neural systems. Factors such as shape similarity (homomorphy), manipulability, and sensory mode of transaction (whether the entity is learned and operated primarily through vision or through both vision and touch) have been identified as important determinants of whether recognition of certain types of stimuli will be disrupted by a particular brain lesion (Farah, McMullen, & Meyer 1991; Humphreys, Riddoch, & Price 1997; Small et al. 1995; Tranel et al. 1997b).

Prosopagnosia. Prosopagnosia (or face agnosia) refers to the inability to recognize familiar faces (Damasio, Tranel, & Damasio 1990b; De Renzi 1997). The condition has been noted since the turn of the century and has been a popular focus of scientific inquiry (Bodamer 1947; Meadows 1974), especially considering its relative rarity. Disproportionate scientific attention can be attributed to the fact that prosopagnosia has proved to be a highly informative paradigm for studying the neural substrates of visual learning and recognition (Damasio et al. 1990b; De Renzi 1997; Farah 1990). Investigations of this condition have yielded insights about issues ranging from hemispheric laterality to nonconscious brain processes.

In prototypical instances of prosopagnosia, patients cannot recognize the faces of family members, of close friends, or even of themselves in a mirror. Upon seeing those faces, the patients do not experience a sense of familiarity and evidently have no inkling that those faces are known to them. Behaviorally, they appear to respond to a highly familiar face in the same way that a normal individual would respond to the face of a complete stranger. Prosopagnosia typically covers both the retrograde and anterograde compartments, so that patients can no longer recognize the faces of previously known individuals and are also unable to learn new ones. The impairment is modality-specific, however, being entirely confined to vision. Thus, when they hear the voice of a person whose face was unrecognized, prosopagnosic patients make an accurate identification. Also, prosopagnosia must be distinguished carefully from disorders of face naming. An inability to name faces of persons who are otherwise recognized as familiar (which is rather commonplace in everyday experience) does not constitute prosopagnosia.

The recognition impairment in prosopagnosia occurs at the most subordinate taxonomic level – that is, at the level of identification of unique faces. Prosopagnosics are fully capable of recognizing faces *as faces*. Also, most prosopagnosics can recognize facial expressions and can make accurate determinations of gender and age based on face information (Humphreys, Donnelly, & Riddoch 1993; Tranel, Damasio, & Damasio 1988). These dissociations highlight several intriguing separations in the neural systems dedicated to processing different types of conceptual knowledge, such as knowledge about the meaning of stimuli, knowledge of emotion, and so on.

Although face agnosics will recognize any number of visual entities at the basic object level (e.g., they recognize cars as cars, buildings as buildings, and dogs as dogs), they will often fail to recognize these items at the more subordinate level of unique identity. Also, like the problem with faces, they are unable to recognize the specific identity of particular cars, buildings, and so forth. These impairments underscore the notion that the core defect in face agnosia is the inability to disambiguate fully individual visual stimuli. In fact, cases have been reported in which the most troubling problem for the patient was in classes of visual stimuli other than human faces – for example, a farmer who lost his ability to recognize individual dairy (e.g. Holstein) cows, or a bird watcher who became unable to distinguish various subtypes of birds (see Assal, Favre, & Anderes 1984; Bornstein, Sroka, & Munitz 1969).

As we have mentioned, prosopagnosic patients can often recognize identity based on movement. This means not only that their perception of movement is intact but also that they can evoke appropriate memories from the perception of unique patterns of movement. Combined with the finding that recovery of identity from motion can be impaired by lesions in superior occipitoparietal regions, these findings underscore the separable functions of the dorsal and ventral visual systems. The dorsal system is specialized for spatial placement, movement, and "where" capacities; the ventral system is specialized for form detection, shape recognition, and "what" capacities (Rao, Rainer, & Miller 1997; Ungerleider & Mishkin 1982).

Despite an inability to recognize familiar faces overtly (e.g., based on self-report), prosopagnosic patients often have accurate "covert" or nonconscious discrimination of those faces. They may, for example, generate discriminatory electrodermal responses to familiar faces (Bauer 1984; Bauer & Verfaellie 1986; Tranel & Damasio 1985, 1988). Preserved covert face discrimination has been demonstrated in other experimental paradigms, such as reaction time and forced choice procedures (De Haan, Bauer, & Greve 1992) and an oculomotor task (Rizzo, Hurtig, & Damasio 1987). In the electrodermal paradigm, covert face discrimination

has even been demonstrated for faces from the anterograde compartment (Tranel & Damasio 1988), indicating that the brain can continue to learn new visual information even without conscious influence.

In the paradigmatic presentation of prosopagnosia, known as *associative* prosopagnosia, the recognition impairment is relatively pure in the sense that it is confined to the visual modality and occurs in the setting of normal visual perception, thus conforming to the strict definition of associative agnosia. Associative prosopagnosia is most commonly caused by bilateral damage in inferior occipital and temporal visual association cortices in the occipitotemporal junction area (Damasio, Damasio, & Van Hoesen 1982). More rarely, unilateral right-sided lesions to this same region produce the condition (De Renzi et al. 1994).

Most patients with associative prosopagnosia also have achromatopsia, which is an acquired disturbance of color perception. The combination of the defects is due to the contiguity of the neural processing systems for form and color, which makes them susceptible to concurrent damage by one lesion. Also, if a left-sided occipitotemporal lesion encompasses both the occipitotemporal region and the left periventricular region – the white matter beside, beneath, and behind the occipital horn – then a reading impairment (alexia) is likely to coexist with the prosopagnosia.

Inferential Context

The development and refinement of modern neuroimaging techniques over the past two decades, including computed tomography (CT) in about 1973 and magnetic resonance imaging (MRI) a decade later, has had a profound impact on neuropsychology and behavioral neurology – both for clinical and scientific implementations. On the clinical side, such techniques have shifted the focus of bedside and laboratory testing of mental status from asking "where is the lesion?" and toward characterizing in detail the nature of the patient's cognitive strengths and weaknesses. The neuroimaging procedures nearly always answer the question of where a lesion is located, so mental status testing can now focus on quantifying such higher-order aspects of the patient's cognition and behavior as memory, speech, decision making, attention, and concentration. Finer-grained analyses of cognitive and behavioral functions – and more attention to rehabilitation – have been facilitated by this change in emphasis.

On the scientific side, modern neuroimaging techniques have triggered an explosion of research at the level of large-scale cognitive and neural systems. Suddenly, a very powerful tool existed for localizing brain lesions in humans in vivo; when used in conjunction with careful cognitive experimentation, this opened the way for a tremendous proliferation of brain–behavior research. With the addition of sophisticated theoretical formulations (Crick & Koch 1990; Damasio 1989a,b; Edelman 1987; Kosslyn & Koenig 1995;

Singer et al. 1990; see also Poggio & Glaser 1993), the stage was set for a rapid accrual of both new and confirmatory findings regarding the neural underpinnings of various cognitive functions. This trend has gathered even more force with the recent development of functional neuroimaging techniques, especially positron emission tomography (PET) and functional magnetic resonance imaging (fMRI), which have opened the way for detailed investigation of the cognitive operations of the normal human brain.

Neuropsychology and behavioral neurology have also benefitted in recent years from the incorporation of various psychophysiological techniques into the armamentarium of experimental approaches. This development is illustrated in studies of attention, perception, memory, and consciousness. For example, as noted in the previous section, electrodermal activity has been used to index nonconscious processing of faces in patients with prosopagnosia. In another intriguing example, electrophysiological evidence has demonstrated that subjects can analyze information meaningfully (albeit at a subconscious level) during the so-called attentional blink (Luck, Vogel, & Shapiro 1996).

Psychophysiological techniques have been particularly important in the investigation of the neural correlates of emotion and feeling (for reviews, see Andreassi 1995; Cacioppo et al. 1993; Cacioppo & Tassinary 1990; Ekman & Davidson 1994; Hugdahl 1995; Nadel & Lane in press). The cross-fertilization between neuropsychology and psychophysiology has also led to advances in the understanding of the neural basis of psychophysiological processes per se (Tranel & Damasio 1994).

THE LESION METHOD

For more than a century, the lesion method has been the principal paradigm for scientific inquiry into brain–behavior relationships. This method remains a rich source – and arguably the most powerful source – of knowledge regarding the neural underpinnings of cognition and behavior (Damasio & Damasio 1994; Damasio & Damasio 1989). The lesion method refers to an approach whereby (i) a focal area of brain damage is correlated with the development of a defect in some aspect of cognition or behavior and (ii) an inference is made that the damaged brain region is part of the neural substrate for the impaired function. In humans, obviously, the scientist does not have true control over the lesion and must rely instead upon the availability of suitable experimental lesions. This need not compromise the power of the approach *provided* it is applied in the context of several important parameters.

We believe (see Damasio & Damasio 1997) there are five prerequisites for optimal laboratory practice of the lesion method:

1. the availability of detailed structural imaging of the human brain in vivo;

2. a reliable method for neuroanatomical analysis of lesions;

3. a suitable pool of subjects from which to draw, allowing selection of experimental and control subjects in such a way as to remove the confounding influences of factors such as age, education, IQ, and socioeconomic status;

4. the availability of methods for reliable cognitive measurements; and

5. testable hypotheses concerning the neural basis for specific cognitive and behavioral functions.

So long as these prerequisites are satisfied, the lesion method can produce important new insights into brain–behavior relationships.

Neuroanatomical analysis of brain lesions has been greatly facilitated not only by the availability of fine-grained neuroimaging techniques but also by the development of analysis techniques that allow precise and reliable mapping of brain lesions. The template system developed by Damasio and Damasio (1989) is an example of such a technique; recently, this system has been replaced by an even more powerful approach based on a technique known as BRAINVOX (Frank, Damasio, & Grabowski 1997). BRAINVOX involves three-dimensional reconstruction of the human brain from high-resolution MRI; this allows the investigator to identify, in vivo, every major gyrus and sulcus of the brain, to slice and reslice the brain in whatever incidence necessary for anatomical analysis, and to define and quantify – in three dimensions – the degree of overlap of brain lesions from various subjects. Lesion commonalities between brain-damaged subjects can be characterized at a level of precision far greater than previously available, allowing rigorous probing of putative brain–behavior relationships. Lesion overlaps can function as either the independent or the dependent variable (see Damasio et al. 1996 and Tranel et al. 1997a for examples of this approach).

Traditionally, the lesion method was implemented primarily in case studies; this imposed certain limitations on the findings, especially if they proved difficult to replicate. However, this weakness has been substantially remedied with more recent work involving large groups of brain-damaged subjects, where conclusions have been derived based on subject groups comparable in size to those used in traditional psychological experiments (Damasio et al. 1996; Tranel et al. 1994b, 1997a). Striking case studies will continue to fuel new hypotheses and insights regarding brain–behavior relationships, and the astute clinician–scientist will take advantage of opportunities to explore interesting new leads in individual patients. Even so, the days of relying almost exclusively on single cases are well behind us.

FUNCTIONAL IMAGING

The emergence of functional imaging techniques, especially PET and fMRI, has allowed the development of intuitively appealing paradigms in which mental functions of the brain can be studied directly in normal individuals by using methods in which carefully localized physiological changes can be associated with experimentally induced changes in neuronal activity (Posner et al. 1988; Raichle 1997). Both PET and fMRI can be used with normal subjects, and thus many of the major limitations of the lesion method are bypassed. Imaging techniques have become enormously popular in the past few years (Frith et al. 1991; Grabowski et al. 1995; McCarthy 1995; Petersen et al. 1988; Roland 1993) – especially fMRI, which is noninvasive and readily accessible to nonmedical scientists. At the core of both techniques is the measurement of blood flow to local areas of the brain. The logic is straightforward: as neural tissue becomes more "active," demands for blood will increase; PET and fMRI allow precise measurement of these changes in blood flow.

In order to conclude that a particular brain region activated during a PET or fMRI experiment is related to a particular psychological function, it is necessary to design a cognitive task in which engagement of the function can be linked unequivocally to brain activation (increased blood flow). The prevailing approach to this challenge has been what is know as the "subtraction method." Fundamentally, this involves a comparison between two conditions: a baseline, in which the subject is resting or engaged in some simple task, and an experimental "activation" condition, in which the subject is doing everything in the baseline plus some particular task. By subtracting the blood flow changes in the baseline condition from those in the experimental condition, the investigator can get a notion of which changes are specific to the task (and its cognitive demands) in the experimental condition.

Both PET and fMRI hold great promise for the future of cognitive neuroscience. There are limitations of these techniques (in terms of spatial and temporal resolution), and most of the findings to date from functional imaging studies have served primarily to confirm what was already known from lesion studies. However, that these techniques can be used in normal subjects confers a major advantage to the investigator, and there is every reason to believe that these approaches will eventually lead to important new discoveries regarding the neural underpinnings of higher-order human behavior. Functional imaging techniques also promise to play a very important role in the study of brain-damaged individuals – for example, in exploring how plasticity and recovery of function are modulated by the neural tissue surrounding a lesion or in homologous areas of the hemisphere opposite to the lesion (Engelien et al. 1995; Naeser 1994; Weiller et al. 1995).

COGNITIVE EXPERIMENTATION

At the heart of reliable and valid application of any technique for studying brain–behavior relationships – and

of the clinical practice of behavioral neurology and neuropsychology – is a carefully designed and well-controlled cognitive experiment. Following the tradition of the eminent neuropsychologists who founded the field during the middle part of this century (Benton 1988; Newcombe 1969; Teuber 1968; Weiskrantz 1968; Zangwill 1964), modern clinical and experimental neuropsychologists continue to develop and refine a wide variety of cognitive tasks that can be used to measure precisely higher-order functions of the brain such as memory, perception, attention, speech, emotion, and decision making. The specification of detailed methods for conducting neuropsychological evaluation has contributed also (see Lezak 1995; McKenna & Warrington 1996; Milberg, Hebben, & Kaplan 1996; Reitan & Wolfson 1996; Tranel 1996).

The refinement of neuropsychological assessment and cognitive experimentation follows a long tradition in clinical psychology of careful, standardized measurement of psychological functions. The principal consideration is that the measurements take into account a variety of demographic factors that are common and often potent influences on performance in cognitive tasks, including age, gender, and educational and occupational background. Over the past few decades, the field of clinical neuropsychology has provided a wealth of information to deal with this challenge (Benton et al. 1983; Lezak 1995; Spreen & Strauss 1991). This information has allowed individual case application as required in clinical diagnosis and has also facilitated the power of experimental applications by allowing the removal of unwanted variability in dependent measures. The net result has been a severalfold increase in the power of cognitive experiments. This is especially important in functional imaging studies in normal subjects, where effect sizes tend to be far smaller than those typical of lesion studies.

Concluding Comments

The fields of neuropsychology and behavioral neurology have grown exponentially over the past two decades. Twenty years ago, it was possible to read virtually all of the major journals in these fields, journals with such broad titles as *Brain* and *Neuropsychologia*. Now, there are journals devoted to highly specific levels of the central nervous system (e.g., *Hippocampus* and *Cerebral Cortex*), and it can be a challenge to read even the tables of contents of many relevant journals. As emphasized repeatedly in early sections of this chapter, the development of powerful imaging techniques – first the structural ones including CT and MR, and now the functional ones including PET and fMRI – has been a key catalyst in this explosion. The role of the techniques is even reflected in some of the journal titles, for example, *Human Brain Mapping* and *NeuroImage*.

The rapid growth of the field and the prodigious adoption of new imaging techniques notwithstanding, it seems that many of the most important discoveries in neuropsychology and behavioral neurology will continue to derive from astute observations of patient behavior following brain disease. In this vein, the role of the clinician in these fields remains as important as ever. In our view, the model of clinician–scientist that harks back to the days of the great pioneers (e.g. Sperry, Milner, Hecaen, Geschwind, Newcombe, and Benton) will remain quite viable, even if many of the investigations are eventually carried out by scientists who have no direct contact with patients. Finally, it is highly encouraging to note that neuropsychology and behavioral neurology have enjoyed a mutually beneficial relationship with the field of psychophysiology. Psychophysiology has furnished important techniques for exploring previously untapped aspects of brain function that often were not amenable to direct observation. Moreover, the field provides methodological rigor and experimental sophistication that have enhanced the power of scientific exploration of brain–behavior relationships (Hugdahl 1995; Ohman & Soares 1997).

NOTE

This research was supported by Program Project Grant NINDS NS19632.

REFERENCES

Adolphs, R., Cahill, L., Schul, R., & Babinsky, R. (1997). Impaired declarative memory for emotional material following bilateral amygdala damage in humans. *Learning and Memory, 4,* 291–300.

Adolphs, R., Tranel, D., Damasio, H., & Damasio, A. R. (1994). Impaired recognition of emotion in facial expressions following bilateral damage to the human amygdala. *Nature, 372,* 669–72.

Adolphs, R., Tranel, D., Damasio, H., & Damasio, A. R. (1995). Fear and the human amygdala. *Journal of Neuroscience, 15,* 5879–91.

Alexander, M. P., & Freedman, M. (1984). Amnesia after anterior communicating artery rupture. *Neurology, 34,* 752–9.

Anderson, S. W., & Tranel, D. (1989). Awareness of disease states following cerebral infarction, dementia, and head trauma: Standardized assessment. *The Clinical Neuropsychologist, 3,* 327–39.

Andreassi, J. L. (1995). *Psychophysiology: Human Behavior and Physiological Response,* 3rd ed. Hillsdale, NJ: Erlbaum.

Assal, G., Favre, C., & Anderes, J. P. (1984). Non-reconnaissance d'animaux familiers chez un paysan. *Rev. Neurol., 140,* 580–4.

Babinski, J. (1914). Contribution a l'etude des troubles mentaux dans l'hemiplegie organique cerebrale (agnosognosie). *Rev. Neurol., 27,* 845–7.

Baddeley, A. D. (1992). Working memory. *Science, 255,* 566–9.

Bauer, R. M. (1984). Autonomic recognition of names and faces in prosopagnosia: A neuropsychological application of the guilty knowledge test. *Neuropsychologia, 22,* 457–69.

Bauer, R. M., & Verfaellie, M. (1986). Electrodermal discrimination of familiar but not unfamiliar faces in prosopagnosia. *Brain and Cognition, 8,* 240–52.

Bechara, A., Damasio, A. R., Damasio, H., & Anderson, S. W. (1994). Insensitivity to future consequences following damage to human prefrontal cortex. *Cognition, 50,* 7–12.

Bechara, A., Damasio, H., Tranel, D., & Damasio, A. R. (1997). Deciding advantageously before knowing the advantageous strategy. *Science, 275,* 1293–5.

Bechara, A., Tranel, D., Damasio, H., Adolphs, R., Rockland, C., & Damasio, A. R. (1995). Double dissociation of conditioning and declarative knowledge relative to the amygdala and hippocampus in humans. *Science, 269,* 1115–18.

Bechara, A., Tranel, D., Damasio, H., & Damasio, A. R. (1996). Failure to respond autonomically to anticipated future outcomes following damage to prefrontal cortex. *Cerebral Cortex, 6,* 215–25.

Benton, A. L. (1988). Neuropsychology: Past, present and future. In F. Boller & J. Grafman (Eds.), *Handbook of Neuropsychology,* vol. 1, pp. 3–27. New York: Elsevier.

Benton, A. L., Hamsher, K., Varney, N. R., & Spreen, O. (1983). *Contributions to Neuropsychological Assessment.* New York: Oxford University Press.

Benton, A. L., & Sivan, A. B. (1993). Disturbances of body schema. In K. M. Heilman & E. Valenstein (Eds.), *Clinical Neuropsychology,* 3rd ed., pp. 123–40. New York: Oxford University Press.

Benton, A., & Tranel, D. (in press). Historical notes on reorganization of function and neuroplasticity. In H. S. Levin & J. Grafman (Eds.), *Neuroplasticity and Reorganization of Function after Brain Injury.* New York: Oxford University Press.

Bisiach, E., & Luzzatti, C. (1978). Unilateral neglect of representation space. *Cortex, 14,* 129–33.

Blumer, D., & Benson, D. F. (1975). Personality changes with frontal and temporal lobe lesions. In D. F. Benson & D. Blumer (Eds.), *Psychiatric Aspects of Neurologic Disease,* pp. 151–69. New York: Grune & Stratton.

Bodamer, J. (1947). Prosopagnosie. *Arch. Psychiatr. Nervenkr., 179,* 6–54.

Bornstein, B., Sroka, H., & Munitz, H. (1969). Prosopagnosia with animal face agnosia. *Cortex, 5,* 164–9.

Breiter, H. C., Etcoff, N. L., Whalen, P. J., Kennedy, W. A., Rauch, S. L., Buckner, R. L., Strauss, M. M., Hyman, S. E., & Rosen, B. R. (1996). Response and habituation of the human amygdala during visual processing of facial expression. *Neuron, 17,* 875–87.

Brickner, R. M. (1934). An interpretation of frontal lobe function based upon the study of a case of partial bilateral frontal lobectomy. *Research Publication of the Association for Research in Nervous and Mental Disease, 13,* 259–351.

Broca, P. (1865). Sur la faculte du langage articule. *Bull. Soc. Anthropol., 6,* 337–93.

Butters, N., & Stuss, D. T. (1989). Diencephalic amnesia. In F. Boller & J. Grafman (Eds.), *Handbook of Neuropsychology,* vol. 3, pp. 107–48. Amsterdam: Elsevier.

Cacioppo, J. T., Klein, D. J., Berntson, G. G., & Hatfield, E. (1993). The psychophysiology of emotion. In R. Lewis & J. M. Haviland (Eds.), *Handbook of Emotion,* pp. 119–42. New York: Guilford.

Cacioppo, J. T., & Tassinary, L. G. (Eds.) (1990). *Principles of Psychophysiology: Physical, Social, and Inferential Elements*. Cambridge University Press.

Cahill, L., Babinsky, R., Markowitsch, H. J., & McGaugh, J. L. (1995). The amygdala and emotional memory. *Nature, 377,* 295–6.

Calder, A. J., Young, A. W., Rowland, D., Perrett, D. I., Hodges, J. R., & Etcoff, N. L. (1996). Facial emotion recognition after bilateral amygdala damage: Differentially severe impairment of fear. *Cognitive Neuropsychology, 13,* 699–745.

Cermak, L. S., & O'Connor, M. (1983). The anterograde and retrograde retrieval ability of a patient with amnesia due to encephalitis. *Neuropsychologia, 21,* 213–34.

Cohen, J. D., Perlstein, W. M., Braver, T. S., Nystrom, L. E., Noll, D. C., Jonides, J., & Smith, E. E. (1997). Temporal dynamics of brain activation during a working memory task. *Nature, 386,* 604–8.

Cohen, N. J., & Eichenbaum, H. (1993). *Memory, Amnesia, and the Hippocampal System*. Cambridge, MA: MIT Press.

Cohen, N. J., & Squire, L. R. (1981). Retrograde amnesia and remote memory impairment. *Neuropsychologia, 19,* 337–56.

Corkin, S. (1965). Tactually guided maze learning in man: Effects of unilateral cortical excisions and bilateral hippocampal lesions. *Neuropsychologia, 3,* 339–51.

Corkin, S. (1984). Lasting consequences of bilateral medial temporal lobectomy: Clinical course and experimental findings in HM. *Seminars in Neurology, 4,* 249–59.

Courtney, S. M., Ungerleider, L. G., Keil, K., & Haxby, J. V. (1997). Transient and sustained activity in a distributed neural system for working memory. *Nature, 386,* 608–11.

Crick, F. H., & Koch, C. (1990). Towards a neurobiological theory of consciousness. *Seminars in Neuroscience, 2,* 263–75.

Curran, T., & Schacter, D. L. (1997). Amnesia: Cognitive neuropsychological aspects. In T. E. Feinberg & M. J. Farah (Eds.), *Behavioral Neurology and Neuropsychology*, pp. 463–71. New York: McGraw-Hill.

Damasio, A. R. (1985). Disorders of complex visual processing: Agnosias, achromatopsia, Balint's syndrome, and related difficulties of orientation and construction. In M. M. Mesulam (Ed.), *Principles of Behavioral Neurology*, pp. 259–88. Philadelphia: Davis.

Damasio, A. R. (1989a). Time-locked multiregional retroactivation: A systems-level proposal for the neural substrates of recall and recognition. *Cognition, 33,* 25–62.

Damasio, A. R. (1989b). The brain binds entities and events by multiregional activation from convergence zones. *Neural Computation, 1,* 123–32.

Damasio, A. R. (1994). *Descartes' Error: Emotion, Reason, and the Human Brain*. New York: Grossett/Putnam.

Damasio, A. R. (1995). Toward a neurobiology of emotion and feeling: Operational concepts and hypotheses. *The Neuroscientist, 1,* 19–25.

Damasio, A. R. (1996). The somatic marker hypothesis and the possible functions of the prefrontal cortex. *Philosophical Transactions of the Royal Society of London, Ser. B, 351,* 1413–20.

Damasio, A. R., & Anderson, S. W. (1993). The frontal lobes. In K. M. Heilman & E. Valenstein (Eds.), *Clinical Neuropsychology*, 3rd ed., pp. 409–60. New York: Oxford University Press.

Damasio, A. R., & Damasio, H. (1993). Cortical systems underlying knowledge retrieval: Evidence from human lesion studies. In T. A. Poggio & D. A. Glaser (Eds.), *Exploring Brain Functions: Models in Neuroscience*, pp. 233–48. New York: Wiley.

Damasio, A. R., & Damasio, H. (1994). Cortical systems for retrieval of concrete knowledge: The convergence zone framework. In C. Koch (Ed.), *Large-Scale Neuronal Theories of the Brain*, pp. 61–74. Cambridge, MA: MIT Press.

Damasio, A. R., Damasio, H., Tranel, D., & Brandt, J. (1990a). Neural regionalization of knowledge access: Preliminary evidence. *Symposia on Quantitative Biology, 55,* 1039–47.

Damasio, A. R., Damasio, H., & Van Hoesen, G. W. (1982). Prosopagnosia: Anatomic basis and behavioral mechanisms. *Neurology, 32,* 331–41.

Damasio, A. R., Eslinger, P., Damasio, H., Van Hoesen, G. W., & Cornell, S. (1985a). Multimodal amnesic syndrome following bilateral temporal and basal forebrain damage. *Archives of Neurology, 42,* 252–9.

Damasio, A. R., Graff-Radford, N. R., Eslinger, P. G., Damasio, H., & Kassell, N. (1985b). Amnesia following basal forebrain lesions. *Archives of Neurology, 42,* 263–71.

Damasio, A. R., Tranel, D., & Damasio, H. (1990b). Face agnosia and the neural substrates of memory. *Annual Review of Neuroscience, 13,* 89–109.

Damasio, A. R., Tranel, D., & Damasio, H. (1990c). Individuals with sociopathic behavior caused by frontal damage fail to respond autonomically to social stimuli. *Behavioural Brain Research, 41,* 81–94.

Damasio, H., & Damasio, A. R. (1989). *Lesion Analysis in Neuropsychology*. New York: Oxford University Press.

Damasio, H., & Damasio, A. R. (1997). The lesion method in behavioral neurology and neuropsychology. In T. E. Feinberg & M. J. Farah (Eds.), *Behavioral Neurology and Neuropsychology*, pp. 69–82. New York: McGraw-Hill.

Damasio, H., Grabowski, T. J., Tranel, D., Hichwa, R. D., & Damasio, A. R. (1996). A neural basis for lexical retrieval. *Nature, 380,* 499–505.

Davis, M. (1992). The role of the amygdala in conditioned fear. In J. P. Aggleton (Ed.), *The Amygdala: Neurobiological Aspects of Emotion, Memory, and Mental Dysfunction*, pp. 255–306. New York: Wiley-Liss.

De Haan, E. H. F., Bauer, R. M., & Greve, K. W. (1992). Behavioral and physiological evidence for covert recognition in a prosopagnosic patient. *Cortex, 28,* 27–95.

Deluca, J., & Diamond, B. J. (1995). Aneurysm of the anterior communicating artery: A review of neuroanatomical and neuropsychologic sequelae. *Journal of Clinical and Experimental Neuropsychology, 17,* 100–21.

De Renzi, E. (1997). Prosopagnosia. In T. E. Feinberg & M. J. Farah (Eds.), *Behavioral Neurology and Neuropsychology*, pp. 245–55. New York: McGraw-Hill.

De Renzi, E., Perani, D., Carlesimo, G. A., Silveri, M. C., & Fazio, F. (1994). Prosopagnosia can be associated with damage confined to the right hemisphere: An MRI and PET study and a review of the literature. *Neuropsychologia, 32,* 893–902.

Dolan, R. J., & Fletcher, P. C. (1997). Dissociating prefrontal and hippocampal function in episodic memory encoding. *Nature, 388,* 582–5.

Edelman, G. (1987). *Neural Darwinism*. New York: Basic Books.

Ekman, P., & Davidson, R. J. (Eds.) (1994). *The Nature of Emotion*. New York: Oxford University Press.

Engelien, A., Silbersweig, D., Stern, E., Huber, W., Doring, W., Frith, K., & Frackowiak, R. S. J. (1995). The functional anatomy of recovery from auditory agnosia: A PET study of sound categorization in a neurological patient and normal controls. *Brain, 118,* 1395–1409.

Eslinger, P. J., & Damasio, A. R. (1985). Severe disturbance of higher cognition after bilateral frontal lobe ablation: Patient EVR. *Neurology, 35,* 1731–41.

Farah, M. J. (1990). *Visual Agnosia.* Cambridge, MA: MIT Press.

Farah, M. J., McMullen, P. A., & Meyer, M. M. (1991). Can recognition of living things be selectively impaired? *Neuropsychologia, 29,* 185–93.

Flourens, P. (1846). *Phrenology Examined* (translated by Charles de Lucena Meigs). Philadelphia: Hogan & Thompson.

Frank, R. J., Damasio, H., & Grabowski, T. J. (1997). BRAIN-VOX: An interactive, multimodal visualization and analysis system for neuroanatomical imaging. *NeuroImage, 5,* 13–30.

Frith, C. D., Friston, K., Liddle, P. F., & Frackowiak, R. S. J. (1991). A PET study of word finding. *Neuropsychologia, 29,* 1–12.

Gabrieli, J. D. E., Brewer, J. B., Desmond, J. E., & Glover, G. H. (1997). Separate neural bases of fundamental memory processes in the human medial temporal lobe. *Science, 276,* 264–6.

Gabrieli, J. D. E., Corkin, S., Mickel, S. F., & Growden, J. H. (1993). Intact acquisition and long-term retention of mirror-tracing skill in Alzheimer's disease and in global amnesia. *Behavioral Neuroscience, 107,* 899–910.

Gazzaniga, M. S. (1987). Perceptual and attentional processes following callosal section in human. *Neuropsychologia, 25,* 119–33.

Geschwind, N. (1965). Disconnexion syndromes in animals and man. *Brain, 88,* 237–94, 585–644.

Goldman-Rakic, P. S. (1987). Circuitry of primate prefrontal cortex and regulation of behavior by representational memory. In F. Plum (Ed.), *Handbook of Physiology: The Nervous System,* pp. 373–417. Bethesda, MD: American Physiological Society.

Grabowski, T. J., Damasio, H., Frank, R. J., Brown, C. K., Boles-Ponto, L. L., Watkins, G. L., & Hichwa, R. D. (1995). Neuroanatomical analysis of functional brain images: Validation with retinotopic mapping. *Human Brain Mapping, 2,* 134–48.

Graff-Radford, N. R., Tranel, D., Van Hoesen, G. W., & Brandt, J. P. (1990). Diencephalic amnesia. *Brain, 113,* 1–25.

Harlow, J. M. (1868). Recovery from the passage of an iron bar through the head. *Publications of the Massachusetts Medical Society, 2,* 327–47.

Hebb, D. O., & Penfield, W. (1940). Human behavior after extensive bilateral removals from the frontal lobes. *Archives of Neurology and Psychiatry, 44,* 421–38.

disorders. In K. M. Heilman & E. Valenstein (Eds.), *Clinical Neuropsychology,* 3rd ed., pp. 279–336. New York: Oxford University Press.

Hodges, J. R. (1995). Retrograde amnesia. In A. Baddeley, B. A. Wilson, & F. N. Watts (Eds.), *Handbook of Memory Disorders,* pp. 81–107. New York: Wiley.

Hugdahl, K. (1995). *Psychophysiology: The Mind–Body Perspective.* Cambridge, MA: Harvard University Press.

Humphreys, G. W., Donnelly, N., & Riddoch, M. J. (1993). Expression is computed separately from facial identity, and it is computed separately for moving and static faces: Neuropsychological evidence. *Neuropsychologia, 31,* 173–81.

Humphreys, G. W., Riddoch, M. J., & Price, C. J. (1997). Top-down processes in object identification: Evidence from experimental psychology, neuropsychology and functional anatomy. *Philosophical Transactions of the Royal Society of London, Ser. B., 352,* 1275–82.

Hyman, B. T., Damasio, A. R., Van Hoesen, G. W., & Barnes, C. L. (1984). Alzheimer's disease: Cell specific pathology isolates the hippocampal formation. *Science, 225,* 1168–70.

Jackson, J. H. (1870). A study of convulsions. *Transactions, St. Andrews Medical Graduate Association, 3,* 162–204.

Jackson, J. H. (1873). On the anatomical and physiological localisation of movement in the brain. *Lancet, 1,* 84–5, 162–4, 232–4.

Jonides, J., Smith, E. E., Koeppe, R. A., Awh, E., Minoshima, S., & Mintun, M. A. (1993). Spatial working memory in humans as revealed by PET. *Nature, 363,* 623–5.

Jurgens, U. (1982). Amygdalar vocalization pathways in the squirrel monkey. *Brain Research, 241,* 189–96.

Kapur, N. (1993). Focal retrograde amnesia in neurological disease: A critical review. *Cortex, 29,* 217–34.

Kapur, N., Ellison, D., Parkin, A. J., Hunkin, N. M., Burrows, E., Sampson, S. A., & Morrison, E. A. (1994). Bilateral temporal lobe pathology with sparing of medial temporal lobe structures: Lesion profile and pattern of memory disorder. *Neuropsychologia, 32,* 23–38.

Kling, A. S., & Brothers, L. A. (1992). The amygdala and social behavior. In J. P. Aggleton (Ed.), *The Amygdala: Neurobiological Aspects of Emotion, Memory, and Mental Dysfunction,* pp. 353–77. New York: Wiley-Liss.

Kling, A., Steklis, H. D., & Deutsch, S. (1979). Radiotelemetered activity from the amygdala during social interactions in the monkey. *Experimental Neurology, 66,* 88–96.

Kopelman, M. D. (1992). The neuropsychology of remote memory. In F. Boller & J. Grafman (Eds.), *Handbook of Neuropsychology,* vol. 8, pp. 215–38. Amsterdam: Elsevier.

Kosslyn, S. M., & Koenig, O. (1995). *Wet Mind: The New Cognitive Neuroscience.* New York: Free Press.

LaBar, K. S., LeDoux, J. E., Spencer, D. D., & Phelps, E. A. (1995). Impaired fear conditioning following unilateral temporal lobectomy in humans. *Journal of Neuroscience, 15,* 6846–55.

Lashley, K. S. (1929). *Brain Mechanisms and Intelligence: A Quantitative Study of Injuries to the Brain.* University of Chicago Press.

Lashley, K. S. (1950). In search of the engram. *Symposium of the Society for Experimental Biology, 4,* 454–82.

LeDoux, J. E., Cicchetti, P., Xagoraris, A., & Romanski, L. M. (1990). The lateral amygdaloid nucleus: Sensory interface of the amygdala in fear conditioning. *Journal of Neuroscience, 10,* 1062–9.

Lewicki, P., Hill, T., & Czyzewska, M. (1992). Nonconscious acquisition of information. *American Psychologist, 47,* 796–801.

Lezak, M. (1995). *Neuropsychological Assessment,* 3rd ed. New York: Oxford University Press.

Lissauer, H. (1890). Ein Fall von Seelenblindheit nebst einem Beitrag zur Theorie derselben. *Arch. Psychiatr. Nervenkr., 21,* 22–70.

Luck, S. J., Vogel, E. K., & Shapiro, K. L. (1996). Word meanings can be accessed but not reported during the attentional blink. *Nature, 383,* 616–18.

Luria, A. R. (1969). Frontal lobe syndromes. In P. G. Vinken & G. W. Bruyn (Eds.), *Handbook of Clinical Neurology,* vol. 2, pp. 725–57. Amsterdam: North-Holland.

Markowitsch, H. J., Calabrese, P., Haupts, M., Durwen, H. F., Liess, J., & Gehlen, W. (1993). Searching for the anatomical basis of retrograde amnesia. *Journal of Clinical and Experimental Neuropsychology, 15,* 947–67.

Markowitsch, H. J., Calabrese, P., Wuerker, M., Durwen, H. F., Kessler, J., Babinsky, R., Brechtelsbauer, D., Heuser, L., & Gehlen, W. (1994). The amygdala's contribution to memory – A study on two patients with Urbach–Wiethe disease. *Neuroreport, 5,* 1349–52.

McCarthy, G. (1995). Functional neuroimaging of memory. *The Neuroscientist, 1,* 155–63.

McCarthy, G., Blamire, A. M., Puce, A., Nobre, A. C., Bloch, G., Hyder, F., Goldman-Rakic, P., & Shulman, R. G. (1994). Functional magnetic resonance imaging of human prefrontal cortex activation during a spatial working memory task. *Proceedings of the National Academy of Sciences U.S.A., 91,* 8690–4.

McKenna, P., & Warrington, E. K. (1996). The analytical approach to neuropsychological assessment. In I. Grant & K.M. Adams (Eds.), *Neuropsychological Assessment of Neuropsychiatric Disorders,* 2nd ed., pp. 43–57. New York: Oxford University Press.

Meadows, J. C. (1974). The anatomical basis of prosopagnosia. *Journal of Neurology, Neurosurgery and Psychiatry, 37,* 489–501.

Milberg, W. P., Hebben, N., & Kaplan, E. (1996). The Boston process approach to neuropsychological assessment. In I. Grant & K. M. Adams (Eds.), *Neuropsychological Assessment of Neuropsychiatric Disorders,* 2nd ed., pp. 58–80. New York: Oxford University Press.

Milner, B. (1972). Disorders of learning and memory after temporal lobe lesions in man. *Clinical Neurosurgery, 19,* 421–46.

Milner, B., Petrides, M., & Smith, M. L. (1985). Frontal lobes and the temporal organization of memory. *Human Neurobiology, 4,* 137–42.

Mishkin, M. (1978). Memory in monkeys severely impaired by combined but not separate removal of amygdala and hippocampus. *Nature, 273,* 297–8.

Mishkin, M. (1982). A memory system in the monkey. *Philosophical Transactions of the Royal Society of London, Ser. B, 98,* 85–95.

Morris, J. S., Frith, C. D., Perrett, D. I., Rowland, D., Young, A. W., Calder, A. J., & Dolan, R. J. (1996). A differential neural response in the human amygdala to fearful and happy facial expressions. *Nature, 383,* 812–15.

Murray, E. A., & Gaffan, D. (1994). Removal of the amygdala plus subjacent cortex disrupts the retention of both intramodal and crossmodal associative memories in monkeys. *Behavioral Neuroscience, 108,* 494–500.

Nadel, L., & Lane, R. (Eds.) (in press). *The Interface of Emotion and Cognitive Neuroscience.* New York: Oxford University Press.

Naeser, M. A. (1994). Neuroimaging and recovery of auditory comprehension and spontaneous speech in aphasia with some implications for treatment in severe aphasia. In A. Kertesz (Ed.), *Localization and Neuroimaging in Neuropsychology,* pp. 245–95. New York: Academic Press.

Nahm, F. K. D., Tranel, D., Damasio, H., & Damasio, A. R. (1993). Cross-modal associations and the human amygdala. *Neuropsychologia, 31,* 727–44.

Newcombe, F. (1969). *Missile Wounds of the Brain: A Study of Psychological Deficits.* Oxford University Press.

Newcombe, F., & Ratcliff, G. (1989). Disorders of visuospatial analysis. In F. Boller & J. Grafman (Eds.), *Handbook of Neuropsychology,* vol. 2, pp. 333–56. Amsterdam: Elsevier.

Nyberg, L., Cabeza, R., & Tulving, E. (1996). PET studies of encoding and retrieval: The HERA model. *Psychonomic Bulletin and Review, 3,* 135–48.

O'Connor, M., Verfaellie, M., & Cermak, L. (1995). Clinical differentiation of amnesic subtypes. In A. Baddeley, B. A. Wilson, & F. N. Watts (Eds.), *Handbook of Memory Disorders,* pp. 53–80. New York: Wiley.

Öhman, A., & Soares, J. J. F. (1997). Emotional conditioning to masked stimuli: Expectancies for aversive outcomes following non-recognized fear-relevant stimuli. *Journal of Experimental Psychology: General, 127,* 69–82.

Petersen, S. E., Fox, P. T., Posner, M. I., Mintun, M., & Raichle, M. E. (1988). Positron emission tomographic studies of the cortical anatomy of single-word processing. *Nature, 331,* 585–9.

Petrides, M., Alivisatos, B., Evans, A. C., & Meyer, E. (1993). Dissociation of human mid-dorsolateral from posterior dorsolateral frontal cortex in memory processing. *Proceedings of the National Academy of Sciences U.S.A., 90,* 873–7.

Poggio, T. A., & Glaser, D. A. (Eds.) (1993). *Exploring Brain Functions: Models in Neuroscience.* New York: Wiley.

Posner, M. I., Petersen, S. E., Fox, P. T., & Raichle, M. E. (1988). Localization of cognitive operations in the human brain. *Science, 240,* 1627–31.

Raichle, M. E. (1997). Functional imaging in behavioral neurology and neuropsychology. In T. E. Feinberg & M. J. Farah (Eds.), *Behavioral Neurology and Neuropsychology,* pp. 83–100. New York: McGraw-Hill.

Ramachandran, V. S., Hirstein, W. S., Armel, K. C., Tecoma, E., & Iragui, V. (1997). The neural basis of religious experience. *Society for Neuroscience Abstracts, 23,* 1316.

Rao, S. C., Rainer, G., & Miller, E. K. (1997). Integration of what and where in the primate prefrontal cortex. *Science, 276,* 821–4.

Reitan, R. M., & Wolfson, D. (1996). Theoretical, methodological, and validational bases of the Halstead–Reitan neuropsychological test battery. In I. Grant & K. M. Adams (Eds.), *Neuropsychological Assessment of Neuropsychiatric Disorders,* 2nd ed., pp. 3–42. New York: Oxford University Press.

Rempel-Clower, N. L., Zola, S. M., Squire, L. R., & Amaral, D. G. (1996). Three cases of enduring memory impairment after bilateral damage limited to the hippocampal formation. *Journal of Neuroscience, 16,* 5233–55.

Rizzo, M. (1989). Astereopsis. In F. Boller & J. Grafman (Eds.), *Handbook of Neuropsychology,* vol. 2, pp. 415–27. Amsterdam: Elsevier.

Rizzo, M. (1993). "Balint's syndrome" and associated visuospatial disorders. In C. Kennard (Ed.), *Bailliere's International Practice and Research,* pp. 415–37. London: Saunders.

Rizzo, M., & Hurtig, R. (1987). Looking but not seeing: Attention, perception, and eye movements in simultanagnosia. *Neurology, 37,* 1642–8.

Rizzo, M., Hurtig, R., & Damasio, A. R. (1987). The role of scanpaths in facial recognition and learning. *Annals of Neurology, 22,* 41–5.

Robertson, I. H., & Marshall, J. C. (Eds.) (1993). *Unilateral Neglect: Clinical and Experimental Studies.* Hillsdale, NJ: Erlbaum.

Roland, P. E. (1993). *Brain Activation.* New York: Wiley-Liss.

Sartori, G., Job, R., Miozzo, M., Zago, S., & Marchiori, G. (1993). Category-specific form-knowledge deficit in a patient with herpes simplex virus encephalitis. *Journal of Clinical and Experimental Neuropsychology, 15,* 280–99.

Schacter, D. L., Harbluk, J. L., & McLachlan, D. R. (1984). Retrieval without recollection: An experimental analysis of source amnesia. *Verbal Learning and Verbal Behavior, 23,* 593–611.

Schenk, T., & Zihl, J. (1997). Visual motion perception after brain damage: I. Deficits in global motion perception. *Neuropsychologia, 35,* 1289–97.

Scott, S. K., Young, A. W., Calder, A. J., Hellawell, D. J., Aggleton, J. P., & Johnson, M. (1997). Impaired auditory recognition of fear and anger following bilateral amygdala lesions. *Nature, 385,* 254–7.

Scoville, W. B., & Milner, B. (1957). Loss of recent memory after bilateral hippocampal lesions. *Journal of Neurology, Neurosurgery, and Psychiatry, 20,* 11–21.

Singer, W., Gray, C., Engel, A., Konig, P., Artola, A., & Brocher, S. (1990). Formation of cortical cell assemblies. *Symposium on Quantitative Biology, 55,* 939–52.

Small, S. L., Hart, J., Nguyen, T., & Gordon, B. (1995). Distributed representations of semantic knowledge in the brain. *Brain, 118,* 441–53.

Smith, E. E., Jonides, J., & Koeppe, R. A. (1996). Dissociating verbal and spatial working memory using PET. *Cerebral Cortex, 6,* 11–20.

Smith, E. E., Jonides, J., Koeppe, R. A., Awh, E., Schumacher, E. H., & Minoshima, S. (1995). Spatial versus object working memory: PET investigations. *Journal of Cognitive Neuroscience, 7,* 337-56.

Sperry, R. W. (1968). The great cerebral commissure. *Scientific American, 210,* 42–52.

Spreen, O., & Strauss, E. (1991). *A Compendium of Neuropsychological Tests: Administration, Norms, and Commentary.* New York: Oxford University Press.

Spurzheim, J. G. (1815). *The Physiognomical System of Drs. Gall and Spurzheim; Founded on an Anatomical and Physiological Examination of the Nervous System in General, and of the Brain in Particular; and Indicating the Dispositions and Manifestations of the Mind.* London: Baldwin, Cradock, & Joy.

Squire, L. R. (1992). Memory and hippocampus: A synthesis from findings with rats, monkeys, and humans. *Psychological Review, 99,* 195–231.

Squire, L. R., & Alvarez, P. (1995). Retrograde amnesia and memory consolidation: A neurobiological perspective. *Current Opinion in Neurobiology, 5,* 169–77.

Squire, L. R., & Moore, R. Y. (1979). Dorsal thalamic lesion in a noted case of human memory dysfunction. *Annals of Neurology, 6,* 503–6.

Squire, L. R., & Shimamura, A. (1996). The neuropsychology of memory dysfunction and its assessment. In I. Grant & K. M. Adams (Eds.), *Neuropsychological Assessment of Neuropsychiatric Disorders,* 2nd ed., pp. 232–62. New York: Oxford University Press.

Stuss, D. T., & Benson, D. F. (1986). *The Frontal Lobes.* New York: Raven.

Teuber, H. L. (1968). Alteration of perception and memory in man: Reflections on methods. In L. Weiskrantz (Ed.), *Analysis of Behavioral Change,* pp. 274–328. New York: Harper & Row.

Teuber, H. L., Milner, B., & Vaughan, H. G. (1968). Persistent anterograde amnesia after stab wound of the basal brain. *Neuropsychologia, 6,* 267–82.

Thompson, R. F. L. (1986). The neurobiology of learning and memory. *Science, 233,* 941–7.

Tranel, D. (1996). The Iowa–Benton school of neuropsychological assessment. In I. Grant & K. M. Adams (Eds.), *Neuropsychological Assessment of Neuropsychiatric Disorders,* 2nd ed., pp. 81–101. New York: Oxford University Press.

Tranel, D., Anderson, S. W., & Benton, A. L. (1994a). Development of the concept of "executive function" and its relationship to the frontal lobes. In F. Boller & J. Grafman (Eds.), *Handbook of Neuropsychology,* vol. 9, pp. 125–48. Amsterdam: Elsevier.

Tranel, D., & Damasio, A. R. (1985). Knowledge without awareness: An autonomic index of facial recognition by prosopagnosics. *Science, 228,* 1453–4.

Tranel, D., & Damasio, A. R. (1988). Nonconscious face recognition in patients with face agnosia. *Behavioural Brain Research, 30,* 235–49.

Tranel, D., & Damasio, A. R. (1993). The covert learning of affective valence does not require structures in hippocampal system or amygdala. *Journal of Cognitive Neuroscience, 5,* 79–88.

Tranel, D., & Damasio, A. R. (1995). Neurobiological foundations of human memory. In A. D. Baddeley, B. A. Wilson, & F. N. Watts (Eds.), *Handbook of Memory Disorders,* pp. 27–50. New York: Wiley.

Tranel, D., Damasio, A. R., & Damasio, H. (1988). Intact recognition of facial expression, gender, and age in patients with impaired recognition of face identity. *Neurology, 38,* 690–6.

Tranel, D., Damasio, A. R., Damasio, H., & Brandt, J. P. (1994b). Sensorimotor skill learning in amnesia: Additional evidence for the neural basis of nondeclarative memory. *Learning and Memory, 1,* 165–79.

Tranel, D., & Damasio, H. (1994). Neuroanatomical correlates of electrodermal skin conductance responses. *Psychophysiology, 31,* 427–38.

Tranel, D., Damasio, H., & Damasio, A. R. (1997a). A neural basis for the retrieval of conceptual knowledge. *Neuropsychologia, 35,* 1319–27.

Tranel, D., & Hyman, B. T. (1990). Neuropsychological correlates of bilateral amygdala damage. *Archives of Neurology, 47,* 349–55.

Tranel, D., Logan, C. G., Frank, R. J., & Damasio, A. R. (1997b). Explaining category-related effects in the retrieval of conceptual and lexical knowledge for concrete entities: Operationalization and analysis of factors. *Neuropsychologia, 35,* 1329–39.

Tulving, E., Markowitsch, H. J., Craik, F. I. M., Habib, R., & Houle, S. (1996). Novelty and familiarity activations in PET studies of memory encoding and retrieval. *Cerebral Cortex, 6,* 71–9.

Ungerleider, L. G., & Mishkin, M. (1982). Two cortical visual systems. In D. J. Ingle, M. A. Goodale, & R. J. W. Mansfield (Eds.), *Analysis of Visual Behavior,* pp. 549–86. Cambridge, MA: MIT Press.

Van Hoesen, G. W., & Damasio, A. R. (1987). Neural correlates of cognitive impairment in Alzheimer's disease. In V. Mountcastle & F. Plum (Eds.), *Handbook of Physiology: Higher Functions of the Nervous System,* pp. 871–98. Bethesda, MD: American Physiological Society.

Victor, M., Adams, R. D., & Collins, G. H. (1989). *The Wernicke–Korsakoff Syndrome and Related Neurologic Disorders Due to Alcoholism and Malnutrition,* 2nd ed. Philadelphia: Davis.

Warrington, E. K., & McCarthy, R. A. (1994). Multiple meaning systems in the brain: A case for visual semantics. *Neuropsychologia, 32,* 1465–73.

Warrington, E. K., & Shallice, T. (1984). Category specific semantic impairments. *Brain, 107,* 829–54.

Weiller, C., Isensee, C., Rjntjes, M., Huber, W., Muller, S., Bier, D., Dutschka, K., Woods, R. P., Noth, J., & Diener, H. C. (1995). Recovery from Wernicke's aphasia: A positron emission tomographic study. *Annals of Neurology, 37,* 723–32.

Weintraub, S., & Mesulam, M. M. (1989). Neglect: Hemispheric specialization, behavioral components and anatomical correlates. In F. Boller & J. Grafman (Eds.), *Handbook of Neuropsychology,* vol. 2, pp. 357–74. Amsterdam: Elsevier.

Weiskrantz, L. (Ed.) (1968). *Analysis of Behavioral Change.* New York: Harper & Row.

Wernicke, C. (1874). *Der aphasische Symptomencomplex.* Wroclaw, Poland: Cohn & Weigert.

Wilson, F. A. W., O'Scalaidhe, S. P., & Goldman-Rakic, P. S. (1993). Dissociation of object and spatial processing domains in primate prefrontal cortex. *Science, 260,* 1955–8.

Young, A. W., Aggleton, J. P., Hellawell, D. J., Johnson, M., Broks, P., & Hanley, J. R. (1995). Face processing impairments after amygdalotomy. *Brain, 118,* 15–24.

Zald, D. H., & Pardo, J. V. (1997). Emotion, olfaction and the human amygdala: Amygdala activation during aversive olfactory stimulation. *Proceedings of the National Academy of Sciences U.S.A., 94,* 4119–24.

Zangwill, O. L. (1964). Intelligence in aphasia. In A. V. S. Reuck & M. O'Connor (Eds.), *Disorders of Language,* pp. 261–74. Boston: Little, Brown.

Zola, S. (1997). Amnesia: Neuroanatomic and clinical aspects. In T. E. Feinberg & M. J. Farah (Eds.), *Behavioral Neurology and Neuropsychology,* pp. 447–61. New York: McGraw-Hill.

Zola-Morgan, S., Squire, L. R., & Amaral, D. G. (1986). Human amnesia and the medial temporal region: Enduring memory impairment following a bilateral lesion limited to field CA1 of the hippocampus. *Journal of Neuroscience, 6,* 2950–67.

Zola-Morgan, S., Squire, L. R., Amaral, D. G., & Suzuki, W. A. (1989). Lesions of perirhinal and parahippocampal cortex that spare the amygdala and hippocampal formation produce severe memory impairment. *Journal of Neuroscience, 9,* 4355–70.

CHAPTER SIX

THE PUPILLARY SYSTEM

JACKSON BEATTY & BRENNIS LUCERO-WAGONER

The pupil is the opening through which light enters the eye and begins the process of visual perception. The diameter of that opening is determined by the relative contraction of two opposing sets of muscles within the iris, the sphincter and dilator pupillae, and is determined primarily by the light and accommodation reflexes. But in addition to reflexive control of pupillary size there are also tiny, cognitively related, visually insignificant fluctuations in pupillary diameter that appear to serve no functional purpose whatsoever. These miniature pupillary movements – usually less than 0.5 mm in extent – appear to be attenuated reflections of changes in brain activation systems that underlie human cognition.

Fortunately for cognitive psychophysiologists, these exceedingly tiny pupillary movements are too small to be of visual consequence. Perhaps because they have no evolutionary cost, they have been spared removal by the sure knife of evolution. These small but ubiquitous pupillary fluctuations form the basis of *cognitive pupillometry*, providing a unique psychophysiological index of dynamic brain activity in human cognition.

We begin by summarizing the brief history of cognitive pupillometry. Next we introduce the concept of pupillary movements as a psychological reporter variable, directly analogous to the reporter genes used with great benefit in molecular biology. We then summarize the anatomy, physiology, and pharmacology of pupillary movements, followed by an overview of the methods by which they are measured.

The heart of the chapter consists of a systematic review of the empirical literature utilizing task-evoked pupillary responses in the study of human cognitive processes. A common graphic format is used in presenting these results so that diverse experimental findings may be directly compared. The result is a consistent depiction of intensity variations in human cognitive processing as reflected by task-evoked pupillary responses. We conclude with a few small suggestions for future pupillometric studies and the role that they may play in cognitive neuroscience more generally.

Historical Background

LARGE-SCALE PUPILLARY MOVEMENTS IN CLINICAL NEUROLOGY

Large-scale changes in pupillary diameter have played a useful role in the daily practice of clinical neurology since the inception of this medical specialty. Large-scale changes of the pupil are conveniently defined as being apparent to a trained observer without the need for specialized measurement or recording apparatus. Large-scale abnormalities in pupillary diameter are usually either static or slowly changing and are indicative of peripheral or central nervous system (CNS) lesions or the use of psychopharmacologically active substances.

Chronic pupillary constriction is indicative of interruption to the sympathetic pathway leading to the sympathetically innervated dilator muscles of the iris (Bickerstaff & Spillane 1989). Such lesions may occur in the hypothalamus, the brainstem, the lateral upper thoracic spinal cord, the sympathetic ganglia, or the peripheral sympathetic fibers leading to the eye. Extremely constricted, pinpoint pupils are also produced by opiate narcotics such as morphine (Jaffe & Martin 1985).

In contrast, chronic pupillary dilation is produced by disruption of the parasympathetic input that ultimately activates the sphincter pupillae, which constrict the pupil. Disruption may occur anywhere from the pretectal nuclei and the nucleus Edinger–Westphal of the midbrain, through the pathway of the oculomotor (III) nerve to the ciliary ganglion of the orbit. The most common lesions

John T. Cacioppo, Louis G. Tassinary, and Gary G. Berntson (Eds.), *Handbook of Psychophysiology*, 2nd ed. © Cambridge University Press 2000. Printed in the United States of America. ISBN 62634X. All rights reserved.

are produced by vascular accidents of the midbrain, herniation produced by space-occupying tumors, or carotid artery aneurysm (Bickerstaff & Spillane 1989). Pupillary dilation is also produced by ingestion of neuroactive compounds such as atropine.

SMALL-SCALE PUPILLARY MOVEMENTS IN COGNITIVE PSYCHOPHYSIOLOGY

Unlike neurology, cognitive psychophysiology is concerned not with localizing neural lesions in clinical patients but rather with understanding the cognitive functions of the human brain. For this purpose, the examination of large-scale pupillary movements is uninstructive. However, there are small-scale, rapid fluctuations in pupillary diameter that are reflective of the dynamic CNS changes that underlie human cognition. The largest of these cognitively driven movements are about 0.5 mm in pupillary diameter, making them difficult to detect by unaided observation. Instead, precise pupillometric recording methods are employed to study the small-scale dynamic pupillary movements that reflect the cognitive activity of the human brain (Beatty 1982a,b; Goldwater 1972).

The fact that pupillary dilation accompanies cognitive processing was suggested in neurology well over a hundred years ago. Schiff (1875; Schiff & Foa 1874) documented that pupillary dilations are evoked by a variety of nonvisual stimuli. Shortly thereafter, W. Heinrich (1896) measured pupillary dilations evoked by cognitive processing in a study of pupillary movements evoked in mental multiplication tasks.

By the turn of the century (1911), Oswald Bumke could assert with confidence that "every active intellectual process, every psychical effort, every exertion of attention, every active mental image, regardless of content, particularly every affect just as truly produces pupil enlargement as does every sensory stimulus" (translated in Hess 1975, pp. 23–4).

However, for reasons that are not at all clear, this body of pupillometric knowledge remained confined to the German neurological literature. American psychophysiology was not aware of this phenomenon until the 1960s, when Hess and Polt (1964) published essentially a reconfirmation of Heinrich's earlier finding of pupillary dilations produced by mental arithmetic. This publication in *Science* was the impetus for the subsequent body of work that is the subject of this chapter.

PSYCHOPHYSIOLOGICAL REPORTER VARIABLES

Pupillary movements have had a curious status in psychophysiological research: they appear to reflect peripheral autonomic factors that are unrelated in any obvious way to central cognitive processes, yet they nonetheless empirically reflect variations in central processing load with extraordinary precision (Beatty 1982b, 1986; Goldwater 1972). "The implication," wrote Just and Carpenter (1993, p. 312), "is that the pupillary response is only a correlate of cognitive intensity, hence the marker is indirect and not causally linked" – a conclusion with which we agree completely.

But is noncausality a problem? How can a measure with so little apparent face validity be useful in psychophysiological research? We believe that noncausality is in no sense a problem. Rather, the use of pupillary movements in cognitive psychophysiology is analogous in several important ways to the use of reporter genes in molecular biology, where correlational measurement has speeded the study of the genome and its regulation (Alberts et al. 1998; Wood 1995). We suggest that explicit recognition of the properties of task-evoked pupillary response as a reporter variable in psychophysiology might facilitate the study of the biological basis of human cognition. Similar arguments have been made previously by Cacioppo and Tassinary (1990) in their discussion of the psychophysiological inference problem.

In molecular cell biology, reporter genes are DNA sequences that encode proteins of no intrinsic interest *except that* the reporter proteins are easily detected when expressed. Reporter genes are attached to the genome in the immediate vicinity of a gene of interest and thus provide an easily measured correlate of the gene being studied (Alberts et al. 1998).

A number of reporter gene sequences and their associated proteins are routinely employed in molecular biology. In a particularly dramatic example of reporter gene technology, Okabe and colleagues (1997) inserted the DNA sequence for an enhanced version of the green fluorescent protein, which produces bioluminescence in the Victoria jellyfish, into the mouse genome in a position that assures its expression throughout the whole body of the mouse, from embryonic stages through adulthood. The result is an extraordinarily vivid marker for use in genetic studies: wherever and whenever this reporter gene is expressed, the mouse glows bright green.

In psychophysiology, we rarely have the luxury of inserting markers of any sort into the human brain to study human cognitive function. Yet we should learn from the molecular biologists and openly exploit any naturally occurring psychophysiological reporter variables that are reliably correlated with central nervous system events of interest to cognitive neuroscience. It is our belief that task-evoked pupillary responses are important psychophysiological reporter variables deserving of further study.

Physical Context

Pupillary movements are determined by the state of the iridic musculature under the direct control of both the sympathetic and parasympathetic branches of the autonomic nervous system. The coupling of pupillary movements to cognitive processes, however, must occur at much higher levels within the human nervous system.

PUPILLARY ANATOMY

The general structure of the eye is often compared to a camera: each has a lens to refract and focus incoming light rays as well as an adjustable aperture that serves to regulate the amount of light admitted. In the eye, the aperture is the pupil – the opening in a pigmented structure called the iris, which contains two antagonistic smooth muscle groups, the sphincter and dilator muscles. Each of these muscles is innervated by a different component of the autonomic nervous system. The sphincter muscles, which constrict the iris, are under sympathetic control; the dilator muscles, which serve to open the iris, receive input from the sympathetic nervous system. At any moment in time, the size of the pupil is the integrated result of the ratio of activity occurring in the pathways innervating these two muscle groups, as seen in Figure 1.

As early as 1911, the illustrious physiologist C. S. Sherrington described the reciprocal nature of the muscles of the iris: as the agonist dilator muscles are activated, motor output to the antagonistic sphincter muscles is reduced. In Sherrington's words, "the inhibition is not peripheral but central, that is, it has its seat not in the muscle but in the nervous centre about the starting point of the final common path. The muscle relaxes because the motor discharge from that centre is abated" (quoted in Loewenfeld 1993).

The mechanics of this reciprocal system is complex. Until Loewenfeld's elegant series of experiments on a single macaca mullata monkey (Loewenfeld 1958), it had been believed that parasympathetic inhibition was simply the consequence of activity along the adrenergic sympa-

thetic pathway via the cervical sympathetic or other nerves. Loewenfeld demonstrated that parasympathetic inhibition persists after the sympathetic nerve is cut and that stimulation of the cervical sympathetic chain is insufficient to block the light reflex, whereas low-intensity electrical stimulation of the thalamus or hypothalamus readily prevents its occurrence. The inhibitory influences on the postganglionic parasympathetic neurons thus come not from the periphery but from suppression of the parasympathetic motor nucleus in the midbrain, which is then unable to send constricting impulses to the periphery. This result follows what Sherrington had postulated more than fifty years earlier in his law of reciprocal innervation.

The electrophysiological research of Bonvallet and Zbrozna (1963) directly demonstrated the two opposing systems. When the sympathetic agonist is activated, the motor nucleus of the antagonist is inhibited. These investigators recorded electrical activity in the cortex, the sympathetic chain, and the short parasympathetic ciliary nerves in a flaxidil-immobilized cat with a thoracic-level transection of the spinal cord. Immediately following stimulation of the pontine-mesencephalic reticular formation, several events occurred: cortical arousal, activity along the cervical sympathetic nerve to the dilator muscles, and inhibition of parasympathetic activity in the postganglionic ciliary nerve serving the constrictor muscles. Stimulation of sensory nerves entering above the level of the transection had identical effects.

PUPILLARY MOVEMENTS

Some pupillary movements are primarily optical in nature. For example, the pupillary light reflex serves to regulate the amount of light entering the eye. The accommodation response, or near reflex, involves a series of movements that result in changes in the curvature of the lens to control the depth of field. In addition, there are pupillary movements that are not related to luminance levels or to the distance between a visual image and the fovea of the retina; instead, they are related to sensory, mental, and emotional events. Of special interest to psychophysiologists are those changes in pupil diameter that are the systematic indicators of attention and mental effort (Kahneman 1973). These small but reliable changes in pupil diameter are superimposed on the diameter of the pupil, which is determined by the two optical reflexes and the organism's tonic state of arousal. These types of pupillary movements are described next.

Pupillary Hippus

Clinical neurologists and ophthalmologists often comment on the phenomenon of pupillary hippus or pupillary unrest – the rhythmic but irregular (usually < 0.04-Hz) constrictions and dilations of the pupil that occur

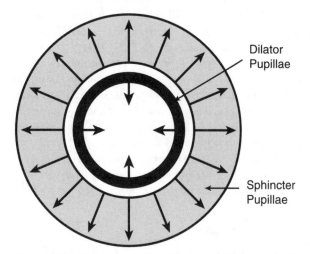

Figure 1. Muscles of the iris. Two opposing muscle groups within the iris of the human eye determine the aperture of the pupil. The sphincter muscles of the iris constrict the pupil when they contract, whereas constriction of the dilator muscles increases pupillary diameter.

Dilator
Pupillae

Sphincter
Pupillae

independently of eye movements or changes in illumination (McLaren, Erie, & Brubaker 1992). These movements are called pupillary hippus, after the Greek *hippos* meaning horse; the term was probably chosen to convey the notion of a galloping horse's gait. Hippus is a normal condition of the human pupil, although pathological hippus does occur. Pupillary hippus must be the result of central rather than peripheral muscular factors, since these rhythmic movements are always consensual. It has been suggested that hippus may actually reflect the brain processes that underlie task-evoked pupillary responses but are triggered by spontaneous, otherwise unobserved thought.

Pupillary Light Reflex

The pupil is a dynamic structure that changes in diameter in response to luminance levels. In bright light the pupil is small and constricted, whereas in dim light it is dilated and relaxed. The amount of light that enters the eye is proportional to the diameter of the pupil, which changes in size to accommodate variations in luminance at a ratio of approximately 16 to 1. The range of these pupillary movements is quite broad and varies from species to species. In humans, pupil diameter can vary from less than 1 mm to more than 9 mm; in the cat, the range extends from 0.5 mm to more than 13 mm.

The pupillary light reflex can serve as an important diagnostic indicator of neurological status. Under normal circumstances, presentation of a bright light produces consensual constriction of the pupil. These constrictions can occur within 0.2 sec, with peak response occurring from 0.5 to 1.0 sec later. Since it is sensitive also to reductions in luminance levels, the pupil correspondingly dilates in darkness. Either absence of the light reflex or nonconsensual light reflexes may be indicative of lesions in subcortical structures.

The parasympathetic neural pathway subserving the pupillary light reflex is relatively simple and involves a six-neuron arc (Loewy 1990). Three of the cells in this arc are located in the retina itself: the retinal photoreceptors (rods and cones), which synapse on bipolar cells that in turn send their output to third-order neurons, the ganglion cells. Ganglion cell axons form the optic nerve, which carries visual information to both cortical and subcortical projection sites. The optic nerve fibers associated with the light reflex are conveying information from a subset of W-type retinal ganglion cells that are responsive to luminance levels. Cells in homonymous hemiretinae project to the olivary, medial, and posterior pretectal nuclei located at the juncture of the diencephalon and the midbrain (Barlow & Levick 1969). Cells in the olivary pretectal nucleus have been characterized as luminance detectors and are associated with pupilloconstriction. Olivary pretectal cells project to the lateral visceral cell column of the Edinger–Westphal nucleus, from which preganglionic fibers project to the ciliary ganglion via the III cranial nerve, the

oculomotor (Kourouyan & Horton 1997). Postganglionic fibers are then distributed to the sphincter muscles via the short fibers of the ciliary nerve to produce pupillary constriction (Loewenfeld 1993). Clarke and Ikeda (1985) averred that the pupilloconstrictions of the light reflex are almost entirely reliant upon parasympathetic control, because superior cervical sympathectomy has little effect on the nature or occurence of the light reflex. The cells that produce the dilations observed in dark settings are located in the posterior pretectal nucleus (Clarke & Ikeda 1985). These darkness-sensitive cells follow a similar path to the ciliary ganglion via the oculomotor (III) nerve and are thought to produce the pupillary dilations observed in low luminance.

The Accommodation Response

An unfocused foveal image and binocular disparity are the stimuli that elicit the accommodation response (Cumming & Judge 1986). Loewy (1990) described the accommodation response as requiring three muscular adjustments: contraction of the ciliary muscle and release of tension on the zonule fibers to increase the curvature of the lens; constriction of the iris sphincter to produce pupillary constriction; and contraction of the medial rectus muscle, controlled by the oculomotor (III) nerve, to converge the eyes. The *afferent* pathways involved in accommodation are not known. Jampel (1960) provided evidence of involvement of the Y-retinal ganglion cell pathway that has a series of cortico-cortico projections from Brodmann's area 17 to the middle temporal region located along the surface of the superior temporal sulcus near the anterior limit of the occipital lobe. Although this cortical area lacks direct connections with the oculomotor complex, stimulation of cells in this region produces all three aspects of the accommodation response, and animals with middle temporal lesions show deficits in detecting and grasping near objects (Ungerleider et al. 1984).

The *efferent* pathways concerned with the accommodation response are similar to those involved in the light reflex. There is some evidence that the accommodation fibers, which leave the Edinger–Westphal nucleus via the oculomotor nerve, innervate the eye directly and without synapse in the ciliary ganglion (Jaeger & Benevento 1980; Ruskell & Griffiths 1979; Westheimer & Blair 1973).

PUPILLARY REFLEX DILATIONS

All somatic and visceral afferents and all central connections associated with arousal responses may serve as afferents for the pupillary reflex dilation, which is also called the psychosensory reflex (Loewenfeld 1993). Any sensory occurrence – whether tactile, auditory, gustatory, olfactory, or noxious – evokes a pupillary reflex dilation. Exceptions to this are light stimuli and accommodations to near visual stimuli, both of which produce pupil constrictions. However, one should not assume that pupillary reflex dilations occur only to external sensory events, because emotions, mental processes, increases in intentional efforts, and motor output also produce systematic changes in pupillary diameter. It is thus not surprising that there is no single, dedicated afferent path subserving pupillary reflex dilations. Several factors determine the magnitude of these pupillary dilations – for example, the individual's tonic state of arousal, the emotional effect of the stimulus, and luminance levels.

The pupillary (or psychosensory) reflex is subserved by both sympathetic and parasympathetic inputs. Loewenstein and Loewenfeld (1969) have written that the efferent sympathetic fibers that innervate all visceral organs arise in the hypothalamic motor regions of the diencephalon. The radially oriented and sympathetically innervated dilator muscles of the iris are but one aspect of this complex sympathetic system. The first-order neurons of the pupillary dilator path descend from the posterior and lateral hypothalamus and travel through the brainstem to the cervico-thoracic spinal cord. These discrete, first-order neurons synapse on preganglionic cells in the grey matter of the cord known as the cilio-spinal center of Budge.

Preganglionic second-order neurons then take an afferent course and exit the ciliospinal center via the ventral roots, primarily at T2 but also at T1. These fibers continue without synapse to the superior cervical ganglion, where they synapse on the third-order neurons. There are species differences in the course of fibers from this point, but in humans it is thought that these fibers extend rostrally in the internal carotid nerve for a short distance from the

superior cervical ganglion, at which point they deviate into the middle ear with the carotico-tympanic fibers and cross the tympanic plexus. After emerging from the middle ear, the fibers pass into the cranium, enter the cavernous plexus, and approach the Gasserian ganglion without synapse to enter the ophthalmic branch of the trigeminal nerve. The pupillary dilator fibers then pass into the nasociliary nerve to reach the iris muscles via the long ciliary fibers; see Figure 2.

Cell bodies for the parasympathetic constricting fibers of the pupil reside in the Edinger–Westphal nucleus of the oculomotor complex located in the mesencephalon. Fibers of these cell bodies course rostrally to the ciliary ganglion as part of the oculomotor (III) nerve. Postganglionic fibers are then distributed to the annular constricting muscles of the iris via the short ciliary fibers.

PUPILLARY PHARMACOLOGY

The fibers of the iris sphincter muscle, like other sphincters, are arranged concentrically. These muscle fibers receive cholinergic input from the parasympathetic nervous system and produce constriction of the pupil. Cholinergic agonists and antagonists have predictable effects on the sphincter pupillae; compounds that are acetylcholine (ACh) agonists produce miosis or pupillary constrictions, whereas ACh antagonists produce mydriasis or pupil dilation. For example, pilocarpine, which has a molecular structure similar to ACh, produces miosis by depolarizing the effector cells directly. Carbachol, another ACh agonist, evokes pupillary constrictions by initiating spontaneous release of ACh at preganglionic cholinergic nerve endings. In contrast, ACh antagonists reduce activity along the parasympathetic pathways innervating the iris and decrease the activity of the constrictor muscles, which reduces opposition of the dilator muscles. Under these circumstances, the dilator muscles contract and open the iris, resulting in mydriasis (Thompson 1996). Atropine, which reduces cholinergic activity by competing with the neural transmitter at the effector sites, and botulinum toxin, whose mechanism of action is to prevent release of ACh, both result in mydriasis.

The dilator pupillae are arranged radially, like the spokes of a bicycle wheel. Contraction of these muscle fibers serves to enlarge the diameter of the pupil and necessarily reduce the size of the iris. Although there is some evidence for inhibitory cholinergic input to the dilator muscles (Ehinger 1967; Paulson & Kapp 1967), they are traditionally thought to be activated primarily via alpha-adrenergic input from the sympathetic nervous system. Thus, noradrenergic agonists and antagonists will produce dilation or constriction of the pupil respectively. Ephedrine, an adrenergic agonist, causes spontaneous release of norepinephrine from the synaptic endfoot and directly stimulates the receptor. With increased activity at

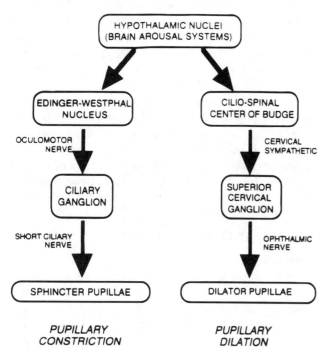

Figure 2. Neural structures and pathways that control pupillary diameter.

the effector site, the pupil dilates. Cocaine, a topical anesthetic for the conjunctiva and a powerful uptake blocker, also produces mydriasis as norepinephrine accumulates in the synaptic cleft. Adrenergic antagonists like thymoxamine (a noradrenergic receptor blocker) reduce activity at the neuromuscular junction, so that the sphincter muscle incurs reduced opposition and miosis results.

Inferential Context: Task-Evoked Pupillary Responses Are Reporter Variables

Nonreflexive phasic pupillary movements are of interest to cognitive psychophysiology for one and only one reason: they function as empirically based reporter indicators for brain processes that underlie the dynamic, intensive aspects of human cognition. In order to understand the use of task-evoked pupillary responses in cognitive psychophysiology, it is necessary to review the methods by which they are measured and analyzed.

BIOMETRICS: MEASURING PUPILLARY MOVEMENTS

Historically, pupil diameter was measured by employing motion picture photography (Hess & Polt 1964; Kahneman & Beatty 1966). This methodology requires photographing the pupil with a macrofocusing motion picture camera and preferably infrared film that allows recording at low luminance levels. Either 16 mm or 35 mm film may be employed; the former is less costly but the latter provides greater resolution. Filming begins with photographing a millimeter rule placed at a distance from the camera that corresponds to the distance at which the pupil will be photographed. The iris is then centered in the frame and the pupil is photographed at a 0.5–1.0-sec rate. Pupillometric measures are obtained by projecting the image of the iris onto a large surface, and measures are extracted with an ordinary ruler. These measures are scaled according to the standard rule appearing at the start of the film.

Infrared motion picture measurement is both labor- and time-intensive for the experimenter. Janisse (1977) reported that 20,000 measurements would not be unusual, citing an instance in which more than 100,000 separate measurements were taken. More recent technologies employ high-resolution infrared-sensitive video cameras that allow continuous monitoring of the dynamic changes in pupil diameter. Most video pupillometers employ a headrest to stabilize the image of the pupil with respect to the camera, although complex devices are also available that provide eye- and head-tracking systems that allow free movement of the head. For both simple and complex devices, the output of the video camera is sent to a hardware interface that contains pattern recognition circuits that automatically determine the boundary of the pupil in the video image. Pupil area or vertical pupil diameter is then computed electronically. The output of the pattern recognition hardware can be sent to a strip chart recorder, or (preferably) the analog signal is digitized and stored on computer for later analysis. A number of these devices are available commercially and have been described elsewhere (Alexandridis, Leendertz, & Barbur 1991; Nguyen & Stark 1993). Nguyen and Stark (1993) described an economical pupillometric system whose essential feature is a computer with a "frame grabber" to process the output of an infrared-sensitive video camera. In conjunction with the hardware, they describe a set of algorithms that allow precise measurement of pupil size and eye position in real time.

Once the data are acquired and stored on disk, they should be inspected for eye blink, movement artifacts, or accommodation responses. All artifact detection should be conducted blind with respect to experimental condition, response, and behavioral outcome. Artifacts typically appear as either discontinuities or constrictions in the pupil record. If small anomalies are detected in noncritical portions of the trial then it is reasonable to correct them by linear interpolation, a process that does not substantially alter the data. When large artifacts appear, or when small artifacts occur in critical areas of the pupillometric record, it is best to eliminate that trial from further analysis. Data that have been edited and are artifact-free may then be analyzed by single trial or averaged. Trials may be averaged conventionally – that is, averaged with respect to a temporal event – or backward-averaged by realigning trials using the occurrence of a behavioral response as the temporal reference (Richer, Silverman, & Beatty 1983).

The technologies described here are equally useful for the measurement of changes in pupil diameter that are elicited by the light reflex, accommodation response, or task-evoked pupillary responses. Because the light reflex and accommodation responses are quite large in magnitude relative to the changes that are evoked by mental or sensory events, precautions must be taken to avoid masking the small task-evoked pupillary responses (TEPRs) with responses produced by optic reflexes. To do so, care should be taken to equate the luminance levels of all visual stimuli. Accommodation responses can be minimized by providing participants with a distant fixation point. Under all circumstances, participant-initiated trials are preferred because they minimize the occurrence of blinks in the record.

PSYCHOMETRICS: COMPUTING TEPRs

After the data have been edited according to the principles just described, all artifact-free pupil records may then be averaged. The pupillometric data are then analyzed similarly to event-related potentials recorded from the scalp. Usually, baseline pupil diameter is established at trial onset or at some other relevant premeasurement interval. The baseline value is then subtracted from the peak dilation or average pupil diameter in the trial epoch of interest. The pupil values obtained reflect changes in pupil diameter evoked by the events that served as stimuli.

There are three measures that are typically extracted from each interval of interest: mean pupil dilation, peak dilation, and latency to peak. The methods for extracting summary values, described here, are applicable when the data have been digitized and stored on computer. *Mean pupil dilation* is calculated by first establishing the baseline interval. Assuming a typical sampling rate of 50 Hz (20 points per second) and a baseline period of 500 msec, the first ten data points in the record would be summed and averaged to obtain the average pupil diameter in the 500-msec baseline interval. Mean pupil dilation in the measurement epoch is obtained by averaging the relevant number of data points in the measurement interval and subtracting the mean diameter obtained in the baseline period. There are several sources of bias to consider when using mean pupil diameter, including trials that vary in length across participants. For example, pupil dilations may be measured during a maximum memory span task. In this case, trial durations will vary as a function of the size of an individual participant's span. Thus, the number of data points contributing to a mean will vary across participants. A second source of bias arises when the mean dilations are computed for overlapping intervals of interest. When such sources of bias are present, it is best to employ peak dilation as the index of amplitude.

Peak dilation is defined as the maximal dilation obtained in the measurement interval of interest. It is calculated similarly to mean dilation: first, mean diameter in the baseline interval is established. Baseline diameter is then subtracted from the single maximum value in the measurement interval. Because this measure is based on a single value, it is more vulnerable to random variations than is the measure of mean diameter. It is, however, independent of the number of data points occurring in the measurement interval. *Latency to peak* reflects the amount of time elapsed between start of the measurement interval and emergence of the peak dilation.

TEPRs AS A GENERAL MEASURE OF PROCESSING LOAD

The idea that task-evoked pupillary responses may provide a dynamic neurophysiological index of momentary information processing load was first suggested to American psychophysiology by Hess and Polt (1964) in a small but widely read research report. Hess and Polt photo-

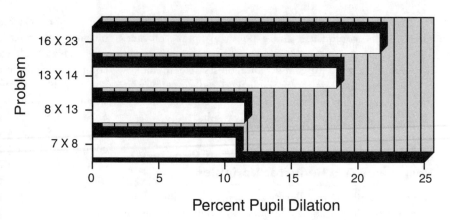

Figure 3. Pupillary dilations during mental multiplication: the original Hess and Polt (1964) finding. A simple but convincing demonstration that pupillary movements reflect an essential physiological aspect of cognitive processing was provided by Hess and Polt, who measured pupillary dilations as subjects mentally calculated the product of two numbers provided by the experimenter. They reported their results as percent pupillary dilation. Today, pupillary movements are conventionally reported as changes in diameter (in millimeters), since this measure appears to be independent of baseline pupillary diameter for a wide range of baseline values (Beatty 1982b).

graphically measured pupil size in five people who were mentally calculating the product of two small numbers in four problems of varying difficulty. Thus, the entire experiment consisted of twenty experimental trials. Yet their results were extraordinarily clear. Each subject's pupils dilated as each product was mentally calculated. Further, the extent of the observed dilation was nearly perfectly monotonically related to the difficulty of the calculation. These results are shown in Figure 3.

The robust nature of even very small TEPR has been repeatedly established in subsequent experiments (e.g. Beatty & Wagoner 1978). The specific finding of pupillary dilations varying directly with problem difficulty in a mental multiplication task has also been replicated by Ahern and Beatty (1979, 1981) in the context of studying individual differences in pupillary responding as a function of intelligence (see Figure 4).

It should be noted that Hess and Polt reported their findings in units of percent dilation over baseline pupillary diameter, but the baseline diameters themselves were not reported. Subsequent investigators have adopted a different convention in quantifying the TEPR, reporting both baseline diameter and pupillary dilation in millimeters. This convention is not only more complete, it is also more appropriate since all available evidence indicates that the extent of the pupillary dilation evoked by cognitive processing is independent of baseline pupillary diameter over a wide range of baseline values. Thus, if the baseline diameter is small – as it probably was in the Hess and Polt experiment, given the conditions of illumination they employed – then the pupil response expressed as a percentage

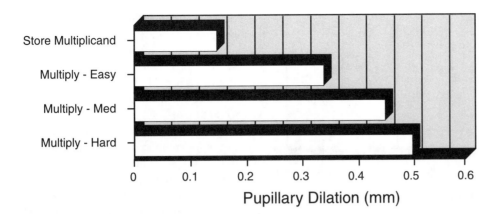

Figure 4. TEPR amplitude in mental multiplication as a function of problem difficulty. Ahern and Beatty replicated the original Hess and Polt finding as part of a larger study of individual differences in intelligence and pupillary movements. (See Beatty 1982b for these data.)

will be much larger than would be measured in percentage units at lower illumination with a large baseline diameter.

This conclusion is supported strongly by the findings of Bradshaw (1969). Bradshaw measured TEPR in seven subjects using a simple reaction task with either a long or short warned foreperiod under two levels of illumination (25 or 0.56 ftL at the fixation screen) to manipulate baseline pupillary diameter. Pupillary diameter was larger by 33% with the darker screen illumination, nearly doubling pupillary area. Yet there was "little evidence of any change in peak (TEPR) amplitude or shape" (Bradshaw 1969, p. 271) for responses at either of the two warning conditions. Similarly, administration of amphetamine in this same task produced a small increase in baseline pupillary diameter (from 3.8 to 4.2 mm) but no change in either the TEPR or reaction time (Bradshaw 1970).

Because TEPR amplitude appears to be independent of baseline pupillary diameter, it is possible to directly compare the amplitude of TEPRs obtained in different laboratories with varying conditions of illumination using absolute dilation amplitude as a common metric. This idea was first suggested by Kahneman (1973) in his influential monograph *Attention and Effort*. Kahneman argued that task-evoked pupillary dilations could serve psychology as a converging psychophysiological measure of mental effort, an idea later refined by Norman and Bobrow (1975) in their concept of a unitary central processing resource.

Beatty (1982b) tested this idea in a meta-analysis of the cognitive pupillometry literature and found that the results of this literature as a whole were coherent. Across a variety of qualitatively different cognitive domains, TEPR amplitude appeared to provide a consistent index of the presumed cognitive demands of each task. It appeared to be empirically demonstrable that TEPR amplitude acts as a psychophysiological reporter variable or psychophysiological marker for task-evoked cognitive activation.

Finally, it has been suggested that the pupil dilates to pleasant and constricts to unpleasant stimuli and thus might serve as a psychophysiological measure of emotional valence. This hypothesis stemmed from the widely cited early report by Hess and Polt (1960) that seemed to demonstrate a bidirectional pupillary response to affectively loaded photographs. This conclusion has not been supported by subsequent, carefully controlled pupillometric studies (e.g. White & Maltzman 1978). Further, the pleasantness hypothesis has been criticized on a variety of methodological grounds by a number of reviewers of the pupillometric literature, who have marshalled strong support for the cognitive activation hypothesis instead (Beatty 1982b; Goldwater 1972; Janisse 1977).

TEPRs and Perception

Among the most basic of all cognitive tasks is the detection of weak sensory signals. Once conceived as a threshold problem, the process of signal detection is now widely recognized to be probabilistic in nature and has been well described by statistical decision theory (Green & Swets 1966). In this formulation, a weak sensory signal generates some amount of evidence of its presence. This evidence is compared with a criterion and a decision is then made. The value of the criterion is determined by nonsensory factors, such as the a priori probability of a signal and the various rewards and costs of the various decision outcomes (e.g., correct detection of a signal, correct report of signal absence, incorrect report of a signal in its absence, or incorrect missing of a signal).

The first pupillometric treatment of this problem was reported by Hakerem and Sutton (1966), who studied detection using an increment in the duration of a pulse illumination in a monocularly viewed *Ganzfeld*. They report the presence of a stimulus-evoked pupillary dilation on trials in which the stimulus was detected that was absent on trials in which the same stimulus was not "seen," as shown in Figure 5.

Beatty and Lucero-Wagoner (1975) explicitly employed a decision-theoretic framework in their pupillometric analysis of the signal detection task. They studied a standard

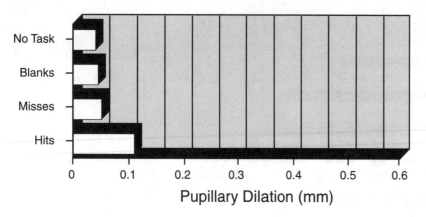

Figure 5. TEPR amplitude in a signal detection task. Hakerem and Sutton (1966) provided the first analysis of pupillary movements in sensory signal detection, reporting their data within the theoretical framework of the threshold model of perception.

auditory signal detection task (cf. Green & Swets 1966) with a 100-msec, 1-kHz sinusoid against a background of white noise. The use of auditory rather than visual stimuli prevented contamination of the TEPR by pupillary movements resulting from the light reflex. Beatty and Lucero-Wagoner also employed a four-alternative rating scale of response in order to assess a range of criterion values. They reported that TEPR amplitude varied as a monotonic function of the likelihood ratio across four stimulus–response conditions (certain hits, uncertain hits, uncertain correct rejections, and certain correct rejections). Thus, the largest responses appeared for certain hits and the smallest for certain correct rejections, with the two uncertain categories having intermediate values. Such a result would be expected if the TEPR reflected the processing of varying amounts of weak sensory signals that are present on any given trial. Thus, targets detected with certainty would result from the presence of relatively large amounts of sensory data, and nonsignal trials rejected with certainty would occur when virtually no sensory evidence was available for processing. This interpretation is consistent with Norman and Bobrow's (1975) characterization of signal detection as a data-limited task. These pupil-

lometric findings also argue against any interpretation of the pupillary response as a reflection of test anxiety or similar emotional reaction to the possibility of error, since TEPR amplitude does not vary directly with subjective uncertainty. See Figure 6.

Signal discrimination is computationally more complex than signal detection and involves additional cognitive processes. In simultaneous discrimination, two sensory signals must be analyzed simultaneously and compared with respect to some underlying dimension. In successive discrimination using the method of constant stimuli, relevant properties of the second (comparison) stimulus must be compared with a stored representation of the first (standard) stimulus. This was the procedure used by Kahneman and Beatty (1967) in their pupillometric analysis of pitch discrimination, which used eleven frequencies of tones that were compared with a 850-Hz standard tone. The comparison stimuli varied between 820 Hz and 880 Hz in 6-Hz steps. In this situation, the amplitude of the TEPR evoked by the comparison stimulus varies monotonically with its similarity to the standard stimulus (or the difficulty of the sequential discrimination), as shown in Figure 7. The additional cognitive demands induced by signal discrimination result in systematically larger task-evoked pupillary responses than occur in signal detection.

TEPRs and Memory

Pupillometric analysis was extended to the study of short-term memory and a long-term memory retrieval in

Figure 6. TEPR amplitude in signal detection as a function of decision category and certainty. Beatty and Lucero-Wagoner (1975) utilized statistical decision theory's signal detection model in a study of the detection of weak auditory signals. Using a four-category rating scale permitted the assessment of pupillary dilations evoked by detection judgments reaching different internal criterion levels. These results suggest that TEPR magnitude in this task reflects the accumulation of sensory evidence leading to a decision of signal present.

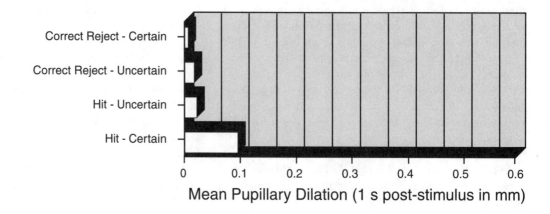

the early experiments of Kahneman and Beatty. The Kahneman and Beatty (1966) study was motivated by the striking findings of Hess and Polt (1964) on mental multiplication and pupillary dilation. In the first of a series of pupillometric studies, Kahneman and Beatty (1966) tested subjects with three paced auditory serial recall tasks. In the first, pupillary dilations were measured in the common digit span task for digit strings of three, four, five, six, and seven items presented and repeated at the rate of one item per second. Pupillary diameter systematically dilated as each stimulus digit was presented, reached a maximum between presentation and reporting, and declined to baseline after the last item was reported from short-term memory. Peak pupillary dilation varied as a function of the number of digits in the target string, as shown in Figure 8.

Kahneman and Beatty also examined the effect of item difficulty on pupillary dilation and performance using two additional serial tasks. The first was a four-item word span in which a string of high-frequency monosyllabic nouns were presented instead of digits. The second was a digit transformation task in which the subject heard a string of four digits (as in the four-item digit span) but was required to add 1 to each digit heard and report the transformed digit string. These three four-item tasks differed markedly from each other in difficulty, as indicated by mean span for correct performance in each task (digit span, 7.8 correct items; word span, 5.7 items; digit transformation, 4.5 items). These differences in task-induced processing load were also reflected in the amplitude of the task-evoked pupillary responses, as shown in Figure 9.

In one of the first applications of dual-task methodology in the measurement of mental processing load (see also Gopher & Donchin 1986; Norman & Bobrow 1975), Kahneman, Beatty, and Pollack (1967) examined the effects of the four-item digit transformation task on concurrent performance of a visual target detection task and the task-evoked pupillary response. The top half of Figure 10 presents pupillary dilation in the digit transformation task as a function of time. As in Kahneman and Beatty (1966), pupillary diameter increases as each digit is presented, reaching a maximum as the first transformed item of the string is reported. Pupillary diameter then decreases, returning to baseline after completion of report.

Performance on the visual target detection task mirrors these results, providing converging evidence that the amplitude of the task-evoked pupillary response is a reporter

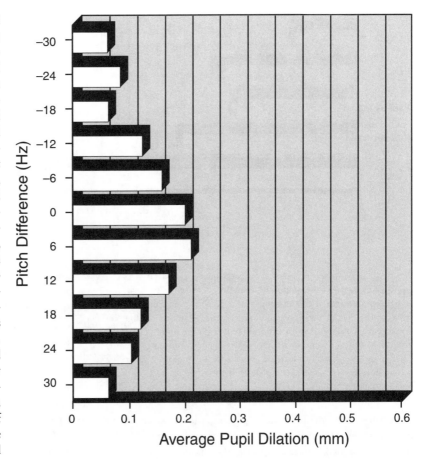

Figure 7. TEPR amplitude in signal discrimination. Kahneman and Beatty (1967) examined pupillary dilations evoked in a successive auditory discrimination task. The magnitude of the task-evoked pupillary response during the decision period of each trial varied with the similarity between the standard and comparison stimuli.

index of central information processing load. Errors in the target detection task follow the curve of the TEPR, reaching a peak at the beginning of transformation report. These results are shown in the bottom half of Figure 10.

If the task-evoked pupillary response is in fact a reporter of central processing load or processing intensity, then what would happen if central processing resources are fully saturated? Peavler (1974) examined this question by presenting subjects with strings of five, nine, or thirteen digits for immediate paced recall, the task previously employed by Kahneman and Beatty (1966). The three string lengths were randomly intermixed, so that subjects could not anticipate string length on any given trial. Under these conditions, pupillary diameter increased with each digit present until the maximum digit span (about seven or eight items) was reached. At this point, the task-evoked pupillary response reached an asymptotic value for the task. Peavler's results provide evidence that overloading the capacity of the human short-term memory system does not result in any additional pupillary dilation. These results are shown in Figure 11.

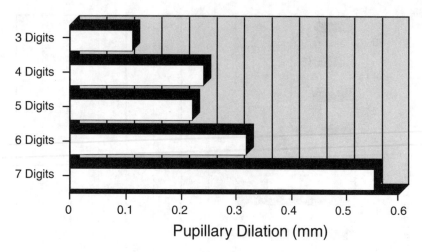

Figure 8. TEPR amplitude in a short-term memory task. In a paced auditory digit-span task, pupillary diameter increases as each successive digit is presented to the subject and reaches maximum dilation between the end of digit presentation and the beginning of digit report. Peak pupillary dilation varies directly with the number of digits held in short-term memory for immediate report. During the report itself, pupillary diameter decreases with each digit spoken, returning to baseline diameter at the completion of the trial. (Data from Kahneman & Beatty 1966.)

It should be mentioned in passing that Peavler's data also provide strong evidence against the idea that TEPRs in cognitive tasks index emotional, anxiety-related variables commonly associated with the autonomic nervous system. Emotional activation (if any) produced by performance failure should peak after digit span overload, but this is precisely the point in the task at which no additional dilation is present.

More recently, Granholm and colleagues (1997) reported a replication and extension of Peavler's original overload study. Like Peavler, Granholm et al. reported that the amplitude of the TEPR increases as each digit is presented, up to the span of digit memory (about 7 ± 2 digits). But unlike Peavler's finding that the pupil reached an asymptote in the 13-digit condition, pupillary diameter in Granholm's data decreased from maximum as the subject became overloaded. Granholm et al. attributed this discrepancy to a difference in instructions in the two experiments, not-

ing that Peavler explicitly told his subjects that some strings would be too long to remember perfectly (but to try nonetheless to reproduce as many digits as possible on every trial). Thus, Peavler's subjects may have adopted a "strategy of maintaining active rehearsal of the maximum number of digits possible [i.e., 7 ± 2] and ignoring further input" (Granholm et al. 1997, p. 460). Thus, the asymptote of the TEPR that Peavler observed may reflect a continued constant engagement in the memory task on the part of his subjects.

Finally, the same type of pupillary responses that reflect processing load in the storage and recall of digit strings in short-term memory (STM) occur in long-term memory (LTM) as well. We have all had the experience of dialing a telephone number from the fleeting short-term memory established by a telephone information operator or automated system, an action that seems subjectively to be much more difficult than simply dialing an already well-known number. Beatty and Kahneman (1966) measured TEPRs in a close analog of this familiar situation; their subjects verbally produced the seven-digit number in response to hearing an unfamiliar string or a one-word cue for a number that each knew well. Perhaps surprisingly, a larger TEPR was evoked when the telephone number was recalled from the subject's own long-term memory than when it was supplied by the experimenter, as shown in Figure 12. This finding suggests that TEPR in the LTM task reflects the load imposed by LTM retrieval in addition to that imposed by the processes of response organization and production, which is common to both the LTM and STM conditions.

Figure 9. TEPR amplitude for differing item types and memory tasks. Maximum pupillary dilation in the short-term memory task depends upon the types of information being processed and the nature of that processing. Kahneman and Beatty (1966) found that TEPR amplitude for four words was greater than for four digits. The largest dilations were produced by the four-item digit transformation task, which required recoding of the output string and not simply repetition. In these tasks, TEPR amplitude varied inversely with span length.

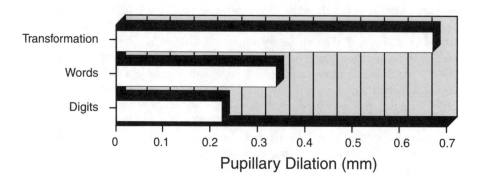

TEPRs and Responding

Richer, Silverman, and Beatty (1983) recorded pupillary dilations during the performance of simple and disjunctive (Go–No-Go) responses. In the simple reaction task (experiment 1), the foreperiod was either short (1 sec) or long (3 sec). Waveforms for the two conditions showed steady dilations that begin approximately 1.5 sec prior to the imperative stimulus and peak about 1 sec after stimulus presentation. The time course of these preparatory dilations is paralleled in the electrophysiological literature by the contingent negative variation (CNV), a slow negative potential measured from the scalp. Rohrbaugh, Syndulko, and Lindsley (1976) reported that the response-related component of the CNV also precedes movement by approximately 1.5 sec. Rate of dilation was inversely proportional to the length of the foreperiod, but neither peak dilation nor latency to peak differentiated short- and long-foreperiod trials.

Experiment 2 required a disjunctive reaction in which one of two stimuli are presented at S2. The Go stimulus required execution of a speeded response, whereas the No-Go stimulus mandated that no motoric output occur. Participants performed in both an immediate- and a delayed-response condition. In the immediate-response condition, subjects were presented with a warning tone of 860 Hz (S1), which was followed 1.5 sec later by a tone (S2) of either 600 Hz or 1,110 Hz. In the delayed-response condition, participants withheld any responses mandated by S2 until the presentation of S3, an 860-Hz tone. The delayed-response paradigm is especially valuable because it allows the separation of dilations due to response selection and preparation from those due to response execution.

In comparing immediate- and delayed-response conditions, small but reliable dilations are observed following S2 for all four trial types. Dilations to Go trials are greater than dilations to No-Go stimuli in both immediate- and delayed-response conditions. Further inspection of the data show that there are large dilations associated with the immediate No-Go trials and smaller dilations for the delayed No-Go trials. This suggests that there is a response-related process involved in the suppression of a response. This process may reflect either central organization and preparation of the response or peripheral motor adjustments.

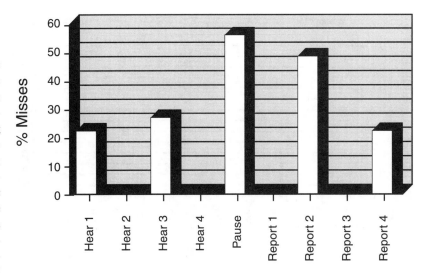

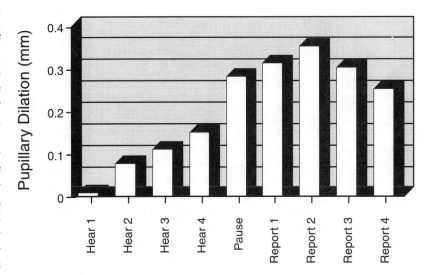

Figure 10. Two measures of processing load in the four-digit transformation task. Kahneman and colleagues (1967) measured both the TEPR and second-task interference produced by the four-digit transformation task. The upper panel presents the percentage of missed detections in a visual target detection task performed simultaneously with the digit transformation task. Targets were presented at one of five temporal positions in the paced trial. The bottom panel shows pupillary dilation during the performance of the two tasks.

To determine whether the dilations seen in the immediate No-Go trials were due to response execution processes, Richer and associates varied the probability of occurrence of Go and No-Go trials. They rationalized that if motor preparation is common to both Go and No-Go trials then the preparatory process should be sensitive to changes in likelihood of the response. Increasing the probability that a response will be required should increase the amplitude of the No-Go dilations, while the dilations associated with Go trials should not be affected because the demand associated with execution of the task has not changed.

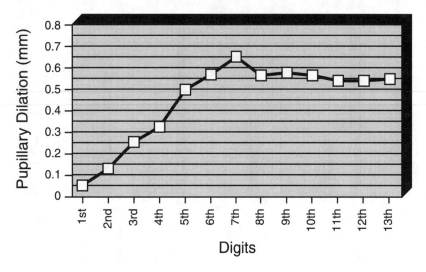

Figure 11. Pupillary response and short-term memory overload. These data from Peavler (1974) show pupillary dilation when the memory span of the subjects is exceeded but the subjects endeavor to report the largest number of sequential digits possible. These data suggest that the amplitude of the TEPR reaches an asymptote that corresponds to the behavioral limit of the short-term memory system.

Participants performed a task identical to the immediate-response paradigm just described, but the probability of occurrence of an overt response was manipulated between 0.33 and 0.66. As predicted, the amplitude of the No-Go trials increased as their likelihood decreased. There was no effect of probability on the pupil dilations generated by the Go trials. The absence of a probability effect in Go trials suggests that these dilations represent the maximum processing demands associated with the task. The nondecisional component of the dilations associated with No-Go trials reflects motor preparation processes, with amplitude of the response reflecting the proportion of preparation completed.

To examine the time course and amplitude of pupil responses that attend the preparation and execution of simple movements, Richer and Beatty (1985) asked participants to execute self-paced finger flexions. Participants produced either a single key press, a double key press with the right index finger, double key presses involving both index fingers, or a sequence of key presses with the index, ring, and middle finger in a counterbalanced order. Both peak pupil diameter and latency to peak were found to vary with

complexity of movement. These dilations began 1.5 sec before response execution and peaked 0.5 sec after the response.

In a second experiment, Richer and Beatty determined that force of movement systematically affects the magnitude of movement-related pupillary responses. When participants pressed a microswitch activated by a 100-g load, average peak pupillary dilations were 0.28 mm. The more forceful movements required to activate a microswitch with a 1,250-g load produced average peak dilations of 0.38 mm.

Readiness potentials recorded from the scalp during similar finger movements have a time course similar to the preparatory dilations seen in Richer and Beatty's first experiment. Like pupillary diameter, these readiness potentials appear approximately 1 sec prior to movement and vary in amplitude with the force of the movement required (Becker et al. 1976; Kutas & Donchin 1974). Slow preparatory responses are also seen in the electromyogram (Brunia & Vingerhoets 1980), and heart rate deceleration has been found to index response preparation (Coles & Strayer 1985). Such parallels between certain event-related potential components and autonomic variables such as the TEPR may be of use in providing an interpretation of the electrophysiological readiness potentials, at least under some conditions.

TEPRs and Probability

The pupil response to probability also has parallels in the electrophysiological event-related potentials recorded from the scalp. These brain potentials consist of a series of positive and negative components that have been associated with certain psychological processes. The components appearing within 100 msec of stimulus presentation are taken to reflect stimulus characteristics. The late-occurring components (evident 100 msec or more poststimulus) have

Figure 12. TEPR amplitude in short- and long-term memory. Beatty and Kahneman (1966) measured TEPR amplitude as subjects produced seven-digit telephone numbers in response to hearing a novel number presented for the first time or hearing a verbal cue for a well-known telephone number that subjects had supplied before the testing session. Larger TEPRs were produced when numbers had to be extracted from long-term memory before they were produced.

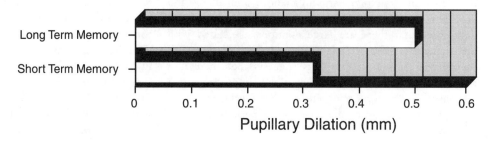

been shown to be sensitive to higher-order psychological processes such as attention. Friedman and colleagues (1973) demonstrated that both the P300 component (which appears approximately 300 msec after stimulus presentation) and pupil dilations have inverse relationships to stimulus probability: less-frequent stimuli produce higher-amplitude P300 and pupil responses.

Qiuyuan and associates (1985) conducted a series of three experiments to assess the effects of stimulus probability and task relevance (target vs. nontarget) on task-evoked pupillary responses. In each of the three experiments, participants heard Bernoulli series of 50 tones of 50-msec duration presented at 1.5-sec intervals. For each level of stimulus probability, the participant's task was to count the number of stimuli of a given type (the targets).

In their first experiment, Qiuyuan et al. employed probabilities of 0.2, 0.5, and 0.8. An inverse relationship was found between pupil amplitude and probability. Dilations to both targets and nontargets were found to be larger in amplitude and longer in latency when their probability of occurrence was 0.2 than when their respective probabilities of occurrence were 0.5 or 0.8. For a given level of stimulus probability, TEPRs to targets were similar to nontargets. These results differentiate the task-evoked pupillary response from the P300, which is seemingly insensitive to nontargets (Pritchard 1981).

In the second experiment, the participant's task was once again to count the target tones. In this instance, however, target probabilities were restricted to 0.1, 0.2, and 0.3. A significant effect of probability was seen for targets but not for nontargets for this restricted range of probabilities. Peak amplitude and latency to peak increased as target probability decreased from 0.3 to 0.1. The amplitude and latency for nontargets did not change as a function of their complementary probabilities of 0.7, 0.8, and 0.9.

In a third experiment, Qiuyuan et al. established that the TEPR need not be stimulus driven. For this experiment, tones were either presented or omitted with target probabilities of either 0.1 or 0.3. As in the second experiment, probability affected peak dilations to targets but not nontargets; greater amplitudes to targets were elicited by a probability of 0.1 than by a probability of 0.3. More interestingly, the magnitude of the pupillary response was greater for trials in which the tone was omitted than for those trials in which the tone was presented. This effect of target type (omitted vs. tonal) interacted with probability in such a way that dilations to omitted targets were greater when the probability of target occurrence was 0.1 than when the probability of target occurrence was 0.3. These results suggest that pupil dilations are elicited not only by external stimuli but also by an orienting response or a stimulus mismatch, as described by Sokolov (1960). Thus, the P300 and the TEPR may be complementary reflections of central processes associated with orientation to a task-important stimulus.

TEPRs and Language

Pupillometric studies of language processing have been both plentiful and productive, perhaps in part because language (and its symbolism) is the essential distinguishing feature of the human brain (Deacon 1997) and because there are well-developed linguistic models of the human language system (Pinker 1994). Task-evoked pupillary responses have been employed to investigate language processing dynamics from the levels of letter perception, syntax, and processing of semantic content – all with compelling findings.

Beatty and Wagoner (1978) built upon the seminal reaction time studies of Michael Posner (see e.g. Posner 1978) to examine the processing dynamics of visual letter matching. In a pair of related experiments, Beatty and Wagoner measured TEPRs as subjects viewed pairs of visually presented letters and were required to make Same–Different judgments about the pair presented. In the first experiment, subjects were requested to render a judgment of Same if the two letters shared the same name. Thus, the letter pairs *AA, aa,* and *Aa* are all examples of Same pairs (whereas *Ae* would be categorized as Different). Following Posner's logic, a Same judgment could be reached for the examples *AA* and *aa* after processing only the physical attributes of the printed letters, whereas judging the example *Aa* as Same requires an additional computational step – the extraction of each symbol's name code – an inferred processing step that increases reaction time (Posner 1978). Beatty and Wagoner reported that physically identical letter pairs evoke a smaller TEPR than do letter pairs identical only at the level of naming.

In a second experiment, subjects were requested to render Same or Different judgments using a category rule: determining whether the phoneme represented by the printed letters were vowels or consonants. In this experiment, there were three types of pairs that should be judged as Same: *AA* (visually identical), *Aa* (phonetically identical), and *Ae* (categorically identical). As before, the amplitude of the TEPR clearly reflects the extent of processing required to reach a correct decision of Same, as shown in Figure 13. Task-evoked pupillary response amplitude is indeed a sensitive and reliable reporter of even very small (but well-specified) differences in the structure of cortical language processing and decision.

Schluroff (1982) presented a striking set of data relating TEPR amplitude to syntactic complexity of English sentences. Schluroff asked his subjects to rate the comprehensibility of a series of auditorily presented sentences, and TEPRs were measured during sentence presentation. All sentences were parsed using Syntako, a transformational grammar of English, and from these derivations a quantitative measure of Yngve (1960) sentence depth or complexity was calculated. Schluroff reported that mean pupillary dilation during sentence presentation correlated

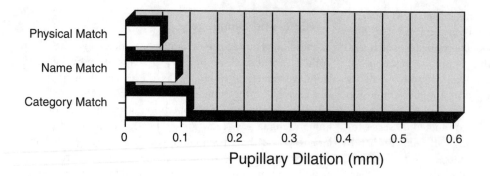

Figure 13. TEPR amplitudes vary with level of language processing. Here, subjects performed category judgments for letter pairs that could be identical at the orthographic, phonemic, or category level. The amplitude of the TEPR varied with the complexity of the processing required by each judgment.

+0.82 with Yngve syntactic complexity, accounting for 67% of the variance in TEPR amplitude. This correlation was not significantly reduced by covariation with sentence length. Schluroff's seminal investigation provides a strong demonstration of the close relation between quantitative aspects of syntactic sentence structure and the computational demands imposed by the language processing system of the normal human brain.

Schluroff and colleagues (1986) extended this pupillometric analysis of syntax in an ingenious study of syntactic ambiguity, presenting subjects with sentences (such as "Peter chased the man on the motor bike") that are ambiguous in the active voice but are disambiguated when transformed into the passive voice (as either "The man was chased by Peter on the motor bike" or "The man on the motor bike was chased by Peter"). The first rendering is verb-oriented (since the relative clause refers to the action denoted by the verb) whereas the second interpretation is object-oriented, with the phrase referring to the object of the sentence. Object-oriented readings of such ambiguous sentences are syntactically simpler than verb-oriented readings (Schluroff et al. 1986), which leads to a prediction concerning ambiguity resolution and TEPR amplitude.

In the foregoing example, both the verb-oriented and object-oriented resolutions of the syntactic ambiguity are sensible; thus, this example is not strongly biased toward object- or verb-oriented resolution. But other examples of syntactically ambiguous sentences are highly biased toward a single alternative. Schluroff proposed that highly biased syntactically ambiguous sentences are easier to process since they are disambiguated by semantic factors.

Schluroff tested these ideas by visually presenting subjects with a series of syntactically ambiguous sentences of high or low bias and requiring them to transform the ambiguous active form to an unambiguous passive form while changes in pupillary diameter were measured. Principal components analysis was employed to identify three main factors contributing to the TEPR: factor 1 loaded on pupillary diameter as subjects transformed the sentence into the passive voice; factor 2 covered the period of the task in which the sentence is read; and factor 3 was related to baseline pupillary diameter.

Pupillary dilation during the actual transformation of the sentence from active to passive voice, as reflected in factor 1, indicates that verb-oriented transformations impose a greater cognitive load than do the simpler, object-oriented transformations. Furthermore, low-bias sentences produced larger-amplitude pupillary responses than did high-bias sentences, as Schluroff predicted, suggesting mediation of syntactic complexity by semantic interpretation.

Just and Carpenter (1993) also used pupillometric methods to study the cognitive load imposed by syntactic structure in sentence processing. They examined sentences with center-embedded relative clauses, which impose significant demands on short-term memory.

The sentence "The reporter that the senator attacked admitted the error" is an example of an object-relative center-embedded clause because the leading noun of the sentence, "reporter," is the object of the clause. This particular construction imposes a large load on short-term memory. In contrast, subject-relative center-embedded clauses such as "The reporter that attacked the senator admitted the error" are much easier to process, since (i) the leading noun of the sentence is near the beginning of the relative clause and (ii) the agent of the sentence and agent of the clause is the same. This is evident from previous experiments of word-by-word sentence reading times in which subjects take 25 msec longer to make a lexical decision about the verb in object-relative versus subject-relative clauses (Ford 1983).

Just and Carpenter presented subjects with a series of sentences similar to the preceding example – intermixed with other superficially similar filler sentences – and required them to judge the truth of a comprehension probe that followed presentation of the sentence. They found that the TEPR amplitude was greater for the sentences with object-relative (versus subject-relative) center-embedded relative clauses, as shown in Figure 14. Further, the peak of the TEPR was delayed by 116 msec in the object-relative as compared with the subject-relative clause items. Thus, increased syntactic complexity results not only in more errors of comprehension and longer processing times but also in increased central processing demands, as indicated by larger-amplitude task-evoked pupillary responses.

Increases in the semantic demands of sentence processing also result in increases of the TEPR. Hyönä, Tommola, and Alaja (1995) reported two experiments measuring pupillary responses in simultaneous interpretation and translation of semantic content between Finnish and English. The first experiment measured averaged pupillary diameter for large passages of text as Finnish subjects passively listened to English text, shadowed English text, or simultaneously translated English text into their native Finnish. They report mean pupillary diameters for the three conditions of 4.20 mm (listening), 4.72 mm (shadowing), and 5.22 mm (interpreting).

In a second experiment, Hyönä, Tommola, and Alaja modified their tasks for single words (rather than long passages of text), permitting the computation of TEPRs. Stimulus words were also scaled for ease of translation using data from a preliminary experiment. Hyönä et al. confirmed and extended the findings of their first experiment, as shown in Figure 15. Increasing semantic processing of single words by variations in task demands produced an orderly increase in TEPR amplitude. The smallest dilations were produced by word listening. Shadowing produced intermediate dilations, and the largest dilations were evoked by simultaneous translation. Further, words that were more difficult produced larger TEPRs in each of the three task conditions.

Taken as a whole, the experimental literature relating task-evoked pupillary responses to theory-based measures of linguistic processing is remarkably robust and reliable. Indeed, TEPRs appear to provide an exquisitely sensitive measure for assessing processing demands imposed in human language processing tasks.

Figure 14. TEPR amplitude for sentences of differing syntactic structures. Sentences with syntactically more complex object-relative clauses evoked larger task-evoked pupillary responses than did sentences with simpler subject-relative clauses.

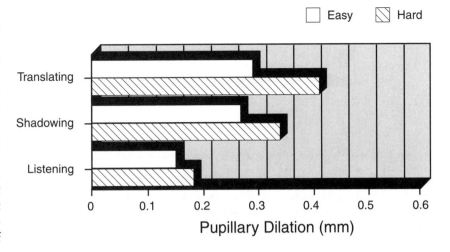

Figure 15. TEPR amplitude in bilingual language tasks. Here, subjects were required to listen passively to single English words, shadow English words, or translate English words into the listener's native Finnish. TEPR amplitude reflected the complexity of the processing task. For each task, the more difficult words elicited the larger responses.

TEPRs and Attention

Perhaps one of the slipperiest fundamental concepts in all of cognitive psychophysiology is that of *attention*. William James's century-old definition of attention still holds well today. He viewed attention as "the taking possession by the mind, in clear and vivid form, of one out of what seem several simultaneously possible objects or trains of thought. Focalization, concentration, of consciousness are of its essence" (James 1890, pp. 403–4).

Two studies have used pupillometric methods to explicitly examine human attention. Beatty (1988) looked for pupillometric evidence of selective attentional processes as subjects monitored one of two channels (a series of 800-Hz tone bursts presented to one ear or 1,500-Hz tone bursts presented to the other) for targets (tone bursts of 860 or 1,575 Hz, respectively). Interstimulus intervals (ISIs) were randomly generated to produce an average ISI of 333 msec and average of one target every 10 sec. Subjects were required to detect targets on either the high- or low-pitch channel on different blocks of trials.

These conditions generated some of the smallest task-evoked pupillary responses ever published, which are shown in Figure 16. There were no visible TEPRs for nontarget

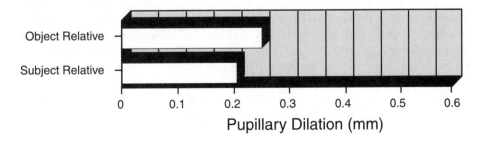

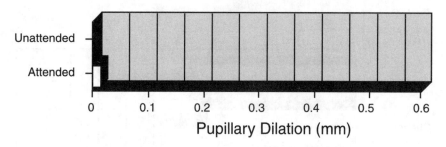

Figure 16. Amplitude of the TEPR in auditory selective attention. When subjects selectively monitor one of two auditory channels to detect slightly deviant target stimuli, an exceedingly small but reliable TEPR is evident for nontarget stimuli on the attended channel. No pupillary response is observed for nontargets on the unattended channel.

stimuli in the unattended channel while 0.015-mm peak TEPRs were present for nontarget stimuli in the attended channel. (Signal stimuli, naturally, generated large TEPRs as well as overt behavioral responses.) These results are similar to those previously reported by Hink, Van Voorhis, and Hillyard (1977) for event-related potentials.

Task-evoked pupillary responses in a sustained attention or vigilance task have also been reported. Beatty (1982a) measured pupillary movements as students monitored a series of 1-kHz 50-msec tone bursts presented at 3.2-sec intervals for a period of 48 min. Their task was to detect infrequent targets (tone bursts at −3 dB). These conditions produced a classic vigilance decrement. Signal detection analysis revealed that subjects became both decreasingly sensitive and increasingly conservative in their judgment criteria as a function of time in the task. Amplitude of the TEPR mirrored this change in sensitivity as it also decreased with time in the task.

Taken with the literature just summarized, TEPR amplitude appears to quantitatively reflect the state of central attentional processes. It is our opinion that pupillometry provides a unique and powerful methodology for the study of human attention that has yet to be fully exploited.

TEPRs and Individual Differences

The question of individual differences in cognitive abilities has also received attention in the pupillometric literature. Ahern (see Ahern & Beatty 1979, 1981) asked if college students of differing psychometric intelligence would exhibit differences in the amplitude of TEPRs during cognitive processing. They examined a group of 43 UCLA students with (combined verbal and quantitative) Scholastic Aptitude Test scores of either below 950 (low-intelligence group) or above 1350 (high-intelligence group). Four cognitive tests were used to search for between-group TEPR differences: mental multiplication, digit span, vocabulary, and sentence comprehension. In all but the vocabulary test, increasing task difficulty resulted in increased TEPR amplitude, confirming that these tests were in accord with previously published results.

Between-group intelligence differences in TEPR amplitude emerged in the tests for mental multiplication, digit span, and sentence comprehension. Task-evoked pupillary responses were smaller for subjects in the high-intelligence group than for their counterparts in the low-intelligence group. (Pupillary responses were essentially identical for both groups in the vocabulary test.) These results suggest that the cognitive processes of individuals with high psychometric intelligence are more efficient and less demanding of attention or resources. Whether this presumed heightened efficency is innate or the product of practice and overlearning is a question not addressed by the pupillometric data.

RELATION BETWEEN TEPRs AND OTHER PSYCHOPHYSIOLOGICAL VARIABLES

Kahneman and associates (1969) provided comparative data concerning task-evoked pupillary responses and co-occurring changes in heart rate and skin resistance. Investigators measured the pupillary diameter, heart rate, and skin resistance of ten subjects performing a four-item digit task at three levels of difficulty: add 0, 1, or 3 to each digit. The results are shown in Figure 17.

Kahneman et al. reported similar changes in all three psychophysiological systems, suggesting that the common origin of these effects is relatively high within the central nervous system. But of the three response systems, the responses of the pupillary system were most reliable and significant for the size of the observed data sample. This finding is in accord with the frequent observation of high statistical reliability with very small sample sizes common in pupillometric research (cf. the highly systematic and significant data obtained from only twenty experimental trials by Kahneman & Beatty 1966). These and other data indicate that the pupillary system is a very sensitive, low-noise system for psychophysiological measurement.

RELATION BETWEEN TEPRs AND BRAIN ACTIVITY

Perhaps even more interesting than the concordance of task-evoked pupillary responses with other autonomic psychophysiological indicators is evidence that TEPR amplitude also covaries with cortical activation. Just et al. (1996) described an elegant experiment using positron emission tomography (PET) to measure the extent of activation in Broca's and Wernicke's areas of the left cerebral hemisphere in a sentence comprehension task similar to that studied pupillometrically by Just and Carpenter (1993). Just et al. (1996) presented subjects with superficially similar sentences of equal length that differed in syntactic construction and short-term memory load. In the least demanding syntactic structure, two related active clauses were conjoined (e.g., "The reporter attacked the senator and admitted the error"). More demanding were sentences with a subjective-relative clause ("The reporter that attacked the senator admitted the error"). The most demanding syntactic structure contained an object-relative clause ("The reporter that the senator attacked admitted the error"). As in the earlier study, the subject's comprehension of each sentence was tested with a true–false comprehension probe ("The reporter attacked the senator; true or false?"). These conditions had been shown previously to yield increasingly large task-evoked pupillary responses.

The PET data revealed that increasing syntactic complexity in this sentence comprehension task increased the area of task-evoked cortical activation most prominently in Wernicke's area, but also in Broca's area as well as homologous regions of the right cerebral hemisphere (Figure 18). In all cases, the additional activation appeared as expansion of the regions activated by the simplest sentences. Additional, new areas were never recruited as syntactic complexity increased.

These data of Just et al. (1996) are particularly important for the purposes of this chapter in that they provide a unique, parallel evaluation of specific regional cortical activation patterns in a task previously characterized more generally using pupillometry. Their results are clear and conclusive elaboration of the task-evoked specific cortical events that occur concomitantly with the task-evoked pupillary response in a behaviorally well-controlled and linguistically well-defined high-level cognitive task. Such data speak directly to the importance of pupillometric methods in the psychophysiological study of human cognitive processes.

Epilogue

Pupillometry has served psychophysiology well in the study of the dynamics of human cognitive processing. This literature is remarkably consistent and without significant contradictions. The TEPR meets Kahneman's three criteria for a psychophysiological measure of processing load. Task-evoked pupillary responses have been shown to index accurately the within-task variations in task demands that result from changes in task parameters. Further,

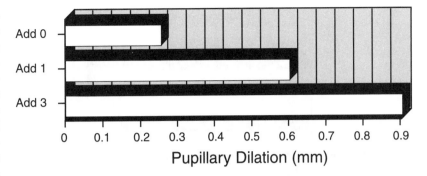

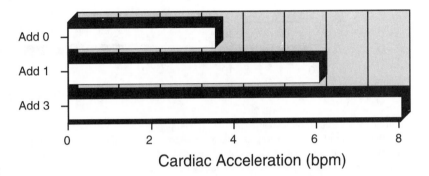

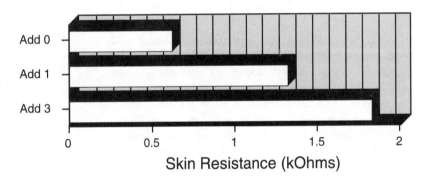

Figure 17. Concordant responses in three psychophysiological systems. Similar patterns of results of varying the difficulty of the digit repetition/transformation task are seen in pupillary dilation, cardiac acceleration, and skin resistance, arguing for the high-level central nervous system origin of these psychophysiological responses.

they relate between-task differences in processing load evoked by qualitatively different mental tasks in a reasonable and consistent fashion. Finally, TEPR amplitude is responsive to individual differences in cognitive abilities, as reflected in studies of intelligence and processing load.

Given the sensitivity, reliability, and consistency of TEPRs as a measure of cognitive load, it is somewhat surprising that the pupillometric psychophysiological literature is not large. We suspect that pupillometry is not widely employed in cognitive psychophysiology because the pupil lacks face validity as a measure of brain function. If a similar pattern of findings were produced by an electrophysiological indicator of cortical origin, we suspect that

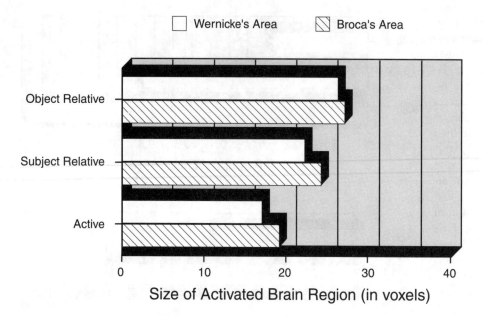

Figure 18. Brain activation responses mirror prior pupillary response data. The extent of activation in two language-related regions of the dominant cerebral hemisphere, Broca's and Wernicke's areas, directly reflects the processing load imposed by auditorily presented sentences that differ in syntactic structure. This pattern of results (Just et al. 1996) is predictable from previous pupillometric findings (Just & Carpenter 1993).

it would be widely pursued as a chosen methodology in cognitive psychophysiological research.

For this reason, in this chapter we offer the argument that the TEPR should be viewed as a reporter variable for human cognitive processes in much the same way as reporter genes are used in studying the molecular biology of the cell. In both cases, correlation is quite sufficient and the lack of causality is irrelevant. We hope that this reasoning will encourage others to join in the pupillometric study of cognitive processes.

REFERENCES

Ahern, S. K., & Beatty, J. (1979). Pupillary responses during information processing vary with scholastic aptitude test scores. *Science, 205,* 1289–92.

Ahern, S. K., & Beatty, J. (1981). Physiological evidence that demand for processing capacity varies with intelligence. In M. P. Friedman, J. P. Das, & N. O'Connor (Eds.), *Intelligence and Learning,* pp. 121–8. New York: Plenum.

Alberts, B., Bray, D., Johnson, A., & Lewis, J. (1998). *Essential Cell Biology: An Introduction to the Molecular Biology of the Cell.* New York: Garland.

Alexandridis, J. A., Leendertz, J. A., & Barbur, J. L. (1991). Methods for studying the behavior of the pupil. *Journal of Psychophysiology, 5,* 223–39.

Barlow, H. B., & Levick, W. R. (1969). Changes in the maintained discharge with adaption level in the cat retina. *Journal of Physiology (London), 202,* 699–718.

Beatty, J. (1982a). Phasic not tonic pupillary responses vary with auditory vigilance performance. *Psychophysiology, 19,* 167–72.

Beatty, J. (1982b). Task-evoked pupillary responses, processing load, and the structure of processing resources. *Psychological Bulletin, 91,* 276–92.

Beatty, J. (1986). The pupillary system. In M. G. H. Coles, E. Donchin, & S. M. Porges (Eds.), *Psychophysiology: Systems, Processes, and Applications,* pp. 43–50. New York: Guilford.

Beatty, J. (1988). Pupillometric signs of selective attention in man. In G. C. Galbraith, M. L. Kietzman, & E. Donchin (Eds.), *Neurophysiology and Psychophysiology: Experimental and Clinical Applications,* pp. 138–43. Hillsdale, NJ: Erlbaum.

Beatty, J., & Kahneman, D. (1966). Pupillary changes in two memory tasks. *Psychonomic Science, 5,* 371–2.

Beatty, J., & Lucero-Wagoner, B. (1975). Pupillary measurement of sensory and decision processes in a signal-detection task. Paper presented at the meeting of the Psychonomic Society (Denver).

Beatty, J., & Wagoner, B. L. (1978). Pupillometric signs of brain activation vary with level of cognitive processing. *Science, 199,* 1216–18.

Becker, W., Iwase, K., Jurgens, R., & Kornhuber, H. H. (1976). Brain potentials preceding slow and rapid hand movements. In W. C. McCallum & J. R. Knott (Eds.), *The Responsive Brain,* pp. 99–102. Bristol, U.K.: Wright.

Bickerstaff, E. R., & Spillane, J. A. (1989). *Neurological Examination in Clinical Practice.* Oxford, U.K.: Blackwell.

Bonvallet, M., & Zbrozna, A. (1963). Les commandes reticulaires du systeme autonome et en particulier de l'innervation sympathetique et parasympathique de la pupille. *Archives of Italian Biology, 101,* 174–207.

Bradshaw, J. L. (1969). Background light intensity and the pupillary response in a reaction time task. *Psychonomic Science, 14,* 271–2.

Bradshaw, J. L. (1970). Pupil size and drug state in a reaction time task. *Psychonomic Science, 18,* 112–13.

Brunia, C. H. M., & Vingerhoets, A. J. J. M. (1980). CNV and EMG preceding a plantar flexion of the foot. *Biological Psychology, 11,* 181–91.

Caccioppo, J. T., & Tassinary, L. G. (1990). Inferring psychological significance from physiological signals. *American Psychologist, 45,* 16–28.

Clarke, R. J., & Ikeda, J. (1985). Luminance and darkness detectors in the olivary and posterior pretectal nuclei and their relationship to the pupillary light reflex in the rat. I. Studies with steady luminance levels. *Experimental Brain Research, 57,* 224–32.

Coles, M. G. H., & Strayer, D. L. (1985). The psychophysiology of the cardiac cycle time effect. In J. F. Orlebeke, G. Mulder, & L. J. P. van Doornen (Eds.), *Psychophysiology of Cardiovascular Control. Methods, Models, and Data,* pp. 517–34. New York: Plenum.

Cumming, B. G., & Judge, J. S. (1986). Disparity-induced and blur-induced convergence eye movement and accommodation in the monkey. *Journal of Neurophysiology, 55,* 896–914.

Deacon, T. W. (1997). *The Symbolic Species: The Co-evolution of Language and the Brain.* New York: Norton.

Ehinger, B. (1967). Double innervation of the feline iris dilator. *Archives of Ophthalmology and Visual Science, 77,* 541–5.

Ford, M. (1983). A method for obtaining measures of local parsing complexity throughout sentences. *Journal of Verbal Learning and Verbal Behavior, 22,* 203–18.

Friedman, D., Hakerem, G., Sutton, S., & Fliess, J. L. (1973). Effect of stimulus uncertainty on the pupillary dilation response and the vertex evoked potential. *Electroencephalography and Clinical Neurophysiology, 34,* 475–84.

Goldwater, B. C. (1972). Psychological significance of pupillary movements. *Psychological Bulletin, 77,* 340–55.

Gopher, D., & Donchin, E. (1986). Workload – An examination of the concept. In K. R. Boff, L. Kaufman, & J. P. Thomas (Eds.), *Handbook of Perception and Human Performance, Volume II: Cognitive Processes and Performance,* pp. 41.1–41.49. New York: Wiley.

Granholm, E., Morris, S. K., Sarkin, A. J., Asarnow, R. F., & Jeste, D. V. (1997). Pupillary responses index overload of working memory resources in schizophrenia. *Journal of Abnormal Psychology, 106,* 458–67.

Green, D. M., & Swets, J. (1966). *Signal Detection Theory and Psychophysics.* New York: Wiley.

Hakerem, G., & Sutton, S. (1966). Pupillary response at visual threshold. *Nature, 212,* 485–6.

Heinrich, W. (1896). Die Aufmerksamkeit und die Funktion der Sinnesorgane. *Zeitschrift für Psychologie und Physiologie der Sinnesorgane, 9,* 342–88.

Hess, E. (1975). *The Tell-Tale Eye.* New York: Van Nostrand.

Hess, E. H., & Polt, J. M. (1960). Pupil size as related to interest value of visual stimuli. *Science, 132,* 349–50.

Hess, E. H., & Polt, J. M. (1964). Pupil size in relation to mental activity during simple problem solving. *Science, 143,* 1190–2.

Hink, R. F. Van Voorhis, S. T., & Hillyard, S. A. (1977). The division of attention and the human auditory evoked potential. *Neuropsychologia, 15,* 597–605.

Hyönä, J., Tommola, J., & Alaja, A.-M. (1995). Pupil dilation as a measure of processing load in simultaneous interpretation and other language tasks. *Quarterly Journal of Experimental Psychology, 48A,* 598–612.

Jaeger, R. J., & Benevento, L. A. (1980). A horseradish peroxidase study of the innervation of the internal structures of the eye. *Investigative Ophthalmology and Visual Science, 19,* 575–83.

Jaffe, J. H., & Martin, W. R. (1985). Opioid analgesics and antagonists. In A. G. Gilman, L. S. Goodman, T. W. Rall, and F. Murad (Eds.), *Goodman and Gilman's The Pharmacological Basis of Therapeutics,* 7th ed., pp. 491–531. New York: Macmillan.

James, W. (1890). *The Principles of Psychology,* vol. 1. New York: Dover.

Jampel, R. S. (1960). Convergence, divergence, pupillary reactions and accommodation of the eyes from faradic stimulation of the macaque brain. *Journal of Comparative Neurology, 115,* 371–99.

Janisse, M. P. (1977). *Pupillometry.* Washington, DC: Hemisphere.

Just, M. A., & Carpenter, P. A. (1993). The intensity dimension of thought: Pupillometric indices of sentence processing. *Canadian Journal of Experimental Psychology, 47,* 310–39.

Just, M. A., Carpenter, P. A., Keller, T. A., Eddy, W. F., & Thulborn, K. R. (1996). Brain activation modulated by sentence comprehension. *Science, 274,* 114–16.

Kahneman, D. (1973). *Attention and Effort.* Englewood Cliffs, NJ: Prentice-Hall.

Kahneman, D., & Beatty, J. (1966). Pupil diameter and load on memory. *Science, 154,* 1583–5.

Kahneman, D., & Beatty, J. (1967). Pupillary responses in a pitch discrimination task. *Perception and Psychophysics, 2,* 101–5.

Kahneman, D., Beatty, J., & Pollack, I. (1967). Perceptual deficit during a mental task. *Science, 157,* 218–19.

Kahneman, D., Tursky, B., Shapiro, D., & Crider, A. (1969). Pupillary, heart rate, and skin resistance changes during a mental task. *Journal of Experimental Psychology, 79,* 164–7.

Kourouyan, H. D., & Horton, J. C. (1997). Transneuronal retinal input to the primate Edinger–Westphal nucleus. *Journal of Comparative Neurology, 381,* 68–80.

Kutas, M., & Donchin, E. (1974). Studies of squeezing: Handedness, responding hand, and asymmetry of readiness potential. *Science, 186,* 545–8.

Loewenfeld, I. E. (1958). Mechanisms of reflex dilation of the pupil. Historical review and experimental analysis. *Documenta Ophthalmologica, 12,* 185–448.

Loewenfeld, I. E. (1993). *The Pupil: Anatomy, Physiology, and Clinical Applications,* vols. I, II. Ames: Iowa State University Press / Detroit: Wayne State University Press.

Loewenstein, O., & Loewenfeld, I. E. (1969). The pupil. In H. Dawson (Ed.), *The Eye,* vol. 3, pp. 255–337. New York: Academic Press.

Loewy, A. D. (1990). Autonomic control of the eye. In A. D. Loewy & K. M. Spyer (Eds.), *Central Regulation of Autonomic Functions.* New York: Oxford University Press.

McLaren, J. W., Erie, J. C., & Brubaker, R. F. (1992). Computerized analysis of pupillograms in studies of alertness. *Investigative Ophthalmology and Visual Science, 33,* 671–6.

Nguyen, A. H., & Stark, L. W. (1993). Model control of image processing: Pupillometry. *Computerized Medical Imaging and Graphics, 17,* 21–33.

Norman, D. A., & Bobrow, D. J. (1975). On data limited and resource limited processes. *Cognitive Psychology, 7,* 44–64.

Okabe, M., Ikawa, M., Kominami, K., Nakanishi, T., & Nishimune, Y. (1997). "Green mice" as a source of ubiquitous green cells. *FEBS Letters, 407,* 313–19.

Paulson, G. W., & Kapp, J. P. (1967). Dilatation of the pupil in the cat via the oculomotor nerve. *Archives of Ophthalmology, 77,* 536–40.

Peavler, W. S. (1974). Pupil size, information overload, and performance differences. *Psychophysiology, 11,* 559–66.

Pinker, S. (1994). *The Language Instinct.* New York: Morrow.

Posner, M. I. (1978). *Chronometric Explorations of Mind.* Hillsdale, NJ: Erlbaum.

Pritchard, W. S. (1981). Psychophysiology of P300. *Psychological Bulletin, 89,* 506–40.

Qiuyuan, J., Richer, F., Wagoner, B. L., & Beatty, J. (1985). The pupil and stimulus probability. *Psychophysiology, 22,* 530–4.

Richer, F., & Beatty, J. (1985). Pupillary dilations in movement preparation and execution. *Psychophysiology, 22,* 204–7.

Richer, F., Silverman, C., & Beatty, J. (1983). Response selection and initiation in speeded reactions: A pupillometric analysis. *Journal of Experimental Psychology: Human Perception and Performance, 9,* 360–70.

Rohrbaugh, J. W., Syndulko, K., & Lindsley, D. B. (1976). Brain wave components of the contingent negative variation in humans. *Science, 191,* 1055–7.

Ruskell, F. L., & Griffiths, T. (1979). Peripheral nerve pathway to the ciliary muscle. *Experimental Eye Research, 10,* 319–30.

Schiff, J. M. (1875). *La pupille consideré comme esthésiomètre* (translated by R. G. de Choisity). Paris: J. B. Bailliére.

Schiff, J. M. & Foa, P. (1874). La pupille considerée comme esthésiomètre (translated by R.G. de Choisity). *Marseille Médical, 2,* 736–41.

Schluroff, M. (1982). Pupil responses to grammatical complexity of sentences. *Brain and Language, 17,* 322–44.

Schluroff, M., Zimmermann, T. E., Freeman, R. B., Jr., Hofmeister, K., Lorscheid, T., & Weber, A. (1986). Pupillary responses to syntactic ambiguity of sentences. *Brain and Language, 27,* 322–44.

Sokolov, E. N. (1960). Neuronal models and the orienting reflex. In M. A. B. Brazier (Ed.), *The Central Nervous System and Behavior.* New York: Macy Foundation.

Thompson, H. S. (1996). Autonomic control of the pupil. In D. Robertson, P. A. Low, & R. J. Polinsky (Eds.), *Primer on the Autonomic Nervous System.* New York: Academic Press.

Ungerleider, K. D., Desimone, R., Galkin, T. W., & Mishkin, M. (1984). Subcortical projections of area MT in the macaque. *Journal of Comparative Neurology, 223,* 368–86.

Westheimer, G., & Blair, S. M. (1973). The parasympathetic pathways to internal eye muscles. *Investigative Ophthalmology and Visual Science, 12,* 193–7.

White, G. L., & Maltzman, I. (1978). Pupillary activity while listening to verbal passages. *Journal of Research in Personality, 12,* 361–9.

Wood, K. V. (1995). Marker proteins for gene expression. *Current Opinion in Biotechnology, 6,* 50–8.

Yngve, V. H. (1960). A model and hypothesis for language structure. *Proceedings of the American Philosophical Society, 104,* 444–66.

CHAPTER SEVEN

THE SKELETOMOTOR SYSTEM
Surface Electromyography

LOUIS G. TASSINARY & JOHN T. CACIOPPO

The principal function of the nervous system is the co-ordinated innervation of the musculature. Its fundamental anatomical plan and working principles are understandable only on these terms. (Sperry 1952, p. 298)

Adaptive success finally accrues not to brains but to brain–body coalitions embedded in ecologically realistic environments. (Clark 1997, p. 98)

Introduction

The sophistication of the skeletomuscular system enables the vast repertoires of adaptive reflexes and skilled actions characteristic of behavior. The electrophysiological signals associated with active muscles have been of interest for centuries, owing to the complexity of their organization and dynamics, their clinical applications, and their value as indices of and possible contributors to behavioral processes.

In this chapter, we provide an introduction specifically to psychophysiological research on the skeletomotor system.[1] We begin by reviewing the history of this research and by articulating some of the major issues, limitations, and advantages of surface electromyography (EMG) as a noninvasive measure of muscular activity. We then review briefly the physiological basis of EMG and summarize guidelines for surface EMG recording in humans. We continue with a discussion of the social context for EMG recording and of psychophysiological principles, paradigms, and applications that have emerged from research on the skeletomotor system.

A major theme in this chapter is that technical competence in recording EMG activity is necessary for securing scientifically meaningful data. As Claude Bernard (1865) commented:

In scientific investigation, minutiae of method are of highest importance.... [A] bad method or defective processes of research may cause the gravest errors, and may retard science by leading it astray. In a word, the greatest scientific truths are rooted in details of experimental investigation which form, as it were, the soil in which these truths must develop. (Bernard 1865/1949, pp. 14–15)

Such competence is necessary, but it is not sufficient. Analyzing any muscular act is complex psychophysiologically; similar limb displacements or feature distortions can be achieved by distinctly different muscular actions, and control over these actions can be exerted at many levels of the neuraxis. At the behavioral level, muscular acts do not always occur as intended, are sometimes nonobvious, may mislead, and are typically polysemous. Thus, for EMG signals to be of theoretical significance, one must consider conjointly the historical, physical, social, and inferential contexts in which these signals are acquired.

Historical Context

At least two distinct themes can be identified in the development of electromyography in psychophysiology. The first is the history of the physiology of the muscles, which derives from writings of early Greek philosophers and physicians and from the field of neurophysiology, whose origin can be traced to Francesco Redi's deduction in 1666 that the shock of the electric ray fish (*Torpedo torpedo*) emanated from specialized muscle tissue (see Wu 1984). The second is the history of psychophysiological research, which began in earnest with the work of such figures as Duchenne (1862/1990), Spencer (1870), Darwin (1872/1873), and James (1890), all of whom emphasized relatively subtle patterns of muscular actions as a way of characterizing and understanding human behavior generally.

John T. Cacioppo, Louis G. Tassinary, and Gary G. Berntson (Eds.), *Handbook of Psychophysiology*, 2nd ed. © Cambridge University Press 2000. Printed in the United States of America. ISBN 62634X. All rights reserved.

MUSCLE PHYSIOLOGY

According to Fulton (1926), the history of muscle physiology can be broken into partially overlapping phases. The first period, lasting roughly from the fourth century B.C. until the seventeenth century, was characterized by sporadic investigations into the causes of animal movement. In his books *De Motu Animalium* and *De Incessu Animalium,* Aristotle provided clear descriptions of coordinated motor acts (e.g., locomotion and the importance of the mechanism of flexion). Claudius Galen, about half a century later, observed that a muscle is still capable of contracting even after surgical removal from the body and also noted correctly that muscles can only contract or relax. This level of knowledge remained relatively unchanged until the publication in 1664 of *De ratione motus musculorum* by William Croone.[2] In this seminal monograph, Croone proposed that muscular contraction might be produced by a process of fermentation within the muscle rather than by the flow of *spiritus animi* into the muscle, an explanation first proposed by Erasistratus around the beginning of the third century B.C. and left essentially unchallenged until Croone's work (Fulton & Wilson 1966).

Direct evidence for a relationship between muscle contraction and electricity was not obtained until the late eighteenth century, when the Galvanis conducted a series of studies on muscular contractions evoked by the discharge of static electricity (Green 1953). They discovered that the muscles of a frog's legs were activated merely by touching them with metal rods, noted that the intensity of the contraction depended on the type of metal used, and interpreted these observations to mean that electricity was stored in muscle. Alessandro Volta initially endorsed this hypothesis and yet – after subsequent reflection and experimentation – argued later that the muscle contractions resulted from electrical current generated because dissimilar metals touched the muscle preparation (Pupilli 1953). Using nerves from a severed spinal cord rather than metal rods, Luigi Galvani repeated their experiments and again found that the muscles contracted when brought into contact with the severed nerve. Alexander von Humboldt subsequently replicated these findings using a large variety of animals, but the notoriety accorded Volta for his many inventions minimized the impact of these observations for almost 40 years (Fulton 1926).

It was not until the early nineteenth century that a sensitive instrument for measuring small electric currents (i.e., the galvanometer) was invented. In 1833, Carlo Matteucci used such a device to demonstrate an electrical potential between an excised frog's nerve and its damaged muscle. Du-Bois Reymond, a student of the renowned physiologist Johannes Müller, built upon Matteucci's then-recent publication, eventually publishing the results of an extensive series of investigations on the electrical basis of muscular contraction as well as providing the first in vivo evidence of electrical activity in human muscles during voluntary contraction (Basmajian & De Luca 1985).

The study of the thermodynamics of muscle contraction owes a debt to another of Müller's students, Hermann Ludwig Ferdinand von Helmholtz. Fueled by the desire to abolish the notion of vital forces underlying muscular actions, von Helmholtz began an investigation into the chemical transformations occurring in frog muscle during contraction. Put simply, he reasoned that the heat of combustion combined with the transformation of food material should produce a quantity of heat measurable at the muscle surface during contraction. By stimulating an isolated muscle through its nerve and employing a sensitive thermocouple, he was able to demonstrate a rise in temperature during contraction. This demonstration not only provided the experimental basis for his classic paper on the conservation of energy; it also proved instrumental in focusing subsequent investigations on the central problem of understanding the physiochemical processes involved in converting neural energy to mechanical work (Hill 1959).

Based on experimental observations using electrical stimulation, muscle physiologists during the eighteenth and early nineteenth century attributed graded muscular responses to graded variations in the intensity of the stimulation. Until late in the nineteenth century, many investigators erroneously inferred from the strong correlation between the intensity of exogenous electrical stimulation and the intensity of contraction that the actual size of the neural impulses was proportional to the stimulus intensity. However, experimental work around the turn of the century (e.g. Lucas 1909) challenged this belief, strongly suggesting that graded muscular responses resulted from the firing of individual contractile units rather than from variation in the size of the nerve impulse. Direct evidence for the "all-or-none" character of the response of muscle fibers was finally obtained by Frederick Pratt and his colleagues in the early 1900s (Pratt 1917; Pratt & Eisenberger 1919). They applied graded electrical stimulation to individual muscle fibers while simultaneously photographing the spatial displacement of mercury droplets sprinkled previously over the muscle surface, and they observed that additional fibers contracted coincident with each quantal step in the displacement of a mercury droplet.[3] The foundations of modern electromyography were finally laid in the 1930s with publications of Adrian and Bronk (1929), Jacobson (1927), and Lindsley (1935) and with the prelusion of the differential amplifier (Mathews 1934).

SKELETOMOTOR ACTIVATION AND PATTERNING

Detecting myoelectric signals using surface electrodes remained difficult throughout the nineteenth and early twentieth centuries. Electrically stimulating a muscle cutaneously was considerably simpler, however. Perhaps best known for this work was Guillaume Duchenne de Boulogne, who used this technique in the mid-nineteenth century to investigate the dynamics and function of the human facial muscles in vivo (Duchenne 1862/1990). Not surprisingly, Charles Darwin corresponded with Duchenne in an effort to evaluate his own observations about facial expressions and emotion (Cuthbertson 1990).

Darwin's interest in muscular action was based upon his belief that many behaviors were in part inherited. He focused his inquiry on the expression of emotions in man and animals to buttress this belief and presaged contemporary studies of the patterns of muscle contractions and facial actions that are undetectable to the naked eye with his conclusion that, "whenever the same state of mind is induced, however feebly, there is a tendency through the force of habit and association for the same movements to be performed, though they may not be of the least use" (Darwin 1872/1873, p. 281).

The somatic elements of William James's (1884) theory of emotions and the various motor theories of thinking prevalent at the turn of the century (e.g. Washburn 1916) further fueled interest in objective measures of subtle or fleeting muscle contractions. Among the more creative procedures used to magnify tiny muscular contractions were sensitive pneumatic systems used to record finger movements during conflict situations (Luria 1932) as well as elaborate lever-based systems to record subtle tongue movements during thinking (Thorson 1925). However, more sensitive and specific noninvasive recordings had to await the development of metal surface electrodes, vacuum-tube amplifiers, and the cathode-ray oscilloscope early in this century; these enabled the pioneering work of Edmund Jacobson (1927, 1932) on electrical measurements of muscle activity during imagery. The results of these studies and others (e.g. Davis 1938) demonstrated that EMG responses were evoked by psychologically relevant tasks (e.g., recalling a poem), were minute and highly localized, and often occurred in the part of the body that one would use had the task called for an overt response. This work was subsequently criticized primarily for not definitively achieving mentally quiescent comparison periods (see e.g. Humphrey 1951; Max 1937), but successful replications of this early work using different comparison tasks have been reported (McGuigan 1966, 1978).

ENDURING ISSUES

Subsequent research using surface EMG has extended these early observations, documenting patterns of covert skeletomotor activity that differentiate both within and between emotional and cognitive processes (see reviews by Cacioppo et al. 1993a; Fridlund & Izard 1983; McGuigan 1978; Tassinary & Cacioppo 1992) as well as between normal and clinical populations (e.g. Hazlett, McLeod, & Hoehn-Saric 1994; Orr et al. 1993; van Boxtel, Goudswaard, & Janssen 1983a; Whatmore & Ellis 1959). The enduring important issues in this research include the extent to which recorded EMG responses reflect specific or global activation, as well as to what extent they reflect characteristics of the situation, the individual, or the processing task. Not surprisingly, it has proven advantageous to monitor multiple EMG responses across time using sophisticated designs with multiple control conditions and to employ time-locked recording procedures. For example, Cacioppo, Bush, and Tassinary (1992b) examined simultaneously the effect of communicative intent and stimulus valence, using both social and asocial stimuli, on EMG activity at five discrete sites on the face. Their results suggest (i) that facial EMG activity continues to be modulated by both affective and communicative processes even when it is too subtle to produce a clearly perceptible expression and (ii) that muscles in the brow and periocular regions are more responsive differentially to both processes than are muscles in either the forehead, cheek, or perioral regions.

Two general features of the physical architecture of the skeletomotor system also present some enduring inferential challenges to surface EMG recording. First is the sheer number of muscles. Most of the striated muscles are bilaterally symmetrical in pairs, with several hundred distinct muscles throughout the human body. The general distribution of these muscles across the body, as depicted in Morris and Anson (1966), is as follows: 37 bilaterally symmetrical muscle pairs in the head and face; 29 pairs in the neck and shoulder girth; 54 pairs in the shoulders, arms, and hands; 21 pairs in the spinal region; 15 pairs in the thoracoabdominal region; 9 pairs in the pelvic outlet; and 62 pairs in the hips, thighs, legs, and feet. Second is the alluring aggregate simplicity of the muscle as a functional unit. That is, from such a perspective, each striated muscle can be characterized as a linear actuator whose potential states are limited to onset of contraction, offset of contraction, and relaxation (Tomovic & Bellman 1970). Even so, the structural arrangements of the striated muscles as agonist–antagonist pairs, or through their interdigitation, expand dramatically the number of actions that can be achieved using these deceptively simple elements. The relatively small number of muscles in the head and face, for instance, has been estimated to enable the encoding of some 6,000 to 7,000 appearance changes (Izard 1971; see Figure 1).

The challenges that derive from these architectural features are several. First, it is feasible to obtain measurements over only a small number of muscles in the human body in any given experiment. Yet because the action of the striated muscles is multiply determined, monitoring activity from a single site may provide only global or ambiguous information about the associated psychological or behavioral process. For instance, Ekman (1982) observed that emotions (with the possible exception of happiness) cannot be identified by the activity of a single muscle, echoing an earlier

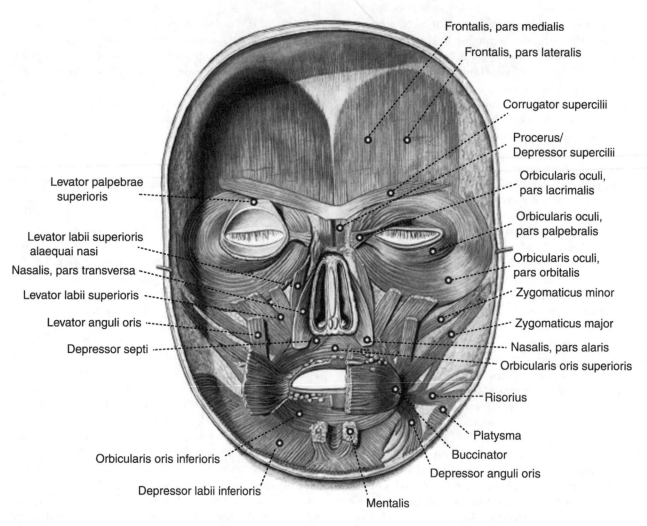

Figure 1. Schematic representation of the facial musculature, as viewed from behind the face (modified from Figure 137 of Pernkopf 1980). Overt facial expressions are based on contractions of this underlying musculature sufficiently intense to result in perceptible dislocations of skin and landmarks. More common perceptible effects of strong contractions of the depicted facial muscles include the following, divided into the major regions of the face. Muscles of the lower face: *depressor anguli oris,* pulls lip corners downward; *depressor labii inferioris,* depresses lower lip; *orbicularis oris (superioris* and *inferioris),* tightens, compresses, protrudes, and/or inverts lips; *mentalis,* elevates chin boss and protrudes lower lip; *platysma,* wrinkles skin of neck and may draw down both lower lip and lip corners. Muscles of the middle face: *buccinator,* compresses and tightens cheek, forming dimples; *levator labii superioris alaequai nasi,* raises center of upper lip and flares nostrils; *nasalis pars alaris,* tightens or flares the ala of the nose; *nasalis pars transversa,* produces transverse wrinkles across the nose and may pull down the medial part of the brows; *depressor septi,* pulls down septum and protrudes upper lip; *levator labii superioris,* raises upper lip and flares nostrils, exposing canine teeth; *zygomaticus major,* pulls lip corners up and back; *zygomaticus minor,* draws the upper lip backward, upward, and outward; *risorius,* retracts the lip corners. Muscles of the upper face: *corrugator supercilii,* draws brows together and downward, producing vertical furrows between brows; *procerus/depressor supercilii,* pulls medial part of brows downward and may wrinkle skin over bridge of nose; *frontalis pars lateralis,* raises outer brows, producing horizontal furrows in lateral regions of forehead; *frontalis pars medialis,* raises inner brows, producing horizontal furrows in medial region of forehead; *levator palpebrae superioris,* raises and pulls back upper eyelid; *orbicularis oculi pars orbitalis,* tightens skin surrounding eye, causing "crow's-feet" wrinkles; *orbicularis oculi pars palpebrae,* tightens skin surrounding eye, causing lower eyelid to rise; *orbicularis oculi pars lacrimalis,* compresses the lachrymal sac and facilitates effective tearing. Descriptions are consistent with those in Daniels and Worthingham (1986), Ekman and Friesen (1978), Gray (1901/1977), Izard (1971), Kendall and McCreary (1980), and Weaver (1977).

call for the necessity of recording from more than one muscle group during emotional reactions (Lindsley 1951).

Second, many movements can be achieved by the actions of different or differently activated striated muscles. Electromyographic responses may therefore appear unreliable if the focus is solely on the behavioral output

rather than the mechanisms by which these movements were achieved (Gans & Gorniak 1980; Kelso et al. 1984). Third, the imperfect selectivity of surface electrodes and the close proximity of the various striated muscles make it difficult to pinpoint exactly which muscles are contracting. Hence, when using surface electrodes, it is typically appropriate to refer to EMG signals as reflecting activity from sites or regions (e.g., the *zygomaticus major* muscle region). Fourth, surface EMG recording, although noninvasive, can be obtrusive and potentially reactive. Electrodes attached to the surface of the skin with wires connected to preamplifiers can restrict an individual's movement or make the individual tense, self-conscious, or sensitive to experimental demand characteristics. Finally, although acknowledged standards do exist for the placement of surface electrodes to detect activity in particular muscles or muscle regions (Fridlund & Cacioppo 1986; Zipp 1982), these have not been adopted universally (see Andreassi 1995, p. 149; McGuigan 1994, p. 225) and so comparisons across laboratories or across individuals and sessions within laboratories remain somewhat problematic.

Progress has been made in overcoming many of these limitations (see e.g. De Luca & Knaflitz 1992; Fridlund & Cacioppo 1986; Kumar & Mital 1996; Tassinary, Cacioppo, & Geen 1989), and this progress is reviewed in the sections that follow. In addition, surface EMG recording offers several unique advantages that complement the study of overt behavior through traditional means. First, EMG responses, in contrast to measures such as response latencies or verbal reports, can be collected continuously without the individual participant's attention or labor. Second, with the assistance of computers, the detection and quantification of EMG signals as a measure of muscle activation can be performed more sensitively, reliably, and quickly than can fine-grain analyses of overt behavior (Tuomisto, Johnston, & Schmidt 1996; cf. Cohn et al. in press; Himer et al. 1991). Third, analyses of subtle somatic patterns and their time course may provide a means of differentiating underlying mechanisms of control over similar overt behaviors (Ghez 1991b).

Finally, many subtle psychological processes or events are not accompanied by visually perceptible actions or significant visceral changes (Graham 1980; Rajecki 1983). Darwin (1872/1873, p. 12) recognized this limitation in the study of emotional expressions, stating that "the study of expression is difficult, owing to the movements being often extremely slight, and of a fleeting nature." It is now clear that fast or low-level changes in EMG activity can occur without leading to any visible movements. Facial expressions, for instance, result from displacements of skin and connective tissue – due to the contraction of muscles that create folds, lines, and wrinkles in the facial skin – and the movement of landmarks such as the brows and corners of the mouth (Rinn 1991). Although muscle activation must occur if these facial distortions are to be achieved, it is possible for muscle activation to occur in the absence of any overt action if the activation is weak or transient or if the overt response is very rapid, suppressed, or aborted (Cacioppo et al. 1992b). This holds for nonfacial striated muscles as well (see Coles et al. 1985; de Jong et al. 1990; McGarry & Franks 1997).

In the face, the uncoupling of muscle activation and observable movement is due in part to the structure and elasticity of the facial skin, fascia, and adipose tissue, as well as to the unique architecture of the facial musculature. The muscles of expression are attached to other muscles and bones or to a superficial musculoaponeurotic system (SMAS) (Kikkawa, Lemke, & Dortzbach 1996; Mitz 1976) that extends throughout the cervicofacial area. Not unlike a loose chain, the facial muscles can be pulled a small distance (i.e., contracted slightly) before exerting a significant force on the points to which they are anchored. In addition, the elasticity of the SMAS, facial skin, and adipose tissue forms a complex low-pass mechanical filter, attenuating the visible effects of very brief or slight contractions yet allowing the displacement and bulging of the face due to sustained or moderate contractions (Gousain et al. 1996; Partridge 1966; Waters 1992).

In summary, measures of EMG and of observable muscular actions each have unique advantages and disadvantages. Neither is necessarily better or more capable of capturing completely the information provided by the other. A general congruence between the results based on EMG recordings and those obtained through fine-grain analyses of overt behavior is to be expected, given the physiological basis of the surface EMG (see what follows). Therefore, the wealth of information that exists regarding nonverbal behavior during such processes as sleeping, thinking, communicating, dissimulating, and feeling (Feldman & Rime 1991; Russel & Fernández-Dols 1997; Tyron 1991) provides a rich theoretical resource for research on subtler, more fleeting responses or on underlying mechanisms.

Yet EMG recordings and fine-grain behavioral observations do not coincide completely. As noted, EMG recordings can reveal muscular activity or patterns of activity too small or fleeting to evoke detectable movements or whose corresponding muscle contractions are counteracted by contraction of an antagonist. Ekman (1982) reported an illustrative study conducted by Ekman, Schwartz, and Friesen. Surface EMG recordings and high-quality video recordings were secured simultaneously as individuals deliberately intensified the contraction of specific facial muscles (the *corrugator supercilii* and medial *frontalis*). Results revealed that measurements of facial feature distortions using Ekman and Friesen's (1978) Facial Action Coding System (FACS) and measurements from surface EMG over these muscle regions were highly correlated ($r = +0.85$). Nevertheless, reliable EMG signals emerged at levels lower than could reliably be detected visually. Tassinary and associates (Girard et al. 1997) examined in more detail the relationship between surface EMG activity recorded over the *corrugator supercilii* muscle region and FACS measurements while subjects deliberately furrowed their brows. They discovered (i) that FACS-coded movement onsets were associated with average EMG levels over three times higher than those associated with movement offsets and (ii) that FACS-coded onsets and offsets were also influenced by the relative speed of the movement. These results speak well for the validity of facial EMG measurement and also for the possibility of tracking at least limited features of moment-by-moment psychological processes even in the absence of a visually detectable motor response. Moreover, because individuals may be less likely or able to control momentary or minute muscular contractions that do not result in observable actions, discrepancies between EMG responses underlying covert versus overt responses may be of special interest (Cacioppo & Tassinary 1989). Indeed, Freeman (1948) argued decades ago that this was the primary theoretical advantage of EMG for psychophysiological research; that is, somatic responses could be tracked throughout their development and thereby reveal the continuous seam binding apparently discrete overt behavior. We return to these issues following a discussion of the technical aspects of the surface EMG.

Physical Context

Not quite a century ago, Baines (1918) argued that appropriate technical considerations should precede the collection or interpretation of data related to electrophysiological phenomena. In their survey of the EMG literature, Basmajian and De Luca (1985, p. 6) strongly concurred, observing that "this call still echoes among the numerous abuses that have been promulgated throughout the past seven decades."

An understanding of the physical system being studied and the bioelectrical principles underlying its responses serve several important purposes. These include the development of operational definitions and procedures, the ability to discriminate signal from artifact, the maintenance of a safe environment for both experimenters and research participants (see Chapter 35 of this volume), and the guidance of inferences based on physiological data (see Chapter 1). In this section, therefore, we review the physical basis of the surface EMG and outline principles and technical issues involved in obtaining valid measures of EMG activity.

THE ANATOMICAL AND PHYSIOLOGICAL BASIS OF THE SURFACE ELECTROMYOGRAM

Muscles perform many different functions (Smith & Kier 1989). Their orchestrated activation maintains posture, causes reflexive movements, and produces both spontaneous and voluntary movements that occur across many different scales of space and time. A schematic of the central organization and control of the several hundred striated muscles in the human body is presented in Figure 2.[4]

Fundamentally, muscle is a tissue that both generates and transmits force. Striated muscle, in particular, is a hierarchical material made up of a very large number of parallel fibers whose diameters are orders of magnitude smaller than a millimeter and yet may be up to several centimeters in length (see Figure 3). The term "striated" comes from the fact these fibers are actually bundles of thinner structures, known as *fibrils,* which have repeating cross-striations (known as Z-lines or Z-bands) throughout their length. Electron microscopy reveals that between these striations (an area know as the *sarcomere*) are a series of thick and thin filaments bound together by a system of molecular cross-linkages. The thick filaments are made up of the protein myosin and lie in the center of the sarcomere between the thin filaments. The thin filaments are composed of the proteins actin, tropomyosin, and troponin, are discontinuous, and are attached at either end of the sarcomere. During contraction, conformational changes in the cross-linkages lead to only very slight changes in the length of the filaments but cause substantial changes in the distance between Z-bands as the thick filaments slide in between the thin filaments (Schmidt-Nielsen 1997).

Each striated muscle is innervated by a single motor nerve whose cell bodies are located primarily in the anterior horn of the spinal cord or, in the case of the muscles of the head, in the cranial nerves of the brainstem. All behavior – that is, all actions of the striated muscles regardless of the brain processes involved – results from neural signals traveling along these motor nerves. For this reason, the set of lower motor nerves has been designated the final common pathway (Sherrington 1906/1923).

The motor nerve traveling to the muscle consists of axons of numerous individual motoneurons, referred to collectively as a motoneuron pool. Each motoneuron axon divides into a number of small branches, termed axon fibrils, just before reaching the muscle; each axon fibril, in turn, forms a junction, called a motor endplate, on an individual muscle fiber. Each motoneuron innervates a number of interspersed muscle fibers within a muscle, and each muscle fiber is usually innervated by only one motoneuron. The spatial distribution of motor endplates on the muscle surface is not random but forms at most a few clusters (typically only one); these are referred to as *innervation zones*. An important functional consequence of this structure is that muscle fibers do not contract individually; instead, the entire set of muscle fibers innervated by a single motoneuron contracts in consonance. Therefore, the most elementary functional unit within the final common pathway is the motoneuron cell body, its axon, its axon fibrils, and the individual muscle fibers innervated by these axon fibrils. This functional physiological entity is called the *motor unit,* a concept proposed by Liddell & Sherrington (1925) and subsequently quantified by Eccles and Sherrington (1930); see Figure 4.

The axons of the motoneurons within a motoneuron pool vary in diameter, and this structural feature has important functional consequences. Generally, the smaller the diameter of a motoneuronal axon, the smaller the number of axon fibrils, the smaller the number of muscle

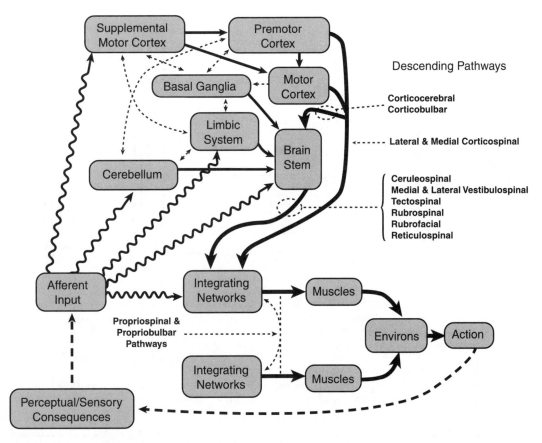

Figure 2. Major components of motor system. Solid lines represent efferent pathways, dashed lines represent feedback pathways, and wavy lines represent afferent pathways. Converging arrows do not necessarily imply convergence on same individual neurons. Neither crossing of pathways nor details of specific connections within brain areas are indicated. Note that arrows denote strong influences; they do not imply direct (monosynaptic) connections. Note also that the list of descending pathways is representative, not exhaustive. The thalamus and hypothalamus have been omitted for clarity. (Modified and redrawn from Figure 2 of Cacioppo, Tassinary, & Fridlund 1990b.)

fibers it innervates, and the smaller the size of its cell body. Hence, activation of muscle via small motoneurons produces smaller and more precise actions than activation of the same muscle by the depolarization of large motoneurons. In addition, the smaller the diameter of the motoneuron, the lower the critical firing threshold of its cell body and the more fatigue-resistant (i.e., greater glycolytic capacity) are the muscle fibers it innervates. These relationships constitute the "size principle" (Henneman 1980), which contributes to our ability to control force in a smooth and graded fashion. More specifically, the initial force of contraction produced by a muscle is attributable to small motoneurons discharging intermittently and then discharging more frequently. Stronger muscle contractions are attributable to the depolarization of increasingly large motoneurons within the motoneuron pool concurrent with increases in the firing rates of the smaller motoneurons already active. As muscle contraction approaches maximal levels, further increases in force are attributable primarily to the entire pool of motoneurons firing more rapidly. This cascade of processes appears to be regulated by unidimensional increases in the aggregate neural input to the motoneuronal pool, a process referred to as "common drive" (De Luca & Erim 1994; Erim et al. 1996).[5]

The number of muscle fibers innervated per motoneuron, known as the *innervation ratio,* varies even more dramatically across than within muscles. Consistent with the principles just outlined, muscles with low innervation ratios are capable of producing actions more rapidly and with greater precision than are muscles with high innervation ratios. For example, the small extrinsic muscles of the eye, which are capable of very fast and fine movements, have innervation ratios of about 10:1, whereas the relatively large and more slowly acting postural muscles, such as the gastrocnemius (i.e., superficial foot extensor muscle of the calf), have innervation ratios of about 2,000:1 (Ghez 1991a).

The depolarization of a motoneuron results in the quantal release of acetylcholine at the motor endplates. The activating neurotransmitter acetylcholine is quickly metabolized by the enzyme acetylcholinesterase so that continuous efferent discharges are required for continued propagation of muscle action potentials (MAPs) and fiber contraction. Nonetheless, the transient excitatory potential within a motor endplate can lead to a brief (e.g.,

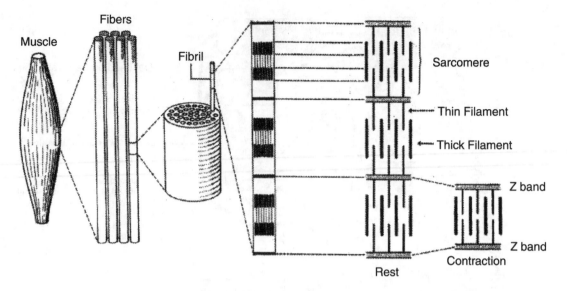

Figure 3. Diagram of the structure of muscle with increasing magnification going from left to right. The bottom right corner of the figure illustrates the microgeometric changes that occur with contraction. (Modified from Figure 10.7 of Schmidt-Nielsen 1997.)

1-msec) depolarization of the resting membrane potential of the muscle cell and a MAP that is propagated bidirectionally across the muscle fiber with constant velocity and undiminished amplitude. The MAP travels rapidly along the surface of the fiber and flows into the muscle fiber itself via a system of T-tubules, thus ensuring that the contraction (known as a twitch) involves the entire fiber. The physiochemical mechanism responsible for the twitch involves a complex yet well-characterized self-regulating calcium-dependent interaction between the actin and myosin molecules.

A small portion of the changing electromagnetic field confederated with these processes passes through the extracellular fluids to the skin, and it is these voltage fluctuations that constitute the major portion of the surface EMG signal. The voltage changes that are detected in surface EMG recording do not emanate from a single MAP but rather from MAPs traveling across many muscle fibers within a motor unit (i.e., motor unit action potential, or MUAP) and, more typically, from MAPs traveling across numerous motor fibers due to the activation of multiple motor units. Thus, the EMG provides a direct measure not of tension, muscular contraction, or movement but rather of the electrical activity associated with these events. More specifically, the surface EMG signal represents the ensemble electromagnetic field detectable at the surface of the skin at a given moment in time. Normally, neither the details of the individual MAPs nor the precise muscular origins of the signal are recoverable (see Khan, Bloodworth, & Woods 1971). Reliable, valid, and sensitive information about the aggregate actions (or inactions) of motoneuron pools across time can nonetheless be obtained by careful attention to the elements of surface EMG recording and

analysis (see e.g. Cacioppo, Marshall-Goodell, & Dorfman 1983a; De Luca & Knaflitz 1992; Lippold 1967).

SIGNAL DETECTION

As we have just outlined, the ensemble surface EMG signal emanating from the muscle is the result of the spatiotemporal summing of a quasi-random train of MUAPs. The aggregate signal is characterized by a frequency range of several hertz to over 500 Hz and by amplitudes ranging from fractions of a microvolt to over a thousand microvolts. These frequency and amplitude characteristics are broader than most bioelectrical signals of interest to psychophysiologists, and they overlap a variety of disparate bioelectrical signals (e.g., the electroencephalogram and the electrocardiogram) as well as the ubiquitous external 50/60-Hz signals emanating from most AC-powered equipment (Marshall-Goodell, Tassinary, & Cacioppo 1990). Consequently, the detection of EMG signals from a localized muscle region requires careful attention to noise reduction and grounding practices, electrode site preparation and placement, and appropriate differential preamplification and preliminary signal conditioning in order to eliminate extraneous electrical noise, minimize the detection of irrelevant bioelectrical signals, and enhance the signal-to-noise ratio.

Noise Reduction and Grounding

Noise has been defined by many authors as simply any unwanted signal. In the present context, it is important to note that EMG signals can be obscured by noise from many sources. These include but are not limited to external electrical sources, physiological responses whose frequency and amplitude characteristics overlap those for EMG recording, EMG signals emanating from task-irrelevant muscles (i.e., cross-talk), and EMG signals from target sites that result from "irrelevant" actions presumed to be minimized

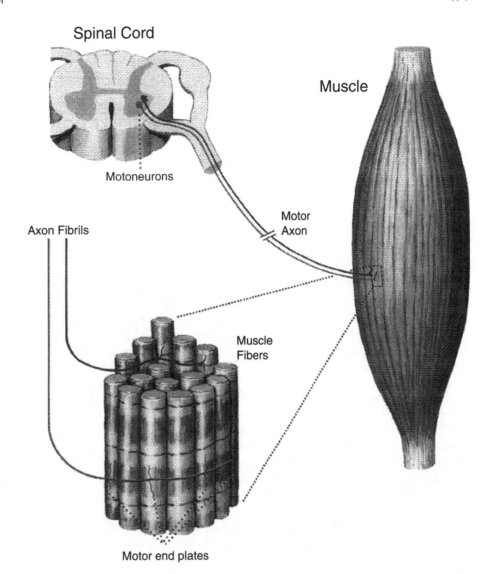

Figure 4. Diagram of two motor units. (Modified from slide 3705 of Netter 1991.)

or eliminated by the design of the experiment (e.g., movement artifacts).

The most problematic exogenous electrical noise in the laboratory is narrowband noise, because it arises from several common sources, radiates through walls and air, and overlaps in frequency with the EMG signal. For example, 50/60-Hz noise emanates from AC power lines, lights, relays, and transformers. Televisions, video monitors, and most computer terminals use cathode-ray tubes (CRTs), and these tend to generate high-frequency electrical noise (ranging from 15 kHz to several megahertz). Although many EMG preamplifiers include filters to eliminate such noise, filters are neither completely selective nor entirely effective. Special-purpose notch filters, for example, attenuate frequencies to a varying degree on both sides of 50/60 Hz – a bandwidth that can represent a significant portion of the total power in an EMG signal – and strong signals in the high-frequency range can appear under the "alias" of small signals in the EMG bandwidth. It is therefore important to minimize electrical noise prior to amplifi-

cation. This can be done through appropriate placement and shielding of equipment and careful grounding of the research participant and laboratory equipment (Bramsley et al. 1967; Fridlund & Cacioppo 1986; McGuigan 1979). Wideband noise (white noise) is usually attributable to the Brownian motion intrinsic to electronic devices. This noise is unavoidable but can be minimized by keeping electrode impedances low, ensuring that amplifier filters are set tightly to the proper bandwidth, and using calibrated high-grade equipment.

With respect to grounding, a research participant affixed with electrodes should be grounded at one and only one point on her or his body; ideally, any equipment touched by the participant should be nonconductive. If multichannel recordings are to be made, the grounds for each channel should be strapped together and a single ground electrode attached. This procedure further minimizes 50/60-Hz noise in the recordings and enhances the safety of the participant by eliminating the possibility of ground loops (i.e., unintended current flow due to imperfect grounding).

Biological noise includes all endogenous signals that are not part of the bioelectrical signal of interest. In the sections that follow, we outline several procedures for minimizing biological noise. However, the careful and correct placement of a ground electrode does not prevent artifacts from cross-talk, one of the primary sources of biological noise. Put simply, this is because the impedance into the ground electrode tends to exceed the access impedance of the volume-conductive tissues between the spurious current source and the recording electrode(s). Additional details and discussions are provided by Basmajian and De Luca (1985) and Loeb and Gans (1986).

Electrode Selection and Placement

Psychophysiologists, nearly without exception, use surface rather than needle or fine-wire electrodes for EMG recording. This is due primarily to the noninvasive nature of surface recording and to the fact that the research questions posed thus far by psychophysiologists involve muscles or sets of muscles rather than motor units within muscles. Surface EMG electrodes are less sensitive to exact anatomical placement because they detect the summated MAPs from an indeterminate cluster of motor units rather than a single unit.[6] This aggregate response develops in an orderly manner such that surface EMG recordings correlate well with the overall level of contraction of muscle groups underlying and near the electrodes, especially when limb movement is constrained and contractions are neither minimal nor maximal (Lawrence & De Luca 1983; Lippold 1967).

Because most EMG amplifiers are AC coupled, the electrical stability of the electrodes is not as important as, for instance, when recording skin conductance (see Chapter 8 of this volume). Nonpolarizing electrodes such as silver–silver chloride electrodes, however, can be used very effectively in nearly all recording situations. Tin, stainless steel, gold, or the platinum family of noble metals can be used effectively in many recording situations, although the lack of chemical equilibrium at the metal–electrolyte junction makes this class of electrode inherently more noisy and susceptible to artifact. In addition, stainless steel may be contraindicated when recording low-frequency low-amplitude signals (Cooper, Osselton, & Shaw 1980). As a result, the silver–silver chloride electrode is – in most research applications – the electrode of choice.

Surface electrodes can be constructed to be either active or passive. If passive, the electrode consists simply of a detection surface. If active, the input impedance of the electrode is made artificially high using proximal microelectronics.[7] Essentially, these microelectronics consist of a low-gain differential preamplifier with very high input and very low output impedances built into the electrode housing. Locating the first stage of high-impedance amplification as close as possible to the detection surfaces renders this class of electrodes relatively insensitive to the vagaries of the electrode–skin interface, and the low output impedance minimizes artifacts due to any movement of the cable connecting the electrode to the main amplifier. However, these advantages are obtained at the cost of increased noise levels, higher expense, and typically much greater mass. Surface electrodes are also available in a variety of sizes. Electrodes with small detection surfaces and housings allow closer interelectrode spacing and consequently higher selectively. Such factors as the electrode size, electrode positioning, and interelectrode distance over a particular site can affect the detected EMG signals and hence should be held constant across experimental conditions. For example, a smaller spacing shifts the bandwidth to higher frequencies and lowers the amplitude of the signal.

Fridlund and Cacioppo (1986) found that electrodes with 0.5-cm–diameter detection surfaces and 1.5-cm–diameter housings are used commonly for limb and trunk EMG recording and that miniature electrodes with 0.25-cm–diameter detection surfaces and 0.5- or 1.0-cm–diameter housings are used for facial EMG recording. They and others (Basmajian & De Luca 1985) advocated – based on a variety of criteria – the use of a 1.0-cm interdetector surface spacing whenever possible. Given a circular detection surface, however, the interdetector surface spacing is limited by the diameter of the electrodes. This is unfortunate because, ceteris paribus, the larger the size of the detection surfaces, the larger the amplitude of the signal that will be detected and the smaller the electrical noise that will be generated at the skin–detector interface. Some investigators have advocated the use of a rectangular rather than a circular detection surface based on the reasoning that a "bar" will, in general, intersect more fibers (De Luca 1997). To our knowledge, no empirical research has addressed explicitly this issue of detection surface geometry, but the theoretical arguments are persuasive. Regardless of the optimal detection surface geometry, only closely spaced electrodes and differential amplification can yield spatially selective surface EMG recordings. For example, using only these two basic procedures, a recent study of the human nasal musculature demonstrated a remarkable degree of specificity with passive surface EMG electrodes (Bruintjes et al. 1996).

Specification of surface electrode placements over target muscle groups is important to ensure that findings are comparable across individuals, sessions, or laboratories. Several studies offer empirically and anatomically derived recommendations for EMG recording for facial, masticatory, and articulatory muscle activity using subdermal electrodes (Compton 1973; Fridlund & Cacioppo 1986; Isley & Basmajian 1973; O'Dwyer et al. 1981; Seiler 1973; Vitti et al. 1975), and additional studies have examined the reliability of EMG measurements in relatively large, well-defined muscles (Gans & Gorniak 1980; Komi & Buskirk 1970; Martin 1956). This research supports a general principle of electrode orientation for spatially sensitive and specific differential recording over a given muscle region. Put directly, electrodes should be placed (i) proximal and oriented parallel to voltage gradients of interest and (ii) distal and oriented perpendicular to voltage gradients of extraneous signal sources (e.g., other muscles). Successful implementation of this principle is limited by the severity of interfering signals, the availability of reliable anatomical landmarks, and the presence of task-related complications (e.g., obstruction of vision).

Davis (1952) was the first to offer recommendations for recording the muscle activity involved in movements of the limbs, neck, jaw, lower lip, and eyebrows. Davis, however, presented no evidence for the choice of particular sites over others, and he occasionally based placements on incorrect anatomical assumptions (Fridlund & Cacioppo 1986); thus, only those regarding limb and neck placements are currently recommended (Zipp 1982).

Tassinary and colleagues (1989) provided relevant data for the *corrugator supercilii*, *depressor supercilii*, and *zygomaticus major* muscle regions, regions that have proven informative in studies of emotion. Based on anatomical data regarding the location of these muscles (see Figure 1), several experiments were conducted to isolate the sites for surface EMG recording that met the general principles outlined here. Participants twice posed a series of facial actions and expressions while facial EMG activity was recorded. The activity of a specific muscle or set of muscles was verified using the FACS. The surface recording sites identified as providing both sensitive and relatively selective measures of activation of specific muscle regions are illustrated in the top panel of Figure 5.

Tassinary and associates (1987) provided relevant data for recording over the perioral muscle region and, in particular, for detecting silent language processing. Five sites in the perioral region were compared for their ability to differentiate facial actions due to the activation of discrete facial muscles in the perioral region. In addition to four sites located over the *mentalis, orbicularis oris superioris, orbicularis oris inferioris,* and *depressor anguli inferioris* (see Figure 1), a standard electrode site (i.e., "chin") – recommended by Davis (1952) and routinely used in sleep research (see Chapter 25) to measure general perioral EMG activity – was included. Activation of specific muscles or sets of muscles was again achieved by poses and was verified using the FACS. Following their correct performance of the poses on two separate occasions, participants were asked to read affectively neutral passages silently, subvocally, and aloud. Only EMG responses recorded over the *mentalis, orbicularis oris inferior,* and "chin" muscle regions differentiated quiescent baseline activity from silent reading. Of these three sites, only the site over the *orbicularis oris inferior* muscle re-

gion demonstrated high discriminant validity when poses activating this versus proximal superficial muscles were contrasted.[8]

Site Preparation

Surface EMG electrodes can be attached to the skin in a variety of ways, but the most common is via double-sided adhesive tape. A highly conductive medium (paste or gel) is used routinely between skin and the detection surface. This medium serves to stabilize the interface between the skin and each detection surface through minimizing movement artifacts (by establishing an elastic connection between the detection surface and the skin), reducing interelectrode impedances (by forming a conductive pathway across the hornified layers of the skin), and stabilizing the hydration and conductivity of the skin surface.

Prior to the application of the conductive medium and electrodes, the designated site on the skin surface is usually cleaned (to remove dirt and oil) and is typically abraded gently to lower interelectrode impedances to 5 or 10 kΩ. The electrodes are then commonly affixed in a bipolar configuration, as illustrated in Figure 5. The proximity of the ground electrode to the EMG sites being monitored is less important than the impedance of the skin–ground contact in helping to minimize extraneous electrical noise in EMG recording. Consequently, care and reflection can and should be used to ensure a stable and low-impedance connection to ground. For example, based on the importance of the skin–ground impedance, Turker, Miles, and Le (1988) invented a "lip clip" that required no skin preparation and took advantage of the exceptionally low impedance of the oral mucosa, albeit at the cost of being somewhat obtrusive. Regardless of the chosen site, however, one and only one ground electrode should be used and all inputs should be configured to share this ground. Finally, to avoid obstructing movement, care should be given to the orientation of electrode collars and wires. Electrode wires, for instance, should be draped and secured to minimize distraction, annoyance, or obstruction of movement or vision.

Preamplification and Signal Conditioning

Electromyographic signals are "small" in two ways: they have low voltage and low current. An amplifier supplies both voltage gain (turning low into high voltages), which can be controlled by the investigator, and current gain, a function of the ratio of the input and output impedances of the amplifier. Electromyographic signals are amplified using differential amplifiers wherein the difference signal between two electrodes (with respect to a third, ground electrode) is amplified and carried through the signal processing chain. Any bioelectrical or extraneous electrical signal that is common to both electrodes (the "common mode" signal) is therefore attenuated (Marshall-Goodell et al. 1990).

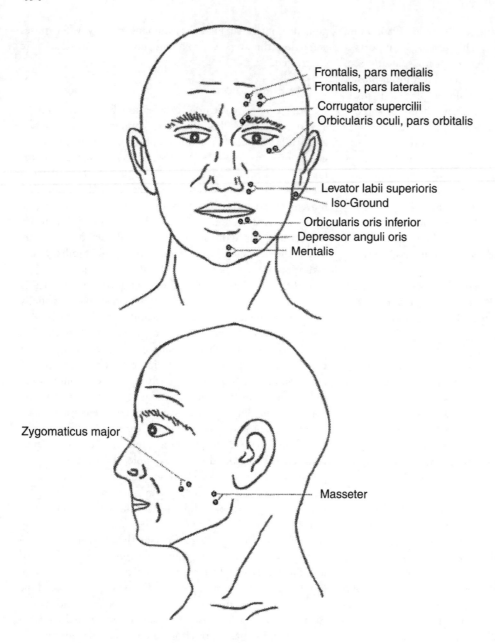

Figure 5. Suggested electrode placements for surface EMG recording of the facial muscles, based on Fridlund and Cacioppo 1986. (Modified and redrawn from Figure 6 of Cacioppo et al. 1990b.)

An older and more traditional method of recording EMG signals is the *monopolar* method, which involves the placement of one electrode over each target site (i.e., muscle or muscle group) of interest. The difference signal between the activity recorded at each target site and a common reference electrode (which, in theory, is in contact with an isoelectric site on the participant's body) is amplified and carried through the signal processing chain. However, the *bipolar* method is now the most commonly used method of recording EMG signals. Electrode pairs are aligned parallel to the course of the muscle fibers, and this alignment – coupled with the high common-mode rejec-

tion capability of modern differential amplifiers – produces relatively sensitive and selective recording of the activity of the underlying muscle groups (Basmajian & De Luca 1985; see also Cooper et al. 1980, chap. 3).

Monopolar or "common reference" recording is characterized by (i) a much more general pickup region than bipolar recording and (ii) an increased sensitivity to variations in the absolute level of electrical activity, assuming the ground electrode reflects an isoelectric state. Bipolar recording, in contrast, is more sensitive to variations in the gradient of electrical activity between the two active electrodes and is less susceptible to cross-talk. An elaboration of traditional bipolar recording, known as double-differential recording, promises to be even more spatially selective (De Luca & Merletti 1988). In the simplest version of this technique, three rather than two detection surfaces are placed in a line over the muscle of interest. Detection surfaces d_1 and d_2 are fed into one differential amplifier, detection surfaces d_2 and d_3 are fed into a second differential amplifier, and the outputs of the two differential amplifiers are fed into yet a third differential amplifier. The argument is that synchronous activity detected in pairs $d_1 - d_2$ and $d_2 - d_3$ indicates a source of electrical activity that did not propagate along the contracting muscle (i.e., cross-talk) and that the addition of the second stage of differential amplification will remove such influences. This particular technique can be seen as a simple unidimensional linear spatial filter, and both theoretical and experimental research suggest that even greater spatial resolution in surface EMG recording is possible with more complex weighted electrode arrays (Disselhorst-Klug, Silny, & Rau 1997; Lynn et al. 1978).

A schematized representation of a sequence of raw EMG signals is presented in the upper panel of Figure 6. As noted in the preceding, some filtering of the raw EMG signal is performed to increase the signal-to-noise ratio, decrease 50/60-Hz and ECG/EEG artifact, and reduce cross-talk. The primary energy in the bipolar recorded surface EMG signal lies between approximately 10 Hz and 200 Hz (Hayes 1960; van Boxtel, Goudswaard, & Shomaker 1984). Between 10 Hz and 30 Hz, this power is due primarily to the firing rates of motor units; beyond 30 Hz, it is due to the shapes of the aggregated motor unit action potentials (Basmajian & De Luca 1985). Attenuating the high frequencies in the EMG signal (e.g., using 500-Hz low-pass filters) reduces amplifier noise but rounds the peaks of detected motor unit action potentials. Retaining sharp signal peaks may be important for waveform or spectral analysis but is less critical for obtaining overall estimates of muscle tension. Attenuating the low frequencies (e.g., using 90-Hz high-pass filters) reduces 50/60-Hz noise from AC power lines, EEG (electroencephalogram) and ECG (electrocardiogram) artifacts, and (to some extent) cross-talk attributable to the intervening tissue's preferential transmission of low frequencies, but it also eliminates a significant and sizable portion of the EMG signal. Use of an overly restricted EMG signal passband may result in inaccurate appraisal of the level and form of EMG activity or in failure to detect small changes in the level of EMG activity. Hence, selection of an EMG detection passband must proceed based on susceptibility to artifact, presence of extraneous electrical noise at the source and high-frequency noise internal to the amplifier, consideration of the amplitude of the EMG signals to be detected, need to minimize cross-talk, and variations across conditions in muscular fatigue. A passband from 10 Hz to 500 Hz is satisfactory for most psychophysiological recording situations; if low-frequency artifact and cross-talk are problematic then a 20-Hz or 30-Hz high-pass filter may be used (possibly in combination with the double-differential recording technique), but the investigator should realize one consequence

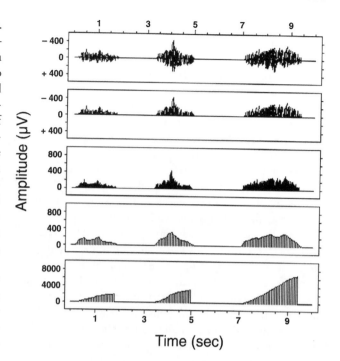

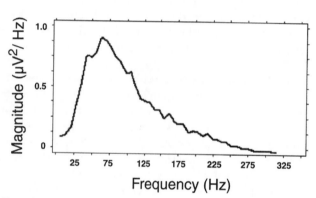

Figure 6. Common alternative representations of the surface EMG signal. The top five panels depict three distinct nonfatigued responses. Going from top to bottom: the first represents "raw" (amplified and bandpass-filtered only) waveforms; the second, half-wave rectified waveforms; the third, full-wave rectified waveforms; the fourth, smoothed waveforms; and the fifth, true integrated waveforms. The bottom panel depicts what one of the responses might look like if represented in the frequency domain. (Modified from Figure 7 in Cacioppo et al. 1990b.)

of this selection is that weak signals from the target muscle may also be attenuated.[9]

The two most common signal conditioning techniques are integration and smoothing, terms that are often confused. True *integration* is the temporal summation or accumulation of EMG activity, whereas *smoothing* typically refers to performing integration with a built-in signal decay via low-pass filtering or some type of signal averaging. Because the total energy in the EMG signal in any epoch of time is roughly equivalent to the rectified and smoothed EMG response, considerable economy in terms of data acquisition and signal processing can be achieved by rectification and smoothing prior to digitization – as long as the frequency components of the raw signal are not of interest.

The most frequently used on-line "smoother" in psychophysiological research remains the *contour following* integrator, an electronic device consisting primarily of a precision rectifier connected to a simple first-order low-pass filter. Its output represents a running average of ongoing EMG activity by providing a varying voltage proportional to the envelope of the EMG signal. Short time constants provide sensitivity to momentary fluctuations in EMG signals and so are useful when measuring a rapidly changing EMG signal. A long time constant blurs rapid changes and hence the associated output can severely underestimate or overestimate EMG signal amplitude at any given moment as well as compromise precise measurements of response onset and offset. Conversely, if EMG signals that vary slowly are of primary interest, relatively short time constants may be too sensitive to momentary EMG fluctuations and the economic advantages of smoothing will be sacrificed. Despite the popularity of simple contour following integrators, a variety of more sophisticated quantitations that overcome many of these limitations have been available generally for over a decade (Paynter filters, pulsed sampling integrators, etc.; see Loeb & Gans 1986).

Many investigators have performed frequency analyses on surface EMG recordings to determine whether there are shifts in the EMG spectra (i.e., changes in magnitude or power across frequency) as a function of some psychological or physiological variable. A particularly robust finding is that shifts in the central tendency of the EMG spectra (e.g., median frequency) are associated with muscle fatigue (Merletti 1994; Mulder & Hulstijn 1984; van Boxtel, Goudswaard, & Janssen 1983b). The persistent lack of attention to spectral analyses of the surface EMG in psychophysiology is primarily due to the fact that sophisticated spectral analyses have proven no more sensitive to psychological processes than relatively inexpensive amplitude and time-based analyses (Dollins & McGuigan 1989; McGuigan et al. 1982).

Signal Representation

Electromyographic activity unfolds over time and, like many other psychophysiological responses, the complexity of the raw signal enjoins data reduction. Whether represented in the time, amplitude, or frequency domains, the first step involves the conversion of the digitized signal to a descriptive (e.g., physiological) unit of measurement. The numbers assigned to EMG signals of different amplitudes depend on: (1) the electrical unit chosen for description of the signal, (2) the accuracy of the calibration procedure and amplifier's gain setting, and (3) the type of integration method and length of time constant or reset criterion used. Here we focus on the first two factors; interested readers can consult Fridlund and Cacioppo (1986) and Basmajian and De Luca (1985) for additional details.

EMG Activity as a Voltage–Time Function. EMG signals can be viewed as a voltage–time function, where the ordinate represents bounded signal amplitudes and the abscissa represents discrete intervals of time. The quantification of the amplitudes at each unit of time is determined by the direction and magnitude of the measured voltage and is expressed typically in units of microvolts (μV). The EMG voltage–time envelope, like the motor unit action potential, is bipolar and asymmetrical about electrical zero.

Most psychophysiological research using EMG has focused on some variation of EMG signal amplitude as the dependent variable. Simple averaging of the raw EMG amplitudes is uninformative, however, because the nature of the signal ensures that the average expected value is zero. Counting or averaging the peaks in the EMG signal, or tallying its directional changes or zero crossings, are relatively easy methods to implement and are useful for gauging differences in EMG activity if a sufficiently high sampling rate is used (Loeb & Gans 1986, chap. 17). Lippold (1967) maintained that the total energy in an EMG signal at a given moment in time, or what he referred to as the integrated EMG signal, represents overall muscular contraction more accurately than the number or average amplitude of peaks in the EMG signal. Subsequent research has largely corroborated Lippold's assertion for cases where limb movements are constrained and contractions are not extreme (Basmajian & De Luca 1985; Goldstein 1972). However, the phrase "integrated EMG" has been used in this research to refer to the output of several different quantification techniques. Two of the most common parameters in contemporary research are the arithmetic average of the rectified and smoothed EMG signal and the root-mean-square (rms) of the raw EMG signal.[10] Both processing techniques transform the EMG voltage–time function into a waveform that is nonnegative and bounded in time and amplitude. The moment-by-moment amplitude of this function represents an estimate of the total energy of the signal across time; the mean amplitude of this voltage–time function represents the average level of electrical energy emanating from the underlying muscle region(s) during a given recording epoch; and the integral of this function (e.g., the sum of the amplitudes) represents the total electrical activity (i.e., the size of the response) emanating from the underlying muscle region(s) during the recording epoch.

One unfortunate consequence of the traditional focus on the amplitude domain of the EMG signal is that the form of the response across time has been largely ignored (cf. Cacioppo et al. 1988; Hess et al. 1989). A notable exception is Malmo's (1965) use of "EMG gradients" (Davis & Malmo 1951), defined as a "progressively rising level of voltage reflecting gradually rising tension in the specific muscle group on which the electrodes are placed" (Malmo 1975, p. 34). Electromyographic gradients are still used successfully to assess variations across time in tonic muscle tension; these gradients are depicted by plotting EMG amplitude for two or more consecutive recording epochs (Braathen & Svebak 1994; Rimehaug & Svebak 1987).

Baselines. As in psychophysiology generally, it is often desirable to obtain response measures that are uncontaminated by the basal (prestimulus) level of activity. The notion of basal activity, however, can be ambiguous when applied to EMG signals. This is because the true physiological baseline for EMG activity is zero; hence, the lowest empirical baseline for EMG recording is actually the level of noise in the recording system.

In laboratory practice, muscles seldom show zero activity because the alert research participant is rarely completely relaxed. It is therefore important to consider the EMG activity that exists in the absence of experimental stimuli in order to assess individual differences and also to help achieve a measure of the experimental treatments free from prestimulus EMG activity. In assessing basal EMG activity, care is required to avoid any confounding of measurements with task-irrelevant activity (e.g., adaptation, fatigue, apprehension). The procedures commonly used include recording during prestimulus periods and recordings during pseudotrials (Johnson & Lubin 1972; see also Chapter 32 of this volume). The use of pseudotrials has the advantage that assessments are obtained under conditions that – except for the lack of experimental stimuli – are identical to the experimental trials.

A closed-loop baseline procedure offers an alternative to the use of pseudotrials (McHugo & Lanzetta 1983). Briefly, the presentation of experimental stimuli or treatments is programmed to be contingent on acceptably low levels of somatic activity across the recording sites. Task-specific EMG responses are thus quantified while minimizing the confounding effects of extraneous muscular activity or basal differences in somatic activity across treatments, a procedure that is reminiscent of Jacobson's (1932) use of progressive relaxation in studies of EMG and imagery. A closed-loop baseline procedure also has the advantage over simple change scores in that time series and waveform moment analyses (Dorfman & Cacioppo 1990) can be performed with fewer restrictions. A potential liability of the closed-loop procedure is that both the speed and accuracy with which acceptably low levels of EMG activity are achieved may be partially a function of experimental condition or idiosyncratic strategies, and designs employing this procedure may shape participants inadvertently in subtle ways that complicate interpretation. For this reason, most EMG-based psychological investigations have not employed the closed-loop baseline procedure, although some variant of it is used routinely in investigations of physiological constructs such as muscle fatigue (Roy et al. 1997).

Standard Scores. Obtaining measures of the response free from the influence of prestimulus levels is complicated. Perhaps the oldest procedure is to subtract an index of prestimulus period activity from that same index calculated during the stimulus or poststimulus period. However, this procedure is unproblematic only if the prestimulus state does not itself vary systematically as a function of experimental condition. Significant systematic differences across conditions in prestimulus period EMG activity contraindicate the use of this simple procedure.

Standard scores, range-corrected scores, and percent change scores have all been used in an attempt to achieve a common metric less subject to the vagaries of the simple change score. For example, standardizing EMG scores within sites and participants continues to be used widely in order to reduce participant and site variability. Bush, Hess, and Wolford (1993) reported the results of an extensive computer simulation study that examined the influence of common transformations and outliers on statistical power in simple pretest–posttest within-subject designs. In summary, they found that the Z-score metric did consistently better than nearly all other common transformations vis-à-vis both consistency with the raw data and the ability to detect true differences. Despite the compelling nature of these results, it is important to note that they are based on theoretical rather than empirical distributions (cf. Fridlund, Schwartz, & Fowler 1984). It is also well known in psychophysiology that such "simple" transformations can have surprising consequences (e.g., the long-standing debate over when to use heart period vs. heart rate; see Graham 1978). Consequently, we reiterate the caution expressed previously by Cacioppo et al. (1990b) and by Fridlund and Cacioppo (1986) with respect to the pro forma application of any nonlinear transformation. For the sake of replicability, the application of any nonlinear transformation of EMG signals for purely statistical reasons should be accompanied by both an explicit justification (Levey 1980) and an acknowledgment of any differences in the ordering of the untransformed versus transformed means.

Social Context

Psychophysiological research was once thought to be exempt from the laboratory artifacts that have led others to consider the physical and social context in which the research was conducted (Rosenthal & Rosnow 1969). The vulnerability of physiological responses to instructional sets (Sternbach 1966), intentional distortions (Ekman 1985; Honts et al. 1996), ethnicity (Rankin & Campbell 1955; Vrana & Rollock 1998), and social presence (Cacioppo et al. 1990a; Geen & Bushman 1989) vitiates this notion. Nowhere is this vulnerability more apparent in psychophysiology than in studies of the skeletomotor system (Cacioppo, Petty, & Tassinary 1989). The evidence clearly suggests that vigilance with respect to these factors can contribute to the construction of more sensitive, artifact-free psychophysiological experimentation and hence to stronger inferences (Cacioppo, Marshall-Goodell, & Gormezano 1983b; Gale & Baker 1981).

Social factors have been found also to moderate the influence of nonsocial factors on physiological responding. This point, too, is perhaps clearest in studies of skeletomotor response. The expression of a person's joy following successful completion of a task, for instance, can be magnified, attenuated, or masked because of the presence of others, and comprehensive psychophysiological theories must accommodate such moderating influences (see Cacioppo & Petty 1986 and Chapter 23 of this volume).

SOCIAL FACTORS AS LABORATORY ARTIFACTS

Gale and Baker (1981) noted that experimenter–participant interactions are particularly important in psychophysiology because the procedures may involve touching, partial removal of clothing, skin abrasion, and the application and removal of sensors. This somewhat unique and extended interaction may result in participants becoming anxious, distracted, or aware of the experimenter's expectations, so significant laboratory artifacts may be introduced.

Demand Characteristics

To the extent that participants can discern the experimental hypotheses and manipulate their actions accordingly, EMG studies are vulnerable to experimental demand confounds (Orne 1962). Fridlund and Izard (1983) argued that many facial EMG studies of emotion and emotional imagery could be interpreted in terms of demand characteristics. Specifically, they reasoned that placing multiple electrodes on a person's face could make the person acutely aware of her or his facial expressions. Participants who desired to please the experimenter or to "contribute to science" might alter their expressions in accordance with what they believed were the experimental hypotheses. Particularly susceptible, they suggested, were studies in which the experimental hypothesis was obvious, such as the early studies of facial EMG activity during emotional imagery (e.g. Schwartz 1975). Not all prior research using facial EMG to study emotion was susceptible to this interpretation (see Cacioppo & Petty 1979a), and more recent studies whose designs minimize experimental demands have continued to find that subtle emotions can be discriminated using facial EMG (Cacioppo et al. 1992b; Dimberg 1997; Greenwald, Cook, & Lang 1989; Hess, Banse, & Kappas 1995; McHugo, Lanzetta, & Bush 1991).

Although experimental demands do not appear to be necessary for facial EMG patterning to emerge during emotions, they nevertheless remain a potential source of bias. Procedures contrived to minimize such biases include: (1) providing participants with plausible alternative hypotheses; (2) employing cover stories that divert attention away from the physiological recording; (3) utilizing engaging experimental tasks; (4) placing multiple nonfunctional sensors over other areas of the body to reduce the salience of the functional sensors; and (5) designing the laboratory setting to be comfortable and free of unnecessary equipment. The level of experimental demand can also be assessed directly, either (i) through a "funnel" debriefing procedure that involves gradually revealing more and more of the hypothesis to participants while gauging their awareness of the hypothesis or (ii) by including a simulation condition in which the EMG study is described explicitly to a naive group of participants who are then asked to predict how they would or should respond in such a situation.[11]

Evaluation Apprehension

Naive participants may be apprehensive about participating in research involving the use of electrodes and electrical recording equipment. Such apprehension, although possibly of interest in its own right, may create a level of tension or hypervigilance in the participant that is unrepresentative and that can obscure the effects of the experimental treatments. This apprehension is in addition to the potential apprehension that participants may feel about being evaluated by experimenters who are presumably experts in human behavior. Rosenthal (1966) suggested that such evaluation apprehension might also lead participants to distort their actions in a socially desirable fashion. If an experimenter's behavior or experimental treatment makes participants especially anxious or aware that they are being evaluated, then the data may be significantly biased.

Procedures for minimizing evaluation apprehension, in addition to those outlined in the preceding section, include: (1) providing a tour of portions of the laboratory to prospective participants (to brief them on the tasks and procedures involved in the study) prior to seeking informed consent or scheduling them for participation; (2) allowing time before the beginning of the experimental procedures for participants to adapt to the laboratory; (3) using buffer trials or tasks to allow adaptation to the experimental procedure; (4) employing a closed-loop baseline to ensure participants are not unduly tense or aroused prior to initiating the next trial; and (5) minimizing the sense participants may have that they are being scrutinized by automating procedures, assuring them that their responses are anonymous, and using unobtrusive monitoring methods (e.g., hidden cameras; see Kappas, Hess, & Kleck 1990) during the experiment.

Individual Difference Variables

Finally, various attributes of individual participants can affect EMG measures and are thus important to assess or control by means of the experimental design. These attributes include age, intramuscular temperature (which can be affected by muscle activity as well as ambient temperature), muscle strength, and expressiveness (Allport & Vernon 1933; Goldstein 1972; Manstead 1991).

SOCIAL FACTORS AS DETERMINANTS

In the previous section, we saw that the nature of the interaction between the experimenter and participant is both a source of bias in psychophysiological research and a means for its solution. In this section, we briefly review illustrative research demonstrating how social factors can also moderate the influence of nonsocial factors on EMG responses.

Audience Effects

The classic observations of Charles Darwin (1872/1873) suggested that facial expressions of emotion were universal. Most members of both the scientific community and the lay public, however, would undoubtedly agree that felt emotions are not always accompanied by perceptible expressions. According to an influential "neurocultural" model proposed by Paul Ekman (1972) to explain communalities and idiosyncrasies in facial expressions, a given emotion will not always be displayed in the same fashion owing to the influence of personal habits, situational pressures, and cultural norms. In an early study on such "display rules," groups of Japanese or American students were exposed to a disgusting film while being videotaped unobtrusively or with an authoritarian experimenter present (Friesen 1972). Results revealed that both the Japanese and American students displayed revulsion while viewing the film in solitude, but the Japanese students masked their feelings of revulsion by smiling during the film when the experimenter was present. A recent study of racial bias suggests the opposite dissociation between expression and self-report may occur when examining covert responses (Vanman et al. 1997). In the context of a cooperative task, European-American participants tended to report more liking for African-American partners while simultaneously showing greater increases in the EMG activity recorded over the brow region, a result indicative of greater negative affect and interpreted by the authors as evidence of racial prejudice. The ability of affective stimuli to evoke small but reliable changes in facial EMG activity even in the absence of awareness (Tassinary et al. 1984; Wexler et al. 1992), when combined with the possibility that minute levels of activity may be imperceptible to both observers and producers (Epstein 1990; Max 1932), provides a plausible explanation for why such covert responses may be less susceptible to audience effects.

The influence of an observer on people's facial expressions of emotion emphasizes the multiple roles played by behavioral responses. Because the skeletomotor system is the only means individuals have of approaching, avoiding, or modifying elements in their physical environment, one

might expect that overt somatic responses in part reflect or serve to gratify certain goals or desires. An individual who accidentally touches a hot platter is likely to exhibit a rapid withdrawal, just as an individual who smells a foul odor is likely to express disgust and either quickly stop breathing or rapidly exhale (Tassinary 1985).

The skeletomotor system is also an individual's primary means of communication and of effecting change in the social environment. It is not surprising, therefore, that overt somatic responses such as facial expressions can be affected strongly by the perceived presence of observers. Kraut and Johnson (1979), for instance, related the observed frequency of smiling to simultaneously occurring events in a wide range of naturalistic settings (e.g., bowling alleys, public walkways, hockey arenas). Their results indicated that people were most likely to smile while speaking with other people; they were significantly less likely to smile perceptibly to a presumably positive event (e.g., bowling a strike) when their faces were unobserved than observed. Related findings were reported by Chovil (1991), Fridlund (1991), Gilbert, Fridlund, and Sabini (1987), and Jaencke (1996). Fridlund (1994) argued forcefully that such results provide strong evidence against the two-factor neurocultural model and strong evidence for a one-factor behavioral ecology model. However, a wide variety of results (e.g. Cacioppo et al. 1992b; Davis et al. 1995; Geen 1992; Hess et al. 1995; Vanman et al. 1997) suggest that a more rather than less inclusive and sophisticated model is necessary, and this prevision is consistent with the multitude of neural systems contributing to the coordination and control of the facial musculature (Fanardjian & Manvelyan 1987; Jenny & Saper 1987).

Facial expressions of emotion are not the only somatic responses that are affected by the presence of observers. Chapman (1974), for instance, monitored EMG activity over the forehead region as participants listened to a story while either unobserved, watched by a concealed observer, or watched by an unconcealed observer. Chapman found that EMG activity over the forehead region was higher during the story when the participant was observed than when unobserved and also slightly (though not significantly) higher when the observer was present than when concealed. Groff, Baron, and Moore (1983) further demonstrated that the presence of observers led to more vigorous motor responses. These data fit well with observations dating as far back as the late 1890s (Triplett 1898) demonstrating that an individual's performance on a task can be altered dramatically simply by moving the task from a nonsocial to a social context. Zajonc (1965) organized much of this research with his proposal that the presence of conspecifics lowered the threshold for the single most likely response to a task (see reviews by Bond & Titus 1983; Geen & Gange 1977). The important point here is that not only performance but also physiological responses such as EMG activity have been found to vary as a function of the presence of observers (see Cacioppo & Petty 1986, pp. 658–64).

The presence of others has also been shown to lessen rather than heighten the vigor of somatic responses when their presence renders the subject anonymous or unaccountable for her or his performance. Latane, Williams, and Harkins (1979) dubbed this effect "social loafing." In an illustrative series of studies, Latane et al. (1979) instructed participants to clap or shout as loudly as possible. On some trials, participants were led to believe their individual performance was being monitored, whereas on other trials they were led to believe their performance was being pooled with those of varying numbers of other participants. On all trials, participants heard a masking noise through headphones as they clapped or shouted, so they could not tell how loudly they or others were performing. Results revealed that participants expended more physical effort (i.e., clapped or shouted more loudly) when they believed they were personally accountable for their performance than when they were able to diffuse their responsibility for performing the task. Hence, the presence of others can enhance or reduce muscular response magnitude depending on whether the presence of others increases or decreases the threat of social sanctions or embarrassment based on one's performance.

Mimicry

Mimicry refers in this context to the elicitation of a localized motor response through witnessing the same response being performed by another. Evidence for motor mimicry includes such demonstrations as wincing at another's pain (Vaughan & Lanzetta 1980), straining at another's effort (Markovsky & Berger 1983), and spontaneously imitating another's evident emotion (Dimberg 1982, 1990; Lundqvist & Dimberg 1995). Motor mimicry in psychology has traditionally been conceptualized as primarily intrapersonal, representing either primitive empathy, a conditioned emotional response based on one's direct experience, or an expression of vicarious emotion (Allport 1968) and as such is closely related to the concept of emotional contagion (Hatfield, Cacioppo, & Rapson 1993; cf. Hess, Phillipot, & Blairy in press). Consistent with this framework, Dimberg (1982, 1990) reported that subtle decreases in EMG activity over the *corrugator supercilii* muscle region and increases in EMG activity over the *zygomaticus major* muscle region were observed when participants viewed pictures of smiling faces, whereas the opposite pattern of facial EMG activity was observed when participants viewed pictures of angry faces. Lanzetta and his colleagues (Englis, Vaughan, & Lanzetta 1982; Lanzetta & Englis 1989) provided evidence that counterempathic as well as empathic processes can result in subtle changes in facial EMG activity.

Studies by Bavelas and colleagues (1986, 1988) suggest the form and intensity of *visible* motor mimicry is influenced strongly by the communicative significance of the mimesis. For instance, in their earlier study, the victim of what appeared to be a painful injury was either increasingly or decreasingly visible to the observing participant. Results revealed that the pattern and timing of the observer's motor mimicry was affected significantly by the visibility of the victim. In sharp contrast to research demonstrating the interpersonal and emotional significance of mimicry, the evidence to date is decidedly against the notion that there are significant cognitive consequences to such mimicry (Graziano et al. 1996). Thus, the research on mimicry is consistent with the preceding suggestion that social factors can influence somatic responding in the service of interpersonal (i.e., communicative) goals as well as personal feelings and emotions.

Inferential Context

An understanding of the physiological basis of surface EMG, the electrical principles underlying its measurement, and the social context moderating its expression is essential for conducting meaningful research, but it is clearly not sufficient. As Shapiro and Crider (1969, p. 3) noted:

In the most concrete sense, physiological variables are measures of nothing but themselves, and cannot be taken as ready-made indicators of ... psychological constructs. A response measure, whether of overt or covert functioning, has meaning only in the context of observation.

General discussions of the issues involved in moving from physiological data to psychological or behavioral inferences have been provided in Chapter 1 of this volume. In this section, we review briefly several general paradigms in psychophysiological studies of EMG activity. In so doing, we also highlight some of the information about cognitive, emotional, and behavioral processes that has come from EMG studies.

PSYCHOPHYSIOLOGICAL PARADIGMS

One of the challenges in psychophysiological research involving surface EMG is to create paradigms that allow strong inferences (Platt 1964) about psychological constructs based on somatic responses. Cacioppo et al. (1990b) proposed that much of the variety and complexity in the experimental paradigms in this area can be characterized in terms of the function (independent vs. dependant variable) and the proximal origin (endogenous vs. exogenous) of a somatic response. The result is four generic paradigms, referred to as the outcome, the conditional probability, the reflex probe, and the manipulated response paradigms (see Figure 7). Within these general paradigms, answers have been sought to questions regarding the psychological, behavioral, and health significance of somatic activity and the extent to which skeletomotor activity reflects specific or

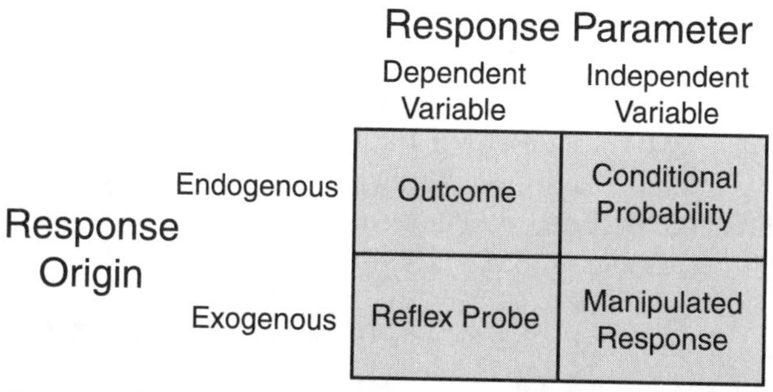

Response Parameter

	Dependent Variable	Independent Variable
Endogenous	Outcome	Conditional Probability
Exogenous	Reflex Probe	Manipulated Response

Response Origin

Figure 7. Classification scheme for typical psychophysiological paradigms involving the use of surface EMG. (Modified and redrawn from Figure 8 in Cacioppo et al. 1990b.)

global activation; phasic, tonic, or modulated thresholds for activation; and characteristics of the stimulus situation or the individual's disposition.

Outcome Paradigms

Outcome paradigms continue to be the most prevalent in psychophysiology. The essence of such paradigms is that a psychological or behavioral process is manipulated while one or more physiological (e.g. EMG) responses are monitored. Edmund Jacobson's (e.g. 1932) pioneering EMG studies mentioned at the beginning of this chapter are cases in point as are any studies based on subtractive or additive factors methodology (Cacioppo & Petty 1986; Sternberg 1969).

For over half a century, studies conducted within this general paradigm on phasic EMG responses have found that reliable and oftentimes minute patterns of EMG activity accompany thought, emotion, and imagery despite large variations within and between individuals. Cacioppo and Petty (1981a) provided a useful summary of this research through the use of a small set of empirical generalizations. They concluded that there are foci of somatic activity in which changes signalize particular psychological processes (e.g., emotion and the mimetic muscles, language processes and the musculature employed in speech) and that these changes can be (a) inhibitory as well as excitatory, (b) patterned temporally as well as spatially, and (c) less evident as the distance of measurement from the focal point increases. In addition, likely candidates for significant foci can be identified a priori either by observing generally the actions involved in the production of the behavioral process of interest or by analyzing the overt reactions that initially characterize such a process but appear to drop out with practice.

In an illustrative study, Shaw (1940) instructed subjects to lift or imagine lifting weights. Not surprisingly, the amplitude of EMG activity over the preferred arm increased as subjects lifted heavier and heavier weights. More interestingly, this same trend held when subjects merely imagined lifting the weights, and these effects have since been replicated and extended many times (e.g. Bakker, Boschker, &

Chung 1996). Similarly, Schwartz and his colleagues (1976) reported that clinically depressed subjects displayed higher levels of EMG activity over the brow muscle region (*corrugator supercilii*) and lower levels of EMG activity over the cheek muscle region (*zygomaticus major*) when they imagined unpleasant experiences than when they imagined pleasant ones. Nondepressed subjects displayed patterns similar to those produced by the depressed subjects, but the pattern accompanying pleasant imagery was accentuated and the pattern accompanying unpleasant imagery was attenuated in the normal subjects.[12] Numerous studies conducted over the past two decades have expanded upon these basic findings and consistently demonstrated that affect-laden events, whether imagined or perceived, result in patterned changes in the facial musculature (Cacioppo et al. 1986a; Lang et al. 1993; Sirota & Schwartz 1982). Occasional failures to find such effects have also been reported (Malcolm, Von, & Horney 1989).

Although most EMG research in psychophysiology has focused primarily on specific phasic changes in EMG activity, a parallel tradition of research has focused on general or tonic changes in tension, activation, or arousal (see reviews by Duffy 1962; Freeman 1931; Malmo 1975; van Boxtel & Jessurun 1993). For instance, Germana (1974) suggested that, although skilled or habitual actions are characterized by a well-orchestrated patterning of skeletomotor activity, response uncertainty leads to a general activation of the musculature. He speculated that general activation across functionally disparate muscle regions signifies extensive preparation for overt behavior, and he proposed that both novel and partially conditioned stimuli are the most likely to produce response uncertainty. It is interesting to note that recent research provides partial support for Germana's suggestion that generalized somatic activation during response uncertainty reflects an equalization of response probabilities (see e.g. Chapter 3 of this volume), and this suggestion has been incorporated into a recent heuristic model of emotion (Cacioppo, Berntson, & Klein 1992a) via the proposal that psychologically relevant somatic activity may range from completely undifferentiated tonic activation to emotion-specific patterns of phasic activation.

Malmo (1965, 1975), while also interested in general or tonic somatic activation during task performance, focused specifically on observed temporal EMG gradients within a site as providing a means to quantify the unfolding of general activation across time. Malmo and others (e.g. Bartoshuk 1955; Davis & Malmo 1951; Wallerstein 1954) observed reliable gradients in a variety of muscles, whether task-relevant or otherwise. The steepness of these gradients throughout the entire course of the sequence was interpreted to be monotonically related to the stress or effort involved throughout the experimental task.

Research with respect to motivational states has tended to focus on the significance of EMG gradients in the task-irrelevant musculature (Rimehaug & Svebak 1987). In an illustrative study, participants played one of two versions of a video game that required they stop a "ball" from passing across the screen by maneuvering a video "bat" to intercept the ball (Svebak, Dalen, & Storfjell 1981). In the easy version, an unimpeded ball bounced across the screen in approximately 3 sec; in the difficult version, the ball traveled at approximately twice this rate. Both versions required the subject to engage in continuous performance for 150 sec, and EMG activity was recorded over the forearm flexor of the passive arm during baseline and task periods. Results revealed the EMG gradient associated with the difficult game to be significantly steeper than that associated with the easy game. Van Boxtel and Jessurun (1993) also reported strong EMG gradients recorded from the forehead, brow, and lip muscle regions during performance on difficult and extended tasks. They concluded that such activity provides a sensitive index of the degree of exerted mental effort.

In a similar vein but on a shorter time scale, Davis (1940) recorded EMG activity over several muscle regions (e.g., forearm extensors) as participants performed a choice reaction time task under unwarned, fixed foreperiod, or variable foreperiod conditions. Davis observed that (a) EMG activity was higher in the foreperiod when the participant was warned as opposed to unwarned, (b) EMG activity began to rise approximately 200–400 msec following the warning signal and continued to rise until the overt response was completed, and (c) EMG activity was higher (and reaction time shorter) with a fixed than variable foreperiod. Davis concluded that the EMG responses during the foreperiod reflected preparation for the upcoming response. In a similar paradigm, van Boxtel, Damen, and Brunia (1996) recorded EMG activity over several pericranial muscle regions as participants performed a fixed foreperiod simple reaction time task involving either an auditory or visual reaction signal. The responses were performed with the hand or foot. Throughout the warning interval they observed that: (a) neck muscle EMG activity remained relatively unchanged; (b) forehead, brow, and lip EMG activity systematically increased; and (c) periocular, cheek, and temple EMG activity systematically decreased. Van Boxtel et al. interpreted this pattern of activation in the task-irrelevant pericranial musculature to be in the service of increasing perceptual sensitivity rather than facilitating response preparation.

There is thus no more consensus within the EMG field than within other fields of psychophysiology regarding which measure best reflects general motivation, tension, or activation. Meyer (1953) suggested that eye-blink rate provided the best overall measure of generalized tension, and Meyer, Bahrick, and Fitts (1953) reported that individuals who score high on anxiety inventories also have high blink rates. Rossi (1959) found a similar relationship between manifest anxiety scores and EMG activity over the forearm extensors. Similarly, Davis, Malmo, and Shagass (1954)

administered white-noise blasts at 1-min intervals to both normals and individuals with anxiety disorders. Results revealed that, although the noise blast evoked a slightly larger EMG response over the forearm extensor region in the anxious than normal individuals, the more significant difference occurred during recovery following the stressor. The elevation in EMG activity in normal subjects was sharply delimited, returning to basal levels within seconds of the termination of the noise burst, whereas the elevation in EMG in the anxious subjects lingered.

Fridlund and associates (1986) replicated and extended these findings using EMG measures over the head, neck, and limbs. Participants first rested quietly for 15 min and then were exposed to 5 min of 105-dB binaural white-noise stimulation. Participants who were more anxious exhibited higher levels of EMG activity, primarily over the head and neck preceding the stimulus and more generally during the stimulus. An idiographic principal components analysis of EMG activity during these periods failed to reveal evidence for a general, intercorrelated tensional factor; instead, the EMG elevations in the highly anxious subjects consisted largely of uncorrelated response bursts. This pattern of EMG responses was interpreted to indicate a state of heightened activation or a lower threshold for activation. Consistent with this interpretation, Britt and Blumenthal (1992) reported that the latencies of auditory startle responses in participants low in state anxiety were intensity-dependent, whereas those high in state anxiety responded with equal latency regardless of stimulus intensity.

Woodworth and Schlosberg (1954, pp. 173–9) suggested that EMG activity, particularly in the neck region (e.g., splenius, upper trapezius), may be a somewhat unique indicator of the level of activation owing to the possibility that a disproportionate share of proprioceptive impulses to the central nervous system originate in this muscle region. This suggestion is interesting in light of the sparse evidence for the notion of a coherent tensional factor (see e.g. Fridlund, Fowler, & Pritchard 1980). In accord with this suggestion, Eason and White (1961) had subjects perform a variety of vigilance tasks (e.g., rotary tracking) while recording EMG activity over the splenius, upper trapezius, lower trapezius, and the deltoid and biceps of the right arm. The major finding in these studies was that the general level of EMG activity (most consistently that recorded over the neck muscles) varied as a function of the effort subjects expended on tasks. Waersted and Westgaard (1996) recorded surface EMG activity from 20 different sites while participants performed a complex two-choice reaction time task designed to demand continuing attention yet require minimal activity. The major finding in this study was that attention-related activity was most clearly observed over the frontalis and upper trapezius muscle regions.

In summary, substantial increases in task difficulty, the subjective effort expended on tasks, and stress have been found to lead to elevated EMG activity during preparatory periods as well as during the performance of effortful engaging tasks. In addition, an inhibition of EMG activity over irrelevant musculature is sometimes observed during such tasks, particularly when the response to the task is well practiced (Germana 1974; Goldstein 1972; Chapter 19 of this volume). Although these findings are inconsistent with a simple-minded view of general tension or arousal, such a view has been questionable for over a half a century:

The literature of muscle tonus has been burdened in the past and is still being burdened by observations which have not taken into account the functional significance of tonic activity. Tonic manifestations have been sought for indiscriminately in all muscles, at all times, and not infrequently the operative procedure of the investigator has caused the very tonicity he has sought for to vanish. (Fulton 1926, p. 384)

Double Dissociation Design. Whether changes in EMG activity reflect particular actions or rather general somatic attitudes often has important theoretical implications. The double dissociation design (Teuber 1955) is considered to be one of the more powerful in this regard. This experimental design is so named because (a) one or more treatments that should evoke a specific response is (are) contrasted with one or more treatments that should not evoke the expected response, and (b) one or more measures of the target response are included as well as one or more measures of a nontarget response. The former establishes discriminant validity of the treatments, whereas the latter demonstrates the discriminant validity of the responses.

To illustrate, there has long been a hypothesis that silent language processing is associated with increased activation of the speech (e.g., perioral) musculature (McGuigan 1978). As McGuigan (1970) noted previously, there are a number of studies demonstrating that EMG activity over the perioral musculature increased from basal levels when individuals engaged in silent language processing. These results alone are not particularly informative because such a psychophysiological outcome could be attributed to aspects of the task that had nothing to do with speech processing per se. A slight tensing of lips, for example, might be associated with orthographic or auditory processing or possibly to general increases in tension or arousal due to concerns about task performance. The inclusion of nonspeech as well as speech tasks addresses the first of these interpretational problems, and the measurement of EMG activity over nontarget as well as target sites addresses the second.

In most applications of the double dissociation paradigm, different subjects or stimuli are used to achieve treatments that theoretically should and should not evoke a specific somatic action or pattern. In a particularly comprehensive series of studies, McGuigan and Bailey (1969) recorded EMG activity over the chin, tongue, and forearm muscle regions while subjects silently read, memorized

prose, listened to prose, listened to music, and attentively listened to "nothing." Results revealed that EMG activity over the perioral musculature was uniquely associated with the performance of silent language tasks.

Double Dissociation with Constant Stimuli. Although the outcome observed by McGuigan and Bailey (1969) is consistent with the hypothesis that silent language processing leads to increased perioral EMG activity, Cacioppo and Petty (1979b, 1981b) noted that the grounds for such an inference would be strengthened further if the participants and the physical characteristics of the target stimuli were held constant within the double dissociation paradigm. To achieve this refinement, EMG activity was monitored over the inferior *orbicularis oris* and the superficial forearm flexor muscle regions while participants evaluated a series of trait adjectives presented visually. The treatment conditions were altered by varying systematically the dimension of evaluation rather than by varying either participants or stimuli. Specifically, for half of the trait adjectives participants were asked to evaluate the stimulus semantically ("Is the following descriptive of you?"); for the other half they were asked to evaluate the stimulus graphemically ("Is the following printed in uppercase letters?"). Results revealed EMG activity over the perioral region to be greater during the semantic task, whereas EMG activity over the nonpreferred forearm did not differ as a function of task. Because the type of stimulus presented or type of participant tested was held constant, the inference appears more secure that silent language semantic processing involving short-term memory leads to increased EMG activity over the perioral muscle region.

It must be noted, however, that inferences derived from outcome paradigms are tentative at best when using even the most rigorous of designs. The data obtained from additive and subtractive factors designs in general, as well as double dissociation designs in particular, are indeterminate to the extent that continuous causal functions are dichotomized arbitrarily (Cook & Campbell 1979, p. 12), the underlying mechanisms are nonlinear (McClelland 1979), or relevant factors have been overlooked (Cacioppo, Petty, & Morris 1985). The more recent controversy over the evidence for multiple memory systems (Knowlton & Squire 1993; Nosofsky & Zaki 1998) illustrates clearly the diagnostic limitations of interpretations based solely on the results from such designs.

Conditional Probability

Most psychologists, like many psychophysiologists, have sought to use physiological data to infer psychological or behavioral constructs such as anxiety, emotion, deception, and depression. Typically, the target physiological events have been identified as those that have been shown to vary as a function of the theoretical construct of interest. Electromyographic activity over the forehead region has been of interest, for example, because anxiety, tension, and mental effort are often accompanied by increased EMG activity over this site. However, knowing that the manipulation of a psychological or behavioral factor leads to this particular skeletomotor response does not logically imply that this response indexes the psychological or behavioral factor (see Cacioppo & Tassinary 1990). Put succinctly, the probability of event A given event B cannot be assumed to equal the probability of event B given event A, and the former cannot even be derived unless both the latter and the probability of event B given the *absence* of event A are known. Put more concretely, the utility of a skeletomotor response to serve as an index of a theoretical construct is weakened by the occurrence of such responses in the absence of the construct of interest (see Chapter 1).

Although one cannot logically identify all possible factors that might influence a target response or response pattern, its ability to index a theoretical construct can be defined as the extent to which the construct of interest is present given the presence of the target response or response pattern. That is, one can block on the presence or absence of a skeletomotor response (or on variations of this response) and analyze the extent to which the construct of interest is evident. In so doing, an endogenous skeletomotor response pattern functions as the independent rather than the dependent variable.

Cacioppo et al. (1988) utilized a conditional probability paradigm to examine the extent to which specific forms of EMG response over the brow region indexed particular emotions evoked during an interview. Previous research has demonstrated that mild negative imagery and unpleasant sensory stimuli tend to evoke greater EMG activity over the brow (*corrugator supercilii*) and less EMG activity over the cheek (*zygomaticus major*) and ocular (*orbicularis oculi*) muscle regions than mild positive imagery and pleasant sensory stimuli. This previous research did not address whether facial EMG responses provided a sensitive and specific index of particular emotions, however, because there are a multiplicity of events that can affect facial EMG activity. To address this question directly, Cacioppo et al. (1988) obtained both facial EMG and audiovisual recordings while individuals were interviewed about themselves. A while later, individuals were asked to describe what they had been thinking during specific segments of the interview marked by distinctive EMG responses over the brow region in the context of ongoing but stable levels of activity elsewhere in the face. Consistent with the notion that the expressive components of emotion are "sometimes brought unconsciously into momentary action by ludicrously slight causes" (Darwin 1872/1873, p. 184), inconspicuous EMG responses over the *corrugator supercilii* muscle region were observed to covary with subtle variations in emotion during the interview even though the overt facial expressions evinced by subjects were rated similarly across conditions by observers. Furthermore, it was reasoned that certain forms of EMG activity in the context of an interview, such as brief jagged bursts rather than sustained smooth mounds, would be especially predictive of variations in emotion due primarily to theoretical differences in the probability of such responses in the absence of emotion. *Videlicet,* smooth modulations in EMG activity over the brow region were hypothesized to reflect paralinguistic signaling and emotional expression equally, whereas abrupt modulations in EMG activity over the same region were hypothesized to be much less likely to be associated with paralinguistic signaling. Support for this reasoning was also found. These results illustrate the power of the conditional probability paradigm and provide evidence that specific patterns of facial EMG response can actually index variations in emotion, at least within this limited context.

It is interesting that a classic study by Max (1935) can also be viewed within this paradigm. Max hypothesized that EMG activity would increase during dreaming and that this activity would be evident in the fingers of deaf-mutes because fingers are intimately involved in the production of sign language. In a test of this reasoning, EMG activity was recorded over the arm and finger muscles of both hearing and deaf participants as they slept. A general decrease in EMG activity was observed in both groups as they approached sleep, and occasional bursts of EMG activity were observed over the finger muscles during their sleep. When the latter occurred, participants were awakened and were asked to report if and about what they had been dreaming. As predicted, EMG activity over the finger muscles was associated with dreaming in the deaf-mute participants but not in the participants with normal hearing and speech.

More recently, Shimizu and Inoue (1986) completed a study of sleep and dreams that bears on the utility of perioral EMG activity as a marker of silent language processing in participants with normal hearing and speech. Electroencephalographic, electro-oculographic (EOG), perioral EMG, and nonoral EMG activity were recorded during sleep. Participants were awakened during either rapid eye movement (REM) or stage-2 sleep, as determined by inspection of the EEG and EOG recordings. When participants reported dreaming they were asked whether or not they had been speaking in their dreams. Dream recall during REM sleep occurred in approximately 80% of the awakenings; it occurred during stage-2 sleep in approximately 28% of the awakenings. Awakenings without dream recall were excluded from further analyses, as were awakenings preceded by phasic discharges in the perioral musculature that were accompanied by any whispering or vocalization. Results revealed that when phasic discharges over the perioral musculature were observed within the 30 sec preceding the awakening, subjects reported having been speaking in their dreams in 88% of the awakenings from REM sleep and 71% of the awakenings during stage-2 sleep. Moreover, when phasic discharges over the perioral musculature were not observed within the 30 sec preceding the awakening, subjects reported having been speaking in their dreams in only 19% of the awakenings from REM sleep and in none of the awakenings during stage-2 sleep.

In summary, previous research has indicated (a) that situations in which participants report emotional reactions are accompanied by patterned EMG activity in the facial musculature, (b) that effortful tasks requiring cognitive resources influence the EMG activity in task-irrelevant muscles, and (c) that silent language processing is accompanied by EMG activity in the perioral musculature. The research reviewed in this section further suggests that autochthonous EMG activity can be used to mark episodes of affect and silent language processing in some limited contexts.

Reflex Probe Paradigms

Reflexes generally refer to any automatic reaction of the nervous system to stimuli impinging upon the body or arising within it (Merton 1987).[13] Although there have been clear analytical attempts to define the concept of the reflex in precise logical and empirical terms from within both physiology (Sherrington 1906/1923) and psychology (Skinner 1931), the definition of the reflex and the functional significance of reflexes in the intact organism remain active topics of research (see e.g. Berkinblit, Feldman, & Fukson 1986).

From a physiological perspective, reflexes can be defined as a discrete type of behavior mediated by a reflex arc, thus providing both functional and structural constraints on the definition (Gallistel 1980). Structurally, a *reflex arc* is an anatomical entity consisting of:

1. receptors tuned to transduce specifiable classes of environmental stimuli into neural signals;
2. sensory neurons that conduct the output signals from the receptors to the central nervous system (CNS);
3. mediators – either a single synapse or a small set of interneurons – that relay the sensory output to an appropriate subset of motoneurons or neurohumoral cells;
4. motoneurons or neurohumoral cells that conduct the signal from the CNS to particular effectors; and
5. the effectors themselves, which impact on the environment as a function of neural and/or hormonal input.

Functionally, four conditions must be met in order for a particular behavior to be classified as reflexive. First, the effector response to any single sensory stimulus of sufficient intensity to actually elicit a response must rise to a single peak and then decline rapidly. Second, response duration and amplitude must be determined strictly by the intensity of the elicitor and current states of the intervening synapses and effector organs. Third, signal conduction can proceed in only one direction ("the irreversibility of conduction"). And finally, the actual result of the activation of the effectors cannot directly modify subsequent

effector output (i.e., there should be no feedback from the effectors to any part of the reflex arc).

From a psychological perspective, Skinner proposed that the concept of the reflex is fundamentally both behavioral and statistical and that it reduces simply to "the observed correlation of the activity of an effector (i.e., a response) with the observed forces affecting a receptor (i.e., a stimulus)" (Skinner 1931, p. 438). He argued that the functional attributes (unlearned, unconscious, and involuntary) of reflexes, as well as any physiological attributes so often claimed to define a reflex, were actually incidental properties of the class of reflexes that were first discovered and investigated by neurophysiologists. Generalizing the concept beyond its historical beginnings, he partitioned the experimental study of the reflex into two parts. First, there is the investigation of the correlation between a specifiable stimulus class (S) and response class (R) – that is, the latency, threshold, and range of variation in S and R over which the correlation holds. Second, there is the investigation of variations in these characteristics as a function of third variables. This latter investigation would include assessing changes in reflex strength (i.e., the magnitude of the correlation) as a function of external variables such as deprivation, gender, and prior conditioning history.

Since the turn of the century, the scientific study of the reflex has proceeded in two directions. Disciplines concerned with the control of movement (e.g., neurophysiology, physiological psychology, psychology) have generally followed the tradition of Sherrington and examined reflexes as integral to the regulation of behavior. Predicated on this view of the reflex as a relatively invariant unit of behavior, the accompanying research and theory focuses on specifying the rules by which reflexes combine to generate coordinated, goal-directed movements.

In neurology and psychophysiology, however, the reflex is viewed in a manner more consistent with the behaviorist generalization of the concept articulated by Skinner. In the field of neurology this conceptualization led initially to widespread confusion, with the early part of the century referred to as an open season for the "hunting of the reflex" (Wartenberg 1946). During this time, any stimulus–response correlation was fair game to be named and reified. An unfortunate result was that many reflexes were "discovered" by one author after another, each time renamed and claimed to be unique. However, it is now possible to use the parameters of reflex responses as *markers* of CNS function owing to increasingly detailed information about the neural circuits mediating specific reflexes (Davis 1989; Ongerboer de Visser 1983) and the development of standardized testing conditions (Bickerstaff 1980).

As a tool in the investigation of psychological processes, surface electromyography provides an ongoing record of muscular activity while minimally interfering with the behavior under study. However, the unique advantage of the reflex probe paradigm is that it allows estimation of changes in the excitability of spinal and brainstem motor structures that may not be manifest in either overt behavior or in peripheral EMG activity. The use of the reflex as a probe into ongoing psychological processes further exemplifies the examining of variations in reflex characteristics as a function of third variables. Although Skinner (1931) intended this experimental procedure to be used to quantify the influences of external variables on the reflex behavior of intact organisms, the same logic allows one to use variations in reflex strength as an indicant of internal psychological processes as well. In the former case, the focus is on the description of behavior; in the latter, one infers the operation either of intervening variables or hypothetical constructs.

Early investigations of reflexes revealed that psychological factors (i.e., attention) affected aspects of reflex responsivity. Clinical neurologists looked upon these influences as nuisance variables, factors that could increase the likelihood of both false positives and false negatives in their diagnosis of CNS function. Even so, the enormous potential to use such procedures in psychophysiological investigations was apparent from the turn of the century (Dodge 1911; Sherrington 1906/1923). Surprisingly, for reasons that remain somewhat unclear (see Ison & Hoffman 1983), the use of this technique remained sporadic until the mid-1960s.

The power of the reflex probe paradigm for psychophysiological inference was first seen most clearly in the work on attention (Anthony 1985), activation, and response preparation (Brunia & Boelhouwer 1988; see also Chapter 19). More recently, it has been conscripted to reveal the motivational substrate of affective processes (e.g. Bradley, Cuthbert, & Lang in press; see also Chapter 22).

Anthony (1985) reviewed numerous experiments on the modulation of the blink reflex by manipulations affecting attention. The general conclusion from such studies is that the amplitude and/or latency of the blink can be used in specific situations to measure how attention is allocated to different sensory modalities. Specifically, in paradigms in which the subject is warned of an impending target stimulus, the amplitude of the blink is reliably enhanced or suppressed in the warning interval as a function of the match or mismatch, respectively, between the modalities of the two stimuli. In addition, reliable changes in the degree of facilitation or inhibition across the warning interval suggest that the selective allocation of attention may begin as early as the onset of the warning stimulus but that the rate of allocation speeds up dramatically about 2 sec before the onset of the target stimulus.

Brunia and Boelhouwer (1988) reviewed a large and well-established body of experiments on the modulation of Achilles tendon, Hoffman, and blink reflex amplitude as a function of a wide range of tasks. They concluded that such changes in amplitude are a function of both aselective (i.e., activation) and selective (i.e., response preparation) processes, and they associated these hypothetical processes with major pathways in the central nervous system. Aselective activation effects are hypothesized to be the result of activity in the reticulo-spinal and reticulo-bulbar pathways, and selective preparation effects are hypothesized to be the result of activity in the cortico-spinal and cortico-bulbar pathways (see Figure 2). Brunia and Boelhouwer also presented evidence to suggest that three distinct independent phases in the reflex amplitude function exist in the interval between the presentation of a warning stimulus and the execution of a movement, arguing that these empirically defined phases can be linked to the information processing operations of stimulus evaluation, motor preparation, and response execution. Finally, they presented evidence of situations in which changes in reflex amplitude (a) are redundant with nonprobed surface EMG activity (after the onset of the imperative stimulus), (b) stand in contraposition to surface EMG activity (during the foreperiod in an already activated muscle), and (c) occur in the absence of surface EMG activity (during the foreperiod in task-irrelevant muscles and, after practice, in the task-relevant muscles as well). See also Davis (1940) and van Boxtel et al. (1996).

Over the past decade, the reflex probe technique (specifically, the blink reflex) has been employed increasingly in psychophysiology to investigate basic affective processes, although much earlier investigations do exist (see Burtt & Tuttle 1925). Bradley et al. (in press) review the literature to date and evaluate the theoretical implications of this research. Although the exact time course of both affective and attentional modulation of the blink reflex are variable and task-dependent (Vanman et al. 1996), sufficient consistency across studies exists to support the proposition that reflex modulation by affective valence occurs principally in the context of contemplative situations that both enthrall and induce. Viewed in this manner, augmented blink amplitudes observed during the perception of menacing events signalize the prefatory activation of defense or avoidance responses. Conversely, attenuated blink amplitudes observed during the perception of enticing events signalize the prefatory activation of consummatory or approach responses.

In summary, the reflex probe paradigm has proved useful when simply recording surface EMG activity has appeared to be either insensitive or polysemous. In these contexts, variations in reflex amplitudes have been used to track the allocation of attention, the recruitment of motivational systems, and the preparation for action. It is important to note, however, that this paradigm is inherently more intrusive, potentially less efficient, and only possibly more sensitive than either of the previous two paradigms. The decision regarding which paradigm to use in a given application depends heavily on the nature of the question asked as well as on the social context of the experiment.

Manipulated Response

Questions about the contributions of skeletomotor actions to psychological states or processes have also been addressed by manipulating skeletomotor actions to achieve the desired configuration, verifying the configuration using some observational procedure such as the FACS, and measuring the outcome variables of interest (e.g., subjective states, autonomic responses). Although skeletomotor actions have occasionally been manipulated through explicit operant conditioning procedures (Hefferline, Keenan, & Harford 1959; Hutchinson et al. 1977; Kleinke & Walton 1982; Laurenti-Lions et al. 1985), the most common approaches have been to instruct subjects either to exaggerate or suppress general skeletomotor configurations (Cacioppo et al. 1992b; McCanne & Anderson 1987) or to achieve a particular pose by unobtrusively varying the actions of individual muscles (Larsen, Kasimatis, & Frey 1992; Strack, Martin, & Stepper 1988).

Muscle-by-Muscle Induction. In an illustrative study utilizing the muscle-by-muscle induction variant of this general approach, Levenson, Ekman, and Friesen (1990) instructed participants to contract individual muscles until prototypes of the expressions of happiness, sadness, fear, anger, disgust, or surprise were constructed. The construction of each emotional expression was preceded by the construction of a nonemotional expression. Each expression was held for 10 sec and was subsequently verified (using the FACS) as having been achieved. Averaged data during emotional faces minus that during nonemotional ones revealed that: (a) the anger face was associated with elevated heart rate, skin conductance levels, and palmar skin temperature; (b) the fear and sad faces were associated with elevated heart rate and skin conductance levels; (c) the disgust face was associated with elevated skin conductance levels; and (d) the happy and surprise faces were associated with relatively unchanged levels of heart rate, finger temperature, and skin conductance.

Results obtained using the muscle-by-muscle induction paradigm have occasionally been inconsistent and are often open to alternative explanations (see Boiten 1996; Tourangeau & Ellsworth 1979). Methodological issues that may contribute to inconsistent results and flawed interpretations include (a) improper controls for somatic tension or effort, (b) floor and ceiling effects in emotional responding, and (c) the inherent difficulties associated with specifying and constructing appropriate expressions with naturalistic durations and trajectories while simultaneously controlling for the intensity and the inconspicuousness of the facial configurations. Relevant commentaries and reviews have been provided by Cacioppo et al. (1993a), Cappella (1993), Hager and Ekman (1981), Laird (1984), Levenson (1992), Matsumoto (1987), and Zajonc & McIntosh (1992).

Exaggeration–Suppression. Vaughan and Lanzetta (1981) employed the exaggeration–suppression variant of this paradigm to assess the possible influence of facial expressions on vicarious emotional arousal. Subjects were exposed to a videotaped model displaying pain, ostensibly from receiving electric shocks. One group of subjects was instructed to inhibit any facial expressions when the model was shocked, a second group was instructed to amplify their facial expressions when the model was shocked, and a third (control) group received no instructions about modulating their facial expressions. Results revealed that the "amplify" group exhibited larger skin conductance responses, heart rate increases, and facial EMG activity in response to the model's display of pain than the other two groups, which did not differ from one another.

Wells and Petty (1980) tested the hypothesis that affect-pertinent bodily movements might similarly influence attitudinal responses toward a persuasive appeal. Specifically, head movements (nodding in agreement or wagging in disagreement) were chosen for study because of their strong association with agreeing and disagreeing responses in a wide variety of cultures (Eibl-Eibesfeldt 1972). Participants were led to believe that they were participating in consumer research on the sound quality of stereo headphones when listeners were engaged in movement (e.g., walking, dancing, jogging). One group of participants was asked to move their heads up and down (nod condition), a second was asked to move their heads from side to side (wag condition), and a third (control) group was told nothing about head movements. Amidst listening to a purported campus radio program, participants heard either an editorial in favor of raising tuition or one in favor of reducing tuition. Results revealed that – although participants believed the appropriate level of tuition was higher following the increase-tuition than following the decrease-tuition editorial – those in the nod condition advocated both more tuition than participants in the wag condition following the increase-tuition message as well as relatively less tuition following the decrease-tuition message; in both instances, judgments by those in the control condition fell between these two. Vertical head movements thus led to greater agreement with the message in both cases than did horizontal head movements. A conceptual replication and extension of this work by Cacioppo, Priester, and Berntson (1993b) found similar compatibility effects for arm flexion and extension, a finding reminiscent of a related compatibility effect reported by Hugo Münsterberg over a century ago (cited in Beebe-Center 1932, p. 339).

Although such motor–attitude compatibility effects appear to be reliable, neither the Wells and Petty (1980) nor the Cacioppo et al. (1993b) studies were designed specifically to explicate the mechanism underlying this phenomenon (e.g., peripheral feedback vs. cognitive balance). However, the results of a study (Foerster & Strack 1997) designed explicitly to address a possible mechanism were decidedly in favor of a cognitive explanation. Briefly, overt movements (e.g., head nod and wag) compatible with the incidental encoding of positive and negative adjectives led to better subsequent recognition and also required less processing capacity than did incompatible movements.

Applications

As described throughout this chapter, surface EMG has proven valuable in studying a wide variety of basic psychological and behavioral processes. This technique has also proven useful in a range of more applied contexts. In what follows we list a few general areas to illustrate the breadth of its application.

DETECTION OF DECEPTION

The physiological detection of deception, both in research and forensic settings, routinely involves monitoring autonomic reactions to a series of test questions. Regardless of the test used (control question, concealed knowledge, relevant–irrelevant), the validity of the test depends on the ability of a pattern of physiological responses to index deceit sensitively and specifically (see Chapter 28). Not surprisingly, the possibility that countermeasures might be used to defeat or distort the polygraph exam has raised concerns about its usefulness (Lykken 1998; Reid & Inbau 1977). By pressing their toes hard against the floor or biting their tongues, for example, examinees can generate autonomic responses that foil the polygraph exam (Honts, Hodes, & Raskin 1985). In an attempt to prevent such physical countermeasures from undermining the validity of the exam, Honts, Raskin, and Kircher (1987) recorded surface EMG activity from the examinee's *gastrocnemius* and *temporalis* (i.e., jaw-closing muscle of the temple) during a typical exam. Such measurement enabled the detection of 80% of the research participants who used either tongue biting or toe pressing to defeat the exam, thus auguring the addition of surface EMG to the list of physiological measures used in the routine detection of deception. Surprisingly, over a decade has passed since this seminal publication yet surface EMG measurement (in both research and forensic polygraphy) remains the exception. We believe this is likely because surface EMG is perceived (incorrectly) to be a recondite technique that is applicable only to the use of physical countermeasures and because more recent studies have demonstrated that mental countermeasures are equally effective in defeating either the control question test or the concealed knowledge test (Honts, Raskin, & Kircher 1994; Honts et al. 1996). As such, it finds application as a manipulation check (Honts et al. 1994) but is not used routinely to improve the predictive validity of the lie detection test.

POLYSOMNOGRAPHY

For at least the past 40 years, it has been known that sleep is not a unitary phenomenon but rather a multistage process. In general, the transition from wakefulness to sleep is accompanied by a decrease in alpha activity (8–13 Hz), a general slowing of EEG activity, a prominence of activity in the theta range (3–7 Hz), and the occurrence of vertex sharp waves. During the transition between wakefulness and stage 1, slow horizontal eye movements occur, blink rate declines, and muscle tonus is generally reduced relative to waking levels (Perry & Goldwater 1987). Stage-2 sleep is typically defined by the sporadic presence of two unique EEG waveforms (K-complexes and spindles) and the relative absence of delta activity (0.5–2 Hz). Stages 3 and 4, also known as "slow-wave" sleep, are typically differentiated from stage 2 and from each other by the relative proportion of delta activity. Rapid eye movement (REM) sleep is defined by the occurrence of a relatively low-voltage, mixed-frequency EEG, the absence of K-complexes and spindles, the presence of sporadically occurring eye movements, and markedly decreased tonus in the pericranial musculature (Ancoli-Israel 1997; Pivik 1986).

The facial muscles are somewhat unique with respect to the rest of the musculature because they appear, paradoxically, to show distinctly decreasing tonus as a function of sleep depth (Jacobsen et al. 1964, 1965) and also to be responsive precisely to the processing of both internal (Shimizu & Inoue 1986) and external (Sumitsuji et al. 1980) stimuli. This clear differentiation of tonic levels from phasic activity enabled a team of researchers (Leifting et al. 1994) to use chin EMG alone to differentiate between wakefulness and sleep (using tonic EMG levels) and between quiet (non-REM) and paradoxical (REM) sleep (using phasic EMG parameters) in young infants. In addition, an investigation of the influence of sleep on the muscles of the upper airway (Wheatley et al. 1993) revealed that a decided drop in the tonic level of activity in the *nasalis par alaris* muscle occurred coincident with the onset of stage-2 sleep. Surface EMG has also been used effectively to study (a) leg spasms in nocturnal myoclonus ("restless legs syndrome"), (b) abdominal actions in airway apneas (breathing difficulties due to paradoxical sleep-related epiglottal collapse), and (c) nocturnal bruxism (tooth grinding) (see Hauri & Orr 1982 and Chapter 25 of this volume).

HEADACHE AND STRESS REDUCTION

A popular use of surface EMG is in clinical biofeedback for tension headache and stress reduction. This use stemmed from a clinical report by Budzynski and Stoyva (1969), who used EMG activity from a bilateral forehead site over the frontalis. In a typical clinical regimen, patients hear tones or clicks – whose pitch or rate varies with the envelope of the smoothed, rectified electromyogram – and learn to lower the tone or click rate by relaxing their muscles. Such a procedure was promulgated as a treatment for muscle contraction ("tension") headache, but this procedure was soon extended to general stress management (Stoyva & Budzynski 1974).

The rash of frontalis EMG biofeedback studies published in biofeedback's halcyon days consisted mostly of case reports and uncontrolled clinical trials (for a review see Alexander & Smith 1979), and the claimed incremental efficacy over simple relaxation or meditation techniques remains controversial. The 1980s witnessed a devaluation of muscle tension's role in tension headache (Chun 1985) and an increased emphasis on vascular dysfunction, secondary ischemia, and nocigenic metabolites in the etiology (Pikoff 1984). The past decade, however, has seen a revival in the use of surface EMG in both the diagnosis and treatment of tension headaches. For example, EMG levels in the neck and forehead of children prone to severe headache have been reported to be both higher and more variable than those of matched groups of controls during the performance of cognitive tasks (Pritchard 1995), with similar results reported for adults (Bansevicius & Sjaastad 1996). Studies have also found trapezius or frontalis EMG biofeedback training to be significantly more effective in the treatment of tension headaches than simple progressive relaxation therapy (Arena et al. 1995).

Psychosomatic medicine researchers in the 1940s and 1950s were interested in painful, idiopathic muscular contractions occurring in stress or conflict (see Malmo 1965 for a review), and these examples of symptom specificity have occasionally been treated with EMG biofeedback to relax the muscles. Recent studies suggest that the mean level of surface EMG activity is actually unrelated to the development of pain during stressful conditions (Bansevicius, Westgaard, & Jensen 1997). Electromyographic activity recorded surreptitiously during rest periods, however, is particularly predictive of future muscle pain (Veiersted 1994).

PHYSICAL MEDICINE AND REHABILITATION

The use of EMG biofeedback in physical medicine was pioneered by John Basmajian in the early 1960s, and it soon led to the widespread use of surface EMG to enhance recovery of function in muscles that were rendered nonfunctional by stroke, illness, and accidents (Basmajian & De Luca 1985). In the rehabilitation setting, feedback derived from the surface EMG signal is used either to relax or tense spastic muscles (e.g., chronic unilateral neck spasms, spastic cerebral palsy; see DeBacher 1979) or to activate atrophied or functionally denervated muscles (e.g., hemiplegia from stroke; Basmajian et al. 1975). Following facial anastomosis surgery (graft of a facial nerve branch from the functional side of the lower face to the nonfunctional side, often after a stroke has induced hemiparesis), biofeedback is often used to restore bilateral symmetry to the hemiparetic face.

Electromyographic biofeedback in rehabilitation is now standard procedure. With respect to diagnosis, there are also promising results in the use of the surface EMG signal to classify muscle impairments in persons with lower back pain (Oddsson et al. 1997; Roy et al. 1997). These techniques are based on (i) the phenomenon of the compression of the power spectral density spectrum of the EMG signal toward lower frequencies during sustained contractions and (ii) the fact that this change is associated with the metabolic concomitants of muscle fatigue. Using the different ways in which EMG median frequency parameters change as a function of contraction duration and muscle site, as well as the symmetry of activation during the early part of the contraction, these investigators have shown the surface EMG signal to perform significantly better than conventional clinical parameters at correctly classifying patients with and without lower back pain.

MISCELLANEOUS

Surface EMG is a noninvasive, precise way of measuring muscular contraction in an ongoing fashion in situations where observation is too imprecise, awkward, or costly. In addition to the uses just detailed, surface EMG continues to be used profitably to:

1. quantify muscle tension in ergonomics (see Kumar & Mital 1996 for a review), such as evaluating computer "mouse" use (Harvey & Peper 1997) or evaluating the comfort of automobile headrests (Lamotte et al. 1996);
2. measure precisely the onset, magnitude, and offset of responses in reaction time tasks, including incipient responses that precede the overt response (McGarry & Franks 1997);
3. discern the specific muscles that maintain posture, coordinate gait, and participate in highly skilled acts (Trepman et al. 1994); and
4. enable the continuous discrimination of adequate versus inadequate anesthesia during surgery (see Paloheimo 1990 for a review).

With the decreasing expense of the instrumentation required for sensitive and precise EMG measurement, the availability of guidelines and standards, and the emergence of conceptual frameworks and paradigms to aid in the interpretation of EMG responses, surface EMG promises to find even wider application.

Conclusion

The skeletomotor system has been central to the field of neurophysiology since Francesco Redi's indirect observation in 1666 that living muscles generate electrical current. The centrality of the skeletomotor system within the field of psychology is illustrated by Herbert Spencer's early suggestion that the "Will" (i.e., an idea or image) comprises the waiting musculature:

In a voluntary act of the simplest kind, we can find nothing beyond a mental representation of the act, followed by the performance of it – a rising of that incipient psychical change which constitutes at once the tendency to act and idea of the act, into the complete psychical change which constitutes the performance of the act, in so far as it is mental. (Spencer 1870, p. 497)

Theories proposed in the early part of this century attempted to explain many psychological processes entirely in terms of peripheral skeletomotor actions. This resulted in an exciting and active period for psychophysiology, but the disconfirmation of categorical predictions made by these motor theories was inevitable given the simplicity of the theories and the newness of the technology. Consequently, this premature peak of activity was followed by a downturn in interest in transient or weak skeletomotor actions during the middle of this century. Nonetheless, many interesting results from this early period have been replicated and extended. Coupled with advances in signal acquisition and analysis, these data are increasingly being incorporated into sophisticated theoretical frameworks based on a more complete understanding of the integrated actions of the central and peripheral nervous systems. The major directions we foresee in the coming decade include:

1. further refinement of the spatial and temporal patterning that characterizes specific organismic–environmental transactions;
2. continuing research on incipient actions of the skeletomotor system and their dynamic relation to ongoing psychological processes;
3. a broadening of the reflex probe paradigm to include transcranial magnetic stimulation of the motor cortex (e.g. Meyer et al. 1994);
4. the development of unobtrusive "smart" sensors (Fischer, Kautz, & Kutsch 1996; Picard 1997); and
5. the continued diagnostic and therapeutic use of EMG in psychopathology, rehabilitative medicine, and ergonomics.

We began this chapter with two quotations. The first, from Roger Sperry, stated that to understand the brain we need to understand the body. The second, from Andy Clark, stated that to understand the organism we need to understand the environment. All indications are that psychophysiological investigations using surface EMG will continue to play a significant role in facilitating such an integrated understanding.

NOTES

The chapter represents a major revision and update of a previous chapter by Cacioppo et al. (1990b). Preparation of this chapter was supported in part by a Presidential Faculty Fellowship to L.G.T. The authors extend their gratitude to Dr. Melanie Ihrig for her many discerning comments and suggestions, to Ms. Jill Joseph and Ms. Nadine Connolly for their editorial assistance, and to Ms. Vannapa Pimviriyakul for her assistance in the preparation of the figures.

1. Additional information on electromyography generally can be found in Basmajian and De Luca (1985), Johnson and Pease (1997), Loeb and Gans (1986), or Ludin (1995).
2. Within four decades (through a bequest in his will), Dr. William Croone, one of the original founders of the Royal Society of London, established a lecture series at the Society on the physiology of muscular motion. The Croonian Lecture remains the Royal Society's premier lecture in the biological sciences.
3. Interested readers may wish to consult Fulton (1926), Huxley (1980), Keynes and Aidley (1992), or Needham (1971) for more in-depth coverage of the history of muscle physiology.
4. A detailed description of the central organization and control of the motor system, although important, is beyond the scope of the present chapter. Interested readers may consult Kandel, Schwartz, and Jessell (1991).
5. Although the size principle provides an elegant explanation for many phenomena related to the "voluntary" control of force, there is some evidence that the principle may not hold when multi–degree-of-freedom muscles are involved, a phenomenon referred to as task-dependent muscle partitioning (see Abbs, Gracco, & Blair 1984; Desmedt & Godaux 1981).
6. Placement with respect to the innervation zone of the muscle is, however, an important consideration because both the amplitude and frequency spectrum of the EMG signal vary as a function of this spatial relationship.
7. Further discussion of these two different classes of surface electrodes can be found in Basmajian and De Luca (1985).
8. This is to be expected for the "chin" site because the distance between the electrodes is sufficiently large that recordings over this region should be sensitive but non-selective.
9. One important implication is that a failure to find significant treatment differences in EMG activity could be due to the selection of an inappropriate recording bandpass and not to an actual absence in EMG activity across treatments. Thus, it is often advisable to use a wide bandpass during recording and subsequently apply filters to copies of the stored data.
10. The rms of the EMG signal is calculated by summing the squares of each EMG amplitude within a specified interval of time and then extracting the square root. The rms is superior to mean rectified amplitude as a measure of sinusoidal alternating current, and Basmajian and De Luca (1985) have extended this argument to motor unit action potentials as well. It is of interest to note that the measures of mean amplitude, rms amplitude, and total electrical energy are closely related mathematically, with each emphasizing a different aspect of the amplitude distribution of a waveform. Interested readers may wish to consult Dorfman and Cacioppo (1990).

11. For instance, Cacioppo et al. (1986b) placed a small set of electrodes on the head and neck as well as on the face and body of their participants, who were told that this array of sensors was placed around their brain to help isolate and identify the involuntary neural processes involved in processing pictoral stimuli. To the extent that the electrodes on the body and the nonfunctional electrodes on the neck and head diverted attention from voluntary facial actions (and debriefing suggested they did), this explanation was both accurate factually and successful at minimizing experimental demand.

12. Similar differences between depressed and nondepressed groups had been observed earlier by Whatmore and Ellis (1959) during periods of relaxation.

13. Readers interested in the history of the reflex are encouraged to consult the monographs by Fearing (1930), Liddell (1960), and Swazy (1969).

REFERENCES

Abbs, J. H., Gracco, V. L., & Blair, C. (1984). Functional muscle partitioning during voluntary movement: Facial muscle activity for speech. *Experimental Neurology, 85,* 469–79.

Adrian, E. D., & Bronk, D. W. (1929). The discharge of impulses in motor nerve fibers. Part II. The frequency of discharge in reflex and voluntary contractions. *Journal of Physiology, 67,* 119–51.

Alexander, A. B., & Smith, D. D. (1979). Clinical applications of EMG biofeedback. In R. I. Gatchel & K. P. Price (Eds.), *Clinical Applications of Biofeedback: Appraisal and Status,* pp. 112–33. New York: Pergamon.

Allport, G. W. (1968). The historical background of modern social psychology. In G. Lindzey & E. Aronson (Eds.), *The Handbook of Social Psychology,* 2nd ed. Menlo Park, CA: Addison-Wesley.

Allport, G. W., & Vernon, P. E. (1933). *Studies in Expressive Movement.* New York: Macmillan.

Ancoli-Israel, S. (1997). The polysomnogram. In M. R. Pressman & W. C. Orr (Eds.), *Understanding Sleep: The Evaluation and Treatment of Sleep Disorders,* pp. 177–91. Washington, DC: American Psychological Association.

Andreassi, J. L. (1995). *Psychophysiology: Human Behavior and Response,* 3rd ed. Hillsdale, NJ: Erlbaum.

Anthony, B. I. (1985). In the blink of an eye: Implications of reflex modification for information processing. *Advances in Psychophysiology, 1,* 167–218.

Arena, J. G., Bruno, G. M., Hannah, S. L., Meador, K., et al. (1995). A comparison of frontal electromyographic biofeedback training, trapezius electromyographic biofeedback training, and progressive relaxation therapy in the treatment of tension headache. *Headache, 35,* 411–19.

Baines, A. E. (1918). *Studies in Electro-physiology (Animal and Vegetable).* London: Routledge.

Bakker, F. C., Boschker, M. S. J., & Chung, T. (1996). Changes in muscular activity while imagining weight lifting using stimulus or response propositions. *Journal of Sport and Exercise Psychology, 18,* 313–24.

Bansevicius, D., & Sjaastad, O. (1996). Cervicogenic headache: The influence of mental load on pain level and EMG of the shoulder-neck and facial muscle. *Headache, 36,* 372–8.

Bansevicius, D., Westgaard, R. H., & Jensen, C. (1997). Mental stress of long duration: EMG activity, perceived muscle tension, fatigue, and pain development in pain-free subjects. *Headache, 37,* 499–510.

Bartoshuk, A. (1955). Electromyographic gradients as indicants of motivation. *Canadian Journal of Psychology, 9,* 215–30.

Basmajian, J. V., & De Luca, C. J. (1985). *Muscles Alive: Their Functions Revealed by Electromyography,* 5th ed. Baltimore: Williams & Wilkins.

Basmajian, J. V., Kukulka, C. G., Narayan, M. G., & Takebe, K. (1975). Biofeedback treatment of foot-drop after stroke compared with standard rehabilitation technique: Effects on voluntary control and strength. *Archives of Physical Medicine and Rehabilitation, 56,* 231–6.

Bavelas, J. B., Black, A., Chovil, N., Lemery, C. R., & Mullett, J. (1988). Form and function in motor mimicry: Topographic evidence that the primary function is communicative. *Human Communication Research, 14,* 275–99.

Bavelas, J. B., Black, A., Lemery, C. R., & Mullett, J. (1986). "I show how you feel": Motor mimicry as a communicative act. *Journal of Personality and Social Psychology, 50,* 322–9.

Beebe-Center, J. G. (1932). *The Psychology of Pleasantness and Unpleasantness.* New York: Van Nostrand.

Berkinblit, M. B., Feldman, A. G., & Fukson, O. I. (1986). Adaptability of innate motor patterns and motor control mechanisms. *Behavioral and Brain Sciences, 9,* 585–638.

Bernard, C. (1949). *An Introduction to the Study of Experimental Medicine* (translated by H. C. Greene). New York: Shuman. [Original work published 1865.]

Bickerstaff, E. R. (1980). *Neurological Examination in Clinical Practice,* 4th ed. Oxford, U.K.: Blackwell.

Boiten, F. (1996). Autonomic response patterns during voluntary facial action. *Psychophysiology, 33,* 123–31.

Bond, C. F., & Titus, L. J. (1983). Social facilitation: A meta-analysis of 241 studies. *Psychological Bulletin, 94,* 265–92.

Braathen, E. T., & Sveback, S. (1994). EMG response patterns and motivational styles as predictors of performance and discontinuation in explosive and endurance sports among talented teenage athletes. *Personality and Individual Differences, 17,* 545–56.

Bradley, M., Cuthbert, B. N., & Lang, P. J. (in press). Affect and the startle reflex. In M. E. Dawson, A. Schell, & A. Boehmelt (Eds.), *Startle Modification: Implications for Neuroscience, Cognitive Science, and Clinical Science.* Cambridge University Press.

Bramsley, G. R., Bruun, G. Buchthal, F., Guld, C., & Petersen, H. S. (1967). Reduction of electrical interference in measurements of bioelectrical potentials in a hospital. *Acta Polytechnica Scandanavia Electrical Engineering Series, 15,* 1–37.

Britt, T. W., & Blumenthal, T. D. (1992). The effects of anxiety on motoric expression of the startle response. *Personality and Individual Differences, 13,* 91–7.

Bruintjes, T. D., van Olphen, A. F., Hillen, B., & Weijs, W. A. (1996). Electromyography of the human nasal muscles. *European Archives of Otorhinolaryngology, 253,* 464–9.

Brunia, C. H. M., & Boelhouwer, A. J. W. (1988). Reflexes as tools: A window in the central nervous system. *Advances in Psychophysiology, 3,* 1–67.

Budzynski, T. H., & Stoyva, I. M. (1969). An instrument for producing deep muscle relaxation by means of analog information feedback. *Journal of Applied Behavior Analysis, 2,* 231–7.

Burtt, H. E., & Tuttle, W. W. (1925). The patellar tendon reflex and affective tone. *American Journal of Psychology, 36,* 553–61.

Bush, L. K., Hess, U., & Wolford, G. (1993). Transformations for within-subject designs: A Monte Carlo investigation. *Psychological Bulletin, 101,* 147–58.

Cacioppo, J. T., Berntson, G., & Klein, D. J. (1992a). What is an emotion? The role of somatovisceral afference, with special emphasis on somatovisceral "illusions." *Review of Personality and Social Psychology, 14,* 63–98.

Cacioppo, J. T., Bush, L. K., & Tassinary, L. G. (1992b). Microexpressive facial actions as a function of affective stimuli: Replication and extension. *Personality and Social Psychology Bulletin, 18,* 515–26.

Cacioppo, J. T., Klein, D. J., Berntson, G., & Hatfield, E. (1993a). The psychophysiology of emotion. In M. Lewis & J. M. Haviland (Eds.), *Handbook of Emotions,* pp. 119–42. New York: Guilford.

Cacioppo, J. T., Losch, M. L., Tassinary, L. G., & Petty, R. E. (1986a). Properties of affect and affect-laden information processing as viewed through the facial response system. In R. A. Peterson, W. D. Hoyer, & W. R. Wilson (Eds.), *The Role of Affect in Consumer Behavior: Emerging Theories and Applications,* pp. 87–118. Lexington, MA: Heath.

Cacioppo, J. T., Marshall-Goodell, B. S., & Dorfman, D. D. (1983a). Skeletal muscular patterning: Topographical analysis of the integrated electromyogram. *Psychophysiology, 20,* 269–83.

Cacioppo, J. T., Marshall-Goodell, B. S., & Gormezano, I. (1983b). Social psychophysiology: Bioelectrical measurement, experimental control, and analog-to-digital data acquisition. In J. T. Cacioppo & R. E. Petty (Eds.), *Social Psychophysiology: A Sourcebook,* pp. 666–92. New York: Guilford.

Cacioppo, J. T., Martzke, J. S., Petty, R. E., & Tassinary, L. G. (1988). Specific forms of facial EMG response index emotions during an interview: From Darwin to the continuous flow hypothesis of affect-laden information processing. *Journal of Personality and Social Psychology, 54,* 592–604.

Cacioppo, J. T., & Petty, R. E. (1979a). Attitudes and cognitive response: An electrophysiological approach. *Journal of Personality and Social Psychology, 37,* 2181–99.

Cacioppo, J. T., & Petty, R. E. (1979b). Lip and nonpreferred forearm EMG activity as a function of orienting task. *Biological Psychology, 9,* 103–13.

Cacioppo, J. T., & Petty, R. E. (1981a). Electromyograms as measures of extent and affectivity of information processing. *American Psychologist, 36,* 441–56.

Cacioppo, J. T., & Petty, R. E. (1981b). Electromyographic specificity during covert information processing. *Psychophysiology, 18,* 518–23.

Cacioppo, J. T., & Petty, R. E. (1986). Social processes. In M. G. H. Coles, E. Donchin, & S. Porges (Eds.), *Psychophysiology: Systems, Processes, and Applications,* pp. 646–79. New York: Guilford.

Cacioppo, J. T., Petty, R. E., Losch, M. E., & Kim, H. S. (1986b). Electromyographic activity over facial muscle regions can differentiate the valence and intensity of affective reactions. *Journal of Personality and Social Psychology, 50,* 260–8.

Cacioppo, J. T., Petty, R. E., & Morris, K. (1985). Semantic, evaluative, and self-referent processing: Memory, cognitive effort, and somatovisceral activity. *Psychophysiology, 22,* 371–84.

Cacioppo, J. T., Petty, R. E., & Tassinary, L. G. (1989). Social psychophysiology: A new look. *Advances in Experimental Social Psychology, 22,* 39–91.

Cacioppo, J. T., Priester, J. T., & Berntson, G. (1993b). Rudimentary determinants of attitudes: II. Arm flexion and extension have differential effects on attitudes. *Journal of Personality and Social Psychology, 65,* 5–17.

Cacioppo, J. T., Rourke, P. A., Marshall-Goodell, B. S., Tassinary, L. G., & Baron, R. S. (1990a). Rudimentary physiological effects of mere observation. *Psychophysiology, 27,* 177–86.

Cacioppo, J. T., & Tassinary, L. G. (1989). The concept of attitude: A psychophysiological analysis. In H. L. Wagner & A. S. R. Manstead (Eds.), *Handbook of Psychophysiology: Emotion and Social Behaviour.* Chichester, U.K.: Wiley.

Cacioppo, J. T., & Tassinary, L. G. (1990). Inferring psychological significance from physiological signals. *American Psychologist, 45,* 16–28.

Cacioppo, J. T., Tassinary, L. G., & Fridlund, A. (1990b). The skeletomotor system. In J. T. Cacioppo & L. G. Tassinary (Eds.), *Principles of Psychophysiology,* pp. 325–84. Cambridge University Press.

Cappella, J. N. (1993). The facial feedback hypothesis in human interaction: Review and speculation. *Journal of Language and Social Psychology, 12,* 13–29.

Chapman, A. J. (1974). An electromyographic study of social facilitation: A test of the "mere presence" hypothesis. *British Journal of Psychology, 65,* 123–8.

Chovil, N. (1991). Social determinants of facial displays. *Journal of Nonverbal Behavior, 15,* 141–54.

Chun, W. X. (1985). An approach to the nature of tension headache. *Headache, 25,* 188–9.

Clark, A. (1997). *Being There: Putting Brain, Body, and World Together Again.* Cambridge, MA: MIT Press.

Cohn, J. F., Zlochower, A. J., Lien, J., & Kanade, T. (in press). Automated face analysis by feature point tracking has high concurrent validity with manual FACS coding. *Psychophysiology.*

Coles, M. G. H., Gratton, G., Bashore, T. R., Eriksen, C. W., & Donchin, E. (1985). A psychophysiological investigation of the continuous flow model of human information processing. *Journal of Experimental Psychology: Human Perception and Performance, 11,* 529–53.

Compton, R. W. (1973). Morphological, physiological, and behavioral studies of the facial musculature of the Coati (Nasua). *Brain, Behavior, and Evolution, 7,* 85–126.

Cook, T. D., & Campbell, D. T. (1979). *Quasi-Experimentation: Design and Analysis Issues for Field Settings.* Boston: Houghton-Mifflin.

Cooper, R., Osselton, J. W., & Shaw, J. C. (1980). *EEG Technology,* 3rd ed. London: Butterworth.

Cuthbertson, R. A. (1990). The highly original Dr. Duchenne. In R. A. Cuthbertson (Ed. & Trans.), *The Mechanism of Human Facial Expression,* pp. 225–41. Cambridge University Press.

Daniels, L., & Worthingham, C. (1986). *Muscle Testing: Techniques of Manual Examination,* 5th ed. Philadelphia: Saunders.

Darwin, C. (1873). *The Expression of the Emotions in Man and Animals*. New York: Appleton. [Original work published 1872.]

Davis, J. F. (1952). *Manual of Surface Electromyography*. Montreal: Laboratory for Psychological Studies, Allan Memorial Institute of Psychiatry.

Davis, J. F., & Malmo, R. B. (1951). Electromyographic recording during interview. *American Journal of Psychiatry, 107*, 908–16.

Davis, J. F., Malmo, R. B., & Shagass, C. (1954). Electromyographic reaction to strong auditory stimulation in psychiatric patients. *Canadian Journal of Psychology, 8*, 177–86.

Davis, M. (1989). Neural systems involved in the fear-potentiated startle. *Annals of the New York Academy of Sciences, 563*, 165–83.

Davis, R. C. (1938). The relation of muscle action potentials to difficulty and frustration. *Journal of Experimental Psychology, 23*, 141–58.

Davis, R. C. (1940). *Set and Muscular Tension* (Science Series no. 10). Bloomington: Indiana University Press.

Davis, W. J., Rahman, M. A., Smith, L. J., Burns, A., Senecal, L., McArthur, D., Halpern, J. A., Perlmuter, A., Sickels, W., & Wagner, W. (1995). Properties of human affect induced by static color slides (IAPS): Dimensional, categorical and electromyographic analysis. *Biological Psychology, 41*, 229–53.

DeBacher, G. (1979). Biofeedback in spasticity control. In J. V. Basmajian (Ed.), *Biofeedback Principles and Practice for Clinicians*. Baltimore: Williams & Wilkins.

de Jong, R., Coles, M. G., Logan, G. D., & Gratton, G. (1990). In search of the point of no return: The control of response processes. *Journal of Experimental Psychology: Human Perception and Performance, 16*, 164–82.

De Luca, C. J. (1997). The use of surface electromyography in biomechanics. *Journal of Applied Biomechanics, 13*, 135–63.

De Luca, C. J., & Erim, Z. (1994). Common drive of motor units in regulation of muscle force. *Trends in Neuroscience, 17*, 299–305.

De Luca, C. J., & Knaflitz, M. (1992). *Surface Electromyography: What's New?* Torino, Italy: C.L.U.T. Editrice.

De Luca, C. J., & Merletti, R. (1988). Surface myoelectric signal cross-talk among muscles of the leg. *Electroencephalography and Clinical Neurophysiology, 69*, 568–75.

Desmedt, J. E., & Godaux, E. (1981). Spinal motoneuron recruitment in man: Rank deordering with direction but not with speed of movement. *Science, 214*, 933–6.

Dimberg, U. (1982). Facial reactions to facial expressions. *Psychophysiology, 19*, 643–7.

Dimberg, U. (1990). Gender differences in facial reactions to facial expressions. *Biological Psychology, 30*, 151–9.

Dimberg, U. (1997). Social fear and expressive reactions to social stimuli. *Scandinavian Journal of Psychology, 38*, 171–4.

Disselhorst-Klug, C., Silny, J., & Rau, G. (1997). Improvement of spatial resolution in surface-EMG: A theoretical and experimental comparison of different spatial filters. *IEEE Transactions on Biomedical Engineering, 44*, 567–74.

Dodge, R. B. (1911). A systematic exploration of a normal knee jerk, its technique, the form of muscle contraction, its amplitude, its latent time and its theory. *Zeitschrift für Allgemeine Physiologie, 12*, 1–58.

Dollins, A. B., & McGuigan, F. J. (1989). Frequency analysis of electromyographically measured covert speech behavior. *Pavlovian Journal of Biological Science, 24*, 27–30.

Dorfman, D., & Cacioppo, J. T. (1990). Waveform moment analysis: Topographical analysis of nonrhythmic waveforms. In J. T. Cacioppo and L. G. Tassinary (Eds.), *Principles of Psychophysiology*, pp. 661–707. Cambridge University Press.

Duchenne, G. B. (1990). *The mechanism of human facial expression* (edited and translated by R. A. Cuthbertson). Cambridge University Press. [Original work published 1862.]

Duffy, E. (1962). *Activation and Behavior*. New York: Wiley.

Eason, R. G., & White, C. T. (1961). Muscular tension, effort, and tracking difficulty: Studies of parameters which affect tension levels and performance efficiency. *Perceptual and Motor Skills, 12*, 331–72.

Eccles, J. C., & Sherrington, C. S. (1930). Number and contraction values of individual motor-units examined in some muscles of the limb. *Proceedings of the Royal Society, 106B*, 326–57.

Eibl-Eibesfeldt, I. (1972). Similarities and differences between cultures in expressive movement. In R. A. Hinde (Ed.), *Nonverbal Communication*. Cambridge University Press.

Ekman, P. (1972). Universal and cultural differences in facial expressions of emotion. In J. Cole (Ed.), *Nebraska Symposium on Motivation*, vol. 19, pp. 207–18. Lincoln: University of Nebraska Press.

Ekman, P. (1982). Methods for measuring facial action. In K. R. Scherer & P. Ekman (Eds.), *Handbook of Methods in Nonverbal Behavior Research*, pp. 45–90. Cambridge University Press.

Ekman, P. (1985). *Telling Lies: Clues to Deceit in the Marketplace, Politics, and Marriage*. New York: Norton.

Ekman, P., & Friesen, W. V. (1978). *Facial Action Coding System (FACS): A Technique for the Measurement of Facial Actions*. Palo Alto, CA: Consulting Psychologists Press.

Englis, B. G., Vaughan, K. B., & Lanzetta, J. T. (1982). Conditioning of counter-empathic emotional responses. *Journal of Experimental Social Psychology, 18*, 375–91.

Epstein, L. H. (1990). Perception of activity in the *zygomaticus major* and *corrugator supercilii* muscle regions. *Psychophysiology, 27*, 68–72.

Erim, Z., De Luca, C. J., Mineo, K., & Aoki, T. (1996). Rank-ordered regulation of motor units. *Muscle and Nerve, 19*, 563–73.

Fanardjian, V. V., & Manvelyan, L. R. (1987). Mechanisms regulating the activity of facial nucleus motoneurons – IV. Influences from brainstem structures. *Neuroscience, 20*, 845–53.

Fearing, F. (1930). *Reflex Action: A Study in the History of Physiological Psychology*. Baltimore: Williams & Wilkins.

Feldman, R. S., & Rime, B. (1991). *Fundamentals of Nonverbal Behavior*. Cambridge University Press.

Fischer, H., Kautz, H., & Kutsch, W. (1996). A radiotelemetric 2-channel unit for transmission of muscle potentials during free flight of the desert locust, *Schistocerca Gregaria*. *Journal of Neuroscience Methods, 64*, 39–45.

Foerster, J., & Strack, F. (1997). Motor action in retrieval of valenced information: A motor congruence effect. *Perceptual and Motor Skills, 85*, 1419–27.

Freeman, G. L. (1931). Mental activity and the muscular processes. *Psychological Review, 38*, 428–47.

Freeman, G. L. (1948). *The Energetics of Human Behavior.* Ithaca, NY: Cornell University Press.

Fridlund, A. J. (1991). Sociality of solitary: Potentiation by an implicit audience. *Journal of Personality and Social Psychology, 60,* 229–40.

Fridlund, A. J. (1994). *Human Facial Expression: An Evolutionary View.* San Diego: Academic Press

Fridlund, A. J., & Cacioppo, J. T. (1986). Guidelines for human electromyographic research. *Psychophysiology, 23,* 567–89.

Fridlund, A. J., Fowler, S. C., & Pritchard, D. A. (1980). Striate muscle tensional patterning in frontalis EMG biofeedback. *Psychophysiology, 17,* 47–55.

Fridlund, A. J., Hatfield, M. E., Cottam, G. L., & Fowler, S. C. (1986). Anxiety and striate-muscle activation: Evidence from electromyographic pattern analysis. *Journal of Abnormal Psychology, 95,* 228–36.

Fridlund, A. J., & Izard, C. E. (1983). Electromyographic studies of facial expressions of emotions and patterns of emotions. In J. T. Cacioppo & R. E. Petty (Eds.), *Social Psychophysiology: A Sourcebook,* pp. 243–86. New York: Guilford.

Fridlund, A. J., Schwartz, G. E., & Fowler, S. C. (1984). Pattern recognition of self-reported emotional state from multiple-site facial EMG activity during affective imagery. *Psychophysiology, 21,* 622–37.

Friesen, W. V. (1972). Cultural differences in facial expression in a social situation: An experimental text of the concept of display rules. Doctoral dissertation, University of California, San Francisco.

Fulton, J. F. (1926). *Muscular Contraction and the Reflex Control of Movement.* Baltimore: Williams & Wilkins.

Fulton, J. F., & Wilson, L. G. (1966). *Selected Readings in the History of Physiology,* 2nd ed. Springfield, IL: Thomas.

Gale, A., & Baker, S. (1981). In vivo or in vitro? Some effects of laboratory environments, with particular reference to the psychophysiological experiment. In M. J. Christie & P. G. Mellet (Eds.), *Foundations of Psychosomatics.* Chichester, U.K.: Wiley.

Gallistel, C. R. (1980). *The Organization of Action: The New Synthesis.* Hillsdale, NJ: Erlbaum.

Gans, C., & Gorniak, G. C. (1980). Electromyograms are repeatable: Precautions and limitations. *Science, 210,* 795–7.

Geen, R. G., & Bushman, B. J. (1989). The arousing effects of social presence. In H. Wagner & A. Manstead (Eds.), *Handbook of Social Psychophysiology,* pp. 261–82. Chichester, U.K.: Wiley.

Geen, R. G., & Gange, J. J. (1977). Drive theory of social facilitation: Twelve years of theory and research. *Psychological Bulletin, 84,* 1267–88.

Geen, T. R. (1992). Facial expressions in socially isolated primates: Open and closed programs for expressive behavior. *Journal of Research in Personality, 26,* 273–80.

Germana, J. (1974). Electromyography: Human and general. In R. F. Thompson & M. M. Patterson (Eds.), *Bioelectric Recording Techniques, Part C: Receptor and Effector Processes,* pp. 155–63. New York: Academic Press.

Ghez, C. (1991a). The control of movement. In E. R. Kandel, J. H. Schwartz, & T. M. Jessel (Eds.), *Principles of Neural Science,* 3rd ed., pp. 534–47. New York: Elsevier.

Ghez, C. (1991b). Muscles: Effectors of the motor systems. In E. R. Kandel, J. H. Schwartz, & T. M. Jessel (Eds.), *Principles of Neural Science,* 3rd ed., pp. 548–63. New York: Elsevier.

Gilbert, A. N., Fridlund, A. J., & Sabini, J. (1987). Hedonic and social determinants of facial displays to odors. *Chemical Senses, 12,* 355–63.

Girard, E., Tassinary, L. G., Kappas, A., Gosselin, P., & Bontempo, D. (1997). The covert-to-overt threshold for facial actions: An EMG study. *Psychophysiology, 34,* S38.

Goldstein, J. B. (1972). Electromyography: A measure of skeletal muscle response. In N. S. Greenheld & R. A. Sternbach (Eds.), *Handbook of Psychophysiology,* pp. 329–66. New York: Holt, Rinehart & Winston.

Gousain, A. K., Amarante, M. T. J., Hydem, J. S., & Yousif, N. J. (1996). A dynamic analysis of changes in the nasolabial fold using magnetic resonance imaging: Implications for facial rejuvenation and facial animation surgery. *Plastic and Reconstructive Surgery, 98,* 622–36.

Graham, F. K. (1978). Constraints on measuring heart rate and period sequentially through real and cardiac time. *Psychophysiology, 15,* 492–5.

Graham, J. L. (1980). A new system for measuring nonverbal responses to marketing appeals. *1980 AMA Educator's Conference Proceedings, 46,* 340–3.

Gray, H. (1977). *Anatomy: Descriptive and Surgical,* 15th ed. New York: Bounty Books. [Original work published 1901.]

Graziano, W. G., Smith, S. M., Tassinary, L. G., Sun, C., & Pilkington, C. (1996). Does imitation enhance memory for faces? Four converging studies. *Journal of Personality and Social Psychology, 71,* 874–87.

Green, R. M. (Ed. & Trans.) (1953). *Galvani on Electricity.* Baltimore: Waverly.

Greenwald, M. K., Cook, E. W., & Lang, P. J. (1989). Affective judgment and psychophysiological response: Dimensional covariation in the evaluation of pictorial stimuli. *Journal of Psychophysiology, 3,* 51–64.

Groff, B. D., Baron, R. S., & Moore, D. L. (1983). Distraction, attentional conflict, and drivelike behavior. *Journal of Experimental Social Psychology, 19,* 359–80.

Hager, J. C., & Ekman, P. (1981). Methodological problems in Tourangeau and Ellsworth's study of facial expression and experience of emotion. *Journal of Personality and Social Psychology, 40,* 358–62.

Harvey, R., & Peper, E. (1997). Surface electromyography and mouse use. *Ergonomics, 40,* 781–9.

Hatfield, E., Cacioppo, J. T., & Rapson, R. L. (1993). *Emotional Contagion.* Cambridge University Press.

Hauri, P., & Orr, W. C. (1982). *The Sleep Disorders,* 2nd ed. Kalamazoo, MI: Upjohn.

Hayes, K. J. (1960). Wave analyses of tissue noise and muscle action potential. *Journal of Applied Physiology, 15,* 749–52.

Hazlett, R. L., McLeod, D. R., & Hoehn-Saric, R. (1994). Muscle tension in generalized anxiety disorder: Elevated muscle tonus or agitated movement? *Psychophysiology, 31,* 189–95.

Hefferline, R. F., Keenan, B., & Harford, R. A. (1959). Escape and avoidance conditioning in human subjects without their observation of the response. *Science, 130,* 1338–9.

Henneman, E. (1980). Organization of the motoneuron pool: The size principle. In V. E. Mountcastle (Ed.), *Medical Physiology,* 14th ed., vol. 1, pp. 718–41. St. Louis: Mosby.

Hess, U., Banse, R., & Kappas, A. (1995). The intensity of facial expression is determined by underlying affective state and social situation. *Journal of Personality and Social Psychology, 69*, 280–8.

Hess, U., Kappas, A., McHugo, G. J., & Kleck, R. E. (1989). An analysis of the encoding and decoding of spontaneous and posed smiles: The use of facial electromyography. *Journal of Nonverbal Behavior, 13*, 121–37.

Hess, U., Phillipot, P., & Blairy, S. (in press). Facial mimicry. In P. Phillipot, R. Feldman, & E. Coats (Eds.), *The Social Context of Nonverbal Behavior*. Cambridge University Press.

Hill, A. V. (1959). The heat production of muscle and nerve, 1848–1914. *Annual Review of Physiology, 21*, 1–18.

Himer, W., Schneider, F., Koest, G., & Heimann, H. (1991). Computer-based analysis of facial action: A new approach. *Journal of Psychophysiology, 5*, 189–95.

Honts, C. R., Devitt, M. K., Winbush, M., & Kircher, J. C. (1996). Mental and physical countermeasures reduce the accuracy of the concealed knowledge test. *Psychophysiology, 33*, 84–92.

Honts, C. R., Hodes, R. L., & Raskin, D. C. (1985). Effects of physical countermeasures on the physiological detection of deception. *Journal of Applied Psychology, 79*, 177–87.

Honts, C. R., Raskin, D. C., & Kircher, J. C. (1987). Effects of physical countermeasures and their electromyographic detection during polygraph tests for deception. *Journal of Psychophysiology, 1*, 241–7.

Honts, C. R., Raskin, D. C., & Kircher, J. C. (1994). Mental and physical countermeasures reduce the accuracy of polygraph tests. *Journal of Applied Psychology, 79*, 252–9.

Humphrey, G. (1951). *Thinking*. New York: Wiley.

Hutchinson, R. R., Pierce, G. E., Emley, G. S., Proni, T. J., & Sauer, R. A. (1977). The laboratory measurement of human anger. *Biobehavioral Reviews, 1*, 241–59.

Huxley, A. F. (1980). *Reflections on Muscle*. Liverpool, U.K.: Liverpool University Press.

Isley, C. L., & Basmajian, J. V. (1973). Electromyography of the human cheeks and lips. *Anatomical Record, 176*, 143–8.

Ison, J. R., & Hoffman, H. S. (1983). Reflex modification in the domain of startle: II. The anomalous history of a robust and ubiquitous phenomenon. *Psychological Bulletin, 94*, 3–17.

Izard, C. E. (1971). *The Face of Emotion*. New York: Appleton-Century-Crofts.

Jacobsen, A., Kales, A., Lehmann, D., & Hoedmaker, F. S. (1964). Muscle tonus in human subjects during sleep and dreaming. *Experimental Neurology, 10*, 418–24.

Jacobsen, A., Kales, A., Zweizig, J. R., & Kales, J. (1965). Special EEG and EMG techniques for sleep research. *American Journal of EEG Technology, 18*, 5–10.

Jacobson, E. (1927). Action currents from muscular contractions during conscious processes. *Science, 66*, 403.

Jacobson, E. (1932). Electrophysiology of mental activities. *American Journal of Psychology, 44*, 677–94.

James, W. (1884). What is an emotion? *Mind, 9*, 188–205.

James, W. (1890). *The Principles of Psychology*. New York: Holt.

Jaencke, L. (1996). Facial EMG in an anger-provoking situation: Individual differences in directing anger outwards or inwards. *International Journal of Psychophysiology, 23*, 207–14.

Jenny, A. B., & Saper, C. B. (1987). Organization of the facial nucleus and corticofacial projection in the monkey: A reconsideration of the upper motor neuron facial palsy. *Neurology, 37*, 930–9.

Johnson, E. W., & Pease, W. S. (Eds.) (1997). *Practical Myography*, 3rd ed. Baltimore: Williams & Wilkins.

Johnson, L. C., & Lubin, A. (1972). On planning psychophysiological experiments: Design, measurement, and analysis. In N. S. Greenheld & R. A. Sternbach (Eds.), *Handbook of Psychophysiology*, pp. 125–58. New York: Holt, Rinehart & Winston.

Kandel, E. R., Schwartz, J. H., & Jessell, T. M. (1991). *Principles of Neural Science*, 3rd ed. New York: Elsevier.

Kappas, A., Hess, U., & Kleck, R. E. (1990). The periscope box: A nonobtrusive method of providing an eye-to-eye video perspective. *Behavior Research Methods, Instruments and Computers, 22*, 375–6.

Kelso, J. A. S., Tuller, B., Vatikiotis-Bateson, E., & Fowler, C. A. (1984). Functionally specific articulatory cooperation following jaw perturbations during speech: Evidence for coordinative structures. *Journal of Experimental Psychology: Human Perception and Performance, 10*, 812–32.

Kendall, P. T., & McCreary, E. K. (1980). *Muscles: Testing and Function*, 3rd ed. Baltimore: Williams & Wilkins.

Keynes, R. D., & Aidley, D. J. (1992). *Nerve and Muscle*, 2nd ed. Cambridge University Press.

Khan, S. D., Bloodworth, D. S., & Woods, R. H. (1971). Comparative advantages of bipolar abraded skin surface electrodes over bipolar intramuscular electrodes for single motor unit recording in psychophysiological research. *Psychophysiology, 8*, 635–47.

Kikkawa, D. O., Lemke, B. N., & Dortzbach, R. K. (1996). Relations of the superficial musculoaponeurotic system to the orbit and characterization of the orbitomalar ligament. *Ophthalmic Plastic and Reconstructive Surgery, 12*, 77–88.

Kleinke, C. L., & Walton, J. H. (1982). Influence of reinforced smiling on affective responses in an interview. *Journal of Personality and Social Psychology, 42*, 557–65.

Knowlton, B. J., & Squire, L. R. (1993). The learning of categories: Parallel brain systems for item memory and category knowledge. *Science, 262*, 1747–9.

Komi, P. V., & Buskirk, E. R. (1970). Reproducibility of electromyographic measurements with inserted wire electrodes and surface electrodes. *Electromyography, 10*, 357–67.

Kraut, R. E., & Johnson, R. E. (1979). Social and emotional messages of smiling: An ethological approach. *Journal of Personality and Social Psychology, 37*, 1539–53.

Kumar, S., & Mital, A. (Eds.) (1996). *Electromyography in Ergonomics*. London: Taylor & Francis.

Laird, J. D. (1984). The real role of facial response in the experience of emotion: A reply to Tourangeau and Ellsworth, and others. *Journal of Personality and Social Psychology, 47*, 909–17.

Lamotte, T., Priez, A., Lepoivre, E., Duchene, J., et al. (1996). Surface electromyography as a tool to study head rest comfort in cars. *Ergonomics, 39*, 781–96.

Lang, P. J., Greenwald, M. K., Bradley, M. M., and Hamm, A. O. (1993). Looking at pictures: Affective, facial, visceral, and behavioral reactions. *Psychophysiology, 30*, 261–73.

Lanzetta, J. T., & Englis, B. G. (1989). Expectations of cooperation and competition and their effects on observers' vicarious emotional responses. *Journal of Personality and Social Psychology, 56*, 543–54.

Larsen, R. J., Kasimatis, M., & Frey, K. (1992). Facilitating the furrowed brow: A unobtrusive test of the facial feedback hypothesis applied to unpleasant affect. *Cognition and Emotion, 6*, 321–38.

Latane, B., Williams, K. D., & Harkins, S. G. (1979). Many hands make light the work: The causes and consequences of social loafing. *Journal of Personality and Social Psychology, 37,* 822–32.

Laurenti-Lions, L., et al. (1985). Control of myoelectrical responses through reinforcement. *Journal of the Experimental Analysis of Behavior, 44,* 185–93.

Lawrence, J. H., & De Luca, C. J. (1983). Myoelectrical signal vs. force relationship in different muscles. *Journal of Applied Physiology, 54,* 1653–9.

Leifting, B., Bes, F., Fagioli, I., and Salzarulo, P. (1994). Electromyographic activity and sleep states in infants. *Sleep, 17,* 718–22.

Levenson, R. W. (1992). Autonomic nervous system differences among emotions. *Psychological Science, 3,* 23–7.

Levenson, R. W., Ekman, P., & Friesen, W. (1990). Voluntary facial action generates emotion-specific autonomic nervous system activity. *Psychophysiology, 27,* 363–84.

Levey, A. B. (1980). Measurement units in psychophysiology. In I. Martin & P. H. Venables (Eds.), *Techniques in Psychophysiology.* Chichester, U.K.: Wiley.

Liddell, E. G. T. (1960). *The Discovery of the Reflexes.* Oxford, U.K.: Clarendon.

Liddell, E. G. T., & Sherrington, C. S. (1925). Recruitment and some other features of reflex inhibition. *Proceedings of the Royal Society of London (Biology), 97,* 488–518.

Lindsley, D. B. (1935). Electrical activity of human motor units during voluntary contraction. *American Journal of Physiology, 114,* 90–9.

Lindsley, D. B. (1951). Emotion. In S. S. Stevens (Ed.), *Handbook of Experimental Psychology,* pp. 473–516. New York: Wiley.

Lippold, O. C. J. (1967). Electromyography. In P. H. Venables & I. Martin (Eds.), *Manual of Psychophysiological Methods,* pp. 245–98. New York: Wiley.

Loeb, G. E., & Gans, C. (1986). *Electromyography for Experimentalists.* University of Chicago Press.

Lucas, K. (1909). The "all-or-none" contraction of amphibian skeletal muscle. *Journal of Physiology, 38,* 113–33.

Ludin, H. P. (Ed.) (1995). Electromyography. In *Handbook of Electroencephalography and Clinical Neurophysiology* (Revised Series), vol. 5. Amsterdam: Elsevier.

Lundqvist, L. O., & Dimberg, U. (1995). Facial expressions are contagious. *Journal of Psychophysiology, 9,* 203–11.

Luria, A. R. (1932). *The Nature of Human Conflicts.* New York: Liveright.

Lykken, D. (1998). *A Tremor in the Blood: Uses and Abuses of the Lie Detector,* 2nd ed. New York: Plenum.

Lynn, P. A., Bettles, N. D., Hughes, A. D., & Johnson, S. W. (1978). Influences of electrode geometry on bipolar recordings of the surface electromyogram. *Medical and Biological Engineering and Computing, 16,* 651–60.

Malcolm, R., Von, J. M., & Horney, R. A. (1989). Correlations between facial electromyography and depression. *Psychiatric Forum, 15,* 19–23.

Malmo, R. B. (1965). Physiological gradients and behavior. *Psychological Bulletin, 64,* 225–34.

Malmo, R. B. (1975). *On Emotions, Needs, and Our Archaic Brain.* New York: Holt, Rinehart & Winston.

Manstead, A. S. R. (1991). Expressiveness as an individual difference. In R. S. Feldman & B. Rimé (Eds.), *Fundamentals of Nonverbal Behavior,* pp. 285–328. Cambridge University Press.

Markovsky, B., & Berger, S. M. (1983). Crowd noise and mimicry. *Personality and Social Psychology Bulletin, 9,* 90–6.

Marshall-Goodell, B., Tassinary, L. G., & Cacioppo, J. T. (1990). Principles of bioelectrical measurement. In J. T. Cacioppo & L. G. Tassinary (Eds.), *Principles of Psychophysiology,* pp. 113–48. Cambridge University Press.

Martin, I. (1956). Levels of muscle activity in psychiatric patients. *Acta Psychologica, 12,* 326–41.

Mathews, B. H. C. (1934). A special purpose amplifier. *Journal of Physiology (London), 81,* 28.

Matsumoto, D. (1987). The role of facial response in the experience of emotion: More methodological problems and a meta-analysis. *Journal of Personality and Social Psychology, 52,* 769–74.

Max, L. W. (1932). Myoesthesis and "imageless thought." *Science, 76,* 235–6.

Max, L. W. (1935). An experimental study of the motor theory of consciousness: III. Action-current responses in deaf mutes during sleep, sensory stimulation and dreams. *Journal of Comparative Psychology, 19,* 469–86.

Max, L. W. (1937). An experimental study of the motor theory of consciousness: IV. Action-current responses in the deaf during awakening, kinaesthetic imagery and abstract thinking. *Journal of Comparative Psychology, 24,* 301–44.

McCanne, T. R., & Anderson, J. A. (1987). Emotional responding following experimental manipulation of facial electromyographic activity. *Journal of Personality and Social Psychology, 52,* 759–68.

McClelland, J. L. (1979). On the time relations of mental processes: An examination of systems in cascade. *Psychological Review, 86,* 287–330.

McGarry, T., & Franks, I. (1997). A horse race between independent processes: Evidence for a phantom point of no return in the preparation of a speeded motor response. *Journal of Experimental Psychology: Human Perception and Performance, 23,* 1533–42.

McGuigan, F. J. (1966). *Thinking: Studies of Covert Language Processes.* New York: Appleton-Century-Crofts.

McGuigan, F. J. (1970). Covert oral behavior during the silent performance of language. *Psychological Bulletin, 74,* 309–26.

McGuigan, F. J. (1978). *Cognitive Psychophysiology: Principles of Covert Behavior.* Englewood Cliffs, NJ: Prentice-Hall.

McGuigan, F. J. (1979). *Psychophysiological Measurement of Covert Behavior: A Guide for the Laboratory.* Hillsdale, NJ: Erlbaum.

McGuigan, F. J. (1994). *Biological Psychology: A Cybernetic Science.* Engelwood Cliffs, NJ: Prentice-Hall.

McGuigan, F. J., & Bailey, S. C. (1969). Longitudinal study of covert oral behavior during silent reading. *Perceptual and Motor Skills, 28,* 170.

McGuigan, F. J., Dollins, A., Pierce, W., Lusebrink, V., & Corus, C. (1982). Fourier analysis of covert speech behavior. *Pavlovian Journal of Biological Science, 17,* 49–52.

McHugo, G., & Lanzetta, J. T. (1983). Methodological decisions in social psychophysiology. In J. T. Cacioppo & R. E. Petty (Eds.), *Social Psychophysiology: A Sourcebook,* pp. 630–65. New York: Guilford.

McHugo, G., Lanzetta, J. T., & Bush, L. (1991). The effect of attitudes on emotional reactions to expressive displays of political leaders. *Journal of Nonverbal Behavior, 15,* 19–41.

Merletti, R. (1994). Surface electromyography: Possibilities and limitations. *Journal of Rehabilitative Science, 7,* 24–34.

Merton, P. A. (1987). Reflexes. In R. L. Gregory (Ed.), *The Oxford Companion to the Mind.* New York: Oxford University Press.

Meyer, B. U., Werhahn, K., Rothwell, J. C., Roericht, S., & Fauth, C. (1994). Functional organization of corticonuclear pathways to motoneurons of lower facial muscles in man. *Experimental Brain Research, 101,* 465–72.

Meyer, D. R. (1953). On the interaction of simultaneous responses. *Psychological Bulletin, 20,* 204–20.

Meyer, D. R., Bahrick, H. P., & Fitts, P. M. (1953). Incentive, anxiety, and the human blink rate. *Journal of Experimental Psychology, 45,* 183–287.

Mitz, V. (1976). The superficial musculo-apneurotic system (SMAS) in the parotid and cheek area. *Plastic and Reconstructive Surgery, 58,* 80–8.

Morris, H., & Anson, B. J. (1966). *Human Anatomy: A Complete Systematic Treatise,* 12th ed. New York: McGraw-Hill.

Mulder, T., & Hulstijn, W. (1984). The effect of fatigue and repetition of the task on the surface electromyographic signal. *Psychophysiology, 21,* 528–34.

Needham, D. M. (1971). *Machina Carnis: The Biochemistry of Muscular Contraction in Its Historical Development.* Cambridge University Press.

Netter, F. (1991). *Anatomy, Physiology and Metabolic Disorders. Part 1: Musculoskeletal System* (Ciba Collection), vol. 8, pp. 57–75. West Sussex, U.K.: Wiley.

Nosofsky, R. M., & Zaki, S. R. (1998). Dissociations between categorization and recognition in amnesic and normal individuals: An exemplar-based interpretation. *Psychological Science, 9,* 247–55.

Oddsson, L. I. E., Giphart, J. E., Buijs, R. J. C., Roy, S. H., Taylor, H. P., & De Luca, C. J. (1997). Development of new protocols and analysis procedures for the assessment of LBP by surface EMG techniques. *Journal of Rehabilitation Research and Development, 34,* 415–26.

O'Dwyer, N. J., Quinn, P. T., Guitar, B. E., Andrews, G., & Neilson, P. D. (1981). Procedures for verification of electrode placement in EMG studies of orofacial and mandibular muscles. *Journal of Speech and Hearing Research, 241,* 273–88.

Ongerboer de Visser, B. W. (1983). Anatomical and functional organization of reflexes involving the trigeminal system in man: Jaw reflex, blink reflex, corneal reflex, and exteroceptive suppression. In J. E. Desmedt (Ed.), *Motor Control Mechanisms in Health and Disease,* pp. 727–38. New York: Raven.

Orne, M. T. (1962). On the social psychology of the psychological experiment: With particular reference to demand characteristics and their implications. *American Psychologist, 17,* 776–83.

Orr, S. P., Pitman, R. K., Lasko, N. B., & Herz, L. R. (1993). *Journal of Abnormal Psychology, 102,* 152–9.

Paloheimo, M. (1990). Quantitative surface electromyography (qEMG): Applications in anaesthesiology and critical care (Suppl. 93). *Acta Anaesthesiologica Scandinavica, 34,* 1–83.

Partridge, L. D. (1966). Signal handling characteristics of load-moving muscle in man. *American Journal of Physiology, 210,* 1178–91.

Pernkopf, E. (1980). *Atlas of Topographical and Applied Human Anatomy* (translated by H. Monsen), 2nd ed., vol. 1. Philadelphia: Saunders.

Perry, T. J., & Goldwater, B. C. (1987). A passive behavioral measure of sleep onset in high-alpha and low-alpha subjects. *Psychophysiology, 24,* 657–65.

Picard, R. W. (1997). *Affective Computing.* Cambridge, MA: MIT Press.

Pikoff, H. (1984). Is the muscular model of headache still viable? *Headache, 24,* 186–98.

Pivik, T. (1986). Sleep: Physiology and psychophysiology. In M. Coles, E. Donchin, & S. Porges (Eds.), *Psychophysiology: Systems, Processes, and Applications.* New York: Guilford.

Platt, J. R. (1964). Strong inference. *Science, 146,* 347–53.

Pratt, F. H. (1917). The all-or-none principle in graded response of skeletal muscle. *American Journal of Physiology, 44,* 517–42.

Pratt, F. H., & Eisenberger, J. P. (1919). The quantal phenomena in muscle: Methods with further evidence of the all-or-none principle in graded response for the skeletal fibre. *American Journal of Physiology, 49,* 1–54.

Pritchard, D. (1995). EMG levels in children who suffer from severe headache. *Headache, 35,* 554–6.

Pupilli, G. C. (1953). Introduction. In R. M. Green (Ed. & Trans.), *Galvani on Electricity,* pp. ix–xx. Cambridge, U.K.: Elizabeth Licht.

Rajecki, D. W. (1983). Animal aggression: Implications for human aggression. In R. G. Geen & E. J. Donnerstein (Eds.), *Aggression: Theoretical and Empirical Reviews,* vol. 1, pp. 189–211. New York: Academic Press.

Rankin, R. E., & Campbell, D. (1955). Galvanic skin response to negro and white experimenters. *Journal of Abnormal and Social Psychology, 51,* 30–3.

Reid, J. E., & Inbau, F. E. (1977). *Truth and Deception: The Polygraph ("Lie Detector") Technique.* Baltimore: Williams & Wilkins.

Rimehaug, T., & Sveback, S. (1987). Psychogenic muscle tension: The significance of motivation and negative affect in perceptual-cognitive task performance. *International Journal of Psychophysiology, 5,* 97–106.

Rinn, W. E. (1991). Neuropsychology of facial expression. In R. Feldman & B. Rimé (Eds.), *Fundamentals of Nonverbal Behavior.* Cambridge University Press.

Rosenthal, R. (1966). *Experimenter Effects in Behavior Research.* New York: Appleton-Century-Crofts.

Rosenthal, R., & Rosnow, R. (Eds.) (1969). *Artifact in Behavioral Research.* New York: Academic Press.

Rossi, A. M. (1959). An evaluation of the manifest anxiety scale by the use of electromyography. *Journal of Experimental Psychology, 58,* 64–9.

Roy, S. H., De Luca, C., Emley, M., Oddsson, L. I. E., Buijis, R. J. C., Levins, J., Newcombe, D. S., & Jabre, J. F. (1997). Classification of back muscle impairment based on the surface electromyographic signal. *Journal of Rehabilitation Research and Development, 34,* 405–14.

Russel, J. A., & Fernández-Dols, J. M. (Eds.) (1997). *The psychology of facial expression.* Cambridge University Press.

Schmidt-Nielsen, K. (1997). *Animal Physiology: Adaptation and Environment,* 5th ed. Cambridge University Press.

Schwartz, G. E. (1975). Biofeedback, self-regulation, and the patterning of physiological processes. *American Scientist, 63,* 314–24.

Schwartz, G. E., Fair, P. L., Salt, P., Mandel, M. R., & Klerman, G. L. (1976). Facial muscle patterning to affective imagery in depressed and nondepressed subjects. *Science, 192,* 489–91.

Seiler, R. (1973). On the function of facial muscles in different behavioral situations: A study based on the muscle morphology and electromyography. *American Journal of Physical Anthropology, 38,* 567–72.

Shapiro, D., & Crider, A. (1969). Psychophysiological approaches to social psychology. In G. Lindzey & E. Aronson (Eds.), *The Handbook of Social Psychology,* 2nd ed., vol. 3. Reading, MA: Addison-Wesley.

Shaw, W. A. (1940). The relation of muscular action potentials to imaginal weight lifting. *Archives of Psychology, 247,* 1–50.

Sherrington, C. S. (1923). *The Integrative Actions of the Nervous System.* New Haven, CT: Yale University Press. [Original work published 1906.]

Shimizu, A., & Inoue, T. (1986). Dreamed speech and speech muscle activity. *Psychophysiology, 23,* 210–15.

Sirota, A., & Schwartz, G. (1982). Facial muscle patterning and lateralization during elation and depression imagery. *Journal of Abnormal Psychology, 91,* 25–34.

Skinner, B. F. (1931). The concept of the reflex in the description of behavior. *The Journal of General Psychology: Experimental, Theoretical, Clinical, and Historical Psychology, 5,* 427–57.

Smith, R. R., & Kier, W. M. (1989). Trunks, tongues, and tentacles: Moving with skeletons of muscle. *American Scientist, 77,* 28–35.

Spencer, H. (1870). *Principles of Psychology,* 2nd ed. London: Williams & Norgate.

Sperry, R. (1952). Neurology and the mind–brain problem. *American Scientist, 40,* 291–312.

Sternbach, R. A. (1966). *Principles of Psychophysiology.* New York: Academic Press.

Sternberg, S. (1969). The discovery of processing stages: Extensions of Donder's method. *Acta Psychologica, 30,* 276–315.

Stoyva, J., & Budzynski, T. (1974). Cultivated low arousal: An anti-stress response? In L. V. DiCara (Ed.), *Recent Advances in Limbic and Autonomic Nervous System Research,* pp. 370–94. New York: Plenum.

Strack, F., Martin, L. L., & Stepper, J. (1988). Inhibitory and facilitatory conditions of the human smile: A nonobtrusive test of the facial feedback hypothesis. *Journal of Personality and Social Psychology, 54,* 768–77.

Sumitsuji, N, Nan'no, H., Kuwata, Y., & Ohta, Y. (1980). The effects of the noise due to the jet airplane to the human facial expression (EMG study), EEG changes and their manual responses at the various sleeping stages of the subjects. *Electromyography and Clinical Neurophysiology, 20,* 49–72.

Svebak, S., Dalen, K., & Storfjell, O. (1981). The psychological significance of task-induced tonic changes in somatic and autonomic activity. *Psychophysiology, 18,* 403–9.

Swazy, J. P. (1969). *Reflexes and Motor Integration: Sherrington's Concept of Integrative Action.* Cambridge, MA: Harvard University Press.

Tassinary, L. G. (1985). Odor hedonics: Psychophysical, respiratory and facial measures. Doctoral dissertation, Dartmouth College, Hanover, NH.

Tassinary, L. G., & Cacioppo, J. T. (1992). Unobservable facial actions and emotion. *Psychological Science, 3,* 28–33.

Tassinary, L. G., Cacioppo, J. T., & Geen, T. R. (1989). A psychometric study of surface electrode placements for facial electromyographic recording: I. The brow and cheek muscle regions. *Psychophysiology, 26,* 1–16.

Tassinary, L. G., Cacioppo, J. T., Geen, T. R., & Vanman, E. (1987). Optimizing surface electrode placements for facial EMG recordings: Guidelines for recording from the perioral muscle region. *Psychophysiology, 24,* 615–16.

Tassinary, L. G., Orr, S. P., Wolford, G., Napps, S. E., & Lanzetta, J. T. (1984). The role of awareness in affective information processing: An exploration of the Zajonc hypothesis. *Bulletin of the Psychonomic Society, 22,* 489–92.

Teuber, H. L. (1955). Physiological psychology. *Annual Review of Psychology, 6,* 267–94.

Thorson, A. M. (1925). The relation of tongue movements to internal speech. *Journal of Experimental Psychology, 8,* 1.

Tomovic, R., & Bellman, R. (1970). A systems approach to muscle control. *Mathematical Biosciences, 8,* 265–77.

Tourangeau, R., & Ellsworth, P. C. (1979). The role of facial response in the experience of emotion. *Journal of Personality and Social Psychology, 37,* 1519–31.

Trepman, E., Gellman, R. E., Solomon, R., Murthy, K. R., Micheli, L. J., & De Luca, C. (1994). Electromyographic analysis of standing posture and demi-plié in ballet and modern dancers. *Medicine and Science in Sports and Exercise, 26,* 771–82.

Triplett, N. (1898). The dynamogenic factors in pacemaking and competition. *American Journal of Psychology, 9,* 507–33.

Tuomisto, M. T., Johnston, D. W., & Schmidt, T. F. H. (1996). The ambulatory measurement of posture, thigh acceleration, and muscle tension and their relationship to heart rate. *Psychophysiology, 33,* 409–15.

Turker, K. S., Miles, T. S., & Le, H. T. (1988). The lip-clip: A simple, low-impedance ground electrode for use in human electromyography. *Brain Research Bulletin, 21,* 139–41.

Tyron, W. W. (1991). *Activity Measurement in Psychology and Medicine.* New York: Plenum.

van Boxtel, A., Damen, E. J. P., & Brunia, C. H. M. (1996). Anticipatory EMG responses of the pericranial muscles in relation to heart rate during a warned simple reaction time task. *Psychophysiology, 33,* 576–83.

van Boxtel, A., Goudswaard, P., & Janssen, K. (1983a). Absolute and proportional resting EMG levels in muscle contraction and migraine headache patients. *Headache, 23,* 215–22.

van Boxtel, A., Goudswaard, P., & Janssen, K. (1983b). Changes in EMG power spectra of facial and jaw-elevator muscles during fatigue. *Journal of Applied Physiology, 54,* 51–8.

van Boxtel, A., Goudswaard, P., & Shomaker, L. R. B. (1984). Amplitude and bandwidth of the frontalis surface EMG: Effects of electrode parameters. *Psychophysiology, 21,* 699–707.

van Boxtel, A., & Jessurun, M. (1993). Amplitude and bilateral coherency of facial and jaw-elevator EMG activity as an index of effort during a two-choice serial reaction task. *Psychophysiology, 30,* 589–604.

Vanman, E. J., Boehmelt, A. H., Dawson, M. E., & Schell, A. M. (1996). The varying time course of attentional and affective modulation of the startle eyeblink response. *Psychophysiology, 33,* 691–7.

Vanman, E. J., Paul, B. Y., Ito, T. A., & Miller, N. (1997). The modern face of prejudice and structural features that moderate the effect of cooperation on affect. *Journal of Personality and Social Psychology, 73*, 941–59.

Vaughan, K. B., & Lanzetta, J. T. (1981). The effects of modification of expressive displays on vicarious emotional arousal. *Journal of Experimental Social Psychology, 17*, 16–30.

Vaughan, K. B., & Lanzetta, J. T. (1980). Vicarious instigation and conditioning of facial expressive and autonomic responses to a model's expressive display of pain. *Journal of Personality and Social Psychology, 13*, 909–23.

Veiersted, K. B. (1994). Sustained muscle tension as a risk factor for trapezius myalgia. *International Journal of Industrial Ergonomics, 14*, 333–9.

Vitti, M., Basmajian, J. V., Ouelette, P. L., Mitchell, D. L., Eastman, W. P., & Seaborn, R. D. (1975). Electromyographic investigations of the tongue and circumoral muscular sling with fine-wire electrodes. *Journal of Dental Research, 54*, 844–9.

Vrana, S. R., & Rollock, D. (1998). Physiological response to a minimal social encounter: Effects of gender, ethnicity, and social context. *Psychophysiology, 35*, 462–9.

Waersted, M., & Westgaard, R. H. (1996). Attention-related muscle activity in different body regions during VDU work with minimal physical activity. *Ergonomics, 39*, 661–76.

Wallerstein, H. (1954). An electromyographic study of attentive listening. *Canadian Journal of Psychology, 8*, 228–38.

Wartenberg, R. (1946). *The Examination of Reflexes: A Simplification.* Chicago: Year Book Publishers.

Washburn, M. F. (1916). *Movement and Imagery: Outlines of a Motor Theory of the Complexer Mental Processes.* Boston: Houghton-Mifflin.

Waters, K. (1992). A physical model of facial tissue and muscle articulation derived from computer tomography data. *Visualization in Biomedical Computing, 1808*, 574–83.

Weaver, C. V. (1977). Descriptive anatomical and quantitative variation in human facial musculature and the analysis of bilateral asymmetry. *Dissertation Abstracts International* (University Microfilms, no. 77-24, 305).

Wells, G. L., & Petty, R. E. (1980). The effects of overt head-movements on persuasion: Compatibility and incompatibility of responses. *Basic and Applied Social Psychology, 1*, 219–30.

Wexler, B. E., Warrenburg, S., Schwartz, G. E., & Jamner, L. D. (1992). EEG and EMG responses to emotion-evoking stimuli processed without conscious awareness. *Neuropsychologia, 30*, 1065–79.

Whatmore, G., & Ellis, R. M. (1959). Some neurophysiological aspects of depressed states: An electromyographic study. *Archives of General Psychiatry, 1*, 70–80.

Wheatley, J. R., Tangel, D. J., Mezzanotte, W. S., and White, D. P. (1993). Influence of sleep on the alae nasi EMG and nasal resistance in normal man. *Journal of Applied Physiology, 75*, 626–32.

Woodworth, R. S., & Schlosberg, H. (1954). *Experimental Psychology,* rev. ed. New York: Holt.

Wu, C. H. (1984). Electric fish and the discovery of animal electricity. *American Scientist, 72*, 598–607.

Zajonc, R. B. (1965). Social facilitation. *Science, 149*, 269–74.

Zajonc, R. B., & McIntosh, D. N. (1992). Emotions research: Some promising questions and some questionable promises. *Psychological Science, 3*, 70–4.

Zipp, P. (1982). Recommendations for the standardization of lead positions in surface electromyography. *European Journal of Applied Physiology, 50*, 41–54.

CHAPTER EIGHT

THE ELECTRODERMAL SYSTEM

MICHAEL E. DAWSON, ANNE M. SCHELL, & DIANE L. FILION

Prologue

OVERVIEW

Electrodermal activity (EDA) has been one of the most widely used – some might add "abused" – response systems in the history of psychophysiology. A search of the PsychLit computerized database reveals that the use of electrodermal activity in research has remained high and stable over the past several decades. During this time, research involving EDA has been reported in mainstream psychology, psychiatry, and psychophysiology research journals such as the *Archives of General Psychiatry, Biological Psychiatry, Biological Psychology, International Journal of Psychophysiology, Journal of Abnormal Psychology, Journal of Experimental Psychology, Journal of Personality and Social Psychology*, and *Psychophysiology*, but it has also appeared in more surprising venues such as the *International Journal of Eating Disorders, Behavior Therapy, Crisis*, and the *European Journal of Parapsychology*. The wide range of journals in which EDA research is published is reflective of the fact that EDA measures have been applied to a wide variety of questions – ranging from basic research examining attention, information processing, and emotion to more applied clinical research examining predictors and/or correlates of normal and abnormal behavior. The application of EDA measures to a wide variety of issues is due in large part to its relative ease of measurement and quantification combined with its sensitivity to psychological states and processes.

The purpose of this chapter is to provide a tutorial overview of EDA for the interested student, researcher, or practitioner who is not a specialist in this particular system. We begin with a historical orientation and then discuss the physical, inferential, and psychosocial aspects of EDA.

HISTORICAL BACKGROUND

The Discovery of Electrodermal Activity

The empirical study of the electrical changes in human skin began over 100 years ago in the laboratory of Jean Charcot, the French neurologist famous for his work on hysteria and hypnosis. Vigouroux (1879, 1888), a collaborator of Charcot, measured tonic skin resistance levels from various patient groups as a clinical diagnostic sign. In the same laboratory, Féré (1888) found that, by passing a small electrical current across two electrodes placed on the surface of the skin, one could measure momentary decreases in skin resistance in response to a variety of stimuli (visual, auditory, gustatory, olfactory, etc.). The basic phenomenon discovered by Féré is that the skin momentarily becomes a better conductor of electricity when external stimuli are presented. Shortly thereafter, a Russian physiologist named Tarchanoff (1890) reported that one could measure changes in electrical potential between two electrodes placed on the skin without applying an external current (see Bloch 1993 for interesting details regarding these initial discoveries). Hence, Féré and Tarchanoff are said to have discovered the two basic methods of recording electrodermal activity in use today. Recording the skin resistance (or its reciprocal, skin conductance) response relies on the passage of an external current across the skin and hence is referred to as the *exosomatic* method, whereas recording the skin potential response does not involve an external current and hence is referred to as the *endosomatic* method. The present chapter will focus on the exosomatic method of recording skin resistance and conductance because this clearly is the method of choice among contemporary researchers (Fowles et al. 1981).

It is interesting and somewhat humbling to find that the very early investigators identified many of the important aspects of EDA that remain of interest today. For

John T. Cacioppo, Louis G. Tassinary, and Gary G. Berntson (Eds.), *Handbook of Psychophysiology*, 2nd ed. © Cambridge University Press 2000. Printed in the United States of America. ISBN 62634X. All rights reserved.

example, the tonic–phasic distinction was implied in the earliest of these publications. The tonic level of skin resistance or conductance is the absolute level of resistance or conductance at a given moment in the absence of a measurable phasic response, and it is referred to as SRL (skin resistance level) or SCL (skin conductance level). Superimposed on the tonic level are phasic decreases in resistance (increases in conductance), referred to as SRRs (skin resistance responses) or SCRs (skin conductance responses). Similar distinctions are made with skin potential and are referred to as SPL and SPRs. (It should be noted that other terms have been used to refer to EDA phenomena in the history of this response system, particularly psychogalvanic reflex, PGR, and galvanic skin response, GSR.)

Even more humbling is that many of the variables and phenomena intensively studied today were already being investigated in this early research. For example, the ability of various types of sensory stimuli to elicit phasic EDA changes was clearly in evidence. The fact that stronger stimulation would elicit larger responses, as well as the fact that repetitions of the same stimulus would lead to habituation, were noted. Moreover, the effectiveness of mental images, mental effort (e.g., solving arithmetic problems), emotions, and surprise in eliciting EDA also was demonstrated. Individual differences in EDA were observed, and questions regarding the utility of this new measure in distinguishing normal from pathological groups were being raised. Clearly, these early investigators recognized the psychophysiological significance of this newly discovered phenomenon and laid the foundation for more than a century of subsequent research. A detailed historical review of these early articles is provided by Neumann and Blanton (1970); English translations of some of the classic early reports on electrodermal phenomena can be found in Porges and Coles (1976).

Issues in the History of EDA Research

Several issues identified in this early research have continued to be sources of considerable speculation and investigation throughout the history of this response system. One set of such issues concerns the mechanisms and functions of EDA. In terms of peripheral mechanisms, Vigouroux proposed what became known as the "vascular theory" of EDA (Neumann & Blanton 1970). The vascular theory associated changes in skin resistance with changes in blood flow. Tarchanoff favored a "secretory theory" that related EDA to sweat gland activity. This theory was supported later by Darrow (1927), who measured EDA and sweat secretion simultaneously and found the two measures to be closely related. However, the phasic EDR would begin about 1 sec before moisture would appear on the surface of the skin, so it was concluded that activity of the sweat glands, not sweat on the skin per se, was critical for EDA. (Other lines of evidence indicating that sweat glands are the major contributors to EDA have been reviewed by

Fowles 1986, pp. 74–5.) It was generally known at the time that palmar sweat glands are innervated by the sympathetic chain of the autonomic nervous system, so EDA was said to reflect sympathetic activation. In terms of more central physiological mechanisms, work by early investigators such as Wang and Richter indicated that EDA was complexly determined by both subcortical and cortical areas (for a review of this early research, see Darrow 1937). Darrow proposed that "the function of the secretory activity of the palms is primarily to provide a pliable adhesive surface facilitating tactual acuity and grip on objects" (1937, p. 641).

Issues surrounding the proper methods of recording and quantifying EDA also have been important in the history of this response system. Lykken and Venables noted that EDA provides useful data "in spite of being frequently abused by measurement techniques which range from the arbitrary to the positively weird" (1971, p. 656). In fact, we would date the beginning of the modern era of EDA research to the early 1970s, when Lykken and Venables (1971) proposed standardized techniques of recording skin conductance and standardized units of measurement. This was followed shortly by an edited book (Prokasy & Raskin 1973) that was devoted entirely to EDA and contained several useful review chapters, including a particularly outstanding chapter by Venables and Christie (1973). Published around the same time were several other excellent reviews (Edelberg 1972a; Fowles 1974; Grings 1974). More recently, book-length reviews of EDA have been provided by Boucsein (1992) and by Roy and colleagues (1993a); see also Fowles (1986) and Hugdahl (1995).

Another issue of central importance concerns the psychological significance of EDA. From the beginning, this response system has been closely linked with the psychological concepts of emotion, arousal, and attention. Early in this century, Carl Jung added EDA measurements to his word association experiments in order to objectively measure the emotional aspects of "hidden complexes." An American friend joined Jung in these experiments and in 1907 enthusiastically reported: "Every stimulus accompanied by an emotion produced a deviation of the galvanometer to a degree in direct proportion to the liveliness and actuality of the emotion aroused" (Peterson, cited by Neumann & Blanton 1970, p. 470). About half a century later, when the concept of emotion was less in favor, Woodworth and Schlosberg devoted most of one entire chapter of their classic textbook in experimental psychology to EDA, which they described as "perhaps the most widely used index of activation" (1954, p. 137). They supported this indexing relationship by noting that tonic SCL is generally low during sleep and high in activated states such as rage or mental work. The authors also related phasic SCRs to attention, noting that such responses are sensitive to stimulus novelty, intensity, and significance.

Many of these issues have remained important for contemporary psychophysiologists and are discussed in the remainder of this chapter. In the next section we present a summary of the contemporary perspectives regarding the basic physiological mechanisms and proper recording techniques of EDA.

Physical Context

ANATOMICAL AND PHYSIOLOGICAL BASIS

The skin is a selective barrier that serves the functions of preventing entry of foreign matter into the body and selectively facilitating passage of materials from the bloodstream to the exterior of the body. It aids in the maintenance of water balance and of constant core body temperature, functions accomplished primarily through vasoconstriction/dilation and through variation in the production of sweat. As pointed out by Edelberg (1972a), it is not surprising that an organ with such vital and dynamic functions constantly receives signals from control centers in the brain. Edelberg suggested that we "can listen in on such signals by taking advantage of the fact that their arrival at the skin is heralded by measurable electrical changes that we call electrodermal activity" (1972a, p. 368).

There are two forms of sweat glands in the human body: the eccrine, which have been of primary interest to psychophysiologists, and the apocrine, which have been relatively unstudied. The distinction between these two is usually made on the basis of location and function (Robertshaw 1983). Whereas apocrine sweat glands typically open into hair follicles and are found primarily in the armpits and the genital areas, eccrine glands cover most of the body and are most dense on the palms and soles of the feet. The function of the apocrine glands is not yet well understood, and this may account for the subordinate status they currently hold within the field of psychophysiology. However, there have been some recent suggestions in the literature that apocrine glands may be more interesting than was once believed. For example, in mammals such as dogs and monkeys, apocrine glands are believed to produce a secretion that serves – when modified by bacteria on the surface of the skin – as an identifying or sexual scent hormone (pheromone). Some authors (e.g. Jakubovic & Ackerman 1985) have suggested that apocrine glands in humans may serve a similar function. It has also been noted that there is some evidence suggesting that apocrine gland secretion is induced by any emotional stress that causes sympathetic nervous system discharge (Jakubovic & Ackerman 1985). To date, the evidence still appears to be inconclusive, and the responsivity of the apocrine glands to emotional, stressful, or sexually arousing stimuli is still under debate (Shields et al. 1987).

In contrast to the apocrine gland, a great deal is known about the function of the eccrine sweat gland. For example, it is known that the primary function of most eccrine

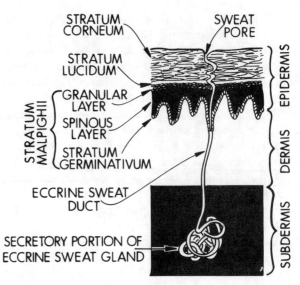

Figure 1. Anatomy of the eccrine sweat gland in various layers of skin. Adapted with permission from Hassett, *A Primer of Psychophysiology.* Copyright 1978 W. H. Freeman and Company.

sweat glands is thermoregulation. However, those located on the palmar and plantar surfaces have been thought of as being more concerned with grasping behavior than with evaporative cooling (Edelberg 1972a), and it has been suggested that they are more responsive to significant or emotional stimuli than to thermal stimuli. Although all eccrine glands are believed to be involved in emotion-evoked sweating, such sweating is usually most evident in these areas primarily because of the high gland density (Shields et al. 1987). The measurement of EDA by psychophysiologists is primarily concerned with this psychologically induced sweating.

Figure 1 shows the basic peripheral mechanisms involved in the production of EDA. The extreme outer layer of the skin, the stratum corneum or horny layer, consists of a dead layer of cells that serves to protect the internal organs. Below the stratum corneum lies the stratum lucidum, and just below that is the stratum Malpighii. The stratum Malpighii actually consists of three cell layers: the granular layer; the spinous layer; and the deepest layer – the *stratum germinativum* – which consists of cells that are continually reproducing and replacing the dead cells on the skin's surface. The eccrine sweat gland itself consists of a coiled compact body that is the secretory portion of the gland and the sweat duct, the long tube that is the excretory portion of the gland. The sweat duct remains relatively straight in its path through the stratum Malpighii and stratum lucidum; it then spirals through the stratum corneum and opens to the surface of the skin as a small pore (Edelberg 1972a).

Many models have been suggested to explain how these peripheral mechanisms relate to the electrical activity of the skin and to the transient increases in skin conductance elicited by stimuli. The dominant view has been a two-effector model summarized by Edelberg (1972a). According to this model, there are two peripheral mechanisms that contribute to EDA: (i) secretion of sweat from the sweat gland and the attendant filling of the sweat duct; and (ii) the activity of a selective membrane that lies somewhere in the epidermis. However, there have been lingering questions about the selective membrane, leading to the proposal of alternative models (Fowles 1986). More recently, Edelberg (1993) concluded that it is not necessary to hypothesize participation of an active membrane in EDA. Instead, one can account for the variety of electrodermal phenomena – including changes in tonic SCL and phasic SCR amplitude and recovery – with a model based on the single effector of the sweat glands (see Edelberg 1993 for details regarding the origins of the original two-effector model and the proposed single-effector model).

To understand how electrodermal activity is related to the sweat glands, it is useful to think of the sweat ducts (the long tubular portion of the gland that opens onto the skin surface) as a set of variable resistors wired in parallel. Columns of sweat will rise in the ducts in varying amounts and in varying numbers of sweat glands, depending on the degree of sympathetic activation. As sweat fills the ducts, there is a more conductive path through the relatively resistant corneum. The higher the sweat rises, the lower the resistance in that variable resistor. Any change in the level of sweat in the ducts changes the values of the variable resistors and yields observable changes in EDA.

Historically, both the sympathetic and parasympathetic divisions of the autonomic nervous system (ANS) were considered as possible mediators of EDA. This is partially due to the fact that the neurotransmitter involved in the mediation of eccrine sweat gland activity is acetylcholine, which is generally a parasympathetic neurotransmitter, rather than noradrenaline, the neurotransmitter typically associated with peripheral sympathetic activation (Venables & Christie 1980). Now, however, it is generally agreed that (i) human sweat glands have predominately sympathetic cholinergic innervation from sudomotor fibers originating in the sympathetic chain but that (ii) some adrenergic fibers also exist in close proximity (Shields et al. 1987). Convincing evidence for the sympathetic control of EDA has been provided by studies measuring sympathetic action potentials in peripheral nerves while simultaneously recording EDA. The results have shown that, within normal ranges of ambient room temperature and subject thermoregula-

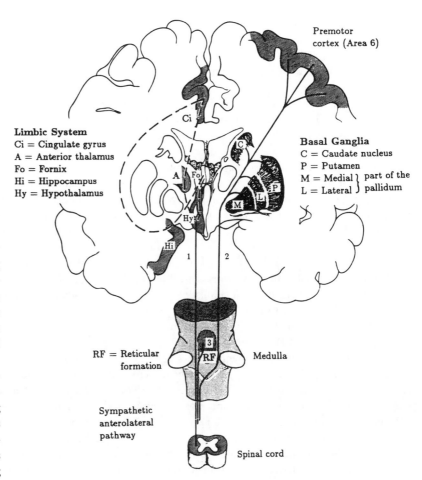

Figure 2. Central nervous system determiners of EDA in humans. See text for discussion of the three pathways shown. Reprinted with permission from Boucsein, *Electrodermal Activity.* Copyright 1992 Plenum Press.

tory states, there is a high correlation between bursts of sympathetic nerve activity and SCRs (Wallin 1981).

Excitatory and inhibitory influences on the sympathetic nervous system are distributed in various parts of the brain, so the neural mechanisms and pathways involved in the central control of EDA are numerous and complex. These mechanisms have been reviewed by Edelberg (1972a) and Venables and Christie (1973) and, more recently, by Boucsein (1992), Hugdahl (1995), Raine and Lencz (1993), Roy, Sequeira, and Delerm (1993b), and Sequeira and Roy (1993).

Boucsein (1992, pp. 30–6) followed the suggestions of Edelberg (1972a) in describing at least two and possibly three relatively independent pathways that lead to the production of SCRs (see Figure 2). The *first* level of EDA control involves ipsilateral influences from the hypothalamus and limbic system (Sequeira & Roy 1993). There is considerable evidence of an excitatory hypothalamic descending control of EDA. Limbic influences are complicated, but there is evidence of excitatory influences from the amygdala and inhibitory effects originating from the hippocampus.

The *second* and highest level of central EDA control involves contralateral cortical and basal ganglion influences (Sequeira & Roy 1993). One cortical pathway involves excitatory control by the premotor cortex (Brodmann area 6) descending through the pyramidal tract, and another involves both excitatory and inhibitory influences originating in the frontal cortex. The *third* and lowest-level mechanism is in the reticular formation in the brainstem (Roy et al. 1993b). Activation of the reticular formation by direct electrical stimulation or sensory stimulation evokes skin potential responses in cats and (presumably) skin conductance responses in humans. An inhibitory EDA system has also been located in the bulbar level of the reticular formation.

Given the roles of the various brain centers just identified, different functional roles of EDA have been hypothesized to be associated with the various central mechanisms (Boucsein 1992; Edelberg 1973; Hugdahl 1995). Electrodermal activity elicited by activation of the reticular formation is likely to be associated with gross movements and increased muscle tone; EDA associated with hypothalamic activity is likely due to thermoregulatory sweating; EDA associated with amygdala activation is likely reflecting affective processes; EDA mediated by the premotor cortex may occur in situations requiring fine motor control; and EDA elicited by prefrontal cortical activity is likely associated with orienting and attention.

Most of the evidence regarding the central pathways that control EDA is derived from animal studies, usually cats (see e.g. Roy et al. 1993b; Wang 1964). More recently, neural mechanisms of human EDA have been studied with neuroimaging techniques (Raine & Lencz 1993), in patients with focal cerebral lesions (Tranel & Damasio 1994), and in patients with direct electrical stimulation of brain structures (Mangina & Beuzeron-Mangina 1996). These lines of research are just beginning and much remains to be done. However, the results are likely to be complex given the multiple central determiners of EDA. As useful as EDA is for indexing psychological processes, it may be more difficult to identify specific brain centers and pathways given its diffuse levels of control.

PHYSICAL RECORDING BASIS

As briefly described earlier, EDA is measured by passing a small current through a pair of electrodes placed on the surface of the skin. The principle invoked in the measurement of skin resistance or conductance is that of Ohm's law, which states that skin resistance (R) is equal to the voltage (V) applied between two electrodes placed on the skin surface divided by the current (I) being passed through the skin; that is, $R = V/I$. If the current is held constant then one can measure the voltage between the electrodes, which will vary directly with skin *resistance*. Alternatively, if the voltage is held constant then one can measure the current flow, which will vary directly with the reciprocal of skin resistance, skin *conductance*.

Lykken and Venables (1971) argued strongly for the direct measurement of skin conductance with a constant-voltage system rather than measuring skin resistance with a constant-current system. This argument was based in part on the fact that skin conductance had been shown to be more linearly related to the number of active sweat glands and their rate of secretion. This is so because the individual sweat glands function as resistors in parallel, and the conductance of a parallel circuit is simply the sum of all of the conductances in parallel. On the other hand, the overall resistance of a parallel circuit is a complex function of each of the individual resistances. Thus, unlike the relationship of SRR and SRL, the SCR is potentially independent of SCL, since a given increment in the number of active sweat glands will produce the same increment in the total conductance of the pathway regardless of the level of basal activity. Boucsein (1992, pp. 208–16) stated that the discussion of this issue often confounds the choice of method of measurement (constant voltage versus constant current) with the choice of units of measurement (conductance versus resistance). He raised thoughtful questions about the bioelectrical assumptions underlying the parallel conduction model. Nevertheless, Boucsein agreed on pragmatic grounds with the recommendation to use constant-voltage methods and skin conductance units (for the sake of standardization in the field).

A description of constant-voltage circuits that allow the direct measurement of skin conductance can be found in Lykken and Venables (1971) as well as in Fowles et al. (1981), and most of the physiological recording systems currently on the market include constant-voltage couplers for the direct recording of skin conductance.

EDA Recording Systems

The decision of whether to record skin conductance or skin resistance and the availability of a constant-voltage coupler for direct recording of skin conductance are important factors that should be considered when choosing an EDA recording system. In addition, serious consideration should be given to the issue of paper-based versus paperless systems.

Paper-based systems provide a continuous on-line hardcopy record of the EDA recording over the experimental session. The advantages of paper-based systems are: (1) they can provide a continuous record of an entire experimental session; (2) they provide an easy means for the experimenter to "flag" important events such as participant movement that may produce artifact in the recording (the experimenter simply writes on the polygraph chart "participant moved here"); and (3) they are not dependent on expensive computer interfaces or complex software, since the EDA can be quantified by "hand scoring" directly from the paper record. However, there are three disadvantages of paper-based systems that have led to the search for alternatives: (1) the cost of polygraph paper, ink, and pens; (2) the potential for malfunction and mess that is invariably associated with a mechanical ink-on-paper system; and, most importantly, (3) the time required for (and potential unreliability of) quantification from the paper record. To deal with the latter issue, most researchers using paper-based systems also collect EDA on a computer using an analog-to-digital converter and specialized computer programs for quantification (see the quantification section later in this chapter). However, this computer sampling is generally carried out on an event-by-event basis rather than as a continuous recording.

In contrast to a paper-based system, a paperless system involves the digitization and storage of EDA by a computer with no on-line hard-copy record. In most paperless systems, a researcher must select the time points at which the computer will sample the EDA. This sampling window has traditionally been event-related, such as following each presentation of an experimental stimulus. In these cases, EDA at all other time points is lost. Fortunately, with expanding computing capability, it is now possible for a paperless system to sample EDA continuously, to allow an experimenter to flag critical events with a keypress, and to provide a continuous printout of an experimental session. Therefore, in choosing an EDA recording system, one must consider its output capabilities (paper only, computer only, or paper and computer) and also its computing capabilities and software issues as well. For example, some manufacturers offer software packages for the acquisition of EDA, some offer software for the quantification of EDA, and some offer both.

In addition to selecting an EDA recording system, special consideration must be given to the choice of recording electrodes, electrode paste, and electrode placement. Silver–silver chloride cup electrodes are the type most typically used in skin conductance recording because they minimize the development of bias potentials and polarization. These electrodes can be easily attached to the recording site through the use of double-sided adhesive collars, which also serve the purpose of helping to control the size of the skin area that comes in contact with the electrode paste. This is an important parameter because it is the contact area, not the size of the electrode, that affects the conductance values.

The electrode paste is the conductive medium between electrode and skin. Probably the most important concern in choosing an electrode paste is that it preserve the electrical properties of the bioelectrical signals of the response system of interest. Since the measurement of EDA involves a small current passed through the skin, the electrode paste interacts with the tissue over which it is placed. For this reason, the use of a paste that closely resembles sweat in its salinity is recommended (Venables & Christie 1980). Instructions for making such paste are given in Fowles et al.

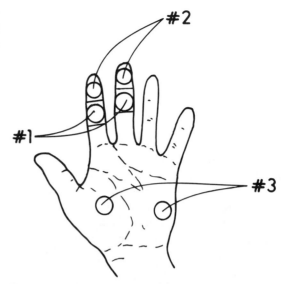

Figure 3. Three electrode placements for recording electrodermal activity. Placement #1 involves volar surfaces on medial phalanges, placement #2 involves volar surfaces of distal phalanges, and placement #3 involves thenar and hypothenar eminences of palms.

(1981, p. 235) and Grey and Smith (1984, p. 553). Commercial ECG or EEG gels should not be used because they usually contain near-saturation levels of sodium chloride and have been shown to significantly inflate measures of skin conductance level (Grey & Smith 1984).

Skin conductance is recorded with both electrodes on active sites (bipolar recording); hence it does not matter in which direction the current flows between the two electrodes. Skin conductance recordings are typically taken from locations on the palms of the hands, with several acceptable placements. The most common electrode placements are the thenar eminences of the palms and the volar surface of the medial or distal phalanges of the fingers (see Figure 3). It should be noted that, although electrodermal activity can be measured from any of these sites, the values obtained are not necessarily comparable. Scerbo and colleagues (1992) made a direct comparison of EDA recorded from the distal and medial phalange sites simultaneously and found that both the elicited SCR amplitude and SCL were significantly higher from the distal recording site. Moreover, the greater level of reactivity at the distal site was found to be directly related to a larger number of active sweat glands at that location (Freedman et al. 1994). Therefore, the distal phalange site is recommended unless there are specific reasons for not using the distal site (e.g., recording from children whose fingertips may be too small for stable electrode attachment, presence of cuts or heavy calluses on the fingertips, etc.).

Another recording issue concerns the hand from which to record. Many laboratories use the nondominant hand for EDA measurements because it is less likely to have cuts or calluses and because it leaves the dominant hand free to perform a manual task. However, this begs the question of whether there are significant laterality differences in EDA. Although differences between left- and right-hand EDA recordings have been reported, the differences reported by different studies are often in opposite directions and the interpretations have been ambiguous (see a review of early literature by Hugdahl 1984). It is tempting to speculate that the prior conflicting findings may be due to the lack of clear distinctions between emotional and nonemotional tasks (Hugdahl 1995). Electrodermal activity in emotional tasks is presumably controlled primarily by the ipsilateral limbic system, whereas EDA in nonemotional tasks may be controlled by the contralateral system (see Figure 2). However, there is not yet any definitive evidence that EDA recorded from one hand gives consistently different results with respect to the effects of experimental variables than that recorded from the other hand.

Because it is critical in EDA recording that the electrical properties of the response system be preserved, the electrode sites for bipolar recording should not receive any special preparation such as cleaning with alcohol or abrading the skin, which might reduce the natural resistive/conductive properties of the skin. However, since a fall in conductance has been noted following the use of soap and water (Venables & Christie 1973) and since the length of time since the last wash will be variable across subjects when they arrive at the laboratory, these authors recommended that subjects be asked to wash their hands with a nonabrasive soap prior to having the electrodes attached. It is recommended that the electrodes be kept on the same hand to avoid ECG (electroencephalographic) artifact and that the placement sites be clean and dry (Venables & Christie 1973).

Inferential Context

QUANTIFICATION PROCEDURES

Figure 4 shows tracings of two hypothetical skin conductance recordings during a 20-sec rest period and then during three repetitions of a simple discrete stimulus (e.g., a mild tone). Several important aspects of EDA can be seen in the figure. First, it can be seen that tonic SCL begins at 10 μS (microsiemens) in the upper tracing and at 5 μS in the lower tracing. Although tonic SCL can vary widely between different subjects and within the same subject in different psychological states, the typical range is between 2 μS and 20 μS with the types of apparatus and procedures described here. Computing the log of SCL can significantly reduce skew and kurtosis in the SCL data and is recommended by Venables and Christie (1980).

It can also be seen in the lower tracing of Figure 4 that the SCL drifts downward from 5 μS to nearly 4 μS during the rest period. It is common for SCL to gradually decrease while subjects are at rest, then rapidly increase

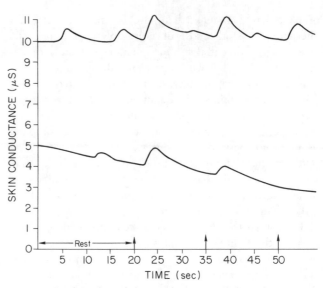

Figure 4. Two hypothetical skin conductance recordings during 20 sec of rest followed by three repetitions of a simple discrete stimulus. Arrows represent the presentation of a stimulus. Reprinted from Dawson & Nuechterlein (1984), "Psychophysiological dysfunctions in the developmental course of schizophrenic disorders," *Schizophrenia Bulletin*, vol. 10, pp. 204–32.

when novel stimulation is introduced, and finally gradually decrease again when the stimulus is repeated.

Phasic SCRs are only a small fraction of the SCL and have been likened to small waves superimposed on the tidal drifts in SCL (Lykken & Venables 1971). If the SCR occurs in the absence of an identifiable stimulus, as shown in the rest phase of Figure 4, it is referred to as a "spontaneous" or "nonspecific" SCR (NS-SCR). The most widely used measure of NS-SCR activity is its rate per minute – typically between 1 and 3 while the subject is at rest. However, responses can be elicited by sighs, deep breaths, and bodily movements, so unless these also are recorded it is impossible to say which responses truly are NS-SCRs.

Presentation of a novel, unexpected, significant, or aversive stimulus will likely elicit what is known as a "specific" SCR. With the exception of responses elicited by aversive stimuli, these SCRs are generally considered to be components of the orienting response. As is also the case with NS-SCRs, one must decide upon a minimum amplitude change in conductance to count as an elicited SCR. A common minimum response amplitude is 0.05 μS, which is a largely arbitrary value that happens to be the minimum change that can be reliably detected through visual inspection of most polygraph paper recordings. This arbitrary minimum is decreasing as computer scoring becomes more popular, because the computer can reliably detect much smaller changes. Another decision regarding scoring of SCRs concerns the latency window of time during which time a response will be assumed to be elicited by the stimulus. Based on frequency distributions of response latencies to simple stimuli, it is common to use a 1–3-sec

TABLE 1. Electrodermal Measures, Definitions, and Typical Values

Measure	Definition	Typical Values
Skin conductance level (SCL)	Tonic level of electrical conductivity of skin	2–20 μS
Change in SCL	Gradual changes in SCL measured at two or more points in time	1–3 μS
Frequency of NS-SCRs	Number of SCRs in absence of identifiable eliciting stimulus	1–3 per min
ER-SCR amplitude	Phasic increase in conductance shortly following stimulus onset	0.2–1.0 μS
ER-SCR latency	Temporal interval between stimulus onset and SCR initiation	1–3 sec
ER-SCR rise time	Temporal interval between SCR initiation and SCR peak	1–3 sec
ER-SCR half recovery time	Temporal interval between SCR peak and point of 50% recovery of SCR amplitude	2–10 sec
ER-SCR habituation (trials to habituation)	Number of stimulus presentations before two or three trials with no response	2–8 stimulus presentations
ER-SCR habituation (slope)	Rate of change of ER-SCR amplitude	0.01–0.05 μS per trial

Key: ER, event-related; NS, nonspecific; SCR, skin conductance response.

or 1–4-sec latency window. Hence, any SCR that begins between one and three (or four) seconds following stimulus onset is considered to be elicited by that stimulus. It is important to select reasonably short latency windows, perhaps even shorter than 1–3 sec, so as to not have the NS-SCR rate contaminate the measurement of elicited SCRs (Levinson, Edelberg, & Bridger 1984).

An important advance in EDA research has been the development of computerized scoring programs. Scoring software is available from the manufacturers of several EDA recording systems, and customized software or shareware is frequently used as well. One example of shareware is SCRGAUGE by Peter Kohlisch, available in Boucsein (1992). Another shareware with a long history is SCORIT 1980 (Strayer & Williams 1982), which is a revision of SCORIT (Prokasy 1974). Interested readers may contact Dr. William C. Williams (BWilliams@EWU.edu) for an updated version of SCORIT 1980.

Computer scoring is significantly less time-consuming than hand scoring and has the advantage of ensuring perfect reliability (the computer will score the same response the same way every time and will apply the same rules to every response). Another advantage of computerized scoring is the availability of sophisticated algorithms such as that proposed by Lim and associates (1997) for discerning individual components of skin conductance responses. As mentioned before, another advantage of computerized acquisition and scoring is that a computer can detect responses that are too small to be scored reliably by hand. Depending on the range of the analog-to-digital converter and the sensitivity of the skin conductance coupler, responses as small as 0.008 μS may be detected and scored. However, whether this is a psychologically or physiologically meaningful change in conductance remains to be determined.

Having decided on a minimum response amplitude and a latency window in which a response will be considered as an "event-related" SCR, one can measure several aspects of the elicited SCR besides its mere occurrence and frequency. Definitions and typical values of the major EDA component measures are given in Table 1 and are shown graphically in Figure 5. For example, size of the SCR is quantified as the amount of increase in conductance measured from the onset of the response to its peak. The size of an elicited SCR typically ranges between 0.2 μS and 1.0 μS.

When a stimulus is repeated several times and an average size of the SCR is to be calculated, one may choose to compute either mean SCR amplitude or mean SCR magnitude. *Magnitude* refers to the mean value computed across all stimulus presentations including those without a measurable response, whereas *amplitude* is the mean value computed across only those trials in which a measurable (nonzero) response occurred (Humphreys 1943). Prokasy and Kumpfer (1973) argued strongly against use of the magnitude measure in large part because it confounds frequency and amplitude, which do not always covary. A magnitude measure can create the impression that the

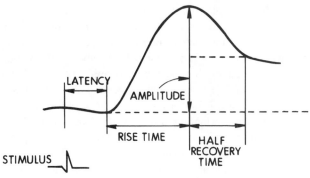

Figure 5. Graphical representation of principal EDA components.

response size is changing when in fact it is the response frequency that is changing. Hence, these authors recommend separate assessments of frequency and amplitude rather than magnitude. However, it is important to note that a complication with the amplitude measure is that the N used in computing average response size can vary depending on how many measurable responses a subject gives, and the data of subjects without any measurable response must be eliminated. Thus, a subject who responds on each of ten stimulus presentations with a response of 0.50 μS will have the same mean SCR amplitude as a subject who responds on only the first stimulus presentation with a response of .50 μS but does not respond thereafter. We concur with Venables and Christie (1980) that there are arguments for and against both amplitude and magnitude; although no absolute resolution is possible, it is important to keep the difference between the two measures clearly in mind. In fact, we recommend that in most situations it is reasonable to compute and compare results obtained with SCR frequency, amplitude, and magnitude.

Like SCL, SCR amplitude and magnitude are frequently found to be positively skewed and also leptokurtotic, so a logarithmic transformation is often used to remedy these problems. If measurements are being made of SCR magnitude, so that zero responses are included, then log(SCR + 1.0) may be calculated, since the logarithm of zero is not defined (Venables & Christie 1980). Another common practice is to use a square root transformation, $\sqrt{SCR}$, to normalize response amplitude data; this does not require the addition of a constant (Edelberg 1972a). In some cases the choice of the square-root or logarithmic transformation should be guided by considerations of achieving or maintaining the homogeneity of variance across several groups (Winer, Brown, & Michels 1991, pp. 356–8). If skew, kurtosis, or homogeneity of variance problems do not exist in a particular set of data, transformations need not be performed.

In addition to response size, one can also measure temporal characteristics of the SCR including onset latency, rise time, and half-recovery time. These temporal characteristics of the SCR waveform are not as commonly quantified as amplitude, and their relationship to psychophysiological processes is not as well understood at this time. The issue of whether SCR recovery time, for example, can provide information independent of other EDA measures and is uniquely responsive to specific psychophysiological processes was suggested by Edelberg (1972b) but was questioned by Bundy and Fitzgerald (1975) and remains unsettled (Edelberg 1993, pp. 14–15; Fowles 1986, pp. 84–7). This is not to say that SCR recovery time is without discriminating power; rather, its qualitatively different informational properties relative to other EDA components is an open issue.

The usual constellation of EDA components is for high SCL, frequent NS-SCRs, large SCR amplitude, short la-

tency, short rise time, and short recovery time to cluster together. However, the correlations among the EDA components generally are not very high, usually less than 0.60 (Lockhart & Lieberman 1979; Venables & Christie 1980). The size and consistency of these relationships is compatible with the hypothesis that many of the EDA components may represent partially independent sources of information, although – as indicated with regard to SCR recovery time – this is a controversial hypothesis. The one exception to the weak relationships among EDA components is the consistently high correlation between SCR rise time and recovery time. Based on this relation, Venables and Christie (1980) suggested that SCR rise time and half-recovery time may be essentially redundant measures and that – since recovery time is not always as available as rise time (owing to subsequent NS-SCRs) – rise time may be the preferred measure.

A problem with quantifying the SCR components occurs when the response to be scored is elicited before an immediately preceding response has had time to recover. It is customary to measure the amplitude of each response from its own individual deflection point (Edelberg 1967; Grings & Lockhart 1965). However, the amplitude as well as the temporal characteristics of the second response are distorted by being superimposed on the recovery of the first response. For example, the measurable amplitude of the second response will be smaller given its occurrence following the first response. The amount of distortion of the second response is a function of the size of the first response and the time since the first response (Grings & Schell 1969). Although there is no good solution to the response interference effect when hand scoring EDA, it can be pointed out that response frequency may be the least distorted component of the response in this situation. In addition, as mentioned earlier, one advantage of computerized scoring of EDA is the availability of more sophisticated scoring algorithms. In this regard, Lim et al. (1997) conducted an investigation in which they applied a multiparameter curve-fitting algorithm to the scoring of overlapping skin conductance responses; they were able to decompose the overall response complex into meaningful components of the separate responses.

Another problem with quantifying the EDA components concerns the existence of large variability due to extraneous individual differences. Thus, whether an SCL of 8 μS is considered high, moderate, or low will depend upon that specific subject's range of SCLs. For example, one can see in Figure 4 that an SCL of 8 μS would be relatively low for the subject depicted in the upper tracing but would be relatively high for the subject depicted in the lower tracing. Similarly, an SCR of 0.5 μS may be relatively large for one person but relatively small for another. Lykken and colleagues (1966) proposed an interesting method to correct for this interindividual variance. The correction procedure involves computing a range for each individual subject and then expressing the subject's momentary value as a proportion of this range. For example, one may compute a subject's minimum SCL during a rest period and a maximum SCL while the subject blows a balloon to bursting; the subject's present SCL can then be expressed as a proportion of his or her individualized range according to the following formula: $(SCL - SCL_{min})/(SCL_{max} - SCL_{min})$.

For SCR data, the minimum SCR can be assumed to be zero and the maximum can be estimated by the presentation of some strong or startling stimulus. Each SCR can then be corrected for individual differences in range simply by dividing each SCR by that subject's maximum SCR. The rationale underlying these procedures is that an individual's maximum and minimum SCL and SCR are due mainly to physiological differences (e.g., thickness of the corneum) that are unrelated to psychological processes. It is the variation within these physiological limits that is normally of psychological interest (Lykken & Venables 1971).

Although the range correction procedure can reduce error variance and increase the power of statistical tests in some data sets, it also can be problematic in others. For example, range correction would be inappropriate in a situation where two groups being compared had different ranges (Lykken & Venables 1971). Also, the range correction procedure relies upon adequate and reliable estimates of maximum and minimum values, yet estimates of these individual extreme values can be unreliable. For this reason, Ben-Shakhar (1985) recommended using within-subject standardized scores to adjust for individual differences because this transformation relies upon the mean, a more stable and reliable statistic than the maximum response. For further discussion of these and other transformation procedures, see Boucsein (1992, pp. 150–7).

Another important aspect of elicited SCRs is their decline in amplitude and eventual disappearance with repetition of the eliciting stimulus (SCR habituation). Habituation is a ubiquitous and adaptive phenomenon whereby subjects become less responsive to familiar and nonsignificant stimuli. There are several methods of quantifying habituation of the SCR (Siddle, Stephenson, & Spinks 1983). One simple method involves counting the number of stimulus repetitions required to reach some predetermined level of habituation (e.g., two or three consecutive trials without measurable SCRs). This "trials-to-habituation" measure is useful and has been widely employed since its use by Sokolov (1963), but it is subject to considerable distortion by the occurrence of a single response. For example, whether an isolated SCR occurs on trial 3 can make the difference between a trials-to-habituation score of "0" (indicative of an atypical nonresponder) and a "3" (indicative of a typical rate of habituation).

Another common measure of habituation is based on the rate of decline of SCR magnitude across trials as assessed by a "trials" main effect or interaction effect within an analysis of variance. However, this measure does not provide information about habituation in individual subjects and moreover can be distorted by differences in initial levels of responding.

A third measure of habituation is based on the regression of SCR magnitude on the log trial number (Lader & Wing 1969; Montague 1963). The regression approach provides a slope and an intercept score (the latter reflecting initial response amplitude), which usually are highly correlated with each other. Covariance procedures have been used to remove the dependency of slope on intercept, providing what Montague (1963) called an "absolute rate of habituation." However, this technique rests on the assumptions that (i) slope and intercept reflect different underlying processes and (ii) the treatment effects under investigation do not significantly affect the intercepts (Siddle et al. 1983). Use of the slope measure also assumes that subjects respond on a sufficient number of trials to compute a meaningful slope measure, which may not be the case for some types of subjects with mild innocuous stimuli. Nevertheless, to the extent that these assumptions can be justified, the slope measure is often preferable because: (1) unlike the analysis-of-variance approach, individual habituation scores can be derived; (2) unlike the trials-to-habituation measure, isolated SCRs have less of a contaminating effect; (3) unlike the trials-to-habituation measure, the slope measure makes fuller use of the magnitude data; and (4) unlike the trials-to-habituation measure, the slope measure can discriminate between subjects who show varying degrees of habituation but who fail to completely stop responding for two or three consecutive trials.

THREE TYPES OF PARADIGMS IN WHICH EDA IS OFTEN USED

Now that the principal EDA components have been identified and defined, we can describe basic experimental paradigms used to study the relationships of these components to psychological states and processes. In this section we will identify three general types of paradigms: those that involve (1) the presentation of discrete stimuli, (2) the presentation of chronic stimuli, and (3) the measurement of individual differences in EDA. In the next section we discuss specific applications and theoretical issues involved in these paradigmatic studies of EDA.

The SCR is elicited by almost any novel, unexpected, potentially important, discrete stimulus in the environment, as well as by the omission of an expected stimulus (Siddle 1991). One of the most widely used paradigms in psychophysiology involves measuring the elicitation and habituation of various indices of the orienting response, of which the SCR is a reliable and easily measurable component. This "orienting response habituation" paradigm typically consists of the repetitive presentation of a simple discrete innocuous stimulus (commonly a 1-sec tone of approximately 75 dB) with interstimulus intervals varying between 20 sec and 60 sec. The initial elicitation and subsequent habituation of the SCR can be measured in this paradigm as a component of the orienting response. The typical finding with this paradigm is that the SCR rapidly declines in amplitude with stimulus repetition and eventually disappears completely. The rate of the decline and disappearance of the SCR varies with such factors as stimulus significance, stimulus intensity, and the length of the interval between stimuli (see review by Siddle et al. 1983). The shape of the response also changes with stimulus repetition as the latency, rise time, and half-recovery time become longer (Lockhart & Lieberman 1979). Moreover, the background tonic SCL generally declines and the frequency of NS-SCRs becomes less. All in all, the picture that emerges is one of a less active and less reactive response system with stimulus repetition.

Next we turn to a paradigm that involves the presentation of a continuous, chronic stimulus or situation such as that involved in performing an ongoing task. Bohlin (1976), for example, required one group of subjects to perform a series of arithmetic problems; a second group of subjects was threatened with delivery of electric shock for poor performance on the arithmetic task. Both groups then were presented a series of discrete innocuous tones during the task so that the elicitation and habituation of SCRs could be measured. It was found that the ongoing task (and threat) (1) increased SCL, (2) reversed the usual decline over time in SCL, (3) increased the overall frequency of NS-SCRs, (4) increased the frequency and magnitude of elicited SCRs, and (5) retarded the rate of elicited SCR habituation (at least with the trials-to-habituation measure). These results demonstrated the sensitivity of these EDA components to simple but powerful manipulations in the ongoing stimulus situation.

The EDA "individual difference" paradigm is fundamentally different from the preceding two paradigms. Here, EDA is assumed to be a relatively stable subject trait related to behavioral and psychological individual differences. Consistent with this assumption is the fact that EDA components exhibit moderate test–retest stability. The test–retest reliability coefficients generally range between 0.50 and 0.70 when measured over a range encompassing a few days to a year or longer (see Freixa i Baque 1982 for a review of early studies; for more recent findings see Fredrikson et al. 1993 or Schell, Dawson, & Filion 1988). Another line of evidence consistent with the assumptions of the individual difference paradigm is that many of the EDA components have a partial genetic influence (Lykken et al. 1988).

Advantages and Disadvantages of the Use of EDA

When one is considering the use of EDA as an indicator of some psychological state or process of interest, it is well to remember that, in the great majority of situations, changes in electrodermal activity do not occur in isolation. Rather, they occur as part of a complex of responses mediated by the autonomic nervous system.

Experimental operations such as those just described that have the effect of increasing SCL and/or NS-SCR rate (e.g. Bohlin 1976) also would generally be expected to increase heart rate level and blood pressure and to decrease finger pulse volume, to mention a few of the more commonly measured ANS responses (Engel 1960; see also Grings & Dawson 1978). Stimuli that elicit an SCR would also be expected to elicit certain components of heart rate response (Bohlin & Kjellberg 1979; Graham & Clifton 1966) and a peripheral vasoconstriction (Uno & Grings 1965), and these response components would ordinarily be increased in magnitude by the same operations that would increase SCR magnitude. The response or responses chosen for monitoring by a particular investigator should reflect such considerations as those discussed next.

Although it is true that operations which alter EDA also typically alter other ANS and nonautonomic response measures, so that the electrodermal response occurs as part of a response complex, it is also true that different components of that response complex may correlate poorly with each other across individuals. The poor intercorrelation across subjects of the different components of the global ANS response pattern reflects in large part what is termed *individual response stereotypy* (Engel 1960; Lacey & Lacey 1958; Wenger et al. 1961). That is, individuals tend (some more strongly than others) to produce the same pattern of relative change across physiological systems, and this pattern differs across individuals. Thus, the decision about which particular physiological response to monitor is an important one.

Before considering examples of the three types of paradigms in which EDA is frequently employed, the reader should consider that, as with any response system, the measurement of EDA has both advantages and disadvantages. It is well to keep these in mind while reviewing specific examples.

For some researchers, EDA may be the response system of choice because, unlike most ANS responses, it provides a direct and undiluted representation of sympathetic activity. As we have pointed out, the neural control of the eccrine sweat glands is entirely under sympathetic control. Therefore, if SCL is observed to increase in a situation or if the SCR is enhanced, then this can be due only to increased tonic or phasic sympathetic activation. If heart rate is observed to slow, on the other hand, this could be due to decreased sympathetic activation of the heart via the cardiac nerves, increased parasympathetic input via the vagus nerve, or some combination of the two. With heart rate, as with most ANS functions (pupil diameter, gastric motility, blood pressure), a change in activity in response to stimuli or situations of psychological significance cannot be unambiguously laid to either sympathetic or parasympathetic activity; it may be due to either one or to a combination of both. Thus, the researcher who wishes an unalloyed measure of sympathetic activity may prefer to monitor EDA, whereas the experimenter who wishes a broader picture of both sympathetic and parasympathetic activity may prefer heart rate (assuming that instrumentation constraints allow only one measure to be recorded). Similarly, if for some reason (perhaps the use of medication with side effects on cholinergic or adrenergic systems) one wishes to monitor a response which is predominately cholinergically mediated at the periphery but which is also influenced by sympathetic activity, then EDA would be the choice.

Another advantage of using SCR is that its occurrence is generally quite discriminable. Thus, on a single presentation of a stimulus, one can determine by quick inspection whether or not an SCR has occurred. In contrast, the presence of a heart rate response to a single stimulus presentation may be difficult to distinguish from ongoing changes in heart rate (HR) that reflect changes in muscle tonus or respiratory sinus arrhythmia. For instance, the triphasic deceleratory–acceleratory–deceleratory HR response that appears in long interstimulus interval classical conditioning or during a long (8.0-sec) reaction time foreperiod (Bohlin & Kjellberg 1979) is often discriminable only when one averages second-by-second HR changes following stimulus presentation over a number of trials, just as one must average over a number of stimulus presentations in order to discriminate the cortical event-related potential (ERP) recorded from the scalp from background electroencephalographic (EEG) activity. This may be disadvantageous for the researcher who has a strong interest in activity occurring on a few individual trials.

In addition to decisions made on the basis of neuroanatomical control and basic response characteristics, an investigator may prefer EDA to other response systems because of the nature of the situation in which the subjects are assessed. Fowles (1988) argued convincingly that HR is influenced primarily by activation of a neurophysiological behavioral *activation* system that is involved in responding during appetitive reward seeking, to conditioned stimuli associated with reward, and during active avoidance. On the other hand, EDA is influenced primarily by activation of a neurophysiological behavioral *inhibition* system that is involved in responding to punishment, to passive avoidance, or to frustrative nonreward. This latter system is viewed as an anxiety system. Thus, if an investigator is studying the reaction of subjects to a situation or to discrete stimuli that elicit anxiety – but in which or to which no active avoidance response can be made – then the electrodermal system should be the physiological system that is most responsive.

For many investigators, an additional advantage of the use of EDA relative to other response systems is that, of all forms of ANS activity, individual differences in EDA are most reliably associated with psychopathological states. In the next section we will discuss in detail the correlates of some of these stable EDA differences between individuals.

Finally, one should bear in mind that, in comparison with many other psychophysiological measures, EDA is relatively inexpensive to record. After initial purchase of the recording system, expenses for each subject are trivial, involving electrode collars and paste and the occasional replacement of electrodes. Electrical shielding of the room or booth in which the subject sits – which is generally needed for noise-free recording of EEG or event-related potentials – is unnecessary, and the costs of using EDA as a response measure are minuscule compared to those of hemodynamic techniques such as PET scans or functional MRI. Furthermore, the techniques used to record EDA are completely harmless and risk-free, and thus they can be used with young children and in research designs that require repeated testing at short intervals of time.

There are also potential disadvantages to the use of EDA as a dependent measure. First, EDA is a relatively slow-moving response system. As mentioned previously, the latency of the elicited SCR is about 1–3 sec, and tonic shifts in SCL produced by changes in arousal, alertness, and so forth require approximately the same time to occur. Thus, an investigator who is interested in tracking very rapidly occurring processes, or stages within a complex process, will not find EDA useful. Such research questions require response measures (e.g., cortical-evoked potentials or prepulse inhibition of the startle blink) that can discriminate among events or processes occurring at intervals of 100 msec or less. Yet even though the SCR cannot index such rapidly occurring processes as sensory gating or stages of stimulus analysis on a real-time basis, the SCR *has* been found to be correlated with real-time measures of these processes. For example, Lyytinen, Blomberg, and Näätänen (1992) observed that the parietal P3a was larger when an SCR was elicited by a novel tone than when it was not elicited. Interestingly, the latter investigators found that the mismatch negativity component of the ERP was not related to elicitation of SCRs, unlike the P3a. This pattern of results suggests that the SCR orienting response is elicited by a controlled cognitive process (indexed by P3a) that is preceded by an early automatic discrimination process (indexed by mismatch negativity).

Electrodermal activity has sometimes been criticized as a measure because it is multiply caused: the elicited SCR is not specific to a single type of event or situation (as, for instance, the N400 ERP component appears to be specifically influenced by semantic expectancy; Kutas 1997). However, the multiple influences on EDA may actually be as much an advantage as a disadvantage. As described throughout this chapter, EDA can be used to index a number of processes, including activation, attention, and the task significance or affective intensity of a stimulus. In using EDA as a response measure, one must simply take care to control experimental conditions – that is, to be sure that one is varying only a single process that may influence EDA at a time. Such experimental control is essential for all attempts to draw clear inferences from results, whether one is recording EDA or, for instance, an electrocortical or hemodynamic measure, given the number of processes that may influence these measures as well.

Thus, like any single response system, EDA has distinct advantages and disadvantages as a response system to monitor. The ideal situation, of course, is one in which the researcher can record more than one response measure. When ANS activity is of primary interest, EDA and heart rate are probably the two most common choices: EDA for its neuroanatomical simplicity, trial-by-trial visibility, and utility as a general arousal/attention indicator; and heart rate for its potential differentiation of more subtle psychological states of interest to the researcher.

Psychosocial Context

In this section, we review in more detail the psychosocial factors that influence EDA results occurring in the three types of paradigms identified earlier: (1) those that involve the presentation of discrete stimuli, (2) those that involve the presentation of chronic stimuli, and (3) those that involve examining the correlates of individual differences in EDA.

EFFECTS OF DISCRETE STIMULI

The stimuli to which the SCR is sensitive are wide and varied; they include stimulus novelty, surprisingness, intensity, emotional content, and significance. It might be argued that, because EDA is sensitive to such a wide variety of stimuli, it is not a clearly interpretable measure of any particular psychological process (Landis 1930). This view is certainly correct in the sense that it is impossible to identify an isolated SCR as an "anxiety" response, or an "anger" response, or an "attentional" response. However, the psychological meaning of an SCR becomes interpretable by taking into account the stimulus condition or experimental paradigm in which the SCR occurred. The better-controlled the experimental paradigm, the more conclusive the interpretation. That is, by having only one aspect of the stimulus change across conditions (e.g., task significance) while eliminating other differences (e.g., stimulus novelty, intensity), one can more accurately infer the psychological process mediating the resultant SCR. Thus, as we will illustrate in the following discussion, the inference of a specific psychophysiological process requires knowledge of both a well-controlled stimulus situation and a carefully measured response.

One discrete stimulus paradigm that relies on the SCR's sensitivity to stimulus significance is the so-called guilty

knowledge test (GKT), a test for detecting deception ("lie detection"). The GKT involves recording SCRs (as well as other physiological responses) while presenting subjects with a series of multiple-choice questions (Lykken 1959). For example, a suspect in a burglary case might be asked to answer "no" to each of the alternatives given for a question concerning details about the burglary. For each question, the correct alternative would be intermixed among other plausible alternatives. The theory behind the technique is that the correct answer to each question will be more psychologically significant to a guilty subject than will the other alternatives, whereas for the innocent subject all of the alternatives would be of equal significance. Therefore, the guilty subject is expected to respond more consistently to the correct alternatives, whereas the innocent subject is expected to respond randomly (Lykken 1959). Lykken (1981) suggested that guilty subjects can be detected nearly 90% of the time and innocent subjects can be correctly classified nearly 100% of the time with a properly constructed GKT. For a discussion of the differing views regarding the accuracy of various techniques for detecting deception, see Jennings, Ackles, and Coles (1991; see also Chapter 28 of this volume).

Tranel, Fowles, and Damasio (1985) developed another type of discrete stimulus paradigm with which to study the effects of significant facial stimuli on SCRs. In their initial investigations, SCRs were recorded from normal college students while being presented a set of slides depicting faces of famous people (e.g., Ronald Reagan, Bob Hope) and faces of unfamiliar people. A total of 55 slides were presented, including 5 initial buffer items, 42 presentations of the nonsignificant stimuli (unfamiliar faces), and 8 intermixed presentations of the significant stimuli (famous faces). Subjects were instructed simply to sit quietly and look at each slide. The results revealed that the average SCR was much larger to slides of significant faces ($X = 1.26\ \mu S$) than to the nonsignificant faces ($X = 0.19\ \mu S$).

Tranel and Damasio (1985) also employed this paradigm with two prosopagnosic patients. Patients with prosopagnosia lose the ability to consciously recognize faces. One patient had a pervasive syndrome and showed a complete failure to consciously recognize any of the faces of famous people (as well as faces of family members, close friends, or even herself). Despite this syndrome, this patient exhibited more frequent as well as larger SCRs to the significant faces than the nonsignificant faces. Bauer (1984) used a paradigm patterned more closely after the GKT with another prosopagnosic patient and also observed SCR discrimination without verbal discrimination.

Although the GKT of Lykken (1959) appears to be quite adequate to detect concealed information (and hence the guilty person) and the paradigm of Tranel et al. (1985) appears adequate to test for recognition of famous faces, one may question whether either paradigm is sufficient to demonstrate the effect of stimulus significance on SCR.

It may be argued that both paradigms confounded relative novelty with relative stimulus significance. If guilty subjects dichotomize items into relevant and irrelevant categories in the GKT (Ben-Shakhar 1977), then the relevant category is presented less often then the irrelevant category and this relative novelty may contribute to the differential SCRs. Likewise, in the studies using slides of famous faces, the significant category of stimuli was presented less often than the nonsignificant category, and this difference in relative novelty may have contributed to the differential SCRs. The number of presentations of significant stimuli should have been equal to that of nonsignificant stimuli in order to unambiguously demonstrate the effect of stimulus significance on SCRs. As mentioned earlier in this section, close control over stimulus properties (e.g., novelty or significance) is necessary in order to infer the psychological processes eliciting the SCR.

Electrodermal activity is commonly measured using a discrete stimulus paradigm known as "discrimination classical conditioning," which highlights the influence of stimulus significance while controlling for stimulus novelty (Grings & Dawson 1973). For example, Dawson and Biferno (1973) employed a discrimination classical conditioning paradigm in which college student subjects were asked to rate their expectancy of the UCS (unconditioned stimulus; here, a brief electric shock) after each presentation of a CS+ and a CS−; tones of 800 Hz and 1,200 Hz were presented equally often and served (respectively) as the reinforced CS+ and the nonreinforced CS−, counterbalanced across subjects. Thus, for each conditioning trial, the subject's expectancy of shock and the associated SCR was recorded. The results, shown in Figure 6, revealed that subjects tended to respond equally to the reinforced CS+ and to the nonreinforced CS− until they became aware of the contingency between the conditioned stimuli and the shock. There was no evidence of SCR discrimination conditioning prior to the development of awareness; however, once the subject became aware, the CS+ became more significant than the CS− and there was an abrupt increase in the magnitude of the SCRs elicited by the CS+.

The SCR discrimination conditioning data suggest that subjects must be consciously aware of the differential stimulus significance before differential SCRs are elicited, whereas the earlier reviewed findings with prosopagnosic patients suggest that conscious awareness is not necessary for SCR discrimination. This apparent contradiction could perhaps be resolved by the hypothesis that conscious awareness is necessary for the initial learning of stimulus significance but not for the later evocation of SCRs to previously learned significant stimuli (Dawson & Schell 1985). However, we should note that the results obtained from one of the prosopagnosic patients studied by Tranel and Damasio (1985) do not appear consistent with this hypothesis. This patient suffered only from anterograde prosopagnosia in that she failed to consciously

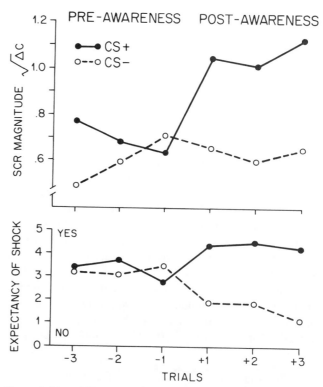

Figure 6. Mean SCR magnitude (top) and mean expectancy of shock (bottom) to the reinforced conditioned stimulus (CS+) and the nonreinforced conditioned stimulus (CS−) on three pre-aware and three post-aware trials. Reprinted with permission from Dawson & Biferno, "Concurrent measurement of awareness and electrodermal classical conditioning," *Journal of Experimental Psychology*, vol. 101, pp. 55–62. Copyright © 1973 by the American Psychological Association.

recognize only new faces experienced since the onset of her prosopagnosia. When this patient was exposed to slides of faces of persons with whom she had contact only since the onset of her illness (physicians, psychologists, etc.), she was unable consciously to recognize these faces yet she still gave more frequent and larger SCRs to these significant faces compared to nonsignificant faces. This provocative finding has essentially been replicated in another patient (Tranel & Damasio 1993), further suggesting that affective associative learning with faces as conditioned stimuli may occur without apparent conscious awareness.

In a related vein, the SCR has been used in the discrimination classical conditioning paradigm to investigate an interesting series of questions concerning "preparedness" and conditioning in normal subjects. The basic idea of preparedness (see Seligman 1970) is that some associations (such as the association between taste and nausea, or perhaps faces and affect) are − because of their survival value for the organism − much more easily and strongly established than others (such as that between an arbitrary tone and a shock). Öhman and his colleagues extended Seligman's concept to human autonomic conditioning, using what have been termed "biologically prepared," "potentially phobic," or "fear-relevant" conditioned stimuli – pictures of spiders, snakes, and angry faces (see McNally 1987; Öhman 1986, 1992). Öhman, Eriksson, and Olofsson (1975) reported that SCRs conditioned to pictures of spiders and snakes using a shock UCS were more resistant to extinction (i.e., were slower to diminish following the absence of the shock UCS) than were SCRs conditioned to neutral stimuli such as pictures of flowers and mushrooms; Öhman and Dimberg (1978) reported the same effect for pictures of angry versus happy faces.

Of particular interest is the finding that cognitive manipulations or processes that would be expected to dramatically reduce the conditioned SCR have a lesser impact on responses conditioned to these potentially phobic stimuli. Such SCRs, for instance, are more resistant to extinction instructions (information given to the subject that the UCS will no longer follow the CS – Hugdahl 1978; Hugdahl & Öhman 1977). Figure 7 shows the acquisition and extinction trials of groups conditioned with fear-relevant (spiders and snakes; left panels) and fear-irrelevant (triangles and circles; right panels) CSs. The lower panel of each pair

shows the effects of extinction instructions on the SCR. The top two panels exhibit the generally greater resistance to extinction of SCRs conditioned to fear-relevant CSs. The lower right panel shows the immediate abolition of the conditioned SCR by the extinction instructions when fear-irrelevant CSs are used. The lower left panel, on the other hand, shows the resistance to the extinction instructions of the SCR conditioned to the fear-relevant CSs. Skin conductance responses conditioned to such stimuli are also retained past the point of cognitive extinction (no greater expectancy of the UCS after the CS+ than after the CS−) when cognitive extinction has been created by the presentation of many nonreinforced trials (Schell, Dawson, & Marinkovic 1991), whether extinction trials are given immediately following acquisition or after a delay of several months. Investigators continue to explore the properties of the SCRs acquired by these stimuli as well as the implications that the unique properties of these stimuli – and the responses conditioned to them – have for theories of emotional learning and clinical phenomena (see e.g. Hugdahl & Johnsen 1993; Öhman et al. 1993).

As mentioned earlier, SCRs elicited by discrete nonaversive stimuli are generally considered to be part of the orienting response (OR) to novel or significant stimuli. We believe that the data reviewed in this section can be interpreted within this theoretical setting. The task of subjects exposed to the GKT is to deceive or conceal knowledge, and the correct item is more relevant to this task than are incorrect alternative items. Thus, subjects orient more to the task-significant items than to the task-nonsignificant items. Likewise, faces of famous people may be perceived as more significant and attention-demanding than the faces of unfamiliar people, and the signal of an impending shock (CS+) is more significant than the signal of no shock (CS−). Thus, the results observed here are consistent with the notion that the SCR is highly sensitive to stimulus significance, although the reader is reminded of the caveat regarding the confounding of stimulus frequency with stimulus significance in some of these paradigms.

There have been several models proposed to account for the elicitation of autonomic ORs such as the SCR (see Siddle et al. 1983 for a review). For example, an influential information processing model was proposed by Öhman (1979). This model distinguishes between automatic preattentive processing and controlled capacity-limited processing. Autonomic orienting is elicited when the preattentive mechanisms call for additional controlled processing. According to this model, there are two conditions under which this call is made. First, the call is made and the OR is elicited when the preattentive mechanisms fail to identify the incoming stimulus because there is no matching representation in short-term memory. Thus, the OR is sensitive to stimulus novelty. Second, the call is made and the OR is elicited when the preattentive mechanisms recognize the stimulus as significant. Thus, the OR represents

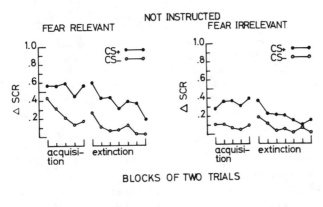

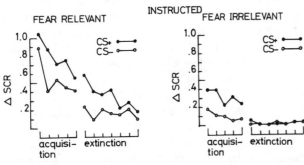

Figure 7. Mean SCR magnitude to the reinforced conditioned stimulus (CS+) and the nonreinforced conditioned stimulus (CS−) during acquisition and extinction for groups conditioned with fear-relevant and fear-irrelevant CSs, groups that either were or were not instructed about the omission of the shock UCS prior to extinction. Reprinted with permission from Hugdahl & Öhman, "Effects of instruction on acquisition and extinction of electrodermal responses to fear-relevant stimuli," *Journal of Experimental Psychology: Human Learning and Memory,* vol. 3, pp. 608–18. Copyright © 1977 by the American Psychological Association.

a transition from automatic to controlled processing based on preliminary preattentive analysis of stimulus novelty and stimulus significance. Others, however, have suggested that the OR occurs when controlled processing resources are actually allocated to the processing of the stimulus, at least where fear-irrelevant stimuli are concerned (Dawson, Filion, & Schell 1989; Öhman 1992).

In conclusion, in this section we have described some of the discrete stimulus paradigms in which EDA is most often measured and has proven to be most useful. Within this description we have emphasized that determining the psychological meaning of any particular SCR is dependent on a well-controlled stimulus situation. In addition, we have described a theoretical model that may be used to account for the SCRs elicited in the paradigms described. Finally, these areas of research examining the SCR to discrete stimuli underscore the point made previously that one advantage of the SCR is that the response can easily be measured on individual presentations of a stimulus. Thus, one may determine whether the response to a "guilty" stimulus in a group of stimuli is greater than to "innocent" stimuli, whether the SCR elicited by a CS+ is greater on the first trial after awareness of the CS–UCS relationship occurs than on the last trial before that awareness occurs, and whether the SCR elicited by a fear-relevant CS+ is greater than the SCR elicited by a CS− on the first trial pair following extinction instructions.

EFFECTS OF CHRONIC STIMULI

We turn now to an examination of the effects of more chronic, long-lasting stimuli or situations as opposed to the brief, discrete stimuli just reviewed. Chronic stimuli might best be thought of as modulating increases and decreases in tonic arousal. Hence, the most useful electrodermal measures in the context of chronic stimuli are SCL and frequency of NS-SCRs, because they can be measured on an ongoing basis over relatively long periods of time.

One type of chronic stimulus situation that will reliably produce increases in electrodermal activity involves the necessity of performing a task. The anticipation and performance of practically any task will increase both SCL and the frequency of NS-SCRs, at least initially. For example, Lacey and colleagues (1963) recorded palmar SCL during rest and during the anticipation and performance of eight different tasks. The tasks ranged from those requiring close attention to external stimuli, such as listening to an irregularly fluctuating loud white noise, to those requiring close attention to internal information processing and rejection of external stimuli, such as solving mental arithmetic problems. The impressive finding for present purposes was that SCL increased in each and every one of the task situations. Typically, SCL increased about 1 μS above resting level during anticipation and then increased another 1 or 2 μS during performance of the task.

Munro and associates (1987) observed that large increases in SCL and NS-SCR frequency were induced by a different task-significant situation. In this case, college student subjects were tested during a 5-min rest period and then during performance of a continuous performance vigilance task. The task stimuli consisted of a series of digits presented visually at a rapid rate of 1/sec with an exposure duration of 48 msec; the subject's task was to press a button whenever the digit "0" was presented. Both the number of NS-SCRs and SCL increased sharply from the resting levels during this demanding task and then gradually declined as the task continued.

The finding that electrodermal activity is reliably elevated during task performance suggests that tonic EDA can be a useful index of a process related to energy regulation or mobilization. An attentional or information processing interpretation of this finding might be that tasks require an effortful allocation of attentional resources and that this is associated with heightened autonomic activation (Jennings 1986). A different (but not necessarily mutually exclusive) explanation would invoke the concepts of stress and affect rather than attention and effortful allocation of resources. According to this view, laboratory tasks are challenging stressors, and a reliable physiological response to stressors is increased sympathetic activation – particularly EDA arousal.

Social stimulation constitutes another class of chronic stimuli that generally produce increases in EDA arousal. Social situations are ones in which the concepts of stress and affect are most often invoked. For example, early research related the EDA recorded during psychotherapeutic interviews to concepts such as "tension" and "anxiety" on the part of both patient and therapist (Boyd & DiMascio 1954; Dittes 1957). In one such study, Dittes measured the frequency of NS-SCRs of a patient during 42 hours of psychotherapy. The results of this study indicated that the frequency of NS-SCRs was inversely related to the judged permissiveness of the therapist, and Dittes concluded that EDA reflects "the anxiety of the patient, or his 'mobilization' against any cue threatening punishment by the therapist" (1957, p. 303).

Schwartz and Shapiro (1973) reviewed electrodermal findings in several areas of social psychophysiology up to 1970. The areas most relevant here are those in which EDA was measured during social interactions. These are situations in which there may occur intense cognitive and affective reaction and therefore large changes in EDA and other physiological responses. For example, in one series of social psychophysiological studies conducted since the Schwartz and Shapiro review, EDA was recorded during marital social interactions (Levenson & Gottman 1983, 1985). The researchers measured SCL (in addition to heart rate, pulse transmission time, and somatic activity) in married couples who were discussing conflict-laden problem areas. It was found that couples from distressed marriages had high "physiological linkage"; that is, there were greater correlations between husbands' and wives' physiological reactions in distressed marriages than those in satisfying marriages during the discussions of problem areas. Moreover, greater physiological arousal, including higher SCL, during the interactions and during baselines was associated with a decline in marital satisfaction over the ensuing three years.

Another series of studies related the effects of stressful social interactions on EDA to the study of relapse among schizophrenia patients. It has been well documented that the emotional attitudes expressed by a family member toward a patient with schizophrenia can be a powerful predictor of later relapse of the patient. That is, patients are at increased risk for relapse if their relatives are critical, hostile, or emotionally over-involved with them at the time of their illness (Brown, Birley, & Wing 1972; Vaughn & Leff 1976; Vaughn et al. 1984). The term "expressed emotion" (EE) is used to designate this continuum of affective attitudes ranging from low EE (less critical) to high EE (more critical) on the part of the relative.

It has been hypothesized that heightened autonomic arousal may be a mediating factor between the continued exposure to a high-EE relative and the increased risk of relapse (Turpin 1983). According to this notion, living with a high-EE family member produces excessive stress and autonomic hyperarousal. Autonomic hyperarousal has been characterized as one of several transient intermediate states that can produce deterioration in the patient's behavior, which in turn can negatively affect people around the patient. Hence, a vicious cycle can be created whereby the increased arousal causes changes in the patient's behavior that have an aggravating effect on the social environment, which serves to increase further autonomic arousal. Unless such a cycle is broken (e.g., by removal from that social environment), it can lead to the return of schizophrenia symptoms and a clinical relapse (Dawson, Nuechterlein, & Liberman 1983; Nuechterlein & Dawson 1984).

One prediction derived from this model is that patients exposed to high-EE relatives should show heightened sympathetic arousal compared to patients exposed to low-EE relatives. The first study to test this prediction obtained rather clear confirmatory results (Tarrier et al. 1979). These investigators measured the EDA of remitted patients living in the community whose relatives' levels of EE had already been determined by Vaughn and Leff (1976). Patients were tested in their homes for 15 minutes without the key relative and for 15 minutes with the key relative present. The frequency of NS-SCR activity of the patients with high-EE relatives and low-EE relatives did not differ when the relative was absent from the testing room, but if the key relative was present then patients with high-EE relatives exhibited higher rates of NS-SCRs than did patients with low-EE relatives. These results indicate that the presence of high-EE and low-EE relatives have differential effects on EDA, which is consistent with the hypothesis that differential autonomic arousal plays a mediating role in the differential relapse rates of the two patient groups.

In a subsequent investigation, Sturgeon and associates (1984) employed similar testing procedures with acutely ill hospitalized patients. In this case, it was found that patients with high-EE relatives exhibited more NS-SCRs than patients with low-EE relatives, whether or not the key relative was present in the testing room. Sturgeon et al. speculated that this pattern of results may indicate that patients from high-EE homes undergo a more sustained elevation of sympathetic arousal than patients from low-EE homes when they experience an exacerbation of schizophrenic symptoms. Another possibility is that the patients knew that the high-EE relatives were at the hospital and anticipated that the relatives would join them. In either event, these studies demonstrate the powerful effects of social stimulation on EDA and the potential importance and applicability of these effects in the area of psychopathology. More complete reviews of these studies and their implications can be found in Turpin, Tarrier, and Sturgeon (1988).

INDIVIDUAL DIFFERENCES IN EDA

We have discussed the utility of EDA as a dependent variable reflecting situational levels of arousal or activation by and attentiveness or responsiveness to individual stimuli. In this section we consider the EDA as a stable trait of the individual – as an individual difference variable. Individual differences in EDA are reliably associated with behavioral differences and psychopathological states of some importance, and we will examine some of these.

Individual differences in the rate of NS-SCRs and the rate of SCR habituation have been used to define a trait called "electrodermal lability" (Crider 1993; Lacey & Lacey 1958; Mundy-Castle & McKiever 1953). Electrodermal *labiles* are those subjects who show high rates of NS-SCRs and/or slow SCR habituation, whereas electrodermal *stabiles* are those who show few NS-SCRs and/or fast SCR habituation. Electrodermal lability is an individual trait that has been found to be relatively reliable over time, and labiles differ from stabiles with respect to a number of psychophysiological variables, including measures of both electrodermal and cardiovascular responsiveness (Kelsey 1991; Schell et al. 1988). In this section we present the behavioral and psychological differences associated with this individual difference in both the normal and abnormal populations.

Electrodermal lability is a trait that has been of interest in psychological research in part because many investigators have reported that labiles outperform stabiles on tasks that require sustained vigilance. When individuals perform a signal detection task that is sustained over time, deterioration across time in the accurate detection of targets is frequently observed, a phenomenon referred to as "vigilance decrement" (Davies & Parasuraman 1982). Numerous experimenters have reported that, when vigilance decrement occurs, it is more pronounced among electrodermal stabiles than among labiles. As time on the task goes by, labiles are apparently better able to keep attention focused on the task and to avoid a decline in performance (Crider & Augenbraun 1975; Hastrup 1979; Munro et al. 1987; Vossel & Rossman 1984). For instance, Munro et al. reported that – with a difficult attentional capacity-demanding detection task – stabiles showed a significant decrement over time in the signal detection measure d', which reflects perceptual sensitivity, whereas labiles did not. Furthermore, the degree of task-induced sympathetic arousal as measured by increases in NS-SCR rate was negatively correlated across subjects with d' decrement.

Researchers investigating such behavioral differences have concluded that electrodermal lability reflects the ability to allocate information processing capacity to target stimuli (Katkin 1975; Lacey & Lacey 1958; Schell et al. 1988). As Katkin (1975, p. 172) concluded, "electrodermal activity is a personality variable that reflects individual differences in higher central processes involved in attending to and processing information." Viewing electrodermal lability in this way suggests that labiles should differ from stabiles in a variety of information processing tasks. Consistent with this view, EDA labile children have been found to generally outperform stabiles on a variety of tasks that require perceptual speed and vigilance (Sakai, Baker, & Dawson 1992).

In addition to the differences between stabiles and labiles in the normal population, reliable abnormalities in electrodermal lability are associated with diagnosable psychopathology. The most common electrodermal abnormality in psychopathological groups is extreme stability in the form of very rapid habituation (or complete absence) of the SCR orienting response, although extreme lability has also been reported in some groups. In the following paragraphs we will summarize EDA abnormalities reported in schizophrenia and depression. A more general discussion of psychophysiological abnormalities in these and other psychopathologies can be found in Chapter 26 of this volume as well as in Zahn (1986).

The most commonly reported EDA abnormality in schizophrenia has been SCR nonresponding and hyporesponding to innocuous tones (see reviews by Bernstein et al. 1982; Dawson & Nuechterlein 1984; Iacono, Ficken, & Beiser 1993; Öhman 1981). In a pathbreaking study on this topic, Gruzelier and Venables (1972) presented a series of nonsignal tones to a large group of schizophrenia patients and to normal controls. Whereas all of the normal controls initially responded to the stimuli and then showed habituation of the SCR, the schizophrenia group showed a bimodal distribution at both extremes of habituation: 54% of the schizophrenia patients failed to give even one SCR, while 42% not only responded but failed to meet the habituation criterion. Gruzelier and Venables (1972) referred to the stabile group as "nonresponders" and to the labile group as "responders."

The high proportion of electrodermal nonresponders in schizophrenia is a very reliable finding. For example, Bernstein et al. (1982) examined a series of fourteen related studies in which samples of American, British, and German schizophrenia patients and normal controls were studied using a common methodology and response scoring criteria. Their consistent finding was that approximately 50% of schizophrenia patients were nonresponders, compared with only 5%–10% of controls. (More recent data, reported and reviewed by Venables & Mitchell 1996, suggest the percentage of SCR nonresponders among normal controls may be close to 25%.) A minority of the studies also reported the existence of a responder subgroup of patients showing slower than normal habituation, but the majority finding is normal rates of habituation in the responder subgroup. The responder–nonresponder distinction is a potentially important one because it may be useful in identifying useful subgroups within the heterogeneous disorder(s) of schizophrenia. For example, nonresponders and responders have been reported to show different symptomology, with responders generally displaying more symptoms such as excitement, anxiety, manic behavior, and belligerence; nonresponders tend to show more emotional withdrawal and conceptual disorganization (Bernstein et al. 1982; Straube 1979). Furthermore, SCR hyporesponsivity has been related to a more severe form of illness (Katsanis & Iacono 1994), lower overall and regionally specific brain metabolism (Hazlett et al. 1993), and poor premorbid adjustment (Öhman et al. 1989), although SCR *hyper*activity also has been associated with higher levels of symptomatology in a group of recent-onset schizophrenia outpatients (Dawson et al. 1992b).

Findings in this area may become clearer by taking into consideration the symptomatic state of the patients at the time of testing. Higher than normal SCL and rates of NS-SCRs have been found in patients while in a psychotic state but not in the same patients while in a symptomatically remitted state (Dawson et al. 1994); see Figure 8. Phasic SCR hyporesponsiveness, on the other hand, was observed in both the psychotic and the remitted state when responsiveness was corrected for overall tonic activation levels. These findings suggest that tonic electrodermal hyperarousal is a state-sensitive symptomatic episode indicator, whereas SCR hyporesponsivity may be an enduring traitlike indicator when corrected for existing arousal level.

Tonic electrodermal hyperactivity may be not only an episode indicator but also an early precursor of symptomatic exacerbation or relapse in schizophrenia. Hazlett and associates (1997b) found elevated EDA in four of five symptomatically completely remitted patients in the week or so prior to a psychotic exacerbation or relapse compared with the levels shown by these same patients in non-prerelapse

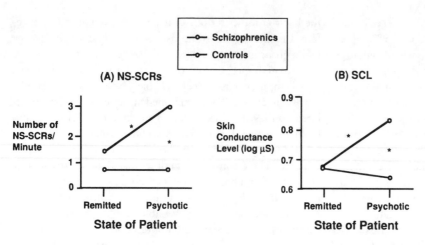

Figure 8. Mean number of nonspecific SCRs per minute (left) and mean SCL (right) obtained from normal controls and patients with schizophrenia when the patients were in remitted and psychotic states. Reprinted with permission from Dawson, Nuechterlein, Schell, Gitlin, & Ventura, "Autonomic abnormalities in schizophrenia: State or trait indicators?" *Archives of General Psychiatry*, vol. 51, pp. 813–24. Copyrighted 1994, American Medical Association.

periods. These findings are consistent with a theoretical model which hypothesizes that sympathetic activation is associated with a "transient intermediate state" that precedes psychotic episodes in vulnerable individuals (Nuechterlein & Dawson 1984). According to this theoretical model, not all such intermediate states will be followed by psychotic exacerbation or relapse. Rather, these states constitute periods of heightened vulnerability and an increased risk of relapse, with the actual occurrence of relapses or exacerbation being influenced by environmental stressors.

Phasic and tonic electrodermal hypoactivity also have been reported for depressed patients (Sponheim, Allen, & Iacono 1995; see also Chapter 26). For example, Mirkin and Coppen (1980) found a higher than normal incidence of SCR nonresponding (67% vs. 13%) in unmedicated depressive inpatients than in controls. Numerous other investigators found EDA hypoactivity in the form of low levels of SCL and/or small SCRs to different classes of stimuli (Dawson, Schell, & Catania 1977; Iacono et al. 1983; Lader & Noble 1975; Ward, Doerr, & Storrie 1983). Although SCR nonresponders have not been treated as a distinct subgroup in depression (as they have in schizophrenia), it should be noted that EDA hypoactivity in terms of both tonic SCL and phasic SCR responsivity has been reported to be more prominent in: psychotic than neurotic depression (Byrne 1975); endogenous than nonendogenous depression (Mirkin & Coppen 1980); and retarded than agitated depression (Lader & Wing 1969). Such hypoactivity has also been associated with overall greater depressive symptomatology (Dawson et al. 1977).

The phasic SCR orienting response deficit observed in both schizophrenia and depression suggests the possibility of a common information processing deficit. Con-

sistent with this possibility, Hazlett and colleagues (1997a) found secondary reaction time abnormalities during a test of SCR orienting in recent-onset schizophrenia patients. The secondary reaction time measure indicated a delay in the allocation of attentional resources in the patients. This abnormality was particularly pronounced in the SCR hyporesponders, consistent with the notion that the SCR deficit is related to an underlying attentional dysfunction in schizophrenia.

However, several lines of evidence suggest that the SCR impairments observed in schizophrenia and depression may reflect different underlying dysfunctions. *First,* Bernstein and his associates (1988, 1995) demonstrated that, although SCR nonresponding is more frequent in both schizophrenia patients and depressive patients than in normal controls, only schizophrenia patients displayed excessive nonresponding with the finger pulse amplitude component of the orienting response. These findings suggest that schizophrenia is associated with a central orienting deficiency, whereas depression may involve a deficit more specific to electrodermal activity (e.g., peripheral cholinergic hypoactivity). *Second,* Bernstein et al. (1988) found that increasing the stimulus significance of the "innocuous" tones served to normalize the elicited SCR on initial trials in schizophrenia but not depression. Although signal stimuli do not always normalize elicited SCRs in schizophrenia (Dawson et al. 1992a; Iacono et al. 1993), these results do suggest that patients with schizophrenia have an orienting dysfunction that can be normalized (at least temporarily), whereas depressed patients have chronic peripheral (cholinergic?) deficits in EDA. *Third,* Lencz, Raine, and Sheard (1996) utilized cluster analysis of MRI and SCR data in patients with schizophrenia, affective disorders (mainly major depression), and controls. They found that SCR hyporesponsivity in schizophrenia was heterogeneous but tended to cluster with reduced prefrontal area and normal lateral ventricles, whereas SCR hyporesponsivity in affective disorder patients clustered more with normal prefrontal area and enlarged ventricles. Thus, schizophrenia patients and depressed patients may be SCR hyporesponsive for different reasons.

There are important lessons for all EDA researchers in this series of studies on psychopathology. The presence or absence of an SCR cannot be interpreted in isolation. In order to reasonably interpret the meaning of the presence or absence of an SCR, one needs to know the stimulus conditions eliciting the response (e.g., signal or nonsignal stimuli), and it is often useful to obtain other behavioral responses (e.g., secondary reaction time), psychophysiological responses (e.g., finger pulse volume), or brain imaging measures (e.g., MRI) in conjunction with the SCR.

Epilogue

Electrodermal activity has proven to be a useful psychophysiological tool with wide applicability. Social and behavioral scientists have found (i) that tonic EDA is useful for investigating general states of arousal and alertness and (ii) that the phasic SCR is useful for studying the multifaceted attentional process and stimulus significance, as well as individual differences that may be related to behavioral differences or psychopathological states. We believe that future research will continue to use EDA in a variety of situations and stimulus conditions to test these theoretical concepts.

Another important direction for future research involves sharpening the "inferential tool" characteristics of EDA itself. That is, basic research is needed to address the specific conditions under which specific EDA components reflect specific psychological and physiological processes and mechanisms. For example, under what stimulus conditions does the SCR amplitude component of the orienting response reflect automatic preattentive cognitive processes versus controlled cognitive processes? Likewise, under what test situations do the tonic and phasic EDA components reflect the different brain systems shown in Figure 2? We certainly hope that the expanding cognitive paradigms and neuroimaging techniques will be applied to elucidate these issues in both normal and abnormal populations, making EDA an even more useful psychophysiological tool.

NOTE

Michael Dawson was supported by a Research Scientist Development Award (K02 MH01086) from the National Institute of Mental Health during preparation of this chapter. We dedicate this chapter to William W. Grings, one of the pioneers in electrodermal activity, who served as mentor to the first two authors and friend to all three.

REFERENCES

Bauer, R. M. (1984). Autonomic recognition of names and faces in prosopagnosia: A neuropsychological application of the guilty knowledge test. *Neuropsychologia, 22*, 457–69.

Ben-Shakhar, G. (1977). A further study of the dichotomization theory of detection of information. *Psychophysiology, 14*, 408–13.

Ben-Shakhar, G. (1985). Standardization within individuals: Simple method to neutralize individual differences in skin conductance. *Psychophysiology, 22*, 292–9.

Bernstein, A., Frith, C., Gruzelier, J., Patterson, T., Straube, E., Venables, P., & Zahn, T. (1982). An analysis of the skin conductance orienting response in samples of American, British, and German schizophrenics. *Biological Psychology, 14*, 155–211.

Bernstein, A. S., Riedel, J. A., Graae, F., Seidman, D., Steele, H., Connolly, J., & Lubowsky, J. (1988). Schizophrenia is associated with altered orienting activity; depression with electrodermal (cholinergic?) deficit and normal orienting response. *Journal of Abnormal Psychology, 97*, 3–12.

Bernstein, A. S., Schnur, D. B., Bernstein, P., Yeager, A., Wrable, J., & Smith, S. (1995). Differing patterns of electrodermal and finger pulse responsivity in schizophrenia and depression. *Psychological Medicine, 25*, 51–62.

Bernstein, A. S., Taylor, K. W., Starkey, P., Juni, S., Lubowsky, J., & Paley, H. (1981). Bilateral skin conductance, finger pulse volume, and EEG orienting response to tones of differing intensities in chronic schizophrenics and controls. *Journal of Nervous and Mental Disease, 169*, 513–28.

Bloch, V. (1993). On the centennial of the discovery of electrodermal activity. In Roy et al. (1993a), pp. 1–6.

Bohlin, G. (1976). Delayed habituation of the electrodermal orienting response as a function of increased level of arousal. *Psychophysiology, 13*, 345–51.

Bohlin, G., & Kjellberg, A. (1979). Orienting activity two-stimulus paradigms as reflected in heart rate. In H. D. Kimmel, E. H. van Olst, & J. F. Orlebeke (Eds.), *The Orienting Reflex in Humans*, pp. 169–98. Hillsdale, NJ: Erlbaum.

Boucsein, W. (1992). *Electrodermal Activity*. New York: Plenum.

Boyd, R. W., & DiMascio, A. (1954). Social behavior and autonomic physiology (A sociophysiologic study). *Journal of Nervous and Mental Disease, 120*, 207–12.

Brown, G., Birley, J. L. T., & Wing, J. K. (1972). Influence of family life on the course of schizophrenia. *British Journal of Psychiatry, 121*, 241–8.

Bundy, R. S., & Fitzgerald, H. E. (1975). Stimulus specificity of electrodermal recovery time: An examination and reinterpretation of the evidence. *Psychophysiology, 12*, 406–11.

Byrne, D. G. (1975). A psychophysiological distinction between types of depressive states. *Australian and New Zealand Journal of Psychiatry, 9*, 181–5.

Crider, A. (1993). Electrodermal response lability-stability: Individual difference correlates. In Roy et al. (1993a), pp. 173–86.

Crider, A., & Augenbraun, C. (1975). Auditory vigilance correlates of electrodermal response habituation speed. *Psychophysiology, 12*, 36–40.

Darrow, C. W. (1927). Sensory, secretory, and electrical changes in the skin following bodily excitation. *Journal of Experimental Psychology, 10*, 197–226.

Darrow, C. W. (1937). Neural mechanisms controlling the palmar galvanic skin reflex and palmar sweating. *Archives of Neurology and Psychiatry, 37*, 641–63.

Davies, D. R., & Parasuraman, R. (1982). *The Psychology of Vigilance*. London: Academic Press.

Dawson, M. E., & Biferno, M. A. (1973). Concurrent measurement of awareness and electrodermal classical conditioning. *Journal of Experimental Psychology, 101*, 55–62.

Dawson, M. E., Filion, D. L., & Schell, A. M. (1989). Is elicitation of the autonomic orienting response associated with allocation of processing resources? *Psychophysiology, 26*, 560–72.

Dawson, M. E., & Nuechterlein, K. H. (1984). Psychophysiological dysfunctions in the developmental course of schizophrenic disorders. *Schizophrenia Bulletin, 10*, 204–32.

Dawson, M. E., Nuechterlein, K. H., & Liberman, R. P. (1983). Relapse in schizophrenic disorders: Possible contributing factors and implications for behavior therapy. In M. Rosenbaum, C. M. Franks, & Y. Jaffe (Eds.), *Perspectives on Behavior Therapy in the Eighties*, pp. 265–86. New York: Springer.

Dawson, M. E., Nuechterlein, K. H., & Schell, A. M. (1992a). Electrodermal anomalies in recent-onset schizophrenia: Relationships to symptoms and prognosis. *Schizophrenia Bulletin, 18,* 295–311.

Dawson, M. E., Neuchterlein, K. H., Schell, A. M., Gitlin, M., & Ventura, J. (1994). Autonomic abnormalities in schizophrenia: State or trait indicators? *Archives of General Psychiatry, 51,* 813–24.

Dawson, M. E., Nuechterlein, K. H., Schell, A. M., & Mintz, J. (1992b). Concurrent and predictive electrodermal correlates of symptomatology in recent-onset schizophrenic patients. *Journal of Abnormal Psychology, 101,* 153–64.

Dawson, M. E., & Schell, A. M. (1985). Information processing and human autonomic classical conditioning. In P. K. Ackles, J. R. Jennings, & M. G. H. Coles (Eds.), *Advances in Psychophysiology,* vol. 1, pp. 89–165. Greenwich, CT: JAI.

Dawson, M. E., Schell, A. M., & Catania, J. J. (1977). Autonomic correlates of depression and clinical improvement following electroconvulsive shock therapy. *Psychophysiology, 14,* 569–78.

Dittes, J. E. (1957). Galvanic skin response as a measure of patient's reaction to therapist's permissiveness. *Journal of Abnormal and Social Psychology, 55,* 295–303.

Edelberg, R. (1967). Electrical properties of the skin. In C. C. Brown (Ed.), *Methods in Psychophysiology,* pp. 1–53. Baltimore: Williams & Wilkins.

Edelberg, R. (1972a). Electrical activity of the skin: Its measurement and uses in psychophysiology. In N. S. Greenfield & R. A. Sternbach (Eds.), *Handbook of Psychophysiology,* pp. 367–418. New York: Holt.

Edelberg, R. (1972b). Electrodermal recovery rate, goal-orientation, and aversion. *Psychophysiology, 9,* 512–20.

Edelberg, R. (1973). Mechanisms of electrodermal adaptations for locomotion, manipulation, or defense. *Progress in Physiological Psychology, 5,* 155–209.

Edelberg, R. (1993). Electrodermal mechanisms: A critique of the two-effector hypothesis and a proposed replacement. In Roy et al. (1993a), pp. 7–29.

Engel, B. T. (1960). Stimulus-response and individual-response specificity. *Archives of General Psychiatry, 2,* 305–13.

Féré, C. (1888). Note on changes in electrical resistance under the effect of sensory stimulation and emotion. *Comptes Rendus des Seances de la Societe de Biologie (Ser. 9), 5,* 217–19.

Fowles, D. C. (1974). Mechanisms of electrodermal activity. In R. F. Thompson & M. M. Patterson (Eds.), *Methods in Physiological Psychology, Part C: Receptor and Effector Processes,* pp. 231–71. New York: Academic Press.

Fowles, D. C. (1986). The eccrine system and electrodermal activity. In M. G. H. Coles, E. Donchin, & S. W. Porges (Eds.), *Psychophysiology: Systems, Processes, and Applications,* pp. 51–96. New York: Guilford.

Fowles, D. C. (1988). Psychophysiology and psychopathology: A motivational approach. *Psychophysiology, 25,* 373–91.

Fowles, D., Christie, M. J., Edelberg, R., Grings, W. W., Lykken, D. T., & Venables, P. H. (1981). Publication recommendations for electrodermal measurements. *Psychophysiology, 18,* 232–9.

Fredrikson, M., Annas, P., Georgiades, A., Hursi, T., & Tesman, Z. (1993). Internal consistency and temporal stability of classically conditioned skin conductance responses. *Biological Psychology, 35,* 153–63.

Freedman, L. W., Scerbo, A. S., Dawson, M. E., Raine, A., McClure, W. O., & Venables, P. H. (1994). The relationship of sweat gland count to electrodermal activity. *Psychophysiology, 31,* 196–200.

Freixa i Baque, E. (1982). Reliability of electrodermal measures: A compilation. *Biological Psychology, 14,* 219–29.

Graham, F. K., & Clifton, R. K. (1966). Heart rate change as a component of the orienting response. *Psychological Bulletin, 65,* 305–20.

Grey, S. J., & Smith, B. L. (1984). A comparison between commercially available electrode gels and purpose-made gel, in the measurement of electrodermal activity. *Psychophysiology, 21,* 551–7.

Grings, W. W. (1974). Recording of electrodermal phenomena. In R. F. Thompson & M. M. Patterson (Eds.), *Bioelectric Recording Technique, Part C: Receptor and Effector Processes,* pp. 273–96. New York: Academic Press.

Grings, W. W., & Dawson, M. E. (1973). Complex variables in conditioning. In Prokasy & Raskin, pp. 203–54.

Grings, W. W., & Dawson, M. E. (1978). *Emotions and Bodily Responses: A Psychophysiological Approach.* New York: Academic Press.

Grings, W. W., & Lockhart, R. A. (1965). Problems of magnitude measurement with multiple GSRs. *Psychological Reports, 17,* 979–82.

Grings, W. W., & Schell, A. M. (1969). Magnitude of electrodermal response to a standard stimulus as a function of intensity and proximity of a prior stimulus. *Journal of Comparative and Physiological Psychology, 67,* 77–82.

Gruzelier, J. H., & Venables, P. H. (1972). Skin conductance orienting activity in a heterogenous sample of schizophrenics: Possible evidence of limbic dysfunction. *Journal of Nervous and Mental Disease, 155,* 277–87.

Hassett, J. (1978). *A Primer of Psychophysiology.* San Francisco: Freeman.

Hastrup, J. L. (1979). Effects of electrodermal lability and introversion on vigilance decrement. *Psychophysiology, 16,* 302–10.

Hazlett, E. A., Dawson, M. E., Buchsbaum, M. S., & Nuechterlein, K. H. (1993). Reduced regional brain glucose metabolism assessed by PET in electrodermal nonresponder schizophrenics: A pilot study. *Journal of Abnormal Psychology, 102,* 39–46.

Hazlett, E. A., Dawson, M. E., Filion, D. L., Schell, A. M., & Nuechterlein, K. H. (1997a). Autonomic orienting and the allocation of processing resources in schizophrenia patients and putatively at-risk individuals. *Journal of Abnormal Psychology, 106,* 171–81.

Hazlett, H., Dawson, M. E., Schell, A. M., & Nuechterlein, K. H. (1997b). Electrodermal activity as a prodromal sign in schizophrenia. *Biological Psychiatry, 41,* 111–13.

Hugdahl, K. (1978). Electrodermal conditioning to potentially phobic stimuli: Effects of instructed extinction. *Behavior Research and Therapy, 16,* 315–21.

Hugdahl, K. (1984). Hemispheric asymmetry and bilateral electrodermal recordings: A review of the evidence. *Psychophysiology, 21,* 371–93.

Hugdahl, K. (1995). *Psychophysiology: The Mind–Body Perspective.* Cambridge, MA: Harvard University Press.

Hugdahl, K., & Johnsen, B. H. (1993). Brain asymmetry and autonomic conditioning: Skin conductance responses. In Roy et al. (1993a), pp. 271–87.

Hugdahl, K., & Öhman, A. (1977). Effects of instruction on acquisition and extinction of electrodermal responses to fear-relevant stimuli. *Journal of Experimental Psychology: Human Learning and Memory, 3,* 608–18.

Humphreys, L. G. (1943). Measures of strength of conditioned eyelid responses. *Journal of General Psychology, 29,* 101–11.

Iacono, W. G., Ficken, J. W., & Beiser, M. (1993). Electrodermal nonresponding in first-episode psychosis as a function of stimulus significance. In Roy et al. (1993a), pp. 239–56.

Iacono, W. G., Lykken, D. T., Peloquin, L. T., Lumry, A. E., Valentine, R. H., & Tuoson, V. B. (1983). Electrodermal activity in euthymic unipolar and bipolar affective disorders. *Archives of General Psychiatry, 40,* 557–65.

Jakubovic, H. R., & Ackerman, A. B. (1985). Structure and function of the skin, Section I: Development, morphology, and physiology. In S. L. Moschella & H. J. Hurley (Eds.), *Dermatology,* vol. 1, pp. 1–74. Philadelphia: Saunders.

Jennings, J. R. (1986). Bodily changes during attending. In M. G. H. Coles, E. Donchin, & S. W. Porges (Eds.), *Psychophysiology: Systems, Processes, and Applications,* pp. 268–89. New York: Guilford.

Jennings, J. R., Ackles, P. K., & Coles, M. G. K. (1991). *Advances in Psychophysiology,* vol. 4. London: Jessica Kingsley.

Katkin, E. S. (1975). Electrodermal lability: A psychophysiological analysis of individual differences in response to stress. In I. G. Sarason & C. D. Spielberger (Eds.), *Stress and Anxiety,* vol. 2, pp. 141–76. Washington, DC: Aldine.

Katsanis, J., & Iacono, W. G. (1994). Electrodermal activity and clinical status in chronic schizophrenia. *Journal of Abnormal Psychology, 103,* 777–83.

Kelsey, R. M. (1991). Electrodermal lability and myocardial reactivity to stress. *Psychophysiology, 28,* 619–31.

Kutas, M. (1997). Views on how the electrical activity that the brain generates reflects the functions of different language structures. *Psychophysiology, 34,* 383–98.

Lacey, J. I., Kagan, J., Lacey, B. C., & Moss, H. A. (1963). The visceral level: Situational determinants and behavioral correlates of autonomic response patterns. In P. H. Knapp (Ed.), *Expression of the Emotions in Man,* pp. 161–96. New York: International Universities Press.

Lacey, J. I. & Lacey, B. C. (1958). Verification and extension of the principle of autonomic response-stereotypy. *American Journal of Psychology, 71,* 50–73.

Lader, M., & Noble, P. (1975). The affective disorders. In P. H. Venables and M. J. Christie (Eds.), *Research in Psychophysiology,* pp. 258–81. New York: Wiley.

Lader, M. H., & Wing, L. (1969). Physiological measures in agitated and retarded depressed patients. *Journal of Psychiatric Research, 7,* 89–100.

Landis, C. (1930). Psychology of the psychogalvanic reflex. *Psychological Review, 37,* 381–98.

Lencz, T., Raine, A., & Sheard, C. (1996). Neuroanatomical bases of electrodermal hypo-responding: A cluster analytic study. *International Journal of Psychophysiology, 22,* 141–53.

Levenson, R. W., & Gottman, J. M. (1983). Marital interaction: Physiological linkage and affective exchange. *Journal of Personality and Social Psychology, 45,* 587–97.

Levenson, R. W., & Gottman, J. M. (1985). Physiological and affective predictors of change in relationships satisfaction. *Journal of Personality and Social Psychology, 49,* 85–94.

Levinson, D. F., Edelberg, R., & Bridger, W. H. (1984). The orienting response in schizophrenia: Proposed resolution of a controversy. *Biological Psychiatry, 19,* 489–507.

Lim, C. L., Rennie, C., Barry, R. J., Bahramali, H., Lazzaro, I., Manor, B., & Gordon, E. (1997). Decomposing skin conductance into tonic phasic components. *International Journal of Psychophysiology, 25,* 97–109.

Lockhart, R. A., & Lieberman, W. (1979). Information content of the electrodermal orienting response. In H. D. Kimmel, E. H. van Olst, & J. F. Orlebeke (Eds.), *The Orienting Reflex in Humans,* pp. 685–700. Hillsdale, NJ: Erlbaum.

Lykken, D. T. (1959). The GSR in the detection of guilt. *Journal of Applied Psychology, 43,* 383–8.

Lykken, D. T. (1981). *A Tremor in the Blood.* New York: McGraw-Hill.

Lykken, D. T., Iacono, W. G., Haroian, K., McGue, M., & Bouchard, T. J. (1988). Habituation of the skin conductance response to strong stimuli: A twin study. *Psychophysiology, 25,* 4–15.

Lykken, D. T., Rose, R. J., Luther, B., & Maley, M. (1966). Correcting psychophysiological measures for individual differences in range. *Psychological Bulletin, 66,* 481–4.

Lykken, D. T., & Venables, P. H. (1971). Direct measurement of skin conductance: A proposal for standardization. *Psychophysiology, 8,* 656–72.

Lyytinen, H., Blomberg, A., & Näätänen, R. (1992). Event-related potentials and autonomic responses to a change in unattended auditory stimuli. *Psychophysiology, 29,* 523–34.

Mangina, C. A., & Beuzeron-Mangina, J. H. (1996). Direct electrical stimulation of specific human brain structures and bilateral electrodermal activity. *International Journal of Psychophysiology, 22,* 1–8.

McNally, R. J. (1987). Preparedness and phobias: A review. *Psychological Bulletin, 23,* 283–303.

Mirkin, A. M., & Coppen, A. (1980). Electrodermal activity in depression: Clinical and biochemical correlates. *British Journal of Psychiatry, 137,* 93–7.

Montague, J. D. (1963). Habituation of the psycho-galvanic reflex during serial tests. *Journal of Psychosomatic Research, 7,* 199–214.

Mundy-Castle, A. C., & McKiever, B. L. (1953). The psychophysiological significance of the galvanic skin response. *Journal of Experimental Psychology, 46,* 15–24.

Munro, L. L., Dawson, M. E., Schell, A. M., & Sakai, L. M. (1987). Electrodermal lability and rapid performance decrement in a degraded stimulus continuous performance task. *Journal of Psychophysiology, 1,* 249–57.

Nuechterlein, K. H., & Dawson, M. E. (1984). A heuristic vulnerability/stress model of schizophrenic episodes. *Schizophrenia Bulletin, 10,* 300–12.

Neumann, E., & Blanton, R. (1970). The early history of electrodermal research. *Psychophysiology, 6,* 453–75.

Öhman, A. (1979). The orienting response, attention and learning: An information processing perspective. In H. D. Kimmel, E. H. Van Olst, & J. F. Orlebeke (Eds.), *The Orienting Reflex in Humans.* Hillsdale, NJ: Erlbaum.

Öhman, A. (1981). Electrodermal activity and vulnerability to schizophrenia: A review. *Biological Psychology, 12,* 87–145.

Öhman, A. (1986). Face the beast and fear the face: Animal and social fears as prototypes for evolutionary analyses of emotion. *Psychophysiology, 23,* 123–45.

Öhman, A. (1992). Orienting and attention: Preferred preattentive processing of potentially phobic stimuli. In B. A. Campbell, H. Hayne, & R. Richardson (Eds.), *Attention and Information Processing in Infants and Adults: Perspectives from Human and Animal Research,* pp. 263–95. Hillsdale, NJ: Erlbaum.

Öhman, A., & Dimberg, U. (1978). Facial expressions as conditioned stimuli for electrodermal responses: A case of "preparedness"? *Journal of Personality and Social Psychology, 36,* 1251–8.

Öhman, A., Eriksson, A., & Olofsson, C. (1975). One-trial learning and superior resistance to extinction of autonomic responses conditioned to potentially phobic stimuli. *Journal of Comparative and Physiological Psychology, 88,* 619–27.

Öhman, A., Esteves, F., Flykt, A., & Soares, J. F. (1993). Gateways to consciousness: Emotion, attention, and electrodermal activity. In Roy et al. (1993a), pp. 137–57.

Öhman, A., Öhlund, L. S., Alm, T., Wieselgren, I. M., Istm, K., & Lindstrom, L. H. (1989). Electrodermal nonresponding, premorbid adjustment, and symptomatology as predictors of long-term social functioning in schizophrenics. *Journal of Abnormal Psychology, 98,* 426–35.

Porges, S. W., & Coles, M. G. H. (Eds.) (1976). *Psychophysiology.* Stroudsburg, PA: Dowden, Hutchinson, & Ross.

Prokasy, W. F. (1974). SCORIT: A computer subroutine for scoring electrodermal responses. *Behavior Research Methods and Instrumentation, 7,* 49–52.

Prokasy, W. F., & Kumpfer, K. L. (1973). Classical conditioning. In Prokasy & Raskin, pp. 157–202.

Prokasy, W. F., & Raskin, D.C. (Eds.). (1973). *Electrodermal Activity in Psychological Research.* New York: Academic Press.

Raine, A., & Lencz, T. (1993). Brain imaging research on electrodermal activity in humans. In Roy et al. (1993a), pp. 115–35.

Robertshaw, D. (1983). Apocrine sweat glands. In L. A. Goldsmith (Ed.), *Biochemistry and Physiology of the Skin,* pp. 642–53. New York: Oxford University Press.

Roy, J. C., Boucsein, W., Fowles, D. C., & Gruzelier, J. H. (Eds.) (1993a). *Progress in Electrodermal Research.* New York: Plenum.

Roy, J. C., Sequeira, H., & Delerm, B. (1993b). Neural control of electrodermal activity: Spinal and reticular mechanisms. In Roy et al. (1993a), pp. 73–92.

Sakai, M. L., Baker, L. A., & Dawson, M. E. (1992). Electrodermal lability: Individual differences affecting perceptual speed and vigilance performance in 9 to 16 year-old children. *Psychophysiology, 29,* 207–17.

Scerbo, A., Freedman, L. W., Raine, A., Dawson, M. E., & Venables, P. H. (1992). A major effect of recording site on measurement of electrodermal activity. *Psychophysiology, 29,* 241–6.

Schell, A. M., Dawson, M. E., & Filion, D. L. (1988). Psychophysiology correlates of electrodermal lability. *Psychophysiology, 25,* 619–32.

Schell, A. M., Dawson, M. E., & Marinkovic, K. (1991). Effects of potentially phobic conditioned stimuli on retention, reconditioning, and extinction of the conditioned skin conductance response. *Psychophysiology, 28,* 140–53.

Schwartz, G. E., & Shapiro, D. (1973). Social psychophysiology. In Prokasy & Raskin, pp. 377–416.

Seligman, M. E. P. (1970). On the generality of the laws of learning. *Psychological Review, 77,* 307–21.

Sequeira, H., & Roy, J. C. (1993). Cortical and hypothalamo-limbic control of electrodermal responses. In Roy et al. (1993a), pp. 93–114.

Shields, S. A., MacDowell, K. A., Fairchild, S. B., & Campbell, M. L. (1987). Is mediation of sweating cholinergic, adrenergic, or both? A comment on the literature. *Psychophysiology, 24,* 312–19.

Siddle, D. (1991). Orienting, habituation, and resource allocation: An associative analysis. *Psychophysiology, 28,* 245–59.

Siddle, D., Stephenson, D., & Spinks, J. A. (1983). Elicitation and habituation of the orienting response. In D. Siddle (Ed.), *Orienting and Habituation: Perspectives in Human Research,* pp. 109–82. Chichester, U.K.: Wiley.

Sokolov, E. N. (1963). *Perception and the Conditioned Reflex.* New York: Macmillan.

Sponheim, S. R., Allen, J. J., & Iacono, W. G. (1995). Selected psychophysiological measures in depression: The significance of electrodermal activity, electroencephalographic asymmetries, and contingent negative variation to behavioral and neurobiological aspects of depression. In G. A. Miller (Ed.), *The Behavioral High-Risk Paradigm in Psychopathology,* pp. 222–49. New York: Springer.

Straube, E. R. (1979). On the meaning of electrodermal nonresponding in schizophrenia. *Journal of Nervous and Mental Disease, 167,* 601–11.

Strayer, D. L., & Williams, W. C. (1982). *SCORIT 1980.* Paper presented at the annual meeting of the Society for Psychophysiological Research (Washington, DC).

Sturgeon, D., Turpin, G., Kuipers, L., Berkowitz, R., & Leff, J. (1984). Psychophysiological responses of schizophrenic patients to high and low expressed emotion relatives: A follow-up study. *British Journal of Psychiatry, 145,* 62–9.

Tarchanoff, J. (1890). Galvanic phenomena in the human skin during stimulation of the sensory organs and during various forms of mental activity. *Pflügers Archiv für die gesammte Physiologie des Menschen und der Tiere, 46,* 46–55.

Tarrier, N., Vaughn, C., Lader, M. H., & Leff, J. P. (1979). Bodily reactions to people and events in schizophrenics. *Archives of General Psychiatry, 36,* 311–15.

Tranel, D., & Damasio, A. R. (1985). Knowledge without awareness: An autonomic index of facial recognition by prosopagnosics. *Science, 228,* 1453–4.

Tranel, D., & Damasio, A.R. (1993). The covert learning of affective valence does not require structures in hippocampal system or amygdala. *Journal of Cognitive Neuroscience, 5,* 79–88.

Tranel, D., & Damasio, H. (1994). Neuroanatomical correlates of electrodermal skin conductance responses. *Psychophysiology, 31,* 427–38.

Tranel, D., Fowles, D. C., & Damasio, A. R. (1985). Electrodermal discrimination of familiar and unfamiliar faces: A methodology. *Psychophysiology, 22,* 403–8.

Turpin, G. (1983). Psychophysiology, psychopathology, and the social environment. In A. Gale & J. A. Edwards (Eds.), *Physiological Correlates of Human Behavior,* pp. 265–80. New York: Academic Press.

Turpin, G., Tarrier, N., & Sturgeon, D. (1988). Social psychophysiology and the study of biopsychosocial models of schizophrenia. In H. Wagner (Ed.), *Social Psychophysiology.* Chichester, U.K.: Wiley.

Uno, T., & Grings, W. W. (1965). Autonomic components of orienting behavior. *Psychophysiology, 1,* 311–21.

Vaughn, C., & Leff, J. P. (1976). The influence of family and social factors on the course of psychiatric illness. *British Journal of Psychiatry, 129,* 125–37.

Vaughn, C. E., Snyder, K. S., Jones, S., Freeman, W. B., & Falloon, I. R. H. (1984). Family factors in schizophrenic relapse: A California replication of the British research on expressed emotion. *Archives of General Psychiatry, 41,* 1169–77.

Venables, P. H., & Christie, M. J. (1973). Mechanisms, instrumentation, recording techniques, and quantification of responses. In Prokasy & Raskin, pp. 1–124.

Venables, P. H., & Christie, M. J. (1980). Electrodermal activity. In I. Martin & P. H. Venables (Eds.), *Techniques in Psychophysiology,* pp. 3–67. Chichester, U.K.: Wiley.

Venables, P. H., & Mitchell, D. A. (1996). The effects of age, sex and time of testing on skin conductance activity. *Biological Psychology, 43,* 87–101.

Vigouroux, R. (1879). Sur le role de la resistance electrique des tissues dans l'electro-diagnostic. *Comptes Rendus Societe de Biologie, 31,* 336–9.

Vigouroux, R. (1888). The electrical resistance considered as a clinical sign. *Progres Medicale, 3,* 87–9.

Vossel, G., & Rossman, R. (1984). Electrodermal habituation speed and visual monitoring performance. *Psychophysiology, 21,* 97–100.

Wallin, B. G. (1981). Sympathetic nerve activity underlying electrodermal and cardiovascular reactions in man. *Psychophysiology, 18,* 470–6.

Wang, G. H. (1964). *The Neural Control of Sweating.* Madison: University of Wisconsin Press.

Ward, N. G., Doerr, H. O., & Storrie, M. C. (1983). Skin conductance: A potentially sensitive test for depression. *Psychiatry Research, 10,* 295–302.

Wenger, M. A., Clemens, T. L., Coleman, M. A., Cullen, T. D., & Engel, B. T. (1961). Autonomic response specificity. *Psychosomatic Medicine, 23,* 185–93.

Winer, B. J., Brown, D. R., & Michels, K. M. (1991). *Statistical Principles in Experimental Design.* New York: McGraw-Hill.

Woodworth, R. S., & Schlosberg, H. (1954). *Experimental Psychology,* rev. ed. New York: Holt.

Zahn, T. P. (1986). Psychophysiological approaches to psychopathology. In M. G. H. Coles, E. Donchin, & S. W. Porges (Eds.), *Psychophysiology: Systems, Processes, and Applications,* pp. 508–610. New York: Guilford.

CHAPTER NINE

CARDIOVASCULAR PSYCHOPHYSIOLOGY

K. A. BROWNLEY, B. E. HURWITZ, & N. SCHNEIDERMAN

Introduction

The discipline of psychophysiology is organized around the study of psychological events and the influence they have on biological processes. Cardiovascular psychophysiology, in particular, examines the impact of such psychological phenomena on functioning of the circulatory system and, as an applied science, focuses on understanding the complex relationships between behavioral stress and cardiovascular-related disease. Technological advancements introduced in the past two decades – in the form of reliable noninvasive methodologies to measure cardiac structure and function and to assess hemodynamic contributions to circulatory control – have enhanced the pursuit of these objectives. As a result, there is a growing appreciation for the unique individual and situational factors that mediate the impact of psychological processes and stress along the health–disease continuum.

The purpose of this chapter is threefold. First, it reviews the structural, mechanical, and electrical bases of cardiovascular functioning; second, it provides an overview of various methodologies currently used in cardiovascular psychophysiological research, with a particular emphasis on issues of reliability and validity; and third, it examines current issues related to the assessment of cardiovascular reactivity and its role in cardiovascular pathology.

Physical Context

ORGANIZATION OF THE CIRCULATORY SYSTEM

The circulatory system is organized into two primary subdivisions: the pulmonary and the systemic circulation. As depicted in Figure 1, the entire system is arranged as a continuous vascular circuit consisting of a pump (heart) together with a network of high-pressure distribution (arteries and arterioles), exchange (capillaries), and low-pressure collection and return (venules and veins) vessels that circulate blood throughout the body (see Tortora & Anagnostakos 1990; Waller & Schlant 1994). The heart muscle (myocardium) is comprised of a left and right pump, each having two chambers – an atrium and a ventricle. Blood is ejected from the left ventricle and traverses the body, delivering nutrients and removing metabolic by-products essential to cell function. Deoxygenated blood returns to the right atrium through the superior and inferior vena cava and passes through the tricuspid valve to the right ventricle. Contraction of the right ventricle directs the blood through the pulmonary artery to the lungs, where blood is reoxygenated and then returned to the left atrium via the pulmonary vein. The bicuspid valve regulates unidirectional flow of this oxygen-rich blood into the left ventricle, and the circuit is completed.

The efficiency with which the heart supplies blood to the body reflects its capacity to contract rhythmically as a unit. This capacity is a function of the multinucleated, striated fibrous structure of cardiac tissue and a specialized conduction system that coordinates sequential excitation and contraction of the atria and ventricles. This arrangement enables cellular depolarization originating in the right atrium to be transmitted rapidly throughout the heart. The process begins with atrial depolarization, during which both ventricles are relaxed, followed by ventricular depolarization, during which the atria repolarize, and a quiescent period, during which all chambers are in repolarization. The contraction phase is referred to as *systole* and the relaxation phase as *diastole*. A full sequence of atrial and ventricular systole and diastole constitutes a single cardiac cycle.

Under normal circumstances, increasing contractile tension in the left ventricle, superimposed on a brief period

John T. Cacioppo, Louis G. Tassinary, and Gary G. Berntson (Eds.), *Handbook of Psychophysiology*, 2nd ed. © Cambridge University Press 2000. Printed in the United States of America. ISBN 62634X. All rights reserved.

during which all cardiac valves are closed, rapidly elevates intraventricular pressure. When intraventricular pressure exceeds the opposing aortic valve pressure, the aorta is thrust open and blood is ejected from the left ventricle. Blood pulses from the heart at high velocity and is slowed by the resistance encountered in smaller arteries and arterioles; pressure decreases until blood flow at the level of the capillaries is steady. The amount of blood passing through a blood vessel at any moment is determined by two factors: blood pressure and resistance to flow. Blood pressure is a measure of the amount of force exerted by blood on a vessel wall and is directly proportional to total blood volume. Resistance is a measure of all factors that oppose blood flow and is dictated by two principal factors: (a) blood viscosity, which is an expression of the ratio of red blood cells and other solutes to fluid; and (b) vessel geometry – resistance to flow is directly proportional to vessel length and inversely proportional to vessel radius. Blood flow is proportional to blood pressure and follows a pressure gradient throughout the body, flowing from regions of high pressure to low pressure. In a young adult human, systemic arterial blood pressure fluctuates between approximately 120 mmHg (systolic) and 80 mmHg (diastolic); pressure dissipates as blood flows from the arterial (~30 mmHg) to the venule (~10 mmHg) side of the capillary bed and returns to the right atrium (~0 mmHg). The average blood pressure, or mean arterial pressure (MAP), at any given moment is a product of the total resistance and the total amount of circulating fluid volume. Although these variables can be measured directly using invasive procedures, measures of cardiac output and total peripheral resistance (TPR) derived noninvasively in the research laboratory by such techniques as impedance cardiography are more than adequate substitutes for assessing cardiovascular functioning.

It is important to keep in mind that blood flow abides by the rule of demand and supply; demand for oxygen by active tissues dictates the rate at which the body circulates hemoglobin and, therefore, blood. Demand is created preferentially by the organs that cannot sustain themselves anaerobically; these organs are the brain, heart, and lungs. The rate at which blood is delivered from the heart is referred to as cardiac output. The amount of blood pumped from the left ventricle per minute (i.e., cardiac output) is the product of stroke volume and the number of beats per minute (i.e., heart rate):

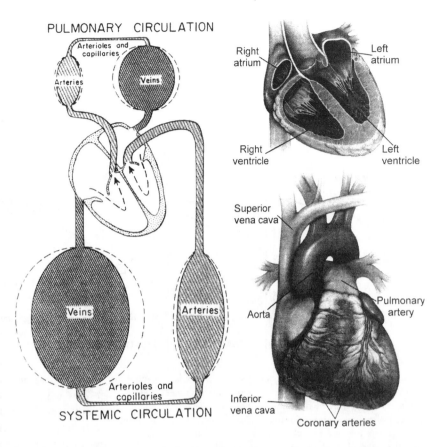

Figure 1. Functional divisions of the circulation are depicted on the left and include the pulmonary circulation, which delivers blood to the lungs for the elimination of carbon dioxide and the acquisition of oxygen. The systemic circulation transports oxygen, other nutrients, and other substances to all tissues of the body. When the right and left atria contract, they propel blood into the respective ventricles. The right ventricle contracts and propels blood toward the lungs through the pulmonary artery, whereas the left ventricle contracts and delivers blood through the aorta to the body's tissues. With the onset of left and right ventricular contraction, the atrioventricular valves close, the aortic and pulmonic valves open, and blood is ejected. A hemisection of the heart is shown on the upper right side of the figure, where the right and left atria and ventricles are indicated. An external view of the heart is shown on the lower right side of the figure, indicating the major blood vessels to and from the heart.

$$\text{cardiac output} = \text{stroke volume} \times \text{heart rate}.$$

Stroke volume may be determined by calculating the difference between end-diastolic volume (EDV), which is the amount of blood that enters a ventricle during diastole, and end-systolic volume (ESV), which is the volume of blood remaining in the ventricle after systole. The EDV, which is typically in the range of 120–130 ml, is directly related to venous pressure and inversely related to the length of ventricular diastole. The ESV, which is typically about 50–60 ml, is influenced both by the force of ventricular contraction and by arterial pressure. In the average adult, resting stroke volume is approximately 70 ml and resting cardiac output normally ranges between 4 and 7 l/min.

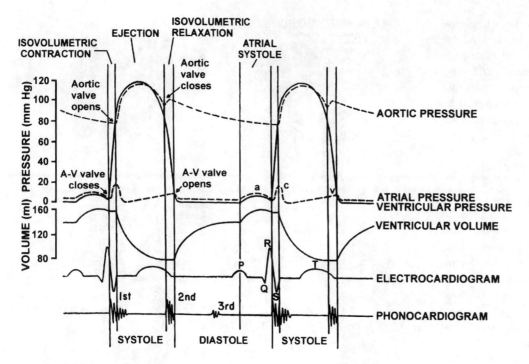

Figure 2. Electromechanical events of two cardiac cycles: changes in aortic, atrial, and ventricular pressure; ventricular volume; the electrocardiogram (ECG); and the phonocardiogram (PCG). A single cycle consists of one relaxation (diastole) and one contraction (systole) period. Aortic pressure falls throughout diastole following opening of the atrioventricular (AV) valve, increases rapidly after the aortic valve opens and blood is ejected. The "a," "c," and "v" waves represent the elevation waves of left atrial pressure. Ventricular pressure is relatively unchanged during diastole but increases dramatically during the isovolumetric contraction period, when the aortic valve is closed. Once ventricular pressure exceeds aortic pressure, the aortic valve opens and ejection occurs (i.e. systole). Ventricular pressure initially increases during systole and then dissipates rapidly. Ventricular volume increases gradually during diastolic passive filling and following depolarization of the SA node (onset of atrial systole), and it decreases rapidly following ejection. The ECG P wave coincides with atrial depolarization and signifies the onset of atrial contraction, which enhances ventricular filling. The ECG QRS wave denotes ventricular depolarization, which signifies ventricular contraction and completion of the cardiac cycle. The point at which ventricular pressure exceeds arterial pressure and the aortic valve opens (allowing blood to be ejected) is marked by the first heart sound on the PCG. Aortic valve closure, marked by the second heart sound of the PCG, coincides with the point at which ventricular pressure drops below aortic pressure.

FUNCTIONING OF THE CIRCULATORY SYSTEM
The Cardiac Cycle

The bulk transport of blood is influenced by mechanical properties of the heart itself. These properties, which act independently of neural control, include the opening and closing of the heart valves and the contraction of cardiac muscle. These events are marked by distinct changes in blood volume and pressure within the various chambers of the heart. For illustrative purposes, it is useful to concep-

tualize these activities by examining the electromechanical events within a cardiac cycle (see Figure 2). The next sections provide an overview of the major electromechanical attributes of the cardiac cycle and highlight issues related to their measurement. For a more detailed review see Guyton (1981), Tortora and Anagnostakos (1990), Strackee and Westerhof (1993), Schlant and Sonnenblick (1994), and Dubin (1996).

Mechanical Events of the Cardiac Cycle. As can be seen in Figure 2, the cardiac cycle can be broken down into three primary stages: (1) atrial systole, (2) ventricular systole, and (3) ventricular diastole. Firing of the sinoatrial (SA) node triggers the first stage, atrial systole. Both atrioventricular valves are closed during this phase, causing both atrial tension and pressure to build as blood fills the atria. Atrial contraction forces deoxygenated blood from the right atrium through the open tricuspid valve into the right ventricle, and oxygenated blood is forced from the left atrium through the open bicuspid valve into the left ventricle. Under normal resting conditions, blood flows passively in these directions without the drive of atrial contraction; thus, this action accounts for the movement of approximately 30% of bulk flow through the heart. The second stage, ventricular systole, occurs in two phases: (i) isometric or isovolumetric contraction, which lasts approximately 50 msec, and (ii) ejection. During isovolumetric contraction, the ventricles contract in the presence of a closed aortic valve, which causes a rapid increase in ventricular pressure despite no appreciable change in ventricular volume. Once ventricular pressure exceeds arterial pressure, the aortic and pulmonary semilunar valves open and blood is ejected from the ventricles. The ejection phase lasts approximately 250 msec and concludes with the closure of the aortic valve. The amount of blood ejected from the heart with each beat is referred to as stroke volume and is roughly 50%–80% of the total ventricular blood volume. The third stage, ventricular diastole, also occurs in two phases. Immediately following ventricular contraction, a brief (50-msec) period of isometric relaxation occurs between closure of the semilunar valves and opening of the atrioventricular valves. Ventricular pressure decreases dramatically and ventricular volume is relatively constant, so blood flows passively back toward the ventricles and the semilunar valves close. Once ventricular pressure declines below atrial pressure, the atrioventricular (AV) valves open and a more pronounced ventricular filling occurs. This period of ventricular filling is often described as having three successive components: (a) rapid filling, which accounts for the majority of blood flow into the ventricles; (b) diastasis, which is attributed to small amounts of blood emptying directly from the vena cavae, coronary sinus, and pulmonary veins into the ventricles through the open AV valves; and (c) slow filling, which coincides with atrial systole. These mechanical events are time-locked with detectable electrical changes in the myocardium, which can be recorded using a standard electrocardiogram (ECG), and with heart sounds, which can be detected with a phonocardiogram (PCG).

Electrical Events of the Cardiac Cycle. The ECG records the electrical impulses that stimulate the heart and cause it to contract. Cardiac cells are said to be "polarized" in the resting state, meaning that the interior is negatively charged relative to the cell surface. Electrical stimulation permits an influx of positively charged ions (predominantly sodium) and causes depolarization of the cells. An advancing wave of depolarization causes the progressive contraction of the cardiac cells, and during repolarization the negative charge within each cell is restored. The successive phases of depolarization and repolarization within each cardiac cycle are detected by ECG electrodes placed on the limbs or body surface and are recorded as deflections in voltage amplitude of the electrical signal. This record can provide fairly detailed information about the integrity of various idiosyncratic properties of the heart. In the following sections, key features of the cardiac conduction system and the ECG waveform are highlighted, and clinical manifestations of various types of cardiac arrhythmias and the techniques available to monitor them in the ambulatory setting are examined.

Atrioventricular Conduction. The conduction system consists of the sinoatrial node, the atrioventricular node, the Bundle of His, and the Purkinje system. A cardiac cycle is initiated within the SA node, a small group of cells within the posterior wall of the right atrium. These unique cells spontaneously depolarize and repolarize at a rate that exceeds the self-excitability rate of other cardiac pacemaker cells. The self-excitation characteristic of the SA

nodal cells is fundamentally linked to their resting membrane potential, which is lower than other cardiac cells. The rate of depolarization in the SA node (105–110/min) exceeds that in the AV node (40–60/min) and Purkinje system (20–40/min). This hierarchy ensures that, under normal circumstances, impulse generation will begin in the SA node and spread throughout the myocardium in a manner that prevents other cardiac cells from generating their own action potentials. Whereas the SA node is the primary pacemaker responsible for intrinsically regulating heart rate, the AV node is the initiating site for ventricular depolarization. In addition, the AV node is responsible for gating the impulse to allow for contraction of the right atrium before ventricular depolarization occurs. Circuitous movement of the impulse is prevented because transit time through the Purkinje fiber system exceeds that of the refractory period for cardiac muscle; thus, AV node cells can not be restimulated within the same cardiac cycle.

Characteristics of the ECG Waveform. A single cardiac cycle is recorded on the ECG as a series of three primary waves, which are designated by letters, and three intervals, which are identified by the waves that mark their beginning and end (Figure 2). Each wave and interval convey explicit information regarding the conduction system and/or the metabolic state of the heart. Atrial depolarization is designated by the P wave, electrical stimulation of the ventricles is recorded as the QRS complex, and repolarization of the ventricles is represented by the T wave. The P-R interval incorporates atrial depolarization, the subsequent pause in the impulse transmission at the AV node, and overall conduction time for passage of the action potential from the atrium to the ventricular muscle. The Q-T interval designates the full sequence of ventricular depolarization and repolarization. The S-T interval originates at the "j point" of the QRS complex (i.e., the end of the S wave, or that point designated by the return of the ECG tracing to its isoelectric baseline) and ends at the completion of ventricular repolarization. Different aspects of the Q-T interval are diagnostically relevant. For example, a change in the duration of the QRS wave indicates a conduction abnormality in the Bundle of His, depression of the S-T segment is associated with myocardial ischemia, and an elongation of the Q-T interval may be related to sudden cardiac death.

Sinus Rhythm and Arrhythmias. Although the intrinsic SA node firing rate is approximately 105 beats per minute (bpm), the heart rate is usually about 60–80 bpm in the average seated adult because of extrinsic neuronal and neuroendocrine factors. In particular, the differences between the intrinsic rate of the heart (105 bpm) and the resting rate (60–80 bpm) is due to the neuronal restraint upon the heart caused by the vagus nerves. An increase in heart rate, such as that occurring during stressful behavioral challenge or exercise, may result from an increase in sympathetic cardiac input or an unloading of vagal cardiac input. In contrast, a resting heart rate level below 60 bpm is not uncommon in the sleeping adult or in an awake, highly conditioned endurance athlete. In the latter case, the tonic heart rate deceleration (bradycardia) may reflect the cumulative effects of an increase in vagal cardiac input and a decrease in both the sympathetic cardiac input and the intrinsic SA node firing rate (McArdle, Katch, & Katch 1986).

Rhythmic dysfunction may occur when the SA node fires at varying intervals, when impulses are generated from sites other than from the SA node, when impulse transmission is blocked within the conduction system, or when abnormal conduction pathways develop. These conditions may be exacerbated during extreme emotional or chemical (e.g., amphetamine) stress and revealed on the ECG as irregularly timed, extra, or skipped beats. Isolated regions of excitation localized in the atria tend to give rise to abnormal P waves, whereas those located in the ventricle tend to augment the amplitude of the R and S waves. Premature ventricular contractions (PVC) can increase risk of cardiac mortality in post–myocardial infarction (MI) patients; however, in asymptomatic individuals they are relatively benign because they do not typically alter the normal sinus rhythm. Depending on their location, blockages in the conduction pathway can (i) elongate particular intervals within or widen the overall QRS complex or (ii) either suppress the normal P wave or produce extra P waves. When an impulse reenters and excites regions of the heart more than once (i.e., circuit reentry), the arrhythmia may be manifest as premature beats or as a sustained tachycardia, depending on the number of reiterations of a given reentry pathway (Hondeghem & Roden 1995). Unusually rapid rhythms that can occur at rest include paroxysmal tachycardia (the sudden onset of heart rate between 150 and 250 bpm), flutter (a single atrial or ventricular ectopic focus firing between 250 and 350 bpm), and ventricular fibrillation (simultaneous firing of multiple ectopic foci resulting in chaotic twitching of the ventricles).

Contractile Properties of the Myocardium. Numerous intrinsic and extrinsic factors regulate the efficiency with which the heart is able to propel blood into the peripheral circulatory system (Smith & Kampine 1990). The primary intrinsic factors, which reflect the contractile properties of the cardiac muscle itself, include preload, afterload, contractility, and heart rate. The principal extrinsic factors that influence contractility fall into three general categories: neurohormonal, chemical and pharmacological, and pathological.

Within physiological limits, the amount of force generated by a contracting muscle is directly related to the extent of precontraction stretch in the muscle. As fiber length increases, muscle tension and force increase independently of any change in time to peak contractile force (Sonnenblick 1962). The implications of these relationships

with respect to the myocardium are formally described by Starling's "law of the heart." According to Starling's law, an increase in precontraction ventricular stretch (i.e. preload) that is associated with increased EDV produces greater peak systolic pressure and greater stroke volume. Because of this relationship, the heart is able to autoregulate cardiac output to accommodate beat-by-beat changes in venous return. In addition, the heart is able to maintain balance between right and left ventricular output and to meet the cardiopulmonary demand associated with different types of challenge (e.g. exercise).

The relationship between arterial pressure and stroke volume is also complexly determined. Loosely defined, stroke volume is enhanced by greater ventricular contraction and is opposed by elevations in arterial pressure. More specifically, ESV is determined in part by the length of myocardial fibers – greater fiber length stretch produces stronger contraction and increases stroke volume. In contrast, an increase in afterload (i.e., the cumulative effects of systemic vascular resistance, blood viscosity and volume, and vascular compliance on resistance to flow) tends to limit or reduce stroke volume. Afterload can be viewed as being analogous to the arterial pressure determinant of ESV, and for this reason TPR and (less adequately) MAP are commonly recognized as indices of afterload.

Myocardial contractility can be conceptualized as either a measure of the work performed by the heart when load forces remain static or as a measure of the actual velocity with which myocardial fibers shorten. Various techniques have been developed to measure contractility on the basis of these two models (i.e., pressure/volume vs. velocity). Since the relationship between ventricular pressure and volume changes as a function of afterload over the cardiac cycle, measurements are typically obtained at four time points: end-diastole, aortic valve opening, end-systole, and mitral valve opening and closing. Simultaneous measurements of volume and pressure at these intervals can be plotted over a series of cardiac cycles to obtain a family of pressure–volume loops. These plots can be used to derive a nonlinear pressure–volume curve, which describes passive ventricular stretch (preload), and a linear pressure–volume curve, which depicts the relationship between end-systolic pressure (ESP) and end-systolic volume (ESV). The slope of the ESP–ESV line subsequently can be used to describe contractility. The independence of this relationship from both preload and afterload forces has been demonstrated both experimentally (Piene & Covell 1981) and clinically (Mehmel et al. 1981). This method of estimating contractility is highly invasive, and the use of beta-adrenergic blockade to preclude extrinsic control of the heart may confound the measurement of other dependent variables in the typical psychophysiological research setting.

The relationship between velocity of cardiac papillary muscle fiber shortening and load was initially described by an inverse hyperbolic function (Sonnenblick 1962). The term V_{max} was coined to refer to the theoretical velocity of fiber shortening at zero load (i.e. contractility). Subsequently, quantitative techniques to characterize V_{max} on the basis of the rate of pressure development (dP/dt) during isovolumetric contraction have been developed. These measurements can be derived invasively using micromanometer-tip catheters or by direct angiographic measurement of the mean velocity of circumferential fiber shortening. Fortunately, they can also be derived using noninvasive echocardiographic measures (see the section entitled "Transthoracic Echocardiography") that are more accessible to the researcher and have proven to be highly correlated with angiographic measures.

Neural Control of the Circulation

In addition to the intrinsic rhythmicity of the myocardium, cardiovascular activity is regulated extrinsically by various local, reflexive, and central nervous system (CNS) mechanisms. The integration of these regulatory factors provides the basis for both the homeostatic and adaptive functions of the cardiovascular system. The following sections focus on (a) the primary CNS mechanisms controlling circulation; (b) the effector branch of the autonomic nervous system (ANS), that portion of the CNS that controls cardiac, smooth muscle, and glandular activity; and (c) cardiovascular reflex mechanisms involved in circulatory control. Reviews of these topics can be found elsewhere (Andresen & Kunze 1994; Levy & Vassalle 1982; Loewy 1982; Randall 1977, 1984; Swanson 1982).

Central Pathways and Mechanisms. Central regulation of the circulation involves structures within the spinal cord, hindbrain, and forebrain. Figure 3 displays a summary of the CNS pathways of cardiovascular control. Axons projecting from the intermediolateral cell column (IML) of the spinal cord connect to the heart and smooth muscle of blood vessels. The ventrolateral medulla (VLM), which is located in the hindbrain, mediates tonic and phasic changes in blood pressure and heart rate. Together with the dorsal motor nucleus of the vagus (DVN), the nucleus ambiguus (NA), and the nucleus tractus solitarius (NTS), these hindbrain structures are key components of the baroreceptor reflex arc.

Two major divisions of the forebrain that are thought to play important roles in the regulation of the cardiovascular system are the hypothalamus and the cerebral cortex. Nuclei within the hypothalamus project along CNS pathways to the brain and spinal cord but also release vasopressin into the portal system of the posterior pituitary, which is then released into the circulation. Vasopressin is involved in blood volume regulation and modulates autonomic reflexes in the lower brainstem and spinal cord. The cerebral cortex is involved in the integration of information (based on sensory input, perception, and emotion) that influences blood pressure and heart rate responses to psychogenic

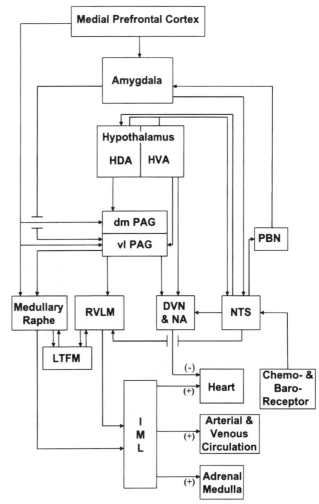

Figure 3. Summary of proposed CNS pathways involved in circulatory regulation. Abbreviations are as follows: HDA/HVA, hypothalamic "defense" and "vigilance" areas; dmPAG/vlPAG, dorsomedial and ventrolateral periaqueductal grey; PBN, parabrachial nucleus of the pons; RVLM, rostral ventrolateral medulla; DVN, dorsal vagal nucleus; NA, nucleus ambiguus; NTS, nucleus tractus solitarius; LTFM, lateral tegmental field of the medulla; IML, intermediolateral cell column of the spinal cord. The sympathetic and parasympathetic branches mediating cardiac and vascular control have cell bodies of origin in the IML and DVN/NA nuclei. Chemo- and baroreceptors provide feedback of chemical and pressure information to the NTS. Reprinted with permission from Winters, McCabe, Green, & Schneiderman, "Stress responses, coping and cardiovascular neurobiology: Central nervous system circuitry underlying learned and unlearned affective responses to stressful stimuli," in McCabe, Schneiderman, & Field (Eds.), *Stress, Coping, and Cardiovascular Disease.* Copyright 2000 Lawrence Erlbaum Associates, Inc.

challenge. The amygdala and other limbic system structures play a critical role in linking stimuli to appropriate emotional responses and, along with the hypothalamus and the periaqueductal gray (PAG) of the midbrain, are involved in regulating the cardiorespiratory components of the "defense" and "vigilance" reactions (see section entitled "Response Patterning"). Specifically, the posterior hypothalamus at sites dorsal and medial to the fornix – labeled as the hypothalamus defense area (HDA) in Figure 3 – and the dorsal PAG are associated with the "defense" or "fight or flight" reaction, which is characterized by increased cardiac output and minimal changes in total peripheral resistance. In contrast, the dorsolateral portion of the posterior hypothalamus – labeled as the hypothalamic vigilance area (HVA) – and the ventrolateral PAG are part of the neurocircuitry that mediates the "vigilance reaction," which is characterized by increased total peripheral resistance, a slowing of the heart rate, and facilitation of the baroreceptor reflex. Collectively, this circuitry underlies affective responses to stressful stimuli and, as such, has a fundamental role in integrating the effects of environmental events on cardiovascular responsiveness (Winters et al. 2000). Much of what is known about central neural networks involved in circulatory control has been derived from retrograde neuroanatomical tracings of specific pathways, electrophysiological recordings to confirm that given structures are components of specific pathways, and immunohistochemical tracings of neurotransmitter pathways. The following paragraphs offer a perspective on their integration at both an anatomical and a behavioral level.

The major cell groups in the forebrain that project to the dorsal vagal complex and the IML are located within the hypothalamus. Projections from the central nucleus of the amygdala, the prefrontal cortex, the nucleus of the stria terminalis, and the lateral and posterior hypothalamic nuclei innervate the NTS. Fibers arising from the IML constitute the primary sympathetic nervous system efferent projections innervating the myocardium and smooth muscle vessels. Vagal cardioinhibitory (parasympathetic) axons projecting from the DVN, along with axons from the NA of the medulla oblongata, exert a direct influence on heart rate and an indirect influence on myocardial contractility.

The primary afferent systems involved in circulatory control consist of the carotid sinus and aortic depressor nerves, which are also known as the "buffer" nerves. The buffer nerves convey information about blood pressure and blood chemistry to the CNS. Transection of these nerves leads to dysregulation of resting blood pressure, pathologic blood pressure lability, and neurogenic hypertension. Carotid sinus nerve projections terminate predominantly in the medial, lateral, dorsolateral, and commissural subnuclei of the NTS and, to a lesser extent, in other NTS subnuclei and brainstem areas (e.g., area postrema, nucleus ambiguus, external cuneate nucleus). Aortic depressor nerve projections are similarly distributed in the solitary complex, with the densest areas of termination being in the interstitial nucleus and dorsolateral aspect. The precise array of active neurotransmitters released from afferent fibers synapsing in the NTS has not been fully elucidated, although norepinephrine (NE), epinephrine (E), and dopamine injections into this region decrease heart rate and blood pressure, and pathologic blood pressure la-

bility develops following destruction of catecholaminergic terminals in the NTS.

Multiple central interconnected pathways have also been described. The hypothalamic-medullary complex, which integrates cardio-respiratory metabolic control, consists of four primary interchange sites. The ventrolateral medulla (VLM), the parabrachial nucleus, the paraventricular nucleus of the hypothalamus (PVH), and the central nucleus of the amygdala share direct and reciprocal projections with the NTS complex and with each other. Evidence for the involvement of these structures in cardiovascular regulation continues to mount. The VLM is involved in regulation of vasomotor tone; stimulation of the central nucleus of the amygdala alters heart rate as well as blood pressure; and lesions of the PVH counteract blood pressure elevations associated with aortic baroreceptor deafferentation. Numerous neurotransmitters are involved in communication within this network, including NE, E, serotonin, enkephalins, dopamine, somatostatin, substance P, and oxytocin, among others. Because of these multilevel connections, structures that receive sensory input from primary sensory nuclei can reciprocate and modulate the functioning of those nuclei. As a consequence, the overall system is plastic and moreover able to "prioritize" information from afferent and efferent circuitry across a range of physiological challenges. The advantages of such an arrangement are evident, for example, during life-threatening events such as hemorrhagic shock or during exercise or stressful behavioral challenge, when baroreceptor sensitivity can be dampened in favor of maintaining an adequate (high) level of arterial pressure.

Cardiovascular changes (e.g., increased blood pressure and skeletal muscle vasodilation) similar to those associated with dynamic exercise can be elicited by electrical stimulation of the motor cortex and of the hypothalamus. Notably, the vasodilatory effect of such stimulation apparently does not occur independent of skeletal muscle contraction or piloerection, suggesting an intricate interplay between the neural and behavioral correlates of arousal (Hilton, Spyer, & Timms 1975). Electrical stimulation of the perifornical region of the hypothalamus, in particular, evokes piloerection and other CNS-mediated circulatory components of fight-or-flight behavior (e.g., dilation of the pupils, increased heart rate and blood pressure, and gastrointestinal vasoconstriction). These cardiovascular effects are thought to be supported by a descending amygdala-hypothalamic-medullary pathway. In contrast, a depressor response (e.g., decreased blood pressure and adrenal output of catecholamines, increased vagal tone and vasoconstriction) can be produced by stimulation of the orbito-frontal cortex, the temporal cortex, the anterior hypothalamus, and the amygdala. Some evidence indicates that the differentiation of the arousal and depressor effects integrated through the hypothalamus may be mediated through the amygdala-fugal and cortico-fugal pathways, respectively.

Efferent Pathways and Mechanisms. There are two principal divisions of the autonomic nervous system: the parasympathetic nervous system (PNS) and the sympathetic nervous system (SNS). Most organs are dually innervated by the PNS and SNS and, as a result, simultaneously receive impulses that both increase and decrease their activity. Hence, depending on the relative input of the PNS and SNS at any moment, the aggregate effect of ANS activation can be either inhibitory or excitatory in nature.

There are several structural and functional differences between the two divisions. For example, efferent parasympathetic neurons originate in the brain and sacral spinal cord and synapse with postganglionic neurons located proximal or within target cells. In contrast, efferent sympathetic nerves arise from thoracic and lumbar regions of the spinal cord, and their postganglionic connections occur in a sympathetic ganglion chain that runs parallel to the vertebral column. Second, the SNS and PNS divisions differ in terms of neurotransmitter and receptor activity at various levels along the ganglionic chain. Acetylcholine (ACh) is released from preganglionic fibers of both divisions and from postganglionic neurons of the PNS; however, the principal postganglionic SNS neurotransmitter is NE. There is one very notable exception to this basic design, which involves SNS innervation of the adrenal medulla. In this case, preganglionic cholinergic SNS fibers act directly on medullary cells that release E and NE into the circulation. These substances then act upon myocardial and vascular cells to influence heart rate and blood flow.

The two divisions are further distinguished at the effector cell site on the basis of receptor type: visceral effector cell activation is mediated by muscarinic-cholinergic receptors in the PNS and by adrenergic receptors in the SNS. Further specificity exists within the SNS, as well, owing to certain selective properties of the two primary classes of adrenergic receptors – alpha (α) and beta (β). Although the distribution of these receptors throughout the body is fairly ubiquitous, differences exist in subclass ($\beta_1, \beta_2, \alpha_1, \alpha_2$) distribution and subclass affinities for E and NE. For example, β_1-adrenoceptors predominate in cardiac tissue, where they mediate the chronotropic (contractile rate) and inotropic (contractile strength) actions of the heart. The majority of these cardiac β_1-adrenoceptors are primarily localized in the ventricles. In comparison, α and β_2-adrenoceptors predominate in vascular smooth muscle, where the α receptors mediate vasoconstriction and the β_2 receptors mediate vasodilation. Nonetheless, β_2-adrenoceptors are found in the SA node, throughout the AV conduction system, and along the intimal surface of coronary arteries (Buxton et al. 1987; Summers et al. 1989). In addition, the plasma concentration of NE exceeds that of E by a factor of about four under resting conditions, yet β_1-adrenoceptors have an equal affinity for NE and E whereas β_2-adrenoceptors have a greater affinity for E. It

is these dynamics of adrenergic receptor–neuroendocrine communication that profoundly affect both the selectivity and specificity of cardiovascular responsiveness to sympathetic activation.

Neural and Hormonal Control of the Heart. Sympathetic innervation of the heart arises from cardiac efferent nerves that originate in the upper thoracic region of the spinal cord in the IML. These SNS preganglionic fibers pass through the middle and inferior cervical ganglion, synapse with postganglionic fibers projecting through the cardiac plexus, and communicate with visceral effectors located primarily in the SA and AV nodes. Efferent cardiac nerve projections originating from opposite sides of the spinal cord tend to have widely overlapping distributions; however, those stemming from the right side play a greater role in chronotropic actions of the heart while those from the left side are generally dedicated to inotropic myocardial control (Randall, Priola, & Ulmer 1963). Synaptic transmission through the ganglion is gated or modulated as a function of different receptor types located on postganglionic neurons (Flacke & Gillis 1969). Specifically, presynaptically released ACh elicits a fast excitatory postsynaptic potential (EPSP) when binding to a postganglionic nicotinic receptor and a slow EPSP when binding to a muscarinic receptor. In addition, ACh can bind to interneuronal small intensely fluorescent (SIF) cells that express muscarinic receptors and produce slow inhibitory postsynaptic potentials (Libet 1977).

Vagal nerve fibers originate from the DVN and NA of the medulla and pass through the superficial and deep cardiac plexus, connect with terminal ganglia, and emerge as postganglionic parasympathetic cardiac fibers (Jordan et al. 1982). The postganglionic effector cells are distributed in a hierarchical fashion within the myocardium, with most being located proximal to the SA and AV nodes, fewer in the atria, and fewer still in ventricular muscle. Consequently, an increase in postganglionic release of ACh by cardiac parasympathetic nerves decreases heart rate primarily by decreasing spontaneous SA nodal firing. In addition, increased release of ACh slows conduction and extends the refractory period of atrial action potentials.

Although the pathways for SNS and PNS innervation of the heart have been described as separate entities, these neural networks actually map onto the heart in close proximity, resulting in coactivated, complex interactions (for a review see Berntson, Cacioppo, & Quigley 1991). Thus, although an increase in heart rate, for example, may be attributed independently either to an increase in SNS or to a decrease in PNS stimulation of the SA node, at any given moment the precise functional status of the heart can reflect reciprocal and nonreciprocal interactions between the two divisions. Activity of the SNS and PNS tend to be mutually antagonistic; however, their structural arrangement, as can be observed in Figure 4, is such that the PNS

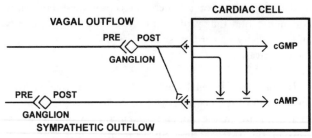

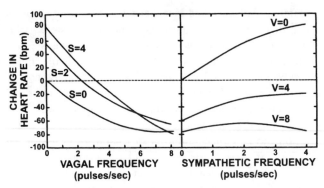

Figure 4. Independent and interactive postganglionic sympathetic nervous system (SNS) and vagal parasympathetic nervous system (PNS) stimulation of the myocardial cell. Norepinephrine released from the SNS promotes the conversion of ATP to cAMP; this in turn facilitates slow calcium channel phosphorylation, thereby increasing mycocellular Ca^2 entry and enhancing myocardial contractility. Acetylcholine (ACh) released from the PNS inhibits adenylate cyclase, which augments cGMP and decreases myocardial cAMP, both of which decrease myocardial contractility. In addition, presynaptic release of ACh can inhibit SNS stimulation, thereby reducing the extent of the positive inotropic response. Reprinted with permission from Berne & Levy, *Cardiovascular Physiology*, 4th ed. Copyright 1981 C. V. Mosby Company.

Figure 5. Heart rate response to simultaneous stimulation of the vagus (parasympathetic) and cardiac sympathetic nerves at varying frequencies (0 to 8 pulses per second). Left panel: Heart rate decreases most dramatically during maximal vagal stimulation in the presence of maximal sympathetic stimulation (S = 4), evidencing the phenomenon of accentuated antagonism. Right panel: Maximal vagal stimulation (V = 8) predominates over maximal sympathetic stimulation (4 pulses/sec), resulting in minimal changes in heart rate. Reprinted with permission from Levy & Zieske, "Autonomic control of cardiac pacemaker activity and atrioventricular transmission," *Journal of Applied Physiology*, vol. 27, pp. 465–70. Copyright 1969 W. B. Saunders Co.

is capable of presynaptically inhibiting SNS stimulation of the heart (Levy 1977). Parasympathetic nervous system activity contributes more than SNS activity to mean heart rate levels (Katona et al. 1982) and heart rate variation (Weinberg & Pfeifer 1986; Wheeler & Watkins 1973), and a concomitant increase in PNS and SNS activity produces deceleration of the heart rate.

The elegant studies in dogs by Levy and colleagues have shown that the chronotropic effect of vagal input to the heart varies inversely with the magnitude and duration of sympathetic stimulation (Henning, Khalil, & Levy 1990; Levy 1977; Yang & Levy 1992). This interactive effect, referred to as "accentuated antagonism," is depicted in Figure 5, which illustrates the effect of simultaneous SNS and PNS stimulation on heart rate. These researchers also demonstrated that vagal stimulation reduces sympathetically driven enhancement of inotropic left ventricular function. Because there is little direct innervation of the ventricles, it may be concluded that the inhibitory effect of vagal stimulation on ventricular contractility is a consequence of the presynaptic antagonism of the prevailing sympathetic drive by the PNS. Thus, it may be inferred that changes in myocardial contractility are the result of "effective" SNS cardiac input (i.e., SNS input that is permitted to pass to the myocardium). The integrity of vagal influences on the myocardium may be assessed by examining the cardiovascular response to facial immersion in water. This maneuver induces a dive reflex that is present in all terrestrial mammals and, as can be seen in Figure 6, includes a large increase in vagal cardiac input. The increase in vagal drive produces a large-magnitude bradycardia that is accompanied by an increase in SNS vascular drive, resulting in peripheral vasoconstriction (Hurwitz & Furedy 1986).

Hormonal control of the heart is mediated by the adrenal medulla. The adrenal medulla is innervated by efferent preganglionic sympathetic fibers that travel in splanchnic nerves and terminate directly in the adrenal gland. Presynaptically released ACh binds to nicotinic receptors on medullary chromaffin cells that, in turn, regulate the release of E and (to a lesser extent) NE into the bloodstream. Early studies indicated that the cardiotropic actions of these circulating substances differed from those of NE released from cardiac efferent nerve endings because the majority of β_1-adrenoceptors, which mediate chronotropy and inotropy, are primarily localized in the ventricles (Baker, Boyd, & Potter 1980). Because of this localization, these receptors receive minimal direct neural input while being optimally exposed to circulating E (Baker & Potter 1980). Nonetheless, this "priming" of the ventricle to circulating E may be offset by the fact that β_1-adrenoceptors themselves are preferentially sensitive to neuronally released NE (Carlsson et al., cited in LeJemtel & Sonnenblick 1994). In contrast, β_2-adrenoceptors located in the SA node preferentially respond to circulating NE. The complex interplay between neuronally released NE versus circulating NE and E is further highlighted under various conditions of stress. For example, the cardiotropic response to exercise is preferentially activated by neuronally released NE, whereas particular types of life-threatening and psychological stress may trigger a preferential release of E into the circulation (Dimsdale & Moss 1980; Glass et al. 1980).

Neural and Hormonal Control of the Vasculature. Resting blood flow in skeletal muscle is approximately 5 ml/min

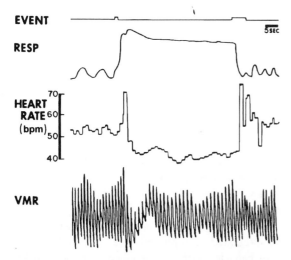

EVENT

RESP

**HEART
RATE
(bpm)**

70
60
50
40

VMR

5sec

Figure 6. The dive reflex includes widespread cardiovascular alterations in which a large bradycardia is accompanied by a selective redistribution of blood flow – away from tissues and organs that can sustain themselves anaerobically and toward the brain, heart, and lungs (which require continuous aerobic supply). A polygraphic tracing is displayed of the dive reflex of a subject during a 40-sec apneic face immersion in 25°C water. The event marker tracing depicts the onset and offset of the immersion. Following full inspiration – marked by the upward deflection of the respiration (RESP) tracing – and then face immersion, the heart rate (HR) decreased markedly below preimmersion resting level. The HR decrease, which is mediated by increased vagal cardiac input, was accompanied by a decrement in finger vasomotor pulse amplitude (VMR), reflecting peripheral vasoconstriction mediated by increased sympathetic activation. Reprinted with permission from Hurwitz & Furedy, "The human dive reflex: An experimental, topographical and physiological analysis," *Physiology and Behavior*, vol. 36, pp. 287–94. Copyright 1986 Elsevier Science.

per 100 g of tissue and may increase dramatically (15-fold) during intense exercise. The maintenance of blood pressure and the adequate distribution of blood flow to meet tissue-specific energy demands are achieved through multiple neurogenic, hormonal, myogenic, and local metabolic mechanisms. The relative contribution of these factors varies between different vascular beds: neurogenic factors are particularly salient in skin but are less important in regulating coronary arteries; their role is comparable to that of autoregulatory factors in skeletal muscle tissue.

Sympathetic nerve terminals located superficially in vascular smooth muscle cells innervate arteriolar, capillary, and venous tissue. When released from these terminals, NE binds with postsynaptic α_1-adrenergic receptors, causing vasoconstriction and thereby increasing arterial vascular resistance and decreasing venous compliance. Hence, the net result of sympathetic stimulation (i.e., an increase in systemic blood pressure) is increased cardiac output and resistance to flow and an increase in venous return of blood to the heart. When released by the adrenal glands, NE elicits response patterns that are analogous to those induced by direct sympathetic nerve stimulation. In contrast, E produces a mixed pattern of vasoactive effects depend-

ing on the target tissue. In skeletal and myocardial tissue, E binds with β_2-adrenoceptors to yield potent vasodilatory effects; in most other tissue, E elicits a vasoconstrictive response.

Hormonal and neural influences on the vasculature are intricately related. For example, the release of NE is autoregulated by presynaptic α_2-adrenoceptors that, when stimulated, inhibit further NE release. In addition, the binding of circulating E to presynaptic β_2-adrenoceptors also inhibits NE release. Moreover, the positive chronotropic effects of NE released directly on the myocardium, which elicit compensatory reductions in blood pressure, are counteracted by the blood pressure–elevating effects of circulating NE. Finally (and as described more thoroughly in the following section), changes in blood pressure trigger pressure-sensitive receptors that signal the DVN/NA brainstem nuclei, bringing about alterations in vagal activity and compensatory changes in heart rate.

Cardiovascular Reflexes. As mentioned previously, CNS control of the circulation is a highly integrated phenomenon. In addition to innervating the heart and vasculature, the CNS also receives information about ongoing changes in blood pressure and other blood-related factors. Intrinsic cardiovascular reflexes relay information about these changes to the CNS and thus play a major role in short-term blood pressure regulation. These reflexive pathways are triggered by mechanical and chemical stimulation of receptors dispersed throughout the cardiovascular system.

Mechanoreceptors. There are two major classes of mechanoreceptors that are responsive to changes in hemodynamic properties (for a review see Smith & Kampine 1990). These are the arterial baroreceptors and the cardiopulmonary receptors. Arterial baroreceptors respond to short-term changes in blood pressure, and cardiopulmonary receptors are stimulated by changes in blood volume and ventricular stretch. Arterial baroreceptors are found primarily in the carotid sinus and the aortic arch, whereas cardiopulmonary receptors are distributed throughout the vena cava, pulmonary artery, atria, and ventricles.

Impulses from carotid sinuses and the aortic arch travel to the brain via glossopharyngeal-carotid sinus and vagal-aortic nerve pathways, respectively. As blood pressure increases, for example, stimulated arterial baroreceptors send impulses via carotid sinus and aortic depressor nerves to the NTS in the medulla, bringing about subsequent reductions in cardiac output and vascular tone to stabilize arterial pressure. The reduction in cardiac output is mediated by primary increases in vagal nerve output (i.e., heart rate deceleration) and by secondary decreases in heart rate, contractility, and sympathetically mediated vasoconstrictor activity (i.e., reduced venous return) (Rompelman 1993). The arterial baroreceptors are stimulated by the rate of change in blood pressure and by the degree of absolute stretch in the vessel wall that is associated with pulse pressure and mean arterial transmural pressure. The sensitivity of arterial baroreceptors to a given incremental change in blood pressure is inversely related to the prevailing level of arterial pressure. In addition, arterial baroreceptors typically are more responsive to acute decreases than to abrupt elevations in blood pressure. Arterial baroreceptors can also make transient changes in their basal functioning relative to changes in steady-state blood pressure levels. Thus, when steady-state blood pressure is elevated for an extended period (e.g., during acute exercise), the functional reference point for the arterial baroreceptor is increased.

As previously mentioned, the cardiovascular system has cardiopulmonary as well as arterial mechanoreceptors. There are three types of atrial cardiopulmonary receptors. The A-type cardiopulmonary receptors are triggered only during atrial systole; B-type cardiopulmonary receptors fire only during atrial filling; and a mixed group of cardiopulmonary receptors respond during atrial systole *and* filling. These receptors are further distinguished by the fact that the B-type are activated by an increase in blood volume whereas the A-type are activated by an increase in atrial tension. Thus, when blood volume increases, the CNS (having been signaled by B-type vagal receptors) reflexively stimulates renal production of urine, decreases pituitary production of antidiuretic hormone, and triggers other circulatory processes that regulate heart rate and blood pressure. Ventricular receptors are stimulated by strong ventricular contraction or by increased stretch. Under these conditions, vagal fibers transmit impulses from these receptors to the medulla, eliciting a reduction in heart rate and vasodilation. These atrial receptor-mediated reflexes may play a role in such conditions as postural hypotension and congestive heart failure (Mancia et al. 1992; Smith & Kampine 1990).

Bainbridge Reflex and Normal Sinus Arrhythmia. Phasic changes in respiration have a gating influence on cardiac vagal efferents: during the expiratory and inspiratory phases of respiration, the heart period lengthens and shortens, respectively (Katona et al. 1970). The oscillatory influence of respiration on heart rate has been referred to as *respiratory sinus arrhythmia* (RSA). Changes in the RSA amplitude correlate with PNS influence on the heart; over the past decade, RSA has received increasing attention in the psychophysiology research setting as a noninvasive index of vagal control. The RSA is influenced by both central and peripheral mechanisms, which include (a) central cardiorespiratory generators that modulate autonomic outflow and produce an intrinsic cardiac rhythm, (b) vagal outflow, and (c) peripheral baroreceptors and chemoreceptors (see Berntson, Cacioppo, & Quigley 1993). Bainbridge (1915), who observed that right atrial distension produces a compensatory increase in heart rate (tachycardia) via a reflex arc, provided one of the first descriptions of these interactive mechanisms. This reflex arc – consisting of afferent myelinated vagal fibers and efferent sympathetic connections to the SA node – is sensitive to changes in venous return, which varies as a function of oscillations in intrapleural pressure throughout the respiratory cycle. In addition, heart rate variability is reflexively regulated by (i) alternate loading and unloading of arterial baroreceptors and cardiopulmonary receptors during the cardiac cycle and (ii) direct connections between respiratory and cardiac centers within the brainstem.

The RSA is a product of both tonic and phasic components of vagal control. These components are highly interdependent, yet they appear to have distinct functional and behavioral sensitivities (Berntson et al. 1993). As such, RSA measures are gaining recognition as tools with which to examine integrated neurophysiological and psychological correlates of behavior within the context of the cardiovascular psychophysiology research paradigm.

Chemoreceptors. Chemoreceptors are specially adapted to respond to changes in blood chemistry. Two subclasses of chemoreceptors (aortic/carotid and ventricular) have been identified. Aortic and carotid chemoreceptors are triggered by decreased blood pressure or blood flow and thus by reduced availability of oxygen; by reduced arterial blood oxygen tension; or by increased arterial blood carbon dioxide tension. In response to any of these triggering events, arterial blood pressure is elevated to facilitate blood circulation and the restoration of oxygen delivery and carbon dioxide removal. In contrast, stimulation of ventricular chemoreceptors produces a hypotensive response. This so-called Bezold–Jarish reflex can be induced pharmacologically by the intracoronary injection of various stimulants such as nicotine, bradykinin, and histamine. In addition, the accumulation of chemotaxic metabolites can trigger this reflex. From a clinical perspective, this reflex may be one pathologic mechanism underlying the hypotensive response observed during cardiogenic shock.

Orthostatic Reflex. Abrupt changes in posture, such as changing from a supine or seated to a standing position, produce a pooling of blood in lower extremities due to gravitational forces. Such abrupt shifts in blood distribution are detected by the arterial baroreceptors, which reflexively trigger an increase in sympathetically mediated vasoconstriction, contractility, and heart rate as well as a decrease in vagal tone. Under normal circumstances, the acute (1–2-sec onset) sympathetic response is accompanied by a more protracted (5–10-min) increase in circulating levels of NE and by a slight increase in peripheral vascular resistance. The complementary response in peripheral resistance is necessary to compensate for a transient decrement that initially occurs in cardiac output. The increase in peripheral resistance aids in maintaining blood pressure until circulation is normalized and stroke volume stabilizes. The blood pressure response to upright postural tilt can be used to assess the contribution of cardiovascular reflex and neuroendocrine pathology to various disease states, such as idiopathic orthostatic hypotension (Hayashida et al. 1996) and diabetes mellitus (Hurwitz et al. 1994b).

Renal Control of Circulation

The renal–body fluid pressure control system is responsible for long-term regulation of blood pressure (CHBPR 1978; DiBona 1989; Guyton 1981). There are two essential distinctions between this system and the short-term mechanisms (mechanoreceptor, chemoreceptor, CNS) previously discussed. First, it is much less sensitive to acute alterations in blood pressure; second, it has an "errorless" self-regulatory feedback gain that enables it to recover completely from profound changes in mean arterial pressure over extended time periods. The basis for blood pressure control via this long-acting system is found in the relationship between MAP and renal excretion of sodium and water. An increase in MAP causes an increase in sodium excretion and water excretion, both of which reduce extracellular fluid and thus lower blood volume. The reduction in blood volume reduces circulatory filling pressure, venous return, and ultimately cardiac output. In turn, reduced venous pressure and cardiac output reduce MAP directly and by triggering autoregulatory reductions in TPR. The system responds in reverse manner to a prevailing decrease in arterial pressure by increasing renal retention of fluid and expanding blood volume. This system is particularly sensitive to changes in MAP above 100 mmHg, which is just above the normal resting level for an average adult.

There are three accessory mechanisms that impact the efficacy of the renal–body fluid pressure control system: the renin-angiotensin system, the aldosterone system, and the sympathetic nervous system. Renin is the converting enzyme that triggers the formation of angiotensin-I, a potent vasoconstrictor, from the liver protein called angiotensinogen. In the lungs, angiotensin-I is converted to angiotensin-II, which subsequently stimulates the production of aldosterone in the adrenal cortex. Both angiotensin-II and aldosterone facilitate the natriuretic and diuretic actions of the kidneys. Therefore, if MAP becomes elevated, then (i) activity in the renin-angiotensin-aldosterone cascade is inhibited and (ii) blood pressure and volume are restabilized via reductions in vasoconstriction and increased sodium and water retention. In concert with these metabolic mechanisms, sympathetic stimulation of renal activity is also decreased in response to a prevailing increase in arterial pressure. This process appears to be linked intricately to both the renocortical release of dopamine and renomedullary endocrine activity (Bell 1987; Su-sic 1988).

MEASUREMENT OF THE CIRCULATORY SYSTEM

Cardiac Function

The noninvasive measurement of cardiac function and structure is essential to understanding cardiovascular physiology in the behaving individual and relating this information to pathological processes underlying cardiovascular disease. Electrical aspects of cardiac activity are measured with the ECG, and methods are available to accomplish this task both under static and ambulatory conditions. Several methodologies are also available for measuring cardiac output and other indices of cardiac function in addition to cardiac structure and vascular blood flow. Generally, these methods can be categorized according to the type of images (two-dimensional vs. three-dimensional) they produce. Overall, three-dimensional (3D) techniques such as magnetic resonance imaging (MRI) and computed tomography (CT) provide images of the heart with greatest resolution and thus yield the most accurate assessment of cardiac functioning. However, these methods are rarely used in psychophysiological research because they employ radioisotopes and X-rays, which place the patient or study participant at some risk and place a limit on the frequency of data sampling in a given protocol. Furthermore, these techniques are more valid under static conditions in which the patient's or participant's mobility is greatly restricted; thus they are not conducive to monitoring cardiac activity while the individual is ambulatory or engages in tasks requiring behavioral responses. Of the two primary 2D techniques designed to assess cardiac function, impedance cardiography and echocardiography, the latter offers a more comprehensive assessment of cardiac function and structure but is more heavily operator-dependent. The following section provides an overview of the principal methodologies employed in research and clinical practice settings to measure these parameters. The distinct advantages and disadvantages associated with each technique are emphasized to illustrate the preferred candidates for use in the psychophysiological research setting.

Monitoring of the ECG. The methodology for monitoring electrical activity of the heart has been used since the early twentieth century (Einthoven, Fahr, & de Waart 1913). Monitoring the heart rhythm and detecting electrical conduction abnormalities of the heart are accomplished by recording the ECG. Recording the ECG involves placing electrodes at strategic locations on the body surface and connecting those electrodes via leads to an electrocardiograph, thus completing an electric circuit between this amplifier and the heart. A lead consists of a pair of terminals, each with a designated polarity, which is connected to recording electrodes. In the typical psychophysiological research setting, heart rhythm is monitored using three unipolar extremity leads placed on the right and left arms and the left leg, or a similar modified three-lead configuration. This configuration, which is based on the principles of Einthoven's equilateral triangle, captures the electrical activity of the heart as a 2D geometric figure. Within a cardiac cycle, a set of positive, negative, and isodiphasic deflections relative to the three unipolar leads characterize conduction of the electrical impulse. In series, these sets of deflections can be used to characterize the heart rhythm. In clinical settings, in which more detailed information is sought regarding electrical conduction and rhythm, a twelve-lead configuration is employed. This configuration includes the limb extremity leads plus a set of chest or precordial leads, which permit the recording of horizontal conduction vectors. Thus, forces in two-dimensional space can represent the three-dimensional heart, and sources of conduction blockage can be detected as vector deflections within that space (Bayes de Luna 1993; Castellanos, Kessler, & Myerburg 1994).

The technology for monitoring a patient's ECG over prolonged periods of time, and more importantly during everyday activities, has been available for over three decades (Holter 1961). The original Holter monitor consisted of a battery-powered slow-speed tape recorder with a synchronized digital clock. Using input from a standard five-lead electrode configuration, this apparatus records the ECG along with event markers indicating the occurrence of specific activities or symptoms of interest in the patient's daily experience. These events are recorded separately in a patient diary and subsequently used to assess the influence of psychosocial and behavioral factors on the patient's cardiac rhythm. More recently, this technology has expanded to include solid-state memory devices that record, amplify, digitize, and store the ECG along with the event markers (Noble & Zipes 1994). These systems incorporate input from two recording ECG leads, permitting the differentiation of supraventricular and ventricular arrhythmias and the identification of S-T segment and T-wave alterations. Microcomputer technology has advanced this methodology to enable the recording of ambulatory data over a period of several days. Alternatively, the technician can program the ambulatory ECG device to record only the occurrence of abnormal cardiac rhythms or instruct the patient to self-initiate readings during symptomatic periods. Data review and analysis can be conducted by a trained observer or by microcomputers, with the latter method tending to result in a smaller margin of error.

Ambulatory ECG techniques have been used to study cardiac impulse and conduction activities in various healthy and patient populations (Kligfield 1989). These studies documented unexpected age-related, gender-related, and occupation-related trends in the prevalence of certain types of arrhythmias, and they revealed a direct relationship between PVC density and increased risk of cardiac mortality. In addition, ambulatory ECG monitoring has been very instrumental in (a) assessing the predictive relationships of various forms of ventricular arrhythmias and conduction abnormalities associated with previous MI and with impending cardiac mortality, (b) bringing to light the contributions of behavioral factors in sudden cardiac death, and (c) teasing apart discrepancies between patient symptoms and arrhythmias.

Impedance Cardiography

Methodology. Impedance cardiography is a relatively unobtrusive, safe, and noninvasive technique for measuring stroke volume and systolic time interval indices of cardiac contractility. In this technique, a constant, low-voltage (1–4-mA), alternating (200–100-kHz) current field is created along the thorax using aluminum-coated Mylar band electrodes (see Figure 7). Alternatively, a spot electrode configuration, which may be more convenient for the experimenter and more comfortable for the subject, can be implemented (see Qu et al. 1986). However, this method has not been adequately standardized and has certain limitations (see section entitled "Limitations"). Since voltage is held constant, deviations in the current flow are attributed to changes in resistance (i.e., impedance Z). Because the red blood cell is the least resistive element in the body and since current passes through the path of least resistance, changes in thoracic blood volume associated with each beat of the heart produce an interpretable change in thoracic resistance (ΔZ). Specifically, the impedance cardiography system generates beat-by-beat changes in output voltage that correspond to changes in stroke volume.

In the last two decades, attempts to measure autonomic mediation of cardiovascular function by impedance cardiography have shown that specific alterations in the rate of change of the thoracic impedance ($d(\Delta Z)/dt$) during systole can reliably estimate indices of myocardial performance (Miller & Horvath 1978; Sherwood et al. 1990). The impedance cardiogram (ICG), as depicted in Figure 8, yields a measure of stroke volume that permits the cardiac output to be derived, and it marks events that signify the onset (B point) and end (X point) of left ventricular ejection. Thus, systolic time interval estimates of cardiac contractility can also be derived.

A growing body of evidence supports the relationship between electrical and mechanical systole as reflecting sympathetic drive on the heart (Larsen, Schneiderman, & Pasin 1986), which shortens the contractile time by influencing both the rate and force of contraction (Winegrad 1982). Four indices of cardiovascular function purported to reflect sympathetic myocardial drive are: (1) the pre-ejection period (PEP); (2) the ratio of electrical systole (QT) to electromechanical systole (QS2); (3) the Heather index (HI), which reflects the maximum velocity of left ventricular ejection; and (4) the acceleration index (ACI), which reflects the acceleration of the rapid systolic ejection phase (Cacioppo, Berntson, & Quigley 1994; Heather 1969; Kizakevich et al. 1989). The PEP is measured as the interval between onset of the ECG Q wave to onset of left ventricular ejection time (LVET); shorter PEP intervals are inversely related to inotropy. The HI and the ACI are measures of contractility that are derived from the ejection velocity (dZ/dt_{max}) of the ICG. The HI is derived by dividing the ejection velocity by the Q-Z peak (i.e., time from onset of electrical systole to the peak of the

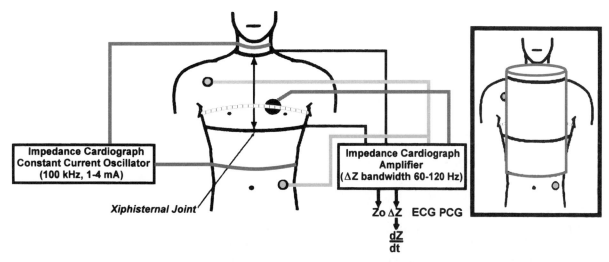

Figure 7. Schematic representation of an impedance cardiography system, illustrating the basic circuit elements of the impedance cardiograph. A constant, sinusoidal, 100-kHz alternating current of 1–4 mA is passed longitudinally through the thorax between electrodes 1 and 4 (lead 1 is located about 3 cm above lead 2, which is located at the base of the neck; lead 3 is placed around the chest at the xiphisternal junction; lead 4 may be placed about 5 cm inferior to lead 3), which are placed 360° around the body. The product of this current and the thoracic impedance generates a voltage measured between the two inner electrodes. The drop in voltage between the inner electrodes that occurs when blood is ejected from the heart is detected by a high-input impedance linear amplifier. The outputs from the impedance cardiograph are the mean thoracic impedance (Z_0) and the change in impedance (ΔZ, bandwidth 60–120 Hz). To obtain the ejection velocity used to derive the stroke volume, the ΔZ is differentiated (dZ/dt) either by electronic circuitry or by computer software with appropriate signal bandwidth (50 Hz). In conjunction with these signals, the electrocardiogram (ECG) and the phonocardiogram (PCG) may be independently obtained to be used for signal processing, which usually includes ensemble averaging (Kelsey & Guethlein 1990). Kubicek introduced the hypothesis that stroke volume could be calculated from the product of the maximal rate of change in thoracic impedance (dZ/dt_{max}) and the duration of left ventricular ejection. In his theoretical model (depicted in the inset), the thorax is considered a cylinder with uniform cross-sectional area and homogeneous conducting material, the blood.

ejection velocity). In contrast, the ACI is derived by dividing the ejection velocity by the B–Z peak (i.e., time from ejection onset to the peak of the ejection velocity). Thus, the ACI is a measure of contractility during the ejection phase, whereas HI reflects both pre-ejection and ejection phase influences. Contractility can be expressed as the ratio of the pre-ejection period to left ventricular ejection time; however, this interpretation must be tempered by known autoregulatory dynamics that influence

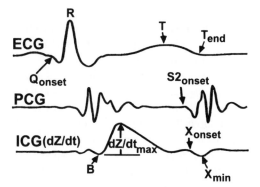

Figure 8. Characteristic electrocardiogram (ECG), phonocardiogram (PCG), and impedance cardiogram (ICG) signals. The ICG is the first derivative of the pulsatile thoracic impedance signal (dZ/dt). In addition, the relevant waveform events used to derive stroke volume, systolic time intervals, and other estimates of cardiac inotropy are depicted.

PEP. For this reason, the PEP/LVET index has been alternatively used indirectly to reflect sympathetically mediated changes in inotropic activity and carries the advantage of adjusting for heart rate variability. Nonetheless, HI may actually be a more sensitive measure of contractility than the PEP/LVET ratio (Baller, Hurwitz, & Nassirian 1983).

Calculation of stroke volume is dependent on several other factors in addition to the voltage decrease (i.e., change in impedance) associated with each heartbeat. The mathematical equation for deriving stroke volume from the ICG signal has undergone several revisions since the publication of Nyober's (1950) equation over four decades ago. A critical issue revolves around the calculation of blood resistivity from hematocrit (Geddes & Sadler 1973). Demeter and colleagues (1993) have shown more valid stroke volume estimates (compared with thermodilution values) when using hematocrit to estimate blood resistivity than when using blood resistivity constants. Currently, the most widely acknowledged formula for estimating stroke volume calculates blood resistivity from the relation of resistivity and hematocrit at 37°C (Kubicek et al. 1966):

$$\text{stroke volume} = [\rho_b(L/Z_0)^2] \times \text{LVET} \times dZ/dt_{max}.$$

In this equation, ρ_b is blood resistivity, L is the distance between the inner recording electrodes, Z_0 is the mean thoracic impedance, LVET is the left ventricular ejection period, and dZ/dt_{max} is the absolute value of the maximum rate of voltage change in the ICG.

The use of the rho (ρ) constant assumes that resistivity is stable throughout the cardiac cycle. However, resistivity actually varies as a function of alterations in red blood cell orientation (random vs. aligned) across the cardiac cycle (Lamberts, Visser, & Zijlstra 1984). In addition to this controversial aspect in the theoretical basis of impedance cardiography, the model of the homogeneously perfused thoracic cylinder (on which Kubicek's equation is based) does not exactly correspond to the actual shape of the thoracic cavity (see Figure 7 inset). Thus, attempts have been made to improve on these equations by introducing a more realistic conical thoracic model. Sramek (1981, 1982) proposed an equation based on the assumption that current flow between electrodes is limited to a truncated cone of homogeneous resistivity. Subsequently, Bernstein (1986) proposed a modified version of Sramek's equation to compensate for differences in body shape. In general, the major limitations of each of these equations stem from oversimplification of real anatomical and physiological parameters and from inherent difficulties in determining the other hemodynamic, cardiac cycle timing, and amplitude variables on which they are based. Consequently, the empirical precision of these equations for estimating stroke volume continues to be debated vigorously and requires extensive validation.

In clinical populations, impedance cardiography awaits broad acceptance, largely because validation studies have generally found consistent patterns of overestimation of low cardiac output values and underestimation of high cardiac output values when compared to standard techniques (see Fuller 1992; Jensen, Yakimets, & Teo 1995). In addition, the Sramek–Bernstein equation has been shown to systematically underestimate stroke volume both in cardiac patients and in healthy individuals (Huang et al. 1990; Perrino et al. 1994; Pickett & Buell 1992; Yakimets & Jensen 1995). In contrast, impedance cardiography using the Kubicek equation has proven to be astonishingly robust in healthy individuals, presenting high correlation coefficients when compared to other, mostly invasive, techniques for stroke volume determination (Sherwood et al. 1990). The following sections summarize the major issues of impedance cardiography validity and reliability as they relate to measurement of cardiac function within healthy populations.

Validity and Reliability. Successful implementation of impedance cardiography in psychophysiological research ultimately depends on accurate instrumentation (Sherwood et al. 1990). Proper electrode placement and signal analysis of the ICG waveform are critical to successful instrumentation, and impedance cardiography has been validated using various techniques. In addition, impedance cardiographs need to incorporate appropriate filtering bandwidths that take into account the spectral bandwidth of the ICG. Am-

plifiers that do not take this into account will attenuate amplitude and waveform aspects of the ICG as a function of the heart rate. Specifically, impedance cardiographs that employ a 50-Hz upper band limit provide greater resolution of the ICG events (Hurwitz et al. 1993a). When precise application of electrodes are employed on test and retest and when enhanced computer processing techniques for ensemble averaging the ICG cycles enable the events within ICG to be precisely measured (Hurwitz et al. 1990; Nagel et al. 1989), impedance cardiography can be a very reliable tool for the assessment of cardiovascular function (Llabre et al. 1993; Saab et al. 1992). Reproducible measurements of stroke volume and systolic time intervals have been obtained under static and dynamic conditions over intervals of up to one year (Ebert et al. 1984; Llabre et al. 1993; Pincomb et al. 1985; Saab et al. 1992; Sherwood et al. 1997; Veigl & Judy 1983).

The LVET is used in the Kubicek equation for calculation of stroke volume. An issue in impedance cardiography scoring of LVET pertains to the scoring of the end of ejection at the X-wave onset versus placing this event at the X-wave minimum. The onset of the X wave correlates more closely in time with the aortic closure than X-wave minimum, but it is more difficult to locate. Placing the event at the X-wave minimum results in longer LVET periods and consequently greater stroke volume estimates (Nagel et al. 1989). Another methodological issue in impedance cardiography concerns the inner electrode distance used in the equation. This is an important issue because, when using the Kubicek stroke volume equation, the electrode distance is squared and is directly proportional to the derived stroke volume value. The method recommended by Kubicek is to use the average of the midaxillary sternal distance and the midline spinal distance between inner electrodes. However, others have found that, when compared with the thermodilution method, ICG-derived stroke volumes are more valid if the shorter midaxillary sternal distance is used (Denniston et al. 1976). Findings from our laboratory indicate that systematic error in ICG-derived stroke volume estimation can be avoided when using X-wave onset to represent the end of left ventricular ejection and when using the midaxillary sternal electrode distance.

Attempts to validate the impedance methodology in humans using standard (dye-dilution; Fick) and 2D imaging (nuclear ventriculography) methods have resulted in favorable correlations of about 0.80 (ranging from 0.48 to 0.97), despite a tendency for impedance-derived values to overestimate stroke volume as much as 25% (Geddes & Baker 1989; Sherwood et al. 1990). In healthy normotensive individuals, high correlations between ICG-derived stroke volume estimates based on the Kubicek equation and simultaneously measured 3D images of left ventricular volumes using computerized tomography (CT) have also been reported under conditions of dobutamine infusion ($r = 0.87$) and placebo infusion ($r = 0.94$) (Hurwitz et al. 1994b). Mean error (±SE) and the absolute value of the error (±SE) between the two methods (i.e., impedance minus CT stroke volume) were also minimal during infusions of placebo (0.6 ± 2 ml and 4.5 ± 1 ml, respectively) and dobutamine (1.5 ± 3 ml and 6.0 ± 2 ml, respectively). The accuracy of these ICG data reflects the stringent methodological conditions under which they were obtained: blood resistivity was estimated using hematocrits from blood samples; the end of LVET was measured at the ICG X-wave onset; and the inner electrode distance as measured on the sternal axis (with the subject standing upright) was used in the estimation of stroke volume. In contrast, when LVET was calculated using the X-wave minimum and the average of the electrode distances on the sternal and spinal axes, increasing error (up to 40%) could be observed with increasing stroke volume. Thus, excellent validity for deriving stroke volume using impedance cardiography can be obtained when methodological factors such as instrumentation, event detection and derivation, and correction factors are appropriately measured.

Impedance cardiogram–derived estimates of stroke volume have also been validated against simultaneously derived ultrasound Doppler measurements. The pulsed Doppler measures the flow velocity from the left ventricular outflow tract, yielding a curve that can be integrated to derive the stroke volume. High correlations have been observed between Doppler and impedance-derived stroke volumes, both at rest ($r = 0.91$) and during behavioral challenge ($r = 0.96$) (Vallenilla et al. 1997). These findings further support the notion that ICG-derived stroke volume can be measured accurately in healthy normotensive men and women, over a broad age range, during pharmacological and behavioral manipulations that alter stroke volume and contractility.

When compared to M-mode echocardiography, impedance cardiography provides sensitive measurements of systolic time intervals under pharmacological and behavioral challenge that alter the shape of the ICG in some individuals. During atropine challenge, for example, changes in LVET as estimated from the combination of the ICG and PCG have been shown to correlate very well with those derived from the M-mode echocardiogram (Stern, Wolf, & Belz 1985). Error associated with estimates of systolic time intervals are indicative of the accuracy by which impedance-derived measures (i.e., B point, X wave) can estimate aortic opening and closure under these conditions. In this light, findings from our laboratory (Kibler et al. 1996, 1997) suggest that: (a) X-wave onset provides a more accurate estimate of aortic closure than X-wave minimum; (b) the error of aortic opening and aortic closure detection during resting baseline is less than 10 msec and does not differ from the error observed during stressful challenge; and (c) hypertensive status does not affect the validity of ICG-derived systolic time intervals. Therefore, when factors such as signal transduction, waveform

processing, and instrumentation are optimized, impedance cardiography using the Kubicek formula appears to provide highly accurate and reliable stroke volume and systolic time interval estimates.

Limitations. Since its introduction into cardiovascular psychophysiological research nearly three decades ago, the theoretical basis and practical techniques and applications of impedance cardiography have been rigorously debated and studied. Through this process, researchers have come to acknowledge several specifications and limitations of the methodology (Sherwood et al. 1990; White et al. 1990b). For instance:

1. impedance cardiographic changes are posited as alterations in aortic flow and thus are linked to changes in left rather than right ventricular ejection (although no conclusive proof of this has been obtained to this point);
2. measures of hematocrit taken during experimental protocols enhance the accuracy of calculating stroke volume, given the randomness with which ρ varies across the cardiac cycle; and
3. ICGs may not provide reliable or valid measures of stroke volume in individuals with certain cardiac abnormalities (e.g., aortic regurgitation) or in individuals with cardiac conduction disturbances.

Until recently, impedance cardiography was limited to the laboratory or clinic setting; however, technology for monitoring the ICG in ambulatory settings is developing (Willemsen et al. 1996). The VU-AMD uses six disposable spot electrodes to record the ICG and ECG, and it can be worn inconspicuously underneath the subject's clothing to permit normal activity throughout the monitoring period. When validated against laboratory devices, the VU-AMD provides highly reliable estimates of stroke volume and cardiac output across a wide range of activities (except bicycle exercise). Continued refinement and validation of this methodology will greatly enhance the ability to study the influence of real-life stress on cardiovascular functioning in the field. These achievements may ultimately be tied into the resolution of present controversies surrounding the validity and limitations of spot electrodes for recording the ICG.

Spot electrode configurations are more desirable than band electrodes in terms of subject comfort; they may also circumvent instrumentation problems (such as those encountered in bed-confined patients or those with surgical incisions in the cervical or thoracic regions) and may be less prone to movement artifact (Sherwood et al. 1990). Spot electrodes placed in the Qu configuration yield comparable systolic time interval estimates relative to those obtained from the band electrodes (Sherwood et al. 1990, 1992; Woltjer et al. 1995). Furthermore, cardiac output values estimated using spot electrodes correlate highly with those obtained via invasive techniques (Bernstein 1986; Zhang et al. 1986). However, mixed results have been reported regarding the agreement between spot- and band-derived estimates of absolute stroke volume and cardiac output values (Boomsma, de Vries, & Orlebeke 1989; Gotshall & Sexson 1994; Woltjer et al. 1995). For example, one study found that stroke volume was differentially estimated in that values derived during challenge conditions but not resting conditions were overestimated when using the spot electrode configuration (Sherwood et al. 1992). Others have suggested using spot electrodes placed in a configuration that emulates the full-band configuration (Sramek 1981). However, these stroke volume values are underestimated compared with full-band configuration values owing to substantially greater levels of mean thoracic impedance (Nagel et al. 1989).

These discrepancies may reflect the fact that full-band electrodes detect a composite of signals from various regions of the thorax that potentially can go undetected by spot configurations such as the Qu method (Patterson, Wang, & Raza 1991). Moreover, the distribution of current across the thorax is less uniform when using spot configurations. Thus, this configuration is more susceptible than the full-band configuration to individual difference factors such as body shape, which may exacerbate difficulties in the uniformity of current spread, and gender, which may influence the impedance cardiographic components (Z_0, dZ/dt_{max}) on which estimates of stroke volume are based (Woltjer et al. 1995).

An important issue underlying the validity of stroke volume values derived using spot electrodes is the effect that discrete configurations have on the homogeneity of the electrical field. After systematically investigating several different current-injecting electrode arrays, Woltjer and colleagues (1996) proposed that a configuration of four voltage-detecting electrodes (one each on the left and right lateral thorax at the level of the xiphoid of the sternum and one each on the left and right base of the neck) and five current-injecting electrodes (four placed in a semicircular pattern on the abdomen, 15 cm caudal to the voltage-detecting electrodes, and one placed on the forehead) provides optimum field homogeneity. To date, no comparable investigation of different voltage-detecting configurations has been conducted. In addition, the clinical significance of the output differences obtained using the semicircular array compared to the band electrode array established by Kubicek has not been determined, and the contribution of the neck region to the overall homogeneity of the electric field remains a controversial issue (Raaijmakers et al. 1997).

Transthoracic Echocardiography

Methodology. Echocardiography involves the use of high-frequency (2.0–7.0-MHz) ultrasound to evaluate functional, structural, and hemodynamic aspects of cardiovascular functioning (see Feigenbaum 1994; Felner & Martin 1994; Pearlman 1994). High-frequency pulses are transmitted from a transducer along a defined path to the heart. As the pulse encounters various acoustic boundaries (i.e., different tissue densities or surfaces), the ultrasonic wave is reflected back toward a receiving crystal. The pattern of the reflected ultrasound produces a distinct tomographic image that can be quantitatively analyzed. The three principal methods of echocardiography imaging are motion (M-mode), two-dimensional (2D), and Doppler. The M-mode method uses a narrow ultrasound beam to produce a one-dimensional, "ice-pick" view of the heart (see Figure 9). The 2D method, as its name implies, is able to generate cross-sectional views of the heart and has the advantage of providing real-time tomographic images of cardiac function and morphology. In particular, structural abnormalities such as valve and regional wall motion impairment are better quantified using 2D methodology. The primary advantage of Doppler echocardiography is that it is a hemodynamic as well as an imaging technique; it is used to detect blood flow velocities and can thus detect pressure gradients across fixed orifices within the heart (see Figure 9). Doppler technology can be used to derive measures of stroke volume, various time intervals related to systolic and diastolic function (e.g., isovolumetric contraction and relaxation, ventricular ejection and filling), and turbulence (i.e., disturbances of flow). There are four subcategories of Doppler, including pulsed wave (PWD), continuous wave (CWD), high–pulse repetition frequency (HPRF), and color flow imaging (CFI). Specialized applications of Doppler technology (e.g., stress, transesophageal, and intravascular echocardiography) have developed and, in practice, Doppler is commonly used in conjunction with 2D echocardiography to provide assessment of structural and functional activities of the heart. The following section focuses on issues related to the validity and reliability of echocardiographic techniques. More thorough reviews of the basic principles, applications, and mathematical and practical issues surrounding echocardiography have been published elsewhere (Hillard 1982; Nanda 1993).

Validity and Reliability. There is a great deal of complexity inherent in the successful orchestration of these techniques. For example, when using M-mode or 2D methods, the echocardiographic technician must be able to locate accurately the placement of the transducer, correctly identify the relevant acoustic boundaries within the target region, and fine-tune the ultrasound waveform to enhance signal clarity and maximize image interpretation. It is thus not surprising that the validity of these measurement techniques is intricately linked to the technician's skill and attention to detail.

Several methods have been used to validate these noninvasive echocardiographic measures. Compared to invasive Fick oximetry and thermodilution procedures, echocardiographic techniques produce clinically acceptable estimates of resting cardiac output and changes in cardiac output

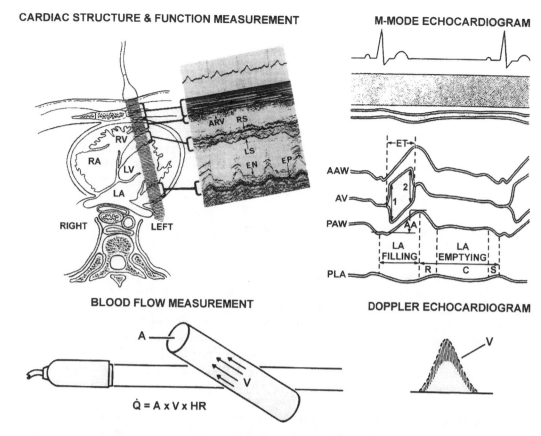

CARDIAC STRUCTURE & FUNCTION MEASUREMENT

M-MODE ECHOCARDIOGRAM

BLOOD FLOW MEASUREMENT

DOPPLER ECHOCARDIOGRAM

$$\dot{Q} = A \times V \times HR$$

during exercise (Christie et al. 1987; Espersen et al. 1995; Marx, Hicks, & Allen 1987). In addition, the sensitivity and specificity for detecting wall motion abnormalities in patients with coronary heart disease using echocardiography is comparable to that based on radionuclide and angiographic techniques (Beleslin et al. 1997; Ho et al. 1997; Oguzhan et al. 1997).

In the clinical setting, echocardiographic techniques are revered for their capacity to produce highly reliable measurements of valvular disease and pericardial effusion. In both the clinic and the research laboratory, measurements of wall and chamber dynamics are moderately reliable and can provide useful information regarding cardiac function in these settings (Felner & Martin 1994). In exercise settings, Doppler recordings of aortic velocity have shown acceptable reproducibility in healthy patients; however, in patients with coronary heart disease and known exercise-induced wall abnormalities, Doppler measurements of transmitral flow velocity show less consistency (Nissen 1994; Pearlman 1994).

Limitations. Echocardiography has multiple strengths and weaknesses, and in many cases they are intertwined. For example, the lack of automated quantitative measurements in 2D echocardiography is a limitation because the process of extrapolating the 2D data to a 3D tomographic context is time-consuming and requires a high level of technical and interpretive skill. Echocardiography is also limited in its use with certain patients because of their

Figure 9. Illustrations of echocardiographic and ultrasonographic data acquisition techniques. *Upper left.* One-dimensional "ice-pick" view of the heart with associated M-mode echocardiogram. Views of the right and left atria (RA, LA), right and left ventricles (RV, LV), the anterior right ventricular wall (ARV), the right and left septa (RS, LS), and the posterior left ventricular endocardium and epicardium (EN, EP) are obtained by angling the ultrasound beam toward the target structure. *Upper right.* M-mode echocardiogram and corresponding functional measurements: ejection time (ET), marked by opening and closing of the aortic valve (AV); onset (1) and end (2) of ejection; amplitude of motion (AA) of the posterior aortic wall (PAW), which reflects left atrial volume changes; the rapid filling (R), conduit (C), and atrial systole (S) phases contributing to left atrial emptying; and the anterior aortic wall (AAW) and posterior left atrial wall (PLA). *Lower left and right.* Diagram of Doppler ultrasonographic measurement of blood flow. Cardiac output (Q̇) is calculated by the product of the cross-sectional area of the vessel/orifice (A) with integrated flow velocity (V) multiplied by the heart rate (HR). Area is measured by either M-mode or two-dimensional echocardiography and velocity by Doppler. Reprinted with permission from Feigenbaum, *Echocardiography,* 5th ed. Copyright 1994 Lea & Febiger.

physique (e.g. obesity) and in patients with severe pulmonary disease.

Artifactual or extraneous ultrasound waveforms can also confound interpretation of echocardiographic recordings. Artifacts can arise from several sources, including: (a) reverberation of the waveform, which usually is misinterpreted as a second acoustic boundary at twice the depth of the target; (b) incorrect use of the echocardiography controls (e.g., gain settings), which may create distortion of the target image; (c) "side-lobe" waveforms, which are generated from weaker beams emanating from the edge of the transducer and can be misinterpreted as actual anatomic structures; and (d) electrical interference from other energy sources in the test environment. Variations in the width of the ultrasound beam can also cause complications in echocardiography. There is some degree of energy spread inherent in all ultrasound beams, and thus some extraneous echoes can be generated from energy that "escapes" the projected beam width and contacts structures juxtaposed to the target axis.

Other Cardiac Imaging Techniques. Several other imaging techniques have been developed to assess cardiac function and anatomy (Brundage 1994; Johnson & Lawson 1996; Johnson & Pohost 1994; Pettigrew 1994; Schelbert 1994; Stanford & Rumberger 1992). These modalities – which provide information about regional and global ventricular function, myocardial perfusion, and metabolic function and viability – have proven most beneficial in the critical care of patients with established heart disease and in evaluating acute MI damage.

Nuclear imaging techniques, such as gated blood pool scanning (GBPS) and radionuclide angiography (RNA), provide reliable measures of: left and right ventricular ejection fractions; end-systolic, end-diastolic, and heart chamber volumes; wall motion; and cardiac output. Ultrafast computed tomography provides highly accurate measurements of ventricular volume, ejection fraction, and flow derived from 3D images of the heart taken sequentially throughout the cardiac cycle. Single-photon emission computerized tomography (SPECT) is a particularly sensitive tool for detecting exercise stress–induced changes in coronary blood supply; and positron emission tomography (PET) is particularly useful in measuring left ventricular ischemia during acute coronary occlusion. In addition, it is now possible to obtain reliable and reproducible measurements of left ventricular function under ambulatory and exercise conditions using the VEST, a portable, miniaturized radionuclide cardiac probe incorporated within a semirigid plastic vest (Goodman et al. 1994; Mortelmans et al. 1991; Wilson et al. 1983). Although evaluation of ventricular function with the VEST has been conducted in a limited number of patients to date, this technology may improve the detection of ischemic events and be useful in determining risk stratification (see Kayden & Burns 1993). Despite the advanced nature of these techniques, their utility in psychophysiological research remains limited because they are more obtrusive and often more expensive than other noninvasive cardiac imaging techniques.

Measurement of Cardiac Parasympathetic Regulation. Although heart rate and its derivatives (e.g., heart rate variability, $HR_{max} - HR_{min}$) are commonly used in research and clinical settings as indices of cardiac PNS activity, none of these measures provide a relatively pure estimate of vagal control because they do not exist independent of SNS and nonneural influences on the heart. Several investigators have suggested, however, that heart rate variation during paced respiration is a sensitive noninvasive method for the diagnosis of parasympathetic cardiac impairment (Ewing et al. 1978; Genovely & Pfeifer 1988; Grossman, Stemmler, & Meinhardt 1990; Stemmler et al. 1991). Nonetheless, measurement of heart rate variation poses its own set of issues and controversy.

Spectral analysis, which is a frequency-domain approach, has been used to partition the heart rate variation occurring in the respiratory frequency band (Chess, Tam, & Calaresu 1975). Of these frequency ranges, the low- to mid-frequency bandwidths are associated with SNS, some PNS, and nonneural cardiac activity, whereas the high-frequency bandwidth best reflects PNS cardiac activity (Akselrod et al. 1981, 1985; Weise, Heydenreich, & Runge 1988). The spectral decomposition of both respiration and heart rate results in similar dominant frequency bands, although heart rate exhibits other prominent frequencies independent of respiration (Akselrod et al. 1985). Spectral analysis enables the quantitative description of the RSA amplitude but requires fairly long sampling periods (i.e., minutes) to produce stable measurement. This requirement prevents the examination of temporal response characteristics when the interest is to examine second-to-second rather than minute-to-minute RSA adjustments – although, if periods shorter than minutes are used, repeated time-locked samples may be aggregated over trial or stimuli (see Berntson et al. 1997).

Two time-domain approaches that lend themselves to the study of dynamic vagal changes are the V-hat (Porges 1985) and peak–valley methods (Grossman et al. 1990). Each of these methods has considerable advantages, although not without some limitations (see Berntson et al. 1997; Litvack et al. 1995). The V-hat technique uses a detrending filtering procedure and a bandpass filter with a bandwidth of 0.12–0.4 Hz (the bandwidth of human adult respiration) to extract the heart period variability in the respiratory band. The V-hat estimate is derived by calculating the natural logarithm of the variance of the filtered heart period time series over any chosen single period or sequential epochs of time. This technique has been validated in numerous studies using animals and humans with pharmacological and invasive techniques (Dellinger, Taylor, & Porges 1987; Jansen & Dellinger 1989; McCabe et al. 1984, 1985; Yongue et al. 1982). It is widely used and generates reliable and physiologically sound findings in clinical and nonclinical studies of adult humans (Donchin et al. 1992; George et al. 1989; Hatch et al. 1986).

A more recent time-domain technique assesses vagal activity by using an adaptive filtering methodology to quantitate the magnitude of vagal–respiratory (i.e., RSA)

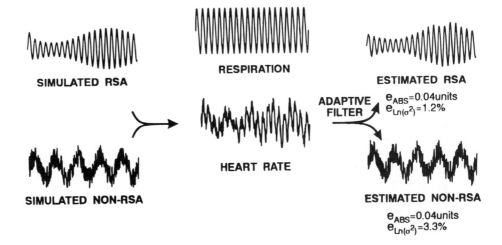

Figure 10. Decomposition of artificially simulated heart rate signals using the adaptive filtering technique is depicted within the context of a validational assessment. The simulated respiratory sinus arrhythmia (RSA) component was obtained by mixing the primary input of respiration (0.19-Hz sinusoid with constant amplitude) with a 0.01-Hz sinusoid and then passing it through a low-pass filter. The heart rate signal was formed by adding the simulated non-RSA (noise plus 0.05-Hz sinusoid) with the simulated RSA. In order to extract the heart rate variation that is most highly correlated with respiration, the respiration signal is used as the reference input to which the adaptive filter is modulated. Thus, the estimated RSA and non-RSA time series were generated by adaptive filtering of the heart rate signal. When comparing these waveforms with the original RSA and non-RSA waveforms, the average relative error is less than 4% (e_{ABS} = absolute error of the estimate; $e_{Ln(\sigma^2)}$ = average relative error in the natural logarithm of the estimated variances of non-RSA and RSA).

and nonrespiratory (i.e., NRSA) influences on heart rate variability and also provides RSA and NRSA measures (see Han et al. 1991; Nagel et al. 1993). This method, as depicted in Figure 10, decomposes the heart rate signal based upon its correlations with the respiration signal and takes into consideration both the magnitude and the phase of each signal. Therefore, a main advantage of adaptive filtering relative to other time-domain methods is that no definition of respiratory spectral bandwidth is necessary, because the RSA will contain only the heart rate that is within the ongoing respiratory frequency. Under changing conditions in which respiration frequency may move outside the assumed respiratory band, V-hat calculations will, by definition, be in error. However, because adaptive filtering makes no such assumptions regarding respiratory bandwidth, it continues to represent the variability in heart rate due to respiration. Note that if the respiratory frequency drops within the mid-frequency band (i.e., 0.05–0.12 Hz) then the resulting RSA may, in part, include information reflecting sympathetic neural input. Of course, this is true of time-domain as well as all other RSA methods. In addition, the adaptive filtering method relies on an accurate depiction within the respiration signal of respiratory frequency, so error in respiratory amplitude will not degrade the RSA estimate.

Another limitation of the V-hat method is that it may include some subset of the heart rate variation that happens to be within the respiratory band but that does not correlate with actual ongoing respiration. It is not known whether this heart rate variation might reflect other processes in addition to vagal cardiac processes. Therefore, to extract the heart rate variation that is most highly correlated with respiration and that can track the changes in cardiovagal input under changing conditions regardless of ongoing respiratory frequency, a continuous signal (RSAᴇ) was developed to assess the temporal characteristics of the adjustments in parasympathetic cardiac input (Han et al. 1991). The RSAᴇ is a continuous measure of the RSA obtained by calculating the envelope of the complex

RSA representation from the adaptive filter (Nagel et al. 1993).

The RSAᴇ is particularly useful in assessing concurrent contributions of the hemodynamic and autonomic branches of cardiovascular regulation during pharmacological challenge with adrenergic agonists. Figure 11 shows that, during a bolus intravenous phenylephrine (α-agonist) infusion, the MAP and estimates of vagal cardiac input (V-hat, RSAᴇ) increased significantly, tracking the substantial decline in heart rate. In contrast, bolus intravenous isoproterenol (β-agonist) infusion resulted in a substantial increase in heart rate, accompanied by a small decrease in MAP. Despite the changes in cardiac function and blood pressure during isoproterenol infusion, there were no significant changes in the RSA indices. Thus, the close correspondence between the RSA measure and MAP during phenylephrine infusion was not present during the isoproterenol infusion, indicating that RSA indices can provide information that is not present in either blood pressure or heart rate alone. Specifically, these data illustrate an increase in parasympathetic drive reflecting the cardiac limb of the baroreceptor reflex to vasoconstrictive increases in blood pressure. Thus, the RSA indices are sensitive measures that track in a

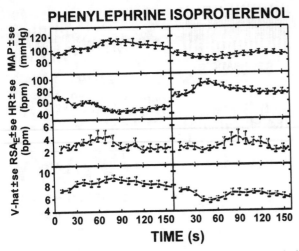

PHENYLEPHRINE ISOPROTERENOL

Figure 11. The mean ± SE response to bolus intravenous phenylephrine and isoproterenol infusions for mean arterial pressure (MAP), heart rate (HR), respiratory sinus arrhythmia envelope (RSAE), and V-hat methods. The RSA and MAP are closely correlated during phenylephrine, but not isoproterenol, infusion; thus, the RSA indices track dynamic changes in vagal cardiac input and provide information not present in either MAP or HR alone.

physiologically sound fashion the dynamic adjustments in cardiovagal input.

The Vascular System

Blood Pressure. Blood pressure is one of the most frequently recorded physiological functions in clinical medicine and psychophysiological research. Most of the different methodologies and instruments used within this broad range of applications are presumed to accurately measure blood pressure. However, indirect measurement techniques are susceptible to many forms of bias and error, and a working knowledge of the pertinent technical considerations and publication guidelines now available is recommended (Pickering 1996; Shapiro et al. 1996). The following section is intended to draw attention to the major methodological issues surrounding blood pressure recording devices principally used in contemporary psychophysiological research and to highlight unique concerns in dealing with special clinical populations and circumstances.

Methods of Blood Pressure Measurement

Intra-arterial. Blood pressure can be measured intra-arterially by inserting a teflon cannula percutaneously into the radial artery. The cannula is connected to a transducer and micromanometers are used to record true wave and pulsatile displacement of fluid. From these measures, reasonably precise determinations of mean arterial pressure (MAP) and pulse pressure – the difference between systolic blood pressure (SBP) and diastolic blood pressure (DBP) – can be made by integrating pressure curves derived simultaneously from various arterial beds. These measurements correspond well with the conventional formula used to estimate MAP using noninvasive techniques:

$$MAP = DBP + (SBP - DBP)/3.$$

Intra-arterial studies have demonstrated that this formula accurately estimates MAP at normal resting levels of heart rate; however, as heart rate increases, diastole is disproportionately shortened relative to systole. Thus, using this formula to determine MAP is subject to error associated with changes in heart rate occurring between the measurement of SBP and DBP. Nonetheless, in the broadest sense, there exists a direct relationship between MAP, flow, and resistance, which can be summarized as

$$MAP = \dot{Q} \times R,$$

where $\dot{Q}$ (flow) and R (resistance) are the cumulative derivatives of all the locally and neurohumorally regulated flow and resistance throughout all body tissues. However, it is neither feasible nor essential that they be measured directly in psychophysiological research to characterize MAP. In fact, because of their invasive nature and because they often are liable to artifact at more distally located recording sites, intra-arterial measurements are rarely used in behavioral medicine paradigms. Typically, with the use of noninvasive impedance cardiographic techniques, $\dot{Q}$ is operationalized as cardiac output and R as TPR.

Auscultatory. The auscultatory method of determining blood pressure involves the use of an inflatable bladder embedded within a blood pressure cuff that is typically placed around the subject's upper arm. The cuff is inflated to occlude the brachial artery and then slowly deflated. A stethoscope is used to detect audible sounds generated with each heartbeat as flow resumes in the artery below the cuff. Korotkoff described the distinct nature of these sounds, which begin as a faint clear tapping sound (phase I) and gradually change in quality and intensity. The SBP is defined as the pressure associated with phase-I sounds, and DBP is typically defined by the disappearance of Korotkoff sounds (phase V). This method has been used in clinical settings for over a century, yet there are still methodological issues surrounding it.

Depending on the characteristics of the subjects being studied, DBP may be better represented by phase IV, which is signaled by an abrupt, distinct muffling of the Korotkoff sounds approximately 5 to 10 mmHg before phase V. Thus, in scientific publications it is important to specify the criteria used to determine DBP. In addition, cuff size and placement can be critical factors in obtaining accurate blood pressure measurements. For example, a cuff that is too small can cause an overestimation of blood pressure. In addition, the mercury column or aneroid manometer used to detect cuff pressure should be in an upright position, parallel to the subject's heart level. Basic human error and biases also come into play, as observers may tend to round off readings toward a particular number (0 or 5) or bias their readings toward normal values. The

London School of Hygiene sphygmomanometer and the Hawksley "zero muddling" sphygmomanometer were developed to reduce observer bias and digit preference in clinical trials. The London School of Hygiene instrument consists of three mercury columns that are concealed from the operator's view during blood pressure measurement. The operator stops the descent of column 1, 2, and 3 to mark Korotkoff phases I, IV, and V (respectively) and views the corresponding levels of mercury post hoc. The zero-muddling instrument randomly adjusts the zero reference point to an unknown level prior to measurement. The observed blood pressure is then corrected to reflect the difference between the random and true zero values. Despite their methodological advantages, neither of these instruments are typically used in the research setting because they are somewhat cumbersome and their accuracy and utility as standard referents for evaluating other automated blood pressure devices have been widely challenged (Conroy et al. 1994; Mackie, Whincup, & McKinnon 1995; O'Brien & O'Malley 1981). Given the variety of instruments that are available to measure blood pressure, technician training and documentation of interobserver reliabilities in published reports will continue to be essential ingredients underlying the validity and reliability of cardiovascular psychophysiological research paradigms.

Many electronic devices for measuring blood pressure have been developed and incorporated into the psychophysiological research setting. The major advantage of these devices is that they permit measurement of a subject's blood pressure without the immediate presence of an observer. Readings can be recorded, amplified to facilitate identification of Korotkoff sounds, outputed digitally, and displayed for visual examination during the recording period. Despite these advantages, the accuracy and reliability of some of these devices (when compared to intra-arterial recordings) vary considerably (van Egmond et al. 1993). Thus, in practice, automated blood pressure readings must be standardized against manual auscultatory readings and, in most cases, a correction factor that captures the average differential between the two methods should be applied before reporting data or making a clinical diagnosis. Recommendations for standardization methodology have been published elsewhere (White et al. 1993).

A general concern related to auscultatory methods concerns the use of intermittent noninvasive readings of SBP and DBP to calculate MAP. Specifically, SBP and DBP are measured on the basis of two distinct pressure waves separated by a variable length of time that is dependent on pulse pressure. In other words, it takes longer to deflate the cuff to obtain a blood pressure measurement of 140/70 compared to 120/70, and that variable length of time can introduce error into the measurement depending on beat-to-beat variations in both the SBP and DBP pressure waves. In addition, subtle differences occur within the SBP and DBP pressure waves and so the relationship between the two is not necessarily stable over time. The implications of these potential sources of error can carry over into the estimation of peripheral resistance when a single value of MAP calculated from auscultatory measurements is associated with a single measure of cardiac output to derive TPR. Therefore, whenever possible, the research design should allow for multiple blood pressure readings over reasonably steady-state conditions in order to minimize the influence of these factors. Alternatively, MAP can be estimated on the basis of a single pressure, rather than separate systolic and diastolic pressures, using oscillometric methods.

Oscillometry. A standard cuff is positioned over the brachial artery and inflated to a pressure between SBP and DBP. As blood pulses under the cuff it generates pressure oscillations in the vessel that are transmitted to the cuff. No pulsations or oscillations can be felt in the radial artery until cuff pressure falls below systolic pressure level. At this point, the distant radial pulse can be felt and distinct oscillations can be seen in the mercury column. These oscillations increase in amplitude and reach a maximum as cuff pressure approaches mean arterial pressure. As cuff pressure further decreases, the oscillations decrease in amplitude. The SBP, MAP, and DBP can be derived, respectively, on the basis of (a) the initial sharp increase in pressure oscillation, (b) the lowest cuff pressure at which maximum cuff oscillation occurs, and (c) the pressure immediately prior to the cessation of oscillations. The primary advantage of this method is that it provides a very accurate mean arterial pressure, which is the best indicator of overall tissue perfusion. The oscillometric technique is particularly useful for measuring blood pressure in young children and shock patients in whom distinct Korotkoff sounds are not easily detected. However, it is less consistent in determining SBP and DBP than the auscultatory method (Fowler et al. 1991; Mauck et al. 1980). The obvious trade-off inherent in this method (less reliant on observer accuracy but more complex in terms of the electrical circuitry needed to determine SBP and DBP) must be taken into consideration by each researcher in designing study protocols.

Special Techniques for Measuring Blood Pressure

Volume Clamp Photoplethysmography. The FINAPRES Continuous Noninvasive Blood Pressure monitor (Ohmeda; Englewood, Colorado) and the PORTOPRES (TNO, Amsterdam) are two devices that measure blood pressure using a small finger cuff applied to the middle phalanx of the middle finger. The cuff contains an inflatable air bladder and a photoplethysmographic volume transducer (consisting of an infrared-transmitting diode and sensor) that are connected to a fast-response servo control system. Blood flow through the vessel is determined on a continuous basis according to the amount of scatter in the infrared light, and blood pressure is determined by fluctuations in cuff pressure as follows. When blood pressure rises, the arterial wall expands and finger volume increases. The transducer measures the volume differential and the device responds instantaneously by increasing the cuff pressure until the original arterial size and blood volume are re-established. The fluctuations in cuff pressure closely follow intra-arterial pressure, and pressure pulsations are of the greatest magnitude when the cuff is at mean arterial pressure. Thus, arterial blood pressure is measured continuously as a function of the external pressure applied through the cuff.

The FINAPRES monitor has been used in psychophysiological research settings for over a decade. It has been validated against intra-arterial and oscillometric methods, and its reliability has been tested in numerous patient and research populations. In general, the FINAPRES is regarded as a suitable method for monitoring blood pressure at rest, during postural tilt, and during exercise (Imholz 1996; Novak, Novak, & Schondorf 1994; Petersen, Williams, & Sutton 1995); however, minor errors in cuff application or positioning of the arm can lead to significant deviations between FINAPRES-measured and intra-arterial blood pressure (Jones et al. 1993). Furthermore, some have contended that prolonged exposure to the finger cuff pressure might facilitate vasoconstriction and thereby confound blood pressure measurement. Indeed, recent findings suggest that (i) the measurement of blood pressure during recovery from behavioral stress may be distorted as a function of nonstop FINAPRES monitoring and (ii) the degree of distortion may be greater in individuals who are higher reactors to the stressful challenge (Ristuccia et al. 1997).

Despite these limitations, this methodology has proven to be a useful tool in the assessment of sympathetic receptor mechanisms associated with hypertension and other cardiovascular pathologies. By combining impedance cardiographic measurements of beat-to-beat changes in heart rate with beat-by-beat changes in MAP, dose–response relationships for isoproterenol (β-agonist) and phenylephrine (α_1-agonist) can be determined. In turn, these dose–response relationships can be used to infer individual differences in receptor responsiveness (see section entitled "Hypertension"). Unfortunately, despite its success, the FINAPRES is no longer commercially available and its long-range application is uncertain.

Tonometry. An additional noninvasive method for deriving beat-by-beat blood pressure is arterial tonometry (Drzewiecki, Melbin, & Noordergraaf 1983). This method is based on the principles of ocular tonometry, which has been routinely used to measure intraocular pressure for many years. In this technique, an array of several independent pressure transducers is pressed against the skin overlying an artery to measure vascular tone during the cardiac cycle. Colin Medical Instruments (San Antonio, Texas) manufactures a tonometric device that employs a pressure sensor grid array that records vascular wall tension in the radial artery. This device provides beat-by-beat

SBP and DBP values as well as the continuous high-fidelity arterial pressure waveform. A standard occluding cuff is used for automatic calibration of the tonometric signal, with cuff inflation occurring only during initial calibration and when recalibration is necessary. Tonometry has practical utility in multiple settings and may be particularly useful for cardiovascular assessment during postural tilt or exercise maneuvers. This approach holds considerable promise for continuous, noninvasive blood pressure monitoring, but the technology is new and there is not yet a substantive literature on the device.

Ambulatory Blood Pressure Monitoring. Noninvasive ambulatory blood pressure monitoring technology has been available since the 1960s. Since that time, substantial improvements in the technology have occurred, including the development of fully automated, lightweight, user-friendly monitors for which standardization and validation specifications are now available (White et al. 1993). These devices can employ auscultatory and/or oscillometric methods for measuring blood pressure; however, a review of several types of devices indicated that those using the auscultatory method are generally more accurate (White, Lund-Johansen, & Omvik 1990a). They can be programmed to collect blood pressure and heart rate measurements at prescribed intervals that are relevant to the particular patient's concerns or researcher's experimental question. The data that are collected can be used to evaluate average blood pressure levels over fairly lengthy time intervals (i.e., day vs. night; home vs. work) or to investigate blood pressure variability within shorter periods of time. Ambulatory measurements relative to clinic measurements of blood pressure are highly reproducible, with negligible 24-hour placebo effects, and have considerable prognostic value (Devereux & Pickering 1991; Mancia et al. 1995; Mancia, Omboni, & Parati 1997; Ohkubo et al. 1997). Therefore, the information derived from this technique can be used to assess: (a) blood pressure patterns during sleep, relaxed wakefulness, and work; (b) the efficacy and diurnal profile of antihypertensive medications, which can be instrumental in establishing the individual patient's dosing regimen; (c) the overestimation of an individual's blood pressure level in the clinic as opposed to more normal readings elsewhere (i.e., "white coat" hypertension), which can lead to overmedication; and (d) the influence of real-life interpersonal stressors and individual behaviors (e.g., diet, smoking, physical activity) on short-term fluctuations in blood pressure.

To ensure the validity and reproducibility of ambulatory blood pressure measurements, certain precautions should be taken. For instance, documentation of postural changes during the monitoring period (Gellman et al. 1990) and proper sampling rates (Llabre et al. 1988) are crucial for deciphering individual and between-group differences in environmental and psychological determinants of ambulatory blood pressure. In addition, clear instructions need to be given to the subject or patient concerning proper arm position during readings, accurate record keeping of diary information, and expectations regarding personal discomfort and distraction while wearing the monitor. There are presently no published guidelines on the treatment of artifactual data (i.e., those beyond the normal range of acceptable, physiologically possible values), so care must be taken to describe artifact editing criteria in scientific reports.

Blood Pressure Measurement in Special Populations. The measurement of blood pressure in obese individuals and infants presents special concerns and challenges for the psychophysiologist and clinician. The central issue is using a blood pressure cuff that properly matches limb circumference (Prineas 1991). Consequently, various cuff designs have been introduced into the marketplace, including multi-bladder cuffs, forearm cuffs, and various portable devices using wrist and finger cuffs. Of these designs, only the Tricuff (Tricuff Pressure Group, Stockholm), which contains three rubber bags of different sizes that can automatically be selected according to the (adult) patient's arm girth, appears to provide any advantage over more traditional designs (Schwartz et al. 1996; Stolt et al. 1993; Tachovsky 1985). Given the inherent individual variability in arm girth, others have suggested a mathematical solution to this issue (i.e., use of standard formulas to correct for measurement error; Maxwell et al. 1982). In neonatal settings, reliable measurements of blood pressure in premature and healthy newborn infants can be obtained with a cuff placed around the infant's calf (Kunk & McCain 1996; Park & Lee 1989). In addition, blood pressure can be measured accurately in infants with newly developed high-fidelity intra-arterial systems (Gevers et al. 1996).

Blood Pressure Measurement during Exercise. Noninvasive measurement of systemic blood pressure during exercise is an important aspect of clinical evaluation of cardiac patients as well as in the psychophysiology laboratory setting, where the assessment of exercise-induced vascular, hormonal, and neural control mechanisms is of interest (see Griffin, Robergs, & Heyward 1997). Manual sphygmomanometry using auscultation is the most commonly used method for determining blood pressure during exercise, although movement artifact and noise greatly compromise the accuracy of this method. Resulting measurement inaccuracies can jeopardize the safety of the patient and the interpretation of research findings. To avoid these complicating factors, some technicians elect to measure blood pressure upon immediate cessation of exercise; however, such maneuvers result in gross underestimation of systemic pressure values induced by the exercise challenge. This underestimation is fundamentally linked to the rapid dissipation of systemic pressure values during the time it takes for a single inflation and deflation of the blood pressure cuff. Automated devices offer some advantage over manual techniques by limiting problems associated with

intertechnician variability and auditory acuity. However, the validity of many of these devices is suspect because manual sphygmomanometry, which is fraught with its own shortcomings, served as the criterion methodology against which they were compared. Nonetheless, several automatic blood pressure monitors provide accurate measurement of exercise SBP when compared with simultaneously derived intra-arterial pressures.

Blood Flow

Coronary Artery Flow. Up to this point, we have addressed the role of the heart as the pump or engine that ensures constant circulation of the body's fuel (oxygen) supply. The integrity of the oxygen supply to the working cardiac muscle is itself an equally important aspect of overall cardiovascular regulation. As previously mentioned, oxygenated blood empties into the left atrium via the pulmonary veins. Then, from the left ventricle, the blood is pumped into the ascending aorta and then on through the great vessels of the heart, which include the right and left coronary arteries. The right coronary artery is dedicated to supplying blood to the right atrium and ventricle. The left coronary artery bifurcates into the left anterior descending branch and left circumflex branch, which supply the left atrium and left ventricle, respectively (Schlant & Sonnenblick 1994).

At rest, the heart is able to draw readily upon the available oxygen in order to supply its energy needs. When the myocardial demand for oxygen increases (e.g., with exercise), the heart meets this need by increasing coronary blood flow rather than increasing its rate of oxygen extraction (Schlant & Sonnenblick 1994). Under normal conditions, coronary blood flow increases proportionally to myocardial demand for oxygen; however, when the integrity of the coronary arteries is compromised, localized or global deficiencies in coronary blood flow can occur and the heart can become arrhythmic and eventually stop pumping (Factor & Bache 1994). Generally, an occlusion must reduce the epicardial arterial lumen to roughly one third its original capacity in order to cause a significant decrease in coronary blood flow. In the presence of occlusive coronary heart disease (CHD), perfusion pressure can drop in the immediate site distal to the atherosclerotic plaque; however, ischemia at that site can be compensated for by an autoregulatory drop in resistance in the distal arteriolar bed. Thus, coronary blood flow is described as being independent of changes in perfusion pressure.

Coronary blood flow can be measured with conventional transthoracic Doppler technology using high-speed (2–5-MHz) ultrasound frequencies (see Figure 9). Frequency spectrum analysis is used to depict flow based on a change in velocity over time, and simultaneous ECG recordings are typically obtained to aid in determining temporal relationships within the cardiac cycle. Recent findings indicate that Doppler methods are sufficiently sensitive to identify abnormal peak systolic blood velocity and diastolic deceleration times in patients with cardiomyopathy (Crowley et al. 1997). In addition, Doppler methods can detect pharmacologically induced decrements in coronary blood flow, such as those associated with acute administration of sublingual nitroglycerin (Crowley & Shapiro 1997) and estradiol (Sbarouni, Kyriakides, & Kremastinos 1997).

Endothelial-Dependent Vasodilation. An intact endothelium is critical to vascular smooth muscle integrity and function. Acetylcholine stimulation causes vascular smooth muscle dilation in a dose-dependent fashion when the endothelium is intact; however, vasoconstriction occurs when the endothelium is damaged. The vasodilatory process involves diffusion of endothelial-derived relaxing factor (EDRF) to the smooth muscle layer, which triggers an increase in cyclic GMP and causes relaxation of the blood vessel. Of the various vasodilator substances that have been identified (e.g., serotonin, substance P, and thrombin), nitric oxide appears to be the predominant EDRF involved in this process (Palmer, Ferrige, & Moncada 1987). When blood flow increases, the endothelium responds by augmenting formation of nitric oxide and facilitating vascular smooth muscle relaxation. Nitric oxide is believed to play a modulating role throughout various stages of atherogenic CHD and congestive heart failure (see Cooke 1996; Dusting 1996). Defective endothelium-dependent regulation of vasomotor tone is a predisposing factor for vasospasm and ischemia in patients presenting with anginal pain, and it leads to impaired coronary blood flow during mental stress (Bult 1996; Wennmalm 1994). Endothelium-dependent vasodilation and the bioavailability of nitric oxide also appear to be *negatively* influenced by coronary risk factors such as smoking, hypercholesterolemia, hypertension, body fatness, and SBP reactivity to behavioral stress and *positively* related to cardiovascular fitness (Celermajer et al. 1994; Quyyumi et al. 1995; Treiber et al. 1997).

Endothelium-dependent vasodilation can be assessed by measuring the change in the diameter of the brachial artery during reactive hyperemia, a maneuver that increases flow through the conduit segment being studied (Lieberman et al. 1994). This stimulus is re-created by occluding flow to the forearm by inflating a cuff placed on the upper arm to suprasystolic pressure for five minutes. Consequently, the downstream forearm resistance vessels dilate; following cuff deflation, reactive hyperemia occurs as brachial artery blood flow increases to accommodate the dilated resistance vessels. Images of the brachial artery are obtained proximal to the antecubital fossa using high-resolution ultrasound. These images are obtained longitudinally, allowing clear visualization of the posterior wall intima-lumen surface and the anterior wall media–adventitial interface. Images are collected for a five-minute period following cuff deflation in order to (a) capture the peak diameter change during reactive hyperemia that occurs approximately one minute after deflation and (b) allow basal conditions to be re-established

(Uehata et al. 1993). Baseline images and those that occur one minute after cuff deflation (corresponding to the end of the T wave on a simultaneous ECG) are selected and digitized. To assure that the blood flow stimulus during reactive hyperemia is comparable, forearm blood flow is measured using Doppler ultrasound and venous occlusion strain gauge plethysmography (Creager et al. 1990).

Plethysmography. Plethysmography is a noninvasive technique for measuring blood flow to an isolated limb segment. The methodology involves placement of one blood pressure cuff (which produces venous occlusion) above the site of interest and a second cuff (which produces both arterial and venous occlusion) beyond the site of interest. In the case of the forearm, for example, a cuff is placed around the biceps area and around the wrist. The biceps (i.e. compression) cuff is inflated to a pressure above venous pressure but below arterial pressure, and the distal cuff is inflated to a suprasystolic level. The plethysmographic device, which senses changes in limb volume, is located between the cuffs. Typically, this device is a mercury-filled Silastic tube that stretches as limb volume expands. Changes in blood flow are derived from changes in electrical resistance along a flow of current through the tube. Alternatively, the limb can be submersed in water in an enclosed container or placed in an airtight chamber. Venous occlusion is then reflected in the amount of displaced water or air captured in an attached column, and total limb volume is reflected by the amount of water or air needed to refill the plethysmograph once the limb has been removed. These latter two methods are attractive because they provide direct measurement of volume related to blood flow. However, they are typically less mobile, harder to maintain, and more sensitive to environmental factors; thus, they are less commonly used than strain gauge techniques. Typically, a protocol will call for alternating cycles of occlusion (5–8 sec) and recovery (8–10 sec) to provide multiple readings of limb volume over the course of several minutes. Drainage of the limb during the recovery phase is facilitated by elevating the limb above the level of the heart.

Strain gauge measurements can be used to derive an indirect estimate of minimum forearm vascular resistance (MFVR) by dividing MAP by forearm blood flow. In turn, MFVR is used as an index of vascular functioning, and abnormalities in MFVR have been interpreted as an index of underlying structural pathology. An important application of this methodology has focused on the investigation of vascular contributions to hypertension. Several studies have revealed greater MVFR in borderline hypertensive compared to normotensive men, leading to the proposal that alterations in vascular structure may precipitate the establishment of essential hypertension (Egan et al. 1987; Sherwood, Hinderliter, & Light 1995a).

Venous Distensibility. The venous system plays an integral role in determining the hemodynamic profile both at rest and in response to stress. Venous distensibility decreases with age (Gascho, Fanelli, & Zelis 1989) and with progressive severity of congestive heart failure (Ikenouchi et al. 1991). Furthermore, venous distensibility is inversely related to plasma renin suppression during saline infusion (Borghi et al. 1988). Thus, decreased integrity of the venous system may contribute to the impaired hemodynamic control underlying various cardiovascular disorders. Assessment of venous distensibility – the change in transmural venous pressure as a function of venous volume – provides a noninvasive measurement of the integrity of the capacitance vessels. There are two primary plethysmographic techniques for assessing venous distensibility, equilibration and limb occlusion.

In the equilibration method, the limb is either submersed in a volume of water or raised above the level of the heart to cause the veins to collapse. In either case, care is taken to establish a stable, low-pressure baseline measure from which changes in venous pressure can be recorded. In a stepwise fashion, transmural pressure is increased by inflation of the compression cuff above the target limb area, and venous distensibility can be represented by plotting incremental changes in limb volume versus corresponding changes in distension pressure. The distension pressure is calculated as the difference between the intravenous and external water pressures. Changes in venous pressure can be characterized in two ways: (1) by using a venous catheter, which directly records changes in venous pressure that occur when arterial blood flows into the limb; or (2) by using a strain gauge, in which case venous pressure changes are presumed to match changes in pressure exerted by the compression cuff. Accuracy of the strain gauge technique is limited by relying on circumference changes to estimate limb volume and by subtle differences that may exist between the compression cuff pressure and actual venous pressure.

Limb occlusion involves inflating the proximal compression cuff to suprasystolic levels for several minutes in order to induce ischemia in the limb segment. Under these conditions of static venous volume, any changes in venous pressure (which are detected via intravenous catheter) can be attributed to reflexive changes in venomotor tone. Although this approach cannot be used to assess structural or humoral influences on venous distensibility, it is useful in the study of reflex neural contributions to venomotor responses to stress (Anderson 1989).

Ultrasonography. Doppler technology can be applied to the measurement of blood velocity (Pearlman 1994). The ultrasonic waveform is scattered by contact with moving red blood cells, and the frequency of the reflected ultrasound beam (i.e., its loudness) increases and then decreases as the blood cells move toward and then away from the ultrasound source. Scattered waves return to the receiving transducer, and the differences in their frequencies are compared to those of the transmitting waveform. The frequency difference is termed a Doppler shift. Blood flow can be described as being either laminar (i.e., adjacent cells are moving in an orderly pattern of similar velocity and direction) or turbulent (i.e., velocity and direction of neighboring cells is variable and disturbed). Doppler measurements can capture an image of flow turbulence and organization according to changes in Doppler shift frequencies.

Doppler methodology has a high specificity and sensitivity for evaluating gradations in carotid artery stenosis. Because the magnitude of the Doppler shift reflects both blood flow velocity and directional change, it is possible to assess the extent to which flow at the site of occlusion has become neutralized, "redirected" via collateral circulation, or even reversed (Dashefsky et al. 1991). Consequently, this technology has advanced our ability to detect lesions at earlier stages of the atherosclerotic disease process and to understand the progressive nature of atherosclerosis and the relationship between artery stenosis, ischemic episodes, and stroke (Moneta et al. 1987; Strandness 1994). Nonetheless, Doppler echocardiography has its own set of limitations. Namely, because Doppler uses low-amplitude signals, it is sometimes difficult to distinguish background noise from the actual ultrasound waveform. In addition, over- and underestimation of velocity can easily occur if the transducer is not held at the correct angular orientation relative to blood flow.

Recent advancements in the development of miniature intraluminal transducers have significantly enhanced ultrasonographic assessment of CHD (Nissen 1994). Intravascular ultrasound yields a 360° intramural anatomical view of lesioned and normal vessel wall segments and thus offers a distinct advantage over traditional angiographic procedures that often underestimate the severity of atherosclerotic lesions. Like other tomographic techniques, intravascular ultrasound imaging is susceptible to distortion due to nonorthogonal placement of the transducer, which can be problematic in small, circular cross-sectional vessels such as the coronary arteries. As long as the patient does not have an unusually small coronary artery diameter, this technique can provide extremely precise information regarding normal and diseased wall morphology in CHD. It can also be used to monitor maladaptive processes following revascularization surgery or cardiac transplantation.

Psychophysiological Context

Recent data indicate that nearly 13 million Americans suffer from coronary heart disease, and an estimated half million deaths are attributed to myocardial infarction each year. To date, significant progress has been made in the behavioral sciences toward identifying and delineating the contributions of behavioral and psychosocial factors to these outcomes. Consequently, biopsychosocial models of cardiovascular disease are being formulated to integrate both disease-promoting (e.g., depression, social isolation, socio-economic stress, hostility, and anger) and cardio-protective (e.g., adaptive coping and social support) factors that interactively influence disease trajectory beyond the scope of more traditional risk factors. The development of these models reflects a melding of findings from laboratory and field-based studies, which have employed a wide variety of pharmacological, behavioral, and real-life stress manipulations and an array of methodological and technical approaches. The following sections provide a brief overview of the major findings derived from the behavioral assessment of pathophysiological markers across the spectrum of cardiovascular disease.

HYPERTENSION

Approximately 43 million American adults have hypertension, which is the most important modifiable risk factor for CHD (see He & Whelton 1997). *Essential* hypertension is a condition marked by persistent elevations in resting blood pressure in the absence of a known organic origin (e.g., renal disease). In the early stages of hypertension, there are marked elevations in cardiac output, heart rate, and plasma NE, together with reduced β-adrenergic responsiveness. Over time, this pattern shifts toward chronic elevations in vascular resistance, vascular α-adrenergic hyperresponsiveness, and less pronounced elevations in NE. Julius (1993) proposed a pathological model of essential hypertension, suggesting that these transitional patterns (e.g., early-stage elevations in cardiac output, later elevations in vascular resistance) reflect an inherent CNS mandate to maintain blood pressure at a given level. Accordingly, prolonged elevations in sympathetic tone (increased NE, blood pressure, and cardiac output) and exaggerated sympathetic reactivity during stress promote vascular hypertrophy. Subsequently, as β-adrenergic receptor activity becomes progressively down-regulated, hypertrophied vessels become increasingly sensitive to α-adrenergic stimulation (e.g., vasoconstriction). Once hypertension is well established, a compensatory reduction in sympathetic tone occurs as blood pressure is maintained predominantly through permanent structural alterations in the vasculature.

Empirical support for this model stems from multiple sources. For example, greater blood pressure, cardiac output, and NE responses to behavioral stress, as well as higher mean forearm vascular resistance (suggestive of vascular hypertrophy), have been observed in prehypertensive and borderline hypertensive men compared with their normotensive counterparts (Light & Obrist 1980; Sherwood et al. 1995a). In addition, enhanced pressor responsivity has been associated prospectively with elevations in resting DBP in normotensive samples (Matthews, Woodall, & Allen 1993), and heightened vascular reactivity to pressor agents is a commonly reported characteristic of established hypertension (Egan at al. 1987).

According to the diathesis–stress model of essential hypertension (Manuck, Kasprowicz, & Muldoon 1990), hyperreactivity to stress is thought to lead to hypertension only in the presence of other predisposing negative psychosocial factors, and individual differences in personality or other stable behavioral traits are viewed as mediators of the reactivity–psychosocial hypertension relationship. Consistent with this model are recent findings of differences in sympathetic reactivity as a function of complex interactions involving ethnicity, family history of hypertension, anger, task demand, and environment.

Ethnicity

Black Americans are two times more likely to be hypertensive than white Americans, and the difference in CHD mortality between these two groups is expanding (Willems et al. 1997). Although the precise etiology of these disparities is not clear, evidence points to ethnic differences in biology, nutrition, environment, and psychophysiological reactivity (Anderson, McNeilly, & Myers 1991; Barnes et al. 1997). In addition to being greater vascular reactors to behavioral and pharmacological challenge (Dysart et al. 1994; Light et al. 1993; MacDonald et al. 1995; Saab et al. 1992; Sherwood & Hinderliter 1993; Sherwood et al. 1995b), blacks tend to excrete less sodium during behavioral stress and their blood pressure profiles appear to be more sensitive to dietary sodium and potassium manipulation (Dimsdale et al. 1987; Dimsdale, Ziegler, & Graham 1988; Light & Turner 1992; West et al. 1997). Notably, although both blacks and whites exhibit attenuated blood pressure reactivity to the cold pressor stimulus during normalization of dietary potassium, this intervention is associated with decreased vascular reactivity in blacks only (Sudhir et al. 1997). Furthermore, the emotional attributes of suppressed hostility and anger and certain types of social support may be particularly salient moderators of blood pressure in blacks as compared to whites (Brownley, Light, & Anderson 1996; Harburg, Blakelock, & Roeper 1979; Livingston, Levine, & Moore 1991). Finally, ambulatory monitoring studies have indicated that α-adrenergic–mediated reactivity measured in the laboratory predicts ambulatory blood pressure in blacks but not whites (Ironson et al. 1989) and that blacks exhibit smaller decreases in ambulatory blood pressure levels when they move from the work to home environment (Gellman et al. 1990). Thus, blacks may be predisposed to a greater hypertensive risk owing to multiple biological and psychosocial factors that include greater exposure to total hemodynamic load throughout a typical day, greater vascular responsivity during behavioral challenge, and greater negative emotional stress.

Family History of Hypertension

To better understand the genetic component of hypertension, numerous studies have attempted to determine if offspring of hypertensive parents are more likely to be high sympathetic reactors than those with normotensive parents. The results from these studies have been somewhat mixed (Anderson et al. 1989; de Visser et al. 1995; Gerin & Pickering 1995; Halstrup, Light, & Obrist 1982), possibly because the influence of family history of hypertension on vascular reactivity in particular is mediated by other factors. Those factors include an individual's resting blood pressure level, gender, and sodium intake, as well as the psychosocial elements of the behavioral task (al'Absi, Everson, & Lovallo 1995; Marrero et al. 1997; Miller, Friese, & Sita 1995a; Miller et al. 1995b).

ATHEROSCLEROSIS

Nearly 50% of mortality in Westernized societies is attributable to atherosclerotic disease. Atherosclerosis results from the accumulation of lipid deposits around atheromatous plaques that form along the intimal lining of arterial walls. Plaques tend to develop at sites where vascular damage has occurred, and the pathogenesis of vascular damage has been linked to platelet aggregation. Lipid deposits restrict blood flow and oxygen delivery and, if sufficiently large, can cause blockage of vessels resulting in ischemic pain. Recent findings indicate that atherosclerotic processes are well established in adolescence and that the prevailing resting blood pressure is a critical determinant in the development of advanced plaques (Barnett et al. 1997; Oalmann et al. 1997). Smoking and hypercholesterolemia are also major risk factors for atherosclerosis, but along with hypertension they account for only half of the variance for developing CHD. Thus, the characterization of other psychological, behavioral, and physiological factors that influence atherosclerosis presents a major challenge in contemporary behavioral research.

Circulating catecholamines influence platelet function directly, so sympathoadrenal hyperactivation is presumed to be one link between psychological stress and atherosclerotic disease (Anfossi & Trovati 1996). Platelet aggregation increases following postural and mental stress (Gebara et al. 1996; Wallen et al. 1997). Furthermore, recent findings indicate that the mental stress–platelet relationship is: (a) more pronounced in angina patients than in normal controls (Wallen et al. 1997); (b) highly selective (i.e., positively related to NE, negatively related to E, and unrelated to MAP; Patterson et al. 1995); and (c) accentuated during periods of increased occupational stress (Frimerman et al. 1997), by the outward expression of anger (Wanneberg et al. 1997), and by an individual's self-awareness of hypertensive status (Mundal & Rostrup 1996). Human platelet membranes predominantly express α-adrenergic receptors, which is consistent with the prevailing relationship between NE and platelet aggregability and which may partly explain the association between vascular reactivity and cardiovascular morbidity.

Disturbances in glucose and lipid metabolism are also related to the development of atherosclerosis and CHD, and these pathological processes may have psychosocial precipitants (NIH 1998). Epidemiological findings point to a constellation of interrelated CHD risk factors that constitute an insulin metabolic syndrome. This constellation of factors (central obesity, glucose intolerance, dyslipidemia, hypertension, and atherosclerosis) seldom occurs in its entirety within a given individual, yet a person who exhibits any one factor is highly likely to exhibit other features of the syndrome. Behaviors that increase insulin resistance (e.g., physical inactivity, excessive caloric intake, and psychosocial stress) also increase these CHD risk factors, whereas behaviors that decrease these risk factors (e.g., aerobic exercise training, weight reduction) tend to enhance insulin sensitivity. Although the precise biobehavioral pathways underlying these associations are not fully clear, they appear to reflect an interactive relationship involving insulin resistance, hyperinsulinemia, and sympathetic hyperactivity. In support of this contention, it has been observed that: (a) hypersecretion of insulin is a normal compensatory response to insulin resistance in individuals with normal glucose tolerance; (b) insulin causes dose-dependent increases in NE and subsequent increases in SBP; and (c) glucose extraction from skeletal muscle (where insulin resistance manifests) is influenced by SNS-mediated vasoconstriction. In addition, psychological stress and certain psychological traits affect insulin resistance and sensitivity both directly and indirectly through their influence on dietary, smoking, and physical activity patterns. For example, insulin resistance is related to sodium loading–induced increases in resting and ambulatory blood pressure as well as to cardiac output and vascular reactivity during stressful behavioral challenge (Gellman et al. 1997; Hurwitz & Schneiderman 1998). Ultimately, this trilogy (insulin resistance, hyperinsulinemia, and sympathetic hyperactivity) may form a positive feedback loop that, over time, promotes structural myocardial and vascular hypertrophy, increased platelet activation, and atherosclerosis (Schneiderman & Skyler 1996). Consistent with this model, impaired glucose metabolism has been observed in ischemic heart disease patients. However, findings demonstrating a lack of relationship between glucose intolerance and severity of coronary atherosclerosis (Seibaek et al. 1997) suggest the need for further examination of this model.

Predicting the progression of atherosclerosis could be particularly useful in the overall prevention of CHD. Behavioral stress testing and assessment of psychological factors may be beneficial in this regard. In 136 medically untreated subjects, SBP response to the Stroop task was predictive of change in extracranial carotid artery plaques at two-year follow-up (Barnett et al. 1997). Similarly, in a population-based sample of 940 Finnish men, low-paying, highly demanding occupations were associated with a significantly greater progression of carotid atherosclerosis (Lynch et al. 1997).

MYOCARDIAL ISCHEMIA

Mental stress has been implicated as a triggering mechanism in myocardial ischemia (see Krantz et al. 1996). Although the precise physiological mechanisms underlying mental stress–induced ischemia remain unclear, recent findings point to sympathetically mediated changes in vascular tone and blood circulation. In 58 patients with ischemia confirmed by ambulatory ECG monitoring, self-report diary measures of tension, sadness, and frustration were associated with a twofold increase in the risk of myocardial ischemia in the subsequent hour, after adjusting for physical activity and time of day (Gullette et al. 1997). In the Psychophysiological Investigations of Myocardial Ischemia (PIMI) study, ischemia was detected in 58% of patients during mental stress testing and in 92% of patients during exercise using radionuclide ventriculography, ECG, and blood pressure monitoring techniques (Goldberg et al. 1996). Notably, in the PIMI study, mental stress–induced ischemia was associated with increases in vascular resistance whereas exercise ischemia was not. Mental stress has also been associated with decreased coronary microcirculation (Dakak et al. 1995). Further studies are needed to delineate the psychological and physiological factors that account for individual differences in exercise and mental stress patterns of ischemia (Lenfant 1997). Candidate mediators include depression, which has been linked to reduced ambulatory heart rate variability in ischemic CAD patients (Krittayaphong et al. 1997), and various stress-sensitive sympathetic neurotransmitters such as NE, which has been shown to correlate with regional differences in coronary blood flow during cold stimulation in cardiac transplant patients but not in normal controls (Di Carli et al. 1997).

ACUTE CARDIAC EVENTS

A growing body of evidence points to intense psychological stress superimposed on a hypertonic sympathetic nervous system as a major precipitating factor in MI and sudden death. In addition to these triggering mechanisms, biobehavioral models of acute cardiac events suggest that individual difference factors (e.g., emotion, neuroendocrine pathways, behavior, and environment) and vulnerability factors interactively influence the occurrence of an adverse event (see Muller et al. 1994). Acute cardiac event risk is elevated with increased anatomical severity of CHD, chronic psychosocial factors (e.g., low socioeconomic status, high hostility), and episodic psychological distress syndromes (e.g., depression) (Kop 1997; Krantz et al. 1996). Furthermore, the psychological triggering of acute cardiac events may vary as a function of gender, age, and other patient characteristics (Behar et al. 1993; Cleophas et al. 1993;

Hallstrom et al. 1986), and post-MI quality of life may be influenced by pre-event depression (Conn, Taylor, & Wiman 1991). The consistency with which psychological factors have been linked to acute cardiac events implicates mental health intervention as a viable strategy to enhance survival and facilitate rehabilitation following such events.

A high degree of circadian variability has been noted in the occurrence of acute cardiac events, with an increased frequency of acute events occurring between 6:00 A.M. and noon (Cooke & Lynch 1994; Willich et al. 1993). This temporal pattern of elevated early morning risk is associated with concomitant elevations in heart rate, neuroendocrine activity, platelet aggregation, physical activity, and mental stress; it may also vary as a function of disease state (Behar et al. 1993) and be influenced by such factors as sleep (Koskenvuo 1987). These observations suggest that management of these disorders must consider individual patient differences and take advantage of temporal relationships among event risk and the pharmacodynamic properties of medications.

The laboratory stress reactivity paradigm and ambulatory ECG monitoring methods have proven useful in understanding genetic factors and the role of mental and physical stress in acute cardiac events. Ambulatory studies have shown that sudden cardiac death is linked to an inherited long Q-T interval syndrome, catecholamine-induced arrhythmias, ventricular dysplasia, and nocturnal hypoxia (Charoenpan et al. 1994; Myrianthefs et al. 1997). In addition, ischemia, left ventricular dysfunction, and exaggerated blood pressure and catecholamine responsiveness during mental stress have been associated with a significantly higher incidence of subsequent fatal and nonfatal cardiac events and other adverse cardiac profiles two to five years later (Jain et al. 1995; Jiang et al. 1996; Manuck et al. 1992). Also, CHD patients have been shown to exhibit greater increases in platelet aggregation during mental stress compared with healthy controls (Grignani et al. 1992). Sudden cardiac death is often precipitated by physical stressors, which may be exacerbated by excessive fatigue and mental stress (Appels & Otten 1992; Sugishita et al. 1988). Furthermore, exercise-induced sudden death, which has been documented both in recreational and laboratory stress-test settings (Rochmis & Blackburn 1971), tend to cluster around the time of peak exercise or the immediate postexercise period, during which time dramatic increases in NE occur (Dimsdale et al. 1984). Collectively, these findings support the notion that sympathoadrenergic hyperresponsiveness may be one mechanism linking stress with sudden cardiac death.

STRESS REACTIVITY, RESPONSE PATTERNING, AND CARDIOVASCULAR RISK

The process by which stressful stimuli influence disease is multifactorial, interactive, and individualistic. Fundamentally, the process involves exposure to some potentially stressful objective event that, pending subjective cognitive appraisal and interpretation, leads to some emotional, physiological, and/or behavioral response. The stress response is mediated by activation of the hypothalamic-pituitary-adrenocortical (HPAC) axis and the sympathetic-adrenomedullary (SAM) system. Activation of the HPAC axis during a stressful event results in an increased release of corticosteroids, permitting increased access to energy stores, and includes increased lipolysis and decreased inflammation. In comparison, SAM system activation during a stressful event results in increased catecholamine release, blood pressure, cardiac output, respiration, and blood flow. Actual differences in stress load or perceived differences in control of the aversive content of the stressor may lead to differential response patterns consequent to the integration of this information at the level of the CNS (Schneiderman 1978; Schneiderman & McCabe 1989).

Animal and human studies have shown that mammals exposed to behavioral stress exhibit differential cardiorespiratory and metabolic response patterns depending on access to and activation of appropriate coping actions. Accordingly, two primary behavioral patterns that may be characterized as activational ("defense") versus inhibitional ("vigilance") have been associated with two SNS patterns. The pattern-1 (activational) response is characterized by increased skeletal muscle vasodilation, cardiac output, SBP, and β_1-adrenergic tone; the pattern-2 (inhibitional) response is characterized by increased skeletal muscle vasoconstriction, DBP, TPR, and α-adrenergic tone.

The stress reactivity paradigm has evolved as a means to explore potential pathophysiological relationships between these differential response patterns and cardiovascular disease risk in humans. A growing body of research indicates that blood pressure reactivity to several behavioral challenges (e.g., mental arithmetic, mirror tracing, evaluative speech) is predictive of resting blood pressure levels years later (Borghi et al. 1986; Matthews et al. 1993; Murphy, Alpert, & Walker 1992). Furthermore, the blood pressure response to cold pressor stimulation, which is associated with a highly reliable vasoconstrictive response (Durel et al. 1993; Hurwitz et al. 1993b; Saab et al. 1993; Sherwood et al. 1997), is predictive of later development of hypertension (Menkes et al. 1989; Woods et al. 1984). It has been argued that the cold pressor task is physical in nature and thus does not provide a meaningful probe with which to examine psychological contributions to cardiovascular pathophysiology. However, recent findings suggest that the elevated blood pressure response to the cold pressor test is essentially due to the psychological properties (e.g., perceived pain) of the task (Peckerman et al. 1991, 1994). Thus, reactivity to the cold pressor stimulus has emerged as a useful tool for evaluating α-adrenergic contributions to cardiovascular regulation in hypertension.

The predictive relationship between cardiovascular reactivity and hypertension has been challenged on the basis that reactivity does not generalize across a wide variety of tasks (McKinney et al. 1985; Parati et al. 1988, 1991; Pickering & Gerin 1990). The generalization issue is interesting and important, but it does not really challenge the association between psychological reactivity and subsequent hypertension development. In defining psychological reactivity, it is important to emphasize the reliability of responses because reactivity is conceived as being a dispositional attribute. Thus, if reactivity is situation-specific, then one would expect individuals who show situation-specific reactivity to a stressor at one time to show comparable situation-specific reactivity at a later time. For this reason, generalization of one task to another is not necessary for the validity of the reactivity hypothesis. Instead, it adds the important insight that different psychological stressors may elicit different patterns of hemodynamic response, demonstrating situational stereotypy. Data consistent with this conceptualization have been obtained from echocardiographic studies relating left ventricular mass to cardiovascular reactivity (Rostrup et al. 1994).

Although blood pressure elevations during psychological stressors are generally associated with either a pattern-1 or a pattern-2 response profile, a mixed pattern of responding may also occur. This mixed pattern may reflect the behavioral task itself and its context, differences in individual history, perceptual and response styles, and other variables (Schneiderman & McCabe 1989). In a community sample of adult white men and women matched for age and body mass, the preparation for evaluative speech elicited pattern 1, in which the increase in blood pressure was supported by increases in cardiac contractility and cardiac output. In contrast, both the mirror tracing and cold pressor tests induced pattern 2, in which the blood pressure increase was supported by an increase in TPR (Hurwitz et al. 1993b). The presentation of the speech induced a mixed pattern of response in which the blood pressure increase was supported by both increased cardiac output and TPR.

A growing body of evidence also suggests that both situational stereotypy and individual response stereotypy may be important in characterizing autonomic responses to psychological stress. A review of empirical studies focused on blood pressure indices of autonomic arousal (Marwitz & Stemmler 1998) revealed a low rate (33%) of individual response specificity (IRS) and IRS stability (15%). However, Saab and colleagues (1992) observed consistent TPR-mediated increases in blood pressure during a battery of stressors in black men – demonstrating individual response stereotypy – compared with distinct situation-specific hemodynamic response patterns to the same stressors in white men. Therefore, it appears that comprehensive hemodynamic assessments of response to stressful behavioral challenge may be essential to disentangling the complex interactions between these factors.

Findings of cardiovascular response stereotypy provide a conceptual foundation for hypothesizing that individual difference variables may be related to CHD pathology. Friedman and Rosenman (1959), for example, described the type-A behavior pattern as an "action-emotion complex" exhibited by an individual who is engaged in a chronic, excessive struggle to achieve poorly defined goals, often against the opposing efforts of others. Based upon this hypothesis, the Western Collaborative Group Study (WCGS) was established as a prospective, epidemiologic study of CHD incidence in more than 3,100 men aged 39–59 years. After 8.5 years, the type-A subjects exhibited 2.25 times the rate of new CHD morbidity as their type-B counterparts (Rosenman et al. 1975), which – after controlling for differences in age, serum cholesterol, systolic blood pressure, and smoking – provided a relative risk of approximately 1.97 (Brand 1978). Reanalysis of the initial epidemiological findings suggested that hostility was a key factor distinguishing type-A from type-B men in the WCGS (Matthews et al. 1977). Subsequent epidemiological studies confirmed that individuals who were high in hostility revealed a higher rate of CHD disease incidence (Barefoot, Dahlstrom, & Williams 1983; Shekelle et al. 1983).

An early psychophysiology study indicated that type-A individuals exceeded type-Bs in magnitude of SBP responses to a video task only if the subjects were harassed (Diamond et al. 1984). Follow-up analyses indicated that only subjects rated high in hostility showed significant SBP reactivity as a function of type-A behavior pattern. Subsequent studies have confirmed and extended findings that high-hostile individuals demonstrate exaggerated blood pressure responses to harassing or emotionally provocative stressors (Suarez et al. 1993; Suls & Wan 1993). Presently, it is not clear whether hostility confers its CHD risk by accelerating the development of atherosclerosis (Barefoot et al. 1994), by precipitating acute events such as MI (Brackett & Powell 1988), or both. Limited cross-sectional data demonstrate greater activation of the SAM system and HPAC axis during laboratory and real-life stress in hostile individuals (see Smith 1992); however, further studies need to be conducted longitudinally and in CHD patient populations to elucidate the precise mechanisms mediating the hostility–CHD association.

Summary

This chapter has provided an overview of the basic anatomy and physiology of the cardiovascular system; it introduced several techniques for measurement of cardiac function and highlighted issues of reliability and validity surrounding these techniques; and it briefly examined the literature on individual differences, response tendencies, and psychosocial factors affecting various processes underlying cardiovascular pathology. Incorporation of ultrasonography and impedance cardiography methods, in particular, into the psychophysiological research arsenal have enhanced our understanding of behavioral influences on both normal and pathological cardiac function. In addition, recent progress in the development of signal processing techniques has provided new insight regarding the interactive nature of parasympathetic and sympathetic cardiac control during behavioral paradigms. Such advancements, coupled with other refinements in noninvasive measurement techniques and the extension of those methodologies into ambulatory settings, will continue to promote a more integrated perspective of the putative etiological and behavioral mechanisms underlying cardiovascular-related disease.

REFERENCES

Akselrod, S., Gordon, D., Madwed, J. B., Snidman, N. C., Shannon, D. C., & Cohen, R. J. (1985). Hemodynamic regulation: Investigation by spectral analysis. *Am. J. Physiol.*, 249, H867–H875.

Akselrod, S., Gordon, D., Ubel, F. A., Shannon, D. C., Berger, A. C., & Cohen, R. J. (1981). Power spectrum analysis of heart rate fluctuation: A quantitative probe of beat-to-beat cardiovascular control. *Science*, 213, 220–2.

al'Absi, M., Everson, S. A., & Lovallo, W. R. (1995). Hypertension risk factors and cardiovascular reactivity to mental stress in young men. *Int. J. Psychophysiol.*, 20, 155–60.

Anderson, E. A. (1989). Measurement of blood flow and venous distensibility. In N. Schneiderman, S. M. Weiss, & P. G. Kaufmann (Eds.), *Handbook of Research Methods in Cardiovascular Behavioral Medicine*, pp. 81–90. New York: Plenum.

Anderson, N. B., Lane, J. D., Taguchi, F., Williams, R. B., & Houseworth, S. J. (1989). Race, parental history of hypertension, and patterns of cardiovascular reactivity in women. *Psychophysiology*, 26, 39–47.

Anderson, N. B., McNeilly, M., & Myers, H. (1991). Autonomic reactivity and hypertension in blacks: A review and proposed model. *Ethn. Dis.*, 1, 154–70.

Andresen, M. C., & Kunze, D. L. (1994). Nucleus tractus solitarius – Gateway to neural circulatory control. *Annu. Rev. Physiol.*, 56, 93–116.

Anfossi, G., & Trovati, M. (1996). Role of catecholamines in platelet function: Pathophysiological and clinical significance. *Eur. J. Clin. Invest.*, 26, 353–70.

Appels, A., & Otten, F. (1992). Exhaustion as precursor of cardiac death. *Br. J. Clin. Psychol.*, 31, 351–6.

Bainbridge, F. A. 1915. The influence of venous filling upon the rate of the heart. *J. Physiol.*, 50, 65–78.

Baker, S. P., Boyd, H. M., & Potter, L. T. (1980). Distribution and function of β-adrenoceptors in different chambers of the canine heart. *Br. J. Pharmacol.*, 68, 57–63.

Baker, S. P., & Potter, L. T. (1980). Biochemical studies of cardiac β-adrenoceptors, and their clinical significance. *Circ. Res.*, 46 (Suppl. I), 34–42.

Baller, L. E., Hurwitz, S. J., & Nassirian, M. (1983). Assessment of contractility from the electrical impedance cardiogram. In C. W. Hall (Ed.), *Biomedical Engineering II: Recent Developments* (Proceedings of the Second Southern Biomedical Engineering Conference), pp. 23–6. New York: Pergamon.

Barefoot, J. C., Dahlstrom, G., & Williams, R. B. (1983). Hostility, CHD incidence, and total mortality: A 25-year follow-up study of 255 physicians. *Psychosom. Med., 45,* 59–63.

Barefoot, J. C., Patterson, J. C., Haney, T. L., Cayton, T. G., Hickman, J. R., Jr., & Williams, R. B. (1994). Hostility in asymptomatic men with angiographically confirmed coronary artery disease. *Am. J. Cardiol., 74,* 439–42.

Barnes, V., Schneider, R., Alexander, C., & Staggers, F. (1997). Stress, stress reduction, and hypertension in African Americans: An updated review. *J. Natl. Med. Assoc., 89,* 464–76.

Barnett, P. A., Spence, J. D., Manuck, S. B., & Jennings, J. R. (1997). Psychological stress and the progression of carotid artery disease. *J. Hypertens., 15,* 49–55.

Bayes de Luna, A. (1993). *Clinical Electrocardiography: A Textbook.* Mount Kisco, NY: Futura.

Behar, S., Halabi, M., Reicher-Reiss, H., Zion, M., Kaplinsky, E., Mandelzweig, L., & Goldbourt, U. (1993). Circadian variation and possible external triggers of onset of myocardial infarction. SPRINT Study Group. *Am. J. Med., 94,* 395–400.

Beleslin, B. D., Ostojic, M., Djordjevic-Dikic, A., Nedeljkovic, M., Stankovic, G., Stojkovic, S., Babic, R., Stepanovic, J., Saponjski, J., Marinkovic, J., Vasiljevic-Pokrajcic, Z., & Kanjuh, V. (1997). Coronary vasodilation without myocardial erection. Simultaneous haemodynamic, echocardiographic and arteriographic findings during adenosine and dipyridamole infusion. *Eur. Heart J., 18,* 1166–74.

Bell, C. (1987). Endogenous renal dopamine and control of blood pressure. *Clin. Exp. Hypertens., 9,* 955–75.

Berne, R. M., & Levy, M. N. (1981). *Cardiovascular Physiology,* 4th ed. St. Louis, MO: Mosby.

Bernstein, D. P. (1986). A new stroke volume equation for thoracic electrical bioimpedance: Theory and rationale. *Crit. Care Med., 14,* 904–9.

Berntson, G. G., Bigger, J. T., Eckberg, D. L., Grossman, P., Kaufman, P. G., Malik, M., Nagaraja, H. N., Porges, S. W., Saul, J. P., Stone, P. H., & van der Molen, M. W. (1997). Heart rate variability: Origins, methods, and interpretive caveats. *Psychophysiology, 34,* 623–48.

Berntson, G. G., Cacioppo, J. T., & Quigley, K. S. (1991). Autonomic determinism: The modes of autonomic control, the doctrine of autonomic space, and the laws of autonomic constraint. *Psychol. Rev., 98,* 459–87.

Berntson, G. G., Cacioppo, J. T., & Quigley, K. S. (1993). Respiratory sinus arrhythmia: Autonomic origins, physiological mechanisms, and psychophysiological implications. *Psychophysiology, 30,* 183–96.

Boomsma, D. I., de Vries, J., & Orlebeke, J. F. (1989). Comparison of spot and band impedance cardiogram electrodes across difference tasks. *Psychophysiology, 26,* 695–9.

Borghi, C., Boschi, S., Costa, F. V., Munarini, A., Mussi, A., & Ambrosioni, E. (1988). Importance of plasma renin activity suppression and venous distensibility on pressor and natriuretic responses to intravenous salt load in borderline hypertension. *Am. J. Hypertens., 1,* 294–7.

Borghi, C., Costa, F. V., Boschi, S., Mussi, A., & Ambrosioni, E. (1986). Predictors of stable hypertension in young borderline subjects: A five-year follow-up study. *J. Cardiovasc. Pharmacol., 8,* S138–S141.

Brackett, C. D., & Powell, L. H. (1988). Psychological and physiological predictors of sudden cardiac death after healing of acute myocardial infarction. *Am. J. Cardiol., 61,* 979–83.

Brand, R. J. (1978). Coronary-prone behavior as an independent risk factor for coronary heart disease. In T. M. Dembroski, S. M. Weiss, J. L. Shields, S. G. Haynes, & M. Feinleib (Eds.), *Coronary-Prone Behavior,* pp. 11–24. New York: Springer-Verlag.

Brownley, K. A., Light, K. C., & Anderson, N. B. (1996). Social support and hostility interact to influence clinic, work, and home blood pressure in black and white men and women. *Psychophysiology, 33,* 434–45.

Brundage, B. H. (1994). Computed tomography of the heart. In Schlant & Alexander, pp. 2325–37.

Bult, H. (1996). Nitric oxide and atherosclerosis: Possible implications for therapy. *Mol. Med. Today, 2,* 510–18.

Buxton, B. F., Jones, C. R., Molenaar, P., & Summers, R. J. (1987). Characterization and autoradiographic localization of beta-adrenoceptor subtypes in human cardiac tissues. *Br. J. Pharmacol., 92,* 299–310.

Cacioppo, J. T., Berntson, G. G., & Quigley, K. S. (1994). Autonomic cardiac control. II. Noninvasive indices and basal response as revealed by autonomic blockades. *Psychophysiology, 31,* 586–98.

Castellanos, A., Kessler, K. M., & Myerburg, R. J. (1994). The resting electrocardiogram. In Schlant & Alexander, pp. 321–56.

Celermajer, D. S., Sorensen, K. E., Bull, C., Robinson, J., & Deanfield, J. E. (1994). Endothelium-dependent dilation in the systemic arteries of asymptomatic subjects relates to coronary risk factors and their interaction. *J. Am. Coll. Cardiol., 24,* 1468–74.

Charoenpan, P., Muntarbhorn, K., Boongird, P., Puavilai, G., Ratanaprakarn, R., Indraprasit, S., Tanphaichitr, V., Likittanasombat, K., Varavathya, W., & Tatsanavivat, P. (1994). Nocturnal physiological and biochemical changes in sudden unexplained death syndrome: A preliminary report of a case control study. *Southeast Asian J. Trop. Med. Public Health, 25,* 335–40.

CHBPR [Council for High Blood Pressure Research] (1978). *Hypertension: Renal, Hormonal, and Neural Mechanisms: Proceedings of the 1977 Annual Meeting.* Dallas, TX: American Heart Association.

Chess, G. F., Tam, R. M. K., & Calaresu, F. R. (1975). Influence of cardiac neural inputs on rhythmic variations of heart period in the cat. *Am. J. Physiol., 228,* 775–80.

Christie, J., Sheldahl, L. M., Tristani, F. E., Sagar, K. B., Ptacin, M. J., & Wann, S. (1987). Determination of stroke volume and cardiac output during exercise: Comparison of two-dimensional and Doppler echocardiography, Fick oximetry, and thermodilution. *Circulation, 76,* 539–47.

Cleophas, T. J., de Jong, S. J., Niemeyer, M. G., Tavenier, P., Zwinderman, K., & Kuypers, C. (1993). Changes in life-style in men under sixty years of age before and after acute myocardial infarction: A case-control study. *Angiology, 44,* 761–8.

Conn, V. S., Taylor, S., & Wiman, P. (1991). Anxiety, depression, quality of life, and self-care among survivors of myocardial infarction. *Issues Ment. Health Nurs., 12,* 321–31.

Conroy, R. M., Atkins, N., Mee, F., O'Brien, E., & O'Malley, K. (1994). Using Hawksley random zero sphygmomanometer as a gold standard may result in misleading conclusions. *Blood Press. 3*, 283–6.

Cooke, H. M., & Lynch, A. (1994). Biorhythms and chronotherapy in cardiovascular disease. *Am. J. Hosp. Pharm., 51*, 2569–80.

Cooke, J. P. (1996). Role of nitric oxide in progression and regression of atherosclerosis. *West. J. Med., 164*, 419–24.

Creager, M. A., Cooke, J. P., Mendelsohn, M. E., Gallager, S. J., Coleman, S. M., Loscalzo, J., & Dzau, V. J. (1990). Impaired vasodilation of forearm resistance vessels in hypercholesterolemic humans. *J. Clin. Invest., 86*, 228–34.

Crowley, J. J., Dardas, P. S., Harcombe, A. A., & Shapiro, L. M. (1997). Transthoracic Doppler echocardiographic analysis of phasic coronary blood flow velocity in hypertrophic cardiomyopathy. *Heart, 77*, 558–63.

Crowley, J. J., & Shapiro, L. M. (1997). Transthoracic echocardiographic measurement of coronary blood flow and reserve. *J. Am. Soc. Echocardiogr., 10*, 337–43.

Dakak, N., Quyyumi, A. A., Eisenhofer, G., Goldstein, D. S., & Cannon, R. O. (1995). Sympathetically mediated effects of mental stress on the cardiac microcirculation of patients with coronary artery disease. *Am. J. Cardiol., 76*, 125–30.

Dashefsky, S. M., Cooperberg, P. L., Harrison, P. B., Reid, J. D., & Araki, D. N. (1991). Total occlusion of the common carotid artery with patent internal carotid artery. Identification with color flow Doppler imaging. *J. Ultrasound Med., 10*, 417–21.

Dellinger, J. A., Taylor, H. L., & Porges, M. S. (1987). Atropine sulfate effects on aviator performance and on respiratory-heart period interactions. *Aviati. Space Environ. Med., 58*, 333–8.

Demeter, R. J., Parr, K. L., Toth, P. D., & Woods, J. R. (1993). Use of noninvasive bioelectric impedance to predict cardiac output in open heart recovery. *Biol. Psychol., 36*, 23–32.

Denniston, J. C., Maher, J. T., Reeves, J. T., Cruz, J. C., Cymerman, A., & Grover, R. F. (1976). Measurement of cardiac output by electrical impedance at rest and during exercise. *J. Appl. Physiol., 40*, 91–5.

Devereux, R. B., & Pickering, T. G. (1991). Relationship between the level, pattern, and variability of ambulatory blood pressure and target organ damage in hypertension. *J. Hypertens., 9 (Suppl. 8)*, S34–S38.

de Visser, D. C., van Hooft, I. M., van Doornen, L. J., Hoffman, A., Orlebeke, J. F., & Grobbee, D. E. (1995). Cardiovascular response to mental stress in offspring of hypertensive parents: The Dutch hypertension and offspring study. *J. Hypertens., 13*, 901–8.

Diamond, E. L., Schneiderman, N., Schwartz, D., Smith, J. C., Vorp, R., & Pasin, R. D. (1984). Harassment, hostility, and type A as determinants of cardiovascular reactivity during competition. *J. Behav. Med., 7*, 171–89.

DiBona, G. F. (1989). Neural control of renal function: Cardiovascular implications. *Hypertension, 13*, 539–48.

Di Carli, M. F., Tobes, M. C., Mangner, T., Levine, A. B., Muzik, O., Chakroborty, P., & Levine, T. B. (1997). Effects of cardiac sympathetic innervation on coronary blood flow. *N. Engl. J. Med., 336*, 1208–15.

Dimsdale, J., Graham, R. M., Ziegler, M. G., Zusman, R. M., & Berry, C. C. (1987). Age, race, diagnosis, and sodium effects on the pressor response to infused norepinephrine. *Hypertension, 10*, 564–9.

Dimsdale, J. E., Hartley, H., Guiney, T., Ruskin, J. N., & Greenblatt, D. (1984). Postexercise peril: Plasma catecholamines and exercise. *JAMA, 251*, 630–2.

Dimsdale, J. E., & Moss, J. M. (1980). Plasma catecholamines in stress and exercise. *JAMA, 243*, 340–2.

Dimsdale, J., Ziegler, M., & Graham, R. (1988). The effect of hypertension, sodium, and race on isoproterenol sensitivity. *Clin. Exper. Hypertens. – Theory Prac., A10*, 747–56.

Donchin, Y., Constantini, S., Szold, A., Byrne, E. A., & Porges, S. W. (1992). Cardiac vagal tone predicts outcome in neurosurgical patients. *Crit. Care Med., 20*, 942–9.

Drzewiecki, G. M., Melbin, J., & Noordergraaf, A. (1983). Arterial tonometry: Review and analysis. *J. Biomech., 16*, 141–52.

Dubin, D. (1996). *Rapid Interpretation of EKGs*, 5th ed. Tampa, FL: Cover Publishing.

Durel, L. A., Kus, L. A., Anderson, N. B., McNeilly, M., Llabre, M. M., Spitzer, S., Saab, P. G., Efland, J., Williams, R., & Schneiderman, N. (1993). Patterns and stability of cardiovascular responses to variations of the cold pressor test. *Psychophysiology, 30*, 39–46.

Dusting, G. J. (1996). Nitric oxide in coronary artery disease: Roles in atherosclerosis, myocardial reperfusion and heart failure. *EXS, 76*, 33–55.

Dysart, J. M., Treiber, F. A., Pflieger, K., Davis, H., & Strong, W. B. (1994). Ethnic differences in the myocardial and vascular reactivity to stress in normotensive girls. *Am. J. Hypertens., 7*, 15–22.

Ebert, T. J., Eckberg, D. L., Vetrovec, G. M., & Cowley, M. J. (1984). Impedance cardiograms reliably estimate beat-by-beat changes of left ventricular stroke volume in humans. *Cardiovasc. Res., 18*, 354–60.

Egan, B., Panis, R., Hinderliter, A., Schork, N., & Julius, S. (1987). Mechanism of increased alpha adrenergic vasoconstriction in human essential hypertension. *J. Clin. Invest., 80*, 812–17.

Einthoven, W., Fahr, G., & de Waart, A. (1913). Uber die Richtung und die manifeste Grosse der Pontetialschwankungen in menchlichen Herzen und uber den Einfluss der Herzlage auf die Form des Elecktrokardiogramms. *Arch. Physiol., 150*, 275–315.

Espersen, K., Jensen, E. W., Rosenborg, D., Thomsen, J. K., Eliasen, K., Olsen, N. V., & Kanstrup, I. L. (1995). Comparison of cardiac output measurement techniques: Thermodilution, Doppler, CO2-rebreathing and the direct Fick method. *Acta Anaesthesiol. Scand., 39*, 245–51.

Ewing, D. J., Campbell, I. W., Murray, A., Neilson, J. M. M., & Clarke, B. F. (1978). Immediate heart-rate response to standing: Simple test for autonomic neuropathy in diabetes. *Br. Med. J., 1*, 145–7.

Factor, S. M., & Bache, R. J. (1994). Pathophysiology of myocardial ischemia. In Schlant & Alexander, pp. 1033–53.

Feigenbaum, H. (1994). *Echocardiography*, 5th ed. Philadelphia: Lea & Febiger.

Felner, J. M., & Martin, R. P. (1994). The echocardiogram. In Schlant & Alexander, pp. 375–422.

Flacke, W., & Gillis, R. A. (1969). Impulse transmission via nicotine and muscarinic pathways in the stellate ganglion of the dog. *J. Pharmacol. Exp. Ther., 163*, 266–76.

Fowler, G., Jamieson, M. J., Lyons, D., Jeffers, T. A., Webster, J., & Petrie, J. C. (1991). Sphygmomanometers in clinical practice and research. In E. O'Brien & K. O'Malley (Eds.), *Handbook of Hypertension, vol. 14: Blood Pressure Measurement*, pp. 72–94. Amsterdam: Elsevier.

Friedman, M., & Rosenman, R. H. (1959). Association of specific overt behavior pattern with blood and cardiovascular findings. *JAMA, 169*, 1286–96.

Frimerman, A., Miller, H. I., Laniado, S., & Keren, G. (1997). Changes in hemostatic function at times of cyclic variation in occupational stress. *Am. J. Cardiol., 79*, 72–5.

Fuller, H. D. (1992). The validity of cardiac output measurement by thoracic impedance: A meta-analysis. *Clin. Invest. Med., 15*, 103–12.

Gascho, J. A., Fanelli, C., & Zelis, R. (1989). Aging reduces venous distensibility and the venodilatory response to nitroglycerin in normal subjects. *Am. J. Cardiol., 63*, 1267–70.

Gebara, O. C., Jimenez, A. H., McKenna, C., Mittleman, M. A., Xu, P., Lipinska, I., Muller, J. E., & Tofler, G. H. (1996). Stress-induced hemodynamic and hemostatic changes in patients with systemic hypertension: Effect of verapamil. *Clin. Cardiol., 19*, 205–11.

Geddes, L. A., & Baker, L. E. (1989). *Principles of Applied Biomedical Instrumentation*, 3rd ed. New York: Wiley.

Geddes, L. A., & Sadler, L. E. (1973). The specific resistance of blood at body temperature. *Med. Biol. Eng., 11*, 336–9.

Gellman, M. D., Ironson, G. H., Marks, J. B., Spencer, S., Czarnecki, E., Durel, L., Skyler, J. S., & Schneiderman, N. (1997). The relationship between insulin resistance and sodium sensitivity using multiple blood pressure measurements [Abstract]. *Ann. Behav. Med., 19*, S67.

Gellman, M., Spitzer, S., Ironson, G., Llabre, M., Saab, P., DeCarlo Pasin, R., Weidler, D. J., & Schneiderman, N. (1990). Posture, place, and mood effects on ambulatory blood pressure. *Psychophysiology, 27*, 544–51.

Genovely, H., & Pfeifer, M. A. (1988). RR-variation: The autonomic test of choice in diabetes. *Diabetes Metab. Rev., 4*, 255–71.

George, D. T., Nutt, D. J., Walker, W. V., Porges, S. W., Adinoff, B., & Linnoiala, M. (1989). Lactate and hyperventilation substantially attenuate vagal tone in normal volunteers. *Arch. Gen. Psychiatry, 46*, 153–6.

Gerin, W., & Pickering, T. G. (1995). Association between delayed recovery of blood pressure after acute mental stress and parental history of hypertension. *J. Hypertens., 13*, 603–10.

Gevers, M., van Genderingen, H. R., Lafeber, H. N., & Hack, W. W. (1996). Accuracy of oscillometric blood pressure measurement in critically ill neonates with reference to the arterial pressure wave shape. *Intensive Care Med., 22*, 242–8.

Glass, D. C., Krakoff, L. R., Contrada, R., Hilton, W. F., Kehoe, K., Mannucci, E. G., Collins, C., Snow, B., & Elting, E. (1980). Effect of harassment and competition upon cardiovascular and plasma catecholamine responses in type A and type B individuals. *Psychophysiology, 17*, 453–63.

Goldberg, A. D., Becker, L. C., Bonsall, R., Cohen, J. D., Ketterer, M. W., Kaufman, P. G., Krantz, D. S., Light, K. C., McMahon, R. P., Noreuil, T., Pepine, C. J., Raczynski, J., Stone, P. H., Strother, D., Taylor, H., & Sheps, D. S. (1996). Ischemic, hemodynamic, and neurohormonal responses to mental and exercise stress. Experience from the Psychophysiological Investigations of Myocardial Ischemia study (PIMI). *Circulation, 94*, 2402–9.

Goodman, L. S., Goodman, J. M., Yang, L., Sloninko, J., Hsia, T., & Freeman, M. R. (1994). Measurement of left ventricular function during arm ergometry using the VEST nuclear probe. *Can. J. Appl. Physiol., 19*, 462–71.

Gotshall, R. W., & Sexson, W. R. (1994). Comparison of band and spot electrodes for the measurement of stroke volume by the bioelectric impedance technique. *Crit. Care Med., 22*, 420–5.

Griffin, S. E., Robergs, R. A., & Heyward, V. H. (1997). Blood pressure measurement during exercise: A review. *Med. Sci. Sports Exer., 29*, 149–59.

Grignani, G., Pacchiarini, L., Zucchella, M., Tacconi, F., Caneveari, A., Soffiantino, F., & Tavazzi, L. (1992). Effect of mental stress on platelet function in normal subjects and in patients with coronary artery disease. *Haemostasis, 22*, 138–46.

Grossman, P., Stemmler, G., & Meinhardt, E. (1990). Paced respiratory sinus arrhythmia as an index of cardiac parasympathetic tone during varying behavioral tasks. *Psychophysiology, 27*, 404–16.

Gullette, E. C., Blumenthal, J. A., Babyak, M., Jiang, W., Waugh, R. A., Frid, D. J., O'Connor, C. M., Morris, J. J., & Krantz, D. S. (1997). Effects of mental stress on myocardial ischemia during daily life. *JAMA, 277*, 1521–6.

Guyton, A. C. (1981). *The Textbook of Medical Physiology*. Philadelphia: Saunders.

Hallstrom, T., Lapidus, L., Bengtsson, C., & Edstrom, K. (1986). Psychosocial factors and risk of ischaemic heart disease and death in women: A twelve-year follow-up of participants in the population study of women in Gothenburg, Sweden. *J. Psychosom. Res., 30*, 451–9.

Halstrup, J. L., Light, K. C., & Obrist, P. A. (1982). Parental hypertension and cardiovascular response to stress in healthy young adults. *Psychophysiology, 19*, 615–22.

Han, K., Nagel, J. H., Hurwitz, B. E., & Schneiderman, N. (1991). Decomposition of heart rate variability by adaptive filtering for estimation of cardiac vagal tone. In J. H. Nagel & W. M. Smith (Eds.), *Bioelectric Phenomena, Electrocardiography, Electromagnetic Interactions, Neuromuscular Systems*, pp. 660–1. New York: IEEE Publishing.

Harburg, E., Blakelock, E. E., & Roeper, P. J. (1979). Resentful and reflective coping with arbitrary authority and blood pressure: Detroit. *Psychosom. Med., 41*, 189–202.

Hatch, J. P., Klatt, K., Porges, S. W., Schroeder-Jasheway, L., & Supik, J. D. (1986). The relation between rhythmic cardiovascular variability and reactivity to orthostatic, cognitive, and cold pressor stress. *Psychophysiology, 23*, 48–56.

Hayashida, K., Nishiooeda, Y., Hirose, Y., Ishida, Y., & Nishimura, T. (1996). Maladaptation of vascular response in frontal area of patients with orthostatic hypotension. *J. Nucl. Med., 37*, 1–4.

He, J., & Whelton, P. K. (1997). Epidemiology and prevention of hypertension. *Med. Clin. North Am., 81*, 1077–97.

Heather, L. W. (1969). A comparison of cardiac output values by the impedance cardiograph and dye dilution techniques in cardiac patients. In W. G. Kubicek, D. A. Witsoe, & R. P. Patterson (Eds.), *Development and Evaluation of an Impedance Cardiographic System to Measure Cardiac Output and Other Cardiac Parameters* (Publication CR 101965), pp. 247–58. Houston, TX: NASA.

Henning, R. J., Khalil, I. R., & Levy, M. N. (1990). Vagal stimulation attenuates sympathetic enhancement of left ventricular function. *Am. J. Physiol., 258*, H1470–H1475.

Hillard, W. (1982). Basic physics of ultrasound. In J. Schapira, Y. Charuzi, & R. M. Davidson (Eds.), *Two-Dimensional Echocardiography*, p. 319. Baltimore: Williams & Wilkins.

Hilton, S. M., Spyer, K. M., & Timms, R. J. (1975). Hind limb vasodilation evoked by stimulation of the motor cortex. *J. Physiol., 252*, 22–3.

Ho, Y. L., Wu, C. C., Huang, P. J., Tseng, W. K., Lin, L. C., Chieng, P. U., Chen, M. F., & Lee, Y. T. (1997). Dobutamine stress echocardiography compared with exercise thallium-201 single-photon emission computed tomography in detecting coronary artery disease – Effect of exercise level on accuracy. *Cardiology, 88*, 379–85.

Holter, N. J. (1961). New method for heart studies: Continuous electrocardiography of active subjects over long periods is now practical. *Science, 134*, 1214–16.

Hondeghem, L. M., & Roden, D. M. (1995). Agents used in cardiac arrhythmias. In B. G. Katzung (Ed.), *Basic and Clinical Pharmacology*, pp. 205–29. Norwalk, CT: Appleton & Lange.

Huang, K. C., Stoddard, M., Tsueda, K., Heine, M. F., Thomas, M. H., White, M., & Wieman, J. (1990). Stroke volume measurements by electrical bioimpedance and echocardiography in healthy volunteers. *Crit. Care Med., 18*, 1274–8.

Hurwitz, B. E., & Furedy, J. J. (1986). The human dive reflex: An experimental, topographical and physiological analysis. *Physiol. Behav., 36*, 287–94.

Hurwitz, B. E., Lu, C.-C., Reddy, S. P., Shyu, L.-Y., Schneiderman, N., & Nagel, J. H. (1993a). Signal fidelity requirements for deriving impedance cardiographic measures of cardiac function over a broad range of heart rate. *Biol. Psychol., 36*, 3–21.

Hurwitz, B. E., Nagel, J. H., Reddy, S. P., Shyu, L.-Y., Leitten, C. L., Keels, D. L., Peckerman, A., & Schneiderman, N. (1994a). Methodology and application of impedance cardiography: Toward study of the dynamic aspects of cardiovascular function. *Third Annual Proceeding of the International Congress of Behavioral Medicine*, p. 24. Amsterdam: International Congress of Behavioral Medicine.

Hurwitz, B. E., Nelesen, R. A., Saab, P. G., Nagel, J. H., Spitzer, S. B., Gellman, M. G., McCabe, P. M., Phillips, D. J., & Schneiderman, N. (1993b). Differential patterns of dynamic cardiovascular regulation as a function of task. *Biol. Psychol., 36*, 75–95.

Hurwitz, B. E., Quillian, R. E., Marks, J. B., Schneiderman, N., Agramonte, R. F., Freeman, C. R., La Greca, A. M., & Skyler, J. S. (1994b). Resting parasympathetic status and cardiovascular response to orthostatic and behavioral challenges in type I insulin-dependent diabetes mellitus. *Int. J. Behav. Med., 1*, 137–62.

Hurwitz, B. E., & Schneiderman, N. (1998). Cardiovascular reactivity and the relation to cardiovascular disease risk. In D. Krantz & A. Baum (Eds.), *Technology and Methodology in Behavioral Medicine*. Mahwah, NJ: Erlbaum.

Hurwitz, B. E., Shyu, L.-Y., Reddy, S. P., Schneiderman, N., & Nagel, J. H. (1990). Coherent ensemble averaging techniques for impedance cardiography. In H. T. Nagle & J. N.

Brown (Eds.), *Computer-Based Medical Systems*, pp. 228–35. Washington, DC: IEEE Computer Society Press.

Ikenouchi, H., Iizuka, M., Sato, H., Momomura, S., Serizawa, T., & Sugimoto, T. (1991). Forearm venous distensibility in relation to severity of symptoms and hemodynamic data in patients with congestive heart failure. *Jpn. Heart J., 32*, 17–34.

Imholz, B. P. (1996). Automated blood pressure measurement during ergometric stress testing: Possibilities of Finapres. *Z. Kardiol., 85 (Suppl. 3)*, 76–80.

Ironson, G. H., Gellman, M. D., Spitzer, S. B., Llabre, M. M., Pasin, R. D., Weidler, D. J., & Schneiderman, N. (1989). Predicting home and work blood pressure measurements for resting baselines and laboratory reactivity in black and white Americans. *Psychophysiology, 26*, 174–84.

Jain, D., Burg, M., Soufer, R., & Zaret, B. L. (1995). Prognostic implications of mental stress-induced silent left ventricular dysfunction in patients with stable angina pectoris. *Am. J. Cardiol., 76*, 31–5.

Jansen, H. T., & Dellinger, J. A. (1989). Comparing the cardiac vagolytic effects of atropine and methylatropine in rhesus macaques. *Pharmacol. Biochem. Behav., 32*, 175–9.

Jensen, L., Yakimets, J., & Teo, K. K. (1995). Issues in cardiovascular care. A review of impedance cardiography. *Heart Lung, 24*, 183–93.

Jiang, W., Babyak, M., Krantz, D. S., Waugh, R. A., Coleman, R. E., Hanson, M. M., Frid, D. J., McNulty, S., Morris, J. J., O'Connor, C. M., & Blumenthal, J. A. (1996). Mental stress-induced myocardial ischemia and cardiac events. *JAMA, 275*, 1651–6.

Johnson, L. L., & Lawson, M. A. (1996). New imaging techniques for assessing cardiac function. *Crit. Care Clinics, 12*, 919–37.

Johnson, L. L., & Pohost, G. M. (1994). Nuclear cardiology. In Schlant & Alexander, pp. 2281–2323.

Jones, R. D., Kornberg, J. P., Roulson, C. J., Visram, A. R., & Irwin, M. G. (1993). The Finapres 2300e finger cuff. The influence of cuff application on the accuracy of blood pressure measurement. *Anaesthesia, 48*, 611–15.

Jordan, D., Khalid, M. E., Schneiderman, N., & Spyer, K. M. (1982). The localization and properties of preganglionic vagal cardiomotor neurons in the rabbit. *Pflugers Arch., 395*, 244–50.

Julius, S. (1993). Sympathetic hyperactivity and coronary risk in hypertension. *Hypertension, 21*, 886–93.

Katona, P. G., McLean, M., Dighton, D. H., & Guz, A. (1982). Sympathetic and parasympathetic cardiac control in athletes and nonathletes at rest. *J. Appl. Physiol., 52*, 1652–7.

Katona, P. G., Poitras, J. W., Barnett, G. O., & Terry, B. S. (1970). Cardiac vagal efferent activity and heart period in the carotid sinus reflex. *Am. J. Physiol., 218*, 1030–7.

Kayden, D. S., & Burns, J. W. (1993). Use of ambulatory monitoring of left ventricular function with the VEST. In J. Blascovich & E. S. Katkin (Eds.), *Cardiovascular Reactivity to Psychological Stress and Disease*, pp. 135–53. Washington, DC: American Psychological Association.

Kelsey, R. M., & Guethlein, W. (1990). An evaluation of the ensemble averaged impedance cardiogram. *Psychophysiology, 27*, 24–33.

Kibler, J. L., Hurwitz, B. E., Reddy, S. P., Nagel, J. H., Peckerman, 'A., Agatston, A. S., Keels, D., & Schneiderman, N.

(1996). Impedance cardiography yields valid systolic time interval measures at rest and during stressful challenge [Abstract]. *Ann. Behav. Med., 28,* S135.

Kibler, J. L., Hurwitz, B. E., Schneiderman, N., Lakhani, M. N., Peckerman, A., Keels, D., Reddy, S. P., Agatston, A. S., & Nagel, J. H. (1997). Hypertensive status does not affect validity of impedance cardiography derived systolic time intervals [Abstract]. *Ann. Behav. Med., 29,* S156.

Kizakevich, P. N., Teague, S. M., Jochem, W. J., Nissman, D. B., Niclou, R., & Sharma, M. K. (1989). Detection of ischemic response during treadmill exercise by computer-aided impedance cardiography. *Proceedings of the 2nd Annual IEEE Symposium on Computer-Based Medical Systems* (IEEE catalog #89CH2755-7), pp. 10–15. Los Alamitos, CA: IEEE.

Kligfield, P. (1989). Ambulatory electrocardiographic monitoring: Methods and applications. In N. Schneiderman, S. M. Weiss, & P. G. Kaufmann (Eds.), *Handbook of Research Methods in Cardiovascular Behavioral Medicine,* pp. 273–91. New York: Plenum.

Kop, W. J. (1997). Acute and chronic psychological risk factors for coronary syndromes: Moderating effects of coronary artery disease severity. *J. Psychosom. Res., 43,* 167–81.

Koskenvuo, M. (1987). Cardiovascular stress and sleep. *Ann. Clin. Res., 19,* 110–13.

Krantz, D. S., Kop, W. J., Santiago, H. T., & Gottdiener, J. S. (1996). Mental stress as a trigger of myocardial ischemia and infarction. *Cardiol. Clin., 14,* 271–87.

Krittayaphong, R., Cascio, W. E., Light, K. C., Sheffield, D., Golden, R. N., Finkel, J. B., Glekas, G., Koch, G. G., & Sheps, D. S. (1997). Heart rate variability in patients with coronary artery disease: Differences in patients with higher and lower depression scores. *Psychosom. Med., 59,* 231–5.

Kubicek, W. G., Karnegis, J. N., Patterson, R. P., Witsoe, D. A., & Mattson, R. H. (1966). Development and evaluation of an impedance cardiac output system. *Aerospace Med., 39,* 248–52.

Kunk, R., & McCain, G. C. (1996). Comparison of upper arm and calf oscillometric blood pressure measurement in preterm infants. *J. Perinatol., 16,* 89–92.

Lamberts, R., Visser, K. R., & Zijlstra, W. G. (1984). *Impedance Cardiography.* Amsterdam: Van Gorcum.

Larsen, P. B., Schneiderman, N., & Pasin, R. D. (1986). Physiological bases of cardiovascular psychophysiology. In M. G. H. Coles, E. Donchin, & S. W. Porges (Eds.), *Psychophysiology: Systems, Processes, and Applications,* pp. 122–65. New York: Guilford.

LeJemtel, T. H., & Sonnenblick, E. H. (1994). Nonglycosidic cardioactive agents. In Schlant & Alexander, pp. 589–94.

Lenfant, C. (1997). Health and behavior research at NHLBI. *APS Observer, 10,* 2, 47.

Levy, M. N. (1977). Parasympathetic control of the heart. In W. C. Randall (Ed.), *Nervous Control of Cardiovascular Function,* pp. 68–94. New York: Oxford University Press.

Levy, M. N., & Vassalle, M. (Eds.) (1982). *Excitation and Neural Control of the Heart.* Bethesda, MD: American Physiological Society.

Levy, M. N., & Zieske, H. (1969). Autonomic control of cardiac pacemaker activity and atrioventricular transmission. *J. Appl. Physiol., 27,* 465–70.

Libet, B. (1977). The role SIF cells play in ganglionic transmission. *Adv. Biochem. Psychopharmacol., 16,* 541–6.

Lieberman, E. H., Gerhard, M. D., Uehata, A., Walsh, B. W., Selwyn, A. P., Ganz, P., Yeung, A. C., & Creager, M. A. (1994). Estrogen improves endothelium-dependent, flow-mediated vasodilation in postmenopausal women. *Ann. Intern. Med., 121,* 936–41.

Light, K. C., & Obrist, P. A. (1980). Cardiovascular reactivity to behavioral stress in young males with and without marginally elevated casual systolic pressures. Comparison of clinic, home, and laboratory measures. *Hypertension, 2,* 802–8.

Light, K. C., & Turner, R. J. (1992). Stress-induced changes in the rate of sodium excretion in healthy black and white men. *J. Psychosom. Res., 36,* 497–508.

Light, K. C., Turner, R. J., Hinderliter, A. L., & Sherwood, A. (1993). Race and gender comparisons: I. Hemodynamic responses to a series of stressors. *Health Psychol., 12,* 354–65.

Litvack, D. A., Oberlander, T. F., Carney, L. H., & Saul, J. P. (1995). Time and frequency domain methods for heart rate variability analysis: A methodological comparison. *Psychophysiology, 32,* 492–504.

Livingston, I. L., Levine, D. M., & Moore, R. D. (1991). Social integration and black intraracial variation in blood pressure. *Ethn. Dis., 1,* 135–49.

Llabre, M. M., Ironson, G. H., Spitzer, S. B., Gellman, M. D., Weidler, D. J., & Schneiderman, N. (1988). How many blood pressure measurements are enough? An application of generalizability theory to the study of blood pressure reliability. *Psychophysiology, 25,* 97–106.

Llabre, M. M., Saab, P. G., Hurwitz, B. E., Schneiderman, N., Spitzer, S., Frame, C. A., & Phillips, D. (1993). The stability of cardiovascular parameters under different behavioral challenges: One-year follow-up. *Int. J. Psychophysiol., 14,* 241–8.

Loewy, A. D. (1982). Central cardiovascular pathways. In O. A. Smith, R. A. Galosy, & S. M. Weiss (Eds.), *Circulation, Neurobiology, and Behavior,* pp. 3–11. New York: Elsevier.

Lynch, J., Krause, N., Kaplan, G. A., Salonen, R., & Salonen, J. T. (1997). Workplace demands, economic reward, and progression of carotid atherosclerosis. *Circulation, 96,* 302–7.

MacDonald, P. A., Evans, J. D., Saab, P. G., Llabre, M. M., & Schneiderman, N. (1995). Hemodynamic responsivity as a function of race, gender, and experimenter characteristics. *Sixteenth Annual Proceedings of the Society for Behavioral Medicine,* p. S119. San Diego: Society of Behavioral Medicine.

Mackie, A., Whincup, P., & McKinnon, M. (1995). Does the Hawksley random zero sphygmomanometer underestimate blood pressure, and by how much? *J. Hum. Hypertens., 9,* 337–43.

Mancia, G., Omboni, S., & Parati, G. (1997). Assessment of antihypertensive treatment by ambulatory blood pressure. *J. Hypertens. (Suppl.), 15,* S43–S50.

Mancia, G., Omboni, S., Parati, G., Ravogli, A., Villani, A., & Zanchetti, A. (1995). Lack of placebo effect on ambulatory blood pressure. *Am. J. Hypertens., 8,* 311–15.

Mancia, G., Seravalle, G., Giannattasio, C., Bossi, M., Preti, L., Cattaneo, B. M., & Grassi, G. (1992). Reflex cardiovascular control in congestive heart failure. *Am. J. Cardiol., 69,* 17G–22G.

Manuck, S. B., Kasprowicz, A. L., & Muldoon, M. F. (1990). Behaviorally evoked cardiovascular reactivity and hypertension:

Conceptual issues and potential associations. *Ann. Behav. Med., 12,* 17–29.

Manuck, S. B., Olsson, G., Hjemdahl, P., & Rehnqvist, N. (1992). Does cardiovascular reactivity to mental stress have prognostic value in postinfarction patients? A pilot study. *Psychosom. Med., 54,* 102–8.

Marrero, A. F., al'Absi, M., Pincomb, G. A., & Lovallo, W. R. (1997). Men at risk for hypertension show elevated vascular resistance at rest and during mental stress. *Int. J. Psychophysiol., 25,* 185–92.

Marwitz, M., & Stemmler, G. (1998). On the status of individual response specificity. *Psychophysiology, 35,* 1–15.

Marx, G. R., Hicks, R. W., & Allen, H. D. (1987). Measurement of cardiac output and exercise factor by pulsed Doppler echocardiography during supine bicycle ergometry in normal young adolescent boys. *J. Am. Coll. Cardiol., 10,* 430–4.

Matthews, K. A., Glass, D. C., Rosenman, R. H., & Bortner, R. W. (1977). Competitive drive, pattern A, and coronary heart disease: A further analysis of some data from the Western Collaborative Group Study. *J. Chron. Dis., 30,* 489–98.

Matthews, K. A., Woodall, K. L., & Allen, M. T. (1993). Cardiovascular reactivity to stress predicts future blood pressure status. *Hypertension, 22,* 479–85.

Mauck, G. W., Smith, C. R., Geddes, L. A., & Bourland, J. D. (1980). The meaning of the point of maximum oscillations in cuff pressure in the indirect measurement of blood pressure. *J. Biomech Eng., 102,* 28–33.

Maxwell, M. H., Waks, A. U., Schroth, P. C., Karam, M., & Dornfeld, L. P. (1982). Error in blood-pressure measurement due to incorrect cuff size in obese patients. *Lancet, 2,* 33–6.

McArdle, W. D., Katch, F. I., & Katch, V. L. (1986). *Exercise Physiology: Energy, Nutrition, and Human Performance.* Philadelphia: Lea & Febiger.

McCabe, P. M., Yongue, B. G., Porges, S. W., & Ackles, P. K. (1984). Change in heart period, heart-period variability, and a spectral analysis estimate of respiratory sinus arrhythmias during aortic nerve stimulation in rabbits. *Psychophysiology, 21,* 149–58.

McCabe, P. M., Yongue, B. G., Porges, S. W., & Ackles, P. K. (1985). Changes in heart period, heart-period variability, and a spectral analysis estimate of respiratory sinus arrhythmia in response to pharmacological manipulations of the baroreceptor reflex in cats. *Psychophysiology, 22,* 195–202.

McKinney, M. E., Miner, M. H., Rüddel, H., McIlvain, H. E., Witte, H., Buell, J. C., Elliot, R. S., & Grant, L. B. (1985). The standardized mental stress protocol: Test–retest reliability and comparison with ambulatory blood pressure monitoring. *Psychophysiology, 22,* 453–63.

Mehmel, H. C., Stockins, B., Ruffman, K., von Olshaussen, K., Schuler, G., & Kubler, W. (1981). The linearity of the end-systolic pressure-volume relationship in man and its sensitivity for assessment of left ventricular function. *Circulation, 63,* 1216–22.

Menkes, M. S., Matthews, K. A., Krantz, D. S., Lundberg, U., Mead, L. A., Qagish, B., Liang, K. Y., Thomas, C. B., & Pearson, T. A. (1989). Cardiovascular reactivity to the cold pressor test as a predictor of hypertension. *Hypertension, 14,* 524–30.

Miller, J. C., & Horvath, S. M. (1978). Impedance cardiography. *Psychophysiology, 15,* 80–91.

Miller, S. B., Friese, M., & Sita, A. (1995a). Parental history of hypertension, sodium loading and cardiovascular response to stress. *Psychosom. Med., 57,* 381–9.

Miller, S. B., Turner, J. R., Sherwood, A., Brownley, K. A., Hinderliter, A. L., & Light, K. C. (1995b). Parental history of hypertension and cardiovascular response to stress in black and white men. *Int. J. Behav. Med., 2,* 339–57.

Moneta, G. L., Taylor, D. C., Nicholls, S. C., Bergelin, R. O., Zierler, R. E., Kazmers, A., Clowes, A. W., & Strandness, D. E., Jr. (1987). Operative versus nonoperative management of symptomatic high-grade internal carotid artery stenosis: Improved results with endarterectomy. *Stroke, 18,* 1005–10.

Mortelmans, L., Cabera, E. Z., Dorny, N., Thoeng, J., Wauters, M., van de Werf, F., VanHaecke, J., de Roo, M., & de Geest, H. (1991). Left ventricular function changes during pharmacological and physiological interventions and routine activities monitored in healthy volunteers by a portable radionuclide probe (VEST). *Int. J. Card. Imaging, 7,* 79–87.

Muller, J. E., Abela, G. S., Nesto, R. W., & Tofler, G. H. (1994). Triggers, acute risk factors and vulnerable plaques: The lexicon of a new frontier. *J. Am. Coll. Cardiol., 23,* 809–13.

Mundal, H. H., & Rostrup, M. (1996). Blood platelet responses to laboratory stress in young men. The effect of awareness of high blood pressure. *Am. J. Hypertens., 9,* 12–17.

Murphy, J. K., Alpert, B. S., & Walker, S. S. (1992). Ethnicity, pressor reactivity, and children's blood pressure: Five years of observations. *Hypertension, 20,* 327–32.

Myrianthefs, M., Cariolou, M., Eldar, M., Minas, M., & Zambartas, C. (1997). Exercise-induced ventricular arrhythmias and sudden cardiac death in a family. *Chest, 111,* 1130–4.

Nagel, J. H., Han, K., Hurwitz, B. E., & Schneiderman, N. (1993). Assessment and diagnostic applications of heart rate variability. *Biomed. Eng. – Applications, Basis & Communication, 5,* 147–58.

Nagel, J. H., Shyu, L. Y., Reddy, S. P., Hurwitz, B. E., McCabe, P. M., & Schneiderman, N. (1989). New signal processing techniques for improved precision of noninvasive impedance cardiography. *Ann. Biomed. Eng., 17,* 517–34.

Nanda, N. C. (1993). *Doppler Echocardiography,* 2nd ed. Philadelphia: Lea & Febiger.

NIH [National Institutes of Health] (1998). National Heart, Lung, and Blood Institute Report of the Task Force on Behavioral Research in Cardiovascular, Lung, and Blood Health and Disease. www.nhlbi.nih.gov/resources/index.htm.

Nissen, S. E. (1994). Intravascular ultrasound. In Schlant & Alexander, pp. 2273–8.

Noble, R. J., & Zipes, D. P. (1994). Long-term continuous electrocardiographic recording. In Schlant & Alexander, pp. 873–80.

Novak, V., Novak, P., & Schondorf, R. (1994). Accuracy of beat-to-beat noninvasive measurement of finger arterial pressure using the Finapres: A spectral analysis. *J. Clin. Monit., 10,* 118–26.

Nyober, J. (1950). Electrical impedance plethysmography. *Circulation, 2,* 811–87.

Oalmann, M. C., Strong, J. P., Tracy, R. E., & Malcom, G. T. (1997). Atherosclerosis in youth: Are hypertension and other coronary heart disease risk factors already at work? *Pediatr. Nephrol., 11,* 99–107.

O'Brien, E., & O'Malley, K. (1981). *Essentials of Blood Pressure Measurement*. Edinburgh, U.K.: Churchill Livingstone.

Oguzhan, A., Kisacik, H. L., Ozdemir, K., Altunkeser, B. B., Durmaz, T., Altinyay, E., Kural, T., Korkmax, S., Kir, M., Kutuk, E., & Goksel, S. (1997). Comparison of exercise stress testing with dobutamine stress echocardiography and exercise technetium-99m isonitrile single photon emission computerized tomography for diagnosis of coronary artery disease. *Jpn. Heart J., 38*, 333–44.

Ohkubo, T., Imai, Y., Tsuji, I., Nagai, K., Watanabe, N., Minami, N., Itoh, O., Bando, T., Sakuma, M., Fukao, A., Satoh, H., Hisamichi, S., & Abe, K. (1997). Prediction of mortality by ambulatory blood pressure monitoring versus screening blood pressure measurements: A pilot study in Ohasama. *J. Hypertens., 15*, 357–64.

Palmer, R. M., Ferrige, A. G., & Moncada, S. (1987). Nitric oxide release accounts for the biological activity of endothelium-derived relaxing factor. *Nature, 327*, 524–6.

Parati, G., Pomidossi, G., Casadei, R., Ravogli, A., Groppelli, A., Cesana, B., & Mancia, G. (1988). Comparison of the cardiovascular effects of different laboratory stressors and their relationship with blood pressure variability. *J. Hypertens., 6*, 481–8.

Parati, G., Trazzi, S., Ravogli, A., Casadei, R., Omboni, S., & Mancia, G. (1991). Methodological problems in evaluation of cardiovascular effects of stress in humans. *Hypertension, 17 (Suppl. III)*, III-50–III-55.

Park, M. K., & Lee, D. H. (1989). Normative arm and calf blood pressure values in the newborn. *Pediatrics, 83*, 240–3.

Patterson, R. P., Wang, L., & Raza, S. B. (1991). Impedance cardiography using band and regional electrodes in supine, sitting, and during exercise. *IEEE Trans. Biomed. Eng., 38*, 393–400.

Patterson, S. M., Krantz, D. S., Gottdiener, J. S., Hecht, G., Vargot, S., & Goldstein, D. S. (1995). Prothrombotic effects of environmental stress: Changes in platelet function, hematocrit, and total plasma protein. *Psychosom. Med., 57*, 592–9.

Pearlman, A. S. (1994). Technique of Doppler and color flow Doppler in the evaluation of cardiac disorders and function. In Schlant & Alexander, pp. 2229–51.

Peckerman, A., Hurwitz, B. E., Saab, P. G., Llabre, M. M., McCabe, P. M., & Schneiderman, N. (1994). Stimulus dimensions of the cold pressor test and the associated patterns of cardiovascular response. *Psychophysiology, 31*, 282–90.

Peckerman, A., Saab, P. G., McCabe, P. M., Skyler, J. S., Winters, R., Llabre, M. M., & Schneiderman, N. (1991). Blood pressure reactivity and perception of pain during the forehead cold pressor test. *Psychophysiology, 28*, 485–95.

Perrino, A., Lippman, A., Ariyan, C., O'Connor, T. Z., & Luther, M. (1994). Intraoperative cardiac output monitoring: Comparison of impedance cardiography and thermodilution. *J. Cardiothorac. Vasc. Anesth., 8*, 24–9.

Petersen, M. E., Williams, T. R., & Sutton, R. (1995). A comparison of noninvasive continuous finger blood pressure measurement (Finapres) with intra-arterial pressure during prolonged head-up tilt. *Eur. Heart. J., 16*, 1641–54.

Pettigrew, R. I. (1994). Magnetic resonance imaging of the heart and great vessels. In Schlant & Alexander, pp. 2339–59.

Pickering, T. (1996). Recommendations for the use of home (self) and ambulatory blood pressure monitoring. American Society of Hypertension Ad Hoc Panel. *Am. J. Hypertens., 9*, 1–9.

Pickering, T. G., & Gerin, W. (1990). Cardiovascular reactivity in the laboratory and the role of behavioral factors in hypertension: A critical review. *Ann. Behav. Med., 12*, 3–16.

Pickett, B. R., & Buell, J. C. (1992). Validity of cardiac output measurement by computer-averaged impedance cardiography, and comparison with simultaneous thermodilution determinations. *Am. J. Cardiol., 69*, 1354–8.

Piene, H., & Covell, J. W. (1981). A force-length-time relationship describes the mechanics of canine left ventricular wall segments during auxotonic contractions. *Circ. Res., 49*, 70–9.

Pincomb, G. A., Lovallo, W. R., Passey, R. B., Whitsett, T. L., Silverstein, S. M., & Wilson, M. F. (1985). Effects of caffeine on vascular resistance, cardiac output and myocardial contractility in young men. *Am. J. Cardiol., 56*, 119–22.

Porges, S. W. (1985). Method and apparatus for evaluating rhythmic oscillations in aperiodic physiological response systems. U.S. Patent No. 4,510,944.

Prineas, R. J. (1991). Measurement of blood pressure in the obese. *Ann. Epidemiol., 1*, 321–6.

Qu, M., Zhan, Y., Webster, J. G., & Tompkins, W. J. (1986). Motion artifact from spot and band electrodes during impedance cardiography. *IEEE Trans. Biomed. Eng., 33*, 1029–36.

Quyyumi, A. A., Dakak, N., Andrews, N. P., Husain, S., Arora, S., Gilligan, D. M., Panza, J. A., & Cannon, R. O. (1995). Nitric oxide activity in the human coronary circulation. Impact of risk factors for coronary atherosclerosis. *J. Clin. Invest., 95*, 1747–55.

Raaijmakers, E., Faes, Th. J. C., Goovaerts, H. G., de Vries, P. M. J. M., & Heethaar, R. M. (1997). The inaccuracy of Kubicek's one-cylinder model in thoracic impedance cardiography. *IEEE Trans. Biomed. Eng., 44*, 70–6.

Randall, W. C. (1977). *Neural Regulation of the Heart*. New York: Oxford University Press.

Randall, W. C. (Ed.) (1984). *Nervous Control of Cardiovascular Function*. New York: Oxford University Press.

Randall, W. C., Priola, D. V., & Ulmer, R. H. (1963). A functional study of distribution of cardiac sympathetic nerves. *Am. J. Physiol., 205*, 1227–31.

Ristuccia, H. L., Grossman, P., Watkins, L. L., & Lown, B. (1997). Incremental bias in Finapres estimation of baseline blood pressure levels over time. *Hypertension, 29*, 1039–43.

Rochmis, P., & Blackburn, H. (1971). Exercise tests. A survey of procedures, safety, and litigation experience in approximately 170,000 tests. *JAMA, 217*, 1061–6.

Rompelman, O. (1993). Rhythms and analysis techniques. In J. Strackee & N. Westerhof (Eds.), *The Physics of Heart and Circulation*, pp. 101–20. Philadelphia: Institute of Physics.

Rosenman, R. H., Brand, R. J., Jenkins, D., Friedman, M., Straus, R., & Wurm, M. (1975). Coronary heart disease in Western Collaborative Group Study. Final follow-up experience of 8-1/2 years. *JAMA, 233*, 872–7.

Rostrup, M., Smith, G., Bjrnstad, H., Westheim, A., Stokland, O., & Eide, I. (1994). Left ventricular mass and cardiovascular reactivity in young men. *Hypertension, 23*, 1168–1171.

Saab, P. G., Llabre, M. M., Hurwitz, B. E., Frame, C. A., Reineke, L. J., Fins, A. I., McCalla, J., Cieply, L. K., & Schneiderman, N. (1992). Myocardial and peripheral vascular responses to behavioral challenges and their stability in black and white Americans. *Psychophysiology, 29,* 384–97.

Saab, P. G., Llabre, M. M., Hurwitz, B. E., Schneiderman, N., Durel, L. A., Wohlgelmuth, W., Massie, C., & Nagel, J. (1993). The cold pressor test: Vascular and myocardial response patterns and their stability. *Psychophysiology, 30,* 366–73.

Sbarouni, E., Kyriakides, Z. S., & Kremastinos, D. T. (1997). Effect of intracoronary estrogen on coronary collateral blood flow velocity. *Am. J. Cardiol., 79,* 666–9.

Schelbert, H. R. (1994). Positron emission tomography. In Schlant & Alexander, pp. 2361–79.

Schlant, R. C., & Alexander, R. W. (Eds.) (1994). *Hurst's The Heart: Arteries and Veins.* New York: McGraw-Hill.

Schlant, R. C., & Sonnenblick, E. H. (1994). Normal physiology of the cardiovascular system. In Schlant & Alexander, pp. 113–51.

Schneiderman, N. (1978). Animal models relating behavioral stress and cardiovascular pathology. In T. M. Dembroski, S. M. Weiss, J. L. Shields, S. G. Haynes, & M. Feinleib (Eds.), *Coronary-Prone Behavior,* pp. 155–82. New York: Springer.

Schneiderman, N., & McCabe, P. M. (1989). Psychophysiologic strategies in laboratory research. In N. Schneiderman, S. M. Weiss, & P. G. Kaufman (Eds.), *Handbook of Research Methods in Cardiovascular Behavioral Medicine,* pp. 349–64. New York: Plenum.

Schneiderman, N., & Skyler, J. S. (1996). Insulin metabolism, sympathetic nervous system regulation, and coronary heart disease prevention. In K. Orth-Gomer & N. Schneiderman (Eds.), *Behavioral Medicine Approaches to Cardiovascular Disease Prevention,* pp. 105–33. Mahwah, NJ: Erlbaum.

Schwartz, W. J., Rayburn, W. F., Turnbull, G. L., & Christensen, H. D. (1996). Blood pressure monitoring during pregnancy. Accuracy of portable devices designed for obese patients. *J. Reprod. Med., 41,* 581–5.

Seibaek, M., Sloth, C., Vallebo, L., Hansen, T., Urhammer, S. A., Burchardt, H., Torp-Pederson, C., Pedersen, O., & Hildebrandt, P. (1997). Glucose tolerance status and severity or coronary artery disease in men referred to coronary arteriography. *Am. Heart J., 133,* 622–9.

Shapiro, D., Jamner, L. D., Lane, J. D., Light, K. C., Myrtek, M., Sawada, Y., & Steptoe, A. (1996). Blood pressure publication guidelines. Society for Psychophysical Research. *Psychophysiology, 33,* 1–12.

Shekelle, R. B., Gale, M., Ostfeld, A. M., & Paul, O. (1983). Hostility, risk of coronary heart disease, and mortality. *Psychosom. Med., 45,* 109–14.

Sherwood, A., Allen, M. T., Fahrenberg, J., Kelsey, R. M., Lovallo, W. R., & van Doornen, L. J. P. (1990). Methodological guidelines for impedance cardiography. *Psychophysiology, 27,* 1–23.

Sherwood, A., Girdler, S. S., Bragdon, E. E., West, S. G., Brownley, K. A., Hinderliter, A. L., & Light, K. C. (1997). Ten-year stability of cardiovascular responses to laboratory stressors. *Psychophysiology, 34,* 185–91.

Sherwood, A., & Hinderliter, A. L. (1993). Responsiveness to α- and β-adrenergic receptor agonists: Effects of race in borderline hypertension compared to normotensive men. *Am. J. Hypertens., 6,* 630–5.

Sherwood, A., Hinderliter, A. L., & Light, K. C. (1995a). Physiological determinants of hyperreactivity to stress in borderline hypertension. *Hypertension, 25,* 384–90.

Sherwood, A., May, C. W., Siegel, W. C., & Blumenthal, J. A. (1995b). Ethnic differences in hemodynamic responses to stress in hypertensive men and women. *Am. J. Hypertens., 8,* 552–7.

Sherwood, A., Royal, S. A., Hutcheson, J. S., & Turner, J. R. (1992). Comparison of impedance cardiographic measurements using band and spot electrodes. *Psychophysiology, 29,* 734–41.

Smith, J. J., & Kampine, J. P. (1990). *Circulatory Physiology: The Essentials.* Baltimore: Williams & Wilkins.

Smith, T. W. (1992). Hostility and health: Current status of a psychosomatic hypothesis. *Health Psychol., 11,* 139–50.

Sonnenblick, E. (1962). Force-velocity relations in mammalian heart muscle. *Am. J. Physiol., 202,* 931–42.

Sramek, B. B. (1981). Noninvasive technique for measurement of cardiac output by means of electrical impedance. *Proceedings of the Fifth International Conference on Electrical Bioimpedance,* pp. 39–42. Tokyo: Business Center for Academic Societies.

Sramek, B. B. (1982). Cardiac output by electrical impedance. *Med. Electronics., 13,* 93–7.

Stanford, W., & Rumberger, J. A. (Eds.) (1992). *Ultrafast Computed Tomography in Cardiac Imaging: Principles and Practice.* Mount Kisco, NY: Futura.

Stemmler, G., Grossman, P., Schmid, H., & Foerster, F. (1991). A model of cardiovascular activation components for studies using autonomic receptor antagonists. *Psychophysiology, 28,* 367–82.

Stern, H. C., Wolf, G. K., & Belz, G. G. (1985). Comparative measurements of left ventricular ejection time by mechano-, echo- and electrical impedance cardiography. *Arzneim.–Forsch./Drug Res., 35,* 1583–6.

Stolt, M., Sjonell, G., Astrom, H., Rossner, S., & Hansson, L. (1993). Improved accuracy of indirect blood pressure measurement in patients with obese arms. *Am. J. Hypertens., 6,* 66–71.

Strackee, J., & Westerhof, N. (Eds.) (1993). *The Physics of Heart and Circulation.* Bristol, U.K.: Institute of Physics.

Strandness, D. E. (1994). Doppler methods for analysis of arterial and venous disorders. In Schlant & Alexander, pp. 2215–18.

Suarez, E. C., Harlan, E., Peoples, M. C., & Williams, R. B., Jr. (1993). Cardiovascular and emotional responses in women: The role of hostility and harassment. *Health Psychol., 12,* 459–68.

Sudhir, K., Forman, A., Yi, S. L., Sorof, J., Schmidlin, O., Sebastian, A., & Morris, R. C., Jr. (1997). Reduced dietary potassium reversibly enhances vasopressor responses to stress in African Americans. *Hypertension, 29,* 1083–90.

Sugishita, Y., Iida, K., Matsuda, M., Ajisaka, R., Ito, I., Koshinaga, J., and Ueno, M. (1988). Sudden death in hypertrophic cardiomyopathy, a guideline to prevention in daily life. *Acta. Cardiol., 43,* 677–88.

Suls, J., & Wan, C. K. (1993). The relationship between trait hostility and cardiovascular reactivity: A quantitative review and analysis. *Psychophysiology, 39,* 615–26.

Summers, R. J., Molnaar, P., Russell, F., Elnatan, J., Jones, C. R., Buxton, B. F., Chang, V., & Hambley, J. (1989). Coexistence and localization of beta 1- and beta 2-adrenoceptors in the human heart. *Eur. Heart. J., 10 (Suppl. B),* B11–B21.

Su-sic, D. (1988). The role of the renal medulla in blood pressure control. *Am. J. Med. Sci., 295,* 234–40.

Swanson, L. W. (1982). Forebrain neural mechanisms involved in cardiovascular regulation. In O. A. Smith, R. A. Galosy, & S. M. Weiss (Eds.), *Circulation, Neurobiology, and Behavior,* pp. 13–22. New York: Elsevier.

Tachovsky, B. J. (1985). Indirect auscultatory blood pressure measurement at two sites in the arm. *Res. Nurs. Health, 8,* 125–9.

Tortora, G. J., & Anagnostakos, N. P. (Eds.) (1990). *Principles of Anatomy and Physiology,* 6th ed. New York: Harper & Row.

Treiber, F., Papavassiliou, D., Gutin, B., Malpass, D., Yi, W., Islam, S., Davis, H., & Strong, W. (1997). Determinants of endothelium-dependent femoral artery vasodilation in youth. *Psychosom. Med., 59,* 376–81.

Uehata, A., Gerhard, M. D., Meredith, I. T., LieBerman, E. H., Selwyn, A. P., Creager, M., Polak, J., Ganz, P., Yeung, A. C., & Anderson, T. J. (1993). Close relationship of endothelial dysfunction in coronary and brachial artery [Abstract]. *Circulation, 88,* I618.

Vallenilla, C. T., Hurwitz, B. E., Bilsker, M. S., Nagel, J. H., Kibler, J. L., Motivala, S. J., Gellman, M. D., & Schneiderman, N. (1997). Stroke volume validation of impedance cardiography compared with pulsed-Doppler echocardiography in healthy men and women [Abstract]. *Ann. Behav. Med., 19,* S156.

van Egmond, J., Lender, J. W. M., Weernink, E., & Thien, T. (1993). Accuracy and reproducibility of 30 devices for self-measurement of arterial blood pressure. *Am. J. Hypertens., 6,* 873–9.

Veigl, V. L., & Judy, W. V. (1983). Reproducibility of haemodynamic measurements by impedance cardiography. *Cardiovasc. Res., 17,* 728–34.

Wallen, N. H., Held, C., Rehnqvist, N., & Hjemdahl, P. (1997). Effects of mental and physical stress on platelet function in patients with stable angina pectoris and healthy controls. *Eur. Heart J., 18,* 807–15.

Waller, B. F., & Schlant, R. C. (1994). Anatomy of the heart. In Schlant & Alexander, pp. 59–111.

Wanneberg, S. R., Schneider, R. H., Walton, K. G., MacLean, C. R., Levitsky, D. K., Mandarino, J. V., Waziri, R., & Wallace, R. K. (1997). Anger expression correlates with platelet aggregation. *Behav. Med., 22,* 174–7.

Weinberg, C. R., & Pfeifer, M. A. (1986). Development of a predictive model for symptomatic neuropathy in diabetes. *Diabetes, 35,* 873–80.

Weise, F., Heydenreich, F., & Runge, U. (1988). Heart rate fluctuations in diabetic patients with cardiac vagal dysfunction: A spectral analysis. *Diabet. Med., 5,* 324–7.

Wennmalm, A. (1994). Endothelial nitric oxide and cardiovascular disease. *J. Intern. Med., 235,* 317–27.

West, S., Stanwyck, C., Brownley, K., Bragdon, E., Hinderliter, A., & Light, K. (1997). Salt restriction increases norepinephrine and cholesterol in blacks more than in whites [Abstract]. *Ann. Behav. Med., 19,* S067.

Wheeler, T., & Watkins, P. J. (1973). Cardiac denervation in diabetes. *Br. Med. J., 4,* 584–6.

White, W. B., Berson, A. S., Robbins, C., Jamieson, M. J., Prisant, L. M., Roccella, E., & Sheps, S. B. (1993). National standard for measurement of resting and ambulatory blood pressures with automated sphygmomanometers. *Hypertension, 21,* 504–9.

White, W. B., Lund-Johansen, P., & Omvik, P. (1990a). Assessment of four ambulatory blood pressure monitors and measurements by clinicians versus intraarterial blood pressure at rest and during exercise. *Am. J. Cardiol., 65,* 60–6.

White, S. W., Quail, A. W., de Leeuw, P. W., Traugott, F. M., Brown, W. J., Porges, W. L., & Cottee, D. B. (1990b). Impedance cardiography for cardiac output measurement: An evaluation of accuracy and limitations. *Eur. Heart J., 11 (Suppl. 1),* 79–92.

Willems, J. P., Saunders, J. T., Hunt, D. E., & Schorling, J. B. (1997). Prevalence of coronary heart disease risk factors among rural blacks: A community-based study. *South. Med. J., 90,* 814–20.

Willemsen, G. H., De Geus, E. J., Klaver, C. H., Van Doornen, L. J., & Carroll, D. (1996). Ambulatory monitoring of the impedance cardiogram. *Psychophysiology, 33,* 184–93.

Willich, S. N., Maclure, M., Mittleman, M., Arntz, H. R., & Muller, J. E. (1993). Sudden cardiac death. Support for a role of triggering in causation. *Circulation, 87,* 1442–50.

Wilson, R. A., Sullivan, P. J., Moore, R. H., Zielonka, J. S., Alpert, N. M., Boucher, C. A., McKusic, K. A., & Strauss, H. W. (1983). An ambulatory ventricular function monitor: Validation and preliminary clinical results. *Am. J. Cardiol., 52,* 601–6.

Winegrad, S. (1982). Calcium release from cardiac sarcoplasm reticulum. *Annu. Rev. Physiol., 44,* 451–62.

Winters, R. W., McCabe, P. M., Green, E. J., & Schneiderman, N. (2000). Stress responses, coping and cardiovascular neurobiology: Central nervous system circuitry underlying learned and unlearned affective responses to stressful stimuli. In P. M. McCabe, N. Schneiderman, T. Field, & A. R. Wellens (Eds.), *Stress, Coping, and Cardiovascular Disease.* Mahwah, NJ: Erlbaum.

Woltjer, H. H., Arntzen, B. W. G. J., Bogaard, H. J., & de Vries, P. M. J. M. (1996). Optimalisation of the spot electrode array in impedance cardiography. *Med. Biol. Eng. Comput., 34,* 84–7.

Woltjer, H. H., van der Meer, B. J. M., Bogaard, H. J., & de Vries, P. M. J. M. (1995). Comparison between spot and band electrodes and between two equations for calculations of stroke volume by means of impedance cardiography. *Med. Biol. Eng. Comp., 33,* 330–4.

Woods, D. L., Sheps, S. G., Elveback, L. R., & Schirger, A. (1984). Cold pressor test as a predictor of hypertension. *Hypertension, 6,* 301–6.

Yakimets, J., & Jensen, L. (1995). Evaluation of impedance cardiography: Comparison of NCCOM3-R7 with Fick and thermodilution methods. *Heart Lung, 24,* 194–206.

Yang, T., & Levy, M. N. (1992). Sequence of excitation as a factor in sympathetic–parasympathetic interactions in the heart. *Circ. Res., 71,* 898–905.

Yongue, B. G., McCabe, P. M., Porges, S. W., Rivera, M., Kelley, S. L., & Ackles, P. K. (1982). The effects of pharmacological manipulation that influence vagal control of the heart on heart period, heart-period varibility and respiration in rats. *Psychophysiology, 19,* 426–32.

Zhang, Y., Qu, M., Webster, J. G., Tompkins, W. J., Ward, B. A., & Bassett, D. R. (1986). Cardiac output monitoring by impedance cardiography during treadmill exercise. *IEEE Trans. Biomed. Eng., 33,* 1037–42.

CHAPTER TEN

RESPIRATION

ANDREW HARVER & TYLER S. LORIG

One man's technique is another man's science.
(Donald W. Shearn, 1972)

Prologue

Respiration is likely the most awkward organ system for the psychophysiologist. If breathing "is truly a strange phenomenon of life, caught midway between the conscious and unconscious" (Richards 1953), then respiratory activity reflects not only voluntary actions arising from the central nervous system but also involuntary processes stemming from homeostatic mechanisms. Breath holding, for example, is accompanied by progressively higher rates of diaphragmatic activity up to the breaking point: voluntary inhibition of respiratory muscle activity is followed by involuntary respiratory efforts (Agostoni 1963).

The duplicity of respiratory control is evident in the ongoing history of research on breathing and behavior. It is well appreciated, for example, that alterations in either the depth or rate of breathing are a source of variance in heart rate and heart rate control (Holmes et al. 1980; Levenson 1979; Obrist et al. 1975; Sroufe 1971; Vandercar, Feldstein, & Solomon 1977), although no consistent value has been attributed to voluntary control of breathing in psychophysiological research (Grossman 1983; Grossman, Karemaker, & Wieling, 1991). On the other hand, respiratory sinus arrhythmia (RSA) – an expression of the covariance between respiratory and heart rate activity – has recently captivated the field (Berntson et al. 1997; Berntson, Cacioppo, & Quigley 1993; Grossman & Kollai 1993; Porges 1995). Enthusiasm over RSA as a mark of parasympathetic state complements the long-standing role of respiration as a mark of autonomic nervous system activity. Respiration period is one of seven variables that Wenger (e.g. Wenger & Cullen 1972) used to estimate "autonomic balance"; five items included in the Autonomic Perception Questionnaire

of Mandler, Mandler, and Uviller (1958) relate to perceived changes in breathing that occur with anxiety; and respiratory signals remain prominent alongside cardiovascular and electrodermal signals in the evaluation of deception (Horowitz et al. 1997; Patrick & Iacono 1991).

Respiration is not a convenient system to record, and surface electrodes are not the primary transducers needed to measure either pulmonary ventilation or gas exchange (Langer et al. 1985a). Most respiratory signals lack a familiar electrophysiological dimension – unlike those recorded from the brain, the heart, and skeletal muscle (but see Bruce 1984; Lansing & Savelle 1989). In one sense, however, respiration underlies the functioning of systems that have attracted greater psychophysiologic research efforts (Figure 1). It provides the *oxygen* that (a) binds with radioactive isotopes to localize mental activity (Posner & Raichle 1997), (b) serves to predict metabolically excessive heart rate responses (Turner, Carroll, & Courtney 1983), and (c) energizes muscle to enable study of response selection and execution (Brener 1987).

INTRODUCTION AND OVERVIEW: THE PLIGHT OF RESPIRATION

The respiratory system consists of the lungs, the conducting airways, parts of the central nervous system concerned with the control of the muscles of respiration (i.e., diaphragm, intercostals, rib cage), and the chest wall (Levitzky 1986); see Figure 2. The main functions of the respiratory system are: (1) to obtain oxygen from the environment and to supply it to the cells; and (2) to remove carbon dioxide from the body produced by cellular metabolism (Comroe 1974; West 1985). The brain and heart together comprise less than 3% of total body weight but account for over 30% of oxygen usage (West 1985). A variety of cardiopulmonary diseases that affect either ventilation,

John T. Cacioppo, Louis G. Tassinary, and Gary G. Berntson (Eds.), *Handbook of Psychophysiology*, 2nd ed. © Cambridge University Press 2000. Printed in the United States of America. ISBN 62634X. All rights reserved.

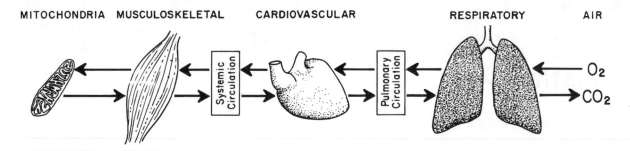

Figure 1. Interaction of the respiratory, cardiovascular, and musculoskeletal systems for transport and exchange of oxygen and carbon dioxide. Reprinted with permission from Mahler, "Pulmonary aspects of aging," in Gambert (Ed.), *Contemporary Geriatric Medicine,* vol. 1, pp. 45–85. Copyright 1983 Plenum Publishing Corp.

gas exchange, or oxygen transport give rise to respiratory insufficiency (Guyton 1981). In asthma, for example, the risk from death during severe airway obstruction is likely the result of severe asphyxia due to inadequate alveolar ventilation (Guyton 1981; Molfino et al. 1991).

Despite the biological significance of breathing, respiration research has occurred mostly in the shadow of interest in the brain, the heart, and electrodermal activity (Sanchez-Hernandez et al. 1996). Respiratory activity is most likely recorded to reduce, through methodological and statistical adjustments, the noise in researchers' cardiovascular and electrodermal signals (Grossman 1983; Stern & Anschel 1968). Respiration not only has been overshadowed by interest in other systems but also has been overlooked by authors in a series of handbooks, texts, and primers published in the 1970s and 1980s. Hassett (1978), for example, points out that there is no chapter on respiration in Greenfield and Sternbach's (1972) *Handbook of Psychophysiology* and that "respiration" does not even appear in the index; similar statements are true for Andreassi's (1980) *Psychophysiology* and for Martin and Venables's (1980) *Techniques in Psychophysiology.* Grings and Dawson (1978) refer the interested reader to Stein and Luparello (1967) for a discussion of respiration. Respiration shares a chapter with the digestive system in Hassett (1978) but earns a separate unit in Stern, Ray, and Davis (1980). More recently, Kaufman and Schneiderman (1986) contributed a chapter entitled "Physiological Bases of Respiratory Psychophysiology" to Coles, Donchin, and Porges's (1986) edited volume, although none of the 75 references listed at the end of that chapter include the journal *Psychophysiology.*

A more inclusive attitude toward respiration research is evident in the 1990s. For example, Stein and Luparello's (1967) contribution was updated (Lorig & Schwartz 1990), several review articles were published (Boiten, Frijda, & Wientjes 1994; Ley 1999; Wientjes 1992), and a special issue of *Biological Psychology* on respiratory psychophysiology was arranged (Wientjes & Grossman 1998). The Assembly on Behavioral Science became the 12th pri-

mary group within the American Thoracic Society in 1991, the International Society for the Advancement of Respiratory Psychophysiology was established in 1993 (Benchetrit & Ley 1995; Ley 1994; Timmons 1994), and in 1996 a section on applied respiratory psychophysiology was formed within the Association for Applied Psychophysiology and Biofeedback. In this chapter, we attempt a review of respiratory psychophysiology to extend these developments that overcome, in part, a perceived history of respiratory neglect.

HISTORICAL BACKGROUND: AFFECT, PERSONALITY, AND PSYCHOSOMATIC DISEASE

The breathing pattern is regulated by well-understood reflexes acting on the brainstem in concert to determine the depth of breathing (tidal volume, V_T), the duration of the phases of the breathing cycle (inspiratory time T_I and expiratory time T_E), and the lung volume at which inspiration begins (end-expiratory volume or EEV) (Remmers 1976). Early in the century, tidal volume and the duration of the phases of breathing in humans were typically derived from measures of airflow (made with a spirometer) or of chest wall movement (made with a strain gauge). Since the 1970s, investigators in pulmonary medicine and in respiratory physiology have routinely used flow meters and pressure transducers to record breathing pattern changes. In behavioral investigations, however, these changes have been inferred largely from gross recordings of abdominal and thoracic displacement throughout the century.

Very little literature relates either to the individuality of the breathing pattern or to the behavioral control of breathing. Nielsen and Roth (1929) developed ten categories, or types, of breathing patterns based on review of 20,000 spirometric tracings and associated the categories with heritable conditions that purportedly affect the respiratory center in predictable ways. For example, the type-B pattern was predominant in individuals with endocrine disturbances and the type-F pattern was evident in obesity. Christie (1935) distinguished the breathing pattern prevalent in anxiety neuroses from that evident in conversion hysteria. Sutherland, Wolf, and Kennedy (1938) suggested a more intimate relationship between personality and respiratory behavior and argued that the "respiratory curve is as constant and characteristic of an individual as is his handwriting." On hindsight, such arguments appear to be based largely on anecdote and single-case studies. On the other hand, a ventilatory personality – *personalité ventilatoire* – is intimated by the relatively stable characteristic of the adult breathing pattern despite a seemingly infinite number of possible combinations of tidal volume and breathing frequency that could serve to maintain adequate alveolar ventilation (for a review see Shea & Guz 1992).

Variations in the pattern of breathing have been associated with emotional state, psychopathology, and psychodynamic conflict for nearly 100 years. Since at least 1916, and the first volume of the *Journal of Experimental Psychology,* experimental interest in the relationship between emotional experience and respiration is evident (see Boiten et al. 1994). Feleky (1916), influenced by contemporary study of McDougall's list of primary emotions and facial expression, argued that emotions are reflected in the muscles of respiration to the same degree that they are reflected in the muscles of the face. Variations in the ratio between inspiratory times and expiratory times (the I : E ratio) for disgust, pleasure, anger, pain, wonder, and fear provided the most compelling evidence for the specificity of emotional expression in the "organ of breathing." The respiratory response to fear received special consideration from earlier psychologists. Blatz (1925) characterized an inspiratory gasp to fear induced by tipping subjects backwards (to 60°) while they sat blindfolded in a chair. Skaggs (1926, 1930) described a "sharp inspiratory movement" in subjects to startle and "excited expectancy" induced by intense noise from a hidden auto horn, a threat of shock, or a "very vigorous shock." Such movement was hypothesized to result from violent contraction of the diaphragm and chest muscles involved in inspiration.

Dudley and colleagues (1964a; Dudley, Martin, & Holmes 1964b; Dudley et al. 1969) conceptualized the biological significance of ventilatory responses to emotional stimuli – including those to life stress, measured as life change units with the "schedule of recent experience" – in terms of personal behavioral and metabolic needs. They hypothesized a continuum of response styles,

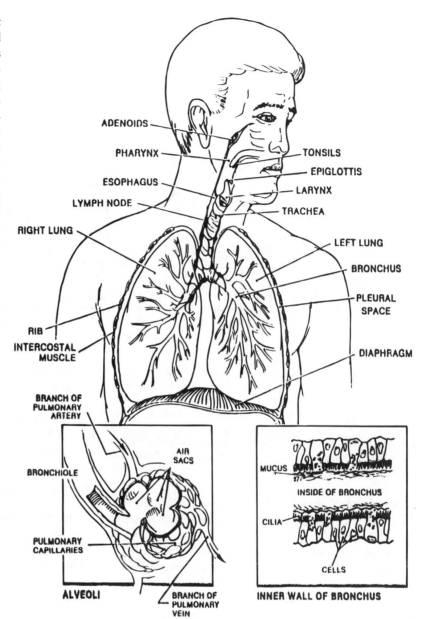

Figure 2. The respiratory system. Reprinted with permission from Luce, *Lung Diseases of Adults.* Copyright 1986 American Lung Association.

ranging from action-oriented to non–action-oriented, by observing changes in respiratory parameters to suggestions of relaxation, depression, anger, anxiety, pain, and exercise in patients with lung disease and in control subjects (see Figure 3). Action-oriented patterns – evident in states of anger, hostility, panic, and euphoria – were associated with hyperventilation and involved increases in breathing frequency and oxygen consumption that serve to prepare the individual metabolically to expend energy. Non–action-oriented patterns were associated with hypoventilation and the conservation of energy and were evident in despair, sadness, deep relaxation, and withdrawal. Current interest

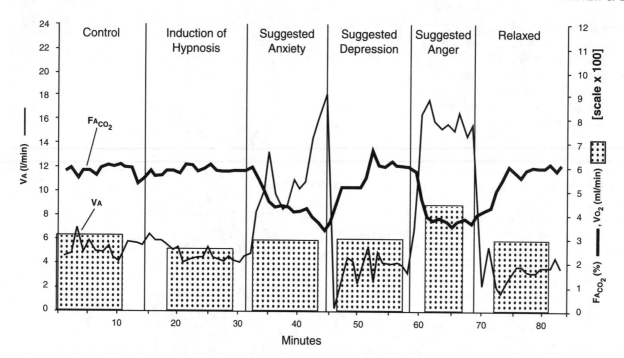

Figure 3. Metabolic changes in a single subject to suggested anxiety, depression, anger, and deep relaxation: V_A = alveolar ventilation (l/min); $F_{A_{CO_2}}$ = fractional concentration (%) of alveolar carbon dioxide; V_{O_2} = oxygen consumption (ml/min). Redrawn with permission from Dudley, Holmes, Martin, & Ripley, "Changes in respiration associated with hypnotically induced emotion, pain, and exercise," *Psychosomatic Medicine*, vol. 26, pp. 645–60. Copyright 1964 Lippincott Williams & Wilkins.

in the psychophysiology of hyperventilation, hyperventilation syndrome, and panic evolved in part from comparable clinical studies (e.g. Fried 1993).

Casual review of the psychodynamic literature confirms that asthma emerges as the respiratory disorder most vulnerable to psychosomatic interpretation (Saul & Lyons 1951; Stein & Luparello 1970). One case study (asthma elicited by an artificial rose) and one theoretical model (equating asthma to a cry for help) are sufficient to illustrate the psychodynamic grip placed on asthma in earlier decades (Dekker, Pelser, & Groen 1957; Franks & Leigh 1959; Stein & Luparello 1970; Turnbull 1962). In these formulations, the vulnerability of patients to an episode of asthma was related to learned or conditioned respiratory responses that lead to wheezing, chest tightness, and dyspnea. Studies demonstrating classical conditioning of respiratory responses in both animals and humans were reviewed by Freedman (1951) and more recently by Ley (1999). Many of these studies share the same procedures and involve pairing an auditory (conditioned) stimulus with a shock (unconditioned) stimulus to produce conditioned increases in respiratory frequency or variations (e.g., inspiratory gasps) in the pattern of breathing. Current research in the psychology of asthma is far removed, however, from both classical conditioning and instrumental learning

models proposed to account for the psychogenic origin and maintenance of asthma and asthmalike responses. A more contemporary concern, for example, relates to asthma self-management and to the behavioral elements that play a role in the control of asthma (Kotses & Harver 1998; Kotses, Lewis, & Creer 1990).

Physical Context

Complete introductions to respiration may be found in a variety of excellent medical textbooks, including those by Comroe (1974), Guyton (1981), Levitzky (1986), Mines (1986), and West (1985).

ANATOMY OF BREATHING

The respiratory system is made up of the structures that are involved in the exchange of oxygen (O_2) and carbon dioxide (CO_2) between the atmosphere and the blood. These structures include the lungs, the airways, parts of the central nervous system that regulate the muscles of respiration, and the chest wall. The chest wall consists of the rib cage, the diaphragm and the intercostal muscles, and the visceral and parietal pleura. The lungs – two irregularly cone-shaped structures – are contained within separate pleural sacs. The right and left lungs differ slightly in their gross anatomy. The right lung is slightly larger, shorter, and broader than the left, and is divided into three lobes (upper, middle, and lower). The left lung is divided into only two lobes (upper and lower). The diaphragm separates the liver from the right lung and, depending on the size of the liver, from the left lung. The left lung is also separated from the stomach and the spleen by the diaphragm.

Inhaled air passes through the nose and mouth and enters the region of the pharynx and epiglottis. During inhalation, the epiglottis is folded up so that the air may enter the larynx and trachea and eventually the lungs. During swallowing, the epiglottis folds down, covering the larynx and preventing food or liquid from entering the airway. Air enters the mouth and nose, passes over the pharynx and larynx, and enters the trachea, which divides into two main branches, the right and left bronchi (Levitzky 1986). The right bronchus is larger in diameter than the left because it supports the larger lung. The bronchi each divide again, and the branching and division of the airways continues for 20–30 generations. No alveoli are present in the conducting zone – the first 16 generations – but they begin to appear in the next several generations (the transitional zone). The final set of branches (the respiratory zone) are lined with alveoli, about 300 million in the two lungs (Comroe 1974; Mines 1986). If we assume an average inspiratory volume of 500 ml and a breathing frequency of 15 breaths/min, then total (or "minute") ventilation is $500 \times 15 = 7,500$ ml/min (West 1985). Because a portion of the inspired air (~ 150 ml) remains in the anatomical dead space (i.e., the conducting zone) on each breath, the volume of fresh gas reaching the respiratory zone each minute (i.e., alveolar ventilation) is about $[(500 - 150) \times 15] = 5,250$ ml/min.

The alveoli are small sack-shaped structures about 100–300 μm in diameter, thin-walled, and highly vascularized. About 1,000 pulmonary capillaries serve each of the 300 million alveoli, resulting in 50–100 m^2 of surface area available for gas exchange. Gas exchange, which takes place by diffusion along a partial pressure gradient, occurs very rapidly. Although the transit time of blood through the pulmonary capillaries is only 0.75 sec, diffusion is so rapid that the partial pressure of oxygen in alveolar air (~ 100 mmHg) and that of mixed venous blood (~ 40 mmHg) reach equilibrium before the blood has passed even halfway along the capillary.

The primary muscle of respiration is the diaphragm, a dome-shaped muscle separating the thorax from the abdomen that provides for the movement of more than two-thirds of the air that enters the lungs during quiet breathing. Unlike the heart, contraction of this specialized muscle is under direct neural (i.e. phrenic) control. When the diaphragm contracts during quiet breathing, the volume of the thorax increases because the abdominal contents are forced down and forward, and the rib cage is lifted. During quiet breathing, the diaphragm descends about a centimeter or so and the shape of the diaphragm dome remains largely unchanged (West 1985). Several other muscle groups play an important role in inspiration in addition to the diaphragm. Contraction of the external intercostals effectively rotates the ribs up and out which serves to increase the volume of the chest cavity and enhance the action of the diaphragm. Both the external and internal intercostal muscles contribute to the rigidity of the thoracic wall by preventing the intercostal spaces from bulging in and out during breathing. Chest wall mechanoreceptors participate in postural adjustments and other compensatory responses mostly by stabilizing the chest wall or by adjusting the strength of respiratory muscle contractions through segmental, spinal reflexes (Shannon 1986; Younes 1995). The scalene and sternomastoid muscles make their contribution during high levels of ventilation. The sternomastoids also serve to anchor the upper ribs during inspiration and provide a foundation for the external intercostals. Expiration is usually a passive return to end-expiratory volume due to the recoil of the lung, but it can be enhanced in high-demand situations. Contraction of the abdominal muscles decreases the distention of the abdomen caused by the diaphragm and forces the diaphragm back to its dome-shaped resting state. Through postinspiratory contraction of the diaphragm, exhalations may be slowed or braked to produce less dramatic or rapidly shifting ventilatory patterns. Various expiratory muscles play important roles in the regulation of breathing during talking, singing, and coughing.

PHYSIOLOGY OF RESPIRATION

Respiration involves four primary processes: pulmonary ventilation (the movement of air in and out of the lungs), diffusion (the exchange of oxygen and carbon dioxide between the alveoli and the blood), transport (the transport of oxygen and carbon dioxide in the blood to and from cells), and regulation (the neural control of breathing).

Levels of Respiration

In one earlier formulation, Comroe (1974) distinguished between "external respiration" and "internal respiration." The former is of usual interest to the physiologist and involves the movement of the lungs, thorax, and air (i.e. ventilation). The latter, of primary interest to the biochemist, involves the cellular processes in tissues that use oxygen and give off carbon dioxide. In between these extremes are the processes involving gas exchange among the alveoli, blood, and cells ("intermediate respiration"). We subsequently emphasize those processes involved in external and intermediate respiration, and we elect to "leave to the biochemists the actual cellular processes that use O$_2$" (Comroe 1974).

Pulmonary Ventilation. Pulmonary ventilation is largely concerned with the mechanics of breathing – that is, the forces that move the lung and chest wall, resulting in the flow of air to and from the alveoli. It is the mechanics of breathing that is largely disturbed in diseases of airflow obstruction. In asthma, for example, an increased burden is placed on the muscles of respiration, which must generate sufficient tension to overcome the increase in resistance and hyperinflation that accompanies bronchoconstriction.

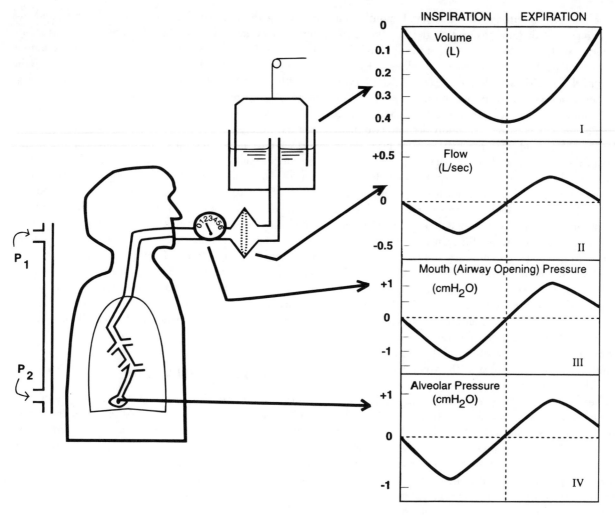

Figure 4. Respiratory volume, airflow, mouth pressure, and alveolar pressure during a single breathing cycle; see text. From Harver & Mahler (1998), "Perception of increased resistance to breathing," in Kotses & Harver (Eds.), *Self-Management of Asthma*, pp. 147–93. Reprinted courtesy of Marcel Dekker Inc.

Air moves into the airways because of a (negative) pressure gradient that develops between the atmosphere and alveoli during inspiration. The cycle of changes in three fundamental forces, or pressures, account for the "bulk flow" of air into the lungs with each breath: atmospheric (P_{ATM}) or airway opening pressure, which is typically measured near the mouth (P_{MO}); alveolar pressure (P_{ALV}); and pleural pressure (P_{PL}). At the end of expiration, when no air is flowing, $P_{MO} = P_{ALV}$ and P_{PL} is about 5 cmH$_2$O lower than P_{ATM}. (In respiratory physiology, pressure is expressed typically in units of cmH$_2$O; 1 cmH$_2$O is equivalent to about 0.75 mmHg). When the muscles of respiration contract, the diaphragm expands the thoracic cage and lowers P_{PL} further. As the airways widen and the alveoli enlarge, the distance between gas molecules increases and P_{ALV} decreases (i.e., $P_{ALV} < P_{MO}$). As alveolar pressure drops, air flows along the pressure gradient created between atmospheric pressure and the relative neg-

ative pressure developed in the alveoli. An average pressure gradient of less than 3 cmH$_2$O moves about 500 ml of air into the lungs.

Three variables are typically recorded in pulmonary ventilation studies: volume (the amount of air moved, in liters); flow (the rate of movement of air, in liters per second); and pleural pressure (the amount of muscle force involved in the production of chest wall movement, in cmH$_2$O). A schematic for the measurement of volume (with a water-sealed spirometer), flow (with a flowmeter, or pneumotachograph), and mouth pressure (with a differential pressure transducer) is depicted in Figure 4. The pressure gradient developed during inspiration is represented also in Figure 4 simply as the difference between the airway opening (P_1) and the alveoli (P_2). The rate of airflow is dependent on the pressure gradient; an airflow rate of 1 l/sec requires a pressure drop along the airways of less than 2 cmH$_2$O.

Resistance and Compliance. The force that must be generated for air to move must be sufficient to overcome the impedances, or "loads," that normally oppose breathing: resistance and compliance. Pulmonary (or total) resistance is composed of the pulmonary tissue resistance caused by the friction encountered as tissues slide over one another during lung expansion and airway resistance caused by the frictional resistance to airflow offered by the respiratory passageways (Cherniack 1983). Resistive loads are due chiefly to the resistance to airflow through the tracheobronchial tree; airway resistance comprises the major component (80%–90%) of pulmonary resistance. Resistance (in units of cmH$_2$O/l/sec) is the ratio between respiratory pressure (in cmH$_2$O) and the rate of flow (in l/sec) produced by that pressure. Because the rate of airflow is determined by the mouth–alveolar pressure gradient, airway resistance (R_{AW}) is measured as the drop in pressure between the alveoli and the mouth (measured in cmH$_2$O) divided by flow ($\dot{V}$):

$$R_{AW} = \frac{P_{MO} - P_{ALV}}{\dot{V}}. \tag{1}$$

The major sites of airway resistance are the upper airway and the medium-sized bronchi; less than 20% of total airway resistance is attributed to airways less than 2 mm in diameter. Normal airway resistance values vary between 2 and 4 cmH$_2$O/l/sec; values from 2 to 15 times as great may be observed in acute asthma, where the size of the airway is critically important. Decreases in the size of the airway (as occurs in acute bronchoconstriction) lead to increases in resistance to breathing. Reducing the airway's radius by half leads to a 16-fold increase in resistance (Comroe 1974).

At the end of a normal breath (i.e., at functional residual capacity), the tendency of the chest wall to spring out in an inspiratory direction is equal to the tendency of the lungs to "recoil" or collapse in an expiratory direction. At maximal inspiration, there is a marked tendency of the system to recoil toward a smaller volume; at maximal expiration, the net force is in an inspiratory direction. The distensibility or compliance (C_L) of the lungs or chest wall or both can be expressed as the volume change (in liters) produced by a unit of change in transpulmonary pressure (in cmH$_2$O), measured under static conditions:

$$C_L = \frac{\Delta l}{\Delta cmH_2O}. \tag{2}$$

Lung elastance or stiffness is proportional to the force required to expand the lungs against its elastic recoil forces. The stiffer the lung, the less its compliance (West 1985). For example, in emphysema an applied pressure of 5 cmH$_2$O may result in 2 l of air ($C_L = 0.4$ l/cmH$_2$O), but in pulmonary fibrosis the same pressure change may result in only 0.5 l of air ($C_L = 0.1$ l/cmH$_2$O) (Cherniack 1983). Chest wall compliance depends on the rigidity and shape of the thoracic cage and may be decreased, for example, in diseases that affect the bony thorax such as scoliosis (Mines 1986). Diminished respiratory function during normal aging can be explained (at least in part) by decreases in lung elasticity, decreases in respiratory muscle strength, and increases in thoracic cage stiffness (Mahler 1983).

Load Compensation and Load Perception. Over the course of about a decade – from 1974 to 1985 – several conferences and symposia highlighted two goals that have stimulated ongoing study of resistive and elastic loads (e.g. Altose & Zechman 1986; Pengelly, Rebuck, & Campbell 1974). One goal relates to the regulation of ventilation (i.e., load compensation) and in the consequences for respiratory homeostasis of disturbances in the mechanics of breathing in lung disease. The other purpose relates to the sensation of dyspnea and in the quantification of the relationship between mechanical perturbations and respiratory sensations (i.e., load perception). Load perception studies, which evolved from load compensation studies, serve to bridge ventilatory regulation and the study of respiratory sensation (Harver & Mahler 1998b).

A primary goal of load compensation experiments is to uncover the intrinsic muscle responses and neural mechanisms acting on the brainstem that mediate breathing pattern responses to acute or chronic disturbances in the mechanics of breathing. In his exhaustive review, Younes (1995) concluded that two primary mechanisms (the intrinsic properties of the respiratory muscles and chemical feedback) and two secondary mechanisms (increases in intercostal activity and a reflex that shortens expiration during inspiratory loads) account for compensatory responses to added loads. The large interindividual differences in load responses observed commonly in conscious humans, he further concluded, are due largely to "noncompensatory" behavioral (i.e. voluntary) responses – following conscious perception of an added load – that serve to minimize abnormal respiratory sensations. In this context, Cherniack and colleagues suggested that the ventilatory pattern may be determined to reduce respiratory sensory input and to minimize perceived respiratory discomfort (Cherniack 1996; Oku et al. 1993).

Diffusion and Transport. Dry air is composed of oxygen (O$_2$; 20.93%), carbon dioxide (CO$_2$; 0.04%), and nitrogen (N; 79.03%). The partial pressure, or tension, these elements exert independently on a closed container at sea level (barometric pressure = 760 mmHg) would be 159.1, 0.3, and 600.6 mmHg or torr (in honor of the inventor of the barometer, Evangelista Torricelli), respectively. Inspired air becomes saturated with water vapor as soon as it enters the nose, mouth, and pharynx. In the lungs, the partial pressure (P) of alveolar levels of O$_2$, CO$_2$, N, and water vapor in humans at sea level are 104, 40, 569, and 47 torr, respectively. An alveolar P_{O_2} of about 100 torr and a P_{CO_2} of about 40 torr are perceived to best meet the needs of the body for oxygen supply, carbon dioxide removal, and regulation of blood acidity (Comroe 1974).

The main purpose of ventilation is to enable the optimal composition of alveolar gas, the compartment of gas lying between atmospheric air and alveolar capillary air (Comroe 1974). Alveolar ventilation – the volume of fresh air entering the alveoli on each breath, or per minute – is always less than total ventilation, and it varies as a function of the anatomic dead space, the alveolar dead space (i.e., the volume of gas entering underperfused alveoli), tidal volume, and breathing frequency. Alveolar ventilation is sufficient for oxygen metabolism when it matches oxygen use with oxygen supply. Alveolar hyperventilation results when more oxygen is supplied (P_{O_2} rises) and more carbon dioxide is removed (P_{CO_2} falls) than the metabolic rate requires. Hypoventilation results when less oxygen is supplied (P_{O_2} decreases) and less carbon dioxide is removed (P_{CO_2} rises) than the metabolic rate requires.

Blood that is low in oxygen and high in carbon dioxide is pumped by the right ventricle of the heart through the pulmonary artery to the lungs. In the pulmonary capillaries, carbon dioxide is exchanged for oxygen. The blood leaving the lungs is rich in oxygen and relatively low in carbon dioxide, and it is distributed to the rest of the body by the left side of the heart. Tissue metabolism depletes the O_2 and increases the level of CO_2 in the blood, which is then returned to the right half of the heart to be pumped again to the lungs (Figure 5). About 300 ml of oxygen

is diffusing continuously from the alveoli into pulmonary capillary blood each minute; about 250 ml/min of carbon dioxide is continuously diffusing from mixed venous blood into the alveoli.

Diffusion. The movement of O_2 and CO_2 between the alveoli and capillary blood is accomplished passively through the process of diffusion. The factors that determine the rate of diffusion of a gas through the alveolocapillary barrier are summarized in Fick's law of diffusion:

$$\dot{V}_{gas} = \frac{A}{T} \times D \times (P_1 - P_2), \tag{3}$$

where $\dot{V}_{gas}$ = the volume of gas diffusing through the barrier (ml/min); A = the surface area of the barrier; T = thickness of the barrier, or diffusion distance; D = the diffusing coefficient of the gas; and $(P_1 - P_2)$ = the partial pressure difference of the gas across the barrier. The diffusion of oxygen occurs rapidly. In a normal alveolus, it is 80% complete in 0.002 sec if the diffusion distance is 0.5 mm (Comroe 1974). The pressure differences responsible for the diffusion of oxygen across the barrier depends upon many complex factors, including the **S**-shaped oxyhemoglobin (HbO_2) dissociation curve.

Transport. The heart would need to pump about 83 liters of blood per minute if the need for oxygen were met only through the levels of physically dissolved oxygen in the blood. But maximum cardiac output in adults during severe exercise reaches only about 25 l/min (Levitzky 1986). Toward this end, blood contains hemoglobin, which enables whole blood to take up 65 times as much oxygen as plasma at a P_{O_2} of 100 torr (Comroe 1974). The HbO_2 dissociation curve characterizes well-appreciated effects of P_{O_2}, blood temperature, and blood pH on the amount of oxygen that binds to (and is released by) hemoglobin.

The proportion of hemoglobin that is bound to oxygen is expressed in terms of percent saturation. Between P_{O_2} values of about 70 and 100 torr, there is little change in the association, or loading, of O_2 with Hb; a decrease from 100 to 70 torr decreases saturation to only 94.1% (Comroe 1974). The part of the HbO_2 dissociation curve below 60 torr might be called the "tissue" or dissociation part (Levitzky 1986). Tissues continuously use O_2 and lower the P_{O_2} in and around cells below the P_{O_2} of capillary blood (Comroe, 1974). At P_{O_2} levels between 10 and 40 torr – as exist in metabolically active tissue – the dissociation (unloading) of bound O_2 from Hb is marked. For example, Hb can hold only 75% of its oxygen at a P_{O_2} of 40 torr and only 9.6% of its oxygen at a P_{O_2} of 10 torr. The acidification of blood – as occurs, for example, with increases in P_{CO_2} – results in the release of much more oxygen than normal (i.e., the Bohr effect). A proper type and quantity of Hb are necessary for optimal loading and unloading of oxygen, and the heart and vessels are necessary to deliver the proper amount of oxygenated blood to all tissues in proportion to their need.

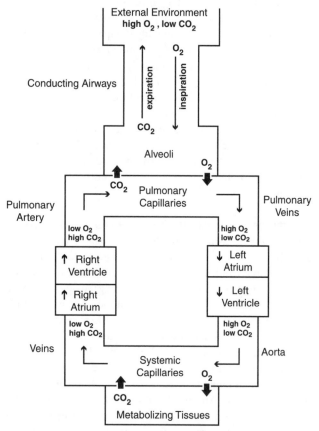

Figure 5. Schematic representation of gas exchange between the tissues of the body and the environment. Redrawn with permission from Levitzky, *Pulmonary Physiology,* 2nd ed. Copyright 1986 The McGraw-Hill Companies.

Tissue metabolism influences tissue P_{O_2} in two ways: (1) the more active the tissue, the higher the local P_{CO_2} and temperature leading to vasodilation, increases in blood flow, and dissociation of O_2 from HbO_2 in capillary blood; (2) the greater the use of O_2, the lower the tissue P_{O_2} and the sharper the concentration gradient for diffusion (Comroe 1974). In functional magnetic resonance imaging (fMRI), the relative activity of various brain areas can be mapped because hemoglobin slightly changes its paramagnetic properties after it has released its oxygen, allowing researchers to distinguish between hemoglobin with oxygen and hemoglobin without oxygen.

The primary product of cell metabolism is CO_2, which is carried to the lungs in venous blood and eliminated in the expired gas. In this context, the lungs are the most important organ in the body for maintaining acid–base balance. Carbon dioxide molecules diffuse from active tissue into capillary blood plasma. In the lungs, the alveolar P_{CO_2} (40 torr) is lower than the P_{CO_2} of mixed venous blood flowing into the pulmonary capillaries (46 torr). Each breath removes about 350 ml of air containing 5%–6% CO_2.

Oxygen, Hypoxemia, and Neuropsychological Function. The body provides only a small reserve of oxygen to overcome acute periods of hypoxia or asphyxia. The total oxygen store of about 1,500 ml would be sufficient to sustain life for about six minutes if it were distributed appropriately. In humans, cessation of blood flow to the brain results in a loss of function in 4–6 sec, a loss of consciousness in 10–20 sec, and permanent brain damage in 3–5 min (West 1985).

Respiration usually increases in proportion to metabolic demand (e.g., as arterial P_{O_2} falls), although the body's sensitivity to arterial P_{O_2} levels is much less acute than its sensitivity to alveolar P_{CO_2} levels. Chemosensitive cells in aortic bodies – attached to the arch of the aorta and in carotid bodies near the division of the common carotid artery – respond to decreases in arterial P_{O_2}. Hypoxia, a decrease in P_{O_2} below normal levels, may result from variations in the level of oxygen in the inspired air, in alveolar air, in the blood, or in the tissues. The amount of O_2 available to tissues depends upon blood flow, the amount of oxygen in the blood, and the unloading of bound oxygen from hemoglobin. Hypoxemia usually refers to a significant and specific decrease in O_2 saturation of hemoglobin. In patients with cardiopulmonary disease, the most frequent cause of hypoxemia is uneven alveolar ventilation in relation to alveolar blood flow (i.e., an uneven matching of gas and blood).

Subtle to moderate neuropsychological deficits that potentially reflect effects of subacute or chronic diffuse hypoxia have been observed in hypoxemic patients with chronic obstructive pulmonary disease (Prigatano & Grant 1988). Results compiled from the Halstead–Reitan neuropsychological test battery, which was administered to patients participating in two large clinical trials (supported by the National Heart, Lung, and Blood Institute in the late 1970s) to determine the effectiveness of nighttime oxygen, revealed subtle to moderate levels of impairment in abstract reasoning, complex perceptual motor skills, concentration, problem solving, and short-term memory. In the nocturnal oxygen therapy trial (NOTT), 77% of the 203 tested patients exhibited clinically significant neuropsychological impairment. The observed level of neuropsychological impairment was associated with the severity of hypoxemia (i.e., with *arterial* P_{O_2}, Pa_{O_2}). Analyses of the combined pool of NOTT and the intermittent positive pressure breathing data (302 patients and 99 controls) showed that more severely hypoxemic patients (mean $Pa_{O_2} = 44$ mmHg) performed more poorly than those with either moderate (mean $Pa_{O_2} = 54$ mmHg) or mild (mean $Pa_{O_2} = 68$ mmHg) hypoxemia (Prigatano & Grant 1988).

Control of Breathing

Breathing is regulated automatically by sets of interactive medullary neurons located bilaterally in or near the nucleus of the solitary tract (dorsal respiratory group) and the nuclei ambiguus and retroambiguus (ventral respiratory group). The dorsal respiratory group (DRG) consists primarily of inspiratory cells. The DRG receives afferent input from pulmonary stretch and pulmonary irritant receptors; the nucleus of the solitary tract serves as the primary projection site for glossopharyngeal and vagal afferents. The ventral respiratory group (VRG) consists of both inspiratory and expiratory cells and is driven by the activity of the DRG. The medulla is not only necessary but also sufficient for involuntary breathing (Grodins & Yamashiro 1978). Normal periodic breathing derives from the intrinsic oscillation of respiratory center activity (i.e., of the "respiratory pattern generator").

Most axons from cells of the respiratory pattern generator cross in the medulla and descend in the ventral and lateral columns to spinal segmental levels. The cells in the DRG seem to serve the upper motor neurons of many muscles of respiration and extend to the phrenic motor neurons of the diaphragm (Mines 1986). The cells of the VRG project to intercostal, abdominal, and auxiliary muscles of respiration. Impulses mediating the voluntary control of breathing arise from the motor and premotor cortex and descend in the corticospinal tracts (Grodins & Yamashiro 1978). The activity of the medullary oscillator is modulated by neural inputs from pontine areas (e.g., both the pneumotaxic and apneustic centers) and by mechanical and chemical stimuli. The state of alertness, or level of wakefulness, also acts as an important stimulus to respiration. For example, in deep sleep the sensitivity to P_{CO_2} levels – which rise from 40 to 46 torr – is diminished. One recent model of ventilatory control (Pack & Gottschalk 1993) that emphasizes a state-dependent input for breathing (i.e., a wakefulness stimulus) is depicted in Figure 6.

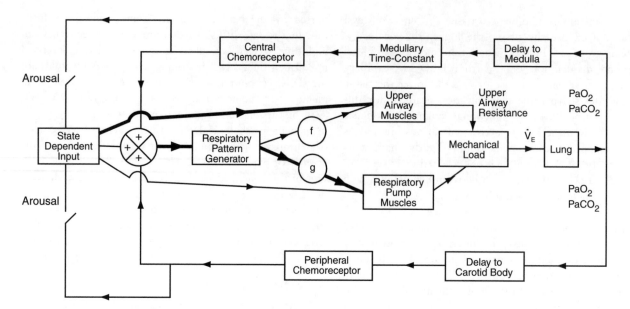

Figure 6. Block diagram of the ventilatory control system incorporating a state-dependent input (wakefulness stimulus) and arousal. Ventilation is determined by neural drive not only to the upper airway muscles (function f) but also to the respiratory muscles, including the diaphragm (function g). The wakefulness stimulus is envisaged to have a proportionately greater effect on the activity of the upper airways. Redrawn with permission from Pack & Gottschalk, "Mechanisms of ventilatory periodicities," *Annals of Biomedical Engineering*, vol. 21, pp. 537–44. Copyright 1993 Biomedical Engineering Society.

Pulmonary Inputs. The pulmonary receptors include slowly adapting stretch receptors (SARs), rapidly adapting irritant receptors (RARs), and the type-J (juxtapulmonary-capillary) receptors (see Kubin & Davies 1995). Stretch receptors are evident in airway smooth muscles and are activated by lung distension. Irritant receptors in the nasal mucosa, upper airways, and tracheobronchial tree are activated by a wide range of mechanical and chemical substances including noxious gases, smoke, dust, histamine, and cold air. The type-J receptors (pulmonary and bronchial C-fibers) in the walls of the alveoli or capillaries respond to pulmonary vascular congestion and edema. Vagal afferents carry information from lung receptors about physiological processes occurring in the lungs and airways that result in adaptive changes in the pattern of breathing as occur in coughing, swallowing, and vomiting (Kubin & Davies 1995). In addition, the lung receptors are involved in the reflex regulation of the breathing pattern as well as breath-to-breath modulation of bronchomotor tone. For example, activation of SARs results in bronchodilation through inhibition of efferent vagal activity; mechanical or chemical stimulation of RARs results in reflex bronchoconstriction. Reflex bronchoconstriction also results from stimulation of type-J receptors following increases in pulmonary vascular congestion, as occurs for example in cases of left heart failure (Paintal 1977).

Chemoreceptive Inputs. Both peripheral and central chemoreceptors respond to low arterial P_{O_2}, high arterial P_{CO_2}, and low arterial pH. The peripheral receptors, located in the carotid and aortic bodies, sense decreases in P_{O_2} and, to a lesser extent, increases in P_{CO_2}. The ventilatory response to hypoxia arises solely from the peripheral chemoreceptors (Levitzky 1986). Receptor response is sufficiently rapid and sensitive to relay information about breath-to-breath alterations in blood chemistry to the medullary respiratory center (Levitzky 1986), although the threshold for hypoxia is less predictable than for hypercapnia. Decreased inspired O_2 does not reliably stimulate marked increases in ventilation until arterial P_{O_2} falls to 50–60 torr and HbO_2 falls to about 80%.

The most important factor in the control of ventilation is arterial P_{CO_2}; a rise of only 2 mmHg is capable of producing a doubling of ventilation in some subjects (Mines 1986; West 1985). The most important chemosensitive receptors are located centrally and superficially (no deeper than 0.2 mm) on the ventral surface of the medulla at the level of cranial nerves 8–11 (Mines 1986). Carbon dioxide diffuses freely from the blood across the blood–brain barrier into the cerebrospinal fluid, where it reacts with water to form hydrogen ions that in turn affect medullary centers to stimulate ventilation. Low concentrations of CO_2 in inspired air are easily tolerated, but higher levels ($\sim$ 5%–10% CO_2 inspired air) lead to restlessness, faintness, and dulling of consciousness. At higher levels (> 15% CO_2 inspired air), tremors, muscular rigidity, and unconsciousness occur (Levitzky 1986).

Proprioceptive Inputs. Respiratory muscles contain a rich supply of afferents (including muscle spindles, tendon organs, and slowly adapting receptors in costovertebral joints) that are sensitive to changes in muscle length and muscle tension, although many fundamental questions remain concerning the influence of these muscle receptors in the

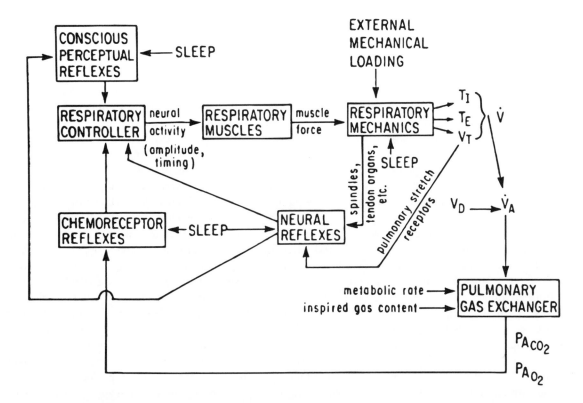

Figure 7. Conceptual diagram showing reflex loops involved in breathing pattern regulation and their relationship to the respiratory mechanics. Reprinted with permission from "Mechanical factors in breathing pattern regulation in humans," *Annals of Biomedical Engineering*, vol. 9, pp. 409–24. Copyright 1981 Biomedical Engineering Society.

control of breathing, load compensation, and load perception (Campbell & Newsom Davis 1970; Jammes & Speck 1995; Shannon 1986). Respiratory mechanoreceptors, especially those of the chest wall, participate in postural adjustments and the compensatory response to mechanical perturbations mostly by stabilizing the chest wall or by adjusting the force of respiratory muscle contractions through segmental, spinal reflexes (Shannon 1986; Younes 1995). Chest wall proprioceptors seem to have little direct effect on ventilatory control under normal conditions, but neurophysiological studies show that respiratory muscle afferents project to pons, thalamus, and cortex (Eldridge & Chen 1996). Davenport and Reep (1995) reviewed ascending pathways for respiratory muscle afferents to account for cortical-evoked potentials elicited by electrical or mechanical stimulation of phrenic and intercostal muscle afferents.

Regulation of the Breathing Pattern. Ventilation is adjusted automatically to maintain O_2 and CO_2 homeostasis in response to environmental, metabolic, and pathophysiological processes, and such adjustments are affected by the mechanics of breathing (i.e., by airway resistance, lung and chest wall compliance, and the mechanical advantage of the respiratory muscles) that change, even during normal breathing, with each inflation and deflation (Cherniack & Altose 1981). Accordingly, a recurrent interest in respiratory physiology relates to the control of breath-to-breath variations in a range of ventilatory parameters, including tidal volume (V_T), the duration of the phases of the breath-

ing cycle (inspiratory time, T_I, and expiratory time, T_E), total cycle time (T_{TOT}), breathing frequency (f), mean inspiratory flow rate (V_T/T_I), and end-expiratory volume (EEV). A historical difference is evident in the goals of those physiologists concerned with the "mechanical" control of breathing and those concerned with the "chemical" control of breathing. The former tended to ignore humoral factors, electing to emphasize the mechanisms underlying the regulation of the breathing cycle; the latter tended to ignore the respiratory cycle, electing to emphasize achieved ventilation. In contemporary physiology, such distinction is more methodological than theoretical. One integrative model showing the potential influences of mechanics upon the regulation of the breathing pattern and encompassing both neural and chemical reflexes is depicted in Figure 7.

Interest in the reflex regulation of the rate and depth of individual breaths derives, in part, from the observations of Hering and Breuer in 1868 (see Comroe 1974). They hypothesized that the breathing pattern turned on vagal reflexes (i.e., increases in pulmonary stretch receptor activity during lung inflation) that served to inhibit central inspiratory activity, thereby limiting tidal volume. The Hering–Breuer reflex, however, is not readily evident in humans over the normal tidal volume range. Clark and von Euler (1972) hypothesized that tidal volume increases during inspiration until a threshold curve for inspiratory termination is achieved (Daubenspeck 1981). In their model, volume and inspiratory time were determined by how quickly volume increases (i.e., by the slope of mean inspiratory flow, V_T/T_I), and expiratory time was determined to be linearly dependent on the preceding inspiration. The rate of inflation, in turn, seemed to depend mainly on the chemical drive for breathing (Clark & von Euler 1972).

Many models of ventilatory control have emphasized the manner in which the respiratory pattern generator is organized to optimize, in some way, breath-to-breath variations in the ongoing operation of the "respiratory pump" (Cherniack 1996; Oku et al. 1993). Gad, in 1880, hypothesized that the Hering–Breuer reflex served to regulate the respiratory muscles in such a way that the greatest alveolar ventilation occurred for the least muscular effort (see Comroe 1974). In 1925, Rohrer proposed a model of respiratory control based on respiratory energetics and intimated that the cost of alveolar ventilation varied with the particular f–V_T combination selected (see Daubenspeck 1981). In this context, Hey and colleagues (1966) demonstrated that the effects of various stimuli (hypercapnia, hypoxia, exercise) on alterations in the rate and depth of breathing followed a single straight-line relationship between ventilation and tidal volume (i.e., the "Hey plot"). The work of breathing approaches a minimum when V_T is set to 400 ml and breathing frequency is set to about 15/min (Comroe 1974). Although it is well appreciated that the work or energy cost of breathing can affect ventilatory responses, it is not yet clear that it plays a significant role in optimizing ventilation or breathing patterns either in normal subjects or in patients with lung disease (Cherniack 1996).

Behavioral Control of Breathing. Markedly limited research relates to the behavioral control of breathing in humans. Evidence for sustained interest in the voluntary control of breathing in psychophysiological research is lacking (Sanchez-Hernandez et al. 1996), and physiologists have attended mainly to brainstem mechanisms serving ventilation by using heavily anesthetized animal preparations, although recent work reflects notable departures from this tradition (see e.g. Cherniack 1996; Eldridge & Chen 1996). We subsequently review five areas of research on breathing that not only involve (to some degree) forebrain processes but also represent ongoing areas of convergence for behavioral and biomedical respiratory researchers.

Constancy of the Individual Breathing Pattern. Tobin and colleagues (1983a,b) measured the breathing pattern through respiratory inductive plethysmography in young and old subjects and in a variety of patient groups to determine the range of values evident in the supine position during quiet breathing. Mean levels of frequency (16.2 ± 2.8 breaths/min), tidal volume (383 ± 91 ml), minute ventilation (6.01 ± 1.39 l/min), and inspiratory duration (1.62 ± 0.31 sec) were virtually equivalent in young (20–50 years) and old

(60–81 years) subjects, though overall rhythmicity was more irregular in the elderly (Tobin et al. 1983b). Asymptomatic smokers exhibited increases in breathing frequency (V_T) and minute ventilation when compared with nonsmokers (Tobin et al. 1983a). Heightened respiratory drive – evident as increases in mean inspiratory flow rate (V_T/T_I) – was a common nonspecific finding in smokers and in patients with symptomatic asthma, chronic obstructive pulmonary disease, restrictive lung disease, and pulmonary hypertension (Tobin et al. 1983a).

Although variation in V_T/T_I is the rule in subjects during normal breathing (Daubenspeck & Farnham 1982), evidence for characteristic individual breathing patterns – especially in terms of the profile of airflow obtained through harmonic analysis (Figure 8) – was derived from respiratory measurements made in 16 adults on two occasions, four to five years apart (Benchetrit et al. 1989). Similarities in the shape of airflow profiles in monozygotic twins, although less than that obtained within individuals, are also evident (Shea et al. 1989, 1993). Shea, Benchetrit, Guz, and colleagues have speculated that the stability of the individual breathing pattern within persons, as well as the similarity of airflow profiles between identical twins, could result from an inherent property of the respiratory pattern generator, a genetically based sensitivity to inspired CO_2, the pattern of innervation of the respiratory musculature, the size and structure of the ventilatory apparatus, pulmonary and/or proprioceptive inputs, cortical influences upon breathing, or any combination of these factors (Benchetrit et al. 1989; Shea & Guz 1992). Recent animal work suggests that as few as two genes determine differences in respiratory timing between two inbred strains of mice; accordingly, a limited number of genes are likely present – in the human genome – that control differences in individual breathing patterns (Tankersley et al. 1997).

Behavioral Adjustments to Added Loads. Breathing pattern responses to added resistive and elastic loads are affected by both neural reflexes and behavioral reactions following conscious perception of altered breathing mechanics (Daubenspeck & Rhodes 1995). The interindividual differences in load responses observed in conscious humans appear to be due largely to behavioral (i.e. voluntary) responses that serve to minimize abnormal respiratory sensations (Younes 1995). Freedman and Campbell (1970) suggested almost 30 years ago that the stability of ventilation with maximally tolerable loads appeared to be directed toward reducing subjective discomfort. More recently, it has been suggested that the ventilatory pattern may be optimized to reduce respiratory sensory input and thereby to minimize uncomfortable breathing sensations (Cherniack 1996; Oku et al. 1993). But many uncertainties surround the way in which individuals actually respond to respiratory sensations. For example, respiratory sensations may not always fulfill a role in optimizing the breathing

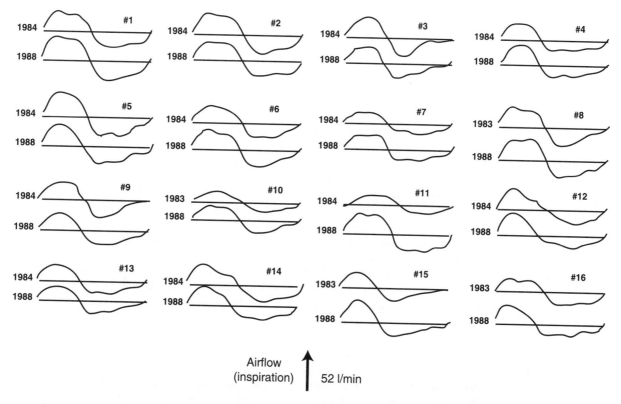

Airflow
(inspiration) ↑ 52 l/min

Figure 8. Average patterns of inspiratory and expiratory airflow from individual subjects obtained on two occasions, 4–5 years apart. The shapes were derived from harmonic analysis of the digitized airflow signal (approximately 50 breaths per subject) and are plotted in normalized time. Redrawn with permission from Benchetrit, Shea, Dinh, Bodocco, Baconnier, & Guz, "Individuality of breathing patterns in adults assessed over time," *Respiration Physiology*, vol. 75, pp. 199–210. Copyright 1989 Elsevier Science.

pattern on the basis of either gas exchange or comfort (Shea, Banzett, & Lansing 1996).

Breath Holding. Variations in breath-holding times have been attributed to both physiological and psychological processes for nearly 100 years (Bartlett 1977; Schneider 1930). One conclusion reached from studies conducted in the 1920s is that "men who fail to hold their breath for less than 30 or 45 seconds do so because they are not willing, or are mentally and nervously unable, to withstand the symptoms induced" (Schneider 1930). Breath-holding time is inversely proportional to P_{CO_2}, which rises linearly throughout the breath hold; it is shortened by hypoxia and, for any given level of P_{CO_2} and P_{O_2}, is directly proportional to lung volume (Godfrey & Campbell 1968). Nonchemical factors that arise from the absence of normal respiratory movement contribute substantively to the unpleasant sensations that increase with increases in breath-holding time (Godfrey & Campbell 1968). Distraction – performing either a psychomotor task or a mental arithmetic task – results in reliable increases in breath-holding times (Alpher, Nelson, & Blanton 1986; Bartlett 1977). Such effects are not inconsistent with the hypothesis that competition between internal and external events affects the distribution of attentional resources and, accordingly, the salience of symptoms (Pennebaker 1982). Distraction may serve to reduce awareness of unpleasant respiratory sensations, including the perception of effort (Thornby, Haas, & Axen 1995).

Breathing and Sleep. Behavioral control of respiration is evident during sleep, and respiration may serve as a sensitive measure of information processing during sleep. Badia

and colleagues (1984; Badia, Harsh, & Balkin 1986) demonstrated that subjects instructed during waking to produce a deep inspiration (sufficient to cause a 50% increase in breathing amplitude) following presentation of an auditory signal did exhibit a high probability of responding to the signal in all stages of sleep. Such control, moreover, was enhanced when responding was reinforced (Badia et al. 1984). Respiration may also serve as a sensitive measure of sleep onset. Ogilvie and Wilkinson (1984), for example, demonstrated orderly relationships between reaction time and relative changes in the breathing pattern that complemented more traditional EEG (electroencephalographic) assessments of sleep onset.

Modification of Ventilatory Mechanics. Breathing behavior can be brought under stimulus control through either classical or instrumental conditioning procedures. Studies demonstrating conditioning of respiratory responses in both animals and humans were reviewed by Freedman (1951) and more recently by Ley (1999). Ongoing interest in the psychophysiology of asthma, the treatment of panic and anxiety disorders, and breathing-related complaints (as occur, for example, in multiple chemical sensitivity) have stimulated more recent demonstrations of: (a) conditioned changes in total respiratory resistance in young adults using a differential conditioning procedure (Miller & Kotses 1995); (b) conditioned increases in total cycle time in an experiment involving pairing of an auditory stimulus with a hypoxic stimulus (Gallego & Perruchet 1991); and (c) conditioned increases in breathing frequency in an experiment involving pairing of an odor (ammonia) stimulus with 7.4% CO_2 inspired air (Van den Bergh et al. 1995).

The application of biofeedback to the control of asthma represents a distinct phase of research and theory on the perception and control of respiratory responses, since it serves to link past demonstrations that physiological responses can be brought under stimulus control through either classical or instrumental conditioning procedures with current efforts to affect perceived increases in the resistance to breathing (see Harver & Katkin 1998). Biofeedback training for asthma has involved both direct and indirect attempts to alter lung function through instrumental, or operant, procedures (Kotses 1998; Kotses & Glaus 1981). In direct approaches, feedback is provided to improve a specific measure of lung function. The effectiveness of feedback – based on either forced expiratory volume in one second (FEV_1) or peak expiratory flow rate (PEFR) – is inconclusive because the studies performed to date have not provided evidence that lung function was reliably altered by a biofeedback treatment. On the other hand, feedback based on total respiratory resistance (R_{TOT}) has provided evidence of conditioned R_{TOT} responding in asthmatics (Janson-Bjerklie & Clarke 1982; Kotses & Glaus 1981; Mass, Dahme, & Richter 1993). In indirect approaches, training is provided to improve lung function by reducing levels of skeletal muscle tension. The control of asthma obtained through general relaxation is not enhanced by the addition of biofeedback training for general relaxation, but specific reductions in facial muscle tension lead to improvements in lung function and to better attitudes toward asthma (Kotses 1998; Kotses & Glaus 1981).

Social Context

Compared with other response systems, little systematic work has isolated the recurrent issues relevant to the conduct of respiration research. Similarly, the singular contributions of respiration for understanding psychological processes remain largely ill-defined. On the other hand, the perceived value of respiration for health and behavior is evident.

MEASUREMENT ISSUES IN RESPIRATORY PSYCHOPHYSIOLOGY

Two variables influence respiratory recordings: apparatus and instructions. Golla and Antonovich (1929) observed that "any attempt to breathe through an open mouthpiece or mask, that is to say a piece of apparatus which centres the subject's attention on his breathing, invariably gives rise to an abnormal type of respiration." Although precise measures of breath-to-breath variations in ventilation are enabled when subjects breathe on a mouthpiece with a noseclip in place, breathing to and from a spirometer or pneumotachograph induces increases in tidal volume, decreases in breathing frequency, and unpredictable changes in ventilation as compared with breathing monitored with alternative and less "invasive" procedures (Askanazi et al. 1980; Gilbert et al. 1972; Maxwell, Cover, & Hughes 1985).

Instructions to subjects reliably affect respiratory function, especially when the instructions establish expectancies created by experimenter suggestions. Faulkner (1941) reported narrowing of the right main bronchus to unpleasant suggestions and widening of the bronchus to pleasant suggestions in a man who had developed difficulty in swallowing subsequent to a financial strain. A series of inhalation studies have subsequently been devoted to the so-called suggestion effect (for a review see Kotses 1998). In these studies, research participants were told to expect either bronchodilation or bronchoconstriction following inhalation of aerosolized solutions containing either allergens or neutral substances. In some studies, either bronchodilating or bronchoconstricting agents were administered along with suggestions that were either consistent with or opposite to their intended physiological effects. In general, improvement in respiratory function followed suggestions of bronchodilation, and deterioration in respiratory function followed suggestions of bronchoconstriction. Effects of suggestion on respiratory function are not limited to patients with lung disease; suggestion effects have also been observed in healthy adults (Kotses et al. 1987a). Kotses and colleagues (Kotses, Hindi-Alexander, & Creer 1989) argued that the negative effects of suggestion derived from *anticipation* of the administration of the substance (i.e., threat of aversive stimulation) and not from the administration itself. More recently, experimenter expectancy has been shown to act jointly with instructions to subjects to increase airflow resistance in response to suggestion (Wigal et al. 1997).

A final set of observations related to the effects of instructions on respiration serves to emphasize the interactions between the voluntary and involuntary nature of respiratory control that have affected enthusiasm for respiration research in psychology: instructions to subjects to "breathe normally" oftentimes yield breathing patterns that are arrhythmic and irregular, appearing practiced or otherwise unnatural!

PSYCHOLOGICAL PROCESSES AND BREATHING

For nearly a century, investigation of the relationship between psychological processes and respiration has conformed mostly to a traditional psychophysiological model: subjects are presented affective stimuli or are asked to perform a behavioral task, and respiratory responses are recorded during the course of these manipulations to determine effects of psychological quantities on breathing. It is likely that greater value has not been ascribed to the study of respiration in psychophysiological research in part because the voluntary nature of breathing is presumed to mask the value of respiration as a metric of either central or autonomic nervous system processes. However, areas of emerging convergence between behavioral and biomedical researchers, including recent respiratory psychophysiological research (Cherniack 1996; Oku et al. 1993; Plassman, Lansing, & Foti 1987; Shea & Guz 1992; Wientjes, Grossman, & Gaillard 1998), demonstrate that "behaviorally-controlled processes in higher brain centers play a much more significant role in the regulation of breathing than previously suspected" (Wientjes & Grossman 1998).

Emotion. Perhaps the most long-standing interest in respiration for psychologists relates to the study of emotion and of affective processes (Boiten 1998; Boiten et al. 1994). Feleky (1916) was able to discriminate among the list of primary emotions advocated by McDougall by using the ratio of inspiratory times to expiratory times (the I : E ratio), and irregularities in the breathing pattern have been associated with attempts at deception at least since the investigation of a series of thefts in a women's dormitory (Winter 1936). Dudley and colleagues (1969) examined breathing during emotional states such as anger in normal subjects and found that breathing rate increased and depth of inspiration decreased compared with baseline levels. Following periods of rapid breathing, subjects took long inspirations followed by long expirations. Similar "sighs" were often observed when subjects were instructed to relax. Changes in respiration are readily apparent during laughter (Svebak 1975), and changes in respiration are prominent in states of arousal. In quoting Darwin, Dudley et al. (1969, p. 87) recalled that "Men during numberless generations have endeavored to escape from their enemies or danger by headlong flight, or by violent struggling with them; and such great exertions will have caused the heart to beat rapidly, the breathing to be hurried, the chest to heave, and the nostrils to be dilated."

The capacity of music to affect the ventilatory rhythm derives, in part, from its affective qualities. Haas, Distenfeld, and Axen (1986), for example, demonstrated that rhythmic, melodious music induced rhythmic respiratory oscillations whereas dissonant music did not. Such observations are similar to other forms of entrainment and, in a curious way, to reports of the use of rhythmic music in nonindustrialized tribes to drive respiratory patterns in religious ceremonies. Lyon (1994) reviewed several reports wherein chanting and music were used to produce over-breathing and, finally, trancelike states during ceremonial dancing. !Kung bushmen, for instance, use overbreathing to "transform consciousness," deemed necessary for healing to occur. The breathing pattern of the dancers involves rapid and deep inhalations followed by long exhalations. Such a pattern is comparable to the one exploited by neurologists to evoke paroxysmal EEG activity in individuals thought to suffer seizure disorders, suggesting that more than autonomic arousal may account for the psychological phenomena experienced during overbreathing.

Stress, Anxiety, and Hyperventilation. The anticipation or application of aversive events, including mental arithmetic, results in patterns of respiratory activation typical of a broad range of autonomic nervous system and motor responses; these include increases in breathing frequency, increases in ventilation, and increases in total respiratory resistance (Bechbache et al. 1979; Cohen et al. 1975; Kotses, Westlund, & Creer 1987b; Mador & Tobin 1991; Rigg et al. 1977; Shea 1996; Suess et al. 1980). Variations in stress-related respiratory responses are associated with stress-related cardiovascular responses (Grossman 1983).

The effects of anxiety on breathing are well known (Barlow 1988; Bass & Gardner 1985; Bechbache et al. 1979; Christie 1935; Suess et al. 1980; Timmons & Ley 1994) and were described at the turn of the century by Freud (1894/1962). Christie (1935) observed that anxious patients complained of an "inability to get enough air into the lungs" and "a sense of oppression or suffocation." These subjective experiences were consistent with the behavioral manifestations of sighing and atypical respirations common in anxious patients.

Anxiety is frequently linked to hyperventilation and hyperventilation syndrome and to panic and panic disorder. Hyperventilation is a physiologic state and refers to breathing that is in excess of metabolic requirements (Gardner 1994). Because ventilation remains high in relation to the rate of CO_2 production, hyperventilation results in reduced levels of P_{CO_2} (i.e., in hypocapnia). Hyperventilation can occur in the absence of anxiety, but anxiety can exacerbate the hyperventilation (Bass & Gardner 1985). Bass (1997) reported that 136 articles on "hyperventilation syndrome" were published since 1966, but called into question the validity of the disorder. On the other hand, he concluded that hyperventilation was not an unimportant source of symptoms evident in a variety of cardiopulmonary disorders.

The perception of ambiguous and unpleasant sensations serves to exacerbate the symptoms evident in panic disorder. Of agoraphobic patients, for example, 61% complained of hyperventilation symptoms and 80% of those subjects said that the fear of an attack led them to avoid social situations (Garssen, van Weendeendaal, & Bloemink 1983). Most authors agree that, in panic, some precipitating event leads to increased stress and a variety of physiological reactions, including increased breathing. Individuals sensitive to their breathing continue to become concerned about their physiological state and, in a classic feedforward loop, exhibit further hyperventilation and an array of symptoms including shortness of breath, dizziness, chest tightness, and chest pain. The event itself becomes anxiety-provoking, and individuals become fearful of repeating the incident, effectively making the next event seem more stressful and thereby continuing the feedforward nature of the cascade.

Attention, Wakefulness, and Control of Breathing. Flexman, Demaree, and Simpson (1974) observed higher detection rates to visual stimuli in a signal detection task presented during expiration as compared with those presented during inspiration; they hypothesized that inspiration interfered with attentional processes. In the same year, Beh and Nix-James (1974) observed that reaction times in an auditory task were longer for stimuli presented during expiration as compared with those presented during inspiration; these researchers hypothesized that a readiness to respond was enhanced during the more active phase of breathing. Subsequently, Gallego and colleagues (Gallego, Perruchet, & Camus 1991) assessed more fully the attentional control of breathing by comparing reaction times to stimuli presented during inspiration or expiration and with either spontaneous or controlled breathing. No differences in reaction times were observed for stimuli delivered during either inspiration or expiration when subjects adopted a spontaneous pattern of breathing. On the other hand, reaction times were significantly increased during periods of controlled breathing (i.e., when attentional resources were compromised) as opposed to those obtained during spontaneous breathing.

Wakefulness, sleep, and other states (e.g., meditation) differentially affect the control of breathing (Wallace, Benson, & Wilson 1971). We noted previously that current models of ventilatory control emphasize a state-dependent input for breathing (Pack & Gottschalk 1993). State-dependent effects vary not only as a function of wakefulness and sleep (Pack et al. 1992) but also as a function of environmental demands. For example, reliable increases in breathing frequency and in ventilation are observed in subjects when they are seated quietly with their eyes open as compared to when they are seated quietly with their eyes closed (Asmussen 1977; Shea et al. 1987). Similarly, reliable increases in breathing frequency and ventilation are observed in subjects when seated quietly and listening to a story compared to when they are seated in a quiet room (Shea et al. 1987). Relatedly, subjects hyperventilate – without awareness – when imagining exercise (Gallego et al. 1996). Gallego et al. (1996) hypothesized that the automatic increase in breathing frequency that accompanied imagined exercise may reflect the contribution of higher nervous centers to exercise hyperpnea.

APPLICATIONS

Respiration, Stress, and Fitness

Reductions in autonomic nervous system responses to laboratory stressors are evident in subjects who adopt a slow (8 breaths/min) respiratory rate (Harris et al. 1976; McCaul, Solomon, & Holmes 1979). The purported value of relaxation training for reducing stress and anxiety is well appreciated, and many therapies emphasize various forms of breathing "retraining" in order to augment benefits rising from reductions in somatomotor activity (Fried 1993; Timmons & Ley 1994). On the other hand, controlled investigations that demonstrate the value of breathing retraining for treatment of panic, hyperventilation, and other respiratory disorders – alone or in combination with other relaxation or cognitive practices – are largely absent (see Barlow 1988; Gallego 1998).

Unlike the limited research devoted to breathing pattern training and stress, a developing literature relates to interactions among oxygen consumption, stress, and fitness. To perform exercise, the increased transport of oxygen to the exercising muscles must be rapid, adequate, and sustained (Wasserman 1981). Accordingly, heart rate and cardiac output increase predictably, in healthy subjects, in proportion to metabolic demand. Cardiovascular activity that exceeds physiologic requirements is "metabolically inappropriate" (Obrist 1981). The dissociation between cardiac and metabolic parameters is evident in both men and women engaged in behaviorally challenging tasks (Stoney, Langer, & Gelling 1986; Turner & Carroll 1985) and is mediated primarily by β-adrenergic influences (see e.g. Langer et al. 1985b). Fit individuals – those who achieve high levels of maximum oxygen consumption during aerobic exercise – evidence smaller sympathetic effects on both the myocardium and blood vessels during laboratory stress than do less fit individuals (Crews & Landers 1987; van Doorren & de Gues 1989). Even so, the value of aerobic training for reducing psychophysiological stress reactions – as well as the mechanism that could serve to mitigate the inappropriate response to acute stress in fit individuals – remains to be elucidated (see de Geus et al. 1990; McCubbin et al. 1992; Steptoe et al. 1990).

Respiratory Sensations and Dyspnea

Dyspnea is a term used to characterize a subjective experience of "breathlessness" or breathing discomfort that is marked by qualitatively distinct sensations that vary in intensity. The experience derives from (and has implications for) physiological, psychological, and social interactions (see Harver & Mahler 1998a). The conditions in which the symptom of dyspnea is a primary complaint are many and varied, but the singular feature of these circumstances has yet to be elucidated. Patients with either cardiac or pulmonary disease – including those with congestive heart failure, anemia, chest trauma, airway disease, fibrosis of

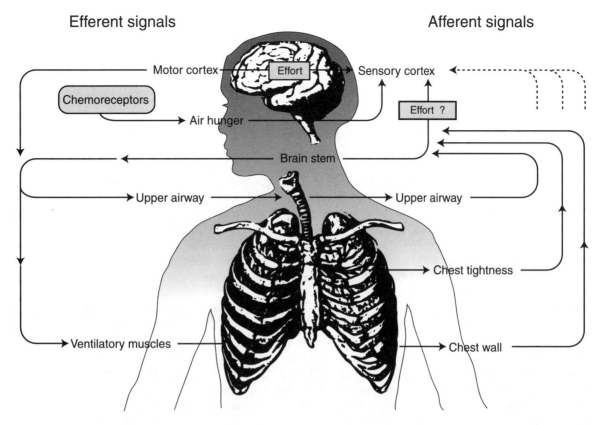

Efferent signals   Afferent signals

Figure 9. Efferent and afferent signals that contribute to the sensation of dyspnea. The sense of effort is believed to arise from collateral motor commands to the ventilatory muscles. Chest tightness probably results from stimulation of vagal irritant receptors. Although afferent information likely passes through the brainstem before reaching the sensory cortex, the dashed lines indicate uncertainty about whether some afferents bypass the brainstem and project directly to the sensory cortex. Redrawn with permission from Manning & Schwartzstein, "Pathophysiology of dyspnea," *New England Journal of Medicine*, vol. 333, pp. 1547–53. Copyright © 1995 Massachusetts Medical Society. All rights reserved.

the lungs, gas exchange abnormalities, pulmonary circulation defects, pulmonary edema, and metabolic acidosis – complain of either acute or chronic episodes of dyspnea. Dyspnea occurs in many other conditions as well, including neuromuscular disorders, skeletal deformities, panic, hyperthyroidism, obesity, vigorous exercise, and pregnancy (Mahler 1998).

An area of consensus among clinicians and researchers is that dyspnea is a sensory experience, likely perceived in accordance with the same processes implicated in the perception of external stimuli (Tobin 1990). An awareness of a sensation – of ventilatory increases, ventilatory difficulty, or ventilatory need (Campbell & Guz 1981) – permeates all definitions of dyspnea (Harver & Mahler 1990). Although new insight to afferent nerve fibers that mediate sensory experience is encouraging (Shea et al. 1996), explaining how disturbances in physiological processes give rise to unpleasant perceptual experiences, or combine in unpleasant sensations linked to dyspnea, remains a formidable challenge (Manning & Schwartzstein 1995). Efferent and afferent signals hypothesized to play a role in the genesis of dyspnea are summarized in Figure 9.

Load perception studies, which evolved from load compensation studies, serve as a bridge between physiological research programs and those related to the quantification of the relationship between the perceived magnitude of respiratory sensations and the physical intensity of respiratory stimuli (Harver & Mahler 1998b). Over 125 papers published since 1962 have examined psychophysical properties of respiratory sensations, and several recent chapters and reviews have surveyed various numbers of these studies (Davenport & Revelette 1996; Harver & Mahler 1990, 1998b; Lansing & Banzett 1996; Zechman & Wiley 1986).

Breathing and the Cortex

Event-Related Potentials (ERPs) to Added Loads. A potentially powerful method for enhancing understanding of sensory-perceptual correlates of respiratory sensations involves analysis of central respiratory-related signals. For decades, relationships between sensory stimulation and perceptual responses have been elucidated with ERPs. Application of such noninvasive neurophysiological techniques to respiratory sensations have been concerned mostly with responses to respiratory occlusion (i.e., complete obstruction of the airway). Davenport and colleagues (1986) first recorded ERPs to inspiratory occlusion and found that potentials elicited to occlusions in a passive attention paradigm were not evident on unoccluded inspirations. Subsequently, Revelette and Davenport (1990) observed that mid-inspiratory occlusions resulted in potentials that were shorter in latency and larger in amplitude compared with those resulting from occlusions presented at the onset of inspiration. More recently, Davenport, Colrain, and Hill (1996) reported bilateral responses to inspiratory occlusions in children and speculated that such activity could arise from one of several populations of respiratory mechanoreceptors.

Harver and colleagues (1995) first examined P300 in response to respiratory occlusion in young (20–30 years) and old (50–70 years) healthy subjects, in both Ignore and Attend conditions. The P300 was shorter in latency and larger in amplitude in the Attend condition than in the Ignore condition, and P300 latencies were longer and amplitudes were smaller in older subjects than in younger subjects. The relationships between P300 latency to both inspiratory and expiratory occlusion and age – recorded from these and other subjects, including patients with obstructive lung disease – are presented in Figure 10. In separate multiple regression analyses using age and measures of lung function as predictors, both age and lung function emerged as significant and independent predictors of P300 latency to inspiratory (multiple $R = 0.52$) and expiratory (multiple $R = 0.53$) occlusion.

In two experiments, Bloch-Salisbury and colleagues recorded ERPs to resistive loads presented briefly (~ 200 msec) at the onset of inspiration. In one study (Bloch-Salisbury, Harver, & Squires 1998), both the latency and amplitude of the ERP components varied systematically as a function of stimulus magnitude (in a manner comparable to that observed in ERP paradigms using auditory and visual stimuli) and were related, in part, to behavioral judgments obtained during the stimulus periods. In the other study (Bloch-Salisbury & Harver 1994), ERPs to each of two levels of resistive and elastic loads (equated for subjective magnitude) were examined. Subjects detected equivalent numbers of loads but classified loads correctly as either "resistive" or "elastic" at chance levels. The ERP latencies, however, were sensitive to load type even though the added loads were not distinguishable subjectively: latencies for both N2 and P300 were shorter to resistive than to elastic loads, a finding consistent with perceptual processing of mechanical dynamics (Davenport & Revelette 1996).

Positron Emission Tomography (PET). A series of PET investigations has enabled identification of brain areas involved in the execution of purposeful breathing (Colebatch et al. 1991; Fink et al. 1996; Ramsay et al. 1993). Colebatch et al. (1991) observed significant increases in regional cerebral blood flow (rCBF) in five brain areas during production of a specific inspiratory volume and breathing frequency: right premotor cortex, supplementary motor area, the cerebellum, and both right and left superolateral primary motor cortices. These brain areas had previously been shown to be activated with simple, repetitive arm and hand movements. Volitional expiration induced increases in rCBF in areas that overlapped (but were more extensive than) those for volitional inspiration (Ramsay et al. 1993). Fink et al. (1996) examined rCBF changes in subjects to three levels of added inspiratory resistance (i.e., to three levels of increasing respiratory muscle force). Breathing against external inspiratory loads revealed significant neuronal activations, as before, in superolateral motor cortex and in supplementary and premotor areas (i.e., in structures involved in motor preparation and programming). Additional force-related activations were evident in inferolateral sensorimotor cortex (facial and upper airway muscles?), in medial parietal cortex (task-related changes in sensory input?), and in dorsal prefrontal cortex (volition?).

Nasal Flow, Odors, and the Cortex. The subject of breathing's relationship to olfaction is often neglected, probably because most humans neglect the abundance of olfactory information in the environment. It has recently been suggested (Lorig 1999) that neglect of the ambient olfactory environment is the result of the evolution of language among humans. In spite of this inattention to odors, there is abundant evidence that humans constantly monitor the olfactory environment and that odor information is important to a variety of functions. For instance, McClintock's early findings of odor-induced menstrual synchrony (McClintock 1971) have been supported (Preti et al. 1986) and extended to include synchrony induced by male odors (Stern & McClintock 1998). Lorig and associates (1991) found that concentrations of the odor galaxolide, even though below detection thresholds, altered EEG and visual search performance as well as P200 and P300 in an auditory "oddball" task. Even when recognized in the environment, odors convey far more information than is apparent. In one study, several different odorants were administered to subjects as EEG were recorded (Lorig & Schwartz 1988). The odors, while perceptually indistinguishable, produced marked EEG differences. These findings indicated that, at a neurophysiological level, the odors were processed quite differently and (presumably) conveyed different information.

Respiration is, of course, necessary for normal olfaction to occur. A number of investigators, in order to reduce variability in the stimulus, have presented olfactory stimuli in a manner that does not require active inhalation (see Kobal & Hummel 1991). Subjects certainly report olfactory sensations but, as Laing (1983) points out, natural sniffing produces the best identification and lowest olfactory thresholds. The reasons for natural sniffing's superiority may not be entirely mechanical. Freeman and Schneider (1982) noted that new patterns of electrical activity on the olfactory bulbs of rabbits were generated as a function of

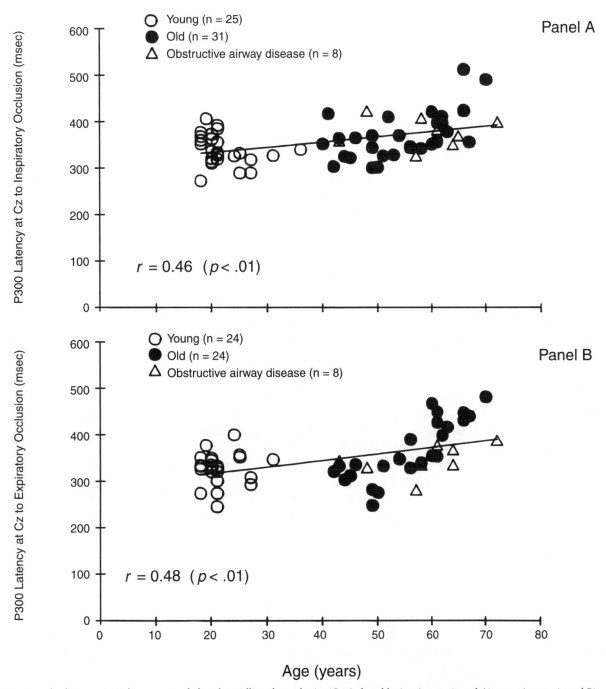

Figure 10. Scatter plot between P300 latency recorded at the midline electrode site (Cz) induced by inspiratory (panel A) or expiratory (panel B) occlusion of the airway, and age. As in other sensory modalities, there is a systematic increase in the latency of the endogenous event-related potential to added loads with increasing age. From Harver & Mahler (1998), "Perception of increased resistance to breathing," in Kotses & Harver (Eds.), *Self-Management of Asthma*, pp. 147–93. Reprinted courtesy of Marcel Dekker Inc.

inspirations in the absence of odors. These findings suggest the possibility that, in addition to providing the ventilation required to pull odor molecules over the olfactory mucosa, inspiratory patterns may prime, poll, or cue neural regions related to smell. Lorig and colleagues (1996) tested this hypothesis using human chemosensory event-related potentials (CSERP). They presented odors (butanol) in and out of phase with respiration and found different patterns

of CSERPs when subjects were inhaling versus exhaling. Such findings strongly suggest that nasal inhalations lead to altered processing of olfactory information. These findings were recently substantiated by Sobel et al. (1998) using functional magnetic resonance imaging. Their studies indicated that nasal inhalations (sniffing) produced activity in piriform cortex and medial and posterior orbito-frontal areas. Adding odorant to the air led to activity in lateral and anterior orbito-frontal gyri of the frontal lobe. These data make it clear that respiration, in addition to its mechanical constituents, cues or primes neural resources for olfaction and possibly other types of processes.

Inferential Context

EXPERIMENTAL TECHNIQUE: QUANTIFICATION OF RESPIRATION

An intimidating number of respiratory responses can be recorded from willing subjects, including not only those related to variations in the pattern of the individual breathing cycle but also those related to gas exchange. Our efforts to review those measures of long-standing interest to behavioral researchers are organized in terms of the primary processes of respiration reviewed earlier: pulmonary ventilation, gas exchange, and regulation.

Pulmonary Ventilation. Behavioral scientists have generally adopted a casual view of respiratory measurement. Woodworth and Schlosberg (1956), for example, declared that since breathing "is a massive response, there is little trouble in recording it"; they outlined the variety of "gasometers" and "modern artificial respirators" available to measure volume-related changes in breathing. However, it has been distension of the abdomen or expansion of the thorax that have been employed most frequently in investigations of respiratory activity in psychological research. Recordings of chest wall movement are generally noninvasive and reliable, and they provide information about respiratory rate and breathing amplitude. Such recordings are accomplished through the use of low-cost transducers and general-purpose amplifiers.

Several types of strain gauges have been used to quantify changes in breathing in psychological research. Most techniques involve beltlike devices that are strapped around the abdomen, the thorax, or both body segments (Cromwell et al. 1973; Stern et al. 1980). Typically, the output of the strain gauge is directed to a Wheatstone bridge to produce a voltage that is proportional to the variations in resistance that accompany each inspiration (inflation) and expiration (deflation). Few guidelines direct the appropriate placement of these transducer systems, but investigators generally position transducers to maximize their sensitivity. Mercury strain gauges consist of thin tubing containing mercury (Shapiro & Cohen 1965). At each end of the tube, electrodes allow recording of the changes in resistance that accompany changes in the diameter of the tubing. During inspiration, for example, expansion of the chest wall stretches the tubing and increases the resistance of the conducting medium. Because these transducers must be stretched to achieve adequate sensitivity, care is warranted to minimize the risk of rupture of the tubing and leakage of the mercury. Mechanical strain gauges do not share this

risk but may instead reduce chest wall compliance or serve to increase chest wall recoil.

Aneroid bellows, or air-pressure pneumographs, are also commonly used in psychological research. The bellows are connected to a band that is fitted around the abdomen or thorax. Expansion of the chest stretches the bellows and reduces the pressure within the tubing that can, in turn, be recorded readily with a pressure transducer. Although this method can be effective, researchers must attend to possible leaks in the system. Because most bellows are constructed of rubber, aging and oxidation may result in small breaks that serve to compromise the accuracy of the recordings. Piezoelectric transducers are less likely to suffer age-related deteriorations and serve as yet another option for assessing breathing. A piezoelectric crystal is fastened to an elastic strap. Stretching of the strap produces mechanical deformation of the piezo, and the voltage consequently produced by the crystal can be recorded by general purpose DC amplifiers or AC amplifiers with long time constants. A "proximity" transducer suitable for measuring breathing rate has also been described (Casali, Wierwille, & Cordes 1983).

Impedance pneumography involves the placement of electrodes on the thorax and serves as an alternative to the belts and tubes for measuring chest wall movement. Impedance pneumography is based on the functional relationship between transthoracic impedance and the volume of air within the thorax (Stein & Luparello 1967). The movement of air in and out of the lungs results in cyclic variations in the impedance of the chest wall to an applied alternating electrical current; impedance increases, for example, during chest wall expansion (Baker, Geddes, & Hoff 1965).

Strain gauges and similar recording devices can provide estimates of simple time-dependent respiratory parameters (e.g., breathing frequency, T_I and T_E) but do not provide volume-dependent respiratory parameters (e.g., V_T, V_T/T_I, or ventilation). Moreover, the independent contributions of thoracic and abdominal compartments to total respiratory volume are well recognized (Konno & Mead 1967), so recordings of only thoracic or only abdominal changes do not provide adequate estimates of relative breathing amplitude. These same caveats apply – and perhaps even more so – to breathing pattern records obtained with a variety of devices that may be attached near the mouth or nose and are sensitive to the difference in temperature between inspired and expired air. Thermistors are small and often bulb-shaped probes that change their resistive characteristics depending upon temperature fluctuations. Like any resistive device, these probes depend upon a constant voltage and use an amplifier to measure the drop in voltage caused by changes in resistance. Thermocouples are voltage-generating probes that increase or decrease their output as a function of temperature. These devices require only an amplifier, since they create their own voltage. Both thermistors and thermocouples have the same advantages and disadvantages. For example, both types of probes are easily placed on the face, are durable and reliable, and are easily interfaced to most amplifiers available in a psychophysiology laboratory. On the other hand, both types of probes often respond slowly to changes in absolute temperature and depend, moreover, on the cooperation of subjects to breathe continuously through either their mouth only or nose only.

The extended dependence on movement and temperature recordings of respiration in psychological research is evident in sporadic research, conducted over the course of about five decades, on the effects of auditory stimulation on respiration (see Harver & Kotses 1987). For example, estimates of changes in breathing amplitude and respiratory rate to auditory signals have been derived from recordings obtained with impedance pneumography (McCollum, Burch, & Roessler 1969), mercury strain gauges (Poole, Goetzinger, & Rousey 1966; Rousey & Reitz 1967), pneumographs (Davis, Buchwald, & Frankman 1955; Gautier 1972; Skaggs 1926), and thermistors (Steinschneider 1968). Perhaps more striking than the differences between the recording procedures employed in the various studies was the virtually nonoverlapping scoring procedures used to define variations in breathing amplitude and breathing rate in these investigations.

An alternative recording device, the respiratory inductive plethysmograph (Cohn et al. 1982), is based on chest wall movement and enables accurate and reliable measurement of both time-dependent and volume-dependent respiratory responses. The respiratory inductive plethysmograph was developed to provide noninvasive monitoring of ventilation in research, clinical, and ambulatory settings. The device consists of two coils, which are sewn into elastic bands encircling the rib cage (RC) and abdomen (ABD) and are connected to an oscillator module (see Tobin et al. 1983b). Changes in cross-sectional area of the RC and ABD compartments alter the self-inductance of the coils and the frequency of their oscillations, which, after appropriate calibration with spirometry (SP), reflect tidal volume. The device is calibrated by using values for RC, ABD, and SP volumes in the following equation:

$$RC/SP + ABD/SP = 1. \qquad (4)$$

Unfortunately, very few behavioral researchers have adopted the respiratory impedance plethysmograph as their preferred method for recording chest wall movement.

Accurate calibration of the respiratory impedance plethysmograph requires a spirometer, which provides an accurate and direct measurement of the volume (and rate) of air flow to and from the lungs. Spirometry is most closely associated with the measurement of respiratory volumes and capacities and the detection of abnormal lung function in clinical settings. Many texts, manuals, and chapters have described the assortment of tests and measures that are used to document both normal and abnormal lung function (e.g. Kaufman & Schneiderman 1986; Stein & Luparello 1967; West 1982).

Both discrete and continuous measures of airway resistance are of increasing interest to respiratory psychophysiologists (see Ritz, Wiens, & Dahme 1998). Because airway resistance is defined as the pressure difference between the alveoli and the mouth divided by flow, direct assessment of airway resistance requires more elaborate solutions than those needed for recording chest wall movement. For instance, alveolar pressure can be measured only indirectly. Such measurements are normally obtained through the technique of whole body plethysmography, first described by DuBois, Botelho, and Comroe (1956). A subject sits in an airtight booth and pants against a flowmeter while flow, box pressure, and airway opening pressure are measured. The process is then repeated with the flowmeter occluded (i.e., when no air is flowing) so that $P_{MO} = P_{ALV}$. Finally, P_{MO} is plotted against the simultaneous changes in flow obtained during the first maneuver and against box pressure obtained during the second maneuver, and P_{ALV} is deduced through application of Boyle's law (Antonisen 1986; Comroe 1974). An older method for measuring airway resistance involves rapid interruptions of airflow (10/sec) during normal breathing by a shutter placed in a mouthpiece. The pressure measured at the airway opening immediately after an occlusion is assumed to provide a reasonable estimate of alveolar pressure just before occlusion (Antonisen 1986; Jackson, Milhorn, & Norman 1974). Another method is to connect the individual to a source of forced air oscillations, such as a loudspeaker, and apply low-frequency pulses to the airway. Respiratory resistance can be determined by relating the extremes of flow and corresponding pressure variations produced by the oscillations (Fisher, DuBois, & Hyde 1968; Goldman et al. 1970; Lándsér et al. 1976; West 1982).

Gas Exchange. We reviewed earlier a developing literature related to interactions among oxygen consumption, stress, and fitness. In most studies, gas exchange (oxygen consumption and carbon dioxide production) was recorded with a metabolic "cart" common to exercise physiology laboratories. It is unlikely that individual psychophysiologists would be independently able to afford either the cost or maintenance of these units. On the other hand, both oxygen and carbon dioxide analyzers can be purchased separately and configured by the experimenter to test a variety of research questions (see e.g. Langer et al. 1985a).

In subjects with normal lungs, arterial P_{CO_2} is very close to end-tidal P_{CO_2}, which can be measured by continuous sampling from the nostril or mouth with a capnogram, a unit dedicated to the analysis of breath-to-breath variations in the rate of CO_2 production (Gardner 1994). Fried (1993) described in detail the ongoing clinical interest in (and broad-based applications of) capnometry in the assessment and treatment of breathing-related disorders. An especially novel approach to respiratory CO_2 gas analysis is the use of a transdermal probe (for a review see Wientjes 1992). These probes heat the skin and sense CO_2 levels in the capillary beds. Transcutaneous P_{CO_2} measures are valid but tend to overestimate the partial pressure of CO_2 in arterial blood. In addition, the response time of the sensor to a change in arterial P_{CO_2} is excessive, ranging between 30 sec and 300 sec (Wientjes 1992). Accordingly, the value of transcutaneous monitoring of P_{CO_2} in the laboratory remains to be determined.

Respiratory Neural Output. The output of the respiratory centers appears first as a neural signal, then as electromyographic (EMG) activity, then as muscle tension, then as pressure, and then finally as gas flow and ventilation (Milic-Emili, Grassino, & Whitelaw 1981). Each stage of activity requires a different device for its measurement. The measurement of respiratory EMG activity with surface electrodes is perhaps the most familiar stage in the analysis of respiratory system output for psychophysiologists. Pauly (1957) studied the EMG activity of the diaphragm and intercostal muscles during breathing by placing EMG surface electrodes on the chest wall. He concluded that EMG was a reliable and useful technique for measurement of some aspects of breathing. For instance, respiratory rate and phase were readily quantifiable. Other respiratory parameters such as volume were more difficult to interpret, and artifacts were especially problematic using this approach. Because of the proximity to the heart, electrocardiographic (ECG) artifacts were especially large. Additionally, rotational movements of the torso could also produce increased EMG even though these movements are less likely to produce artifacts in strain gauge–type recordings. More recently, Lansing and Savelle (1989) characterized the distribution of diaphragm potentials over the chest surface, and Whitelaw and Feroah (1989) characterized the pattern of inspiratory intercostal muscle activity in humans.

Diaphragmatic EMG activity can be recorded directly from electrodes that are positioned at the junction of the esophagus and stomach with gastroesophageal catheters (Lourenco & Mueller 1967). Several authors have described the development and implementation of single catheters designed for the simultaneous measurement of transdiaphragmatic pressures and diaphragmatic EMG (Önal et al. 1981). Direct recordings of diaphragmatic EMG can be used to dissociate neural from mechanical adjustments to added resistive and elastic loads (Kobylarz & Daubenspeck 1992). Electrodes have also been designed for intraoral surface recordings of genioglossus muscle activity (Doble et al. 1985).

Facial muscles are also associated with breathing. When the mouth is closed, the nares open wider (dilator nares) during inhalations. Sasaki and Mann (1976) placed concentric needle electrodes in the *alae nasi* and recorded electrical activity during mouth-closed breathing; they found that this form of EMG measurement could also be a reliable indicator of rate and phase of breathing.

EXPERIMENTAL DESIGN: STUDIES OF RESPIRATION

Few standards have evolved to enable behaviorally oriented respiration research. For example, there are no publication guidelines available to promote "best practices" in respiratory psychophysiology. Accordingly, we elect to offer three simple recommendations to those individuals inclined to consider studies of respiration.

First, researchers who include respiration as a dependent measure of interest in their studies should not be reluctant to develop as great an understanding of the physiology of the system as possible. Behavioral scientists can ill afford to ignore important developments in respiratory physiology (see also Wientjes 1992; Wientjes et al. 1998). Second, researchers should be fully sensitive to the limits of their instrumentation practices and minimize, whenever possible, the use of unconventional scoring algorithms.

Finally, procedures should be designed to accommodate the inherent oscillations of the respiratory rhythm and the rather long period of the cycle. The entire cycle tends to last about five seconds, and this could interfere with measurements that are collected in sequential blocks of trials. Since one respiratory phase follows the other, the assumption of independence may be compromised if successive blocks of trials follow each other immediately. Thus, if one block ended with an inspiration, the next must begin with expiration. If there is a short delay between successive blocks then this restriction is eliminated. It is also possible to use respiration to segment the trials of an experiment. For instance, under some conditions it may be useful to administer stimuli only during the inspiratory phase of the respiratory cycle (Lorig et al. 1996). In those cases, the investigator may randomly administer stimuli and, off-line, segment the administrations into inspired and expired categories. If this approach is taken, there is little control over the portion of the inhalation or exhalation in which the stimulus is delivered. A better approach may be recording respiration to determine the cycle and then delivering stimuli when the desired respiratory event occurs.

Epilogue

We have attempted to review the state of respiration in psychophysiological research. Wientjes & Grossman's (1998) claim – that respiratory psychophysiology has become more a subdiscipline of physiology than of psychology – is echoed in our efforts. For example, our emphasis on several lines of respiratory research adopting psychological principles such as learning and perception, including those related to the individuality of the breathing pattern and to the optimization of the breathing pattern, have been generated mostly by respiratory physiologists and pulmonary physicians. Behavioral scientists, in turn, have yet to adopt the assessment strategies that embrace important aspects of respiratory behavior (Wientjes et al. 1998).

UNANSWERED QUESTIONS

The duplicity of respiratory control is evident in the ongoing history of research on breathing and behavior, but no consistent value has been attributed to voluntary control of breathing in psychophysiology. Concerted efforts are needed to determine the value of understanding the voluntary and involuntary regulation of the breathing pattern, and such efforts may extend to other respiratory parameters in addition to the mechanics of the breathing cycle. For example, high resting end-tidal CO_2 levels tend to be a stable individual characteristic that is accompanied by a tendency to worry and to experience negative events (Dhokalia, Parsons, & Anderson 1998). It is likely that the perceived history of respiratory neglect (see e.g. Woodworth & Schlosberg 1956) relates, in part, to a perception that respiration does not serve as a metric of either central or autonomic nervous system processes. Ongoing efforts that serve to question such an assumption are likely to continue (Anderson, Coyle, & Haythornthwaite 1992; Wientjes & Grossman 1998).

Very little research relates to the role of modification or learning in the regulation of breathing, even though voluntary breathing can become automatic and voluntary changes in breathing can become habitual, requiring little or no attention. Results from the many dozens of load perception studies conducted by respiratory physiologists and pulmonary clinicians serve to affirm the hypothesis that ventilation is affected by behavior and may serve to reduce respiratory sensory input and minimize perceived respiratory discomfort. The idea that voluntary changes in breathing can become automatic or habitual suggests at least two important research questions:

1. What is the role of learning in the control of breathing?
2. Is there a distinction between "adaptation" (decreases in peripheral sensitivity) and "habituation" (decreases in central responsivity) to unpleasant respiratory sensory experience?

Finally, among many other unanswered questions are those that emphasize more clinically relevant concerns. For example, greater articulation is required of the relationship between airflow obstruction and alterations in blood chemistry on the one hand, and cognitive function, evoked potentials, symptom perception, and emotional behaviors on the other hand. What are the environmental effects, including variations in the quality of indoor air, on these same quantities?

FUTURE DIRECTIONS

The future of any field is difficult to predict. It is likely, however, that respiration research will continue to move out from behind the shadow of interest in the brain, the heart, and electrodermal activity. In this way, new light will shine on our understanding of the role of physiological processes in human experience.

NOTE

We thank Murray D. Altose and Harry Kotses for helpful comments provided on the manuscript.

REFERENCES

Agostoni, E. (1963). Diaphragm activity during breath holding: Factors related to its onset. *Journal of Applied Physiology, 18,* 30–6.

Alpher, V. S., Nelson, R. B., & Blanton, R. L. (1986). Effects of cognitive and psychomotor tasks on breath-holding span. *Journal of Applied Physiology, 61,* 1149–52.

Altose, M. D., & Zechman, F. W. (1986). Loaded breathing: Load compensation and respiratory sensation. *Federation Proceedings, 45,* 114–22.

Anderson, D. E., Coyle, K., & Haythornthwaite, J. A. (1992). Ambulatory monitoring of respiration: Inhibitory breathing in the natural environment. *Psychophysiology, 29,* 551–7.

Andreassi, J. L. (1980). *Psychophysiology: Human Behavior and Physiological Response.* New York: Oxford University Press.

Antonisen, N. R. (1986). Tests of mechanical function. In N. S. Cherniack & J. G. Widdicombe (Eds.), *Handbook of Physiology, Section 3: The Respiratory System,* vol. III, pp. 753–84. Bethesda, MD: American Physiological Society.

Askanazi, J., Silverberg, P. A., Foster, R. J., Hyman, A. I., Milic-Emili, J., & Kinney, J. M. (1980). Effects of respiratory apparatus on breathing pattern. *Journal of Applied Physiology, 48,* 577–80.

Asmussen, E. (1977). Regulation of respiration: The black box. *Acta Physiologia Scandinavica, 99,* 85–90.

Badia, P., Harsh, J., & Balkin, T. (1986). Behavioral control over sleeping respiration in normals for ten consecutive nights. *Psychophysiology, 23,* 409–11.

Badia, P., Harsh, J., Balkin, T., Cantrell, P., Klempert, A., O'Rourke, D., & Schoen, L. (1984). Behavioral control of respiration in sleep. *Psychophysiology, 21,* 494–500.

Baker, L. E., Geddes, L. A., & Hoff, H. E. (1965). Quantitative evaluation of impedance pneumograph in man. *American Journal of Medical Electronics, 4,* 73–7.

Barlow, D. H. (1988). *Anxiety and Its Disorders: The Nature and Treatment of Anxiety and Panic.* New York: Guilford.

Bartlett, D., Jr. (1977). Effects of Valsalva and Mueller maneuvers on breath-holding time. *Journal of Applied Physiology, 42,* 717–21.

Bass, C. (1997). Hyperventilation syndrome: A chimera? *Journal of Psychosomatic Research, 42,* 421–6.

Bass, C., & Gardner, W. (1985). Emotional influences on breathing and breathlessness. *Journal of Psychosomatic Research, 29,* 599–609.

Bechbache, R. R., Chow, H. H. K., Duffin, J., & Orsini, E. C. (1979). The effects of hypercapnia, hypoxia, exercise and anxiety on the pattern of breathing in man. *Journal of Physiology, 293,* 285–300.

Beh, H. C., & Nix-James, D. R. (1974). The relationship between respiration phase and reaction time. *Psychophysiology, 11,* 400–2.

Benchetrit, G., & Ley, R. (1995). Abstracts of papers presented at International Society for the Advancement of Respiratory Psychophysiology (ISARP). Inaugural meeting and 13th International Symposium on Respiratory Psychophysiology. *Biological Psychology, 41,* 83–102.

Benchetrit, G., Shea, S. A., Pham Dinh, T., Bodocco, S., Baconnier, P., & Guz, A. (1989). Individuality of breathing patterns in adults assessed over time. *Respiration Physiology, 75,* 199–210.

Berntson, G. G., Bigger, T., Jr., Eckberg, D. L., Grossman, P., Kaufmann, P. G., Malik, M., Nagaraja, H. N., Porges, S. W., Saul, J. P., Stone, P. H., & van der Molen, M. W. (1997). Heart rate variability: Origins, methods, and interpretive caveats. *Psychophysiology, 34,* 623–48.

Berntson, G. G., Cacioppo, J. T., & Quigley, K. S. (1993). Respiratory sinus arrhythmia: Autonomic origins, physiological mechanisms, and psychophysiological implications. *Psychophysiology, 30,* 183–96.

Blatz, W. E. (1925). The cardiac, respiratory, and electrical phenomena involved in the emotion of fear. *Journal of Experimental Psychology, 8,* 109–32.

Bloch-Salisbury, E., & Harver, A. (1994). Effects of detection and classification of resistive and elastic loads on endogenous event-related potentials. *Journal of Applied Physiology, 77,* 1246–55.

Bloch-Salisbury, E., Harver, A., & Squires, N. K. (1998). Event-related potentials to inspiratory flow-resistive loads in young adults: Stimulus magnitude effects. *Biological Psychology, 49,* 165–86.

Boiten, F. A. (1998). The effects of emotional behaviour on components of the respiratory cycle. *Biological Psychology, 49,* 29–51.

Boiten, F. A., Frijda, N. H., & Wientjes, C. J. E. (1994). Emotions and respiratory patterns: Review and critical analysis. *International Journal of Psychophysiology, 17,* 103–28.

Brener, J. (1987). Behavioural energetics: Some effects of uncertainty on the mobilization and distribution of energy. *Psychophysiology, 24,* 499–512.

Bruce, E. N. (1984). Techniques for electromyography of respiratory muscles. *Techniques on the Life Sciences: Techniques in Respiratory Physiology, P408,* 1–19.

Campbell, E. J. M., & Guz, A. (1981). Breathlessness. In T. F. Hornbein (Ed.), *Regulation of Breathing,* part 2, pp. 1181–95. New York: Marcel Dekker.

Campbell, E. J. M., & Newsom Davis, J. (1970). Respiratory sensation. In E. J. M. Campbell, E. Agostoni, & J. Newsom Davis (Eds.), *The Respiratory Muscles: Mechanics and Neural Control,* 2nd ed., pp. 291–306. Philadelphia: Saunders.

Casali, J. G., Wierwille, W. W., & Cordes, R. E. (1983). Respiratory measurement: Overview and new instrumentation. *Behavior Research Methods and Instrumentation, 15,* 401–5.

Cherniack, N. S. (1996). Respiratory sensation as a respiratory controller. In L. Adams & A. Guz (Eds.), *Respiratory Sensation,* pp. 213–30. New York: Marcel Dekker.

Cherniack, N. S., & Altose, M. D. (1981). Respiratory responses to ventilatory loading. In T. F. Hornbein (Ed.), *Regulation of Breathing,* part 2, pp. 905–64. New York: Marcel Dekker.

Cherniack, R. M. (1983). Mechanics of breathing. *Seminars in Respiratory Medicine, 4,* 171–83.

Christie, R. V. (1935). Some types of respiration in the neuroses. *Quarterly Journal of Medicine, 4,* 427–32.

Clark, F. J., & von Euler, C. (1972). On the regulation of depth and rate of breathing. *Journal of Physiology, 222,* 267–95.

Cohen, H. D., Goodenough, D. R., Witkin, H. A., Oltman, P., Gould, H., & Shulman, E. (1975). The effects of stress on components of the respiration cycle. *Psychophysiology, 12,* 377–80.

Cohn, M. A., Rao, A. S. V., Broudy, M., Birch, S., Watson, H., Atkins, N., Davis, B., Stott, F. D., & Sackner, M. A. (1982). The respiratory inductive plethysmograph: A new noninvasive monitor of respiration. *Clinical Respiratory Physiology, 18,* 643–58.

Colebatch, J. G., Adams, L., Murphy, K., Martin, A. J., Lammertsma, A. A., Tochon-Danguy, H. J., Clark, J. C., Friston, K. J., & Guz, A. (1991). Regional cerebral blood flow during volitional breathing in man. *Journal of Physiology, 443,* 91–103.

Coles, M. G. H., Donchin, E., & Porges, S. W. (Eds.) (1986). *Psychophysiology: Systems, Processes, and Applications.* New York: Guilford.

Comroe, J. H. (1974). *Physiology of Respiration,* 2nd ed. Chicago: Year Book Medical Publishers.

Crews, D. J., & Landers, D. M. (1987). A meta-analytic review of aerobic fitness and reactivity to psychosocial stressors. *Medicine and Science in Sports and Medicine, 19,* S114–S120.

Cromwell, L., Weibell, F. J., Pfeiffer, E. A., & Usselman, L. B. (1973). *Biomedical Instrumentation and Measurements.* Englewood Cliffs, NJ: Prentice-Hall.

Daubenspeck, J. A. (1981). Mechanical factors in breathing pattern regulation in humans. *Annals of Biomedical Engineering, 9,* 409–24.

Daubenspeck, J. A., & Farnham, M. W. (1982). Temporal variation in the V_T–T_I relationship in humans. *Respiration Physiology, 47,* 97–106.

Daubenspeck, J. A., & Rhodes, E. (1995). Effect of perception of mechanical loading on human respiratory pattern regulation. *Journal of Physiology, 79,* 83–93.

Davenport, P. W., Colrain, I. M., & Hill, P. (1996). Scalp topography of the short-latency components of the respiratory-related evoked potential in children. *Journal of Applied Physiology, 80,* 1785–91.

Davenport, P. W., Friedman, W. A., Thompson, F. J., & Franzen, O. (1986). Respiratory-related cortical potentials evoked by inspiratory occlusion in humans. *Journal of Applied Physiology, 60,* 1843–8.

Davenport, P. W., & Reep, R. L. (1995). Cerebral cortex and respiration. In J. A. Dempsey & A. I. Pack (Eds.), *Regulation of Breathing,* 2nd ed., pp. 365–88. New York: Marcel Dekker.

Davenport, P. W., & Revelette, W. R. (1996). Perception of respiratory mechanical events. In L. Adams & A. Guz (Eds.), *Respiratory Sensation,* pp. 101–23. New York: Marcel Dekker.

Davis, R. C., Buchwald, A. M., & Frankman, R. W. (1955). Autonomic and muscular responses and their relation to simple stimuli. *Psychological Monographs, 69.*

de Gues, E. J. C., van Doornen, L. J. P., de Visser, D. C., & Orlebeke, J. F. (1990). Existing and training induced differences in aerobic fitness: Their relationship to physiological response patterns during different types of stress. *Psychophysiology, 27,* 457–78.

Dekker, E., Pelser, H. E., & Groen, J. (1957). Conditioning as a cause of asthmatic attacks. *Journal of Psychosomatic Research, 2,* 97–108.

Dhokalia, A., Parsons, D. J., & Anderson, D. E. (1998). Resting end-tidal CO_2 association with age, gender, and personality. *Psychosomatic Medicine, 60,* 33–7.

Doble, E. A., Leiter, J. C., Knuth, S. L., Daubenspeck, J. A., & Bartlett, D. (1985). A noninvasive intraoral electromyographic electrode for genioglossus muscle. *Journal of Applied Physiology, 58,* 1378–82.

DuBois, A. B., Botelho, S. Y., & Comroe, J. H. (1956). A new method for measuring airway resistance in man using a body plethysmograph: Values in normal subjects and in patients with respiratory disease. *Journal of Clinical Investigation, 35,* 327–35.

Dudley, D. L., Holmes, T. H., Martin, C. J., & Ripley, H. S. (1964a). Changes in respiration associated with hypnotically induced emotion, pain, and exercise. *Psychosomatic Medicine, 26,* 46–57.

Dudley, D. L., Martin, C. J., & Holmes, T. H. (1964b). Psychophysiologic studies of pulmonary ventilation. *Psychosomatic Medicine, 26,* 645–60.

Dudley, D. L., Martin, C. J., Masuda, M., Ripley, H. S., & Holmes, T. H. (1969). *Psychophysiology of Respiration in Health and Disease.* New York: Appleton-Century-Crofts.

Eldridge, F. L., & Chen, Z. (1996). Respiratory sensation: A neurophysiological perspective. In L. Adams & A. Guz (Eds.), *Respiratory Sensation,* pp. 19–67. New York: Marcel Dekker.

Faulkner, W. B. (1941). Influence of suggestion on size of bronchial lumen. *Northwest Medicine, 40,* 367–8.

Feleky, A. (1916). The influence of the emotions on respiration. *Journal of Experimental Psychology, 1,* 218–41.

Fink, G. R., Corfield, D. R., Murphy, K., Kobayashi, I., Dettmers, C., Adams, L., Frackowiak, R. S. J., & Guz, A. (1996). Human cerebral activity with increasing inspiratory force: A study using positron emission tomography. *Journal of Applied Physiology, 81,* 1295–1305.

Fisher, A. B., DuBois, A. B., & Hyde, R. W. (1968). Evaluation of the forced oscillation technique for the determination of resistance to breathing. *Journal of Clinical Investigation, 47,* 2045–57.

Flexman, J. E., Demaree, R. G., & Simpson, D. (1974). Respiratory phase and visual signal detection. *Perception and Psychophysics, 16,* 337–9.

Franks, C. M., & Leigh, D. (1959). The theoretical and experimental application of a conditioning model to a consideration of bronchial asthma in man. *Journal of Psychosomatic Research, 4,* 88–98.

Freedman, B. (1951). Conditioning of respiration and its psychosomatic implications. *Journal of Nervous and Mental Disease, 113,* 1–19.

Freedman, S., & Campbell, E. J. M. (1970). The ability of normal subjects to tolerate added inspiratory loads. *Respiration Physiology, 10,* 213–35.

Freeman, W. J., & Schneider, W. (1982). Changes in the spatial patterns of rabbit olfactory EEG with conditioning to odors. *Psychophysiology, 19,* 44–56.

Freud, S. (1894/1962). On the grounds for detaching a particular syndrome from neurasthenia under the description of "anxiety neurosis." In *Standard Edition of the Complete Psychological Works of Sigmund Freud,* vol. III. London: Hogarth.

Fried, R. (1993). *The Psychology and Physiology of Breathing in Behavioral Medicine, Clinical Psychology, and Psychiatry.* New York: Plenum.

Gallego, J. (1998). Review of *Behavioral and Psychological Approaches to Breathing Disorders* (Timmons & Ley, Eds.). *Biological Psychology, 49,* 223–6.

Gallego, J., Denot-Ledunois, S., Vardon, G., & Perruchet, P. (1996). Ventilatory responses to imagined exercise. *Psychophysiology, 33,* 711–19.

Gallego, J., & Perruchet, P. (1991). Classical conditioning of ventilatory responses in humans. *Journal of Applied Physiology, 70,* 676–82.

Gallego, J., Perruchet, P., & Camus, J. (1991). Assessing attentional control of breathing by reaction time. *Psychophysiology, 28,* 219–27.

Gardner, W. N. (1994). Diagnosis and organic causes of symptomatic hyperventilation. In B. H. Timmons and R. Ley (Eds.), *Behavioral and Psychological Approaches to Breathing Disorders,* pp. 99–123. New York: Plenum.

Garssen, B., Van Weendeendaal, W., & Bloemink, R. (1983). Agoraphobia and the hyperventilatory syndrome. *Behavior Research Therapy, 21,* 643–9.

Gautier, H. (1972). Respiratory and heart rate responses to auditory stimulations. *Physiology and Behavior, 8,* 327–32.

Gilbert, R., Auchincloss, J. H., Brodsky, J., & Boden, W. (1972). Changes in tidal volume, frequency, and ventilation induced by their measurement. *Journal of Applied Physiology, 33,* 252–4.

Godfrey, S., & Campbell, E. J. M. (1968). The control of breath holding. *Respiration Physiology, 5,* 385–400.

Goldman, M., Knudson, R. J., Mead, J., Peterson, N., Schwaber, J. R., & Wohl, M. E. (1970). A simplified measurement of respiratory resistance by forced oscillation. *Journal of Applied Physiology, 28,* 113–16.

Golla, F. L., & Antonovich, S. (1929). The respiratory rhythm in its relation to the mechanism of thought. *Brain, 52,* 491–509.

Greenfield, N. S., & Sternbach, R. A. (1972). *Handbook of Psychophysiology.* New York: Holt, Rinehart & Winston.

Grings, W. W., & Dawson, M. E. (1978). *Emotions and Bodily Responses: A Psychophysiological Approach.* New York: Academic Press.

Grodins, F. S., & Yamashiro, S. M. (1978). *Respiratory Function of the Lung and Its Control.* New York: Macmillan.

Grossman, P. (1983). Respiration, stress, and cardiovascular function. *Psychophysiology, 20,* 284–300.

Grossman, P., Karemaker, J., & Wieling, W. (1991). Prediction of tonic parasympathetic cardiac control using respiratory sinus arrhythmia: The need for respiratory control. *Psychophysiology, 28,* 201–16.

Grossman, P., & Kollai, M. (1993). Respiratory sinus arrhythmia, cardiac vagal tone, and respiration: Within- and between-individual relations. *Psychophysiology, 30,* 486–95.

Guyton, A. C. (1981). *Textbook of Medical Physiology,* 6th ed. Philadelphia: Saunders.

Haas, F., Distenfeld, S., & Axen, K. (1986). Effects of perceived musical rhythm on respiratory pattern. *Journal of Applied Physiology, 61,* 1185–91.

Harris, V. A., Katkin, E. S., Lick, J. R., & Habberfield, T. (1976). Paced respiration as a technique for the modification of autonomic response to stress. *Psychophysiology, 13,* 386–91.

Harver, A., & Katkin, E. S. (1998). Modification of respiratory perceptions: A self-management perspective. In H. Kotses & A. Harver (Eds.), *Self-Management of Asthma,* pp. 407–33. New York: Marcel Dekker.

Harver, A., & Kotses, H. (1987). Effects of auditory stimulation on respiration. *Psychophysiology, 24,* 26–34.

Harver, A., & Mahler, D.A. (1990). The symptom of dyspnea. In D. A. Mahler (Ed.), *Dyspnea,* pp. 1–53. Mount Kisco, NY: Futura.

Harver, A., & Mahler, D. A. (1998a). Dyspnea: Sensation, symptom, and illness. In D. A. Mahler (Ed.), *Dyspnea,* pp. 1–34. New York: Marcel Dekker.

Harver, A., & Mahler, D. A. (1998b). Perception of increased resistance to breathing. In H. Kotses & A. Harver (Eds.), *Self-Management of Asthma,* pp. 147–93. New York: Marcel Dekker.

Harver, A., Squires, N. K., Bloch-Salisbury, E., & Katkin, E. S. (1995). Event-related potentials to airway occlusion in young and old subjects. *Psychophysiology, 32,* 121–9.

Hassett, J. (1978). *A Primer of Psychophysiology.* San Francisco: Freeman.

Hey, E. N., Lloyd, B. B., Cunningham, D. J. C., Jukes, M. G. M., & Bolton, D. P. G. (1966). Effects of various respiratory stimuli on the depth and frequency of breathing in man. *Respiration Physiology, 1,* 193–205.

Holmes, D. S., Solomon, S., Frost, R. O., & Morrow, E. F. (1980). Influence of respiratory patterns on the increases and decreases in heart rates in heart rate biofeedback training. *Journal of Psychosomatic Research, 24,* 147–53.

Horowitz, S. W., Kircher, J. C., Honts, C. R., & Raskin, D. C. (1997). The role of comparison questions in physiological detection of deception. *Psychophysiology, 34,* 108-15.

Jackson, A. C., Milhorn, H. T., Jr., & Norman, J. R. (1974). A reevaluation of the interrupter technique for airway resistance measurement. *Journal of Applied Physiology, 36,* 264–8.

Jammes, Y., & Speck, D. F. (1995). Respiratory control and respiratory muscle afferents. In J. A. Dempsey & A. I. Pack (Eds.), *Regulation of Breathing,* 2nd ed., pp. 543–82. New York: Marcel Dekker.

Janson-Bjerklie, S., & Clarke, E. (1982). The effects of biofeedback training on bronchial diameter in asthma. *Heart and Lung, 11,* 200–7.

Kaufman, M. P., & Schneiderman, N. (1986). Physiological bases of respiratory psychophysiology. In M. G. H. Coles, E. Donchin, & S. W. Porges (Eds.), *Psychophysiology: Systems, Processes, and Applications,* pp. 107-21. New York: Guilford.

Kobal, G., & Hummel, T. (1991). Olfactory evoked potentials in humans. In T. Getchel, R. Doty, L. Bartoshuk, & J. Snow (Eds.), *Smell and Taste in Health and Disease,* pp. 255–75. New York: Raven.

Kobylarz, E. J., & Daubenspeck, J. A. (1992). Immediate diaphragmatic electromyogram responses to imperceptible mechanical loads in conscious humans. *Journal of Applied Physiology, 73,* 248–59.

Konno, K., & Mead, J. (1967). Measurement of the separate volume changes of rib cage and abdomen during breathing. *Journal of Applied Physiology, 22,* 407–22.

Kotses, H. (1998). Emotional precipitants of asthma. In H. Kotses & A. Harver (Eds.), *Self-Management of Asthma,* pp. 35–61. New York: Marcel Dekker.

Kotses, H., & Glaus, K. D. (1981). Applications of biofeedback to the treatment of asthma: A critical review. *Biofeedback and Self-Regulation, 6,* 573–93.

Kotses, H., & Harver, A. (Eds.) (1998). *Self-Management of Asthma.* New York: Marcel Dekker.

Kotses, H., Hindi-Alexander, M., & Creer, T. L. (1989). A reinterpretation of psychologically induced airway changes. *Journal of Asthma, 26,* 53–63.

Kotses, H., Lewis, P., & Creer, T. L. (1990). Environmental control of asthma self-management. *Journal of Asthma, 27,* 375–84.

Kotses, H., Rawson, J. C., Wigal, J. K., & Creer, T. L. (1987a). Respiratory airway changes in response to suggestion in normal individuals. *Psychosomatic Medicine, 49,* 536–41.

Kotses, H., Westlund, R., & Creer, T. L. (1987b). Performing mental arithmetic increases total respiratory resistance in individuals with normal respiration. *Psychophysiology, 24,* 678–82.

Kubin, L., & Davies, R. O. (1995). Central pathways of pulmonary and airway vagal afferents. In J. A. Dempsey & A. I. Pack (Eds.), *Regulation of Breathing,* 2nd ed., pp. 219–84. New York: Marcel Dekker.

Laing, D. G. (1983). Natural sniffing gives optimum odor perception in humans. *Perception, 12,* 99–117.

Lándsér, F. J., Nagels, J., Demedts, M., Billiet, L., & van de Woestijne, K. P. (1976). A new method to determine frequency characteristics of the respiratory system. *Journal of Applied Physiology, 41,* 101–6.

Langer, A. W., Hutcheson, J. S., Charlton, J. D., McCubbin, J. A., Obrist, P. A., & Stoney, C. M. (1985a). On-line minicomputerized measurement of cardiopulmonary function on a breath-by-breath basis. *Psychophysiology, 22,* 50–8.

Langer, A. W., McCubbin, J. A., Stoney, C. M., Hutcheson, J. S., Charlton, J. D., & Obrist, P. A. (1985b). Cardiopulmonary adjustments during exercise and an aversive reaction time task: Effects of beta-adrenoceptor blockade. *Psychophysiology, 22,* 59–68.

Lansing, R. W., & Banzett, R. B. (1996). Psychophysical methods in the study of respiratory sensation. In L. Adams & A. Guz (Eds.), *Respiratory Sensation,* pp. 69–100. New York: Marcel Dekker.

Lansing, R. W., & Savelle, J. (1989). Chest surface recording of diaphragm potentials in man. *Electroencephalography and Clinical Neurophysiology, 72,* 59–68.

Levenson, R. W. (1979). Cardiac-respiratory-somatic relationships and feedback effects in a multiple session heart rate control experiment. *Psychophysiology, 16,* 367–73.

Levitzky, M. G. (1986). *Pulmonary Physiology,* 2nd ed. New York: McGraw-Hill.

Ley, R. (1994). Breathing-related disorders. *Current Opinion in Psychiatry, 7,* 486–9.

Ley, R. (1999). The modification of breathing behavior: Pavlovian and operant control in emotion and cognition. *Behavior Modification, 23,* 441–79.

Lorig, T. S. (1999). On the similarity of odor and language processing. *Neuroscience and Biobehavioral Reviews, 23,* 391–8.

Lorig, T. S., Huffman, E., DeMartino, A., & DeMarco, J. (1991). The effects of low concentration odors on EEG activity and behavior. *Journal of Psychophysiology, 5,* 69–77.

Lorig, T. S., Matia, D. C., Peszka, J. J., & Bryant, D. N. (1996). The effects of active and passive stimulation on chemosensory event-related potentials. *International Journal of Psychophysiology, 23,* 199–205.

Lorig, T. S., & Schwartz, G. E. (1988). Brain and odor I: Alteration of human EEG by odor administration. *Psychobiology, 16,* 281–4.

Lorig, T. S., & Schwartz, G. E. (1990). The pulmonary system. In J. T. Cacioppo & L. G. Tassinary (Eds.), *Principles of Psychophysiology: Physical, Social, and Inferential Elements,* pp. 580–98. Cambridge University Press.

Lourenco, R. V., & Mueller, E. P. (1967). Quantification of electrical activity in the human diaphragm. *Journal of Applied Physiology, 22,* 598–600.

Luce, J. M. (1986). *Lung Diseases of Adults.* New York: American Lung Association.

Lyon, M. L. (1994). Emotion as mediator of somatic and social processes: The example of respiration. In W. M. Wentworth & J. Ryan (Eds.), *Social Perspectives on Emotion,* vol. 2, pp. 83–108. Greenwich, CT: JAI.

Mador, J., & Tobin, M. J. (1991). Effect of alterations in mental activity on the breathing pattern in healthy subjects. *American Review of Respiratory Disease, 144,* 481–7.

Mahler, D. A. (1983). Pulmonary aspects of aging. In S. R. Gambert (Ed.), *Contemporary Geriatric Medicine,* vol. 1, pp. 45–85. New York: Plenum.

Mahler, D. A. (Ed.) (1998). *Dyspnea.* New York: Marcel Dekker.

Mandler, G., Mandler, J. M., & Uviller, E. T. (1958). Autonomic feedback: The perception of autonomic activity. *Journal of Abnormal and Social Psychology, 56,* 367–73.

Manning, H. L., & Schwartzstein, R. M. (1995). Pathophysiology of dyspnea. *New England Journal of Medicine, 333,* 1547–53.

Martin, I., & Venables, P. H. (Eds.) (1980). *Techniques in Psychophysiology.* Chichester, U.K.: Wiley.

Mass, R., Dahme, B., & Richter, R. (1993). Clinical evaluation of a respiratory resistance biofeedback training. *Biofeedback and Self-Regulation, 18,* 211–23.

Maxwell, D. L., Cover, D., & Hughes, J. M. B. (1985). Effect of respiratory apparatus on timing and depth of breathing in man. *Respiration Physiology, 61,* 255–64.

McCaul, K. D., Solomon, S., & Holmes, D. (1979). Effects of paced respiration and expectations on physiological and psychological responses to threat. *Journal of Personality and Social Psychology, 37,* 564–71.

McClintock, M. K. (1971). Menstrual synchrony and suppression. *Nature, 291,* 244–5.

McCollum, M., Burch, N. R., & Roessler, R. (1969). Personality and respiratory responses to sound and light. *Psychophysiology, 6,* 291–300.

McCubbin, J. A., Cheung, R., Montgomery, T. B., Bulbulian, R., & Wilson, J. F. (1992). Aerobic fitness and opioidergic inhibition of cardiovascular stress reactivity. *Psychophysiology, 29,* 687-97.

Milic-Emili, J., Grassino, A. E., & Whitelaw, W. A. (1981). Measurement and testing of respiratory drive. In T. F. Hornbein (Ed.), *Regulation of Breathing,* part 2, pp. 675–743. New York: Marcel Dekker.

Miller, D. J., & Kotses, H. (1995). Classical conditioning of total respiratory resistance in humans. *Psychosomatic Medicine, 57,* 148–53.

Mines, A. H. (1986). *Respiration Physiology,* 2nd ed. New York: Raven.

Molfino, N. A., Nannini, L. J., Martelli, A. N., & Slutsky, A. S. (1991). Respiratory arrest in near-fatal asthma. *New England Journal of Medicine, 324,* 285–8.

Nielsen, J. M., & Roth, P. (1929). Clinical spirography: Spirograms and their significance. *Archives of Internal Medicine, 43,* 132–8.

Obrist, P. A. (1981). *Cardiovascular Psychophysiology: A Perspective.* New York: Plenum.

Obrist, P. A., Galosy, R. A., Lawler, J. E., Gaebelein, C. J., Howard, J. L., & Shanks, E. M. (1975). Operant conditioning of heart rate: Somatic correlates. *Psychophysiology, 12,* 445–55.

Ogilvie, R. D., & Wilkinson, R. T. (1984). The detection of sleep onset: Behavioral and physiological convergence. *Psychophysiology, 21,* 510–20.

Oku, Y., Saidel, G. M., Altose, M. D., & Cherniack, N. S. (1993). Perceptual contributions to optimization of breathing. *Annals of Biomedical Engineering, 21,* 509–15.

Önal, E., Lopata, M., Ginzburg, A. S., & O'Connor, T. D. (1981). Diaphragmatic EMG and transdiaphragmatic pressure measurements with a single catheter. *American Review of Respiratory Disease, 124,* 563–5.

Pack, A. I., Cola, M. F., Goldszmidt, A., Ogilvie, M. D., & Gottschalk, A. (1992). Correlation between oscillations in ventilation and frequency content of the electroencephalogram. *Journal of Applied Physiology, 72,* 985–92.

Pack, A. I., & Gottschalk, A. (1993). Mechanisms of ventilatory periodicities. *Annals of Biomedical Engineering, 21,* 537–44.

Paintal, A. S. (1977). Thoracic receptors connected with sensation. *British Medical Bulletin, 33,* 169–74.

Patrick, C. J., & Iacono, W. G. (1991). A comparison of field and laboratory polygraphs in the detection of deception. *Psychophysiology, 28,* 632–8.

Pauly, J. E. (1957). Electromyographic studies of human respiration. *Chicago Medical School Quarterly, 18,* 80–8.

Pengelly, L. D., Rebuck, A. S., & Campbell, E. J. M. (Eds.) (1974). *Loaded Breathing.* Edinburgh, U.K.: Churchill Livingstone.

Pennebaker, J. W. (1982). *The Psychology of Physical Symptoms.* New York: Springer-Verlag.

Plassman, B. L., Lansing, R. W., & Foti, K. (1987). Inspiratory muscle movements to airway occlusion during learned breathing movements. *Journal of Neurophysiology, 57,* 274–88.

Poole, R., Goetzinger, C. P., & Rousey, C. L. (1966). A study of the effects of auditory stimuli on respiration. *Acta Otolaryngologica, 61,* 143–52.

Porges, S. W. (1995). Orienting in a defensive world: Mammalian modifications of our evolutionary heritage. A polyvagal theory. *Psychophysiology, 32,* 301–18.

Posner, M. I., & Raichle, M. E. (1997). *Images of Mind.* New York: Freeman.

Preti, G., Cutler, W. B., Garcia, C. R., Huggins, G. R., & Lawkey, H. J. (1986). Human axillary secretions influence women's menstrual cycles: The role of donor extract of females. *Hormones and Behavior, 20,* 474–82.

Prigatano, G. P., & Grant, I. (1988). Neuropsychological correlates of COPD. In A. J. McSweeny & I. Grant (Eds.), *Chronic Obstructive Pulmonary Disease: A Behavioral Perspective,* pp. 39–57. New York: Marcel Dekker.

Ramsay, S. C., Adams, L., Murphy, K., Corfield, D. R., Grootoonk, S., Bailey, D. L., Frackowiak, R. S. J., & Guz, A. (1993). Regional cerebral blood flow during volitional expiration in man: A comparison with volitional inspiration. *Journal of Physiology, 461,* 85–101.

Remmers, J. E. (1976). Analysis of ventilatory response. *Chest, 70 (Suppl. 1),* 134–7.

Revelette, W. R., & Davenport, P. W. (1990). Effects of timing of inspiratory occlusion on cerebral evoked potentials in humans. *Journal of Applied Physiology, 68,* 282–8.

Richards, D. W., Jr. (1953). The nature of cardiac and pulmonary dyspnea. *Circulation, 7,* 15–29.

Rigg, J. R. A., Inman, E. M., Saunders, N. A., Leeder, S. R., & Jones, N. L. (1977). Interaction of mental factors with hypercapnic ventilatory drive in man. *Clinical Science and Molecular Medicine, 52,* 269–75.

Ritz, T., Wiens, S., & Dahme, B. (1998). Stability of total respiratory resistance under multiple baseline conditions, isometric arm exercise and voluntary deep breathing. *Biological Psychology, 49,* 187–213.

Rousey, C. L., & Reitz, W. E. (1967). Respiratory changes at auditory and visual thresholds. *Psychophysiology, 3,* 258–61.

Sanchez-Hernandez, A., Pedraja, M. J., Quiñones-Vidal, E., & Martinez-Sanchez, F. (1996). A historic-quantitative approach to psychophysiological research: The first three decades of the journal *Psychophysiology* (1964–1993). *Psychophysiology, 33,* 629–36.

Sasaki, C. T., & Mann, D. G. (1976). Dilator naris function. *Archives of Otolaryngology, 102,* 365–7.

Saul, L. J., & Lyons, J. W. (1951). The psychodynamics of respiration. In H. A. Abramson (Ed.), *Somatic and Psychiatric Treatment of Asthma,* pp. 93–103. Baltimore: Williams & Wilkins.

Schneider, E. C. (1930). Observations on holding the breath. *American Journal of Physiology, 94,* 464–70.

Shannon, R. (1986). Reflexes from respiratory muscles and costovertebral joints. In N. S. Cherniack & J. G. Widdicombe (Eds.), *Handbook of Physiology, Section 3: The Respiratory System,* vol. II, pp. 431–47. Bethesda, MD: American Physiological Society.

Shapiro, A., & Cohen, H. D. (1965). The use of mercury capillary length gauges for the measurement of the volume of thoracic and diaphragmatic components of human respiration: A theoretical analysis and a practical method. *Transactions of the New York Academy of Sciences, 27,* 634–49.

Shea, S. A. (1996). Behavioral and arousal-related influences on breathing in humans. *Experimental Physiology, 81,* 1-26.

Shea, S. A., Banzett, R. B., & Lansing, R. W. (1996). Respiratory sensations and their role in the control of breathing. In L. Adams & A. Guz (Eds.), *Respiratory Sensation,* pp. 923–57. New York: Marcel Dekker.

Shea, S. A., Benchetrit, G., Pham Dinh, T., Hamilton, R. D., & Guz, A. (1989). The breathing pattern of identical twins. *Respiration Physiology, 75,* 211–24.

Shea, S. A., & Guz, A. (1992). Personnalité ventilatoire – An overview. *Respiration Physiology, 87,* 275–91.

Shea, S. A., Pham Dinh, T., Hamilton, R. D., Guz, A., & Benchetrit, G. (1993). Breathing patterns of monozygous twins during behavioral tasks. *Acta Genet. Med. Gemellol., 42,* 171–84.

Shea, S. J., Walter, J., Pelley, C., Murphy, K., & Guz, A. (1987). The effect of visual and auditory stimuli on resting ventilation in man. *Respiration Physiology, 68,* 345–57.

Skaggs, E. B. (1926). Changes in pulse, breathing, and steadiness under conditions of startledness and excited expectancy. *Journal of Comparative Psychology, 6,* 303–18.

Skaggs, E. B. (1930). Studies in attention and emotion. *Journal of Comparative Psychology, 10,* 375–419.

Sobel, N., Prabhakaran, V., Desmond, J. E., Glover, G. H., Goode, R. L., Sullivan, E. V., & Gabrielli, J. D. E. (1998). Sniffing and smelling: separate subsystems in the human olfactory cortex. *Nature, 392,* 282–6.

Sroufe, L. A. (1971). Effects of depth and rate of breathing on heart rate and heart rate variability. *Psychophysiology, 8,* 648–55.

Stein, M., & Luparello, T. J. (1967). Measurement of respiration. In C. C. Brown (Ed.), *Methods in Psychophysiology,* pp. 75–94. Baltimore: Williams & Wilkins.

Stein, M., & Luparello, T. J. (1970). Psychosomatic aspects of respiratory disorders. *Postgraduate Medicine, 47,* 137–41.

Steinschneider, A. (1968). Sound intensity and respiratory responses in the neonate. *Psychosomatic Medicine, 30,* 534–41.

Steptoe, A., Moses, J., Mathews, A., & Edwards, S. (1990). Aerobic fitness, physical activity, and psychophysiological reactions to mental tasks. *Psychophysiology, 27,* 264–74.

Stern, K., & McClintock, M. K. (1998). Regulation of ovulation by human pheromones. *Nature, 392,* 177–9.

Stern, R. M., & Anschel, C. (1968). Deep inspirations as stimuli for responses of the autonomic nervous system. *Psychophysiology, 5,* 132–41.

Stern, R. M., Ray, W. J., & Davis, C. M. (1980). *Psychophysiological Recording.* New York: Oxford University Press.

Stoney, C. M., Langer, A. W., & Gelling, P. D. (1986). The effects of menstrual cycle phase on cardiovascular and pulmonary responses to behavioral and exercise stress. *Psychophysiology, 23,* 393–402.

Suess, W. M., Alexander, A. B., Smith, D. D., Sweeney, H. W., & Marion, R. J. (1980). The effects of psychological stress on respiration: A preliminary study of anxiety and hyperventilation. *Psychophysiology, 17,* 535–40.

Sutherland, G. F., Wolf, A., & Kennedy, F. (1938). The respiratory "fingerprint" of nervous states. *Medical Record, 148,* 101–3.

Svebak, S. (1975). Respiratory patterns as predictors of laughter. *Psychophysiology, 12,* 62–5.

Tankersley, C. G., Fitzgerald, R. S., Levitt, R. C., Mitzner, W. A., Ewart, S. L., & Kleeberger, S. R. (1997). Genetic control of differential baseline breathing pattern. *Journal of Applied Physiology, 82,* 874–81.

Thornby, M. A., Haas, F., & Axen, K. (1995). Effect of distractive auditory stimuli on exercise tolerance in patients with COPD. *Chest, 107,* 1213–17.

Timmons, B. H. (1994). A brief history of the annual International Symposium on Respiratory Psychophysiology and summary of the 1993 workshops. *Biofeedback and Self-Regulation, 19,* 97–101.

Timmons, B. H., & Ley, R. (Eds.) (1994). *Behavioral and Psychological Approaches to Breathing Disorders.* New York: Plenum.

Tobin, M. J. (1990). Dyspnea: Pathophysiological basis, clinical presentation, and management. *Archives of Internal Medicine, 150,* 1604–13.

Tobin, M. J., Chadha, T. S., Jenouri, G., Birch, S. J., Gazeroglu, H. B., & Sackner, M. A. (1983a). Breathing patterns: Diseased subjects. *Chest, 84,* 286–94.

Tobin, M. J., Chadha, T. S., Jenouri, G., Birch, S. J., Gazeroglu, H. B., & Sackner, M. A. (1983b). Breathing patterns: Normal subjects. *Chest, 84,* 202–5.

Turnbull, J. W. (1962). Asthma conceived as a learned response. *Journal of Psychosomatic Research, 6,* 59–70.

Turner, J. R., & Carroll, D. (1985). Heart rate and oxygen consumption during mental arithmetic, a video game, and graded exercise: Further evidence of metabolically-exaggerated cardiac adjustments? *Psychophysiology, 22,* 261–7.

Turner, J. R., Carroll, D., & Courtney, H. (1983). Cardiac and metabolic responses to "Space Invaders": An instance of metabolically-exaggerated cardiac adjustment? *Psychophysiology, 20,* 544–9.

Van den Bergh, O., Kempynk, P. J., Van de Woestijne, K. P., Baeyens, F., & Eelen, P. (1995). Respiratory learning and somatic complaints: A conditioning approach using CO_2-enriched air inhalation. *Behaviour Research and Therapy, 33,* 517–27.

Vandercar, D. H., Feldstein, M. A., & Solomon, H. (1977). Instrumental conditioning of human heart rate during free and controlled respiration. *Biological Psychology, 5,* 221–31.

van Doornen, L. J. P., & de Gues, E. J. C. (1989). Aerobic fitness and the cardiovascular response to stress. *Psychophysiology, 26,* 17–28.

Wallace, R. K., Benson, H., & Wilson, A. F. (1971). A wakeful hypometabolic physiologic state. *American Journal of Physiology, 221,* 795–9.

Wasserman, K. (1981). Physiology of gas exchange and exertional dyspnea. *Clinical Science, 61,* 7–13.

Wenger, M. A., & Cullen, T. D. (1972). Studies of autonomic balance in children and adults. In N. S. Greenfield & R. A. Sternbach (Eds.), *Handbook of Psychophysiology,* pp. 535–69. New York: Holt, Rinehart & Winston.

West, J. B. (1982). *Pulmonary Pathophysiology – The Essentials,* 2nd ed. Baltimore: Williams & Wilkins.

West, J. B. (Ed.) (1985). *Best and Taylor's Physiological Basis of Medical Practice,* 11th ed. Baltimore: Williams & Wilkins.

Whitelaw, W. A., & Feroah, T. (1989). Patterns of intercostal muscle activity in humans. *Journal of Applied Physiology, 67,* 2087–94.

Wientjes, C. J. E. (1992). Respiration in psychophysiology: Methods and application. *Biological Psychology, 34,* 179–203.

Wientjes, C. J. E., & Grossman, P. (1998). Respiratory psychophysiology as a discipline: Introduction to the special issue [Editorial]. *Biological Psychology, 49,* 1–8.

Wientjes, C. J. E., Grossman, P., & Gaillard, A. W. K. (1998). Influence of drive and timing mechanisms on breathing pattern and ventilation during mental task performance. *Biological Psychology, 49,* 53–70.

Wigal, J. K., Stout, C., Kotses, H., Creer, T. L., Fogle, K., Gayhart, L., & Hatala, J. (1997). Experimenter expectancy in resistance to respiratory air flow. *Psychosomatic Medicine, 59,* 318–22.

Winter, J. E. (1936). A comparison of the cardio-pneumo-psychograph and association methods in the detection of lying in cases of theft among college students. *Journal of Applied Psychology, 20,* 243–8.

Woodworth, R. S., & Schlosberg, H. (1956). *Experimental Psychology,* rev. ed. New York: Holt.

Younes, M. (1995). Mechanisms of respiratory load compensation. In J. A. Dempsey & A. I. Pack (Eds.), *Regulation of Breathing,* 2nd ed., pp. 867–922. New York: Marcel Dekker.

Zechman, F. W., Jr., & Wiley, R. L. (1986). Afferent inputs to breathing: Respiratory sensation. In N. S. Cherniack & J. G. Widdicombe (Eds.), *Handbook of Physiology, Section 3: The Respiratory System,* vol. II, pp. 449–74. Bethesda, MD: American Physiological Society.

CHAPTER ELEVEN

THE GASTROINTESTINAL SYSTEM

ROBERT M. STERN, KENNETH L. KOCH, & ERIC R. MUTH

Prologue

OVERVIEW

Why do many people report gastrointestinal (GI) symptoms during stress? This and related questions about brain–gut interactions have interested investigators at least as far back as 1833, when Beaumont described his experiments on a fistulated patient, Alexis St. Martin. In the case of St. Martin, his fistula (an external opening into the stomach) was created by an accidental gunshot wound. Beaumont reported that upsetting emotions suppressed gastric secretion and delayed gastric emptying in his subject. Between 1840 and 1870, several physiologists created fistulas in dogs, based on Beaumont's work, and found that an intact vagus is needed for normal brain–gut interaction. This was an important finding because it tells us that one pathway by which the brain and gut communicate is via the vagus nerve or parasympathetic nervous system. Today we use the term "cephalic-vagal reflex" to refer to, for example, the anticipatory stomach contractions that occur when we think about eating Thanksgiving dinner. More about the cephalic-vagal reflex will follow in a later section of this chapter, but we should keep in mind that brain–gut interaction is a two-way street. That is, not only does brain activity affect GI activity, but GI activity also affects activity in the brain. An example of the latter (which will be discussed in some detail) is the effect of changes in stomach activity on the sensation of nausea.

During the first half of the twentieth century, gastrointestinal scientists and clinicians were deeply committed to an interactive brain–gut view of gastrointestinal functioning and thus had much to say to psychophysiologists. Wolf and Wolff (1943) wrote a fascinating book about their experiences over many years with their fistulated subject Tom. Their basic findings were that when Tom was fearful or depressed his gastric activity decreased, but when he was angry or hostile his gastric activity increased. Cannon studied the effects of various emotions on GI activity and published several books on the topic, including *Digestion and Health* (1936), which contains chapters on the nature of appetite and hunger and on indigestion from pain, worry, and excitement. Alvarez, perhaps the best-known gastroenterologist of the century, stressed the interaction of psychological and physiological factors in GI functioning in all of his writings, both scientific and popular. His book, *Nervousness, Indigestion, and Pain* (1943), is highly recommended reading for psychophysiologists.

During the second half of the twentieth century, gastroenterologists developed many new techniques for measuring the activity of the GI system and adhered, in general, to a medical model. Unlike Alvarez, who stated that "to understand a man's stomach, one must understand the man," gastroenterologists relied more and more on the results of laboratory tests of the GI system and ignored the "man." This meant that there was little interaction between gastroenterologists and psychophysiologists, or psychologists of any type. Moreover, since most of the new tests of GI activity were invasive, most psychophysiologists could not make use of them outside of a medical center. Fortunately, the pendulum has been swinging back during the past few years, and an interdisciplinary group of scientists and clinicians trained in gastroenterology, psychophysiology, epidemiology, and clinical psychology have recently formed an association called the Functional Brain–Gut Research Group.

As a consequence of the paucity of interaction heretofore between gastroenterologists and psychophysiologists, no psychophysiological studies of absorption are known to the authors, and few studies of gastric acid secretion have been conducted by psychophysiologists. However, several studies of motor activity, particularly in the more easily

John T. Cacioppo, Louis G. Tassinary, and Gary G. Berntson (Eds.), *Handbook of Psychophysiology*, 2nd ed. © Cambridge University Press 2000. Printed in the United States of America. ISBN 62634X. All rights reserved.

accessible two ends of the GI tract – the esophagus and rectum, but also the stomach – have been conducted. In this chapter we review psychophysiological studies that have measured gastric motor activity; the major emphasis will be on the motor activity of the stomach as measured with a noninvasive technique first used by Alvarez in 1921: the electrogastrogram (EGG).

Electrogastrography refers to the recording of electrogastrograms, which reflect gastric myoelectrical activity as it is recorded from the abdominal surface with electrodes placed on the skin. Electrogastrograms are more or less sinusoidal waves recurring at a rate of three cycles per minute (cpm) in healthy humans. This predominant frequency is usually discernable by visual inspection of the signal, but computer analysis is essential for quantitative study of EGG recordings.

The stomach is also the source of abnormally fast or slow (usually dysrhythmic) myoelectrical signals, the tachygastrias and bradygastrias. Acute or chronic shifts from normal 3-cpm EGG signals to the gastric dysrhythmias are associated with a variety of clinical syndromes and symptoms, particularly nausea. In contrast to these abnormalities in frequency, the amplitude, duration, waveform, and wave propagation characteristics of the EGG have been infrequently studied.

Psychophysiological and pathophysiological investigations of EGG characteristics in health and disease are increasing in number. The International EGG Society was established in 1995, and at least four companies now sell EGG hardware and software, including ambulatory models.

HISTORICAL BACKGROUND

During the first half of this century and prior to the availability of computerized literature searches, scientists working independently frequently discovered similar measures, phenomena, or relationships. The EGG was discovered by at least three independent investigators: Walter Alvarez, a gastroenterologist; I. Harrison Tumpeer, a pediatrician; and R. C. Davis, a psychophysiologist.

On October 14, 1921, after considerable experimentation with rabbits at the University of California in San Francisco, Alvarez (1922) recorded the first human EGG from an elderly woman with a hernia who was so thin that Alvarez could observe 3-cpm gastric contractions corresponding to the 3-cpm sinusoidal waves that were clearly seen in the EGG. Alvarez did not publish additional studies with EGG during his long and productive career, probably because of the technical difficulties inherent in recording such a weak signal prior to the development of vacuum-tube amplifiers.

The second investigator to discover the EGG is not as well known as Alvarez. In 1926, I. Harrison Tumpeer, a pediatrician working at Michael Reese Hospital in Chicago, reported in a note (Tumpeer & Blitzsten 1926) that, while he was attempting to record the EGG, "Alvarez of California published his results." In this same note and in a subsequent publication (Tumpeer & Phillips 1932), Tumpeer mentioned successfully recording the EGG from a 5-week-old child who was suffering from pyloric stenosis. Tumpeer described the EGG as looking like an ECG (electrocardiogram) with a slowly changing baseline. Tumpeer mentioned that cardiologists in 1926 often noted a changing baseline in the ECGs that they could not explain. Thus, the EGG had been recorded, but perhaps not recognized as such, since the time of the first ECG at the turn of the century.

In the mid-1950s, R. C. Davis, one of the founders of the Society for Psychophysiological Research, began a series of exploratory studies with the EGG. When he began his investigations he was not aware of the earlier EGG work of Alvarez or Tumpeer; thus, he was the third discoverer of the EGG. Davis, like Alvarez, was primarily interested in the interactive effects of psychological and physiological factors on gastric functioning. Davis published two papers before his untimely death in 1961, papers that stimulated several other investigators to begin doing EGG research.

In a 1957 paper (Davis, Garafolo, & Gault 1957), Davis and his co-workers described their attempt to validate the EGG using simultaneous recordings from needle electrodes, a mine detector that picked up the movements of a steel ball in the subject's GI tract, and the EGG. They used needle electrodes that were insulated except at the tip so that they could rule out cutaneous tissue as the source of the EGG signal.

In a 1959 paper (Davis, Garafolo, & Kveim 1959), Davis and his co-workers described their continuing study of the validation of the EGG using swallowed balloons as well as their studies of the effects of eating on the EGG. They reported that the activity of the stomach is at its lowest point when the stomach is empty, a controversial finding in light of the reports of so-called hunger contractions by Cannon and Carlson (Cannon & Washburn 1912; Carlson 1916). After recording the EGG from many fasted subjects – both with and without a balloon in the stomach – Davis concluded that hunger contractions are rare and are usually stimulated by the introduction of a balloon into the stomach. This is a good example of one of the advantages of using psychophysiological methods; namely, noninvasive recording techniques do not interfere with the behavior being studied. All other methods of recording stomach activity either require putting something inside the stomach – which stimulates it to contract – or are dangerous to use for extended periods (e.g., X-rays or fluoroscopy).

Physical Context: Anatomy and Physiology of the Gastrointestinal Tract with Particular Emphasis on the Stomach

The GI system extends from the mouth to the rectum and includes the mouth, esophagus, stomach, small intestine, large intestine, and rectum. The three functions of the

GI system are movement of food through the alimentary tract, secretion of substances that aid in digestion or protect the alimentary tract, and absorption of the digestive end-products.

The GI tract may be viewed as a series of muscular tubes that have been modified to perform region-specific digestive functions: transit of food from esophagus to stomach, mixing and emptying of ingested foods from the stomach into the duodenum, and absorption of micronutrients from the small intestine. Other specialized tubes (i.e., the cecum, the ascending, transverse, and descending colon, and the rectum) conserve water, electrolytes, and nutrients and evacuate wastes. These functions require exquisite control and integration of relevant neural, muscular, mucosal, and hormonal systems within the GI tract.

The purpose of this section is to describe briefly the anatomy and physiology of the stomach. Although basic similarities exist between the anatomy and physiology of the stomach and other regions of the GI tract, each region has its own function-specific modifications. The interested reader is referred to the volume edited by Johnson and colleagues (1987) for a review of the physiology of these other regions of the GI tract.

GASTRIC ANATOMY

The stomach lies in the upper quadrant of the abdomen, although there is a wide range of variability in its shape and form (Figure 1). The body and antrum, however, are rotated toward the midline such that the antrum is near the epigastric region. As is shown in Figure 1, the esophagus enters the stomach in the fundic region; the antrum is connected to the first portion of the duodenum, the duodenal bulb, via the pylorus.

The stomach has three major regions: the fundus, body, and antrum. The stomach wall has three layers: outermost is the serosa; innermost is the mucosa, which secretes acid and pepsin; and the thickest layer is the muscular portion, which itself has three layers – an outer longitudinal layer, an inner circular layer, and in some areas an oblique layer (see Figure 1).

The muscular wall of the stomach contains extensive neural elements, both extrinsic and intrinsic. Extrinsic nerves are pre- and postganglionic parasympathetic fibers from the vagus nerve and postganglionic neurons from the sympathetic splanchnic nerves. These extrinsic neural circuits are closely integrated with the intrinsic nervous system of the stom-

ach and of all regions of the GI tract, the enteric nervous system.

The enteric nervous system is a collection of nerve cell bodies in plexi located between the circular and longitudinal muscle layers, that is, the myenteric plexus (Auerbach's plexus) and submucosal plexus (see Figure 1). The myenteric and submucosal plexi are the largest, but seven discrete plexi have been described. Postganglionic parasympathetic neurons, internuncial neurons, and sensory neurons are present within the plexi. At least ten different types of enteric neurons have been identified by immunohistochemical methods (Furness & Costa 1980). It has been estimated that there are 10^9 neurons in the enteric nervous system, a number similar to that in the spinal cord. Fibers from the sympathetic neurons synapse on myenteric plexus neurons and innervate the circular muscle layer. Thus, the muscular layers of the stomach, particularly the circular muscle layers, have rich neural integration that allows for the fine control of muscular contraction required for normal digestive function. The interested reader may refer to review articles on neural control of gastric motility (Meyer 1987; Roman & Gonella 1987).

Figure 1. Stomach and its principal regions. Inset shows major layers of gastric wall. Origin of gastric pacesetter potentials (gastric electrical slow waves) is indicated by stippled region on gastric body. Reprinted with permission from Stern & Koch, *Electrogastrography*. Copyright 1985 by Praeger, an imprint of Greenwood Publishing Group, Inc., Westport, CT.

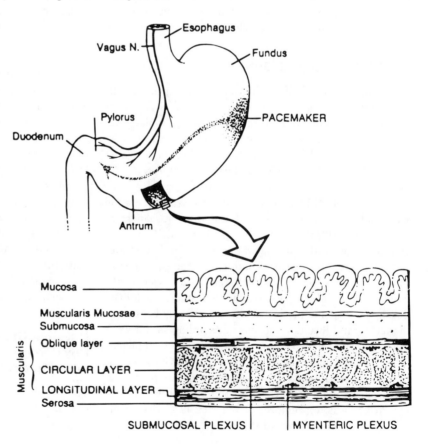

GASTRIC PHYSIOLOGY

Postprandial Gastric Physiology

The major physiological activities of the stomach are to receive ingested foodstuffs and to mix the foodstuffs into suspensions until they are appropriate for emptying and further digestion in the small intestine.

Normal reception of ingested food requires the gastric fundus to relax and to accommodate the particular ingested volume. These muscular activities of the stomach are termed receptive relaxation and accommodation and are accomplished via vagal efferent activity (Roman & Gonella 1987). Moreover, because nearly 90% of vagal fibers are sensory, it is assumed that sensory vagal traffic modulates ongoing vagal efferent activity.

After ingestion, solid foods are moved from the gastric fundus into the gastric body and antrum for mixing and emptying. This period is called the *lag phase* because it precedes actual emptying of the nutrient suspensions from the stomach into the duodenum (Lavigne et al. 1978; Meyer et al. 1976). In contrast to solids, nonnutrient liquids such as water have no lag phase. Before emptying, solids are normally mixed and reduced to 0.1–1-mm–diameter particles and suspended in gastric juice (Meyer et al. 1981).

The stomach accomplishes the work of mixing and emptying through a series of smooth rhythmic contractions at the rate of three cycles per minute. This phase in the digestive process, known as *peristalsis,* commences in the gastric body and moves through this region into the antrum, where the waves dissipate in the prepyloric region. As a result of these wavelike contractions, small food particles already in suspension are carried through the open pyloric sphincter into the duodenum (Meyer et al. 1981, 1986). The pyloris and the duodenum may contract to create resistance to gastric emptying, or it may relax to promote *gastroduodenal synchrony* and so enhance gastric emptying (Meyer 1987). The hydrodynamics of the suspension itself may determine which particles are emptied and their rate of emptying (Meyer et al. 1986).

Control of the mixing and emptying of gastric content is complex. In addition to physical properties of the gastric contents and the various neural-muscular responses, the release of gastrointestinal hormones (e.g., gastrin, secretin, cholecystokinin, enteroglucagon, gastric inhibitory polypeptide, somatostatin, vasoactive intestinal polypeptide, and motilin, to name a few of the more than 20 GI hormones and candidate hormones) is believed to modulate the contractile responses of the stomach and to affect overall gastric emptying rates. However, specific actions of most GI hormones on gastric motility in humans remain to be determined.

The rate at which foodstuffs are emptied from the stomach is dependent on many factors, including the volume of ingested material, caloric density (i.e., fat, protein, or carbohydrate), osmolality, temperature, acidity, and viscosity. These factors are adjusted by chemo- and mechanoreceptors in the stomach and duodenum and by the variety of hormones released by the specific foodstuffs (Meyer 1987).

Emptying of liquids is thought to be controlled by fundic tone. That is, after the ingestion of a liquid such as water, fundic pressure is greater than duodenal pressure; the pressure gradient between fundus and duodenum provides the force necessary to empty the liquid from the stomach (Meyer 1987). Other studies indicate that the antrum has a more active role in the emptying of liquids (Camilleri et al. 1985; Stemper & Cooke 1975).

Gastric Physiology during Fasting

During the interdigestive state (e.g., an overnight fast), the stomach completes its digestive function and participates in a stereotyped periodic sequence of contractile events termed the *interdigestive complex.* The complex is divided into three phases: phase I is a period of quiescence lasting approximately 20 min; phase II is a period of irregular contractile activity of the body and antrum lasting about 80–90 min; and phase III is a 5–10-min period of regular and intense 3-cpm contractions of the gastric body and antrum. The antral contractions are peristaltic, moving into the duodenum and subsequently through the small bowel. Phase-III activity occurs approximately every 90–110 min in humans during prolonged fasts and has been associated with bursts of pancreatic and biliary secretions and elevations in plasma motilin levels (Code & Marlett 1975; Lee et al. 1978; Meyer 1987; Schlegel & Code 1975; Vantrappen et al. 1979).

From a physiological viewpoint, phase-III contractions have been shown to empty fibrous meal residue from the stomach (Schlegel & Code 1975). The phase-III contractions may serve a similar function in the small intestine and have been termed the "intestinal housekeeper."

RELATIONSHIP BETWEEN GASTRIC MOTOR ACTIVITY AND GASTRIC MYOELECTRIC ACTIVITY

The gastric contractions that occur at 3 cpm during the mixing and emptying of meals are the result of coordinated electromechanical coupling of circular layer smooth muscle cells. We next explore the electrical and mechanical events within the smooth muscle that underlie the mechanical work performed by the stomach.

Gastric Slow Waves

Gastric slow waves are the electrical events that control gastric contractions. The slow waves result from spontaneous depolarizations of the longitudinal muscle in the region of the juncture of the fundus and body on the greater curvature (see Figure 1). The outer layer of the circular muscle layer may participate in the genesis of

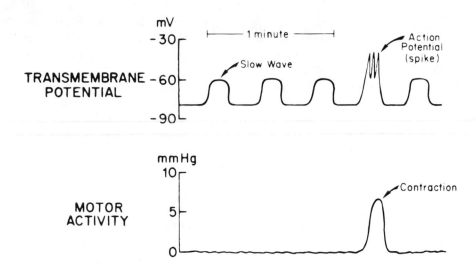

Figure 2. Relationship among slow waves, action or spike potentials, and contractile or motor activity in stomach. Rhythmic slow waves are not associated with appreciable contractile activity. In contrast, when spike potentials are linked to slow waves and occur on slow-wave plateaus, contraction of circular muscle occurs. Reprinted with permission from Feldman & Schiller, "Disorders of gastrointestinal motility associated with diabetes mellitus," *Annals of Internal Medicine,* vol. 98, pp. 378–84. Copyright 1983 American College of Physicians.

slow waves. From this region, the pacemaker area, the depolarization wave front moves circumferentially and distally toward the distal antrum (see Figure 1). The normal slow-wave frequency in humans is 3 cpm (Abell & Malagelada 1985; Couturier et al. 1972; Hamilton et al. 1986; Hinder & Kelly 1977; Kwong et al. 1970). The slow wave does not move into the fundic area, which is electrically silent. The slow wave is a spontaneous event, sodium-mediated and omnipresent, that is associated with very low-amplitude contractile activity (Morgan, Schmalz, & Szurszewski 1978; You & Chey 1984).

The slow wave coordinates the frequency and propagation velocity of gastric contractions in the body antrum. That is, the slow wave brings the circular muscle layer near the point of depolarization; if physical, neural, and/or hormonal signals are appropriate for contraction, then the depolarization threshold is reached and circular muscle contraction occurs (Figure 2). Because circular muscle contractions are linked with the slow wave, the circular muscle contractions occur at the slow-wave frequency (3 cpm in humans) and the contractions propagate at the slow-wave velocity (0.8–4 cm/sec). For these reasons the slow waves have also been referred to as pacesetter potentials and electrical control activity (Meyer 1987; Roman & Gonella 1987).

Slow waves are considered myogenic phenomena, but extrinsic neural input may modulate the rhythmicity of depolarization. For example, after vagotomy in dogs and humans, the slow-wave frequency may be disrupted for

weeks (Kelly, Code, & Elveback 1969; Stoddard, Smallwood, & Duthie 1981). The precise origins and controls of slow-wave activity are unknown.

Gastric Spike Potentials

The electrical events underlying circular smooth muscle contractions are plateau and spike potentials (see Figure 2). Depolarizations of the circular muscle, in contrast to the longitudinal muscle, are very fast (i.e. spikes). The spikes may or may not occur on plateau potentials, which are associated with the slow wave. The spikes reflect fluxes of calcium passing through the circular muscle membrane. Contractions of the circular muscle may increase tone and/or intraluminal pressure, particularly if they form concentric ring contractions. Such strong contractions may be recorded with strain gauges, intraluminal pressure transducers, or perfused catheters. Gastric contractions that are not concentric may be difficult to record using intraluminal devices, but they can be recorded by strain gauges positioned on the muscle itself (You & Chey 1984).

In summary, gastric slow waves are present at all times and control the frequency and propagation velocity of spike potentials (i.e., circular muscle contractions) when the latter are elicited by the appropriate stimuli. Gastric slow waves and spike potentials are the myoelectric components of gastric contractions. It is these contractions that perform the work of mixing and emptying foodstuffs. Slow waves and spike potentials from the stomach may be recorded from electrodes sewn to the serosa or from electrodes applied to the gastric mucosa. Because slow waves occur within a conducting medium (i.e., the body), they are also recorded with fidelity from electrodes positioned on the skin – that is, via EGG (Abell & Malagelada 1985; Brown et al. 1975; Familoni et al. 1987; Hamilton et al. 1986). Figure 3 shows gastric myoelectric activity recorded from serosal and cutaneous electrodes during motor quiescence (Figure 3A) and during gastric peristalsis (Figure 3B).

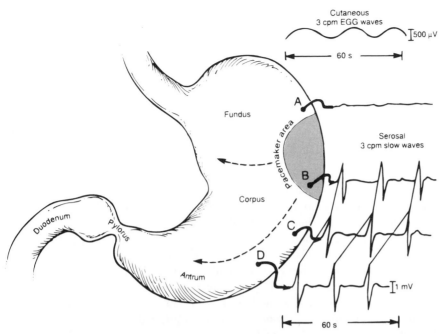

Figure 3A. Gastric myoelectrical activity during motor quiescence. The antral peristaltic contractions that produce flow of gastric content are controlled by gastric electrical slow waves. The fundus does not have pacemaker activity, as shown by electrode A. Pacesetter potentials begin in the pacemaker area located in the proximal gastric body along the greater curve, as shown by the gray area. Slow waves spread circumferentially and distally from the pacemaker region and migrate through the antrum (as shown by serosal electrodes B, C, D). The slow wave migration ends at the pylorus. As the slow wave dissolves in the terminal antrum, another slow wave begins to migrate distally from the pacemaker region. Thus, as shown in the figure, three slow waves will propagate from proximal to distal stomach every 60 sec (yielding 3-cpm slow waves). As shown in A, the cutaneous electrogastrogram (EGG) reflects the dipole created by the migrating slow wave, which occurs every 20 sec. Reprinted with permission from Koch & Stern, "Electrogastrography," in Kumar & Wingate (Eds.), *An Illustrated Guide to Gastrointestinal Motility*, pp. 290–307. Copyright 1993 Churchill Communications Europe.

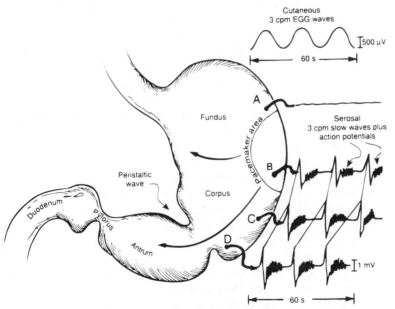

Figure 3B. Gastric myoelectrical activity during gastric peristalsis. Action potentials occur during gastric circular muscle contraction; these potentials are linked to the gastric slow waves or pacesetter potentials, as shown in the extracellular recordings from the serosa electrodes (B, C, D). As the slow wave linked with action potentials migrates distally along the gastric body and antrum, one gastric peristaltic wave occurs and one EGG wave is recorded, as measured from the surface electrodes. Thus, gastric peristalses normally occur at a rate of 3 cpm. During gastric peristaltic contractions, the EGG amplitude is generally increased (compared with Figure 3A). Reprinted with permission from Koch & Stern, "Electrogastrography," in Kumar & Wingate (Eds.), *An Illustrated Guide to Gastrointestinal Motility*, pp. 290–307. Copyright 1993 Churchill Communications Europe.

Psychological Context

MEASUREMENT MILIEU

Subjects are instructed what and when to eat prior to an EGG recording session, since the contents of the stomach will affect the EGG. For most studies, subjects are instructed to fast for at least four hours prior to the experimental session. In other studies, subjects are asked to come to the lab after an overnight fast and are given a standard small breakfast (e.g., two pieces of toast and juice). When the subject arrives at the lab, the procedure required to record EGG is explained as part of the total information needed by the subject in order to give informed consent. Many subjects show apprehension when told that electrodes will be applied to the skin of their abdomen. Some of the apprehension may be caused by concerns about evaluation, but two other factors that are frequently expressed by the subjects are fear of electric shock from the electrodes (a problem in all psychophysiological studies) and embarrassment at having hair on the abdomen shaved, the area abraded, and electrodes applied. An attempt is made to reduce evaluation apprehension and to ensure the subject that he or she cannot receive a shock. To reduce possible embarrassment, female experimenters apply EGG electrodes to female subjects.

APPLICATIONS OF EGG RECORDING TO PSYCHOLOGY AND MEDICINE

Applications that have been described in the psychological and medical literature to date include the following areas: eating, stress and anxiety, motion sickness, and GI disorders.

Eating and Sham Feeding

A number of investigators have reported effects of nutrient meals on EGG patterns. Yogurt or pancake meals increase the amplitude of the 3-cpm EGG wave – as we would expect, since the presence of food in the stomach is the natural stimulus for it to contract (Geldof, van der Schee, & Grashuis 1986). Initially, the increase in amplitude occurs at a slower frequency, 2.2–2.5 cpm (a so-called frequency dip); after approximately 10–15 min, the EGG frequency gradually shifts back to the 3-cpm range. Smout, van der Schee, and Grashuis (1980b) and Jones and Jones (1985) reported finding similar increases in the amplitude of the 3-cpm EGG following eating. Ingestion of whole milk has also been shown to increase the amplitude of 3-cpm EGG waves (Hamilton et al. 1986). A technetium-labeled omelet meal evokes a complex series of events, including increased 3-cpm waves in the first 15 min after ingestion and a subsequent increase in the 1–2-cpm EGG activity during the linear phase of gastric emptying (Koch et al. 1991b). Uijtdehaage, Stern, and Koch (1992) reported that eating a small breakfast not only increased the power of normal 3-cpm EGG but also increased respiratory sinus arrhythmia (a measure of parasympathetic nervous system activity) and inhibited motion sickness symptoms. Nonnutrient meals such as water loads also stimulate 3-cpm waves of increased amplitude and a brief frequency dip (Koch & Stern 1993).

More recently, Chen, Davenport, and McCallum (1993a) investigated the effect of a fat preload on gastric myoelectric activity in healthy humans using EGG. They reported that fat preload significantly decreased the postprandial 3-cpm EGG amplitude, implying a decrease in gastric contractility. In a related study, Chen and colleagues (1995) looked at the effect of cholecystokinin (CCK) on postprandial gastric myoelectric activity. It is generally accepted that CCK released endogenously by a meal delays gastric emptying and inhibits additional eating. Chen et al. (1995) found that CCK given at a physiological concentration significantly decreased postprandial EGG amplitude, as did a fat preload, but did not affect the frequency or regularity of the EGG.

Stern and associates (1989) used a sham feeding procedure to examine the cephalic-vagal reflex, a response that was mentioned in the introduction to this chapter. Previous research by several authors had shown that food or even the presence of nonnutritive substances in the stomach stimulate an increase in the amplitude of the 3-cpm EGG. The question asked by Stern and colleagues was whether the sight, smell, and taste of food would do the same thing to the EGG. Following a 15-min baseline period, subjects were required to chew and expectorate a hot dog and roll. After another baseline period, subjects were given a second hot dog to eat normally. The effect on the EGG of eating the hot dog was, as expected, a large increase in the amplitude of the 3-cpm EGG wave that lasted several minutes. The effect on the EGG of sham feeding was an equally large but short-lasting increase in the amplitude of the EGG, as can be seen in Figure 4A. Figure 4A depicts this finding for one subject in the form of a running spectral analysis: EGG frequency is plotted on the x axis, time is plotted on the y axis, and power or spectral intensity is the third dimension. Spectral analysis will be described in more detail in the section entitled "Quantification of the EGG." It was of interest to note that two subjects who later reported that the experience of chewing and expectorating the hot dog was "disgusting" showed a decrease rather than an increase in the amplitude of their EGG during sham feeding (see Figure 4B).

Following this serendipitous finding, we conducted another study (Jokerst et al. 1997) in which one group of subjects was given pleasant food (a cooked hot dog) to chew and spit, whereas a second group was given an unpleasant food – an uncooked tofu dog – to chew and spit. The hot-dog group showed a significant increase in 3-cpm activity and the tofu group did not. This result supported

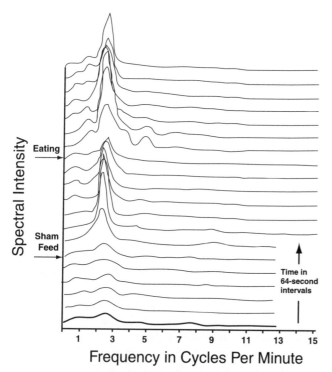

Figure 4A. Running spectral analysis of the EGG of a subject who reported that the experience of sham feeding was not disgusting. Note the low level of activity at approximately 2.5 cpm before sham feeding and the increase in power during sham feeding and during eating. Redrawn with permission from Stern, Crawford, Stewart, Vasey, & Koch, "Sham feeding: Cephalic-vagal influences on gastric myoelectric activity," *Digestive Diseases and Sciences*, vol. 34, pp. 521–7. Copyright 1989 Plenum Publishing Corp.

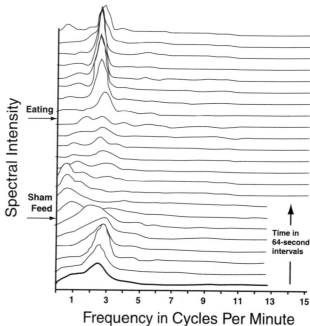

Figure 4B. Running spectral analysis of the EGG from a subject who reported that the experience of sham feeding was disgusting. This subject showed an increase in power at approximately 2.8 cpm before sham feeding and a decrease during sham feeding. The subject showed the typical increase in power during eating. Redrawn with permission from Stern, Crawford, Stewart, Vasey, & Koch, "Sham feeding: Cephalic-vagal influences on gastric myoelectric activity," *Digestive Diseases and Sciences*, vol. 34, pp. 521–7. Copyright 1989 Plenum Publishing Corp.

our initial finding that the cephalic-vagal reflex, as measured by the power in the EGG 3-cpm wave, depends on the subjective palatability of the food. We think that this is a good example of the sensitivity of the EGG to cognitive processing. A potential application of this finding is to use the EGG response to the sham feeding of pleasant food to track the progress during therapy of individuals with eating disorders. Assuming that subjects with certain types of eating disorders cognitively appraise eating as less than pleasant, we would expect them *not* to show an increase in EGG 3-cpm activity during sham feeding. Quantification of the cephalic-vagal reflex, as measured by the EGG 3-cpm activity, might provide a more valid measure of recovery than weight gain or the judgment of a therapist.

Do patients with anorexia nervosa or unexplained nausea and vomiting respond with an increase in the amplitude of their 3-cpm EGG following the actual eating of pleasant food? Abell and associates (1985a) have reported that several of their anorexic subjects failed to show an increase in amplitude of their 3-cpm EGG following eating, and some showed tachygastria (4–9 cpm). Geldof and colleagues (1983) found that 49% of their patients with unexplained nausea and vomiting showed tachygastria as well as the

absence of the normal increase in EGG amplitude after eating.

Stress, Pain, and Mood

At the beginning of this chapter we raised the question of why many people report GI symptoms when they are under stress. We think of the GI system as a buffer between an individual and his or her environment. When extra energy is needed for fight or flight, the GI system slows down or shuts down, and not only fight or flight but also anxieties and worries slow down our GI system. In terms of the activity of the autonomic nervous system (one of the pathways for communication between the brain and the GI system), fight, flight, anxiety, and worry are all usually associated with an increase in activity in the sympathetic branch (SNS) of the autonomic nervous system. Numerous studies have shown that an increase in SNS activity decreases stomach activity; conversely, stomach activity increases in response to increases in activity in the parasympathetic branch (PNS) of the autonomic nervous system. The cephalic-vagal reflex is an example of this relationship. However, one complication is that not much is known about the changes in PNS activity that are associated with different psychological states for different people or about the relationship between SNS and PNS activity. For a discussion of this important issue see the paper by Berntson et al. (1994). As we will see in the examples that follow, some individuals in a particular stress situation might show an increase in SNS and little change in PNS (or even an increase in PNS) activity whereas, in a different stress situation, some individuals might show an increase in SNS activity and a decrease in PNS activity. We should remember that the normal functioning of the GI system is not crucial for momentary survival, as is the case with the cardiovascular system. Wide swings in functioning of the GI system have been documented, and these extreme responses may be perceived as GI symptoms.

Stewart (1987) studied the effects of brief exposure to two laboratory stressors on EGG activity. In this experiment, 42 fasted undergraduates were subjected to two days of laboratory stress testing. A computer-paced version of the Stroop color–word conflict task served as the stressor task for one session and was matched with reading a history essay as an innocuous control task. Viewing an industrial training film that depicted a series of three mutilating injuries served as the other stressor task; it was matched with viewing a documentary on the modern Olympics as its control task. Stroop stress produced an attenuation of EGG 3-cpm activity but no change in level of tachygastria activity. The stress film produced no change in either 3-cpm or tachygastria power. Subjective reports of stress, arousal, gastric, and somatic symptoms all showed marked increases following involvement with the stress but not control tasks.

Muth and associates (1998) studied the effect on the EGG of two tasks, reaction time–shock avoidance and cold face stress. As expected, the reaction time (RT) task produced shorter cardiac interbeat intervals (IBIs) than baseline, and placing a cool bag of water on the face produced longer IBIs than baseline. These manipulation checks supported the experimenters' assumption that the RT task would increase SNS activity while the cold face stress would increase PNS activity. Analyses of the EGG data indicated that there was significantly greater normal 3-cpm activity during the cold face stress than during the RT task. Moreover, there was greater tachygastria during RT than during the cold face stress. These findings are in agreement with the results of motion sickness studies (see next section), which have shown that increased PNS activity increases 3-cpm EGG activity and decreases symptoms of motion sickness. On the other hand, subjects who experience motion sickness show an increase in SNS activity, a decrease in PNS activity, and tachygastria (Stern & Koch 1994).

Stern and colleagues (1991) examined the effects of another stressor, the cold pressor test, on EGG activity. The procedure used was similar to that used by Thompson, Richelson, and Malagelada (1982), who reported a significant decrease in gastric emptying as a response to cold stress. In our experiment, subjects who had recently eaten were asked to put their hand into a container of ice water (4°C) for 1 min, take it out for 15 sec, put it back for 1 min, and so on, for a total of 20 min. The results were similar to those reported by Stewart (1987) for the effects of the Stroop stress and were what would be predicted by the gastric emptying results of Thompson et al. (1982). There was a significant attenuation of EGG 3-cpm activity starting the moment the subject's hand was immersed in ice water (see Figure 5). Tachygastria was not seen as a response to the cold pressor test, a procedure that induces pain and not just stress.

Changes in EGG as a function of the subject's mood is a relatively unexplored area, which is somewhat surprising since there have been many articles written suggesting that emotional functioning (or mood) is closely related to motor hyper- and/or hypoactivity in the GI system, particularly the stomach. In a preliminary study, Stewart, Chen, and McCallum (1991) used the Profile of Mood States to examine the relationship between positive and negative mood states and the 3-cpm amplitude. They reported that more than half of the variance in amplitude of the 3-cpm activity was accounted for by current mood functioning, with relatively lower amplitude associated with negative mood states such as depression and greater amplitude related to positive mood states such as vigor. This was a follow-up to a previous study (Stewart, Hurm, & Valenzuela 1989) in which the authors reported finding that low positive affect was significantly correlated with delayed gastric emptying.

Figure 5. Running spectral analysis of the EGG of a subject who put his hand in cold water. Note the inhibition of 3-cpm power when the subject put his hand in the ice water and the gradual recovery. Reprinted with permission from Stern, Vasey, Hu, & Koch, "Effects of cold stress on gastric myoelectic activity," *Journal of Gastrointestinal Motility,* vol. 3, pp. 225–8. Copyright 1991 Blackwell Science Ltd.

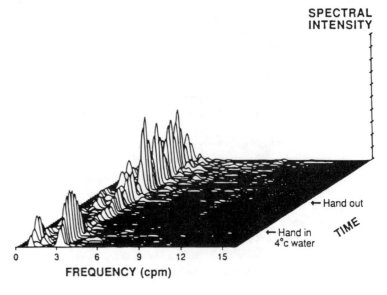

SPECTRAL INTENSITY

← Hand out

← Hand in 4°c water

TIME

FREQUENCY (cpm)

0   3   6   9   12   15

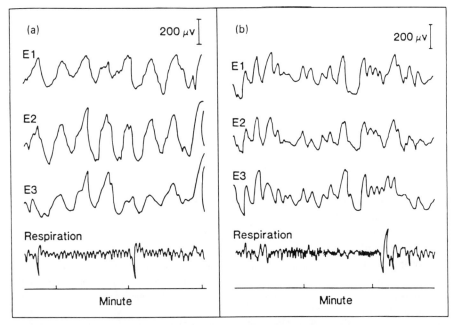

Figure 6A. (a) EGG activity recorded from upper, middle, and lower electrodes (E1–E3) prior to drum rotation; the EGG frequency is 3 cpm. (b) EGG from same subject after start of drum rotation. Note presence of tachygastria (6 cpm). Tachygastria began at 4 min; subject reported nausea at 6 min and requested that drum rotation be stopped at 11 min. Reprinted with permission from Stern, Koch, Leibowitz, Lindblad, Shupert, & Stewart, "Tachygastria and motion sickness," *Aviation Space and Environmental Medicine,* vol. 56, pp. 1074–7. Copyright 1985.

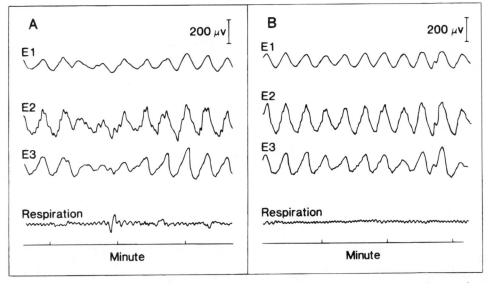

Figure 6B. (A) The EGG activity prior to drum rotation; the EGG frequency is 3 cpm. (B) The EGG from the same subject 7 min after start of drum rotation. Subject reported no symptoms of motion sickness, and EGG frequency remained at 3 cpm during 15 min of drum rotation. Reprinted with permission from Stern, Koch, Leibowitz, Lindblad, Shupert, & Stewart, "Tachygastria and motion sickness," *Aviation Space and Environmental Medicine,* vol. 56, pp. 1074–7. Copyright 1985.

Motion Sickness

In the first experiment attempting to relate changes in gastric myoelectric activity to the development of symptoms of motion sickness, Stern and associates (1985) obtained EGGs from 21 healthy human subjects who were seated within an optokinetic drum, the rotation of which produced vection (illusory self-motion). Fourteen subjects developed symptoms of motion sickness during vection, and in each the EGG frequency shifted from the normal 3 cpm to 4–9 cpm (tachygastria). An EGG recording for one of these subjects is shown in Figure 6A. In six of seven asymptomatic subjects, the 3-cpm EGG pattern was unchanged during vection; a portion of one of these EGG recordings is shown in Figure 6B. It was concluded that the sensory mismatch created by the illusory self-motion produced tachygastria and symptoms of motion sickness in susceptible subjects. In a follow-up study (Stern et al. 1987), 15 healthy subjects were exposed to the rotation of the same drum. Ten subjects showed a shift of the dominant frequency of their EGG from 3 cpm to 4–9 cpm during drum rotation and reported symptoms of motion sickness. A comparison of running spectral analyses and symptom reports revealed a close correspondence over time between tachygastria and the development of symptoms of motion sickness.

One of the most common symptoms of motion sickness is nausea, so it is interesting to note that, during tachygastria, gastric motility decreases or even completely shuts down. The reason why this is of interest is that Wolf (1943) showed that stressful situations (e.g., putting cold water in one ear, swinging, rotating the head, and situations involving fear) inhibited gastric motor activity *and* provoked nausea. (The advantage of our current use of the EGG in similar studies is that it is noninvasive; Wolf's subjects had a balloon positioned in their stomach to record gastric pressure changes.) Wolf grappled with a problem inherent in all studies that relate some bodily change to a sensation – in his case, the relationship of inhibited gastric motor activity to the sensation of nausea. To what extent is the altered bodily change essential to the occurrence of the sensation? In a series of ingenious experiments (albeit with only three subjects), Wolf gave his subjects a combination of two drugs that prevented the inhibition of gastric motor activity, exposed the subjects to stress situations that had previously provoked nausea, and found that no nausea was reported. Wolf concluded as follows: "The fact that nausea may be prevented, despite strong nauseating stimuli, by controlling with drugs the pattern of gastric motility indicates that gastric relaxation and hypomotility are essential to the occurrence of nausea" (1943, p. 882).

In our lab, 50% of healthy European-American and African-American subjects and 80%–90% of Asian and Asian-American subjects developed tachygastria and motion sickness while sitting inside a rotating optokinetic drum. We have studied this differential susceptibility to motion sickness for over ten years and recently published a review article that summarizes our findings (Stern & Koch 1996).

GI Disorders

Russian investigators have been using the EGG to diagnose GI disorders since the 1960s (e.g., Krapivin & Chernin 1967; Sobakin, Smirnov, & Mishin 1962). More recently, a group of French investigators (Murat et al. 1985) reported the successful application of the EGG to the study of digestive pathology. Gaultier and Baille (1982) used biofeedback of the EGG to increase the rate of gastric emptying. According to the authors, twelve training sessions were necessary before the patients improved enough to be taken off medication. In China, an electrogastrograph designed and manufactured at Anhui College of Traditional Chinese Medicine has been used in numerous hospitals and clinics and on more than 1,000 patients to diagnose GI disorders and to measure the therapeutic effects of acupuncture (Xu & Zhou 1983).

Figure 7. EGGs and running spectral analyses from a patient with diabetic gastroparesis, nausea, and vomiting. Part A (month 0) shows a flatline pattern EGG signal (inset) and 6-cpm peaks in the spectral plot (baseline) when patient had significant nausea; Part B (month 6) shows a 3-cpm EGG pattern in the same patient after six months of treatment with domperidone. Many regular peaks at 3 cpm are seen in the running spectral plot. The patient's symptoms resolved. Reprinted with permission from Koch, Stern, Stewart, & Vasey, "Gastric emptying and gastric myoelectrical activity in patients with diabetic gastroparesis: Effect of long-term domperidone treatment," *American Journal of Gastroenterology*, vol. 84, pp. 1069–75. Copyright 1989.

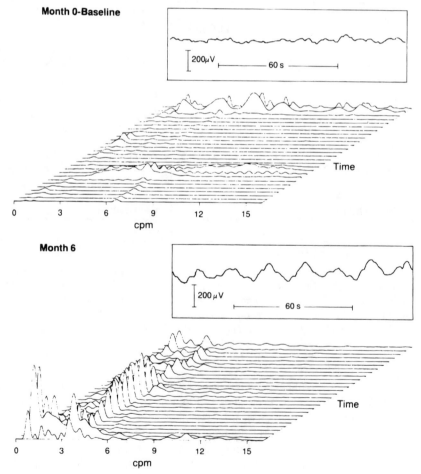

During the past decade, the most significant contribution of EGG recording to gastroenterology has been the finding that acute or chronic gastric dysrhythmias (such as tachygastrias or bradygastrias) appear to be markers of gastric neuromuscular dysfunction from diverse causes. Some of the clinical syndromes in which tachygastrias have been recorded are described next.

Gastroparesis

Obstructive Gastroparesis. Gastroparesis due to a fixed obstructive lesion, such as pyloric outlet obstruction or duodenal obstruction from peptic disease due to adhesions, has been associated with normal 3-cpm EGG activity (Koch et al. 1991a). In these cases of obstructive lesions, the normal 3-cpm gastric myoelectrical activity suggested the possibility that the gastroparesis was *not* due to neural or muscular dysfunction. Thus, a 3-cpm EGG pattern in a patient with documented gastroparesis suggests the possibility of a mechanical cause of the gastroparesis.

Diabetic Gastroparesis. Tachygastrias have been recorded in patients with symptomatic diabetic gastroparesis. Koch and colleagues (1989) showed that treatment with domperidone, a prokinetic drug, converted gastric dysrhythmias to normal 3-cpm EGG rhythms (see Figure 7). This pharmacologic "gastroversion" from tachygastria and bradygastria to normal 3-cpm gastric electrical activity was associated with significant improvement in symptoms. Hamilton et al. (1986) recorded gastric dysrhythmias in some diabetics who exhibited no upper gastrointestinal symptoms, but Abell et al. (1991) found many tachygastrias that were associated with gastroparesis. Further studies are needed to determine the gastric electrical and contractile activities in diabetics with and without gastroparesis.

Idiopathic Gastroparesis. Tachygastrias have been recorded with mucosal electrodes in patients with idiopathic gastroparesis (Bortolotti et al. 1990). These electrical recordings were obtained in the fasting state. Tachygastrias during fasting and also after a water load were reported in patients with idiopathic gastroparesis (Koch et al. 1992). We have observed that metoclopramide converts tachygastria associated with idiopathic gastroparesis to a normal 3-cpm electrical activity and that cisapride converts bradygastria to normal 3-cpm EGG patterns.

Ischemic Gastroparesis. Tachygastria and gastroparesis due to chronic mesenteric ischemia were described in two patients by Liberski and colleagues (1990). The gastric dysrhythmia and gastroparesis were completely reversed following mesenteric revascularization. In five additional patients, the gastric dysrhythmias converted to a normal 3-cpm rhythm and gastric emptying became normal within three to six months after revascularization (unpublished observations).

Intestinal Pseudo-Obstruction.

This term comprises a diverse variety of disorders involving damage to the muscular and/or neural elements of the gastrointestinal tract. Tachygastrias have been reported in the neuropathic form of intestinal pseudo-obstruction in children, and EGG recordings from the myopathic form have revealed chaotic gastric tachyarrhythmias (Bisset, Devane, & Milla 1989). In an adolescent with intestinal pseudo-obstruction, regular 9-cpm tachygastrias were recorded when gastroparesis was present; treatment with metoclopramide resulted in improved symptoms, conversion of the tachygastria to a predominant 3-cpm gastric electrical pattern, and normalization of gastric emptying.

Nausea of Pregnancy and Hyperemesis Gravidarum.

Tachygastrias were found in the majority of 32 women who had nausea during the first trimester of pregnancy (Koch et al. 1990). The four pregnant women who did not have nausea on the study day had normal 3-cpm myoelectrical activity. Furthermore, six women returned for EGG recordings after their deliveries; their EGGs showed normal 3-cpm rhythm compared with gastric dysrhythmias and nausea during the first trimester.

Functional Dyspepsia – Dysmotility Type (with Normal Gastric Emptying).

The symptoms of functional dyspepsia are vague and include early satiety, upper abdominal discomfort, nausea, and the absence of any obvious cause for these symptoms. Thirty to fifty percent of these patients have gastric dysrhythmias and delayed gastric emptying. Koch et al. (1992) reported that 9 of 13 subjects with functional dyspepsia and *normal* gastric emptying studies had gastric dysrhythmias; two had tachygastrias and seven had bradygastrias. Gastric dysrhythmias have been reported in children with functional dyspepsia, and in many cases cisapride treatment converted the gastric dysrhythmias to normal 3-cpm signals (Cucchiara et al. 1992).

Gastric Ulcers.

Many patients with gastric ulceration have upper abdominal burning discomfort. Some patients also have considerable nausea associated with gastric ulcers. Geldof and colleagues (1989) showed that patients with acute gastric ulcers and nausea had tachygastrias (as recorded with cutaneous electrodes), whereas those subjects with no nausea had normal 3-cpm rhythms.

Inferential Context

QUANTIFICATION OF THE EGG
Early Attempts

R. C. Davis developed procedures for hand-scoring EGG records in 30-sec segments for amplitude, frequency, and displacement (see Russell & Stern 1967 for details). Amplitude was the favored measure in precomputer times because deviations were more obvious than with other measures. We are still interested in the amplitude of the EGG, but we must caution the reader that it does vary from subject to subject and, within the same subject, from site to site; also, the interpretation of EGG amplitude changes is still controversial (Dubois & Mizrahi 1994; Mintchev & Bowes 1996; Mintchev, Kingma, & Bowes 1993). Frequency is of greatest interest to contemporary workers in this area, and spectral analysis will be discussed in the next section. "Displacement" was Davis's term for very slow changes in the EGG. We now believe that some of what Davis called displacement was caused by inadequate techniques (e.g., electrode or amplifier drift) and some was ultraslow-wave activity, 0.5–2.0 cpm. Several investigators have noted the presence of ultraslow-wave activity in the EGG (e.g. Hölzl, Loffler, & Muller 1985; Stern et al. 1987).

Spectral Analysis

Spectral analysis typically uses the fast Fourier transform (FFT) to convert a signal in the time domain into the frequency domain. The FFT uses a series of coefficients describing the amplitudes and phase relationships of its independent sinusoidal waveforms. This transformation is analogous to a prism transforming white light into the visible spectrum of colors.

The output of a spectral analysis is the squared magnitude of the Fourier transform and is typically graphed as a curve showing the strength, or power, of the frequencies into which the original signal can be decomposed. Although power has a very specific meaning in mathematics and physics, we may think of it as an index of the amplitude of the sine waves of a particular frequency that would be required in order to re-create the EGG record. In the analysis of EGG recordings, we are usually interested in the power within the following three frequency bands: 0–2.25, 2.5–3.5, and 3.75–9.75 cycles per minute. The exact cut-offs for these bands vary in the literature because the frequency resolution (bin-width) of the FFT is equal to the sampling rate divided by the number of samples in a window. Hence, varying sampling rates and window size will produce slightly different bandwidths based on the spectral resolution in the frequency domain. The first frequency band represents the often found but poorly understood ultraslow rhythm referred to as bradygastria. The second encompasses the normal electrical rhythm of the healthy human gastric antrum (3 cpm). The third includes frequencies commonly associated with nausea and is referred to as tachygastria when regular and gastric tachyrhythmia when dysrhythmic.

Spectral analysis is currently the most commonly used method of analyzing the EGG (see Smallwood & Brown 1983) and the method favored by the authors. Van der Schee et al. (1982) described an extension of this method that makes use of running spectral analysis to depict EGG data. Running spectral analysis, with overlapping power spectra displayed as a function of time, yields both frequency and time information. The more conventional spectral analysis provides power only as a function of frequency, not time. With running spectral analysis, frequency, power, and time can all be depicted two-dimensionally with either a pseudo-3D display or a grayscale plot. Figures 4, 5, and 7 show examples of pseudo-3D displays.

A brief description follows of the procedure used to transform raw EGG data into a pseudo-3D display. The first step in any quantification procedure is to ensure that quality data are being analyzed. In fact, Kingma (1989) argues that high-quality analysis techniques are available for analyzing the EGG yet high quality recordings are often lacking. Hence, time must be taken to ensure the quality of EGG recordings before complex analysis procedures are undertaken. Because of the relatively slow electrical changes that are associated with EGG, only a very electrically stable electrode can be used; silver–silver chloride (Ag–AgCl) electrodes are recommended. The optimal recording sites will depend on the nature of the signal desired: for example, largest possible amplitude; lowest artifact from ECG, respiration, and subject movement; or position of the subject's internal organs, particularly the antrum of the stomach and the diaphragm (Mirizzi & Scafoglieri 1983). For single-channel recording of most subjects, the greatest EGG amplitude will be obtained with bipolar electrodes: one electrode on the subject's left side, approximately 6 cm from the midline and just below the lowest rib, and the other on the midline just above the umbilicus. The location of these electrodes will not affect the frequency of the EGG but will affect the amplitude and waveform.

The amplifying and recording system should filter out signals below 0.5 cpm and above 15 cpm. With these filter settings one can record ultraslow rhythms (0.5–2.0 cpm) but still eliminate shifts in baseline due to DC potentials. Frequencies higher than 30 cpm are filtered out to avoid domination of the gastric signal by ECG. Respiration can also obscure the EGG since its frequency range falls near that of tachygastria. Rather than remove respiratory signals with analog filters at the time of the recording, it is preferable to remove them later with more precise and flexible digital filters or by using a separate respiration tracing to visually select and exclude data that contain respiration artifact.

From the polygraph the EGG signal is channeled to an analog-to-digital (A-D) converter, where it is digitized into a series of numerical values representing discrete voltage levels of the input signal. Thus, the analog EGG signal is converted to a digital time series that can then be subjected to a wide range of analyses. The A-D conversion units typically allow sampling at a wide range of speeds. Given an EGG signal that has had frequencies faster than 15 cpm or 0.25 Hz attenuated at the time of recording, a sampling rate of at least 1 Hz is required. Since most FFT procedures require a number of points equal to a power of 2, a noninteger sampling rate may be chosen to fulfill this requirement. For example, a sampling rate of

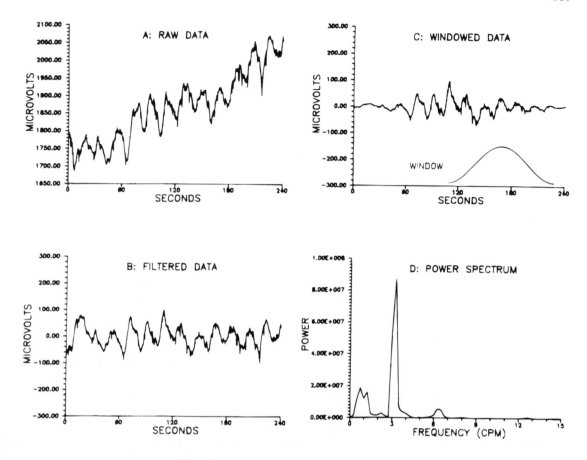

4.267 Hz yields 256 data points per minute. However, today's computers are capable of calculating more complex discrete or prime factor algorithms that allow for a wider variety of sampling rates. In any case, we recommend a sampling rate of at least 4 Hz because of the potential for aliasing the high-frequency components (such as ECG) that may be present in the EGG. Even when the EGG signal is subjected to a high-frequency filter with a relatively low cut-off (e.g. 0.25 Hz), some ECG may still be present, though greatly attenuated. A high sampling rate (e.g. 4.267 Hz) allows complete resolution of all frequencies remaining in the EGG and thus prevents aliasing of these frequencies.

Once the EGG signal has been digitized, it must be pre-processed in order to best meet the assumptions of spectral analysis. Because the dominant frequency in the EGG is relatively slow, we recommend the use of at least 4-min data windows. Thus, at 4.267 samples per second, a 4-min segment would be composed of 1,024 data points. It is generally desirable in spectral analysis to center data around a mean of zero. This is easily accomplished by subtracting the mean of the segment from each data point. Additionally, the EGG is likely to contain some very slow components that reflect a shifting baseline or other undetermined factors. Such extremely low frequency shifts and simple linear trends should be removed to provide a clean spectrum. A high-pass digital filter that attenuates frequen-

Figure 8. (A) Raw EGG segment showing slow drift in baseline. (B) Same segment after zero centering and removal of slow drift via high-pass filtering. (C) Segment after Hamming window was applied (Hamming window is shown below windowed waveform). (D) Power spectrum of windowed data segment. Reprinted with permission from Stern, Koch, & Vasey, "The gastrointestinal system," in Cacioppo & Tassinary (Eds.), *Principles of Psychophysiology*. Copyright 1990 Cambridge University Press.

cies below 0.01 Hz will effect such trend removal. One can also remove simple linear trends by fitting a least-squares regression line and subtracting it from the data segment.

Figure 8 illustrates the processing of the EGG. A raw digitized EGG segment of 4-min duration and composed of 1,024 data points is presented in part A. This data segment shows an obvious baseline shift. The segment was first zero-centered and then the baseline shift was removed using a high-pass filter (part B). Next, this data segment was windowed in order to reduce leakage (part C). Windowing is the application of a weighting function that tapers the beginning and end of the data segment to zero. Thus, the middle of the segment is unaltered, or multiplied by a weight of 1, while the ends are multiplied by weights that gradually approach zero. This is necessary because there is leakage in the power spectrum when a signal terminates abruptly. The window shown in part C of the figure gradually tapers a signal to zero at each end of the segment and greatly reduces this leakage. The window applied in this example is a Hamming window, but many other windows may be chosen depending on the characteristics of the signal (see Lin & Chen 1994 for a discussion of various windowing techniques for use with EGG). Generally, such windows as the Hamming, Hanning, and Tukey–Blackman all provide comparable results when used with the EGG.

After pre-processing, the data segment is Fourier transformed and the spectral density estimates are calculated. The spectrum of our data segment is shown in part D of Figure 8. These density estimates reflect the power at the various frequency components of the data segment. In our example, this Fourier transformation provides 512 power estimates for the frequency range 0–2.134 Hz, which yields resolution of frequencies at intervals of 0.0042 Hz or 0.25 cpm. These values were derived because spectral analysis provides information on frequencies only up to half the sampling rate, which was 4.267 Hz in the example. These estimates may be averaged together to provide more stable estimates of power.

In order to produce a running spectral analysis, one overlaps consecutive data segments by, for example, 75%. In other words, segment 1 includes minutes 1–4, segment 2 includes minutes 2–5, and so forth. Thus, one minute of new information is provided in each consecutive power spectrum. These overlapping power spectra can be plotted in a pseudo-3D fashion to allow easy viewing of changes in power at various frequencies as a function of time (see Figures 4, 5, and 7).

Running spectral analyses do provide a useful way to view frequency and power changes over time, but it is important to note that transient changes in the EGG may go unnoticed if they are small. If such transient changes are large enough then they will be evident, but only as a gradual change and with the peak in spectral density appearing in the pseudo-3D display several minutes after it occurred in real time. Thus, running spectral analysis may not be appropriate for experiments in which very short-duration, stimulus-induced changes are expected. For such cases, adaptive spectral analysis methods are recommended (Chen & McCallum 1991; Chen, Stewart, & McCallum 1993c; Chen et al. 1990; Lin & Chen 1994).

Similarly, spectral analysis is useful only when the EGG signal contains a significant amount of cyclical activity. This is usually the case for 3-cpm activity. However, some gastric phenomena occur intermittently and may not appear in a spectral plot. This is not a problem for most studies examining only the 3-cpm activity, because any segment of normal EGG is likely to contain a strong cyclical component. However, the issue is less clear for phenomena such as tachygastria. We have experienced no difficulty in quantifying this phenomenon through spectral analysis. When bursts of tachygastria are seen during motion sickness, they are typically one or more minutes in duration and are seen quite clearly in running spectral plots of 4-min epochs (Stern et al. 1987). However, there may

indeed be more appropriate methods of analysis for quantification of very brief-duration, intermittent phenomena (see e.g. Hölzl et al. 1985 for a discussion of so-called zoom FFTs and Lin & Chen 1994 for a discussion of the exponential distribution).

Once spectral power estimates have been calculated, data reduction is usually performed. Our lab typically calculates percentage of total power estimates for the bradygastria, normal 3-cpm, and tachygastria bands mentioned previously. This is accomplished by summing the power estimates for a given band, dividing this sum by the total spectral power, and multiplying by 100%. However, when looking at changes in percentage of power as a function of, say, exposure to a stressor, the calculations of percentage of 3-cpm activity and tachygastria can be grossly distorted if there is a large change in the amount of bradygastria. Various other methods of data reduction can be found in the literature. Chen and McCallum (1991) proposed focusing on the frequency peak that contains the dominant power of the EGG signal. It is possible to analyze changes not only in the power of this peak but also in the frequency of the dominant peak. Smout, Jebbink, and Samsom (1994) suggested an instability factor, which is essentially a measure of the frequency variability of this dominant peak. The best method for reducing the EGG frequency and power data obtained from an FFT is still unsettled. All the methods mentioned here have merit, so in most cases it will depend on the question to be answered. No matter what analysis method is used, it is critical that quality raw recordings be obtained with high signal-to-noise ratio. In addition, data from healthy subjects during normal psychophysiological states should be recorded for comparison purposes.

RELATIONSHIP OF THE EGG TO GASTRIC MYOELECTRIC ACTIVITY AND GASTRIC MOTOR ACTIVITY

EGG and Gastric Myoelectric Activity

Nelsen and Kohatsu (1968) simultaneously recorded EGGs and the electrical activity from electrodes implanted on the serosal surface of the stomach in 13 patients. They found an excellent correspondence between the frequency of the signals obtained from the EGG and the internal electrodes; they did not compare the amplitudes of the signals. A more recent comparison of EGG and serosal recordings from dogs (Smout et al. 1980b) indicated a perfect correspondence between the frequency of the signals.

In an effort to study the relationship of the EGG to internal electrical activity of the stomach without resort to surgery, several investigators have compared the EGG to simultaneously recorded mucosal signals, which are obtained from swallowed electrodes (i.e., electrodes inside the stomach). Hamilton and colleagues (1986) compared EGG and mucosal signals from 20 human subjects during fasting, after ingesting milk, and (in one case) during a period of spontaneous dysrhythmia. They summarized their findings as follows:

We did find that the surface recordings were of similar visual form as those obtained directly from the mucosa simultaneously. In addition, frequency analysis determined that the two simultaneously obtained signals were of the same frequency. Finally when the rare arrhythmic events occurred, they were detected in both the mucosal and cutaneous signals. Therefore, the signal obtained from the skin does seem to accurately reflect the BER as measured directly from the stomach mucosa. (1986, p. 37)

Abell and Malagelada (1985) used magnetic force to maintain internal electrodes in opposition with the gastric wall and then compared signals obtained from the mucosal electrodes with those obtained from the EGG. They also reported that frequency analysis showed very good correspondence between the internal and EGG signals. More recently, Mintchev, Otto, and Bowes (1997) made simultaneous serosal and EGG recordings from dogs in whom they had created dysrhythmias by surgical means. They reported that the EGG could be used to detect severely abnormal gastric myoelectric activity 93% of the time and mild abnormalities 74% of the time.

EGG and Gastric Motor Activity. Until the mid-1960s, investigators who used the EGG assumed that they were recording, from the surface of the skin, voltage changes that were due to the contractions of the smooth muscle of the stomach; that is, they assumed a one-to-one relationship between the EGG and the contractions of the stomach. In 1968, however, Nelsen and Kohatsu presented a different view of the source of the EGG signal. They stated that the EGG was a function of gastric slow-wave activity, or pacesetter potentials. Nelsen and Kohatsu (and others) have claimed that the surface-recorded EGG reflects the waxing and waning of pacesetter potentials of the stomach but not gastric contractions. Yet they did present evidence indicating that, when contractions do occur, they are time-locked to the slow wave and thus to the EGG.

Beginning in 1975, Smallwood and his colleagues published a number of studies (e.g. Smallwood 1978; Smallwood & Brown 1983) in which they examined the frequency of the EGG and made numerous advances in techniques for analysis of the EGG signal. In some studies (e.g. Brown et al. 1975) they compared the EGG signal with intragastric pressure recordings; their findings were the same as those of Nelsen and Kohatsu (1968). When contractions occurred, they occurred at the same frequency as the EGG signals, and whereas the EGG showed 3-cpm activity almost continuously for most subjects, contractions as recorded with intragastric pressure instruments did not.

It should be noted that the simultaneous presence of 3-cpm EGG and the absence of changes in intragastric pressure does not necessarily indicate that the EGG is unrelated to contractions, as suggested by Nelsen and Kohatsu (1968), Brown et al. (1975), and others. The possibility exists that the EGG is a more sensitive measure of gastric contractile activity than the pressure-sensitive probes. That is, the EGG may reflect increases in electrical activity (i.e., spike activity) during low-level contractile events that do not alter gastric intraluminal pressure. In fact, Vantrappen and colleagues (1983) indicated that low-amplitude 5-cpm motor activity is always present in the dog. In addition, You and Chey (1984) showed that the 5-cpm pacesetter potentials in dogs correlated well with low-amplitude contractions (recorded by strain gauges sewn to serosa) yet poorly with intraluminal pressure changes.

From 1980 to present, published reports have appeared that suggest not only that the EGG provides information about frequency of contractions but also, indeed, that the amplitude of the EGG is related to the degree of contractile activity (Smout 1980; Smout, van der Schee, & Grashuis 1980a,b). One of the major contributions of Smout and his colleagues was to point out that the amplitude of the EGG increases when a contraction occurs. They concluded that the pacesetter potential and the second potential, which is related to contractions, are reflected in the EGG. Abell, Tucker, and Malagelada (1985b) conducted a study in which they compared the EGG signal from healthy human subjects with intraluminal pressure and the electrical signal recorded from the mucosal surface of the stomach. They summarized their findings as follows: "Antral phasic pressure activity, when present, was accompanied by an increase in amplitude and/or a change in shape of both the internal and external EGG" (p. 86).

Koch and Stern (1985) reported a perfect correlation of EGG waves and peristaltic antral contractions observed during simultaneous EGG–fluoroscopy recordings in four healthy subjects. Hamilton et al. (1986) reported that fluoroscopy revealed contractions in the antrum that correlated with three- and fourfold increases in amplitude of the EGG.

The relationship of the amplitude of EGG waves to contractions is complex and not totally understood at this time. However, in addition to the studies mentioned, there is considerable indirect evidence linking amplitude changes in the EGG with strength of contractile activity. For example, in situations where increased contractile activity would be expected (e.g., eating, after swallowing barium), EGG amplitude increases (Hamilton et al. 1986; Jones & Jones 1985; Koch, Stewart, & Stern 1987). And in patients with diabetic gastroparesis, where one would expect weak contractility activity, Hamilton et al. (1986) found no increase in the amplitude of EGG after eating.

Can EGG amplitude alone be used to infer reliably the presence or absence of GI contractions? No, not at this time. It is possible that, with improved methods of measuring contractile activity, we shall later find that all myoelectric activity is accompanied by some contractile activity (see Morgan et al. 1978; Vantrappen et al. 1983; You & Chey 1984) and that the amplitude of the EGG is related to the intensity or strength of contractile activity. A significant question then becomes: Can the amplitude of the EGG be used to determine whether the accompanying gastric contractile activity is of sufficient strength to do the motor work of the stomach (i.e., mixing and propelling)?

Several investigators (e.g. Bruley des Varannes et al. 1991; Dubois & Mizrahi 1994) have examined the possibility of using the EGG as an indirect measure of gastric emptying. Chiloiro and associates (1994) simultaneously recorded gastric emptying using ultrasound and the power in the normal 3-cpm EGG from healthy subjects; the correlations ranged from 0.68 to 0.96. Other investigators (e.g. Chen, Richards, & McCallum 1993b) have demonstrated a negative relationship between the presence of dysrhythmias in the EGG and gastric emptying. And Bortolotti et al. (1990) have demonstrated the presence of tachygastria in patients suffering from idiopathic gastroparesis – that is, patients with severely delayed gastric emptying with no known cause.

In summary, the frequency of the EGG is identical to the frequency of gastric pacesetter potentials recorded from the mucosal or serosal surface of the stomach. There is, however, less general agreement as to the interpretation of the EEG amplitude. Indirect evidence from several studies has demonstrated that amplitude increases during an increase in contractile activity, but the amplitude of the EGG alone cannot be used to determine the presence or absence of contractions.

Epilogue

UNANSWERED QUESTIONS

Why *do* many people complain of GI symptoms when they are under stress? This is the question that we raised at the beginning of this chapter and one that we referred back to, but the question is still largely unanswered. During the 1940s, psychoanalytically oriented writers made two suggestions. The first was that, phylogenetically, the GI system is old and very primitive; if one is unable (for whatever reason) to express anger, fear, hatred, and the like through appropriate means, then an attempt may be made to express oneself through the GI system. The second suggestion was that, since security and sustenance often go together in infancy, if in later life security is threatened then the organ system that regulates sustenance – the GI system – may malfunction. We find both of these suggestions thought-provoking but – since neither can be empirically tested – we don't think they can help us answer the question of why people complain of GI symptoms when they are experiencing stress.

We take more of a functionalist position on this question and, as stated earlier, we think of the GI system as a sort of buffer between the organism and the environment. When extra energy is needed for fighting with or fleeing from a saber-toothed tiger, the GI system shuts down. In our lab and in others, the EGG has been used to document and quantify the shutting down of the stomach. Two distinct patterns of EGG activity have been identified that are associated with a decrease in normal motor activity of the stomach: a flat line (the absence of cyclic activity) and tachygastria. We know that tachygastria is associated with the experience of nausea, but we don't know much about the association of the absence of cyclic activity in the EGG and GI symptoms. This is an unexplored area. Perhaps symptoms are only experienced after the passage of a certain period of time. Or perhaps unpleasant symptoms are experienced only if one eats while one's stomach is shut down.

We know that eating or thinking about eating pleasant food both increase the amplitude of normal 3-cpm activity in the EGG of asymptomatic subjects. Disgusting food does not have this effect. These recent studies raise important methodological questions that have not been systematically studied. For example, how fast does gastric myoelectric activity, as measured with EGG, change? That is, can we expect to see a measurable change in the EGG following the presentation of a brief discrete stimulus? How long would a given stimulus have to be presented before we would expect to see a change in the EGG? In general, we view the GI system as being slow to respond compared with other biological systems, since momentary adjustments in activity are not essential to survival. However, data on this issue are lacking.

FUTURE DIRECTIONS

Because of its noninvasive nature, EGG will continue to aid basic researchers in their quest for additional information about gastric myoelectric activity, gastric motility, and their relationship in normal and pathophysiological conditions.

Applied research by gastroenterologists using the EGG is increasing rapidly, owing largely to the ease and reliability of its use in detecting gastric dysrhythmias and the recently established relationship between gastric dysrhythmias and upper-GI disorders, including delayed gastric emptying and nausea. Much of this research has been supported by pharmaceutical companies, and we anticipate that this will continue. A related exciting new area that requires EGG recording in order to assess results is electrical pacing of the stomach. Research is currently being carried out (on dogs and on a small number of humans) in cases (a) where the stomach has ceased to contract, (b) of gastric paresis, and (c) where drugs have not been helpful. A less dramatic but related area of research that we have planned is biofeedback of EGG for individuals with gastric dysrhythmias in an effort to restore normal 3-cpm activity and thereby relieve nausea.

The recent increase in the use of the EGG by gastroenterologists has brought with it refinements in both hardware and software, including ambulatory units that have flown on NASA shuttle flights. We predict that – given the availability of this new equipment – more psychophysiologists will soon be using the EGG to study the effects of stress and the effects of emotions such as disgust.

REFERENCES

Abell, T. L., Camilleri, M., Hench, V. S., & Malagelada, J. R. (1991). Gastric electromechanical function and gastric emptying in diabetic gastroperesis. *European Journal of Gastroenterology and Heptology, 3,* 163–7.

Abell, T. L., Lucas, A. R., Brown, M. L., & Malagelada, J. R. (1985a). Gastric electrical dysrhythmias in anorexia nervosa (AN). *Gastroenterology, 88A,* 1300.

Abell, T. L., & Malagelada, J. R. (1985). Glucagon-evoked gastric dysrhythmias in humans shown by an improved electrogastrographic technique. *Gastroenterology, 88,* 1932–40.

Abell, T. L., Tucker, R., & Malagelada, J. R. (1985b). Simultaneous gastric electro-manometry in man. In R. M. Stern & K. L. Koch (Eds.), *Electrogastrography,* pp. 78–88. New York: Praeger.

Alvarez, W. C. (1922). The electrogastrogram and what it shows. *Journal of the American Medical Association, 78,* 1116–19.

Alvarez, W. C. (1943). *Nervousness, Indigestion, and Pain.* New York: Hoeber.

Beaumont, W. (1833/1959). *Experiments and Observations on the Gastric Juice and the Physiology of Indigestion.* New York: Dover.

Berntson, G. G., Cacioppo, J. T., Binkley, P. F., Uchino, B. N., Quigley, K. S., & Fieldstone, A. (1994). Autonomic cardiac control. III. Psychological stress and cardiac response in autonomic space as revealed by pharmacological blockades. *Psychophysiology, 31,* 599–608.

Bisett, W. M., Devane, S. P., & Milla, P. J. (1989). Gastric antral dysrhythmias in children with idiopathic intestinal pseudo-obstruction. *Journal of Gastrointestinal Motility, 1,* 53.

Bortolotti, M., Sarti, P., Barara, L., & Brunelli, F. (1990). Gastric myoelectrical activity in patients with chronic idiopathic gastroparesis. *Journal of Gastrointestinal Motility, 2,* 104–8.

Brown, B. H., Smallwood, R. H., Duthie, H. L., & Stoddard, C. J. (1975). Intestinal smooth muscle electrical potentials recorded from surface electrodes. *Medical Biological Engineering, 13,* 97–103.

Bruley des Varannes, S., Mizrahi, M., Curran, P., Kandasamy, A., & Dubois, A. (1991). Relation between postprandial gastric emptying and cutaneous electrogastrogram in primates. *American Journal of Physiology, 261,* 248–55.

Camilleri, M., Malagelada, J. R., Brown, M. L., Becker, G., & Zinsmeister, A. R. (1985). Relation between antral motility and gastric emptying of solids and liquids in humans. *American Journal of Physiology, 249,* G580–G585.

Cannon, W. B. (1936). *Digestion and Health.* New York: Norton.

Cannon, W. B., & Washburn, A. L. (1912). An explanation of hunger. *American Journal of Physiology, 29,* 441–54.

Carlson, A. J. (1916). *The Control of Hunger in Health and Disease.* University of Chicago Press.

Chen, J. D. Z., Davenport, K., & McCallum, R. W. (1993a). Effects of fat preload on gastric myoelectrical activity in normal humans. *Journal of Gastrointestinal Motility, 5,* 281.

Chen, J. D. Z., Lin, Z. Y., Parolisi, S., & McCallum, R. W. (1995). Inhibitory effects of cholecystokinin on postprandial gastric myoelectric activity. *Digestive Diseases and Sciences, 40,* 2614–22.

Chen, J., & McCallum, R. W. (1991). Electrogastrogram: Measurement, analysis and prospective applications. *Medical and Biological Engineering and Computing, 29,* 339–50.

Chen, J., Richards, R., & McCallum, R. W. (1993b). Frequency components of the electrogastrogram and their correlations with gastrointestinal motility. *Medical and Biological Engineering and Computing, 31,* 60–7.

Chen, J., Stewart, W. R., & McCallum, R. W. (1993c). Adaptive spectral analysis of episodic rhythmic variations in gastric myoelectric potentials. *IEEE Trans. Biomed. Eng., 40,* 128–35.

Chen, J., Vandewalle, J., Sansen, W., Vantrappen, G., & Janssens, J. (1990). Adaptive spectral analysis of cutaneous electrical signals using autoregressive moving average modeling. *Medical and Biological Engineering and Computing, 28,* 531–6.

Chiloiro, M., Riezzo, G., Guerra, V., Reddy, S. N., & Girgio, I. (1994). The cutaneous electrogastrogram reflects postprandial gastric emptying in humans. In J. Z. Chen & R. W. McCallum (Eds.), *Electrogastrography: Principles and Applications,* pp. 293–306. New York: Raven.

Code, C. F., & Marlett, J. A. (1975). The interdigestive myoelectric complex of the stomach and small bowel of dogs. *Journal of Physiology, 246,* 289–309.

Couturier, D., Roze, C., Paologgi, J., & Debray, C. (1972). Electrical activity of the normal human stomach: A comparative study of recordings obtained from serosal and mucosal sites. *Digestive Diseases and Sciences, 17,* 969–76.

Cucchiara, S., Minella, R., Riezzo, G., Vallone, P., Castellone, F., & Auricchio, S. (1992). Reversal of gastric electrical dysrhythmias by cisapride in children with functional dyspepsia: Report of three cases. *Digestive Diseases and Sciences, 37,* 1136–40.

Davis, R. C., Garafolo, L., & Gault, F. P. (1957). An exploration of abdominal potentials. *Journal of Comparative and Physiological Psychology, 50,* 519–23.

Davis, R. C., Garafolo, L., & Kveim, K. (1959). Conditions associated with gastrointestinal activity. *Journal of Comparative and Physiological Psychology, 52,* 466–75.

Dubois, A., & Mizrahi, M. (1994). Electrogastrography, gastric emptying, and gastric motility. In J. Z. Chen & R. W. McCallum (Eds.), *Electrogastrography: Principles and Applications,* pp. 247–56. New York: Raven.

Familoni, B. O., Bowes, K. L., Kingma, Y. J., & Cote, K. R. (1987). Can transcutaneous electrodes diagnose gastric electrical abnormalities? *Digestive Diseases and Sciences, 32,* 909.

Feldman, M., & Schiller, L. (1983). Disorders of gastrointestinal motility associated with diabetes mellitus. *Annals of Internal Medicine, 98,* 378–84.

Furness, J. B., & Costa, M. (1980). Types of nerves in the enteric nervous system. *Neuroscience, 5,* 1–20.

Gaultier, C., & Baille, J. (1982). Cognitive mediations in biofeedback. *Agressologie, 23,* 285–97.

Geldof, H., van der Schee, E. J., & Grashuis, J. L. (1986). Accuracy and reliability of electrogastrography (EGG). *Gastroenterology, 90,* 1425.

Geldof, H., van der Schee, E. J., Smout, A. J. P. M., van de Merwe, J. P., van Blankenstein, M., & Grashuis, J. L. (1989). Myoelectrical activity of the stomach in gastric ulcer patients: An electrogastrographic study. *Gastrointestinal Motility, 1,* 122–30.

Geldof, H., van der Schee, E. J., van Blankenstein, M., & Grashuis, J. L. (1983). Gastric dysrhythmia; an electrogastrographic study. *Gastroenterology, 84,* 1163.

Hamilton, J. W., Bellahsene, B. E., Reichelderfer, M., Webster, J. H., & Bass, P. (1986). Human electrogastrograms. Comparison of surface and mucosal recordings. *Digestive Diseases and Sciences, 31,* 33–9.

Hinder, R. A., & Kelly, K. A. (1977). Human gastric pacesetter potentials: Site of origin and response to gastric transection and proximal vagotomy. *American Journal of Physiology, 133,* 29–33.

Hölzl, R., Loffler, K., & Muller, G. M. (1985). On conjoint gastrography or what the surface gastrograms show. In R. M. Stern & K. L. Koch (Eds.), *Electrogastrography: Methodology, Validation, and Applications,* pp. 89–115. New York: Praeger.

Johnson, L. R., Christensen, J., Jacobsen, E. D., & Schultz, S. G. (Eds.) (1987). *Physiology of the Gastrointestinal Tract.* New York: Raven.

Jokerst, M. D., Levine, M., Stern, R. M., & Koch, K. L. (1997). Modified sham feeding with pleasant and disgusting foods: Cephalic-vagal influences on gastric myoelectric activity. *Gastroenterology, 112,* A755.

Jones, K. R., & Jones, G. E. (1985). Pre- and postprandial EGG variation. In R. M. Stern & K. L. Koch (Eds.), *Electrogastrography: Methodology, Validation, and Applications,* pp. 168–81. New York: Praeger.

Kelly, K. A., Code, C. F., & Elveback, L. R. (1969). Patterns of canine gastric electrical activity. *American Journal of Physiology, 217,* 461–70.

Kingma, Y. J. (1989). The electrogastrogram and its analysis. *CRC Crit. Rev. Biomed. Eng., 17,* 105–24.

Koch, K. L. (1993). Stomach. In M. M. Schuster (Ed.), *Atlas of Gastrointestinal Motility,* pp. 158–76. Baltimore: Williams & Wilkins.

Koch, K. L., Bingaman, S., Sperry, N., & Stern, R. M. (1991a). Electrogastrography differentiates mechanical vs. idiopathic gastroparesis in patients with nausea and vomiting. *Gastroenterology, 100,* A99.

Koch, K. L., Medina, M., Bingaman, S., & Stern, R. M. (1992). Gastric dysrhythmias and visceral sensations in patients with functional dyspepsia. *Gastroenterology, 102,* A937.

Koch, K. L., & Stern, R. M. (1985). The relationship between the cutaneously recorded electrogastrogram and antral contractions in man. In R. M. Stern & K. L. Koch (Eds.), *Electrogastrography: Methodology, Validation, and Applications,* pp. 116–31. New York: Praeger.

Koch, K. L., & Stern, R. M. (1993). Electrogastrography. In D. Kumar & D. Wingate (Eds.), *An Illustrated Guide to Gas-trointestinal Motility,* pp. 290–307. London: Churchill Communications Europe.

Koch, K. L., Stern, R. M., Bingaman, S., & Eggli, D. (1991b). Satiety, stomach volume and gastric myoelectrical activity during solid-phase gastric emptying: A study of healthy individuals. *Journal of Gastrointestinal Motility, 3,* 187.

Koch, K. L., Stern, R. M., Stewart, W. R., & Vasey, M. W. (1989). Gastric emptying and gastric myoelectrical activity in patients with diabetic gastroparesis: Effect of long-term domperidone treatment. *American Journal of Gastroenterology, 84,* 1069–75.

Koch, K. L., Stern, R. M., Vasey, M. W., & Dwyer, A. (1990). Gastric dysrhythmias and nausea of pregnancy. *Digestive Diseases and Sciences, 35,* 961–8.

Koch, K. L., Stewart, W. R., & Stern, R. M. (1987). Effects of barium meals on gastric electromechanical activity in man: A fluoroscopic-electrogastrophic study. *Digestive Diseases and Sciences, 32,* 1217–22.

Krapivin, B. V., & Chernin, V. V. (1967). Study of the motor function of the stomach by the electrogastrographic method in patients with peptic ulcer. *Soviet Medicine, 30,* 57–60.

Kwong, N. K., Brown, B. H., Whittaker, G. E., & Duthie, H. L. (1970). Electrical activity of the gastric antrum in man. *British Journal of Surgery, 12,* 913–16.

Lavigne, M. E., Wiley, Z. D., Meyer, J. H., Martin, P., & MacGregor, I. L. (1978). Gastric emptying rates of solid food in relation to body size. *Gastroenterology, 74,* 1258–60.

Lee, K., Chey, W., Tai, H., & Yajima, H. (1978). Radioimmunoassay of motilin: Validation and studies on the relationship between plasma motilin and interdigestive myoelectric activity in the duodenum of dog. *Digestive Diseases and Sciences, 23,* 789–95.

Liberski, S. M., Koch, K. L., Atnip, R. G., & Stern, R. M. (1990). Ischemic gastroparesis: Resolution of nausea, vomiting and gastroparesis after mesenteric artery revascularization. *Gastroenterology, 99,* 252–7.

Lin, Z., & Chen, J. Z. (1994). Comparison of three running spectral analysis methods. In J. Z. Chen & R. W. McCallum (Eds.), *Electrogastrography: Principles and Applications,* pp. 75–98. New York: Raven.

Meyer, J. H. (1987). Motility of the stomach and gastroduodenal junction. In L. R. Johnson, J. Christensen, E. D. Jacobsen, & S. G. Schultz (Eds.), *Physiology of the Gastrointestinal Tract,* pp. 613–30. New York: Raven.

Meyer, J. H., Gu, Y. G., Dressman, J., & Amidon, G. (1986). Effect of viscosity and flow rate on gastric emptying of solids. *American Journal of Physiology, 250,* G161–G164.

Meyer, J. H., MacGregor, I. L., Gueller, R., Martin, P., & Cavalieri, R. (1976). 99Tc-tagged chicken liver as a marker of solid food in the human stomach. *American Journal of Digestive Diseases, 21,* 296–304.

Meyer, J. H., Ohashi, H., Jehn, D., & Thompson, J. B. (1981). Size of liver particles emptied from the human stomach. *Gastroenterology, 80,* 1489–96.

Mintchev, M. P., & Bowes, K. L. (1996). Extracting quantitative information from digital electrogastrograms. *Medical and Biological Engineering and Computing, 34,* 244–8.

Mintchev, M. P., Kingma, Y. J., & Bowes, K. L. (1993). Accuracy of cutaneous recordings of gastric electrical activity. *Gastroenterology, 104,* 1273–80.

Mintchev, M. P., Otto, S. J., & Bowes, K. L. (1997). Electrogastrography can recognize gastric electrical uncoupling in dogs. *Gastroenterology, 112,* 2006–11.

Mirizzi, N., & Scafoglieri, V. (1983). Optimal direction of the electrogastrographic signal in man. *Medical and Biological Engineering and Computing, 21,* 385–9.

Morgan, K. G., Schmalz, P. F., & Szurszewski, J. H. (1978). The inhibitory effects of vasoactive intestinal polypeptide on the mechanical and electrical activity of canine antral smooth muscle. *Journal of Physiology, 282,* 437–50.

Murat, J., Martin, A., Stevanovic, D., Beloncle, M., & Masson, J. M. (1985). Electroenterography: Application to digestive pathology. In R. M. Stern & K. L. Koch (Eds.), *Electrogastrography: Methodology, Validation, and Applications,* pp. 215–25. New York: Praeger.

Muth, E. R., Thayer, J. F., Stern, R. M., Friedman, B. H., & Drake, C. (1998). The effect of autonomic nervous system activity on gastric myoelectrical activity: Does the spectral reserve hypothesis hold for the stomach? *Biological Psychology, 71,* 265–78.

Nelsen, T. S., & Kohatsu, S. (1968). Clinical electrogastrography and its relationship to gastric surgery. *American Journal of Surgery, 116,* 215–22.

Roman, C., & Gonella, J. (1987). Extrinsic control of digestive tract motility. In L. R. Johnson, J. Christensen, E. D. Jacobsen, & S. G. Schultz (Eds.), *Physiology of the Gastrointestinal Tract,* pp. 507–53. New York: Raven.

Russell, R. W., & Stern, R. M. (1967). Gastric motility: The electrogastrogram. In P. H. Venables & I. Martin (Eds.), *Manual of Psychophysiological Methods,* pp. 218–43. Amsterdam: North-Holland.

Schlegel, J. F., & Code, C. F. (1975). The gastric peristalsis of the interdigestive housekeeper. In G. Vantrappen (Ed.), *Proceedings from the Fifth International Symposium on Gastrointestinal Motility,* p. 321. Herentals, Belgium: Typoff.

Smallwood, R. H. (1978). Analysis of gastric electrical signals from surface electrodes using phase-lock techniques. Part 2: System performance with gastric signals. *Medical and Biological Engineering and Computing, 16,* 513–18.

Smallwood, R. H., & Brown, B. H. (1983). Noninvasive assessment of gastric activity. In P. Rolfe (Ed.), *Noninvasive Physiological Measurements,* vol. II. London: Academic Press.

Smout, A. J. P. M. (1980). Myoelectric activity of the stomach: Gastroelectromyography and electrogastrography. Thesis, Erasmus University, Rotterdam.

Smout, A. J. P. M., Jebbink, H. J. A., & Samsom, M. (1994). Acquisition and analysis of electrogastrographic data: The Dutch experience. In J. Z. Chen & R. W. McCallum (Eds.), *Electrogastrography: Principles and Applications,* pp. 3–30. New York: Raven.

Smout, A. J. P. M., van der Schee, E. J., & Grashuis, J. L. (1980a). What is measured in electrogastrography? *Digestive Diseases and Sciences, 25,* 179–87.

Smout, A. J. P. M., van der Schee, E. J., & Grashuis, J. L. (1980b). Postprandial and interdigestive gastric electrical activity in the dog recorded by means of cutaneous electrodes. In J. Christensen (Ed.), *Gastrointestinal Motility,* pp. 187–94. New York: Raven.

Sobakin, M. A., Smirnov, I. P., & Mishin, L. N. (1962). Electrogastrography. *IRE Trans. Biomed. Electr., 9,* 129–32.

Stemper, T. J., & Cooke, A. R. (1975). Gastric emptying and its relationship to antral contractile activity. *Gastroenterology, 69,* 649–53.

Stern, R. M., Crawford, H. E., Stewart, W. R., Vasey, M. W., & Koch, K. L. (1989). Sham feeding: Cephalic-vagal influences on gastric myoelectric activity. *Digestive Diseases and Sciences, 34,* 521–7.

Stern, R. M., & Koch, K. L. (Eds.) (1985). *Electrogastrography: Methodology, Validation, and Applications.* New York: Praeger.

Stern, R. M., & Koch, K. L. (1994). Using the electrogastrogram to study motion sickness. In J. Z. Chen & R. W. McCallum (Eds.), *Electrogastrography: Principles and Applications,* pp. 199–218. New York: Raven.

Stern, R. M., & Koch, K. L. (1996). Motion sickness and differential susceptibility. *Current Directions in Psychological Science, 5,* 115–20.

Stern, R. M., Koch, K. L., Leibowitz, H. W., Lindblad, I., Shupert, C., & Stewart, W. R. (1985). Tachygastria and motion sickness. *Aviation Space and Environmental Medicine, 56,* 1074–7.

Stern, R. M., Koch, K. L., Stewart, W. R., & Lindblad, I. M. (1987). Spectral analysis of tachygastria recorded during motion sickness. *Gastroenterology, 92,* 92–7.

Stern, R. M., Koch, K. L., & Vasey, M. W. (1990). The gastrointestinal system. In J. T. Cacioppo & L. G. Tassinary (Eds.), *Principles of Psychophysiology: Physical, Social, and Inferential Elements.* Cambridge University Press.

Stern, R. M., Vasey, M. W., Hu, S., & Koch, K. L. (1991). Effects of cold stress on gastric myoelectric activity. *Journal of Gastrointestinal Motility, 3,* 225–8.

Stewart, W. R. (1987). Stress-induced alterations in gastric myoelectric activity as measured with the electrogastrogram. Dissertation, Penn State University, University Park, PA.

Stewart, W. R., Chen, J., & McCallum, R. W. (1991). Mood and gastric slow wave amplitude. *Gastroenterology, 100,* A498.

Stewart, W. R., Hurm, K. D., & Valenzuela, G. A. (1989). Low positive affect and gastric hypomotility. *Psychophysiology, 26,* S58.

Stoddard, C. J., Smallwood, R. H., & Duthie, H. L. (1981). Electrical arrhythmias in the human stomach. *Gut, 22,* 705–12.

Thompson, D. G., Richelson, E., & Malagelada, J. R. (1982). Perturbation of gastric emptying and duodenal motility through the central nervous system. *Gastroenterology, 83,* 1200–6.

Tumpeer, I. H., & Blitzsten, P. W. (1926). Registration of peristalsis by the Einthoven galvanometer. *American Journal of Diseases of Children, 31,* 454–5.

Tumpeer, I. H., & Phillips, B. (1932). Hyperperistaltic electrographic effects. *American Journal of Medical Science, 184,* 831–6.

Uijtdehaage, S. H. J., Stern, R. M., & Koch, K. L. (1992) Effects of eating on vection-induced motion sickness, cardiac vagal tone and gastric myoelectric activity. *Psychophysiology, 29,* 193–201.

van der Schee, E. J., Smout, A. J. P. M., & Grashuis, J. L. (1982). Applications of running spectrum analysis to electrogastrographic signals recorded from dog and man. In M. Wienbeck

(Ed.), *Motility of the Digestive Tract*, pp. 241–50. New York: Raven.

Vantrappen, G., Hostein, J., Janssens, J., Vanderweerd, M., & De Wever, I. (1983). Do slow waves induce mechanical activity? *Gastroenterology, 84,* 1341.

Vantrappen, G., Janssens, J., Peeters, T. L., Bloom, S. R., Christofides, N. D., & Hellemans, J. (1979). Motility and the interdigestive migrating motor complex in man. *Digestive Diseases and Sciences, 24,* 497–500.

Wolf, S. (1943). Relation of gastric function to nausea in man. *Journal of Clinical Investigations, 22,* 877–82.

Wolf, S., & Wolff, H. G. (1943). *Human Gastric Function*. New York: Oxford University Press.

Xu, G., & Zhou, Y. (1983). Modulated effect of acupuncture on gastroelectrical activity. *Acupuncture Research, 8,* 1–6.

You, C. H., & Chey, W. Y. (1984). Study of electromechanical activity of the stomach in humans and in dogs with particular attention to tachygastria. *Gastroenterology, 86,* 1460–8.

CHAPTER TWELVE

THE SEXUAL RESPONSE SYSTEM

JAMES H. GEER & ERICK JANSSEN

Prologue

OVERVIEW

Sexual psychophysiology can be distinguished from other branches of sex research by its use of a particular methodology. The approach utilizes electrophysiological measures, principally of genital responding, to assess sexual arousal and response patterns. When most effectively applied, this approach entails the systematic exploration of the interdependence between cognitive, affective, and behavioral processes in association with physiological activation of the sexual response system (Rosen & Beck 1988). In this sense, sexual psychophysiology can be used to help clarify and understand the interplay of interpersonal and environmental events and their effects on the sexual response system. Conversely, it seeks to understand the effects of the response system (i.e., genital reactions and response) on the interpretation of interpersonal and environmental events. In some sense, sexual psychophysiology has always been the stepchild of research into the physiological events that are part of the broad emotional landscape of humans. This has occurred principally because things sexual have always been accompanied by judgments of an ethical and moral nature. This background of ethics and morality forms an important part of the context that permeates sex research and sexual psychophysiology.

HISTORICAL BACKGROUND

The truism that we stand on the shoulders of giants holds in this area of research as it does in all of science. These individuals not only have provided the findings that stimulated further study but have also opened the eyes of the scientific community to the feasibility of quality sex research. Three names that are important when considering the early history of sex research are Richard von Krafft-Ebbing, Havelock Ellis, and Sigmund Freud, who all pointed out the importance of sexuality in the understanding of human behavior. Krafft-Ebbing, using the clinical case history as his data, provided the medical community with instances of sexual deviance that forced the medical community to consider sexuality seriously. Havelock Ellis, in his extensive collection of material on sexual behavior, attempted to identify the scope of sexual behavior and to examine its prevalence. His was the first attempt to put things sexual into a normative framework and not to relegate sexuality to items of curiosity and prurient interest alone. Freud, who placed sexuality at the center of human motivation and personality, forced upon the scientific and clinical community the consideration of sexual behavior.

Following these initial efforts was a scattering of work on the direct study of sexual responding. The earliest report that we identified was published in Germany in 1896. In that paper (Mendelsohn 1896), there was a description of "pulse curves" (electrocardiograms) recorded during intercourse. We would next point to the report (Magoun 1981) that the father of behaviorism, J. B. Watson, directly observed sexual responding. Magoun reports that these efforts resulted in serious personal problems for Watson, who apparently stopped that work because of those concerns. Two medical texts were produced early in the century that described genital responding during sexual arousal. These included the popular marriage manual *Ideal Marriage* by Van de Velde (1926) and Dickinson's (1933) *Human Sex Anatomy*. It is unclear how important these early studies were in promoting research in sexual psychophysiology. What we do know is that they predated the next giants in the field: Alfred Kinsey, and William Masters and Virginia Johnson.

John T. Cacioppo, Louis G. Tassinary, and Gary G. Berntson (Eds.), *Handbook of Psychophysiology*, 2nd ed. © Cambridge University Press 2000. Printed in the United States of America. ISBN 62634X. All rights reserved.

Without a doubt, Kinsey and his colleagues and Masters and Johnson provided the context that both encouraged and permitted further studies of sexuality. Kinsey, in a point not often recognized by scholars, provided a description of the responses that occur during sexual arousal and responding. In *Sexual Behavior in the Human Female*, Kinsey et al. (1953) gave a rather detailed description of some 20 different physiological changes that accompany sexual behavior, including pulse rate, blood pressure, peripheral blood flow, respiration, genital secretions, and central nervous system changes. Kinsey also provided charts of heart rate, blood pressure, and electroencephalographic changes that occur during sexual activity.

Perhaps more importantly than an early description of genital responding during sexual arousal was the impact of Kinsey's work on society in general. His findings, while challenged by many, made it clear that humans are sexual beings. There is a very wide range of sexual activities, and both genders are active. This flew in the face of moral teachings and folklore. Perhaps most importantly for our purposes, Kinsey demonstrated that sexuality could be incorporated into the body of natural science.

Western society, primarily that in the United States, had just begun to assimilate the two works by Kinsey when, in 1966, William Masters and Virginia Johnson published their milestone book *Human Sexual Response*. In that book they described in detail their findings concerning the nature of the human sexual response. They reported on the observation of 694 individuals during both intercourse and masturbation. They summarized their work by presenting a descriptive model of human sexual response. That now well-known four-stage model of sexual arousal, with its accompanying specification of the physiological events that accompany each stage, has been the stimulus for much psychophysiological research. Although of less direct relevance to this work, their next book, *Human Sexual Inadequacy* (1970), also had a profound impact on the field of sexuality. In particular, the report of very high success rates in the treatment of many sexual dysfunctions marked the beginning of sex therapy as a separate clinical field of practice.

The history of research on the psychophysiology of sexual responding within the first half of the twentieth century was dominated by the use of extragenital measures such as heart rate, respiration, blood pressure, sweat gland activity, and body temperature to index sexual arousal. In 1971, Zuckerman reviewed that literature and concluded that, because of their lack of specificity, extragenital measures of sexual responding were not very useful in assessing sexual arousal. Zuckerman's review of the literature – coupled with Masters and Johnson's (1966) report that myotonia and vasocongestion (particularly that occurring in the genitals) were the two major indicators of sexual arousal in humans – accounts for the trend in the field toward using direct genital measures to assess sexual arousal and response patterns.

Physical Context

ANATOMICAL SUBSTRATE

Before beginning a discussion of the methodologies of measuring responses obtained from the genitals, some background material may be of value. We begin with a brief discussion of some aspects of genital anatomy and responding, limiting our discussion to those aspects that are relevant to this chapter.

Men

In men, the external sex organs consist of the penis and the scrotum, which contains the sperm-producing testes. Figure 1 contains drawings of the male pelvic region in

Figure 1. Cross-section of male pelvic region and cross-section of penis.

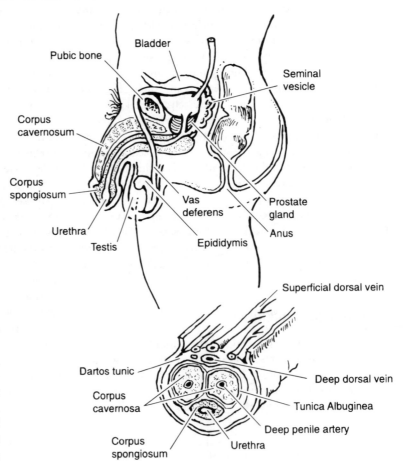

cross-section and a cross-section of the penis. There are three cylindrical spongelike bodies of erectile tissue in the penis: the two lying dorsally are called the corpora cavernosa and the one lying ventrally is called the corpus spongiosum. The corpora cavernosa are surrounded by a thick fibrous sheath, the tunica albuginea, and share a perforated septum that allows them to function as a single unit. The three corpora contain small irregular compartments (vascular spaces) separated by bonds of smooth muscle tissue. These bodies become engorged with blood during erection. The function of the corpora cavernosa is purely erectile. The corpus spongiosum and glans also act as a urinary conduit and an organ of ejaculation. On erection, the corpus spongiosum and the glans develop a modest turgidity but never become rigid enough to shut off urethral lumen. Along with its sensory function, the glans swells appreciably during arousal and ejaculation.

With the exception of several minor branches from the scrotal and epigastric arteries, the blood supply to the penis is furnished by the two internal pudendal arteries. Each pudendal artery branches off to become a complex of arteries that supply the penis. Of particular interest is the cavernous (or deep) artery of the penis, which follows the length of the penis and terminates at the glans. In its course, the deep artery gives off many branches to the corpus spongiosum and, most importantly, to the helical arteries. The numerous helical arteries provide the arteriovenous shunts that are integral to the mechanism of erection. From the helical arteries arise short-end arteries with bulbous tips that open into the cavernous spaces. Numerous anastomotic channels unite the veins of the penis at various junctions. *Polsters* appear as a split in the internal elastic lamella of certain blood vessels, with the intervening space filled with longitudinal muscle and connective tissue fibers; they are present in both arteries and veins and constitute a variable amount of the lumen.

Previous theories of erection (Conti 1952; Weiss 1972) implicated the polsters as important structures in the mechanism of erection. It was postulated that the contraction or relaxation of the muscle or connective tissue in the polsters resulted in dilating or contracting the lumen of the vessel. It was assumed that erection was effected by (a) opening of the shunts, aided by active relaxation of the polsters in the arteries leading to the cavernous spaces; coincident with (b) active contraction of polsters within the arteries to the somatic parts of the penis and the veins draining the penis. However, a study by Newman and Northup (1981) suggested that polsters exert only a passive impedance to flow. These authors further suggested that polsters apparently represent a response to aging and stress that may be related to the incidence of arteriosclerosis (Newman & Northup 1981). Conti, Virag, and von Niederhausern (1988) confirmed earlier findings and found polsters in penile arteries, but they left open their role in erection: null, complementary, or primordial. According

to Andersson and Wagner (1995), this is a reasonable summing up of available evidence. It appears, therefore, that the increased arterial inflow – and subsequent shunting of the increased arterial blood via the helical arteries – is adequate to induce erection and that polsters are at best minimally involved.

From this point of view, erection is essentially a hydrodynamic manifestation, weighing arterial inflow against venous outflow. Many investigators now believe that the principal cause for the increase in arterial flow to the penis is decreased vascular resistance in the penile corpora, and an increasing number of studies have explored the role of corporeal smooth muscle tissue in this process. Cavernosal tissue is spongelike and composed of a meshwork of interconnected cavernosal spaces. The smooth muscle cells of the corpus cavernosum are connected by gap junctions, which are believed to play an important role in the control of smooth muscle activity (Andersson & Wagner 1995). The most plausible theory at this time is that the cavernous smooth muscles of the corpora, which are in a tonically contracted state when the penis is flaccid, relax during the initiation of penile erection (Melman 1992). This lowers the corporal vascular resistance and results in increased blood flow to the penis. Venous return is diminished by means of a passive occlusion of the penile veins against the tunica albuginea.

Women

Figure 2 shows a view of the external female genitals and a cross-sectional view of the pelvic region. The external female genital area is known as the vulva. The entire genital area has been found to be rich in nerve endings and heavily vascularized. The layer of fatty tissue covering the junction of the pubic bones at the top of this area is known as the mons pubis. The labia majora, also known as the outer lips, consist of two large folds of tissue extending downward from the mons and surrounding the genital area. The labia minora, or inner lips, lie just inside the labia majora. The labia minora enclose an area called the vestibule, which contains the clitoris, the urethral opening, and the vaginal opening. The portion of the labia minora that covers the clitoris is known as the prepuce, or the clitoral hood. During sexual arousal, both the clitoris and the labia minora become engorged. The labia minora have been observed by Masters and Johnson (1966) to increase in diameter by two to three times during sexual excitement. They consequently become a little everted, exposing their inner surfaces (Bancroft 1989). The clitoris is composed of the clitoral shaft, the crura, and the clitoral head or glans. It has a body formed from two corpora cavernosa and a single corpus spongiosum. Erectile tissue of the clitoral shaft becomes engorged with blood during sexual arousal in much the same way as does the male penis.

The organ that has been the principal focus of psychophysiological measurement in women has been the vagina. The vagina is a collapsed canal that is more a potential than a permanent space. It consists of a flat and scalelike epithelium serviced by blood vessels and lymphatics and is surrounded by a sheath of smooth muscle (Levin 1992). The vagina has numerous transverse folds. They are believed to help provide accordionlike distensibility and are more prominent in the lower third of the vagina (Droegemueller 1992). The vascular system of the vagina is supplied with an extensive anastomotic network throughout its length. The blood supply originates with the uterine artery, the internal iliac artery, and the vaginal artery. The vaginal artery consists of multiple arteries on each side of the pelvis and branches to both the anterior and posterior surfaces of the vagina. Vasocongestion occurs during sexual arousal, and it appears that vaginal lubrication occurs as a result of changes associated with this. Vaginal vasocongestion is viewed to be the result of increased arterial inflow that is not matched by venous drainage. The engorgement of the vagina raises the pressure inside the capillaries and creates an increase in transudation of plasma through the vaginal epithelium. This vaginal lubricative fluid flows through the epithelium onto the surface of the vagina, initially forming sweat-like droplets that coalesce to form a lubricative film that covers the vaginal wall (Levin 1992). Vascular responding of the erectile tissues of the introitus and extending to the clitoris is, as with the penis, controlled by the nerves that pass through the nervi erigentes from the sacral plexus. In comparison to men, much less is known about the vascular mechanisms involved in the female genital response. Although it is possible that similar specialized vascular mechanisms are involved, there is no functional equivalent of the hydraulic system of the male penis in the human vagina (Bancroft 1989).

NEURAL/HUMORAL CONTROL
Neurophysiology of Erection

Weiss (1972) presented a dual-innervation model of erection that relies on both psychogenic and reflexogenic control of erection. According to this model, the reflexogenic component consists of a sacral parasympathetic pathway, whereas the psychogenic pathway is sympathetic in origin. The evidence for the two distinct mechanisms stems mainly from observations in men with spinal cord injury and experimental spinal transections in animals. It has been demonstrated, for example, that in men with high transections of the spinal cord (i.e., at levels above thoracic segment T9; Brindley 1991), reflexogenic erections can be elicited. In most of these men, an erection can be induced by direct stimulation of the penis, but central stimuli (e.g., sexual fantasies) do not result in an erectile response. At the other extreme, many men with lesions impairing the reflex arc at sacral segments 2 to 4 (S2–S4) still experience psychogenic erections. In neurologically intact men, the two pathways are thought to interact such that psychogenic stimuli such as sexual fantasy can enhance genital responding by diminishing the amount of tactile genital stimulation necessary to produce an erection. By the same token, other central processes can operate in the reverse direction to inhibit reflexive arousal (Janssen et al. 1994b; Weiss 1972).

Figure 2. External female genitals and cross-section of pelvic region.

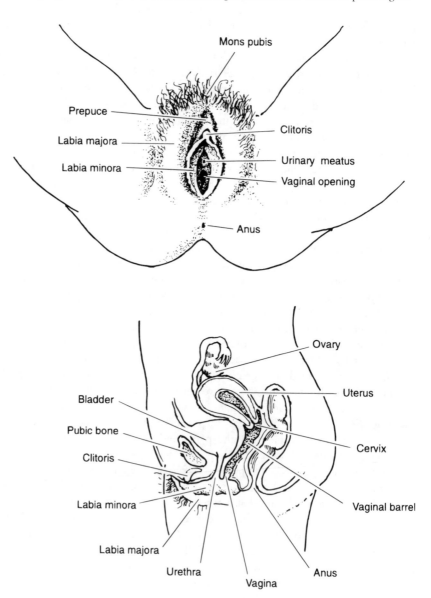

For years, the cholinergic, parasympathetic component of erection has been viewed to be the primary efferent system for generating penile erection. Although cholinergic nerves indeed are present in the penis and are involved in the control of erection, more recent evidence suggests that they play a less important role than initially thought. The blood vessels and the smooth muscles of the penis are innervated by nerves from three parts of the peripheral nervous system: the sympathetic, the parasympathetic, and the somatic. It is now widely accepted that normal erection requires participation of all these systems. Parasympathetic nerve endings are sparse within the corpora cavernosa, and their primary role is believed to be the initiation of vasodilatation in the penile blood vessels and of increased blood flow to the cavernous tissue. Sympathetic pathways have been found to mediate antierectile as well as erectile effects. Modulation of adrenergic activity is viewed to be one influence on the contractile state of the smooth muscles in the penis (Andersson & Wagner 1995). Indeed, histological studies have revealed that the penile corpora are richly endowed with alpha-adrenergic receptors. Brindley (1983) produced reflex erection in the laboratory by local injection of alpha-adrenoceptor blockers (phenoxybenzamine, phentolamine). Also, injections of papaverine, a smooth muscle relaxant, have been shown to produce reflex erections. Although cholinergic and adrenergic mechanisms are important, they are not believed to be in full control of erection. For this reason, researchers have begun to explore the role of nonadrenergic noncholinergic neurotransmitters. In studies reported by Ottesen and associates (1987), a vasoactive intestinal polypeptide (VIP) has been implicated in the mediation of erection. Other studies have focused on the role of (among other agents) prostaglandins and nitric oxide. The latter is believed to exert the most significant role in the physiology of the penis. At present, although its synthesis and action in the penis are regulated by many other factors, nitric oxide is considered to be the principal mediator of corporeal smooth muscle relaxation (Burnett 1997).

Neurophysiology of Vaginal Arousal

As for vascular mechanisms, considerably less is known about the neurophysiology of vaginal arousal than is known about the neural control of penile erection. The vaginal epithelium, blood vessels, and smooth muscle are innervated by the sympathetic and parasympathetic divisions of the autonomous nervous system. The striated muscles that surround the vagina are innervated by the somatic nervous system (Levin 1992). The clitoris, which contains a number of nerve endings similar to those found in the male penis (Bancroft 1989), is innervated through the terminal branch of the pudendal nerve.

Early speculation about the type of innervation of the female genitalia focused on acetylcholine as the primary neurotransmitter. However, this idea seems to have been based on the erroneous transfer of conclusions obtained from animal experiments, and it has been refuted by the findings of studies evaluating the effects of atropine in women (Levin 1992). Aside from cholinergic and adrenergic nerves, a number of peptides with neurotransmitter or neuromodulator roles have been located in the female genital tissues. Among these are nitric oxide and VIP, neurotransmitters that have also been found in the male genitals. According to Levin (1998), the available data point to VIP as the possible major neurotransmitter controlling vaginal blood flow and lubrication during sexual arousal. In his discussion on the role of nitric oxide (NO), he concludes: "While NO has been strongly implicated as an essential neurotransmitter in penile erection mechanisms of human males, there is no evidence, as yet, that it is involved in controlling human vaginal blood flow" (Levin 1998). Indeed, Hoyle and colleagues (1996), in a study with pre- and postmenopausal women, failed to find nitric oxide synthase, the enzyme that manufactures nitric oxide, in approximately half of the women.

Hormonal Control of the Sexual Response System

That sexual arousal involves mediation of the central nervous system, autonomic nervous system, and hormonal system has been well documented. It has also been noted that there are species and sex differences in the dependence of sexual arousal on the neocortex and hormones (Beach 1958). A brief description of some of the hormonal effects upon the response system is warranted.

Male hormones (often referred to as *androgens*) are defined as those that have masculinizing effects; female hormones, as those that have feminizing effects. Although both males and females produce both types of hormones, males produce more masculinizing hormones and females produce more feminizing hormones. In humans, sex hormones are produced throughout life with an increase at puberty. Even though the level of sex hormones in the bloodstream has less effect on the sexual activity of humans than of other animals, the sex hormones still have an influence on sexual behavior. For men, sexual interest tends to be highest during the ages when androgen levels are highest (about 15 to 25). Also, men with low androgen levels generally have less-than-average frequencies of erection and sexual activity (Kalat 1984). With women, a marked decrease in sexual response was shown in about one third of women after removal of the sex organs (Zussman et al. 1981, cited in Kalat 1984), presumably due to decreased levels of both estrogens and androgens. Androgen replacement has been shown to be effective in restoring sexual activity in both women (Burdine, Shipley, & Papas 1957, cited in Kalat 1984) and men (Bancroft 1995a). Bancroft (1989) suggested that sexual interest is more variably influenced by hormone levels in women than in men.

A number of studies have examined the effects of anti-androgens and exogenous androgens in men. There is also some literature on the effects of sexual activity or erotic stimuli on hormone levels. However, the most relevant evidence on the role of sex hormones in men comes from androgen replacement studies in hypogonadal men. These studies have shown that, within weeks after androgen withdrawal, a decline in sexual desire occurs. A more complex picture emerges with regard to androgen effects on erectile function. Erections during sleep (nocturnal penile tumescence or NPT) are substantially reduced by androgen depletion and restored with androgen replacement. On the other hand, erections to visual erotic stimuli have been found to continue in spite of androgen withdrawal. These findings have led to the distinction between androgen-dependent and -independent erectile responsiveness in men, with measurement of NPT being seen as a window into the neurophysiological substrate of central arousal (Bancroft 1989). The findings of more recent studies suggest that the relationship between the two proposed classes of erectile responsiveness is more complicated than initially believed. Whereas the earlier evidence was restricted to the effects on penile circumference, newer findings suggest that erections to visual erotic stimuli are affected in terms of degree of rigidity and duration of response (Bancroft 1995a). As the effects of androgen replacement are much greater with NPT than with the response to visual sexual stimuli, the distinction between androgen-dependent and -independent erectile responsiveness remains useful and warrants further study. However, although pertinent to our understanding of neurophysiological mechanisms relating hormone systems to sexual responsiveness, the findings from hypogonadal studies are not thought to apply to sexual responsivity in men with normal androgen levels. It is widely assumed that there is a threshold level of circulating testosterone above which an increase will have no additional effects. Variations in androgen levels are not believed to lead to variations in sexual behavior and responsiveness unless the hormonal variation is below threshold level, as in hypogonadal men, or in boys around puberty (Bancroft 1989).

The majority of studies on the relationship between reproductive hormones and sexual behavior and responsiveness in women have assessed these variables across the menstrual cycle. In his discussion of the available literature, Bancroft (1989) concluded that, "with the possible exception of estrogens and vaginal function, there is as much evidence against as for the role of hormones in female sexuality." The more variable findings in women may (according to this author) be attributed to methodological deficiencies, social and psychological differences between men and women, and to a possibly greater genetic–behavioral variability of hormone–behavior responsiveness in women. As far as psychophysiological responsivity is concerned, a similarly complex picture emerges. The evidence that subjective and physiological levels of sexual response may vary across the menstrual cycle is inconsistent and inconclusive (Meuwissen & Over 1992). Several studies have found that the level of subjective sexual arousal evoked by fantasy, erotic film, and audiotaped stories remains stable across phases of the menstrual cycle. Hoon, Bruce, and Kinchelow (1982) and Meuwissen and Over (1992) found that vaginal blood volume levels as measured by a vaginal plethysmograph (described later in this chapter) were stable across phases. Results regarding changes in pulse amplitude in response to erotic stimuli have been less consistent. Whereas Meuwissen and Over (1992) and Schreiner-Engel et al. (1981) found pulse amplitude responses to be higher in the premenstrual phase than in the periovulatory phase, Hoon et al. (1982) and Morrell et al. (1984) did not find any differences between phases of the menstrual cycle. Slob and colleagues (1990), who measured labial temperature to index genital responses, found no relationship between phases of the menstrual cycle and either changes in temperature or subjective sexual arousal to erotic film presentations. In contrast, Slob, Ernste, and van der Werff-ten Bosch (1991) did find differences, but only during the first of two measurement sessions. Women tested for the first time in their follicular phase were sexually more aroused, both physiologically and subjectively, than women tested for the first time during their luteal phase. Thus the available data leave us with an inconclusive and incomplete picture of the relationship between sexual arousal and menstrual cycle phases. Among the methodological factors that may have occasioned this lack of consistency are differences in the method used for determining cycle phase, variations in experimental design, and differences in subject characteristics (Hedricks 1994). Although no clear-cut answer can be given regarding the extent of possible effects of menstrual cycle phase, the potential for laboratory confounding clearly exists and so controls for menstrual phase are advised.

Social Context

MEASUREMENT MILIEU
Confidentiality

The American Psychological Society has formulated guidelines for the ethical treatment of participants in research (American Psychological Association 1992). These apply "in spades" to research on sexuality. Due to the highly personal nature of the inquiry, researchers must be particularly sensitive to the individual concerns of their participants in an endeavor to ensure both the confidentiality of the data and the comfort and well-being of research or clinical participants. Concerned researchers need to recognize that, because laboratory recording using genital devices will be conducted on a sensitive area and in a setting that is very far removed from the natural environment, care must be taken to avoid negative reactions by participants. It has been reported (Rosen 1976) that male erection measures in the laboratory can create performance anxiety with patients undergoing treatment for sexual dysfunction. It is reasonable to assume that the same would hold true for females in a similar situation.

Fully informed voluntary consent coupled with well-trained experimenters is the best line of defense for both confidentiality and participant welfare issues. A widely used practice is to have participants come to an informational session in which all aspects of the research are described. Particularly important is the clear and understandable description of the details concerning measurement of genital responding and any collection of information concerning the participant's sexual practices or attitudes. This session ends without the participant being asked to make a decision as to whether or not he or she will enter the study. The participant then leaves the experimental facility and is contacted, by phone, several days later and given the opportunity to volunteer for the research. This procedure minimizes pressure to become involved in the research and optimizes meeting the criteria of fully informed voluntary consent.

Another problem is that the need for fully informed voluntary consent means that participants cannot be studied without their having considerable information concerning the nature of the experiment and the stimuli that will be employed. It would be inappropriate to expose individuals to explicit sexual material without their advance knowledge. This means that participants in sex research are told a great deal about the nature of the stimuli to which they will be exposed. In turn, this means that they will have developed expectations concerning the nature of the study, and the influence of such expectations is unknown. It has been informally observed that men waiting for the delivery of erotic stimuli have shown genital responding prior to the presentation of that stimuli. Such responding must arise from the expectations generated by the individual participant. In a related vein, Amoroso and Brown (1973) reported that demand characteristics of sex research can create artifacts in both physiological and subjective assessments of sexual arousal. Their study found that participants attached to electrical recording devices rated stimuli more erotic that participants rating the same stimuli outside the specific laboratory setting. In another study, Hicks (1970) showed that different experimenter moods and behaviors produced different physiological records and subjective reports. It is not possible to avoid these problems and maintain the very high ethical standards that must accompany sex research. Only further study of the actual effects of these variables will tell us how important they are and if they substantially influence research outcomes.

We describe in greater detail elsewhere how to deal with the issue of sterilizing genital transducers. Obviously there is a risk if the device is not carefully and completely cleansed and sterilized. It is incumbent upon any responsible investigator to ensure that participants run absolutely no risk of contamination; anything less would be unacceptable.

Volunteer Biases

Volunteer biases have been a point of concern for the sex researcher. Wolchik, Braver, and Jensen (1985) studied the effects of increasingly intrusive measures of sexual arousal on volunteer rate and type of volunteer. They compared sexual behaviors and attitudes of volunteers and nonvolunteers across increasingly intrusive experimental conditions. They also examined gender differences in volunteer rates across these same conditions. They found that female volunteers were more sexually experienced than female nonvolunteers, that volunteers of both sexes displayed more sexual curiosity than nonvolunteers, and that male volunteers had experienced more sexual difficulties and had been exposed to more erotica than male nonvolunteers. In addition, males were more likely to volunteer than females. It was found that the more intrusive the method of investigation, the lower the rate of volunteers. Strassberg and Lowe (1995) reported that volunteers for plethysmographic research had higher levels of sexual experience and lower levels of sex guilt. A study by Bogaert (1996) also identified differences between volunteers and nonvolunteers that were quite similar to those reported by other investigators. What was new in this study was that the personality variable of "sensation seeking" was higher in volunteers and that social conformity and some measures of rule-following were lower. Such findings make it clear that generalizing research on volunteers to the entire population must be done with limitations in view.

The question, of course, is not whether there are differences between volunteers and the general population but whether or not these differences influence research outcomes. There is no definitive answer to that question. By definition, we do not collect information on genital responding from nonvolunteers, so the question of how nonvolunteers might respond is moot. As Bogaert (1996) noted, the impact of such variables likely varies as a function of the research question being addressed. What is of some interest is that a fair portion (10%–20%) of volunteers are relatively unsophisticated and relatively inexperienced yet do participate in sex research measuring genital responses. In a related vein, Laan and Everaerd (1995) noted that their participant population contains a significant portion (22%) who have experienced sexual abuse. The assumption that volunteer populations will represent only those who have had positive sexual experiences is not tenable. These various findings suggests less bias than might otherwise be expected if one were to assume that only experienced participants who like sex volunteer for research involving genital measures.

Political Issues

Political issues powerfully influence research in sexuality. As Laumann et al. (1994, p. xxviii) noted, "there are those on both sides of the political spectrum who oppose the gathering and publicizing of information about sex." We support the position of Laumann and colleagues, who state: "We contend that orchestrated ignorance about basic human behavior has never been wise public policy. Anti-intellectualism and fear are not convincing arguments against inquiry and knowledge" (1994, p. xxviii). To the scholar, opting for ignorance over information seems a folly; yet that is exactly what the sex researcher is occasionally faced with.

This concern boils down to the practical issue that there are important questions that we can not and, perhaps, should not study. As an obvious example, it is most unlikely that scholars will rigorously investigate sexual behavior in children. This restriction flows naturally from the moral and legal issues that would be involved. In a highly controversial matter that is related to children's sexual activity, there has been some examination of the issues surrounding the question of whether or not children are harmed by adult–child sexual contacts (Sandfort 1992). As Sandfort noted, even asking the question raises cries of outrage and shame from professionals and the public alike. If one believes that adult sexual behavior and attitude formation result at least in part from childhood experiences, it is extremely difficult to see how the many questions that flow from that perspective will be studied.

It is clear that social variables influence sexuality. Ever since the pioneering work of Alfred Kinsey and his colleagues (Kinsey, Pomeroy, & Martin 1948; Kinsey et al. 1953), the role of societal variables in sexuality has been widely acknowledged. The demonstrated importance of such variables (e.g., religiosity, social class, educational level) on human sexual response is powerful and undisputed evidence of the influence of social factors in sexuality. We can note that much sex research is directed at examining cultural differences in order to explicate the role of societal factors (Davenport 1987; Kon 1987). To the researcher, these facts mean that care must be taken to evaluate or control social variables in studies. It could well be argued that cultural and societal factors are among the most interesting in the field of sexuality, and their presence adds a richness to the area of study. Far from abandoning research on sexuality because it is powerfully influenced by social variables, we should seize the opportunity to examine these variables and so further our understanding of their influence.

COMPARATIVE PROCESSES

Within- and Between-Subject Approaches

Most research on the psychophysiology of sexuality has used as a validating criterion the relationship between sub-

jective and physiological responses. Those measures that show low correlations are generally considered less important and useful. Evaluating the relationship between genital measures and the experiential state of the individual is heavily influenced by the research approach, the most common of which is the between-subject approach. From this perspective, a stimulus (e.g., an erotic videotape) is shown to an individual who is later asked to rate the highest level of sexual arousal experienced during the film's presentation. The data that are entered into a correlation computation are (a) the subjective rating and (b) the maximum genital response obtained during the stimulus presentation. These two data points are collected across a set of subjects and a correlation is computed. The question being addressed is based on the assumption that each individual can accurately assess his or her subjective feeling state. The resultant statistic assesses the degree to which the two measures covary to a single stimulus presentation; it tells us nothing about individual differences in the relationship between genital and subjective feeling states. Yet the variable – that is, individual differences in the correlation between subjective experience and physiological change – has the potential to provide important information.

The common between-subject design using a single erotic stimulus fails also to answer this question: What is the relationship between the intensity of the stimulus and the response to that stimulus? Using a single rating and a single stimulus would be analogous to seeking the relationship between the perceived intensity and the physical intensity of a light when only one level of the light is presented; it is necessary to use a range of stimulus intensities. Korff and Geer (1983) conducted such a study in women. They computed the correlation between stimulus intensity (photos that varied in erotic value) and genital change in women. Korff and Geer's within-subject methodology yielded high intraindividual correlations. Perhaps more importantly, they found that the correlation could be used as a dependent variable: the mean correlation between genital change and ratings of arousal was raised from 0.48 to 0.89 by the simple instruction to attend to what the body was doing. This finding brought into question the view that the relationship between genital change and subjective experience was lower for women than men (see Laan & Everaerd 1995 for a more detailed review of this topic). The within-subject design permits use of the relationship as a dependent variable and opens the possibility of a range of investigations asking how the relationship itself may vary across conditions.

Answering the simple question, "What is the correlation between the subjective experience of sexual arousal and the genital changes that occur during that arousal?" is actually not so simple. The correlation itself is not immutable but is a function of variables that have only begun to be explored. Additionally, the correlation may be an individual difference of genuine interest – one that not only may vary among individuals but may well vary within the individual in interesting ways.

A final point that upon reflection is obvious yet often is not made salient concerns the use of experimental outcomes to establish between-group differences. For example, should the nature of the relationship between variables differ as a function of participant gender, it is not necessary to have measurement units in common in order to discuss the results. Likewise, should genital change increase over time for one gender and decrease over time for the other gender, the measurement units need not be identical for that finding to be meaningful. Thus, between-group designs can help identify differences that might otherwise go unidentified.

Male–Female Differences

A topic of interest to the public as well as to students and researchers is the nature of gender differences. The senior author has just published a paper that begins to sketch some of the differences that occur when considering cognitive variables in sexuality (Geer & Manguno 1997). It would appear that, across the entire field of sexuality, gender differences are the norm rather than the exception. The issue is particularly complicated when we consider sexual psychophysiology. There are two principal reasons why the question is complex. First is the nature of the physiological events themselves; second, the presence of gender differences in response biases. We first consider the physiological aspects of the problem.

The simple fact is that one can not directly compare male and female genital measures. Attempts to develop identical measures (using e.g. the anal probe) have not solved the problem. Changes in vaginal vascular responses cannot be compared with changes in penile responding; they are two widely different measures on different anatomical structures. One possible solution to this problem is to use some type of standard score as a metric into which each of the variables can be transformed. It would then be possible to compare and contrast standard scores between the genders. This strategy incorporates a number of hidden assumptions regarding which we have no evidence either for or against. For example, the standard score forces a normal distribution upon the data; this may be a false assumption, as may be the assumption of linearity of changes. Is a standard score change of 10 the same at the lower end of the distribution as it is at the upper end or even the middle? There are no available data to answer these questions. The standardized score technique might prove useful, but we don't have enough information to assess its appropriateness.

The second complexity concerns the problem of response biases. We all know that sexuality is a topic that is surrounded by emotionality. When attempting to map genital response to psychological events, care must be taken

to assure that the subject is providing accurate and reliable data. Two simple examples will demonstrate how we know that serious gender bias exists in data collected on sexual phenomena. The first is the well-known fact that, regarding the incidence of intercourse, males and females report substantially different numbers of partners (Laumann et al. 1994). Unless one is willing to assume there are a few women who are sexual partners to a great number of men, there is a problem in the data. It is not our goal to offer solutions to this problem but only to note that there appears to be a systematic difference in reporting of sexual activity between the genders. Be it a gender-linked memory distortion or a deliberate over- or underestimate by the genders, it points to a systematic bias. A second (and more casual) observation that makes this point has been made by the senior author in informal classroom surveys in courses on sexuality. Upon asking college students to rate their level of "sex drive" as compared to other members of their gender who are peers, women report a relatively normal distribution with about 50% above the mean. For males, however, about 80% report themselves "well above" the mean. Such findings make clear that there are substantial gender biases in reporting sexual behavior. Using the same scale does not mean that the results are equivalent. The issues of response contamination by demand characteristics and social desirability biases must be carefully considered. There is no easy answer to evaluating these biases. It does require, however, that investigators use caution when interpreting data gathered via subjective reports.

RANGE OF APPLICATIONS

Sexual psychophysiology has often been used in studies evaluating its effectiveness in the detection and diagnosis of sexual dysfunctions and problematic sexual behaviors. It also has been used to track the effectiveness of various treatment strategies. We have chosen not to review the findings based upon clinical diagnostic labels. Rather, we have chosen to note the two categories of clinical use to which genital psychophysiology has been applied. A thorough review of the clinical findings is beyond this chapter's focus; the interested reader should consult Rosen and Beck (1988), Buvat et al. (1990), Everaerd (1993), or Morokoff (1993). In addition, we recommend the 1995 *Journal of Consulting and Clinical Psychology* (Special Section: Contemporary Issues in Human Sexuality), which contains several relevant papers.

The first of the two categories into which we place applied work using genital measures is studies evaluating arousal and response, including erectile dysfunctions and problems of low sexual desire or interest. The second general category encompasses dysfunctions in which the individual reports problematic sexual interests or behavior preferences. In agreement with the American Psychiatric

Association and the American Psychological Association, we do not include "same-gender preferences" (i.e. homosexuality) in this category.

Arousal and Response Problems

One of the most obvious places to use measures of genital responding as a diagnostic tool is in males who experience erectile disorders. One of the more critical issues involved in the diagnosis of erectile dysfunction has been whether the problem stems from physiological or psychological mechanisms. As is typically the case in behavioral science, one can not precisely differentiate between these categories of causation. Even if we accept the psychogenic–biogenic dichotomy as useful, the answer turns out that both sets of factors are involved. For example, in a study of 117 male patients, Melman, Tiefer, and Pederson (1988) reported that 29% of dysfunctional cases were primarily biogenic in origin, 40% primarily psychogenic, 15% primarily biogenic worsened by psychogenic factors, and 10% primarily psychogenic worsened by biogenic factors (6% had erectile problems of unknown origin). The numbers of individuals with various etiological attributions assigned often reflect the biases of investigators or different base rates of biogenic versus psychogenic cases in their patient population as much as the reality of causation in the general population.

Everaerd (1993) noted that two categories of assessment paradigms have been used to evaluate males with erectile dysfunctions. The waking assessment paradigm consists of presenting erotic stimuli to the patient and determining if a "normal" penile response occurs. The nocturnal assessment paradigm consists of recording during sleep to determine if a normal NPT (nocturnal penile tumescence) response occurs. Sakheim, Barlow, and Beck (1985) reported 80% diagnostic accuracy in identifying functional versus organically impaired men using a waking assessment paradigm. Janssen and colleagues (1994a) found similarly high predictive values using a procedure in which patients were presented with combinations of visual, tactile, and cognitive stimuli. This accuracy rate is equivalent to most reports using the NPT assessment. Rosen and Beck (1988) reported that males with psychogenic dysfunction showed lower correlations (than asymptomatic subjects) between penile response to erotica and subjective report. As Everaerd pointed out, this may add to the range of diagnostic strategies available. The problem is that a lack of response to erotic stimuli could result from either psychogenic or biogenic variables; therefore, in the awake nonresponding subject, the nature of the interfering etiological factor cannot be determined.

The nocturnal assessment was developed in an attempt to more accurately discriminate between psychogenic and biogenic factors in erectile dysfunction. Working from the fact that the normal male shows spontaneous erections during sleep, it was assumed that if a dysfunctional individual showed normal NPT responses then the erectile system is operative and thus the problem must be psychogenic. However, there is considerable individual variance (Wincze et al. 1980). Everaerd estimated diagnostic accuracy for the NPT in the sleep lab to be about 80%. The NPT assessment procedure is quite expensive and creates a practical issue concerning its application. Buvat et al. (1990) noted some of the many complications in interpreting the NPT.

There has been only limited psychophysiological assessment of males with premature ejaculation as a presenting problem. If it is assumed that this is a problem of arousal, genital measures should be useful in identifying the problem. However, thus far no clear-cut genital response differences have been identified in this population (Rowland et al. 1997; Spiess, Geer, & O'Donohue 1984). For example, Rowland and colleagues found subjective and perceived response differences but none in the penile response, although this finding may have been influenced by their use of a noncontinuous measure, the Erectiometer. The lack of penile responding differences suggests a reformulation of the problem, one that de-emphasizes the role of atypical arousal in the etiology. In a move in that direction, Metz and associates (1997) suggested that, as with erectile failure, the premature ejaculator population may be meaningfully divided into categories of biogenic and psychogenic causation.

All of the described work evaluated males. Relatively speaking, little evidence exists concerning women with arousal dysfunctions. Wincze, Hoon, and Hoon (1976) reported reduced vaginal blood volume (VBV) in dysfunctional women. In contrast, Morokoff and Heiman (1980) – using vaginal pulse amplitude – found no differences between nonclinical women and clinical groups experiencing low arousal and anorgasmia. Palace and Gorzalka (1990) found enhanced VBV for nonclinical individuals to a combination of anxiety and erotic stimuli. Finally, Palace and Gorzalka (1992) reported reduced VBV in dysfunctional women as well as reduced subjective levels of arousal. These conflicting patterns of results may reflect differences in procedures or in the physiological measure used. This is an area of research that is in dire need of further study.

As noted previously, a variable of possible interest in these studies is the "individual difference" variable of the relationship between genital measures and subjective ratings of arousal; Rosen and Beck (1988) reported on the usefulness of this relation as a measure of individual differences. It is possible – given the importance of the role of cognitive factors in sexual responding – that this information is particularly relevant. We would encourage further evaluation of the subjective–genital relationship in clinical populations.

Specific Object Preferences

The second category of sexual dysfunction that has been evaluated are problems associated with sexual object preferences. From the simple suggestion that individuals will show arousal (and thus genital responding) to what for them is effective stimulation, the use of genital measures to assess and track treatment of such problems follows naturally. Genital responding has been used both to diagnose and track the progress of treatment of individuals whose sexual preferences involve children. Similarly, the sexual aggressor or rapist has been studied using the genital methodology. The basic question evaluated is: Do these individuals show enhanced genital responding when exposed to stimuli (e.g., photos or videotapes) relevant to the interest under study? The most general answer to that question is Yes. Finkelhor summarized the work on individuals with child preferences by saying, "As a whole, the above studies seem to establish the fact that some pedophiles have arousal preference for children, but whether or not all child molesters, including incest offenders, have such a preference is not clear" (1986, p. 101). As with erectile dysfunctions, the preferences appear to hold up in group effects but may or may not hold for the individual.

The same appears to be true for the sexual aggressor or rapist. Barbaree, Marshall, and Lanthier (1979) developed a statistic they called the "rape index" based on genital responding. The index was obtained by dividing the mean percent of erection to rape cues by the average percent of erection to cues of consenting heterosexual activity. They reported significant correlations with the frequency of previously reported rapes as well as with the tendency to commit violent rapes. However, as remarked by Laws and Holmen, "We are continually astonished at the creativity in circumventing our procedures shown by supposedly uncreative, undereducated, and undersocialized sex offenders" (1978, p. 344). In other words, there is presently no accepted way to detect faking. Particularly it seems that offenders (as well as others) can inhibit genital responding. There is solid experimental evidence (e.g. Geer & Fuhr 1976) that distraction can block or greatly reduce genital responding, which suggests that those who wished to do so could minimize their response to stimuli by relatively simple techniques (e.g., counting backward).

Of importance is the finding by Hall, Hirschman, and Oliver (1995) that 25% of their male participants showed sexual arousal to pedophilic stimuli equal to or greater than that found to adult erotic stimuli – and this in participants who reported no pedophilic behavior. Likewise, Lohr, Adams, and Davis (1997) reported that, although men with sexually coercive histories showed greater penile responding to coercive cues, males with no such history also yielded some arousal to those same cues. These findings make clear the fact that arousal to a particular stimulus category does not necessarily correspond with behavior. In women there are anecdotal and clinical reports of rape victims responding with vaginal lubrication while terrorized during a sexual assault. Laan et al. (1994) found that women responded with equal genital arousal to male-

oriented versus female-oriented erotica, even though the women reported subjectively that they found the female-oriented more arousing. Hence, care must be taken before one accepts genital responding as the "gold standard" of sexual arousal. Sexual arousal is a complexly determined phenomenon, expressing itself in multiple response systems that are not always tied closely together.

Inferential Context

MENSURATION AND QUANTIFICATION

The following discussion of how genital measures relate to physiological events will cover only those that are most widely used. We begin with a consideration of measures of the male genital response.

Male Genital Measurement Devices

The earliest genital devices were developed for the monitoring of male erection. The first of these devices was a simple electromechanical transducer (Ohlmeyer, Brilmayer, & Hullstrong 1944). The device consisted of a circular ring that fit around the participant's penis and provided a simple binary signal of the presence or absence of erection. Current research in male sexual arousal relies primarily on continuous measures of penile volume, circumference, and rigidity. We now turn our attention to those measures.

Volume. Figure 3 presents a schematic diagram of Freund's (1963) air volumetric plethysmograph. This device uses the general principle of volumetric plethysmography, in which a body part is enclosed in a sealed container with air or fluid. Less widely used variants of this technique have been described by Fisher, Gross, and Zuch (1965), who used water instead of air, and McConaghy (1974). The plethysmograph is positioned on the participant by the experimenter, who places a sponge-rubber ring and a plastic ring with an inflatable cuff over the penis. A glass cylinder with a funnel at the top is then fitted over the other components, and the cuff is inflated with air. Changes in the size of the penis result in displacement of air, which can be detected by a pressure transducer.

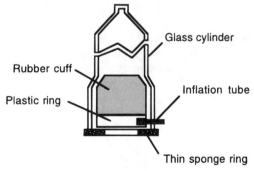

Figure 3. A schematic diagram of Freund's (1963) air volumetric plethysmograph.

Volumetric devices can be calibrated and scored in terms of absolute penile volume. Volumetric plethysmography has the advantage of offering high sensitivity. A limitation of this technique, however, is that it does not allow for the determination of the source of change. For example, the device cannot be used to discriminate between changes in volume due to increases in penile length versus penile circumference. In addition, the apparatus is relatively complex, cumbersome, and sensitive to temperature and movement artifacts.

Circumference. A diagram of the strain gauge as originally described by Fisher et al. (1965) is shown in Figure 4. This device, known as a mercury-in-rubber strain gauge, was adapted from a similar transducer used by Shapiro and Cohen (1965). The device consists of a hollow rubber tube filled with mercury and sealed at the ends with platinum electrodes that are inserted into the mercury. The electrodes are attached to a bridge circuit for connection to a polygraph or computer. The operation of the mercury-in-rubber strain gauge depends upon penile circumference changes that cause the rubber tube to stretch or shorten, thus altering the cross-sectional area of the column of mercury within the tube. The resistance of the mercury inside the tube varies directly with its cross-sectional area, which in turn is reflective of changes in the circumference of the penis. Variations of the mercury-in-rubber gauge have been described by Bancroft, Jones, and Pullan (1966), Jovanovic (1967), and Karacan (1969).

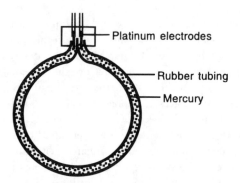

Figure 4. Schematic diagram of the mercury-in-rubber penile strain gauge.

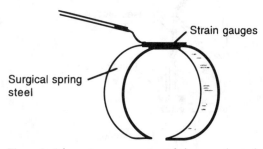

Figure 5. Schematic representation of electromechanical penile strain gauge developed by Barlow and co-workers (1970).

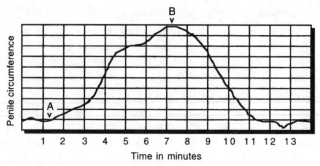

Figure 6. Example of recording from penile strain gauge. Elevation from point A to point B represents penile circumference changes over a particular time span.

Another widely used type of penile strain gauge is the electromechanical strain gauge, developed by Barlow and co-workers (1970) and depicted in Figure 5. This device is made of two arcs of surgical spring material joined with two mechanical strain gauges. These gauges are flexed when the penis changes in circumference, producing changes in their resistance. The resistance changes are in turn coupled through a bridge circuit to a polygraph or computer. The electromechanical gauge does not fully enclose the penis. For this reason, it is more sensitive to movement artifacts and less suitable for studies on nocturnal penile tumescence than the mercury-in-rubber gauge. However, mechanical strain gauges are quite sensitive and more rugged than their rubber counterparts. Figure 6 represents a typical recording of penile circumference as rendered by a strain gauge device.

Comparison Studies on Volume and Circumference Measures. To date, three studies have been reported comparing volumetric and circumferential measures. Freund, Langevin, and Barlow (1974) compared Freund's volumetric device with Barlow's electromechanical strain gauge. They presented a group of men with 48 slides of male and female nudes. Their results indicated that, compared with circumference measurement, volumetric plethysmography is more sensitive to changes in penile tumescence and is better at discriminating between different response levels. However, considering the type of stimuli used and the absence of a check for habituation, their conclusion most likely pertains to differences between relatively low response levels. In another study, McConaghy (1974) compared his adaptation of the volumetric device with a mercury strain gauge. He showed his subjects 10-second shots of male and female nudes, which were inserted in a sexually neutral film. In his report, McConaghy provided some example recordings but no descriptive or other statistical analyses. In 1987, Wheeler and Rubin compared the mercury gauge and Freund's volumetric device using erotic film excerpts. In contrast to Freund et al. (1974), they did not find any evidence for a higher sensitivity of the volumetric device. In addition, the authors reported that the volumetric device was more difficult to use and displayed considerably more artifacts than the strain gauge. The absence of systematic differences between the two measures in the study of Wheeler and Rubin (1987) may have been a result of the film stimuli they used, which likely induced higher response levels than the series of slides used by Freund and colleagues. In reviewing the available data, it seems that the two measures mainly differ in sensitivity at low response levels.

Owing to the relative ease of their use in contrast with volumetric devices, penile strain gauges have become increasingly popular in laboratory use. Although only two studies have as yet examined and compared the properties of the two types of strain gauge in vivo, several in vitro (i.e., laboratory simulation) studies have shown that both the mercury-in-rubber and the electromechanical strain gauge demonstrate very linear outputs, high test–retest reliability, high stability over time, and minor sensitivity to temperature changes (Earls & Jackson 1981; Farkas et al. 1979; Janssen et al. 1997; Karacan 1969; Richards et al. 1985, 1990). Nowadays, the mercury-in-rubber type of strain gauge is also available in versions filled with an indium-gallium alloy, which is considered to be even less sensitive to temperature changes than mercury (Richards et al. 1985).

A potential concern with the use of circumferential measures is the suggestion that penile circumference may show a slight decrease at the onset of sexual arousal (Abel et al. 1975; Laws & Bow 1976; McConaghy 1974), which may represent a problem in that it may be incorrectly interpreted as a decrease in sexual response. Further, it has also been noted that strain gauges may be unreliable at the upper end of the tumescence curve (Earls et al. 1983). This may represent a limitation if the measures are to be used for determining the full range of erectile capacity.

Laws (1977), who was the first to compare the two strain gauges in vivo, found discrepancies in measurement with the two devices. Unfortunately, he obtained data from only one participant. Recently, Janssen et al. (1997) compared the two penile strain gauges (using indium-gallium instead of mercury for the rubber gauge) in a group of 25 sexually functional men. In addition, they compared two different calibration methods. Typically, both gauges are calibrated using a graduated circular cone. Janssen and colleagues hypothesized that, given the fact that the penis is formed principally by two cylindrical bodies, the shape of its cross-sectional area is probably more accurately described as an oval than as a circle. The two gauges are prone to be differentially affected by the shape of the calibration device. In contrast to the mercury gauge, the electromechanical gauge does not fully enclose the penis. Thus, penile circumference as assessed by this gauge is in fact estimated, using the calibration device as a model. If a penis approximates an oval shape in cross-section, then the electromechanical gauge can be expected to overestimate its circumference when calibrated on a circular device. The authors found that the electromechanical gauge calibrated on the circular device indeed reported greater circumference changes. Circumference changes were not different for the two gauges when the oval calibration device was used. In addition, their findings suggested that the electromechanical gauge is more sensitive to changes in penile circumference during initial stages of erection than the other strain gauge, a conclusion that is consistent with findings of earlier studies examining the output of the two gauges in vitro (Earls & Jackson 1981; Richards et al. 1985).

Rigidity. One of the first attempts to measure penile rigidity was made by Karacan and colleagues (1978), who reported the use of "buckling pressure" as a dependent variable in penile responding. This method uses a device that measures the axial force required for the bending of the penis. Typically, this procedure is coupled with visual inspections by both the technologist and the participant, and sometimes photographs of the penis are taken. There is, to date, no information on the validity and reliability of this method (Schiavi 1992). Other single measurement methods for indexing rigidity include stamp tests, the snap gauge, and the Erectiometer. In particular, the latter method has been successfully applied in research on erectile and ejaculation dysfunctions. The Erectiometer is a felt band, calibrated in millimeters, with a sliding collar fastened to one end. When the penis increases in circumference with sufficient force it will pull the band through the collar. There are two types available, one requiring a force equivalent to 250 g to expand and the other requiring 450 g. This method is easy to use and inexpensive, but it does not provide continuous readings.

Bradley and associates (1985) described an instrument designed to measure continuously both circumference and radial rigidity. This device has been modified and is now commercially available as the Rigiscan Plus monitor. The Rigiscan consists of a recording unit that can be strapped around the waist or the thigh. The device can operate in ambulatory mode or be connected to a PC. It has two loops, one placed around the base of the penis and the other around the shaft just behind the corona. Each loop contains a cable that is tightened at discrete time intervals. Circumference is measured at 15-sec intervals, using a linear force of 1.7 N. The Rigiscan takes its first rigidity measure when a 20% increase in circumference is detected. This is repeated every 30 sec. To measure rigidity, the loops tighten a second time after circumference is measured, with a greater force of 2.8 N. The rigidity of a noncompressible shaft (i.e., no loop shortening to the higher force) is given as 100%.

The Rigiscan represents the first feasible attempt to measure rigidity continuously and has gained wide acceptance, particularly in clinical research settings. However, some basic questions related to its validity and reliability have yet to be explored. For example, there are no published in vitro data available on the test–retest reliability of the Rigiscan. Information on the reliability of the device over longer periods of usage is pertinent because – in contrast to strain gauges, where routine calibration allows for the test of linearity over time and where replacement is viable – a Rigiscan monitor is typically used for a number of years. The importance of developing a stable calibration method for the Rigiscan is stressed by the finding of Munoz, Bancroft, and Marshall (1993) that different Rigiscan devices can record different degrees of rigidity. In their study, Munoz et al. developed a "system" that provided a relatively constant circumference with variable rigidity. Using this system, they found that the Rigiscan underestimated circumference – in particular, at lower levels of rigidity. This finding was confirmed by an in vivo comparison between the performance of the Rigiscan and a mercury-in-rubber strain gauge in the measurement of NPT (Munoz et al. 1993).

The unique procedure used by the Rigiscan to measure tumescence and rigidity raises another methodological question: the potential reactivity of the measurement itself. The extent to which tightening of the loops may actually induce or modify sexual responses – in the absence of or in interaction with experimental or clinical manipulations – has not yet been assessed. With regard to this issue, Munoz et al. (1993) found fewer NPT episodes in a group of men with erectile problems when a mercury-in-rubber strain gauge was used together with a Rigiscan as compared to nights during which only the strain gauge was used. The authors attributed these differences to methodological (e.g. placement) factors.

The arguments that have been put forward in support of the development and use of rigidity measures have face validity and merit the continued exploration of ways to measure this characteristic. In essence, these arguments are twofold: (1) penile circumference is not a reliable predictor of penile rigidity, and (2) penile rigidity is the ultimate and behaviorally relevant measure of erectile capacity. Regarding the first assertion, two studies have been cited frequently. Wein and associates (1981) reported that significant changes in penile circumference occurred in 23% of normal control patients without sufficient increases in penile rigidity for vaginal penetration. Earls, Morales, and Marshall (1988) reported finding discrepancies between circumference and participants' perception of erectile sufficiency for intromission. Wein et al. (1981), however, based their conclusions on a measure of rigidity (buckling force) that is considered to lack proper validation (Schiavi 1992). As for the second study, it is well established that the perception of erectile responses is biased in patient groups (Janssen & Everaerd 1993; Sakheim et al. 1987). The more important point to be made, however, is that initial studies would be expected to converge on the relationship between circumference and rigidity as measured by the Rigiscan. Remarkably, only one study to date has reported correlations between the Rigiscan's circumference and rigidity

measures. Levine and Carroll (1994) studied NPT responses in 44 sexually functional men, with a wide age range, and analyzed the data of 113 nights of recording. They reported correlations of $r = 0.87$ and $r = 0.88$, respectively, between Rigiscan's time–intensity measures of tip tumescence and rigidity and of base tumescence and rigidity.

As for the second issue, the argument is that the key problem in erectile dysfunction is not the lack of increasing volume but the lack of stiffness (Giesbers et al. 1987). Therefore, from a clinical perspective, penile rigidity is regarded as a more crucial variable than circumferential expansion. The question of whether or not erectile capacity is normal is commonly described in terms of whether erections are "adequately rigid for penetration." The question of what level of rigidity satisfies this criterion has not yet been answered. Ultimately, for intercourse to occur, the amount of penile rigidity that is necessary will depend on how much pressure is required to penetrate. Wabrek and colleagues (1996) and Wagner, Wabrek, and Dalgaard (1986) gathered normative data on vaginal penetration pressure, which was defined as the pressure required to introduce a probe of a specific size into the vagina. They found that penetration pressure varied among positions (e.g., supine versus kneeling) and that vaginal penetration pressure was lower during conditions of sexual stimulation. The findings of these studies indicate that, at present, any clinical criterion for deciding whether an erection is "sufficiently" rigid for penetration is in essence a predictor and not an absolute measure of erectile functionality in sexual interactions with a partner.

Other Measures of Genital Response in Men. Less widely used measures involve the assessment of penile temperature, penile arterial pulse amplitude, and penile EMG (electromyography). Thermistor measurement devices have been designed to detect temperature changes that may accompany penile tumescence changes. Solnick and Berrin (1977) compared thermistor measures of tumescence with circumference measures. The results showed a relatively high concordance between temperature changes and penile circumference, findings that were supported by results of Webster and Hammer (1983).

Bancroft and Bell (1985) developed a reflectance photometer for noninvasive measurement of penile arterial pulse amplitude. The essential components of this device are similar to those used in the vaginal photometer, described later in this chapter. It has been suggested that penile pulse amplitude may provide an index of arterial inflow related to generalizable penile tumescence (Rosen & Beck 1988). However, the currently available data are insufficient to warrant a judgment on the usefulness of the penile photometer.

Wagner and Gerstenberg (1988) first described electrical activity in the cavernous tissues of the penis. Using needle electrodes to obtain EMG recordings, they found that the perception of visual sexual stimuli resulted directly in decreased smooth muscle activity (Gerstenberg et al. 1989; Wagner & Gerstenberg 1988; Wagner, Gerstenberg, & Levin 1989). Although this approach shows potential for becoming one of the more sensitive measures of male genital response, and in particular of the neurophysiological mechanisms involved in its activation, at present the reliability of the technique is still controversial. Various investigators have failed to reproduce the original findings in patient groups. More problematic, however, is that interpretation of the signal is hampered by lack of information on its characteristic features and by the absence of standardized recording techniques. Because of the low level of electrical activity in the penis and the consequently high level of amplification needed, the recording of penile EMG is susceptible to sources of interference such as pelvic and penile muscle contractions, cross-talk due to cardiac action, and (through its effects on placement of the electrodes) respiration (Jünemann et al. 1994). Work on a consensus in measuring penile EMG using needle electrodes is in progress (Sasso et al. 1997). The noninvasive alternative to this procedure – recording penile EMG using surface electrodes – has been less well studied and also may be expected to be sensitive to endogenous and exogenous sources of interference.

Female Measures

The development of genital measurement devices for women was stimulated by the Masters and Johnson (1966) report of vaginal vasocongestion being a relatively invariant concomitant of sexual arousal and by Zuckerman's (1971) report, which stated that the lack of genital measurement in women was an obstacle to research on sexuality.

In 1967, Palti and Bercovici reported that they mounted a light source and photoelectric cell on a vaginal speculum to detect vaginal pulse waves. Although the device reliably yielded a record of vaginal pulse waves, the method has not been adopted for use in sex research. Other early attempts to measure genital responses in women included a device designed to measure vaginal pH as an indicator of lubrication (Shapiro et al. 1968), yet attempts to measure vaginal pH or vaginal lubrication have been technically difficult and intrusive (Wagner & Levin 1978). Furthermore, Wagner and Levin (1984) reported that sexual arousal can induce changes in the surface pH of one part of the participant's vagina while having little effect elsewhere. A mechanical strain gauge was developed to measure clitoral enlargement, but the device has not proved to be applicable to the general female population (Karacan, Rosenbloom, & Williams 1970). In 1971, Jovanovic developed a balloon-like device that was filled with water and then inserted through the cervix into the uterus. This device, designed to measure uterine contractions, has many problems, including the tendency to extrude the device and pain associated with its placement (Rosen & Beck 1988). The following

approaches are currently the most widely used to measure genital responses in women.

Oxygenation and Thermal Clearance. First we discuss the sophisticated measures obtained from a device developed and described by Levin and Wagner (1978), in which a heated oxygen probe is used to detect changes in oxygen pressure (P_{O_2}) that is transduced across the walls of the vagina. The device consists of an oxygen electrode and a suction cup that are held on the vaginal wall by a partial vacuum generated in the cup. It is assumed that the more blood present in the tissues, the greater the amount of oxygen perfused across the vaginal epithelium. Using this device, it is possible to determine rather precisely the level of oxygen in the blood of the tissues located beneath the device. The actual dependent variable used is oxygen pressure, expressed in terms of millimeters of mercury.

The device that measures oxygen pressure can also measure heat dissipation into the tissues under the transducer. This method uses as the dependent variable the amount of energy (in milliwatts) required to keep the temperature of a heated thermistor constant. The heated oxygen probe has proven to be of value in the advancement of our understanding of the mechanisms underlying genital arousal in women (see Levin 1992 for a review). Further, one advantage of the device is that it is relatively free of movement artifacts. Disadvantages are its expense, the relative obtrusiveness of the measurement procedure, and the need to limit duration of measurement sessions to protect the vaginal mucosa from damage caused by heat and the suction needed to hold the device against the vaginal wall (Levin 1992).

Another device using thermal clearance as a method to index genital arousal, the vaginal blood flowmeter (Shapiro et al. 1968), consists of two thermistors mounted on a diaphragm ring that is placed against the cervix. One thermistor is placed in contact with the vaginal wall and is heated slightly above intravaginal temperature. The second thermistor is placed so as to avoid contact with the vaginal wall and thus record intravaginal temperature. As with the unit developed by Levin and Wagner (1978), the current necessary to maintain a constant temperature difference between the two thermistors reflects dissipation of heat into the vaginal wall. Fisher and colleagues (1983) reported data on patterns of sexual arousal during sleep and waking hours using the Shapiro et al. (1968) device. The data indicated that the vaginal blood flowmeter is sensitive to the effects of erotic stimulation in the waking state. The nighttime data were complex and require further investigation. The main disadvantages of the flowmeter are that it is a relatively delicate device and requires custom fitting of the diaphragm.

Temperature. Fisher and Osofsky (1967) and Fisher (1973) used a thermistor probe to measure vaginal temperature as

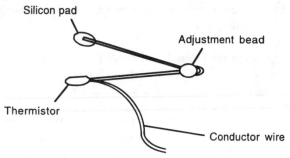

Figure 7. Diagram of labial thermistor clip developed by Henson et al. (1978).

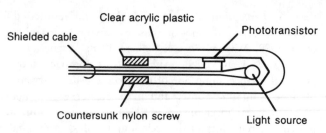

Figure 8. Schematic representation of the vaginal photometer.

an indicator of sexual arousal in women. These studies indicated that vaginal temperature generally reflects core temperature and is relatively insensitive to changes in arousal. In contrast, Fugl-Meyer, Sjogren, and Johansson (1984) described a radiotelemetric method for measuring vaginal temperature using a battery-powered transducer mounted on a diaphragm ring. They reported decreases in vaginal temperature, measured during masturbation as well as intercourse, that were speculated to be due to vaginal wall edema during sexual arousal (Wagner & Levin 1978). Advantages of the device include absence of movement artifacts and usability in natural settings. In view of the conflicting reports, however, replication is needed before the utility of vaginal temperature as a measure of arousal is fully ascertained.

Figure 7 depicts the transducer designed by Henson, Rubin, and Henson (1978) for measuring labial temperature. This device consists of three surface temperature probes designed to measure temperature changes from individually determined baselines. One of the thermistors monitors ambient room temperature. The other two thermistors are employed to monitor changes in surface skin temperature: one is attached to the labia minora by means of a brass clip; the other is attached to an extragenital site (i.e., the chest) and provides a reference temperature. Labial temperature for nine of the ten participants in the study of Henson and colleagues (1978) was shown to increase in response to their viewing an erotic film. Slob et al. (1990, 1991) also found an increase in labial temperature in the majority of participants during the viewing of erotic stimuli. Slob et al. (1990) compared women with and without diabetes mellitus and found initial labial temperature to be lower in the diabetic women than in the nondiabetic women. Apparent differences in responsivity between the two groups disappeared when participants were matched on initial labial temperature.

Pulse Amplitude and Blood Volume. The most widely used method for monitoring vaginal blood flow is vaginal photoplethysmography. This technique uses a vaginal photometer, originally developed by Sintchak and Geer (1975) and improved by Hoon, Wincze, and Hoon (1976). The device, shown in Figure 8, is made of clear acrylic plastic and

is shaped like a menstrual tampon. Embedded in the front end of the probe is a light source that illuminates the vaginal walls. Light is reflected and diffused through the tissues of the vaginal wall and reaches a photosensitive cell surface mounted within the body of the probe. Changes in the resistance of the cell correspond to changes in the amount of back-scattered light reaching the light-sensitive surface. It is assumed that a greater back-scattered signal reflects increased blood volume in the vaginal blood vessels (Levin 1992). Hoon et al. (1976) introduced an improved model of the vaginal photometer that substituted an infrared LED (light-emitting diode) for the incandescent light source and a phototransistor for the photocell. These innovations reduced potential artifacts associated with blood oxygenation levels, problems of hysteresis, and light history effects. The vaginal photometer is designed so that it can be easily placed by the participant. A shield can be placed on the probe's cable so that depth of insertion and orientation of the photoreceptive surface is known and held relatively constant (Geer 1983; Laan, Everaerd, & Evers 1995).

The photometer yields two analyzable signals. The first is the DC signal, which is thought to provide an index of the total amount of blood (Hatch 1979), often abbreviated as VBV (vaginal blood volume). The second signal available from the photometer is AC-coupled. This signal, the AC or vaginal pulse amplitude (VPA) signal, provides information on vaginal pulse wave and reflects phasic changes in the vascular walls that are dependent upon pressure changes within the vessels (Jennings, Tahmoush, & Redmont 1980). Figure 9 depicts the pulse wave components as rendered by the vaginal photometer under experimental conditions.

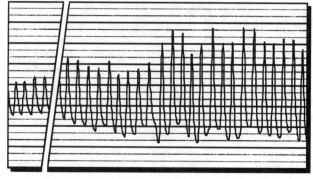

Figure 9. Example of AC or pulse-wave component obtained from vaginal photometer.

Although both measures have been found to reflect responses to erotic stimuli, the exact nature and source of the two signals is unknown. The interpretation of their relationship with underlying vascular mechanisms is hindered by the lack of a sound theoretical framework (Levin 1992) and of a calibration method that would allow transformation of the signals into known physiological events. At present, most researchers describe their findings in relative measures such as millimeters of pen deflection or change in microvolts. Levin (1998) stated that one of the basic assumptions underlying use of the plethysmograph is that changes in VBV and VPA always reflect local vascular events. However, in his discussion of findings from studies on the effects of exercise and orgasm on VBV and VPA, he suggested that the signals are likely to reflect rather complex interactions between sympathetic and parasympathetic regulatory processes and between circulatory and vaginal blood pressure. According to Levin (1992), vaginal blood flow changes could partly reflect increases in circulatory blood pressure that occur with sexual arousal.

The correspondence between the VPA and VBV components has been found to vary across studies. For example, Heiman (1976) reported relatively high correlations (between 0.4 and 0.6) between the two signals. However, she also found evidence indicative of correlations being lower at lower levels of sexual arousal. Meston and Gorzalka (1995) also reported a high correlation between VPA and VBV, yet they found a nonsignificant correlation between the two signals in a condition where a sexual film was preceded by exercise. Furthermore, Heiman (1977) found correlations between VPA and subjective sexual arousal to be higher than correlations between VBV and subjective arousal. These findings have led to a further exploration of the issue of which signal is the most sensitive and specific to sexual arousal. Geer, Morokoff, and Greenwood (1974) found that whereas VPA increased contingent upon the progression of an erotic film, no such variance was found in the VBV measure; they concluded that VPA was the more sensitive measure. Heiman (1977) and Osborne and Pollack (1977) arrived at a similar conclusion: Heiman on the basis of the higher correlations she found between VPA and subjective arousal, and Osborne and Pollack on the basis of their findings that only VPA discriminated between responses to hard-core and "erotically realistic" stories. It should be noted, however, that these studies provide only indirect support for the conclusion that VPA is the more sensitive measure. That is, they rely partly on implicit assumptions about the relationship between vaginal blood flow and variables such as subjective arousal and stimulus content.

Laan et al. (1995) were the first to test the sensitivity and specificity of the two measures concurrently. Although earlier studies (e.g. Geer et al. 1974) had established the differential sensitivity to erotic and nonerotic stimuli, only one study (Hoon et al. 1976) compared the effects of sexual and other, nonsexual, emotional stimuli; unfortunately, only VBV was measured in that study. Laan et al. (1995) investigated the specificity of the two signals by comparing responses of sexually functional women to sexual, anxiety-inducing, sexually threatening, and neutral film excerpts. The authors reported fairly high correlations between VPA and VBV, but found that the correspondence between the two signals was highly dependent upon the type of stimulus used. In contrast to VPA, VBV was found to be sensitive to the sex stimulus but not to the sexual threat stimulus. Participants did, however, report feelings of sexual arousal to the sexual threat stimulus. In addition, a striking difference between the two signals was that VBV, and not VPA, showed a marked decrease during the presentation of the anxiety stimulus, coinciding with an increase in skin conductivity and heart rate. These latter findings indicate that VBV is less specific to sexual arousal than VPA. In general, the results demonstrate response specificity of vaginal vasocongestion to sexual stimuli.

The findings of Laan et al. (1995) are potentially quite important to the study of the effects of anxiety on women's sexual response. In such studies it is common to induce anxiety prior to presenting participants with a sexual stimulus. Laan et al. (1995) found that, in sexually functional women, anxiety reduces VBV. If this finding holds for women with sexual dysfunctions, anxiety would also lead to a reduction in VBV in patient groups. Thus, the effect of anxiety could be incorrectly interpreted as having a facilitative effect on subsequent sexual responding when what is actually observed is a change from a lowered baseline to normal response levels. This possibility points to the relevance of controlling for stability of pre-exposure VBV levels and for the potential occurrence of negative change scores during nonsexual emotional stimulus presentations. More importantly, since the two signals provide nonoverlapping information, assessment of both signals should be preferred in this type of research because it allows for a more precise determination regarding what portion of total variance is explained by each variable.

Comparison Studies on Temperature versus Pulse Amplitude and Blood Volume. The literature comparing the various devices that measure genital responses in women is scant. To date, only one study has compared the measurement of vaginal temperature with vaginal blood flow (Gillian & Brindley 1979). However, in that study, an atypical photometer with more than one photocell was used. No studies exist on the direct comparison of heat oxygenation measures and vaginal plethysmography. In contrast, various studies have been reported on the relationship between labial temperature and vaginal blood flow measures. Henson and Rubin (1978) and Henson, Rubin, and Henson (1982) compared changes in VBV and labial temperature in response to sexual films. Both measures were found to increase reliably during stimulation, although there were large individual differences. Henson and Rubin (1978) found a very low, nonsignificant correlation between VBV and labial temperature. Further, only correlations between labial temperature and subjective arousal were significant. On the basis of this result, the authors suggested that physiological changes in the labia might be more easily perceived than intravaginal changes. Although vaginal responses tended to decrease more quickly after the sexual stimulus presentation, neither instrument returned to prestimulus baseline levels. In two other studies, Henson, Rubin, and Henson (1979a,b) compared labial temperature with both the VPA and VBV signals of the vaginal plethysmograph. The purpose of the study of Henson et al. (1979b) was to determine intrasubject consistency across two recording sessions. Although there was considerable consistency over sessions with regard to response patterns and amplitudes, labial temperature was the most consistent on both parameters. In the second study, Henson et al. (1979a) found high correlations between subjective arousal and both VPA and labial temperature changes. Vaginal blood volume was found to correlate less strongly with subjective arousal and was found to return to baseline more slowly than either VPA or labial temperature. These findings support the previously mentioned recommendation of VPA as a more sensitive measure of sexual arousal than VBV.

In their publications, Henson, Rubin, and Henson commented on the advantages and disadvantages of each device. For example, Henson et al. (1979b) noted that ambient temperature control is a requirement for use with the labial clip but not with the vaginal transducer. In contrast, movement artifacts are more common with the vaginal probe, and reliable measurement with the thermistor is not precluded by the menses. We are not aware of any published reports of vaginal photometer readings during menses. Levin (1998) asserted that measurements are readily invalidated because the vaginal photometer slides easily over the lubricated epithelium, illuminating new areas of tissue. According to him, VBV seems especially affected by this. It would seem that the shield, whose function is to stabilize probe placement, would mitigate against this artifact. Another important difference between the two devices is that a common absolute unit of measurement (°C) is used with the labial clip, whereas changes in vaginal blood flow are relative. Thus, the values obtained during the recording of vaginal blood flow are dependent on the electronic circuitry and the level of amplification used. Further, it is not yet known to what extent factors related to individual variations in anatomy and to physiological characteristics – such as resting levels of vaginal muscular tone and vaginal moistness – may affect the amplitude of the signal. Finally, although sensitivity of the probe to temperature appears to be minimal, it is in fact the temperature of the light source that is most often discussed. It is not implausible to suggest that vaginal

temperature can alter the probe's output, thus confounding the data (Beck, Sakheim, & Barlow 1983). Rogers et al. (1985), in a study on genital arousal during sleep, used a measure of integrated VPA and muscle contraction pressure that enabled the detection of movement and muscle contractions. It may prove valuable to extend the current design of the vaginal plethysmograph with additional measures of muscle contraction pressure and vaginal temperature.

Cross-Sex Measurement Devices

The desire to develop devices that will allow direct comparison of the sexes has been the impetus for the development of several genital measurement devices. Unfortunately, it often has not been recognized that the problem is much more complex than simply developing similar measures from similar locations. In general, investigators have ignored psychometric considerations. For example, it has been shown that vaginal vascular responses continue for 15 minutes or so following masturbatory induced orgasm (Geer & Quartararo 1976). Since that time course is much longer than that of penile detumescence, it appears likely that the time course for pelvic vasocongestion differs between the sexes. It follows that simple correlations are inadequate to study sex differences or similarities. The issues of cross-sex differences in subjective ratings and in the nature of the relationship between physiological and subjective indices also contribute to the complexity of cross-sex comparisons. We discussed this point in more detail in the section on social context. In spite of these complexities, several investigators have worked on developing devices to facilitate cross-sex comparisons.

Intra-Anal Pressure and Blood Volume. Bohlen and Held (1979) described a device designed to monitor intra-anal pressure changes and pulse waves. The authors suggested that it could be used to directly compare sexual responses in men and women. The design of the anal probe is based on the observation that genital changes associated with the experience of sexual arousal are a result of increased blood volume and muscle tension throughout the pelvic area, and this includes anal responding (Masters & Johnson 1966). The anal probe consists of an LED-transistor photometer and pressure transducer encased within a body constructed of silicone rubber tubing. Electrical signals reflecting anal pulse wave activity and muscle tension are fed directly to the recording system. An adaptation of this design was used by Carmichael and colleagues (1994) to measure both anal electromyographic activity and blood flow during orgasm in sexually functional men and women. They found that, although men and women did not differ in anal muscle tone during baseline testing, higher initial levels of blood flow were measured in women. During both sexual arousal and orgasm, men had significantly higher levels of anal blood flow and muscle activity.

Temperature. Thermistors have been used to measure genital temperature in both sexes. Since the measurements are obtained from different anatomical structures, we do not include that methodology under the male–female category. We do, however, wish to consider thermography here since it has been proposed as a methodology that can be used in cross-sex comparisons (Seeley et al. 1980). Thermography is a method of detecting and measuring heat from various regions of the body and transforming them into signals that can be recorded photographically. The result is a picture of heat patterns of a particular region. By analyzing thermograms, it is possible to detect subtle elevations in temperature due to cellular and metabolic changes. The methodology is not frequently used because it is costly and intrusive (participants must be unclothed when measures are taken). In the study by Seeley et al. (1980), thermographic pictures of a male participant engaging in masturbation and pictures of a female participant engaging in masturbation were compared. Their results suggested that thermography did reflect sexual arousal in the tested conditions. However, the relationship of temperature to physiological events in the various genital structures, regardless of the methodology by which it is obtained, is unclear; studies have not been performed that directly relate thermographic data to vascular responses.

SIGNAL RECORDING AND PROCESSING: GENERAL ISSUES

In contrast to many other areas of psychophysiological research, at present no guidelines exist for the measurement of sexual arousal. Although it is beyond doubt that choices related to methodology are made conscientiously, the current lack of standardization of signal recording, processing, and analysis complicates the evaluation and comparison of research findings. Standardization is further complicated by the fact that a number of different measurement devices are used in sexual research. Although amplification and filtering of signals are not likely to be consequential sources of variance in findings across studies, signal processing and analysis are. The detection of artifacts is not standardized, and the procedures used are often not described in research publications. It would be a step forward if authors would provide their readers with information about, for instance, the proportion of data points that were removed by the researcher because of movement or other artifacts.

Another source of error in sexual response measurement is related to variations in device placement. In contrast with clinical research, devices are usually put in place by participants in the psychophysiological lab. Placement (or pretest inspection of placement) by the experimenter is likely to increase measurement accuracy and reliability. However, these procedures are not an infallible safeguard against inaccurate or unreliable readings. A well-placed electromechanical gauge that fits well on a flaccid penis may prove too small for an erect penis. Similarly, a properly placed mercury-in-strain gauge may move and get twisted during the process of erection and thus cause compression of the rubber tubing, leading to excessively high output levels. Thus, with measures such as the penile strain gauges, improper device selection or placement cannot always be prevented. The same is true for measurement devices used in studies of sexual arousal in women. Placement of the vaginal plethysmograph can be standardized, as noted previously, by using a shield (Geer 1983, Laan et al. 1995). This practice is recommended. A placement shield, however, will not prevent inaccurate readings due to (phasic or tonic) muscle contractions. As for labial clips, less is known about the effects of variations in placement and how changes in volume of the labia during sexual arousal may affect the output of the device. In view of this, we wish to emphasize the importance of checking genital response data for outliers before performing statistical analyses, regardless of whether visual inspection was part of the procedure.

Several other aspects of the methodology of psychophysiological sex research require further study. These include issues related to baseline establishment, checks for the applicability of the law of initial values (LIV), calibration, and what variables to use for analysis. Also, more work is needed on the development of criteria for the selection of sexual stimuli and on the validation of measures of subjective sexual arousal. We will not discuss all of these issues here but instead limit ourselves to a brief discussion of the LIV as it applies to genital measures.

A few studies have examined whether LIV applies to the measurement of genital responses in women (Meuwissen & Over 1993) and men (Julien & Over 1981). For men, in a study using the mercury-in-rubber gauge, no consistent evidence was obtained that stimulation levels or change scores varied with prestimulus baseline values (Julien & Over 1981). Note, however, that in this study there was a period of guided relaxation before baseline measures were obtained and that the authors failed to report how repeated measurements influenced LIV. Meuwissen and Over (1993) reported that baseline levels of VPA were generally positively correlated with difference scores. For VBV, the correlations were inconsistent in direction and small in magnitude. According to Jin (1992), LIV should be reconceptualized to mean that: (a) within the middle range of initial states, higher initial values will be related to greater reactivity; and (b) when an initial value reaches its upper limit, a tendency to reversed responses may occur. It is thought that the presence, magnitude, and direction of LIV are dependent on a combination of constitutional factors and homeostatic mechanisms (Jin 1992). Although the LIV can account for a portion of the variance in psychophysiological sex studies, the LIV may have little utility as an empirical generalization (Berntson, Cacioppo, & Quigley

1991). Before sex researchers adopt specific statistical techniques to deal with differences in initial levels, more research is needed on how LIV relates to constitutional and physiological factors. To give an example, in men it would be relevant to explore what proportion of LIV is affected by baseline tumescence levels (physiological) versus what proportion by differences in penile size (constitutional).

As briefly mentioned in the section on social context, genital devices should be sterilized. To expand upon that point here, there are standardized sterilization procedures that kill viruses. Activated glutaraldehyde 3.4%, sold commercially as Cidexplus, works as a chemical sterilant, a high-level disinfectant, or an intermediate-level disinfectant, depending on the immersion time used. The Centers for Disease Control recommends a minimum of high-level disinfection for items that touch mucous membranes. High-level disinfection destroys all pathogenic microorganisms (bacteria, fungi, and viruses) except for endospores. For Cidexplus, this level of disinfection translates into an immersion time of 20 min. Longer soaking is unnecessary and may cause damage to measurement devices.

MODELS OF SEXUAL AROUSAL

We have chosen to place models of sexuality into three categories. First we consider the well-known stage models that offer a description of the events that occur during the typical sexual response cycle. As Rosen and Beck (1988) pointed out, these are variants on the two-stage model of excitement and orgasm that dates back to Havelock Ellis. The best known of these models are the Masters and Johnson (1966) four-stage model and the Helen Singer Kaplan (1977, 1979) three-stage model. The second category we use describes models applying psychological mechanisms that are suggested by the information processing approach (IPA) to understanding human behavior. This category has been heavily influenced by the cognitive revolution in psychology and is reflected in contemporary theories of emotion. The best-known of these models as applied to sexuality are suggestions by Barlow (1986) and the adoption of the IPA by Everaerd, Geer, and their colleagues. This section is not exhaustive, but it covers the psychosexual models that we believe are currently most influential. The final category to be discussed is the increased interest of applying an evolutionary perspective to sexuality. While not speaking directly to psychophysiological concepts, this approach provides valuable heuristics that can be studied with psychophysiological methodologies. We will not discuss neuroanatomical models.

Masters and Johnson's Model of the Sexual Response Cycle

Masters and Johnson (1966) proposed a four-phase descriptive model of the responses that occur in humans during sexual behavior. The sequential phases are excitement,

plateau, orgasmic, and resolution. Masters and Johnson (1966) described the genital and extragenital responses associated with each phase, emphasizing two generalized responses to sexual stimulation: vasocongestion and myotonia. The former has proven more useful in research. They report no data on the subjective experiences that accompanied the sexual stimulation.

The first phase (excitement) describes the initial response to "effective" sexual stimulation. In this formulation the model is reflexive in that the stages follow when effective stimulation is present. (An independent definition of effective stimulation is not offered.) During the excitement phase, there is continuous increase in the level or intensity of arousal. If effective stimulation is continued, the individual next will enter the plateau phase. This phase, which consists of high-level arousal at a relatively constant intensity, will – with continued effective stimulation – ultimately result in orgasm. However, cessation of stimulation during the plateau or excitement phases results in eventual return to prestimulation levels. The orgasmic phase, which signals the end of the plateau phase, is of brief duration and represents the involuntary reaching of maximal sexual tension. Males report that a period of ejaculatory inevitability develops at the beginning of the orgasmic phase. The resolution phase, which follows the orgasmic phase, is characterized by a loss of tension, which leads to an eventual return to prestimulation levels. Masters and Johnson note that there are substantial individual differences in sexual response cycles. An interesting aspect of the model is that it emphasizes similarities between men and women. See Masters and Johnson (1966) for a detailed description of the responses they report as occurring during the four phases in the sexual response cycle.

Although few would dispute the importance of this model, it has been subjected to serious criticism. There is scant evidence of a clearly identifiable plateau phase. Of particular interest to the psychophysiologist is that Masters and Johnson failed to describe adequately the methods used to collect their psychophysiological data, making it impossible to replicate their studies. In addition, the physiological data were neither quantified nor presented in a form that permitted evaluation by others. Finally, we note that questions have been raised concerning the universality of the model (Rosen & Rosen 1981; Tiefer 1991).

Kaplan's Three-Stage Model

Reacting to the lack of motivational concepts in the Masters and Johnson model, Helen Singer Kaplan (1977, 1979) proposed an alternative three-stage model in which motivational concepts played a central role. The first stage in this model is *desire,* described by Kaplan as follows: "When this system is active, a person is 'horny.' He may feel genital sensations, or he may feel vaguely sexy, interested in sex, open to sex, or even just restless" (1979, p. 10). Her second phase, *excitement,* is quite similar to that of Masters and Johnson; the third phase is *orgasm*, characterized by reflexive pelvic muscle contractions. Kaplan suggested that the first phase involves central nervous system events with the second and third phases being reflexive spinal events. The importance of this model is reflected by its influence on the diagnostic formulations of the American Psychiatric Association's manuals since DSM III.

Emotion Models from Information Processing Approaches

The basic point made by the IPA is that it is useful to conceptualize humans as active information processors and not just a set of reflexive (albeit complex) responses to stimuli. It would be inaccurate to suggest that the IPA rejects concepts such as classical conditioning. However, in this approach, conditioning is only a part of the complex interactions that determine behavior: in the processing of stimuli, alterations and changes are made by the individual that function to determine responses. Contemporary experimental psychology is heavily dependent upon this general model, and it is fair to say that contemporary emotion theories borrow heavily from the concepts found in the IPA.

Everaerd (1988) made the point that sex is an emotion. What may be surprising is that contemporary emotion theories, for the most part, have ignored the emotions surrounding sexuality. This may be partly due to their focus on the negative emotional states and partly due also to a desire to avoid the controversies that surround sex. We would hope that the text edited by Parkinson and Colman (1995), which contains a chapter on sexual motivation by Bancroft (1995b), represents a change in the recognition of sexuality as an important segment of the spectrum of human emotion. Bower (1981, 1992) and Lang (1984) drew heavily upon the IPA and attendant network theories in their emotion models. In Bower's model, cognitive variables play a central role in the explanations of such phenomena as state-dependent learning. Lang also drew heavily upon network concepts yet, importantly for the psychophysiologist, included behavioral and physiological concepts in his formulations. In his more recent work on psychophysiology, Lang (1994) developed closer ties to sexual phenomena as offering an index to the valence of the emotional state being experienced by the individual. We will not describe either of these models in detail, since they do not deal expressly with sexuality.

Barlow's Interactive Model of Sexual Arousal

Barlow and colleagues (Barlow 1986; Cranston-Cuebas & Barlow 1990) proposed an interactive model of sexual arousal emphasizing cognitive-affective processes in the mediation of sexual arousal. That model focuses particularly on the perception of physiological arousal and the processing of erotic cues. They suggest that the sexual arousal experience begins with the individual's perception of external expectations of sexual arousal. Concepts such as appraisal have played an important role in cognitive models that speak to individual perceptual responding, but that idea is not incorporated in Barlow's model. The model suggests that the individual responds to the external situation with either positively or negatively valenced emotion. This emotional response influences the salience of certain features of the erotic stimulation. Attentional focus on salient features, when influenced by a positive response to the erotic situation, serves to enhance sexual arousal. Salient features then serve to increase the focus upon erotic cues. The positive affective response also acts to trigger autonomic arousal. Attention to autonomic arousal results in further processing of erotic cues, thus heightening arousal in a feedback loop. Continued processing of erotic cues ultimately leads to sexual approach behavior. Conversely, when influenced by a negative emotional response to the erotic situation, attention is focused on the negative aspects of the situation, ultimately producing avoidance behavior. Under these latter conditions, sexual arousal does not occur. By combining cognitive-affective and physiological features of sexual response, this type of model holds genuine promise of yielding substantial theoretical progress.

The Information Processing Approach Applied to Sexuality

Everaerd and Geer and their colleagues have directly applied the IPA to sexuality. Janssen and Everaerd (1993) and Laan and Everaerd (1995), in reviewing male and female sexual arousal, referred repeatedly to concepts derived from the IPA. Geer and Manguno (1997) described the role of cognitive factors in gender differences and noted a wide range of data and findings that flow from the IPA. The IPA is not a theory but rather a set of heuristics that guide research. It directs the investigator to aim research efforts at certain sets of variables and offers a range of research paradigms to explore those variables. Important concepts include attentional variables, which examine what stimuli are admitted to the system for processing. For example, there is evidence (Janssen & Everaerd 1993) that nonconscious sexual stimuli affect genital responding. Other research has shown that sexual stimuli are processed differently than other emotional stimuli and are processed differently by the two genders (Geer & Manguno 1997). Laan and Everaerd (1995) reported evidence for the idea that women's subjective experience of sexual arousal is determined more by appraisal of the situation than by genital feedback.

The IPA focuses attention upon encoding variables that are important in acting to ensure that stimuli entering the system are passed on for further processing. Concepts such as memory storage and retrieval processes direct the interested investigator to explore these concepts further. It is our belief that the IPA provides a useful set of heuristics and paradigms for examining sexuality. The implications for psychophysiology are powerful and impressive. The advantage that the study of genital responding holds is the specificity of the genital response: although there is an independence of genital responding to subjective or cognitive events, there is also amazing specificity. Certainly there is no other domain in emotion and psychophysiology in which the response system is as closely tied to the feeling state and stimuli under study.

Evolution Theory

We would be remiss if we did not mention a third approach in our discussion of models in sexuality. There has been a burgeoning of interest in evolutionary theory and its application to understanding sexuality (Allgeier & Wiederman 1994). The contribution of evolutionary thinking begins perhaps with the simple idea that all living organisms are equipped with mechanisms that ensure perpetuation of their species. Given that sexual behavior is involved in all human reproduction, it follows that sexuality has been influenced by evolutionary concepts. Albertus Magnus noted in the thirteenth century that "pleasure is attached to intercourse so that it will be more desired, and thus generation will continue" (quoted in Kitchell and Resnick in press). This is the basic premise that suggests that living animals are "prewired" to find sexual behavior rewarding.

However, this foundational notion has not been the focus of the evolutionary perspective; instead, the focus has been upon a more limited set of phenomena. Allgeier and Wiederman (1994) described three areas that have been the principal focus of interest in evolutionary approaches to sexuality: mate selection strategies; gender differences in jealousy; and characteristics that are associated with attractiveness. It is not our intention to review these areas and their predictions from evolutionary theory but only to note that this perspective appears to be gaining in importance. Psychophysiological methodologies can provide a useful tool for exploring some of the available predictions.

Epilogue

UNANSWERED QUESTIONS

It is tempting to suggest that we don't have any real answers at this time and that all is up for grabs. From the very long view, that is bound to be the case, but as prisoners of our own time we should hesitate before denigrating contemporary work. Still, there are obvious questions upon which we could collect meaningful data.

In males there is little empirical evidence of the role of feedback from the genitals and how it interacts with other processes to help determine behavior. Laan and Everaerd (1995) argue that, for women, feedback plays a minor role.

Harking back to the early views of James and Lange, there is a continuing interest in peripheral feedback. Lang's (1994) work, as well as contemporary perspectives in emotion theory, emphasizes the importance of examining the role of feedback.

We note that very little has been done from a lifespan developmental perspective. Changes in genital responding over the lifespan is a topic that cries for research. We have already noted how important the study would be during the formative years of sexual interests. As noted, research on the formation of sexual interests and preferences around the time of puberty may be a topic that cannot be rigorously investigated. Another very general topic with many unanswered questions is the role of hormones in determining genital response. This is a problem area that requires sophisticated methodologies from diverse research domains and thus is very difficult to attack. Yet the potential for quality outcomes makes the effort and risks worthwhile.

One last unanswered question, alluded to earlier, is how to conceptualize and deal with the fact that sexuality is often surrounded with both positively and negatively valenced emotions. The individual who feels guilty while engaging in some forbidden act is the prototype for such an experience. Emotion theories do not deal well with such phenomena. Although there has been some data showing that anxiety can both inhibit and facilitate sexual arousal, we have as yet to do a credible job of conceptualizing the simultaneous occurrence of both positively and negatively valenced emotional states.

THE FUTURE

The success of future research lies, we believe, in the amalgamation of interdisciplinary efforts. Specifically, the explosion of methodologies for assessing brain function will have a powerful impact. As methodologies become increasingly available to study individual brain functioning in naturalistic settings, our theories and conceptualizations will be altered dramatically. This does not mean that psychophysiology will become lost in the shuffle. It appears that peripheral feedback is important, so information from only central events will not present the full picture.

In a similar vein, increasing attention to the views of experimental cognitive psychologists – who may have new and sophisticated paradigms for examining cognitive processes – will play an increasingly important role in the study of sexuality. The combination of studying brain function, cognitive processing functioning, and peripheral feedback will provide the study of sexuality with powerful methodologies and paradigms.

Finally, we believe that the increasing emphasis on biological variables will support increased attention to the evolutionary concepts and their importance in understanding sexuality. We believe that genital responding will provide an index that will support continued study and advancement of these concepts.

In the current zeitgeist (at least in the United States) of increased political and religious conservatism, research on sexual matters is not always welcomed by the community at large. The competent and ethical sex researcher must provide a context in which research not only provides new and important information but also convinces all of the value of that contribution.

REFERENCES

Abel, G. G., Blanchard, E. B., Barlow, D. H., & Mavissakalian, M. (1975). Identifying specific erotic cues in sexual deviations by audiotaped descriptions. *Journal of Applied Behavior Analysis, 8*, 247–60.

Allgeier, E. R., & Wiederman, M. W. (1994). How useful is evolutionary psychology for understanding contemporary human sexual behavior? *Annual Review of Sex Research, 5*, 218–56.

American Psychological Association (1992). Ethical principles of psychologists and code of conduct. *American Psychologist, 47*, 1597–1611.

Amoroso, D. M., & Brown, M. (1973). Problems in studying the effects of erotic material. *Journal of Sex Research, 9*, 187–95.

Andersson, K. E., & Wagner, G. (1995). Physiology of penile erection. *Physiological Review, 75*, 191–236.

Bancroft, J. (1989). *Human Sexuality and Its Problems.* Edinburgh, U.K.: Churchill Livingstone.

Bancroft, J. (1995a). Are the effects of androgens on male sexuality noradrenergically mediated? Some consideration of the human. *Neuroscience and Biobehavioral Reviews, 2*, 1–6.

Bancroft, J. (1995b). Sexual motivation and behaviour. In B. Parkinson & A. M. Colman (Eds.), *Emotion and Motivation,* pp. 58–75. New York: Longman.

Bancroft, J., & Bell, C. (1985). Simultaneous recording of penile diameter and penile arterial pulse during laboratory-based erotic stimulation in normal subjects. *Journal of Psychosomatic Research, 29*, 303–13.

Bancroft, J., Jones, H. G., & Pullan, B. P. (1966). A simple transducer for measuring penile erection with comments on its use in the treatment of sexual disorder. *Behavior Research and Therapy, 4*, 239–41.

Barbaree, H. E., Marshall, W. L., & Lanthier, R. (1979). Deviant sexual arousal in rapists. *Behavior Therapy and Research, 17*, 215–22.

Barlow, D. H. (1986). Causes of sexual dysfunction: The role of anxiety and cognitive interference. *Journal of Consulting and Clinical Psychology, 54*, 140–57.

Barlow, D. H., Becker, R., Leitenberg, H., & Agras, W. (1970). A mechanical strain gauge for recording penile circumference change. *Journal of Applied Behavior Analysis, 6*, 355–67.

Beach, F. A. (1958). Neural and chemical regulation of behavior. In H. F. Harlow & C. N. Woolsey (Eds.), *Biological and Biochemical Bases of Behavior.* Madison: University of Wisconsin Press.

Beck, J. G., Sakheim, D. K., & Barlow, D. H. (1983). Operating characteristics of the vaginal photoplethysmograph: Some implications for its use. *Archives of Sexual Behavior, 12*, 43–58.

Berntson, G. G., Cacioppo, J. T., & Quigley, K. S. (1991). Autonomic determinism: The modes of autonomic control, the doctrine of autonomic space and the laws of autonomic constraint. *Psychological Review, 98*, 459–87.

Bogaert, A. F. (1996). Volunteer bias in human sexuality research: Evidence for both sexuality and personality differences in males. *Archives of Sexual Behavior, 25*, 125–40.

Bohlen, J. G., & Held, J. P. (1979). An anal probe for monitoring vascular and muscular events during sexual response. *Psychophysiology, 16*, 318–23.

Bower, G. H. (1981). Mood and memory. *American Psychologist, 36*, 129–48.

Bower, G. H. (1992). How might emotions affect memory? In S. A. Christianson (Ed.), *Handbook of Emotion and Memory,* pp. 3–31. Hillsdale, NJ: Erlbaum.

Bradley, W. E., Timm, G. W., Gallagher, J. M., & Johnson, B. K. (1985). New method for continuous measurement of nocturnal penile tumescence and rigidity. *Urology, 26*, 4–9.

Brindley, G. S. (1983). Cavernosal alpha-blockade: A new technique for investigating and treating erectile impotence. *British Journal of Psychiatry, 143*, 332–7.

Brindley, G. S. (1991). Mechanisms of erection and causes of impotence: Neurophysiology. In R. S. Kirby, C. C. Carson, & G. D. Webster (Eds.), *Impotence: Diagnosis and Management of Male Erectile Dysfunction,* pp. 27–31. Oxford, U.K.: Butterworth-Heinemann.

Burnett, A. L. (1997). Nitric oxide in penis: Physiology and pathology. *Journal of Urology, 157*, 320–4.

Buvat, J., Herbaut, M. B., Lemaire, A., Marcolin, G., & Quittelier, E. (1990). Recent developments in the clinical assessment and diagnosis of erectile dysfunction. *Annual Review of Sex Research, 1*, 265–308.

Carmichael, M. S., Warburton, V. L., Dixen, J., and Davidson, J. M. (1994). Relationships among cardiovascular, muscular, and oxytocin responses during human sexual activity. *Archives of Sexual Behavior, 23*, 59–79.

Conti, G. (1952). L'erection du penis humain et ses bases morphologico-vasculaires. *Acta Anatomica, 14*, 217.

Conti, G., Virag, R., & von Niederhausern, W. (1988). The morphological basis for the polster theory of penile vascular regulation. *Acta Anatomy, 133*, 209–12.

Cranston-Cuebas, M. A., & Barlow, D. H. (1990). Cognitive and affective contributions to sexual functioning. *Annual Review of Sex Research, 1*, 119–61.

Davenport, W. H. (1987). An anthropological approach. In J. H. Geer & W. T. O'Donohue (Eds.), *Theories of Human Sexuality,* pp. 197–236. New York: Plenum.

Dickinson, R. L. (1933). *Human Sex Anatomy.* Baltimore: Williams & Wilkins.

Droegemueller, W. (1992). Anatomy. In A. L. Herbst, D. R. Mishell, M. A. Stenchever, & W. Droegemueller (Eds.), *Comprehensive Gynecology,* pp. 43–78. St. Louis: Mosby Year Book.

Earls, C. M., & Jackson, D. R. (1981). The effects of temperature on the mercury-in-rubber strain gauge. *Journal of Applied Behavioural Analysis, 3*, 145–9.

Earls, C. M., Marshall, W. L., Marshall, P. G., Morales, A., & Surridge, D. H. (1983). Penile elongation: A method for the screening of impotence. *Journal of Urology, 139*, 90–2.

Earls, C. M., Morales, A., & Marshall, W. L. (1988). Penile sufficiency: An operational definition. *Journal of Urology, 139,* 536–8.

Everaerd, W. (1988). Commentary on sex research: Sex as an emotion. *Journal of Psychology and Human Sexuality, 2,* 3–15.

Everaerd, W. (1993). Male erectile disorder. In W. O'Donohue & J. H. Geer (Eds.), *Handbook of Sexual Dysfunctions: Assessment and Treatment,* pp. 201–24. Boston: Allyn & Bacon.

Farkas, G. M., Evans, I. M., Sine, L. F., Eifert, G., Wittlieb, E., & Vogelmann-Sine, S. (1979). Reliability and validity of the mercury-in-rubber strain gauge measure of penile circumference. *Behavior Therapy, 10,* 555–61.

Finkelhor, D. (1986). *A Sourcebook on Child Sexual Abuse.* London: Sage.

Fisher, C., Cohen, H. D., Schiavi, R. C., Davis, D., Furman, B., Ward, K., Edwards, A., & Cunningham, J. (1983). Patterns of female sexual arousal during sleep and waking: Vaginal thermo-conductance studies. *Archives of Sexual Behavior, 12,* 97–122.

Fisher, C., Gross, J., & Zuch, J. (1965). Cycle of penile erection synchronous with dreaming (REM) sleep. *Archives of General Psychiatry, 12,* 27–45.

Fisher, S. (1973). *The Female Orgasm.* New York: Basic Books.

Fisher, S., & Osofsky, H. (1967). Sexual responsiveness in women: Psychological correlates. *Archives of General Psychiatry, 17,* 214–26.

Freund, K. (1963). A laboratory method for diagnosing predominance of homo- or hetero-erotic interest in the male. *Behaviour Research and Therapy, 1,* 85–93.

Freund, K., Langevin, R., & Barlow, D. (1974). Comparison of two penile measures of erotic arousal. *Behaviour Research and Therapy, 12,* 355–9.

Fugl-Meyer, A. R., Sjogren, K., & Johansson, K. (1984). A vaginal temperature registration system. *Archives of Sexual Behavior, 13,* 247–60.

Geer, J. H. (1983). Measurement and methodological considerations in vaginal photometry. Paper presented at the meeting of the International Academy of Sex Research (Harriman, NY).

Geer, J. H., & Fuhr, R. (1976). Cognitive factors in sexual arousal: The role of distraction. *Journal of Consulting and Clinical Psychology, 44,* 238–43.

Geer, J. H., & Manguno, G. M. (1997). Gender differences in cognitive processes in sexuality. *Annual Review of Sex Research, 9,* 90–124.

Geer, J. H., Morokoff, P., & Greenwood, P. (1974). Sexual arousal in women: The development of a measurement device for vaginal blood volume. *Archives of Sexual Behavior, 3,* 559–64.

Geer, J. H., & Quartararo, J. (1976). Vaginal blood volume responses during masturbation and resultant orgasm. *Archives of Sexual Behavior, 5,* 403–13.

Gerstenberg, T. C., Nordling, J., Hald, T., & Wagner, G. (1989). Standardized evaluation of erectile dysfunction in 95 consecutive patients. *Journal of Urology, 141,* 857–62.

Giesbers, A. A. G. M., Bruins, J. L., Kramer, A. E. J. L., & Jonas, U. (1987). New methods in the diagnosis of impotence: Rigiscan penile tumescence and rigidity monitoring and diagnostic papaverine hydrochloride injection. *World Journal of Urology, 5,* 173–6.

Gillian, P., & Brindley, G. S. (1979). Vaginal and pelvic floor responses to sexual stimulation. *Psychophysiology, 16,* 471–81.

Hall, G. C. N., Hirschman, R., & Oliver, L. L. (1995). Sexual arousal and arousability to pedophilic stimuli in a community sample of normal men. *Behavior Therapy, 26,* 681–94.

Hatch, J. P. (1979). Vaginal photoplethysmography: Methodological considerations. *Archives of Sexual Behavior, 8,* 357–74.

Hedricks, C. A. (1994). Sexual behavior across the menstrual cycle: A biopsychosocial approach. *Annual Review of Sex Research, 5,* 122–72.

Heiman, J. R. (1976). Issues in the use of psychophysiology to assess female sexual dysfunction. *Journal of Sex and Marital Therapy, 2,* 197–204.

Heiman, J. R. (1977). A psychophysiological exploration of sexual arousal patterns in females and males. *Psychophysiology, 14,* 266–74.

Henson, C., Rubin, H. B., & Henson, D. (1979a). Women's sexual arousal concurrently assessed by three genital measures. *Archives of Sexual Behavior, 8,* 459–69.

Henson, D. E., & Rubin, H. B. (1978). A comparison of two objective measures of sexual arousal of women. *Behaviour Research and Therapy, 16,* 143–51.

Henson, D., Rubin, H., & Henson, C. (1978). Consistency of the labial temperature change measure of human female eroticism. *Behavior Research and Therapy, 16,* 125–9.

Henson, D. E., Rubin, H. B., & Henson, C. (1979b). Analysis of the consistency of objective measures of sexual arousal in women. *Journal of Applied Behavior Analysis, 12,* 701–11.

Henson, D. E., Rubin, H. B., & Henson, C. (1982). Labial and vaginal blood volume responses to visual and tactile stimuli. *Archives of Sexual Behavior, 11,* 23–31.

Hicks, R. G. (1970). Experimenter effects on the physiological experiment. *Psychophysiology, 7,* 10–17.

Hoon, P., Bruce, K., & Kinchelow, G. (1982). Does the menstrual cycle play a role in erotic arousal? *Psychophysiology, 19,* 21–6.

Hoon, P. W., Wincze, J. P., & Hoon, E. F. (1976). Physiological assessment of sexual arousal in women. *Psychophysiology, 13,* 196–204.

Hoyle, C. H., Stones, R. W., Robson, T., Whitley, K., & Burnstock, G. (1996). Innervation of vasculature and microvasculature of the human vagina by NOS and neuropeptide-containing nerves. *Journal of Anatomy, 188,* 633–44.

Janssen, E., & Everaerd, W. (1993). Determinants of male sexual arousal. *Annual Review of Sex Research, 4,* 211–45.

Janssen, E., Everaerd, W., van Lunsen, H., & Oerlemans, S. (1994a). Validation of a psychophysiological waking erectile assessment (WEA) for the diagnosis of male erectile disorder. *Urology, 43,* 686–95.

Janssen, E., Everaerd, W., van Lunsen, H., & Oerlemans, S. (1994b). Visual stimulation facilitates penile responses to vibration. *Journal of Consulting and Clinical Psychology, 62,* 1222–8.

Janssen, E., Vissenberg, M., Visser, S., & Everaerd, W. (1997). An in vivo comparison of two circumferential penile strain gauges: Introducing a new calibration method. *Psychophysiology, 34,* 717–20.

Jennings, J. R., Tahmoush, A. J., & Redmont, D. P. (1980). Noninvasive measurement of peripheral vascular activity. In I. R. Martin & P. H. Venables (Eds.), *Techniques in Psychophysiology.* New York: Wiley.

Jin, P. (1992). Toward a reconceptualization of the law of initial value. *Psychological Bulletin, 111,* 176–84.

Jovanovic, U. J. (1967). Some characteristics of the beginning of dreams. *Psychologie Fortschung, 30,* 281–306.

Julien, E., & Over, R. (1981). Male sexual arousal and the law of initial value. *Psychophysiology, 18,* 709–11.

Jünemann, K. P., Scheepe, J., Persson-Jünemann, C., Schmidt, P., Abel, K., Zwick, A., Tschada, R., & Alken, P. (1994). Basic experimental studies on corpus cavernosum electromyography and smooth-muscle electromyography of the urinary bladder. *World Journal of Urology, 12,* 266–73.

Kalat, J. W. (1984). *Biological Psychology,* 2nd ed. Hillsdale, CA: Wadsworth.

Kaplan, H. S. (1977). Hypoactive sexual desire. *Journal of Sex and Marital Therapy, 3,* 3–9.

Kaplan, H. S. (1979). *Disorders of Sexual Desire.* New York: Brunner/Mazel.

Karacan, I. (1969). A simple and inexpensive transducer for quantitative measurements of penile erection during sleep. *Behavior Research Methods and Instrumentation, 1,* 251–2.

Karacan, I., Rosenbloom, A., & Williams, R. L. (1970). The clitoral erection cycle during sleep. *Psychophysiology, 7,* 338.

Karacan, I., Salis, P. J., Ware, J. C., Dervent, B., Williams, R. L., Scott, F. B., Attia, S. L., & Beutler, L. E. (1978). Nocturnal penile tumescence and diagnosis in diabetic impotence. *American Journal of Psychiatry, 135,* 191–7.

Kinsey, A. C., Pomeroy, W. B., & Martin, C. E. (1948). *Sexual Behavior in the Human Male.* Philadelphia: Saunders.

Kinsey, A. C., Pomeroy, W. B., Martin, C. E., & Gebhardt, P. H. (1953). *Sexual Behavior in the Human Female.* Philadelphia: Saunders.

Kitchell, K. F., Jr., & Resnick, I. M. (in press). *Albertus Magnus on Animals: A Medieval Summa Zoologica.* Baltimore: Johns Hopkins University Press.

Kon, I. S. (1987). An anthropological approach. In J. H. Geer & W. T. O'Donohue (Eds.), *Theories of Human Sexuality,* pp. 257–86. New York: Plenum.

Korff, J., & Geer, J. H. (1983). The relationship between sexual arousal experience and genital response. *Psychophysiology, 20,* 121–7.

Laan, E., & Everaerd, W. (1995). Determinants of female sexual arousal: Psychophysiological theory and data. *Annual Review of Sex Research, 6,* 32–76.

Laan, E., Everaerd, W., van Bellen, G., & Hanewald, G. (1994). Women's sexual and emotional responses to male- and female-produced erotica. *Archives of Sexual Behavior, 23,* 153–70.

Laan, E., Everaerd, W., & Evers, A. (1995). Assessment of female sexual arousal: Response specificity and construct validity. *Psychophysiology, 32,* 476–85.

Lang, P. J. (1984). Cognition in emotion: Concept and action. In C. E. Izard, J. Kagan, & R. B. Zajonc (Eds.), *Emotions, Cognitions and Behavior,* pp. 192–228. Cambridge University Press.

Lang, P. J. (1994). The varieties of emotional experience: A meditation on James–Lange theory. *Psychological Review, 101,* 211–21.

Laumann, E. O., Gagnon, J. H., Michael, R. T., & Michaels, S. (1994). *The Social Organization of Sexuality: Sexual Practices in the United States.* University of Chicago Press.

Laws, D. R. (1977). A comparison of the measurement characteristics of two circumferential penile transducers. *Archives of Sexual Behavior, 6,* 45–51.

Laws, D. R., & Bow, R. A. (1976). An improved mechanical strain gauge for recording penile circumference changes. *Psychophysiology, 13,* 596–9.

Laws, D. R., & Holmen, M. L. (1978). Sexual response faking by pedophiles. *Criminal Justice and Behavior, 5,* 343–56.

Levin, R. J. (1992). The mechanisms of human female sexual arousal. *Annual Review of Sex Research, 3,* 1–48.

Levin, R. J. (1998). Assessing human female sexual arousal by vaginal plethysmography: A critical examination. *Sexologies: European Journal of Medical Sexology, 6,* 26–31.

Levin, R. J., & Wagner, G. (1978). Haemodynamic changes of the human vagina during sexual arousal assessed by a heated oxygen electrode. *Journal of Physiology, 275,* 23–4.

Levine, L. A., & Carroll, R. A. (1994). Nocturnal penile tumescence and rigidity in men without complaints of erectile dysfunction using a new quantitative analysis software. *Journal of Urology, 152,* 1103–7.

Lohr, B. A., Adams, H. E., & Davis, J. M. (1997). Sexual arousal to erotic and aggressive stimuli in sexually coercive and non-coercive men. *Journal of Abnormal Psychology, 106,* 230–42.

Magoun, H. W. (1981). John B. Watson and the study of human sexual behavior. *Journal of Sex Research, 17,* 368–78.

Masters, W. H., & Johnson, V. E. (1966). *Human Sexual Response.* New York: Little, Brown.

Masters, W. H., & Johnson, V. E. (1970). *Human Sexual Inadequacy.* New York: Little, Brown.

McConaghy, N. (1974). Measurements of change in penile dimensions. *Archives of Sexual Behavior, 3,* 381–8.

Melman, A. (1992). Neural and vascular control of erection. In R. C. Rosen & S. R. Leiblum (Eds.), *Erectile Disorders: Assessment and Treatment,* pp. 141–70. New York: Guilford.

Melman, A., Tiefer, L., & Pederson, R. (1988). Evaluation of first 406 patients in urology department based center for male sexual dysfunction. *Urology, 32,* 6–10.

Mendelsohn, M. (1896). Ist das Radfahren als eine Gesundheitsgemässe uebung anzusehen und aus ärztlichen Gesichtspunkten zu empfehlen? *Deutsche Medicinische Wochenschrift, 22,* 383–4.

Meston, C. M., & Gorzalka, B. B. (1995). The effects of sympathetic activation on physiological and subjective sexual arousal in women. *Behaviour Research and Therapy, 3,* 651–64.

Metz, M. E., Pryer, J. L., Nesvacil, L. J., Abuaazhab, F., & Koznar, J. (1997). Premature ejaculation: A psychophysiological review. *Journal of Sex and Marital Therapy, 2,* 3–23.

Meuwissen, I., & Over, R. (1992). Sexual arousal across phases of the human menstrual cycle. *Archives of Sexual Behavior, 21,* 101–19.

Meuwissen, I., & Over, R. (1993). Female sexual arousal and the law of initial value: Assessment at several phases of the menstrual cycle. *Archives of Sexual Behavior, 22,* 403–13.

Morokoff, P. J. (1993). Female sexual arousal disorder. In W. T. O'Donohue and J. H. Geer (Eds.), *Handbook of Sexual Dysfunctions: Assessment and Treatment,* pp. 157–99. Boston: Allyn & Bacon.

Morokoff, P. J., & Heiman, J. K. R. (1980). Effects of erotic stimuli on sexually functional and dysfunctional women. Multiple measures before and after sex therapy. *Behavior Research and Therapy, 18,* 127–37.

Morrell, M. J., Dixen, J. M., Carter, S., & Davidson, J. M. (1984). The influence of age and cycling status on sexual arousability in women. *American Journal of Obstetric Gynecology, 148,* 66–71.

Munoz, M. M., Bancroft, J., & Marshall, I. (1993). The performance of the Rigiscan in the measurement of penile tumescence and rigidity. *International Journal of Impotence Research, 5,* 69–76.

Newman, H. F., & Northup, J. D. (1981). Mechanisms of human penile erection: An overview. *Urology, 17,* 399–408.

Ohlmeyer, P., Brilmayer, H., & Hullstrong, H. (1944). Periodische organge im Schlaf II. *Pflügers Archiv für die gesammte Physiologie, 249,* 50–5.

Osborne, C. A., & Pollack, R. H. (1977). The effects of two types of erotic literature on physiological and verbal measures of female sexual arousal. *Journal of Sex Research, 13,* 250–6.

Ottesen, B., Pedersen, B., Nielsen, J., Dalgaard, D., Wagner, G., & Fahrenkrug, J. (1987). Vasoactive intestinal polypeptide (VIP) provokes vaginal lubrication in normal women. *Peptides, 8,* 797–800.

Palace, E. M., & Gorzalka, B. B. (1990). The enhancing effects of anxiety on arousal in sexually dysfunctional and functional women. *Journal of Abnormal Psychology, 99,* 403–11.

Palace, E. M., & Gorzalka, B. B. (1992). Differential patterns of arousal in sexually functional and dysfunctional women: Physiological and subjective components of sexual response. *Archives of Sexual Behavior, 21,* 135–59.

Palti, Y., & Bercovici, B. (1967). Photoplethysmographic study of the vaginal blood pulse. *American Journal of Obstetrics and Gynecology, 97,* 143–53.

Parkinson, B., & Colman, A. (Eds.) (1995). *Emotion and Motivation.* New York: Longman.

Richards, J. C., Bridger, B. A., Wood, M. M., Kalucy, R. S., & Marshall, V. R. (1985). A controlled investigation into the measurement properties of two circumferential penile strain gauges. *Psychophysiology, 22,* 568–71.

Richards, J. C., Kalucy, R. S., Wood, M. M., & Marshall, V. R. (1990). Linearity of the electromechanical penile plethysmograph's output at large expansions. *Journal of Sex Research, 27,* 283–7.

Rogers, G. S., Van de Castle, R. L., Evans, W. S., & Critelli, J. W. (1985). Vaginal pulse amplitude response patterns during erotic conditions and sleep. *Archives of Sexual Behavior, 14,* 327–42.

Rosen, R. C. (1976). Genital blood-flow measurement: Feedback applications in sexual therapy. *Journal of Sex and Marital Therapy, 2,* 184–96.

Rosen, R. C., & Beck, J. G. (1988). *Patterns of Sexual Arousal.* New York: Guilford.

Rosen, R. C., & Rosen, L. R. (1981). *Human Sexuality.* New York: Knopf.

Rowland, D. L., Cooper, S. E., Slob, A. K., & Houtsmuller, E. J. (1997). The study of ejaculatory response in men in the psychophysiological laboratory. *Journal of Sex Research, 34,* 161–6.

Sakheim, D. K., Barlow, D. H., Abrahamson, D. J., & Beck, J. G. (1987). Distinguishing between organogenic and psychogenic erectile dysfunction. *Behaviour Research and Therapy, 25,* 379–90.

Sakheim, D. K., Barlow, D. H., & Beck, J. G. (1985). Diurnal penile tumescence: A pilot study of waking erectile potential in sexual functional and dysfunctional men. *Sexuality and Disability, 4,* 68–97.

Sandfort, T. G. M. (1992). The argument for adult–child sexual contact: A critical appraisal and new data. In W. O'Donohue & J. H. Geer (Eds.), *Handbook of Sexual Dysfunctions: Theory and Research,* pp. 38–48. Boston: Allyn & Bacon.

Sasso, F., Stief, C. G., Gulino, G., Alcini, E., Jüneman, K. P., Gerstenberg, T., Merckx, L., & Wagner, G. (1997). Progress in corpus cavernosum electromyography (CC-EMG): Third international workshop on corpus cavernosum electromyography (CC-EMG). *International Journal of Impotence Research, 1,* 43–5.

Schiavi, R. C. (1992). Laboratory methods for evaluating erectile dysfunction. In R. C. Rosen & S. R. Leiblum (Eds.), *Erectile Disorders: Assessment and Treatment,* pp. 55–71. New York: Guilford.

Schreiner-Engel, P., Schiavi, R. C., Smith, H., & White, D. (1981). Sexual arousability and the menstrual cycle. *Psychosomatic Medicine, 43,* 199–214.

Seeley, F., Abramsen, P., Perry, L., Rothblatt, A., & Seeley, D. (1980). Thermogenic measures of sexual arousal: A methodological note. *Archives of Sexual Behavior, 9,* 77–85.

Shapiro, A., & Cohen, H. (1965). The use of mercury capillary length gauges for the measurement of the volume of thoracic and diaphragmatic components of human respiration: A theoretical analysis and a practical method. *Transactions of the New York Academy of Sciences, 26,* 634–49.

Shapiro, A., Cohen, H., DiBianco, P., & Rosen, G. (1968). Vaginal blood flow changes during sleep and sexual arousal in women [Abstract]. *Psychophysiology, 4,* 349.

Sintchak, G., & Geer, J. H. (1975). A vaginal plethysmograph system. *Psychophysiology, 12,* 113–15.

Slob, A. K., Ernste, M., & van der Werff-ten Bosch, J. (1991). Menstrual cycle phase and sexual arousability in women. *Archives of Sexual Behavior, 20,* 567–77.

Slob, A. K., Koster, J., Radder, J. K., & van der Werff-ten Bosch, J. (1990). Sexuality and psychophysiological functioning in women with diabetes mellitus. *Journal of Sex and Marital Therapy, 2,* 59–69.

Solnick, R., & Berrin, J. E. (1977). Age and male erectile responsiveness. *Archives of Sexual Behavior, 6,* 1–9.

Spiess, W., Geer, J. H., & O'Donohue, W. (1984). Premature ejaculation: A psychophysiological and psychophysical investigation of ejaculatory latency. *Journal of Abnormal Psychology, 94,* 242–5.

Strassberg, D. S., & Lowe, K. (1995). Volunteer bias in sexuality research. *Archives of Sexual Behavior, 24,* 369–82.

Tiefer, L. (1991). Historical, scientific, clinical, and feminist criticisms of "the human sexual response cycle" model. *Annual Review of Sex Research, 2,* 1–23.

Van de Velde, T. H. (1926). *Ideal Marriage: Its Physiology and Technique.* New York: Random House.

Wabrek, A. J., Whitaker, K. F., McCahill, D., & Woronick, C. L. (1986). Vaginal penetration pressure: A pilot study. *World Congress of Sexology – Proceedings,* 55–61.

Wagner, G., & Gerstenberg, T. (1988). Human in vivo studies of electrical activity of corpus cavernosum (EACC). *Journal of Urology, 139 (part 2),* 327A.

Wagner, G., Gerstenberg, T., & Levin, R. (1989). Electrical activity of corpus cavernosum during flaccidity and erection of the human penis: A new diagnostic method? *Journal of Urology, 142,* 723–5.

Wagner, G., & Levin, R. (1978). Vaginal fluid. In E. Hafez & T. Evans (Eds.), *The Human Vagina.* Amsterdam: Elsevier.

Wagner, G., & Levin, R. J. (1984). Human vaginal pH and sexual arousal. *Fertility and Sterility, 41,* 389–94.

Wagner, G., Wabrek, A. J., & Dalgaard, D. (1986). Vaginal penetration pressure: A parameter in impotence diagnosis? *World Journal of Urology, 4,* 250–1.

Webster, J. S., & Hammer, D. (1983). Thermistor measurement of male sexual arousal. *Psychophysiology, 20,* 111–15.

Wein, A. J., Fishkin, R., Carpiniello, V. L., & Malooy, T. R. (1981). Expansion without significant rigidity during nocturnal penile tumescence testing: A potential source of misinterpretation. *Journal of Urology, 126,* 343–4.

Weiss, H. D. (1972). The physiology of human penile erection. *Annals of Internal Medicine, 76,* 793–9.

Wheeler, D., & Rubin, H. B. (1987). A comparison of volumetric and circumferential measures of penile erection. *Archives of Sexual Behavior, 16,* 289–99.

Wincze, J. P., Hoon, E. F., & Hoon. P. W. (1976). Physiological responsivity of normal and sexually dysfunctional women during erotic stimulus exposure. *Journal of Psychosomatic Research, 20,* 445–51.

Wincze, J. P., Venditti, E., Barlow, D., & Mavissakalian, M. (1980). The effects of a subjective monitoring task in the physiological measure of genital response to erotic stimuli. *Archives of Sexual Behavior, 9,* 533–45.

Wolchik, S. A., Braver, S. L., & Jensen, K. (1985). Volunteer bias in erotica research: Effects of intrusiveness of measure and sexual background. *Archives of Sexual Behavior, 14,* 93–107.

Zuckerman, M. (1971). Physiological measures of sexual arousal in the human. *Psychological Bulletin, 75,* 297–329.

CHAPTER THIRTEEN

STRESS HORMONES IN PSYCHOPHYSIOLOGICAL RESEARCH

Emotional, Behavioral, and Cognitive Implications

WILLIAM R. LOVALLO & TERRIE L. THOMAS

Historical Context

In 1936, Hans Selye reported a historic series of studies on severe stress in rats. Exposure to bacterial infection, toxic chemicals, and other life-threatening insults consistently caused adrenal gland enlargement with high levels of corticosterone secretion, atrophy of the immune organs, and gastric ulcers. All three components of this nonspecific stress response are caused by prolonged activation of the hypothalamic-pituitary-adrenocortical axis (HPAC), resulting in secretion of stress levels of adrenocorticotropin (ACTH) and glucocorticoids. In spite of these harmful effects, glucocorticoids in normal levels are necessary for sustaining life (Munck, Guyre, & Holbrook 1984).

We now recognize that the HPAC, along with its central nervous system (CNS) controls, supports all of our behaviors with needed metabolic resources, in concert with the actions of the catecholamines – norepinephrine and epinephrine. The HPAC operates in states ranging from sleep to severe stress, and it responds to our private thoughts and emotions. This complete integration of hormonal outflow with our thoughts and feelings makes the study of stress hormones an ideal venue for the pursuit of psychophysiological research.

SCOPE AND PURPOSE

In this chapter we will discuss the stress hormones, emphasizing their modulation by emotionally salient stimuli, including mental and social stressors. We will describe their biological characteristics and the neural basis of their responsiveness to psychological stimulation. We will next consider the relationship between their metabolic and circadian variations and psychologically induced changes. We will then consider research designs to achieve maximum

sensitivity to psychogenic variations. Finally, we will comment on practical issues in the collection, handling, and storage of biological specimens for the quantification of stress hormone changes.

Because the HPAC is central to the stress response, this chapter will say more about cortisol than about catecholamines. The stress literature is too large to provide a full review; instead, we will provide selected examples of work illustrating key themes. Certain topics, such as gender- and age-related differences in stress hormone response, will be dealt with only briefly. Finally, some topics – such as hormone interactions with obesity and insulin resistance (Björntorp 1996), posttraumatic stress disorders (Yehuda et al. 1991), and depression – will not be covered. Although endogenous opioids are also secreted during stress, they are beyond the scope of this chapter. Excellent coverage is provided in McCubbin, Kaufmann, and Nemeroff (1993). Information on related topics (e.g., thyroid hormones, gonadal hormones, stress-related peptides) is available from other sources (Weiner 1992). A recent review of stress hormones and their behavioral response characteristics may be found in Folkow (1993).

HISTORY OF THE STRESS CONCEPT

Claude Bernard (1865/1961), a founder of physiology, noted that life depends on the body's ability to regulate its internal environment within narrow limits, providing individual cells with appropriate levels of nutrients and removing their waste products. Walter Cannon, holder of the first chair in physiology at Harvard University, used the term *homeostasis* to characterize the processes maintaining these life-sustaining actions (Cannon 1929). In this tradition, Hans Selye was concerned with severe challenges to homeostasis, ones that could result in death if not properly countered, and he made the first extensive use of the term

John T. Cacioppo, Louis G. Tassinary, and Gary G. Berntson (Eds.), *Handbook of Psychophysiology*, 2nd ed. © Cambridge University Press 2000. Printed in the United States of America. ISBN 62634X. All rights reserved.

"stress" (Selye 1956). In this manner, the study of stress is part of the more general topic of systemic regulation.

Selye became concerned with this topic when he learned in medical school that all diseases have two components: specific symptoms that characterize the disease in question, and nonspecific changes that occur regardless of the particulars of the disorder. Against the medical wisdom of the day, he believed that this generalized response was fundamental to the body's ability to withstand assaults to its integrity. The dictionary defines stress as the mental or bodily tension that results from factors that tend to alter the existing equilibrium. A *stressor* is any agent causing such disequilibrium, and a stress response is the total set of reactions to the stressor (*Webster's Ninth New Collegiate Dictionary* 1988). Following his focus on general characteristics of disease, Selye defined stress as the sum of nonspecific changes produced by the body in the course of adapting to severe challenge. He termed this the "general adaptation syndrome."

Because some stimuli have the direct ability to damage tissue, they are considered physical stressors. Such stressors can operate in the absence of consciousness. On the other hand, some stressors challenge our equilibrium because of their *perceived* potential for harm, and these are considered psychological stressors (Lazarus & Folkman 1984). These operate only in conscious organisms, although conditions that lead to them may not be in consciousness (see Lovallo 1997, pp. 76ff). With either type of stressor, the system will engage in physiological and behavioral adaptations in striving to return to a state of minimal challenge.

Changing Perspectives on HPAC Function

Selye viewed the nonspecific stress response as an unvarying reflex (Selye 1956). Mason (1968) introduced a major shift in this concept. He noted that naïve animals produced large glucocorticoid responses when exposed to novel procedures, but that future exposures resulted in progressively diminished reactions. HPAC activity was also seen to be sensitive to social conditions among rodents and primates. Mason argued that HPAC responses, and the stressfulness of a stimulus, could not be purely reflexive but instead are modifiable by experience, the nature of the environment, and the challenge itself. The stressfulness of an event is not a simple property of the stimulus but results from cognitive and emotional reactions by the organism (Lazarus & Folkman 1984; Lovallo 1997, pp. 75–100). As we will see, certain stimuli are more likely to produce HPAC responses than others, and individuals differ in their reactivity to such stimuli. Therefore, HPAC responses demonstrate both stimulus–response specificity and individual response stereotypy (Stern & Sison 1990).

Most recently, we have recognized that adrenal secretions are more than a simple output that indicates the stressfulness of the organism–environment interaction. We now appreciate the interconnections between metabolic regulation, the emotions, and cognition. More generally, psychophysiological investigators should view the stress hormones as active agents for physical and psychological change in the organism. Mounting profound defenses during stress has consequences on how thoughts and emotions are later managed by the CNS (see McGaugh & Cahill 1997; Sapolsky, Krey, & McEwen 1986). Epinephrine and cortisol contribute to the maintenance of normal cognitive function and to memory formation in particular. On the other hand, prolonged high levels of cortisol can damage the hippocampus, resulting in cell loss and decrements in memory. Because the stress hormones have a dual role – as response elements and causal agents – they become a vitally important system for psychophysiologists to incorporate into studies of stress, emotional responses, and cognitive processes.

Physical Context: The Glucocorticoids

Cortisol is the primary hormone secreted by the adrenal cortex. It has two states – one serving normal metabolic and diurnal functions, and one coming into play in times of stress. The HPAC normally produces sufficient quantities of glucocorticoid to allow normal tissue regulation, termed its *permissive* function (Munck et al. 1984). During stress, high levels of cortisol are produced to exert *regulatory* control over stress-related processes that would otherwise prove injurious. For example, an immune response can be fatal unless regulated by stress levels of glucocorticoids secreted during infection.

METABOLIC AND DIURNAL PHYSIOLOGY OF CORTISOL SECRETION

Apart from its role as a stress hormone, cortisol is essential for normal functions, including growth and development as well as diurnal variations in metabolism and fuel homeostasis.

Biosynthesis and Tissue Actions of the Adrenal Steroids

The adrenal corticosteroids are synthesized from cholesterol taken from low-density lipoproteins. Cortisol, a key regulator of glucose metabolism, is considered a *glucocorticoid*. There are two principal glucocorticoids, cortisol (found in humans and other species) and corticosterone (produced in rats, mice, and others). Their effects are very similar, although cortisol is more potent, based on several criteria of receptor action. An extensive review of the biochemistry of the glucocorticoids may be found in Martin (1985, pp. 215–69).

Another adrenal steroid, aldosterone, is a *mineralocorticoid* that controls electrolyte and water balance in conjunction with the kidney. Although not a primary participant in the stress response, it shares its receptor with cortisol, accounting for the complex roles played by cortisol in CNS regulation (Arriza et al. 1987).

Tissue Compartments and Transport of Cortisol

Cortisol is transported in the blood and freely enters all tissues. The unbound, biologically active cortisol fraction passes through the parotid gland into the saliva and also through the kidney into the urine. Cortisol crosses the blood–brain barrier, allowing it to reach all parts of the CNS, and enters the cerebrospinal fluid via the choroid plexus to reach important regulatory sites on the amygdala, hippocampus, and hypothalamus that lie adjacent to the ventricles. It also reaches the anterior pituitary through the systemic circulation.

Tissue Regulation and Receptor Systems for the Corticosteroids

The adrenal steroids have receptors in every nucleated cell type in the body. Cortisol crosses the cell membrane to combine with its receptors in the cytoplasm. This receptor complex enters the cell nucleus, where its primary action is to induce or inhibit expression of a wide range of regulatory genes (Cake & Litwack 1975). Dramatic evidence of cortisol's importance for normal function is seen in animals deprived of its benefits by adrenalectomy and also in medical conditions resulting from its under- or overproduction. Some signs of glucocorticoid excess or deficiency are given in Table 1.

Rats deprived of their adrenal glands are not viable for long, but under careful maintenance they show greatly reduced motor activity, inability to undertake sustained exercise, poor temperature regulation, deficient food intake, and impaired circulation. Immune system function can be exaggerated, resulting in autoimmune disorders. Centrally mediated changes include altered sensory processes and impaired learning and memory (Russell & Wilhelmi 1954). Humans with adrenal insufficiency (Addison's disease) show these same changes and report altered sensorium and moods, feelings of paranoia, and other delusions. Excess cortisol, as in Cushing's disease, can cause elevated glucose in blood and urine, excessive food intake, loss of bone density and muscle mass, shrinkage of the thymus and lymph nodes, and impaired immune function. Psychological changes also occur in this state of excess, including mood swings and depression (Starkman & Schteingart 1981).

Secretory Characteristics

Cortisol is secreted as periodic pulses regulated by the frequency and amplitude of ACTH pulses arising from the pituitary (Veldhuis et al. 1990). Most importantly, cortisol has a pronounced diurnal pattern (as shown in Figure 1), with a peak beginning just prior to awakening, a nadir in the late evening and early morning, and additional rises during the day related to meal times (Van

TABLE 1. Effects of Glucocorticoid Dysregulation

Function	Deficiency	Excess
Global		
Mortality	↑	↑
Stress tolerance	↓↓	↑
Energy balance		
Appetite	↓	↑
Blood glucose	↓	↑
Weight	↓	↑
Autonomic regulation		
Synthesis of α and β recep.	↓	
Temperature regulation	↓	
Water balance	↓	
Blood volume	↓	
Blood pressure	↓	↑
Pressor regulation	↓	
Cardiac function	↓	
Vascular permeability	↑	
Immune and blood		
Clotting	↓	↑
Red cell count	↓	
Lymphocyte count	↑	↓
Immune function	↓	↓
Thymus	↑	↓
Lymph nodes	↑	↓
Autoimmunity	↑	↓
Behavioral and CNS		
Exertion	↓	
Locomotion	↓	
EEG		↓
Sensory threshold	↓	↑
Learning	↓	↓
Memory	↓	↓
Mood swings		↑
Euphoria		↑
Depression	↑	↑
Anger		↑

Key: ↓ = decreased or disrupted, ↑ = increased or above normal; EEG, electroencephalogram.

Cauter 1989; Van Cauter et al. 1992). Its diurnal cycle is tied to the sleep-wake cycle rather than to the light–dark cycle (Spith-Schwalbe et al. 1993); it is reversed in nocturnal species and disrupted by sleep deprivation and changes in sleep patterns. These secretory characteristics present a challenge to the interpretation of measurements of cortisol in psychophysiological research, and recommendations for dealing with this issue are made in a later section.

Control of Cortisol Secretion

Cortisol's secretion is regulated by three primary structures: the pituitary gland, the hypothalamus, and the hippocampus; see Figures 2 and 3.

The positive signal for the secretion of cortisol begins at the paraventricular nucleus (PVN) of the hypothalamus. The PVN has a high concentration of specialized neurons that produce the neuropeptide known as *corticotropin releasing factor* (CRF). These CRF neurons project to the median eminence of the hypothalamus, where their axonal processes form specialized junctions with the portal capillaries of the pituitary stalk (Vale et al. 1981). The portal vein carries CRF to the anterior pituitary, where corticotroph cells produce the complex protein pro-opiomelanocortin. Corticotropin releasing factor cleaves this protein into ACTH and the opioid agonist, beta-endorphin, and the two are then released in identical quantities into the systemic circulation (Guillemin et al. 1977). Each pulse of ACTH circulates to the adrenal cortex where it causes an increased rate of cortisol synthesis, resulting in a pulse of cortisol being released into the bloodstream.

Negative Feedback Regulation of Cortisol Secretion

Cortisol secretion is regulated by negative feedback at the pituitary, hypothalamus, and hippocampus, as shown in Figure 3 (Jacobson & Sapolsky 1991; Kovacs et al. 1987).

These sites each have different feedback dynamics, resulting in highly sensitive regulation. At the pituitary, the rate of pro-opiomelanocortin synthesis is rapidly slowed at the cell nucleus. At the hypothalamus, CRF gene expression is inhibited by mechanisms sensitive to cortisol level and its rate of change. The result is a modulation in the rate at which the pituitary secretes ACTH pulses. The negative feedback relationship changes over the day. Adrenal cortex sensitivity is highest in the morning, and the feedback sensitivity of the system is lowest at that time (Dallman et al. 1987). These dynamics may account for

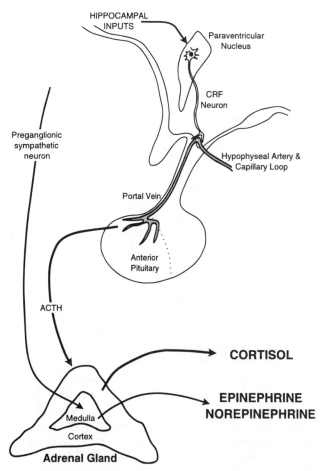

Figure 2. The hypothalamic-pituitary-adrenocortical axis. ACTH, adrenocorticotropic hormone; CRF, corticotropin releasing factor.

the greatly increased rate of cortisol secretion in the early morning hours.

The classical understanding of the regulation of glucocorticoid secretion by the pituitary and the hypothalamus underwent substantial modification when McEwen and colleagues reported that corticosterone in vivo was taken up in significant quantities by binding sites located in the rat hippocampus (McEwen, Weiss, & Schwartz 1968). The discovery of active receptor sites led to the recognition of the hippocampus as the highest site of negative feedback for glucocorticoid regulation.

The hippocampus is considered the primary point of negative feedback regulation of cortisol during normal activity and periods of stress (Jacobson & Sapolsky 1991). The hippocampus has more corticosteroid receptors than any other region. During normal activity, its stimulation inhibits glucocorticoid secretion, and its ablation tonically increases their secretion (Bouille & Bayle 1973). The circadian rhythm is

Figure 1. Idealized human 24-hour plasma cortisol curve. Prominent increase in secretion occurs in the hours near awakening, with a significant evening nadir from bedtime until 2:00–3:00 A.M.

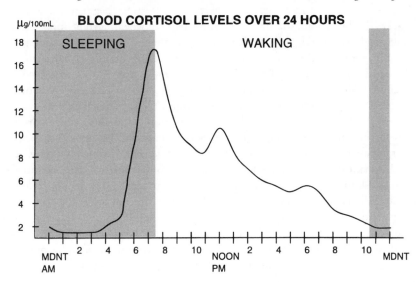

BLOOD CORTISOL LEVELS OVER 24 HOURS

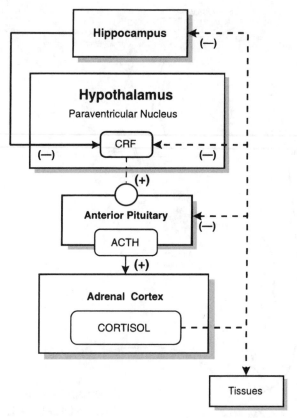

Figure 3. Regulation of cortisol secretion. The paraventricular nucleus (secreting corticotropin releasing factor) and the anterior pituitary (secreting adrenocorticotropin) are responsible for the activation of cortisol secretion by the adrenal cortex. Regulation is shown as negative feedback by cortisol at the anterior pituitary, hypothalamus, and hippocampus. ACTH, adrenocorticotropin; CRF, corticotropin releasing factor.

flattened by destruction of the fornix connecting the hippocampus to the hypothalamus, suggesting a failure to inhibit secretion at the nadir of the diurnal cycle (Moberg et al. 1971). During stress, secretion of high levels of cortisol is inhibited by hippocampal stimulation (DuPont et al. 1972).

It is noteworthy that the hippocampus is a key limbic system structure, important for the establishment of long-term, declarative memories (Scoville & Milner 1957); this leads to the insight that cortisol secretion is linked to both emotional and cognitive processes (Wolkowitz et al. 1990).

Adrenal Corticosteroid Receptors

Receptors for the adrenal steroid hormones in the rat are identified as the mineralocorticoid (MR, or type-I receptor) and the glucocorticoid (GR, or type-II receptor) (Reul & De Kloet 1985). The GR has a single steroid binding domain that is specific to glucocorticoid. The MR has a binding domain with an affinity for aldosterone and glucocorticoid. As a result, glucocorticoids alone act at the GR; both substances act on the MR, but with differing responses.

The presence of two receptor types with domains having high affinity (MR) and low affinity (GR) for corticosterone suggests a graded regulation of CRF gene expression over a wide range of concentrations. Both GR and MR occur in the hippocampus, and their 10–20-fold difference in binding affinities in the rat has led some workers to postulate that MRs regulate diurnal variations and normal metabolic secretion of the glucocorticoids and that GRs regulate their stress-related secretion (Dallman et al. 1987).

STRESS PHYSIOLOGY OF CORTISOL SECRETION

The picture of cortisol secretion presented here does not account for its regulation during psychological stress. In order to appreciate the responsiveness of the HPAC to events originating as perceptions and evaluations, it is necessary to incorporate the activities of the cerebral cortex and its relationships to the limbic system structures associated with emotions and their physiological patterning.

In considering the initial events in the process of psychological stress, we refer to the model of Lazarus and Folkman (1984), who propose that the key element in generating a psychological stress response is a two-stage appraisal process. In the first stage, a perceived event is evaluated for its threat value. The threat value of an event depends on how much it interferes with the person's commitment to a course of action or beliefs about how the environment is structured. In this view, when an event has been judged a threat to well-being, the individual undertakes a second-stage appraisal to consider courses of action and coping resources. This second stage of appraisal can therefore result in diminished or enhanced judgments of global threat, according to the known or perceived effectiveness of the coping resources at hand. We note that this model subsumes processes occurring both in and out of awareness, based on the individual's history of conditioning (see Lovallo 1997, pp. 76–80).

In either case, psychological stress begins with events initiated by the cerebral cortex, where current inputs can be highly synthesized and evaluated in light of experience. Such events must be processed by high-level association cortex. Three areas of unimodal association cortex considered critical to this process are the inferior temporal gyrus (for visual information), the superior temporal gyrus (conveying auditory information), and the insular cortex (providing somesthetic information). Polymodal associations, and the establishment of fully formed percepts in awareness, depend on the frontal cortex. For example, complex visual features such as identity of an object and its physical location depend on frontal areas for their integration (Rao, Rainer, & Miller 1997). In Figure 4 we present a schematic model of how events, and the thoughts and percepts they give rise to, may result in stress responses (for a discussion see Lovallo 1997, pp. 75–100).

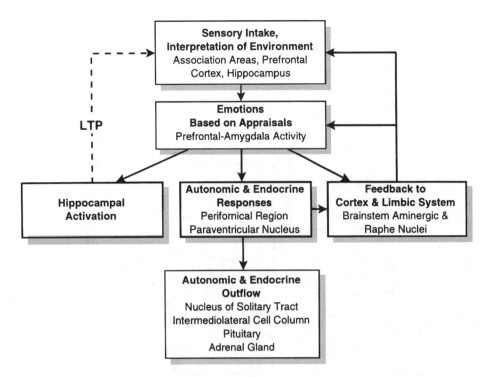

Figure 4. Central nervous system structures and processes thought to be involved in the generation of physiological responses to psychological stress. The activity of the amygdala is emphasized as having three key consequences during stress: hippocampal activation, autonomic and neuroendocrine responses, and enhanced feedback to the cortex by aminergic nuclei of the brainstem reticular formation. LTP, long-term potentiation.

The next step in the initiation of psychological stress calls for connecting the percept with bodily responses that result from emotional coloring of the evaluative process (for a useful review, see Feldman, Conforti, & Weidenfeld 1995). This step depends on the amygdala, an almond-sized structure located just anterior to the hippocampus that is known to be necessary for the formation of aversive associations to novel places and events (Rolls 1992). Damasio (1994) presented striking cases of patients with lesions of the subcallosal frontal cortex (disrupting frontal–amygdaloid connections) who are notably lacking in emotional responses to events they grasp intellectually. Such patients show deficiencies in the production of autonomic responses while making high-risk decisions in a simulated gambling situation (Bechara et al. 1997). Damasio and his colleagues argued that the formation of emotions in conjunction with ongoing events requires intact pathways between the frontal cortex and the temporal-lobe limbic structures, the amygdala in particular.

In Figure 5 we present an expanded model of HPAC function that incorporates the role of the amygdala during stressful events. The cortical areas and processes just described are seen to involve the lateral and basal nuclei of the amygdala. The lateral nucleus receives highly processed inputs from the inferior and superior temporal gyri, the insular cortex, and the prefrontal and orbital cortexes (Halgren 1992). In turn, the basal nucleus projects to both association and primary projection areas. This cortical-amygdaloid circuit is very likely to be a critical link in the initiation of emotionally based evaluations of events. It is also probable that the hippocampus participates in this process by assisting in the activation of stored memories.

The amygdala has a significant degree of input to the hippocampus but receives relatively few fibers in return. This leads to the speculation that the hippocampus acts in response to signals from amygdala (Amaral et al. 1992).

The next stage in connecting events and evaluations with autonomic and endocrine responses is mediated by the very important connection from the amygdala to the hypothalamus. This connection is, in part, a multisynaptic pathway from the central nucleus of the amygdala, via the stria terminalis, to the bed nucleus of the stria terminalis and then to the lateral hypothalamus-perifornical region (Smith, DeVito, & Astley 1990) and to the PVN. The set of connections just described accounts for a chain of events by which cortical events, including environmental and endogenous stimuli in conjunction with evaluative processes, can result in the beginnings of an emotional response and its accompanying hormonal output.

Figure 5 also shows an expanded model of glucocorticoid regulation, including its relationships with activities of the cortex and limbic system. A population of PVN neurons is shown that contains arginine vasopressin (AVP) along with CRF. Studies with isolated pituitary corticotrophs show that they secrete three- to fourfold more ACTH when CRF and AVP are both present relative to CRF alone. In rats subjected to severe and prolonged stress,

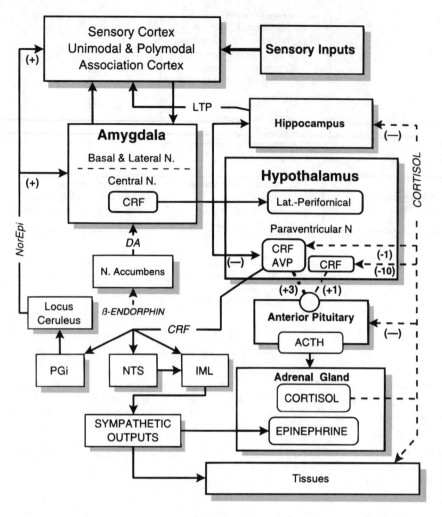

negative feedback than during normal circumstances.

The foregoing discussion is consistent with Munck, Guyre, and Holbrook's (1984) proposal that cortisol has two distinct families of functions. Cortisol's metabolic and diurnal functions are driven by signals from the hypothalamus with highly sensitive negative feedback control. During psychological stress, secretion is enhanced by input from the amygdala and negative feedback is much less effective.

Exposure of neurons to high glucocorticoid levels has a cost, however. The occupancy of GR and MR by cortisol during stress can result in impairment and possible loss of hippocampal neurons. This led to the formulation of the glucocorticoid *cascade* hypothesis: The loss of cells in a critical feedback site such as the hippocampus may leave the system less able to regulate cortisol output diurnally and in response to normal metabolic demands, resulting in chronically high levels of cortisol and hence increased hippocampal vulnerability to further stress-related neuron loss (Sapolsky et al. 1986). This may have both systemic and cognitive consequences.

Figure 5. HPAC function in relation to higher nervous system processes. The interactions of the amygdala and frontal cortex determine outputs via the central nucleus that are activational at the paraventricular nucleus and stimulate the activity of a population of CRF neurons that cosynthesize and cosecrete AVP. Activity of this population of neurons is about three times as potent at producing ACTH secretion (+3), and it is less sensitive to cortisol's negative feedback (−1). Beta-endorphin causes nucleus accumbens to activate dopaminergic pathways that modulate CRF neurons in central nucleus of amygdala. AVP, arginine vasopressin; CRF, corticotropin releasing factor; DA, dopamine; IML, intermediolateral cell column; LTP, long-term potentiation; NorEpi, norepinephrine; NTS, nucleus of the solitary tract; PGi, nucleus paragigantocellularis.

the proportion of paraventricular CRF neurons shifts from approximately 50% CRF-only to 90% of the CRF-AVP type. These findings suggest that the secretion of stress levels of cortisol is associated with activation of these CRF-AVP neurons by the amygdala. An additional feature of Figure 5 concerns negative feedback sensitivity of the CRF and CRF-AVP neurons. The effectiveness of cortisol at diminishing the output of these two sets of neurons is respectively 10:1. As a result, the output of cortisol during states of stress may be less easily dampened by

THE CENTRAL CRF SYSTEM

Corticotropin releasing factor acts as a neuropeptide at the portal circulation, but it also acts as a neurotransmitter in an elaborate system of neurons reactive to exogenous challenge and endogenous distress. The CRF fiber system has a key role in central integration of behavior, autonomic activity, and HPAC function (Swanson et al. 1983). It is responsive to conditions that produce stress responses, its stimulation by injection of CRF produces all of the major components of the "fight or flight" response (Hilton 1982), and its blockade prevents the formation of this response. Activation of this fiber network results in integrated hormonal and sympathetic nervous system outflow to the periphery and inhibition of parasympathetic outflow. It is regulated in part by cortisol feedback to the subpopulation of CRF neurons that has glucocorticoid receptors and in part from neural sources.

So pervasive is the role of the CRF system in regulating all components of the fight-or-flight response that some investigators believe that "recent results identify the CRF-41 neuronal system as a widespread and complex system that appears to be dedicated, perhaps uniquely among chemically defined neurons, to a single task: the regulation and coordination of the body's endocrine, autonomic, metabolic, behavioral, and emotional responses to stressful stimuli" (Petrusz & Merchenthaler 1992).

Anatomical Distribution of the CRF System

The greatest aggregation of CRF-producing neurons is in the PVN. Major accumulations occur also in the prefrontal, insular, and cingulate cortexes – areas that communicate closely with the lateral nucleus of the amygdala in the formation of emotional responses to evaluation of external events and internal sensations. A dense accumulation of CRF cell bodies is also found in the central nucleus of the amygdala, and lesser accumulations occur in the septum, lateral amygdala, and hippocampus. CRF-carrying fiber connections exist among these areas, serving to integrate their functions during periods of stress.

Important projections of PVN CRF neurons travel to the brainstem (Figure 5). One set enters the pons and synapses with cells of the nucleus paragigantocellularis – a large, complex, primitive integrator of motor responses and the primary source of fibers projecting to the locus ceruleus (Aston-Jones et al. 1986). The locus ceruleus sends noradrenergic fibers to the entire CNS, and these are a source of ascending cerebral activation (Curtis, Drolet, & Valentino 1993). Another set of PVN fibers projects to the intermediolateral cell column of the spinal cord, the pathway for all sympathetic preganglionic fibers, and to the nucleus of the solitary tract, where cardiovascular sympathetic reflexes are organized. For this reason, descending outflow to sympathetically innervated structures, including the adrenal medulla, is influenced by activity of CRF neurons arising from the PVN.

The distribution of CRF receptors also occurs mainly in systems serving the stress response. As expected, CRF receptors occur in the anterior pituitary (De Souza & Kuhar 1986). Moderate to high densities of CRF receptors occur in: all layers of the cortex; the basal ganglia; lateral nucleus of the amygdala; the pons and nuclei of several cranial nerves; and the medulla, including the nucleus of the solitary tract, which organizes cardiovascular sympathetic activity.

Pharmacologic Effects of CRF Administration

Injection of physiological quantities of CRF into the cerebrospinal fluid results in integrated behavioral and physiological changes suggestive of stress responses, including:

1. increased ACTH release (Rivier & Vale 1985);
2. increased sympathetic nerve firing;
3. increased epinephrine, norepinephrine, and glucose in the circulation (Brown et al. 1982);
4. increased firing of the brainstem locus ceruleus (Valentino, Foote, & Aston-Jones 1983);

5. the classic fight-or-flight circulatory pattern, consisting of increased arterial pressure and cardiac output and decreased peripheral resistance (Davis 1992);
6. decreased parasympathetic activity;
7. increased motor activity; and
8. decreased food and water intake and sexual activity (Petrusz & Merchenthaler 1992).

Functional Characteristics of the CRF System

The functional characteristics of the central CRF system are revealed in part by the effects of adrenalectomy, which leads to loss of feedback from peripheral cortisol and a consequent up-regulation of CRF activity in areas subject to negative feedback. Adrenalectomy produces greatly increased numbers of CRF-containing storage vesicles in neurons of the PVN as well as lesser increases in the central nucleus of the amygdala, the bed nucleus of the stria terminalis, and the spinal cord (Merchenthaler 1984). This sensitivity of CRF neurons to the absence of cortisol suggests that cortisol has a feedback role, not only on its own secretion via the hippocampus and hypothalamus but also on structures involved with the formation of emotions, such as the amygdala and amygdaloid outflow to the hypothalamus (Joëls & De Kloet 1989).

The stress-integrative role of the CRF system is also revealed by applying endogenous and exogenous stressors and then noting expression of immediate-early genes, an indicator of increased neuronal metabolism (Melia et al. 1994). During stress, immediate-early gene expression occurs in noradrenergic, dopaminergic, and serotonergic cell groups of the pons and medulla – neuron populations that are involved in mood regulation, attention, and reward systems.

The responsiveness of the CRF system to endogenous stressors is illustrated by the effects of rapid pharmacologic withdrawal in cannabinoid-dependent rats. Within minutes of induced withdrawal, immediate-early gene expression was found in CRF-expressing neurons of the hippocampus, nucleus accumbens, central nucleus of the amygdala and bed nucleus of the stria terminalis, the PVN, the locus ceruleus, and the nucleus of the solitary tract; these expressions are followed by CRF increases, behavioral signs of distress, and increased plasma corticosterone (Rodriguez de Fonseca et al. 1997). Another endogenous stressor capable of activating the CRF system is the initiation of an immune response by tissue inflammation. In this case, inflammatory cytokines are transported to the PVN where they stimulate CRF gene expression, resulting in stress-related activation of the HPAC.

Summary

Glucocorticoid regulation reveals two overlapping sets of central controls: one for normal metabolism and diurnal functions and another for periods of stress.

During stress, cortisol's secretion and sensitivity to feedback are both biased to allow higher circulating concentrations to occur. The stress secretion of cortisol is under control of a highly integrated system of CRF-synthesizing neurons. The CRF system – integrating activities of the hypothalamus, anterior pituitary, brainstem aminergic and serotonergic nuclei, and the amygdala – is well positioned to respond to stressors of many types. Psychologically meaningful stimuli can activate this system by way of the amygdala, with consequent variation from person to person and from time to time as a function of learning history and varying interpretations of the situation.

It is perhaps not coincidental that the principle site for negative feedback regulation of glucocorticoid secretion is the hippocampus. This suggests intimate connections between emotions, endocrine regulation, and cognition. Hand-in-hand with the hippocampus, the critical role of the amygdala in activating stress responses indicates that these structures form an important juncture at which experience is translated into bodily responses. Finally, the role of cortisol as a modifier of CNS structures and cognitive functions appears to be a key topic for future investigation.

Physical Context: The Catecholamines

Along with the glucocorticoids, the catecholamines – norepinephrine, epinephrine, and dopamine – play a key role in both normal homeostasis and in sympathetically mediated responses to stress. They also act as neurotransmitters in the central nervous system, where they affect glucocorticoid regulation and modulate alertness and affect.

The importance of the sympathetic nervous system for systemic regulation was amply demonstrated by the work of Walter Cannon (1929), who noted that sympathetically mediated activity accompanied many emotional disturbances and so set the stage for an enduring interest in the role of sympathetic patterning in behavioral stress (Cannon 1928). At the time, sympathetic nervous system activity was known to be accompanied by elevations in a circulating substance later identified by von Euler (1948) as norepinephrine.

Since then, the measurement of catecholamines has been used to estimate sympathetic nervous system activity in clinical states and in response to emotional stimuli. Most psychophysiological studies have measured changes over time and across stimulus conditions in order to assess physiological components of cognitive, emotional, and other behavioral states.

The catecholamines have similar structures to and a degree of cross-reactivity with their respective receptors, although dopamine is not considered a stress hormone. The peripheral actions of norepinephrine and epinephrine are summarized in Table 2.

SOURCES AND FATE OF THE PERIPHERAL CATECHOLAMINES

The sources of circulating catecholamines are the sympathetic nerves and the adrenal medulla. The metabolic fates of the catecholamines are indicated in Figure 6.

Sources of Catecholamine in Circulation

Norepinephrine in circulation reflects sympathetic nervous system activity by way of the adrenal medulla and sympathetic nerve endings. Nearly all the norepinephrine secreted by the adrenal medulla enters circulation. At sympathetic nerve terminals, norepinephrine secretion is nearly proportional to rates of nerve firing (Blombery & Heinzow 1983), and 10%–20% of this enters the circulation (Esler et al. 1985). The pool of circulating norepinephrine at any given time has the following sources: lungs (30%), kidneys (25%), skeletal muscle (22%), liver and related circulation (6%), skin (5%), heart (3%), and adrenal glands (2%) (Esler et al. 1985).

Epinephrine presents a relatively simpler picture; the sole source of circulating epinephrine is the adrenal medulla, although it undergoes several fates including uptake by tissues and metabolic degradation.

At any given time, the amount of catecholamine in circulation is the product of its rate of entry and its rate of removal (Esler et al. 1988). The balance of entry and removal often varies in the very states that are of interest in psychophysiological investigations. For example, mental arithmetic causes increased sympathetic nervous system outflow and decreased renal blood flow. As a result, plasma norepinephrine will rise owing to an unknown combination of increased spillover from sympathetic nerves and slower removal via the kidneys. The effect of decreased clearance is potentially significant. Esler has shown that, during the physical challenge of head-up tilt (a stimulus that increases sympathetic activity), the increase in plasma norepinephrine due to decreased renal flow was twice that due to increased spillover (Esler et al. 1988). This indicates the complexity of inferring increased sympathetic nervous system activity from plasma measurements of norepinephrine.

Sources of Blood Sampling

An additional consideration for psychophysiological research concerns the most appropriate site from which to obtain blood samples. Data provided by Esler (Esler et al. 1988) based on studies using radiolabeled norepinephrine and sampling from several venous and arterial withdrawal sites have shown that radioactivity counts, and therefore norepinephrine concentrations, will vary by a factor of 2.8 across sites. The researchers concluded that no single sampling site represents the blood pool as a whole. Methodological issues are discussed in further detail in a later section.

HORMONAL VERSUS NEUROEFFECTOR ACTIONS OF THE CATECHOLAMINES

A hormone is defined as "a product of living cells that circulates in body fluids ... and produces a specific effect on the activity of cells remote from its point of origin" (*Webster's Ninth New Collegiate Dictionary* 1988). By this definition, epinephrine found in circulation is a true hormone secreted by the adrenal medulla and acting on a range of tissues at noninnervated beta-adrenoreceptors. Beta-1 receptors are located in the heart, and they act to increase the rate and force of contractions; beta-2 receptors are located primarily in the walls of blood vessels, where they act to relax smooth muscle cells.

Norepinephrine has limited hormonal effects. The alpha-adrenoreceptors of the blood vessels are anatomically distant from the blood supply, and their neuroeffector junctions are very narrow. They are activated by norepinephrine released from the prejunctional nerve terminal but not by the norepinephrine in circulation. Although textbooks often imply that circulating norepinephrine is responsible for vascular tonus – infused norepinephrine does raise vascular resistance – the necessary plasma concentrations of 1,800–2,000 pg/ml are well above physiological levels and are rarely, if ever, achieved in the psychophysiological laboratory. Similarly, the beta-1-adrenoreceptors of the heart are insensitive to physiological levels of plasma norepinephrine. "The norepinephrine in plasma represents transmitter overflow rather than circulating hormone, and under most circumstances it is devoid of metabolic and cardiovascular effects" (Esler et al. 1988). The lack of hormonal action by norepinephrine is consistent with the many studies reporting null correlations between catecholamine levels and cardiovascular activity (e.g. Kirschbaum, Pirke, & Hellhammer 1993). Note that others have reported effects of infused norepinephrine on neutrophil counts and renin release (DeChamplain et al. 1966; Sloand, Hooper, & Izzo 1989). A partial listing of the hormonal and neuroeffector actions of the catecholamines is given in Table 2.

Social and Psychological Context: The Psychophysiology of Stress Hormone Secretion

The existence of reliable relationships between emotions and endocrine patterns has been recognized for some time. In the aftermath of World War II and the attendant interest in how to predict performance under conditions of

TABLE 2. Effects of Catecholamines on Adrenergic Receptors in Selected Tissues

Tissue	Function	Receptor Type
Hormonal Actions		
Heart	↑ Contractility	beta-1, Non-Inv
	↑ Pacemaker frequency	beta-1, Non-Inv
	↑ Conduction velocity	beta-1, Non-Inv
Arteries		
Skeletal muscle	↑ Dilation	beta-2, Non-Inv
Heart	↑ Dilation	beta-2, Non-Inv
Veins	↑ Constriction	beta-2, Non-Inv
Bronchioles	↑ Dilation	beta-2, Non-Inv
Gut	↓ Motility	beta-2, Non-Inv
	↑ Sphincter constriction	beta-2, Non-Inv
Spleen	↓ Contraction	beta-2, Non-Inv
Exocrine glands		
Parotid	↓ Secretion	beta-2, Non-Inv
Adipose tissue	↑ Lipolysis	beta-2, Non-Inv
Liver	↑ Glycogenolysis	beta-2, Non-Inv
	↑ Gluconeogenesis	beta-2, Non-Inv
Neurotransmitter Actions		
Heart	↑ Contractility	beta-1, Inv
	↑ Pacemaker frequency	beta-1, Inv
	↑ Conduction velocity	beta-1, Inv
Arteries	↑ Constriction	alpha, Inv
Veins	↑ Constriction	alpha, Inv
Bronchioles	↑ Dilation	alpha, Inv
Gastrointestinal tract	↓ Motility	alpha, Inv
	↑ Sphincter constriction	alpha, Inv
Spleen	↑ Contraction	alpha, Inv
Iris radial muscle	↑ Contraction	alpha, Inv
Exocrine glands		
Sweat	↑ Secretion	alpha, Inv

Key: Inv, innervated receptor; Non-Inv, noninnervated receptor.
Notes: Noninnervated receptors are responsive to hormonal actions of epinephrine; innervated receptors are responsive to the neuroeffector actions of norepinephrine. Adapted from Moran (1975).

fear, Lazarus noted that conditions of extreme demand accompanied by strong negative emotions resulted in a deterioration of performance (Lazarus, Deese, & Osler 1952). Lazarus later argued that stressful situations are ones in which the person's motivated behavior is thwarted by the circumstances (Lazarus & Folkman 1984). Conditions of high motivation accompanied by frustration, failure, or extreme danger were seen as stressful and being accompanied by negative emotional states. Conditions favoring motivated behavior and successful achievement of goals were seen as nonstressful and conducive to positive emotions. In this framework, loss of control over the environment became a critical determinant of psychological stress reactions (Averill 1973).

The themes of control, success, positive emotions, and feelings of activation versus loss of control, failure, negative

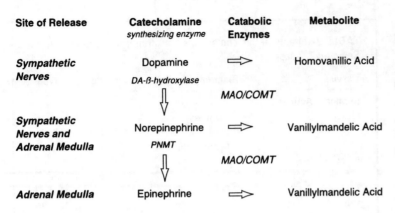

Site of Release	Catecholamine *synthesizing enzyme*	Catabolic Enzymes	Metabolite
Sympathetic Nerves	Dopamine	⇒	Homovanillic Acid
	DA-β-hydroxylase	MAO/COMT	
Sympathetic Nerves and Adrenal Medulla	Norepinephrine	⇒	Vanillylmandelic Acid
	PNMT	MAO/COMT	
Adrenal Medulla	Epinephrine	⇒	Vanillylmandelic Acid

Figure 6. Biosynthetic and degradative pathways for the catecholamines. MAO, monoamine oxidase; COMT, catechol-o-methyltransferase.

emotions, and feelings of fruitless effort appear in several forms. Henry and Stephens (1977) showed that socially dominant animals had catecholamine output with normal cortisols, whereas those that were subordinate had catecholamine activity with high cortisol output. Others distinguished between a defensive, fearlike "cortisol factor" and a successlike "catecholamine factor" in endocrine measures and self-reports of men undergoing stressful military training procedures (Ellertsen, Johnsen, & Ursin 1978; Rose, Poe, & Mason 1967).

Frankenhaeuser (1980) noted that persons reporting behavioral control efforts *without* distress were likely to show high catecholamine excretion with normal cortisol output; distress, frustration, and low control involved both cortisol and catecholamine output. Self-report items loading on an "effort" factor (effort, concentration, stimulation, and the inverses of tiredness and boredom) and a "distress" factor (distress, irritation, tiredness, impatience, tenseness, and the inverse of pleasantness) appear to represent clusters of positive and negative emotion reports, respectively (Lundberg & Frankenhaeuser 1980). Extensive coverage is available in Ursin, Baade, and Levine (1978).

To summarize these viewpoints: cortisol release seems to be selectively associated with negative emotions accompanying failure or efforts without reward whereas catecholamine secretion is found in conditions of high behavioral effort with or without success. This provides a useful organizing framework for examining endocrine function in relation to conditions perceived as stressful and nonstressful.

PSYCHOLOGICAL FACTORS AFFECTING STRESS HORMONE RELEASE

As noted in our discussion of the biology of glucocorticoid and catecholamine secretion, these substances have significant metabolic functions apart from their connections to emotional states. For example, prolonged exercise results in increased catecholamine and cortisol secretion to metabolically support muscular exertion and cardiovascular activity (Smith et al. 1976). Brief bouts of maximal exercise do not increase circulating cortisol if the duration does not challenge the fuel homeostasis of the individual (Sung et al. 1990). Therefore, we might say that physical stressors will evoke catecholamine and cortisol changes in proportion to metabolic expenditure.

The stress hormones are also responsive to cognitive and affective stimulation in the absence of metabolic demand. During a mental arithmetic task, the subject performs mental calculations rapidly and accurately under human supervision or an automated monitor. The task produces significant increases in cortisol and catecholamine release (al'Absi et al. 1994; Williams et al. 1982) with minimal physical demands, so we can think of it as a purely psychological stressor, requiring a high degree of effort and producing moderate frustration and mild aversiveness (al'Absi et al. 1994). Similar endocrine reactions are evoked by public speaking in the lab (Sgoutas-Emch et al. 1994) or work on the frustrating Stroop color–word interference task (Kirschbaum et al. 1993; McCann et al. 1993). All of these challenges produce cortisol and catecholamine secretion in relation to cognitive effort and negative emotions evoked by potential failure and social disapproval. Such demonstrations illustrate that endocrine changes evolving to support metabolic demands can be evoked by top-down processes associated with the cognitive demands and affective overtones of the situation. This formulation is consistent with our earlier discussion of the particular role of the amygdala in responding to conditions of real or implied threat and its ability to stimulate the PVN of the hypothalamus.

In our research we have conducted two studies that are useful in illustrating activation versus distress effects on catecholamines and cortisol. In the first study, healthy male volunteers worked on a difficult 15-min reaction time task to avoid presentation of noise bursts (115 dBA) and electric shocks (3.5 mA) (Lovallo, Pincomb, & Wilson 1986b). Under these aversive circumstances, we observed a significant rise in both norepinephrine and cortisol secretion over 15 min. Self-reports using Frankenhaeuser's scale (Lundberg & Frankenhaeuser 1980) showed significant increases in both activation and distress (Figure 7).

In the second study, subjects worked on a nearly identical reaction time task in order to earn monetary bonuses (Lovallo, Pincomb, & Wilson 1986c). These rewarding circumstances were associated with significant reports of increased effort similar to the aversive study but significantly lower reports of distress. Norepinephrine increased significantly, in an amount similar to the aversive study, but cortisol did not change from baseline (Figure 7; see also Lovallo et al. 1990).

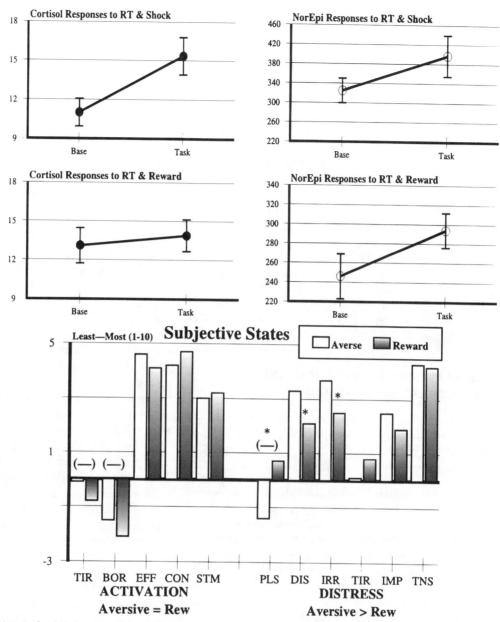

Figure 7. Cortisol, norepinephrine, and subjective states in response to a reaction time task motivated by threat of noise and shock (upper panels) and by monetary reward (lower panels). The norepinephrine response was present to both stressors; cortisol response occurred only to the aversive task (upper left panel). Subjective reports show the tasks did not differ in causing feelings of activation or effort. The aversive task was rated as more distressing (DIS) and irritating (IRR) and less pleasant (PLS). Data represent the most reactive individuals based on median split of heart rate response to a different stressor.

Because the subjects were semirecumbent during both studies, we consider the norepinephrine changes to be related to cognitive effort rather than a bottom-up demand for increased systemic blood flow, as in exercise. Similarly, the cortisol secretion was associated with the anticipation of aversive stimulation much more than with its actual presentation; the aversive study included four shocks and eight noise bursts – for 12 sec of aversive stimulation in 15 min (1.3% of the total task time).

In a study using simulated public speaking, we found that cortisol secretion was correlated with negative emotions (using the "profile of mood states") but not with positive affect (al'Absi et al. 1997). We recently performed a more stringent test of the cortisol–negative affect relationship (Buchanan, al'Absi, & Lovallo 1999). Male subjects were tested on: a neutral-affect rest day; a negative-affect high-activation day with a 30-min speech stressor; and a positive-affect high-activation day viewing a 30-min video that contained material judged to be positively affective and highly activating (subjective reports were in accord with these expectations). Cortisol was elevated only during the speech stressor (Figure 8).

Consistent with HPAC responses to distress in the lab, findings indicate that daily stressors (Brantley et al. 1988), anticipation of a painful tooth extraction (Goldstein et al. 1982), and school exam stress (Francis 1979; Lovallo et al. 1986a; Malarkey et al. 1995b) may yield increases in cortisol and catecholamine (Sausen et al. 1992) secretion.

These findings suggest that cortisol is preferentially responsive to subjective states of fear, frustration, and related negative emotions. In contrast, the catecholamines reflect sympathetic activation supporting metabolic processes during states of activation, regardless of the emotional valence. Attempts have been made to distinguish epinephrine as being more psychologically reactive than norepinephrine. There are occasional reports of increased epinephrine without norepinephrine in threatening situations (e.g. Frankenhaeuser & Rissler 1970; Sausen et al. 1992), but findings have been inconsistent. This may be due to technical difficulties in measuring epinephrine, resulting in a paucity of reliable results. These difficulties are discussed in the section entitled "Design Considerations in Psychophysiological Studies of Catecholamines."

INTERACTIONS BETWEEN HPAC AND CATECHOLAMINE ACTIVATION

There are points of interaction between the HPAC and the sympathetic nervous system that suggest that – during fight-or-flight states – the activity of the two branches of the stress response may be integrated as follows.

1. Selye (1936) showed that his HPAC-based stress response was greatly diminished in rats deprived of endogenous epinephrine by removal of the adrenal medulla.
2. Ventricular administration of CRF leads to activation of the HPAC and sympathetic outflow (Irwin et al. 1988).
3. The HPAC may be activated directly by systemic epinephrine entering the pituitary circulation (Proulx et al. 1984).
4. The PVN increases CRF secretion during beta-adreno-receptor activity at brainstem sites (Richardson Morton et al. 1990).
5. Catecholamine synthesis, sympathetic nervous activity, and the beta-adrenoreceptor complex depend on the tonic presence of cortisol (Davies & Lefkowitz 1984).
6. The HPAC may enhance the actions of catecholamines (Szabo et al. 1988).

The lateral hypothalamus-perifornical area, which is crucial to the cardiovascular component of the fight-or-flight response in rodents and primates (Smith et al. 1990), is closely associated with the PVN, and both send fibers to sympathetic output pathways. We and others have noted significant evidence of coincident cardiovascular and cortisol activation during fear-associated tasks in humans, especially among those persons with the greatest sympathetically mediated cardiovascular response tendencies

(Lovallo et al. 1990; Uchino et al. 1995). However, these response systems are not strictly coupled at their outputs, for the blockade of the HPAC response to combined public speaking and mental arithmetic stress leaves the catecholamine response undisturbed (Malarkey, Lipkus, & Cacioppo 1995a).

SENSITIVITY TO INDIVIDUAL DIFFERENCES

Although cortisol and catecholamines are reliably responsive to certain stimulus conditions in grouped data, there are substantial differences between individuals in how they react to both aversive and rewarding challenges (see e.g. Lovallo et al. 1990). Such individual differences may be important if there are health consequences to frequent or sustained stress hormone activation (Berger et al. 1987).

Cortisol reactivity differences have a significant heritability component (Kirschbaum et al. 1992a), suggesting a genetic basis. Borderline hypertensive young men produce larger cortisol responses than low-risk controls when exposed to a novel laboratory environment (al'Absi & Lovallo 1993) and to mental arithmetic stress (al'Absi et al. 1994). These men did not differ in self-reports of effort or distress, suggesting a constitutionally based sensitivity to novel situations. However, some differences in reactivity are clearly determined by psychological traits. Cynical hostility, a stable trait measured by the Cook–Medley Hostility Scale from the Minnesota Multiphasic Personality Inventory, predicts greater cortisol activity at work but not at home (Pope & Smith 1991), suggesting more stressful social interactions during work hours.

Such reactivity may therefore be due to differences in hypothalamic activity or in psychological responses to appropriate challenges, depending on the character of the group in question (see Lovallo 1997, pp. 145–64).

Sex Differences in Stress Hormone Activity

In younger subjects (20–29 years of age), women have lower 24-hr plasma cortisol concentrations than men and lower peak morning values, and women show larger age-related increases in basal output (Van Cauter, Leproult, & Kupfer 1996). Women may also evidence increases in stress hormone reactivity as a function of menopause (see Saab et al. 1989). Women have consistently smaller stress catecholamine responses than men in the laboratory and workplace (Frankenhaeuser et al. 1978; Johansson & Post 1974), although this may be less true of women who have assumed nontraditional roles (Frankenhaeuser, Lundberg, & Chesney 1991). Much of the earlier work on gender differences in stress hormone response is reviewed thoroughly by Saab (1989). Men and women show equal cortisol responses to CRF injection (Kirschbaum, Wust, & Hellhammer 1992b), suggesting equivalent pituitary and adrenal responsiveness. This implies that greater male responsiveness may be due to brain structures at or above the hypothalamus or to differential sensitivity of feedback receptor systems. A broad conclusion from such work is that men are more reactive to challenging or threatening cues, although this gender difference may vary with the task or social demands of the experiment (Kirschbaum et al. 1995a).

SOCIAL FACTORS AND STRESS HORMONE SECRETION

Social challenges – typified by potential for negative evaluations by significant others, loss of status among equals, and low controllability – can provoke substantial stress hormone responses. Simulated public speaking produces reliable cortisol responses in the laboratory (al'Absi et al. 1997; Kirschbaum et al. 1995a). Young physicians speaking before an audience of older colleagues produced significant increases in epinephrine (Dimsdale & Moss 1980) and norepinephrine (Taggart, Carruthers, & Somerville 1973), and soldiers undergoing an oral exam by superior officers showed significant increases in ACTH and cortisol (Meyerhoff, Oleshansky, & Mougey 1988).

Gender Differences in Hormonal Response to Social Stress

Several studies, but not all, indicate larger cortisol responses to public speaking challenge among men (see Kirschbaum et al. 1992b). On the other hand, women seem to be more responsive to the social nuances of the task situation, such as expressions of support and threats of withdrawal. For example, during a structured marital conflict task, newlywed women were reactive to their husbands' signs of involvement versus withdrawal, while the men responded to the situation as a whole but not to the interpersonal nuances (Kiecolt-Glaser et al. 1996). In a study of social support, young males appeared to benefit from the presence of their girlfriends during public speaking and mental arithmetic stress. In contrast, the women actually had larger stress cortisol responses in the presence of their boyfriends (Kirschbaum et al. 1995a). Such findings indicate that the psychophysiological relationships between stressful events, social processes, and stress hormone secretion are likely to be quite different for men and women, although both sexes are reactive to social cues.

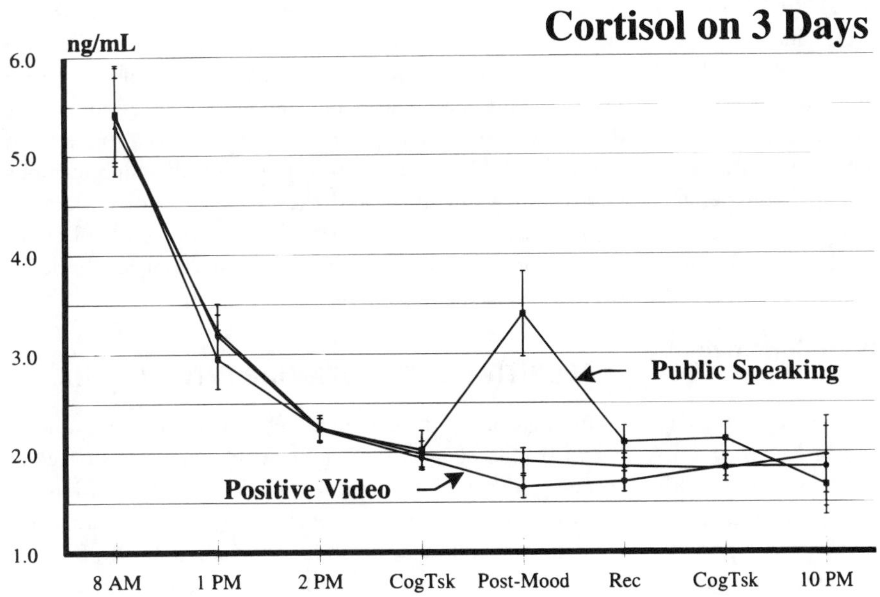

An extensive review of social support and effects on stress hormones is available in Uchino, Cacioppo, and Kiecolt-Glaser (1996). The preliminary indications of gender differences in the influence of socially meaningful stimuli on endocrine homeostasis is clearly an understudied but potentially important area for psychophysiological research.

STRESS HORMONE EFFECTS ON BEHAVIOR

While the bulk of the literature on stress hormones concerns the hormone response to behavioral manipulations, there is an important and growing literature on the impact of the stress hormones themselves on emotions and behavior. These findings are critical because they graphically demonstrate the influence of biological activity on functions traditionally associated with the psychological realm.

Glucocorticoid Effects on Fear- and Anxiety-Related Behavior

Activation of the central CRF system mimics the effects of negative emotional states. Administration of CRF directly into the ventricles in rats results in: defensive behaviors (Takahashi et al. 1989); increased freezing (Sherman & Kalin 1986); decreased exploration (Berridge & Dunn 1989); increased acoustic startle response (Liang et al. 1992); and decreased mating (Rivier & Vale 1984) – all signs consistent with fear- and anxietylike states. Chronic high levels of corticosterone in rats will potentiate the effect of an acute intraventricular dose of CRF (Lee, Schulkin, & Davis 1994). Recent work implicates the hippocampal MR (high affinity) receptor in such effects (Smythe et al. 1997), although it is likely that the amygdala is also involved (Lee et al. 1994). These studies suggest that CRF and glucocorticoid activity are

Figure 8. Cortisol activity (ng/ml) from 8:00 A.M. to 10:00 P.M. with a laboratory protocol from 1:00 P.M. to 3:00 P.M. on a stress day compared with days of rest and positive mood induction. Only the stressor increased cortisol; the positive mood induction lowered cortisol relative to rest.

Cortisol on 3 Days

not only expressions of fear and anxiety but can actually potentiate such behaviors. Note that there are also conditions under which acute glucocorticoid administration can exert anxiolytic effects (File, Vellucci, & Wendlandt 1979). Collectively, these studies indicate that there are clear mechanisms by which the initiation of an emotional response at the central nervous system (a top-down process) can be augmented or regulated by the peripheral portion of that response in a bottom-up fashion.

Cognitive–Glucocorticoid Interactions

Cortisol, often viewed primarily as an indicator of stress, is also an active agent for modification of CNS structure and function. The presence of both MRs and GRs in hippocampus, amygdala, and hypothalamus suggests that corticosteroids may significantly affect behavior (Martignoni et al. 1992; McEwen & Sapolsky 1995). The most dramatic example of glucocorticoid-induced behavioral change is the observation that young rats exposed to high levels of corticosterone suffer loss of hippocampal neurons due to excitatory neuropeptide actions (McEwen & Sapolsky 1995).

Stress levels of glucocorticoids, resulting in occupancy of low-affinity GR, have three effects on hippocampal neurons: (1) temporary reduction in long-term potentiation, possibly accounting for post-stress and diurnal variations in working memory; (2) suppression of hippocampal neurogenesis; and (3) potential atrophy of apical dendrites (McEwen 1997). In contrast, occupancy of high-affinity MR by low glucocorticoid concentrations prolongs long-term potentiation (Pavlides et al. 1995).

Human clinical research supports a hippocampal link between cortisol and cognition. Cortisol-related cognitive deficits and loss of hippocampal volume have been observed in Cushing's disease, depression, normal aging, and Alzheimer's disease (DeLeon et al. 1988; Meaney et al. 1995; Rubinow et al. 1984; Starkman et al. 1992). Elderly volunteers showing high cortisol levels that increased over several years had impaired spatial memory in a full-size walking maze (Lupien et al. 1995), and impaired declarative memory related to their degree of hippocampal atrophy (Lupien et al. 1998). Others have reported a relationship between cognitive deficits, loss of hippocampal volume, and presumed severe HPAC activation due to childhood physical and sexual abuse or traumatic wartime stress (Bremner et al. 1993, 1995a,b).

Acute Effects of Glucocorticoids on Cognitive Function

In three studies we have seen that – when subjects were exposed to a stressful mental arithmetic task – their cortisol response was inversely related to performance, with Pearson r values in the range of −0.40 (al'Absi et al. 1994, 1997; al'Absi, Hugdahl, & Lovallo 1998); see Figure 9. These results suggest that cortisol was having an acute ef-

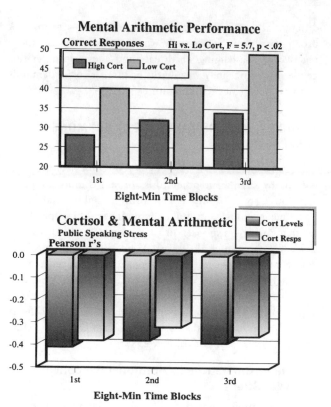

Figure 9. Mental arithmetic performance as a function of cortisol activity. Subjects performed three 8-min mental arithmetic tasks in succession, either before or after undergoing a 24-min public-speaking challenge. Top panel: Subjects with larger cortisol responses, by a median split, had fewer correct responses in each segment of the mental arithmetic task. Lower panel: Correct items on mental arithmetic items were negatively correlated with cortisol levels during the entire stress period (left bars) or in response to the speech stressor (right bars).

fect on memory. Support for this hypothesis comes from the finding that high cortisol secretion to a mixed mental arithmetic and speech stressor resulted in poor retention of word lists over a 5-min recall interval (Kirschbaum et al. 1996). Oral administration of cortisol, relative to a placebo, led to impaired performance on tests of declarative memory and spatial learning but not on a test of procedural memory (Kirschbaum et al. 1996; see also Veltman & Gaillard 1993). The known role of the hippocampus in declarative memory, and the impairment of declarative memory during endogenous and exogenous cortisol exposure, suggests a cognitive impact of cortisol feedback on the hippocampus in humans.

COGNITIVE–CATECHOLAMINE INTERACTIONS

In addition to glucocorticoid effects on memory, a number of studies suggest that epinephrine enhances storage of events in declarative memory (McGaugh 1983). Memory performance is improved when epinephrine is administered to rats following training (McGaugh 1989). Because epinephrine does not cross the blood–brain barrier, this must be an indirect effect mediated by peripheral structures. McGaugh and colleagues have shown that this effect is mediated by peripheral beta-adrenoreceptors. Propranolol, a nonspecific beta-receptor blocker, reduces recall of material from a narrative slide show (Cahill et al. 1994), and this effect appears to depend on beta-adrenoreceptors on afferent fibers of the vagus nerve that project to the nucleus of the solitary tract (Liang, Juler, & McGaugh 1986; Williams & McGaugh 1993). This important brainstem cardiovascular regulatory nucleus has afferents to the amygdala. Blockade of these inputs by administration of beta blockers prevents formation of memories of rewarded relationships (McGaugh & Cahill 1997).

This relatively recent work showing the important effects of the stress hormones on emotion and cognition will undoubtedly yield much more important information on the two-way interaction between the central nervous system and responses traditionally thought of as bodily responses. More generally, the earlier view of the stress response as a reflexive set of outputs is seen to have intimate connections with our perceptions of the world, our emotional reactions, cognitive states, and the registration of our experience.

Inferential Context: Issues in Research Design and Methods

Psychophysiological investigations of stress hormone activity will most frequently be concerned with changes in secretion in relation to some behavioral, emotional, or cognitive stimulus condition. In some cases, changes in contrasting groups are compared.

What follows is a compilation of information on stress hormone research based on published information and our own experience in psychophysiological investigations. This sort of methodological discussion is always a blending of art and science, and our recommendations should be considered in light of the reader's experience and the unique circumstances prevailing in a given research project. Finally, since psychophysiologists will usually find themselves working with an endocrinologist or clinical chemist, the experience of the collaborator will be invaluable. This section is intended in part as an aid to communication with other investigators.

DESIGN CONSIDERATIONS IN PSYCHOPHYSIOLOGICAL STUDIES OF CORTISOL

Availability in Blood, Saliva, and Urine

In blood, about 3%–5% of the total cortisol is the unbound, biologically active fraction, while the remainder is bound to the proteins albumin and transcortin (also called corticosteroid-binding globulin or CBG). However, CBG binding characteristics are not static and the ratio of free to bound cortisol is not constant; for example, elevated free fatty acids following high fat intake can alter the affinity and number of CBG binding sites (Haourigui et al. 1995), thus altering peak cortisol values and half-life. The presence of only unbound cortisol in saliva and urine make these sample sources valuable in assessing the biologically active fraction free of CBG changes.

Secretion, Clearance, and Sample Timing

The single most important consideration in study design is the diurnal variation of cortisol secretion (Figure 1). Averaged plasma values may range from 1 μg/dl during sleep to 18 μg/dl at awakening. This 18-fold variation dictates that diurnal cycle be controlled, usually by testing all subjects at the same time of day. We and others have greatly enhanced the sensitivity of our study designs by testing all subjects on one day with the intended experimental manipulations and also on an alternate day during which they rest while samples are taken, time-locked to the schedule of the experimental day (Figure 8) (al'Absi et al. 1997; McCann et al. 1993).

Stressor onset will activate a cortisol response in as few as 10–15 min for a potent stressor, such as mild electric shock (Lovallo et al. 1985), whereas moderate mental stressors may take 20–30 min. Owing to the slow response of the HPAC, stressors of longer duration ($\geq$ 15 min) are more likely to result in a reliable cortisol response than brief ones.

The liver is the major site of cortisol metabolism (Wortmann et al. 1971), although cortisol is also broken down in adipose tissue and kidney (Weidenfeld et al. 1982; Whitworth et al. 1989). Half-life following oral or intravenous administration is approximately 105 $\pm$ 30 min for serum and about 70 $\pm$ 9 min for saliva (Tunn et al. 1992).

Sample sources also vary in their time windows, and this will influence the choice of specimen source in the context of the goals of the study. Saliva and blood provide information about cortisol dynamics prevailing over the prior 45 min. Urine provides a time-integrated sample source representing dynamics for the entire period of collection. The timing and frequency of sampling involve choosing intervals likely to allow the peak response to be discriminated from background noise in the data. In most cases, laboratory studies use blood or saliva whereas studies outside the lab use either saliva or urine.

Sources of Experimental Confounding

Cortisol and catecholamine excretion rates in urine vary significantly with the seasons of the year (Malarkey et al. 1995b). Studies measuring stress hormones in the same persons over long periods or comparing persons tested at widely differing times may benefit from use of statistical techniques to control for such sources of variation.

Gender differences and hormonal changes also deserve special mention. As noted earlier, men produce more cortisol across the diurnal cycle and are more stress-reactive than women. Furthermore, cortisol responsivity in women may vary with menstrual phase (Tersman, Collins, & Eneroth 1991), although this is not a universal finding (Choi & Salmon 1995). Another confound is hormonal change due to pregnancy or oral contraceptive use, which can change CBG levels and so affect total plasma cortisol, with unknown effects on the unbound fraction. Women on oral contraceptives may have elevated basal plasma cortisol levels (Brien 1975) and reduced stress responsiveness (Kirschbaum, Pirke, & Hellhammer 1995b).

Cortisol production and stress reactivity can also be influenced by age (Brandtstadter et al. 1991; Seeman & Robbins 1994), sleep cycles, and sleep stage structure (Follenius et al. 1992; Van Cauter et al. 1996); increased with increasing body weight (Strain et al. 1980) or by smoking (Kirschbaum, Wust, & Strasburger 1992c); show enhanced responsivity with hypertension risk (al'Absi et al. 1994); and altered by psychological factors – suppressed in post-traumatic stress disorder (Yehuda et al. 1991) and elevated in depression (Young et al. 1991).

Glucocorticoid-containing medications can change the response characteristics of the adrenal gland, and heavy meals can cause a transient rise in blood cortisol. While these factors can appear daunting, they merely highlight the necessity of having clear research objectives and a well-thought out design when obtaining hormonal measures; they point also to the need for appropriate control groups.

Our experience has been that satisfactory results can be obtained in studies of cortisol response in humans that incorporate the following features:

1. time-of-day controls by using a rest day to contrast with the stress day;
2. adherence to the same time of testing for all subjects;
3. testing only subjects who work during the day and have a normal sleep schedule;
4. avoiding low blood sugar by instructing subjects in pretest dietary practices or providing a light meal in the lab during long protocols; and
5. using the least invasive technique compatible with the goals of the study.

Collection and Quantification in Saliva

Saliva is a convenient and unobtrusive specimen source for cortisol measurement (Kirschbaum & Hellhammer 1989). Its increasing use over the past ten years suggests widespread acceptance, simplicity, and safety. Because subjects can provide their own samples, saliva (along with urine) is useful for studies done outside the lab. Unbound cortisol passes rapidly from the bloodstream through the parotid glands via passive intracellular diffusion, reaching equilibrium within 5 min (Landon et al. 1984). Concentration is not influenced by saliva flow rate, and excellent correlations are reported between saliva cortisol and unbound cortisol extracted from serum or plasma following

intravenous injection (Aardal & Holm 1995; Riad-Fahmy et al. 1982).

Collection has been greatly simplified by use of the "Salivette" (Sarstedt, Newton, NC), a readily available, low-cost device consisting of a sterilized cotton pledget in a small beaker within a 5-ml test tube. Samples are obtained by placing the pledget into the mouth for 2 min and allowing it to become saturated. Swabs are then placed back into the Salivette for centrifuging and storage.

Another device used for saliva collection is an "oral diffusion sink" (see Wade 1992). This currently has limited availability, but it has the desirable feature of accumulating saliva over a period of hours at a constant rate through a permeable membrane into a small capsule and so allowing time-integrated sampling, similar to urine collection. However, the device must be secured against loss or swallowing by attaching a loop of dental floss to a tooth, limiting its practicality in field work.

Since only the unbound cortisol fraction reaches saliva, concentrations will be low (1–6 ng/ml), necessitating the use of a highly sensitive detection technique. Plasma radioimmunoassay (RIA) kits, modified for saliva, are most frequently used (see Kirschbaum et al. 1989 for kit comparisons). A technique combining automated HPLC (high-performance liquid chromatography) and polarization fluorescence is also available (Okumura et al. 1995). Specifics of collection may depend on the assay being used, so consult with the laboratory performing your assays before beginning data collection.

Collection and Quantification in Blood

Although measures of cortisol in serum or plasma have long been considered the "gold standard," there are three drawbacks for psychophysiological research. Chief among these is the necessity of venipuncture and the attendant emotional reaction to the anticipation and actual needle stick. This problem is compounded if repeated samples are required. Therefore, an indwelling catheter placed 45–60 min prior to the first blood draw is recommended, although some investigators use a sample immediately after venipuncture, before a response can develop. A second difficulty is that any type of puncture requires a trained phlebotomist, attention to standard "universal safety precautions," and careful handling to avoid the transmission of disease (see Chapter 35 of this volume). Finally, serum or plasma measures typically are for total cortisol rather than the biologically active, unbound fraction. Although free cortisol cannot be measured directly in blood, it can be estimated (see Mendel 1989).

Collection and Quantification in Urine

Measures of urinary free cortisol have shown good correlations with circulating blood levels (Trainer et al. 1993). For research on exposure to chronic environmental or life stressors, urinary measures may be the most informative.

Typically, total 24-hr urine samples are considered best for this purpose, although shorter sampling times are possible and may be more practical. A compromise is to break the 24-hr collection into the sleep hours and several periods while awake. While this imposes more burden on the subjects to collect separate aliquots, the result is a 24-hr integrated sample providing some diurnal characteristics, a useful method if the stressor is more active at one time of day. The most common problem is that subjects often object to carrying and voiding into a urine collection container. Refrigeration is not necessary during the day of collection.

During assay, creatinine must also be measured to take into account variations in water clearance, giving a ratio of microgram of cortisol per gram of creatinine. Older methods of quantification expressed the excretion of cortisol in units of μg/l/24h.

The most popular method for detecting urinary cortisol is HPLC, although several RIA kits and other methods have been used (Lamb, Noonan, & Burrin 1994; Nahoul et al. 1992). Urinary levels are reportedly higher in males (96–295 nmol/24h) than females (29–196 nmol/24h) (Lamb et al. 1994), although the cause of the difference is unclear (see Makin 1996; Taylor & Raven 1996a,b).

Handling and Storage

Handling and storage of blood, urine, or saliva for cortisol quantification are rather straightforward. Since cortisol is an extremely stable compound, samples can remain at room temperature for several hours or be frozen until processing. If shipping is necessary, we normally pack the storage tubes on dry ice, although this is not strictly necessary if delivery is by overnight courier. All of the major delivery services provide special handling for blood, urine, or saliva.

DESIGN CONSIDERATIONS IN PSYCHOPHYSIOLOGICAL STUDIES OF CATECHOLAMINES
Availability in Blood, Saliva, and Urine

All catecholamines in bodily fluids are found in the unbound state. At rest, epinephrine can range from 30–100 pg/ml in arterial plasma (antecubital venous plasma being 50% of this), while norepinephrine can vary from 150–500 pg/ml (Esler et al. 1990). They are found in blood or urine unchanged or as metabolites. Catecholamines also appear in the saliva.

Secretion and Clearance

The catecholamines are degraded by monoamine oxidase throughout the body and by catechol-o-methyltransferase, which is abundant in brain, liver, and kidney. They and their metabolites are excreted through saliva or urine (Figure 6). Norepinephrine is released in proportion to sympathetic nerve firing, with perhaps 10%–20% overflowing into the circulation while the rest is taken up by the nerve terminals. All of the catecholamine secreted by the adrenal cortex enters the circulation. Therefore, changes in blood levels are rough indices of the changes in activity of the sympathetic nervous system over time. Steptoe (1987) suggested that catecholamines in urine are useful indicators of global sympathetic activity prevailing over the time of collection, and we agree.

Sources of Experimental Confounding

There are many factors that can alter catecholamine concentrations (for reviews see Goldstein 1984; Hart et al. 1989).

Emotionally induced catecholamine activation is difficult to estimate with certainty because many organs contribute to the circulating pool (Esler et al. 1984, 1988, 1990). Emotional responses can also act as confounds during baseline measurements. Precautions should be taken to keep conditions constant and relaxing, and sufficient time (usually 30 min) should be allotted after venipuncture to allow the initial response to dissipate prior to taking a baseline sample. Posture and movement can also be significant confounds at this time. The circulation half-life of catecholamines is on the order of minutes, further necessitating fast and efficient sampling technique during the study proper.

As in the case of cortisol, catecholamines have seasonal variations that call for appropriate attention according to the study design (Malarkey et al. 1995b). A special mention should be given regarding the influence of drugs and foods on plasma catecholamine levels. Any medications affecting the heart or blood pressure (e.g., vasodilators or diuretics) can have either direct or indirect effects on catecholamine levels. Commonly consumed drugs such as caffeine, nicotine, or alcohol can increase norepinephrine levels. In addition, dihydrocaffeic acid, a noncaffeine constituent of both caffeinated and decaffeinated coffee, can give a false reading during HPLC assay detection (see the section on assay techniques), so these common beverages should not be ingested for 18 hours before blood sampling (Goldstein 1984). Diet also influences norepinephrine levels, with carbohydrate ingestion increasing nerve firing rates (Macdonald & Webber 1993).

Collection and Quantification in Saliva

Collection of saliva for measurement of catecholamines is not recommended at this time. One study tested whether salivary catecholamine levels are affected by changes in peripheral sympathetic nervous system activity. Despite having subjects perform strenuous physical activity, which resulted in a large increase in plasma catecholamines, no change was registered in comparable salivary samples (Schwab, Heubel, & Bartels 1992). Therefore, for documentation of transitory changes in sympathetic activity, plasma is still the best specimen source. Urine is most useful for time-integrated sampling.

Collection and Quantification in Blood

Catecholamines in psychophysiological research are most commonly derived from plasma extracted from blood sampled by simple venipuncture or by indwelling catheter, although the latter is recommended. Careful studies of norepinephrine concentrations have shown that no single peripheral site is fully representative of the mean level of norepinephrine in the central circulation. For example, increased blood flow to the sampling site could reduce concentrations, washing out an effect, while decreased flow could elevate regional values. Arterial and venous levels of norepinephrine and epinephrine from a given area (e.g. forearm) can be quite different, although they show a high correlation at rest ($r \geq 0.96$; Renard et al. 1987). In addition, catecholamines have a circadian rhythm, increasing slightly during the day. For these reasons, repeated sampling and relatively large sample sizes may be necessary to reliably detect trends (Ziegler 1989).

A useful technique for minimizing catecholamine concentration differences between arterial and venous blood is to enhance flow through the tissues of the extremity being sampled. For example, if blood is being taken from a forearm vein, it is possible to create an arterialized sample source by gently warming the hand and forearm with a heating pad to fully dilate the resistance vessels. This will provide a peripheral venous source more closely representative of arterial blood (see McCann et al. 1993).

Although some investigators measure catecholamines using a radioenzymatic assay procedure, HPLC is by far the most frequently used assay technique. However, HPLC requires rather large sample volumes (≥ 1 ml plasma or approximately 2 ml whole blood). Another consideration is contamination. As mentioned, caffeinated and decaffeinated coffee can give false readings in HPLC assays. In addition, contaminants can come from any of the blood collection apparatus, sample tubes, syringes, reagents, or the HPLC equipment. Goldstein (1984) gave a nice summary of proper controls and checks for possible sample contamination.

Collection and Quantification in Urine

Catecholamines and their metabolites can also be measured from urine. Urinary measures show good reliability from day to day when adequate samples are obtained (Curtin, Walker, & Schulz 1996), the concentrations are higher than in plasma, and infusion studies have shown them to mirror blood levels accurately (Moleman et al. 1992). Sampling is rarely for less than 6-hr periods, but shorter intervals of 75 min have been used successfully (Forsman 1981). One important consideration is that, since kidney is a major site of norepinephrine production, urinary levels may partially reflect local production and so

potentially mask more subtle general systemic changes (Ziegler 1989). Other design considerations are the same as for blood sampling. Quantification is the same as for plasma samples.

Handling and Storage

Handling and storage of biological samples for catecholamine quantification are moderately difficult, and there are wide variations in the recommended procedures. The best course of action for the researcher is to collaborate with a reliable laboratory and adhere to their guidelines. However, several excellent articles review such considerations as the use of buffered solutions, storage temperature, and degradation rate (Brent, Hall, & Henry 1985; Goldstein 1984; Pettersson, Hussi, & Janne 1980; Weir et al. 1986; Ziegler 1989).

UNITS OF MEASURE

The Systéme Internationale (SI) unit for biochemical concentrations is mol/l (the molecular weight of a substance in mg/l), usually expressed simply as mol. In practice, however, values are frequently reported in earlier metric units, such as μg/dl (or μg/100ml) in blood, mg/l in urine, and ng/ml in saliva. The SI units can be converted to metric and vice versa using appropriate factors (based on molecular weights) and attending to the units of concentration in question. For example: The molecular weight of cortisol is 362.5 g/mol, the metric–SI conversion factor is 0.3625, and the SI–metric conversion factor is $1/0.3625 = 2.759$; hence nmol $\times$ 0.3625 = ng/ml and μg/dl $\times$ 2.759 = nmol. In the case of epinephrine, the molecular weight is 183.2, the metric–SI conversion factor is 0.1832, and the SI–metric conversion factor is $1/0.1832 = 54.58$. Norepinephrine has a molecular weight of 169.18; its metric–SI conversion factor is 0.1692 and its SI–metric conversion factor is 59.10.

ASSAY TECHNIQUES

Because these techniques may require specialized equipment, licensure for the handling of radioactive material, and extensive experience, it is recommended that the researcher collaborate with a proficient laboratory and follow their recommendations for sample handling and storage. However, it is worthwhile to have a basic understanding of the various techniques available.

Radioimmunoassay (RIA)

These assays are based on the binding of an antibody to the compound being measured. To measure cortisol levels in your sample, a known amount of highly specific antibody and radioactively labeled cortisol is added to a standard amount of sample. The cortisol in the specimen and the radioactively labeled cortisol compete for binding sites on the antibody. The portion of the mixture that is bound to the antibody is then separated out, and cortisol can be quantified by measuring the radioactivity with a gamma counter. Thus you will end up with a negative correlation between amount of radioactivity remaining and level of endogenous cortisol present in your sample. It is useful to incorporate all samples from a single subject in a single batch for processing and to use kits from the same manufacturer for the duration of a study.

High-Performance Liquid Chromatography (HPLC)

In HPLC, the sample is mixed with a "carrier" that allows the chemical constituents of the sample to separate under high pressure. Each constituent moves at a known rate through a separator "column" within the HPLC unit (based on empirical standards), and the quantity present is converted into a graph. This technique is generally considered to have good specificity and reliability, but it can be prohibitively expensive for certain compounds (e.g. cortisol) and is known to be extremely demanding of quality control, requiring extensive training and expertise.

Other Assay Techniques

Other techniques are available, but the two just listed are those most frequently cited and thus most widely accepted and standardized. Other techniques have been used with some success. For example, the enzyme-linked immunosorbent assay (ELISA) involves incubating a sample on a microtiter plate with antibody. A second antibody linked to peroxidase allows the development of color, the amount of which is inversely proportional to the amount of cortisol present. Since it does not require the use of any radioactive reagent, it is safer and more economical to use than RIAs. However, it requires a type of spectrophotometer not widely in use and does not yet have the sensitivity of an RIA (Kuhn 1989).

Fluorescence polarization immunoassay (FPIA) technology using a proprietary TDxFLx System (Abbott) is also becoming more common. This method combines competitive binding immunoassay methodology similar to the RIA with fluorescence polarization technology, thus also eliminating the necessity of radioactive labeling. Instead, a fluorophore tracer attached to a large antibody molecule binds to the cortisol. Polarized light is rapidly switched on and off, causing selective fluorescence of the antibody-bound cortisol; this allows it to be quantified by measurement of the specific wavelength of light emitted.

Discussion

Our understanding of the endocrine component of the stress response has passed through three major stages: fixed reflex (Selye), modification with experience (Mason), and cognitive interaction. Cortisol has pervasive effects on every system in the body, notably the CNS and particularly limbic and cognitive areas. Since glucocorticoids pass the blood–brain barrier, high levels during states of stress or other conditions of excess may exert profound long-term effects on humans. Epinephrine, acting on peripheral receptors, may enhance memory formation. These findings suggest that the study of cortisol and epinephrine forms a perfect synthesis of two major branches of psychophysiology: the study of psychological interactions with bodily responses and the study of physical processes related to cognition.

The recent findings of altered memory performance with acute rises in cortisol and of structural effects on the hippocampus in long-term glucocorticoid exposure suggest that psychophysiologists should engage in intensive efforts to examine mechanisms associated with alterations in emotional and cognitive processes. The development of increasingly powerful tools for noninvasive measurement allows a wide range of potential brain studies to be undertaken that will reflect the acute and long-term impact of cortisol on emotional and cognitive processes.

Although the catecholamines do not pass the blood–brain barrier, they exert significant peripheral effects. Epinephrine may act indirectly on memory, as noted. More generally, catecholamine secretion may have important effects on health by altering dispositions for cardiovascular diseases, obesity, and diabetes. The study of stress catecholamine secretion is therefore of importance in the fields of psychophysiology and health psychology.

Future work may profitably concentrate on both methodological and conceptual issues. These include: (1) developing reliable, standardized psychological challenges capable of increasing endogenous cortisol production; (2) establishing standards concerning frequency and forms of sampling; (3) developing a base of information on gender and age differences in reactivity; (4) undertaking extensive cognitive research on relevant clinical groups; and (5) exploring the interactions of catecholamines and cortisol in altering cognitive processes.

NOTES

Supported by Grant HL-32050 from the National Heart, Lung, and Blood Institute (Bethesda, MD), the John D. and Catherine T. MacArthur Foundation, and the Medical Research Service of the Department of Veterans Affairs.

The authors thank Dr. Paul J. Mills and the editors for their generous discussions and review of earlier drafts of this chapter, Mireille L'Hermite-Balriaux for discussing hormonal laboratory methods, and Tony Buchanan for his research on the cognitive effects of epinephrine.

REFERENCES

Aardal, E., & Holm, A.-C. (1995). Cortisol in saliva – reference ranges and relation to cortisol in serum. *Eur. J. Clin. Chem. Clin. Biochem., 33,* 927–32.

al'Absi, M., Bongard, S., Buchanan, T., Pincomb, G. A., Licinio, J., & Lovallo, W. R. (1997). Cardiovascular and neuroendocrine adjustment to public speaking and mental arithmetic stressors. *Psychophysiology, 34, 266–75.*

al'Absi, M., & Lovallo, W. R. (1993). Cortisol concentrations of borderline hypertensive men exposed to a novel experimental setting. *Psychoneuroendocrinology, 18, 355–63.*

al'Absi, M., Hugdahl, K., & Lovallo, W. R. (1998). Adrenocortical stress responses in relation to cognitive performance and hemisphere asymmetry. *Psychophysiology, 35 (Suppl.),* S15.

al'Absi, M., Lovallo, W. R., McKey, B. S., & Pincomb, G. A. (1994). Borderline hypertensives produce exaggerated adrenocortical responses to mental stress. *Psychosom. Med., 56,* 245–50.

Amaral, D. G., Price, J. L., Pitkänen, A., & Carmichael, S. T. (1992). Anatomical organization of the primate amygdaloid complex. In J. P. Aggleton (Ed.), *The Amygdala: Neurobiological Aspects of Emotion, Memory, and Mental Dysfunction,* pp. 1–66. New York: Wiley-Liss.

Arriza, J. L., Weinberger, C., Cerelli, G., Glaser, T. M., Handelin, B. L., Housman, D. E., & Evans, R. M. (1987). Cloning of human mineralocorticoid receptor complimentary DNA: Structural and functional kinship with the glucocorticoid receptor. *Science, 237, 268–75.*

Aston-Jones, G., Ennis, M., Pieribone, R. A., Nickell, W. T., & Shipley, M. T. (1986). The brainstem nucleus locus coeruleus: Restricted afferent control of a broad efferent network. *Science, 234, 734–7.*

Averill, J. R. (1973). Personal control over aversive stimuli and its relation to stress. *Psychol. Bull., 80, 286–303.*

Bechara, A., Damasio, H., Tranel, D., & Damasio, A. R. (1997). Deciding advantageously before knowing the advantageous strategy. *Science, 275, 1293–4.*

Berger, M., Bossert, S., Krieg, J., Dirlich, G., Ettmeier, W., Schreiber, W., and von Zerssen, D. (1987). Interindividual differences in the susceptibility of the cortisol system: An important factor for the degree of hypercortisolism in stress situations? *Biol. Psychiatry, 22, 1327–39.*

Bernard, C. (1961). *An Introduction to the Study of Experimental Medicine* (H. C. Greene, Trans.). New York: Collier. [Original work published in 1865.]

Berridge, C. W., & Dunn, A. J. (1989). Restraint-stress-induced changes in exploratory behavior appear to be mediated by norepinephrine-stimulated release of CRF. *J. Neurosci., 9,* 3513–21.

Björntorp, P. (1996). Behavior and metabolic disease. *Int. J. Behav. Med., 3, 285–302.*

Blombery, P. A., & Heinzow, B. G. J. (1983). Cardiac and pulmonary norepinephrine release and removal in the dog. *Circ. Res., 53, 688–94.*

Bouille, C., & Bayle, J. C. (1973). Effects of limbic stimulation or lesions on basal and stress-induced hypothalamic-pituitary-adrenocortical activity in the pigeon. *Neuroendocrinology, 13,* 264–77.

Brandtstadter, J., Baltes Gotz, B., Kirschbaum, C., & Hellhammer, D. (1991). Developmental and personality correlates of adrenocortical activity as indexed by salivary cortisol: Observations in the age range of 35 to 65 years. *J. Psychosom. Res., 35, 173–85.*

Brantley, P. J., Dietz, L. S., McKnight, G. T., Jones, G. N., & Tulley, R. (1988). Convergence between the Daily Stress Inventory and endocrine measures of stress. *J. Consult. Clin. Psychol., 56, 549–51.*

Bremner, J. D., Randall, P., Scott, T. M., Bronen, R. A., Seibyl, J. P., Southwick, S. M., Delaney, R. C., McCarthy, G., Charney, D. S., & Innis, R. S. (1995a). MRI-based measurement of hippocampal volume in patients with combat-related posttraumatic stress disorder. *Am. J. Psychiatry, 152, 973–81.*

Bremner, J. D., Randall, P., Scott, T. M., Capelli, S., Delaney, R., McCarthy, G., & Charney, D. S. (1995b). Deficits in short-term memory in adult survivors of childhood abuse. *Psychiatry Res., 59, 97–107.*

Bremner, J. D., Scott, T. M., Delaney, R. C., Southwick, S. M., Mason, J. W., Johnson, D. R., Innis, R. B., McCarthy, G., & Charney, D. S. (1993). Deficits in short-term memory in posttraumatic stress disorder. *Am. J. Psychiatry, 150, 1015–19.*

Brent, P. J., Hall, S., & Henry, D. A. (1985). Stability of norepinephrine in blood. *Clin. Chem., 31, 659–60.*

Brien, T. G. (1975). Cortisol metabolism after oral contraceptives: Total plasma cortisol and the free cortisol index. *Br. J. Obstet. Gynaecol., 82, 987–91.*

Brown, M. R., Fisher, L. A., Spiess, J., Rivier, C., Rivier, J., & Vale, W. (1982). Corticotropin releasing factor: Actions on the sympathetic nervous system and metabolism. *Endocrinology, 111, 928–31.*

Buchanan, T. W., al'Absi, M., & Lovallo, W. R. (1999). Cortisol fluctuates with increases and decreases in negative affect. *Psychoneuroendocrinology, 24, 227–41.*

Cahill, L., Prins, B., Weber, M., & McGaugh, J. L. (1994). Beta-adrenergic activation and memory for emotional events. *Nature, 371, 702–4.*

Cake, M. H., & Litwack, G. (1975). The glucocorticoid receptor. *Biochem. Actions Horm., 3, 319–90.*

Cannon, W. B. (1928). The mechanism of emotional disturbance of bodily functions. *N. Engl. J. Med., 198, 165–72.*

Cannon, W. B. (1929). *Bodily Changes in Pain, Hunger, Fear, and Rage,* 2nd ed. New York: Appleton.

Choi, P. Y. L., & Salmon, P. (1995). Stress responsivity in exercisers and non-exercisers during different phases of the menstrual cycle. *Soc. Sci. Med., 41, 769–77.*

Curtin, F., Walker, J.-P., & Schulz, P. (1996). Day-to-day intraindividual reliability and interindividual differences in monoamines excretion. *J. Affective Disord., 38, 173–8.*

Curtis, A. L., Drolet, G., & Valentino, R. J. (1993). Hemodynamic stress activates locus ceruleus neurons of unanesthetized rats. *Brain Res. Bull., 31, 737–44.*

Dallman, M. F., Akana, S. F., Cascio, C. S., Darlington, D. N., Jacobson, L., & Levin, N. (1987). Regulation of ACTH secretion: Variations on a theme of B. *Recent Prog. Horm. Res., 43, 113–73.*

Damasio, A. R. (1994). *Descartes' Error: Emotion, Reason, and the Human Brain.* New York: Putnam.

Davies, A. O., & Lefkowitz, R. J. (1984). Regulation of β-adrenergic receptors by steroid hormones. *Ann. Rev. Physiol., 46, 119–30.*

Davis, M. (1992). The role of the amygdala in conditioned fear. In J. P. Aggleton (Ed.), *The Amygdala: Neurobiological Aspects of Emotion, Memory, and Mental Dysfunction,* pp. 255–305. New York: Wiley-Liss.

DeChamplain, J., Genest, J., Veyrat, R., & Boucher, R. (1966). Factors controlling renin in man. *Arch. Intern. Med., 117,* 355–63.

DeLeon, M. J., McRae, T., Tsai, J., George, A., Marcus, D., Freedman, M., Wolf, A., & McEwen, B. (1988). Abnormal cortisol response in Alzheimer's disease linked to hippocampal atrophy. *Lancet, 2,* 391–2.

De Souza, E. B., & Kuhar, M. J. (1986). Corticotropin-releasing factor receptors in the pituitary gland and central nervous system. *Methods Enzymol., 124,* 560–90.

Dimsdale, J. E., & Moss, J. (1980). Short-term catecholamine response to psychological stress. *Psychosom. Med., 42,* 493–7.

DuPont, A., Bastarache, E., Endroczi, E., & Fortier, C. (1972). Effect of hippocampal stimulation on the plasma thyrotropin (THS) and corticosterone responses to acute cold exposure in the rat. *Can. J. Physiol. Pharmacol., 50,* 364–77.

Ellertsen, B., Johnsen, T. B., & Ursin, H. (1978). Relationship between the hormonal responses to activation and coping. In H. Ursin, E. Baade, & S. Levine (Eds.), *Psychobiology of Stress: A Study of Coping Men,* pp. 243–8. New York: Academic Press.

Esler, M. D., Hasking, G. J., Willett, I. R., Leonard, P. W., & Jennings, G. L. (1985). Noradrenaline release and sympathetic nervous system activity. *J. Hypertens., 3,* 117–29.

Esler, M., Jennings, G., Korner, P., Willett, I., Dudley, F., Hasking, G., Anderson, W., & Lambert, G. (1988). Assessment of human sympathetic nervous system activity from measurements of norepinephrine turnover. *Hypertension, 11,* 3–20.

Esler, M., Jennings, G., Lambert, G., Meredith, I., Horne, M., & Eisenhofer, G. (1990). Overflow of catecholamine neurotransmitters to the circulation: Source, fate, and functions. *Physiol. Rev., 70,* 963–85.

Esler, M., Jennings, G., Leonard, P., Sacharias, N., Burke, F., Johns, J., & Blombery, P. (1984). Contribution of individual organs to total noradrenaline release in humans. *Acta Physiol. Scand., 527 (Suppl.),* 11–16.

Feldman, S., Conforti, N., & Weidenfeld, J. (1995). Limbic pathways and hypothalamic neurotransmitters mediating adrenocortical responses to neural stimuli. *Neurosci. Biobehav. Rev., 19,* 235–40.

File, S. E., Vellucci, S. V., & Wendlandt, S. (1979). Corticosterone – An anxiogenic or anxiolytic agent? *J. Pharm. Pharmacol., 31,* 300–5.

Folkow, B. (1993). Physiological organization of neurohormonal responses to psychosocial stimuli: Implications for health and disease. *Ann. Behav. Med., 15,* 236–44.

Follenius, M., Brandenberger, G., Bandesapt, J. J., Libert, J. P., & Ehrhart, J. (1992). Nocturnal cortisol release in relation to sleep structure. *Sleep, 15,* 21–7.

Forsman, L. (1981). Note on estimating catecholamines in urine sampled after 75 minutes of mental work and inactivity. *J. Psychosom. Res., 25,* 223–5.

Francis, K. T. (1979). Psychologic correlates of serum indicators of stress in man: A longitudinal study. *Psychosom. Med., 41,* 617–28.

Frankenhaeuser, M. (1980). Psychobiological aspects of life stress. In S. Levine & H. Ursin (Eds.), *Coping and Health,* pp. 203–23. New York: Plenum.

Frankenhaeuser, M., Lundberg, U., & Chesney, M. (1991). *Women, Work and Health: Stress and Opportunities.* New York: Plenum.

Frankenhaeuser, M., Rauste-von Wright, M., Collins, A., von Wright, J., Sedvall, G., & Swahn, C.-G. (1978). Sex differences in psychoneuroendocrine reactions to examination stress. *Psychosom. Med., 40,* 334–43.

Frankenhaeuser, M., & Rissler, A. (1970). Effects of punishment on catecholamine release and efficiency of performance. *Psychopharmacologia, 17,* 378–90.

Goldstein, D. S. (1984). Sample handling and preparation for liquid chromatography and electrochemical assays for plasma catecholamines. In A. M. Krstulovic (Ed.), *Quantitative Analysis of Catecholamines and Related Compounds,* pp. 126–36. New York: Wiley.

Goldstein, D. S., Dionne, R., Sweet, J., Gracely, R., Brewer, B., Gregg, R., & Keiser, H. R. (1982). Circulatory, plasma catecholamine, cortisol, lipid, and psychological responses to a real-life stress (third molar extractions): Effects of diazepam sedation and of inclusion of epinephrine with the local anesthetic. *Psychosom. Med., 44,* 259–72.

Guillemin, R., Vargo, T., Rossier, J., Minick, S., Ling, N., Rivier, C., Vale, W., & Bloom, F. (1977). Beta-endorphin and adrenocorticotropin are secreted concomitantly by the pituitary gland. *Science, 197,* 1367–9.

Halgren, E. (1992). Emotional neurophysiology of the amygdala within the context of human cognition. In J. P. Aggleton (Ed.), *The Amygdala: Neurobiological Aspects of Emotion, Memory, and Mental Dysfunction,* pp. 191–228. New York: Wiley-Liss.

Haourigui, M., Sakr, S., Martin, M. E., Thobie, N., Girard-Globa, A., Benassayag, C., & Nunez, E. A. (1995). Postprandial free fatty acids stimulate activity of human corticosteroid binding globulin. *Am. J. Physiol., 269,* E1067–E1075.

Hart, B. B., Stanford, G. G., Ziegler, M. G., Lake, C. R., & Chernow, B. (1989). Catecholamines: Study of interspecies variation. *Crit. Care Med., 17,* 1203–22.

Henry, J. P., & Stephens, P. M. (1977). *Stress, Health and the Social Environment: A Sociobiological Approach to Medicine.* New York: Springer.

Hilton, S. M. (1982). The defence-arousal system and its relevance for circulatory and respiratory control. *J. Exp. Biol., 100,* 159–74.

Irwin, M., Hauger, R. L., Brown, M., & Britton, K. T. (1988). CRF activates autonomic nervous system and reduces natural killer cytotoxicity. *Am. J. Physiol., 255,* R744–R747.

Jacobson, L., & Sapolsky, R. (1991). The role of the hippocampus in feedback regulation of the hypothalamic-pituitary-adrenocortical axis. *Endocr. Rev., 12,* 118–34.

Joëls, M., & De Kloet, E. R. (1989). Effects of glucocorticoids and norepinephrine on the excitability in the hippocampus. *Science, 245,* 1502–5.

Johansson, G., & Post, B. (1974). Catecholamine output of males and females over a one-year period. *Acta Physiol. Scand., 92,* 557–65.

Kiecolt-Glaser, J. K., Newton, T., Cacioppo, J. T., MacCallum, R. C., Glaser, R., & Malarkey, W. B. (1996). Marital conflict and endocrine function: Are men really more physiologically affected than women? *J. Consult. Clin. Psychol., 64,* 324–32.

Kirschbaum, C., & Hellhammer, D. H. (1989). Salivary cortisol in psychobiological research: An overview. *Neuropsychobiology, 22,* 150–69.

Kirschbaum, C., Klauer, T., Filipp, S.-H., & Hellhammer, D. H. (1995a). Sex-specific effects of social support on cortisol and subjective responses to acute psychological stress. *Psychosom. Med., 57,* 23–31.

Kirschbaum, C., Pirke, K.-M., & Hellhammer, D. H. (1993). The "Trier Social Stress Test" – A tool for investigating psychobiological stress responses in a laboratory setting. *Neuropsychobiology, 2,* 76–81.

Kirschbaum, C., Pirke, K.-M., & Hellhammer, D. H. (1995b). Preliminary evidence for reduced cortisol responsivity to psychological stress in women using oral contraceptive medication. *Psychoneuroendocrinol., 20,* 509–14.

Kirschbaum, C., Strasburger, C. J., Jammers, W., & Hellhammer, D. H. (1989). Cortisol and behavior: 1. Adaptation of a radioimmunoassay kit for reliable and inexpensive salivary cortisol determination. *Pharmacol. Biochem. Behav., 34,* 747–51.

Kirschbaum, C., Wolf, O. T., May, M., Wippich, W., & Hellhammer, D. (1996). Stress- and treatment-induced elevations of cortisol levels associated with impaired declarative memory in healthy adults. *Life Sci., 58,* 1475–83.

Kirschbaum, C., Wust, S., Faig, H.-G., & Hellhammer, D. (1992a). Heritability of cortisol responses to human corticotropin-releasing hormone, ergometry, and psychological stress in humans. *J. Clin. Endocrinol. Metab., 75,* 1526–30.

Kirschbaum, C., Wust, S., & Hellhammer, D. (1992b). Consistent sex differences in cortisol responses to psychological stress. *Psychosom. Med., 54,* 648–57.

Kirschbaum, C., Wust, S., & Strasburger, C. J. (1992c). "Normal" cigarette smoking increases free cortisol in habitual smokers. *Life Sci., 50,* 435–42.

Kovacs, G. L., Fekete, M., Szabó, G., & Telegdy, G. (1987). Action of ACTH-corticosteroid axis on the central nervous system. *Front. Horm. Res., 15,* 79–127.

Kuhn, C. (1989). Adrenocortical and gonadal steroids in behavioral cardiovascular medicine. In N. Schneiderman, S. M. Weiss, & P. G. Kaufman (Eds.), *Handbook of Research Methods in Cardiovascular Behavioral Medicine,* pp. 185–204. New York: Plenum.

Lamb, E. J., Noonan, K. A., & Burrin, J. M. (1994). Urine-free cortisol excretion: Evidence of sex-dependence. *Ann. Clin. Biochem., 31,* 455–8.

Landon, J., Smith, D. S., Perry, L. A., & Al-Ansari, A. A. K. (1984). The assay of salivary cortisol. In G. F. Read, D. Riad-Fahmy, R. F. Walker, & K. Griffiths (Eds.), *Immunoassays of Steroids in Saliva,* pp. 300–7. Cardiff, Wales: Alpha Omega.

Lazarus, R. S., Deese, J., & Osler, S. F. (1952). The effects of psychological stress upon performance. *Psychol. Bull., 49,* 293–317.

Lazarus, R. S., & Folkman, S. (1984). *Stress, Appraisal and Coping.* New York: Springer.

Lee, Y., Schulkin, J., & Davis, M. (1994). Effect of corticosterone on the enhancement of the acoustic startle reflex by corticotropin releasing factor (CRF). *Brain Res., 666,* 93–8.

Liang, K. C., Juler, R. G., & McGaugh, J. L. (1986). Modulating effects of posttraining epinephrine on memory: Involve-

ment of the amygdala norepinephrine system. *Brain Res., 368,* 125–33.

Liang, K. C., Melia, K. R., Miserendino, M. J. D., Falls, W. A., Campeau, S., & Davis, M. (1992). Corticotropin-releasing factor: Long lasting facilitation of the acoustic startle reflex. *J. Neurosci., 12,* 2303–12.

Lovallo, W. R. (1997). *Stress and Health: Biological and Psychological Interactions.* Thousand Oaks, CA: Sage.

Lovallo, W. R., Pincomb, G. A., Brackett, D. J., & Wilson, M. F. (1990). Heart rate reactivity as a predictor of neuroendocrine responses to aversive and appetitive challenges. *Psychosom. Med., 52,* 17–26.

Lovallo, W. R., Pincomb, G. A., Edwards, G. L., Brackett, D. J., & Wilson, M. F. (1986a). Work pressure and the Type A behavior pattern: Exam stress in male medical students. *Psychosom. Med., 48,* 125–33.

Lovallo, W. R., Pincomb, G. A., & Wilson, M. F. (1986b). Heart rate reactivity and Type A behavior as modifiers of physiological response to active and passive coping. *Psychophysiology, 23,* 105–12.

Lovallo, W. R., Pincomb, G. A., & Wilson, M. F. (1986c). Predicting response to a reaction time task: Heart rate reactivity compared with Type A behavior. *Psychophysiology, 23,* 648–56.

Lovallo, W. R., Wilson, M. F., Pincomb, G. A., Edwards, G. L., Tompkins, P., & Brackett, D. (1985). Activation patterns to aversive stimulation in man: Passive exposure versus effort to control. *Psychophysiology, 22,* 283–91.

Lundberg, U., & Frankenhaeuser, M. (1980). Pituitary-adrenal and sympathetic-adrenal correlates of distress and effort. *J. Psychosom. Res., 24,* 125–30.

Lupien, S., DeLeon, M., DeSanti, S., Convit, A., Tasshish, C., Nair, N. P., Thakur, M., McEwen, B. S., Hauger, R. L., & Meaney, M. J. (1998). Cortisol levels during human aging predict hippocampal atrophy and memory deficits. *Nature Neuroscience, 1,* 69–73.

Lupien, S., Ngô, T., Rainville, C., Nair, N. P. Y., Hauger, U. L., & Meaney, M. J. (1995). Spatial memory as measured by a human maze in aged subjects showing various patterns of cortisol secretion and memory function. *Soc. Neurosci. Abst., 21,* 1709.

Macdonald, I. A., & Webber, J. (1993). Catecholamine-induced thermogenesis: Effects of diet composition and nutritional status. *Internatl. J. Obesity, 17 (Suppl. 3),* S63–S67.

Makin, H. L. J. (1996). Origins of the sex difference in human urinary free cortisol excretion [Comment]. *Ann. Clin. Biochem., 33,* 471–2.

Malarkey, W. B., Lipkus, W. B., & Cacioppo, J. T. (1995a). The dissociation of catecholamine and hypothalamic-pituitary-adrenal responses to daily stressors using dexamethasone. *J. Clin. Endocrinol. Metab., 80,* 2458–63.

Malarkey, W. B., Pearl, D. K., Demers, L. M., Kiecolt-Glaser, J. K., & Glaser, R. (1995b). Influence of academic stress and season on 24-hour mean concentrations of ACTH, cortisol, and β-endorphin. *Psychoneuroendocrinology, 20,* 499–508.

Martignoni, E., Costa, A., Sinforiani, D., Liuzzi, A., Chiodini P., Mauri, M., Bono, G., & Nappi, G. (1992). The brain as a target for adrenocortical steroids: Cognitive implications. *Psychoneuroendocrinology, 17,* 343–54.

Martin, C. R. (1985). *Endocrine Physiology.* Oxford University Press.

Mason, J. W. (1968). Organization of psychoendocrine mechanisms. *Psychosom. Med., 30*, 791–808.

McCann, B. S., Carter, J., Vaughan, M., Raskind, M., Wilkinson, C. W., & Veith, R. C. (1993). Cardiovascular and neuroendocrine responses to extended laboratory challenge. *Psychosom. Med., 55*, 497–504.

McCubbin, J. A., Kaufmann, P. G., & Nemeroff, C. B. (Eds.) (1993). *Stress, Neuropeptides, and Systemic Disease.* New York: Academic Press.

McEwen, B. S. (1997). Atrophy of the human hippocampus. *Mol. Psychiatry, 2*, 255–62.

McEwen, B. S., & Sapolsky, R. M. (1995). Stress and cognitive function. *Curr. Opinion Neurobiol., 5*, 205–16.

McEwen, B. S., Weiss, J. M., & Schwartz, L. S. (1968). Selective retention of corticosterone by limbic structures in rat brain. *Nature, 220*, 911–12.

McGaugh, J. L. (1983). Hormonal influences on memory. *Ann. Rev. Psychol., 34*, 13508–14.

McGaugh, J. L. (1989). Involvement of hormonal and neuromodulatory systems in the regulation of memory storage. *Ann. Rev. Neurosci., 12*, 255–87.

McGaugh, J. L., & Cahill, L. (1997). Interaction of neuromodulatory systems in modulating memory storage. *Behav. Brain Res., 83*, 31–8.

Meaney, M. J., O'Donnell, D., Rowe, W., Tannenbaum, B., Steverman, A., Walker, M., Nair, N. P., & Lupien, S. (1995). Individual differences in hypothalamic-pituitary-adrenal activity in later life and hippocampal aging. *Exp. Gerontol., 30*, 229–51.

Melia, K. R., Ryabinin, A. E., Schroeder, R., Bloom, F. E., & Wilson, M. C. (1994). Induction and habituation of immediate early gene expression in rat brain by acute and repeated restraint stress. *J. Neurosci., 14*, 5929–38.

Mendel, C. (1989). The free hormone hypothesis: A physiologically based mathematical model. *Endocrinol. Rev., 10*, 232–74.

Merchenthaler, I. (1984). Corticotropin-releasing factor (CRF)-like immunoreactivity in the rat central nervous system: Extrahypothalamic distribution. *Peptides, 5 (Suppl. 1)*, 53–69.

Meyerhoff, J. L., Oleshansky, M. A., & Mougey, E. H. (1988). Psychologic stress increases plasma levels of prolactin, cortisol, and POMC-derived peptides in man. *Psychosom. Med., 50*, 295–303.

Moberg, G. P., Scapagnini, U., DeGroot, J., & Ganong, W. F. (1971). Effect of sectioning the fornix on diurnal fluctuation in plasma corticosterone levels in the rat. *Neuroendocrinology, 7*, 11–15.

Moleman, P., Tulen, J. H. M., Blankestijn, P. J., Man in 't Veld, A. J., & Boomsma, F. (1992). Urinary excretion of catecholamines and their metabolites in relation to circulating catecholamines. *Arch. Gen. Psychiatry, 49*, 568–72.

Moran, N. C. (1975). Adrenergic receptors. In R. O. Greep & E. B. Astwood (Eds.), *Handbook of Physiology, Section 7: Endocrinology*, vol. 6, pp. 447–72. Washington, DC: American Physiological Society.

Munck, A., Guyre, P. M., & Holbrook, N. J. (1984). Physiological functions of glucocorticoids in stress and their relation to pharmacological actions. *Endocr. Rev., 5*, 25–44.

Nahoul, K., Patricot, M.-C., Moatti, J.-P., & Revol, A. (1992). Determination of urinary cortisol with three commercial immunoassays. *J. Steroid Biochem. Mol. Biol., 43*, 573–80.

Okumura, T., Nakajima, Y., Takamatsu, T., & Matsuoka, M. (1995). Column-switching high-performance liquid chromatographic system with a laser-induced fluorimetric detector for direct, automated assay of salivary cortisol. *J. Chromatog. B: Biomed. Applications, 670*, 11–20.

Pavlides, C., Watanabe, Y., Magariños, A. M., & McEwen, B. S. (1995). Opposing roles of Type I and Type II adrenal steroid receptors in hippocampal long-term potentiation. *Neuroscience, 68*, 387–94.

Petrusz, P., & Merchenthaler, I. (1992). The corticotropin-releasing factor system. In C. B. Nemeroff (Ed.), *Neuroendocrinology*, pp. 129–83. Boca Raton, FL: CRC Press.

Pettersson, J., Hussi, E., & Janne, J. (1980). Stability of human plasma catecholamines. *Scand. J. Clin. Lab. Invest., 40*, 297–303.

Pope, M. K., & Smith, T. W. (1991). Cortisol excretion in high and low cynically hostile men. *Psychosom. Med., 53*, 386–92.

Proulx, L., Giguere, V., Lefevre, G., & Labrie, F. (1984). Interactions between catecholamines, CRF and vasopressin in the control of ACTH secretion in the rat. In E. Usdin, R. Kvetnansky, & J. Axelrod (Eds.), *Stress: The Role of Catecholamines and Other Neurotransmitters*, vol. 1, pp. 211–24. New York: Gordon & Breach.

Rao, S. C., Rainer, G., & Miller, E. K. (1997). Integration of what and where in the primate prefrontal cortex. *Science, 276*, 821–4.

Renard, M., Sterling, I., Giot, J.-M., & Bernard, R. (1987). Relevance of forearm samples for plasma catecholamine determinations. *Hypertension, 10*, 237.

Reul, J. M. H. M., & De Kloet, E. R. (1985). Two receptor systems for corticosterone in rat brain: Microdistribution and differential occupation. *Endocrinology, 117*, 2505–11.

Riad-Fahmy, D., Read, G. R., Walker, R. F., & Griffiths, K. (1982). Steroids in saliva for assessing endocrine functions. *Endocr. Rev., 3*, 367–95.

Richardson Morton, K. D., Van de Kar, L. D., Brownfield, M. S., Lorens, S. A., Napier, T. C., & Urban, J. H. (1990). Stress-induced renin and corticosterone secretion is mediated by catecholaminergic nerve terminals in the hypothalamic paraventricular nucleus. *Neuroendocrinology, 51*, 320–7.

Rivier, C., & Vale, W. (1984). Influence of corticotropin-releasing factor on reproductive function in the rat. *J. Endocrinol., 114*, 2409–11.

Rivier, C., & Vale, W. (1985). Effects of corticotropin-releasing factor, neurohypophyseal peptides, and catecholamines on pituitary function. *Proc. Fed. Exp. Biol. Med., 44*, 189–95.

Rodriguez de Fonseca, F., Carrera, M. R. A., Navarro, M., Koob, G. F., & Weiss, F. (1997). Activation of corticotropin-releasing factor in the limbic system during cannabinoid withdrawal. *Science, 276*, 2050–4.

Rolls, E. T. (1992). Neurophysiology and functions of the primate amygdala. In J. P. Aggleton (Ed.), *The Amygdala: Neurobiological Aspects of Emotion, Memory, and Mental Dysfunction*, pp. 143–65. New York: Wiley-Liss.

Rose, R. M., Poe, R. O., & Mason, J. W. (1967). Observations on the relationship between psychological state, 17-OHCS excretion, and epinephrine, norepinephrine, insulin, BEI, estrogen and androgen levels during basic training. *Psychosom. Med., 29*, 544–54.

Rubinow, D., Post, R., Savard, R., & Gold, P. (1984). Cortisol hypersecretion and cognitive impairment in depression. *Arch. Gen. Psychiatry, 41,* 279–83.

Russell, J. A., & Wilhelmi, A. E. (1954). Physiology of the adrenal cortex. In F. D. W. Lukens (Ed.), *Medical Uses of Cortisone,* pp. 1–45. New York: Blakiston.

Saab, P. G. (1989). Cardiovascular and neuroendocrine responses to challenge in males and females. In N. Schneiderman, S. M. Weiss, & P. G. Kaufman (Eds.), *Handbook of Research Methods in Cardiovascular Behavioral Medicine,* pp. 453–81. New York: Plenum.

Saab, P. G, Matthews, K. A., Stoney, C. M., & McDonald, R. H. (1989). Premenopausal and postmenopausal women differ in their cardiovascular and neuroendocrine responses to behavioral stressors. *Psychophysiology, 26,* 270–80.

Sapolsky, R. M., Krey, L. C., & McEwen, B. S. (1986). The neuroendocrinology of stress and aging: The glucocorticoid cascade hypothesis. *Endocr. Rev., 7,* 284–301.

Sausen, K. P., Lovallo, W. R., Pincomb, G. A., & Wilson, M. F. (1992). Cardiovascular responses to occupational stress in medical students: A paradigm for ambulatory monitoring studies. *Health Psychol., 11,* 55–60.

Schwab, K. O., Heubel, G., & Bartels, H. (1992). Free epinephrine, norepinephrine and dopamine in saliva and plasma of healthy adults. *Eur. J. Clin. Chem. Clin. Biochem., 30,* 541–4.

Scoville, W. B., & Milner, B. (1957). Loss of recent memory after bilateral hippocampal lesions. *J. Neurol. Neurosurg. Psychiatry, 20,* 11–21.

Seeman, T. E., & Robbins, R. J. (1994). Aging and hypothalamic-pituitary-adrenal response to challenge in humans. *Endocr. Rev., 15,* 233–60.

Selye, H. (1936). Thymus and adrenals in the response of the organism to injuries and intoxications. *Br. J. Exp. Pathol., 17,* 234–48.

Selye, H. (1956). *The Stress of Life.* New York: McGraw-Hill.

Sgoutas-Emch, S. A., Cacioppo, J. T., Uchino, B. N., Malarkey, W., Pearl, D., Kiecolt-Glaser, J. K., & Glaser, R. (1994). The effects of an acute psychological stressor on cardiovascular, endocrine, and cellular immune responses: A prospective study of individuals high and low in heart rate reactivity. *Psychophysiology, 31,* 264–71.

Sherman, J. E., & Kalin, N. (1986). I.c.v.-CRF alters stress induced freezing without affecting pain sensitivity. *Pharmacol. Biochem. Behav., 30,* 801–7.

Sloand, J. A., Hooper, M., & Izzo, J. L., Jr. (1989). Effects of circulating norepinephrine on platelet, leukocyte and red blood cell counts by α_1-adrenergic stimulation. *Am. J. Cardiol., 63,* 1140–2.

Smith, E. E., Guyton, A. C., Manning, R. D., & White, R. J. (1976). Integrated mechanisms of cardiovascular response and control during exercise in the normal human. *Prog. Cardiovasc. Dis., 28,* 421–43.

Smith, O. A., DeVito, J. L., & Astley, C. A. (1990). Neurons controlling cardiovascular responses to emotion are located in lateral hypothalamus-perifornical region. *Am. J. Physiol., 259,* R943–R954.

Smythe, J. W., Murphy, D., Timothy, C., & Costall, B. (1997). Hippocampal mineralocorticoid, but not glucocorticoid, receptors modulate anxiety-like behavior in rats. *Pharmacol. Biochem. Behav., 56,* 507–13.

Spith-Schwalbe, E., Uthgenannt, D., Voget, G., Kern, W., Born, J., & Fehm, H.-L. (1993). Corticotropin-releasing hormone-induced adrenocorticotropin and cortisol secretion depends on sleep and wakefulness. *J. Clin. Endocrinol. Metab., 77,* 1170–3.

Starkman, M. N., Gebarski, S. S., Berent, S., & Schteingart, D. E. (1992). Hippocampal formation volume, memory dysfunction, and cortisol levels in patients with Cushing's syndrome. *Biol. Psychiatry, 32,* 756–65.

Starkman, M. N., & Schteingart, D. E. (1981). Neuropsychiatric manifestations of patients with Cushing's syndrome. *Arch. Intern. Med., 141,* 215–19.

Steptoe, A. (1987). The assessment of sympathetic nervous function in human stress research. *J. Psychosom. Res., 31,* 141–52.

Stern, R. M., & Sison, C. E. E. (1990). Response patterning. In J. T. Cacioppo & L. G. Tassinary (Eds.), *Principles of Psychophysiology,* pp. 193–215. Cambridge University Press.

Strain, G. W., Zumoff, B., Strain, J. J., Levin, J., & Fukushima, D. K. (1980). Cortisol production in obesity. *Metabolism, 29,* 980–5.

Sung, B. H., Lovallo, W. R., Pincomb, G. A., & Wilson, M. F. (1990). Effects of caffeine on blood pressure response during exercise in normotensive healthy young men. *Am. J. Cardiol., 65,* 909–13.

Swanson, L. W., Sawchenko, P. E., Rivier, J., and Vale, W. (1983). Organization of ovine corticotropin-releasing factor immunoreactive cells and fibers in the rat brain: An immunohistochemical study. *Neuroendocrinology, 36,* 165–86.

Szabo, B., Hedler, L., Schurr, C., & Starke, K. (1988). ACTH increases noradrenaline release in the rabbit heart. *Naunyn Schmiedebergs Arch. Pharmacol., 338,* 365–72.

Taggart, P., Carruthers, M., & Somerville, W. (1973). Electrocardiograms, plasma catecholamines, and lipids and their modification by oxprenolol when speaking before an audience. *Lancet, 2,* 341–6.

Takahashi, L. K., Kalin, N. H., Vanden Burgt, J. A., & Sherman, J. E. (1989). Corticotropin-releasing factor modulates defensive withdrawal and exploratory behavior in rats. *Behav. Neurosci., 103,* 648–54.

Taylor, N., & Raven, P. (1996a). Origins of the sex difference in human urinary free cortisol excretion. *Ann. Clin. Biochem., 33,* 174–6.

Taylor, N., & Raven, P. (1996b). Author's reply. *Ann. Clin. Biochem., 33,* 471–2.

Tersman, Z., Collins, A., & Eneroth, P. (1991). Cardiovascular responses to psychological and physiological stressors during the menstrual cycle. *Psychosom. Med., 53,* 185–97.

Trainer, P. J., McHardy, K. C., Harvey, R. D., & Reid, I. W. (1993). Urinary free cortisol in the assessment of hydrocortisone replacement therapy. *Horm. Metab. Res., 25,* 117–20.

Tunn, S., Mollmann, H., Barth, J., Derendorf, H., & Krieg, M. (1992). Simultaneous measurement of cortisol in serum and saliva after different forms of cortisol administration. *Clin. Chem., 38,* 1491–4.

Uchino, B. N., Cacioppo, J. T., & Kiecolt-Glaser, J. K. (1996). The relationship between social support and physiological processes: A review with emphasis on underlying mechanisms and implications for health. *Psychol. Bull., 119,* 488–531.

Uchino, B. N., Cacioppo, J. T., Malarkey, W., & Glaser, R. (1995). Individual differences in cardiac sympathetic control predict endocrine and immune responses to acute psychological stress. *J. Pers. Soc. Psychol., 69,* 736–43.

Ursin, H., Baade, E., & Levine, S. (Eds.) (1978). *Psychobiology of Stress: A Study of Coping Men.* New York: Academic Press.

Vale, W., Spiess, J., Rivier, C., & Rivier, J. (1981). Characterization of a 41-residue ovine hypothalamic peptide that stimulates secretion of corticotropin and beta-endorphin. *Science, 213,* 1394–7.

Valentino, R. J., Foote, S. L., & Aston-Jones, G. (1983). Corticotropin-releasing factor activates noradrenergic neurons of the locus ceruleus. *Brain Res., 270,* 363–7.

Van Cauter, E. (1989). Physiology and pathology of circadian rhythms. In C. R. W. Edwards & D. W. Lincoln (Eds.), *Recent Advances in Endocrinology and Metabolism,* pp. 109–34. Edinburgh, U.K.: Churchill Livingstone.

Van Cauter, E., Leproult, R., & Kupfer, D. J. (1996). Effects of gender and age on the levels and circadian rhythmicity of plasma cortisol. *J. Clin. Endocrinol. Metab., 81,* 2468–73.

Van Cauter, E., Shapiro, E. T., Tillil, H., & Polonsky, K. S. (1992). Circadian modulation of glucose and insulin responses to meals: Relationship to cortisol rhythm. *Am. J. Physiol., 262,* E467–E475.

Veldhuis, L. D., Iranmanesh, A., Johnson, M. L., & Lizarralde, G. (1990). Amplitude, but not frequency, modulation of adrenocorticotropin secretory bursts gives rise to the nyctohemeral rhythm of the corticotropic axis in man. *J. Clin. Endocrinol. Metab., 71,* 452–63.

Veltman, J. A., & Gaillard, A. W. K. (1993). Indices of mental workload in a complex task environment. *Neuropsychobiology, 28,* 72–5.

von Euler, U. S. (1948). Identification of the sympathomimetic ergone in adrenergic nerves of cattle (sympathin N) with laevo-noradrenaline. *Acta Physiol. Scand., 16,* 63–74.

Wade, S. E. (1992). An oral-diffusion-sink device for extended sampling of multiple steroid hormones from saliva. *Clin. Chem., 38,* 1878–82.

Webster's Ninth New Collegiate Dictionary (NeXT digital ed.) (1988). Springfield, MA: Merriam-Webster.

Weidenfeld, J., Siegel, R. A., Levy, J., & Chowers, I. (1982). In vitro metabolism of cortisol by human abdominal adipose tissue. *J. Steroid Biochem., 17,* 357–60.

Weiner, H. (1992). *Perturbing the Organism: The Biology of Stressful Experience.* University of Chicago Press.

Weir, T. B., Smith, C. C. T., Round, J. M., & Betteridge, D. J. (1986). Stability of catecholamines in whole blood, plasma, and platelets. *Clin. Chem., 32,* 882–3.

Whitworth, J. A., Stewart, P. M., Burt, D., Atherden, S. M., & Edwards, C. R. W. (1989). The kidney is the major site of cortisone production in man. *Clin. Endocrinol., 31,* 355–61.

Williams, C. L., & McGaugh, J. L. (1993). Reversible lesions of the nucleus of the solitary tract attenuate the memory modulating effects of post training epinephrine. *Behav. Neurosci., 107,* 955–62.

Williams, R. B., Jr., Lane, J. D., Kuhn, C. M., Melosh, W., White, A. D., & Schanberg, S. M. (1982). Type A behavior and elevated physiological and neuroendocrine responses to cognitive tasks. *Science, 218,* 483–5.

Wolkowitz, O. M., Reus, V. I., Weingartner, H., Thompson, K., Breier, A., Doran, A., Rubinow, D., & Pickar, D. (1990). Cognitive effects of corticosteroids. *Am. J. Psychiatry, 147,* 1297–1303.

Wortmann, W., Touchstone, J. C., Knapstein, P., Dick, G., & Nappes, G. (1971). Metabolism of 1,2-^{3}H-cortisol perfused through liver in vivo. *J. Clin. Endocrinol., 33,* 597–603.

Yehuda, R., Giller, E. L., Southwick, S. M., Lowy, M. T., & Mason, J. W. (1991). Hypothalamic-pituitary-adrenal dysfunction in posttraumatic stress disorder. *Biol. Psychiatry, 30,* 1031–48.

Young, E. A., Haskett, R. F., Murphy-Weinberg, V., Watson, S. J., & Akil, H. (1991). Loss of glucocorticoid fast feedback in depression. *Arch. Gen. Psychiatry, 48,* 693–9.

Ziegler, M. G. (1989). Catecholamine measurement in behavioral research. In N. Schneiderman, S. M. Weiss, & P. G. Kaufman (Eds.), *Handbook of Research Methods in Cardiovascular Behavioral Medicine,* pp. 167–83. New York: Plenum.

CHAPTER FOURTEEN

REPRODUCTIVE HORMONES

CHARLES T. SNOWDON & TONI E. ZIEGLER

Historical Background

Hormones are chemical messages. Most hormones are secreted by the endocrine glands, ductless glands located throughout the body that release their products into the bloodstream, affecting tissues in other parts of the body. Early in this century, both the endocrine system and the nervous system were known to regulate body function but were thought to be distinct from one another. The nervous system was considered to be the high-speed information track transmitting by electric stimuli, whereas the endocrine system worked at a much slower pace but enacted long-term changes in the body. However, the nervous system carries information not only by neural impulses from one cell to another; nerve endings may also release chemical transmitters that, under some circumstances, circulate in the blood and can be considered endocrine gland products or hormones (Moore 1978). Thus, to study hormones, it is essential to understand both endocrinology and neuroscience. This chapter examines both the endocrine and neural aspects of reproductive hormone action on behavior.

The concept of a hormone and the endocrine glands is so complex that it has taken until the middle of the twentieth century to understand endocrinology and to develop efficient methods to measure hormones and neural secretions. In order to recognize a gland or group of tissue as part of the endocrine system, information in four areas was needed: (1) an anatomical recognition that a group of tissue was glandular; (2) a method to detect internal secretions from the gland; (3) preparations of extracts to test that the substances produced in the gland influenced other parts of the body; and (4) isolation of the pure hormone, determining its structure and synthesis (Doisy 1936).

In prehistoric times, men would eat the organs of their enemies after battle, drink their blood, or devour the extracts of the enemy's organs to obtain their bravery, thereby ingesting hormones that would act on their own bodies. Since early times, infertility has been a source of shame and worry, and endocrine dysfunctions have been recorded since antiquity. Ancient societies made reference to gigantism, acromegaly, goiters, dwarfs, and diabetes – all of which are manifestations of endocrine disorders. Scholars in ancient Egypt, Greece, China, and India were interested in the workings of the body. Early suggestions of internal secretions that affected health and behavior can be traced back to Pythagoras of Samos (580–489 B.C.), who had studied in Egypt and influenced the Greek physicians. Pythagoras combined the doctrine of the four "elements" (earth, fire, air, and water, where an imbalance of these four elements caused disease in an individual) with the four "qualities" (dry, moist, hot, and cold), which produced the four "humors" of the body (blood, phlegm, yellow bile, and black bile). Combinations of these sets of four were used to explain disease and the physiological action of drugs (see Garrison 1929).

Anatomical description of the gonads and some understanding of their influence on the body has long been noted. Many of the early societies had a moderate understanding of the reproductive system (for a review, see Medvei 1982), and contraception was effected by both herbal and physical remedies. Ovaries were described as far back as Aristotle's time (384–322 B.C.), and ovariectomy was described in Aristotle's *History of Animals* as a method to increase strength and endurance as well as a contraceptive device for animals. Ovariectomies may have been performed by the Egyptians with the understanding that ovaries were part of the process of conception.

The importance of the testicles was well known. Early scholars debated the source of the genetic material of the offspring but many agreed with Aristotle that the testicles were the source of male genetic material and determined

John T. Cacioppo, Louis G. Tassinary, and Gary G. Berntson (Eds.), *Handbook of Psychophysiology*, 2nd ed. © Cambridge University Press 2000. Printed in the United States of America. ISBN 62634X. All rights reserved.

the sex of the child. Castration was practiced on a large scale, not only on slaves and defeated enemies, but also by the priesthood of various cults and on male attendants in harems. Castrated males, or eunuchs, were known to be sterile and thus were sought after by women for love affairs because there was no danger of pregnancy (Medvei 1982). Hippocratic writings indicate that the menstrual cycle was known and note that timing intercourse to the tenth day after the beginning of the period would increase one's chances for conception (Himes 1936). Few advancements in understanding reproduction and hormones occurred from the time of Hippocrates (460–370 B.C.), Aristotle, and their disciples until the sixteenth century.

The Renaissance brought about intensive studies of anatomy with contributions by great artists, such as Leonardo da Vinci (1452–1519), Michelangelo Buonarotti (1475–1564), and Rafael of Urbino (see Knox 1852). Organs were described anatomically but their functions were unknown. With the advent of microscopes in the seventeenth century, many advances in understanding the reproductive organs were made. The first descriptions of spermatozoa were made by Antonj van Leeuwenhoek and were referred to as "little animals of the sperm" or "animalcules" (van Leeuwenhoek 1679). Detailed descriptions of ovaries from animals and humans were made from observations by scientists such as Marcello Malphighi (1628–1694) and Regner de Graaf (1641–1673), who described the ovarian follicles and corpus luteum. The essential contribution of the ovaries to the process of conception was beginning to be realized.

Historically, the circulation of the blood through the arteries and veins was first described by William Harvey in the early seventeenth century, but another 250 years passed before the use of the circulatory system for sending messages from one organ of the body to another was widely realized (Medvei 1982). The concept that glands secreted substances into the circulation that then influenced other parts of the body was first published by de Bordeu in 1775. De Bordeu called the substances "emanations" and reported that they were derived from all organs of the body, which is actually more accurate than the restricted view held in the early 1900s that a few specific organs acted as endocrine glands.

Experimentation that demonstrated the secretion of hormones and truly initiated the study of endocrinology was the transplantation work of John Hunter in the late 1700s aimed at understanding the "vital principle" that would explain the continued support of transplanted tissue. Hunter's first experiments were on the transplantation of spurs in fowl. When the spur of a hen was transplanted to a cock, it grew to the size of a cock's spur; however, the small spur of a young cock would not grow if transplanted to a hen. Hunter also experimented with removing one ovary or testis in animals and determined that sex-specific characteristics continued, whereas total castra-

tion prevented the regrowth of antlers in the stag. Thus, the influence of gonadal hormones on secondary sexual characteristics was demonstrated. Hunter and his contemporaries did not understand the endocrine implications of these important experiments. During the eighteenth century, the ovary was understood to be the female counterpart to the male's testis, but how and where fertilization occurred was still unknown (Medvei 1982).

By the mid-1800s, several investigators had described the anatomy of glands, indicating that secretions of certain glands may enter the venous system and thereby have access to the entire body (Rolleston 1936; Vulpian 1856). Experimental evidence came when Arnold Berthold (1849) published his explanation of the experiments of cock testicle transplants into hens, with the testicular influence occurring via the blood system. Unfortunately, the paper was not cited until the beginning of the twentieth century. In the late 1800s, one accepted theory of testicular influence over secondary sexual characteristics was through the connections between the brain and the testis (Curling 1856). The first use of hormone replacement occurred when the French neurologist and physiologist Charles Brown-Sequard (1817–1894) injected endocrine gland extracts from animals into humans to increase energy or, in the case of testicular injections, to rejuvenate "intellectual work and physical powers" (Brown-Sequard 1889). These original experiments with animal testicular extracts were done by the physicians on themselves with reported increase in "strength, vigor and mental activity as well as increased contractility of the bladder" (Brown-Sequard 1889). The procedure was called "organotherapy" and, within a few years, these techniques became an acceptable mode of therapeutics (Borell 1976). Although interest in the testicular extract injections began to fade, treatment with thyroid extracts became a useful method of restoring thyroid function in humans (Murray 1891). Injections of adrenal extracts were found to increase blood pressure (Abel & Crawford 1897).

Understanding the pituitary as a major director of the endocrine glands was very difficult. Anatomical descriptions of the pituitary with its glandular and neural components were reported beginning in the late 1800s through the early 1900s (Duret 1874; Howell 1898; Popa & Fielding 1930), although it was still considered to be an organ without a known function (Rolleston 1936). Evidence that the pituitary was necessary for the life of an animal came after extensive studies of removing the pituitaries from animals (Crowe, Cushing, & Homans 1910). Removal of the neural component was not life-threatening, whereas removal of the anterior pituitary was (Crowe et al. 1910). Disruption of the pituitary caused cessation of growth, water and mineral metabolism imbalance (Vassale & Sacchi 1892), and atrophy of the gonads (Crowe et al. 1910). Pituitary tumors added to the knowledge of the importance of the pituitary and some of its functional significance (Cushing 1909).

Isolation, purification, and synthesis of hormones began in the early 1900s. Adrenaline (epinephrine) was the first hormone to be isolated (Aldrich 1901) and synthesized (Stolz 1904). Other hormones – such as the estrogens, androgens, and corticosteroids – were extracted, isolated, and synthesized in the 1920s and 1930s (Dodds et al. 1938; Moore, Gallagher, & Koch 1929; Reichstein 1936). During this time, large quantities of estrogens were discovered in the urine of women, small amounts in the urine of men, and tremendous amounts in the urine of pregnant mares. Extracts from pregnant mare urine are now the most popular hormone replacement for postmenopausal women (PREMARIN = PREgnant MARe urINe).

In the 1950s, the neural connections to the endocrine system were discovered. Harris (1955) suggested that the release of the pituitary hormones was controlled by humoral factors, probably of hypothalamic origin. Extracts made from the hypothalamus were found to release some of the anterior pituitary hormones. After this, the race was on to isolate and identify the structure of the many releasing factors of the hypothalamus. Schally and Guillemin, who worked independently of each other, competed to be the first to isolate and determine the structure of a releasing hormone. The race led to the structure of thyrotropin releasing hormone, first reported by Schally's lab. As summarized in *Science*, "This race was monumental in that it lasted for 21 years, involved the creation of two rival teams of experts, and required investing time, money, and reputation in a venture seemed doomed to failure" (Wade 1978). The two scientists were using techniques barely adequate for the job, were facing skepticism by their colleagues, and were threatened with withdrawal of government funding if they didn't provide proof of a releasing hormone in a hurry (Wade 1978). The two labs were responsible for identifying thyrotropin releasing hormone, gonadotropin releasing hormone, and somatostatin. For their perseverance, in 1978 they also shared the Nobel Prize in medicine.

The other major breakthrough was the development of methods to measure hormones. The development of specialized tests made it possible to measure minute amounts of circulating and excreted hormones. The first methods of measurement were by bioassays, which measure the functional response of an organism, target organ, tissue, or group of cells to a hormone (Heist & Poland 1992). For instance, the mouse Leydig cell bioassay for luteinizing hormone (LH) employs dispersed Leydig cells from post-pubertal male mice testis. The dispersed cells are target cells that are stimulated by the gonadotropin molecules (LH or chorionic gonadotropin, CG) present in the sample (blood or urine) and produce a dose–response increase in testosterone production (Ellinwood & Resko 1980). Another bioassay uses the steroid-primed uterus of the rat to study oxytocin-induced contraction of the uterus.

There are many types of bioassays for determining the biological activity of hormones. In most cases, how-

ever, bioassays have been replaced by radioimmunoassays (RIA) – except when a difference between the biological response and the immune response is found. The use of RIA has provided not only an increase in sensitivity but also an increase in specificity. The RIA technique was first developed to measure insulin in humans by Yallow and Berson (1959), who discovered that hormones can exhibit antigenic properties when the molecular weight of the molecule is high enough. In cases were the molecular weight is low, such as with steroids, then the molecule is conjugated to a higher–molecular weight molecule. Techniques for labeling organic compounds were already available. The underlying principle of RIA consists of combining a radiolabeled hormone with an antibody made specifically for the hormone of interest. The labeled hormone and the antibody produce an antigen–antibody complex where the molecules are bound tightly to each other (Figure 1). When an unlabeled hormone (found in blood, urine, feces, or saliva) is added to the system, it competes with the labeled hormone for binding to the antibody, and a displacement of radioactivity can be measured. The higher the amount of radioactivity measured, the less of the target hormone in the sample. Radioimmunoassays have been used extensively since the 1960s to measure hormone concentration and can measure less than a picogram per milliliter of sample (10^{-12} g/ml).

Recently, other methods of measuring hormones have been developed. Owing to the cost of safe handling and disposal of radioactive wastes, alternative methods are

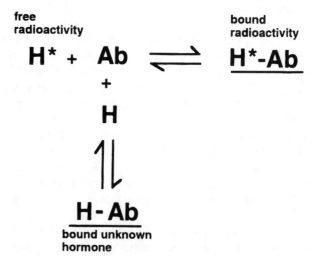

Figure 1. The principle of a competitive binding assay. Labeled hormone (H*), either radioactive or enzymatic, is combined with a specific antibody (Ab) made against the hormone (H) to produce labeled antigen–antibody complexes. Unlabeled hormone also binds with specific antibody and produces antigen–antibody complexes. By separating the bound from the free, a ratio can be calculated to determine the percent bound. Standard amounts of the hormone can be used to create a standard curve and thereby interpret the concentration of the hormone of interest in the sample. (Figure adapted from Yallow 1992, in Wilson & Foster (Eds.), *Textbook of Endocrinology*, p. 1636.)

employed when available. One of the more popular methods is the use of enzyme immunoassays (EIA) to measure hormones. The EIA works on the same principle as the RIA except the hormone has an enzyme tag instead of a radioactive tag. These assays are rapid and easy to perform. The endpoint uses a color change measurable by spectrophotometry. The EIAs have been shown to be just as sensitive as RIAs and, in some cases, even more sensitive (Munro & Stabenfeldt 1984). Other methods of measuring hormones make use of the chemical characteristics of the hormones. Chemical luminescence, fluorescence, chemical detection, and ultraviolet detection of HPLC-separated hormones are all methods that are being used to identify or quantitate hormones.

A major conceptual advance came when Phoenix and colleagues (1959) introduced the important distinction between the organizational and activational effects of hormones by showing that fetal or perinatal stimulation by certain hormones (or the absence of certain hormones at this time) had long-term effects on behavior. Hormones serve to "organize" the nervous system in particular ways that may or may not be influenced by the subsequent short-term activational effects of hormones. Any attempt to understand how reproductive hormones affect behavior must consider the potential organizational effects of early hormonal experience.

Another recent advance is the recognition that relatively few of the phenomena associated with reproductive hormones are influenced solely by hormonal activity. There is abundant evidence of a bi-directionality or interaction of control. Behavioral and social events are as likely to influence reproductive hormones as the hormones are likely to influence behavior. This recognition has led to the development of a new field, socioendocrinology (Ziegler & Bercovitch 1990). Many of our assumptions about how reproductive hormones work must be tempered by detailed knowledge of prior social and behavioral experience, and many of our assumptions about how reproductive hormones control behavior must be re-evaluated in appropriate social contexts.

Critical to the development of socioendocrinology has been research with nonhuman animals. Many of our insights about the interaction of hormones and human behavior and our questions about what to study stem from initial research on animals, such as Lehrman's (1965) classic work on the delicate interplay of hormones and behavior on reproduction and parental care in ring doves and Phoenix et al.'s (1959) paper on organizational effects of hormones on sex-typical behavior in guinea pigs. Many of the social influences on and interactions with reproductive hormones to be discussed here were discovered first in controlled studies with nonhuman animals. Although the major focus of what follows will be on phenomena of interest and relevance to humans, we will draw extensively on research from animals.

Physical Context: Anatomy and Physiology of the Neuroendocrine System

HYPOTHALAMUS AND PITUITARY

Although the control of the endocrine system by the brain was one of the last areas to be discovered, the brain is a logical place to start describing the structures of the system. The brain's influence over the endocrine system is mediated through the hypothalamus (for review see Riskind & Martin 1989). This structure forms an extension of the brainstem and is considered to be a phylogenetically ancient structure. Anatomically, the hypothalamus is found below the thalamus and forms the walls and lower part of the third ventricle of the brain (Figure 2). The third ventricle is part of the fluid canal system that flows into the spinal cord. Links from other areas of the brain to the hypothalamus allow for sociobehavioral, visceral, and autonomic controls of hormone production. The hypothalamus is located directly above the optic chiasm and consists of areas referred to as the tuber cinereum, the infundibulum (also called the median eminence), and the mammillary bodies. Clusters of neurons are located here that secrete neurohormones for regulating the activity of the pituitary (Figure 2). The nerve clusters are named by position: supraoptic nucleus (SON), paraventricular nucleus (PVN), suprachiasmatic nucleus (SCN), ventromedial nucleus (VMN), dorsomedial nucleus (DMN), medial preoptic area (MPOA), arcuate nucleus (ARC), anterior nucleus, and the posterior nucleus. These clusters of neurons contain cell bodies whose axons extend into the infundibulum (see Figure 2). Some of the axons extend into the neural or anterior pituitary, while some of the neurons produce regulatory hormones that are transported from the median eminence to the anterior pituitary by the hypothalamic-pituitary portal circulation. This is a rich vascular supply that allows transport of the hypothalamic regulatory hormones, neuropeptides, and neurotransmitters to the anterior pituitary. It is anatomically possible for blood flow to be reversed in the portal system, allowing the pituitary hormones to influence the functional activity of several neural centers and so produce an ultrashort-loop feedback (Thorner et al. 1992).

The pituitary is divided into two parts: the anterior pituitary and posterior pituitary (also called the adenohypophysis and neurohypophysis, respectively). The anterior lobe is composed of three divisions: pars distalis, pars intermedia, and pars tuberalis (for extensive details, see Thorner et al. 1992). The hormone-producing cells are located in the pars distalis. The pars intermedia is very small and rudimentary in humans. Pars tuberalis is the upward extension of the anterior lobe and its attachment to the pituitary stalk. The posterior pituitary is an extension of the hypothalamus consisting of the infundibulum, the infundibular stem, and the neural lobe. Two hormones,

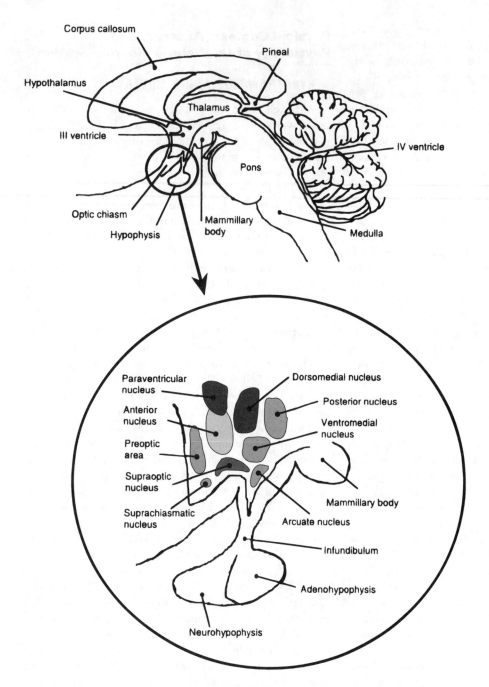

Figure 2. Major parts of the brain. Circled part in the top diagram illustrates the position of the hypothalamus and pituitary. The hypothalamus and pituitary are shown in the enlarged circle. The hypothalamus is divided into nuclei named for their position. Nerve fibers extend from the hypothalamus into the infundibulum. Production and storage of LH, FSH, GH, TSH, ACTH, and prolactin occur in the adenohypophysis. Vasopressin and oxytocin are produced in the hypothalamus and stored in the neurohypophysis.

arginine vasopressin (AVP) and oxytocin (OT), are synthesized in the supraoptic nucleus and paraventricular area of the hypothalamus, transported through elongated axons, and stored in the posterior lobe. From there they can be released into the peripheral circulation. The anterior pituitary synthesizes the following hormones: adrenocorticotropin hormone (ACTH), growth hormone (GH), prolactin (PRL), thyroid stimulating hormone (TSH), luteinizing hormone (LH), and follicle stimulating hormone (FSH); in the pars intermedia, melanocyte stimulating hormone (MSH) is produced in many mammals but not in adult humans. These hormones regulate the hormones produced in the endocrine glands located throughout the body. Table 1 shows the relationships between the hypothalamus, pituitary, and target gland hormones.

Hypothalamic control of pituitary hormones may effect a positive or an inhibitory release of hormones, as occurs with dopamine's inhibition of prolactin release.

The anterior pituitary releases its hormones in a pulsatile fashion into the bloodstream, wherein they travel to their target glands and exert their effect. The hormones in the target glands can feed back to both the hypothalamus and the pituitary. In this way, the hormonal production of the endocrine glands can be continuously monitored and regulated by the brain. The control of pituitary hormones is more complex than demonstrated in Table 1. For example, thyroid releasing hormone also can stimulate the release of prolactin from the pituitary, and dopamine causes an inhibition of prolactin release. Oxytocin stored in the posterior pituitary can stimulate the release of prolactin (Mori et al. 1990). Although gonadotropin releasing hormone stimulates the release of both LH and FSH, the quantity of release of both these pituitary hormones changes during the ovarian cycle: at ovulation, LH is released as a large surge; during menses and with the onset of follicular growth, FSH is released while LH is maintained at basal levels in the bloodstream. Additionally, there are over 16 different neurotransmitters that contribute to regulating LH and prolactin. Neurons located in many areas of the brain send axons to the hypothalamus (or have cell bodies in the nuclear complexes in the hypothalamus) and can regulate the production of releasing hormones (see Kordon et al. 1994 for extensive review).

Neurotransmitters are involved in controlling the secretion of the releasing hormones and are secreted from neurons, which in turn may be linked to other neuronal inputs or to sensory neurons that are receptive to endogenous and exogenous cues. Neurotransmitters may have an inhibitory or a stimulatory effect on the releasing hormones. There are two categories of neurotransmitters: small-molecule neurotransmitters and neuropeptides (or neuromodulators). The neurotransmitters mediate rapid reactions, whereas neuropeptides tend to modulate slower, ongoing brain functions. Small-molecule neurotransmitters include: acetylcholine; the amino acids such as glutamate, aspartate, GABA, and glycine; the catecholamines such as dopamine, norepinephrine, and epinephrine; and the bioamines serotonin and histamine (Purves et al. 1997). The neuropeptides include the enkephalins, endorphins, cholecystokinin (CCK), vasoactive intestinal peptide (VIP), neuropeptide-Y, AVP, OT, and angiotensin-II.

The main feedback control of anterior pituitary hormones comes from the release of steroids from the target endocrine glands. The major endocrine glands of the body include the adrenal gland, the thyroid gland, the gonads

TABLE 1. Hypothalamic and Pituitary Hormones and Their Feedback Control from the Glands

Hypothalamic Hormone	Pituitary Hormone	Target Gland	Feedback Hormone
TRH	TSH	Thyroid	T_4 and T_3
GnRH	LH	Gonads	E_2 (women), T (men), P
	FSH	Gonads	Inhibin and (?) E_2 and T
SS	GH	Multiple	IGF 1
GHRH	GH	Multiple	IGF 1
DA, OT, TRH	PRL	Breast	?
		Gonads + ?	E_2, T, P
CRH	ACTH	Adrenal	Cortisol
AVP	ACTH	Adrenal	Cortisol
DA, CRH, GABA	MSH	Skin	
		Fetal adrenal	?

Key: ACTH, adrenocorticotropin; AVP, arginine vasopressin; CRH, corticotropin releasing hormone; DA, dopamine; E_2, estradiol; GABA, gamma amino butyric acid; GH, growth hormone; GnRH, gonadotropin releasing hormone; IGF, insulinlike growth factor; LH, luteinizing hormone; MSH, melanocyte stimulating hormone; OT, oxytocin; PRL, prolactin; SS, somatostatin; T, testosterone; TRH, thyrotropin releasing hormone; TSH, thyroid stimulating hormone.
Source: Adapted from Thorner et al. (1992).

(ovaries and testes), the pancreas, the pineal, and the placenta. Steroids secreted from these glands are released into the bloodstream to exert their effect on many tissues. They also reach the pituitary and the hypothalamus to exert the negative feedback loop to control their own secretion. For instance, ACTH released from the pituitary circulates through the blood until it reaches the adrenals. There, ACTH binds the receptors for the hormone and initiates the synthesis and/or release, into the bloodstream, of cortisol, which affects a variety of tissues in the body. Cortisol also feeds back to the pituitary and – through direct interactions with corticotropin releasing hormone and ACTH – decreases the output of ACTH and thereby the release of cortisol. The gonads exert the same type of negative feedback. Estradiol, however, exerts both a positive and negative feedback on the brain and pituitary at different times during the ovarian cycle.

NEUROHYPOPHYSIS HORMONES: OXYTOCIN AND ARGININE VASOPRESSIN

The nona-peptides, oxytocin (OT) and arginine vasopressin (AVP), are very closely related structurally yet serve distinct physiological roles. Both hormones consist of nine amino acids folded into a ring through a disulfide bridge, with a terminal tripeptide side chain. The hormones differ by only two amino acids. Classically, OT is known for its control of milk release from the mammary gland and the contractions of the uterus during labor; AVP (once referred to as antidiuretic hormone) is involved with water balance.

Actually, these hormones serve many other functions within the body. Both hormones appear to be involved in the processes of learning and memory (Engelmann et al. 1996). Both OT and AVP are released from the anterior pituitary into the bloodstream, but they also serve a role in interneuronal communication. Both substances are released synaptically from axon terminals, dendrites, and somata of hypothalamic neurons. Central actions include a variety of autonomic, endocrine, and behavioral effects (Engelmann et al. 1996). Concentration of AVP and OT in the extracellular fluid of discrete brain areas is several orders of magnitude higher than peripheral levels in the blood or urine.

The role of oxytocin as a maternal hormone is without doubt. Oxytocin is not only responsible for milk let-down during nursing but is known for its induction of contractions during labor. Synthetic oxytocins are used for stimulating contractions during difficult labors in humans. Oxytocin facilitates mother–infant interactions and has an inhibitory effect on aggressive behavior in rats (Giovenardi et al. 1997). Pair-bond formation in monogamous prairie voles appears to be influenced by oxytocin released centrally in the brain (Carter 1998). In adult animals, oxytocin may facilitate social contact and attachment as well as the regulation of parasympathetic functions. Oxytocin exerts an inhibitory effect on corticotropin releasing hormone-mediated ACTH secretion in human males. Oxytocin has also been reported to have effects on female sexual receptivity (lordosis in rodents) and on penile erection and male mounting behavior (Rao 1995).

Arginine vasopressin (AVP), on the other hand, may be working in the opposite direction by regulating defensive behaviors such as arousal, attention, or vigilance – increased aggressive behaviors with an increase in sympathetic functions (Carter & Altemus 1997). In monogamous male prairie voles, however, AVP induces pair-bond formation and promotes parental behavior (Wang, Ferris, & De Vries 1994). Arginine vasopressin works to induce the contraction or relaxation of certain types of smooth muscle, and it promotes the movement of water and sodium across responsive epithelial tissues, especially the kidney (Hadley 1992). Finally, AVP is highly responsive to the osmolality of the blood.

THE STRUCTURE OF THE GLANDS

The major glands secreting hormones in the body are listed in Table 2, but many tissues in the body secrete chemical messengers. At least ten hormones are recognized in the gastrointestinal tract alone. Other tissues that release chemical messengers are skin, liver, kidney, heart, plasma, and various tissues releasing growth factors considered to be hormones. For the purposes of this chapter, we will concentrate on describing the adrenal glands and the gonads with their communication to the hypothalamus and pituitary.

Adrenals

The adrenals are located directly above the kidneys and are only one tenth the size of the kidneys. Each adrenal consists of two functionally distinct endocrine glands. The cortex is the steroid-secreting gland consisting of cells grouped into the zona glomerulosa, zona fasciculata, and zona reticularis. The zona glomerulosa produces mineralocorticoids such as aldosterone, which promote sodium retention and potassium excretion and so aid regulation of extracellular fluid volume (Bartter, Liddle, & Duncan 1956). The zona fasciculata and zona reticularis secrete the glucocorticoids and androgens, including dihydroepiandrosterone (DHEA) and androstenedione. The major glucocorticoid in humans is cortisol, whose functions will be described shortly. The medulla is the other endocrine gland and is derived from the neural crest. Epinephrine is the predominant catecholamine released from the medulla. The close anatomical coupling and functional interrelations between the adrenal cortex and medulla suggest that these two tissues may constitute an integrated functional unit (Hadley 1992).

Cortisol is well known for its role in the stress response, and many investigators study the response of cortisol to both physical and emotional stress. Cortisol, however, also plays a critical role in regulating metabolism and modulating the responses of many hormones and growth factors. Chronic levels – higher or lower than the physiological levels – lead to disease states. Cortisol increases hepatic glucose production and so affects lipid metabolism. Excess corticosteroids can suppress the immune response of an individual, decrease bone formation, decrease calcium absorption, and increase blood pressure. Since cortisol and aldosterone are structurally similar, in disease states cortisol will exhibit both glucocorticoid and mineralocorticoid activity. Superphysiological levels of cortisol can modulate the mood of an individual as well as influence sleep patterns, cognition, and the reception of sensory input (McEwen 1979). Cortisol has an inhibitory influence on the reproductive system. During stress, the secretion of hypothalamic gonadotropin releasing hormone (GnRH) and also the pituitary release of luteinizing hormone and follicle stimulating hormone (FSH) are inhibited. Beta-endorphin and corticotropin releasing hormone inhibit GnRH release; stress causes the pituitary to be less sensitive to GnRH and the glucocorticoids inhibit ovarian sensitivity to LH (Sapolsky 1992).

The control of glucocorticoids and mineralocorticoids differs. Adrenal glucocorticoid synthesis and secretion are controlled by pituitary ACTH whereas aldosterone secretion is controlled by the renin-angiotensin system, which is activated by hypovolemia (low blood pressure) and plays an important role in maintaining body water balance and sodium balance. In turn, ACTH is controlled by the hypothalamic release of CRH. The glucocorticoids provide a

TABLE 2. Endocrine Glands in Mammals and the Major Known Hormones

Gland	Secreted Hormone
Anterior pituitary	Growth hormone
	Prolactin
	Melanophore stimulating hormone
	Adrenocorticotopin
	Luteinizing hormone
	Follicle stimulating hormone
	Thyroid stimulating hormone
Posterior pituitary	Arginine vasopressin
	Oxytocin
Thyroid gland	Thyroxin
	Calcitonin
Adrenal cortex	Glucocorticoids
	Corticosterone
	Cortisol
	Dehydroepiandrosterone
	Mineralocorticoids
	Aldosterone
Adrenal medulla	Epinephrine
	Norepinephrine
	Enkephalins
	Endorphins
Kidney	Renin
Liver	Preangiotensin
Pancreas	Insulin
	Glucagon
Stomach and intestines	Gastrin
	Secretin
	Cholecystokinin
	Gastric inhibitory peptide
	Vasoactive intestinal peptide
	Chymodenin
	Motilin
	Neurotensin
	Substance P
	Gastrin releasing peptide
Pineal	Melatonin
Ovary	Estrogens
	Estradiol
	Estrone
	Progesterone
	Androgens
	Inhibin
Testes	Androgens
	Testosterone
	Dihydrotestosterone
	Androstenedione

negative feedback system: circulating glucocorticoids reach the pituitary, hypothalamus, or even higher brain centers and thereby reduce the release of ACTH and hence of cortisol. Release of ACTH from the brain is pulsatile and has a circadian rhythm cycle length of about 24 hours. How stress causes the cascade of hormonal events is unknown, but it is thought to occur through the release of CRH and AVP. Moreover, the androgens appear to have an additional but unknown control over secretion of CRH and AVP.

Epinephrine is synthesized and stored in the adrenal medulla. Although it is released centrally from neurons like other catecholamines, it is the primary catecholamine known to be released peripherally. The adrenal medulla is under the direct control of the central nervous system. Functionally, catecholamines are neurochemical transducers that convert electrical neural activity into physiological response. The effects of catecholamines are induced rapidly and dissipate quickly, unlike the slower and more prolonged effects of most hormones. The role of catecholamines is to maintain the constancy of the body's internal environment. Decreases in blood pressure, blood glucose levels, or oxygen availability lead to increases in catecholamines, which increase in response to stressors of external or internal origin, real or imagined. Catecholamines have an immediate response to stressors, whereas the glucocorticoids have a slower but longer response. Measurement of plasma and urinary epinephrine reflect adrenal medulla function. An increase in plasma epinephrine level or urinary epinephrine excretion is good evidence of adrenomedullary stimulation. However, the duration and intensity of a stimulation is most easily determined from urinary epinephrine excretion. The half-life of plasma epinephrine is so short and the basal concentrations so small that most assays are not sensitive enough.

In summary, the adrenal glands have both an endocrine and a neural component. The main function of the adrenals is to maintain homeostasis. By secreting epinephrine via the adrenal medulla and glucocorticoids via the adrenal cortex, the body responds rapidly to a change in homeostasis with release of neurally controlled epinephrine – or more slowly and for a longer duration with release of the endocrine controlled glucocorticoids. The adrenals also secrete small amounts of gonadal steroids that can be especially important with regard to changes in or failure of gonadal function.

Ovaries

The ovaries control reproduction in the female. It is here that ova are produced and the hormones that regulate female sexual life are synthesized. Development of the ovum and synthesis of steroid hormones are both under control of the hypothalamo-pituitary-ovarian axis. Figure 3 shows the reproductive organs of the human female. The ovaries lie laterally and posteriorly in the pelvic wall, attached to the posterior surface of the broad ligament by a peritoneal fold termed the mesovarian. The ovary consists of three regions: the cortex, containing the germinal epithelium and the follicles; the central medulla, consisting of stroma; and a hilum, where the attachment of the ovary

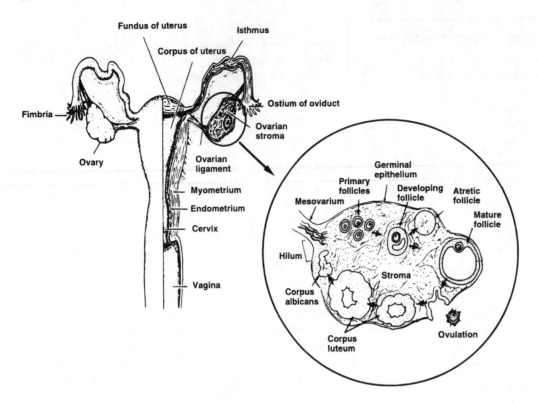

Figure 3. The reproductive organs of the human female. An enlargement of the ovary and the process of ovulation are shown in the circle. (Parts of this figure were adapted from Niswender & Nett 1988, in Knobil & Neill (Eds.), *The Physiology of Reproduction*, p. 490.)

to the mesovarian occurs (Carr 1992). The primordial follicles lie near the periphery of the cortex and contain the primordial germ cells that give rise to the oocytes. The number of oocytes are fixed by birth in the female at about one million per ovary. The stroma consists of connective and interstitial tissue. The primordial follicles begin the process of meiosis within the embryo and became arrested in the prophase by birth of the fetus. After puberty, the endocrine system initiates further maturation of the follicles.

During each ovarian cycle, six to twelve primary follicles develop into secondary follicles. The size of the oocyte and the number of layers of the granulosa cells that surround the ovum increase. At this stage, a zona pellucida is formed and granulosa cells begin to develop. Usually, only one or two follicles will continue to develop beyond this stage at each ovarian cycle. Those that do not develop go through a process of atresia and eventually disappear. As a selected follicle continues to develop, the granulosa cells continue to mature and the interstitial tissue surrounding the follicle differentiates into the theca layers: theca externa and theca interna. As the follicle enlarges, a single large vesicle is formed. A mature follicle is also called a Graafian follicle. The mechanisms controlling the rupture of the mature follicle and the actual ovulation are still

uncertain, but they are initiated by release of luteinizing hormone from the pituitary. The LH causes rapid secretion of follicular steroid hormones and begins the conversion to secreting progesterone. At this time, the outside capsule of the follicle (theca externa) begins secreting proteolytic enzymes, weakening the capsular wall and increasing follicular swelling. A rapid growth of new blood vessels occurs in the follicle wall, and prostaglandins are secreted in the follicular tissues. The prostaglandins act like local hormones and cause vasodilation of the blood vessels (Guyton & Hall 1996). Plasma flows into the follicle, increasing the swelling, and the follicle ruptures. During ovulation, the fimbria of the uterine tubes (Fallopian tubes) spread over most of the medial surface of the ovary and provide wavelike movements to draw in the ova. From here the ova move down the uterine tubes, where fertilization takes place. After fertilization, the embryo moves into the fundus of the uterus where implantation and growth takes place to form the fetus. If fertilization does not take place, then prostaglandins are secreted (by the endometrium of the uterus in some species and by the ovary in others) to initiate the luteolysis of the corpus luteum.

After the follicle ruptures, it fills up with blood, forming the corpus hemorrhagicum. Both granulosa cells and thecal cells begin to increase in number. The granulosa cells begin to accumulate large quantities of cholesterol by a process termed luteinization. The corpus luteum is now formed; it will remain large for about 14 days and begin to regress.

Ovarian steroids are derived from the follicle and corpus luteum. The steroids consist of three types: estrogens, androgens, and progestogens. During the follicular phase of the cycle, estrogens are considered the major steroids secreted from the ovary; during the luteal phase (formation of the corpus luteum) and during pregnancy, progesterone is the major steroid hormone secreted. The ovarian steroids, like all steroids (including cortisol), are derived from cholesterol. Estradiol is biosynthesized from cholesterol via steroidogenic pathways, shown in Figure 4. The thecal cells synthesize the androgens androstenedione and testosterone from cholesterol via pregnenolone. The predominant pathway is through dihydroepiandrosterone. The androgens are transferred to the granulosa cells, where they are aromatized to estrogens. During follicular maturation, the ability of granulosa cells to aromatize androgens into estradiol increases. Low levels of estradiol exert a negative feedback on pituitary LH. Peak levels of estradiol feed back to the hypothalamus and pituitary to initiate the release of gonadotropin releasing hormone, which in turn releases LH and FSH. With the LH–FSH surge, progesterone biosynthesis begins in the granulosa cells. Large quantities of cholesterol form and are synthesized to progesterone and 17-hydroxyprogesterone. Progesterone acts on the hypothalamus to decrease LH and FSH secretion. As progesterone levels decline, the pituitary gonadotropins resume secreting and initiate the next set of follicle growth. Other hormones found within the ovary also help to regulate the pituitary's influence on the ovary. For example, follicular activin exerts a positive release on FSH, and follicular inhibin and follistatin exert an inhibitory release on pituitary FSH.

At puberty, estrogens stimulate the continued development of the vagina, uterus, and oviducts. Secondary sexual characteristics developed at this time are due to estrogen secretion. However, ovarian androgens are also responsible for some of the changes that occur during puberty, such as pubic and axillary hair growth, acne, and sebaceous gland activity. Estrogen secretion also causes the fat distribution and mammary growth typical of developing females. Whereas estradiol is primarily secreted from the follicle, estrone is mainly secreted from extraglandular conversion of androstenedione in peripheral tissues such as skin and fat.

Progesterone is responsible for preparing and maintaining the reproductive tract for the embryo during pregnancy. It inhibits uterine contractions, increases the viscosity of the cervical mucus, promotes glandular development of the breast, and increases body temperature. The sequence of estrogen-primed tissue with increasing levels of progesterone has been implicated in triggering sexual behavior in many mammals.

Steroids and other hormones regulate specific target tissues by interacting with specific receptors. The hormone-specific receptors are located in plasma membranes, in the cell cytosol (cytoplasm), or in the nucleus. Hormone receptors, such as estradiol receptors, may bind with other substances that resemble estradiol. Many compounds have estrogenlike effects on the body when bound to estrogen receptors. Estrogenlike compounds (e.g. synthetic diethylstilbestrol) or naturally occurring plant estrogens can mediate estrogen effects in the body producing physiological responses (Miksicek 1993).

Ovulation occurs on average once every 28 days in the nonpregnant woman. However, there are many social and stressful events that can influence the length of the ovarian cycle or the onset of puberty (see subsequent sections for more details).

Testes

The testes produce the sperm necessary for fertilization of the female ovum, and they also produce the steroid hormones that interact with the pituitary and hypothalamus to regulate sperm production and male sexual activity (Griffin & Wilson 1992). The testes lie outside the abdominal cavity within the scrotal sac. Descent of the testes from the abdominal cavity (where development takes place) occurs during the latter two thirds of gestation. In the adult male, the testes have two components necessary for sexual function: in Figure 5, the structures of the seminiferous tubules and the steroid-producing Leydig cells are demonstrated. The tubules produce and transport the sperm to the excretory–ejaculatory ducts. Steroid-producing cells are located outside the seminiferous tubules and are called Leydig cells. They possess lipid droplets full of cholesterol, which serves as a substrate for testosterone synthesis. Testosterone is metabolized from cholesterol by conversion to pregnenolone with subsequent 17-hydroxylation synthesis (through dihydroepiandrosterone and androstenedione) to testosterone, as occurs in the ovary (Figure 4). Dihydroepiandrosterone and androstenedione are also endproducts of the Leydig cells, but in small amounts and with low physiological potencies. Storage of testosterone within the Leydig cells is low, since the newly synthesized testosterone diffuses quickly into the blood from nearby capillary cells (Hadley 1992).

The seminiferous tubules are filled with Sertoli cells, which give rise to the spermatocytes. The FSH interacts with receptors on the Sertoli cells to cause the synthesis of an androgen-binding protein (ABP), which is secreted into the lumen of the seminiferous tubules. The Leydig cells respond to LH stimulation and produce testosterone. Although testosterone diffuses into the capillaries and into the blood system, it is also actively transported into the seminiferous tubules where it becomes bound to ABP within the Sertoli cells. The spermatocytes begin the process of maturation under the influence of testosterone. Mature sperm are stored in the epididymis, where they develop the potential for fertilization and motility.

The GnRH is released in an episodic manner into the hypophyseal portal system, causing LH and FSH release in a pulsatory manner. The rate of secretion of

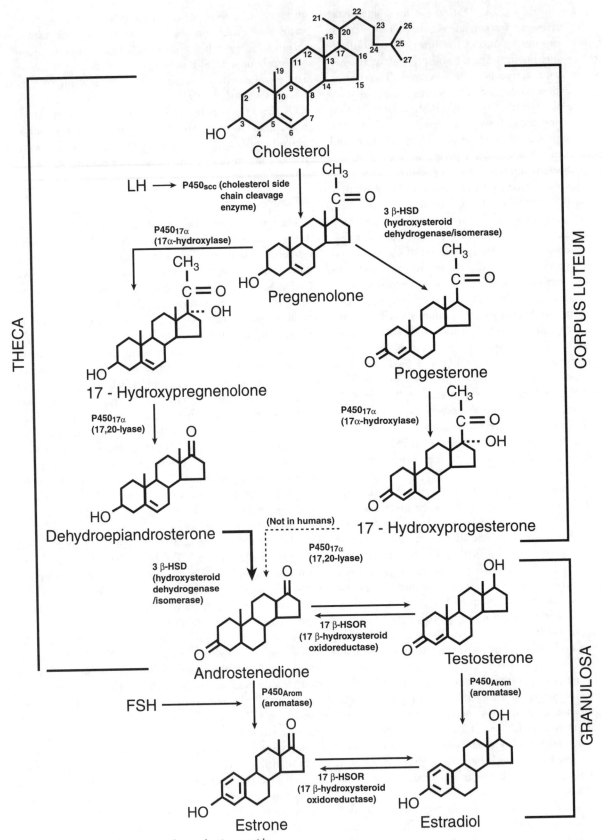

Figure 4. Steroidogenic pathway of reproductive steroids.

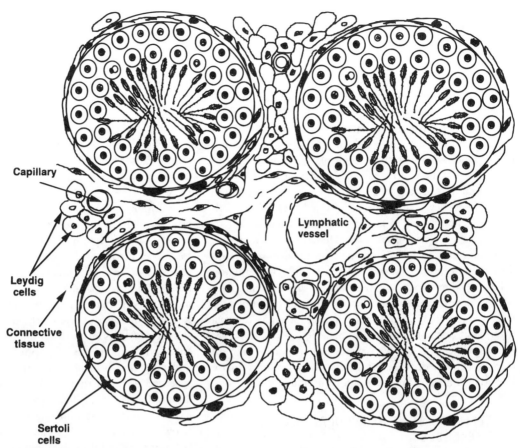

Figure 5. Diagram of the testicular tissue in man, showing the arrangement of the Sertoli cells with spermatocytes and the interstitial tissue containing the Leydig cells (where testosterone is produced).

LH is controlled by the action of gonadal steroids on the hypothalamus and the pituitary. Both testosterone and estradiol exert a negative feedback on LH. Testosterone can be converted to estradiol in the brain and pituitary. The ratio of testosterone to estradiol appears to influence the release of FSH (Sherins, Paterson, & Brightwell 1982), which is also controlled by negative feedback from inhibin produced by the Sertoli cells under the influence of FSH.

Although testosterone is the main steroid secreted by the testes, it actually serves as a precursor, or prohormone, for the formation of two types of active metabolites that have a higher biological activity than testosterone and provide the means for androgen effects on the body. Testosterone can be reduced by 5 alpha-reductase to dihydrotestosterone (the conversion can take place in the prostate and seminal vesicles or in peripheral tissues). This steroid mediates the growth-promoting, differentiative, and functional aspects of male sexual development. Alternatively, testosterone can be aromatized to estrogens in extraglandular tissues. The estrogens can either act in concert with the androgens or (most often) have the opposite effect of androgens. Androgens can act directly on the brain to affect the male's behavior; acting on other androgen-sensitive tissues

(including accessory sex organs), androgens may affect behavior indirectly.

Sexual development into male or female proceeds from the establishment of genetic sex at time of conception. Genetic sex governs development of gonadal sex, which in turn regulates development of phenotypic sex. The phenotypic sex is the differentiation of internal and external sex organs and the attainment of adult secondary sexual characteristics. The gonads and accessory glands develop toward the female in mammals unless influenced by the Y chromosome (Roberts 1988). The Y chromosome triggers the genital ridges in the embryo to develop into testes rather than ovaries. The differentiation toward the male gonadal and body phenotype requires the inductive actions of gonadal androgens. Female ovarian and genital development may be considered an essentially autonomous process requiring no hormonally active inductive substances. Removal of the gonads from undifferentiated embryos of either sex results in development of a female genotype (Bardin & Catterall 1981). The timing of androgen exposure to the brain is important for physiological and behavioral processes. Deprivation of testosterone in the male animal during his species-specific critical time of brain differentiation will result in a female pattern of sexual dimorphic behavior.

Social Context

INTRODUCTION

The study of reproductive hormones is important for psychophysiologists for several reasons. Many of the most interesting behavioral phenomena of life (behavioral sex differences, courtship, sex, parental care, aggression, cognition) are to some degree influenced by reproductive hormones, and psychological research plays an important role in discovering the relative role of the hormones versus environmental and social factors influencing these phenomena.

There are seven broad areas reviewed here: What is the role of genes, hormones, and social environment on the development of sex differences? What is the interaction of hormones and social environment on puberty and reproductive maturation? How do hormones influence affiliative behavior, courtship, and pair bonding? Do hormones influence behavior across the ovarian cycle, and how do social interactions influence ovarian function? What is the relative role of hormones and social behavior on parental care? Are there sex differences in aggression and do these result from hormonal differences? Finally, how do reproductive hormones influence memory and cognition?

DEVELOPMENT OF BEHAVIORAL SEX DIFFERENCES

There is great diversity in how sex is determined biologically, and within mammals there are many places where sex determination can go awry. In mammals, the ovum always contains an X chromosome and the sperm can be either X or Y, meaning that the sperm of the father determines the sex of the offspring. In birds, however, males are homogametic (with two Z chromosomes) and ova contain either W or Z chromosomes, meaning that mothers determine the sex of their offspring (Breedlove 1992). In some reptiles there are no sex chromosomes, and sex is determined by the temperature at which eggs are incubated (Bull & Vogt 1979). Some species of fish are sequentially hermaphroditic (female then male or male then female) – changing sex in response to the social structure of the group – or simultaneously hermaphroditic (trading sex roles and gametes during a sexual interaction; Demski 1987).

In mammals, the Y chromosome contains a gene that stimulates fetal testes development, and secretions from the fetal testes lead to differentiation of male external genitalia and internal accessory organs. In the absence of testicular hormones, female external genitalia and internal accessory organs develop. Thus, being female is the default value in mammalian fetal development (Eve had to precede Adam).

Research on rats and guinea pigs demonstrated that manipulation of fetal or perinatal hormone levels influenced the development of sex-typical behavior. Injections of testosterone to fetal females produced malelike behavior

in adults. Subsequently, female rats injected with estrogen displayed masculine behavior. How could this happen? Testosterone can be converted into estrogen by an aromatase enzyme found in the hypothalamus. In rodents, alpha-feto-protein binds plasma estrogen in female fetuses, preventing exposure of the brain to estrogen. Testosterone is not bound to alpha feto-protein and makes its way to the brain, where it is aromatized locally into estrogen and masculinizes neural structures (Breedlove 1992). This protein is not found in primates, so the aromatization of testosterone to estrogen does not explain masculinization of primates.

Hormonal manipulations in nonhuman primates have used (a) injection of testosterone to females at various stages of fetal development and (b) administration of drugs to block testosterone secretion in males. Injections of testosterone to fetal females for 35–80 days masculinized the degree of rough-and-tumble play and double-foot clasp mounts, both male-typical behaviors (Goy 1970; Goy & Resko 1972). Goy, Bercovitch, and McBrair (1988) used short-term doses of testosterone that did not lead to masculinized genitalia and still reported increases in rough play and mounting behavior. Injections of diethylstilbestrol, a synthetic estrogen that often has masculinizing effects on human females, had little effect on male behavior but did have a limited masculinizing effect on female macaques (Goy & Deputte 1996). Wallen, Maestripieri, and Mann (1995) injected fetal male monkeys with a gonadotropin releasing hormone antagonist to block testosterone secretion and found no effects on male behavioral development.

Social environments have important influences on sex-role development. Goldfoot and associates (1984) reared rhesus macaques in isosexual groups – five females together or five males together – and found aspects of behavior typical to each sex within the isosexual groups. Thus, in all-female groups, some showed malelike mounting and reduced femalelike presenting; the opposite was found in the all-male groups. One dimorphic behavior, rough play, was limited to males regardless of social condition. Wallen (1996) concluded that, with the exception of rough play (which remains consistent as a male-typical behavior), all other sexually dimorphic behavior in rhesus macaques can be modulated by social experience and group composition.

Let us now consider early hormonal influences on humans. There are several hormonal disorders that provide analogs to the experiments with monkeys. Androgen-insensitive males have normal testes that secrete testosterone, but the receptor tissues are insensitive to testosterone. As a result, internal accessory organs and external genitalia are female. Because the testes and adrenal glands secrete small amounts of estrogen, these androgen-insensitive males develop breasts and other female secondary sex characteristics at puberty. Generally, they discover they are genetic males only when they fail to menstruate at puberty and seek medical advice. These genetic males identify themselves as female, suggesting the importance of sexual anatomy on sexual identification (Breedlove 1992).

A second disorder occurs when the enzyme needed to convert testosterone to dihydrotestosterone (5-alpha-reductase) is missing. Dihydrotestosterone is needed for the masculinization of external genitalia. A genetic male is born with testes inside the labia and an enlarged clitoris instead of a penis. In the Dominican Republic there is a population where this genetic disorder is relatively common. Children are typically reared as girls, but with the surge of testosterone at puberty leading to secondary sex characteristics, the children start taking on male roles and wearing male clothes (Imperator-McGinley et al. 1979). The culture appears to support the social transition from girlhood to young manhood.

Fetal females can be exposed to exceptional levels of testosterone through congenital adrenal hyperplasia (CAH) when the adrenal gland lacks the enzyme needed to convert androstenedione to cortisol. Cortisol is not sufficient to stop production of ACTH, and thus the adrenal gland produces high levels of androgens. Some synthetic progestins and estrogens (e.g. diethylstilbestrol, used to sustain pregnancies in women with a history of hormonal insufficiency) also have androgenic effects.

The results are that genitals are often ambiguous at birth, with an enlarged clitoris that may resemble a penis and fused labia that resemble a scrotum. There has been considerable controversy over the effects of this early masculinization and about appropriate treatment. Ehrhardt and Money (1967) described the androgenized girls as being more tomboyish and athletic, preferring male playmates and male clothes and preferring career to marriage. But these tomboys of the 1960s sound like ideal feminist girls of the 1990s. Early masculinization may affect several aspects of behavior. Zucker and colleagues (1996) studied a group of women with CAH and used as controls unaffected cousins or sisters of similar age. The CAH women recalled more cross-gender role behavior and less comfort with their sense of "femininity" in childhood. As adults, the CAH women had lower rates of heterosexual fantasy and fewer sexual relations with men than the controls. However, there were no differences between CAH and control women in relationship status or sexual relations with women. Three women lived in a male gender role, two having been reared as boys and one having switched gender role during adolescence.

Meyer-Bahlburg and associates (1996) studied four CAH women who lived as males. Each of the gender-change subjects had more masculine childhood gender-role behavior, each was sexually attracted only to females, and each had changed gender gradually with the change extending well into adulthood. A combination of gender-atypical behavioral image, a gender-atypical body image, and sexual attraction to women was involved in the gender change.

In summary, there is no simple role for reproductive hormones in sociosexual development. The social structure of rearing groups, the responses of parents to genital development, and individual differences appear to play important roles. The prenatal hormonal environment predisposes responses by caretakers toward infants and influences development. As Wallen concluded his review: "Social context and biological predispositions are indispensable components in the development of behavioral sex differences" (1996, p. 377).

INFLUENCES ON PUBERTY AND FERTILITY

The social regulation of puberty has been well studied in rodents, where evidence of pheromonal control of reproductive maturation is clear (Vandenbergh 1987). A female mouse exposed to the odor of an adult male reaches puberty sooner than expected, and a young female exposed to the odors of cycling females reaches puberty much later than expected. These social influences on reproduction have been tested in natural environments where the population density of mice on freeway cloverleafs has been manipulated experimentally. In areas with high population density, female mice reach puberty at a much later age than do mice in a low-density population (Vandenbergh 1987). Thus the social regulation of puberty has a direct effect on regulating population density in rodents. (These effects do not seem evident in humans.)

Social regulation of fertility is also common in cooperatively breeding mammals, where only one or two females breed while the other females do not (canids, Moehlman & Hofer 1997; voles, Carter, Getz, & Cohen-Parsons 1986; dwarf mongoose, Creel et al. 1992; naked mole rats, Faulkes & Abbott 1997; marmosets and tamarins, Snowdon 1996 and French 1997). We followed the reproductive hormones of 31 postpubertal cotton-top tamarin females housed in intact families and found no evidence of ovulation (Snowdon 1996), yet in golden lion tamarins French and Stribley (1987) found that mothers and daughters show synchronous estrogen cycles. In common marmosets (Saltzman et al. 1997) and pygmy marmosets (Carlson, Ziegler, & Snowdon 1997), some females ovulate within the natal family but do not become pregnant. Transfer of scents from the mother to a daughter newly paired with a novel male delayed the onset of ovulation compared with control females (Barrett, Abbott, & George 1990; Savage, Ziegler, & Snowdon 1988). Stimulation by a novel male is also important (Widowski et al. 1990). Females removed from their mother and housed with a brother failed to ovulate, but the mere sight, sound, or smell of a novel male was sufficient to induce ovulation (Widowski et al. 1992).

Puberty acceleration and delay in rodents and reproductive inhibition in cooperatively breeding mammals may seem to have little relevance to human reproduction, but there do exist social influences on human reproductive functioning. Intense physical training by gymnasts, ballet dancers, or runners can lead to a delay in menarche or to anovulatory cycles in women already past menarche (Dale, Gerlach, & Wilhite 1979; Frisch, Wyshak, & Vincent 1980).

Surbey (1990), studying a large sample in Ontario, found that girls who experienced absence of father or of both parents prior to menarche reached puberty 4–5 months sooner than girls in biparental families. There were no differences in terms of family size, birth order, socioeconomic status, body weight, or height between girls in biparental families versus girls in father-absent families. Girls with stepfathers matured two months sooner than other girls. This result supports the novel-male result with tamarins. Girls whose fathers were absent *after* 10 years of age did not differ in age of menarche from biparental girls. Mothers and daughters were highly correlated in age of menarche. The number of stressful life events was negatively correlated with age of menarche, but when stress was removed by partial correlation there was still a significant effect of years with father. Thus, maternal age of menarche, years of contact with father, and stressful life events each affect the age of puberty in girls. Gerra and colleagues (1993) found lower basal luteinizing hormone levels in adolescent girls from divorced families compared with girls in intact families. After exercise stress, girls from divorced families had lower responses of growth hormone and prolactin, suggesting other hormonal disorders in children of single-parent families.

AFFILIATION, BONDING, AND COURTSHIP

Although sexual behavior and parental care have been well studied, the precursors of courtship and pair bonding have rarely been studied (but see Carter 1998). In many species sexual contact is relatively brief, but in humans (and in several other socially monogamous or cooperatively breeding species) there is a long-term relationship established between mates. Such bonds can be evaluated by several methods: brief separations and reunions to see if affiliation is increased on reunions, intruder challenges when same-sex and opposite-sex intruders are presented, and tests to choose between one's mate and another individual. These types of tests have been used to evaluate a mother–infant bond but less often to study the relationship between a pair of adults.

Recently, there has been increased interest in the hormonal correlates of pair bonding and affiliation. One influence is the finding that female prairie voles, a monogamous species showing strong pair bonds, have increased oxytocin levels following the extensive vaginal cervical stimulation resulting from mating. After a prolonged mating bout, females have formed strong partner preferences. Intracerebral injections of oxytocin can facilitate pair-bond formation in female voles, and administration of oxytocin inhibitors can block pair formation (Carter 1998).

In male voles, vasopressin administration influences partner choice and also leads to increased levels of territory defense and mate guarding. Preliminary evidence shows that increased levels of vasopressin may influence parental care in male prairie voles (Wang & Insel 1996). The distribution of vasopressin receptor sites in the brain differs between monogamous and polygynous species of voles, and similar differences as a function of breeding system are found in the distribution of oxytocin receptors in female voles (Wang & Insel 1996).

Adrenal steroid levels (corticosterone) are higher in monogamous voles than in polygynous voles (Carter 1998), and oxytocin reduces levels of adrenal steroids in both rodents and humans (Carter & Altemus 1997); this suggests that one consequence of pair bonding is reduction of stress hormones (Carter 1998). Relatively little is known about the hormonal basis of pair bonding in nonhuman and human primates. However, in the monogamous titi monkey, Mendoza and Mason (1997) found that (i) pairs spend much time in physical contact and (ii) adrenal hormones rise to very high levels when pair mates are separated and return to normal levels at pair reunion. Little is known about the role of oxytocin and vasopressin in primates, but Wang et al. (1997) found fibers in the brains of common marmosets – monogamous primates – that show distributions of reactivity to vasopressin and oxytocin similar to those in monogamous voles. Future research using minimally invasive methods is needed to evaluate the importance of oxytocin and vasopressin on pair bonding in primates.

SEXUAL BEHAVIOR AND CHANGES OVER THE MENSTRUAL CYCLE
Role of Hormones in Sexual Behavior

Reproductive hormones appear to be important for copulatory behavior in many species. Removal of gonads prior to puberty may produce a failure to express sexual behavior, and removal of gonads after puberty can also reduce or eliminate sexual activity. Yet in primates (both human and nonhuman), sexual arousal and sexual behavior may continue for years after castration. Although testes size decreases and testosterone levels decline in men over 60, men over 80 can be sexually active. Correlations between testosterone and sexual activity are weak (Carter 1992). Males who are hypogonadal due to Kallman's syndrome (a deficiency of gonadotropin releasing hormone) have very low testosterone levels and do not experience puberty without hormonal supplementation; they also show low interest in sex, low sexual activity, and few nocturnal erections or emissions. When testosterone is administered, sexual interest does not appear within a year of injections. Although testosterone is not essential for sexual activity or interest, reduced testosterone levels generally correlate with lower sexual activity. Both surgical castration and administration of the antiandrogen cyproterone acetate (CPA) can reduce sexually directed aggression in male sex offenders (Bradford 1988). Low rates of recidivism occur after CPA administration, and Bradford (1988) argued that consensual adult heterosexual relations are not affected by CPA.

Removal of ovaries or menopause can reduce sexual activity, but the effects may be indirect because estrogen influences vaginal lubrication. In general, little is known about the effects of reproductive steroids on female sexuality (Carter 1992).

Carter (1992) suggested that oxytocin be considered in future studies of sexual behavior. Oxytocin is released during the contractions of the orgasmic response in humans of both sexes and during ejaculation in other species. Steroids, particularly estrogen and testosterone, can modulate oxytocin binding and release in the brain. Stimulation of breasts and other parts of the body during foreplay also releases oxytocin. Oxytocin may play a role in sexual satiation, in sperm transport into the uterus, and in promoting social bond formation in humans as it does in other species (Carter 1998). Simple physical contact can lead to increased oxytocin release correlated with feelings of well-being (Uvnas-Moberg 1997).

Changes in Behavior over the Ovarian Cycle

In many species, females communicate their ovulatory status by showing swellings of the genitals (chimpanzees, baboons) or marked changes in behavior (hamsters, rats, cats). However, in several monogamous species – including humans – physical or behavioral evidence of ovulation is not evident. This "concealed ovulation" has been described as adaptive for females of species that need to co-opt fathers for infant caretaking (Burley 1979). Traditional theory has held that male mammals will have greatest reproductive success by mating with as many females as possible and deserting them before infants are born. Female mammals with greater parental certainty and the obligatory costs of gestation and lactation can easily be stuck with infant care – so long as mothers can successfully rear infants alone (see Snowdon 1997 for a summary and an alternative view). Monogamous and cooperatively breeding species typically require helpers in addition to mothers to rear infants successfully, and concealed ovulation represents a way to "trick" males into staying long enough to engage in infant care. If the female is continuously receptive to copulation and conceals ovulation, males never know when a female becomes pregnant.

Two lines of evidence counter the idea of concealed ovulation. First, ovulation may be concealed from scientists but not from males of the species involved. In the monogamous cotton-top tamarin, Ziegler and associates (1993) transferred odors from ovulating females each day to recipient pairs. On the day of the donor female's ovulation, her scent induced higher rates of male erection and mounting of his own partner than did the donor female's scent from the remaining days of her cycle. In the pygmy marmoset, Converse and colleagues (1995) showed elevated rates of male olfactory interest in females at the time of ovulation. Females were also less aggressive toward their mates, suggesting a greater willingness to copulate at ovulation (although copulations do occur throughout the cycle).

In polygynous species, where sexual behavior is expected to be more under hormonal control, several studies have reported copulations throughout the female cycle. However, mating depends on whether the female is able to control or pace sexual behavior. When captive monkeys and apes are paired within a small area, one observes rates of copulation higher than seen in the wild, and copulation occurs over the entire ovulatory cycle. When females are given control over whether to allow sexual access by males, copulation rates are much lower and more tightly linked to the time of ovulation (Graham & Nadler 1990). Moreover, cage size affects the timing of mating patterns. Wallen (1990) reported lower levels of mating as well as mating more tightly linked to ovulation in large environments, where presumably the female has more control over mating. In rats there is evidence that female-paced matings are different from those where females cannot control mating (McClintock 1984).

Female hormonal state is critical for sexual behavior and for social integration of rhesus monkey males into a group. Wallen and Tannenbaum (1997) found that females initiated proximity to males and groomed males only during the time of peak estradiol levels, times when ejaculations were most likely. They introduced ten adolescent males to a group of six ovariectomized adult females and found, over a period of 2.5 years, no social interactions between males and females. Females were then injected with estradiol and within a weekend were grooming and mating with the males. Affiliation with males remained high even after hormonal therapy was stopped. In a follow-up study, Tannenbaum and Wallen (1997) reported that novel males were more easily integrated into a female group during the breeding season (when female estrogen levels are high) than in the nonbreeding season. Elevated estrogen facilitates social interactions with and social integration of males into macaque groups.

Wallen (1990) distinguished between desire and ability, and he noted that nonhuman primate females can mate independent of hormonal state. Thus, only female initiations of sexual activity are valid indices of motivation. Pfaus (1996) made a similar point with respect to human sexual behavior. The consummatory act of copulation must be carefully distinguished from the appetitive phase, and the appetitive phase must be clearly differentiated according to which partner initiates. Tremendous effort has been expended to determine whether humans have concealed ovulation and whether sexual initiation or enjoyment changes with the ovarian cycle. Several problems have been identified in conducting such studies. Women who were told the purpose of a study – examining changes in sexual behavior over the cycle – reported high levels of arousal shortly before menstruation, whereas those uninformed about the goals of the study reported greater enjoyment close to ovulation (Englander-Golden et al. 1980). One study measured urinary luteinizing hormone to determine ovulation and found an increase in sexual activity at ovulation. Subsequently, the authors had to change their conclusions when the LH was divided by creatinine to control for differences in urine volume (Hedricks, Schramm, & Udry 1994).

A careful study of sexual behavior over the ovulatory cycle must: (1) eliminate subjects using oral contraception, since oral contraceptives inhibit the cyclic fluctuations of ovarian hormones; (2) be aware that fear of pregnancy due to contraceptive failure may alter sexual patterns; and (3) distinguish clearly between which partner initiated sex and between initiation and acceptance of copulation. Furthermore, initiation (representing the appetitive or desire phase) must be clearly distinguished from enjoyment (the consummatory phase). Mateo and Rissman (1984) avoided some of these problems by studying lesbians, where contraceptives were not necessary and fear of conception was unlikely to be a factor. They found a significant increase in sexual initiations and orgasms by both partners at midcycle, although ovulation was not determined.

Some studies suggest that testosterone may be important in female sexual responses. Morris and associates (1987) reported a midcycle increase in testosterone that correlated with the frequency of sexual initiation. Sherwin, Gelfand, and Brender (1985) – in a study of premenopausal women with ovariectomies – found that administration of testosterone increased sexual desire, arousal, and frequency of sexual fantasies, whereas administration of estrogen and progesterone did not.

There are many interesting questions concerning the role of reproductive hormones on female sexual desire and responsiveness, and there are few studies concerning whether humans conceal ovulation. Careful attention to the conceptual distinctions raised in the animal literature, coupled with use of hormonal assays to determine when ovulation really occurs (rather than simply inferring ovulation from menstruation), should lead to appropriate future research on human sexual behavior.

Menstrual Synchrony

Menstrual cycle synchrony has been demonstrated in women who are close friends living in a college dormitory (McClintock 1971). More recent studies have implicated the factors of close bonding or friendship, as well as time spent together, as affecting cycle synchrony (Goldman & Schneider 1987; Weller & Weller 1993, 1995).

Looking at menstrual synchrony under optimal conditions, Weller and Weller (1997) studied Bedouin women living in Israel. In Bedouin families, women live together in close quarters and often share sleeping quarters. The society is sexually segregated, with little contact between sexes. Housing conditions are similar across all subjects and there is little use of oral contraceptives. Under these conditions, there was strong evidence of menstrual synchrony among all women in the family, among sisters who shared the same sleeping quarters, and among those who were close friends; however, there was no correlation between the degree of synchrony and either time spent together or degree of friendship.

McClintock (1971, 1984) suggested that olfactory cues provide the most plausible mechanisms for menstrual synchrony. Olfactory chemical cues from men can also affect the length of ovarian cycles. Axillary secretions of men have been shown to reduce the variability in menstrual cycle lengths in women. Women's axillary secretions were found to synchronize the onset of the menstrual cycle in recipient women (Preti et al. 1986), and women show increased sensitivity to certain odors at ovulation (Le Magnen 1952).

The effects found even in an optimal study (like that of the Bedouin women) are small: a 20%–25% shift toward synchrony from random expectations. Menstruation is easy to document, and it is used as a substitute for ovulation. But since ovulation has not been measured directly and because there is likely to be variation among women in when they ovulate relative to menstruation, the next generation of studies should measure whether there is ovulatory rather than menstrual synchrony. There are several functional explanations for synchrony based on polygamous mating in species like rats, sheep, other ungulates, and polygynous primates where females can control mate choice through synchronous ovulation, but these explanations do not seem useful for explaining synchrony within families (Weller & Weller 1997). Menstrual synchrony in humans remains an intriguing phenomenon in search of a function.

Ovarian Hormones and Stress

There is evidence that physiological responses to stress are modulated by ovarian hormones. A study of premenopausal and postmenopausal middle-aged women found that postmenopausal women showed increases over baseline in heart rate during three stress tasks as well as increased systolic blood pressure in one of the tasks (Saab, Stoney, & McDonald 1989). A similar study of pregnant versus nonpregnant women found reduced diastolic blood pressure in response to serial subtraction, mirror image tracing, and isotonic hand-grip tasks in pregnant women compared with their prepregnant responses and compared with a nonpregnant control group (Matthews & Rodin 1992). The increased ovarian hormones of pregnancy and of premenopausal compared with postmenopausal women are likely to be involved in modulating the stress response. However, a study by some of the same authors looking at the performance of women in stress tests over the menstrual cycle found no effects of menstrual cycle on heart rate or blood pressure responses (Stoney et al. 1990).

PARENTAL CARE
Maternal Care

There is an extensive literature on the mechanisms of maternal care in a variety of species (Rosenblatt 1992; Rosenblatt & Snowdon 1996). Rosenblatt (1992) described three distinct patterns of maternal behavior in mammals as follows.

1. *Nesting* – where infants may be left on their own for various periods of time while mothers forage and return intermittently to provide food. This is found in many rodents, many carnivores, and some prosimians.
2. *Leader–follower* – where infants are highly precocial and must follow mothers within a few hours after birth. This pattern is found among ungulates.
3. *Clinging–carrying* – found in marsupials and many primates. In the absence of a pouch, nonmarsupial infants must have motor skills to hold on to mothers during rapid locomotion.

Conceptually, it is important to distinguish between the onset and the maintenance of maternal care. The onset of maternal care appears to be influenced by the hormones of pregnancy and parturition. Thus, progesterone and estrogen are present at high levels through pregnancy and progesterone declines just before parturition, leading to increased levels of prolactin (to prepare the mammary tissue) and oxytocin, which stimulates uterine contractions and the milk let-down response from the nipple. Each of these hormones has been demonstrated to be involved in controlling the onset of maternal behavior, though the patterns and effects often vary across species.

Because estrogen, progesterone, and oxytocin levels drop before parturition, it appears that maternal behavior is maintained by stimuli from the infant rather than by any hormonal mechanism. Olfactory, auditory, and visual cues, nipple stimulation, and tactile contact with infants are all important stimuli for maintaining maternal care. Rabbits nurse infants only once a day, but even this brief nursing contact appears essential early in lactation to maintain maternal behavior. In sheep, where infants must follow mothers, oxytocin levels producing uterine contractions at parturition appear critical for forming a bond between mother and infant and facilitating maternal recognition of her infant based on its odors.

Surprisingly little evidence is available on the mechanisms influencing maternal behavior in primates. Pryce and colleagues (1988) showed (in red-bellied tamarins) that the quality of infant care shown by first-time mothers was dependent upon the levels of estrogen in late pregnancy. In females showing the normal pattern of elevated estrogen through the end of pregnancy, maternal care was adequate, but in females with reduced levels of estrogen prior to birth, maternal care was poor. These mothers seemed to be fearful and rejected their infants. For mothers with ex-

tensive infant care experience, on the other hand, there was no relationship between estrogen levels in late pregnancy and maternal quality. Pryce, Doebeli, and Martin (1993) found that treatment of nulliparous common marmosets with the hormones of late pregnancy (progesterone and estrogen) increased motivation toward infant care. Marmosets and tamarins often require experience with caring for someone else's infants in order to be competent parents, but there is still a high level of poor parental care, especially with first-born infants (see Snowdon 1996 for review). Pryce (1996) developed a motivational model that integrates social learning, maternal experience, hormonal changes, and infant stimuli as factors in maternal care. Infant stimuli can elicit attraction, aversion, anxiety, and neophobia, with negative motivational states being high in females without prior infant experience. Preadult infant care experience changes the valence of infant stimuli toward more positive motivational states. Furthermore, hormonal changes in late pregnancy (e.g., high levels of progesterone, estrogen, and prolactin) also lead to increased attraction to infant stimuli coupled with increased anxiety responses to infant crying. With the reinforcement that results from direct contact with infants and with learning which behaviors reduce crying, long-term memories are formed that make a mother less dependent on hormonal stimuli with successive infants.

This model, coupled with cognition about one's own infant, may apply to human mothers as well (Corter & Fleming 1990). Pregnancy does not make women more interested in other people's babies, and first-time mothers report less responsiveness to their own fetus – especially early in pregnancy – compared with experienced mothers. Many mothers showed the greatest responsiveness to infant stimuli and learned to discriminate their infant from others within a short period after parturition, suggesting that the hormones of late pregnancy play only an indirect role. Experienced mothers were more responsive to infant cries than first-time mothers, but only outside the period of postpartum hormonal changes (Corter & Fleming 1990). Fleming and associates (1997) found in both longitudinal and cross-sectional studies that feelings of nurturance grew during pregnancy and increased after parturition. These changes were not directly related to changes in pregnancy hormones, but the estrogen/progesterone ratio in late pregnancy did predict postpartum attachment. Women with low attachment had higher estrogen/progesterone ratios during weeks 20–35 of pregnancy than did women with high infant attachment, although there were no hormonal differences between these two groups at the end of pregnancy or postpartum. Both estrogen and progesterone serve to prime prolactin secretion. Fleming (1990) reported a significant positive correlation between cortisol levels before or after nursing and the amount of affectionate interactions with infants. She speculated that cortisol may arouse the mother, making her more attentive to cues from the infant, and that cortisol may lead mothers to recognize infant odors and vocalizations more readily, leading to stronger bonding.

One hormone that logically should be important in maternal behavior is prolactin, but there are few studies of prolactin levels and maternal care in human or nonhuman primates. Fleming (1990) reported that breast-feeding mothers (who should have higher prolactin levels) showed more affection toward infants, left the infants alone less often, and responded more contingently to infants than did mothers who bottle-fed infants. Warren and Shortle (1990) reported an increase in maternal responsiveness correlated with prolactin levels, and they found that prolactin levels in women increased with successive births. In cotton-top tamarins, we found that prolactin levels during the two weeks before parturition predicted the amount of infant care shown by females postpartum (S. Saini, C. T. Snowdon, & T. E. Ziegler, unpublished data). Tamarin mothers can control the time of their next ovulation through how they nurse. Mothers who tended to nurse both twins simultaneously ovulated significantly sooner after parturition than mothers who tended to nurse their twins sequentially (Ziegler et al. 1990).

Nonmaternal Infant Care

In many species that are socially monogamous, fathers and older siblings play important roles in infant care and often are necessary for the survival of infants (Savage et al. 1997; Snowdon 1996). Monogamy is generally thought to result when maternal effort is not sufficient to rear infants successfully, especially during extreme variations in temperature or food availability. Species where older siblings delay their own reproduction to assist in the care of younger siblings are described as cooperative breeders. The social structure of most human families is socially monogamous, so examination of the mechanisms leading to infant care by nonmaternal group members in birds and mammals has direct relevance to human parental care systems.

Ziegler (in press) reviewed studies on socially monogamous and cooperatively breeding birds, rodents, and primates, and she found several common themes. Prolactin levels are elevated in caregivers, both biological parents and nonreproductive helpers, in cooperatively breeding birds and primates. In female mammals, maternal hormones and stimuli from the infant appear to influence maternal care and prolactin levels, whereas in males stimuli from the pregnant female and from infants appear to be important.

Dixson and George (1982) reported that common marmoset males had elevated prolactin levels when caring for infants. We measured urinary prolactin before and after the birth of infants in male cotton-top tamarins. Fathers had significantly higher prolactin levels than nonfathers, and experienced fathers had higher prolactin levels than first-time fathers or sons who assist in infant care. The prolactin levels of first-time fathers and of sons were elevated over males paired with nonpregnant females. There was a highly significant correlation ($r = 0.92$) between the number of births a father had experienced and his prolactin levels. But there was no correlation with the amount of infant care behavior shown, since experienced fathers also had helpers available to care for infants. Nursing mothers also had postpartum prolactin levels similar to fathers, whereas mothers with miscarriages or infant deaths showed declining prolactin levels by the third week postpartum. Surprisingly, both first-time and experienced fathers had elevated prolactin levels in the weeks before their mates gave birth, suggesting that some communication between mates occurs during pregnancy to prepare males for infant care (Ziegler, Wegner, & Snowdon 1996b; Ziegler in press).

Ziegler (in press) noted a reciprocal relationship between testosterone and prolactin in many species. Males that care for infants have low testosterone levels while prolactin levels are elevated. Preliminary data (F. B. Bercovitch, personal communication) show that rhesus monkeys who rarely show direct paternal care – but who do tolerate infants – had high levels of testosterone in the mating season but low levels of testosterone with higher prolactin levels in the birth season. Further research on the role of prolactin and testosterone in other species of male primates, especially in human fathers, is critical.

AGGRESSION AND DOMINANCE

Aggression and dominance behaviors are commonly thought to be more typical of males than females and thus under the influence of testosterone. However, the importance and role of testosterone in human aggression is controversial. There have been several typologies that distinguish among different functional aspects of aggression, with the broadest distinction being between offensive aggression or dominance (thought to be under the control of testosterone) and defensive aggression (which is not linked with testosterone).

Albert, Walsh, and Jonik (1993) argued that testosterone is directly involved with offensive aggression in nonhuman species, yet after reviewing several hundred studies they concluded that there are no consistent differences in testosterone levels between men who exhibit high versus low aggressiveness. Abnormal states such as hypogonadism or castration in men or hirsutism in females (where testosterone levels may be 200% above normal female levels) show neither increases of offensive aggression with increased testosterone nor decreased aggression with decreased testosterone. Albert et al. (1993) concluded that there are many similarities between defensive aggression in humans and that displayed by nonhuman species, where mechanisms other than testosterone appear to be similar across species. However, most studies have not been done over long periods of time. More recent studies that cover longer time periods do show effects of hormone levels on aggression. Users of anabolic androgenic steroids showed higher levels of verbal aggression, indirect aggression, and impulsiveness than controls (Galligani, Renek, & Hansen 1996). Although this study contradicts Albert et al. (1993), there were no data on these users prior to steroid use. Those likely to use steroids may already be more aggressive and impulsive.

Mazur and Booth (1998) reached the opposite conclusion. They argued that a single measure of testosterone can predict dominant or antisocial aggressive behaviors. The anticipation of competition leads to increases in testosterone, and after competition testosterone increases in winners and decreases in losers. Mazur and Booth (1998) developed a reciprocal model where testosterone levels vary as a function of the cumulative dominance interactions a man experiences along with his history of winning and losing, with testosterone being both a cause and a consequence of dominance interactions. This is an intriguing model that can only be evaluated by longitudinal studies with adequate sample sizes. One longitudinal study of more than 4,000 U.S. Air Force veterans found small but statistically significant negative correlations between testosterone and both education and income. Men with higher testosterone levels were more likely to be arrested for traffic violations and theft. Most interesting was an increase in testosterone just before and after a divorce and a decrease in testosterone with marriage (Mazur & Booth 1998). Even though the correlations were significant, they were quite low and explained a small amount of variance.

Two sources of evidence question a simple model relating testosterone to offensive aggression. First, several studies of nonhuman species indicate that aggression is influenced by social, environmental, and cognitive variables. Second, there is increasing evidence (with human and nonhuman species) of dominance and offensive aggression by females that cannot easily be explained by testosterone.

Testing conditions often influence the outcome of contests. Castrated male woodrats fight as vigorously as intact males when tested in neutral arenas (Caldwell, Glickman, & Smith 1984); castrated mice with no previous fighting experience do poorly, but males castrated after experiencing fights show normal levels of aggression (Scott & Fredericson 1951). As we have noted, Wallen (1996) concluded that most aggressive behaviors (with the exception of rough-and-tumble play, which is under androgenic influence) are primarily influenced by social variables. Thus, even in nonhuman males, social and environmental variables are at least as important as hormones.

Recent data question our common assumptions about sex differences in offensive aggression. Because it has been assumed that there was little variance in female reproductive success but high variance in male success, offensive aggression was thought to benefit males more than females.

There are species of cooperatively breeding mammals where only one or two females reproduce while the remaining females do not. In one of these species, the golden lion tamarin, two independent studies have found high levels of sex-specific aggression. Male–male aggression was as common as female–female aggression, but the latter was often lethal whereas the former was not (Inglett et al. 1989; Kleiman 1979). De Waal (1982) described sex differences in aggression among chimpanzees. Males frequently engaged in dominance interactions but were readily reconciled after fighting. Females engaged in aggressive interactions much less often, but when they did fight were less likely to reconcile and more likely to harm each other. An analysis of long-term field data shows that dominant female chimpanzees have greater lifetime reproductive success – with more total offspring and with daughters reaching reproductive age earlier than daughters of subordinate females (Pusey, Williams, & Goodall 1997). Thus, for tamarin and chimpanzee females, dominance contests are of critical importance. In some species, females are dominant to males (hamsters, Floody 1983; spotted hyenas, Frank 1986).

An epidemiological study of human couples found that females were more likely to initiate aggression than males. Magdol et al. (1997) studied all members of the 1972 birth cohort in a city in New Zealand at age 21. Of the women, 37% reported initiating aggression in the home compared with 22% of the men. Severe aggression was initiated by 18.6% of the women but by only 5.7% of the men. Men who committed severe aggression were more likely to be deviant on social and mental health measures, whereas highly aggressive women were psychologically normal. This study contradicts popular beliefs about human aggression, and it is unbiased – sampling an entire birth cohort in a population rather than using court or hospital records. The authors explained the results in terms of social norms. Men are reared to avoid being aggressive toward females and know they are more likely to be prosecuted if they do act aggressively. Women do not have these constraints and will be held less accountable by society and the legal system. Although this study suggests that aggression is an "equal opportunity" behavior within the home that cannot be explained simply by testosterone, there is little evidence that women are as aggressive as men outside the family. In general, though, aggressive behavior is most likely the product of social, developmental, environmental, and cognitive variables interacting with hormones.

EFFECTS OF HORMONES ON COGNITION

There has been considerable controversy concerning the degree to which there are gender differences in cognition, with meta-analyses of a large number of studies generally reporting small effect sizes for both verbal ability (Hyde & Linn 1988) and mathematical ability (Hyde, Fennema, & Lamon 1990). Nonetheless, there are some specific sex differences where the effects, though small, appear to be consistent (Hampson & Kimura 1992). Women tend to do better in tests of verbal abilities, perceptual speed and accuracy, and fine motor tasks, whereas males do better on spatial abilities, quantitative abilities, and tests of physical strength. Hampson and Kimura (1992) reported that left-hemisphere brain damage has a more devastating effect on verbal IQ in men than in women, suggesting possible sex differences in lateralization. Women perform better on tests of spatial ability at menstruation, when estrogen and progesterone levels are low, compared with performance at the time of ovulation, when hormonal levels are high (Hampson & Kimura 1992). Verbal tasks that involve reading lists, counting, or repeating syllables tend to show higher levels of performance at ovulation than at other times in the cycle. There were very small menstrual cycle effects on more complex verbal tasks (Hampson & Kimura 1992).

Studies of variation over the menstrual cycle test activational effects of hormones on performance but do not evaluate possible organizational effects. Hines and Sandberg (1996) studied women exposed to diethylstilbestrol during fetal development and found no differences between them and their untreated sisters on measures of verbal fluency, perceptual speed, or associative memory.

Estrogen levels influence synaptic connections in the hippocampus, the brain area associated with formation of memory. Sherwin (see Wickelgren 1997) found that women being treated with an estrogen blocker to suppress fibroid tumors showed a decrease in verbal intelligence and also found improvement in women treated with estrogen compared with those taking a placebo. A few early trials with Alzheimer's patients show improvements in verbal memory and attention with estrogen administration (Wickelgren 1997). Studies of postmenopausal women with or without estrogen replacement therapy have shown that estrogen facilitates verbal memory but has no effect on visuospatial memory (Sherwin 1997). Girls with congenital adrenal hyperplasia (which produces elevated testosterone) have lower verbal IQ but higher visuospatial performance than control girls (Sherwin 1997). In most of these studies, the effects are relatively small but still suggestive that estrogen may facilitate verbal memory and that estrogen replacement therapy might be therapeutic in preventing or delaying the effects of Alzheimer's disease.

Inferential Context

Many methods can be used to determine hormone concentrations. Likewise, there are several types of samples that can be collected from the participant. Any body fluid will contain hormones, although not all hormones will be found in every type of body fluid. Hormones are released from the glands into the circulatory system, where they can contact any tissue in the body. Hormones may be measured in blood, saliva, ventricles of the brain, cerebral spinal fluid, scent secretions, urine, and feces. Selecting the type of body fluid to collect depends on the nature of the questions to be addressed, the type of invasiveness that is permissible, the location of the individual (e.g., out-of-the-way areas vs. hospitals) and how frequently samples are needed (daily vs. weekly). There are advantages and disadvantages to each type of body fluid used. For example, steroids are very small molecules and can therefore be found in any body fluid. Steroids can diffuse through cellular membranes and through tight junctions between cells, provided they are not conjugated. Protein hormones, however, are much larger molecules and cannot diffuse between cells. Therefore, measurements of the protein hormones are limited to blood and urine or in brain fluids, where they are released. The advantages and disadvantages of using blood, saliva, urine, or feces will be described next.

BLOOD

Advantages. Measurement of hormone levels in the blood of animals and humans has been the most routine method used. Blood levels have been recorded for the majority of hormones for men and women and are run routinely in hospital and research laboratories. Normative blood values for humans are known for most hormones. Samples can be collected throughout the day if there is a need to understand the changes in circulating hormones. All other methods of hormone measurement are usually compared with the pattern and levels of circulating hormones. Circulating hormones will reflect rapid changes in hormones in response to a stimulus, whereas other measurements may be delayed relative to timing in blood. For instance, circulating cortisol will increase within minutes in response to an acute stressor such as capture and restraint.

Disadvantages. Measurement of circulating hormones requires venipuncture and needles. In small animals or human infants, venipuncture may cause undue stress. Blood samples give a point level of the hormone at the time of collection of the sample. Some hormones fluctuate considerably in the blood (owing to differential release systems) or have diurnal rhythms that will change the hormone level. For instance, prolactin levels in the blood are known to change within minutes in response to factors such as sleep, exercise, stress, and sexual interactions. A cortisol response to social stressors, which influence cortisol changes over time, may best be seen in samples (e.g., urine or feces) that likewise accumulate the steroid over time. In small organisms, repeated blood sampling can deplete red blood cells.

SALIVA

Advantages. Saliva samples can be collected noninvasively on cooperating animals and humans without any restraint. Noninvasive sampling eliminates some of the ethical issues relating to studies directed at various age groups, infants and the elderly, and the handicapped (physically and mentally). The concentrations of steroids in saliva may correlate directly with the free levels of circulating steroids. Samples can be taken daily or more frequently without physical effects on the subject.

Disadvantages. Protein hormones are not found in saliva, which limits measurement to steroid hormones. Most saliva steroid levels represent the free portion of circulating steroids and not total levels (a proportion of circulating steroids can be bound to specific or nonspecific blood proteins and thus is not available for binding to receptors). Enzymes within the saliva can metabolize steroids, changing their structure and hence our ability to measure them. Additionally, bacteria within the oral cavity can metabolize the steroids. False high values can occur if small amounts of blood enter the oral cavity due to lesions in the mouth. Conjugated steroids such as dihydroepiandrosterone cannot be measured in saliva, since the conjugates will not filter into the saliva.

URINE

Advantages. Steroids, protein hormones, catecholamines, and neuropeptides can be found in the urine. Their levels will reflect an accumulation over time, since hormones are filtered by the kidneys and stored in the bladder until urination. First morning void urine provides a concentrated sample that may represent an overnight accumulation. Collection procedures can be noninvasive and can be performed daily. Indexing with creatinine levels controls for variability in fluid excreted. Any disease-related alterations in hormone metabolism can be monitored in the urine. Steroid hormones are usually found in very high amounts in the urine owing to the accumulation over time.

Disadvantages. Many of the hormones may be metabolized by the liver prior to excretion into the urine, so metabolites must be identified that accurately reflect the circulating hormones. Many of the steroid hormones are conjugated to glucuronides and sulfates prior to excretion. In this form, the steroids are unmeasurable by most antibodies and must be liberated prior to analysis. Some of the protein hormones have a short half-life and therefore small levels may appear in the urine. For example, prolactin has a half-life of 12 min whereas LH has a half-life of 45 min (Yen & Jaffe 1978). Peak levels of hormones (such as the LH peak) found in the blood may be found the following day in the urine. Samples may need the addition of stabilizers such as glycerol before freezing to protect the protein hormones.

FECES

Advantages. Feces may be collected freely from free-ranging organisms where close contact is not possible. Steroid levels are found in large amounts in the feces. The fecal excretion of steroids reflects an accumulation over time and therefore adjusts for fluctuations in the hormones throughout the day.

Disadvantages. Most steroids are metabolized into many different steroids prior to excretion into the feces. The liver conjugates many of the steroids prior to release into the intestines. Some steroids, such as estradiol, are highly conjugated and may recirculate before being fully excreted. No protein hormones or catecholamines can be measured in the feces.

METABOLISM OF STEROIDS AND ANALYSES

The measurement of steroids in the blood has been thought to be fairly straightforward, and it should represent the pure steroids released from the endocrine glands. However, recent research has shown that some steroids, such as estradiol and estrone, can be conjugated quickly after release into the circulation and interconverted (Ruoff & Dziuk 1994). A majority of estradiol can be converted to estrone and its conjugates within 5 min of its release (Ruoff & Dziuk 1994). Therefore, the measurement of pure steroids in circulation may not always accurately assess the total amount of steroid unless conjugated steroids are also measured. Women and some primate species (e.g., the common marmoset) have very high levels of estrone sulfite in circulation throughout the ovarian cycle (Harlow, Hearn, & Hodges 1984; Nunez et al. 1977).

Steroid metabolites are a result of conversions of circulating steroids in the liver, although the stomach, intestines, and some peripheral tissues can also metabolize steroids. The liver filters the steroids from the blood and inactivates them by conjugation. Conjugation is the process by which sulfate esters or glucuronates are attached to the steroid, primarily by reduction of the A-ring double bond and the 3-keto group. The addition of sulfate or glucuronide acids renders the steroids water-soluble, whence they can be removed from circulation by kidney filtration or released into the intestines by bile. Conjugation can be simple (e.g. monoconjugates) or complex, as with di- or triconjugates consisting of both glucuronides and sulfates.

When measuring steroids by an immune reaction (as in RIAs or EIAs), the antibody does not always recognize the steroid in its conjugated form (Hodges & Eastman 1984). Direct assays sometimes use antibodies that measure the steroid conjugated to a single glucuronide or sulfate but do not recognize the steroid when it is di- or triconjugated. It therefore becomes necessary to break the steroid apart from its conjugates before measuring by antibody–antigen reaction. Without determining the level of conjugation, measurements of the steroid may be underestimated. Since the level of conjugation may also change during different phases of the ovarian cycle and pregnancy (Hodges &

Eastman 1984), measurement of total steroid can provide a more complete profile of the steroids during functional changes.

A technique called "sequential hydrolysis and solvolysis" is a method that allows for the separation of free steroids and those that are conjugated to simple or complex conjugates (Ziegler et al. 1996a). This method first extracts the free steroids by ether extraction. The remaining fluid is then subjected to hydrolysis by beta-glucuronidase in order to break the simple glucuronides and sulfates in an overnight incubation. The newly liberated steroids are then extracted from the aqueous solution. The remaining solution is then subjected to solvolysis with ethyl acetate in an acid environment. The steroids of interest from the three extractions are then measured, and the proportion of steroid found in each fraction can be determined. Those steroids that are found primarily as free steroids can be measured directly. For steroids found primarily as simple conjugates, direct assay may be performed with antibodies that measure steroids conjugated to a sulfate or glucuronide. When steroids are found as complex conjugates, solvolysis will be needed before the steroid can be measured.

There are several ways to determine which steroid metabolites represent the excreted steroid from the endocrine gland. One of the most informative methods uses radiolabeled steroids injected into an animal; urine and feces are collected for the next five days until all the radioactivity has been eliminated (Ziegler et al. 1989). In this manner, the proportion of steroids that are excreted into the urine and feces can be determined. Through high-pressure liquid chromatography (HPLC) analysis, the actual steroids and their metabolites can be identified. When injecting labeled hormones is not possible, the injection of pure steroid (unlabeled) can be performed. With this technique, the steroid can be injected into the organism of interest; urine and/or feces are collected before and following the injection. The HPLC separation and analysis can reveal which steroid metabolites were elevated after the injection and so identify those steroids metabolized from the injected steroid. If neither of the foregoing techniques is feasible and no invasive injections are possible, then HPLC separation and ultraviolet detection of the steroids found in the sample can provide information on the most appropriate metabolites to measure. For example, HPLC separation and analysis determined that cortisol appeared in the urine of cotton-top tamarins as cortisol and cortisone, both of which are measurable by the same antibody (Ziegler, Scheffler, & Snowdon 1995).

Epilogue and Future Directions

The study of reproductive hormones should become an important part of psychophysiology. The interplay between psychology and physiology is clear in the topics discussed here: sex role development, social regulation of puberty and fertility, courtship, affiliation, sexual behavior, parental care, aggression, and cognition. Several directions for future research emerge.

1. There is currently considerable controversy about how to rear children with hormonal anomalies that lead to ambiguous genitalia. More long-term research is needed on the consequences of surgical "correction" (coupled with hormonal therapy) used to provide concordance with genetic sex and on the environmental, social, and hormonal variables that affect gender identity. Surgical correction of genital anatomy is a drastic procedure with long-term consequences, and long-term hormonal therapy can have a variety of health-related consequences, so it is important to have a solid psychophysiological basis on which to make these decisions.

2. There are a few studies that demonstrate differences in age of menarche as a function of family demography and stressful family events, but there is some disagreement over whether it is the absence of a father per se or rather the stressful event of losing a parent through death or divorce that influence the onset of puberty. The finding of a correlation between age of menarche in mothers and daughters suggests a genetic component to the age of puberty that may covary with family demography if, say, early-menarche females are more prone to divorce. We have little data on the social and hormonal consequences to girls reared by their fathers, and these data will be critical in assessing the mechanisms of early menarche. We know of no data on how family structure or family dynamics affect puberty in boys, and there are no models of nonhuman animals to guide hypothesis development.

3. Until recently, much attention has been focused on aggressive behavior with little attention given to processes of affiliation or pair bonding. Studies of nonhuman animals showing that neuropeptides like oxytocin and vasopressin are involved in pair bonding and partner preference (perhaps in direct response to tactile stimulation that results from courtship and copulatory behavior) raise exciting possibilities. Although it is unlikely that hormonal effects would override social and environmental aspects of mate choice and pair bonding in human and nonhuman primates, these peptides may play an important role in maintaining a couple's affiliation with each other until psychological and social processes can be activated. Since there is a high rate of divorce in Western human societies, better understanding of the role of copulation and other tactile stimulation in maintaining a pair bond would be useful.

4. Two models of sexual behavior based on studies of nonhuman primates have been presented. In cooperatively breeding and socially monogamous primates such as marmosets and tamarins, long-term relationships develop and copulation occurs throughout the ovulatory cycle and during pregnancy, although there is also evidence that females communicate their reproductive state to partners.

In contrast, the promiscuously breeding rhesus macaques accept new males only during the breeding season; the females initiate copulation only when estrogen levels are high, although in small groups or pairs (and in small enclosures) they tolerate copulations with males outside of ovulation. Which of these models, if either, is relevant to human sexual behavior? Do women communicate their ovulatory state to partners? Do women initiate sexual activity more frequently during ovulation? Are new relationships more likely to be formed at the time of ovulation than at other times? Is there greater sexual satisfaction or greater orgasm at ovulation? With current noninvasive methods and low-cost assays, hormonal sampling can be conducted more frequently. Future studies relating behavior to ovulation should use direct measurement of ovulation rather than relying on inferences from menstruation. Future studies need to separate female-initiated from partner-initiated sex and need to control for fear of conception or of contraceptive failure. Studies on the cues used to produce menstrual synchrony and to communicate ovulatory state to partners will require great ingenuity.

5. The hormonal basis of human parental behavior should be further examined. We have only a few studies of hormonal involvement in maternal behavior and none on male parental behavior, despite an extensive nonhuman animal literature and well-developed models of hormonal–social interactions in parental care. Pryce's (1996) model of maternal care identifies emotional, motivational, hormonal, social, and experiential variables that explain maternal care in nonhuman primates. The same model should have applicability to the study of human maternal and paternal behavior. What roles do prenatal pregnancy classes and maternal permission to care for newborn infants have on fathers' hormones and interest in infant care? As we move toward two-career families and increasingly depend more upon fathers and extrafamily caregivers, a better understanding of how hormones interact with parental behavior – and also of which experiential and social variables will lead to quality infant care – will be necessary. Finally, little is known about the effects that infants have on caregivers. Can infants manipulate the hormonal state of caregivers to increase the quality of care provided?

6. Much focus on aggressive behavior has been on males and on the role of testosterone. But the studies of testosterone on aggression show generally small effects. Longer-term studies and more subtle models that include social and experiential effects may be needed. Dihydrotestosterone is involved in masculinizing genitalia and has greater biological activity than testosterone, yet it is rarely studied in the context of aggression. Little research has been done on the controls of dominance and aggression in females, and further study is needed. There appears to be greater potential for female aggression within the family than outside, suggesting that social context will be an important variable for studies of aggression.

7. There is an emerging literature showing small but significant effects of estrogen on memory, especially in increasing dendritic growth in the hippocampus. This research has important implications for treatment of Alzheimer's disease and for other memory deficits associated with aging. Does estrogen replacement therapy at menopause provide a buffer to later memory loss? What are the trade-offs between potentially increased memory versus the negative side effects of estrogen therapy? What role would estrogen play in memory processes in men? There are suggestions of a role of oxytocin in the formation of social attachments and social memory, and this suggests an exciting area for future study.

8. Some of the most compelling recent research on hormones has involved neuropeptides: oxytocin, vasopressin, and prolactin, as well as dopamines and catecholamines. Many of the effects can be seen only in highly invasive studies involving monitoring of brain levels of these hormones and neurotransmitters. We need advances in techniques to find peripheral measures reflecting central processes affected by these hormones. Recent advances in brain imaging techniques applied to nonhuman animals allow visualization of the activity of brain areas under different treatments of hormones or modulators and their agonists and antagonists. These methods can lead to noninvasive ways of inferring neurohormonal functioning in human participants. Much of the research to date has focused on the effects of single hormones. More detailed research is needed on how these peptides interact with each other and with other hormones to influence behavior.

9. The role of prenatal stress on sexual development and the relationship between stress, reproduction, and the immune system needs further study. Cortisol is treated as a stress hormone and can have direct effects on reproductive physiology, but cortisol also reflects energy mobilization and interacts in complex ways with reproductive hormones. Do cortisol levels covary with the energetic demands on reproductive females? Do pair bonding and copulation reduce stressful levels of cortisol or do the increased levels of cortisol found in some animals at the time of mating reflect the energetic costs of finding or attracting a mate? What energetic costs are involved in human mate choice and attraction and how do these costs affect reproductive functioning? What role does mate competition play in male aggression and the levels of testosterone found? Does mating or pair bonding reduce testosterone and aggression? These interactions need to be explored further.

10. The last decade has seen major advances in the development of methodology for measuring hormones and their metabolites. We need a similar advance in the design of behavioral studies that can exploit these measurement methods to better understand the interplay between psychology and physiology. Many behavioral studies do not fully exploit the possibilities that hormonal techniques

provide. Urine samples collected through the menstrual cycle can pinpoint ovulation precisely, and the cost of these assays is now quite low. Samples of hormones and behavior should be collected before and after naturally occurring or experimental events. The varieties of courtship, mating, parental, and aggressive behaviors found in studies of nonhuman animals should be considered in developing alternative hypotheses for studying humans. We should not let ourselves be limited by a particular animal model in developing hypotheses. The importance of social and environmental context is taken seriously in most research in psychophysiology, and it has been shown to be important in studies of the effects of reproductive hormones on nonhuman animals. These contextual effects, often first identified in basic research with nonhuman animals, need to be applied in the design of hormonal research with human participants.

NOTE

Our research and the preparation of this chapter were supported by USPHS grants MH 00,177 and MH 35,215. We thank Catherine Marler and the editors for a critical review of the chapter.

REFERENCES

Abel, J. J., & Crawford, A. C. (1897). On the blood-pressure raising constituent of the suprarenal capsule. *Johns Hopkins Hosp. Bull., 8,* 151–7.

Albert, D. L., Walsh, M. L., & Jonik, R. H. (1993). Aggression in humans: What is its biological foundation? *Neurosci. Biobehav. Rev., 17,* 405–25.

Aldrich, T. B. (1901). A preliminary report on the active principle of the suprarenal gland. *Am. J. Physiol., 5,* 457–61.

Bardin, C. W., & Catterall, J. F. (1981). Testosterone: A major determinant of extragenital sexual dimorphism. *Science, 211,* 1285–94.

Barrett, J., Abbott, D. H., & George, L. M. (1990). Extension of reproductive suppression by pheromonal cues in subordinate female marmoset monkeys (*Callithrix jacchus*). *J. Reprod. Fert., 90,* 411–18.

Bartter, F. C., Liddle, G. W., & Duncan, L. E., Jr. (1956). The regulation of aldosterone secretion in man: The role of fluid volume. *J. Clin. Invest., 35,* 1306–15.

Berthold, A. A. (1849). Transplantation der Hoden. *Arch. Anat., Physiol. Wiss. Med.,* pp. 42–6.

Borell, M. (1976). Brown-Sequard's organotherapy and its appearance in America at the end of the nineteenth century. *Bull. Hist. Med., 50,* 309–20.

Bradford, J. M. W. (1988). Organic treatment for the male sex offender. *Ann. New York Acad. Sci., 528,* 193–202.

Breedlove, S. M. (1992). Sexual differentiation of brain and behavior. In J. B. Becker, S. M. Breedlove, & D. Crews (Eds.), *Behavioral Endocrinology,* pp. 39–68. Cambridge, MA: MIT Press.

Brown-Sequard, C. E. (1889). De quelques régles générales relatives à l'inhibition. *Arch. Physiol. Norm. Pathol., 5e, Ser. 1,* 739–46.

Bull, J. J., & Vogt, R. C. (1979). Temperature dependent sex-determination in turtles. *Science, 206,* 1186–8.

Burley, N. (1979). The evolution of concealed ovulation. *Am. Nat., 114,* 835–58.

Caldwell, G. S., Glickman, S. E., & Smith, E. R. (1984). Seasonal aggression independent of seasonal testosterone in woodrats. *Proc. Nat. Acad. Sci. USA, 81,* 5255–7.

Carlson, A. A., Ziegler, T. E., & Snowdon, C. T. (1997). Ovulatory patterns of pygmy marmosets in intact and motherless families. *Am. J. Primatol., 43,* 347–55.

Carr, B. R. (1992). Disorders of the ovary and female reproductive tract. In J. D. Wilson & D. W. Foster (Eds.), *Textbook of Endocrinology,* 8th ed., pp. 733–98. Philadelphia: Saunders.

Carter, C. S. (1992). Hormonal influences on human sexual behavior. In J. B. Becker, S. M. Breedlove, & D. Crews (Eds.), *Behavioral Endocrinology,* pp. 131–42. Cambridge, MA: MIT Press.

Carter, C. S. (1998). Neuroendocrine perspectives on social attachments and love. *Psychoneuroendocrin., 23,* 779–818.

Carter, C. S., & Altemus, M. (1997). Integrative functions of lactational hormones in social behavior and stress management. *Ann. New York Acad. Sci., 807,* 164–74.

Carter, C. S., Getz, L. L., & Cohen-Parsons, M. (1986). Relationships between social organization and behavioral endocrinology in a monogamous mammal. *Adv. Stud. Behav., 16,* 109–45.

Converse, L. J., Carlson, A. A., Ziegler, T. E., & Snowdon, C. T. (1995). Communication of ovulatory state to mates by female pygmy marmosets, *Cebuella pygmaea. Anim. Behav., 49,* 615–21.

Corter, C. M., & Fleming, A. S. (1990). Maternal responsiveness in humans: Emotional, cognitive and biological factors. *Adv. Stud. Behav., 19,* 83–136.

Creel, S. R., Creel, N. M., Wildt, D. E., & Montfort, S. L. (1992). Behavioral and endocrine mechanisms of reproductive suppression in Serengeti dwarf mongooses. *Anim. Behav., 43,* 231–45.

Crowe, J., Cushing, H. W., & Homans, J. (1910). Experimental hypophysectomy. *Bull. Johns Hopkins Hosp., 21,* 127–69.

Curling, T. B. (1856). *A Practical Treatise on the Diseases of the Testis,* 2nd ed. London: John Churchill.

Cushing, H. W. (1909). Partial hypophysectomy for acromegaly with remarks on the function of the hypophysis. *Ann. Surg., 50,* 1003–17.

Dale, E., Gerlach, D. H., & Wilhite, A. L. (1979). Menstrual dysfunction in distance runners. *Obstet. Gynecol., 54,* 47–53.

de Bordeu, T. (1775). Recherches sur les Maladies chroniques. VI. In *Analyse medicinale du sang,* pp. 379–82. Paris: Rouault.

Demski, L. S. (1987). Diversity of reproductive patterns in teleost fishes. In D. Crews (Ed.), *Psychobiology of Reproductive Behavior: An Evolutionary Perspective,* pp. 1–27. Englewood Cliffs, NJ: Prentice-Hall.

deWaal, F. B. M. (1982). *Chimpanzee Politics: Power and Sex among the Apes.* New York: Harper & Row.

Dixson, A. F., & George, L. (1982). Prolactin and parental behavior in a male New World primate. *Nature, 229,* 551–3.

Dodds, J. C., Goldberg, L., Lawson, W., & Robinson, R. (1938). Oestrogenic activity of certain synthetic compounds. *Nature, 141,* 247–8.

Doisy, E. A. Sex hormones. (1936). Porter Lectures delivered at the University of Kansas School of Medicine (Lawrence).

Duret, H. (1874). Recherches anatomiques sur la circulation de l'encéphale. *Arch. Physiol. Norm. Pathol., 16,* 73.

Ellinwood, W. E., & Resko, J. A. (1980). Sex differences in biologically active and immunoreactive gonadotropins in the fetal circulation of rhesus monkeys. *Endocrinol., 107,* 902–7.

Engelmann, M., Wotjak, C. T., Neumann, I., Lidwig, M., & Landgraf, R. (1996). Behavioral consequences of intracerebral vasopressin and oxytocin: Focus on learning and memory. *Neurosci. Biobehav. Rev., 20,* 341–58.

Englander-Golden, P., Chung, H.-S., Whitmore, M. R., & Dientsbier, R. A. (1980). Female sexual arousal and the menstrual cycle. *J. Human Stress, 6,* 42–8.

Ehrhardt, A. A., & Money, J. (1967). Progestin-induced hermaphroditism: IQ and psychosexual identity in a study of ten girls. *J. Sex. Res., 3,* 83–100.

Faulkes, C. G., & Abbott, D. H. (1997). The physiology of a reproductive dictatorship: Regulation of male and female reproduction by a single breeding female in colonies of naked mole rats. In N. G. Solomon & J. A. French (Eds.), *Cooperative Breeding in Mammals,* pp. 302–34. Cambridge University Press.

Fleming, A. S. (1990). Hormonal and experiential correlates of maternal responsiveness in human mammalian mothers. In N. A. Krasnegor & R. S. Bridges (Eds.), *Parenting: Biochemical, Neurobiological and Behavioral Determinants,* pp. 184–208. New York: Oxford University Press.

Fleming, A. S., Ruble, D., Krieger, H., & Wong, P. Y. (1997). Hormonal and experiential correlates of maternal responsiveness during pregnancy and the puerpium in human mothers. *Horm. Behav., 31,* 145–58.

Floody, O. R. (1983). Hormones and aggression among female mammals. In B. B. Svare (Ed.), *Hormones and Aggressive Behavior,* pp. 39–89. New York: Plenum.

Frank, L. G. (1986). Social organization of the spotted hyena, *Crocuta crocuta.* II. Dominance and reproduction. *Anim. Behav., 34,* 1510–27.

French, J. A. (1997). Proximate regulation of singular breeding in callitrichid primates. In N. G. Solomon & J. A. French (Eds.), *Cooperative Breeding in Mammals,* pp. 34–75. Cambridge University Press.

French, J. A., & Stribley, J. A. (1987). Ovarian cycles are synchronized between and within social groups of lion tamarins (*Leontopithecus rosalia*). *Am. J. Primatol., 12,* 469–78.

Frisch, R. E., Wyshak, G., & Vincent, L. (1980). Delayed menarche and amenorrhea of ballet dancers. *New England J. Med., 303,* 17–19.

Galligani, N., Renck, A., & Hansen, S. (1996). Personality profiles of men using anabolic steroids. *Horm. Behav., 30,* 170–5.

Garrison, F. M. (1929). *Introduction to the History of Medicine,* 4th ed. Philadelphia: Saunders.

Gerra, G., Caccavari, R., Delsignore, R., Passeri, M., Fertonani Affini, G., Maestri, D., Monica, C., & Brambilla, F. (1993). Parental divorce and neuroendocrine changes in adolescents. *Acta. Psychiatr. Scand., 87,* 350–4.

Giovenardi, M., Padoin, M. F., Cadore, L. P., & Lucion, A. B. (1997). Hypothalamic paraventricular nucleus, oxytocin, and maternal aggression in rats. *Ann. New York Acad. Sci., 807,* 606–9.

Goldfoot, D. A., Wallen, K., Neff, D. A., McBrair, M. C., & Goy, R. W. (1984). Social influences on the display of sexually dimorphic behavior in rhesus monkeys: Isosexual rearing. *Arch. Sex Behav., 13,* 395–412.

Goldman, S. E., & Schneider, H. G. (1987). Menstrual synchrony: Social and personality factors. *J. Soc. Behav. Pers., 2,* 243–50.

Goy, R. W. (1970). Early hormonal influences on the development of sexual and sex-related behavior. In F. O. Schmitt (Ed.), *The Neurosciences: Second Study Program,* pp. 196–207. New York: Rockefeller University Press.

Goy, R. W., Bercovitch, F. B., & McBrair, M. C. (1988). Behavioral masculinization is independent of genital masculinization in prenatally androgenized female rhesus macaques. *Horm. Behav., 22,* 552–71.

Goy, R. W., & Deputte, B. L. (1996). The effects of diethylstilbestrol (DES) before birth on the development of masculine behavior in juvenile female rhesus monkeys. *Horm. Behav., 30,* 379–86.

Goy, R. W., & Resko, J. A. (1972). Gonadal hormones and behavior of normal and pseudohermaphroditic nonhuman female primates. *Rec. Prog. Horm. Res., 28,* 707–33.

Graham, C. E., & Nadler, R. D. (1990). Socioendocrine interactions in great ape reproduction. In T. E. Ziegler & F. B. Bercovitch (Eds.), *Socioendocrinology of Primate Reproduction,* pp. 33–58. New York: Wiley-Liss.

Griffin, J. E., & Wilson, J. D. (1992). Disorders of the testes and the male reproductive tract. In J. D. Wilson & D. W. Foster (Eds.), *Textbook of Endocrinology,* 8th ed., pp. 799–852. Philadelphia: Saunders.

Guyton, A. C., & Hall, J. E. (1996). *Textbook of Medical Physiology,* 9th ed. Philadelphia: Saunders.

Hadley, M. E. (1992). Neurohypophysial hormones. In *Endocrinology,* pp. 153–78. Englewood Cliffs, NJ: Prentice-Hall.

Hampson, E., & Kimura, D. (1992). Sex differences and hormonal influences on cognitive function in humans. In In J. B. Becker, S. M. Breedlove, & D. Crews (Eds.), *Behavioral Endocrinology,* pp. 357–98. Cambridge, MA: MIT Press.

Harlow, C. R., Hearn, J. P., & Hodges, J. K. (1984). Ovulation in the marmoset monkey: Endocrinology, prediction and detection. *J. Endocrin., 103,* 17–24.

Harris, G. W. (1955). *Neural Control of the Pituitary Gland.* London: Arnold.

Hedricks, C. A., Schramm, W., & Udry, J. R. (1994). Effects of creatinine correction to urinary LH levels on the timing of the LH peak and distribution of coitus within the human menstrual cycle. *Ann. New York Acad. Sci., 709,* 204–6.

Heist, E. K., & Poland, R. E. (1992). Bioassay methods. In C. B. Nemeroff (Ed.), *Neuroendocrinology,* pp. 21–38. Boca Raton, FL: CRC Press.

Himes, N. E. (1936). *Medical History of Contraception.* New York: Gamut.

Hines, M., & Sandberg, E. C. (1996). Sexual differentiation of cognitive abilities in women exposed to diethylstilbestrol (DES) prenatally. *Horm. Behav., 30,* 354–63.

Hodges, J. K., & Eastman, S. A. K. (1984). Monitoring ovarian function in marmosets and tamarins by the measurement of urinary estrogen metabolites. *Am. J. Primatol., 6,* 187–97.

Howell, W. H. (1898). Physiological effects of extracts of the hypophysis cerebri and infundibular body. *J. Exp. Med., 3,* 245–58.

Hyde, J. S., Fennema, E., & Lamon, S. J. (1990). Gender differences in mathematics performance: A meta-analysis. *Psych. Bull., 107*, 139–55.

Hyde, J. S., & Linn, M. C. (1988). Gender differences in verbal ability: A meta-analysis. *Psych. Bull., 104*, 53–69.

Imperator-McGinley, J., Peterson, R. E., Gautier, T., & Sturla, E. (1979). Androgens and the evolution of male sexual identity among male pseudohermaphrodites with 5 alpha reductase deficiency. *New England J. Med., 300*, 1233–7.

Inglett, B. J., French, J. A., Simmons, L. G., & Vires, K. W. (1989). Dynamics of intrafamily aggression and social reintegration in lion tamarins. *Zoo. Biol., 8*, 67–78.

Kleiman, D. G. (1979). Parent–offspring conflict and sibling competition in a monogamous primate. *Am. Nat., 114*, 753–60.

Knox, R. (1852). *Great Artists and Great Anatomists*. London: Renshaw.

Kordon, C., Drouva, S. V., Escalera, G. M., & Weiner, R. I. (1994). Role of classic and peptide neuromediators in the neuroendocrine regulation of luteinizing hormone and prolactin. In E. Knobil & J. D. Neill (Eds.), *The Physiology of Reproduction*, 2nd ed., pp. 1621–59. New York: Raven.

Lehrman, D. S. (1965). Interaction between the internal and external environments in the regulation of the reproductive cycle of the ring dove. In F. A. Beach (Ed.), *Sex and Behavior*, pp. 355–80. New York: Wiley.

Le Magnen, J. (1952). Les phenomenes olfacto-sexuels chez l'homme. *Arch. Sci. Physiol., 6*, 125–60.

Magdol, L., Moffitt, T. E., Caspi, A., Newman, D. L., Fagan, J., & Silva, P. A. (1997). Gender differences in partner violence in a birth cohort of 21 year olds: Bridging the gap between clinical and epidemiological approaches. *J. Clin. Consult. Psych., 65*, 68–78.

Mateo, S., & Rissman, E. F. (1984). Increased sexual activity during the mid-cycle portion of the human menstrual cycle. *Horm. Behav., 18*, 249–55.

Matthews, K. A., & Rodin, J. (1992). Pregnancy alters pressure responses to psychological and physical change. *Psychophys., 29*, 232–40.

Mazur, A., & Booth, A. (1998). Testosterone and dominance in men. *Behav. Brain Sci., 21*, 353–97.

McClintock, M. K. (1971). Menstrual synchrony and suppression. *Nature, 229*, 244–5.

McClintock, M. K. (1984). Group mating in the domestic rat as a context for sexual selection: Consequences for the analysis of sexual behavior and neuroendocrine response. *Adv. Stud. Behav., 14*, 2–50.

McEwen, B. S. (1979). Influences of adrenocortical hormones on pituitary and brain function. In F. D. Baxter & G. G. Rousseau (Eds.), *Glucocorticoid Hormone Action*, pp. 467–92. New York: Springer-Verlag.

Medvei, V. C. (1982). *A History of Endocrinology*. Lancaster, U.K.: MTP Press.

Mendoza, S. P., & Mason, W. A. (1997). Attachment relationships in New World primates. *Ann. New York Acad. Sci., 807*, 203–9.

Meyer-Bahlburg, H. F. L., Gruen, R. S., New, M. I., Bell, J. J., Morishima, A., Shimshi, M., Bueno, Y., Vargas, I., & Baker, S. W. (1996). Gender change from female to male in classical congenital adrenal hyperplasia. *Horm. Behav., 30*, 319–32.

Miksicek, R. J. (1993). Commonly occurring plant flavonoids have estrogenic activity. *Molec. Pharmacol., 44*, 37–43.

Moehlman, P. D., & Hofer, H. (1997). Cooperative breeding, reproductive suppression and body mass in canids. In N. G. Solomon & J. A. French (Eds.), *Cooperative Breeding in Mammals*, pp. 76–128. Cambridge University Press.

Moore, C. R., Gallagher, T. F., & Koch, F. C. (1929). The effects of extracts of testis in correcting the castrated condition in the fowl and in the mammal. *Endocrinol., 13*, 367–74.

Moore, R. Y. (1978). Neuroendocrine regulation of reproduction. In S. S. C. Yen & R. B. Jaffe (Eds.), *Reproductive Endocrinology: Physiology, Pathophysiology and Clinical Management*, pp. 3–33. Philadelphia: Saunders.

Mori, M., Vigh, S., Miyata, A., Yoshihara, T., Oka, S., & Arimura, A. (1990). Oxytocin is the major prolactin releasing factor in the posterior pituitary. *Endocrinol., 125*, 1009–13.

Morris, N. M., Udry, J. R., Khan-Dawood, F., & Dawood, M. Y. (1987). Marital sex frequency and midcycle female testosterone. *Arch. Sex Behav., 16*, 27–37.

Munro, C., & Stabenfeldt, G. (1984). Development of a microtiter plate enzyme immunoassay for the determination of progesterone. *J. Endocrinol., 101*, 41–9.

Murray, G. R. (1891). Note on the treatment of myxedema by hypodermic injections of an extract of the thyroid gland of a sheep. *Br. Med. J., 2*, 796–7.

Niswender, G. D., & Nett, T. M. (1988). The corpus luteum and its control. In E. Knobil & J. D. Neill (Eds.), *The Physiology of Reproduction*, pp. 489–525. New York: Raven.

Nunez, M., Aedo, A. R., Landgren, B. M., Cekan, S. Z., & Dicfalusy, E. (1977). Studies on the pattern of circulating steroids in the normal menstrual cycle. 6. Levels of oestrone sulphate and oestradiol sulphate. *Acta Endocrin., 86*, 621–33.

Pfaus, J. G. (1996). Homologies of animal and human sexual behavior. *Horm. Behav., 30*, 187–200.

Phoenix, C. H., Goy, R. W., Gerall, A. A., & Young, W. C. (1959). Organizing action of prenatally administered testosterone propionate on the tissues mediating mating behavior in the female guinea pig. *Endocrinology, 65*, 369–82.

Popa, G. & Fielding, V. (1930). A portal circulation from the pituitary to the hypothalamic region. *J. Anat., 65*, 88–91.

Preti, G., Cutler, W. B., Garcia, C. R., Huggins, G. R., & Lawley, H. J. (1986). Human axillary secretions influence women's menstrual cycles: The role of donor extract of females. *Horm. Behav., 20*, 474–82.

Pryce, C. R. (1996). Socialization, hormones and the regulation of maternal behavior in nonhuman simian primates. In J. S. Rosenblatt & C. T. Snowdon (Eds.), *Parental Care: Evolution, Mechanisms and Adaptive Strategies*, pp. 423–73. San Diego: Academic Press.

Pryce, C. R., Abbott, D. H., Hodges, J. K., & Martin, R. D. (1988). Maternal behavior is related to prepartum urinary estradiol levels in red-bellied tamarin monkeys. *Physiol. Behav., 44*, 717–26.

Pryce, C. R., Dobeli, M., & Martin, D. R. (1993). Effects of sex steroids on maternal motivation in the common marmoset (*Callithrix jacchus*): Development and application of an operant system with maternal reinforcement. *J. Comp. Psych., 107*, 99–115.

Purves, D., Augustine, G. J., Fitzpatrick, D., Katz, L. C., LaMantia, A. S., & McNamara, J. O. (Eds.) (1997). *Neuroscience*. Sunderland, MA: Sinauer Associates.

Pusey, A., Williams, J., & Goodall, J. (1997). The influence of dominance rank on the reproductive success of female chimpanzees. *Science, 277,* 828–31.

Rao, G. M. (1995). Oxytocin induces intimate behaviors. *Ind. J. Med. Sci., 49,* 261–6.

Reichstein, T. (1936). Constituents of the adrenal cortex. *Helv. Chim. Acta, 19,* 402–12.

Riskind, P. N., & Martin, J. B. (1989). Functional anatomy of the hypothalamic-anterior pituitary complex. In L. J. Degroot (Ed.), *Endocrinology,* 2nd ed., vol. 1, pp. 97–107. Philadelphia: Saunders.

Roberts, L. (1988). Zeroing in on the sex switch. *Science, 239,* 21–3.

Rolleston, Sir H. D. (1936). *The Endocrine Organs in Health and Disease with an Historical Review.* Oxford University Press.

Rosenblatt, J. S. (1992). Hormone–behavior relations in the regulation of parental behavior. In J. B. Becker, S. M. Breedlove, & D. Crews (Eds.), *Behavioral Endocrinology,* pp. 219–59. Cambridge, MA: MIT Press.

Rosenblatt, J. S., & Snowdon, C. T. (1996). *Parental Care: Evolution, Mechanisms and Adaptive Significance.* San Diego: Academic Press.

Ruoff, W. L., & Dziuk, P. J. (1994). Circulation of estrogens introduced into the rectum or duodenum in pigs. *Domes. Anim. Endocrin., 11,* 383–91.

Saab, P. G., Stoney, C. M., & McDonald, R. H. (1989). Premenopausal and postmenopausal women differ in their cardiovascular and neuroendocrine responses to behavioral stressors. *Psychophys., 26,* 270–80.

Saltzman, W., Severin, J. M., Schultz-Darken, N. J., & Abbott, D. H. (1997). Behavioral and social correlates of escape from suppression of ovulation in female common marmosets housed with the natal family. *Am. J. Primatol., 41,* 1–21.

Sapolsky, R. (1992). Neuroendocrinology of the stress response. In J. B. Becker, S. M. Breedlove, & D. Crews (Eds.), *Behavioral Endocrinology,* pp. 287–324. Cambridge, MA: MIT Press.

Savage, A., Snowdon, C. T., Giraldo, H., & Soto, H. (1997). Parental care patterns and vigilance in wild cotton-top tamarins (*Saguinus oedipus*). In M. Norconk, A. Rosenberger, & P. A. Garber (Eds.), *Adaptive Radiations of Neotropical Primates,* pp. 187–99. New York: Plenum.

Savage, A., Ziegler, T. E., & Snowdon, C. T. (1988). Sociosexual development, pair-bond formation and maintenance, and mechanisms of fertility suppression in female cotton-top tamarins (*Saguinus oedipus*). *Am. J. Primatol., 14,* 345–59.

Scott, J. P., & Fredericson, E. (1951). The causes of fighting in mice and rats. *Physiol. Zool., 24,* 273–309.

Sherins, R. J., Paterson, A. P., & Brightwell, D. (1982). Alteration in the plasma testosterone : estradiol ratio: An alternative to the inhibin hypothesis. *Ann. New York Acad. Sci., 383,* 295–306.

Sherwin, B. B. (1997). Estrogen and memory: Evidence from clinical studies. Paper presented at the Society of Behavioral Neuroendocrinology (May, Baltimore).

Sherwin, B. B., Gelfand, M. M., & Brender, W. (1985). Androgen enhances sexual motivation in females: A prospective, cross-over study of sex steroid administration in the surgical menopause. *Psychosom. Med., 4,* 339–51.

Snowdon, C. T. (1996). Infant care in cooperatively breeding species. In J. S. Rosenblatt & C. T. Snowdon (Eds.), *Parental Care: Evolution, Mechanisms and Adaptive Strategies,* pp. 643–89. San Diego: Academic Press.

Snowdon, C. T. (1997). The "nature" of sex differences: Myths of male and female. In P. A. Gowaty (Ed.), *Feminism and Evolutionary Biology,* pp. 276–93. New York: Chapman & Hall.

Stolz, F. (1904). *Ber. Deutsche Chem. Ges., 37,* 4149–54.

Stoney, C. M., Owens, J. F., Matthews, K. A., Davis, M. C., & Caggiula, A. (1990). Influences of the normal menstrual cycle on physiologic functioning during behavioral stress. *Psychophys., 27,* 125–35.

Surbey, M. K. (1990). Family composition and the timing of human menarche. In T. E. Ziegler & F. B. Bercovitch (Eds.), *Socioendocrinology of Primate Reproduction,* pp. 11–32. New York: Wiley-Liss.

Tannenbaum, P. L., & Wallen, K. (1997). Sexually initiated affiliation facilitates rhesus monkey integration. *Ann. New York Acad. Sci., 807,* 578–82.

Thorner, M. O., Vance, M. L., Horvath, E., & Kovacs, K. (1992). The anterior pituitary. In J. D. Wilson & D. W. Foster (Eds.), *Textbook of Endocrinology,* 8th ed., pp. 221–310. Philadelphia: Saunders.

Uvnas-Moberg, K. (1997). Physiological and endocrine effects of social contact. *Ann. New York Acad. Sci., 807,* 146–63.

Vandenbergh, J. G. (1987). Regulation of puberty and its consequences on population dynamics in mice. *Am. Zool., 27,* 891–8.

van Leeuwenhoek, A. (1679). Observations de natis e semine genitali animalculis. *Philos. Trans. R. Soc., 12,* 1040.

Vassale, G., & Sacchi, E. (1892). Sulla Distruzione della ghiandola pituitaria. *Riv. Sper. Freniat., 18,* 525–61.

Vulpian, E. F. A. (1856). Note sur quelques reactions propres a la substance des capsules surrenales. *C. R. Acad. Sci. Paris, 43,* 663–5.

Wade, N. (1978). Guillemin and Schally. *Science, 200,* 279–82, 411–14, 510–13.

Wallen, K. (1990). Desire and ability: Hormones and the regulation of female sexual behavior. *Neurosci. Biobehav. Rev., 14,* 233–41.

Wallen, K. (1996). Nature needs nurture: The interaction of hormonal and social influences on the development of behavioral sex differences in rhesus monkeys. *Horm. Behav., 30,* 364–78.

Wallen, K., Maestripieri, D., & Mann, D. R. (1995). Effects of neonatal testicular suppression with a GnRH antagonist on social behavior in group-living rhesus monkeys. *Horm. Behav., 18,* 431–50.

Wallen, K., & Tannenbaum, P. L. (1997). Hormonal modulation of sexual behavior and affiliation in rhesus monkeys. *Ann. New York Acad. Sci., 807,* 185–202.

Wang, Z., Ferris, C. F., & De Vries, G. J. (1994). Role of septal vasopressin innervation in paternal behavior in prairie voles (*Microtus ochrogaster*). *Proc. Nat. Acad. Sci. USA, 91,* 400–4.

Wang, Z., & Insel, T. R. (1996). Parental behavior in voles. In J. S. Rosenblatt & C. T. Snowdon (Eds.), *Parental Care: Evolution, Mechanisms and Adaptive Significance,* pp. 361–84. San Diego: Academic Press.

Wang, Z., Moody, K., Newman, J. D., & Insel, T. (1997). Vasopressin and oxytocin immunoreactive neurons and fibers in the forebrain of male and female common marmosets (*Callithrix jacchus*). *Synapse, 27,* 14–25.

Warren, M. P., & Shortle, B. (1990). Endocrine correlates of human parenting: A clinical perspective. In N. A. Krasnegor & R. S. Bridges (Eds.), *Mammalian Parenting: Biochemical, Neurobiological and Behavioral Determinants,* pp. 209–26. New York: Oxford University Press.

Weller, A., & Weller, L. (1993). Menstrual synchrony between mothers and daughters and between roommates. *Physiol. Behav., 53,* 943–9.

Weller, A., & Weller, L. (1995). The impact of social interaction factors on menstrual synchrony in the workplace. *Psychoneuroendocrin., 20,* 21–31.

Weller, A., & Weller, L. (1997). Menstrual synchrony under optimal conditions. Bedouin families. *J. Comp. Psych., 111,* 143–51.

Wickelgren, I. (1997). Estrogen stakes claim to cognition. *Science, 276,* 675–8.

Widowski, T. M., Porter, T. A., Ziegler, T. E., & Snowdon, C. T. (1992). The role of males on the initiation, but not the maintenance, of ovarian cycling in cotton-top tamarins (*Saguinus oedipus*). *Am. J. Primatol., 26,* 97–108.

Widowski, T. M., Ziegler, T. E., Elowson, A. M., & Snowdon, C. T. (1990). The role of males in stimulation of reproductive function in female cotton-top tamarins (*Saguinus o. oedipus*). *Anim. Behav., 40,* 731–41.

Yallow, R. S. (1992). Radioimmunoassay of hormones. In J. D. Wilson & D. W. Foster (Eds.), *Textbook of Endocrinology,* 8th ed., pp. 1635–45. Philadelphia: Saunders.

Yallow, R. W., & Berson, S. A. (1959). Assay of plasma insulin in human subjects by immunological methods. *Nature, 184,* 1648–9.

Yen, S. C., & Jaffe, R. B. (1978). *Reproductive Endocrinology: Physiology, Pathophysiology and Clinical Management.* Philadelphia: Saunders.

Ziegler, T. E. (in press). Hormones associated with non-maternal infant care: A review of mammalian and avian studies. *Folia Primatol.*

Ziegler, T. E., & Bercovitch, F. B. (1990). *Socioendocrinology of Primate Reproduction.* New York: Wiley-Liss.

Ziegler, T. E., Epple, G., Snowdon, C. T., Porter, T. A., Belcher, A. M., & Kuderling, I. (1993). Detection of the chemical signals of ovulation in the cotton-top tamarin (*Saguinus oedipus*). *Anim. Behav., 45,* 313–22.

Ziegler, T. E., Scheffler, G., & Snowdon, C. T. (1995). The relationship of cortisol levels to social environment and reproductive functioning in female cotton-top tamarins (*Saguinus oedipus*). *Horm. Behav., 29,* 407–24.

Ziegler, T. E., Scheffler, G., Wittwer, D. J., Schultz-Darken, N. J., Snowdon, C. T., & Abbott, D. H. (1996a). Metabolism of reproductive steroids during the ovarian cycle in two species of callitrichids, *Saguinus oedipus* and *Callithrix jacchus,* and estimation of the ovulatory period from fecal steroids. *Biol. Reprod., 54,* 91–9.

Ziegler, T. E., Sholl, S. A., Scheffler, G., Haggerty, M. A., & Lasley, B. L. (1989). Excretion of estrone, estradiol and progesterone in the urine and feces of the female cotton-top tamarin (*Saguinus oedipus oedipus*). *Am. J. Primat., 17,* 185–95.

Ziegler, T. E., Wegner, F. H., & Snowdon, C. T. (1996b). Hormonal responses to parental and nonparental conditions in male cotton-top tamarin, *Saguinus oedipus,* a New World primate. *Horm. Behav., 30,* 287–97.

Ziegler, T. E., Widowski, T. M., Larson, M. L., & Snowdon, C. T. (1990). Nursing does affect the duration of the post-partum to ovulation interval in the cotton-top tamarin (*Saguinus oedipus*). *J. Reprod. Fert. 90,* 563–70.

Zucker, K. J., Bradley, S. J., Oliver, G., Blake, J., Fleming, S., & Hood, J. (1996). Psychosexual development of women with congenital adrenal hyperplasia. *Horm. Behav., 30,* 300–18.

CHAPTER FIFTEEN

PSYCHOLOGICAL MODULATION OF CELLULAR IMMUNITY

BERT N. UCHINO, JANICE K. KIECOLT-GLASER, & RONALD GLASER

Recent advances in immunology, clarification and the psychophysiology of stress, continued progress in the discovery of emotional factors in relation to physical disease, and the finding of apparent immunological disturbances in conjunction with mental illness lead to this attempt at a theoretical integration of the relation of stress, emotions, and immunological dysfunction (especially autoimmunity), and disease, both physical and mental. At this stage, far more questions will be raised than answered. (Solomon & Moos 1964, p. 657).

Prologue

OVERVIEW

It has been over 33 years since the groundbreaking paper by Solomon and Moos (1964) on psychosocial influences on immune function was published. Despite much progress over the years, there are still many exciting but unanswered questions (Ader, Felten, & Cohen 1991; Cohen & Herbert 1996). This area of research was coined *psychoimmunology* in the seminal paper by Soloman and Moos (1964) and was later termed *psychoneuroimmunology* (PNI) by Ader and Cohen (1981). Research in PNI focuses on bidirectional interactions among the central nervous system (CNS), endocrine system, and immune system (Solomon 1987). The major aim of this chapter is to provide a detailed overview of important physical, social, and inferential elements involved in PNI research, especially in regard to cellular immunity (see Chapter 16 of this volume for an overview of humoral immunity).

HISTORICAL BACKGROUND

The major source of morbidity and mortality for a large part of recorded history was due to infectious diseases. As reviewed by Silverstein (1989), long before the mechanisms of pestilence were discovered it was known that those who had survived an infectious disease were relatively safe from future infections from the same agent.[1] Such observations were utilized by Edward Jenner, who developed one of the first effective vaccination procedures for smallpox. However, immunology as a science has its roots in the landmark experimental vaccination study of Louis Pasteur, who demonstrated in 1880 that specific immunity could be induced via modified pathogens that no longer posed a biological threat. Pasteur's experimental studies were able to explain in a more mechanistic fashion the earlier findings of Jenner.

Around the time of Pasteur's findings, one of the major historical debates in immunology was being staged and would continue for several decades. The debate centered on whether cellular (e.g. phagocyte) or humoral (e.g. antibody) immunity could best explain protection against infections. Those aligned with the humoral camp dated back to Galen, who emphasized the importance of humors in health and disease. However, in 1884 Elie Metchnikoff advanced his theory of phagocytosis, which suggested the importance of cellular processes as a first line of defense against invading organisms. As is often the case with ideas that challenge existing paradigms, his theory met with fierce resistance, particularly from German researchers. Interestingly, Silverstein (1989) suggests that this debate may have also been fueled by the ongoing international politics between the major camps of humoralists (Germany) and cellularists (France). Around 1888 it was found that serum free of cells had the ability to kill certain microorganisms. The following years witnessed emerging support for the importance of serum complement, which seemed more consistent with humoral perspectives of immunity. In addition, the research by von Behring and Kitasato

John T. Cacioppo, Louis G. Tassinary, and Gary G. Berntson (Eds.), *Handbook of Psychophysiology*, 2nd ed. © Cambridge University Press 2000. Printed in the United States of America. ISBN 62634X. All rights reserved.

demonstrated the importance of antibody (Ab) in protection from diptheria and tetanus and signaled the perceived decline of cellular mechanisms, with subsequent researchers focusing primarily on the humoral arm of the immune system for the next 50 years.

It was the emergence of several findings that were not readily interpretable solely in the context of humoral immunity that enabled the eventual acceptance of the importance of cellular mechanisms. For instance, the finding that graft rejection was mediated by genetics and the demonstration of immunologic tolerance were difficult to explain from the perspective of humoral immunity. The end result of this historic debate was the acceptance that both cellular and humoral arms of the immune system were important for protection against infectious diseases and at least certain forms of malignant disease.

It is within this tradition that the immune system had historically been conceptualized as relatively autonomous in its regulation, reflecting specific and nonspecific responses to antigen (Ag) that emphasized both cellular and humoral responses. It is only relatively recently that CNS influences on immune function have been recognized in basic immunology texts (e.g. Roitt, Brostoff, & Male 1993, secs. 9.5–9.6). However, there are many exemplars of early researchers who were foresighted in their conceptualization of the immune system. For instance, Ishigami (1919) reported case studies suggesting that anxiety on the part of tuberculosis patients was associated with a poorer prognosis owing to immune system changes. Ishigami conducted a series of studies showing that glucose and EPI inhibited phagocytosis and might therefore be important factors influencing a link between anxiety and immunity. Ishigami (1919) speculated that the higher tuberculosis mortality rates in Japan's student population may be due, in part, to the increased stress and anxiety in such individuals.

Ishigami's studies were not representative of most immunological research at the time. However, the last 20 years have seen a dramatic increase in conceptually similar research that emphasizes the bidirectional relationships among the CNS, endocrine, and immune systems (Ader et al. 1991; Solomon & Moos 1964). Before we examine such research, we provide a detailed overview of basic cellular immune processes.

Physical Context: The Immune System

INTRODUCTION

The immune system is critical for the body's defense against viruses, bacteria, and other foreign invaders, as well as malignant diseases (for reviews see Abbas, Lichtman & Pober 1994; Roitt et al. 1993; Schindler 1991; *Scientific American* 1993). Most pathogens and some tumor cells express surface molecules (antigens) that are different from "self" and are capable of inducing an immune response. There are two main components of the immune system: innate or natural immunity and specific or acquired immunity. *Innate* immunity generally refers to immune responses that are immediately available to protect the host even prior to exposure to a pathogen. These responses are relatively nonspecific (Abbas et al. 1994). Examples are the phagocytic cells such as neutrophils. Natural killer (NK) cells are also cells that are ready to kill virus-infected cells even before the infection takes place. In comparison, *specific* immunity is generally characterized by Ag recognition and stimulation. The response is specific and results in amplification of T- and B-lymphocyte populations as well as the production of memory cells that can be more quickly activated upon subsequent exposure to the same pathogen (Abbas et al. 1994).

There are at least five defining features of the specific immune response (Abbas et al. 1994). First, immune responses are specific for distinct Ags or pathogens. Lymphocytes recognize specific surface epitopes on Ags via membrane receptors. Second, immune responses are amazingly diverse. For instance, the typical individual has a lymphocyte repertoire that can discriminate at least 10^9 antigenic epitopes. Third, following initial exposure to Ag, immune responses are characterized by memory in which subsequent exposure to Ag (secondary immune response) leads to a larger, more rapid and effective immune response. The secondary immune response is made possible via a subset of memory lymphocytes that survive for long periods of time (as long as decades) in the absence of the Ag. Fourth, most normal immune responses are self-limiting following elimination of Ag. Finally, the immune response is remarkable in its ability to discriminate self from nonself. As a result, the immune system is typically able to recognize and mount an immune response to diverse Ags but not self Ags. Such immunological unresponsiveness is known as tolerance. Classically, specific immune responses can be characterized as cell-mediated or humoral. In this chapter we will focus on cell-mediated immunity but emphasize that, although separable, these are not independent aspects of the immune system.

The primary lymphoid organs are the thymus, bone marrow, and fetal liver. All hematopoietic cells appear to originate from bone marrow and fetal liver. The thymus is the site of T-cell maturation and it is there that self-tolerance is "learned." Immature T-cells are both $CD4^+$ and $CD8^+$. The CD, or cluster of differentiation, refers to surface molecules that are associated with a particular cell lineage or stage of maturation and allows for the quantification of distinct lymphocyte populations. For instance, the $CD4^+$ molecule is associated with helper T-cells, whereas the $CD8^+$ molecule is associated with suppressor/cytotoxic T-cells. In the thymus, a process of positive selection occurs when immature T-cells bind with

TABLE 1. Description of Major Cells Associated with the Cellular Immune Response

Cell Type	Surface Marker	Origin	Function
Helper T-cells	CD4+	Thymus	Proliferation upon contact with AG (MHC class-II restricted); coordinates different effector mechanisms of immune response via release of cytokines (e.g. IL-2)
Suppressor T-cells	CD8+	Thymus	Suppression or down-regulation of the immune response
Cytotoxic T-cells	CD8+	Thymus	MHC class-I restricted; elimination of virus-infected or malignant cells; activated by cytokines (e.g. IFN-γ)
NK cells	CD16+, CD56+, CD57+	Unknown	Nonspecific lysis of virus-infected or malignant cells; activated by cytokines (e.g., IL-2, IFN-γ)
Macrophages		Bone marrow	Delayed type hypersensitivity; activated by cytokines (e.g. IFN-γ); Ag presentation; production of IL-1; aids in T-cell proliferation

Key: Ag, antigen; CD, cluster of differentiation; IFN, interferon; IL, interleukin; MHC, major histocompatibility complex; NK, natural killer.

either CD4+ or CD8+ molecules. T-cells that do not bind are eliminated. In addition, a process of negative selection occurs as T-cells that react to self molecules are eliminated.

The secondary lymphoid organs are the spleen, lymph nodes, and mucosa associated lymphoid tissue (e.g., Peyer's patches). Both primary and secondary lymphoid organs act as filters for the lymphatic system, which provides a microenvironment for Ag–immune cell interactions. The spleen provides an important site for immune responses to Ag in blood, whereas the lymph nodes provide an important site for immune responses to Ag in lymph.

The major cell populations of the cell-mediated immune response consist of helper T-cells, cytotoxic T-cells, suppressor T-cells, and NK cells.[2] Helper T-cells serve to coordinate the different immune effector responses, whereas suppressor T-cells appear to turn off or down-regulate the immune response. Activation of helper T-cells occurs via their interactions with antigen presenting cells (APCs); these include cells such as macrophages and dendritic cells (e.g., Langerhans cells) that process the Ag and present it to helper T-cells in the context of major histocompatibility complex (MHC) class-II molecules. Briefly, MHC molecules (i.e., class-I and class-II) are membrane-associated gene products of the MHC. The MHC is a genetic region in all mammals whose normal biological function is signaling between lymphocytes and cells with MHC molecules. The MHC class-II molecules are distributed on cells involved in the immune response (e.g. APCs). These class-II molecules are synthesized in the endoplasmic reticulum, bind to peptides, and migrate to the cell surface. These peptides may then be displayed by APCs for recognition by helper T-cells, which in turn coordinate the different effector responses. See Table 1.

Helper T-cells have been classified into two types: Th1 and Th2 (Mosmann & Coffman 1989). These helper T-cells secrete different cytokines that help to coordinate different effector responses. Cytokines are glycoprotein hormones produced by cells of the immune system (and other cells as well) and serve to regulate diverse aspects of immunity (Dinarello & Mier 1987). For instance, Th1 helper T-cells produce interleukin-2 (IL-2), an important T-cell growth factor. Th1 cells also secrete interferon-gamma (IFN-γ), which leads to macrophage and NK cell activation; IFN-γ also has antiviral properties. In contrast, Th2 cells secrete IL-4, IL-5, and IL-10, which modulate B-cell class switching and Ab production. Once activated, each Th subset tends to inhibit expression of the other effector responses; for example, IL-10 inhibits IFN-γ production, whereas IFN-γ inhibits the production of Th2 cytokines.

Cytotoxic T-cells have the ability to lyse virus-infected and some malignant cells and to recognize specific Ags in the context of MHC class-I molecules, which are distributed on all nucleated cells and are synthesized in the cytosol of cells. The class-I molecules bind to peptides that have been degraded inside the cell and then migrate to the cell surface. In healthy cells these peptides are self-proteins. However, a virus-infected cell and some tumor cells will display foreign peptides that allow cytotoxic T-cells to destroy the cell.

Natural killer cells are large, granular lymphocytes that are capable of nonspecifically lysing tumor and virus-infected cells. How NK cells recognize particular surface structures associated with infected cells is not understood. NK cells are abundant in the spleen and found in both blood and lymphoid tissue. They are responsive to cytokines – for example, IL-2, tumor necrosis factor (TNF-α), and IFN-γ – that serve to enhance their cytolytic capacity. There may be some specificity in their response in antibody-dependent cell-mediated cytotoxicity (ADCC) reactions, as NK cells can recognize target cells coated with IgG via their CD16 receptors.

Cell lysis by cytotoxic T-cells and NK cells occurs through a variety of mechanisms. Natural killer cells and some cytotoxic T-cells have vesicles that contain perforin, a pore-forming protein that polymerizes in the target cell membrane leading to osmotic lysis. Other cytotoxic T-cells can release lymphotoxin, TNF-α, and other cytotoxic factors that can damage target cells and lead to apoptosis (i.e., programmed cell death).

NEURAL/IMMUNE MODULATION

However, it is now obvious that the immune response depends not only on anatomical, physiological and biochemical properties of lymphatic cells, but also on a variety of nonlymphatic components, cellular or molecular, of the lymphatic microenvironment. Consequently, our understanding of the mode by which the immune system operates will remain very imperfect without the exploration of immune responses in relation to the nervous and endocrine system. (Jankovic & Isakovic 1973, p. 361)

An exciting development in modern immunology is research demonstrating significant interactions among the CNS, endocrine, and immune systems (Ader et al. 1991). Historically, the immune system was thought to operate in relative isolation from the neuroendocrine environment. It is now evident that immune cells have receptors for a variety of hormones – including EPI, norepinephrine (NE), adrenocorticotrophic hormone (ACTH), cortisol, opioids, growth hormone, prolactin, and estrogen – that provide a pharmacological basis for neuromodulation (Carr 1991; Plaut 1987). It is important to note that such hormones have also been shown to modulate directly aspects of the cellular immune response (Ader et al. 1991).

Relatively recent research provides evidence for reciprocal influences between the CNS and immune system (Besedovsky & Del Rey 1991; Maier, Watkins, & Fleshner 1994). For instance, activated macrophages release IL-1, which acts on the CNS to produce fever and the release of central corticotropin releasing hormone or CRH (Blalock 1989). Furthermore, lymphocytes appear to produce hormones such as ACTH, growth hormone, and prolactin (Sabjarwal et al. 1992; Smith & Blalock 1981).

In the following section we will focus on the influence on immunity of the sympathetic nervous system (SNS), hypothalamic-pituitary-adrenal (HPA) axis, and opioids, since these neuroendocrine hormones are likely to be of most interest to psychophysiologists. Readers interested in other hormonal influences on immunity (e.g., growth hormone, prolactin, sex hormones) are referred to the comprehensive review by Ader et al. (1991).

Modulation of the Cellular Immune Response via the SNS

Williams, Snyderman, and Lefkowitz (1976) provided initial evidence that lymphocytes express adrenergic receptors. Subsequent studies have found these adrenergic receptors to be primarily of the β_2 subtype, although evidence also exists for α_2 receptors (Plaut 1987). Such findings provide an important pharmacological basis for neuroendocrine activation. However, different subsets of lymphocytes appear to have a greater density of adrenergic receptors and hence may be more susceptible to influences from the SNS. For instance, the density of β-adrenergic receptors is greater on CD8$^+$ T-cells and NK cells than on CD4$^+$ T-cells (Khan et al. 1986; Maisel et al. 1989, 1990; Van Tits et al. 1990). These data are consistent with studies reporting greater increases in CD8$^+$ T-cells and NK cells in the periphery following infusions of EPI or during exercise (Crary et al. 1983a,b; Landmann et al. 1985; Maisel et al. 1990; Murray et al. 1992; Tvede et al. 1993; Van Tits et al. 1990). It should be noted, however, that a sizable percentage of NK cells (i.e., 30%–50%) also possess low-density CD8$^+$ molecules. In fact, Schedlowski and colleagues (1996) used more comprehensive staining techniques and found that the rise in CD8$^+$ cells was primarily the result of increases in NK cells with such CD8$^+$ molecules.

There appear to be relatively direct and indirect mechanisms by which the SNS may influence cellular immunity. Felten and colleagues have shown that sympathetic nerve fibers innervate both primary and secondary lymphoid organs (Felten et al. 1987; Felten & Felten 1991; Williams et al. 1981), providing a direct mechanism by which the SNS may influence aspects of cellular immunity. In fact, Felten and Olschowka (1987) found synapticlike contacts between SNS fibers and spleenic lymphocytes. Destruction of lymphoid sympathetic fibers via treatment with 6-hydroxydopamine appears to potentiate immune responses to Ag. These observations have led some to argue that the SNS exerts a tonic inhibitory influence on lymphoid immune processes.

A relatively indirect way in which the SNS may influence immunity is via hormones from the adrenal medulla, particularly EPI. In vivo infusions of EPI result in decreases in the proliferative response to mitogens and increases in NK cell activity, an effect that appears primarily mediated by a β_2 adrenergic mechanism (Nomoto, Karasawa, & Uehara 1994; Schedlowski et al. 1993, 1996; Van Tits et al. 1990). One partial explanation for the decreased proliferative response to mitogens and increased NK cell activity is differences in cell trafficking during SNS activation (Crary et al. 1983b; Tvede et al. 1993). For instance, there may be a lower number of CD4$^+$ T-cells and a higher number of NK cells following SNS activation and this may account, in part, for the decreased proliferative response of peripheral blood leukocytes (PBLs). A more complicated pattern of data exists for the in vitro proliferative response of mitogens and NK cell activity following direct incubation with SNS hormones (Hadden, Hadden, & Middleton 1970; Hatfield, Petersen, & DiMicco 1986; Hellstrand, Hermodsson, & Strannegard 1985; Madden & Livnat 1991).

Modulation of the Cellular Immune Response via the HPA Axis

Early studies provided initial evidence for the importance of the HPA axis on the cellular immune response. For instance, hypothalamic lesions inhibited delayed skin hypersensitivity and increased survival time from anaphylactic shock (Jankovic & Isakovic 1973; Korneva & Khai 1963; Luparello, Stein, & Park 1964; Stein, Schiavi, & Camerino 1976). Furthermore, administration of HPA hormones (e.g., cortisone or ACTH) into rabbits and mice increased the survival time of skin grafts, suggesting an inhibition of the cellular immune response involved in graft rejection (Billingham, Krohn, & Medawar 1951; Medawar & Sparrow 1956).

Subsequent research has documented functional receptors for CRH, ACTH, and glucocorticoids on lymphocytes and macrophages (Clarke & Bost 1989; Crabtree, Munck, & Smith 1980a,b; Smith et al. 1987; Webster et al. 1990; Werb, Foley, & Munck 1978). As noted earlier, recent studies also suggest that lymphocytes produce hormones such as ACTH and prolactin (Harbour-McMenamin, Smith, & Blalock 1985; Sabjarwal et al. 1992; Smith & Blalock 1981; Smith et al. 1986). Although the significance of such hormonal production is unclear, theoretically these hormones may act in either an autocrine or paracrine fashion during an immune response (Blalock 1989; Sabjarwal et al. 1992).

The major influence of HPA hormones on cellular immune processes appears to be inhibitory (Munck & Guyre 1991). In vivo infusions of HPA hormones tend to decrease the absolute number of lymphocytes in circulating blood, an effect that appears to reflect a transitory redistribution of lymphocytes into lymphoid compartments (Cupps & Fauci 1982). At higher concentrations, however, glucocorticoids may lead to apoptosis of T-cells (Brunetti et al. 1995). Accompanying the alterations in lymphocyte counts is a decrease in the proliferative response to mitogens following in vivo administrations of HPA hormones (Clarke et al. 1977; Fauci & Dale 1974). Glucocorticoids appear to exert part of their effects on the immune response by inhibiting aspects of Ag presentation (Baus et al. 1996; Moser et al. 1995).

In vitro studies have provided converging evidence for a direct inhibitory influence of HPA hormones, since preincubation of PBLs with glucocorticoids tends to decrease the proliferative response to mitogens as well as NK cell activity (Gatti et al. 1987; Holbrook, Cox, & Horner 1983; Parrillo & Fauci 1978; Pedersen & Beyer 1986; Wiegers et al. 1993, 1994). These effects were blocked by the specific glucocorticoid receptor antagonist RU-486 (Wiegers et al. 1993, 1994).

HPA hormones may indirectly suppress in vivo cellular immune function in at least two ways. Central administration of CRH reliably decreases the proliferative response to mitogens (Johnson et al. 1994; Labeur et al. 1995) and splenic NK cell activity (Irwin et al. 1989). Although central CRH activates the HPA axis, it also activates the autonomic nervous system (ANS), and the influence of central CRH on splenic NK cell activity appears to be mediated by activation of the ANS (Irwin et al. 1989; Irwin, Hauger, & Brown 1992). A possible explanation for these effects is changes in cell trafficking in response to SNS hormones as NK cells are released from lymphoid compartments into the periphery (Crary et al. 1983b).

HPA hormones also appear to modulate cytokine production (Munck & Guyre 1991; Munck, Guyre, & Holbrock 1984). The cytokines IL-2 and IFN-γ enhance the cytolytic activity of NK cells (Dinarello & Mier 1987). Note in particular that HPA hormones such as ACTH appear to inhibit the synthesis of both IL-2 and IFN-γ (Arya, Wong-Staal, & Gallo 1984; Johnson et al. 1984; Kelso & Munck 1984).

Modulation of the Cellular Immune Response via Opioids

Opium addicts are more at risk for the development of infectious diseases (Tubaro et al. 1983). One explanation for such findings is the possibility that opium may have an inhibitory influence on immune function. Indeed, early evidence suggested the presence of opioid receptors on cells of the immune system. Wybran and colleagues (1979) found that in vitro incubation of PBLs with morphine was associated with a decrease in the percentage of active T-cells, an effect that was blocked by pretreatment with naloxone. Subsequent studies appear to have characterized diverse subclasses (e.g., ε, κ, μ) of opioid receptors on cells of the immune system (Carr et al. 1988, 1989; Mehrishi & Mills 1983; for reviews see Carr 1991; Carr, Rogers, & Weber 1996; Sibinga & Goldstein 1988). B-lymphocytes also appear to secrete β-endorphinlike hormones, a process that depends on the secretion of IL-1 from monocytes (Kavelaars, Ballieux, & Heijnen 1989, 1990; Lolait et al. 1984).

Given the diverse opioid receptors identified on lymphocytes, it is perhaps predictable that the influence of the opioids on cellular immunity would be complex. Such data were foreshadowed by the early study from Wybran et al. (1979), who found opposing in vitro effects of morphine and met-enkephalins on the percentage of active T-cells. In general, in vitro effects of β-endorphins have been a decrease in the proliferative response of PBLs to phytohemagglutinin (PHA) (McCain et al. 1982) and an increase in the proliferative response of splenic lymphocytes to PHA and Concanavalin A (Con A) (Gilman et al. 1982; Shahabi, Heagy, & Sharp 1996). Moreover, the effects just reported were not blocked by an opioid receptor antagonist (e.g. naloxone). It is interesting that Shahabi et al. (1996) found that the increased response of spleenic lymphocytes to Con A was blocked by a δ-opiate receptor antagonist but not by a μ-opiate receptor antagonist. These data suggest that distinct receptor subclasses may be responsible for some of the heterogeneity in prior in vitro studies of opioid hormones.

In vivo studies suggest that infusion of morphine or implantation of morphine pellets has been associated with a decrease in the proliferative response to mitogens (Bayer et al. 1990; Bryant, Bernton, & Holaday 1987; Bryant & Roudebush 1990). These effects appear partially antagonized by an opioid antagonist (Bayer et al. 1990; Bryant & Roudebush 1990). However, at least one study found evidence for compartment specificity as blood and spleenic lymphocyte proliferation, but not mesenteric lymph node lymphocyte proliferation, were decreased by in vivo administrations of morphine (Lysle et al. 1993). A subsequent study by Fecho, Dykstra, and Lysle (1993) reported that the decrease in spleenic lymphocyte proliferation to Con A was blocked by β-antagonists, suggesting SNS mediation of this effect. This mechanism could not account for the decrease in blood lymphocyte proliferation to Con A observed, which led the authors to suggest that hormones of the HPA axis might be mediating the influence of morphine on blood lymphocyte proliferation to mitogens.

There appear to be differential in vivo and in vitro effects of opioids on NK cell activity. Many in vitro studies have found an increase in NK cell activity following incubation with opioids such as β-endorphins, met-enkephalins, and leu-enkephalins (Faith et al. 1984; Kay, Allen, & Morley 1984; Mandler et al. 1986; Mathews et al. 1983). Most of these effects were blocked by the opioid antagonist naloxone or naltrexone. These studies suggest that direct opioid activation of NK cells is associated with a potentiation of NK cell activity. In contrast, in vivo effects of opioid agonists appear to indicate a decrease in spleenic NK cell activity that is blocked by naltrexone (Bayer et al. 1990; Fecho et al. 1993; Freier & Fuchs 1994; Lysle et al. 1993; Shavit et al. 1986; Weber & Pert 1989).

Activation of the SNS and HPA are two potential indirect mechanisms that may be responsible for the in vivo effects of morphine on NK cell activity (Fecho et al. 1993). Fecho and et al. (1993) did not find evidence for an SNS mechanism in the morphine-induced decrease in spleenic NK cell activity. In comparison, Freier and Fuchs (1994) reported relatively strong evidence that the decrease in spleenic NK cell activity via morphine was mediated by hormones of the HPA axis. These researchers found that in vivo morphine administration was associated with increased corticosterone levels. In addition, in vitro incubation of corticosterone with spleenic lymphocytes decreased NK cell activity. More important was the finding that RU-486, a glucocorticoid receptor antagonist, blocked the morphine-induced decrease in spleenic NK cell activity.

Frier and Fuchs (1994) argued that morphine activates central opioid receptors, which in turn stimulate the HPA axis. The resulting rise in corticosterone produces the decrease in spleenic NK cell activity.

Social Context: Psychosocial Implications

Psychoneuroimmunology as a discipline has the clear potential to inform our understanding of psychosocial processes at multiple levels of analysis. In this section, we review the literature on stress and immunity to highlight the conceptual utility of human PNI research. However, human PNI research requires attention to relatively unique methodological issues related to the immune system. We begin by discussing such methodological issues.

MEASUREMENT MILIEU

Depending on the research question, different methodological issues are of import to human PNI research. In many PNI studies, the first question is typically *whether* conceptually relevant psychosocial processes are related to immune function. Subsequent studies may then address the question of *why* such relationships occur. For instance, research on stress-induced changes in immune function has clearly established a relationship between psychosocial stressors and immune function (Herbert & Cohen 1993). Research is now characterizing the mechanisms (e.g., hormonal, behavioral) responsible for these associations at different levels of analysis (Daruna & Morgan 1990; Ironson et al. 1997). When possible, the simultaneous collection of such mechanistic data within and across levels of analysis provides an excellent means by which competing hypotheses can be evaluated (Cacioppo & Berntson 1992; Platt 1964).

There are a number of potentially important methodological issues in relating psychosocial processes to immune function that need to be considered in both correlational and experimental designs (see Kiecolt-Glaser & Glaser 1988a for a review). For instance, depressed or distressed individuals are more likely to self-medicate with alcohol or other drugs (Grunberg & Baum 1985), have poorer nutritional status (Gregory & Smeltzer 1983), and have sleep disturbances (Gregory & Smeltzer 1983). These health-related behaviors have definitely been linked to alterations in immune function (Chandra & Newberne 1977; Irwin et al. 1994; Jaffe 1980; Palmblad 1981). An assessment of or screening for these variables is important so that researchers can evaluate the impact of these factors and/or reduce error variance. In many studies, the reduction of error variance is crucial, owing to the measurement error inherent in some immunological assays and the high costs for large-sample human studies. Both of these factors tend to decrease the power of many PNI studies. We next review important methodological factors that warrant careful consideration in human PNI research. We should note, however, that the potential influence of these factors and hence decisions about design (e.g., exclusion criteria) will depend on one's research question.

Alcoholic Consumption. Alcohol intake may influence immunity (MacGregor 1986). In our laboratories, we routinely screen individuals who report drinking ten or more alcoholic beverages a week, or who report more than ten alcoholic drinks in the past week using standard equivalents for alcohol (e.g., 5 oz of wine is equivalent to one 12-oz ounce serving of beer or 1 oz of whiskey). This tends to be a conservative exclusionary criterion, given that many substance abusers underestimate their intake (Grunberg & Baum 1985). There are a number of scales for assessing alcohol abuse in the clinical range (e.g. Selzer 1971). The combination of such scales and biological indices of consumption (e.g., mean corpuscular volume) provides a relatively accurate assessment of alcohol abuse (Skinner et al. 1986).

Nutrition. One of the easiest methods for assessing recent nutrition is to examine self-reported weight changes. This method of assessment, however, is relatively insensitive to the nutritional content of the participant's diet. With the help of a nutritionist, a food diary methodology might be employed for these purposes, but such issues as when individuals report data (e.g., retrospectively or currently) can influence its accuracy and validity (Block 1982). One simple and efficient way to assess nutritional status is by the measurement of certain plasma proteins. Different protein markers can provide information on relatively short- and longer-term nutritional status. For example, plasma transferrin levels have a half-life of about eight days and can provide information on relatively recent nutritional changes. In comparison, plasma albumin levels have a half-life of about 2–3 weeks and provide information on longer-term nutritional status.

Smoking and Caffeine Intake. Both smoking and caffeine consumption have effects on cardiovascular and neuroendocrine function (Chang et al. 1984; Lane 1994). In addition, these health behaviors can modulate stress-induced physiological changes (Lane & Williams 1985; Perkins et al. 1992). However, the assessment of caffeine can be difficult because of differences in brewing procedures, dosage differences, and variable amounts found in foods and over-the-counter drugs (Dews 1984). In our laboratories, we often exclude tobacco users to reduce variability in neuroendocrine and immune measures. We also typically ask individuals to report caffeine intake in an average week, past week, and last 24 hours using a specific standard of comparison (e.g., cup of coffee, tea).

Sleeping Patterns. Irwin et al. (1994) reported that partial sleep deprivation (i.e., 3 A.M. to 7 A.M.) was sufficient to decrease NK cell activity. The sleep-induced decrease in NK cell activity was reversible by one night of regular sleep. These data highlight the importance of assessing sleep patterns in PNI studies (also see Irwin, Smith, & Gillin 1992). In our studies with medical students, we typically assessed sleep patterns in the three nights prior to low-stress periods to compare with the sleep patterns during the examination periods. Although there are usually reliable differences in sleep patterns, the absolute amounts are not large and typically are not related to immunological measures. There are a number of brief sleep assessment scales that might be used in PNI studies (e.g. Buysse et al. 1989; Hoch et al. 1987). For instance, the Pittsburgh sleep quality index (Buysse et al. 1989) assesses sleep quality and disturbances over a one-month interval; it has good diagnostic sensitivity and specificity in distinguishing good and poor sleepers.

Physical Activity. Exercise is associated with transient increases in many neuroendocrine hormones shown to influence immune function. For instance, EPI, NE, and β-endorphins are typically elevated following exercise (Murray et al. 1992; Simon 1991; Tvede et al. 1993). Therefore, it may be important to ask participants to refrain from strenuous exercise just prior to their participation in PNI studies. A related issue is the influence of more regular exercise patterns on longer-term immune alterations. Relatively less data exist on such relationships (Simon 1991). However, several recent interventions with HIV+ populations suggest that aerobic conditioning can attenuate stress-induced alterations in immunity (e.g. LaPerriere et al. 1990) and that aerobic fitness may also influence a quicker recovery from both psychological and physiological stressors (Brooks & Long 1987). The reliable assessment of exercise patterns via self-report measures has been difficult (Laporte, Montoye, & Caspersen 1985). However, the questionnaire reported by Washburn and Montoye (1986) might prove useful in human PNI studies.

Health Status and Medication Use. Acute conditions that might influence immunity should be assessed or screened. For instance, individuals with recent surgery might be excluded because the anesthetics or surgical trauma have adverse effects on immune function (Lukomska et al. 1983). Individuals with a recent episode of an infectious disease are also reasonable to exclude because of short-term alterations in cellular immunity (Lumio et al. 1983).

The potential exclusion of participants with chronic conditions needs to be carefully considered. As much as 86% of older adults have one or more chronic conditions, and such populations are of particular interest to PNI researchers owing to age-related declines in aspects of cellular immunity (Goodwin, Searles, & Tung 1982). Some of these chronic conditions require medication that might influence immunity. For instance, beta blockers appear to have adverse effects on the in vitro proliferative response to mitogens (Goodwin, Messner, & Williams 1979; Goodwin et al. 1982). These drugs may also influence stress-induced alterations in immunity via modulation of SNS activity. When using such populations it may be useful to exclude participants who are on medications that have direct influences on immune function (e.g., corticosteroid therapy, beta blockers) or to match treatment and control groups based on these medications. One issue that warrants careful consideration is that striving to obtain a relatively healthy or medication-free population may yield subject samples that are less representative of their respective population with increasing age (Krauss 1980; Metter et al. 1992).

Blood Samples and Laboratory Assays. If possible, blood should be sampled from participants at approximately the same time of day to control for diurnal variability in some assays. We suggest that matching the exact time of day is probably less important than ensuring that blood samples are taken within the same 1–3-hr period. In addition, the day in which blood is taken and the assay performed can contribute significant sources of variance. The "measurement occasion" can account for up to 85% of the variability of some functional assays (Schleifer et al. 1989). It is thus important that these measurement variables be matched between treatment and control groups. For instance, one would not want to collect all blood draws for depressed individuals on Monday and nondepressed individuals on Friday. Schleifer and colleagues (1993) demonstrated that analysis of partial variance may be a useful statistical tool to control for day-to-day variability in some immune assays.

Another important issue is the length of time that the blood sample is allowed to sit before performing the assay (Fletcher et al. 1987). This is particularly relevant when samples are sent to a commercial laboratory, which may assay some samples immediately or wait up to 24 hours for others in an attempt to aggregate assays and optimize technicians' time.

In human PNI research, blood is typically drawn from the arm. Depending on the type of assays, 30–60 cc (1–2 oz) of blood is needed. It is therefore important to screen for individuals who may be blood or needle phobics so that fainting, nausea, and dizziness are minimized. When a number of blood samples are necessary over a period of several hours, the use of an indwelling catheter is recommended on order to minimize the physical and emotional stress of repeated venipuncture. Adaptation periods of 30 min or longer are recommended following catheter insertion to accommodate transient alterations in neuroendocrine measures that might influence immunity (Baum & Grunberg 1995).

It is also advisable to buy sufficient quantities of laboratory supplies (e.g., mitogens, media) at the beginning of each study. This decision may have consequences for variability in some immune measures. For instance, in two studies we found a tenfold difference in the relative values obtained for IFN-γ using different lots of Con A to stimulate lymphocyte production of cytokines (Glaser et al. 1986, 1987). Of course, such influences can masquerade as changes over time if the investigator is not sensitive to these issues.

There are additional issues involved in the interpretation of measures of immune function that may be useful to discuss. Many functional assays do not have a "normative" value associated with the assay. Differences in laboratory protocols can easily produce different absolute values for some functional assays. For instance, differences in the time that mitogens are incubated with lymphocytes (e.g., 48 hours vs. 72 hours) can influence the values obtained for such assays. Therefore, standardization within a laboratory is extremely important so that relative differences in immune assays are replicable. There is also no single generally accepted measure of immune function. As a result, the interpretation of a single measure of immune function as representing a down-regulation may be difficult to justify. Studies that measure multiple aspects of immune function will be in a stronger position to make such conclusions by examining the pattern of immune changes across assays.

INTER- AND INTRAINDIVIDUAL PROCESSES AND APPLICATIONS

There are at least two related areas in which PNI has made significant contributions. As noted earlier, our understanding of immunity at a systems level would be far more rudimentary without consideration of the relationships among the CNS, endocrine, and immune systems. In particular, PNI has tremendous implications for our understanding of how psychosocial processes might influence health outcomes via immunological mechanisms. Perhaps the most detailed analysis to this point is the possibility that stress may influence health via alterations in immunity. In the following section, we review human studies on the effects of stress on aspects of the cellular immune response and its implications for health. We first discuss in detail laboratory paradigms of immune alterations to acute psychological stress. We then examine studies linking longer-term or chronic stress to immunity and the health implications of such psychosocially mediated immune alterations.

Acute Laboratory Stress and Immunity

The use of standardized tasks for eliciting cardiovascular reactivity in the laboratory has served as a model for PNI researchers, who have examined short-term immune changes to psychological stress. Such laboratory paradigms have demonstrated reliable changes in physiological function that appear to provide information on an individual's reactions to daily hassles and stressors (Matthews et al. 1992; Pollak 1991). In an earlier review of nine laboratory reactivity studies published up to 1992, Kiecolt-Glaser et al. (1992) came to several tentative conclusions. First, acute laboratory stress leads to reliable increases in NK cell numbers and a decreased proliferative response to the mitogen Con A, with some evidence for increased CD8[+] T-cells with longer stressors. Second, these immunological changes may be *mediated* by stress-induced increases in SNS activity. Third, these changes in immune function appear to be *moderated* by individual differences in cardiovascular or catecholinergic reactivity. Last, these findings appear to reflect short-term alterations in immunity.

There have been at least twenty recently published studies that have served to reinforce and/or clarify the preliminary conclusions of the Kiecolt-Glaser et al. review (see Table 2). Most of these studies have reported reliable stress-induced increases in CD8[+] T-cells and NK cells (Benschop et al. 1994; Cacioppo et al. 1995; Herbert et al. 1994; Marsland et al. 1995; Matthews et al. 1995; Mills et al. 1995a,b; Sgoutas-Emch et al. 1994); decreases in Con A and PHA responses of PBLs (Cacioppo et al. 1995; Delahanty et al. 1996; Herbert et al. 1994; Marsland et al. 1995; Matthews et al. 1995; Sgoutas-Emch et al. 1994; Stone et al. 1993; but see Uchino et al. 1995); and increases in NK cell activity (Benschop et al. 1994; Cacioppo et al. 1995; Delahanty et al. 1996; Matthews et al. 1995; Sgoutas-Emch et al. 1994; Uchino et al. 1995; but see Naliboff et al. 1995a,b). These studies clearly demonstrate that acute stress alters lymphocyte trafficking and cellular immune function.

Kiecolt-Glaser and colleagues (1992) suggested that these short-term alterations in immune function may be mediated by changes in SNS activation, as such results were similar to those seen following acute EPI infusion (Crary et al. 1983a,b). Two recent pharmacological blockade studies are consistent with this possibility. Benschop et al. (1994) found that the administration of propanolol, a nonselective β-adrenergic blocker, eliminated stress-induced increases in NK cells and NK cell activity. Bachen and colleagues (1995) replicated the effects of Benschop et al. (1994) and provided further evidence that SNS blockade (i.e., labetalol, a nonselective α- and β-adrenergic blocker) attenuated the stress-related decrease in the proliferative response of PBLs to Con A and PHA. Although the effects of adrenergic blockade on the proliferative response of PBLs to mitogens were not found by Benschop et al. (1994), this discrepancy might be due to the fact that Bachen and colleagues used a combined α- and β-adrenergic antagonist whereas Benschop and colleagues used a β-adrenergic antagonist. Activation of α-adrenergic mechanisms has been linked to a decreased in vitro proliferative response of PBLs to mitogens (Heilig et al. 1993).

Many of the studies detailed in Table 2 have revealed further evidence for the hypothesis that acute stress-induced alterations in immune function may be moderated by individual differences in cardiovascular and/or catecholaminergic reactivity (Cacioppo et al. 1995; Delahanty et al. 1996; Herbert et al. 1994; Knapp et al. 1992; Manuck et al. 1991; Matthews et al. 1995; Sgoutas-Emch et al. 1994; Stone et al. 1993; Uchino et al. 1995; Zakowski et al. 1992). In one of the first studies to demonstrate such a statistical interaction, Manuck and colleagues (1991) classified individuals as high- or low-SNS reactors. High-SNS reactors were above the median on three of the five measures of heart rate (HR), systolic blood pressure (SBP), diastolic blood pressure (DBP), NE, and EPI. The remaining participants were classified as low-SNS reactors. Results revealed that high-SNS reactors showed a greater decrease in the proliferative response to mitogens and a greater increase in CD8[+] cells than low-SNS reactors (also see Herbert et al. 1994; Matthews et al. 1995; Stone et al. 1993). These data are consistent with the adrenergic blockade studies just reviewed. It is interesting that Manuck and colleagues (1991) did not find any SNS group differences in cortisol response, suggesting that the HPA was not responsible for the pattern of results reported by these authors.

Although it appears as if SNS activation may influence aspects of stress-induced immune changes, these general classifications do not allow for an examination of the relatively specific ANS pathways that are activated during acute stress (Cacioppo et al. 1995; Uchino et al. 1995). For instance, heart rate is governed by both the SNS and parasympathetic nervous system. The underlying autonomic substrates of HR reactivity may vary reciprocally, coupled (e.g., coactivated) or uncoupled (Berntson, Cacioppo, & Quigley 1993). Ignoring such specific sources of variability may obscure reliable relationships between the ANS and immune function. In addition, measures of the ANS may differ in their operating characteristics (e.g., threshold, gain, asymptote), which might provide further insight into how the ANS modulates aspects of immunity (Cacioppo et al. 1992).

Research has begun to shed additional light on the complex autonomic and endocrine pathways potentially responsible for short-term stress-induced changes in immune function. It is relatively clear that the SNS is one mechanism mediating stress-induced changes in immunity. The potential role of HPA hormones in mediating such short-term changes is less clear. Lovallo and associates (1990) found that high- but not low-HR reactors showed significant increases in plasma cortisol to stress. Because of the widespread influence of HPA hormones on immune function, Sgoutas-Emch et al. (1994) identified individuals as low or high in HR reactivity to a speech stressor. Approximately three weeks later, they retested the low- and high-HR reactors and examined cardiovascular, endocrine, and immune responses to a mental arithmetic stressor. Consistent with past research, results revealed that the HR reactivity classification was stable across sessions and that high- but not low-HR reactors showed increased cortisol

TABLE 2. Acute Laboratory Stress and Cellular Immune Responses

Authors	Participants (Age, in Years) [Stressor]	Design	Immune Measures	Neuroend.–Immune Interactions	Main Results
Landmann et al. (1984)	11 men, 4 women (Mdn age = 20) [8 min Stroop task]	WS factor: Epoch (pre, post)	B-cells, CD3, CD4, CD8, granulocytes, leukocytes, monocytes, NK cells	Yes	Inc. NK cells, B-cells, monocytes to stressor. Neg. correlation between EPI and ratio of helper/suppressor cells at rest and after stress
Weisse et al. (1990)	22 men (M age = 28) [30 min shock w/noise]	WS factor: Epoch (pre, post) BS factor: Controllability (cont., no-cont.)	B-cells, CD3, CD4, CD8, granulocytes, monocytes, Con A, PHA	No data collected	Cont. group had greater dec. in monocytes and Con A than no-cont. group
Brosschot et al. (1991)	12 men, 13 women (M age = 23) [30 min uncont. interpersonal stress]	WS factor: Epoch (pre, post) BS factor: Group (stress, no stress)	CD4, CD8, NK cells	No data collected	Stress associated with dec. percent CD4 cells and inc. percent NK cells
Manuck et al. (1991)	25 men (ages 18–30) [20 min Stroop and math task]	WS factor: Epoch (pre, post) BS factors: Group (stress, no stress); SNS reactor (low, high)	CD4, CD8, B-cells, PHA	Yes	In response to stress, high-SNS reactors had greater dec. in PHA and inc. in CD8 than low-SNS reactors
Naliboff et al. (1991)	12 younger women (M age = 31), 11 older women (M age = 71) [12 min math or neutral film]	WS factors: Epoch (pre, post); Session (stress, no stress film) BS factor: Age (younger, older)	B-cells, CD3, CD4, CD8, NK cells, NK cell activity	No data reported	Inc. CD8, NK cells to stressor. Younger group showed greater inc. in NK cell activity to stress than older group
Bachen et al. (1992)	44 men (ages 19–25) [21 min Stroop task]	WS factor: Epoch (pre, post) BS factor: Group (stress, no stress)	B-cells, CD3, CD4, CD8, NK cells, PHA	Yes	Stress group showed dec. CD4, PHA and inc. CD8, NK cells. Qualitative analyses suggest that stress-induced changes in CD8 and PHA were more pronounced in high-SNS than low-SNS reactors
Brosschot et al. (1992)	86 men (M age = 41) [30 min uncont. interpersonal stress]	WS factor: Epoch (pre, post) BS factor: Group (stress, no stress)	CD3, CD4, CD8, HLA-DR, leukocytes, monocytes, NK cells, AG, PHA, PWM	No data collected	Stress group had inc. CD8, NK cells

Study	Subjects	Design	Immune measures	Control	Results
Knapp et al. (1992)	10 men, 10 women (ages 18–30) [40 min recall of maximally pos. or neg. experience]	WS factors: Epoch (pre, post); Emotion (pos., neg.)	CD3, CD4, CD8, lymphocytes, monocytes, Con A, PHA, PWM, NK cell activity	Yes	Neg. and pos. recall associated with dec. Con A and PHA During neg. condition, HR reactivity negatively related to PHA response to stress During neg. condition, HR reactivity positively related to number of lymphocytes and NK cell activity in response to stress During neg. condition, SBP reactivity positively related to NK cell activity in response to stress
Sieber et al. (1992)	55 men (ages 18–26) [20 min noise]	WS factor: Epoch (pre, post) BS factor: Group (esc. noise, inesc. noise–resp., inesc. noise–no resp., no noise)	CD3, CD4, CD8, NK cells, monocytes, lymphocytes, NK cell activity	No data collected	Inesc. noise–no resp. associated with NK cell activity compared with other groups
Zakowski et al. (1992)	29 men (M age = 31) [30 min view and recall of "gruesome" film]	WS factor: Epoch (pre, post) BS factor: Group (stress, no stress)	Granulocytes, monocytes, lymphocytes, IL-1, IL-2, Con A, PHA	Yes	Stress group showed dec. in Con A High-SBP reactors (film and recall periods) showed smaller Con A response to stress High-SBP and -DBP reactors (film period) showed dec. Con A response to stress High-SBP reactors (recall period) showed greater Con A response to stress
Stone et al. (1993)	43 men (M age = 23) [20 min Stroop and math tasks]	WS factor: Epoch (pre, post) BS factor: Group (low ANS, high ANS, no stress)	Con A, PHA	Yes	Stress group showed dec. in Con A High-ANS reactors group had greater dec. in Con A to stress than low-ANS reactors and no-stress groups
Benschop et al. (1994)	31 men (M age = 23) [20 min tone avoidance and memory search tasks]	WS factor: Epoch (pre, post) BS factor: Blockade (propanolol, placebo)	CD3, CD4, CD8, NK cells, lymphocytes, PHA, NK cell activity	Yes	Placebo group showed greater stress-induced inc. in NK cells and NK cell activity than propanolol group
Futterman et al. (1994)	16 men actors (M age = 35); 8 men, 1 woman non-actor (M age = 29) [20 min mood induction]	WS factors: Epoch (pre, post); Mood intensity (low, high); Mood valence (pos., neg.) BS factor for baseline only: Group (Actor, non-actor/actress)	CD3, CD4, CD8, NK cells, NK cell activity, PHA	Yes	Overall, mood manipulation associated with inc. CD8, NK cells, and NK cell activity Previous effects eliminated while statistically controlling for HR reactivity (except CD57 cells) Pos. mood associated with inc. in PHA and neg. mood associated with dec. in PHA (high dose)

(continued)

TABLE 2 *(continued)*

Authors	Participants (Age, in Years) [Stressor]	Design	Immune Measures	Neuroend.–Immune Interactions	Main Results
Herbert et al. (1994)	22 men, 19 women (M age = 22) [21 min Stroop task]	WS factor: Epoch (pre, 5-min task, post) BS factor: Group (low card. reactor, high card. reactor, no stress)	B-cells, CD4, CD8, NK cells, PHA	Yes	Stress group had greater inc. in CD8 and NK cells and greater dec. in PHA than no-stress group High card. reactors in stress group had greater inc. in CD8 and NK cells and greater dec. in PHA than low reactors in stress group or no-stress group
Sgoutas-Emch et al. (1994)	Prescreen: 44 men (ages 18–31) Main study: 22 low- and high-HR reactors during prescreen [Prescreen: 6 min speech task Main study: 12 min math task]	WS factor: Epoch (pre, post) BS factor: HR reactor (low, high)	CD4, CD8, NK cells, Con A, PHA, NK cell activity	Yes	Stressor resulted in dec. Con A and inc. CD8, NK cells, and NK cell activity High-HR reactors showed greater stress-induced inc. in cortisol and NK cell activity than low-HR reactors
Bachen et al. (1995)	52 men (ages 18–30) [18 min Stroop, math, and speech tasks]	WS factor: Epoch (pre, post) BS factor: Group (stress, no stress); Blockade (labetalol, placebo)	B-cells, CD4, CD8, NK cells, Con A, PHA, NK cell activity	Yes	Placebo stress group had greater inc. in NK cells and NK cell activity and greater dec. in Con A and PHA than other three groups
Benschop et al. (1995)	70 men (M age = 41) [30 min interpersonal stressor]	WS factor: Epoch (pre, post) BS factor: Group (stress, no stress)	NK cells	Yes	Stress associated with inc. NK cells HR, SBP, and DBP reactivity associated with inc. NK cells in both stress and no-stress conditions
Cacioppo et al. (1995)	22 women (M age = 67) [12 min math and speech tasks]	WS factor: Epoch (pre, 6-min task, post) BS factor: Group (stress, no stress)	CD3, CD4, CD8, NK cells, Con A, PHA, NK cell activity	No data reported	Stressor led to dec. in percent of CD4 and Con A; inc. in percent of CD8, NK cells, and inc. NK cell activity
Caggiula et al. (1995)	29 women in follicular stage (ages 20–30) [11 min mirror tracing, speech, and Stroop tasks]	WS factor: Epoch (pre, post) BS factor: Group (stress, no stress)	B-cells, CD3, CD4, CD8, IL-1β prod., IL-2 prod., IgG prod., IgM prod., granulocytes, monocytes, lymphocytes, NK cells, PHA, PWM, NK cell activity	See Matthews et al. (1995)	Stress associated with dec. in percent CD4, IgM prod., PHA, and PWM Stress associated with inc. in lymphocytes, B-cells, CD3, NK cells, and NK cell activity

Study	Sample [Task]	Factors	Immune measures	Data reported	Results
Marsland et al. (1995)	30 men (ages 18–30) [2 sessions (2 weeks apart) of 5 min speech task]	WS factors: Epoch (pre, post); Session (1, 2)	B-cells, CD3, CD4, CD8, NK cells, Con A, PHA	No data reported	In both sessions, stressor led to inc. CD8, NK cells and dec. B-cells, Con A, PHA
Matthews et al. (1995)	19 women (ages 20–35) [11 min mirror tracing, speech, and Stroop tasks]	WS factor: Epoch (pre, post) BS factor: SNS reactor (low, high)	B-cells, CD3, CD4, CD8, IL-1β prod., IL-2 prod., IgG prod., IgM prod., granulocytes, monocytes, lymphocytes, NK cells, PHA, PWM, NK cell activity	Yes	High-SNS reactors had greater inc. in NK cells and NK cell activity and dec. in percent CD4 than low-SNS reactors EPI, SBP, and HR reactivity associated with greater inc. NK cells to stress EPI and HR reactivity associated with greater inc. in NK cell activity to stress
Mills et al. (1995a)	24 men (M age = 30) [2 sessions (6 weeks apart) of 6 min speech task]	WS factors: Epoch (pre, post); Session (1, 2)	CD3, CD4, CD8, NK cells	No data collected	In both sessions, stress led to inc. CD3, CD8, NK cells
Mills et al. (1995b)	20 women (M age = 31) [2 sessions (6 weeks apart) of 6 min speech task]	WS factor: Epoch (pre, post); Session (1, 2)	CD3, CD4, CD8, NK cells	No data reported	In both sessions, stressor led to inc. CD8, NK cells
Naliboff et al. (1995a)	20 men (M age = 28) [12 min math task]	WS factors: Task (math, video); Drug (naloxone, saline) BS factor: Card. reactor (low, high)	B-cells, CD3, CD4, CD8, NK cells, NK cell activity	Yes	Math (stress) associated with greater inc. in CD8, NK cells, and NK cell activity than video (no stress) No effects of nalaxone on stress-induced immune changes No effects for low vs. high card. reactors on immune changes
Naliboff et al. (1995b)	20 men (M age = 29) [Role-play task (M = 6 min)]	WS factors: Epoch (pre, post); Condition (stress, no stress)	B-cells, CD3, CD4, CD8, NK cells, NK cell activity, adjusted NK cell activity	Yes	Stress group showed inc. CD8 and NK cells compared with no-stress group Stress group showed dec. CD4, B-cells, and adjusted NK cell activity compared with no-stress group HR and SBP reactivity to stress positively related to inc. NK cells
Uchino et al. (1995)	23 women (M age = 19) [12 min math task]	WS factor: Epoch (pre, post)	Con A, PHA, NK cell activity	Yes	Inc. in NK cell activity to stressor SBP reactivity predicted greater stress-induced cortisol and NK cell activity Shorter PEP was associated with greater cortisol and NK cell activity to stress Path analyses revealed that influence of PEP on NK cell activity to stress was mediated by SBP reactivity

(continued)

TABLE 2 *(continued)*

Authors	Participants (Age, in Years) [Stressor]	Design	Immune Measures	Neuroend.–Immune Interactions	Main Results
Delahanty et al. (1996)	31 men (M age = 29) [6 min math or 6 min cold pressor task]	WS factor: Epoch (pre, instruction, 2-min task, 5-min post) BS factor: Group (math, cold pressor, no stress)	Con A, PWM, NK cell activity	Yes	Math group showed inc. of NK cell activity during task while other groups did not change significantly Math and cold pressor groups showed dec. in Con A and PWM during task that recovered faster in cold pressor group (Con A) HR and DBP reactivity predicted inc. NK cell activity to stress HR reactivity predicted dec. peak Con A response to stress
Gerritsen et al. (1996)	Study 1: 17 men, 22 women (M age = 23); Study 2: 23 men, 36 women (M age = 21) [30 min speech preparation and 5 min speech to "expert" audience]	Study 1: WS factor: Epoch (pre, post) Study 2: WS factor: Epoch (pre, prep, post) BS factor: Group (stress, no stress)	B-cells, CD3, CD4, CD8, HLA-DR, NK cells, NK cell activity, Pdb/iona, PHA, PWM	No data reported	In both studies, stress associated with inc. NK cells and NK cell activity (relative to no stress in study 2) In both studies, stress associated with dec. percent CD4 cells (relative to no stress in study 2)
Liang et al. (1997)	24 right-handed boys (ages 14–16) [5 min scanning task, 8 min social competence interview]	WS factor: Epoch (pre, post)	B-cells, CD3, CD4, CD8, NK cells, NK cell activity, PWM, TT	No data reported	Stressor associated with inc. B-cells, CD3, CD4, TT

Key: AG, antigen cocktail; ANS, autonomic nervous system; BS, between-subjects; card., cardiovascular; CD, cluster of differentiation; Con A, concanavalin A; cont., controllable; DBP, diastolic blood pressure; dec., decrease; EPI, epinephrine; esc., escapable; HR, heart rate; HLA, human leukocyte antigen; IgG, immunoglobulin gamma; IgM, immunoglobulin meu; IFN, interferon; IL, interleukin; inc., increase(d); inesc., inescapable; M, mean; Mdn, median; min, minute; NE, norepinephrine; neg., negative; neuroend., neuroendocrine; NK, natural killer; Pdb/iona, phorboldibutyrate/ionomycin; PEP, pre-ejection period; PHA, phytohemagglutinin; pos., positive; prep, preparation; prod., production; PWM, pokeweed mitogen; resp., response; SBP, systolic blood pressure; SNS, sympathetic nervous system; TT, tetanus toxoid; uncont., uncontrollable; WS, within-subjects.

responses during acute stress. Moreover, high-HR reactors also evidenced increased NK cell activity during stress compared to low-HR reactors (see also Delahanty et al. 1996; Knapp et al. 1992). Analyses of catecholamine responses did not reveal the same pattern of results, suggesting that HR reactivity was serving as a relatively specific marker of HPA activation and may be a second mechanism coordinating aspects of immune changes during acute stress.

Subsequent studies by our laboratories have revealed that the sympathetic substrate of HR reactivity (i.e., pre-ejection period) but not the parasympathetic substrate (i.e., respiratory sinus arrhythmia) was specifically associated with stress-induced increases in NK cell activity (Cacioppo et al. 1995; Uchino et al. 1995; see Cacioppo et al. 1994 for validation of these autonomic measures). We also found that blood pressure responses to acute stress predicted changes in NK cell activity (see also Delahanty et al. 1996; Knapp et al. 1992) and hypothesized that cardiac sympathetic activation, as indexed by pre-ejection period (PEP), may influence NK cell activity via SBP reactivity due to mechanical (e.g., increased vascular pressure) or soluble immune factors (Ottaway & Husband 1992). Mediational analyses utilizing a path-analytic model revealed support for this hypothesis (see Uchino et al. 1995).

The association between cardiac sympathetic control and NK cell activity responses to short-term psychological stress were apparently not mediated by the activation of the HPA, as suggested by Sgoutas-Emch et al. (1994). As depicted in Figure 1, the most likely mechanism for short-term immune changes observed in acute laboratory studies appears to be SNS activation. We should note, however, that the potential role of the HPA axis in relatively acute stress should not be ignored, especially in light of the limitations inherent in these studies (e.g., moderate stress levels, short-term duration). In addition, the coactivation of cortisol in high but not low cardiac sympathetic reactors may be a mechanism with significant implication for longer-term immune alterations in chronically stressed individuals. Consistent with the possibility

that these laboratory paradigms may provide information on an individual's response to daily hassles and stressors, we found that PEP and cortisol reactivity to acute psychological stress predicted a decline in the T-cell response to an influenza vaccination in older adults (data reported in Cacioppo 1994). As we shall review, these data suggest that activation of the HPA axis may play a relatively larger role in more chronic stress.

Chronic Stress and Immunity

Chronic stress may be the result of long-term exposure to stressors. However, according to Baum, O'Keefe, and Davidson (1990) this definition does not account for why relatively short-term events can have long-term consequences (e.g., the Three-Mile Island incident). In such cases, chronic stress may result from lasting perceptions of stress that are driven by ruminative thinking (Baum 1990). Thus, chronic stress may be defined in either fashion, with a "perfect" chronic stressor involving long-term exposure *and* lasting perceptions of stress (e.g., caregiving for a family member with dementia).

The literature on chronic stress and immunity suggests a down-regulated immune response in more chronically stressed populations (Herbert & Cohen 1993; O'Leary 1990; Schneiderman & Baum 1992). Aspects of immune function are decreased in survivors of natural or human disasters (Ironson et al. 1997; McKinnon et al. 1989; Solomon et al. 1997); caregivers for patients with Alzheimer's disease (AD) (Kiecolt-Glaser et al. 1987b, 1991, 1995, 1996; but see Irwin et al. 1991); marital discord (Kiecolt-Glaser et al. 1987a, 1988); bereavement (Bartrop et al. 1977; Kemeny et al. 1995; Schliefer et al. 1983), and individuals with high life stress (Jabaaij et al. 1993; Petry, Weems, & Livingstone 1991; Zautra et al. 1989).

As an exemplar, Kiecolt-Glaser and colleagues (1991) found that long-term caregiving for a family member with AD was associated with lower levels of cellular immunity, as indexed by decreased PBL response to mitogens and increased Ab titers to latent Epstein–Barr virus (EBV), compared with demographically matched control participants. Moreover, these changes did not appear to "rebound" upon termination of the chronic stressor. Caregivers whose family members had been deceased on the average of two years still showed signs of a down-regulated immune response (Esterling et al. 1994). It is important to note that these data do not necessarily indicate that such potentially negative changes in immunity are uniform across individuals. For instance, psychosocial resources such as social support may moderate immune changes in chronically stressed individuals. Kiecolt-Glaser and colleagues (1991) also reported that chronically stressed individuals with low social support showed the most negative alterations in cellular immunity.

Although one should proceed cautiously when generalizing the results of these different operationalizations of chronic stress, it appears that chronic stress is more reliably

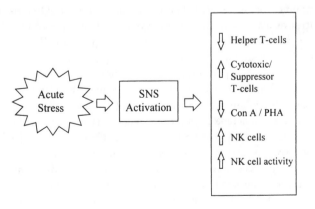

Figure 1. The mediational influence of the sympathetic nervous system linking acute stress to alterations in immune function.

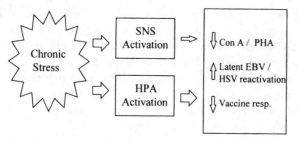

Figure 2. A neuroendocrine mediational model linking chronic stress to alterations in immune function.

related to decreases in functional rather than quantitative measures of cellular immunity (Bartrop et al. 1977; Kiecolt-Glaser et al. 1987a, 1991; Kiecolt-Glaser & Glaser 1995; Jabaaij et al. 1993; Kemeny et al. 1995; Schleifer et al. 1983). As depicted in Figure 2, we propose that although SNS activation may play a role in chronic stress and immunity, the HPA axis may account for a major part of these cellular immune changes. Chronic stress (especially uncontrollable stress) results in HPA activation in both animal and human models (Calabrese, Kling, & Gold 1987; Frankenhaeuser 1986; Mason 1975; Sapolsky, Krey, & McEwen 1986; Seeman & Robbins 1994), and HPA hormones inhibit many aspects of cell-mediated immunity (Munck & Guyre 1991). Chronic stress may also be linked to a down-regulation of adrenergic receptors that limit SNS influences on immunity (Dimsdale et al. 1994). In comparison, chronic stress has been associated with a down-regulation of hippocampal glucocorticoid receptors that terminate the cortisol response (Sapolsky, Krey, & McEwen 1984). These findings have led to the suggestion that the kinetics of the cortisol response may be extended in chronically stressed populations with deleterious consequences (Sapolsky et al. 1986; Seeman & Robbins 1994). However, none of these studies on chronic stress and immunity in humans appears to have directly examined the mediational role of neuroendocrine hormones on these cellular immune changes (see Baron & Kenny 1986).

It is noteworthy that psychosocial interventions appear useful in modulating at least some components of the immune response (Kiecolt-Glaser et al. 1985). These interventions include chronically stressed populations such as cancer patients (Andersen, Kiecolt-Glaser, & Glaser 1994; Fawzy et al. 1990a,b; Kiecolt-Glaser et al. 1985) and HIV+ individuals (LaPerriere et al. 1990). In one of the first studies demonstrating a direct effect of a psychosocial intervention on immunity, Kiecolt-Glaser and colleagues (1985) found that relaxation training increased NK cell activity and decreased Ab titers to latent herpes simplex virus (HSV) in an older adult population. (Ab titers to latent HSV reflect the steady-state expression of the latent virus and the status of the virus-specific T-cell response.) Fawzy and colleagues (1990a,b) evaluated the effects of a six-week structured group intervention that consisted of education, problem-solving skills, and stress management such as re-

laxation and support in stage-I or -II cancer patients. The structured group intervention was associated with increases in aspects of cellular immunity such as percent NK cells and NK cell activity six months later compared with the control condition. Note especially that a six-year follow-up revealed lower mortality rates in individuals assigned to the group intervention relative to the control condition.

The study by Fawzy and colleagues (1990a,b) suggests that psychosocial alterations in immune function may have significant health consequences. Clearly, questions regarding the biological significance of psychosocially mediated immune alterations in humans is an important area of inquiry for health-related PNI research. Animal models have provided relatively consistent evidence that stressors may influence the development of tumor growth and viral infections (Ben-Eliyahu et al. 1991; Bonneau et al. 1991a,b; Habu et al. 1984; Riley 1981; Sklar & Anisman 1981; Visintainer, Volpicelli, & Seligman 1982). In Table 3 we detail recent human studies suggesting that psychosocial factors may result in biologically significant immune changes with health consequences (Cohen, Tyrrell, & Smith 1991; Glaser et al. 1992; Kiecolt-Glaser et al. 1995, 1996). These biological endpoints include viral infections and clinically diagnosed colds (Cohen et al. 1991), vaccination to hepatitis-B and influenza virus (Glaser et al. 1992; Kiecolt-Glaser et al. 1996), and wound healing (Kiecolt-Glaser et al. 1995). All of these studies were prospective designs that included controls for standard demographic variables and/or health-related behaviors. Thus, although more data are needed, direct evidence is beginning to emerge on the health consequences of psychosocial factors via immunological mechanisms.

Inferential Context

MEASUREMENT AND QUANTIFICATION
Biometrics

There is no single measure of immune function, yet researchers in the field of PNI have utilized various measures to index its aspects. A distinction has typically been made between quantitative and functional measures of the immune system (Kiecolt-Glaser & Glaser 1988b). Quantitative measures can include percentages of certain immune cells such as helper T-cells, suppressor/cytotoxic T-cells, and NK cells. With the addition of complete blood counts, measures of cell percentages can be converted to absolute counts. The examination of absolute counts is important because they can serve as a marker of disease progression in immunodeficient populations (e.g., HIV+ individuals). A recent review by Herbert and Cohen (1993) also suggests that psychosocial processes may be more closely related to absolute cell counts than cell percentages. Most importantly, one needs to correct functional measures (e.g., cytokine levels) for number of cells in order to determine if a change in observed function is simply due to a corresponding change in cell numbers.

TABLE 3. Stress-Associated Immune Modulations: Implications for Health

Authors	Participants (Age, in Years) [Psychosocial Factor(s)]	Design	Immune Measures (Outcomes)	Main Results
Cohen et al. (1991)	154 men, 266 women (M age = 34) [Psychological stress]	Prospective viral challenge (common cold) study Assessment period (pre challenge, post challenge)	Biological infections, clinical colds	Psychological stress associated in a dose–response manner with increased infections and clinical colds, controlling for standard variables and health practices
Glaser et al. (1992)	25 men, 23 women 2nd-year medical students (M age = 23) [Anxiety, perceived stress, social support]	Prospective Hep-B vaccination study Assessment period (first injection of Hep-B, second injection 1 month later, and booster injection at 6 months)	Ab titers to Hep-B, T-lymphocyte response to Hep-B (Seroconversion)	No participant was Ab positive for Hep-B before vaccination Participants who seroconverted after first inoculation were less anxious and stressed than later seroconverters Statistical controls for Ab titers and T-lymphocyte response during second inoculation revealed that stress, anxiety, and social support positively associated with a summary index of Ab titers and T-lymphocyte response to Hep-B during third inoculation
Kiecolt-Glaser et al. (1995)	13 AD caregivers (M age = 62), 13 matched controls (M age = 60) [Chronic stress of caregiving]	Prospective wound healing study Assessment period (1 week post punch biopsy, every 2–8 days until wound healed)	IL-1β (Number of days to complete wound healing; size of wound)	Complete wound healing took almost 24% longer in caregivers (48 days) than controls (39 days) Caregivers had lower IL-1β levels in response to stimulation than controls Differences in caregivers and controls did not appear to be a result of health-related behaviors
Kiecolt-Glaser et al. (1996)	14 men, 18 women AD caregivers (M age = 73), 14 men, 18 women matched controls (M age = 73) [Chronic stress of caregiving]	Prospective influenza vaccination study Assessment period (pre inoculation, 3.5–6 week post inoculation, 3 month post inoculation – successful responders only, 6 month post inoculation – successful responders only)	CD3$^+$, CD4$^+$, CD8$^+$, macrophages (Monocytes, IL-1β prod., IL-6 prod., influenza-specific IL-2 response)	Caregivers and controls had comparable influenza vaccine histories and baseline levels of Ab titers Caregivers were less likely to respond successfully to vaccination than controls; this difference was especially evident in participants over 70 years old IL-1β and IL-2 levels were lower in successful responding caregivers than controls at 3- and 6-month follow-up Differences in caregivers and controls did not appear to be a result of health-related behaviors

Key: Ab, antibody; AD, Alzheimer's disease; CD, cluster of differentiation; Hep-B, Hepatitis B; IL, interleukin; M, mean; NK, natural killer; prod., production.

From the white blood cells, immune cell types are identified using commercially available monoclonal Abs. Specific monoclonal antibodies are used for the identification of certain "markers" on cell surfaces. T-cells can be identified by the CD3$^+$ molecule that is present on the T-cell receptor. Subsets of T-cells can also be identified: CD4$^+$ cells distinguish helper T-cells, whereas CD8$^+$ cells distinguish suppressor/cytotoxic T-cells. Natural killer cells may also be quantified as $CD3^-$, $CD16^+$, or $CD56^+$. Quantification of these specific cell types can be performed by flow cytometry.

Cellular immune function is also widely studied from a functional perspective through the use of in vitro methods. One common measure is the blastogenic response of lymphocytes to mitogens (e.g., Con A, PHA) or specific (e.g. viral) Ag. In these assays, lymphocytes and mitogen/Ag are incubated together for a period of time. As lymphocytes proliferate in response to the mitogen, the use of radioactive thymidine to measure the level of DNA in the dividing cells allows the measurement of lymphocyte proliferation. Blastogenesis provides an in vitro model for lymphocyte proliferation in response to pathogens; greater proliferation is typically interpreted as a better cellular immune response. Another common functional assay is NK cell activity, which measures the ability of NK cells to lyse a target cell (e.g., tumor cell). In this assay, the target cells are labeled with ^{51}Cr and incubated with NK cells (PBLs). As the NK cells lyse the target cells, ^{51}Cr is released into solution; NK cell activity is determined by the amount of radioactivity of the sample after incubation. Greater NK cell activity is also thought to represent a better immune response.

One of the hallmarks of immunity is "memory" – whereby pathogens eradicated from the host are met with a more effective immune response upon subsequent exposure. This memory is possible owing to the presence of memory T- and B-cells, which may survive for long periods of time. However, some pathogens have complex strategies that help them to avoid elimination from the body. Latent herpes viruses (e.g., EBV, HSV) avoid elimination by going latent and "hiding" – relatively inactive – in certain cells. The exposed individual is infected for life but the cellular immune response is usually successful at keeping the virus in check. However, individuals with compromised cellular immune responses (e.g., HIV+ populations and patients on immunosuppressive therapies) may experience reactivation of one or more of these latent viruses. In such cases, Ab titers to the virus provide for a measure of the virus-specific cellular immune response. For these measures, increased Ab titers to latent viruses suggest poorer cellular immunity because the cellular immune response is relatively less effective in controlling the steady-state expression of latent viruses. Ab titers to latent viruses appear to be among the more sensitive measures in PNI research to psychosocial influences (Herbert & Cohen 1993; Kiecolt-Glaser & Glaser 1995).

Thus far we have limited our discussion to the more common approaches to measuring the cellular immune response in human PNI research. There are at least two related measurement issues that deserve attention, given recent trends. One general issue in PNI research relates to the problematic interpretation of any single measure of immune function (e.g., decreases in response of PBLs to

Con A, production of INF-γ by PBLs in vitro) as representing a down-regulation of immune function. It is possible that a composite of measures of cellular immunity may provide a better overall characterization of an individual's immune status with implications for health. According to this model, the separate measures combine to influence the composite, so that changes to one aspect may have cascading consequences. For instance, Kiecolt-Glaser and colleagues (1991) found that chronically stressed caregivers of AD patients – caregivers who showed the largest decrements in immunity on a composite measure conceptually linked to cellular immune responses (i.e., Ab titers to latent EBV, response of PBLs to Con A and PHA) – were low in social support. Of course, if one is attempting to model potential mechanisms, a conceptual disaggregation of the composite may provide insight into what stage(s) of the immune response is influenced by psychosocial processes.

In order to demonstrate the biological significance of psychosocial processes, recent human PNI research is beginning to examine the primary and secondary immune responses to antigens. One typically has no prior immunologic exposure to a "new" Ag, whereas one typically has a more vigorous immune response to additional exposure to the same Ag (see the studies listed in Table 3). It is clear that cytokines play an important role in directing and modulating aspects of cellular immunity to such challenges (Detrick & Hooks 1997; Dinarello & Mier 1987). Cytokine production can typically be measured via bioassays or immunoassays such as ELISA (Detrick & Hooks 1997).

Researchers in PNI are also starting to investigate psychosocial modulation of cytokines such as IL-2 and INF-γ in order to model potential mechanisms. For instance, Kiecolt-Glaser and colleagues (1996) examined the influence of chronic stress on immune responses to an influenza virus vaccination in older adults. Results revealed that caregivers had a poorer Ab response to vaccination than demographically matched control participants. An examination of cytokine profiles revealed that IL-1β and IL-2 responses to the vaccination were lower in caregivers than controls. It is important to note that both cytokines play a key role in T-cell activation. In addition, IL-2 enhances the cytolytic function of cytotoxic T-cells. Thus, Kiecolt-Glaser and colleagues (1996) found evidence for the potential pathways responsible for the poorer Ab response in these chronically stressed caregivers.

Psychometrics

An important issue to consider in PNI research is the psychometric properties of the immunological assessments. In this regard, it is conceptually important to distinguish between measurement reliability and temporal stability. Measurement reliability refers to the accurate assessment of the physiological state at one point in time. In comparison, temporal stability refers to a dispositional characterization of physiological function (i.e., stability of the physiological assessment across different situations and occasions). Adequate measurement reliability is necessary but not sufficient for temporal stability. The distinction between measurement reliability and temporal stability is important for at least two reasons. First, it bears on the replicability and generalizability of research findings across occasions, people, and places. Second, if psychosocial factors are to have effects on disease processes with a long-term etiology, the physiological assessments should be characterized by adequate temporal stability. The assessment context (e.g., specific tasks), population (e.g., phobics), and techniques (e.g., specificity of tracers in radioimmunoassay) may all influence an individual difference assessment of cellular immune function. As an example, a needle stick is often associated with relatively short-term elevations in catecholamines. Because of the measurement reliability of current techniques (Baum & Grunberg 1995), the catecholamine changes due to venipuncture would be accurately assessed at that moment. However, this may be a poor index of an individual's catecholamine response across time and situations.

The measurement reliability of immunological data varies across assays and laboratories. Issues such as the day on which an individual's immunological data are analyzed can contribute significant variance for some assays. Considerable work has been done to assure the measurement reliability of some assays across laboratories and times – for example, percentages of T-lymphocytes and subpopulations (Gelman et al. 1993; Paxton et al. 1989; Schenker et al. 1993). Similarly, studies performed after implementation of quality control procedures to establish reliability and reduce daily variability of NK cell lysis show that NK cell activity is also characterized by adequate measurement reliability (Whiteside & Herberman 1994). Only a handful of studies have examined the temporal reliability of common measures of cellular immune function, especially changes in cellular immune function during stress (see Chapter 31 of this volume for a general review of psychometric issues).

Marsland and associates (1995) reported data on the three-week temporal stability of several quantitative and functional immune measures in response to a stressful speech task. The researchers found that most baseline quantitative measures of immunity (e.g., $CD4^+$, $CD8^+$ T-cells) evidenced significant temporal stability ($0.22 \leq r \leq 0.75$). Moreover, immune responses to acute stress were also associated with significant temporal stability for most quantitative measures ($0.25 \leq r \leq 0.53$), as well as changes in the proliferative response of PBLs to PHA ($r = 0.50$, $p < 0.005$).

Two separate studies of males and females (Mills, Haeri, & Dimsdale 1995a; Mills et al. 1995b) reported significant six-week test–retest scores for baseline quantitative measures of $CD4^+$ T-cells ($r = 0.57, 0.61$), $CD8^+$ T-cells ($r = 0.70, 0.50$), and $CD4^+/CD8^+$ cell ratio ($r = 0.92, 0.90$). Residualized change scores for NK cells (i.e. $CD56^+$) and the $CD4^+/CD8^+$ ratio of T-cells ($r = 0.55, 0.60$) in response to acute stress also evidenced significant temporal reliability. In contrast to Marsland and colleagues, the test–retest correlation for $CD8^+$ cells in response to acute stress was not significant in either study; this may reflect the longer test–retest interval utilized by Mills and colleagues.

Llabre and colleagues (1991) discussed the conditions under which simple change scores or residualized change scores might contain more measurement error. In general, the measurement reliability of these change scores depends, in part, on r_{xy} (i.e., the correlation between pretask and task values) and SD_x/SD_y. When $r_{xy} > SD_x/SD_y$ there is more measurement error inherent in residualized change scores than simple change scores (Llabre et al. 1991; Zimmerman & Williams 1982a,b). However, prior research emphasizing the poor reliability of simple change scores (e.g., Chronbach & Furby 1970) has assumed equal variances in x and y (i.e., $SD_x/SD_y = 1$). Under such conditions, residualized change scores typically provide greater reliability, since the upper bound of a correlation is 1. In most psychophysiological studies, SD_x/SD_y is typically less than 1 because task values usually contain more variability than baseline values; the same appears to be true of laboratory PNI reactivity studies (Cacioppo et al. 1995). Thus, in practice, simple change scores appear to produce reliability levels that are equal to residualized change scores (Kasprowicz et al. 1990). Because of the lack of studies comparing these indices of changes in PNI studies, it would be helpful for future research to report data on both simple change and residualized change scores.

According to psychometric theory, several assessments of an individual across times and situations are likely to provide a more accurate individual difference assessment of immune function. Consistent with this possibility, Fletcher and associates (1997) found that the proliferative responses of PBLs to PHA, pokeweed mitogen, and NK cell activity were characterized by adequate generalizability coefficients ($G > 0.70$), which increased when assessments were aggregated across times ($G \geq 0.85$). Unfortunately, the high costs of immunological assays make repeated determinations difficult in many circumstances. Although the data reviewed here suggest that measures of immune response are characterized by adequate-to-good temporal reliability, additional data are needed to examine an individual difference assessment of immune function.

Unanswered Questions and Future Directions

We have attempted to cover the important physical, social, and inferential elements involved in PNI research. As evidenced by this chapter, progress in PNI research has been rapid as advances in areas such as psychology, endocrinology, neuroscience, and immunology have fueled continued growth. However, there are important questions that warrant increased attention in future research.

Perhaps the most common criticism of human PNI research is the question of health consequences of psychosocially mediated immune changes (Borysenko 1987; Cohen & Herbert 1996; Kemeny et al. 1992). There is a growing body of evidence suggesting that such immune alterations may have an influence on diseases such as cancer and infectious illnesses (Cohen et al. 1991; Glaser et al. 1992; Kiecolt-Glaser et al. 1996; see also Kiecolt-Glaser & Glaser 1995) as well as wound healing (Kiecolt-Glaser et al. 1995; Marucha, Kiecolt-Glaser, & Favegehi 1997). Future research is needed, however, to more firmly establish this critical link, and well-designed prospective studies will be helpful in providing more definitive data on this issue.

There are significant questions raised by the basic research on neuroendocrine-immune interactions. In some cases, discrepancies are apparent in comparing in vitro and in vivo data. In vitro data, much like tightly controlled laboratory studies, allow for the isolation of direct influences of hormones on immune function. However, such data may be a simplistic model of neuroendocrine-immune interactions in vivo, where multiple mediating processes may be involved. An examination of both models will provide for a more complete understanding of neuroendocrine–immune interactions.

It is also clear that *where* immune cells are sampled may contribute significant variance. For instance, different patterns appear for some neuroendocrine–immune interactions when lymphocytes are sampled from peripheral blood or the spleen (Cunnick et al. 1992; Fecho et al. 1993; Lysle et al. 1993). For instance, Cunnick et al. (1992) found that foot shock in rats resulted in decreased Con A response of leukocytes in both blood and spleen. However, the mechanisms or antecedent processes were different for blood and spleenic Con A reductions. The decreased blood proliferative response of cells to Con A was reduced in adrenalectomized rats, suggesting mediation via corticosterone. In comparison, the decreased spleenic Con A response appeared mediated by catecholamines, since β-adrenergic antagonists reduced this effect. These reported differences may be attributable to (a) differing proportion of specific immune cells in compartments that may have different sensitivity to selected hormones or (b) greater hormonal release in specific compartments of immunity.

The temporal reliability of common measures of immunity warrants future inquiry. The few studies that exist suggest that many quantitative and some functional measures of resting and stress-induced immune change may be temporally stable. Increasing the reliability of immune measures presents a significant challenge given that repeated measurement – which would enable greater reliability through aggregation – is often prohibitive owing to the high cost of many immune assays. The simultaneous collection of such data in larger-scale prospective studies may prove valuable in examining this issue.

Research on cardiovascular reactivity to acute psychological stress has revealed important psychosocial moderators of cardiovascular reactivity such as coping responses (Gerin et al. 1992b; Sherwood, Dolan, & Light 1990), trait hostility (Christensen & Smith 1993; Lepore 1995), and social support (Gerin et al. 1992a; Kamarck, Manuck, & Jennings 1990; Lepore, Allen, & Evans 1993; Uchino & Garvey 1997). These data are, by and large, lacking in human PNI research. Future studies are needed to examine conceptually relevant psychosocial moderators of stress-induced immune changes, since these data may have important implications for interventions aimed at altering immunity in at-risk populations.

NOTES

Preparation for this chapter was supported by a James A. Shannon Director's Award 1 R55 AG13968 from the National Institute on Aging, a program project grant AG-11585 from the National Institute on Aging, grants R37 MH42096 and R07 MH50538 from the National Institute of Mental Health, and University Research Committee grant no. 21560 from the University of Utah. We would like to thank Heather Llenos for her technical assistance on aspects of this chapter.

1. The following section on the history of immunity is summarized from the historical perspective of Silverstein (1989). Readers interested in a more detailed overview are referred to this very readable account of the history of immunology.
2. We should note that there is considerable controversy regarding suppressor cells. For instance, it is unknown whether such cells are a distinct subset of lymphocytes or rather cytotoxic T-cells that serve dual roles (Abbas et al. 1994).

REFERENCES

Abbas, A. K., Lichtman, A. H., & Pober, J. S. (1994). *Cellular and Molecular Immunology.* London: Saunders.

Ader, R., & Cohen, N. (1981). *Psychoneuroimmunology.* New York: Academic Press.

Ader, R., Felten, D. L., & Cohen, N. (1991). *Psychoneuroimmunology.* New York: Academic Press.

Andersen, B. L., Kiecolt-Glaser, J. K., & Glaser, R. (1994). A biobehavioral model of cancer stress and disease course. *American Psychologist, 49,* 389–404.

Arya, S. K., Wong-Staal, F., & Gallo, R. C. (1984). Dexamethasone-mediated inhibition of human T cell growth factor and γ-interferon messenger RNA. *Journal of Immunology, 133,* 273–6.

Bachen, E. A., Manuck, S. B., Cohen, S., Muldoon, M. F., Raible, R., Herbert, T. B., & Rabin, B. S. (1995). Adrenergic blockade ameliorates cellular immune responses to mental stress in humans. *Psychosomatic Medicine, 57,* 366–72.

Bachen, E. A., Manuck, S. B., Marsland, A. L., Cohen, S., Malkoff, S. B., Muldoon, M. F., & Rabin, B. S. (1992).

Lymphocyte subset and cellular immune responses to brief experimental stress. *Psychosomatic Medicine, 54,* 673–9.

Baron, R. M., & Kenny, D. A. (1986). The moderator–mediator distinction in social psychological research: Conceptual, strategic, and statistical considerations. *Journal of Personality and Social Psychology, 51,* 1173–82.

Bartrop, R., Lazarus, L., Luckhurst, E., Kiloh, L. G., & Penny, R. (1977). Depressed lymphocyte function after bereavement. *Lancet, 1,* 834–6.

Baum, A. (1990). Stress, intrusive imagery, and chronic distress. *Health Psychology, 9,* 653–75.

Baum, A., & Grunberg, N. (1995). Measurement of stress hormones. In S. Cohen, R. C. Kessler, & L. U. Gordon (Eds.), *Measuring Stress: A Guide for Health and Social Scientists,* pp. 175–92. New York: Oxford University Press.

Baum, A., O'Keefe, M. K., & Davidson, L. M. (1990). Acute stressors and chronic response: The case of traumatic stress. *Journal of Applied Social Psychology, 20,* 1643–54.

Baus, E., Andris, F., Dubois, P. M., Urbain, J., & Leo, O. (1996). Dexamethasone inhibits the early steps of antigen receptor signaling in activated T lymphocytes. *Journal of Immunology, 156,* 4555–61.

Bayer, B. M., Daussin, S., Hernandez, M., & Irvin, L. (1990). Morphine inhibition of lymphocyte activity is mediated by an opioid dependent mechanism. *Neuropharmacology, 29,* 369–74.

Ben-Eliyahu, S., Yirmiya, R., Liebeskind, J. C., Taylor, A. N., & Gale, R. P. (1991). Stress increases metastatic spread of a mammary tumor in rats: Evidence for mediation by the immune system. *Brain, Behavior, and Immunity, 5,* 193–205.

Benschop, R. J., Godaert, G. L. R., Geenan, R., Brosschot, J. F., De Smet, M. B. M., Olff, M., Heijnen, C. J., & Ballieux, R. E. (1995). Relationships between cardiovascular and immunological changes in an experimental stress model. *Psychological Medicine, 25,* 323–7.

Benschop, R. J., Nieuwenhuis, E. E. S., Tromp, E. A. M., Godaert, G. L. R., Ballieux, R. E., and van Doornen, L. J. P. (1994). Effects of β-adrenergic blockade on immunologic and cardiovascular changes induced by mental stress. *Circulation, 89,* 762–9.

Berntson, G. G., Cacioppo, J. T., & Quigley, K. S. (1993). Cardiac psychophysiology and autonomic space in humans: Empirical perspectives and conceptual implications. *Psychological Bulletin, 114,* 296–322.

Besedovsky, H. O., & Del Rey, A. (1991). Physiological implications of the immune-neuro-endocrine network. In R. Ader, D. L. Felten, & N. Cohen (Eds.), *Psychoneuroimmunology,* pp. 589–608. New York: Academic Press.

Billingham, R. E., Krohn, P. L., & Medawar, P. B. (1951). Effect of cortisone on survival of skin homografts in rabbits. *British Medical Journal, 1,* 1157–63.

Blalock, E. J. (1989). A molecular basis for bidirectional communication between the immune and neuroendocrine systems. *Physiological Reviews, 69,* 1–31.

Block, G. (1982). A review of validations of dietary assessment methods. *American Journal of Epidemiology, 115,* 492–506.

Bonneau, R. H., Sheridan, J. F., Feng, N., & Glaser, R. (1991a). Stress-induced suppression of herpes simplex virus (HSV)-specific cytotoxic T lymphocyte and natural killer cell activity and enhancement of acute pathogenesis following local HSV infection. *Brain, Behavior, and Immunity, 5,* 170–92.

Bonneau, R. H., Sheridan, J. F., Feng, N., & Glaser, R. (1991b). Stress-induced effects on cell mediated innate and adaptive memory components of the murine immune response to herpes simplex virus infection. *Brain, Behavior, and Immunity, 5,* 274–95.

Borysenko, M. (1987). The immune system: An overview. *Annals of Behavioral Medicine, 9,* 3–10.

Brooks, S. T., & Long, B. C. (1987). Efficiency of coping with a real-life stressor: A multimodal comparison of aerobic fitness. *Psychophysiology, 24,* 173–80.

Brosschot, J. F., Benschop, R. J., Godaert, G. L. R., De Smet, M. B. M., Olff, M., Heijnen, C. J., & Ballieux, R. E. (1992). Effects of experimental psychological stress on distribution and function of peripheral blood cells. *Psychosomatic Medicine, 54,* 394–406.

Brosschot, J. F., Smelt, D., De Smet, M., Heijnen, C. J., Olff, M., Ballieux, R. E., & Godaert, G. L. R. (1991). Effects of experimental psychological stress on T-lymphocytes and NK cells in man: An exploratory study. *Journal of Psychophysiology, 5,* 59–67.

Brunetti, M., Martelli, N., Colasante, A., Piantelli, M., Musiani, P., & Aiello, F. B. (1995). Spontaneous and glucocorticoid-induced apoptosis in human mature T lymphocytes. *Blood, 86,* 4199–4205.

Bryant, H. U., Bernton, E. W., & Holaday, J. W. (1987). Immunosuppressive effects of chronic morphine treatment in mice. *Life Sciences, 41,* 1731–8.

Bryant, H. U., & Roudebush, R. E. (1990). Suppressive effects of morphine pellet implants on *in vivo* parameters of immune function. *Journal of Pharmacology and Experimental Therapeutics, 255,* 410–14.

Buysse, D. J., Reynolds, C. F., Monk, T. H., Berman, S. R., & Kupfer, D. J. (1989). Pittsburgh sleep quality index: A new instrument for psychiatric practice and research. *Psychiatry Research, 28,* 193–213.

Cacioppo, J. T. (1994). Social neuroscience: Autonomic, endocrine, and immune responses to stress. *Psychophysiology, 31,* 113–28.

Cacioppo, J. T., & Berntson, G. G. (1992). Social psychological contributions to the decade of the brain: Doctrine of multilevel analysis. *American Psychologist, 47,* 1019–28.

Cacioppo, J. T., Berntson, G. G., Binkley, P. F., Quigley, K. S., Uchino, B. N., & Fieldstone, A. (1994). Autonomic cardiac control II: Basal response, noninvasive indices, and autonomic space as revealed by autonomic blockade. *Psychophysiology, 31,* 586–98.

Cacioppo, J. T., Malarkey, W. B., Kiecolt-Glaser, K. G., Uchino, B. N., Sgoutas-Emch, S. A., Sheridan, J. F., Berntson, G. G., & Glaser, R. (1995). Heterogeneity in neuroendocrine and immune responses to brief psychological stressors as a function of autonomic cardiac activation. *Psychosomatic Medicine, 57,* 154–64.

Cacioppo, J. T., Uchino, B. N., Crites, S. L., Snydersmith, M. A., Smith, G., Berntson, G. G., & Lang, P. J. (1992). Relationship between facial expressiveness and sympathetic activation in emotion: A critical review, with emphasis on modeling underlying mechanisms and individual differences. *Journal of Personality and Social Psychology, 62,* 110–28.

Caggiula, A. R., McAllister, C. G., Matthews, K. A., Berga, S. L., Owens, J. F., & Miller, A. L. (1995). Psychological stress and immunologial responsiveness in normally cycling, follicular-stage women. *Journal of Neuroimmunology, 59,* 103–11.

Calabrese, J. R., Kling, M. A., & Gold, P. W. (1987). Alterations in immunocompetence during stress, bereavement, and depression: Focus on neuroendocrine regulation. *American Journal of Psychiatry, 144,* 1123–34.

Carr, D. J. J. (1991). The role of endogenous opioids and their receptors in the immune system. *Proceedings of the Society of Experimental Biology and Medicine, 198,* 710–20.

Carr, D. J. J., DeCosta, B. R., Kim, C.-H., Jacobson, A. E., Guarcello, V., Rice, K. C., & Blalock, J. E. (1989). Opioid receptors on cells of the immune system: Evidence for δ- and κ-classes. *Journal of Endocrinology 122,* 161–8.

Carr, D. J. J., Kim, C.-H., DeCosta, B., Jacobson, A. E., Rice, K. C., & Blalock, J. E. (1988). Evidence for a δ-class receptor on cells of the immune system. *Cellular Immunology, 116,* 44–51.

Carr, D. J. J., Rogers, T. J., & Weber, R. J. (1996). The relevance of opioids and opioid receptors on immunocompetence and immune homeostasis. *Proceedings of the Society for Experimental Biology and Medicine, 213,* 248–57.

Chandra, R. K., & Newberne, P. M. (1977). *Nutrition, Immunity, and Infection.* New York: Plenum.

Chang, F. E., Richards, S. R., Kim, M., & Malarkey, W. B. (1984). 24 hour prolactin profiles and prolactin responses to dopamine in the long distance runner. *Journal of Clinical Endocrinology and Metabolism, 59,* 631.

Christensen, A. J., & Smith, T. W. (1993). Cynical hostility and cardiovascular reactivity during self-disclosure. *Psychosomatic Medicine, 55,* 193–202.

Chronbach, L. J., & Furby, L. (1970). How should we measure "change" – Or should we? *Psychological Bulletin, 74,* 68–80.

Clarke, B. L., & Bost, K. L. (1989). Differential expression of functional adrenocorticotropic hormone receptors by subpopulations of lymphocytes. *Journal of Immunology, 143,* 464–9.

Clarke, J. R., Gagnon, R. F., Gotch, F. M., Heyworth, M. R., Maclennan, I. C. M., Truelove, S. C., & Waller, C. A. (1977). The effect of prednisolone on leucocyte function in man: A double blind controlled study. *Clinical Experimental Immunology, 28,* 292–301.

Cohen, S., & Herbert, T. B. (1996). Health psychology: Psychological factors and physical disease from the perspective of human psychoneuroimmunology. *Annual Review of Psychology, 47,* 113–42.

Cohen, S., Tyrrell, D. A. J., & Smith, A. P. (1991). Psychological stress and susceptibility to the common cold. *New England Journal of Medicine, 325,* 606–12.

Crabtree, G. R., Munck, A., & Smith, K. A. (1980a). Glucocorticoids and lymphocytes I. Increased glucocorticoid receptor levels in antigen-stimulated lymphocytes. *Journal of Immunology, 124,* 2430–5.

Crabtree, G. R., Munck, A., & Smith, K. A. (1980b). Glucocorticoids and lymphocytes II. Cell cycle-dependent changes in glucocorticoid receptor content. *Journal of Immunology, 125,* 13–17.

Crary, B., Borysenko, M., Sutherland, D. C., Kutz, I., Borysenko, J. Z., & Benson, H. (1983a). Decrease in mitogen responsiveness of mononuclear cells from peripheral blood after epinephrine administrations in humans. *Journal of Immunology, 130,* 694–7.

Crary, B., Hauser, S. L., Borysenko, M., Kutz, I., Hoban, C., Ault, K. A., Weiner, H. L., & Bensen, H. (1983b). Epinephrine-induced changes in the distribution of lymphocyte subsets in peripheral blood of humans. *Journal of Immunology, 131,* 1178–81.

Cunnick, J. E., Lysle, D. T., Kucinski, B. J., & Rabin, B. S. (1992). Stress-induced alterations of immune function: Diversity of effects and mechanisms. *Annals of the New York Academy of Sciences, 650,* 283–7.

Cupps, T. R., & Fauci, A. S. (1982). Corticosteroid-mediated immunoregulation in man. *Immunological Review, 65,* 133–55.

Daruna, J. H., & Morgan, J. E. (1990). Psychosocial effects on immune function: Neuroendocrine pathways. *Psychosomatics, 31,* 4–12.

Delahanty, D. L., Dougall, A. L., Hawken, L., Trakowski, J. H., Schmitz, J. B., Jenkins, F. J., & Baum, A. (1996). Time course of natural killer cell activity and lymphocyte proliferation in response to two acute stressors in healthy men. *Health Psychology, 15,* 48–55.

Detrick, B., & Hooks, J. J. (1997). Cytokines in human immunology. In M. S. Leffell, A. D. Donnenberg, & N. R. Rose (Eds.), *Handbook of Human Immunology,* pp. 233–66. New York: CRC Press.

Dews, P. B. (1984). *Caffeine.* New York: Springer-Verlag.

Dimsdale, J. E., Mills, P., Patterson, T., Ziegler, M., & Dillon, E. (1994). Effects of chronic stress on beta-adrenergic receptors in the homeless. *Psychosomatic Medicine, 56,* 290–5.

Dinarello, C. A., & Mier, J. W. (1987). Lymphokines. *New England Journal of Medicine, 317,* 940–5.

Esterling, B. A., Kiecolt-Glaser, J. K., Bodnar, J. C., & Glaser, R. (1994). Chronic stress, social support, and persistent alterations in the natural killer cell response to cytokines in older adults. *Health Psychology, 13,* 291–9.

Faith, R. E., Liang, H. J., Murgo, A. J., & Plotnikoff, N. P. (1984). Neuroimmunomodulation with enkephalins: Enhancement of human natural killer (NK) cell activity *in vitro. Clinical Immunology and Immunopathology, 31,* 412–18.

Fauci, A. S., & Dale, D. C. (1974). The effect of in vivo hydrocortisone on subpopulations of human lymphocytes. *Journal of Clinical Investigation, 53,* 240–6.

Fawzy, F. I., Cousins, N., Fawzy, N. W., Kemeny, M. E., Elashoff, R., & Morton, D. (1990a). A structured psychiatric intervention for cancer patients. I. Changes over time in method of coping and affective disturbances. *Archives of General Psychiatry, 47,* 720–5.

Fawzy, F. I., Kemeny, E., Fawzy, N. W., Elashoff, R., Morton, D., Cousins, N., & Fahey, J. L. (1990b). A structured psychiatric intervention for cancer patients. II. Changes over time in immunological measures. *Archives of General Psychiatry, 47,* 729–35.

Fecho, K., Dykstra, L. A., & Lysle, D. T. (1993). Evidence for beta adrenergic receptor involvement in the immunomodulatory effects of morphine. *Journal of Pharmacology and Experimental Therapeutics, 265,* 1079–87.

Felten, D. L., Ackerman, K. D., Wiegand, S. J., & Felten, S. Y. (1987). Noradrenergic sympathetic innervation of the spleen: I. Nerve fibers associate with lymphocytes and macrophages in specific compartments of the splenic white pulp. *Journal of Neuroscience Research, 18,* 28–36.

Felten, S. Y., & Felten, D. L. (1991). Innervation of lymphoid tissue. In R. Ader, D. Felten, & N. Cohen (Eds.), *Psychoneuroimmunology*, pp. 27–69. New York: Academic Press.

Felten, S. Y., & Olschowka, J. (1987). Noradrenergic sympathetic innervation of the spleen: II. Tyrosine hydroxylase (TH)-positive nerve terminals form synapticlike contacts on lymphocytes in the splenic white pulp. *Journal of Neuroscience Research, 18,* 37–48.

Fletcher, M. A., Baron, G. C., Ashman, M. R., Fischl, M. A., & Klimas, N. G. (1987). Use of whole blood methods in assessment of immune parameters in immunodeficiency states. *Diagnostic Clinical Immunology, 5,* 69–81.

Fletcher, M. A., Klimas, N. G., Morgan, R., & Gjerset, G. (1997). Lymphocyte proliferation. In N. Rose (Ed.), *Manual of Clinical Laboratory Immunology*, pp. 313–19. Washington, DC: American Association for Microbiology.

Frankenhaeuser, M. (1986). A psychobiological framework for research on human stress and coping. In M. H. Appley & R. Trumbull (Eds.), *Dynamics of Stress: Physiological, Psychological, and Social Perspectives*, pp. 101–16. New York: Plenum.

Freier, D. O., & Fuchs, B. A. (1994). A mechanism of action for morphine-induced immunosuppression: Corticosterone mediates morphine-induced suppression of natural killer cell activity. *Journal of Pharmacology and Experimental Therapeutics, 270,* 1127–33.

Futterman, A. D., Kemeny, M. E., Shapiro, D., & Fahey, J. L. (1994). Immunological and physiological changes associated with induced positive and negative mood. *Psychosomatic Medicine, 56,* 499–511.

Gatti, G., Masera, R., Cavallo, R., Sartori, M. L., Delponte, D., Carignola, R., Salvadori, A., & Angeli, A. (1987). Studies on the mechanism of cortisol inhibition of human natural killer cell activity: Effects of calcium entry blockers and calmodulin antagonists. *Steroids, 49,* 601–16.

Gelman, R., Cheng, S.-C., Kidd, P., Waxdal, M., & Kagan, J. (1993). Assessment of the effects of instrumentation, monoclonal antibody, and fluorochrome on flow cytometric immunophenotyping: A report based on 2 years of the NIAID DAIDS flow cytometry quality assessment program. *Clinical Immunology and Immunopathology, 66,* 150–62.

Gerin, W., Pieper, C., Levy, R., & Pickering, T. G. (1992a). Social support in social interaction: A moderator of cardiovascular reactivity. *Psychosomatic Medicine, 54,* 324–36.

Gerin, W., Pieper, C., Marchese, L., & Pickering, T. G. (1992b). The multi-dimensional nature of activity coping: Differential effects of effort and enhanced control on cardiovascular reactivity. *Psychosomatic Medicine, 54,* 707–19.

Gerritsen, W., Heijnen, C. J., Wiegant, V. M., Bermond, B., & Fridja, N. H. (1996). Experimental social fear: Immunological, hormonal, and autonomic concomitants. *Psychosomatic Medicine, 58,* 273–86.

Gilman, S. C., Schwartz, J. M., Milner, R. J., Bloom, F. E., & Feldman, J. D. (1982). β-endorphin enhances lymphocyte proliferative responses. *Proceedings of the National Academy of Sciences U.S.A., 79,* 4226–30.

Glaser, R., Kiecolt-Glaser, J. K., Bonneau, R., Malarkey, W., & Hughes, J. (1992). Stress-induced modulation of the immune response to recombinant hepatitis B vaccine. *Psychosomatic Medicine, 54,* 22–9.

Glaser, R., Rice, J., Sheridan, J., Pertel, R. L., Stout, J., Speicher, C. E., Pinsky, D., Kotur, H., Post, A., Beck, H., & Kiecolt-Glaser, J. K. (1987). Stress-related immune suppression: Health implications. *Brain, Behavior, and Immunity, 1,* 7–20.

Glaser, R., Rice, J., Speicher, C. E., Stout, J. C., & Kiecolt-Glaser, J. K. (1986). Stress depresses interferon production by leukocytes concomitant with a decrease in natural killer cell activity. *Behavioral Neuroscience, 100,* 675–8.

Goodwin, J. S., Messner, R. P., & Williams, R. C. (1979). Inhibitors of T-cell mitogenesis: Effects of mitogen dosage. *Cellular Immunology, 45,* 303–8.

Goodwin, J. S., Searles, R. P., & Tung, K. S. K. (1982). Immunological responses of a healthy elderly population. *Clinical and Experimental Immunology, 48,* 403–10.

Gregory, M. D., & Smeltzer, M. A. (1983). *Psychiatry: Essentials of Clinical Practice*. Toronto: Little, Brown.

Grunberg, N. E., & Baum, A. (1985). Biological commonalities of stress and substance abuse. In S. Shiffman & T. A. Wills (Eds.), *Coping and Substance Abuse*, pp. 25–62. Orlando: Academic Press.

Habu, S., Akamatsu, K., Tamaoki, N., & Okumura, K. (1984). In vivo significance of NK cells on resistance against virus (HSV-1) infections in mice. *Journal of Immunology, 133,* 2743–7.

Hadden, J. W., Hadden, E. M., & Middleton, E. (1970). Lymphocyte blast transformation. I. Demonstration of adrenergic receptors in human peripheral lymphocytes. *Cellular Immunology, 1,* 583–95.

Harbour-McMenamin, D., Smith, E. M., & Blalock, J. E. (1985). Bacterial lipopolysaccharide induction of leukocyte-derived corticotropin and endorphins. *Infections and Immunity, 48,* 813–17.

Hatfield, S. P., Petersen, B. H., & DiMicco, J. A. (1986). Beta adrenoceptor modulation of the generation of murine cytotoxic T lymphocytes in vitro. *Journal of Pharmacology and Experimental Therapeutics, 239,* 460–6.

Heilig, M., Irwin, M., Grewal, I., & Sercarz, E. (1993). Sympathetic regulation of T-helper cell function. *Brain, Behavior, and Immunity, 7,* 154–63.

Hellstrand, K., Hermodsson, S., & Strannegard, O. (1985). Evidence for a β-adrenoceptor-mediated regulation of human natural killer cells. *Journal of Immunology, 134,* 4095–9.

Herbert, T. B., & Cohen, S. (1993). Stress and immunity in humans: A meta-analytic review. *Psychosomatic Medicine, 55,* 364–79.

Herbert, T. B., Cohen, S., Marsland, A. L., Bachen, E. A., Rabin, B. S., Muldoon, M. F., & Manuck, S. B. (1994). Cardiovascular reactivity and the course of immune response to an acute psychological stressor. *Psychosomatic Medicine, 56,* 337–44.

Hoch, C. C., Reynolds, C. F., Kupper, D. J., Berman, S. R., Houck, P. R., & Stack, J. A. (1987). Empirical note: Self-report versus recorded sleep in healthy seniors. *Psychophysiology, 24,* 293–9.

Holbrook, N. J., Cox, W. I., & Horner, H. C. (1983). Direct suppression of natural killer activity in human peripheral blood leukocyte cultures by glucocorticoids and its modulation by interferon. *Cancer Research, 43,* 4019–25.

Ironson, G., Wynings, C., Schneiderman, N., Baum, A., Rodriguez, M., Greenwood, D., Benight, C., Antoni, M.,

LaPerriere, A., Huang, H. S., Klimas, N., & Fletcher, M. A. (1997). Posttraumatic stress symptoms, intrusive thoughts, loss, and immune function after Hurricane Andrew. *Psychosomatic Medicine, 59,* 128–41.

Irwin, M., Brown, M., Patterson, T., Hauger, R., Mascovich, A., & Grant, I. (1991). Neuropeptide Y and natural killer cell activity: Findings in depression and Alzheimer caregiver stress. *FASEB, 5,* 3100–7.

Irwin, M., Hauger, R., & Brown, M. (1992). Central corticotropin-releasing hormone activates the sympathetic nervous system and reduces immune function: Increased responsivity in the aged rat. *Endocrinology, 131,* 1047–53.

Irwin, M., Hauger, R. L., Brown, M., & Britton, K. T. (1989). CRF activates autonomic nervous system and reduces natural killer cytotoxicity. *American Journal of Physiology, 255,* R744–R747.

Irwin, M., Mascovich, A., Gillin, J. C., Willoughby, R., Pike, J., & Smith, T. L. (1994). Partial sleep deprivation reduces natural killer cell activity in humans. *Psychosomatic Medicine, 56,* 493–8.

Irwin, M., Smith, T. L., & Gillin, J. C. (1992). Electroencephalographic sleep and natural killer activity in depressed patients and control subjects. *Psychosomatic Medicine, 54,* 10–21.

Ishigami, T. (1919). The influence of psychic acts on the progress of pulmonary tuberculosis. *American Review of Tuberculosis, 2,* 470–84.

Jabaaij, L., Grosheide, P. M., Heijtink, R. A., Duivenvoorden, H. J., Ballieux, R. E., & Vingerhoets, J. J. M. (1993). Influence of perceived psychological stress and distress on antibody response to low dose rDNA Hepatitis B vaccine. *Journal of Psychosomatic Research, 18,* 591–605.

Jaffe, J. H. (1980). Drug addiction and drug abuse. In A. G. Gilman, L. S. Goodman, & A. Gilman (Eds.), *The Pharmacological Basis of Therapeutics,* 6th ed. New York: Macmillan.

Jankovic, B. D., & Isakovic, K. (1973). Neuro-endocrine correlates of immune response: Effect of brain lesions on antibody production, arthus reactivity and delayed hypersensitivity in the rat. *International Archives of Allergy and Applied Immunology, 45,* 360–72.

Johnson, H. W., Torres, B. A., Smith, E. M., Dion, L. D., & Blalock, J. E. (1984). Regulation of lymphokine (γ-interferon) production by corticotropin. *Journal of Immunology, 132,* 246–50.

Johnson, R. W., von Borell, E. H., Anderson, L. L., Kojic, L. D., & Cunnick, J. E. (1994). Intracerebroventricular injection of corticotropin-releasing hormone in the pig: Acute effects on behavior, adrenocorticotropin secretion, and immune suppression. *Endocrinology, 135,* 642–8.

Kamarck, T. W., Manuck, S. B., & Jennings, J. R. (1990). Social support reduces cardiovascular reactivity to psychological challenge: A laboratory model. *Psychosomatic Medicine, 52,* 42–58.

Kasprowicz, A. L., Manuck, S. B., Malkoff, S. B., & Krantz, D. S. (1990). Individual differences in behaviorally evoked cardiovascular response: Temporal stability and hemodynamic patterning. *Psychophysiology, 27,* 605–19.

Kavelaars, A., Ballieux, R. E., & Heijnen, C. J. (1989). The role of IL-1 in the corticotropin-releasing factor and arginine-vasopressin-induced secretion of immunoreactive β-endorphin by human peripheral blood mononuclear cells. *Journal of Immunology, 142,* 2338–42.

Kavelaars, A., Ballieux, R. E., & Heijnen, C. J. (1990). β-endorphin secretion by human peripheral blood mononuclear cells: Regulation by glucocorticoids. *Life Sciences, 46,* 1233–40.

Kay, N., Allen, J., & Morley, J. E. (1984). Endorphin stimulates normal human peripheral blood lymphocyte natural killer activity. *Life Sciences, 35,* 53–9.

Kelso, A., & Munck, A. (1984). Glucocorticoid inhibition of lymphokine secretion by alloreactive T lymphocyte clones. *Journal of Immunology, 133,* 784–91.

Kemeny, M. E., Solomon, G. F., Morley, J. E., & Herbert, T. L. (1992). Psychoimmunology. In C. B. Nemeroff (Ed.), *Psychoneuroimmunology,* pp. 563–91. London: CRC Press.

Kemeny, M. E., Weiner, H., Duran, R., Taylor, S. E., Visscher, B., & Fahey, J. L. (1995). Immune system changes after the death of a partner in HIV-positive gay men. *Psychosomatic Medicine, 57,* 547–54.

Khan, M. M., Sansoni, P., Silverman, E. D., Engleman, E. G., & Melmon, K. L. (1986). Beta-adrenergic receptors on human suppressor, helper, and cytolytic lymphocytes. *Biochemical Pharmacology, 35,* 1137–42.

Kiecolt-Glaser, J. K., Cacioppo, J. T., Malarkey, W. B., & Glaser, R. (1992). Acute psychological stressors and short-term immune changes: What, why, for whom, and to what extent? *Psychosomatic Medicine, 54,* 680–5.

Kiecolt-Glaser, J. K., Dura, J. R., Speicher, C. E., Trask, O. J., & Glaser, R. G. (1991). Spousal caregivers of dementia victims: Longitudinal changes in immunity and health. *Psychosomatic Medicine, 53,* 345–62.

Kiecolt-Glaser, J. K., Fisher, L. D., Ogrocki, P., Stout, J. C., Speicher, C. E., & Glaser, R. (1987a). Marital quality, marital disruption, and immune function. *Psychosomatic Medicine, 49,* 13–34.

Kiecolt-Glaser, J. K., & Glaser, R. (1988a). Methodological issues in behavioral immunology research with humans. *Brain, Behavior, and Immunity, 2,* 67–78.

Kiecolt-Glaser, J. K., & Glaser, R. (1988b). Immunological competence. In E. A. Blechman & K. D. Brownell (Eds.), *Handbook of Behavioral Medicine for Women,* pp. 195–205. New York: Pergamon.

Kiecolt-Glaser, J. K., & Glaser, R. (1995). Psychoneuroimmunology and health consequences: Data and shared mechanisms. *Psychosomatic Medicine, 57,* 269–74.

Kiecolt-Glaser, J. K., Glaser, R., Gravenstein, S., Malarkey, W. B., & Sheridan, J. (1996). Chronic stress alters the immune response to influenza virus vaccine in older adults. *Proceedings of the National Academy of Sciences U.S.A., 93,* 3043–7.

Kiecolt-Glaser, J. K., Glaser, R., Shuttleworth, E. C., Dyer, C. S., Ogrocki, P., & Speicher, C. E. (1987b). Chronic stress and immunity in family caregivers of Alzheimer's disease victims. *Psychosomatic Medicine, 49,* 523–35.

Kiecolt-Glaser, J. K., Glaser, R., Williger, D., Stout, J., Messick, G., Sheppard, S., Ricker, D., Romisher, S. C., Briner, W., Bonnell, G., & Donnerberg, R. (1985). Psychosocial enhancement of immunocompetence in a geriatric population. *Health Psychology, 4,* 25–41.

Kiecolt-Glaser, J. K., Kennedy, S., Malkoff, S., Fisher, L., Speicher, C. E., & Glaser, R. (1988). Marital discord and immunity in males. *Psychosomatic Medicine, 50,* 213–29.

Kiecolt-Glaser, J. K., Marucha, P. T., Malarkey, W. B., Mercado, A. M., & Glaser, R. (1995). Slowing of wound healing by psychological stress. *Lancet, 346*, 1194–6.

Knapp, P. H., Levy, E. M., Giorgi, R. G., Black, P. H., Fox, B. H., & Heeren, T. C. (1992). Short-term immunological effects of induced emotion. *Psychosomatic Medicine, 54*, 133–48.

Korneva, E. A., & Khai, L. M. (1963). The effect of the destruction of areas within the hypothalamic region on the process of immunogenesis [English translation]. In S. Locke, R. Ader, H. Besedovsky, N. Hall, G. Solomon, & T. Strom (Eds.), *Foundations of Psychoneuroimmunology*, pp. 11–20. New York: Aldine.

Krauss, I. K. (1980). Between- and within-group comparisons in aging research. In L. A. Poon (Ed.), *Aging in the 1980s: Psychological Issues*, pp. 542–51. Washington, DC: American Psychological Association.

Labeur, M. S., Arzt, E., Wiegers, G. J., Holsboer, F., & Reul, J. M. H. M. (1995). Long-term intracerebroventricular corticotropin-releasing hormone administration induces distinct changes in rat splenocyte activation and cytokine expression. *Endocrinology, 136*, 2678–88.

Landmann, R. M. A., Durig, M., Gudat, F., Wesp, M., & Harder, F. (1985). Beta-adrenergic regulation of the blood lymphocyte phenotype distribution in normal subjects and splenectomized patients. *Advances in Experimental Medicine and Biology, 186*, 1051–62.

Landmann, R. M. A., Muller, F. B., Perini, C. H., Wesp, M., Erne, P., & Buhler, F. R. (1984). Changes in immunoregulatory cells induced by psychological and physical stress: Relationship to plasma catecholamines. *Clinical Experimental Immunology, 58*, 127–35.

Lane, J. D. (1994). Neuroendocrine responses to caffeine in the work environment. *Psychosomatic Medicine, 546*, 267–70.

Lane, J. D., & Williams, R. B. (1985). Caffeine affects cardiovascular responses to stress. *Psychophysiology, 22*, 648–55.

LaPerriere, A. R., Antoni, M. H., Schneiderman, N., Ironson, G., Klimas, N., et al. (1990). Exercise intervention attenuates emotional distress and natural killer cell decrements following notification of positive serologic status for HIV-1. *Biofeedback and Self-Regulation, 15*, 229–42.

Laporte, R. E., Montoye, H. J., & Caspersen, C. J. (1985). Assessment of physical activity in epidemiologic research: Problems and prospects. *Public Health Reports, 100*, 131–46.

Lepore, S. J. (1995). Cynicism, social support, and cardiovascular reactivity. *Health Psychology, 14*, 210–16.

Lepore, S. J., Allen, K. A., & Evans, G. W. (1993). Social support lowers cardiovascular reactivity to an acute stressor. *Psychosomatic Medicine, 55*, 518–24.

Liang, S., Jemerin, J. M., Tshann, J. M., Wara, D. W., & Boyce, T. W. (1997). Life events, frontal electroencephalogram laterality, and functional immune status after acute psychological stressors in adolescents. *Psychosomatic Medicine, 59*, 178–86.

Llabre, M. M., Spitzer, S. B., Saab, P. G., Ironson, G. H., & Schneiderman, N. (1991). The reliability and specificity of delta versus residualized change as measures of cardiovascular reactivity to behavioral challenges. *Psychophysiology, 28*, 701–11.

Lolait, S. J., Lim, A. T. W., Toh, B. H., & Funder, J. W. (1984). Immunoreactive β-endorphin in a subpopulation of mouse spleen macrophages. *Journal of Clinical Investigations, 73*, 277–80.

Lovallo, W. R., Pincomb, G. A., Brackett, D. J., & Wilson, M. F. (1990). Heart rate reactivity as a predictor of neuroendocrine responses to aversive and appetitive challenges. *Psychosomatic Medicine, 52*, 17–26.

Lukomska, B., Waldemar, L., Engeset, A., & Kolstad, P. (1983). The effect of surgery and chemotherapy on blood NK cell activity in patients with ovarian cancer. *Cancer, 51*, 465–9.

Lumio, J., Welin, M.-G., Hirvonen, P., & Weber, T. (1983). Lymphocyte subpopulations and reactivity during and after infectious mononucleosis. *Medical Biology, 61*, 208–13.

Luparello, T. J., Stein, M., & Park, C. D. (1964). Effect of hypothalamic lesions on rat anaphylaxis. *American Journal of Physiology, 207*, 911–14.

Lysle, D. T., Coussons, M. E., Watts, V. J., Bennett, E. H., & Dykstra, L. A. (1993). Morphine-induced alterations of immune status: Dose dependency, compartment specificity and antagonism by naltrexone. *Journal of Pharmacology and Experimental Therapeutics, 265*, 1071–8.

MacGregor, R. R. (1986). Alcohol and immune defense. *JAMA, 256*, 1474–9.

Madden, K. S., & Livnat, S. (1991). Catecholamine action and immunologic reactivity. In R. Ader, D. L. Felten, & N. Cohen (Eds.), *Psychoneuroimmunology*, pp. 283–310. New York: Academic Press.

Maier, S. F., Watkins, L. R., & Fleshner, M. (1994). Psychoneuroimmunology: The interface between behavior, brain, and immunity. *American Psychologist, 49*, 1004–17.

Maisel, A. S., Fowler, P., Rearden, A., Motulsky, H. J., & Michel, M. C. (1989). A new method for isolation of human lymphocyte subsets reveals differential regulation of β-adrenergic receptors by terbutaline treatment. *Clinical Pharmacology and Therapeutics, 46*, 429–39.

Maisel, A. S., Harris, T., Rearden, C. A., & Michel, M. C. (1990). β-adrenergic receptors in lymphocyte subsets after exercise: Alterations in normal individuals and patients with congestive heart failure. *Circulation, 82*, 2003–10.

Mandler, R. N., Biddison, W. E., Mandler, R., & Serrate, S. A. (1986). β-endorphin augments the cytolytic activity and interferon production of natural killer cells. *Journal of Immunology, 136*, 934–9.

Manuck, S. B., Cohen, S. C., Rabin, B., Muldoon, M. F., & Bachen, E. A. (1991). Individual differences in cellular immune response to stress. *Psychological Science, 2*, 111–15.

Marsland, A. L., Manuck, S. B., Fazzari, T. V., Stewart, C. J., & Rabin, B. S. (1995). Stability and individual differences in cellular immune responses to acute psychological stress. *Psychosomatic Medicine, 57*, 295–8.

Marucha, P. T., Kiecolt-Glaser, J. K., & Favegehi, M. (1997). Mucosal wound healing is impaired by examination stress. *Psychosomatic Medicine, 60*, 362–5.

Mason, J. W. (1975). Emotion as reflected in patterns of endocrine integration. In L. Levi (Ed.), *Emotions: Their Parameters and Measurement*, pp. 143–81. New York: Raven.

Mathews, P. M., Froelich, C. J., Sibbitt, W. L., & Bankhurst, A. D. (1983). Enhancement of natural cytotoxicity by β-endorphin. *Journal of Immunology, 130*, 1658–62.

Matthews, K. A., Caggiula, A. R., McAllister, C. G., Berga, S. L., Owens, J. F., Flory, J. D., & Miller, A. L. (1995). Sympathetic reactivity to acute stress and immune response in women. *Psychosomatic Medicine, 57*, 564–71.

Matthews, K. A., Owens, J. F., Allen, M. T., & Stoney, C. M. (1992). Do cardiovascular responses to laboratory stress relate to ambulatory blood pressure levels?: Yes, in some of the people, some of the time. *Psychosomatic Medicine, 54,* 686–97.

McCain, H. W., Lamster, I. B., Bozzone, J. M., & Grbic, J. T. (1982). β-endorphin modulates human immune activity via non-opiate receptor mechanisms. *Life Sciences, 31,* 1619–24.

McKinnon, W., Weisse, C. S., Reynolds, C. P., Bowles, C. A., & Baum, A. (1989). Chronic stress, leukocyte subpopulations, and humoral response to latent viruses. *Health Psychology, 8,* 389–402.

Medawar, P. B., & Sparrow, E. M. (1956). The effects of adrenocortical hormone, adrenocorticotrophic hormone and pregnancy on skin transplantation immunity in mice. *Journal of Endocrinology, 14,* 240–56.

Mehrishi, J. N., & Mills, I. H. (1983). Opiate receptors on lymphocytes and platelets in man. *Clinical Immunology and Immunopathology, 27,* 240–9.

Metter, E. J., Walega, D., Metter, E. L., Pearson, J., Brant, L. J., Hiscock, B. S., & Fozard, J. L. (1992). How comparable are healthy 60- and 80-year old men? *Journals of Gerontology: Medical Sciences, 47,* M73–M78.

Mills, P. J., Haeri, S. L., & Dimsdale, J. E. (1995a). Temporal stability of acute stressor-induced changes in cellular immunity. *International Journal of Psychophysiology, 19,* 287–90.

Mills, P. J., Ziegler, M. G., Dimsdale, J. E., & Parry, B. L. (1995b). Enumerative immune changes following acute stress: Effects of the menstrual cycle. *Brain, Behavior, and Immunity, 9,* 190–5.

Moser, M., De Smedt, T., Sornasse, T., Tielemans, F., Chentoufi, A. A., Muraille, E., Van Mechelen, M., Urbain, J., & Leo, O. (1995). Glucocorticoids down-regulate dendritic cell function *in vitro* and *in vivo*. *European Journal of Immunology, 25,* 2818–24.

Mosmann, T. R., & Coffman, R. L. (1989). TH1 and TH2 cells: Different patterns of lymphokine secretion lead to different functional properties. *Annual Review of Immunology, 7,* 145–73.

Munck, A., & Guyre, P. M. (1991). Glucocorticoids and immune function. In R. Ader, D. L. Felten, & N. Cohen (Eds.), *Psychoneuroimmunology,* pp. 447–74. New York: Academic Press.

Munck, A., Guyre, P. M., & Holbrook, N. J. (1984). Physiological function of glucocorticoids in stress and their relation to pharmacological actions. *Endocrine Reviews, 5,* 25–44.

Murray, D. R., Irwin, M., Rearden, A., Ziegler, M., Motulsky, H., & Maisel, A. S. (1992). Sympathetic and immune interactions during dynamic exercise. Mediation via a β₂-adrenergic-dependent mechanism. *Circulation, 86,* 203–13.

Naliboff, B. D., Benton, D., Solomon, G. F., Morley, J. E., Fahey, J. L., Bloom, E. T., Makinodan, T., & Gilmore, S. L. (1991). Immunological changes in young and old adults during brief laboratory stress. *Psychosomatic Medicine, 53,* 121–32.

Naliboff, B. D., Solomon, G. F., Gilmore, S. L., Benton, D., Morley, J. E., & Fahey, J. L. (1995a). The effects of the opiate antagonist naloxone on measures of cellular immunity during rest and brief psychological stress. *Journal of Psychosomatic Research, 39,* 345–59.

Naliboff, B. D., Solomon, G. F., Gilmore, S. L., Fahey, J. L., Benton, D., & Pine, J. (1995b). Rapid changes in cellular immunity following a confrontational role-play stressor. *Brain, Behavior, and Immunity, 9,* 207–19.

Nomoto, Y., Karasawa, S., & Uehara, K. (1994). Effects of hydrocortisone and adrenaline on natural killer cell activity. *British Journal of Anaesthesia, 73,* 318–21.

O'Leary, A. (1990). Stress, emotion, and human immune function. *Psychological Bulletin, 108,* 363–82.

Ottaway, C. A., & Husband, A. J. (1992). Central nervous influences in lymphocyte migration. *Brain, Behavior, and Immunity, 6,* 97–116.

Palmblad, J. (1981). Stress and immunologic competence: Studies in man. In R. Ader (Ed.), *Psychoneuroimmunology,* pp. 229–57. New York: Academic Press.

Parrillo, J. E., & Fauci, A. S. (1978). Comparison of the effector cells in human spontaneous cellular cytotoxicity and antibody-dependent cellular cytotoxicity: Differential sensitivity of effector cells to in vivo and in vitro corticosteroids. *Scandinavian Journal of Immunology, 8,* 99–107.

Paxton, H., Kidd, P., Landay, A., Giorgi, J., Flomenberg, N., Walker, E., Valentine, F., Fahey, J., & Gelman, R. (1989). Results of the flow cytometry ACTG quality control program: Analysis and findings. *Clinical Immunology and Immunopathology, 52,* 68–84.

Pedersen, B. K., & Beyer, J. M. (1986). Characterization of the in vitro effects of glucocorticoids on NK cell activity. *Allergy, 41,* 220–4.

Perkins, K. A., Grobe, J. E., Fonte, C., & Breus, M. (1992). "Paradoxical" effects of smoking on subjective stress versus cardiovascular arousal in males and females. *Pharmacology Biochemistry and Behavior, 42,* 301–11.

Petry, L. J., Weems, L. B., & Livingstone, J. N. (1991). Relationship of stress, distress, and the immunologic response to a recombinant hepatitis B vaccine. *Journal of Family Practice, 32,* 481–6.

Platt, J. R. (1964). Strong inference. *Science, 146,* 347–53.

Plaut, M. (1987). Lymphocyte hormone receptors. *Annual Review of Immunology, 5,* 621–69.

Pollak, M. H. (1991). Heart rate reactivity to laboratory tasks and ambulatory heart rate in daily life. *Psychosomatic Medicine, 53,* 1–12.

Riley, V. (1981). Psychoneuroendocrine influences on immunocompetence and neoplasia. *Science, 212,* 1100–9.

Roitt, I., Brostoff, J., & Male, D. (1993). *Immunology.* London: Mosby.

Sabjarwal, P., Glaser, R., Lafuse, W., Varma, S., Liu, Q., Arkins, S., Kooijman, K., Kutz, L., Kelley, K. W., & Malarkey, W. B. (1992). Prolactin synthesized and secreted by human peripheral blood mononuclear cells: An autocrine growth factor for lymphoproliferation. *Proceedings of the National Academy of Sciences U.S.A., 89,* 7713–16.

Sapolsky, R. M., Krey, L. C., & McEwen, B. S. (1984). Stress down-regulates corticosterone receptors in a site-specific manner in the brain. *Endocrinology, 114,* 287–92.

Sapolsky, R. M., Krey, L. C., & McEwen, B. S. (1986). The neuroendocrinology of stress and aging: The glucocorticoid cascade hypothesis. *Endocrine Reviews, 7,* 284–301.

Schedlowski, M., Falk, A., Rohne, A., Wagner, T. O. F., Jacobs, R., Tewes, U., & Schmidt, R. E. (1993). Catecholamines induce alterations of distribution and activity of human natural killer (NK) cells. *Journal of Clinical Immunology, 13,* 344–51.

Schedlowski, M., Hosch, W., Oberbeck, R., Benschop, R. J., Raab, H., & Schmidt, R. E. (1996). Catecholamines modulate human NK cell circulation and function via spleen-independent β_2-adrenergic mechanisms. *Journal of Immunology, 156,* 93–9.

Schenker, E. L., Hultin, L. E., Bauer, K. D., Ferbas, J., Margolick, J. B., & Giorgi, J. V. (1993). Evaluation of a dual-color flow cytometry immunophenotyping panel in a multicenter quality assurance program. *Cytometry, 14,* 307–17.

Schindler, L. W. (1991). Understanding the immune system. Document no. 92-529, U.S. Department of Health and Human Services, Washington, DC.

Schleifer, S. J., Eckholdt, H. M., Cohen, J., & Keller, S. E. (1993). Analysis of partial variance (APV) as a statistical approach to control day to day variation in immune assays. *Brain, Behavior, and Immunity, 7,* 243–52.

Schleifer, S. J., Keller, S. E., Bond, R. N., Cohen, J., & Stein, M. (1989). Depression and immunity: Role of age, sex, and severity. *Archives of General Psychiatry, 46,* 81–7.

Schleifer, S. J., Keller, S. E., Camarino, E., Thornton, J. C., & Stein, M. (1983). Suppression of lymphocyte stimulation following bereavement. *JAMA, 250,* 374–7.

Schneiderman, A. B., & Baum, A. (1992). Acute and chronic stress and the immune system. In N. Schneiderman, P. McCabe, & A. Baum (Eds.), *Stress and Disease Processes,* pp. 1–25. Hillsdale, NJ: Erlbaum.

Scientific American (1993). Life, death, and the immune system. *Scientific American, 269,* 52–144.

Seeman, T. E., & Robbins, R. J. (1994). Aging and hypothalamic-pituitary-adrenal responses to challenge in humans. *Endocrine Reviews, 15,* 233–60.

Selzer, M. L. (1971). The Michigan alcohol screening test: The quest for a new diagnostic instrument. *American Journal of Psychiatry, 127,* 165–8.

Sgoutas-Emch, S. A., Cacioppo, J. T., Uchino, B. N., Malarkey, W., Pearl, D., Kiecolt-Glaser, J. K., & Glaser, R. (1994). The effects of an acute psychological stressor on cardiovascular, endocrine, and cellular immune response: A prospective study of individuals high and low in heart rate reactivity. *Psychophysiology, 31,* 264–71.

Shahabi, N. A., Heagy, W., & Sharp, B. M. (1996). β-endorphin enhances concanavalin-A-stimulated calcium mobilization by murine splenic T cells. *Endocrinology, 137,* 3386–93.

Shavit, Y., Depaulis, A., Martin, F. C., Terman, G. W., Pechnick, R. N., Zane, C. J., Gale, R. P., & Liebeskind, J. C. (1986). Involvement of brain opiate receptors in the immune-suppressive effect of morphine. *Proceedings of the National Academy of Sciences U.S.A., 83,* 7114–17.

Sherwood, A., Dolan, C. A., & Light, K. C. (1990). Hemodynamics of blood pressure responses during active and passive coping. *Psychophysiology, 27,* 656–68.

Sibinga, N. E. S., & Goldstein, A. (1988). Opioid peptides and opioid receptors in cells of the immune system. *Annual Review of Immunology, 6,* 219–49.

Sieber, W. J., Rodin, J., Larson, L., Ortega, S., & Cummings, N. (1992). Modulation of human natural killer cell activity by exposure to uncontrollable stress. *Brain, Behavior, and Immunity, 6,* 141–56.

Silverstein, A. M. (1989). *A History of Immunology.* San Diego: Academic Press.

Simon, H. B. (1991). Exercise and human immune function. In R. Ader, D. L. Felten, & N. Cohen (Eds.), *Psychoneuroimmunology,* pp. 869–95. New York: Academic Press.

Skinner, H. A., Holt, S., Sheu, W. J., & Israel, Y. (1986). Clinical versus laboratory detection of alcohol abuse: The alcohol clinical index. *British Medical Journal, 292,* 1703–8.

Sklar, L. S., & Anisman, H. (1981). Stress and cancer. *Psychological Bulletin, 89,* 369–406.

Smith, E. M., & Blalock, J. E. (1981). Human lymphocyte production of corticotropin and endorphin-like substances: Association with leukocyte interferon. *Proceedings of the National Academy of Sciences U.S.A., 78,* 7530–4.

Smith, E. M., Brosnan, P., Meyer, W. J., & Blalock, J. E. (1987). An ACTH receptor on human mononuclear leukocytes: Relation to adrenal ACTH-receptor activity. *New England Journal of Medicine, 317,* 1266–9.

Smith, E. M., Morrill, A. C., Meyer, W. J., & Blalock, J. E. (1986). Corticotropin releasing factor induction of leukocyte-derived immunoreactive ACTH and endorphins. *Nature, 321,* 881–2.

Solomon, G. F. (1987). Psychoneuroimmunology: Interactions between central nervous system and immune system. *Journal of Neuroscience Research, 18,* 1–9.

Solomon, G. F., & Moos, R. H. (1964). Emotions, immunity, and disease: A speculative theoretical integration. *Archives of General Psychiatry, 11,* 657–74.

Solomon, G. F., Segerstrom, S. C., Grohr, P., Kemeny, M., & Fahey, J. (1997). Shaking up immunity: Psychological and immunologic changes after a natural disaster. *Psychosomatic Medicine, 59,* 114–27.

Stein, M., Schiavi, R. C., & Camerino, M. (1976). Influence of brain and behavior on the immune system. *Science, 191,* 435–40.

Stone, A. A., Valdimarsdottir, H. B., Katkin, E. S., Burns, J., Cox, D. S., Lee, S., Fine, J., Ingle, D., & Bovbjerg, D. H. (1993). Effects of mental stressors on mitogen-induced lymphocyte responses in the laboratory. *Psychology and Health, 8,* 269–84.

Tubaro, E., Borelli, G., Croce, C., Cavallo, G., & Santiangeli, C. (1983). Effect of morphine on resistance to infection. *Journal of Infectious Diseases, 148,* 656–66.

Tvede, N., Kappel, M., Halkjoer-Kristensen, J., Galbo, H., & Pedersen, B. K. (1993). The effects of light, moderate and severe bicycle exercise on lymphocyte subsets, natural and lymphokine activity killer cells, lymphocyte proliferative response and interleukin 2 production. *International Journal of Sports Medicine, 14,* 275–82.

Uchino, B. N., Cacioppo, J. T., Malarkey, W., & Glaser, R. (1995). Individual differences in cardiac sympathetic control predict endocrine and immune responses to acute psychological stress. *Journal of Personality and Social Psychology, 69,* 736–43.

Uchino, B. N., & Garvey, T. G. (1997). The availability of social support reduces cardiovascular reactivity to acute psychological stress. *Journal of Behavioral Medicine, 20,* 15–27.

Van Tits, L. J., Michel, M. C., Grosse-Wilde, H., Happel, M., Eigler, F. W., Soliman, A., & Brodde, O. E. (1990). Catecholamines increase lymphocyte β_2-adrenergic receptors via a

β_2-adrenergic, spleen-dependent process. *American Journal of Physiology, 258,* E191–E202.

Visintainer, M. A., Volpicelli, J. R., & Seligman, M. E. P. (1982). Tumor rejection in rats after inescapable or escapable shock. *Science, 216,* 437–9.

Washburn, R. A., & Montoye, H. J. (1986). The assessment of physical activity by questionnaire. *American Journal of Epidemiology, 123,* 563–76.

Weber, R. J., & Pert, A. (1989). The periaqueductal gray matter mediates opiate-induced immunosuppression. *Science, 245,* 188–90.

Webster, E. L., Tracey, D. E., Jutila, M. A., Wolfe, S. A., & De Souza, E. B. (1990). Corticotropin-releasing factor receptors in mouse spleen: Identification of receptor-bearing cells as resident macrophages. *Endocrinology, 127,* 440–52.

Weisse, C. A., Pato, C. N., McAllister, C. G., Littman, R., Breier, A., Paul, S. M., & Baum, A. (1990). Differential effects of controllable and uncontrollable acute stress on lymphocyte proliferation and leukocyte percentages in humans. *Brain, Behavior, and Immunity, 4,* 339–51.

Werb, Z., Foley, R., & Munck, A. (1978). Interaction of glucocorticoids with macrophages. *Journal of Experimental Medicine, 147,* 1684–94.

Whiteside, T. L., & Herberman, R. B. (1994). Role of human natural killer cells in health and disease. *Clinical and Diagnostic Laboratory Immunology, 1,* 125–33.

Wiegers, G. J., Croiset, G., Reul, J. M. H. M., Holsboer, F., & De Kloet, E. R. (1993). Differential effects of corticosteroids on rat peripheral blood T-lymphocyte mitogenesis in vivo and in vitro. *American Journal of Physiology, 265,* E825–E830.

Wiegers, G. J., Reul, J. M. H. M., Holsboer, F., & De Kloet, E. R. (1994). Enhancement of rat splenic lymphocyte mitogenesis after short-term preexposure to corticosteroids in vitro. *Endocrinology, 135,* 2351–7.

Williams, J. M., Peterson, R. G., Shea, P. A., Schmedtje, J. F., Bauer, D. C., & Felten, D. L. (1981). Sympathetic innervation of murine thymus and spleen: Evidence for a functional link between the nervous and immune systems. *Brain Research Bulletin, 6,* 83–94.

Williams, L. T., Snyderman, R., & Lefkowitz, R. J. (1976). Identification of β-adrenergic receptors in human lymphocytes by $(-)$ [^{3}H] alprenolol binding. *Journal of Clinical Investigation, 57,* 149–55.

Wybran, J., Appelboom, T., Famaey, J., & Govaerts, A. (1979). Suggestive evidence for receptors for morphine and methionine-enkephalin on normal human blood T lymphocytes. *Journal of Immunology, 123,* 1068–70.

Zakowski, S. G., McAllister, C. G., Deal, M., & Baum, A. (1992). Stress, reactivity, and immune function in healthy men. *Health Psychology, 11,* 223–32.

Zautra, A. J., Okun, M. A., Robinson, S. E., Lee, D., Roth, S. H., & Emmanual, J. (1989). Life stress and lymphocyte alterations among patients with rheumatoid arthritis. *Health Psychology, 8,* 1–14.

Zimmerman, D. W., & Williams, R. H. (1982a). Gain scores in research can be highly reliable. *Journal of Educational Measurement, 19,* 149–54.

Zimmerman, D. W., & Williams, R. H. (1982b). The relative error magnitude in three measures of change. *Psychometrika, 47,* 141–7.

CHAPTER SIXTEEN

PSYCHOSOCIAL FACTORS AND HUMORAL IMMUNITY

VIRGINIA M. SANDERS, LAURIE ICIEK, & DEBORAH J. KASPROWICZ

It has been proposed that the activity of the immune system is influenced by the host's response to a number of different psychosocial factors, such as stress, motivation, social support, coping style, personality, emotional repression, clinical depression, and anxiety. In addition, the psychosocial factors themselves may be influenced by a number of confounding factors, such as age, gender, ethnicity, socioeconomic status, social environment, nutritional status, and disease. Considerable attention has focused in the last two decades on the mechanisms by which psychosocial factors influence immune status. In this chapter, we will discuss the evidence indicating that psychosocial factors and endogenous biological mediators can influence the humoral immune defense mechanisms in the body. We will also discuss how accurate measurements of both psychosocial and humoral immune parameters can help show that a relationship exists between these two responses in that the state of one influences the state of the other.

Historical Context

Our ability to combat the many microorganisms that gain entry into our bodies daily depends on both nonspecific and specific mechanisms. As early as the pioneering studies of Jenner and Pasteur, it became clear that some host defense mechanisms become activated to protect individuals against the pathogenic effects of microorganisms. It was first discovered that nonspecific mechanisms of defense included those that prevented the spread of microorganisms from their point of entry into the host. The most well-recognized nonspecific mechanism of immune protection involves cell-mediated immune mechanisms involving the phagocytosis of extracellular bacteria by macrophages. However, a number of deadly organisms, such as encapsulated pneumococci, do not adhere well to phagocytic cells. Therefore, specific humoral immune mechanisms

needed to evolve that could promote the adherence of some bacteria to phagocytic cells for efficient phagocytosis and destruction. Likewise, for intracellular antigens such as viruses and parasites, specific humoral immune mechanisms needed to evolve that could neutralize the activity of these organisms before they entered cells. These mechanisms involve the recognition of invading microorganisms by specialized cells called B lymphocytes. After the recognition of the invading pathogen, these B-cells produce immunoglobulin M (IgM) and IgG antibodies that recognize, neutralize, and destroy the invading microorganism.

One of the earliest studies to suggest that a relationship existed between the immune status of an individual and the individual's mental state was a study (Ishigami 1919) that showed, in a series of animal and human experiments, that one's mental state was associated with an increased incidence of tuberculosis infections. Unfortunately, this study was not fully appreciated at the time owing to (a) a lack of knowledge concerning how the immune system functioned and (b) a lack of techniques for critically evaluating immune cell function. This study showed that there was a relationship between the psychosocial factors imposed upon an individual with pulmonary tuberculosis and the phagocytic capacity of cells (within the blood) required for elimination of the microorganism. Ishigami proposed that the high rate of death of young individuals from tuberculosis in Japan was attributable to the "overtaxation of the mind" and the depressive state imposed upon these individuals by an inadequate and unsatisfactory school system that dictated severe entrance examinations and overcrowded learning conditions. Although this study was pioneering in the area now known as psychoneuroimmunology, it was essentially ignored by the scientific community for a number of years.

The high incidence of industrial workers succumbing to the common cold and pneumonia prompted researchers

John T. Cacioppo, Louis G. Tassinary, and Gary G. Berntson (Eds.), *Handbook of Psychophysiology*, 2nd ed. © Cambridge University Press 2000. Printed in the United States of America. ISBN 62634X. All rights reserved.

to study once again the relationship between the mental perception of fatigue and susceptibility to infection with microorganisms. In 1925, Bailey conducted a study to examine the effects of fatigue on animals. He showed that inducing a state of fatigue in rabbits increased disease susceptibility to and mortality from *Streptococcus pneumoniae* as well as the development of extensive pulmonary lesions and death (Bailey 1925). What was most interesting about this study was that the rabbits could be made less susceptible to infection if they were routinely exercised before inducing a state of fatigue. Thus, once again, this study opened the door for scientists to explore the connection between the state of mind and the immune system.

In 1936, the concepts of stress and stressor were introduced by Selye (Selye 1936, 1946). Stress was defined as a biological response to a noxious stimulus, such as heat or cold, that induced activation of the hypothalamic-pituitary-adrenal axis (HPA); the term *stressor* was used to label the noxious stimulus. Selye described the myriad structural changes that occurred during biological response to stress, including the appearance of lymphoid organ atrophy. This finding was among the first to relate a change in HPA activity to a change in immune system architecture. Since then, many researchers have explored this relationship between physical stressors and immune function. However, the list of stressors has expanded to include nonnoxious stimuli such as psychological stress.

By the 1960s, some clinicians began to show that a relationship existed between psychological profiles in individuals afflicted with rheumatoid arthritis, an immune-mediated disease, and their immunologic profile (Solomon & Moos 1964, 1965). However, there was considerable debate over these findings because of the reliability and validity of psychological and immunological measurements that were made. Nonetheless, these studies introduced the area of psychoimmunology to the health science field and, more importantly, emphasized the need for cross-disciplinary approaches to examine this relationship. It was some fifteen years later that a series of experiments were performed to show that animals could be aversively conditioned to be immunosuppressed (Ader & Cohen 1975; Cohen et al. 1979). These studies not only introduced the area of psychoneuroimmunology to the basic health science field but also provided some of the first experimental evidence for a mechanism linking humoral immune system function to a psychological process.

Findings reported in the early 1970s indicated that cell-mediated and humoral immunity seemed to interchange in dominance over one another during the host's response to pathogens (Parish & Liew 1972). However, the extent to which psychosocial distress influences these two types of immunity, and the mechanisms by which cell-mediated and humoral immune status is influenced by the host's response to psychosocial distress, still awaits definition. Yet it is be-

coming clearer that various stressful situations that elicit a psychological stress response are related to changes in humoral immune responsiveness. Although the endogenous molecules that mediate these changes in humoral immune function remain elusive, the likely candidates to serve as mediators include neuroendocrine hormones, opioid peptides, and sympathetic neurotransmitters. An understanding of the mechanisms by which these molecules modulate humoral immune function, coupled with the availability of sensitive and reliable techniques to evaluate humoral immune status, will help us to show more definitively that a relationship exists between psychological and immunological states.

In this chapter, we review and discuss the possible role of the central nervous system (CNS), the hypothalamic-pituitary-adrenal axis (HPA), and the sympathetic nervous system (SNS) in mediating the effect of psychosocial factors on humoral immune function. We also examine the human and animal studies that have addressed the role of psychosocial factors in modulating humoral immune status as well as the current mechanisms and test systems by which antibody is produced and measured.

Physical Context

THE T-HELPER CELL-DEPENDENT ANTIBODY RESPONSE

Many studies have helped to define the specific order of events that are required for T-helper (Th) cell-dependent B-cell antibody production; these have been reviewed extensively (Parker 1993; Vitetta et al. 1989).

Figure 1 outlines the sequence of events leading to antibody production by the B-cell. This figure is presented to emphasize the complexity of the antibody response to antigen and also to make clear that any cellular function along this pathway can be modulated – by neuroendocrine hormones, opioid peptides, and neurotransmitters – if receptors for these modulators are expressed on the cells participating in the response. Initially, antigen is introduced into the immune system. The Ig receptor expressed on the surface of the naive B-cell binds antigen. The resulting antigen–Ig complexes form patches on the B-cell surface and subsequently "cap" at one region on the cell's surface. This capping event triggers receptor endocytosis into endosomal compartments, where antigen dissociates from the Ig molecule. Further processing of the antigen occurs in the lysosomal compartment, where the antigen is degraded into small peptide fragments by lysosomal enzymes. These peptide fragments encounter major histocompatibility complex (MHC) class-II molecules when intracellular vesicles containing the peptides fuse with vesicles containing newly synthesized MHC class-II bound to invariant chain. The binding of a peptide fragment to the MHC class-II groove displaces the invariant chain,

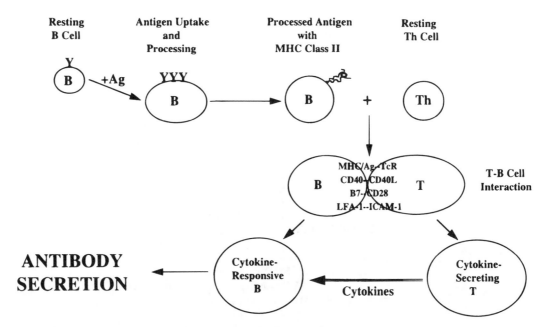

Figure 1. Diagram of the stages of T-cell and B-cell participation in the production of cytokines and antibodies. In this model, the B-cell binds, processes, and re-expresses antigen on the cell surface in association with MHC class-II molecules. The complex of MHC class-II and antigen is recognized by the T-cell receptor associated with a resting Th-cell. The presentation and recognition of MHC/antigen in conjunction with other T-cell– and B-cell–associated adhesion and co-stimulatory molecules allows a physical interaction to occur that is essential for the activation of both cells. The activation of these cells renders the Th-cell capable of producing and secreting cytokines and the B-cell capable of responding to the cytokines. As a result of cytokine stimulation of the activated B-cell, the B-cell is able to further differentiate into an antibody-secreting cell. The intracellular messengers generated as a consequence of cell activation are also shown, as are the adhesion and co-stimulatory molecules that induce and strengthen the interaction between the T-cell and B-cell.

resulting in a peptide–MHC class-II complex that is transported to the cell membrane for expression on the B-cell surface. Following peptide–MHC class-II expression, the B-cell presents the peptide antigen to a MHC class-II–restricted, peptide-specific CD4+ Th cell. It is important to note that, although the literature previously referred to T-cell subsets as T4+ (helper/inducer) and T8+ (suppressor/cytotoxic), we will refer to these subsets using the currently accepted nomenclature of CD4+ and CD8+, respectively.

When the peptide–MHC class-II–expressing B-cell encounters a MHC class-II–restricted, peptide-specific CD4+ Th-cell, several receptor–ligand interactions occur between these two cells that are essential for the process of antibody production to continue. The Th-cell not only activates the B-cell during this cell–cell interaction, it also provides the cytokines necessary for B-cell growth and differentiation into antibody-secreting cells. Two CD4+ Th-cell subsets have been identified and are characterized by the cytokines they secrete following cellular activation. The Th1 cells secrete interferon (IFN-γ) and interleukin (IL-2), while Th2 cells secrete IL-4, IL-5, IL-6, IL-10, and transforming growth factor (TGF-β). The cytokines IFN-γ, IL-4, and TGF-β are involved in determining the antibody isotype produced by B-cells. In vivo and in vitro, IFN-γ–producing Th1 cells induce B-cells to produce IgG$_{2a}$; whereas IL-4–producing Th2 cells induce B-cells to produce IgG$_1$ and IgE, and TGF-β–producing Th2 cells induce B-cells to produce IgA.

A number of cell surface molecules are involved in an antigen-specific, MHC class-II–restricted Th-cell–B-cell interaction. The first receptor–ligand interaction occurs in a specific manner between the T-cell receptor–CD3 complex on the Th-cell and the peptide–MHC class-II complex on the B-cell. The CD4 molecule on the Th-cell plays a role

in determining the specificity of the T-cell receptor–CD3 interaction by binding to a portion of the MHC class-II molecule, thus limiting the interaction of class-II–bearing B-cells to CD4+ Th-cells. One receptor–ligand interaction that is important for stimulation of Th-cell cytokine production is the binding of B7-2 (CD86) on the B-cell to CD28 on the T-cell; CD28 is constitutively expressed on the Th-cell, whereas B7-2 is expressed at low levels on naive splenic B-cells but is up-regulated following B-cell activation.

The interaction between CD40 on the B-cell and CD40L on the T-cell plays an important role in antibody production. CD40–CD40L interactions up-regulate the production of IL-4 by the Th2 cell. Additional receptor–ligand interactions that are important for antibody production include those occurring between intercellular adhesion molecule (ICAM-1) or lymphocyte function–associated (LFA-1) on B-cells and LFA-1 or ICAM-1 on T-cells as well as LFA-3 on B-cells with CD2 on T-cells. Although it is unclear how long an interaction must continue between the B-cell

<u>**Psychosocial Factors**</u>

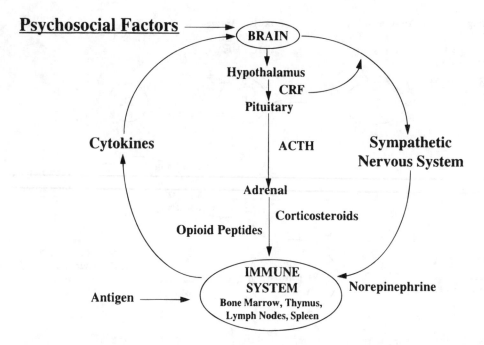

Figure 2. The neuroendocrine–immune communication loop. As an antigen enters the body, the immune system recognizes it and different cells begin an immune response that involves the synthesis and/or release of cytokines. The cytokines affect CNS function and also activate the hypothalamus to secrete corticotropin releasing factor (CRF). CRF induces release of adrenocorticotropin (ACTH), which in turn induces release of glucocorticoids. Glucocorticoids affect immune function but also feed back to inhibit further secretion of both CRF and ACTH. Immune cell and CNS activation induce the release of enkephalin-containing peptides by the adrenal medulla, sympathetic nerve terminals associated with lymphoid organs, and immune cells. CNS activation by cytokines also stimulates the sympathetic nervous system, whose nerve fibers are in close contact with lymphocytes in lymphoid organs. Norepinephrine is released from these nerve terminals and interacts with adrenergic receptors expressed on immune cells. Cytokine secretion is either enhanced or diminished as a consequence of both feedback activity within the loop and the clearance of antigen from the body. Psychosocial factors are proposed to affect the neuroendocrine input into the communication loop.

and Th-cell in order to trigger the B-cell's differentiating into an antibody-secreting cell, the B-cell does require early contact with the Th-cell in order to stimulate and be stimulated by the Th-cell. In summary, the initial interaction between B-cell and Th-cell is important for determining if the B-cell will differentiate into an antibody-secreting cell. Therefore, any mechanism that up-regulates co-stimulatory surface molecules, such as B7-2 on the B-cell, would improve the initial quality of the interaction between the B-cell and Th-cell and consequently result in more B-cells differentiating into antibody-secreting cells.

NEUROENDOCRINE HORMONES AND IMMUNITY

Activation of the HPA is induced by physical stressful stimuli, as first suggested by Selye (1936, 1946), and by psychological stressful stimuli such as academic stress (Malarkey et al. 1995). The pursuit of an understanding of the mechanisms by which the HPA axis is activated to release various biological mediators – and the mechanisms by which these mediators influence immune responsiveness – is an area under much investigation. The reader is referred to Figure 2 for a complete overview of what will be discussed in this section of the chapter.

Interleukin-1 (IL-1) is a biological molecule that is released by an activated immune cell. Interleukin-1 also increases the production of corticotropin releasing hormone (CRH) by neurons located in the paraventricular nucleus of the hypothalamus. These neurons project through the median eminence and terminate on the hypophysial portal vessels that transport CRH to the anterior pituitary to act as a potent secretagogue for adrenocorticotropin (ACTH). The adrenal cortex, in turn, responds to the ACTH by increasing its rate of secretion of glucocorticoids, which exert a suppressive effect on humoral immunity. Glucocorticoids inhibit antigen-specific antibody production after a primary immunization but not after a secondary response (Wallgren, Wilen, & Fossum 1994). Also, various stressors – such as acute alcohol exposure (Han & Pruett 1995) and inescapable shock (Fleshner et al. 1996) – inhibit both cytokine and antibody production via mechanisms that involve elevated levels of glucocorticoids. However, it is interesting to note that corticosteroids are not associated exclusively with immune suppression, and their concentration at the site of action may be important in determining their ability to modulate immune function. For example, the level of stress (which induces corticosteroid release) is an important factor in determining the effect of stress on immunocompetence: moderate stress increases the level of immune responsiveness yet higher levels decrease it (Weiss et al. 1989). In turn, glucocorticoids exert a negative feedback response on the anterior pituitary to reduce the production of ACTH.

Also, both T- and B-lymphocytes release CRH upon activation (Kravchenco & Furalev 1994). It is interesting to note that CRH production by immune cells induces secretion of ACTH by immune cells, leading to an induction of glucocorticoid secretion to feedback and inhibiting CRH secretion by the immune cells. Thus, IL-1 activates the HPA axis at the level of the hypothalamus, and the released CRH acts at the level of either the adrenals or immune system. Specific receptors for CRH are expressed on immune cells (Audhya, Jain, & Hollander 1991; Smith et al. 1986; Webster et al. 1990). The effects of CRH on T-cell and macrophage function are limited to cytokine production and cytokine receptor expression. Specifically, CRH stimulates Th-cell mitogen-induced proliferation and IL-2 receptor expression (Singh 1989), and it augments the production of both IL-2 and IL-1 by mitogen-stimulated Th-cells and macrophages, respectively (Singh & Leu 1990). Moreover, CRH stimulates the locus coeruleus to further activate the HPA and SNS, resulting in T-cell immunosuppression (Rassnick, Sved, & Rabin 1994). The direct effects of CRH to suppress T-cell and macrophage cytokine production may impact on the ability of antigen-activated B-cells to clonally expand into an optimal number of cells to produce antibody. The direct effects of CRH on B-cell function are limited to antigen processing, proliferation, and antibody production. In vitro, CRH exerts a mitogenic effect on rat B-cells as compared with rat T-cells (McGillis et al. 1989) and also inhibits antibody production (Aebischer et al. 1994; Leu & Singh 1993), possibly via an effect of CRH on accessory cells as opposed to a direct effect on B-cells themselves (Aebischer et al. 1994). When CRH is injected into the lateral ventricle of the brain, IgG production in response to a Th-cell–dependent antigen is suppressed if CRH is administered before immunization but remains unaltered if administered after immunization, suggesting an effect of CRH on early B-cell antigen processing events (Irwin 1993). Thus, the actions of CRH within the brain profoundly affect peripheral immune cell function. Furthermore, any drug, disease, or psychosocial factor that might either stimulate or inhibit the functioning of this complicated defense mechanism would likewise be expected to alter immunocompetence.

OPIOID PEPTIDES AND IMMUNITY

Opioid peptides represent a group of neuropeptides that influence immune function. Opioid peptides are categorized as follows: (1) the endorphins, which are encoded by the pro-opiomelanocortin (POMC) gene; (2) the enkephalins, which are encoded by the preproenkephalin-A gene; and (3) the dynorphins, which are encoded by the prodynorphin-B gene. Immunocompetent cells ex-

press receptors for these peptides, synthesize mRNA for POMC and preproenkephalin-A, and secrete endorphins and enkephalins. The role of the endorphins in immune function has been extensively reviewed (Carr & Blalock 1991; Heijnen, Kavelaars, & Ballieux 1991a,b). This chapter will focus primarily on the role of enkephalin-containing peptides on immune function, particularly with regard to their role in modulating the Th-cell–dependent antibody response.

Several sources of the enkephalin-containing peptides include the brain, spinal cord, adrenal medulla, sympathetic ganglia, and sympathetic nerve endings (Clement-Jones & Besser 1984; Fried et al. 1986). Until recently, these tissues were thought to be the only source of endogenously produced enkephalins. Activated murine CD4+ Th-cell lines express mRNA encoding for preproenkephalin-A and secrete met-enkephalin-immunoreactive material (Monstein, Folkesson, & Terenius 1986; Zurawski et al. 1986). Subsequently, preproenkephalin-A mRNA was found to be preferentially expressed by activated Th2 cells (IL-4 secretors) and not by Th1 cells (IL-2/IFN-γ secretors) (Cherwinski et al. 1987). In contrast to T-cells, the production of preproenkephalin-A mRNA by B-cells has not been extensively investigated. Note that B-cell lymphomas – unlike T-cell lymphomas and macrophage cell lines – do not express preproenkephalin-A mRNA (Martin, Prystowsky, & Angeletti 1987). However, basal levels of preproenkephalin-A mRNA in rat splenic B-cells increase after 2.5–5 hr of incubation in culture medium (Rosen et al. 1989) and are further increased if the B-cells are exposed to the B-cell–specific mitogen LPS (lipopolysaccharides). Thus, both T- and B-lymphocytes express preproenkephalin-A mRNA upon activation. These immune cells may influence both immune and nervous system function by releasing opioid peptides that interact with receptors on cells associated with these two organ systems.

In order to characterize the leukocyte population expressing opioid receptors, a number of researchers have performed radioligand binding studies on enriched populations of T- and B-cells (Bidlack, Saripalli, & Lawrence 1992; Carr et al. 1988; Madden et al. 1987). These data suggest that resting immune cells express d-opioid receptors whereas activated immune cells express other subtypes. Upon receptor stimulation, met-enkephalin (0.2–2 mmol) moderately suppresses Th-cell–dependent antibody production (Johnson et al. 1982). The importance of this finding is twofold: first, it demonstrates a direct role for opioid peptides in an immune function; second, it provides direct evidence for a link between the neuroendocrine and immune systems. Initially, the m-opioid receptor was considered to be the primary receptor responsible for mediating these effects on antibody production, and little attention was given to determining if other receptor subtypes were involved. In this regard, agonists selective for the m- and k-opioid receptors (10^{-10}–10^{-5} mol) inhibit the in vitro Th-cell–dependent murine antibody response against sheep erythrocytes, and this inhibition is blocked by naloxone pretreatment (Taub et al. 1991). The m- and k-opioid receptor subtypes are hence both involved in mediating the modulatory effects of opioid peptides on antibody production. Thus, the production and secretion of enkephalin-containing peptides by cells of both the nervous system and immune system suggests a mechanism by which these systems may regulate not only their own activity but each other's activity as well.

THE SYMPATHETIC NEUROTRANSMITTER NOREPINEPHRINE AND IMMUNITY

Over the years, four key discoveries have illustrated a link between the immune system and the SNS, as follows.

1. Discovery that both *primary* lymphoid organs – such as bone marrow and thymus (Bulloch & Pomerantz 1984; Calvo 1968; Felten et al. 1985; Williams & Felten 1981) – as well as *secondary* lymphoid organs – such as spleen, lymph nodes, gut-associated lymphoid tissue, and bronchiole-associated lymphoid tissue (Butter et al. 1988; Reilly, McCuskey, & Meineke 1976; Riegele 1929; Williams & Felten 1981; Williams et al. 1981) are innervated.
2. Identification of the β-2-adrenergic receptor (β_2AR) expressed on the surface of lymphoid cells (Madden, Sanders, & Felten 1995; Sanders 1995; Sanders et al. 1997), showing that the machinery for transducing a norepinephrine signal released within the microenvironment of the cell to the inside of the cell was present on immune cells.
3. Discovery that the sympathetic neurotransmitter norepinephrine is released from the sympathetic nerve terminals in the spleen upon the administration of either antigen or cytokine (Del Rey et al. 1981; Felten et al. 1987; Fuchs, Albright, & Albright 1988; Lorton et al. 1990; Shimizu, Hori, & Nakane 1994).
4. Identification of a role for neurotransmitters in modulating T- and B-lymphocyte functions (Madden, Sanders, & Felten 1995).

A marked decrease in both primary and secondary immune responses is seen following denervation of the lymph nodes and spleen (Livnat et al. 1985). Depletion of peripheral norepinephrine by chemical sympathectomy with 6-hydroxydopamine led to three different conclusions. Chemical sympathectomy of neonatal animals leads to an enhanced antibody response to sheep red blood cells when these animals were analyzed as adults (Besedovsky et al. 1979; Williams et al. 1981). Chemical sympathectomy of adult animals does not alter the Th-cell–dependent antibody response to sheep red blood cells (Miles et al. 1981). And finally, chemical sympathectomy in adult mice leads to a diminished antibody response to various Th-cell–dependent antigens. Thus, the change in Th-cell–dependent

antibody responses following chemical sympathectomy suggests that the SNS may be having a direct effect on cells involved in the antibody response – the T-cell, the B-cell, or both.

A recent study has shown that depletion of norepinephrine by 6-hydroxydopamine in a mouse strain slanted toward a Th1 profile enhances serum levels of both IgG_{2a} and IgG_1 after immunization in vivo and also enhances the ability of spleen cells from these mice to produce both IL-2 and IL-4 after immunization in vitro (Kruszewska, Felten, & Moynihan 1995). Thus, findings suggest that if norepinephrine is released in vivo then it plays a downmodulatory role in Th-cell–dependent antibody production. Such a role for norepinephrine in modulating the level of humoral immunity may explain some of the immunomodulatory effects associated with the exposure of an individual to psychosocial stressors. Therefore, it is important to understand the mechanisms for modulating the ability of Th-cells to deliver both contact- and cytokine-mediated signals.

A recent study examined the role of β_2AR stimulation in modulating Th1/Th2 cell activity when Th-cells were exposed to a β_2AR agonist *before* activation by an antigen-presenting B-cell (Sanders et al. 1997). Results of this study show that exposure of murine Th-cell clones to the β_2AR agonist terbutaline – via a T-cell–B-cell interaction before Th-cell activation – inhibits IFN-γ production by Th1 cells and subsequent IgG_{2a} production by B-cells, but this exposure does not affect IL-4 production by Th2 cells or subsequent IgG_1 production by B-cells. The mechanism responsible for these findings was the differential level of expression of the β_2AR by Th1/Th2 cell clones, such that the ligand binding site of the β_2AR was detectable on the surface of Th1 cells but not on Th2 cells. Hence, these results suggest that the low-to-undetectable level of β_2AR expression by Th2 cells would prohibit the modulation of any Th2 cell function through this receptor. In contrast, the higher level of β_2AR expression by Th1 cells would allow ligands that bind to the β_2AR, such as norepinephrine, to selectively inhibit Th1 cell IFN-γ production and IFN-γ-dependent IgG_{2a} production if β_2AR stimulation occurs *before* cell activation by an antigen-presenting B-cell.

Another recent study shows that murine Th1 and Th2 cell clones continue to differentially express the β_2AR following their activation through the T-cell antigen receptor–CD3 complex using an anti-CD3 monoclonal antibody (Ramer-Quinn, Baker, & Sanders 1997). Furthermore, the level of β_2AR expression is maintained and the affinity of the β_2AR on Th1 cells does not change after activation. As expected, β_2AR agonist exposure of activated Th1 and Th2 cells differentially modulates cytokine production by these effector Th-cell subsets. Whereas exposure of activated Th2 cells to a β_2AR ligand induces no change in Th2 cell cytokine production, exposure of activated Th1 cells decreases IL-2 production (but not IFN-γ). These findings suggest that differential expression of the β_2AR on activated murine Th1 and Th2 clones renders cytokine production by these clones differentially susceptible to the influence of a β_2AR ligand or norepinephrine.

Psychosocial factors influence a number of psychological responses that mediate their effects through activation of the CNS, the HPA, and the SNS, so the possibility exists that these systems also influence immune cell activity and are thus ultimately responsible for mediating the immune effects often associated with individuals experiencing various psychological responses to a variety of psychological factors.

Social Context

PSYCHOLOGICAL FACTORS: ASSOCIATIONS WITH CHANGES IN PARAMETERS OF HUMORAL IMMUNITY

Many studies have shown that a correlation exists between factors that alter psychophysiological states (e.g., mood alterations, depression, chronic stress, and acute stress) and changes in the humoral arm of the immune system. To date, a number of studies have been designed to determine if an association exists between the magnitude of psychological stress and resultant changes in humoral immune responsiveness. It is important to note that most of these studies have measured antibody production against either the endogenously located latent herpes virus, Epstein–Barr virus (EBV), or the exogenously administered influenza virus. Epstein–Barr virus is a latent virus that requires an intact cellular immune response to maintain control over its expression. Therefore, a rise in anti–herpes virus antibody is often used as an indicator of compromised cellular immune status in an individual. On the other hand, an individual exposed to an exogenous virus, such as influenza or hepatitis-B, will tend to mount an antibody response that is more likely to reflect the ability of B-cells to produce antibody with the help of CD4$^+$ Th-cells. Thus, an assessment of humoral immune status may be used as an indicator of the state of both T- and B-lymphocytes at a given time in the response to a stressor.

Most studies have reported changes in the rate and/or magnitude of an antiviral antibody response and included persons that experienced one or more of the following psychosocial stressors: a high number of major stressful life events (Cohen, Tyrrell, & Smith 1991; Stone et al. 1992); a high degree of negative affect (Stone et al. 1987a, 1994); high anxiety or defensive behavior (Esterling et al. 1993); daily problems and psychoneurotic symptoms (Jabaaij et al. 1993, 1996); depression (Maes et al. 1989; Zisook et al. 1994); physical restraint (Feng et al. 1991); mild physical pain (Kusnecov et al. 1992); captivity (Laudenslager et al. 1993); crowding (Edwards & Dean 1977); changes in so-

cial rank or social environment (Cunnick et al. 1991); and emotional repression and coping behavior (Esterling et al. 1990, 1994). The majority of studies show that psychological stressors lead either to an increase in antibody titers against herpes viruses (an indicator for the loss of cellular immune control over expression of the latent virus) or to a decrease in the level of antibody produced against an exogenously administered virus. On the other hand, a few studies show that no change occurs in the antiviral antibody response of subjects exposed to confinement (Husson et al. 1996; Schmitt et al. 1995), physical restraint (Sheridan et al. 1991), or the stress of bereavement when not accompanied by a major depression (Zisook et al. 1994). The latter findings suggest that subtle differences associated with psychological stress may greatly influence the humoral immune status of the afflicted individual.

A number of findings clearly show that stressful situations occurring in everyday life appear to be related to changes in humoral immune function. For example, caregivers of a relative with a progressive dementia experience high levels of distress and also produce high levels of anti–herpes virus antibody (Kiecolt-Glaser et al. 1987b, 1991). On the other hand, a caregiver who is exposed to an exogenous virus (e.g. influenza) tends to produce less antibody (Kiecolt-Glaser et al. 1996). Newlyweds who exhibit negative or hostile behavior show increases in the level of anti-EBV antibody production – unlike those who exhibit positive and supportive behavior and show no change in the level of anti-EBV antibody production (Kiecolt-Glaser et al. 1993). Likewise, marital disruption by separation or divorce leads to a poor anti-EBV antibody response that is more severe in women (Kiecolt-Glaser et al. 1987a) than in men (Kiecolt-Glaser et al. 1988). Academic stress is another well-studied situation for analyzing whether an association exists between the level of psychological stress and changes in immune responsiveness. Increases in anti-EBV antibody production are seen with students who are highly motivated but poor academic performers (Stanislav, Evans, & Niederman 1979), highly stressed and seeking support (Glaser et al. 1993), or very lonely (Glaser et al. 1985). In contrast, a decrease in anti–hepatitis-B antibody production is seen with students who are stressed and anxious as compared with those students seeking social support, who show an increase (Glaser et al. 1992). It is interesting that, in models of stress-induced immune suppression, olfactory cues increase the production of antibodies during a primary response to antigen (Cocke et al. 1993; Komori et al. 1995).

Collectively, these studies have shown changes in the amount of antibody produced, changes in the time course of an antibody response, changes in the number of cells directly involved in humoral immunity (i.e., B-cells and CD4$^+$ Th-cells), and changes in the proliferative response of B- and/or T-cells to mitogens. Although some limitations exist with these studies, a review of their findings is necessary in order to formulate educated hypotheses about psychoneurophysiological and immune interactions and to develop more consistent and intricate experimental designs for addressing such hypotheses.

Mood

On a daily basis, humans are subjected to a variety of positive experiences (e.g., accomplishing a task, being promoted at work) and negative experiences (e.g., losing keys, having an argument with a loved one) that have mood-altering consequences. Concomitant with these events, humans are also exposed on a daily basis to a variety of viral and bacterial pathogens. The secretory immune system – and, in particular, secretory IgA (sIgA), which is present in mucosal membranes – provides the body with a first line of defense against such invading pathogens. With these parameters in mind, a within-subjects analysis strategy was utilized to assess the effect that daily mood changes may have on sIgA production to a novel antigen (Stone et al. 1987b). Subjects in the study were orally administered a novel protein antigen and were asked to keep a daily diary. For a period of eight weeks, secretory IgA specific for the novel antigen was measured three times a week from parotid saliva. The results of this study indicated that the level of sIgA directed against a novel antigen was lower on days in which daily diaries reported a negative mood and that higher levels were found on days in which diaries reported a positive mood. These studies were further confirmed in 1994 with a larger sample size ($N = 96$) over a twelve-week sampling period (Stone et al. 1994).

A second strategy to assess the possibility that daily mood changes influence humoral immune status involved "artificially" inducing alterations in mood state in a laboratory setting. Two previous studies have used this type of strategy to study the effects of "humor" on sIgA production (Dillon, Minchoff, & Baker 1985; Labott et al. 1990). The results of both of these studies indicate that sIgA in saliva increases following the viewing of a humorous videotape. In addition, female viewers who watched a sad videotape and then wept openly showed a significant decrease in sIgA compared with subjects who did not weep openly (Labott et al. 1990).

Two previous studies were conducted to assess the effects of mood changes on T-cell function. In one study (Futterman et al. 1994), male actors who were trained in "method" acting (a technique whereby the actor uses recall of personal experiences and emotions to parallel emotions of the portrayed character) were analyzed to assess the effects of different mood states on T-cell function. Blood samples were taken from subjects at baseline, during the mood induction phase, and during a recovery period. As a potential measure of T-lymphocyte function, the ability of peripheral blood mononuclear cells (PBMC) to proliferate in response to the T-cell mitogen phytohemagglutinin (PHA) was assessed. The findings of this study showed

that PBMC from subjects with positive mood states exhibited a significant increase in the proliferative response to PHA. In contrast, PBMC from subjects with negative mood states exhibited a significant decrease in proliferative responses to PHA. In a broad sense, the data obtained from this study (Futterman et al. 1994) parallel the data obtained for sIgA, suggesting that a positive mood may enhance immune functions whereas a negative mood may decrease immune function. In contrast, a second study – in which both positive and negative mood states were induced in a laboratory setting by having subjects recall positive and negative life experiences – showed that positive and negative moods were *both* associated with decreased proliferative responses to the T-cell mitogens Concanavalin A (Con A) and PHA (Knapp et al. 1992). Together, these two studies suggest that using different methods to elicit mood changes may produce differing effects with regard to T-cell function. This hypothesis can be tested further by having the actors perform both protocols for inducing mood alterations before being subjected to separate immune testing.

All of the studies described here indicate that mood changes are associated with changes in immune function. However, it remains unclear as to whether or not eliciting a mood change by the four types of protocols just outlined results in similar outcomes. Part of this lack of clarity is a result of the immune parameters that were measured (i.e., sIgA vs. T-cell proliferation). To provide a clearer picture, future studies may need to include more than one strategy for evaluating immune cell function. For example, in the study by Stone et al. (1987a), blood samples (in addition to saliva samples) could have been collected and assayed to determine: (1) the concentrations of serum Ig; (2) the absolute number and percentage of B- and CD4$^+$ Th-cells; (3) the proliferative response to the mitogens PHA, Con A, and pokeweed mitogen (PWM); and (4) the T-cell cytokine response following anti-CD3 antibody stimulation in vitro. Also, the subjects under study could be given a novel antigen, after which these four parameters could be assessed prior to, during, and following elicitation of positive and negative moods.

It has been argued that changes in total sIgA could reflect increases in salivary flow and not actual increases in IgA production (Stone et al. 1987b). Thus, it may be informative to examine the effects of mood on other antibody isotypes. With this type of approach, subjects could be given either a novel antigen or a vaccination and then asked to watch humorous films during the induction phase of the immune response. Thereafter, both antigen-specific antibody levels and in vitro T-cell proliferative responses to the antigen could be assessed. Furthermore, infecting subjects with a cold virus after their viewing of a humorous video would help to determine if the increased sIgA actually reflects a protective increase in humoral immunity. In addition to providing new information about a relationship between psychological factors and humoral immunity, these types of studies could be very important therapeutically. For example, if creating a positive mood change with a humorous video or through recall of positive events enhances sIgA or immunoglobulin production in general, then these types of mood-altering strategies may be useful to obtain increased protection against viral and bacterial pathogens.

Depression

Two scenarios emerge upon review of previous studies conducted to look at the correlations between depression and aspects of humoral immunity: (1) depression correlates with immunosuppression, as evidenced by decreases in the absolute number and percentage of B- and T-cells as well as a decrease in the ability of these cells to proliferate in response to mitogens; and (2) depression correlates with immune activation, as illustrated by increases in the absolute number and percentage of B- and T-cells, increases in autoantibody titers, and increases in cytokine production from mitogen-stimulated T-cells. Although these scenarios are somewhat opposed to each other, both indicate concomitant changes in immunity and depressed state. It is possible that some of the differences between the two scenarios are due to the methods used to classify depressed patients, since the studies suggesting a correlation with immunosuppression categorized patients based on Research Diagnostic Criteria (RDC), whereas the Diagnostic and Statistical Manual of Mental Disorders (DSM-III) rating system was used to categorize patients in the studies that suggest a correlation with immune activation. In addition, these latter studies utilized two-color flow cytometric analysis, a technique that may be more sensitive than the "rosette formation" technique used in the studies reporting a suppression in B- or T-cell numbers.

Results from previous studies designed to examine immune parameters in depression are somewhat conflicting (for a review, see Stein, Miller, & Trestman 1991). Much of this conflict may be due to inadequate controls. Therefore, for ease of discourse, a series of well-controlled studies is presented next. Schleifer and colleagues (1984) examined 18 patients hospitalized for major depressive disorder. Blood samples were taken from patients and control subjects, samples from which determinations were made of the absolute number and percentage of B- and T-cells as well as the ability of PBMC to proliferate in response to three mitogens: PHA (T-cell mitogen), Con A (T-cell mitogen), and PWM (T- and B-cell mitogen). Results of this early study showed that depressed patients exhibited decreases in the absolute number of both T- and B-cells but no significant differences in the percentage of T- and B-cells. In addition, the depressed patients showed a significant decrease in the ability of their PBMC to proliferate in response to PHA, Con A, and PWM (when compared with age-, sex-, and race-matched controls). This early study therefore indicated that depression was associated

with a concomitant immunosuppression that involved cells directly involved in the humoral immune response.

In a subsequent study of 15 patients, a significant decrease in the number of circulating T-cells was also reported (Schleifer et al. 1985). However, in contrast to their initial study, there was no difference in either the absolute number of B-cells or in the percentage of T- and B-cells in depressed versus control subjects. Furthermore, lymphocyte responsiveness to the mitogens PHA, Con A, and PWM did not differ between patients and controls. The patients in this second study were assigned a Hamilton Depression Rating Scale (HDRS) score of 18.9, compared to 28 for the first study. Thus, the authors suggested that the differences in immune responsiveness evident between their two studies could be due to differences in the severity of depression experienced by the patient.

In order to clarify the results obtained in the initial studies just described, a larger study ($N = 91$) was conducted (Schleifer et al. 1989). This larger study revealed no significant differences in the absolute number of lymphocytes, lymphocyte percentages, or proliferative responsiveness to mitogens between depressed subjects and (age-, sex-, and race-matched) controls. However, the control group exhibited an age-related increase in CD4$^+$ T-cells and an increase in the proliferative response, whereas these increases were not seen in depressed patients. The effects of age were further supported by a later study that found no differences in the absolute number of B- or CD4$^+$ T-cells or in responsiveness of PBMCs to PHA for depressed patients aged 18–35 (mean age = 21) compared with matched controls (Schleifer et al. 1996). Thus, the authors concluded that the changes that occur in immune parameters during depression are related to subject age and severity of depression.

In contrast to the foregoing studies (Schleifer et al. 1984, 1985, 1989) and others (reviewed by Stein et al. 1991) suggesting that a state of immunosuppression exists in depressed individuals, another pair of studies suggests that a state of immune activation exists (Maes et al. 1992a,b). In the first study (Maes et al. 1992a), two-color flow cytometry was utilized to evaluate lymphocyte populations in patients from three different depression categories: (i) minor depression; (ii) simple major depression; and (iii) major depression with melancholia (based on DSM-III criteria). The results of this initial study indicated the following changes in lymphocyte cell numbers in all three depression groups compared with controls: (1) a trend (not significant) toward an increase in the number of surface Ig-expressing B-cells and CD4$^+$ T-cells; (2) a significant increase in the number of CD4$^+$CD45$^-$ (memory) T-cells in depressed patients; and (3) a significant increase in IL-2R$^+$ cells. In melancholic patients (vs. controls and also vs. the other two depression groups), there was also a significant increase in the total number of lymphocytes and the number of T- and B-cells. Analyses showed no significant differences between age, sex, or smokers versus nonsmokers.

In the second study (Maes et al. 1992b), two-color flow cytometry was utilized to assess the presence of different T-cell subsets in the three depression categories. Results of this study revealed that the number of $CD4^+$ and $CD4^+CD45^-$ (memory) T-cells were significantly higher in melancholic patients. Analysis of T-cell subset percentages revealed a significantly higher percentage of $CD4^+$ T-cells in all depressed patients (most pronounced for melancholics) and a significantly lower percentage of $CD8^+CD57^-$ (suppressor) T-cells in all three depressed categories compared with controls. In addition, there was a trend toward an increased percentage of $CD4^+CD45^-$ (memory) T-cells in melancholics. The $CD4^+/CD8^+$ T-cell ratio was also significantly higher in all depressed subjects. Intercorrelations between the absolute number of immune cell subsets and disease severity showed that the severity of illness was significantly and positively related to both the number of $CD4^+$ naive and $CD4^+$ memory T-cells. From these studies, the authors concluded that important immune cell alterations are associated with depression, including increases in the absolute number and percentage of $CD4^+$ T-cells (partly caused by an up-regulation of $CD4^+CD45^-$ memory T-cells) and a reduction in $CD8^+CD57^-$ suppressor T-cells.

Consistent with the scenario of enhanced humoral immunity, a previous study showed that minor and major depressed patients have significantly higher serum antibody titers to the autoantigens phosphatidylserine and thromboplastin when compared with nondepressed controls (Maes et al. 1993). In addition, following in vitro stimulation with PHA, PBMCs from patients with depression secrete higher levels of the T-cell cytokine IFN-γ (Maes et al. 1994).

Although both sets of data just described suggest that there are changes in immune cell populations (i.e., $CD4^+$ Th-cells and B-cells) in depressed patients that could be responsible for inducing changes in humoral immunity, the actual antibody levels for the depressed patients studied have not been reported. Furthermore, it remains unclear as to whether or not changes in the proliferative responsiveness of PBMC to mitogens actually reflect functional changes in the ability of B-cells to secrete antibody and/or the ability of T-cells to secrete cytokines in vivo. In addition, most of the available data represent only one sample from an individual. Although this type of sampling does allow for interindividual comparison (i.e., depressed vs. nondepressed control), it does not assess changes that may occur *within* an individual owing to daily mood fluctuations or daily stressors.

In order to more clearly address the possible correlation between depression and humoral immunity, further experimentation is necessary. To obtain a clearer picture, these experimental designs should include the following measurements: (1) analysis of total serum Ig levels and isotype profiles; (2) measurement of T-cell cytokine production following in vitro stimulation with anti-CD3 antibody;

and (3) two-color flow cytometric analysis of lymphocyte subsets. It is important that all of these parameters be measured in the same patient. Furthermore, repeated measures of these parameters over time should help to clarify whether part of the immune changes measured are due to variables such as daily mood changes and stressors.

Moreover, a clear understanding of psychoneuroimmune interactions that may occur in depression will also require measurement of neuroendocrine parameters in parallel with measurements of immune parameters. Previous studies have indicated that the following neuroendocrine changes are present in some depressed patients: (1) alterations in CNS neurotransmitter function, as measured by alterations in metabolites of both norepinephrine and serotonin in blood, CSF, and urine (Zis & Goodwin 1982); (2) abnormalities in the HPA axis, as measured by blunted ACTH responses to CRH (Gold et al. 1984; Gold, Goodwin, & Chrousos 1988; Sachar 1982); and (3) abnormalities in autonomic nervous system function, as measured by changes in plasma catecholamine levels (Potter 1984; Rudorfer et al. 1985). Thus, in addition to these immune analyses, future experiments should also include the following measurements: (1) norepinephrine and serotonin metabolites in blood, CSF, and urine; (2) blood cortisol levels; (3) blood catecholamine levels; and (4) ACTH responses to CRH.

Previous studies (Maes et al. 1989; Schleifer et al. 1989) have shown a correlation between decreased proliferation to mitogens and patient age; therefore, it is very important that age-matched controls be utilized in all analyses. As discussed earlier, some of the conflicts in interpretation of the data collected thus far may be due to different methods used to categorize depressed patients. Thus, a study that assays the same parameters yet utilizes different depression categorization methods may provide useful information. Although many previous studies have not included patients with unipolar and bipolar depression, studies should be conducted using such patients as intervariable groups to obtain a better understanding of the effects of depression on humoral immunity. Finally, depression and humoral immunity should be evaluated in patients involved in drug and behavior therapy programs to determine if treatments that decrease depressive symptoms concomitantly change neuroendocrine and humoral immune parameters.

Stress

A number of previous studies have indicated that psychological and physical stress increases the susceptibility of animals and humans to microbial and viral pathogens (for reviews see Biondi & Zannino 1997; Sheridan et al. 1994). Studies conducted to examine the effects of stress on farm and laboratory animals have shown that stress increases disease susceptibility to (and mortality from) a variety of microbial pathogens, including *Escherichia coli* (Gross 1984), *Mycobacterium avium* (Brown et al. 1993) and *tuberculosis* (Tobach & Bloch 1956), *Pasteurella haemolytica*

(Cole et al. 1988), *Staphylococcus aureus* (Previte & Berry 1962), *Streptococcus pneumoniae* (Bailey 1925) and *viridans* (Sherwood et al. 1968), *Mycoplasma gallisepticum* (Gross & Colmano 1969), and *Salmonella typhimurium* (Edwards & Dean 1977).

In addition to bacterial pathogens, animal models have shown that stress is associated both with increases in disease symptoms and with increased mortality following infection with polio virus (Levinson, Milzer, & Lewin 1945), herpes simplex virus (Kusnecov et al. 1992), bovine herpes virus (Filion et al. 1984), vesicular stomatitis virus (Yamada, Jensen, & Rasmussen 1964), Coxsackie virus B3 (Gaitman, Chason, & Lerner 1970; Johnsson et al. 1963), corona virus (Shimizu, Shimizu, & Kodama 1978), Newcastle disease virus (Beard & Mitchell 1987), West Nile virus (Ben-Nathan, Lustig, & Feuerstein 1989), Sindbis virus (Ben-Nathan, Lustig, & Danenberg 1991), and Keystone virus (McLean 1982).

In humans, stress has been associated with increased tuberculosis infections (D'Arcy, Keane, & Clancy 1989; Hawkins, Davies, & Holmes 1955; Holmes et al. 1957; Ishigami 1919) and increases in the development of acute necrotizing gingivitis, an infection caused by indigenous oral bacteria that are not normally pathogenic (Cohen-Cole et al. 1981). Additionally, stress in humans has been associated with increased susceptibility to influenza-B virus (Clover et al. 1989), Epstein–Barr virus (Kasl, Evans, & Niederman 1979), and three viruses associated with the "common cold": rhinovirus, respiratory syncytial virus, and coronavirus (Cohen et al. 1991). Also, in individuals infected with HIV-1, stress is associated with enhanced clinical decline (Goodkin et al. 1992). Although the mechanisms by which stress alters the onset, course, or outcome of infectious disease are still under investigation, a recent review on the association between stress and infectious disease (Biondi & Zannino 1997) suggests that the following mechanisms are likely to be involved: (1) changes in host immunocompetence, including both humoral and cellular parameters; (2) changes in host anatomic and functional barriers; and (3) changes in the virulence of the infecting agent.

Previous studies in animal models have shown that stress alters the antibody response to both bacterial and viral pathogens (see Biondi & Zannino 1997; Sheridan et al. 1994). Although the collected data are more extensive for viral pathogens, one study showed that mice exposed to the stress of crowding mounted a reduced antibody response to the pathogenic bacteria *Salmonella typhimurium* (Edwards & Dean 1977). The data collected from studies using viral pathogens are somewhat more extensive in that a variety of viruses and stressors have been utilized. In one study, exposing chickens to heat stress significantly decreased the level of antibody produced against Newcastle disease virus (Beard & Mitchell 1987). In cotton rats, the induction of stress by administration of the synthetic glucocorticoid prednisolone resulted in both a delay

and a decrease in neutralizing antibody produced against Keystone virus (McLean 1982). Likewise, restraint stress in mice significantly delayed the development of the production of antibody reactive with influenza-A (Feng et al. 1991). In mice, the stress of forced exercise also decreased the neutralizing antibody to Coxsackie virus B3 (Reyes & Lerner 1976). Physical stress delivered by means of electrical foot shock in mice decreased the antibody response produced against HSV (Kusnecov et al. 1992). Restraint stress has also been used in combination with influenza viral infection to show that a decrease occurs in both lymph node and lung mononuclear cellularity and in the level of Th1/Th2 cell cytokine production via a mechanism that involves an increased level of glucocorticoids, since RU486 blocks all effects of the stressor (Dobbs et al. 1996; Hermann, Beck, & Sheridan 1995). In contrast to all of these studies, which indicate that stress either decreases or delays antibody production in response to viral infection, a few studies have reported either no change in antiviral antibody responses or actual increases in antiviral antibody responses (Beard & Mitchell 1987; Chang & Rasmussen 1965; Yamada et al. 1964). At present, the reason for these conflicting sets of data using viral antigens is not clear. It is possible that the differences are due to differences in the animals used for the study, the type of stress administered, or the viruses that were used. As suggested by two previous studies (Feng et al. 1991; McLean 1982), stress may delay antiviral antibody production and so the effect of stress on humoral immune status could be misinterpreted if the antibody production is measured at only one point in time. Thus, although the cumulative antibody levels against a pathogen may be unchanged in stressed individuals, the rate at which these antibodies are made may be the difference between an individual's ability to "fight off" a cold or flu virus early (rather than later) in the course of infection.

The majority of studies examining the effects of stress on the humoral immune response in humans have used natural stress paradigms, such as academic examination stress, bereavement, stress associated with HIV-1 infection, and chronic stress due to caring for a patient with progressive dementia. The majority of the results obtained in these paradigms suggest that stress reduces humoral immunity; however, a few contradictory results have been obtained.

In a 1983 study, the effect of academic stress was examined in 64 first-year dental students (Jemmott et al. 1983). Salivary IgA was measured once during a low-stress period, three times during high-stress periods (examinations), and a final time during a low-stress period. In addition to measuring the intraindividual responses to stress (within-subjects variable), students were asked to take the Thematic Apperception Test; this allowed for a between-subjects comparison (measure of interindividual variability). The test separated students into two categories, those with a great need for power and those with a great need for affiliation. The results showed that sIgA secretion rates were diminished in high-stress periods as compared with low-stress periods. In addition, the between-groups design revealed that secretion of IgA was elevated at all time points in subjects characterized by a great need to establish and maintain warm personal relationships. In those students who exhibited a high inhibited need for power (but not in other subjects), the sIgA secretion did not return to baseline and continued to decline through the final low-stress period.

The effects of academic stress on the ability to mount an immune response to a hepatitis-B vaccination was studied in 48 medical students (Glaser et al. 1992). In this study, students were administered a series of three hepatitis-B vaccinations on the third day of a three-day examination series. To assess the levels of perceived psychological stress, the students filled out a Profile of Mood States (POMS), Perceived Stress Scale (PSS), and an Interpersonal Support Evaluation List (ISEL). The vaccinations were given at time zero, one month later, and six months later. Blood was drawn at each time of vaccination to test for seroconversion. Results of this study revealed that, although all of the students had seroconverted by the six-month interval, only 25% of the students had seroconverted during the one-month interval. Further analysis of the perceived psychological stress data revealed that the students who seroconverted at one month were significantly less anxious than those who seroconverted later. Thus, similar to the findings in mice (Feng et al. 1991), stress may delay the production of antibody in response to viral antigen challenge in humans. The findings of this study suggest that it may be important to monitor seroconversion in individuals who are experiencing stress when they are vaccinated (i.e., health-care workers starting a new job, military personnel who are being transferred overseas, or elderly people who are moving to group care facilities) before exposing them to potential pathogens. In addition, these studies suggest that it may not be advantageous to give students vaccinations on days when they have examinations.

Jabaaij and colleagues (1993) used a recombinant DNA hepatitis vaccine to assess the effects of perceived psychological stress on vaccination efficacy in medical students. The effects of stress on both the initiation phase and the boost phase were examined. One parameter was different, however, from the Glaser et al. (1992) study: students participating in the Jabaaij et al. (1993) study were not experiencing acute stress due to examinations. Results of this study showed that stress reported at month 2 (initiation phase of immune response) had a negative influence on antibody production. Thus, the results from both of these studies indicate that stress has a negative effect on the induction phase of the immune response.

In addition to the two studies just described, the effects of stress on vaccination efficacy were also examined in a third study of medical students (Petry, Weems, & Livingstone 1991). The results of this study showed that subjects who reported high levels of negative perceived stress during the initiation phase had higher peak antibody titers. Although stress appeared to enhance the initiation phase, the booster-phase levels of stress and distress did not significantly correlate with peak antibody titers. It is possible that the results of this study differ from the previous two because its antibody titers were measured nine months after the first vaccination, whereas the former studies measured antibody titers at earlier time points. Studies in both mice and humans (Feng et al. 1991; Glaser et al. 1992) have reported that stress delays antibody production in response to viral antigens. Therefore, if antibody is measured at later time points then this effect of stress may be missed. Another difference between this study and the previous two is that these students filled out questionnaires for assessment of stress at the six-month period only. Assessments of stress that occurred six months prior to filling out a questionnaire may not be accurate. To circumvent this problem, future studies should utilize a protocol in which stress is assessed at the time of each vaccination. Additionally, asking students to keep daily diaries may provide a clearer reflection of their levels of stress.

The effects of chronic stress that is associated with caregiving for a spouse who has a progressive dementia on response to an influenza virus vaccination have also been examined (Kiecolt-Glaser et al. 1996). The results of this study revealed that caregivers showed lower antibody levels to influenza virus than sex-, age-, and socioeconomically matched controls.

In a study devised to examine the effects of stress on the ability to develop an immune response to a novel antigen (Snyder, Roghmann, & Sigal 1990), women were immunized with the novel antigen keyhole limpet hemocyanin (KLH); serum IgG was measured before immunization, three weeks following immunization, and eight weeks following immunization. Although the correlations were not significant, the following trends for antibody production were noted: (1) more stressful events (either good or bad) were correlated with lower antigen-specific IgG at three weeks; (2) more good events correlated with higher levels of IgG at eight weeks; and (3) women who reported more bad stresses exhibited lower IgG at eight weeks.

One commonly occurring stressful event is conjugal bereavement. To determine if the stress of losing a spouse alters immune responsiveness, Schleifer and associates (1983) assessed the absolute number and percentage of B- and T-cells as well as the ability of PBMC to proliferate following mitogen stimulation in a group of men prior to and following the death of their spouses. Results of this study revealed that there were no differences in either the percentage or absolute number of B- and T-cells at one month or two months after the spouse's death. Although there was not a decrease in cells, PBMC proliferation in response to three mitogens (PHA, Con A, and PWM) was significantly decreased at both one and two months following spousal death. This study suggests that suppression of mitogen-induced lymphocyte proliferation was a direct consequence of bereavement and not a consequence of major changes in diet, activity levels, alcohol, tobacco, drug use, or weight changes following death of a spouse. Although serum Ig levels were not reported in this study, the decreased proliferation to PWM – a mitogen that stimulates both B- and T-cells – suggests that the stress of bereavement decreases B-cell function.

In a pilot study of eleven asymptomatic HIV-1 seropositive men, Goodkin and colleagues (1992) assessed the effect of life stressors and coping style on $CD4^+$ T-cell numbers. Results of this study indicated that a significant correlation existed between the occurrence of a major life stressor over the previous year and total lymphocyte count. In addition, the low-stress groups had higher $CD4^+$ T-cell counts than did high-stress groups. Thus, the stress associated with HIV-1 infection may alter an individual's $CD4^+$ Th-cell population, which in turn could decrease antibody production from the B-cells that rely on $CD4^+$ Th-cells for "help."

The majority of the studies presented here indicate that stress has a dampening effect on the humoral immune response in humans. At present, the mechanisms whereby stress leads either to a delay in the mounting of an antibody response or to a decrease in the levels of antibody produced are unclear. Unfortunately, these studies did not use blood and urine samples to assay cortisol and catecholamine levels. Thus, direct connections between these neuroendocrine factors and antibody production cannot be ascertained. Future experimental designs should include such analyses so that the neurophysiological changes associated with stress can be directly linked to changes in immunoglobulin production. Additionally, one strategy that has been used in studies to examine the effects of stress on cellular immune responses involves eliciting stress in a laboratory setting – either by physical means, such as a mild electric shock or audible noise (Weisse et al. 1990), or by inducing mental stress with tasks, such as public speaking or mental arithmetic (Bachen et al. 1995). Future experimental designs that assess the levels of antibody, cortisol, and catecholamines may utilize this type of strategy, along with the administration of a novel antigen, to further understand the connections between stress and antibody production.

PSYCHOLOGICAL INTERVENTION

The findings which suggest that psychological factors such as mood, depression, and stress may have a negative impact on the humoral immune system also suggest that psychological intervention may have beneficial effects on humoral immunity. A few intervention strategies that

are commonly used in the area of psychotherapy include relaxation techniques, exercise, classical conditioning, and self-disclosure. In addition, the degree of social support and personal coping styles are often important factors in effective psychotherapy. Although the effects that these types of psychotherapies have on humoral immunity have not been examined in depth, the studies conducted so far suggest that psychological intervention therapies may provide beneficial effects, particularly in individuals who have dampened humoral immune responses owing to age or HIV-1 infection.

Relaxation

Two studies indicate that relaxation may have a positive effect on the humoral immune system in humans. In the first study, salivary IgA and serum Ig levels were examined in control subjects versus subjects that practiced a daily relaxation technique (Green, Green, & Santoro 1988). Results of this study indicated that, following the first relaxation session, salivary IgA was significantly higher in the relaxation group than in controls. In addition to salivary IgA, serum IgA, IgG, and IgM levels also increased during the relaxation training period (in the relaxation subjects). In a second study, Kiecolt-Glaser and colleagues (1986) examined the effect of relaxation on changes in Th-cell percentages during examination stress. Results indicated that the percentage of Th-cells decreased during examination periods in both the relaxation group and controls. However, further analysis revealed that not all students practiced the relaxation technique with the same frequency (range: 5–50 times). Thus, a regression analysis was used to determine if there was a correlation between the frequency of relaxation practice and the percentage of helper cells. Results of this analysis revealed that an increased frequency of relaxation practice was associated with a higher percentage of Th-cells in the blood during examinations.

Exercise

Previous studies indicate that exercise has a beneficial effect on psychophysiological well-being (for reviews see Morgan 1985; Raglin 1990). Acute or moderate exercise is associated with a decrease in anxiety state and mood alterations. Studies examining the effects of long-term exercise programs have shown pronounced beneficial effects on individuals with both elevated anxiety and depression but only moderate beneficial effects on normal individuals (Raglin 1990). The beneficial effects of long-term exercise programs include reductions in anxiety and depression as well as increases in self-esteem and general psychological well-being (Morgan 1985). Studies on psychoneuroimmune interactions suggest that stress, mood, anxiety, and depression may alter humoral immunity. Thus, therapies such as exercise, which reduce these affective states, may also alter humoral immunity. A review of previous studies (Nieman 1991) suggested that either brief graded maximal or short-term submaximal exercise is associated with increases in serum Ig. This increase in serum Ig does not appear to be due to direct effects on B-cells per se but is likely due to changes in plasma volume levels (i.e., when adjustments are made for changes in plasma volume, no significant increases in serum Ig were evident). Two studies have shown that moderate exercise (i.e., walking for 45 minutes at 60% V_{O_2} max) is associated with increases in serum IgM, IgG, and IgA (Nehlsen-Cannarella et al. 1991a,b). In addition, one study reported that individuals who participated in a ten-week aerobic exercise training program exhibited increases in the number of circulating CD4$^+$ Th-cells and B-cells (LaPerriere et al. 1994a). Although the exact mechanisms whereby exercise alters humoral immunity are currently unknown, two postulated mechanisms are: (a) that noradrenergic sympathetic neural interactions (i.e., release of catecholamines, activation of the HPA axis, release of cortisol, or production of endogenous opiates) influence humoral immune responses; and (b) that antigen stimulation of the humoral immune system increases owing to increased uptake of microorganisms via either higher ventilation rates or decreased mucosal immunity.

The data indicating that exercise decreases anxiety, depression, and other psychological states which may have a negative effect on immunity – and that exercise increases humoral immunity – suggest the possibility that exercise may be a good intervention therapy for individuals infected with HIV-1, who often have decreased immunity as well as increased depression and anxiety. A few studies have been conducted to examine this possibility (see LaPerriere et al. 1994b). The outcomes of these studies suggest that exercise may have beneficial effects for HIV-1 infected individuals, because exercise reduces anxiety, fatigue, anger, and depression (Florijin & Geiger 1991; LaPerriere et al. 1991; Rigsby et al. 1992; Schlenzig, Jager, & Rieder 1989) and either increases (LaPerriere et al. 1991; Rigsby et al. 1992; Schlenzig et al. 1989) or stabilizes the CD4$^+$ Th-cell count (Florijin & Geiger 1991) in HIV-1 infected individuals.

Conditioning

One type of behavioral conditioning involves the illness-induced taste aversion paradigm. In order to condition a taste aversion response, a test animal is given a distinctly flavored solution (i.e., dilute saccharin solution or chocolate milk), which serves as the conditioned stimulus (CS), followed by an intraperitoneal injection of a toxic agent that causes gastrointestinal distress (i.e., cyclophosphamide or lithium chloride), which serves as the unconditioned stimulus (UCS). Since the mid-1970s, a number of studies have been conducted by Ader and others to investigate the effects of behavioral conditioning on both humoral and cell-mediated immune responsiveness (Ader & Cohen 1993; Cohen, Moynihan, & Ader 1994).

In an initial study (Ader & Cohen 1975), the effects of taste aversion conditioning on humoral immune responsive-

ness was assessed by conditioning rats with saccharin (CS) and cyclophosphamide (UCS). Three days after conditioning, the rats were injected with sheep erythrocytes (SRBC), a T-dependent antigen, and allowed to drink saccharin (CS) again. Six days after the administration of the SRBC antigen, serum antibody titers were measured. The results of this study showed that rats receiving saccharin (CS) at the time of or immediately following the SRBC injection had lower hemagglutinating antibody titers. Thus, a conditioned immunosuppression of antibody production had occurred. To further confirm their results, lithium chloride (LiCl) – a drug that causes gastrointestinal distress but pharmacologically is not directly immunosuppressive – was also used as the UCS. When LiCl was used as the UCS and the rats were given SRBC followed by the CS (saccharin), a decrease in antibody titers was (as expected) not seen. This experiment was repeated with similar findings by a second group (Rogers et al. 1976), with the exception that this group found it necessary to have two re-exposures to the CS in order to see a significant decrease in antibody titers. In addition, a later study showed that the timing of the re-exposure to the CS may have a profound effect on its ability to induce immunosuppression of humoral immune responsiveness (Kusnecov, Husband, & King 1988).

Although these studies showed that immunosuppression was linked to a conditioned stimulus, it was unclear as to whether B-cells and/or T-cells were being affected. In an attempt to clarify which population of cells was altered, a conditioning protocol similar to the protocol just described was utilized in concert with both a T-dependent antigen SRBC and a T-independent antigen *Brucella abortus* (*B. abortus*) (Wayner, Flannery, & Singer 1978). The results of this study indicated that T-cell–independent antigen administration resulted in no difference in anti-*B. abortus* antibody titers in the conditioned versus nonconditioned control rats. Thus, this study indicated that T-cells may be the target cell of the conditioned taste aversion. In contrast to the results obtained in rats, a study conducted in mice reported that a conditioned antibody response could be induced with a T-independent antigen (Cohen et al. 1979). Taken together, the data from these two studies suggest that the cell population responding to the conditioned response may be different in different species.

The data obtained from animal models suggest that conditioned immunosuppression may be an alternative therapy for patients with autoimmune diseases who are currently treated with large doses of immunosuppressive agents that possess toxic side effects. Because the reported data implicate both B- and T-cells as targets of the conditioned response, conditioned immunosuppressive therapy may be particularly beneficial in diseases – such as Alzheimer's disease, multiple sclerosis, and systemic lupus erythematosus – in which both B- and T-cells may contribute to pathogenesis. However, it is clear from animal models that further experimentation is necessary with regard to both the number of conditioning training events necessary for beneficial effects and the optimal timing of exposure to the CS.

In 1993, a study was conducted in mice to determine if antigen could be used as the unconditioned stimulus to enhance humoral responses (Ader et al. 1993). In this study, intraperitoneal injections of the antigen KLH (the UCS) were paired with a gustatory chocolate milk drinking solution (the CS). Mice were given either (a) three CS–UCS pairings at three-week intervals, each consisting of intraperitoneal injection of a very low dose of KLH plus the chocolate milk drink, or (b) just the chocolate milk drink. Results of this study showed there was an enhancement of anti-KLH antibody titers when conditioned mice were re-exposed to both the CS and a minimally immunogenic dose of KLH. Thus, the idea that conditioning may enhance antibody production to low doses of antigen suggests some exciting possibilities for its future use in vaccination protocols – especially when the antigen used for vaccination is difficult to obtain owing to limited quantities or limited financial resources.

Self-Disclosure

Previous studies have reported that written disclosure of traumatic experiences may have beneficial effects on health as demonstrated by fewer health center visits (Pennebaker & Beall 1986; Pennebaker, Colder, & Sharp 1990; Pennebaker, Kiecolt-Glaser, & Glaser 1988) and decreases in work absentee rates (Francis & Pennebaker 1992). To examine the effects of self-disclosure on the immune response to a hepatitis-B vaccination, medical students were assigned to two groups: for four consecutive days, one group wrote about traumatic personal events and the other wrote about control topics (Petrie et al. 1995). On the fifth day, students were given an initial hepatitis-B vaccination, followed by booster vaccinations at one- and four-month intervals. Results of this study indicated that students who wrote about traumatic events had significantly higher hepatitis-B antibody titers at both four and six months in comparison to control subjects. Thus, self-disclosure therapies may prove to be a useful tool for enhancing the effectiveness of vaccinations.

Social Support and Coping Styles

A 1992 study suggests that social support may play an important role in an individual's response to a vaccination (Glaser et al. 1992). In this study, designed to determine the effects of examination stress on the ability to generate an immune response to a hepatitis-B antigen, medical students were given a series of three hepatitis vaccinations on days when they had examinations. Results of this study showed that students who reported greater social support also produced higher antibody titers to hepatitis B surface antigen (HpBsAg) and displayed increased peripheral blood leukocyte proliferative responsiveness to HpBsAg peptide

at the time of the third (booster) inoculation. Social support may also be beneficial for HIV-1-infected individuals. A previous study of 49 HIV-1+ male hemophiliacs revealed that a low availability of attachment (AVAT) score was associated with a significant decline in CD4+ T-cell count over a five-year period (Theorell et al. 1995).

A study designed to examine the relationship between stress, social support, coping, and immune function in elderly women revealed that those experiencing high stress exhibited lower CD4+/CD8+ T-cell ratios than women experiencing low stress (McNaughton et al. 1990). The lower CD4+/CD8+ T-cell ratios were partly due to increases in the number of CD8+ T-cells in women experiencing either high stress or less satisfaction with emotional social support. Thus, it appears that not only the quantity but also the quality of social support may be important. In addition, the results of this study showed that CD4+ T-cell number was significantly related to the endorsement of a greater percentage of problem-focused coping. Two previous studies have also indicated that coping styles may alter immunity in HIV-1-infected individuals (Goodkin et al. 1992; Mulder et al. 1995). A study of eleven asymptomatic HIV-1+ males showed that passive coping style and high stress were associated with a decline in total lymphocyte number over a one-year period (Goodkin et al. 1992). Moreover, in both low-stress and high-stress individuals who were active copers, there was a trend (not significant) toward an increased number of CD4+ Th-cells when compared with low- and high-stress individuals who used a passive coping style. A second study of 51 HIV-1-infected men, which included a one-year follow-up, showed that active coping strategy was also associated with a decrease in clinical progression (Mulder et al. 1995).

Although the mechanisms by which intervention strategies (e.g., relaxation, exercise, conditioning, self-disclosure) enhance humoral immunity are not fully understood, the studies presented here suggest that such strategies have beneficial effects on antibody production. Furthermore, the benefits of these therapies may be minor for young, non-stressed, and healthy individuals; they seem to effect the most benefit in those who are experiencing increased levels of stress and are somewhat immunocompromised – such as the elderly and HIV-1-infected individuals. Taken together, these studies suggest that the most beneficial strategies to ward off pathogens include ensuring both a healthy mind and a healthy body (via e.g. psychotherapy to reduce stress levels and regular vaccinations).

NEUROLOGICAL DISORDERS: CORRELATIONS WITH AND POTENTIAL ROLES FOR ANTIBODY WITHIN THE BRAIN

A variety of psychosocial factors that alter both CNS functions – including arms of both the HPA axis and the SNS – and humoral immune responses have been presented in previous sections of this chapter. As discussed, data support the hypothesis that part of this modulation involves alterations in cellular immune functions, which includes a change in cytokine production that (as shown in Figure 2) can modulate CNS function. In addition to cytokines, there is increasing evidence (for reviews see Amaducci, Falcini, & Lippi 1992; Bansil, Cook, & Rohowsky-Kochan 1995; Ganguli et al. 1993; Merrill, Graves, & Mulder 1992) that antibodies may alter CNS function and thus may provide a second mechanism whereby the regulatory loop illustrated in Figure 2 is completed. Two important types of antibody that may alter neurophysiology and neurofunction include brain reactive antibodies and antibodies that are found as part of immune complexes.

Brain reactive antibodies include a group of antibodies – found in serum, cerebrospinal fluid (CSF), and CNS tissue – that can bind brain antigens. One way brain reactive antibodies may alter neurophysiology is by binding directly to important receptors within the central and peripheral nervous system, resulting in (1) a blockade of the receptor, (2) stimulation of the cell via the receptor, or (3) an alteration in the turnover rate of that receptor. Binding of brain reactive antibodies to membrane antigens in the CNS could also result in complement-mediated damage of that particular cell, lysis of the cell, or modification of ion transport. Antibodies that bind to the myelin components within the CNS cause damage and lysis that result in demyelination. When immune complexes form within the CNS, they activate complement on nearby cells, which results in nonspecific lysis of those cells. Additionally, immune complexes may bind to the cerebral vasculature and change blood–brain barrier (BBB) permeability; this, in turn, increases the flow of B-cells, T-cells, and macrophages into the brain, resulting in enhanced inflammation and antibody production within the CNS.

Examples of antibody-mediated neurologic diseases include myasthenia gravis, myasthenic syndrome, "stiff man" syndrome, Guillain–Barre syndrome, and Lambert–Eaton myasthenic syndrome (see Merrill et al. 1992). All of these diseases share at least four criteria that suggest a pathophysiological mechanism mediated by the humoral immune system: (1) antibody is directed against the specific target involved in the pathophysiology of the disease; (2) self-reacting antibody is present in patients with disease but not in controls; (3) disease can be transferred in a laboratory setting using patient antibody; and (4) symptoms of disease are lessened with immunosuppressive treatment such as corticosteroids and plasmaphoresis. In addition to these diseases, antibody has been implicated to play a role in schizophrenia, multiple sclerosis, and Alzheimer's disease. However, the previous data suggest more of a correlation with the presence of antibody and the expression of disease, rather than a direct cause-and-effect paradigm. A review of previous findings is presented next.

Schizophrenia

Some of the earliest support that the humoral immune system plays a role in schizophrenia comes from a 1967 study (Heath et al. 1967) that showed serum IgG from patients with acute schizophrenia altered behavior and EEG (electroencephalogram) recordings when injected intravenously into Macaca rhesus monkeys. Although the serum IgG fraction was psychoactive in monkeys, the serum fractions containing IgM and IgA were not. It is interesting that the psychoactivity of the IgG serum diminished as the symptoms remitted, suggesting a correlation between disease and psychoactive serum IgG.

Since the 1970s, a number of studies (reviewed in Ganguli et al. 1993) have indicated that brain reactive antibodies are present in the CSF and serum of schizophrenic patients. Previous findings have indicated that phospholipid abnormalities are present in the frontal lobe of drug-naive, first-episode schizophrenics (Keshavan et al. 1989); thus, one possible role of antibodies in schizophrenia may be to alter phospholipid metabolism. To address this possibility, a study was conducted to measure serum levels of antibody to the membrane phospholipid cardiolipin in both drug-naive and medicated patients (Chengappa et al. 1991). Results of this study showed that thirteen patients (16.5%) had high IgG-anticardiolipin antibody (ACA) when compared with four controls. However, it should be noted that clinical status (acute vs. remitted) and duration of illness were not related to IgG-ACA levels. Thus, although IgG-ACA is present in some schizophrenic patients, it remains unclear as to whether or not IgG-ACA plays a direct role in altered phospholipid metabolism in schizophrenia.

It has been hypothesized that autoantibody-mediated alterations of the dopaminergic pathway play a role in schizophrenia (Knight 1982). Some proposed mechanisms include autoantibody-mediated stimulation of postsynaptic receptors, autoantibody blockade of neurotransmitter re-uptake, and an autoantibody-potentiated release of neurotransmitter (Knight, Knight, & Ungvari 1992). Although these hypotheses were formulated over ten years ago, the existence of an autoantibody capable of performing these functions has not been reported. However, it remains feasible that such an autoantibody plays a role in the development of schizophrenia and that the relevant brain antigen responsible for inducing autoantibody formation has not yet been identified.

Alzheimer's Disease

Alzheimer's disease (AD) is distinguished neuropathologically by the presence of both senile plaques and neurofibrillary tangles in the frontal and temporal cerebral cortex. Previous studies have shown that the number of plaques and tangles correlates with the degree of mental impairment (Wilcok et al. 1982). Thus, a number of histological studies have been conducted to define the components of both senile plaques and tangles. Results of a number of studies indicate that IgG is present in the senile plaques of AD patients (Eikelenboom & Stam 1982; Ishii & Haga 1975, 1976; Powers et al. 1981). In addition to IgG, at least three studies have found that components of the complement cascade – including C1q, C3, and C4 – are present in senile plaques. The classical complement cascade is activated by antibody–antigen complexes; thus, it is plausible that the IgG found in senile plaques may activate complement which, in turn, may result in either directed or bystander lysis of cells. A previous study showed that the C5b-9 membrane attack complex was present in dystrophic neurites and tangled neurons (McGeer et al. 1989), providing further support that activated complement may play a role in neuronal damage.

Previously it had been shown that antiganglioside antibodies inhibit neuronal regeneration and produce behavioral deficits in rats (Kasarskis et al. 1981). Another study showed that monoclonal antibody to ganglioside binds neurofibrillary tangles from AD patients (Emory, Ala, & Frey 1987). Thus, a sensitive ELISA technique using purified ganglioside as the antigen was utilized to determine if AD patients had serum antibodies to ganglioside (Chapman et al. 1988b). Results of this study indicated that sera from AD patients had IgG antiganglioside antibodies recognizing GM1 ganglioside and that the levels of IgG antiganglioside antibody were higher in AD patients than in age-matched controls. Two other studies showed that antibodies reactive with cholinergic neurons are present in the CSF (Mcrae-Degueurce et al. 1987) and serum (Chapman et al. 1988a) of AD patients. In addition, two studies have shown that serum from AD patients causes complement-mediated lysis of rat cholinergic synaptosomes (Bradford et al. 1989; Foley et al. 1988). These studies suggest that anti-GM1 or cholinergic receptor antibodies may contribute to the disease pathogenesis in AD.

Fillit and colleagues (1987) showed that IgG antibodies that stained the vascular portion of rat and bovine brain tissue were present in sera from 6 out of 16 AD patients but absent in age-matched control sera. Further analysis revealed the sera was binding to vascular heparin sulfate proteoglycans. Proteoglycans are anionic sites that contribute to the charged barrier in the BBB; blocking of these anionic sites may therefore alter BBB function. For these reasons, antibody binding to the vascular proteoglycans may alter BBB function in AD. Consistent with this idea, Alafuzoff and associates (1987) demonstrated BBB alterations in subjects with AD. However, it should be noted that BBB changes were also present in nondemented elderly (Alafuzoff et al. 1987). In addition, not all of the AD patients had antiproteoglycan antibody in their sera (Fillit et al. 1987). Thus it appears that, although changes in the BBB may not be a causative agent in AD, they may contribute to further CNS damage by increasing the flow of B-cells, T-cells, and macrophages into the CNS.

Multiple Sclerosis

Multiple sclerosis (MS) is a demyelinating disease of the central nervous system that exhibits a clinical manifestation ranging from a relapsing–remitting course to a chronic progressive disease. Studies undertaken to examine the immune cell populations present in MS indicate that normal levels of B-cells are present in the peripheral blood of patients with chronic progressive MS and of patients with relapsing–remitting disease during clinical relapses (Reinherz et al. 1980). Although similar levels of B-cells are present, at least one study (Antel et al. 1986) suggested that B-cells may be more active in MS patients, as demonstrated by increased Ig secretion in response to pokeweed mitogen when compared with control subjects. A number of studies have been conducted to investigate a possible humoral component to disease development and progression in MS (see Bansil et al. 1995). These previous studies suggest that the humoral immune system may play a role in the demyelination process.

A number of studies have shown that antibodies to myelin basic protein (MBP) are present in the CSF of MS patients (Gorny, Wroblewska, & Pleasure 1983; Panitch, Hooper, & Johnson 1980; Wajgt & Gorney 1983; Warren & Catz 1987). Furthermore, the levels of anti-MBP have been shown to be elevated in clinically active MS patients (Warren & Catz 1987), providing a correlation between disease state and the level of anti-MBP antibody. Anti-MBP antibody was not detected either in stable MS patients or in patients with other neurologic disorders (Warren & Catz 1987), and previous studies have shown that MBP is a component of circulating immune complexes in both the serum and CSF of MS patients (Coyle 1985; Dasgupta, Catz, & Warren 1983; Warren & Catz 1987). In progressive MS, anti-MBP antibodies are found mainly as part of these immune complexes, whereas elevated levels of free anti-MBP are found in the CSF during disease exacerbation (Warren & Catz 1987).

In addition to anti-MBP antibodies, some studies have indicated that MS patients have increased levels of autoantibodies reactive to CNS antigens in both serum and CSF (Hukkanen et al. 1983; Ryberg 1982). Although these autoantibodies do not appear to be specific for MS and have been found in other neurologic disorders, it is possible that they may contribute to disease by causing further damage to the CNS. Consistent with this idea, other studies have shown that the level of immune complexes are elevated in the serum and CSF in MS patients (Arnadottir et al. 1982; Coyle 1985; Glikmann et al. 1980; Jans et al. 1984; Noronha et al. 1981) and, in at least one study (Noronha et al. 1981), that the level of serum immune complexes is correlated with disease activity. In addition to CNS reactive antibodies, one other study has shown that anti-endothelial cell antibodies are present in MS patients' sera that may cause further damage to the BBB, resulting

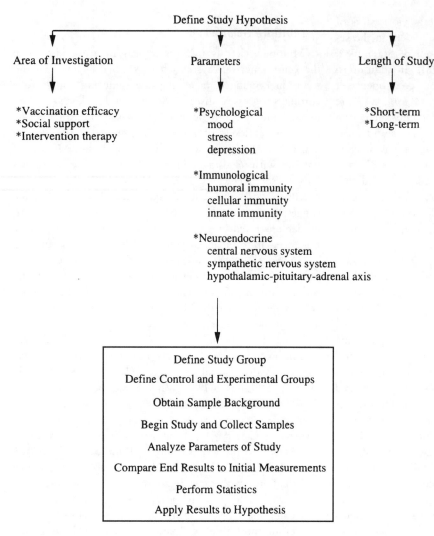

Figure 3. Experimental flow for a psychoneuroimmunology study. The most important component of any study is to define a study hypothesis. The hypothesis should define the following three elements of the study: the area of investigation, the parameters to be examined, and the length of the study. The area of investigation might include vaccine efficacy, social support, or intervention therapy (as discussed in the text). The parameters examined in the study might include psychological, immunological, and neuroendocrine components that are examined at initiation and throughout the duration of the study. A brief outline of a clinical study design is presented in the box. The length of the study will vary depending on the hypothesis and parameters to be tested. Detailed descriptions of several psychoneuroimmunology studies, as well as additional factors that should be incorporated into a thorough study, are presented in the text.

in infiltration of immune cells into the CNS and so precipitating increased CNS damage (Tanaka et al. 1987).

Although clear cause-and-effect mechanisms between antibody and disease have not been shown for schizophrenia, Alzheimer's disease, or multiple sclerosis, the studies reviewed here suggest that antibody may influence the pathophysiology of these diseases. In regard to both Alzheimer's disease (reviewed in Amaducci et al. 1992; McGeer & McGeer 1996) and multiple sclerosis (reviewed

by Bansil et al. 1995; Hohlfeld et al. 1995), there is increasing evidence that T-cells and/or local inflammatory cells of the CNS play a role in disease and contribute to CNS damage. Thus, it is likely that a variety of cells – including T-cells, B-cells, and inflammatory cells – may contribute to disease pathology in these neurological disorders. Note that the functions of the cellular and humoral immune systems can influence each other; for example, the cytokines produced by Th-cells influence the antibody produced by B-cells. In addition, when local inflammations occur in the CNS, they often disrupt the BBB, allowing B-cells to traffic to the brain and become exposed to a variety of CNS antigens. This could result in an increased presentation of CNS antigens to further activate T-cells as well as an increased production of CNS-reactive antibodies. Many current therapies for treating patients with Alzheimer's disease and multiple sclerosis focus on the cellular immune system, including T-cells and inflammatory cells (Bansil et al. 1995; McGeer & McGeer 1996). Based on the data presented here, which support a possible role for antibody in these diseases, future therapeutic strategies should include means for dampening not only the cellular but also the humoral immune responses.

Inferential Context

EXPERIMENTAL DESIGN FOR PNI STUDIES

Although the study of psychoneuroimmunology (PNI) has been ongoing for the past 100 years (Biondi & Zannino 1997), many of the earliest studies in this field merely reported observations that immune function appeared to be modulated by physiological stressors. The general hypothesis was that stress leads to an increased incidence of disease by either prolonging disease symptoms, increasing susceptibility to infection, weakening protective immune mechanisms, or decreasing vaccination efficiency (see Biondi & Zannino 1997; Cohen & Herbert 1996). Many other studies have supported this hypothesis. However, most early studies were not designed to examine psychoneuroimmunomodulation, so the data generated from these studies are controversial in regard to psychoneuroendocrine influences on immune cell function. As outlined in Figure 3, many factors and parameters must be considered in the design of a scientifically sound PNI study.

Development of Hypotheses, Objectives, and Goals

The initial phase of all scientific studies is to establish the study objectives and a hypothesis so that a proper study group can be generated. In regard to a PNI study, it is very important that the initial hypothesis encompass psychological, neuroendocrine, and immune parameters. For example, various psychosocial disorders and interventions have been (and are continuing to be) studied for psychoneuroimmunomodulation. One key area of interest is the study of the effect of intervention or counseling on a diseased patient's immune status (Kiecolt-Glaser & Glaser 1992). Studies in this area have included vaccination efficiency during stress, susceptibility to illness during stress, recurrence of disease, depression and immune status, and aging and immune status (Kiecolt-Glaser & Glaser 1992, 1995). The goal of most of these studies was to determine if social support would improve the immune status of test subjects compared to other test subjects undergoing the same stress but lacking the additional social support. Many of these studies found that the particular immune parameter under investigation could either be modulated during the study or that individuals who participated in group support sessions displayed decreased recurrence of disease, decreased susceptibility to some diseases, and better immune status while caring for an ill relative. However, the neuroendocrine factors contributing to those changes were not always included in the original hypothesis and thus were not always assessed. Therefore, a more inclusive hypothesis for this type of study would be that stress decreases immune function via the hypothalamic-pituitary-adrenal axis and that a high level of social support can negate the effects of stress. As an additional aid for establishing a sound PNI hypothesis, Figure 3 illustrates some important criteria that should be considered.

Selection of Study Groups and Controls

One of the most important criteria for a well-designed PNI study is the selection of a proper or comparable control group. Without a well-designated control group, it is difficult to interpret the data that are obtained. In addition, study subjects should be grouped based on one, several, or many of the following parameters, depending on the objectives of the study: age, gender, lifestyle (e.g., diet, alcohol and caffeine consumption, and smoking), sleep pattern, personality, social status, and disease history (Biondi & Zannino 1997; Cohen & Herbert 1996). The importance of each of these parameters must be defined before the study begins; in most cases, one parameter will be more important than another. For example, immunological status/competency (i.e., the ability to mount an immune/antibody response) has been linked to exer-

cise. If a study is designed to determine the ability of an individual to mount an immune response during and/or following a specific stress response, then the test subjects must be chosen accordingly. If the control group contains individuals who frequently exercise while the experimental group contains subjects who rarely exercise, then the results of an immunological analysis of these subjects may be skewed by factors not properly controlled for in the study. In any scientific study, especially those performed in vivo, it is important to remember that many systems in the body are connected and hence that one system may be influencing other systems. In order to properly control for such events, rigid criteria must be set for test subject selection. It is difficult to draw clear conclusions from many previous studies in the PNI area owing to the lack of control subjects who are matched for age, gender, and lifestyle.

Define Background Levels

Prior to initiation of a PNI study, it is necessary to obtain a background profile for each of the test subjects (Kiecolt-Glaser & Glaser 1992) so that researchers can determine if changes occurred during the experimental testing period. Depending on the specific psychological, neurological, and immunological parameters to be examined, a variety of tests (see Table 1) must be performed to determine each individual's background (resting) levels. To rule out effects of diurnal variation, samples meant to assess background levels should be collected at the same time of day as the test samples. In addition, for studies examining the effects of stress, it may be important to gather two separate background samples: one prior to the first day of study and one on the first day of the study yet prior to application of the stressor.

Sample Collection and Analysis

As reviewed in this chapter, the cellular and humoral immune systems and the CNS, HPA, and SNS are connected in many intricate ways with regulatory mechanisms occurring within and between the individual systems. Therefore, in order to link immunological changes to psychological and neurophysiological changes, it is important that PNI studies include simultaneous analysis of physical, psychological, immune, and neuroendocrine parameters. As discussed previously, a few important physical characteristics that should be recorded for the study group include age, gender, weight, height, diet, lifestyle, and social status. Additional physical parameters that may be important to monitor include nutritional status, vaccine history, disease history, allergic status, number of subjects housed together, and the infectious state of subjects sharing the same house. In addition to physical factors, a number of psychological factors (reviewed earlier) can alter humoral and cellular immunity; these factors include mood changes, depression, stress, degree of social support, and personal motivation. Thus, it is particularly important that these psychological

TABLE 1. Study Parameters of Interest

Parameter	Measure	Sensitivity	Reference
Physical	**Physical Examination**		
Nutritional status	Plasma albumin and transferrin levels	10 nmol/l	Cacioppo et al. 1995
Health evaluation and vaccine history	Height, weight, health practices questionnaire	—	Snyder et al. 1990
Psychological	**Evaluation Forms**		
Stress	Life event checklist	—	Snyder et al. 1990
Depression	Mental health inventory	—	Snyder et al. 1990
	Beck depression inventory		
Social support	Identify support structure	—	Snyder et al. 1990
Motivation	Thematic apperception test	—	Jemmott et al. 1983
Immune	**Blood Sample**		
Percentage of lymphocyte subsets	Flow cytometry with cell-specific markers (macrophage, NK cells, B-cells, CD4$^+$ and CD8$^+$ T-cells)	1.0 μg/ml	Current Protocols in Immunology (CPI)
Immunoglobulin levels (Ig)	ELISA: IgA, IgM, IgG, IgE	0.1–1 ng/ml	CPI
	ELISPOT: # of Ig-secreting cells		
Cellular activity	^{3}H-nucleotide incorporation upon cellular activation with mitogens	Determined by specific activity of isotope	CPI
Cytokine production	ELISA: present in serum	0.1 ng/ml	CPI
	Brefeldin A: present in cells	1.0 μg/ml	
	RNAse Protection: mRNA levels	10 ng RNA	
Cell phenotypes	Flow cytometry with Abs to cellular activation markers	1.0 μg/ml	CPI
Neuroendocrine	**Blood Sample**		
Plasma ACTH	Immunoradiometric assay	0.1 pmol/l	Malarkey et al. 1995
Plasma cortisol	Fluorescent technique	25 nmol/l	Malarkey et al. 1995
Plasma epinephrine and norepinephrine	HPLC	10–20 pg/ml	Cacioppo et al. 1995

states be monitored with questionnaires – either throughout the study or on days when samples are collected for analysis of immune and neuroendocrine parameters.

Previous PNI studies suggested that changes in psychological and neuroendocrine factors alter both the humoral and cellular immune systems (for reviews see Biondi & Zannino 1997; Cohen & Herbert 1996; Kiecolt-Glaser & Glaser 1992). In addition, soluble factors produced during humoral and cellular immune responses may regulate each other. Thus, it is important for initial studies to include measurements of both humoral and cellular immune parameters. Initial analysis of immunity should include:

1. immunofluorescence staining of peripheral blood samples to determine the percentages of B-cells, T-cells (CD4$^+$ and CD8$^+$), NK cells, and macrophages;
2. measurement of both serum and salivary Ig levels by ELISA;
3. measurement of the capacity of peripheral blood T-cells to secrete cytokines following anti-CD3 stimulation;
4. measurement of the ability of T- and B-cells to proliferate in response to mitogens; and
5. measurement of the ability of NK cells to lyse target cells.

In order to obtain a better understanding of which neuroendocrine factor(s) may be altering the immune response, it is important to measure the levels of ACTH, cortisol, epinephrine, and norepinephrine that are present in the blood. Table 1 includes a number of tests to measure these parameters, as well as references for protocols and specific applications to PNI studies that have used these tests. A more in-depth discussion on the analysis of humoral immunity is presented next.

ANALYSIS OF HUMORAL IMMUNITY

Earlier sections of this chapter discussed the process of antibody production in an immune response, as well as the other organ systems that influence this humoral immune response. It is important to understand the mechanism(s) by which antibody is produced and the nonimmune factors that can enhance or inhibit antibody production. However, it is also necessary to understand the techniques that are used to measure the level of antibody produced and to determine specific features about the antibody produced, including antigenic specificity, antibody isotype or class, and affinity of the antibody for its antigen.

This section focuses on techniques that are used to examine antibody production in animal and human systems. In some cases, such as the diagnosis of viral or bacterial infections, human serum can be tested directly for the presence of antibodies to these different antigens (Murakami et al. 1991; Picardo & Guisantes 1981; Schubert & Cornell 1958; Yarchoan et al. 1981). However, if the goal is to define the mechanism by which a disease develops, it may be difficult to study a human model because of the limited reagents and limited sample material available for analysis. To circumvent these limitations, many scientists use mouse models because the mouse mimics many human diseases and the assay reagents are easily accessible. Additional animal model systems utilized in psychoneuroimmunology research include rat, rabbit, and goat (Lingrel et al. 1985; Miyoshi et al. 1985; Peters & Theofilopoulos 1977; Silagi & Schaefer 1986; Talmadge 1985).

Detection of Antibody Production in Animals and Humans

The techniques that will be described here are used to analyze the humoral (antibody) response in both the human and mouse systems. The limitations in human studies stem from the limited study material (usually only serum) versus multiple organs that can be examined in the mouse – such as the spleen and lymph nodes – in addition to serum. Over the past few decades, assay systems have been refined and are now able to detect nanogram to picogram quantities of antibody per milliliter of sample tested, as compared to sensitivity levels of microgram quantities detected in the earlier assay systems (DeLisi 1974; Engvall & Perlman 1971). Although a variety of techniques have been used to measure antibody levels and antibody parameters (de Bruyn & Klein 1976; DeLisi 1974; Lemieux et al. 1993; Lenert, Lenert, & Zanetti 1995; Nilsson 1967; Ouchterlony & Nilsson 1986; Steinman 1982), the authors of this chapter recommend the five techniques described next. To aid in the design of future PNI studies, we will discuss the mechanism of detection, sensitivity of the assay, and advantages and disadvantages of each technique.

Mechanism, Sensitivity, Advantages, and Disadvantages

Radioimmunoassay. The radioimmunoassay (RIA) was developed in 1960 (see Schiffman et al. 1980) and has the greatest sensitivity of all the assays used to measure antibody levels. The radioimmunoassay can be used to test antiserum or purified antibody for its antigenic specificity, isotype, and quantity. Initially, a solid surface (96-well plate) is coated with an antigen or capture antibody. The antiserum sample is then added and allowed to bind to the coated plate. The plate is washed to remove unbound antibody and a radioactively labeled ([125]Iodine) detecting antibody is added. The detecting antibody will bind to specific antibody that has bound to the capture antigen

or antibody. Both the capture antigen–antibody and the detecting antibody that are used can help to define the antigenic specificity and isotype of the antibody present in the antiserum. The level of radioactivity can then be measured using a gamma counter. The experimental samples are compared to a standard curve to determine the amount of antibody present in each sample. The advantages to the RIA are its high sensitivity (0.0001–0.001 μg/ml of sample) and ability to generate a standard curve for quantitative analysis. The greatest disadvantage is the requirement for a radioactively labeled detecting antibody (Schiffman et al. 1980; Spiehler et al. 1975). Therefore, the ELISA (described next) is currently favored because it is just as sensitive but does not use radioactive material.

Enzyme-Linked Immunosorbent Assay (ELISA). The design and sensitivity of the ELISA are similar to the RIA (Engvall & Perlman 1971; Macy, Kemeny, & Saxon 1988). The ELISA can be used to test antiserum or purified antibody for its antigenic specificity, isotype, and quantity. As shown in Figure 4, a solid surface (96-well plate) is coated with an antigen or capture antibody. The antiserum sample is then added and allowed to bind to the coated plate. The plate is washed to remove unbound antibody, and an enzyme-conjugated (alkaline phosphatase, horseradish peroxidase) detecting antibody is added. The detecting antibody will bind to specific antibody that has bound to the capture antigen or antibody, and a soluble substrate is added to the plate. If the enzyme-conjugated detecting antibody is present, it will convert the substrate and result in a colorimetric reaction. The degree of substrate conversion can be measured using an ELISA reader, which determines the optical density of each well. To determine the antibody concentration in each sample well, the optical density readings of the sample wells are compared to the optical density readings of a standard curve. Both the capture antigen–antibody and the detecting antibody can help to define the antigenic specificity and isotype of the bound antibody present in the antiserum. The sensitivity of the ELISA assay also ranges from 0.0001 to 0.001 micrograms per milliliter of sample. The disadvantage of this system is that it requires purified antigens and antibodies for capturing and detecting antibody. The advantages include the ability to determine antigen concentration, isotype, and specificity, its high sensitivity and good reproducibility, and the requirement for small amounts of sample antiserum (Adamkiewicz, Nehls, & Rajewsky 1984; Li 1985).

Jerne Plaque Assay. Unlike the two assays just described, which measure the amount of antibody present in serum or cell supernatant, the Jerne plaque assay determines the number of cells in a population that are secreting antibody (Hubner & Gengozian 1969; Jerne et al. 1974; Kaliss 1971). This technique can be used in conjunction with one of the other assays to determine both the number

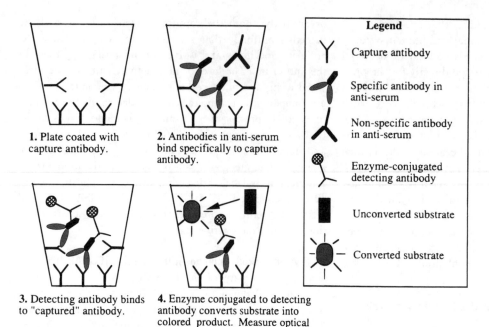

1. Plate coated with capture antibody.

2. Antibodies in anti-serum bind specifically to capture antibody.

3. Detecting antibody binds to "captured" antibody.

4. Enzyme conjugated to detecting antibody converts substrate into colored product. Measure optical density.

Figure 4. Enzyme-linked immunosorbent assay (ELISA). The ELISA assay may be used to detect soluble proteins (e.g. antibody) present in serum. Initially, as shown in step 1, a microtiter plate well is coated with a capture antibody that will specifically bind the soluble protein. In step 2, serum is added to the well, and anything that is recognized by the capture antibody will be bound and remain in the well when it is washed. In step 3, a detecting antibody is added that will also recognize the soluble protein that was bound by the capture antibody. The detecting antibody is usually conjugated to an enzyme. In step 4, when a substrate is added to the well, the enzyme converts the substrate into a soluble colored product. The optical density of the converted substrate is compared to a standard curve (generated with known amounts of the soluble protein) to quantitate the amount of soluble protein present in the well.

of cells in a population that are secreting antibody and how much antibody is being produced by that population of cells. The cells of interest (activated spleen cells, peripheral blood lymphocytes, etc.) are mixed with red blood cells coated with the antigen of interest in a thin layer of agar. Antibody that is secreted by the B-cells will bind to the red blood cells if the antibody is specific for that antigen. Complement is then added to lyse antibody-coated red blood cells. As shown in Figure 5, wells that have secreted antibody specific for the antigen coated on the red blood cells will be surrounded by red blood cell–free regions termed plaques. The plaques can then be counted to determine the number of cells that were secreting antibody directed against the antigen of interest. The advantage to the Jerne plaque assay is that the number of antibody-secreting cells can be determined. Disadvantages include (a) the necessity to count the plaques immediately following the addition of complement and (b) the lack of a standard curve with which to compare and quantify experimental samples. This assay allows for the determination

of antigen specificity, isotype of antibody present, and (in some cases) the affinity of the antibody for its antigen (Kaliss 1971).

ELISPOT. The ELISPOT assay is a modification of the ELISA that uses cells instead of cell supernatants or antiserum to assay for antibody production (Czerkinsky et al. 1983; Sedgwick & Holt 1983). This system allows one to determine not only the number of cells in a population that are producing antibody but also the level of antibody produced by cells in the sample population. As with ELISA, wells are coated with a capture antigen or antibody. Instead of adding antiserum or cell supernatants to the wells, activated cells are added to the wells. The cells are allowed to secrete antibody for a limited period of time. Since the wells are coated with a capture antigen–antibody, antibody secreted by the cells that is specific for the capture antigen–antibody will bind to the plate and remain there when the cells are lysed and the plates are washed. After the plates are washed, an enzyme-linked detecting antibody is added. If antibody from the antiserum has bound to the wells then the detecting antibody will bind to the captured antibody. An insoluble substrate is added to the wells that can be converted by the enzyme conjugated to the detecting antibody. In contrast to the ELISA assay, which employs a soluble substrate to determine antibody concentration using optical density readings, the ELISPOT assay uses an insoluble substrate that will generate "spots" where antibody has been secreted from cells (see Figure 5). These spots can then be counted to determine the number of cells from the starting population that are secreting antibody. One disadvantage to this system is that there is no standard curve to quantify antibody levels. Therefore,

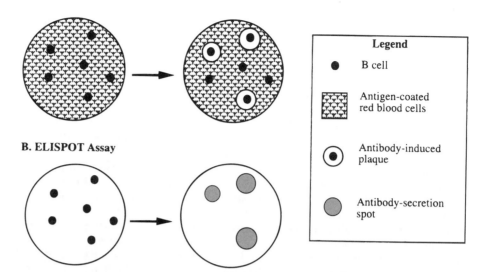

A. Jerne Plaque Assay

B. ELISPOT Assay

Legend

● B cell

▨ Antigen-coated red blood cells

◉ Antibody-induced plaque

● Antibody-secretion spot

Figure 5. Jerne plaque assay and ELISPOT assay. These assays are used to determine the number of cells that are secreting a specific antibody. In panel A, red blood cell–activated B-cells are plated onto either red blood cell monolayers (A) or capture antibody-coated plates (B). B-cells secrete antibody that will bind to either the red blood cells (A) or be captured by the capture antibody that is coated on plate (B). In panel A, complement is added to the red blood cells, and any red cells that are bound by antibody will be lysed by the complement and so create red blood cell–free areas known as *plaques*. In panel B, an enzyme-conjugated detecting antibody is added to wells. This antibody will bind only to antibody that was captured on the plate. A substrate is added to the plate and is converted into an insoluble precipitate. Each cell that secreted antibody of a specific type is then identified as a spot on the plate. With these assays, the plaques or spots are counted using a microscope.

samples must be compared to each other instead of a known standard. The ELISPOT is more practical than the Jerne plaque assay because sample wells can be stored before counting and thus do not require immediate analysis (Czerkinsky et al. 1983; Sedgwick & Holt 1983).

Immunofluorescence. The final technique that will be discussed in this section is immunofluorescence analysis. The surface or intracellular expression of certain proteins can increase or decrease following the activation of immune cells. Analysis using fluorescently tagged antibodies or probes can help identify whether the protein of interest is expressed by the immune cell. Although immunofluorescence is most commonly used in conjunction with flow cytometric analysis to examine protein expression on either the surface or inside of individual immune cells (Havlickova, Pljusnin, & Tumova 1990), it can also be used (in combination with histochemical techniques) to localize protein expression within a tissue sample.

Summary

This chapter described in detail the evidence that neuroendocrine hormones, opioid peptides, and the sympathetic neurotransmitter norepinephrine are involved in modulation of humoral immunity. It is evident that a neuroendocrine–immune relationship indeed exists and that it may influence the physiology and pathophysiology normally associated with each system individually. Data support the hypothesis that a disturbance to one component of the communication loop can influence profoundly the functioning of another component and hence affect both short- and long-term health. Determining the mechanisms by which the multiple systems integrate with each other to function normally will enable us to gain better insight into pathological processes that result from pertur-

bation of the organism as a whole. This will be beneficial with regard to immune changes precipitated in response to either psychosocial factors (such as stress) or the interventions (e.g., relaxation techniques) used to counteract the stress-induced effects. Such insights will aid in the development of new therapeutic approaches and interventions that will more fully contribute to the treatment and prevention of psycho- and immunopathology and also to the enhancement of individual well-being. In order to attain this goal, future research should employ techniques that simultaneously assess immune, psychological, and physiological parameters to determine the mechanisms by which psychoneurophysiological and immune interactions occur.

NOTE

The authors wish to thank Adam Kohm for critical editing of the chapter. We also wish to thank the research funds provided to our laboratory by the National Institutes of Health (AI37326) and the American Cancer Society (IM-798), as well as for career development awards provided to V.M.S. by the American Cancer Society (JFRA-578) and the Schweppe Foundation.

REFERENCES

Adamkiewicz, J., Nehls, P., & Rajewsky, M. F. (1984). Immunological methods for detection of carcinogen-DNA adducts. *IARC Scientific Publications, 59,* 199–215.

Ader, R., & Cohen, N. (1975). Behaviorally conditioned immunosuppression. *Psychosomatic Medicine, 37,* 333–40.

Ader, R., & Cohen, N. (1993). Psychoneuroimmunology: Conditioning and stress. *Annual Review of Psychology, 44,* 53–85.

Ader, R., Kelly, K., Moynihan, J. A., Grota, L. J., & Cohen, N. (1993). Conditioned enhancement of antibody production using antigen as the unconditioned stimulus. *Brain, Behavior, and Immunity, 7,* 334–43.

Aebischer, I., Stampfli, M. R., Zurcher, A., Miescher, S., Urwyler, A., Frey, B., Luger, T., White, R. R., & Stadler, B. M. (1994). Neuropeptides are potent modulators of human in vitro immunoglobulin E synthesis. *European Journal of Immunology, 24,* 1908–13.

Alafuzoff, I., Adolfsson, R., Grundke-Iqbal, I., & Winblad, B. (1987). Blood–brain barrier in Alzheimer dementia and in nondemented elderly. *Acta Neuropathologica (Berlin), 73,* 160–6.

Amaducci, L., Falcini, M., & Lippi, A. (1992). Humoral and cellular immunologic repertoire in Alzheimer's disease. *Annals of the New York Academy of Sciences, 663,* 349–56.

Antel, J. P., Nicholas, M. K., Bania, M. B., Reder, A. T., Arnason, B. G., & Joseph, L. (1986). Comparison of T8[+] cell-mediated suppressor and cytotoxic functions in multiple sclerosis. *Journal of Neuroimmunology, 12,* 215–24.

Arnadottir, T., Kekomaki, R., Lund, G. A., Reunanen, M., & Salmi, A. A. (1982). Circulating immune complexes in patients with multiple sclerosis. A longitudinal study of serum and CSF by C1q and platelet binding tests. *Journal of Neurological Science, 55,* 273–83.

Audhya, T., Jain, R., & Hollander, C. S. (1991). Receptor mediated immunomodulation by corticotropin-releasing factor. *Cellular Immunology, 134,* 77–84.

Bachen, E. A., Manuck, S. B., Cohen, S., Muldoon, M. F., Raible, R., Herbert, T. B., & Rabin, B. S. (1995). Adrenergic blockade ameliorates cellular immune responses to mental stress in humans. *Psychosomatic Medicine, 57,* 366–72.

Bailey, G. H. (1925). The effect of fatigue upon the susceptibility of rabbits to intratracheal injections of type I pneumococcus. *American Journal of Hygiene, 5,* 175–85.

Bansil, S., Cook, S. D., & Rohowsky-Kochan, C. (1995). Multiple sclerosis: Immune mechanism and update on current therapies. *Annals of Neurology, 37,* S87–S101.

Beard, C. W., & Mitchell, B. W. (1987). Effects of environmental temperatures on the serologic responses of broiler chickens to inactivated and viable Newcastle disease vaccines. *Avian Diseases, 31,* 321–6.

Ben-Nathan, D., Lustig, S., & Danenberg, H. D. (1991). Stress-induced neuroinvasiveness of a neurovirulent noninvasive Sindbis virus in cold or isolation subjected mice. *Life Sciences, 48,* 1493–1500.

Ben-Nathan, D., Lustig, S., & Feuerstein, G. (1989). The influence of cold or isolation stress on neuroinvasiveness and virulence of an attenuated variant of West Nile virus. *Archives of Virology, 109,* 1–10.

Besedovsky, H. O., Del Rey, A., Sorkin, E., Da Prada, M., & Keller, H. H. (1979). Immunoregulation mediated by the sympathetic nervous system. *Cellular Immunology, 48,* 346–55.

Bidlack, J. M., Saripalli, L. D., & Lawrence, D. M. P. (1992). Kappa-opioid binding sites on a murine lymphoma cell line. *European Journal of Pharmacology, 227,* 257–65.

Biondi, M., & Zannino, L.-G. (1997). Psychological stress, neuroimmunomodulation, and susceptibility to infectious diseases in animals and man: A review. *Psychotherapy and Psychosomatics, 66,* 3–26.

Bradford, H. F., Foley, P., Docherty, M., Fillit, H., Luine, V. N., McEwen, B., Bucht, G., Winblad, B., & Hardy, J. (1989). Antibodies in serum of patients with Alzheimer's disease cause immunolysis of cholinergic nerve terminals from the rat cerebral cortex. *Canadian Journal of Neurological Science, 16,* 528–34.

Brown, D. H., Sheridan, J., Pearl, D., & Zwilling, B. S. (1993). Regulation of mycobacterial growth by the hypothalamus-pituitary-adrenal axis: Differential responses of *Mycobacterium bovis* BCG-resistant and -susceptible mice. *Infection and Immunity, 61,* 4793–4803.

Bulloch, K., & Pomerantz, W. (1984). Autonomic nervous system innervation of thymic related lymphoid tissue in wild-type and nude mice. *Journal of Comparative Neurology, 228,* 57–68.

Butter, C., Healey, D. G., Agha, N., & Turk, J. L. (1988). An immunoelectron microscopical study of the expression of Class II MHC and a T lymphocyte marker during chronic relapsing experimental allergic encephalomyelitis. *Journal of Neuroimmunology, 20,* 45–51.

Cacioppo, J. T., Malarkey, W. B., Kiecolt-Glaser, J. K., Uchino, B. N., Sgoutas-Emch, S. A., Sheridan, J. F., Berntson, G. G., & Glaser, R. (1995). Heterogeneity in neuroendocrine and immune respones to brief physiological stressors as a function of autonomic cardiac activation. *Psychosomatic Medicine, 57,* 154–64.

Calvo, W. (1968). The innervation of the bone marrow in laboratory animals. *Journal of Anatomy, 123,* 315–28.

Carr, D. J. J., & Blalock, J. E. (1991). Neuropeptide hormones and receptors common to the immune and neuroendocrine systems: Bidirectional pathway of intersystem communication. In R. Ader, N. Cohen, & D. L. Felten (Eds.), *Psychoneuroimmunology,* pp. 573–88. New York: Academic Press.

Carr, D. J. J., Kim, C.-H., De Costa, B., Jacobson, A. E., Rice, K. C., & Blalock, J. E. (1988). Evidence for a delta-class opioid receptor on cells of the immune system. *Cellular Immunology, 116,* 44–51.

Chang, S. S., & Rasmussen, A. F. (1965). Stress induced suppression of interferon production in virus-infected mice. *Nature, 205,* 623–4.

Chapman, J., Bachar, O., Korczyn, A. D., Wertman, E., & Michaelson, D. M. (1988a). Antibodies to cholinergic neurons in Alzheimer's disease. *Journal of Neurochemistry, 51,* 479–85.

Chapman, J., Ben-ami, S., Wertman, E., & Michaelson, D. M. (1988b). Antibodies to ganglioside GM1 in patients with Alzheimer's disease. *Neuroscience Letters, 86,* 235–40.

Chengappa, K. N. R., Carpenter, A. B., Keshavan, M. S., Yang, Z. W., Kelly, R. H., Rabin, B. S., & Ganguli, R. (1991). Elevated IgG and IgM anticardiolipin antibodies in a subgroup of medicated and unmedicated schizophrenic patients. *Biological Psychiatry, 30,* 731–5.

Cherwinski, H. M., Schumacher, J. H., Brown, K. D., & Mosmann, T. R. (1987). Two types of mouse helper T cell clone.

III. Further differences in lymphokine synthesis between Th1 and Th2 clones revealed by RNA hybridization, functionally monospecific bioassays, and monoclonal antibodies. *Journal of Experimental Medicine, 166,* 1229–44.

Clement-Jones, V., & Besser, G. M. (1984). Opioid peptides in humans and their clinical significance. *Peptides, 6,* 323–71.

Clover, R. D., Abell, T., Becker, L. A., Crawford, S., & Ramsey, C. N. (1989). Family functioning and stress as predictors of influenza B infection. *The Journal of Family Practice, 28,* 535–9.

Cocke, R., Moynihan, J. A., Cohen, N., Grota, L. J., & Ader, R. (1993). Exposure to nonspecific alarm chemosignals alters immune responses in BALB/c mice. *Brain, Behavior, and Immunity, 7,* 36–46.

Cohen, N., Ader, R., Green, N., & Bovbjerg, D. (1979). Conditioned suppression of a thymus-independent antibody response. *Psychosomatic Medicine, 41,* 487–91.

Cohen, N., Moynihan, J. A., & Ader, R. (1994). Pavlovian conditioning of the immune system. *International Archives of Allergy and Immunology, 105,* 101–6.

Cohen, S., & Herbert, T. B. (1996). Health psychology: Psychological factors and physical disease from the perspective of human psychoneuroimmunology. *Annual Review of Psychology, 47,* 113–42.

Cohen, S., Tyrrell, D. A. J., & Smith, A. P. (1991). Psychological stress and susceptibility to the common cold. *New England Journal of Medicine, 325,* 606–12.

Cohen-Cole, S., Cogen, R., Stevens, A., Kirk, K., Gaitan, E., Hain, J., & Freeman, A. (1981). Psychosocial, endocrine, and immune factors in acute necrotizing ulcerative gingivitis ("trench-mouth"). *Psychosomatic Medicine, 43,* 91.

Cole, N. A., Camp, T. H., Rowe, L. D., Stevens, D. G., & Hutcheson, D. P. (1988). Effect of transport on feeder calves. *American Journal of Veterinary Research, 49,* 178–83.

Coyle, P. K. (1985). CSF immune complexes in multiple sclerosis. *Neurology, 35,* 429–32.

Cunnick, J. E., Cohen, S., Rabin, B. S., Carpenter, A. B., Manuck, S. B., & Kaplan, J. R. (1991). Alterations in specific antibody production due to rank and social instability. *Brain, Behavior, and Immunity, 5,* 357–69.

Czerkinsky, C. C., Nilsson, L.-A., Nygren, H., Ouchterlony, O., & Tarkowski, A. (1983). A solid-phase enzyme-linked immunospot (ELISPOT) assay for the enumeration of specific antibody-secreting cells. *Journal of Immunological Methods, 65,* 109–21.

D'Arcy, M., Keane, P., & Clancy, L. (1989). Significant life events and pulmonary tuberculosis. *Irish Journal of Psychological Medicine, 6,* 115–17.

Dasgupta, M. K., Catz, I., & Warren, K. G. (1983). Myelin basic protein: A component of circulating immune complexes in multiple sclerosis. *Canadian Journal of Neurological Science, 10,* 239–43.

de Bruyn, A. M., & Klein, F. (1976). The validity of the radial immunodiffusion method for the determination of human IgE. Evaluation of a modified method. *Journal of Immunological Methods, 11,* 311–20.

DeLisi, C. (1974). A theory of precipitation and agglutination reactions in immunological systems. *Journal of Theoretical Biology, 45,* 555–75.

Del Rey, A., Besedovsky, H. O., Sorkin, E., Da Prada, M., & Arrenbrecht, S. (1981). Immunoregulation mediated by the sympathetic nervous system II. *Cellular Immunology, 63,* 329–34.

Dillon, K. M., Minchoff, B., & Baker, K. H. (1985). Positive emotional states and enhancement of the immune system. *International Journal of Psychiatry in Medicine, 15,* 13–18.

Dobbs, C. M., Feng, N., Beck, F. M., & Sheridan, J. F. (1996). Neuroendocrine regulation of cytokine production during experimental influenza viral infection: Effects of restraint stress-induced elevation in endogenous corticosterone. *Journal of Immunology, 157,* 1870–7.

Edwards, E. A., & Dean, L. M. (1977). Effects of crowding of mice on humoral antibody formation and protection to lethal antigenic challenge. *Psychosomatic Medicine, 39,* 19–24.

Eikelenboom, P., & Stam, F. C. (1982). Immunoglobulins and complement factors in senile plaques: An immunoperoxidase study. *Acta Neuropathologica (Berlin), 57,* 239–42.

Emory, C. R., Ala, T. A., & Frey, W. H. (1987). Ganglioside monoclonal antibody (A2B5) labels Alzheimer's neurofibrillary tangles. *Neurology, 37,* 768–72.

Engvall, E., & Perlman, P. (1971). Enzyme-linked immunosorbent assay (ELISA): Quantitative assay of immunoglobulin G. *Immunochemistry, 8,* 871–9.

Esterling, B. A., Antoni, M. H., Fletcher, M. A., Margulies, S., & Schneiderman, N. (1994). Emotional disclosure through writing or speaking modulates latent Epstein–Barr virus antibody titers. *Journal of Consulting and Clinical Psychology, 62,* 130–40.

Esterling, B. A., Antoni, M. H., Kumar, M., & Schneiderman, N. (1990). Emotional repression, stress disclosure responses, and Epstein–Barr viral capsid antigen titers. *Psychosomatic Medicine, 52,* 397–410.

Esterling, B. A., Antoni, M. H., Kumar, M., & Schneiderman, N. (1993). Defensiveness, trait anxiety, and Epstein–Barr viral capsid antigen antibody titers in healthy college students. *Health Psychology, 12,* 132–9.

Felten, D. L., Felten, S. Y., Bellinger, D. L., Carlson, S. L., Ackerman, K. D., Madden, K. S., Olschowka, J. A., & Livnat, S. (1987). Noradrenergic sympathetic neural interactions with the immune system: Structure and function. *Immunological Reviews, 100,* 225–60.

Felten, D. L., Felten, S. Y., Carlson, S. L., Olschowka, J. A., & Livnat, S. (1985). Noradrenergic and peptidergic innervation of lymphoid tissue. *Journal of Immunology, 135,* S755–S765.

Feng, N., Pagniano, R., Tovar, C. A., Bonneau, R. H., Glaser, R., & Sheridan, J. F. (1991). The effect of restraint stress on the kinetics, magnitude, and isotype of the humoral immune response to influenza virus infection. *Brain, Behavior, and Immunity, 5,* 370–82.

Filion, L. G., Willson, P. J., Bielefeldt-Ohmann, H., Babiuk, L. A., & Thomson, R. G. (1984). The possible role of stress in the induction of pneumonic pasteurellosis. *Canadian Journal of Comparative Medicine, 48,* 268–74.

Fillit, H. M., Kemeny, E., Luine, V., Weksler, M. E., & Zabriskie, J. B. (1987). Antivascular antibodies in the sera of patients with senile dementia of the Alzheimer's type. *Journal of Gerontology, 42,* 180–4.

Fleshner, M., Brennan, F. X., Nguyen, K., Watkins, L. R., & Maier, S. F. (1996). RU-486 blocks differentially suppressive effect of stress on in vivo anti-KLH immunoglobulin response. *American Journal of Physiology, 271,* R1344–R1352.

Florijin, Y., & Geiger, A. (1991). Community based physical activity program for HIV-1 infected persons [Abstract]. *Proceedings of the Biological Aspects of HIV Infection Conference* (Amsterdam).

Foley, P., Bradford, H. F., Docherty, M., Fillit, H., Luine, V. N., McEwen, B., Bucht, G., Winblad, B., & Hardy, J. (1988). Evidence for the presence of antibodies to cholinergic neurons in the serum of patients with Alzheimer's disease. *Journal of Neurology, 235,* 466–71.

Francis, M. E., & Pennebaker, J. W. (1992). Putting stress into words: The impact of writing on physiological, absentee, and self-reported emotional well-being measures. *American Journal of Health Promotion, 6,* 280–6.

Fried, G., Terenius, L., Brodin, E., Efendic, S., Dockray, G., Fahenkrug, J., Goldstein, M., & Hokfelt, T. (1986). Neuropeptide Y, enkephalin and noradrenaline coexist in sympathetic neurons innervating the bovine spleen. *Cell and Tissue Research, 243,* 495–508.

Fuchs, B. A., Albright, J. W., & Albright, J. F. (1988). Beta-adrenergic receptor on murine lymphocytes: Density varies with cell maturity and lymphocyte subtype and is decreased after antigen administration. *Cellular Immunology, 114,* 231–45.

Futterman, A. D., Kemeny, M. E., Shapiro, D., & Fahey, J. L. (1994). Immunological and physiological changes associated with induced positive and negative mood. *Psychosomatic Medicine, 56,* 499–511.

Gaitman, B. G., Chason, J. L., & Lerner, A. M. (1970). Augmentation of the virulence of murine Coxsackievirus B-3 myocardiopathy by exercise. *Journal of Experimental Medicine, 131,* 1121–36.

Ganguli, R., Brar, J. S., Chengappa, K. N. R., Yang, Z. W., Nimgaonkar, V. L., & Rabin, B. S. (1993). Autoimmunity in schizophrenia: A review of recent findings. *Annals of Medicine, 25,* 489–96.

Glaser, R., Kiecolt-Glaser, J. K., Bonneau, R. H., Malarkey, W., Kennedy, S., & Hughes, J. (1992). Stress-induced modulation of the immune response to recombinant hepatitis B vaccine. *Psychosomatic Medicine, 54,* 22–9.

Glaser, R., Kiecolt-Glaser, J. K., Speicher, C. E., & Holliday, J. E. (1985). Stress, loneliness, and changes on herpesvirus latency. *Journal of Behavioral Medicine, 8,* 249–60.

Glaser, R., Pearson, G. R., Bonneau, R. H., Esterling, B. A., Atkinson, C., & Kiecolt-Glaser, J. K. (1993). Stress and the memory T cell response to the Epstein–Barr virus in healthy medical students. *Health Psychology, 12,* 435–42.

Glikmann, G., Svehag, S. E., Hansen, E., Hansen, O., Husby, S., Nielson, H., & Farrell, C. (1980). Soluble immune complexes in cerebrospinal fluid of patients with multiple sclerosis and other neurological diseases. *Acta Neurologica Scandinavica, 61,* 333–43.

Gold, P. W., Chrousos, G., Kellner, C., Post, R., Roy, A., Augerinos, P., Schulte, H., & Oldfield, E. (1984). Psychiatric implications of basic and clinical studies with corticotropin-releasing factor. *American Journal of Psychiatry, 141,* 619–27.

Gold, P. W., Goodwin, F. K., & Chrousos, G. P. (1988). Clinical and biochemical manifestations of depression: Relation to the neurobiology of stress. *New England Journal of Medicine, 319,* 413–20.

Goodkin, K., Fuchs, I., Feaster, D., Leeka, J., & Dickson-Rishel, D. (1992). Life stressors and coping style are associated with immune measures in HIV-1 infection – A preliminary report. *International Journal of Psychiatry in Medicine, 22,* 155–72.

Gorny, M. K., Wroblewska, Z., & Pleasure, D. (1983). CSF antibodies to myelin basic protein and oligodendrocytes in multiple sclerosis and other neurological diseases. *Acta Neurologica Scandinavica, 67,* 338–47.

Green, M. L., Green, R. G., & Santoro, W. (1988). Daily relaxation modifies serum and salivary immunoglobulins and psychophysiologic symptom severity. *Biofeedback and Self-Regulation, 13,* 187–99.

Gross, W. B. (1984). Effect of a range of social stress severity on *Escherichia coli* challenge infection. *American Journal of Veterinary Research, 45,* 2074–6.

Gross, W. B., & Colmano, G. (1969). Effect of social isolation on resistance to some infectious agents. *Poultry Science, 48,* 514–20.

Han, Y. C., & Pruett, S. B. (1995). Mechanisms of ethanol-induced suppression of a primary antibody response in a mouse model for binge drinking. *Journal of Pharmacology and Experimental Therapeutics, 275,* 950–7.

Havlickova, M., Pljusnin, A. Z., & Tumova, B. (1990). Influenza virus detection in clinical specimens. *Acta Virologica, 34,* 449–56.

Hawkins, N. G., Davies, R., & Holmes, T. H. (1955). Evidence for psychosocial specificity in pulmonary tuberculosis. *Transactions of the National Tuberculosis Association, 75,* 768–80.

Heath, R. G., Krupp, I. M., Byers, L. W., & Liljekvist, J. I. (1967). Schizophrenia as an immunologic disorder. II. Effects of serum protein fractions on brain function. *Archives of General Psychiatry, 16,* 10–23.

Heijnen, C. J., Kavelaars, A., & Ballieux, R. E. (1991a). Beta-endorphin: Cytokine and neuropeptide. *Immunological Reviews, 119,* 41–63.

Heijnen, C. J., Kavelaars, A., & Ballieux, R. E. (1991b). Corticotropin-releasing hormone and proopiomelanocortin-derived peptides in the modulation of immune function. In R. Ader, N. Cohen, & D. L. Felten (Eds.), *Psychoneuroimmunology,* pp. 429–46. New York: Academic Press.

Hermann, G., Beck, F. M., & Sheridan, J. F. (1995). Stress-induced glucocorticoid response modulates mononuclear cell trafficking during an experimental influenza viral infection. *Journal of Neuroimmunology, 56,* 179–86.

Hohlfeld, R., Meinl, E., Weber, F., Zipp, F., Schmidt, S., Sotgiu, S., Goebels, N., Voltz, R., Spuler, S., Iglesias, A., & Wekerle, H. (1995). The role of autoimmune T lymphocytes in the pathogenesis of multiple sclerosis. *Neurology, 45,* S33–S38.

Holmes, T. H., Hawkins, N. G., Bowerman, C. E., Clark, E. R., & Joffe, J. R. (1957). Psychosocial and physiological studies of tuberculosis. *Psychosomatic Medicine, 19,* 134–43.

Hubner, K. F., & Gengozian, N. (1969). Critical variables of the Jerne plaque technique as applied to rodent antibody-forming systems responding to heterologous red cell antigens. *Journal of Immunology, 102,* 155–67.

Hukkanen, V., Ruutiainen, J., Salmi, A., Reunanen, M., & Frey, H. (1983). Antibodies in cerebrospinal fluid to white matter glycoproteins in multiple sclerosis. *Neuroscience Letters, 35,* 327–32.

Husson, D., Abbal, M., Tafani, M., & Schmitt, D. A. (1996). Neuroendocrine system and immune responses after confinement. *Advances in Space Biology and Medicine, 5,* 93–113.

Irwin, M. (1993). Brain corticotropin-releasing hormone- and interleukin-1-beta-induced suppression of specific antibody production. *Endocrinology, 133,* 1352–60.

Ishigami, T. (1919). The influence of psychic acts on the progress of pulmonary tuberculosis. *American Review of Tuberculosis, 2,* 470–84.

Ishii, T., & Haga, S. (1975). Identification of components of immunoglobulins in senile plaques by means of fluorescent antibody technique. *Acta Neuropathologica (Berlin), 32,* 157–62.

Ishii, T., & Haga, S. (1976). Immuno-electron microscopic localization of immunoglobulins in amyloid fibrils of senile plaques. *Acta Neuropathologica (Berlin), 36,* 243–9.

Jabaaij, L., Grosheide, P. M., Heijtink, R. A., Duivenvoorden, H. J., Ballieux, R. E., & Vingerhoets, A. J. J. M. (1993). Influence of perceived psychological stress and distress on antibody response to low dose rDNA hepatitis B vaccine. *Journal of Psychosomatic Research, 37,* 361–9.

Jabaaij, L., Van Hattum, J., Vingerhoets, J. J., Oostveen, F. G., Duivenvoorden, H. J., & Ballieux, R. E. (1996). Modulation of immune response to rRNA hepatitis B vaccination by psychological stress. *Journal of Psychosomatic Research, 41,* 129–37.

Jans, H., Heltberg, A., Zeeberg, I., Kristensen, J. H., Fog, T., & Raun, N. E. (1984). Immune complexes and the complement factors C4 and C3 in cerebrospinal fluid and serum from patients with chronic progressive multiple sclerosis. *Acta Neurologica Scandinavica, 69,* 34–8.

Jemmott, J. B., Borysenko, M., Chapman, R., Borysenko, J. Z., McClelland, D. C., Meyer, D., & Benson, H. (1983). Academic stress, power motivation, and decrease in secretion rate of salivary secretory immunoglobulin A. *Lancet, 1,* 1400–2.

Jerne, N. K., Henry, C., Nordin, A. A., Fuji, H., Koros, A. M. C., & Lefkovits, I. (1974). Plaque forming cells. Methodology and theory. *Transplantation Reviews, 18,* 130–91.

Johnson, H. M., Smith, E. M., Torres, B. A., & Blalock, J. E. (1982). Regulation of the in vitro antibody response by neuroendocrine hormones. *Proceedings of the National Academy of Sciences U.S.A., 79,* 4171–4.

Johnsson, T., Lavender, J. F., Hultin, E., & Rasmussen, A. F. (1963). The influence of avoidance-learning stress on resistance of mice to Coxsackie B virus in mice. *Journal of Immunology, 91,* 569–75.

Kaliss, N. (1971). Jerne plaque assay for antibody-forming spleen cells: Some technical modifications. *Transplantation, 12,* 146–7.

Kasarskis, E. J., Karpiak, S. E., Rapport, M. M., Yu, R. K., & Bass, N. H. (1981). Abnormal maturation of cerebral cortex and behavioral deficit in adult rats after neonatal administration of antibodies to ganglioside. *Developmental Brain Research, 1,* 25–35.

Kasl, S. V., Evans, A. S., & Niederman, J. C. (1979). Psychosocial risk factors in the development of infectious mononucleosis. *Psychosomatic Medicine, 41,* 445–66.

Keshavan, M. S., Pettegrew, J. W., Panchalingam, K., Kaplan, D., Brar, J., & Campbell, K. (1989). In vivo 31P nuclear magnetic resonance (NMR) spectroscopy of the frontal lobe metabolism in neuroleptic-naive first episode psychoses: Preliminary studies. *Schizophrenia Research, 2,* 122.

Kiecolt-Glaser, J. K., Dura, J. R., Speicher, C. E., Trask, O. J., & Glaser, R. (1991). Spousal caregivers of dementia victims: Longitudinal changes in immunity and health. *Psychosomatic Medicine, 53,* 345–62.

Kiecolt-Glaser, J. K., Fisher, L. D., Ogrocki, P., Stout, J. C., Speicher, C. E., & Glaser, R. (1987a). Marital quality, marital disruption, and immune function. *Psychosomatic Medicine, 49,* 13–34.

Kiecolt-Glaser, J. K., & Glaser, R. (1992). Psychoneuroimmunology: Can psychological interventions modulate immunity? *Journal of Consulting and Clinical Psychology, 60,* 569–75.

Kiecolt-Glaser, J. K., & Glaser, R. (1995). Psychoneuroimmunology and health consequences: Data and shared mechanisms. *Psychosomatic Medicine, 57,* 269–74.

Kiecolt-Glaser, J. K., Glaser, R., Gravenstein, S., Malarkey, W. B., & Sheridan, J. (1996). Chronic stress alters the immune response to influenza virus vaccine in older adults. *Proceedings of the National Academy of Sciences U.S.A., 93,* 3043–7.

Kiecolt-Glaser, J. K., Glaser, R., Shuttleworth, E. C., Dyer, C. S., Ogrocki, P., & Speicher, C. E. (1987b). Chronic stress and immunity in family caregivers of Alzheimer's disease victims. *Psychosomatic Medicine, 49,* 523–35.

Kiecolt-Glaser, J. K., Glaser, R., Strain, E., Stout, J., Tarr, K., Holliday, I., & Speicher, C. E. (1986). Modulation of cellular immunity in medical students. *Journal of Behavioral Medicine, 9,* 5–21.

Kiecolt-Glaser, J. K., Kennedy, S., Malkoff, S., Fisher, L., Speicher, C. E., & Glaser, R. (1988). Marital discord and immunity in males. *Psychosomatic Medicine, 50,* 213–29.

Kiecolt-Glaser, J. K., Malarkey, W. B., Chee, M. A., Newton, T., Cacioppo, J. T., Mao, H.-Y., & Glaser, R. (1993). Negative behavior during marital conflict is associated with immunological down-regulation. *Psychosomatic Medicine, 55,* 395–409.

Knapp, P. H., Levy, E. M., Giorgi, R. G., Black, P. H., Fox, B. H., & Heeren, T. C. (1992). Short-term immunological effects of induced emotion. *Psychosomatic Medicine, 54,* 133–48.

Knight, J. G. (1982). Dopamine receptor stimulating autoantibody: A possible cause of schizophrenia. *Lancet, 2,* 1073–5.

Knight, J., Knight, A., & Ungvari, G. (1992). Can autoimmune mechanisms account for the genetic predisposition to schizophrenia? *British Journal of Psychiatry, 160,* 533–40.

Komori, T., Fujiwara, R., Tanida, M., Nomura, J., & Yokoyama, M. M. (1995). Effects of citrus fragrance on immune function and depressive states. *Neuroimmunomodulation, 2,* 174–80.

Kravchenco, I. V., & Furalev, V. A. (1994). Secretion of immunoreactive corticotropin releasing factor and adrenocorticotrophic hormone by T and B lymphocytes in response to cellular stress factors. *Biochemical and Biophysical Research Communications, 204,* 828–34.

Kruszewska, B., Felten, S. Y., & Moynihan, J. A. (1995). Alterations in cytokine and antibody production following chemical sympathectomy in two strains of mice. *Journal of Immunology, 155,* 4613–20.

Kusnecov, A. V., Grota, L. J., Schmidt, S. G., Bonneau, R. H., Sheridan, J. F., Glaser, R., & Moynihan, J. A. (1992). Decreased herpes simplex viral immunity and enhanced pathogenesis following stressor administration in mice. *Journal of Neuroimmunology, 38,* 129–37.

Kusnecov, A. W., Husband, A. J., & King, M. G. (1988). Behaviorally conditioned suppression of mitogen-induced proliferation and immunoglobulin production: Effect of time span between conditioning and reexposure to the conditioning stimulus. *Brain, Behavior, and Immunity, 2,* 198–211.

Labott, S. M., Ahleman, S., Wolever, M. E., & Martin, R. B. (1990). The physiological and psychological effects of the expression and inhibition of emotion. *Behavioral Medicine, 16,* 182–9.

LaPerriere, A., Antoni, M. H., Ironson, G., Perry, A., McCabe, P., Klimas, N., Helder, L., Schneiderman, N., & Fletcher, M. A. (1994a). Effects of aerobic exercise training on lymphocyte subpopulations. *International Journal of Sports Medicine, 15,* S127–S130.

LaPerriere, A., Fletcher, M. A., Antoni, M. H., Klimas, N. G., Ironson, G., & Schneiderman, N. (1991). Aerobic exercise training in an AIDS risk group. *International Journal of Sports Medicine, 12,* S53–S57.

LaPerriere, A., Ironson, G., Antoni, M. H., Schneiderman, N., Klimas, N., & Fletcher, M. A. (1994b). Exercise and psychoneuroimmunology. *Medicine & Science in Sports & Exercise, 26,* 182–90.

Laudenslager, M. L., Rasmussen, K. L., Berman, C. M., Suomi, S. J., & Berger, C. B. (1993). Specific antibody levels in free-ranging rhesus monkeys: Relationships to plasma hormones, cardian parameters, and early behavior. *Developmental Psychobiology, 26,* 407–20.

Lemieux, R., Verrette, S., Broly, H., & Perron, S. (1993). Direct agglutination of weak D red cells by tetramolecular complexes containing monoclonal IgG anti-D. *Vox Sanguinis, 65,* 141–5.

Lenert, P., Lenert, G., & Zanetti, M. (1995). Human recombinant CD4 and CD4-derived synthetic peptides agglutinate immunoglobulin-coated latex particles. Evidence that residues 25–28 and 35–38 of human CD4 form two separate immunoglobulin binding sites. *Molecular Immunology, 32,* 1399–1404.

Leu, S. J., & Singh, V. K. (1993). Suppression of in vitro antibody production by corticotropin-releasing factor neurohormone. *Journal of Neuroimmunology, 45,* 23–9.

Levinson, S. O., Milzer, A., & Lewin, P. (1945). Effect of fatigue, chilling and mechanical trauma on resistance to experimental poliomyelitis. *American Journal of Hygeine, 42,* 204–13.

Li, C. K. (1985). ELISA-based determination of immunological binding constants. *Molecular Immunology, 22,* 321–7.

Lingrel, J. B., Townes, T. M., Shapiro, S. G., Wernke, S. M., Liberator, P. A., & Menon, A. G. (1985). Structural organization of the alpha and beta globin loci of the goat. *Progress in Clinical and Biological Research, 191,* 67–79.

Livnat, S., Felten, S. Y., Carlson, S. L., Bellinger, D. L., & Felten, D. L. (1985). Involvement of peripheral and central catecholamine systems in neural-immune interactions. *Journal of Neuroimmunology, 10,* 5–30.

Lorton, D., Hewitt, D., Bellinger, D. L., Felten, S. Y., & Felten, D. L. (1990). Noradrenergic reinnervation of the rat spleen following chemical sympathectomy with 6-hydroxydopamine: Pattern and time course of reinnervation. *Brain, Behavior, and Immunity, 4,* 198–222.

Macy, E., Kemeny, M., & Saxon, A. (1988). Enhanced ELISA: How to measure less than 10 picograms of a specific protein (immunogobulin) in less than 8 hours. *FASEB Journal, 2,* 3003–9.

Madden, J. J., Donahoe, R. M., Zwemer-Collins, J., Shafer, D. A., & Falek, A. (1987). Binding of naloxone to human T lymphocytes. *Biochemical Pharmacology, 36,* 4103–9.

Madden, K. S., Sanders, V. M., & Felten, D. L. (1995). Catecholamine influences and sympathetic neural modulation of

immune responsiveness. *Annual Review of Pharmacology and Toxicology, 35,* 417–48.

Maes, M., Bosmans, E., Suy, E., Minner, B., & Raus, J. (1989). Impaired lymphocyte stimulation by mitogens in severely depressed patients. A complex interface with HPA-axis hyperfunction, noradrenergic activity, and the aging process. *British Journal of Psychiatry, 155,* 793–8.

Maes, M., Lambrechts, J., Bosmans, E., Jacobs, J., Suy, E., Vandervorst, C., DeJonckheere, C., Minner, B., & Raus, J. (1992a). Evidence for a systemic immune activation during depression: Results of leukocyte enumeration by flow cytometry in conjunction with monoclonal antibody staining. *Psychological Medicine, 22,* 45–53.

Maes, M., Meltzer, H., Jacobs, J., Suy, E., Calabrese, J., Minner, B., & Raus, J. (1993). Autoimmunity in depression: Increased antiphospholipid autoantibodies. *Acta Psychiatrica Scandinavica, 87,* 160–6.

Maes, M., Scharpe, S., Meltzer, H. Y., Okayli, G., Bosmans, E., D'Hondt, P., Vanden Bossche, B., & Cosyns, P. (1994). Increased neopterin and interferon-gamma secretion and lower availability of L-tryptophan in major depression: Further evidence for an immune response. *Psychiatry Research, 54,* 143–60.

Maes, M., Stevens, W., DeClerck, L., Bridts, C., Peeters, D., Schotte, C., & Cosyns, P. (1992b). Immune disorders in depression: Higher T helper/T suppressor-cytotoxic cell ratio. *Acta Psychiatrica Scandinavica, 86,* 423–31.

Malarkey, W. B., Pearl, D. K., Demers, L. M., Kiecolt-Glaser, J. K., & Glaser, R. (1995). Influence of academic stress and season on 24-hour mean concentrations of ACTH, cortisol, and beta-endorphin. *Psychoneuroendocrinology, 20,* 499–508.

Martin, J., Prystowsky, M. B., & Angeletti, R. H. (1987). Preproenkephalin mRNA in T cells, macrophages, and mast cells. *Journal Neuroscience Research, 18,* 82–7.

McGeer, P. L., Akiyama, H., Itagaki, S., & McGeer, E. G. (1989). Immune system response in Alzheimer's disease. *Canadian Journal of Neurological Science, 16,* 516–27.

McGeer, P. L., & McGeer, E. G. (1996). Anti-inflammatory drugs in the fight against Alzheimer's disease. *Annals of the New York Academy of Sciences, 777,* 213–20.

McGillis, J. P., Park, A., Rubin-Fletter, P., Turck, C., Dallman, M. F., & Payan, D. G. (1989). Stimulation of rat B-lymphocyte proliferation by corticotropin-releasing factor. *Journal Neuroscience Research, 23,* 346–52.

McLean, R. G. (1982). Potentiation of Keystone virus infection in cotton rats by glucocorticoid-induced stress. *Journal of Wildlife Diseases, 18,* 141–8.

McNaughton, M. E., Smith, L. W., Patterson, T. L., & Grant, I. (1990). Stress, social support, coping resources, and immune status in elderly women. *Journal of Nervous and Mental Disorders, 178,* 460–1.

Mcrae-Degueurce, A., Booj, S., Haglid, K., Rosengren, L., Karlsson, J. E., Karlsson, I., Wallin, A., Svennerholm, L., Gottfries, C. G., & Dahlstrom, A. (1987). Antibodies in cerebrospinal fluid of some Alzheimer disease patients recognize cholinergic neurons in the rat central nervous system. *Proceedings of the National Academy of Sciences U.S.A., 84,* 9214–18.

Merrill, J. E., Graves, M. C., & Mulder, D. G. (1992). Autoimmune disease and the nervous system: Biochemical, molecular, and clinical update. *Western Journal of Medicine, 156,* 639–46.

Miles, K., Quintans, J., Chelmicka-Schorr, E., & Arnason, B. G. W. (1981). The sympathetic nervous system modulates antibody response to thymus-independent antigens. *Journal of Neuroimmunology, 1,* 101–5.

Miyoshi, I., Yoshimoto, S., Kubonishi, I., Fujishita, M., Ohtsuki, Y., Yamashita, M., Yamato, K., Hirose, S., Taguchi, H., Niiya, K., et al. (1985). Infectious transmission of human T-cell leukemia virus to rabbits. *International Journal of Cancer, 35,* 81–5.

Monstein, H.-J., Folkesson, R., & Terenius, L. (1986). Proenkephalin A-like mRNA in human leukemia leukocytes and CNS-tissues. *Life Sciences, 39,* 2237–41.

Morgan, W. P. (1985). Affective benefits of vigorous physical activity. *Medicine & Science in Sports & Exercise, 17,* 94–100.

Mulder, C. L., Antoni, M. H., Duivenvoorden, H. J., Kauffmann, R. H., & Goodkin, K. (1995). Active confrontational coping predicts decreased clinical progression over a one-year period in HIV-infected homosexual men. *Journal of Psychosomatic Research, 39,* 957–65.

Murakami, T., Haruki, K., Seto, Y., Kimura, T., Minoshiro, S., & Shibe, K. (1991). Agglutination of human O erythrocytes by influenza A (H1N1) viruses freshly isolated from patients. *Journal of Virological Methods, 32,* 49–56.

Nehlsen-Cannarella, S. L., Nieman, D. C., Balk-Lamberton, A. J., Markoff, P. A., Chritton, D. B., Gusewitch, G., & Lee, J. W. (1991a). The effects of moderate exercise training on immune response. *Medicine & Science in Sports & Exercise, 23,* 64–70.

Nehlsen-Cannarella, S. L., Nieman, D. C., Jessen, J., Chang, L., Gusewitch, G., Blix, G. G., & Ashley, E. (1991b). The effects of acute moderate exercise on lymphocyte function and serum immunoglobulin levels. *International Journal of Sports Medicine, 12,* 391–8.

Nieman, D. C. (1991). The effects of acute and chronic exercise on immunoglobulins. *Sports Medicine, 11,* 183–201.

Nilsson, L. A. (1967). Quantitative determination of serum proteins by Oudin, Mancini and Ouchterlony techniques. *Scandinavian Journal of Clinical Laboratory Investigations, 100,* 10–11.

Noronha, A. B., Antel, J. P., Roos, R. P., & Medof, M. E. (1981). Circulating immune complexes in neurologic disease. *Neurology, 31,* 1402–7.

Ouchterlony, O., & Nilsson, L. A. (1986). *Immunodiffusion and Immunoelectrophoresis* (Handbook of Experimental Immunology, vol. 1). Oxford, U.K.: Blackwell.

Panitch, H. S., Hooper, C. S., & Johnson, K. P. (1980). CSF antibody to myelin basic protein: Measurement in patients with multiple sclerosis and subacute sclerosing panencephalitis. *Archives of Neurology, 37,* 206–9.

Parish, C. R., & Liew, F. Y. (1972). Immune response to chemically modified flagellin. *Journal of Experimental Medicine, 135,* 298–311.

Parker, D. C. (1993). T cell-dependent B cell activation. *Annual Review of Immunology, 11,* 331–60.

Pennebaker, J. W., & Beall, S. (1986). Confronting a traumatic event: Toward an understanding of inhibition and disease. *Journal of Abnormal Psychology, 95,* 274–81.

Pennebaker, J. W., Colder, M., & Sharp, L. K. (1990). Accelerating the coping proccess. *Journal of Personality and Social Psychology, 58,* 528–37.

Pennebaker, J. W., Kiecolt-Glaser, J. K., & Glaser, R. (1988). Disclosure of trauma and immune function: Health implications for psychotherapy. *Journal of Consulting and Clinical Psychology, 56,* 239–45.

Peters, C. J., & Theofilopoulos, A. N. (1977). Antibody-dependent cellular cytotoxicity against murine leukemia viral antigens: Studies with human lymphoblastoid cell lines and human peripheral lymphocytes as effector cells comparing rabbit, goat, and mouse antisera. *Journal of Immunology, 119,* 1089–96.

Petrie, K. J., Booth, R. J., Pennebaker, J. W., Davison, K. P., & Thomas, M. G. (1995). Disclosure of trauma and immune response to a hepatitis B vaccination program. *Journal of Consulting and Clinical Psychology, 63,* 787–92.

Petry, L. J., Weems, L. B., & Livingstone, J. N. (1991). Relationship of stress, distress, and the immunologic response to a recombinant hepatitis B vaccine. *The Journal of Family Practice, 32,* 481–6.

Picardo, N. G., & Guisantes, J. A. (1981). Comparison of three immunological tests for seroepidemiological purposes in human echinococcosis. *Parasite Immunology, 3,* 191–9.

Potter, W. Z. (1984). Psychotherapeutic drugs and biogenic amines: Current concepts and therapeutic implications. *Drugs, 28,* 127–43.

Powers, J. M., Schlaepfer, W. W., Willingham, M. C., & Hall, B. J. (1981). An immunoperoxidase study of senile cerebral amyloidosis with pathogenic considerations. *Journal of Neuropathology and Experimental Neurology, 40,* 592–612.

Previte, J. J., & Berry, L. J. (1962). The effect of environmental temperature on the host–parasite relationship in mice. *Journal of Infectious Diseases, 110,* 201–9.

Raglin, J. (1990). Exercise and mental health: Beneficial and detrimental effects. *Sports Medicine, 9,* 323–9.

Ramer-Quinn, D. S., Baker, R. A., & Sanders, V. M. (1997). Activated Th1 and Th2 cells differentially express the beta-2-adrenergic receptor: A mechanism for selective modulation of Th1 cell cytokine production. *Journal of Immunology, 159,* 4857–67.

Rassnick, S., Sved, A. F., & Rabin, B. S. (1994). Locus coeruleus stimulation by corticotropin-releasing hormone suppresses in vitro cellular immune responses. *Journal of Neuroscience, 14,* 6033–40.

Reilly, F. D., McCuskey, P. A., & Meineke, H. A. (1976). Studies of the hematopoietic microenvironment. VIII. Adrenergic and cholinergic innervation of the murine spleen. *The Anatomical Record, 185,* 109–18.

Reinherz, E. L., Weiner, H. L., Hauser, S. L., Cohen, J. A., Distaso, J. A., & Schlossman, S. F. (1980). Loss of suppressor T cells in active multiple sclerosis: Analysis with monoclonal antibodies. *New England Journal of Medicine, 303,* 125–9.

Reyes, M. P., & Lerner, A. M. (1976). Interferon and neutralizing antibody in sera of exercised mice with Coxsackievirus B-3 myocarditis. *Proceedings of the Society for Experimental Biology and Medicine, 151,* 333–8.

Riegele, L. (1929). Uber die mikroskopische Innervation der Milz. *Z. Zellforsch. Mikrosk. Anat., 9,* 511–33.

Rigsby, L., Dishman, R. K., Jackson, A. W., Maclean, G. S., & Raven, P. B. (1992). Effects of exercise training on men seropositive for the human immunodeficiency virus-1. *Medicine & Science in Sports & Exercise, 24,* 6–12.

Rogers, M. P., Reich, P., Strom, T. B., & Carpenter, C. B. (1976). Behaviorally conditioned immunosuppression: Replication of a recent study. *Psychosomatic Medicine, 38,* 447–51.

Rosen, H., Behar, O., Abramsky, O., & Ovadia, H. (1989). Regulated expression of proenkephalin A in normal lymphocytes. *Journal of Immunology, 143,* 3703–7.

Rudorfer, M. V., Ross, R. J., Linnoila, M., Sherer, M. A., & Potter, W. Z. (1985). Exaggerated orthostatic responsivity of plasma norepinephrine in depression. *Archives of General Psychiatry, 42,* 1186–92.

Ryberg, B. (1982). Anti-brain antibodies in multiple sclerosis: Relation to clinical variables. *Journal of Neurological Science, 54,* 239–61.

Sachar, E. J. (1982). Endocrine abnormalities in depression. In E. S. Paykel (Ed.), *Handbook of Affective Disorders,* pp. 191–201. New York: Guilford.

Sanders, V. M. (1995). The role of adrenoceptor-mediated signals in the modulation of lymphocyte function. *Advances in Neuroimmunology, 5,* 283–98.

Sanders, V. M., Baker, R. A., Ramer-Quinn, D. S., Kasprowicz, D. J., Fuchs, B. A., & Street, N. E. (1997). Differential expression of the beta-2-adrenergic receptor by Th1 and Th2 clones: Implications for cytokine production and B cell help. *Journal of Immunology, 158,* 4200–10.

Schiffman, G., Douglas, R. M., Bonner, M. J., Robbins, M., & Austrian, R. (1980). A radioimmunoassay for immunologic phenomena in pneumococcal disease and for the antibody response to pneumococcal vaccines. *Journal of Immunological Methods, 33,* 133–44.

Schleifer, S. J., Keller, S. E., Bartlett, J. A., Eckholdt, H. M., & Delaney, B. R. (1996). Immunity in young adults with major depressive disorder. *American Journal of Psychiatry, 153,* 477–82.

Schleifer, S. J., Keller, S. E., Bond, R. N., Cohen, J., & Stein, M. (1989). Major depressive disorder and immunity: Role of age, sex, severity and hospitalization. *Archives of General Psychiatry, 46,* 81–7.

Schleifer, S. J., Keller, S. E., Camerino, M., Thornton, J. C., & Stein, M. (1983). Suppression of lymphocyte stimulation following bereavement. *Journal of the American Medical Association, 250,* 374–7.

Schleifer, S. J., Keller, S. E., Meyerson, A. T., Raskin, M. J., Davis, K. L., & Stein, M. (1984). Lymphocyte function in major depressive disorder. *Archives of General Psychiatry, 41,* 484–6.

Schleifer, S. J., Keller, S. E., Siris, S. G., Davis, K. L., & Stein, M. (1985). Depression and immunity: Lymphocyte function in ambulatory depressed patients, hospitalized schizophrenic patients, and patients hospitalized for herniorrhaphy. *Archives of General Psychiatry, 42,* 129–33.

Schlenzig, C., Jager, H., & Rieder, H. (1989). Supervised physical exercise leads to psychological and immunological improvement in pre-AIDS patients [Abstract]. *Proceedings of the 5th International AIDS Conference,* p. 337. Ottawa: International Development Research Centre.

Schmitt, D. A., Peres, C., Sonnenfeld, G., Tkackzuk, J., Arquier, M., Mauco, G., & Ohayon, E. (1995). Immune responses in humans after 60 days of confinement. *Brain, Behavior, and Immunity, 9,* 70–7.

Schubert, J. H., & Cornell, R. G. (1958). Determination of diptheria and tetanus antitoxin by the hemagglutination test in comparison with test in vivo. *Journal of Laboratory and Clinical Medicine, 52,* 737–43.

Sedgwick, J. D., & Holt, P. G. (1983). A solid-phase immunoenzymatic technique for the enumeration of specific antibody-secreting cells. *Journal of Immunological Methods, 57,* 301–9.

Selye, H. (1936). A syndrome produced by diverse noxious agents. *Nature, 138,* 132.

Selye, H. (1946). The general adaptor syndrome and the diseases of adaptation. *Journal of Clinical Endocrinology, 6,* 117–230.

Sheridan, J. F., Dobbs, C., Brown, D., & Zwilling, B. (1994). Psychoneuroimmunology: Stress effects on pathogenesis and immunity during infection. *Clinical Microbiology Reviews, 7,* 200–12.

Sheridan, J. F., Feng, N., Bonneau, R. H., Allen, C. M., Huneycutt, B. S., & Glaser, R. (1991). Restraint stress differentially affects anti-viral cellular and humoral immune responses in mice. *Journal of Neuroimmunology, 31,* 245–55.

Sherwood, B. F., Rowland, D. T., Hackel, D. B., & LeMay, J. C. (1968). Bacterial endocarditis, glomerulonephritis, and amyloidosis in the opossum (*Didelphis virginiana*). *American Journal Pathology, 53,* 115–26.

Shimizu, M., Shimizu, Y., & Kodama, Y. (1978). Effects of ambient temperature on induction of transmissible gastroenteritis in feeder pigs. *Infection and Immunity, 21,* 747–52.

Shimizu, N., Hori, T., & Nakane, H. (1994). An interleukin-1-beta-induced noradrenaline release in the spleen is mediated by brain corticotropin-releasing factor: An in vivo microdialysis study in conscious rats. *Brain, Behavior, and Immunity, 7,* 14–23.

Silagi, S., & Schaefer, A. E. (1986). Successful immunotherapy of mouse melanoma and sarcoma with recombinant interleukin-2 and cyclophosphamide. *Journal of Biological Response Modifiers, 5,* 411–22.

Singh, V. K. (1989). Stimulatory effect of corticotropin-releasing factor neurohormone on human lymphocyte proliferation and interleukin-2 receptor expression. *Journal of Neuroimmunology, 23,* 257–62.

Singh, V. K., & Leu, S.-J. C. (1990). Enhancing effect of corticotropin-releasing neurohormone on the production of interleukin-1 and interleukin-2. *Neuroscience Letters, 120,* 151–4.

Smith, E. M., Morrill, A. C., Meyer, W. J. III, & Blalock, J. E. (1986). Corticotropin releasing factor induction of leukocyte-derived immunoreactive ACTH and endorphins. *Nature, 321,* 881–2.

Snyder, B. K., Roghmann, K. J., & Sigal, L. H. (1990). Effect of stress and other biopsychosocial factors on primary antibody response. *Journal of Adolescent Health Care, 11,* 472–9.

Solomon, G. F., & Moos, R. H. (1964). Emotions, immunity, and disease: A speculative theoretical integration. *Archives of General Psychiatry, 11,* 657–74.

Solomon, G. F., & Moos, R. H. (1965). The relationship of personality to the presence of rheumatoid factor in asymptomatic relatives of patients with rheumatoid arthritis. *Psychiatric Medicine, 27,* 350–60.

Spiehler, V. R., Reed, D., Cravey, R. H., Wilcox, W. P., Shaw, R. F., & Holland, S. (1975). Comparison of results for quantitative determination of morphine by radioimmunoassay, enzyme immunoassay, and spectrofluorometry. *Journal of Forensic Sciences, 20,* 647–55.

Stanislav, V. K., Evans, A. S., & Niederman, J. C. (1979). Psychological risk factors on the development of infectious mononucleosis. *Psychosomatic Medicine, 41,* 445–66.

Stein, M., Miller, A. H., & Trestman, R. L. (1991). Depression, the immune system, and health and illness. *Archives of General Psychiatry, 48,* 171–7.

Steinman, C. R. (1982). Quantitation of submicrogram quantities of DNA by rocket electrophoresis. *Methods in Enzymology, 84,* 181–7.

Stone, A. A., Bovbjerg, D. H., Neale, J. M., Napoli, A., Valdimarsdottir, H., Cox, D., Hayden, F. G., & Gwaltney, J. M. (1992). Development of common cold symptoms following experimental rhinovirus infection is related to prior stressful life events. *Behavioral Medicine, 18,* 115–20.

Stone, A. A., Cox, D. S., Valdimarsdottir, H., Jandorf, L., & Neale, J. M. (1987a). Evidence that secretory IgA antibody is associated with daily mood. *Journal of Personality and Social Psychology, 52,* 988–93.

Stone, A. A., Cox, D. S., Valdimarsdottir, H., & Neale, J. M. (1987b). Secretory IgA as a measure of immunocompetence. *Journal of Human Stress, 13,* 136–40.

Stone, A. A., Neale, J. M., Cox, D. S., Napoli, A., Valdimarsdottir, H., & Kennedy-Moore, E. (1994). Daily events are associated with a secretory immune response to an oral antigen in men. *Health Psychology, 13,* 440–6.

Talmadge, J. E. (1985). Immunoregulation and immunostimulation of murine lymphocytes by recombinant human interleukin-2. *Journal of Biological Response Modifiers, 4,* 18–34.

Tanaka, Y., Tsukada, N., Koh, C. S., & Yanagisawa, N. (1987). Anti-endothelial cell antibodies and circulating immune complexes in the sera of patients with multiple sclerosis. *Journal of Neuroimmunology, 17,* 49–59.

Taub, D. D., Eisenstein, T. K., Geller, E. B., Adler, M. W., & Rogers, T. J. (1991). Immunomodulatory activity of mu- and kappa-selective opioid agonists. *Proceedings of the National Academy of Sciences U.S.A., 88,* 360–4.

Theorell, T., Blomkvist, V., Jonsson, H., Schulman, S., Berntorp, E., & Stigendal, L. (1995). Social support and the development of immune function in human immunodeficiency virus infection. *Psychosomatic Medicine, 57,* 32–6.

Tobach, E., & Bloch, H. (1956). Effect of stress by crowding prior to and following tuberculosis infection. *American Journal of Physiology, 187,* 399–402.

Vitetta, E. S., Fernandez-Botran, R., Myers, C. D., & Sanders, V. M. (1989). Cellular interactions in the humoral immune response. *Advances in Immunology, 45,* 1–105.

Wajgt, A., & Gorney, M. (1983). CSF antibodies to myelin basic protein and to myelin associated glycoprotein in multiple sclerosis: Evidence of the intrathecal production of antibodies. *Acta Neurologica Scandinavica, 68,* 337–43.

Wallgren, P., Wilen, I. L., & Fossum, C. (1994). Influence of experimentally induced endogenous production of cortisol on the immune capacity in swine. *Veterinary Immunology and Immunopathology, 42,* 301–16.

Warren, K. G., & Catz, I. (1987). A correlation between cerebrospinal fluid myelin basic protein and anti-myelin basic protein in multiple sclerosis patients. *Annals of Neurology, 21,* 183–9.

Wayner, E. A., Flannery, G. R., & Singer, G. (1978). Effects of taste aversion conditioning on the primary antibody response to sheep red blood cells and *Brucella abortus* in the albino rat. *Physiological Behavior, 21,* 995–1000.

Webster, E. L., Tracey, D. E., Jutila, M. A., Wolfe, S. A. J., & DeSouza, E. B. (1990). Corticotropin-releasing factor receptors in mouse spleen: Identification of receptor-bearing cells as resident macrophages. *Endocrinology, 127,* 440–52.

Weiss, J. M., Sundar, S. K., Becker, K. J., & Cierpial, M. A. (1989). Behavioral and neural influences on cellular immune responses: Effects of stress and interleukin-1. *Journal of Clinical Psychiatry, 50,* 43–53.

Weisse, C. S., Pato, C. N., McAllister, C. G., Littman, R., Breier, A., Paul, S. M., & Baum, A. (1990). Differential effects of controllable and uncontrollable acute stress on lymphocyte proliferation and leukocyte percentages in humans. *Brain, Behavior, and Immunity, 4,* 339–51.

Wilcok, G. K., Esiri, M. M., Bowen, D. M., & Smith, C. C. (1982). Alzheimer's disease: Correlation of cortical choline acetyl transferase activity with the severity of dementia and histological abnormalities. *Journal of Neurological Science, 57,* 407–17.

Williams, J. M., & Felten, D. L. (1981). Sympathetic innervation of murine thymus and spleen: A comparative histofluorescence study. *Anatomical Record, 199,* 531–42.

Williams, J. M., Peterson, R. G., Shea, P. A., Schmedtje, J. F., Bauer, D. C., & Felten, D. L. (1981). Sympathetic innervation of murine thymus and spleen: Evidence for a functional link between the nervous and immune systems. *Brain Research Bulletin, 6,* 83–94.

Yamada, A., Jensen, M. M., & Rasmussen, A. F. (1964). Stress and susceptibility to viral infections. III. Antibody response and viral retention during avoidance learning stress. *Proceedings of the Society for Experimental Biology & Medicine, 116,* 677–80.

Yarchoan, R., Murphy, B. R., Strober, W., Schneider, H. S., & Nelson, D. L. (1981). Specific anti-influenza virus antibody production in vitro by human peripheral blood mononuclear cells. *Journal of Immunology, 127,* 2588–93.

Zis, A. P., & Goodwin, F. K. (1982). The amine hypothesis. In E. S. Paykel (Ed.) *Handbook of Affective Disorders,* pp. 175–90. New York: Guilford.

Zisook, S., Shuchter, S. R., Irwin, M., Darko, D. F., Sledge, P., & Resovsky, K. (1994). Bereavement, depression, and immune function. *Psychiatry Research, 52,* 1–10.

Zurawski, G., Benedik, M., Kamb, B. J., Abrams, J. S., Zurawski, S. M., & Lee, F. D. (1986). Activation of mouse T-helper cells induces abundant preproenkephalin mRNA synthesis. *Science, 232,* 772–5.

PART THREE

PROCESSES

CHAPTER SEVENTEEN

FROM HOMEOSTASIS TO ALLODYNAMIC REGULATION

GARY G. BERNTSON & JOHN T. CACIOPPO

Introduction

Since the seminal work of Walter Cannon, the concept of homeostasis has been a major force in the historical development of views of autonomic regulation and control. The homeostatic construct also importantly shaped many twentieth-century psychological concepts and theories, including models of reinforcement, motivation, perception, personality, and psychosomatic disorders (Cofer & Appley 1964). The homeostatic construct has been particularly salient in psychophysiology and behavioral medicine because of the putative role of homeostatic processes in the regulation of autonomic and neuroendocrine systems. The present chapter will explore the current status of the homeostatic model as well as the emergence of modern concepts of allostasis and allodynamic regulation.

A second aim of the chapter is to consider the underlying neural systems and mechanisms that give rise to autonomic regulation and hence psychophysiological relationships. A complication in drawing clear psychophysiological relations is that these associations cut across systems and processes that are represented at distinct levels of conceptualization and analysis. One goal of multilevel integrative analyses is to bring the concepts, processes, and terms of the two levels of analysis into registration and so permit a more accurate appreciation of the underlying links and organizations (Cacioppo & Berntson 1992a,b). For example, the construct of fear has a long heuristic tradition in psychology, but brain systems process information and not fear per se. The latter represents a constellation of outputs of brain processes. Rapprochement between psychological and physiological constructs and theories will likely require refinements in conceptualization and quantification within both the physiological and psychological domains. Although an integrative analysis across psychological and physiological levels is still very much a work in progress, psychophysiol-

ogy resides at a critical intersection to pursue this ultimate integration. In considering the psychophysiology of the autonomic nervous system, the present chapter will identify some aspects of a broad framework that may contribute to the emergence of a true neuropsychophysiology.

HOMEOSTASIS AND HOMEODYNAMIC REGULATION

Origins of the Homeostatic Concept

The notion of natural balancing or equilibrium-seeking tendencies may be traced back as early as Hippocrates (Cofer & Appley 1964). The term "homeostasis" and the contemporary negative feedback model of homeostatic regulation have a more recent history. Claude Bernard (1878/1974) reflected on the relative constancy of the internal environment (*milieu intérieur*) of living creatures. This constancy was seen to reflect an organism's ability to stabilize the cellular environment despite powerful entropic forces that threaten to disrupt the biological order essential for life. Mechanisms underlying this constancy permit warm-blooded creatures to live what Bernard termed a "free and independent life" (Bernard 1878/1974, p. 89). Cannon (1929, 1939) extended this perspective, coining the term *homeostasis* to refer to the processes by which the "constancy of the fluid matrix" is maintained. Cannon wrote as follows:

Ordinarily, the variations from the mean position do not reach the dangerous extremes which impair the functions of the cells or threaten the existence of the organism. Before those extremes are reached, agencies are automatically called into service which act to bring back toward the mean position the state which has been disturbed. (1939, p. 39)

This statement captures the important concepts of homeostatic regulation of visceral systems and adaptive

John T. Cacioppo, Louis G. Tassinary, and Gary G. Berntson (Eds.), *Handbook of Psychophysiology,* 2nd ed. © Cambridge University Press 2000. Printed in the United States of America. ISBN 62634X. All rights reserved.

regulation of dimensions (such as blood pressure) that serve to maintain the necessary internal states required for survival. The concept of homeostasis was so central to Cannon's view that he tended to equate adaptive and homeostatic adjustments, and he was prepared to discount autonomic responses that deviated from the homeostatic model. In so doing, however, Cannon implicitly recognized physiological deviations from homeostatic regulation:

[homeostatic] utility is not always complete in details, for at times effects are produced which apparently have little or no value for the organism.... The effects which ... are not useful may reasonably be regarded as incidental, as lying outside the group of sympathico-adrenal agencies which, for the moment, are working for homeostasis. (1939, pp. 298–9)

Cannon's concepts significantly shaped contemporary views of autonomic regulation and control. A related legacy from the Cannon era is that the sympathetic and parasympathetic branches are subject to reciprocal central control. Given a homeostatic perspective – and the fact that the autonomic branches generally exert opposing actions on end organs – the concept of reciprocal control of the autonomic branches was natural. A reciprocal pattern of autonomic control would maximize autonomic resources in the maintenance of a homeostatic set point. The concepts of homeostasis and reciprocal control figured prominently in the development of modern perspectives of autonomic function. These concepts were echoed in Fulton's influential textbook of physiology, which asserts that "The autonomic nerves ... are the regulators concerned with emergency mechanisms, with repair, and with preservation of the constancy of the internal environment" (Fulton 1949, p. 222) and that "In the reflex regulation of the heart rate, the sympathetic and parasympathetic nervous systems are reciprocally linked in their central representations" (p. 668).

Cannon's notions of homeostatic regulation and reciprocal autonomic control continue to be espoused in contemporary textbooks, such as the influential volume *Principles of Neural Science* (Kandel, Schwartz, & Jessell 1991). It is asserted that "sympathetic and parasympathetic pathways are tonically active and operate ... to maintain a steady internal environment in the face of changing external circumstances" (p. 762) and that "most target organs are controlled by coordinated and reciprocal sympathetic and parasympathetic innervation.... [T]he reciprocal control of ... organs by both autonomic divisions is coordinated and necessary for normal function" (p. 770). Among the prototypic homeostatic mechanisms are the baroreceptor reflexes, whereby perturbations in blood pressure initiate powerful reflexive adjustments in vascular tone and cardiac output that tend to oppose this perturbation (Spyer 1990).

The concept of homeostasis has also played an important role in psychophysiological theory. Homeostatic compensatory adjustments were viewed by Lacey as an important contributor to observed patterns of psychophysiological response:

the recorded autonomic response is a function both of the induced magnitude of autonomic activation (as it would be seen in the absence of contrary changes) and of the promptness and vigor of secondarily induced autonomic changes that serve to restrain and limit the effects of the initial disturbance.... Let us be bold about it. This corollary should be made part of the implicit background of every psychophysiological investigation; no conclusions should be drawn in such investigations without explicitly taking the corollary into account. (Lacey 1956, pp. 127–8)

For Lacey, it was this secondary homeostatic dampening that underlies (in part) the "law of initial values," by virtue of the limits or constraints that homeostatic adjustments impose on autonomic responses. Obrist (1981) saw homeostatic processes as contributing more directly to the primary psychophysiological response. In his construct of cardiac-somatic coupling, for example, Obrist (1981) viewed heart rate responses in behavioral contexts as reflecting, at least in part, homeostatic adjustments associated with increased metabolic demands.

Some Mechanisms of Homeostasis

A number of processes contribute to the relative constancy of internal states. These include peripheral processes such as buffering systems of the blood that oppose perturbations in plasma pH and the inherent elasticity of the vasculature that tends to minimize pressor variations due to changes in blood volume. These mechanisms are included in the general class of peripheral *autoregulatory* processes that contribute to stability in physiological dimensions (Guyton 1991; see also Dworkin 1993). An additional example is the role of the kidney in blood pressure regulation. Increases in blood volume and associated blood pressure promote increased renal glomerular filtration and diuresis, leading to a compensatory decrease in vascular volume (Guyton 1991). A wide variety of such peripheral physiological or hormonal mechanisms contribute to homeostatic regulation through autoregulatory processes that are independent of central reflexive control.

In addition to peripheral autoregulatory processes, Cannon emphasized the role of central reflexive mechanisms in the defense of the steady state. It is this set of mechanisms that has generally been of greatest interest in psychophysiology. An important aspect of the homeostatic model is that, by means of visceral feedback, reflexive networks achieve sensitivity to the functional state of a regulated dimension and then issue compensatory responses to restore detected imbalances. Like the thermostatic control of room temperature, homeostatic reflexes may operate as feedback controlled servomechanisms, continually adjusting autonomic outflow to compensate for perturbations in the regulated dimension. This is the classic "feedback control"

TABLE 1. Regulatory Parameters

1. Set Point

The set point is the functional status that is actively regulated, and physiologically defended, by compensatory responses to perturbations. In the absence of overriding perturbations, it can be indexed by the central tendency of the regulated dimension.

2. Operating Characteristics

(a) *Dynamic Range.* The dynamic range characterizes the limits of a compensatory process. It represents the regulatory capacity of the system and is generally expressed as the difference between the maximal and minimal asymptotes of the response (e.g., the maximal and minimal heart rates seen to perturbations of blood pressure associated with the baroreceptor–heart rate reflex).

(b) *Sensitivity (Threshold and Gain).* Sensitivity represents (i) the threshold of perturbation in the regulated dimension that is just capable of initiating compensatory responses and (ii) the magnitude or compensatory capacity of the initiated response. This is often represented as the slope of the response function (e.g., the compensatory change in heart rate to a unit change in blood pressure).

(c) *Linearity.* This refers to the shape of the activation (response) function across the dynamic range of control. Deviations from linearity represent variations in sensitivity along the response function for a given increment in the relevant stimulus (deviation from regulatory level). Response functions in physiological systems are often sigmoidal, but in many cases they may be approximated by a linear function within the typical operating ranges.

(d) *Temporal Dynamics.* Temporal (dynamic) aspects of the control system, including dimensions such as latency, time course, recovery time, frequency response, and phase lag.

(e) *Stability.* The stability of a process is its reliability or reproducibility, for a given set of conditions. Variations may be random (noise), or systematic (e.g., hysteresis resulting from baroreceptor adaptation, so that the heart rate for a given blood pressure may differ for an increasing pressor ramp than for a decreasing ramp).

---

model of homeostasis. There are additional complexities in regulating internal states, but before considering these we consider a typical feedback controlled homeostatic system.

A Typical Homeostatic Mechanism: The Baroreceptor–Heart Rate Reflex

As outlined in Table 1, typical feedback controlled homeostatic systems can be specified by a regulatory level or set point that represents the central tendency of the regulatory system. It is a deviation from this regulated level that constitutes the critical feedback control signal and activates the compensatory response. In addition to the regulatory level, a number of operating characteristics serve to define the features, capabilities, and dynamics of the compensatory processes (see Cacioppo et al. 1992b).

These features and operating characteristics are illustrated in panel A of Figure 1, which depicts the homeostatic baroreceptor–cardiac reflex. As depicted in the figure, an increase in blood pressure (and associated increases in baroreceptor activity) triggers an increase in heart period (decrease in heart rate). This is attributable to a reflexive withdrawal of cardiac sympathetic tone and a reciprocal increase in vagal control of the heart, which (in the aggregate) decrease heart rate and cardiac output. This, together with the withdrawal of sympathetic tone to the vasculature, tends to oppose the pressor perturbation. Homeostatic regulation is rarely perfect, however – a fact well recognized by Cannon. The dynamic range of baroreceptor reflexes limits the ultimate capacity of homeostatic processes to compensate for large perturbations in blood pressure. Moreover, the sensitivity of the

baroreceptor–heart rate reflex (slope of the blood pressure/ heart rate relationship) may be insufficient to fully compensate for perturbations. The latency and persistence of reflex responses may result in transient lags and overshoots in compensatory processes. Noise and hysteresis (related, e.g., to baroreceptor adaptation) may affect the stability and reproducibility of the compensatory response. Some examples of variations in these parameters and their functional consequences on the regulated dimension of blood pressure are illustrated in panels B–D of Figure 1.

BEYOND HOMEOSTASIS: HOMEODYNAMIC REGULATION

Based on the work of Pavlov, Cannon recognized that learned autonomic adjustments could be made in anticipation of, and thus prior to, a visceral perturbation (Cannon 1928). Such anticipatory responses can not be viewed as mere reflexive adjustments to a physiological perturbation. More recently, Dworkin (1993) re-emphasized the potential importance of learning mechanisms in homeostatic regulation (see also Chapter 18 of this volume). Dworkin proposed that by appropriately calibrated conditioned responses, learned autonomic adjustments may minimize or preclude homeostatic disturbances from otherwise perturbing stimuli. Dworkin outlined a sophisticated control theory framework for homeostatic regulation, incorporating anticipatory feedforward components. This model offers an important advance over traditional feedback controlled models of homeostatic regulation. Although not incompatible with the homeostatic concept, the existence

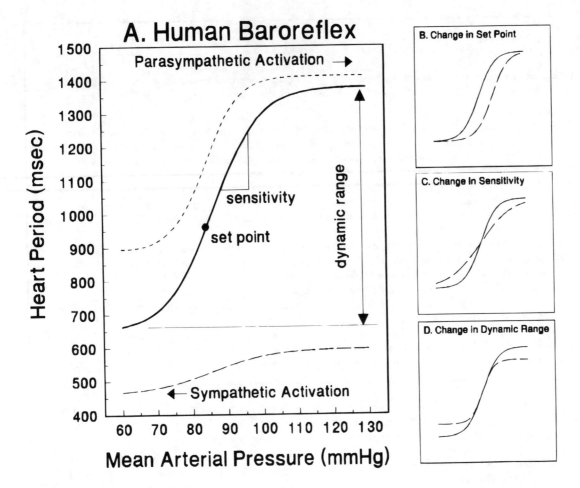

Figure 1. *Panel A.* Baroreceptor–cardiac reflex function in humans. The solid line illustrates changes in heart period with variations in mean arterial pressure. The solid dot depicts the resting blood pressure set point, the slope of the line represents the sensitivity of the reflex, and the distance from the minima to the maxima is the dynamic range. Note that increases in blood pressure yield an increase in parasympathetic activation and a reciprocal decrease in sympathetic activity. The dashed lines illustrate the separate sympathetic and parasympathetic contributions during selective blockades of the other branch. (Data derived from Robinson et al. 1966; see also Berntson et al. 1993.) *Panels B–D.* Schematized reflex functions (solid lines) and consequences (dashed lines) of selective changes in set point (B), sensitivity (C), and dynamic range (D).

of anticipatory controls highlights an important limitation of simple feedback models of homeostatic regulation. In terms of the operating characteristics of Table 1, anticipatory responses would reflect an alteration of the temporal dynamics of the regulatory process.

Other control system operating characteristics (see Table 1) may also be subject to modulation by higher central processes. The notable physiologist Philip Bard (1960) commented on the concurrent increase in blood pressure and heart rate observed during stress, in opposition to the homeostatic baroreceptor–heart rate reflex. Bard speculated that higher brain systems may be capable of modulating lower homeostatic reflexes. It is now clear

that stressors – even those as mild as mental arithmetic – can reduce the sensitivity or otherwise alter the operating characteristics of the baroreceptor–heart rate reflex (Ditto & France 1990; Lawler et al. 1991; Stephenson, Smith, & Scher 1981; Steptoe & Sawada 1989). An alteration in sensitivity of baroreflexes, for example, would impact on the capacity of these reflexes to compensate for a perturbation in blood pressure and hence could lead to secondary restriction in the dynamic range of compensatory responses (see Figure 1). Moreover, dynamic changes in baroreflex function may occur spontaneously, reflecting circadian or other rhythms in homeostatic regulation (Janssen et al. 1992). Additional complexities in homeostatic control reflect that reflexive systems can interact in complex ways with peripheral autoregulatory mechanisms. Sympathetic activity, for example, can alter vascular elasticity and thus affect peripheral autoregulation. Similarly, autoregulatory processes contribute to functional states of the periphery and thus influence visceral feedback and set a background level upon which reflexive adjustments must operate.

In contrast to the relative inflexibility implied by the term homeostasis, the considerations previously outlined suggest that visceral control may be more appropriately viewed as reflecting a pattern of *homeodynamic* regulation, in which operating characteristics may be subject to

TABLE 2. Conceptual Models of Autonomic Regulation

| Set Point | Operating Characteristics | |
	Fixed	Variable
Fixed	Homeostasis	Homeodynamic regulation
Variable	Allostasis	Allodynamic regulation

modification in the face of changing circumstances (see Table 2).

Summary. The findings just outlined suggest that the simple feedback control, set-point model of visceral regulation may not represent adequately the complexity of visceral control. Moreover, the emphasis on static levels and the fixity implied by the term "homeostasis" does not capture appropriately the variability and dynamic features of visceral control systems. A more appropriate construct is that of homeodynamic regulation, which recognizes that regulatory processes do not reflect simple, rigid, negative feedback mechanisms. Rather, regulatory mechanisms are multiple and complex, with lags, limits, and feed-forward components, and may evidence variations in operating characteristics that may themselves be subject to active control. The concept of homeodynamic regulation does imply a regulatory level, but it recognizes that variations around this level may be rather broad and reflective of the operations of multiple dynamic influences. This represents an important conceptual advance over the rigidity and fixity implied by the term homeostasis.

Despite Cannon's tendency to equate constancy with adaptiveness, constancy is not invariably adaptive. Moreover, deviations from a fixed level do not always represent perturbations; they may reflect active alterations in set-point levels.

HETEROSTASIS, ALLOSTASIS, AND ALLODYNAMIC REGULATION

Heterostasis

Although variations in operating characteristics can alter the efficiency, capacity, and time course of regulatory processes, as long as the regulatory set point remained relatively constant these processes could be subsumed under the construct of homeodynamic regulation. Based on studies of the stress response, however, Selye (1973) suggested that regulatory levels or set points are not rigidly fixed but may be actively altered in the face of exogenous challenges or pathogens. For Selye, homeostatic processes may continue to operate at the basic regulatory level, being sensitive to *internal* physiological stimuli that signal deviations from a regulated set point. On the other hand, Selye argued that *exogenous* stimuli could reset regulatory levels, either directly or via a humoral route, to facilitate

resistance or adaptation to the exogenous stressor. Such set-point readjustments could not properly be considered under the rubric of homeostatic or homeodynamic regulation, as they represent active alterations of the regulatory level. In contrast to homeostasis, Selye applied the term "heterostasis" to this class of regulatory adjustment (from the Greek *heteros* meaning "other" and *stasis* meaning "fixity" or "lack of movement").

An illustration of heterostatic regulation is the alteration in body temperature set point associated with a fever. The increase in body temperature during illness does not represent a mere limitation of thermoregulatory processes or a regulatory failure. Rather, the increased temperature of a fever is actively regulated and defended, and reductions in body temperature are met with active compensatory thermogenic processes (e.g., shivering, metabolic thermogenesis, or behavioral thermoregulation; see Stitt 1979 and Werner 1988). The elevation in temperature associated with a fever may be of benefit in mobilizing energy resources to combat infections or other adaptive challenges. Despite its potential adaptive significance, fever is not readily subsumed within the more limited constructs of homeostatic or homeodynamic regulation, because it reflects the adoption of a *new* regulatory set point. Selye (1973) emphasized the role of hormones and the chemical environment in heterostatic regulation. Altered chemical and hormonal conditions associated with exogenous stimuli were seen as contributing to resistance and adaptation by *syntoxic* effects, which render tissues less sensitive to pathogenic stimuli, and/or by *catatoxic* mechanisms that assist in neutralizing or destroying pathogens. Examples of these include the anti-inflammatory effects of adrenocorticoids (syntoxic action) and immunostimulation by cytokines (catatoxic action). As we examine in what follows, modulation of regulatory mechanisms may arise also from central processes, and brain systems likely mediate many of the effects of the exogenous stimuli of Selye.

Allostasis

More recently, Sterling and Eyer (1988) introduced the term *allostasis* (from the Greek *allos,* also meaning "other") to capture the complexities of visceral regulation. Like Selye, these authors recognized that regulatory levels are not fixed but may be flexibly adjusted to meet changing demands. Although allostasis entails the concept of changing regulatory set points, the construct is considerably broader than heterostasis. The allostatic concept of Sterling and Eyer recognizes that many visceral dimensions are regulated by multiple, interacting mechanisms; these mechanisms are seen as subject to a broader range of modulatory influences, whether derived from exogenous challenges or natural endogenous processes. Sterling and Eyer pointed out, for example, that blood pressure is not constant throughout the day; rather, it shows systematic fluctuations associated with diurnal cycles of sleep and waking and with specific patterns of activity during the day. These alterations in set point are not consonant with simple homeostatic or homeodynamic models. Nor do they necessarily involve exogenous agents. Instead, they are seen as reflecting the adaptive readjustment of regulatory levels given changing physiological demands.

There are additional important features of the construct of allostasis, as formulated by Sterling and Eyer (1988). Allostatic regulation was conceptualized as reflecting the operations of higher neural systems, which serve to control and integrate a broad range of more basic "homeostatic" reflexes. Because of this broad control over multiple lower mechanisms, allostatic processes may achieve greater flexibility in maintaining integrative regulation both within and across visceral functions. In the regulation of a given functional endpoint such as blood pressure, higher neural systems can modulate a range of functional dimensions that influence this endpoint. These include heart rate, cardiac contractility, vascular tone, and renal functions; each of these can alter blood pressure and may be adjusted by a combination of autonomic and neuroendocrine influences. One implication of this integrative model is that the endpoint of regulation may not be adequately characterized along a single dimension of visceral function, such as sympathetic outflow, heart rate, or vascular tone. Moreover, given the multiplicity and integrative nature of allostatic control, central abnormalities that contribute to (say) hypertension may not be effectively normalized by clinical treatment of a single visceral parameter (e.g., diuretics or beta blockers). This is because allostatic regulatory processes are speculated to control many response parameters in the regulation of the target visceral dimension. Consequently, "treatment" of one dimension may merely lead to a compensatory alteration in another and so maintain the abnormal regulated state. This concept has substantive implications for health and behavioral medicine, an issue to which we shall return in the section entitled "Inferential Context."

Summary. The term heterostasis was proposed by Selye to reflect the alterations in regulatory levels that may be triggered by exogenous stimuli. The concept of allostasis was subsequently introduced by Sterling and Eyer to represent a wider set of central integrative controls over visceral regulation that involve endogenous and exogenous conditions both. The construct of allostasis may be considered to subsume Selye's more limited concept of heterostasis. The concept of allostasis is particularly significant for psychophysiology, because rostral brain systems that underlie behavioral processes are recognized to contribute to patterns of neuroendocrine and autonomic regulation. Consequently, the optimal approach to understanding and alleviating stress-related psychophysiological disorders is not the mere identification and palliation of peripheral pathology. Rather, the origins of the dysregulation must be sought in central–visceral interactions. Similarly, consideration of the central integrative processes that give rise to physiological responses may help to clarify psychophysiological relations. We shall return to this issue in the "Inferential Context" section.

Allodynamic Regulation

The constructs of homeostasis and homeodynamic regulation both entail a relatively fixed regulatory set point, although the homeodynamic concept explicitly recognizes the dynamic features of regulatory systems and the potential for alteration of operating characteristics (see Table 2). The notion of heterostasis and the broader concept of allostasis similarly assume a regulatory set point, although both emphasize that regulatory levels may be variable rather than fixed. It remains unclear, however, when deviations from a fixed functional level represent an allostaticlike adoption of a new set point. We will consider (under the heading "Physical Context") the possibility that at least some physiological changes associated with behavioral states may reflect the active inhibition of set-point regulation – and not adoption of an altered regulatory level. This is an issue of fundamental importance for conceptions of the nature of visceral control and for its health implications.

As we shall detail, rostral neural systems project directly to lower autonomic motor neurons and brainstem reflex substrates, providing the substrate by which regulatory mechanisms may be bypassed, inhibited, or otherwise modulated. Stressors, for example, appear capable of inhibiting the expression of the baroreceptor–heart rate reflex by altering the regulatory set-point *and* by decreasing the sensitivity and dynamic range of reflexive control (Ditto & France 1990; Lawler et al. 1991; Lundin, Ricksten, & Thoren 1984; Stephenson et al. 1981; Steptoe & Sawada 1989). That is, alterations in cardiovascular function during stress may arise from an active suppression of basic regulatory processes.

In view of these considerations, we introduce as a heuristic starting point the construct of *allodynamic regulation* (see Table 2). This construct is intended to broadly subsume the wide range of regulatory processes represented by the concepts of homeostasis, homeodynamic regulation, heterostasis, and allostasis. In addition, the allodynamic concept recognizes the potential limitations of regulatory processes as well as the possibility that visceral reactions may not always be regulated about a set-point level.

Physical Context

CLASSICAL BARORECEPTOR REFLEX AND HOMEOSTATIC REGULATION

Figure 2 presents a schematic depiction of the basic baroreceptor reflex circuit (Blessing 1997; Guyenet 1990; Spyer 1990). As noted earlier, baroreceptors increase their rate of firing in response to an increase in blood pressure.

This increased baroreceptor afferent activity is conveyed to the nucleus of the tractus solitarius (NTS) in the medulla, the primary visceral receiving area in the brainstem. The NTS issues direct and indirect excitatory projections to vagal motor neurons in the nucleus ambiguus and the dorsal motor nucleus of the vagus, leading to a reflexive increase in parasympathetic outflow. The NTS also projects to the "depressor" area of the caudal ventrolateral medulla (Cvlm), which in turn inhibits sympathoexcitatory neurons of the "pressor" area of the rostral ventrolateral medulla (Rvlm). This leads to a decrease in activity of the sympathetic motor neurons in the intermediolateral cell column of the cord. By this mechanism, baroreceptors achieve reciprocal reflexive control over the sympathetic and parasympathetic outflows and so contribute to the homeostatic feedback regulation of blood pressure.

COMPLEXITIES IN AUTONOMIC CONTROL

This feedback controlled, homeostatic model is elegant in its simplicity; together with the construct of a set point or regulatory level, it might be invoked to account for the relative stability of blood pressure over time. However, this simple model belies the complexity of cardiovascular control. The concept of a fixed blood pressure set point, homeostatically regulated by baroreceptor feedback, is a fiction. Although baroreceptor reflexes certainly serve to oppose transient pressor or depressor perturbations, they cannot account for the relative steady-state stability of blood pressure. Like other interoceptors, baroreceptors are subject to adaptation and thus do not reliably report steady-state levels (Dworkin 1993; see also Chapter 18). The long-term stability of blood pressure can not be attributed to the fixed set point of a simple feedback controlled homeostatic mechanism. The tonic, steady-state level of blood pressure is actually regulated by a variety of factors, including peripheral (autoregulatory) processes, hormonal influences, and brainstem generators of autonomic tone that are at least in part independent of baroreceptor inputs (Blessing 1997; Gebber 1990; Guyenet 1990). Adding to this complexity are the contributions of rostral neural systems and anticipatory modulations of lower autonomic mechanisms.

ROSTRAL INFLUENCES

The central control of autonomic outflow is related in part to rostral neural systems, such as the hypothalamus,

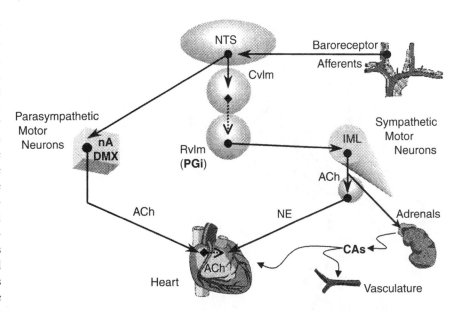

Figure 2. Summary of brainstem systems underlying baroreceptor–cardiac reflex. Baroreceptor afferents project to nucleus tractus solitarius (NTS), which in turn leads to activation of parasympathetic motor neurons in the nucleus ambiguus (nA) and dorsal motor nucleus of the vagus (DMX). The NTS also activates the caudal ventrolateral medulla (Cvlm), which in turn inhibits the rostral ventrolateral medulla (Rvlm), leading to a withdrawal of excitatory drive on the sympathetic motor neurons in the intermediolateral cell column of the cord (IML). Abbreviations: ACh, acetylcholine; CAs, catecholamines; NE, norepinephrine; PGi, paragigantocellularis nucleus (partially coextensive with Rvlm).

amygdala, and cerebral cortex. As illustrated in Figure 3, these structures project to autonomic regulatory substrates in the brainstem, including the NTS and the ventrolateral medulla, as well as to lower central autonomic motor neurons (Buchanan et al. 1994; Cechetto & Saper 1990; Danielsen, Magnuson, & Gray 1989; Hurley et al. 1991; Luiten et al. 1985; Neafsey 1990; Schwaber et al. 1982; Shih, Chan, & Chan 1995; Wallace, Magnuson, & Gray 1992). Of particular relevance for psychophysiology is the fact that many of the rostral sources of these descending projections are limbic and forebrain areas that have been implicated in behavioral processes. Manipulations (i.e., stimulation or lesion) of these rostral structures have been shown to be capable of facilitating, inhibiting, or bypassing basic brainstem autonomic reflexes, thereby potently modulating autonomic outflow in a relatively direct fashion (Inui, Murase, & Nosaka 1994; Inui et al. 1995; Jordan 1990; Koizumi & Kollai 1981; Lewis et al. 1989; Neafsey 1990; Nosaka, Nakase, & Murata 1989; Oppenheimer & Cechetto 1990; Pascoe, Bradley, & Spyer 1989; Spyer 1989, 1990). Stimulation of the central nucleus of the amygdala, for example, can inhibit barosensitive neurons in the rostral ventrolateral medulla (Gelsema, Agarwal, & Calaresu 1989). It is likely that descending influences such as this serve as the basis for observations that psychological

cation in the light of contemporary findings, and it is now apparent that the two autonomic branches can vary reciprocally, coactively, or independently (Berntson, Cacioppo, & Quigley 1991, 1993; Berntson et al. 1994b; Koizumi & Kollai 1992). Descending influences from rostral neural systems are capable of modulating the operating characteristics of brainstem homeostatic mechanisms and can generate highly flexible patterns of autonomic outflow. Hypothalamic stimulation, for example, can evoke each of the basic modes of reciprocal, coactive, or independent changes in the activity of the autonomic branches (Koizumi & Kollai 1981; Powell et al. 1972; Shih et al. 1995). These descending integrative influences likely serve as important substrates for allodynamic regulation of the viscera.

The findings just outlined introduce considerable complexity in the quantification and interpretation of autonomic control. Autonomic control cannot be viewed as lying along a single, reciprocal autonomic continuum extending from sympathetic dominance at one end to parasympathetic dominance at the other. Rather, autonomic control of dually innervated organs is more appropriately represented by a bivariate autonomic plane consisting of orthogonal sympathetic and parasympathetic axes. This is depicted by the model of autonomic space in Figure 4, which shows the chronotropic state of the heart for any given combination of sympathetic and parasympathetic activities.

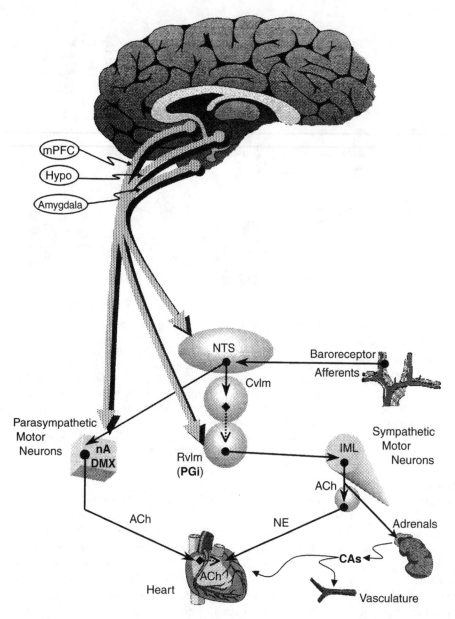

Figure 3. Expansion of the baroreflex circuit of Figure 2, illustrating the ascending and descending pathways to and from rostral neural areas such as the medial prefrontal cortex (mPFC), hypothalamus (Hypo), and amygdala. Ascending systems include routes from the rostral ventrolateral medulla (Rvlm) and the nucleus of the tractus solitarius (NTS) to the locus coeruleus (LC) noradrenergic system, and indirectly to the basal forebrain (BF) cortical cholinergic system. Abbreviations: ACh, acetylcholine; CAs, catecholamines; NE, norepinephrine; PGi, paragigantocellularis nucleus (partially coextensive with Rvlm).

stressors can yield both an increase in blood pressure and heart rate – in direct opposition to the baroreflex.

Although baroreceptor reflexes may exert a classical pattern of reciprocal control over the autonomic branches, rostral systems appear to be much more flexible. The traditional concept of reciprocal central control of the autonomic branches has undergone considerable quali-

ASCENDING INFLUENCES

Of particular relevance for emerging neurobehavioral models of the links between psychological processes and autonomic control is the fact that interactions between rostral and caudal neural systems are bidirectional (see Figure 3). The potential role of visceral afference in higher-level processes has long been of interest to psychologists yet has proven very difficult to characterize and quantify. Although the role of visceral afference in emotion and cognition remains speculative, empirical findings document potent influences of visceral afferent information in central nervous system functions. Consistent with the

Autonomic Space

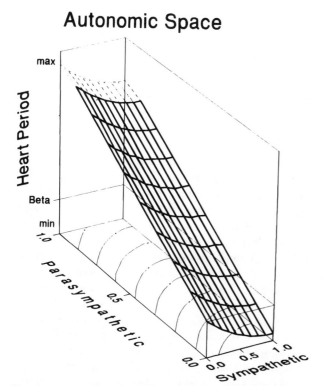

Figure 4. Bivariate autonomic plane and associated chronotropic effector surface. The plane bounded by the parasympathetic and sympathetic axes represents all possible combinations of sympathetic and parasympathetic activities (on a relative scale from 0 to 1). The effector surface overlying the autonomic plane represents the chronotropic state of the target organ, expressed in heart period, for all loci within autonomic space (for details on derivation, see Berntson et al. 1991, 1993). Parasympathetic activation exerts relatively linear effects on heart period, whereas sympathetic activation yields somewhat nonlinear effects. The dotted surface at maximal levels of parasympathetic activation represents the ambiguity in effects at this extreme. For illustrative purposes, the relative lengths of the axes are scaled in proportion to relative dynamic ranges of control of the autonomic branches, and beta represents the "intrinsic" heart period in the absence of autonomic input. The curved lines on the autonomic plane represent isoeffector contours projected from the effector surface onto the autonomic plane. These contour lines illustrate loci on the autonomic plane that yield equivalent chronotropic effects.

baroreceptor hypothesis of Lacey (1959; Lacey et al. 1963; see also the next section, "Psychological Context"), baroreceptor activation has been shown to modulate the afferent transmission of pain signals (Dworkin et al. 1994; Randich & Gebhart 1992). Moreover, baroreceptor and other visceral afferents may influence activity in higher brain systems more directly. Ascending projections from brainstem autonomic substrates project directly to the amygdala and other forebrain areas and are capable of modulating the activity of rostral brain systems (Aston-Jones et al. 1996; Berntson, Sarter, & Cacioppo 1998; Nakata et al. 1991; Shih et al. 1995; Zardetto-Smith & Gray 1995).

As shown in Figure 3, baroreceptor afferents terminate in the nucleus of the tractus solitarius (NTS), the primary visceral receiving area in the brainstem. In addition to

participating in local reflex circuits, baroreceptor afferent activity is relayed via the NTS to the nucleus paragigantocellularis (PGi), which provides a tonic drive on sympathetic motor neurons. Consequently, the PGi (which is coextensive with the rostral ventrolateral medullary pressor area) would be expected to be highly sensitive to the state of activity in the sympathetic branch. The PGi also projects to the locus coeruleus (LC), a structure that has been implicated in arousal and anxiety (Aston-Jones et al. 1996; Berntson et al. 1998); in turn, the LC issues a rostral noradrenergic projection to the limbic system and cerebral cortex. The activity of this noradrenergic pathway would thus be expected to be modulated by the level of sympathetic tone. Sympathetic activation induced by nitroprusside-hypotension, for example, was found to be associated with increases in LC firing, and this effect was shown to be mediated via visceral afferents from the cardiac atrial baroreceptors (Elam, Svensson, & Thoren 1974).

In addition to its direct projections to limbic areas, the locus coeruleus projects to the basal forebrain, which is the primary source of cholinergic innervation of the cortex (for a review, see Sarter & Bruno 1997). This cholinergic projection appears to enhance cortical processing and has been implicated in cognitive and attentional processes (Sarter & Bruno 1997). Decreases in activity of the basal forebrain–cortical cholinergic system due to atrophy of the basal forebrain is considered to be one of the major neuropathological conditions leading to the attentional and cognitive impairments in Alzheimer's disease (Sarter 1994). In contrast, increased activity in this cholinergic system has been suggested to underlie cognitive aspects of anxiety by virtue of the enhanced processing of anxiogenic stimuli (Berntson et al. 1998). In this regard, the prototypic anxiolytic agents – the benzodiazepine receptor agonists such as chlordiazepoxide (Librium) and diazepam (Valium) – may exert their antianxiety actions, at least in part, by attenuating activity in the basal forebrain cholinergic system.

Summary. In the aggregate, these findings at a neurobiological level focus attention on the complex interactions between central systems, autonomic regulation, and peripheral afferent signals. The convergence of visceral afference on common rostral neural systems – together with the hierarchical, integrative control these systems exert on lower autonomic substrates – likely contributes to the broader integration of behavioral and autonomic processes implied by the concept of allodynamic regulation. Homeostatic mechanisms can be highly adaptive, but there are many conditions in which it may not be optimal to maintain a fixed steady state. In view of the limitless adaptive challenges an organism can encounter, it is hardly surprising that evolutionary pressures led to the development of sophisticated learning mechanisms that support behavioral flexibility and adaptability in overcoming these challenges.

It would be most surprising if these same evolutionary pressures ignored the control of autonomic and neuroendocrine functions that provide the visceral support for adaptive response.

Psychological Context

Basic homeostatic reflex mechanisms, such as baroreceptor reflexes, can exert tight reciprocal control over the opposing autonomic branches. Homeostatic (metabolic) demands associated with somatic exercise also yield reciprocal effects on autonomic outflows. The initial effect of exercise is mediated largely by parasympathetic withdrawal, but sympathetic activation is increasingly manifest with progressively higher levels of exertion (Robinson et al. 1966; Rowell 1986). This reciprocal pattern is also apparent in the effects of laboratory isometric handgrip tasks, which have been reported to yield concurrent sympathetic activation and parasympathetic withdrawal (Pollack & Obrist 1988; see also Berntson et al. 1993). For moderate levels of effort, the initial response again appears to be vagal withdrawal, with sympathetic activation appearing at higher levels or over longer periods of effort (Grossman & Kollai 1993; Martin et al. 1974). These homeostatic reflexes likely contribute to psychophysiological responses in behavioral contexts.

THE CARDIAC–SOMATIC HYPOTHESIS: PSYCHOPHYSIOLOGY AND METABOLIC DEMANDS

The relationships between somatic effort, metabolic demand, and autonomic regulation have led to the suggestion that cardiovascular reactions in psychological contexts may be attributable to metabolic factors. Based on the apparent correspondence between the direction and magnitude of cardiac change and subtle variations in somatic response, Obrist proposed that "the metabolically relevant relationship or linkage between cardiac and somatic events is also relevant to behavioral events" (Obrist et al. 1970, p. 570).

Against this backdrop, however, was an emerging recognition that (i) notable cardiac changes in psychological contexts often have metabolically trivial consequences and (ii) cardiac response in psychological contexts often exceeds that expected on the basis of metabolic demands (Obrist 1981; Turner 1994). Moreover, conditioned and unconditioned cardiac responses can be seen in the absence of somatic response in curarized animals (Dworkin & Dworkin 1990) and in paralyzed human subjects (Berntson & Boysen 1990). Cognizant of discrepancies between autonomic and somatic activities, Obrist later revised the concept of cardiac–somatic coupling. In the revised formulation, Obrist (1981) argued that the fundamental linkage between cardiac and somatic events is attributable to a central coupling rather than peripheral metabolic feedback, a view in accord with the homeodynamic model.

According to the revised cardiac–somatic concept, somatic paralysis could yield a dissociation between somatic and cardiovascular reactions because peripheral paralysis would block the skeletal response without disrupting central cardiac–somatic coupling. Consequently, a strong test of the cardiac–somatic hypothesis would require measures of central somatic motor outflows rather than skeletal responses per se. Data relevant to this issue were provided by a study of Dworkin & Dworkin (1990) in which cardiovascular variables and somatic nerve activities were concurrently recorded in a paralyzed rat preparation. Through an array of monitoring and maintenance systems, pharmacologically paralyzed rats were maintained for up to 100 days. During this time, subjects evidenced typical cycles of EEG (electroencephalographic) sleep and wakefulness and displayed characteristic EEG and autonomic responses to environmental stimuli. The somatically paralyzed rats received a sequence of habituation trials to two distinct tone CSs (condition stimuli), a sensitization regimen with a tail-shock UCS (unconditioned stimulus), and then Pavlovian discriminative conditioning. Even under complete paralysis, animals evidenced consistent discriminative conditioning as evidenced by EEG desynchronization, somatic (tibial) nerve activity, and cardiovascular responses. Results revealed a clear dissociation of somatic and autonomic responses. Both the conditioned and unconditioned central somatic responses entailed an increase in tibial nerve activity. From the standpoint of the cardiac–somatic hypothesis, this was consistent with the tachycardia observed as a UR (unconditioned response) to shock but was at variance with the overall bradycardic CR (conditioned response), which was also associated with an increase in somatic nerve activity. In addition, trial-by-trial analyses of the laterality of the responses to the negative CS revealed a moderate concordance – compatible with a central cardiac–somatic linkage – between tibial nerve and vasomotor responses of the homolateral limb. In contrast, even at the local hindlimb level, conditioned somatic and autonomic responses to the positive CS displayed no such concordance, suggesting a separability of central mechanisms of somatic and autonomic control.

Summary. Metabolic effects associated with somatic effort are known to trigger potent reciprocal autonomic adjustments, and the possibility of this contribution must be considered in psychophysiological studies. However, metabolic effects in many behavioral contexts are insufficient or in the wrong direction to account for observed cardiac responses. There is little doubt that central systems orchestrate coordinated somatic and autonomic responses. Yet documented exceptions to the cardiac–somatic model support neither the concept of a universal central linkage between somatic and cardiac responses nor even the *primacy* of somatic responses.

THE NEUROPSYCHOPHYSIOLOGICAL PERSPECTIVE

Basic reciprocal homeostatic reflexes likely contribute to the links between psychological processes and autonomic responses. The allodynamic model and the rostral neuroanatomical systems shown in Figure 3, however, suggest a greater richness in the neurobiological substrates underlying psychophysiological relations. An appreciation for the neurobiology underlying psychophysiology – what we term the *neuropsychophysiological* perspective – affords the basis for a powerful multilevel analysis of the links between psychological processes and visceral functions. The value of the neuropsychophysiological perspective lies in the fact that psychophysiology can both inform and be informed by neurobiological data, constructs, and theories. This general perspective has led to dramatic developments in understanding of the central mechanisms of learning, memory, cognition, and behavior – developments that contributed to a U.S. Congressional declaration of the 1990s as the "decade of the brain." The parallels between the central organization and determinants of behavioral and autonomic output have not always been fully appreciated, however, and this has sometimes led to unrealistic expectations of simple isomorphic relations between psychological processes and autonomic states.

Illustrative is the pessimism expressed by Obrist (1981) over the use of heart rate in the psychophysiological study of behavioral processes. Commenting on the fact that attention to environmental events is often associated with a decrease in heart rate (HR) whereas increased HR is typically observed in active avoidance, Obrist remarked, "both types of conditions have an obvious attentional component. If we assume for the moment that a decrease in HR is indicative of the attentional factor, then it must be overridden by some other aspect of the task during shock avoidance. It is anything but a parsimonious situation and leads to interpretive difficulties" (1981, p. 198). But since attentional responses frequently entail a decrease in behavioral activity, it may be instructive to substitute the term "behavior" for "HR" in the preceding comment. Given our understanding of the multiple determinants of behavior, the mere occurrence of a decrease in behavior cannot be taken to imply attention; nor can an increase in behavior be interpreted as a lack of attention (see Cacioppo & Tassinary 1990). This is insufficient reason to be disillusioned over the study of behavior or, for that matter, heart rate. In both cases, a more productive strategy would be to define and disentangle the multiple determinants and processes operative in a given context and then to clarify the underlying relationships and mechanisms.

Rostral Descending Influences and the Modes of Autonomic Control

Rostral neurobehavioral systems can exert relatively direct and selective influences on central autonomic outflows, and their actions may not adhere to simple principles of homeostasis and reciprocal control. Rather, descending systems are capable of evoking a wide range of autonomic modes of control. This is illustrated by a study of the autonomic origins of cardiac responses to orthostatic and psychological stressors. The autonomic origins of the cardiac responses of human subjects to orthostatic stress (assumption of an upright posture) and to typical psychological stressors (mental arithmetic, reaction time, and a speech stress task) were evaluated by pharmacological blockades that yielded quantitative estimates of the sympathetic and parasympathetic contributions to cardiac response (Berntson et al. 1994a; Cacioppo et al. 1994). At the group level, the orthostatic and psychological stressors yielded an essentially equivalent pattern of heart rate increase, characterized by sympathetic activation and parasympathetic withdrawal. For the orthostatic stressor, the cardiac response reflected a relatively tight reciprocal central control of the autonomic branches, as evidenced by the significant negative correlation between the responses of the autonomic branches across subjects ($r = -0.71$). Although the group response to psychological stressors was similar, there were considerable individual differences in the pattern of response, and there was no significant correlation between responses of the autonomic branches ($r = 0.09$). The individual modes of autonomic response were highly reliable across different psychological stressors, but subjects differed considerably in their pattern of response. As illustrated in Figure 5, some subjects showed primarily sympathetic activation, some showed reciprocal sympathetic activation and parasympathetic withdrawal, and others showed primarily parasympathetic withdrawal.

Individual differences in the pattern of autonomic response may have special relevance to psychophysiological relations. Cardiovascular reactivity to acute laboratory stressors has been reported to predict endocrine and immune responses to stress, with high HR reactors showing greater changes in cortisol and natural killer (NK) cell activity (Bachen et al. 1995; Cacioppo 1994; Cacioppo et al. 1995; Herbert et al. 1994; Manuck et al. 1991; Sgoutas-Emch et al. 1994). However, as shown in Figure 5, there can be sizeable individual differences in the autonomic origins of HR responses to stress, and these distinct autonomic modes of control may have differential implications for neuroendocrine and immune responses. Based on recent findings, it now appears that it is the sympathetic component of the heart rate response – rather than the parasympathetic component or the heart rate response per se – that is most predictive of neuroendocrine and immune reactions to stress (Cacioppo 1994; Cacioppo et al.

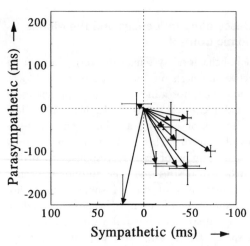

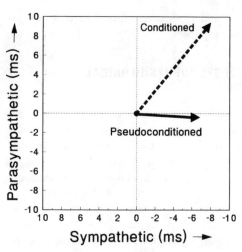

Figure 5. Individual patterns of response to stress depicted on the autonomic plane. The intersection of the dotted lines in the center of the graph represents the basal resting state; the arrows depict the individual response vectors along the sympathetic and parasympathetic axes, with the peak response at the arrowheads. Vectors were derived from independent estimates of the contributions of the autonomic branches under selective pharmacological blockades. Note that some subjects responded primarily with parasympathetic withdrawal, some primarily with sympathetic activation, and some with reciprocal sympathetic activation and parasympathetic withdrawal. These individual response vectors were stable. Three stressors were used (mental arithmetic, a reaction time task, and a speech stressor). The error bars at the tip of each response vector illustrate the standard errors of the response across the three tasks. Units on the axes are milliseconds of heart period. Reprinted with permission from Berntson, Sarter, & Cacioppo, "Anxiety and cardiovascular reactivity: The basal forebrain cholinergic link," *Behavioural Brain Research,* vol. 94, pp. 225–48. Copyright 1998 Elsevier Science.

Figure 6. Autonomic cardiac response vectors to an auditory CS for shock in conditioned and pseudoconditioned rats, depicted on the autonomic plane. Solid dot at the center represents basal resting state; the arrows depict the responses of the autonomic branches to the CS, with the peak response at the arrowheads. Vectors were derived from independent estimates of the contributions of the autonomic branches under selective pharmacological blockades. Response of pseudoconditioned animals (solid arrow) reflected a pattern of sympathetic activation, whereas conditioned animals (dashed arrow) displayed a coactivation of both the sympathetic and parasympathetic branches. Units on the axes are milliseconds of heart period. (Data derived from Iwata & LeDoux 1988; see also Berntson et al. 1993.) Figure reprinted with permission from Berntson, Sarter, & Cacioppo, "Anxiety and cardiovascular reactivity: The basal forebrain cholinergic link," *Behavioural Brain Research,* vol. 94, pp. 225–48. Copyright 1998 Elsevier Science.

1995). This is in keeping with the finding that some immune responses to laboratory stressors can be prevented by selective sympathetic blockade (Bachen et al. 1995; Benschop et al. 1994).

The importance of multiple modes of autonomic control in interpreting psychophysiological relations is further illustrated by a study of cardiovascular conditioned responses. Iwata and LeDoux (1988) observed equivalent cardioacceleratory responses to a fear CS in both conditioned and pseudoconditioned rats. This could lead to the erroneous conclusion that autonomic cardiac control is not sensitive to the learning history of the subjects, and it raises questions concerning the utility of cardiac measures in this paradigm. As illustrated in Figure 6, however, the application of selective pharmacological blockades of the sympathetic and parasympathetic branches revealed that the similar cardioacceleratory responses of the two groups arose from distinct modes of autonomic control. The tachycardia of pseudoconditioned animals arose largely from selective sympathetic activation, as it was virtually eliminated by β-adrenergic blockade and largely unaffected by vagal blockade with atropine. In contrast, the cardioacceleratory response of conditioned animals was *enhanced* by vagal

blockade, being significantly larger than that of pseudoconditioned animals under the identical blockade condition. This suggests that, in the unblocked state, vagal responses may have partially opposed the cardiac manifestation of a greater sympathetic activation in the conditioned animals. Consistent with this interpretation, β-adrenergic blockade not only eliminated the cardioacceleratory response in the conditioned group but also unmasked a sizeable deceleratory response of apparent vagal origin. These findings suggest that the sympathetic response of conditioned animals was in fact appreciably larger but that the cardiac manifestations were dampened by coactivation of the parasympathetic branch. The distinct modes of autonomic control in conditioned and pseudoconditioned animals were not apparent in the unblocked end-organ response, but they were revealed by measures that allowed a physiologically meaningful mapping of the modes of autonomic control.

Summary. Descending projections of rostral neurobehavioral systems confer a high degree of flexibility over patterns of autonomic outflow and can lead to reciprocal, coactive, or independent changes in the activities of the autonomic branches. The allodynamic model incorporates the central integrative nature of behavioral, neuroendocrine, and visceral control, and it affords a more comprehensive framework for psychophysiology than does the more limited construct of homeostasis. The allodynamic model also fosters a neuropsychophysiological perspective, which recognizes that psychophysiology can both inform and be informed by neurobiological analyses.

Ascending Influences and the Role of Visceral Afference in Behavior

As illustrated in Figure 3, there are ample routes by which autonomic tone and associated visceral afference can modulate the activity of rostral neurobehavioral substrates. Over a century ago, William James (1884) proposed that the perception of visceral afferent information may constitute an important component of emotional experience (for a more recent consideration of this issue, see Cacioppo, Berntson, & Klein 1992a). In addition to its potential contribution to emotional experience, a role for visceral afference in cognitive processes was suggested by work of Sokolov (1963) and the Laceys (Lacey 1959; Lacey et al. 1963). The orienting response (OR) and the defensive response (DR) were formulated by Sokolov (1963) as biobehavioral phenomena that subserved perception and learning by amplifying or reducing the effects of stimulation. The generalized autonomic components of the OR and DR were posited to act directly on sense receptors and indirectly via feedback to central mechanisms that control perceptual sensitivity. For Sokolov, the OR served as an information regulator or filter to foster attention to important stimuli and habituation to unimportant stimuli, whereas the DR served the complementary role of sentry or protective filter to foster retreat and protection from provocative stimuli. Paralleling these developments, the Laceys proposed that autonomic feedback to the central nervous system, especially from baroreceptors, can amplify or reduce the effects of environmental inputs. The Laceys proposed that cardiac deceleration during psychological tasks was not only associated with attentional processes but could also foster sensory intake, whereas cardiac acceleration was associated with and fostered sensory rejection.

Research on human subjects with high spinal transections (quadriplegia or tetraplegia) has not yielded strong support for the necessary involvement of visceral activity and associated visceral afference in emotion (Chwalisz, Diener, & Gallagher 1988). Although these transections interrupt descending central influences on sympathetic outflow and associated afferent consequences, they do not eliminate emotional reactivity. This of course does not rule out an important modulatory role of visceral afference in emotion (see Cacioppo et al. 1992a). Moreover, high spinal-cord transections disrupt descending control of sympathetic outflow but eliminate neither parasympathetic responses nor vagally mediated visceral afference. Further, given the modulatory role of norepinephrine and acetylcholine on cortical activation and reactivity, the ascending pathways

of Figure 3 would be expected to enhance cortical/limbic processing generally. Hence, ascending visceral afference may be more likely to prime or bias, rather than strictly determine, affective states. Affective and autonomic reactivity may derive from a cognitive top-down activation (e.g., affective imagery) of the descending system depicted in Figure 3, and the resulting autonomic reactivity may further bias rostral systems toward the processing of affective stimuli via ascending pathways. Alternatively, visceral afference may yield a bottom-up priming of cognitive/affective processing even in the absence of an affective context.

The early study of Schachter and Singer (1962) on emotional priming by epinephrine was consistent with this model, although serious questions have been raised over the generality of these results (Cacioppo et al. 1992a; Reisenzein 1983). More recent work in animals offers substantial support to the view that visceral afference can modulate higher cognitive/emotional processing. Systemic administration of epinephrine or substance P has been reported to potentiate "emotional" memories in rats, and these effects can be blocked or attenuated by subdiaphragmatic vagotomy, by inactivation of the NTS, or by direct infusions of beta blockers into the amygdala (McGaugh, Cahill, & Roozendaal 1996; Nogueira, Tomaz, & Williams 1994; Williams & McGaugh 1993). Visceral afference also appears to play an important role in the allodynamic regulation of body temperature, since the fever associated with behavioral stress or exogenous mitogens has also been reported to be blocked by vagotomy (see Maier, Watkins, & Fleshner 1994; Watkins, Maier, & Goehler 1995). Further work is clearly needed in this area, but the existing data are in accord with the bidirectional interaction among rostral and caudal neural substrates in the control of affective and autonomic reactivity.

Summary. Both ascending and descending neural systems appear to participate in affective states and autonomic control. Although the contributions of descending pathways have been more fully studied, ascending visceral information may prove to be equally important in biasing psychological processes and mediating psychophysiological relations. This has been a particularly difficult issue to address in human studies, but physiological data from animal subjects clearly indicates an important role of ascending systems in cognitive/affective processes and allodynamic regulation. This is an issue where a neuropsychophysiological approach might be especially useful.

Inferential Context

The homeostatic model emerged from the early physiological literature, and it continues as a pervasive organizing construct in both physiology and psychophysiology. There is considerable appeal to the elegant simplicity of the homeostatic construct and the associated reciprocal model of autonomic control. These models do not provide a comprehensive view of autonomic control in behavioral contexts, however, because higher neural systems can modulate or bypass homeostatic mechanisms and reciprocally organized brainstem systems. Deviations from the reciprocal homeostatic model were recognized in the early physiological literature, but it has been the variance observed in psychophysiological studies that has imparted the strongest momentum against these restrictive constructs. The allodynamic model subsumes homeostatic processes and offers a more comprehensive framework for psychophysiology.

The neuropsychophysiological perspective is particularly relevant within the allodynamic framework, as allodynamic systems quintessentially entail central integrative processes. Neuropsychophysiology does not represent a novel perspective and rather is intended to capture the ongoing evolution of the discipline. Fundamentally, psychophysiology entails a multilevel approach to the study of the mind–body problem and the relations between psychological and physiological processes. Psychophysiological theories and data can both inform and be informed by neurobiology. Psychophysiological data provide the ultimate subject matter for neurobehavioral studies as well as the means for validating neurobiological models. At the same time, knowledge of underlying neural mechanisms can inform and constrain psychophysiological theories and also facilitate interpretation of psychophysiological data.

NEUROPSYCHOPHYSIOLOGY: PERIPHERAL MAPPINGS, MEASUREMENT, AND QUANTIFICATION

That the autonomic branches can be separably controlled has substantial implications for psychophysiological theory and measurement. The autonomic space model of Figure 4 suggests that the most meaningful psychophysiological measures of dually innervated organs require attention to the specific autonomic origins of the end-organ state. Although heart rate measures may continue to have utility in psychophysiology, there is an inherent source of variance that is not appropriately parsed by measures of heart rate alone. This variance is relegated to error and tends to obscure lawful psychophysiological relationships.

An additional feature of the model of Figure 4 is the relative linearity between parasympathetic activity and the chronotropic state of the heart, when the latter is expressed in terms of heart period. When expressed as the reciprocal (heart rate), this relationship becomes distinctively nonlinear (hyperbolic). The latter form can exaggerate apparent baseline dependencies and bias estimates of chronotropic level and response (Berntson, Cacioppo, & Quigley 1995). Consequently, heart period is generally preferable as a metric for chronotropic state,[1] especially when the comparisons of interest are quantitative and across subjects or conditions.

The importance of neurophysiologically meaningful measurement of psychophysiological signals is not limited to the heart. Other dually innervated organs (e.g., the iris of the eye) are subject to similar considerations. Pupillary diameter is a joint function of parasympathetically innervated sphincter (pupillary constrictor) muscle and sympathetically innervated radial (dilator) muscle (Loewy 1990; see also Chapter 6 of this volume). Although there is a degree of reciprocity among the autonomic controls of the iris, changes in pupillary diameter can arise from distinct central systems and can be differentially influenced by the autonomic branches (Loewy 1990). Parasympathetic control, for example, is predominant in accommodation and light reflexes, whereas variation in sympathetic activity is the primary determinant of pupillary responses in behavioral and stress contexts.

Even for singly innervated tissues, peripheral psychophysiological mappings are important in deriving meaningful relations with central behavioral states. In peripheral mappings, any unnecessary complexities introduced by methods of measurement or quantification may cloud or obscure psychophysiological relationships. It was this consideration that led to the general recommendation of skin conductance over skin resistance as a metric for electrodermal responses (see Chapter 8). Skin conductance is more linearly related to the number of active sweat glands and their rate of secretion; it hence displays less baseline dependency than resistance measures[2] (Chapter 8; Montagu & Coles 1966; Venables & Christie 1980). Psychophysiological relationships are often complex, and there are many theoretical and empirical challenges in elucidating these relations. Any extraneous variance such as that related to complex or poorly defined peripheral mappings between autonomic outflows and end-organ responses can only further obscure lawful relations.

Careful elucidation of peripheral autonomic–end-organ mappings is important from the perspective of measurement. Equally important are the implications of peripheral mappings for conceptual models and psychophysiological theories. The autonomic space of Figure 4 is not a mere measurement model; it has substantial implications for psychophysiological concepts. In an early yet influential theory, Eppinger and Hess (1915) proposed a classification of people as vagally dominant (vagotonic) or sympathetically dominant (sympathicotonic). This view entailed a bipolar concept of autonomic control together with a dichotomous individual differences model of autonomic balance. The subsequent studies of Wenger (1941) suggested that "autonomic balance" is, at best, continuous rather than dichotomous. More recent studies (outlined in the "Psychological Context" section) reveal that the pattern of autonomic response cannot be characterized along a single continuum but instead requires a bivariate model of autonomic control. These findings mandate a more comprehensive conceptualization of the relations between psychological processes, the modes of autonomic control, and potential dispositional biases in psychophysiological disorders.

NEUROPSYCHOPHYSIOLOGY: CENTRAL MAPPINGS AND THE RELATION BETWEEN PSYCHOLOGICAL PROCESSES AND BRAIN SYSTEMS

The homeostatic framework does not offer a comprehensive account of physiological regulation. A fever associated with illness may be adaptive, but it can not be viewed as a homeostatic response because it represents an actively defended allostatic elevation of body temperature set point. Similarly, the autonomic and neuroendocrine responses associated with psychological stressors do not appear to represent simple homeostatic adjustments. As outlined previously, the stress-induced elevation of heart rate and blood pressure reflects an active inhibition of baroreceptor reflexes and results in a deviation from pressor homeostasis. Although metabolic signals may also contribute to cardiovascular homeostasis and partially override the effects of baroreceptor activity, cardiovascular responses in stress contexts not only deviate from pressor homeostasis but also exceed those required for metabolic homeostasis (Obrist 1981; Turner 1994). These responses may have adaptive value, but they are difficult to envision within a simple homeostatic schema.

The evidence outlined here indicates that rostral neural systems can modulate autonomic control in a fashion that is not easily reconciled with a simple homeostatic model. As illustrated in Figure 3, there are multiple descending neurobehavioral systems that serve to orchestrate and integrate behavioral, autonomic, and neuroendocrine responses. A greater appreciation of the functional contributions of these systems (i.e., a clarification of the mappings between psychological and neural processes) is likely to contribute to the understanding of complex psychophysiological relations. Although neurobehavioral mechanisms are only beginning to be understood, joint studies of psychological and neural functions can be mutually informative. This is illustrated by the utility of brain event-related potentials in clarifying the nature of psychological processes underlying language (see Chapter 21), attention (Hillyard et al. 1995), and evaluative processes (Cacioppo, Crites, & Gardner 1996). Additional developments in brain imaging promise important breakthroughs in understanding the nature and mechanisms of psychological operations and the underlying neural systems and processes that give rise to these operations.

An example of the mutual benefits of an integrative approach across levels of analysis comes from the literature on arousal. Arousal has been an important concept in physiology, psychology, and psychophysiology over the past five decades. Much of the impetus for arousal theories

and for concepts of the role of general arousal in behavior came from work in the 1940s and 1950s on the brainstem reticular formation (for a review see Magoun 1963). Historically, the reticular formation was viewed as a relatively undifferentiated, highly interconnected set of neurons that exerted relatively nonspecific activational effects on rostral neural systems. Results of early stimulation, lesion, and recording studies of the reticular formation led to the construct of an ascending reticular activating system (ARAS), which was believed to regulate the state of arousal of cortical and neurobehavioral systems (Magoun 1963). The ARAS model resonated with psychologists because it was recognized that, apart from associative or structural determinants of behavior, there were important motivational or activational (arousal) contributions (for an extensive review of the early literature, see Cofer & Appley 1964). Moreover, it was noted that arousal associated with one state or condition could energize behaviors more generally (Duffy 1957; Hebb 1955).

The construct of general arousal has an inherent appeal of simplicity and parsimony, which is likely one reason it has been so resilient in the face of contradictory evidence. Even early studies revealed that the effects of "arousal" were not truly generalized and that behavioral and cortical arousal could be dissociated (Bradley & Elkes 1958; Feldman & Waller 1962). Moreover, psychophysiological measures commonly purported to be indices of arousal (e.g., heart rate, electrodermal responses) often do not covary – with each other or with behavioral performance – in a fashion consistent with a generalized arousal process (see e.g. Lacey 1959, 1967). Developments in neuroscience paralleled the emerging recognition of the limitations of the construct of general arousal in psychology and psychophysiology. These developments included a growing appreciation that the reticular formation was not as nonspecific as originally conceived. More refined neuroanatomical methods and neurochemical markers revealed a great deal of specificity within what was classically considered an undifferentiated system. It is now apparent that there are multiple ascending activating systems, each having differential patterns of afferent input, dissimilar projection fields, and distinct neurochemical mediators (Robbins & Everitt, 1995). These include ascending noradrenergic, dopaminergic, cholinergic, and serotonergic systems (the locus coeruleus noradrenergic system and the basal forebrain cholinergic system are depicted in Figure 3). The precise roles of these ascending systems in behavior and autonomic control remain to be fully elucidated, but their functions are differentiated. The mesolimbic dopaminergic system has been implicated in reward, incentive, and behavioral activation (Gray & McNaughton 1996; Robbins & Everitt 1995); the locus coeruleus noradrenergic system in cortical and motivational arousal (Aston-Jones et al. 1996); the cholinergic system in cortical/cognitive processing (Robbins & Everitt 1995; Sarter & Bruno 1997), and the serotonergic system in attention and behavioral inhibition (Gray & McNaughton 1996; Robbins & Everitt 1995). In contrast to the early work on the ARAS, data from psychology, psychophysiology, and neurobiology concur that arousal is not a unitary process.

Research on arousal systems illustrates the mutual benefit of multilevel analyses. Psychological, psychophysiological, and physiological perspectives were each essential for progress in this area. Although psychological concepts of generalized arousal antedated the emergence of the ARAS construct, it required neurophysiological studies on the reticular formation to crystallize this construct and embody it within a neuroanatomical substrate. In the light of current understandings, the ARAS model may seem primitive, but it represented an important conceptual advance at the time. For example, the ARAS offered the first viable psychobiological account for why an organism did not simply lie inert in the absence of evocative environmental stimuli (Hebb 1955). It also warrants comment that even as psychological and psychophysiological data posed the strongest challenges to the concept of general arousal, it was ultimately data from these same disciplines that spearheaded efforts to refine the ARAS construct. Psychological and psychophysiological studies continue to be central to the efforts to define the functional role of ascending activating systems.

NEUROPSYCHOPHYSIOLOGY OF STRESS-RELATED DISORDERS

Psychophysiological disorders have often been viewed as homeostatic dysfunctions (e.g. Cannon 1932; Holmes & Ripley 1955; Selye 1956), and stress has been defined by some researchers as a state of threatened homeostasis (Johnson et al. 1992). The homeostatic construct, however, has been applied so broadly and across such a diverse range of phenomena that its status as an explanatory construct warrants re-examination and refinement. The homeostatic model, for example, has been extended beyond the organism level as a guiding principle of social relations, and the construct of "risk homeostasis" has been suggested to account for the purported increase in driver carelessness with the deployment of airbags and antilock brakes (van Hooff & Filipo 1994; Wilde 1994).

It has long been recognized that psychological factors are associated with the vulnerability to disease, but correlational data cannot establish causal links. Theories have ranged from generalized models of the stress reaction to specific individual differences in constitutional disposition to maladaptive patterns of autonomic response. All these views may be consistent with homeostatic imbalances, but more recent attention has shifted to the potential health implications of allostatic or allodynamic regulation. It is important to recognize that the mere labelling of a condition as a homeostatic or allodynamic dysfunction contributes

little to scientific understanding. For meaningful progress, the origins, mechanisms and implications of dysfunctions must be clarified. The significance of the constructs of homeostasis, allostasis, and allodynamic regulation lies in the strategic guidance they offer for research efforts as well as in the directions and potential mechanisms upon which they focus.

Psychophysiological Disorders as Specific Homeostatic Dysfunctions

Some researchers have considered psychophysiological disorders as manifestations of constitutional dispositions toward specific patterns of autonomic response to stress. An historical example is the Eppinger and Hess (1915) constitutional model, discussed previously. According to this view, exaggerated activity in one of the autonomic branches can bias toward specific disorders such as asthma (parasympathetic) or Raynaud's disease (sympathetic). Also consistent with this notion of a dispositional bias were reports by Moos and Engel (1962) and Malmo (1975) of exaggerated psychophysiological reactivity appearing specifically in organ systems that evidenced psychosomatic dysfunctions. Hypertensive patients, for example, were reported to respond to stress with exaggerated cardiovascular responses, whereas arthritic patients were more likely to show EMG (electromyographic) abnormalities around affected joints. Although these patterns of psychophysiological response could represent consequences of the specific disorders rather than markers of inherent dispositions, some prospective studies are consistent with the dispositional model. The normotensive offspring of hypertensive parents are at risk for the subsequent development of hypertension, and several studies have reported exaggerated cardiovascular reactivity in these individuals even prior to the development of hypertension (Fredrickson & Matthews 1990; Turner 1994).

Additional support for constitutional contributions to hypertension comes from animal models. The spontaneously hypertensive rat (SHR) and the borderline hypertensive rat (BHR) represent potentially important genetic models of hypertension. It has been shown that SHR and BHR animals display exaggerated cardiovascular reactions to challenge stimuli (Kirby et al. 1989); a regimen of behavioral stress can transform a normotensive BHR into a permanently hypertensive animal (Sanders, Knardahl, & Johnson 1989; Sanders & Lawler 1992); and sympathetic activity appears to contribute importantly to the conditions leading to hypertension in these animals (Korner 1995a). These findings are consistent with a dispositional bias interacting within a stress context. Note that SHR rats (and some hypertensive humans) show a lowered sensitivity of baroreceptor reflexes, which could be interpreted to reflect an underlying homeostatic deficit (Head 1994, 1995; Korner 1995c; Watkins, Grossman, & Sherwood 1996). This is intriguing in view of the fact that behavioral stress, which is known to suppress baroreflexes and increase sympathetic outflow, is able to exacerbate the hypertensive condition in the BHR rat. Although this model of homeostatic dysfunction has appeal, it is incorrect – or at least grossly oversimplified. Baroreflexes can buffer short-term changes in blood pressure, but they do not contribute appreciably to long-term pressor regulation. Consequently, a simple deficit in baroreflex control could well be expected to result in short-term blood pressure variability and lability, but not necessarily hypertension. Baroreceptor damage in humans or sino-aortic denervation in animals manifests primarily in labile rather than chronic hypertension; in fact, basal hypotension may be apparent (Franchini & Krieger 1992; Robertson et al. 1993). Moreover, hypertension-related changes in baroreflex sensitivity may be restored with normalization of blood pressure (Head 1995; Moreira, Ida, & Krieger 1990).

These findings do not rule out the possibility that homeostatic deficits contribute to hypertension. However, the origins of hypertension are complex and diverse, and they include renal, cardiac, vascular, neural, and hormonal factors (Cowley et al. 1992; Korner 1995a,b; Korner & Angus 1992; Marche, Hermbert, & Zhu 1995; Pang, Benishin, & Lewanczuk 1991; Pang et al. 1994; Rettig 1993; Sanders et al. 1989; Yamori 1991). As research continues to unravel the mechanisms and interactions underlying clinical hypertension, homeostatic dysfunctions may well be uncovered. The complexity and interactions of the determinants of hypertension are, however, more in keeping with a model of allodynamic regulation.

Generalized Features of Stress: Allostatic Load

In addition to the multitude of specific regulatory deficits that may underlie stress-related disorders, more generalized features of stress have been recognized. For Cannon (1932) these were related to the generalized activation of the sympathetic nervous system. Selye (1956) further developed the generalized model of stress response, but he shifted the focus from the autonomic nervous system to the pituitary adrenocortical system. In addition to potential specific reactions to stressors, Selye (1956) argued that the stressors in general elevate adrenocorticosteroid hormones, a component of what was termed the general adaptation syndrome (GAS). Selye recognized distinct stages in the response to stress, but these were considered to reflect differences in the magnitude and/or duration rather than in the nature of the stress reaction. In Selye's view, autonomic activation contributes to the initial reaction to stress (the alarm stage), but he viewed the adrenocorticosteroid response as representing the generalized and persistent effect of stress (the resistance stage). Adrenocorticosteroids have widespread effects on insulin release and metabolic processes, muscle contractile strength, psychological states, and immune functions. The corticosteroid response was seen as an adaptive mobilization to counter stress challenges through: (a) syntoxic actions, such as anti-inflammatory effects, that minimize tissue damage; and (b) catatoxic actions that enhance bodily defenses. In the GAS model, if the stress is not adequately resolved then defensive resources are ultimately depleted and the individual becomes increasingly susceptible to disease (exhaustion phase).

The generalized consequences of stressors continue to attract attention. Although the negative effects of stress are often the focus of psychophysiological studies, it is important to recognize that stress reactions can confer positive benefits in dealing with adaptive challenges – they can protect and restore vital functions. The adaptive utility of stress reactions were inherent in Selye's (1973) syntoxic and catatoxic features of the stress response. Moderate early stress has been shown to enhance development and improve vigor of the organism, and under some conditions exposure to moderate stress may immunize against subsequent stress effects (Gandelman 1992; Meaney et al. 1996). Severe and prolonged stress, however, can have negative consequences. McEwen and Steller (1993) argued that specific patterns of stress response may vary considerably across individuals and contexts but also show common allostatic features. In contrast to simple homeostatic systems, which are focused on a single dimension (e.g., blood gasses) and regulated around a fixed set point, allostatic systems entail multiple dimensions and are integrated and orchestrated by central, autonomic, and endocrine processes. Within allostatic systems, functional set points are subject to change, and disturbances in one dimension may lead to compensatory fluctuations in another. McEwen and Stellar (1993) proposed that repeated or prolonged allostatic fluctuations extract a physiological cost, a sort of "wear and tear" that they term *allostatic load*. This allostatic load is seen to be cumulative and to dispose toward stress pathology. One example is the consequences of prolonged stress-related elevations in cortisol and resulting increase in insulin secretion, both of which accelerate atherosclerosis and contribute to hypertension (McEwen & Stellar 1993).

Because glucocorticoids represent a common manifestation of stress, and because they modulate a wide range of functions, they assume special importance in the general consequences of stressors and in allostatic load. Adrenal steroid secretion is under the control of pituitary ACTH, which in turn is regulated by hypothalamic corticotropin releasing hormone (CRH). In addition to its role in adrenocortical control, CRH has been implicated as a trigger of the central stress response (Davis, Walker, & Lee 1997; Dunn & Berridge 1990; Gray 1993; Gray & Bingaman 1996). This entire circuit is regulated by an inhibitory glucocorticoid feedback signal that modulates CRH release. One of the consequences of stress is to allostatically alter the operating level of this system, yielding higher basal levels of CRH and glucocorticoid secretion (for reviews see McEwen 1998; Schulkin, McEwen, & Gold 1994). The hippocampus is an important target site of the glucocorticoids, where binding serves to dampen or shut off stress-related CRH release from the hypothalamus. But repeated stress can trigger atrophy of pyramidal dendrites in the hippocampus (via conjoint actions of glucocorticoids and excitatory amino acids), and severe and prolonged stress can lead to loss of hippocampal neurons (McEwen 1998; Uno et al. 1989). This could lead to higher than normal levels of glucocorticoids during stress (Jacobson & Sapolsky 1991) and impose an increased allostatic load due to impaired feedback regulation; this may further contribute to stress pathology. It has been suggested, for instance, that stress-related hippocampal damage may enhance age-related cognitive decline and underlie posttraumatic stress disorder, both of which are associated with hippocampal atrophy (see McEwen 1998).

Summary. Stress reactions may entail both specific and generalized features arising from homeostatic and allodynamic processes. Consequently, stress-related pathology may not be conceptualized adequately within a restricted homeostatic framework. Stress disorders arising from allodynamic disturbances may have multiple origins in complex interacting systems; disturbances in one domain may manifest in another; and compensatory responses can be orchestrated across several functional domains. Consequently, treatment strategies directed to a single perturbed target dimension (e.g., blood pressure) may not be optimal, since they may simply result in compensatory changes in another dimension that could perpetuate the disturbance. An important issue for future research is the extent to which allostatic "load" represents a truly generalized consequence of stress (e.g., from glucocorticoids) and to what extent it may manifest differentially based on the individual and the stress context.

THE ALLODYNAMIC PERSPECTIVE

Homeostatic processes contribute importantly to adaptive function, but the simple feedback controlled homeostatic model – with its fixed operating set point – does not adequately represent the complexity of psychophysiological regulation. Organ systems are complexly controlled and allodynamically regulated by integrative neural, autonomic, and endocrine systems. Regulatory levels and other operating characteristics are not rigidly fixed; they can be adaptively varied to face existing or anticipated demands. Consequently, the allodynamic model affords a more comprehensive framework for psychophysiology than does the homeostatic construct. As we have considered here, the allodynamic model has substantive implications for psychophysiological measurement, constructs of physiological response, theories of psychophysiological relationships, and strategies of clinical intervention.

The neuropsychophysiological perspective is particularly important in studies of allodynamic regulation and dysregulation, since the links between psychological processes and physiological outcomes may be highly complex and dependent on central integrative systems. Studies of these intervening systems can both inform and be informed by psychophysiological relations. Because mappings between terms and concepts among closely related levels of analysis are likely to be simpler than those between more remote levels, the neuropsychophysiological perspective offers a viable bridging strategy for clarifying psychophysiological relations. This perspective does not challenge the importance of contributions from research limited to the psychological, psychophysiological, or neural levels of analysis; rigorous independent research at each of these levels is crucial. On the other hand, the ultimate development of psychophysiology will be substantially enhanced by meaningful interdisciplinary multilevel analyses.

NOTES

1. Although there are nonlinearities in sympathetic effects expressed either in heart rate or heart period, a linear function provides a reasonably good fit for either metric over typical operating ranges. The much broader dynamic range of the parasympathetic branch can result in far greater biases when chronotropic state is expressed in heart rate (Berntson et al. 1995).

2. Individual sweat glands represent parallel resistance paths across the dermis. Ohm's law and Kirchhoff's rules stipulate that parallel resistances add as to the reciprocal, which is to say that the reciprocals (conductances) add linearly. Thus, a given change in resistance of a set of parallel resistors is linearly related to the overall change in conductance but nonlinearly related to the net change in resistance. Related to nonlinear summation of parallel resistances, resistance measures show greater baseline dependencies than do the conductance measures. An additional consideration is the quantitative relation between the level of sympathetic activity and its effect on sweat gland activity. Lidberg and Wallin (1981) showed a reasonably linear relation between sympathetic activity and skin resistance ($r = 0.77$). Although they did not directly compare resistance to conductance measures, it appears (based on the data presented) that the degree of linearity is approximately equivalent for resistance and conductance measures.

REFERENCES

Aston-Jones, G., Rajkowski, J., Kubiak, P., Valentino, R. J., & Shipley, M. T. (1996). Role of the locus coeruleus in emotional activation. *Progress in Brain Research,* 107, 379–402.

Bachen, E. A., Manuck, S. B., Cohen, S., Muldoon, M. F., Raibel, R., Herbert, T. B., & Rabin, B. S. (1995). Adrenergic blockade ameliorates cellular immune responses to mental stress in humans. *Psychosomatic Medicine,* 57, 366–72.

Bard, P. (1960). Anatomical organization of the central nervous system in relation to control of the heart and blood vessels. *Physiological Review, 40 (Suppl. 4)*, 3–21.

Benschop, R. J., Nieuwenhuis, E. E. S., Tromp, E. A. M., Godart, G. L. R., Ballieux, R. E., & van Doornen, L. P. J. (1994). Effects of β-adrenergic blockade on immunologic and cardiovascular changes induced by mental stress. *Circulation, 89,* 762–9.

Bernard, C. (1878/1974). Leçons sur les phénomènes de la vie communes aux animaux et aux végétaux. Paris: B. Baillière et Fils [Lectures on the phenomena of life common to animals and plants] (Translated by H. E. Hoff, R. Guillemin, & L. Guillemin). Springfield, IL: Thomas.

Berntson, G. G., & Boysen, S. T. (1990). Cardiac indices of cognition in infants, children and chimpanzees. In C. Rovee-Collier & L. Lipsitt (Eds.), *Advances in Infancy Research,* vol. 6, pp. 187–220. New York: Ablex.

Berntson, G. G., Cacioppo, J. T., Binkley, P. F., Uchino, B. N., Quigley, K. S., & Fieldstone, A. (1994a). Autonomic cardiac control: III. Psychological stress and cardiac response in autonomic space as revealed by pharmacological blockades. *Psychophysiology, 31,* 599–608.

Berntson, G. G., Cacioppo, J. T., & Quigley, K. S. (1991). Autonomic determinism: The modes of autonomic control, the doctrine of autonomic space, and the laws of autonomic constraint. *Psychological Review, 98,* 459–87.

Berntson, G. G., Cacioppo, J. T., & Quigley, K. S. (1993). Cardiac psychophysiology and autonomic space in humans: Empirical perspectives and conceptual implications. *Psychological Bulletin, 114,* 296–322.

Berntson, G. G., Cacioppo, J. T., & Quigley, K. S. (1995). The metrics of cardiac chronotropism: Biometric perspectives. *Psychophysiology, 32,* 162–71.

Berntson, G. G., Cacioppo, J. T., Quigley, K. S., & Fabro, V. J. (1994b). Autonomic space and psychophysiological response. *Psychophysiology, 31,* 44–61.

Berntson, G. G., Sarter, M., & Cacioppo, J. T. (1998). Anxiety and cardiovascular reactivity: The basal forebrain cholinergic link. *Behavioural Brain Research, 94,* 225–48.

Blessing, W. W. (1997). *The Lower Brainstem and Bodily Homeostasis.* New York: Oxford University Press.

Bradley, P. B., & Elkes, J. (1958). The effect of atropine, hyoseyamine, physostigmine, and neostigmine on the electrical activity of the brain of the conscious cat. *Journal of Physiology (London), 120,* 14.

Buchanan, S. L., Thompson, R. H., Maxwell, B. L., & Powell, D. A. (1994). Efferent connections of the medial prefrontal cortex in the rabbit. *Experimental Brain Research, 100,* 469–83.

Cacioppo, J. T. (1994). Social neuroscience: Autonomic, neuroendocrine, and immune responses to stress. *Psychophysiology, 31,* 113–28.

Cacioppo, J. T., & Berntson, G. G. (1992a). Social psychological contributions to the decade of the brain: Doctrine of multilevel analysis. *American Psychologist, 47,* 1019–28.

Cacioppo, J. T., & Berntson, G. G. (1992b). The principles of multiple, nonadditive and reciprocal determinism: Implications for social psychological research and levels of analysis. In D. N. Ruble, P. R. Costanzo, & M. E. Oliveri (Eds.), *The Social Psychology of Mental Health: Basic Mechanisms and Applications,* pp. 328–49. New York: Guilford.

Cacioppo, J. T., Berntson, G. G., Binkley, P. F., Quigley, K. S., Uchino, B. N., & Fieldstone, A. (1994). Autonomic cardiac control. II. Basal response, noninvasive indices, and autonomic space as revealed by autonomic blockades. *Psychophysiology, 31,* 586–98.

Cacioppo, J. T., Berntson, G. G., & Klein, D. J. (1992a). What is an emotion? The role of somatovisceral afference, with special emphasis on somatovisceral "illusions." *Review of Personality and Social Psychology, 14,* 63–98.

Cacioppo, J. T., Crites, S. L., & Gardner, W. L. (1996). Attitudes on the right: Evaluative processing is associated with lateralized late positive event-related brain potentials. *Personality and Social Psychology Bulletin, 22,* 1205–19.

Cacioppo, J. T., Malarkey, W. B., Kiecolt-Glaser, J. K., Uchino, B. N., Sgoutas-Emch, S. A., Sheridan, J. F., Berntson, G. G., & Glaser, R. (1995). Heterogeneity in neuroendocrine and immune responses to brief psychological stressors as a function of autonomic cardiac activation. *Psychosomatic Medicine, 57,* 154–64.

Cacioppo, J. C., & Tassinary, L. G. (1990). Inferring psychological significance from physiological signals. *American Psychologist, 45,* 16–28.

Cacioppo, J. T., Uchino, B. N., Crites, S. L., Snydersmith, M. A., Smith, G., Berntson, G. G., & Lang, P. J. (1992b). The relationship between facial expressiveness and sympathetic activation in emotion: A critical review, with emphasis on modeling underlying mechanisms and individual differences. *Journal of Personality and Social Psychology, 62,* 110–28.

Cannon, W. B. (1928). The mechanism of emotional disturbance of bodily functions. *New England Journal of Medicine, 198,* 877–84.

Cannon, W. B. (1929). Organization for physiological homeostasis. *Physiological Reviews, 9,* 399–431.

Cannon, W. B. (1932). *The Wisdom of the Body.* New York: Norton.

Cannon, W. B. (1939). *The Wisdom of the Body,* 2nd ed. London: Kegan Paul, Trench, Trubner.

Cechetto, D. F., & Saper, C. B. (1990). Role of the cerebral cortex in autonomic function. In Loewy & Spyer, pp. 208–33.

Chwalisz, K., Diener, E., & Gallagher, D. (1988). Autonomic arousal feedback and emotional experience: Evidence from the spinal cord injured. *Journal of Personality and Social Psychology, 54,* 820–8.

Cofer, C. N., & Appley, M. H. (1964). *Motivation: Theory and Research.* New York: Wiley.

Cowley, A. W., Roman, R. J., Fenoy, F. J., & Mattson, D. L. (1992). Effects of renal medullary circulation on arterial pressure. *Journal of Hypertension 10 (Suppl.),* S187–S193.

Danielsen, E. H., Magnuson, D. J., & Gray, T. S. (1989). The central amygdaloid nucleus innervation of the dorsal vagal complex in rat: A Phaseolus vulgaris leucoagglutinin lectin anterograde tracing study. *Brain Research Bulletin, 22,* 705–15.

Davis, M., Walker, D. L., & Lee, Y. (1997). Roles of the amygdala and the bed nucleus of the stria terminalis in fear and anxiety measured with the acoustic startle reflex. Possible relevance to PTSD. *Annals of the New York Academy of Sciences, 821,* 305–31.

Ditto, B., & France, C. (1990). Carotid baroreflex sensitivity at rest and during psychological stress in offspring of hypertensives and non-twin sibling pairs. *Psychosomatic Medicine, 52,* 610–20.

Duffy, E. (1957). The psychological significance of the concept of "arousal" or "activation." *Psychological Review, 64,* 265–75.

Dunn, A. J., & Berridge, C. W. (1990). Physiological and behavioral responses to corticotropin-releasing factor administration: Is CRF a mediator of anxiety or stress responses. *Brain Research Reviews, 15,* 71–100.

Dworkin, B. R. (1993). *Learning and Physiological Regulation.* University of Chicago Press.

Dworkin, B. R., & Dworkin, S. (1990). Learning of physiological responses: I. Habituation, sensitization, and classical conditioning. *Behavioral Neuroscience, 104,* 298–319.

Dworkin, B. R., Elbert, T., Rau, H., Birbaumer, N., Pauli, P., Droste, C., & Brunia, C. H. (1994). Central effects of baroreceptor activation in humans: Attenuation of skeletal reflexes and pain perceptions. *Proceedings of the National Academy of Sciences U.S.A., 91,* 6329–33.

Elam, M., Svensson, T. H., & Thoren, P. (1974). Differentiated cardiovascular afferent regulation of locus coeruleus neurons and sympathetic nerves. *Brain Research, 358,* 77–84.

Eppinger, H., & Hess, L. (1915). *Vagotonia: A Clinical Study in Vegetative Neurology* (Translated by W. M. Kraus & S. E. Jelliffe). New York: Nervous & Mental Disease Publishing.

Feldman, S. M., & Waller, H. J. (1962). Dissociation of electrocortical activation and behavioral arousal. *Nature, 196,* 1320–2.

Franchini, K. G., & Krieger, E. M. (1992). Carotid chemoreceptors influence arterial pressure in intact and aortic-denervated rats. *American Journal of Physiology, 262,* R677–R683.

Fredrickson, M., & Matthews, K. A. (1990). Cardiovascular responses to behavioral stress and hypertension: A meta-analytic review. *Annals of Behavioral Medicine, 12,* 30–9.

Fulton, J. F. (1949). *Textbook of Physiology,* 16th ed. Philadelphia: Saunders.

Gandelman, R. (1992). *The Psychobiology of Behavioral Development.* New York: Oxford University Press.

Gebber, G. L. (1990). Central determinants of sympathetic nerve discharge. In Loewy & Spyer, pp. 126–44.

Gelsema, A. J., Agarwal, S. K., & Calaresu, F. R. (1989). Cardiovascular responses and changes in neural activity in the rostral ventrolateral medulla elicited by electrical stimulation of the amygdala of the rat. *Journal of the Autonomic Nervous System, 27,* 91–100.

Gray, J. A., & McNaughton, N. (1996). The neuropsychology of anxiety: Reprise. *Nebraska Symposium on Motivation, 43,* 61–134.

Gray, T. S. (1993). Amygdaloid CRF pathways. Role in autonomic, neuroendocrine, and behavioral responses to stress. *Annals of the New York Academy of Sciences, 697,* 53–60.

Gray, T. S., & Bingaman, E. W. (1996). The amygdala: Corticotropin-releasing factor, steroids, and stress. *Critical Reviews in Neurobiology, 10,* 155–68.

Grossman, P., & Kollai, M. (1993). Respiratory sinus arrhythmia, cardiac vagal tone, and respiration: Within- and between-individual relations. *Psychophysiology, 30,* 486–95.

Guyenet, P. G. (1990). Role of the ventral medulla oblongata in blood pressure regulation. In Loewy & Spyer, pp. 134–67.

Guyton, A. C. (1991). Blood-pressure control – Special role of the kidneys and body fluids. *Science, 252,* 1813–16.

Head, G. A. (1994). Cardiac baroreflexes and hypertension. *Clinical and Experimental Pharmacology and Physiology, 21,* 791–802.

Head, G. A. (1995). Baroreflexes and cardiovascular regulation in hypertension. *Journal of Cardiovascular Pharmacology, 26,* S7–S16.

Hebb, D. O. (1955). Drives and the CNS (conceptual nervous system). *Psychological Review, 62,* 243–54.

Herbert, T. B., Cohen, S., Marsland, A. L., Bachen, E. A., Rabin, B. S., Muldoon, M. F., & Manuck, S. B. (1994). Cardiovascular reactivity and the course of immune response to an acute psychological stressor. *Psychosomatic Medicine, 56,* 337–44.

Hillyard, S. A., Mangun, G. R., Woldorff, M. G., & Luck, S. J. (1995). Neural systems mediating selective attention. In M. S. Gazzaniga (Ed.), *The Cognitive Neurosciences,* pp. 665–81. Cambridge, MA: MIT Press.

Holmes, T. H., & Ripley, H. S. (1955). Experimental studies on anxiety reactions. *American Journal of Psychiatry, 111,* 921–9.

Hurley, K. M., Herbert, H., Moga, M. M., & Saper, C. B. (1991). Efferent projections of the infralimbic cortex of the rat. *Journal of Comparative Neurology, 308,* 249–76.

Inui, K., Murase, S., & Nosaka, S. (1994). Facilitation of the arterial baroreflex by the ventrolateral part of the midbrain periaqueductal grey matter in rats. *Journal of Physiology, 477,* 89–101.

Inui, K., Nomura, J., Murase, S., & Nosaka, S. (1995). Facilitation of the arterial baroreflex by the preoptic area in anaesthetized rats. *Journal of Physiology, 488,* 521–31.

Iwata, J., & LeDoux, J. E. (1988). Dissociation of associative and nonassociative concomitants of classical fear conditioning in the freely behaving rat. *Behavioral Neuroscience, 102,* 66–76.

Jacobson, L., & Sapolsky, R. (1991). The role of the hippocampus in feedback regulation of the hypothalamic-pituitary-adrenocortical axis. *Endocrine Review, 12,* 118–34.

James, W. (1884). What is an emotion? *Mind, 9,* 188–205.

Janssen, B. J., Tyssen, C. M., Struijker Boudier, H. A., & Hutchins, P. M. (1992). 24-hour homeodynamic states of arterial blood pressure and pulse interval in conscious rats. *Journal of Applied Physiology, 73,* 754–61.

Johnson, E. O., Kamilaris, T. C., Chrousos, G. P., & Gold, P. W. (1992). Mechanisms of stress: A dynamic overview of hormonal and behavioral homeostasis. *Neuroscience and Biobehavioral Reviews, 16,* 115–30.

Jordan, D. (1990). Autonomic changes in affective behavior. In Loewy & Spyer, pp. 349–66.

Kandel, E. R., Schwartz, J. H., & Jessell, T. M. (1991). *Principles of Neural Science,* 3rd ed. Norwalk, CT: Appleton & Lange.

Kirby, R. F., Callahan, M. F., McCarty, R., & Johnson, A. K. (1989). Cardiovascular and sympathetic nervous system responses to an acute stressor in borderline hypertensive rats (BHR). *Physiology and Behavior, 46,* 309–13.

Koizumi, K., & Kollai, M. (1981). Control of reciprocal and non-reciprocal action of vagal and sympathetic efferents: Study of centrally induced reactions. *Journal of the Autonomic Nervous System, 3,* 483–501.

Koizumi, K., & Kollai, M. (1992). Multiple modes of operation of cardiac autonomic control: Development of the ideas from

Cannon and Brooks to the present. *Journal of the Autonomic Nervous System, 41,* 19–30.

Korner, P. I. (1995a). Cardiovascular hypertrophy and hypertension: Causes and consequences. *Blood Pressure 2 (Suppl.),* 6–16.

Korner, P. I. (1995b). Circulatory control and the supercontrollers. *Journal of Hypertension, 13,* 1508–21.

Korner, P. I. (1995c). Cardiac baroreflex in hypertension: Role of the heart and angiotensin II. *Clinical and Experimental Hypertension, 17,* 425–39.

Korner, P. I., & Angus, J. J. (1992). Structural determinants of vascular resistance properties in hypertension. Haemodynamic and model analysis. *Journal of Vascular Research, 29,* 293–312.

Lacey, J. I. (1956). The evaluation of autonomic responses: Toward a general solution. *Annals of the New York Academy of Sciences, 67,* 123–64.

Lacey, J. I. (1959). Psychophysiological approaches to the evaluation of psychotherapeutic process and outcome. In E. A. Rubinstein & M. B. Parloff (Eds.), *Research in Psychotherapy,* pp. 160–208. Washington, DC: APA.

Lacey, J. I. (1967). Somatic response patterning and stress: Some revisions of activation theory. In M. H. Appley & R. Trumbull (Eds.), *Psychological Stress: Issues in Research,* pp. 4–44. New York: Appleton-Century-Crofts.

Lacey, J. I., Kagan, J., Lacey, B. C., & Moss, H. A. (1963). The visceral level: Situational determinants and behavioral correlates of autonomic response patterns. In P. H. Knapp (Ed.), *Expression of Emotions in Man,* pp. 161–96. New York: International University Press.

Lawler, J. E., Sanders, B. J., Cox, R. H., & O'Connor, E. F. (1991). Baroreflex function in chronically stressed borderline hypertensive rats. *Physiology and Behavior, 49,* 539–42.

Lewis, S. J., Verberne, A. J. M., Robinson, T. G., Jarrott, B., Louis, W. J., & Beart, P. M. (1989). Excitotoxin-induced lesions of the central but not basolateral nucleus of the amygdala modulate the baroreceptor heart rate reflex in conscious rats. *Brain Research, 494,* 232–40.

Lidberg, L., & Wallin, B. G. (1981). Sympathetic skin nerve discharges in relation to amplitude of skin resistance responses. *Psychophysiology, 18,* 268–71.

Loewy, A. D. (1990). Autonomic control of the eye. In Loewy & Spyer, pp. 268–85.

Loewy, A. D., & Spyer, K. M. (Eds.) (1990). *Central Regulation of Autonomic Function.* New York: Oxford University Press.

Luiten, P. G., ter Horst, G. J., Karst, H., & Steffens, A. B. (1985). The course of paraventricular hypothalamic efferents to autonomic structures in medulla and spinal cord. *Brain Research, 329,* 374–8.

Lundin, S., Ricksten, S.-E., & Thoren, P. (1984). Interaction between "mental stress" and baroreceptor reflexes concerning effects on heart rate, mean arterial pressure and renal sympathetic activity in conscious spontaneously hypertensive rats. *Acta Physiologica Scandinavica, 120,* 273–81.

Magoun, H. W. (1963). *The Waking Brain.* Springfield, IL: Thomas.

Maier, S. F., Watkins, L. R., & Fleshner, M. (1994). Psychoneuroimmunology: The interface between behavior, brain, and immunity. *American Psychologist, 49,* 1004–17.

Malmo, R. T. (1975). *On Emotions, Needs, and Our Archaic Brain.* New York: Holt, Rinehart & Winston.

Manuck, S. B., Cohen, S., Rabin, B. S., Muldoon, M. F., & Bachen, E. A. (1991). Individual differences in cellular immune response to stress. *Psychological Science, 2,* 111–15.

Marche, P., Hermbert, T., & Zhu, D. L. (1995). Molecular mechanisms of vascular hypertrophy in the spontaneously hypertensive rat. *Clinical and Experimental Pharmacology and Physiology 1 (Suppl.),* S114–S116.

Martin, C. E., Haver, J. A., Leon, D. F., Thompson, M. E., Reddy, P. S., & Leonard, J. L. (1974). Autonomic mechanisms in hemodynamic responses to isometric exercise. *Journal of Clinical Investigation, 54,* 104–15.

McEwen, B. (1998). Protective and damaging effects of stress mediators: Allostasis and allostatic load. *New England Journal of Medicine, 338,* 171–9.

McEwen, B. S., & Stellar, E. (1993). Stress and the individual: Mechanisms leading to disease. *Archives of Internal Medicine, 153,* 2093–2101.

McGaugh, J. L., Cahill, L., & Roozendaal, B. (1996). Involvement of the amygdala in memory storage: Interaction with other brain systems. *Proceedings of the National Academy of Sciences U.S.A., 93,* 13508–14.

Meaney, M. J., Diorio, J., Francis, D., Widdowson, J., LaPlante, P., Caldji, C., Sharma, S., Seckl, J. R., & Plotsky, P. M. (1996). Early environmental regulation of forebrain glucocorticoid receptor gene expression: Implications for adrenocortical responses to stress. *Developmental Neuroscience, 18,* 49–72.

Montagu, J. D., & Coles, E. M. (1966). Mechanisms and measurement of the galvanic skin response. *Psychological Bulletin, 65,* 261–79.

Moos, R. H., & Engle, B. T. (1962). Psychophysiological reactions in hypertensive and arthritic patients. *Journal of Psychosomatic Medicine, 6,* 227–42.

Moreira, E. D., Ida, F., & Krieger, E. M. (1990). Reversibility of baroreceptor hyposensitivity during reversal of hypertension. *Hypertension, 15,* 791–6.

Nakata, T., Berard, W., Kogosov, E., & Alexander, N. (1991). Effects of environmental stress on release of norepinephrine in posterior nucleus of the hypothalamus in awake rats: Role of sinoaortic nerves. *Life Science, 48,* 2021–6.

Neafsey, E. J. (1990). Prefrontal cortical control of the autonomic nervous system: Anatomical and physiological observations. *Progress in Brain Research, 85,* 147–66.

Nogueira, P. J., Tomaz, C., & Williams, C. L. (1994). Contribution of the vagus nerve in mediating the memory-facilitating effects of substance P. *Behavioural Brain Research, 62,* 165–9.

Nosaka, S., Nakase, N., & Murata, K. (1989). Somatosensory and hypothalamic inhibitions of baroreflex vagal bradycardia in rats. *Pflügers Archiv, 413,* 656–66.

Obrist, P. A., (1981). *Cardiovascular Psychophysiology: A Perspective.* New York: Plenum.

Obrist, P. A., Webb, R. A., Sutterer, J. R., & Howard, J. L. (1970). The cardiac-somatic relationship: Some reformulations. *Psychophysiology, 6,* 569–87.

Oppenheimer, S. M., & Cechetto, D. F. (1990). Cardiac chronotropic organization of the rat insular cortex. *Brain Research, 533,* 66–72.

Pang, P. K., Benishin, C. G., & Lewanczuk, R. Z. (1991). Parathyroid hypertensive factor, a circulating factor in animal and human hypertension. *American Journal of Hypertension, 4*, 472–7.

Pang, P. K., Benishin, C. G., Shan, J., & Lewanczuk, R. Z. (1994). PHF: The new parathyroid hypertensive factor. *Blood Pressure, 3*, 148–55.

Pascoe, J. P., Bradley, D. J., & Spyer, K. M. (1989). Interactive responses to stimulation of the amygdaloid central nucleus and baroreceptor afferent activation in the rabbit. *Journal of the Autonomic Nervous System, 26*, 157–67.

Pollack, M. H., & Obrist, P. A. (1988). Effects of autonomic blockade on heart rate responses to reaction time and sustained handgrip tasks. *Psychophysiology, 25*, 689–95.

Powell, D. A., Goldberg, S. R., Dauth, G. W., Schneiderman, E., & Schneiderman, N. (1972). Adrenergic and cholinergic blockade of cardiovascular responses to subcortical electrical stimulation in unanesthetized rabbits. *Physiology and Behavior, 8*, 927–36.

Randich, A., & Gebhart, G. F. (1992). Vagal afferent modulation of nociception. *Brain Research Reviews, 17*, 77–99.

Reisenzein, R. (1983). The Schachter theory of emotion: Two decades later. *Psychological Bulletin, 94*, 239–64.

Rettig, R. (1993). Does the kidney play a role in the aetiology of primary hypertension? Evidence from renal transplantation studies in rats and humans. *Journal of Human Hypertension, 7*, 177–80.

Robbins, T. W., & Everitt, B. J. (1995). Arousal systems and attention. In M. S. Gazzaniga (Ed.), *The Cognitive Neurosciences*, pp. 703–29. Cambridge, MA: MIT Press.

Robertson, D., Hollister, A. S., Biaggioni, I., Netterville, J. L., Mosqueda-Garcia, R., & Robertson, R. M. (1993). The diagnosis and treatment of baroreflex failure. *New England Journal of Medicine, 329*, 1449–55.

Robinson, B. F., Epstein, S. E., Beiser, G. D., & Braunwald, E. (1966). Control of heart rate by the autonomic nervous system. *Circulation Research, 14*, 400–11.

Rowell, L. B. (1986). *Human Circulation Regulation during Physical Stress.* New York: Oxford University Press.

Sanders, B. J., Knardahl, S., & Johnson, A. K. (1989). Lesions of the anteroventral third ventricle and the development of stress-induced hypertension in the borderline hypertensive rat. *Hypertension, 13*, 817–21.

Sanders, B. J., & Lawler, J. E. (1992). The borderline hypertensive rat (BHR) as a model for environmentally induced hypertension: A review and update. *Neuroscience and Biobehavioral Reviews, 16*, 207–17.

Sarter, M. (1994). Neuronal mechanisms of the attentional dysfunctions in senile dementia and schizophrenia: Two sides of the same coin? *Psychopharmacology, 114*, 539–50.

Sarter, M., & Bruno, J. P. (1997). Cognitive functions of cortical acetylcholine: Toward a unifying hypothesis. *Brain Research Reviews, 23*, 28–46.

Schachter, S., & Singer, J. E. (1962). Cognitive, social, and physiological determinants of emotional state. *Psychological Review, 69*, 379–99.

Schulkin, J., McEwen, B. S., & Gold, P. W. (1994). Allostasis, amygdala, and anticipatory angst. *Neuroscience and Biobehavioral Reviews, 18*, 385–96.

Schwaber, J. S., Kapp, B. S., Higgins, G. A., & Rapp, P. R. (1982). Amygdaloid and basal forebrain direct connections with the nucleus of the solitary tract and the dorsal motor nucleus. *Journal of Neuroscience, 10*, 1424–38.

Selye, H. (1956). *The Stress of Life.* New York: McGraw-Hill.

Selye, H. (1973). Homeostasis and heterostasis. *Perspectives in Biology and Medicine, 16*, 441–5.

Sgoutas-Emch, S. A., Cacioppo, J. T., Uchino, B. N., Malarkey, W., Pearl, D., Kiecolt-Glaser, J. K., & Glaser, R. (1994). The effects of an acute psychological stressor on cardiovascular, endocrine, and cellular immune response: A perspective study of individuals high and low in heart rate reactivity. *Psychophysiology, 31*, 264–71.

Shih, C. D., Chan, S. H., & Chan, J. Y. (1995). Participation of hypothalamic paraventricular nucleus in the locus coeruleus-induced baroreflex suppression in rats. *American Journal of Physiology, 269*, H46–H52.

Sokolov, E. N. (1963). *Perception and the Conditioned Reflex.* New York: Macmillan.

Spyer, K. M. (1989). Neural mechanisms involved in cardiovascular control during affective behavior. *Trends in Neuroscience, 12*, 506–13.

Spyer, K. M. (1990). The central nervous organization of reflex circulatory control. In Loewy & Spyer, pp. 1168–88.

Stephenson, R. B., Smith, O. A., & Scher, A. M. (1981). Baroreflex regulation of heart rate in baboons during different behavioral states. *American Journal of Physiology, 241*, 277–85.

Steptoe, A., & Sawada, Y. (1989). Assessment of baroreceptor reflex function during mental stress and relaxation. *Psychophysiology, 26*, 140–7.

Sterling, P., & Eyer, J. (1988). Allostasis: A new paradigm to explain arousal pathology. In S. Fisher & J. Reason (Eds.), *Handbook of Life Stress, Cognition and Health*, pp. 629–49. New York: Wiley.

Stitt, J. T. (1979). Fever versus hyperthermia. *Federation Proceedings, 38*, 39–43.

Turner, J. R. (1994). *Cardiovascular Reactivity and Stress.* New York: Plenum.

Uno, H., Tarara, R., Else, J. G., Suleman, M. A., & Sapolsky, R. M. (1989). Hippocampal damage associated with prolonged and fatal stress in primates. *Journal of Neuroscience, 9*, 1705–11.

van Hooff, J. A. R. A. M., & Filipo, A. (1994). Social homeostasis and the regulation of emotion. In S. H. M. van Goozen, N. E. Van de Poll, & J. A. Sergeant (Eds.), *Emotions: Essays on Emotion Theory*, pp. 197–217. Hillsdale, NJ: Erlbaum.

Venables, P. H., & Christie, M. J. (1980). Electrodermal activity. In I. Martin & P. H. Venables (Eds.), *Techniques in Psychophysiology*, pp. 3–67. Chichester, U.K.: Wiley.

Wallace, D. M., Magnuson, D. J., & Gray, T. S. (1992). Organization of amygdaloid projections to brainstem dopaminergic, noradrenergic, and adrenergic cell groups in the rat. *Brain Research Bulletin, 28*, 447–54.

Watkins, L., Grossman, P., & Sherwood, A. (1996). Noninvasive assessment of baroreflex control in borderline hypertension: Comparison with the phenylephrine method. *Hypertension, 28*, 238–43.

Watkins, L. R., Maier, S. F., & Goehler, L. E. (1995). Immune activation: The role of pro-inflammatory cytokines in inflammation, illness responses and pathological pain states. *Pain, 63*, 289–302.

Wenger, M. A. (1941). The measurement of individual differences in autonomic balance. *Psychosomatic Medicine, 3,* 427–34.

Werner, J. (1988). Functional mechanisms of temperature regulation, adaptation and fever: Complementary system theoretical and experimental evidence. *Pharmacology and Therapeutics, 37,* 1–23.

Wilde, G. J. S. (1994). *Target Risk: Dealing with the Danger of Death, Disease and Damage in Everyday Decisions.* Toronto: Castor & Columba.

Williams, C. L., & McGaugh, J. L. (1993). Reversible lesions of the nucleus of the solitary tract attenuate the memory-modulating effects of posttraining epinephrine. *Behavioral Neuroscience, 107,* 955–62.

Yamori, Y. (1991). Overview: Studies on spontaneous hypertension-development from animal models toward man. *Clinical and Experimental Hypertension A, 13,* 631–44.

Zardetto-Smith, A. M., & Gray, T. S. (1995). Catecholamine and NPY efferents from the ventrolateral medulla to the amygdala in the rat. *Brain Research Bulletin, 38,* 253–60.

CHAPTER EIGHTEEN

INTEROCEPTION

B. R. DWORKIN

The focus of this chapter is the basic physiological properties of those sensory receptors that monitor the internal state of the body as well as the methods used to study them. Its content is intended to provide an appreciation of the range of biological phenomena that involve interoceptors, to explain the goals and procedures of interoception research, and to offer to researchers some practical suggestions and theoretical guidelines for interoception experiments.[1] The scope of the chapter is well characterized in the following quotation from an 1894 lecture by Pavlov.

In view of the importance of the subject, the greatest handicap should be considered the extremely scanty study of the action of various substances upon the peripheral endings of centripetal nerves. It is evident that in the life of a complex organism the reflex is the most essential and frequent neural phenomenon. With its help a constant, correct, and precise correlation becomes established among the parts of an organism, and among the relationships between the organism as a whole and the surrounding conditions. And the starting point of the reflex is the irritation of the peripheral endings of centripetal nerves. These endings pervade all organs and all tissues. These endings must be visualized as extremely diverse, specific ones, each individually adapted, like the nerve endings of sense organs, to its own specific irritant of mechanical, physical, or chemical nature. Their effectiveness determines at each given moment the magnitude of, and fluctuations in, the activity of the organism. Hence it is clear that many substances, when introduced into the organism, disturb its equilibrium as a result of their interaction, in one form or another, with the peripheral endings which are predominantly sensitive and in readily responsive parts of the animal body. (1940, p. 142)

Sensory Receptors

There are three generally recognized classes of sensory transducers.

1. *Exteroceptors* – such as the photoreceptors of the eye, the hair cells of the cochlea, or the mechanoreceptors of the skin. These are located at or near the body surface and are the basis of exteroception, the perception of mechanical and electromagnetic energy fields in surrounding space.
2. *Proprioceptors* – such as skeletal muscle spindles, Golgi tendon organs, and joint strain receptors. These sense the velocity, orientation, and mechanical tension of the skeleton. They are the basis of proprioception, the perception of the orientation and action of the body in space.
3. *Interoceptors* – such as mechano-, thermo-, and chemo-receptors of the gut; stretch receptors of the atria, carotid arteries, and aorta; chemoreceptors of the carotid sinus; lipid receptors in the portal circulation; and metaboreceptors in the skeletal muscles. These are situated within the body cavities and are the basis of elementary reflexes and of *interoception:* the central neural representation of the blood vessels and visceral organs.

Among the receptors, the first two classes are most readily accessible to stimulation and electrophysiological recording. As a consequence, their microanatomy and biophysical transduction mechanisms are well described, and (to a large extent) their modal selectivity, dynamic response characteristics, and central connections have been analyzed. In contrast, the receptive field, generator structure, and pseudo-dendrite of a typical interoceptor are deep within a body cavity and comparatively inaccessible.

To apply accurate stimuli and to record from an interoceptor's small and often unmyelinated fiber can be quite difficult. Thus, largely because of their inaccessible locations, the detailed properties of interoceptors are less completely known than those of exteroceptors and proprioceptors. Yet anatomically, nearly 90% of the fibers of

John T. Cacioppo, Louis G. Tassinary, and Gary G. Berntson (Eds.), *Handbook of Psychophysiology,* 2nd ed. © Cambridge University Press 2000. Printed in the United States of America. ISBN 62634X. All rights reserved.

the vagus and more than 50% of the fibers of all autonomic nerves are afferent (Norgren 1985, p. 145), and these fibers are thought to convey extensive information from interoceptors to the brain. Functionally, interoceptors are the sensory radix of the elaborate vegetative infrastructure, underpinning and enabling the complex activities of higher animals.

Taxonomy of Interoceptors

The term "interoceptors" includes visceral receptors and more. "Visceral" is from "viscus," meaning an internal organ of the body – especially one (as the heart, liver, or intestine) located in the great cavities of the trunk. For example, the entire small intestine is considered visceral whereas the skeletal muscles are not. Thus defined, the stretch receptors of the gut are all interoceptors, whereas the nearly homologous spindles (which regulate the mechanical function of the skeletal muscles) are not. The spindles and other skeletal mechanoreceptors are instead called proprioceptors. This distinction is logically consistent and reasonably clear. However, adjacent to proprioceptors, the skeletal muscles have other receptors that respond to the metabolic state of the muscle tissue itself. These metaboreceptors fire with elevated lactic acid and diprotonated phosphate ($H_2PO_4^-$) concentrations in the surrounding tissue. Their activation augments muscle sympathetic nerve activity and partially opposes the local vasodilatory effects of metabolic products; thus, they regulate the circulation and ensure that each muscle receives the cardiac output fraction that fits its activity. Metaboreceptors are neither proprioceptors or exteroceptors; they have many properties in common with interoceptors, but are not part of the "viscera" by the usual definition.

The metaboreceptor example points up that, in addition to its anatomy, the receptor's function also must be accounted into the taxonomy. In general, within an organ or tissue there are: (1) those sensory elements that serve a special host organ function – such as photoreceptors of the eye, the hair cells of the cochlea, the spindles of the skeletal muscles, or the stretch and mucosal chemoreceptors of the intestine; and (2) those that subserve more general tissue maintenance functions, as do the various metaboreceptors. Hence, a distinction can be appropriately drawn between receptors serving vegetative and those serving special organ functions.

Thus, to be complete, interoceptors should include all sensory receptors in visceral organs plus other receptors (wherever located) that subserve local tissue metabolic functions. In addition, it is necessary to consider separately certain other cases where the anatomical position of a sensory ending and its effective receptive field do not obviously coincide. For example, some stretch receptors in the mesentery are activated with strong contraction of the muscular layers of adjacent intestine. Although these are indisputably interoceptors and their function seems obvious, there are other more subtle or ambiguous cases. For example, the conscious perception of the heart beat, particularly in arrhythmia, depends (at least in part) on receptors situated in the chest wall and/or overlying skin.[2] Because their receptive field includes visceral structures, should these striate muscle and/or cutaneous receptors appropriately be considered as interoceptors? The general answer probably is No, but in a specific case it may depend on the implications that are to be drawn from the observed effects. (And suppose, for argument, that the receptors in question were located on the pleural membrane instead of the chest wall; would their classification be the same?)

Finally, certain authors have objected to the tacit identification of sensory receptors with one or the other branches of the autonomic nervous system (Jänig & Häbler 1995). This concern is appropriate, and it should be further noted that the peripheral nervous pathway of a receptor cell's afferent process is not always a reliable basis for characterizing a receptor or receptor population. For example, the vagus is mostly composed of visceral afferents yet the vagus is not, in fact, a pure visceral nerve. Fibers from the larynx (via the recurrent laryngeal nerve) enter the vagus at the aortic arch and thence course the full extent of the cervical vagus. Some of these fibers are afferent and project to striate muscle spindles. In addition to these somatic proprioceptive afferents, the vagus also contains a population of general cutaneous sensory fibers derived from its auricular ramus (Brodal 1969, pp. 366–7). Thus, electrical stimulation of the cervical vagus can not be assumed to emulate a pure visceral afferent effect, and electrical activity that is recorded from the vagus may be partially somatic.

In biology, we classify things so that we can make observations on a few members of a class; we then use the result to make useful inferences to the other members of the same class. Definitions, as such, constrain conclusions. If a question concerns, for example, specific hemodynamic effects of low pressure atrial baroreceptors, then the receptor population for study can be readily defined in terms of physiological and anatomical criteria, and the conclusions can be confidently applied back to the appropriate population. However, when more general questions are addressed (e.g., "Is there conscious perception of moderate intestinal dilation?"), the defining criteria become more arguable.

More important than post hoc justification of inferences, definitions guide the design of a convincing experiment. For example, an intestinal perception hypothesis could be tested by applying a signal detection procedure to a balloon in the lumen. But in parts of the intestine, in addition to the stretch receptors of the gut wall, balloon inflation might also distend the overlying abdominal skin. Suppose, in such an experiment, that detection is found to be reliable but that activation of the skin receptors has not been ruled out as a source of the sensory input. Is it then reasonable to infer that, in general, intestinal dilation can be perceived? Probably not, but *why* not? The ready answer is: Because the sensation is obviously from the skin, not the intestine! But then, why are skin receptors not considered to be a legitimate source of visceral sensory input?

To overcome the limitation (on the useful inference class), the intestinal perception experiment would need to incorporate appropriate controls. These could be achieved in two ways: (1) with a differential experiment in which the skin artifact is deliberately included in both the control and experimental stimulations; or (2) by refining the intra-luminal stimulation technique to entirely exclude any skin artifact. In an animal study, inflation of an intraluminal balloon could be compared to "control" inflation of an adjacent extraluminal balloon. The control inflation would stimulate the skin but not the luminal stretch receptors; the intraluminal inflation would stimulate both; and the difference would specifically measure the luminal stretch contribution. This design is satisfactory but requires surgical placement of the control balloon in the abdominal cavity, which is obviously not appropriate in humans.

It is probably quite difficult to dilate an intestinal segment without some possible effect on the overlying skin, but sometimes a more stringent experiment can be used to show that an observation also holds in a less stringent sense. For example, a relatively noninvasive procedure can be used to study differential detection in two adjacent intestinal segments: A catheter with two separately inflatable balloons spaced several centimeters apart (a Barthelheimer tube) can be passed *per os* (via the mouth) into the intestine; the individual balloons are inflated in a controlled quasi-random pattern, while the subject is instructed to attempt to respond to one and only one of the two balloons as the signal. If the experiment shows that the separate inflations can be discriminated then the result would go beyond (and hence definitely include) solid evidence of simple detection. In fact, a procedure of this kind has been successfully used (Àdàm 1967, pp. 127–8) to study the sensory capability of the human duodenum.

It should be noted here that a hazard of using discrimination as the criterion of simple detection is the increased chance of a type-II error, where the null hypothesis is inappropriately accepted. In general, experiments should be designed so as to minimize systematic error, but an indiscriminately draconian standard of evidence can obscure an important phenomenon. Therefore, in stating the conclusions of a highly differential experiment, negative outcomes should be interpreted with the same degree of caution as positive ones.

Ultimately, any acceptable definition depends on the question that it serves, and the question devolves to the relationship between the experimental preparation and the target inference class. Every scientist appreciates that randomization is the crux of statistical inference; a valid proband always must be drawn at random from the applicable universe. In fact, a similar but more general "sampling" principle governs any scientific inference: An experimental preparation must be, as nearly as possible, a *generic* example drawn from the target class. In other words, the properties of the preparation – at least, those properties that arguably are relevant to the putative effect – must be the same for all members of the inference class. For example, consider again the enteric perception experiment: if all intestinal segments were situated such that the overlying skin was stimulated by balloon dilation, the result would be convincingly applicable to all intestinal segments and generally valid; however, because this assumption is almost certainly not true, the inference applies only to those segments where the condition holds. Furthermore, general properties of the physiology and anatomy of the gut dictate that skin stimulation would not likely be a reliable sensory pathway for intestinal distention; thus, in experiments of this kind, sensation in the overlying skin is appropriately considered an experimental artifact.

General Biophysical Properties of Interoceptors

Stimuli have the qualities of anatomical location, physical mode, and time rate of change. Although the receptor of particular sensory fiber is more efficiently activated by certain combinations of these qualities, the selectivity of the receptor itself varies, and most interoceptors are to some degree anatomically diffuse, polymodal, and sensitive to both the level and rate of change of the stimulus.

Selectivity. For any sensory system, stimulus discriminability is ultimately determined by the properties of individual receptors. Studies of skin sensations of awake humans indicate that individual receptors can code a range of stimulus qualities. Intraneural microstimulation of individual afferent units can evoke sensations of intermittent tapping, vibration, or tickle, or a perception of distinctly localized pressure. Quantitatively, depending on the unit stimulated, afferent impulse frequency may determine the magnitude of perceived pressure or the frequency of perceived vibration (Ochoa & Torebjork 1983).

In addition to unit properties, modern sensory physiology – kindled by the work of Adrian, Hartline, Hubel, and Weisel – has confirmed that comparatively simple assemblages of appropriately connected receptors can encode many additional stimulus properties. Thus, in the central visual areas, there are cells that fire differentially to edges moving in a particular direction even though the retina itself has no actual edge-detecting cells. Due to the comparative inaccessibility of the visceral receptive fields and visceral afferent nerve tracts, there are no direct observations of the "complex" sensory capabilities of interoceptors, but most likely the organization is similar. We know, for example, that the anal canal has "shearing" sensitive regions (Jänig & Häbler 1995, tab. 1); that similar shear sensitivity probably occurs in the upper gastrointestinal tract; and that these perceptions probably derive from complex receptive fields composed of simple stretch (pressure) receptors.

For almost all receptors, certain key steps in transduction are common. In particular, although some visual and auditory receptors hyperpolarize to certain stimuli, an adequate stimulus usually depolarizes the membrane potential toward zero. Because maintenance of the negative resting membrane potential depends on metabolically sensitive active processes, the ionic selectivity of the plasma membrane, and the composition of the extracellular environment, depolarization also is an inevitable consequence of any cellular damage or extracellular change that is sufficient to disrupt either metabolism or structure or to affect the Nernst potential of a key ion. Hence, large parametric excursions or moderate nonspecific injury of the surrounding tissue will cause most receptors to begin firing (often rapidly) and to continue to fire, at least until the cell is actually devastated. For similar common biophysical reasons, all receptors are sensitive to ambient electrical currents, and most will also fire with application of mechanical pressure sufficient to produce significant membrane distortion. Beyond these ubiquitous membrane processes, the actual active sites of many transmembrane receptor molecules, which initiate the transduction processes, are also to an extent nonspecific. For example, chemoreceptors respond to both CO_2 and pH, many gustatory receptors respond to several of the basic stimuli, and there are vagal afferent fibers that respond to both cholecystokinin and distention. In addition, the broad and overlapping sensitivity of many "pharmacological" receptor molecules is well documented.

Temporal Properties. Receptors can be broadly characterized by their firing rate as a function of a step change of the stimulus in time. In a qualitative sense there are two separable aspects of this "step response": (i) the accuracy or speed with which the receptor follows the rising edge of the step; and (ii) the stability of the asymptotic firing rate to the steady level of the plateau. In the somatomotor, visual, and auditory systems, receptor response speed is important because it is often the limiting factor in system performance. Yet for the regulation of visceral function, this is rarely the case: for most autonomic reflexes, the speed of the sensory receptor mechanism is relatively fast when compared with the cumulative lag of the proximal stimulus dynamics, central processing, and efferent mechanisms. Thus, *interoceptor response speed is ordinarily not the limiting factor in determining autonomic control properties.*

In contrast to somatosensory, visual, and auditory processes – which engage mostly phasic reflexes acting within seconds – many interoceptors are involved in the feedback-controlled steady-state regulation of the basal value of physiological variables. Consequently, for interoceptors, the stability of the asymptotic firing rate to a constant stimulus is an extremely important issue. In fact, the steady-state response properties of interoceptors (described in what follows) are difficult to reconcile with their putative function within a conventional negative feedback regulatory framework. Exactly how the system actually works remains an open and important question (Dworkin 1993, chaps. 7, 8).

Adaptation is the gradual decline in receptor firing to constant stimulation. Adaptation can be a striking and obvious effect. In the 1950s there were experiments in humans that employed stabilized retinal images produced by special optical projectors (Ditchburn & Ginsborg 1952; Riggs et al. 1953). These experiments showed that "with an essentially motionless retinal image, prolonged fixation results in disappearance of objects from the field of view" (Riggs et al. 1953, p. 500). Complete fading of the image can occur within several seconds. The stabilized image is a particularly graphic example, but receptor adaptation is ubiquitous: in every neural system and at every level of the animal kingdom, adaptation has been found whenever receptor temporal properties have been accurately measured.

Mechanisms of Adaptation. Various biochemical and physical factors account for receptor adaptation. For example, in Pacinian corpuscles (as in certain interoceptors), mechanical high-pass filtering by the surrounding tissue is an important component of the adaptation mechanism (Lowenstein & Mendelson 1965). However, even with removal of the mechanical filtration of the viscous lamellae or capsule, the generator potential of a naked receptor has a duration of less than 100 msec (Lowenstein & Skalak 1966). The usual time scale of adaptation can be appreciated by considering that receptors noted for being *slow* to adapt (e.g., muscle spindle, bee hair-plate, slow crustacean stretch receptors) actually sustain generator potentials for only seconds or minutes.

Whether or not adaptation holds for every membrane-bound receptor (neural or not) is unknown, but in most systems with persistent ligand levels there is "downregulation" or reduced receptor sensitivity of both a fast and slow kind. There are various neurochemical mechanisms of adaptation; however, recovery of sensitivity after long-term ligand exposure probably requires protein synthesis (Axelrod 1974; Axelrod & Reisine 1984; Browning et al. 1976; Deguchi & Axelrod 1973; Gavin et al. 1974; Mallorgra et al. 1980; Strulovici et al. 1984; Terasaki et al. 1978).

Interoceptor Adaptation. All known interoceptors eventually stop firing altogether when exposed to a static stimulus. Thus, the sensory manifestation of adaptation for visceral receptors parallels that of the stabilized image for the retina. In the central nervous system, the representation of any completely constant stimulus gradually and continuously fades, eventually becoming obliterated. Moreover, not only a completely constant stimulus but also the constant component of a variable stimulus eventually disappears. So, for example, although the pulse variation of the blood pressure continues to be indefinitely reflected in corresponding fluctuations in the firing rate of the baroreceptor nerves, the mean arterial pressure (MAP) – the central value around which the pulse pressure varies – gradually disappears from the afferent signal. Table 1 is abstracted from Chernigovskiy (1967, pp. 228–9);[3] it lists the approximate time of adaptation (to a constant stimulus) for a number of carefully studied interoceptors. Again, note the actually rather rapid adaptation times of those receptors that Chernigovskiy saw fit to classify as being "very slow" to adapt. Figure 1 shows the response of a typical "slowly adapting" cardiovascular receptor to a constant stimulus of its receptive surface (Mifflin & Kunze 1982, p. 244).

Interoceptors and Steady-State Physiological Regulation

Interoceptor adaptation poses some intractable and perplexing problems for conventional theories of physiological regulation; because of this, its ubiquity has not been accepted without controversy. Many authors either have ignored evidence of receptor adaptation or attempted to dismiss it as a technical artifact of the isolation and measurement procedure.[4] The classic and very influential analysis of the carotid baroreceptors by Landgren (1952) is typical. For carotid sinus pressures below 100 mmHg he found the usual rapid adaptation; however, above 100 mmHg, the time until "complete" adaptation was much longer. On the basis of this, Landgren surmised that there was a term in the step response that represented a time-invariant pressure-dependent firing rate, wrote the equation for the receptor as frequency $= A(p) + Bt^{-k}$ ($k \approx 0.65$), and explicitly characterized the baroreceptor response to pressures above 100 mmHg as "steady discharge." By including $A(p)$, a purely pressure-dependent term, Landgren implicitly asserted that at higher pressures the baroreceptors did not fully adapt and thus continued to transmit useful pres-

sure information indefinitely. This result challenged the assertion that adaptation was ubiquitous, but Landgren's term "steady discharge" was probably inappropriate. He observed receptors at constant pressure for no more than ten minutes.[5] The firing rate appeared stable at that point and, because of this, Landgren concluded: "The curve approaches a constant asymptotic value."

Given the baroreceptors' putative role in blood pressure regulation, "steady discharge" to a constant pressure was an important issue. Landgren's result was readily accepted as evidence that the baroreceptors indeed had the long-term stability required to regulate blood pressure. By the mid-1950s, however, baroreceptor "resetting" (McCubbin et al. 1956) was experimentally demonstrated, and this raised serious doubts about whether the baroreceptors were involved in tonic blood pressure control.

The controversy about the baroreceptors points out a general problem in interpreting interoceptor adaptation data. In all cases, the temporal response establishes the regulatory limitations of the receptor. For example, if a receptor that adapts to 50% of maximum firing rate in 20 sec is the afferent element of a phasic reflex that requires only a few seconds of firing to initiate, then that receptor is "slowly adapting." For a baroreceptor, an orthostatic response to postural change fits that case well. On the other hand, if the same baroreceptor is assumed to sense mean blood pressure then it needs to maintain its firing rate for very much longer – in certain (quite

TABLE 1. Interoceptor Adaptation Time

Receptors	Adaptation Speed	Adaptation Class
Mechanoreceptors of the carotid sinus (cat)	25% of the initial impulse frequency within 6 sec of stimulation; the initial rapid phase of adaptation is practically absent	Very slow
Mechanoreceptors of the aortic arch (rabbit)	Complete adaptation within 5–10 min	Very slow
Mechanoreceptors of the atrium (cat)		Very slow
Mechanoreceptors of the urinary bladder (dog)	1. Complete adaptation within several fractions of a second (only 10–30 impulses)	Rapid
	2. Incomplete adaptation within 15–25 min	Very slow
Mechanoreceptors of the urinary bladder (cat)	Complete adaptation within fractions of a second	Very rapid
Various types of stretch receptors of the lungs (cat)	Not more than 5% of the initial impulse frequency within 10 sec	
	1. Decrease in impulse frequency by 10%–55% during the 2nd second of stimulation	Slow
	2. Complete or almost complete adaptation by the end of the 1st second of stimulation; these receptors are distinguished by a high threshold	Very rapid

Slowly Adapting

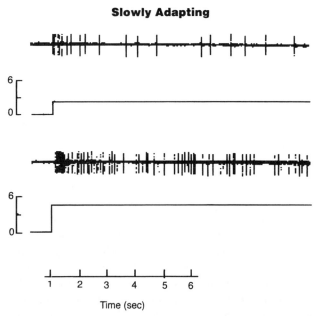

Figure 1. Slowly adapting low-pressure vagal receptor of the rat. The spike record shows the fall-off in firing rate following application and maintenance of a stimulus step. Adaptation occurs with both high- and low-strength stimuli, but complete adaptation is usually more rapid with weaker stimulation. The classification as "slowly adapting" is made relative to other kinds of interoceptors studied under similar conditions (see text).

conventional) conceptions of the regulatory process – possibly even for years. Thus, compared to the time scale of steady-state blood pressure regulation (and this was the important physiological issue), observation of a receptor's response for ten minutes was too brief to make a useful inference.[6]

In sum, all interoceptors appear to adapt within seconds or minutes. Interoceptor adaptation has profound implications for control system models of long-term or steady-state regulation. If the key assumption of the conventional regulatory paradigm – that some receptors continue to faithfully transduce the absolute level of physiological variables for many months and can provide the sensory substrate of long-term central regulation – is valid, then there should be many studies convincingly documenting hours or more of stable transduction by various interoceptors. In fact, there appear to be none whatsoever.

Accommodation

Accommodation occurs when a stimulus change is sufficiently gradual that, because of adaptation, it fails to fully activate a receptor. As such, accommodation is simply another facet of adaptation. It is, however, an especially interesting facet because it illustrates the important regulatory implications of adaptation.

If a receptor adapts then, given an appropriate stimulus change (driving) function, it can be made to fire at a constant frequency. If the driving function is sufficiently gradual then the constant firing frequency can remain close to zero (Gray & Malcolm 1951; Gray & Matthews 1951). In other words, because of accommodation, a stimulus can increase from zero to the physiological maximum without ever changing the receptor's firing rate. A more precise and quantitative way of defining accommodation is in terms of the receptor transfer function: If a time-domain step function response has a Laplace transform, $F(s)$, then its transfer function $T(s)$ is $F(s)$ divided by $1/s$, the transform of a zero-time aligned step. The transform of the output function that describes a particular constant firing frequency R is R/s. It follows that

$$H(s) \cdot T(s) = \frac{R}{s} \quad \text{and so} \quad H(s) = \frac{R}{sT(s)},$$

where $H(s)$ is the Laplace transform of the stimulus or driving function that will cause the receptor to fire continuously at constant frequency R. This relationship can be applied to the step function data for an interoceptor and thereby used to derive a cumulative stimulus drift function that will produce a constant, arbitrarily low, firing rate. For example, for feline right atrial mechanoreceptors, Chapman and Pankhurst (1976) found no evidence of time-invariant firing in the atrial volume receptors; that is, the receptors adapted to a zero firing rate. At above the threshold volume, the firing rate was characterized by

$$\text{frequency} = \frac{12 \text{ Hz}}{1 \text{ ml}} \left(\frac{t}{1 \text{ sec}} \right)^{-0.24};$$

thus, the transfer function for this receptor is

$$T(s) = \frac{12 \text{ Hz}}{\text{ml} \cdot \text{sec}^{-0.24}} \Gamma(0.76) s^{0.24},$$

and the inverse of $H(s)$ for $R = 1$, a firing rate of one impulse per second, is

$$h(t) = \frac{1 \text{ ml}}{12 \Gamma(0.76) \Gamma(1.24)} \left(\frac{t}{1 \text{ sec}} \right)^{0.24},$$

which describes a volume drift curve that will evoke a constant rate of firing over the linear range of the receptor (from threshold to saturation). Solving this equation shows that as much as 0.5 ml of additional atrial volume could accumulate, within only an hour, without ever causing a change in firing rate. Thus, under appropriate circumstances, even an extremely slowly adapting interoceptor can fully accommodate to a rate of volume change that would soon accrue to a substantial physiological error.

Is Adaptation an Experimental Artifact? A possible way to dismiss the physiological implications of interoceptor adaptation is to argue that adaptation is an artifact that results from damage inflicted – in preparation for recording – on a receptor or its nerve. Because direct quantitative measurement of interoceptor adaptation in situ is impractical (for one thing, accurately controlling the stimulation level in an intact animal is difficult), this assertion is extremely hard to prove or refute.

The Russian visceral physiologists had an explicit theoretical commitment to brain-mediated interoceptive regulation of the physiological state (recall Pavlov's comments cited at the start of this chapter). Thus, they found the relentlessness of receptor adaptation particularly vexing and were especially motivated to seek an alternative explanation that would mitigate the adaptation data. Their predicament had two aspects: first, if the primary interoceptor adapts then it is impossible for the brain to continuously acquire information from it; second, in addition to primary adaptation (observed ex situ), there was undeniable evidence for adaptation, resetting, or habituation of many different in situ visceral reflexes.[7] Given these facts (and especially if the second phenomenon is actually a manifestation of the first), these researchers asked, How can the brain have an important role in long-term regulation? Their putative explanations were: (1) primary receptor adaptation, observed ex situ, is an experimental artifact; and (2) adaptation of intact reflexes is due to an active inhibitory process that occurs in the brain, not at the interoceptor. To test these hypotheses, the leading Soviet sensory physiologist Chernigovskiy conducted a famous experiment that attempted to directly challenge the notion that the universally observed adaptation of visceral reflexes is a direct consequence of interoceptor adaptation (Chernigovskiy 1967, pp. 230–4).

The experiment used a loop of intestine and its mesenteric nerves. Distending the segment stimulated mechanoreceptors in the wall, which through afferent nerves to the brain caused a reflexive increase of blood pressure and respiratory rate. The investigators found that, following its increase, the blood pressure gradually returned toward normal as the wall tension was maintained constant for several minutes. This was exactly as expected, and the conventional explanation of this result is that the interoceptors of the gut wall eventually adapt to the constant stretch. In Chernigovskiy's experiment, once adaptation developed and the reflex magnitude diminished, the mesenteric nerve was subjected to transmission block by cooling it to 5°C. As would be expected, the cold block, at that point in the protocol, was without effect on either the blood pressure or respiration. Again, the usual and obvious explanation is that there was no activity on the nerve to be blocked. However, a less readily explained result occurred when the temperature was returned to 37°C and afferent nerve conduction was re-established: blood pressure and respiration again rose, and the change was as large, or even larger, than to the original distention. Chernigovskiy argued that this proved that the receptor had continued to fire undiminished throughout the protocol; that the observed adaptation of the reflex was due only to a process

somewhere central to the block; and – most important for the central regulatory theory – that information from the receptor had, in fact, continued to reach the brain. He said, "Thus, on the basis of these experiments it can be concluded that the apparent cessation of the reflex response takes place not in the least as a result of receptors' adaptation but is due to changes in the excitability of the vasomotor center which develops in the course of the reflex response itself."

These were interesting observations, but Chernigovskiy was almost certainly wrong in his conclusions. Besides the immediate effects of rewarming on the activity of the afferent nerve, which Chernigovskiy claimed (but did not explain how) he adequately controlled, his experiment had other probable pitfalls. In particular, along with stretch afferents, the mixed nerve of the pedicle contains motor, secretory, and vascular fibers; cooling to 5°C would have blocked these efferent fibers and also probably lowered the temperature of the arterial blood supply and thence the tissue of the loop itself. Consequently, the vascular (and possibly thermal and motor) disturbance produced by the cold block would almost certainly have newly activated many different kinds of interoceptors, and the effects of this stimulation would not have become apparent until the afferent nerve was rewarmed.

Nonetheless, Chernigovskiy's experiment was informative for two reasons. First, it illustrated some of the possible ways that interoception experiments can become confounded by failure to isolate pure afferent effects. Second, and more generally, it emphasized that a well-recognized authority on the physiology of interoceptors saw a serious inconsistency between the established ex situ adaptation characteristics of visceral sensory receptors and the participation of the central nervous system in long-term regulation of the physiological state. Clearly, he was sufficiently troubled by this disparity that he attempted a difficult experiment to reconcile interoceptor function with the conventional feedback regulation concepts of the prevalent regulatory theory.

In sum, adaptation is an established feature of all interoceptors that have been adequately studied. The erroneous conclusion that an interoceptor can have time-independent functional activity derives from prematurely curtailing observations or inaccurately measuring the terminal changes in firing rates. In all published cases, observation for periods even remotely comparable to the time scale of steady-state physiological regulation has disclosed evidence of continued monotonically declining firing rates. The direct physiological implications are that, in all cases, information about the absolute stimulus magnitude is gradually distorted by an interoceptor and, after sufficient time, the visceral stimulus (similar to a stabilized visual image) probably fails to register altogether. Similarly, for accommodation, a sufficiently gradual rate of stimulus drift will not change the firing rate of the receptor, and the drift will

elude detection and correction by regulatory mechanisms that depend at some link on sensory neural transduction.

Experimental Methods in Interoceptor Research

The experimental analysis of interoceptor function requires selective activation of the pathway(s) of interest. In general, researchers strive to confine and focus stimulation so that they know exactly what is being stimulated. There are a number of methods for accomplishing this; some can be used in humans, but others – because of their invasive and injurious nature – can only be applied in animal studies. At present there is no interoceptive stimulation method for animals or humans that can be applied without the addition of specific control procedures to verify its effectiveness and/or specificity. The following describes some typical methods, their potential pitfalls, and usual controls.

Direct Nerve Stimulation. In principle, the most precise way to activate a particular fiber or circumscribed group of fibers is to surgically isolate and electrically stimulate them. In practice, however, most sensory fibers are accessible to stimulation only after they have entered mixed nerves; thus, a satisfactory stimulation method depends on detailed knowledge of the relevant anatomy and physiology. For example, in humans the innervation of the tooth pulp is almost exclusively by nociceptive C-fibers, and it is possible to create a relatively pure pain sensation by applying a dental probe electrode to the surface of a tooth (this is the principle of the "pulp tester" used by dentists for many decades). However, with the conventional technique, current leakage to the gingiva reduces the accuracy of the stimulation because the stray current activates mucosal receptors and so produces additional nonpain sensations. Together, these factors degrade the accuracy and specificity of the tooth pain psychophysical function obtained with this method (Zamir & Shuber 1980). However, precise repeatable (within-subject) stimulation of the pulp with a constant stimulation area (and current density) can be achieved with a tooth that has a vital pulp and a stable metal filling. The method involves imbedding the electrical contact in an individually molded and tightly fitted rubber cap that completely insulates the electrode from the mucosa (Lee et al. 1985). It yields far better data than a simple hand-held probe, but it involves extensive preparations and is far more time-consuming. Whether the effort is worthwhile again depends upon the question being asked: for example, does the hypothesis make highly quantitative predictions about pain as distinct from other oral sensations?

In another approach, when diverse pathways are unavoidably activated by an electrical stimulus, selective lesions often can be used to verify those component paths that are needed to produce the observed effect. For example, the general sensory effects of stimulation of the baroafferent pathways have been of increasing interest in recent years (Ghione 1996). The rat vagus includes baroafferent fibers, and Randich and colleagues (1990) – in their study of antinociceptive effects – used electrical stimulation of the whole central vagus as a technically simple means of activating these fibers. Randich controlled nonbaroafferent effects by making selective ibotinic acid lesions in appropriate areas of the brainstem, and he found that lesions placed in regions known to be involved in blood pressure control substantially blunted the antinociceptive effects of vagus stimulation, whereas other located lesions had less or no effect. This method is subject to all of the usual caveats for lesion procedures, but in knowledgeable hands it can effectively help to verify the locus of mixed nerve stimulation effects. Specific lesions or nerve sections also can be used to limit the extent of nonelectrical stimulation methods discussed next.

One issue to be considered with direct electrical stimulation of an afferent pathway is that, in general, the quantitative equivalence between electrical nerve stimulation and natural stimulus parameters is indeterminate. Higher stimulus current cannot be tacitly assumed to mimic stronger natural stimulation (although, as described previously for cutaneous receptors, at a constant suprathreshold current and for certain kinds of individual fibers, the impulse rate of stimulation can have a useful physiological relationship to the properties of a distal stimulus). The general problem with using current strength as a stimulation variable is that, in a whole nerve, increasing current strength is more likely to recruit additional fibers than to more strongly activate those already recruited. In particular, when a nerve consists of a mixture of myelinated and nonmyelinated fibers, the myelinated fibers will be recruited at considerably lower current than the nonmyelinated ones. Thus, it is often possible to selectively activate myelinated fibers but not vice versa. Furthermore, because "current" is determined by the local voltage gradient across the active neural membrane, the geometrical relationship between the stimulating electrode and nerve can strongly affect which fibers are actually stimulated at a particular current. On the whole, the problem of electrically stimulating a mixed nerve is sufficiently complicated that another approach should be employed when the exact identity of the fibers stimulated is crucial – for example, when (to separate specific sensation from pain) large sensory fibers but not C-fibers need to be stimulated.

In the few cases of anatomically distinct nerves that are known to be physiologically homogeneous, electrical stimulation can be a clean and precise technique. Often these stringent requirements are met only in certain species. For example, the baroreceptors of the aortic arch reach the CNS through nerves that travel through the neck along the vagus and sympathetic trunk. These "aortic depressor nerves" (ADNs) are very readily identified in the dog and rabbit but are more elusive in the rat; however, whereas the ADN of both the dog and rabbit also include many fibers from chemoreceptors in the arch, the rat ADN is composed entirely of pressure afferents. When the rat ADN can be successfully isolated, it is apparently a pure baroreceptor input.

The conclusion that a nerve is "pure" depends on several kinds of evidence. In some instances, it is possible to dissect the nerve over the entire course to the actual receptive field; then the effects of various stimuli at the receptors can be directly observed. This has been done for the rat ADN (Numao et al. 1985; Sapru et al. 1981). Another important and often more easily achieved criterion is consistency of the response properties (or sensations) over a range of stimulus strength and rate parameters: responses should monotonically relate to stimulation strength from threshold to saturation. This has also been done for the rat ADN (Dworkin & Dworkin 1995). Monotonicity is potentially a convincing criterion; however, for it to be so, the subject must be capable of expressing a wide range of responses, and all putative extraneous responses must be recorded. For example, the rat ADN enters the superior laryngeal nerve (SLN) near the carotid bifurcation, and the SLN is very much easier to identify and isolate than the much smaller ADN. It is thus technically easier to stimulate baroafferents within the SLN, but the SLN contains numerous laryngeal afferents. Even so, for several typical baroreflex responses (including blood flow), Faber and Brody (1983) showed convincingly monotonic relationships between SLN stimulation parameters and depressor effects. However, because they used anesthetized rats, the effects of the laryngeal afferents were probably blunted or entirely eliminated. When the SLN is stimulated in conscious rats, the mixed effects of stimulation are depressor responses for low levels, often nothing at all for moderate levels, and clear pressor effects for stronger stimulation (Dworkin & Dworkin 1995).

In sum, direct electrical stimulation of afferent nerve tracts can be a useful well-controlled method for interoceptive stimulation.[8] But when modal specificity is important, controls are needed to verify that extraneous pathways are not being inadvertently activated.

Surgically Isolated Receptive Fields. The usual goal of surgical isolation of a receptive field is to create a sensory surface to which stimuli may be applied with greater accuracy, convenience, and specificity than is possible in situ. There are many examples of this method, including the isolated carotid sinus and the isolated intestinal segment. Advantages to using a surgically isolated receptive field are that (a) the stimulus environment can be explicitly controlled and (b) the local sensory apparatus is less likely to be affected by endogenous physiological processes. An isolated intestinal loop is not inadvertently stimulated by the uncontrolled passage of chyme, and the arterial cul de sac

can be stimulated (at an arbitrary pressure) independently of the systemic pressure.

The original carotid sinus cul de sac technique is attributed to Moissejeff (Heymans & Neil 1958, pp. 30–1). It involves ligature of the internal and external carotid arteries (the former being tied cephalic to the sinus, carefully avoiding the carotid sinus nerve) and cannulation of the central stump of the common carotid. Using this method, it is possible – by generating specific pulsatile or static pressures in the cannula – to stimulate the carotid sinus baroreceptors accurately. With a similar preparation, the carotid chemoreceptors also can be independently stimulated by irrigating the isolated sinus at constant pressure. In larger animals (such as the dog) it is possible to create a chronic isolated sinus preparation by anastomosing the common and internal carotid arteries, but for chronic stimulation usually a balloon is inserted into the carotid sinus via an incision in the common carotid artery. The balloon is much easier, but it does have disadvantages. Unless the balloon is constructed to be flaccid at the maximum inflation (something which complicates insertion), the actual pressure in the sinus cannot be accurately gauged; in any case, it is not possible (with a balloon) to apply a stimulation pressure below the systemic arterial value. The balloon method is also less specific, because inflation of the balloon partially disrupts cerebral blood flow. Nonetheless, it has been used to study the effects of carotid stimuli in intact conscious dogs (Àdàm 1967, pp. 42–9; Koch 1932), and it provided some of the earliest evidence that the carotid pressure receptors had general sensory effects that were detectable at the upper reaches of the neuroaxis. The intracarotid balloon is thus a useful technique, and if the animal has an intact Circle of Willis then the net brain blood flow is probably only transiently affected.

The gut is an especially surgically tractable and plastic structure, and numerous ingenious methods have been invented for experimentally modifying its architecture and isolating its various regions. Everyone is familiar with Pavlov's innervated stomach pouches, which he used for collecting specimens of pure gastric juice in studies of the cephalic phase of digestion. Similar pouches and diverticuli can be constructed along the extent of the gastrointestinal tract, including completely isolated loops, which enter and exit at the external skin surface, preserve the nervous and vascular supply, and can continue to be patent and functional for many years if properly maintained.[9] Various stimuli are easily applied to these cul de sacs and/or loops, which are readily distended by balloons or obdurators or are irrigated with solutions of experimental compounds such as acids, fats, or neurotransmitters. The more involved intestinal surgeries are more easily accomplished in the dog or monkey, owing to the strength of their tissues and size of the structures, but it is also possible to make sophisticated surgical rearrangements of the gut in smaller animals such as rabbits or even rats (Bàrdos et al. 1980; Schwartz & Moran 1996).

Observations of intestinal perception in humans are usually carried out with cannulas introduced per os or per anus. At times, researchers have recruited research subjects who have had medically prescribed ileostomy or colonostomy procedures. Using stimuli produced by balloon inflation, Àdàm conducted an extensive series of carefully controlled perceptual experiments with such subjects. Although these are discussed in more detail in a later section, we note here that using a surgically isolated receptive field does not automatically obviate the need for control procedures to exclude the effects of inadvertent stimulation of adjacent sensory structures. For example, distention of a carotid cul de sac or an isolated intestinal loop can inadvertently stretch overlying skin.

Noninvasive or Minimally Invasive Methods for Humans.

These are techniques that are considered to involve only minimal risk for participating human subjects. However, "invasive" has a range of definitions, depending on who the subjects are, who the procedure is performed by, and the extent to which the principal intention of the procedure is therapeutic (versus purely scientific study). To a cardiologist, placing a catheter into the brachial artery of a heart patient may be considered minimally invasive; whereas, in most psychological research, a venous catheter is thought invasive, and even oral administration of approved drugs may be classified as invasive. Intent is possibly also as important as the actual manipulation. Almost everyone considers mild electric shock intended to produce even slight pain to be highly invasive; yet, the same or stronger electric current applied through the same electrodes – with the intention of producing muscle contraction or sweat secretion – might well be considered innocuous or "minimally invasive." In practice, what is "invasive" is determined by local (community) standards, and the arbiter is the legally constituted institutional review board (IRB) to which the investigator is professionally responsible. Virtually all human research must be approved by an IRB, and investigators are strongly advised to consult with the executives of the IRB at the earliest possible stage of research planning in order to obtain an estimate of the probable acceptability of their plans. Often this can save much frustration and wasted time.

Minimally invasive procedures avoid penetration of the skin. Since the locus of stimulation in interoception studies is beneath the skin, and since the skin is richly endowed with sensory receptors, the design problem often devolves to stimulating a structure under the skin without stimulating the skin itself. The proximal parts of the gastrointestinal tract are exceptions; access to the lumen can be achieved per os or per anus with minimal discomfort or risk. Here also, however, if the stimulus involves distention of the lumen then distortion of the overlying skin is a

potential source of extraneous sensation for which appropriate controls must be devised and incorporated.

A novel stimulation technique can sometimes provide the key to an experiment that would otherwise appear to be impossible. Noninvasive stimulation of specific cardiovascular receptors presents an especially difficult problem: not only is access difficult, but the effects of locally applied stimuli propagate to (and influence) distant structures because the vascular system is both anatomically distributed and tightly coupled.

Pharmacological Activation of the Baroreceptors.

Bolus injections of vasoactive drugs are technically the most straightforward methods for stimulating the baroreceptors. The injections are to an extent invasive in that they require venous access, and the drugs used are not without some inherent risk – a too rapid rise in blood pressure can be very dangerous. Nonetheless, the procedures are considered a standard part of medical practice, and the drugs (which are readily available) have been extensively tested in humans.

Vasoactive drugs were first used to experimentally stimulate baroreceptors and study baroreflex gain in the late 1960s. The drug employed was phenylephrine, which has vasoconstrictor actions similar to the naturally occurring adrenergic neurotransmitter norepinephrine. However, phenylephrine is more stable than norepinephrine and is thus more convenient to prepare and administer. The baroreflex gain measurement technique is known as the Oxford method (Smyth et al. 1969).

Vasoconstrictors cause blood pressure to rise by increasing the peripheral resistance; the rise in blood pressure stimulates the high pressure baroreceptors, and the (cardiac inhibitory) baroreflex gain can be assessed by observing the fall in heart rate as a function of the rise in blood pressure. Phenylephrine and similar drugs also have been used in behavioral studies of baroreceptor stimulation in humans (Rockstroh et al. 1988). Vasoactive drugs have the advantage that, if administered through an indwelling venous catheter, the actual administration is indistinguishable (to the subject) from that of an inert substance. For behavioral studies, however, there are two substantial disadvantages to using vasoactive agents to stimulate the baroreceptors. First, most have direct excitatory effects on the CNS (Dworkin et al. 1979). Second, because vasoactive agents act by raising systemic blood pressure, the sympathoinhibitory vascular effects – which are key indices of barostimulation – are not observable.[10]

Lower-Body Negative Pressure (LBNP).

This is a mechanically cumbersome but physiologically straightforward technique for increasing the proportion of the circulating volume that is sequestered in the large veins, primarily those in the legs. The removal of a volume aliquot from the central circulation decreases the net venous return to the heart, reduces cardiac filling, and unloads low pressure receptors in the thoracic vascular bed. The LBNP apparatus consists of a large rigid cylindrical tank with a pneumatic seal at the waist. The entire lower body is enclosed by the tank, whose pressure is reduced with a pump (e.g., a domestic vacuum cleaner) – usually by 10–40 mmHg but sometimes by as much as 70 mmHg. (Larger negative pressures almost always produce syncope, but even pressures as low as −10 mmHg can produce periods of asystole in healthy individuals.) It is probable that low levels of LBNP (< 20 mmHg) selectively activate volume receptors and that higher levels also engage the high-pressure arterial receptors.

The LBNP technique has been used in physiological research to analyze reflex interactions in humans (Eckberg & Sleight 1992, pp. 191–208) and, to some extent, in psychophysiological research for the study of baroreceptor effects on sensory perception. For perceptual studies the method has the obvious disadvantage that the suction also activates receptors of the skin and pelvic organs, and convincing controls for these extraneous stimuli are difficult to implement. It should also be noted that, although apparently noninvasive, LBNP is potentially harmful; there are several reports of extended periods of asystole being induced in healthy volunteers (Eckberg & Sleight 1992, pp. 196–7).

Neck Suction. Distention of a surgically isolated carotid sinus cul de sac is the most widely accepted experimental barostimulation method, and a related (but noninvasive) external pressure stimulation method has been used in humans. The method depends upon the facts that the baroreceptors are actually stretch receptors in the arterial wall and that, although pressure inside the artery normally *pushes* the wall outward, the wall also can be artificially *pulled* outward by extravascular suction applied through an pneumatically sealed collar that encircles the neck. In the usual arrangement, a constant or *static negative* pressure in the "neck chamber" sums with the natural pulsatile intracarotid *positive* pressure and increases the average stretch of the sinus, thus simulating an elevated mean arterial pressure (MAP). The neck chamber has been used extensively to study the peripheral physiology of the human baroreflex, but, as with LBNP, the static pressure neck chamber has a drawback for behavioral studies: the neck suction activates receptors in the skin and deeper neck structures and so may induce perceptual or behavioral effects that are unrelated to barostimulation. In other words, the static chamber is an effective but nonspecific barostimulation method. The usual "first line" strategy for dealing with stimulus nonspecificity is to compare the experimental stimulus with an appropriate control stimulus – for example, suction applied to the skin a distance away from the target receptive field. For neck suction, however, it has not been obvious how to do this in a way that

is satisfactory. Some investigators have used positive neck pressure as the control procedure, but for various reasons this is not very convincing (Elbert et al. 1988; Rockstroh et al. 1988). The detailed solution to this problem is an informative case study in designing a stimulation technique. In general, for any interoceptive stimulation method, there are always several issues that need to be considered, as follows.

1. What is the effective natural stimulus for the target receptors?
2. Where are the target receptors located?
3. What nontarget receptors could be affected?
4. What differences in modal sensitivity exist between the target and nontarget receptors?

For the neck chamber, the first three of these were just discussed. With regard to the fourth, the essential fact was that the baroreceptors are at least as sensitive to changes in pulse pressure as to the mean pressure. Thus, instead of static or constant suction, it is possible to use sequences of brief cardiac cycle–coordinated pressure changes to stimulate or inhibit baroreceptor activity. Eckberg (1976) showed that brief suction pulses applied randomly during various parts of the cardiac cycle differentially affected subsequent P-P wave intervals. However, because suction pulses were random, the barostimulation or inhibition effects they produced were uncontrolled and transitory (lasting for only a single cycle). This was fully satisfactory for Eckberg's purposes, but it limited the utility of the method for psychophysiological studies. In order to stimulate or inhibit the carotid receptors continuously for as long as several minutes, Eckberg's method was augmented by replacing the randomly produced suction pulses with computer generated cardiac cycle–synchronized trains of repeatedly alternating pressure and suction pulses that were phase-locked to an R-wave trigger (Dworkin 1988). Alternating suction during systole with positive pressure during diastole augmented the endogenous carotid sinus pulse pressure (CSPP), whereas reversing the phase relationship (via the valve-operating computer program) created a control condition in which the endogenous CSPP was actually decreased. This "phase-locked neck suction" (PLNS) method produced heart rates about 5%–10% lower during stimulation compared with the control condition. Although the pulse pressure effects of the barostimulation condition (cardiac phase–synchronized suction) and the control condition (cardiac phase–inverted suction) have very different cardiovascular effects, they are indistinguishable to the subject (Furedy et al. 1992).[11]

Comparing PLNS and the original static neck chamber technique points up the advantages as well as some of the hidden costs of specificity. Each method stimulates the baroreceptors, but the static technique is far simpler and somewhat more effective in producing baroreflex activation. On the other hand, the PLNS method is considerably more specific: the stimulation and control conditions differ only in baroreceptor activation. In general, it is not unusual for specificity to be obtained at the price of some loss in potency. For one thing, no procedure is perfectly specific, and an efficient control procedure will probably stimulate the target receptors to some degree. A similar example is found in studies of intestinal pressure sensitivity discussed in a subsequent section.

Regulatory Functions of Interoceptors

The best-studied and most generally accepted role of interoceptors is as afferent components in control loops that regulate the viscera. In fact, interoceptors are the first element of the feedback path of all reflex mechanisms of physiological regulation. In closed-loop control systems, usually within broad parametric limits, the characteristics of the feedback path dictate the dynamics and final level of the regulated variable. Because they occupy this crucial position, interoceptors are directly implicated in many medical conditions, and their properties as simple transducers are pivotal to important areas of basic psychophysiologic research.

For example, all of the following processes involve closed-loop control mechanisms that depend upon information derived from visceral sensory receptors: neural regulation of the circulation; the central control of food and fluid intake, energy balance, and electrolyte metabolism; the sensory substrate of behavioral reward; the afferent mechanisms of conditioned aversions, emotion, and pain; the mechanisms of addiction and the treatment of substance abuse; noncompliance with medical regimens resulting from the aversiveness of treatment-associated side effects; and the pathophysiology of certain psychosomatic conditions.

Specific interoceptors with well-defined reflexogenic effects were not directly observed until the second half of the nineteenth century. In 1866 Cyon and Ludwig found that, in the rabbit, stimulation of the central end of a small nerve that runs along the common carotid artery – adjacent to but separate from the vago-sympathetic trunk – reduced heart rate and blood pressure.[12] They recognized that the "depressor nerve" conveyed sensation, and they proposed that its receptors were in the heart and were part of a regulator of the heart rate and blood pressure. Eighty years later, Bronk and Stella (1935) used the single-fiber method of Adrian (1926) to systematically investigate the properties of the high-pressure baroreceptors. Since then, the baroreceptors have been the most thoroughly studied interoceptors, and it is now well established that (a) the "aortic depressor nerves" described by Cyon and Ludwig actually convey barosensory impulses from receptors in the aortic arch and distal portion of the carotid artery and that (b) these receptors, along with those in the sinus of the carotid bifurcation (which Stella and Bronk studied),

are the afferent limb of the blood pressure regulating buffer reflexes, which stabilize the cardiovascular state. The structural and quantitative dynamic aspects of the baroreflexes have been among the most extensively studied interoceptor mechanisms (Sagawa 1983).

Adrian's technique (Adrian 1926), which has been very important in interoceptor research, involves recording from a small bundle containing a few distinct fibers that have been carefully dissected from a whole nerve. Using this method, Bronk and Stella showed that: (i) for a given fiber over a moderate range of pressures, there is an approximately linear relationship between intrasinus pressure and firing rate; and further that (ii) specific fibers were above threshold and below saturation over only a limited part of the physiological pressure range. Their observations established the important principle of parallel systems of within- and between-fiber (dynamic and channel) coding, which appears to characterize all interoceptors. Figure 2 details the unconditioned physiological reflex.

As discussed previously, most receptors adapt within seconds or minutes; this is a sufficient time for phasic reflexes, such as orthostasis or salivary secretion, to complete a required action. A key property of the negative feedback scheme is that the corrective efferent action of the reflex effectively removes the initiating stimulus from the receptor, and so the receptor returns to its basal state, ready for subsequent reactivation. If the corrective action is not achieved within the time constraint of adaptation, then the receptor will adapt to the residual stimulus and the reflex will become ineffective. If this happens, other mechanisms must be recruited to normalize the physiological state. These mechanisms must be either (a) nonneural and nonadapting or (b) neural and adapting yet functionally different from the conventional negative feedback scheme. The former are well documented and exemplified by pressure diuresis effects in the kidney; the latter are presently not well understood, but they are key to the brain's participation in long-term regulation of such things as blood pressure (Dworkin 1993, chaps. 7, 8).

Interoceptive Conditioned Reflexes. Although the concept of association among stimuli dates to before the British empiricists, the first systematic observations of conditioning in defined reflex systems were by Pavlov in 1897. Pavlovian or classically conditioned responses develop when a sensory conditioned stimulus (CS), which has a weak or no physiological effect, is repeatedly followed by a strong distinct physiological perturbation or unconditioned response (UCR). The UCR is itself produced by application of a second more potent unconditioned stimulus (UCS) that acts at the receptive field of a reflex. The physiological effect of the CS increases with each pairing or trial, and eventually the CS begins to elicit a conditioned response (CR) that mimics the unconditioned physiological reaction. See Figure 3.

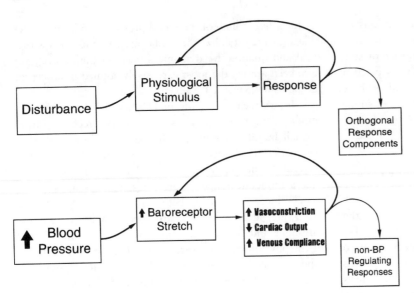

Figure 2. The general scheme of an unconditioned physiological reflex (top) and the specific example of the baroreflex (bottom). The leftmost box represents the initiating events of the Disturbance. These events, along with the nonorthogonal components of the Response, determine the Physiological Stimulus. The events of the Disturbance form a sequence in time, and thus the physiological component of the Disturbance is itself a function of time. In the baroreflex example, a rise in blood pressure distends the blood vessels and thus stretches endings in the vessel walls. This causes depolarization and firing, which is propagated via afferent fibers in the aortic depressor nerve (ADN), the superior laryngeal nerve (SLN), the vagus, and the glossopharyngeal nerve to synapses in the nucleus of the solitary tract (NTS). Fibers from the NTS distribute to the cardioinhibitory and vascular depressor centers of the brainstem, where efferent activity to the heart and blood vessels is modulated. With increased blood pressure, the modulation is achieved by (sympatoinhibitory) reduction of arterial resistance, relaxation of the veins, reduction of the pressure and volume ejected in each cardiac cycle; and (parasympathetic excitatory) slowing of the heart. The net result of this action is a decrease in blood pressure toward the prerise baseline, which restores the stretch on the baroreceptive endings to the original level and thus terminates the reflex activity.

It has been thoroughly accepted for nearly 100 years that conditioning can directly modify visceral function. Pavlov's first conditioned reflexes (secretion of gastric juice and saliva) were both glandular responses; since Pavlov, psychologists and physiologists have established a large literature on classical conditioning of autonomic reflexes, including salivary, sudomotor, cardiac, vascular, pupillary, and gastrointestinal. See Figure 4.

Types of Conditioned Reflexes. The common CSs of the conditioning paradigm are sounds, lights, tastes, and odors. However, various interoceptive stimuli are also effective conditioned stimuli. In fact, on the basis of the sensory mode of the conditioned and unconditioned stimulus, there is a logically complete fourfold classification of conditioned reflexes.

1. *Extero-exteroceptive* conditioned reflexes associate a weak exteroceptive stimulus (e.g., a sound, light, or vibra-

tion) with a stronger, reflex-eliciting, somatosensory stimulus such as electric shock.

The elaboration of extero-exteroceptive conditioned reflexes usually is technically straightforward and reliable; typically, they are both rapidly acquired and stable. These reflexes are most commonly used in research where the focus is on such things as neurophysiological mechanisms of association; the effects of general variables such as stress, diet, or aging on the discrimination, acquisition, retention, or extinction of learning; or in other studies where the need arises for a convenient generic fragment of learned behavior to be used as a dependent variable.

2. *Extero-interoceptive* conditioned reflexes associate a weak exteroceptive stimulus with a stronger, reflex-eliciting, *visceral* stimulus such as food-induced gastric secretion, irritant-induced salivation, or electrical baroreceptor activation.

Extero-interoceptive conditioned reflexes are usually more circumscribed in effect, and both the creation of the unconditioned stimulus and the measurement of the response are ordinarily more technically involved than for extero-exteroceptive reflexes. Pavlov studied extero-interoceptive reflexes as components of the "cephalic" phase of digestion; however, he also extensively used conditioned salivation, as a generic learned response, to study general aspects of association. In recent years, visceral conditioned reflexes have only rarely been used as general indices of behavior; however, there are many recent extero-interoceptive conditioning studies. These have concerned the role of context-conditioned compensatory responses in the development of tolerance to drugs and in adaptation to specific physiological stresses, such as induced shifts in blood pressure (Dworkin & Dworkin 1995), blood glucose, or temperature (Siegel et al. 1987).

3. *Intero-exteroceptive* conditioned reflexes associate an interoceptive stimulus – such as distention of the small intestine, carotid sinus, or renal pelvis – with an externally produced skeletal motor reflex, such as shock-induced paw withdrawal. The usual goal is to estimate the detectability and discriminability of particular interoceptive stimuli. The conditioned response is a substitute for verbal behavior in infrahuman species (and, in certain special cases, with humans). Examples of this paradigm are discussed in what follows with respect to visceral perception. In a variant of this paradigm the response is an operant, such as bar pressing, that is brought under control of an interoceptive stimulus, such as intraintestinal pressure (Slucki et al. 1965).

4. *Intero-interoceptive* conditioned reflexes associate an interoceptive stimulus (such as distention of the small intestine, carotid sinus, or renal pelvis; thermal stimulation of the stomach; or osmotic stimulation of the liver)

with a *visceral* reflex: food-induced gastric secretion, fluid load–induced renal secretion, or activation of the baroreflex. More than 30 years ago, Àdàm wrote:

It seems likely that temporary connections initiated by visceral receptors and affecting both vegetative and somatic functions are being continuously established and extinguished, while never becoming conscious. On the basis of our experimental data we suppose that the unconscious interoceptive sphere, too, has a "memory," i.e., an ability to retain experience, which helps adaptation to changes in the environment. (1967, pp. 139–40)

Outside of Eastern Europe, intero-interoceptive conditioned reflexes have been little studied, and technically they are comparatively quite demanding. Elaborating an intero-interoceptive reflex typically involves performing several separate chronic surgical procedures to prepare access for application of the conditioned and the unconditioned stimuli and for measurement of the response. Nonetheless, the intero-interoceptive reflex is probably of great importance in physiological regulation. In the quotation from Pavlov that began this chapter, the phrase "a constant, correct, and precise correlation becomes established among the parts of an organism" almost certainly refers to intero-interoceptive conditioning.

In fact, normal anatomical juxtaposition of receptors creates many arrangements in which the temporal requirements of conditioning are automatically satisfied. For example, the essence of coordinated gastrointestinal function is that partially processed chyme leaves one segment and enters the next. In principle, intero-interoceptive conditioning could coordinate action among different parts of

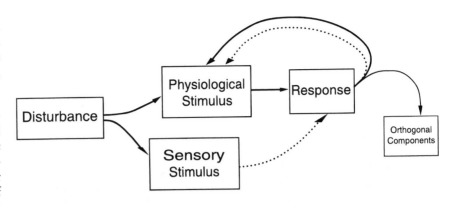

Figure 4. A modified conception of the classical conditioning paradigm for visceral reflexes that emphasizes the interaction between conditioned (dotted path) and unconditioned (solid path) reflexes. This revised scheme and terminology puts the conditioning process into a more biologically consistent framework. The Disturbance is an initiating event that changes the physiological and sensory state. It gives rise to a Sensory Stimulus and a Physiological Stimulus (see Figure 2). The Sensory Stimulus is clearly the same as the conditioned stimulus, but there is ambiguity in the literature concerning the proper physiological identity of the unconditioned stimulus and unconditioned response. The unconditioned and conditioned response together constitute the Response; thus, the Response is the total regulatory reaction of the nervous system to the Disturbance (the Orthogonal Components are other nonregulatory response components) (Dworkin 1993, chap. 3).

the gut. For example, distention in a proximal gut segment could trigger conditioned reflex secretion or motility in a more distal segment. If an oral segment had the necessary receptors, entering chyme could activate these and produce a conditioned stimulus; then, as the chyme entered the next segment, it could produce an unconditioned secretory or motor stimulus that completed the paradigm. Thus, with sufficient repetition (conditioning trials), the distention of the oral segment would trigger digestive activity in the aboral segment, which would effectively anticipate arrival of the chyme and improve its digestion. This intero-interoceptive paradigm parallels the extero-interoceptive paradigm, which Pavlov called the "cephalic phase" of digestion, wherein the sight or aroma of food is the conditioned stimulus that triggers anticipatory salivary or gastric secretion. The Russian physiologists took this general schema quite seriously. Their ideas are highly provocative, but their experimental studies (Bykov 1942/1957, pp. 231–79; Bykov & Kurtsin 1949/1966, pp. 21–78) need to be replicated with better experimental controls and appropriate statistical analyses.

Heterotopic versus Homotopic Conditioning. For the reflexes just described in paragraphs 1 and 4, it is possible

Figure 3. The traditional conception of the relationship among stimuli and responses in the classical conditioning paradigm.

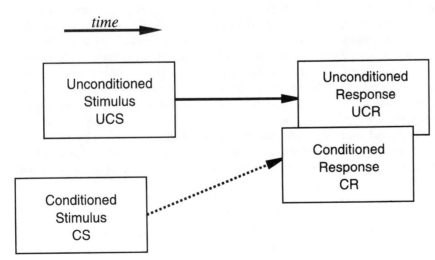

to make the additional logical and biologically important distinction of whether the conditioned and unconditioned stimulus are applied in separate or the same sensory modes. For conventional or *heterotopic* conditioning, the CS and UCS are in *different* sensory modes; for example, the CS can be an auditory tone followed by a UCS of an electric shock to a finger tip. After repeating this stimulus combination many times, or "trials," a withdrawal reaction develops to the sound and the emergence of this new response is evidence of conditioning. For *homotopic* conditioning, both the CS and UCS are applied in the *same* sensory mode. In a roughly parallel example, the CS would be a mild electric current applied to a finger tip and followed by a UCS of a stronger current on the same finger tip; with repetition, the withdrawal reaction to the milder CS current will gradually strengthen from what it was at the start. Here, the quantitative change in the withdrawal response to the weaker current is the measure of conditioning.

There are many commonplace natural adaptations that fit the homotopic extero-exteroceptive paradigm. A simple case is the conditioned response that helps in avoiding burns from objects that are sometimes hot: the CS is the radiated warmth that is first sensed as the fingers approach the object, and the UCS is the pain in the fingers on contact. The heat–pain activates a reflex withdrawal, and gradually with "experience," (i.e., with the accumulation of conditioning trails) the sensation of warmth – that is, the CS by itself – triggers the protective withdrawal. For an example of intero-interoceptive homotopic conditioning, conditioned hyperthermia was produced using a low dose of ethanol as the CS and a higher dose (which produces a clear hypothermia) as the UCS (Greeley et al. 1984). In ethanol thermic conditioning, the UCS is hypothermia, which is due to vasodilatation and consequent heat loss to the environment; the hypothermia activates compensatory metabolic reflexes, which become conditioned to the CS. (For an analysis of the mechanism, see Dworkin 1993, pp. 109–15.)

In fact, at a physiological level, the general properties and underlying neuroanatomy of homotopic conditioning probably closely parallel those of heterotopic conditioning. This is because, for most sensory systems and over a wide stimulus range, coding of stimulus magnitude is not confined to increased firing rate but also involves successive recruitment of higher-threshold receptor populations. For example, there are two classes of heat-sensing receptors in the fingers: warmth receptors, which respond with increasing discharge rate to temperatures between 32°C and 45°C; and heat–pain receptors, which begin to fire only at > 45°C. The baroreceptors also have this kind of intensity–channel coding arrangement. In their seminal study of the carotid receptors, Bronk and Stella found "wide variation in threshold for different receptors" (Bronk & Stella 1932, 1935). Thus, just as do the separate modali-

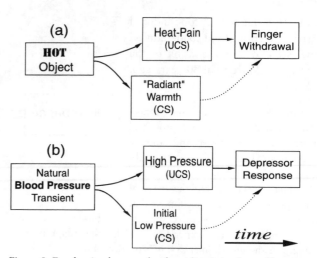

Figure 5. For the simple example of avoiding being burned by a sometimes hot object (a), homotopic conditioning effectively calibrates the sensory threshold of the defensive withdrawal reflex. By similarly calibrating visceral reflexes, such as the example of the baroreflex in (b), interoceptive homotopic conditioning could have an important (but so far unappreciated) role in autonomic regulation.

ties of heterotopic conditioning, the neural representations of the *different strength* homotopic CS and UCS probably enter the CNS over separate axons and project to different synapses. See Figure 5.

In the laboratory, homotopic conditioning has been studied much less than heterotopic – in fact, hardly at all. But there is nothing in conditioning theory that prefers that the CS and UCS be from different sensory modalities; to the contrary, among learning theorists, the usual notion is that the more similar or related are the CS and UCS, the more easily conditioning will occur. In fact, the paucity of research on homotopic conditioning is more likely due to certain practical difficulties in performing the experiments. Although the homotopic CS is a relatively weak stimulus, it measurably activates the reflex when applied in the receptive field of the unconditioned reflex even before any conditioning has taken place. Thus, determining whether homotopic conditioning has occurred requires, at least, the ability to make a reliable quantitative measurement of the change of the conditioned response strength from the beginning and to the end of conditioning. For the comparison to be meaningful, the state of the subject must be stable, the response measurements accurate, and the proximal stimuli constant. Because conditioning takes time, these stringent criteria must be met throughout the many hours (or even several days) of an experiment, and the difficulty in accomplishing all of this is probably why homotopic intero-interoceptive conditioning has not been more extensively investigated by psychophysiologists and regulatory physiologists. See Figure 6.

Early Work on Interoceptive Conditioning. Probably the first explicit description of an interoceptive conditioned reflex was in 1928 by Bykov and Ivanova (Bykov 1942/1957,

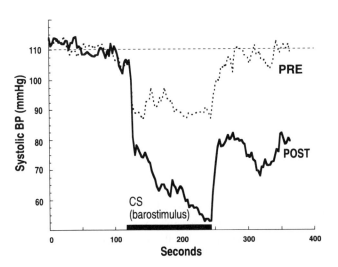

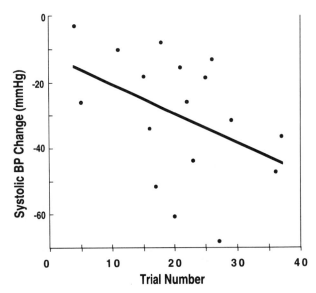

Figure 6. Homotopic conditioning of the baroreflex. Left panel: Response of a 5-Hz electrical stimulus (the CS) applied to the aortic depressor nerve of a rat before and after the CS had been paired with a 25-Hz UCS to the same nerve in a classical conditioning procedure. Right panel: Magnitude of the blood pressure response to the 5-Hz (CS) stimulus as a function of the number of conditioning trials (the conditioned response is a blood pressure decrease).

pp. 246–7). They performed a urinary secretion conditioning experiment in which an unconditioned 200-ml saline stimulus was infused into a dog's stomach directly through a chronic transabdominal fistula. After approximately 25 infusions they observed that the dog secreted urine as soon as the gastric mucosa was wetted – before a physiologically significant amount of saline was introduced. Eventually they found that if saline were briefly introduced and removed before it could be absorbed, urine flow developed that was of smaller magnitude but of similar time course to that caused by the full load. They designated this an intero-interoceptive conditioned reflex because both the conditioned stimulus and unconditioned stimulus were interoceptive stimuli. Figure 7 describes a similar "discriminative" version of this experiment.

In Russian experiments designated as intero-exteroceptive, the conditioned stimulus was interoceptive but the unconditioned stimulus was exteroceptive. For example, the conditioned stimulus of wetting the gastric mucosa was repeatedly paired with an electric shock to the paw, resulting in conditioned paw withdrawal. Airapetyantz (see Bykov 1942/1957, pp. 249–51), another of Bykov's co-workers, demonstrated the formation of a discrimination between 26°C and 36°C intragastric water. After 150 trials in which a salivary unconditioned stimulus followed a 36° but not 26° water infusion, only the 36° conditioned stimulus produced a reliable flow of saliva. Airapetyantz and his associates also did a number of similar experiments with other intestinal interoceptors as conditioned stimuli; for example, they formed discriminated salivary responses to pH and temperature stimuli in isolated intestinal segments.

The general conclusions of the Eastern scientists were that interoceptive conditioned reflexes, when compared with their exteroceptive counterparts, required larger and more variable numbers of trials to become stable. Once formed, however, interoceptive reflexes had the essential characteristics typical of exteroceptive reflexes, including inhibition of delay and susceptibility to disruption by novel stimuli (external inhibition).

What is Necessary for Formation and Consolidation of a Conditioned Response?

The standard conception of the classical conditioning paradigm is shown in Figure 3; Figure 4 extends the paradigm for visceral reflexes to include the feedback mechanisms of regulation and emphasizes that, for visceral reflexes, the conditioned response also can have important regulatory consequences. Nonetheless, both figures presume a similar, relatively uncomplicated, and traditional neurophysiological conception of classical conditioning. Beginning with Pavlov and for the 50 years following him, the central concept was that the temporal contiguity of a neutral stimulus and a reflex formed an association. However, McGaugh's work in the 1960s suggested that learning, especially consolidation (in distinction to formation) of an association, might be affected by pharmacological manipulation of relatively nonspecific central adrenergic and cholinergic mechanisms (McGaugh 1966).

More recently, it has become evident that certain kinds of natural stimuli also might influence consolidation (Mc-Gaugh 1989). There is evidence that aversive stimuli, such as shock, can enhance the retention; that shock also activates central adrenergic mechanisms; and that the amygdala and its major pathway, the striate terminalis, are involved

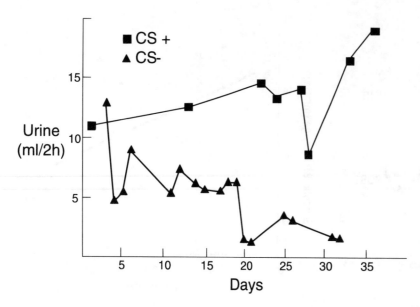

Figure 7. This experiment used two distinctive stimuli. The Active stimulus was a distinctive room where the UCS was administered, and the Differential stimulus was a second, dissimilar room; both rooms were equipped for measuring urine output. In the Active room, water was administered per rectum and urine collected; in the Differential room, urine was collected but no water was administered. The plot shows the daily urine output in the two rooms measured before any water was administered. Initially, the urine output in the differential room was nearly the same as it had been in the active room; this is a typical generalization effect in classical conditioning. As the trials progressed, the rate of urine output in the Differential room fell while urine output in the Active (reinforced) room continued to rise. Bykov described several similar experiments with other dogs, one in which the water load was given by mouth; in another (a discrimination experiment), two distinctive bell sounds were used as conditioned stimuli.

quently and under special circumstances – for example, when the extant central visceral network does not adequately constrain the physiological state within limits that are compatible with the adjustment capacity of nonneural peripheral mechanisms (Dworkin 1993, pp. 118–22). Thus, for central connections to be modified, a net homeostatic imbalance might need to be present in addition to stimulus association. By activating visceral receptors, the imbalance would, in a manner similar to shock or direct neurochemical manipulations, activate central adrenergic mechanisms (Gold 1984), possibly via the amygdala (McGaugh, Cahill, & Roozendaal 1996), and so enable consolidation.

Traditional conceptions of learning distinguish between the classical and operant conditioning paradigms, and the suggestion of a dependence of synaptic modification on "homeostatic imbalance" inevitably brings to mind the operant model's distinctive features of motivation (or drive) and reinforcement (or drive reduction); see Dworkin (1993, chaps. 7, 8). However, there is a substantial difference: in the operant model, the strengthening of a particular response requires, specifically, that the response bring about (or at least be well correlated with) a reduction of the homeostatic imbalance; whereas, in this modified view of classical conditioning, the postulated neurochemical effects of the imbalance need only be present during and/or following the association of the CS and UCS.[13]

Perception of the Viscera and Visceral Influences on Behavior

Historically, "interoception" has had a number of different meanings. In addition to the well-documented regulatory functions already discussed, interoceptors have been attributed more general perceptual functions that parallel those of the receptors of exteroception and proprioception. It is through exteroceptors that we develop a detailed functional model – a conscious perception – of the environment, and it is similarly through proprioceptors that we apprehend the position and motion of the parts of our skeleton in space. The conscious perception of visceral states and the control of autonomic and skeletal behaviors, including verbal reports of visceral stimuli, are also potentially important. But unlike exteroception and proprioception – which, phenomenologically, are clearly valid, robust, and functionally important – there remains some reasonable doubt as to whether conscious perception of the viscera is other than a comparatively fragile laboratory curiosity. There is no doubt that, for most visceral organs, sufficiently strong stimulation produces a conscious perception

in both the pharmacological and shock effects. If these findings prove valid for interoceptive reflexes, such "motivational" influences on conditioning could have implications for the plasticity of regulatory mechanisms.

In the preface to the 1957 English edition of *The Cerebral Cortex and the Internal Organs,* Bykov wrote, "The higher regulating apparatus determines and preserves the unity and integrity of all the complex executive organs and tissues, receiving information through the extero- and interoceptors. The cortex is *at every moment* determining the fate of every reaction of the organism" [emphasis added]. Reading Bykov's book leaves little doubt that he meant there was a continuous formation and extinction of conditioned reflexes, with each successive association slightly changing the visceral regulatory network.

It is possible that this view of an ongoing calculus – continuously reorganizing and adjusting the network to optimum (Dworkin 1993, chaps. 3, 4) – is entirely correct. However, interoceptive conditioning also could be *saltatorial;* that is, new synaptic connections might form, or connection strengths might be modified only infre-

of pain; however, although there has been extensive and excellent work on visceral perception, it is not entirely established whether, under normal circumstances (except for some special cases, such as gastric "hunger"[14] contractions), there is general awareness of sensations from subnoxious stimuli in the deep internal organs. Furthermore, if substantial nonpain conscious awareness of the deep viscera does exist, its function (if any) is unknown.

Typical dictionary definitions distinguish "sensation" as the immediate result of a "sensory input" from "perception," which involves a combination of sensations as well as memory of past sensations. Psychologists often go further in distinguishing perception from discrimination, which is the ability to identify either different stimulus levels or different qualities. This distinction is important, but it is necessary to recognize that a visceral stimulus could have substantial effects on perception and sensation without there being direct perception or discrimination of the stimulus.

For example, baroreceptor activation reduces the arousal level and attenuates both spinal level reflexes and the reported painfulness of noxious stimuli (Dworkin et al. 1994). However, most naive human subjects cannot reliably distinguish baroreceptor activation conditions from control conditions (Furedy et al. 1992); thus, baroreceptor activation is itself probably not directly perceived or discriminated. This is an example of where, without being directly perceived, a visceral stimulus can measurably affect behavior and the perception of other stimuli. Parallel phenomena have been described for the abdominal organs. For example, Kukorelli and Juhàsz (1976, 1977) showed that EEG (electroencephalogram) synchronization and sleep could be induced by levels of subnoxious stimulation of the intestine and abdominal nerves, which probably would not be directly perceived.

The control of ingestion is the most extensively studied and analyzed example of interoception. The first modern observations of intestinal perception were made by Walter B. Cannon with his student Washburn. Using simultaneous kymographic recording of intragastric pressure and behavioral responses, they observed a temporal relationship between gastric contractions and "hunger pangs" (Cannon & Washburn 1912). These observations (in which Washburn was the subject) are illustrated and described in Figure 8. Largely on the basis of these and other "correlational" studies using kymographic or radiographic measures of intestinal movement, Cannon concluded that the experience of hunger derived from the perception of gastric contractions.[15] However, by mid-century a substantial body of data had accumulated that conflicted with Cannon's simple "gastric perception" model of hunger. For example, in humans, most of the stomach can be excised

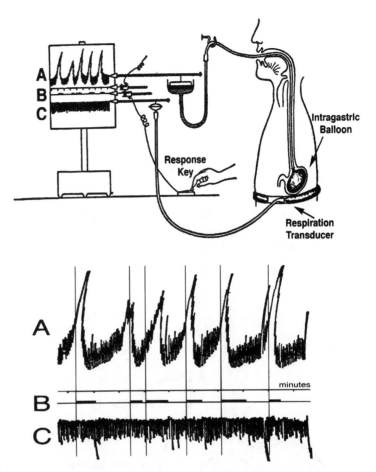

Figure 8. *Top*. Cannon's student, Washburn, learned to swallow a balloon, which registered the contractions of his stomach. Another transducer was placed around his abdomen to register the movement of his abdominal muscles. When Washburn perceived a "hunger pang" he pressed the response key. The entire set of events was recorded on a kymograph, a primitive polygraph device, as a function of time. *Bottom*. The record shows the relationship between the gastric contractions and the "pangs." Cannon made two conclusions from this record: first, that the perception was related to stomach contractions, not to movements of the abdominal wall; second, that the contractions preceded the perception in time. (The original figure did not include the vertical cursors, which have been inserted in this version.) Cannon said that the "hunger pang was not recorded until the contraction had nearly reached its peak"; yet the cursors show that the "pang" marker always begins quite early in the contraction and that the relationship is, in fact, more variable than might be expected from a simple coupling.

or the vagus nerve severed *without* loss of either hunger motivation or the experience of hunger.

Nonetheless, in contrast to the clinical evidence that peripheral signals are not essential to the experience of *hunger*, sophisticated laboratory studies have clearly implicated gastrointestinal stimuli in the interoceptive control of *ingestion* (McHugh & Moran 1985). Hunt showed (i) that the osmotic pressure of the chyme influenced both gastric motility and the rate of gastric emptying and (ii) that energy content and volume were also important control

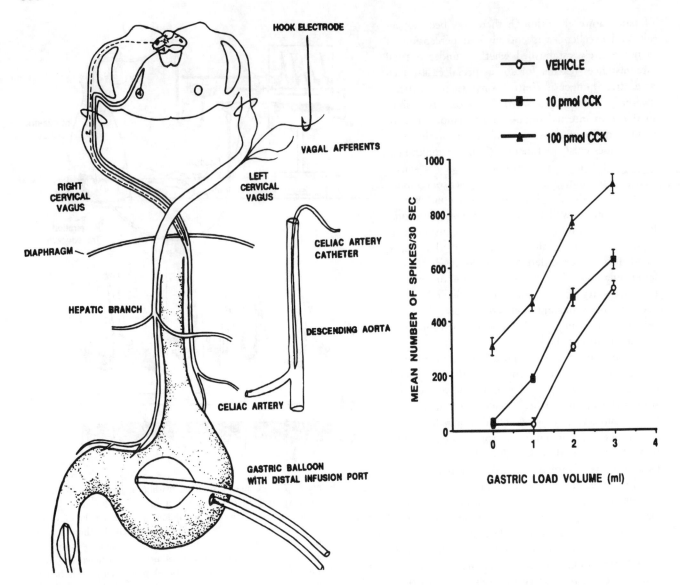

Figure 9. The preparation used by Schwartz and Moran for analysis of the interaction of the effects of cholecystokinin and mechanical (volume) distention on single vagal afferent fibers with receptors in the stomach. The left panel shows the experimental preparation, which enables simultaneous stimulation of gastric mechanoreceptors, infusion of CCK (cholecystokinin) into the celiac artery, and recording of afferent activity in single vagal fibers. The right panel shows the effect of various doses of CCK on the response of vagal afferents. Note that, at higher doses, the effect is clearly additive.

stimuli (Hunt 1961; Hunt & Stubbs 1975). Mei (1978) found specific glucoreceptors in the small intestine. More recent studies of the control of motility, gastric emptying, and satiety have focused on the role of gastric load, mechanical and chemical properties of intestinal contents, and various hormonal receptors – particularly those sensitive to the octapeptide cholecystokinin.

The work of McHugh, Moran, and Schwartz is especially notable in emphasizing the integration of various stimuli by individual interoceptors. For example, Schwartz

and Moran (1996) described the additive effect of cholecystokinin on the firing rate of intraluminal volume sensitive vagal afferents. Using a sophisticated rat preparation (see the left part of Figure 9), they showed that isolated single vagal afferents had polymodal sensitivity, "responding to both mechanical stimulation ... and to exogenous administration of a peptide that is released by the duodenum presence of nutrients." Pretreatment with cholecystokinin caused the vagal gastric mechanosensitive afferents to fire at a higher rate for the same load. At concentrations of cholecystokinin, or at intragastric volumes that individually were too low to activate the afferents, prior application of cholecystokinin produced rapid firing to the volume stimulus (see the right part of Figure 9); thus, operating within a classical regulatory mechanism, cholecystokinin and mechanoreceptor effects apparently summate and enhance the activity of the efferent limb of appropriate digestive reflexes. Because effects of the compound stimulus were effective at levels that individually were ineffective at low stimulus levels, the effects have features of a multiplicative interaction. If the subthreshold levels used in the analysis are in the normal physiological range, then an interaction would have regulatory implications beyond simple summation; however, given the apparent linearity of the combined suprathreshold effects (see Figure 9), it is more probable that the afferents are polymodal and that the cholecystokinin and mechanical receptors are distinct structures that independently produce additive effects. This means that either cholecystokinin *or* gastric load would have similar functional consequences in the CNS; in other words, that neither depends upon the other for reflex activation.

In a conceptualization that is somewhat reminiscent of the Russian school (Bykov 1958; Bykov & Kurtsin 1949/1966), Moran and Schwartz emphasized the general perceptual nature of the complex stimulus patterns that arise in the gut: "Furthermore, we view the constellation of meal-related stimuli arising from several gastrointestinal compartments as comprising a context representative of the internal milieu during a meal.... Thus, it is critical to establish responses to individual properties and then elucidate the integrative capacities of sensory afferents responding to combinations of properties likely to occur in the context of a meal in the gastrointestinal tract" (Schwartz & Moran 1996, p. 49). It remains to be determined whether, in understanding complex integrative processes, this quasi-cognitive formulation has advantages over explicit algebraic control-theoretic or statistically based "autonomic space" (Berntson et al. 1991) formulations of the same effects.

Innate and Learned Conscious Perception. Because stimulation that does not normally reach consciousness still can have detectable behavioral effects, it is arguable that, given the possibility of learning, a nonconscious stimulus could eventually become conscious. For example, if a nonconscious conditioning stimulus affects general arousal or modifies the conscious perception of other stimuli, then a subject with appropriate discrimination training should be able to acquire the capability to estimate and report, at least indirectly, the presence and/or intensity of the conditioning stimulus itself. Discrimination training is known to be helpful in re-establishing bowel continence in adults (Whitehead & Schuster 1983); it is also likely an important factor in the normal development of the perception of bladder and rectal distention, and it is almost certainly involved in the primary establishment of fecal and urinary continence. Experimental results (to be discussed shortly) indicate that the perception threshold for bowel distention can, in fact, be lowered with training.

Whether normal consciousness of interoceptive stimuli – any more so than consciousness of exteroceptive or proprioceptive stimuli – requires discrimination practice is not known. A more biological way of putting this same question is to ask: Does the neuroanatomy of interoception provide access to the neurophysiological substrates of consciousness equivalent to that of exteroception or proprioception? Without doubt, various forms of this question tacitly motivate much of interoception research. At present, however, our neurophysiological and conceptual understanding of what consciousness is (and isn't) is so immature (Dennett 1991) that it is difficult to know where to start seeking an answer. Nonetheless, it is clear that neither interoception nor consciousness are homogeneous classes of phenomena and that both interact with, are affected by, and effect changes in behavior. Thus, even without delving into the nature of consciousness, some useful distinctions can be drawn.

Visceral sensations have obvious and direct effects on behavior, but the selectivity and sensitivity of different tissues varies enormously. For conscious perception and other effects on behavior, the strength of a stimulus and its anatomical site of application interact.

Strong visceral stimuli can function in two ways: First, because various unconditioned defensive reflexes confer a survival advantage, they were selected and well conserved during the evolutionary history of the species. Strong visceral stimuli can promptly activate those simple defensive reflexes that directly and efficiently ameliorate the visceral irritation. Second, in addition to specific reflexes, general mechanisms of behavioral reinforcement and learning evolved also. Acting through these mechanisms, pain or discomfort of visceral origin mobilizes more complex and flexible sequences of behavior. In contrast to the specific reflexes, motivated sequences are not focused and do not immediately ameliorate the initiating stimulus. However, because the reduction of pain or discomfort is a powerful behavioral reinforcer, *for a given individual* those behavioral sequences that reliably antecede pain reduction have a high probability of being selected and strengthened by learning mechanisms.[16]

Distention of the urinary bladder is a straightforward example of both kinds of interoceptor effects: The muscle of the bladder wall (the detrusor) contains mechanoreceptors. Extreme distention strongly activates these receptors and triggers an organized reflex that incites prompt "involuntary" enuresis, whereas moderate bladder distention *motivates* a more elaborate and variable pattern of behavior that potentially leads to better-controlled and more convenient micturition. This sequence is then reinforced by relief of the aversive sensations from the bladder. Another example of both mechanisms is mechanical or chemical stimulation of the nasal mucosa: Strong stimulation by an irritant produces greatly increased serous and mucous secretion and sneezing, which together comprise a protective defensive reflex that can immediately clear the irritant from the upper respiratory tract. Weaker stimulation motivates a more flexible and variable behavior pattern leading to more controlled expulsion of the irritant – for example, by blowing the nose into a handkerchief. Again, the successful sequence is reinforced by relief from the irritation.

In normal individuals, both moderate and strong sensations from the mechanoreceptors of the detrusor are readily perceived, and the presence of a nasal irritant is also easily recognized. However, recognition of the irritant is not ipso facto required to activate simple reflexes, and awareness also may not be prerequisite for the irritant to have a motivational effect (Hefferline & Perera 1963). Instead, the crucial factor is whether the neural activity generated by the receptor reaches the integrative centers where an appropriate effect is initiated.

It could be asserted that bladder distention and nasal irritation are special cases because, although the receptors involved are not actually on the body surface, they are just barely within it. This assertion has some merit, and in general the distinction between exteroception and interoception is often less than comfortably definite. A brief tour through the gastrointestinal tract illustrates this: From the top down, almost everyone would agree that sensations of the lips are not interoception; most would also concur that sensations from the oral mucosa, and maybe even the pharynx, should not be considered interoceptive. At the esophagus, however, the consensus would likely weaken. There are certainly reflexes activated when things go wrong in the esophagus; there can be pain (heartburn) and more moderate sensations as well. We perceive "burning" from too hot a beverage, and often can even sense the passage of a hot bolus down the tube; this is also true for very cold liquids or ice cream. We also are aware when something too large or dry has been swallowed and is having a difficult passage. On the whole, most sensations from the esophagus are unpleasant but not necessarily painful. Esophageal sensations are not as well defined as those from more oral loci: spatial discrimination is less precise, and stimulus qualities are not as distinct. Aside from the special case of sensations associated with hunger, there is little evidence of any entirely nonpainful sensation from receptors in the stomach.

Beginning at the bottom and proceeding orally the sequence is similar: The anus has clear and detailed sensation; the rectum certainly has pain, distention, and probably some amount of temperature sensitivity. Activation of receptors in both regions can both trigger direct reflexes and motivate more complex behaviors (e.g., toilet use). Above the sigmoid flexure, though, perception is again more equivocal. There are some laboratory data showing that (i) below the pain threshold, the colon has sensitivity to distention, and (ii) stimuli in the descending colon that are but several centimeters apart can, after special training, be discriminated. But there is no evidence that different qualities (e.g. temperature) can be discriminated.

The small intestine has an extensive array of sensory receptors: distention or surface irritation activates local peristaltic and other reflexes, which are mediated both by the intrinsic myenteric plexus and extraintestinal intersegmental pathways. For example, stimulating the duodenum or proximal jejunum by distention, acid or lipid, promptly inhibits gastric motility and relaxes the stomach. Nonetheless, evidence of specific subpain level perception in either half of the small intestine is equivocal. Àdàm showed that subnoxious balloon distention of the duodenal wall causes desynchronization of the EEG (Àdàm et al. 1965). He eventually extended this fundamental finding to the differential (two-point) paradigm mentioned previously. The details of these seminal studies were described in his monograph on interoception and behavior (Àdàm 1967), which includes many additional interesting and original examples of interoceptive mechanisms. More recently, to explore the sensibility of distal intestinal segments, Àdàm (1998) studied enterostomy patients. He found that some of these subjects could successfully discriminate moderate degrees of balloon distention of the small intestine; however, the subsequent inclusion of carefully designed control procedures in these studies showed that the apparent interoception was likely due, at least in part, to stretching of the overlying abdominal wall or the skin surrounding the papilla.

To conduct these enterostomy studies, Àdàm constructed a special intraintestinal catheter with an attached annular skin stimulation balloon. Using a similar but modified instrument, Hölzl extended Àdàm's findings to colon stimulation in normal subjects and developed a sophisticated signal detection analysis of the interaction of the skin and intraintestinal stimuli. In patients suffering from irritable bowel, Hölzl found that – depending on the temporal and spatial relationship among the stimuli – skin stimulation can either summate with or mask intestinal stimulation (Hölzl et al. 1994). Hölzl also analyzed these effects in terms of intra- or intersegmental convergence of the sensory fields. His results in normal subjects and patients indicate that detection of stimuli is possible without the subject's awareness but that "localization" requires stimuli sufficiently strong to produce "conscious subjective sensation" (Hölzl et al. 1996).

Concerning the conscious perception of visceral stimuli, in 1967 Görgy Àdàm wrote:

In summarizing, we tend to believe that in man the majority of interoceptive impulses influence behaviour without, however, causing any subjective sensation.... The question might now arise as to whether ... visceral impulses entering consciousness actually occurs in conditions of normal life. It can be assumed that the interoceptive components of functions important for the individual (hunger, thirst) and socially (micturition, defecation) become conditioned in early childhood with exteroceptive stimuli, and the reinforcement of impulses other than these would constitute too great a stress for the higher nervous centers; in other words, to bring into consciousness such internal processes would be pathological. (1967, pp. 139–40)

The intervening thirty years appear not to have substantially contradicted Àdàm's conclusion.

Summary

1. Almost all visceral structures have an extensive array of primary sensory elements. These interoceptors are the sensory radix of the afferent limb of the dynamic visceral reflexes that stabilize the internal milieu. It is well accepted that many different unconditioned interoceptive reflexes have important physiological functions.

2. Interoceptive stimuli can function as conditioned stimuli for visceral and somatic conditioned reflexes, and these intero-exteroceptive or intero-interoceptive reflexes may coordinate various visceral–visceral and visceral–somatic relationships. Interoceptive conditioning is a fruitful subject for further study and could have important implications for autonomic regulation.

3. The special case of the homotopic conditioned reflex, particularly the intero-interoceptive form, could have a role in the calibration of the sensitivity and dynamic characteristics of such visceral regulators as the baroreflex.

4. There is conscious perception of nonnoxious stimuli from certain visceral organs; however, as emphasized throughout this chapter, the validity of this conclusion depends on the definitions of "perception" and "visceral." For the most part, it can probably be said that normal perception of nonnoxious stimuli is limited to special functions, such as hunger, or to special structures, such as the bladder or rectum. There is a strong possibility that conscious perception in special structures – especially those that communicate with the external environment – is not direct and that perception exists (to a large degree) because of learned associations with more perspicuous proprioceptive and exteroceptive stimuli during ontogeny. Aside from the well-recognized special cases, it is not clear that conscious perception of visceral stimuli is important to normal physiological function.

5. Separate from conscious perception, there are well-established effects of nonnoxious interoceptive stimuli on higher CNS function and on behavior. Appropriate interoceptive stimulation can affect satiety, modify reflex activity or pain perception, and produce EEG synchronization and sleep. In addition to their direct consequences, these "nonconscious" CNS effects may be substrates of associative processes involved in the development of conscious visceral perception.

6. All visceral sensory receptors adapt and therefore cannot provide the continuous negative feedback signals required for steady-state regulation through conventional control mechanisms. If interoceptors do participate in long-term regulation, the mechanism remains to be demonstrated. This is also an important area for future investigations.

NOTES

1. Thus, the emphasis is on the physiological implications of visceral sensory mechanisms, not the psychological implications of visceral perception. Excluded are certain subjects dealing with specialized perceptions – for example, the awareness of heart beat (see next note) and a detailed discussion of hunger and satiety. For reviews of the role of the perception of visceral sensation in the control of food intake, see McHugh and Moran (1985) or Schwartz and Moran (1996). Nocioception is discussed in relation to interoceptor properties, but visceral pain (and its mechanism) is an extensive and separate subject.

2. See for example Brenner and Jones (1974) and Paintal (1972). For an excellent and extensive review of heart beat perception, see Jones (1994); for a discussion of probable sources of mediation, see Jones (1994, pp. 156–60).

3. For additional general references on interoceptor properties, see Widdicomb (1974) and Mountcastle (1980).

4. This is a theoretical bias that has been prevalent in autonomic nervous system neurophysiology for many years. As a student, in 1969 I asked the influential neurophysiologist, Detlev Bronk, about the apparent ubiquity of receptor adaptation and its implications for physiological regulation; he insisted that it was not a real phenomenon but rather an artifact of damage inflicted by the dissection required to isolate the receptor.

5. Because the empirically observed firing rates always include some random variability, appropriate statistics must be used to show convincingly that the firing rate actually approaches a final, nonzero, constant level. The assertion that a curve has reached "asymptotic level" means that the regression line fit to data on the terminus of the linear plot has a slope of zero – to within an acceptable error. It is important to appreciate that Landgren did not use appropriate statistical criteria to evaluate the slope of the terminal firing rate, even within the specified ten-minute observation period.

6. Landgren's was an early and pioneering study, but similarly imprecise criteria characterize more recent interoceptor studies also. For example, Mifflin and Kunze (1982) studied slowly and rapidly adapting low-pressure receptors in the left superior vena cava of the rat. For the slow receptors they observed substantial (60%) increases in threshold following 15-min exposures to pressures of 5 mmHg, which agreed with previous results (Kappagoda & Padsha 1980). However, Mifflin and Kunze (1982, p. 243) also made more extended observations of step responses; these, they explicitly claimed, *did* show time-invariant firing. However, when their published data were reanalyzed with standard regression techniques and conservative criteria (Dworkin 1993, p. 139), it was evident that – for these observations also – the firing rate had actually continued to decline substantially during the last ten minutes of observation.

7. Chernogovskiy (1967) gave many examples for intestinal reflexes, but the best documented example in the Western literature is the resetting blood pressure baroreflexes. See McCubbin et al. (1956), Kezdi (1962), Kreiger (1970), Koushanpour and Kelso (1972), and Koushanpour and Kenfield (1981).

8. Direct nerve stimulation can rarely be used in normal humans, but there are occasional opportunities to study patients. For example, stimulation of the carotid sinus nerve is sometimes used to control severe hypertension; some such patients have implanted pacemakers that can be externally controlled.

9. Typical are Thiry–Vella loops, which are completely isolated sections of intestine. They are removed with the circulation and nerve supply intact; the ends are brought through and sutured to the outside of the abdominal wall to form two papillae; and the remainder of the intestine is reconnected with an end-to-end anastomosis. The resultant loop is easily accessible in a unanesthetized animal and, with reasonable care, various pressure, thermal, and chemical stimuli can be applied surreptitiously.

10. Angiotensin II has also been used for baroreceptor stimulation. However, it has few advantages when compared to norepinephrine analogs and has the disadvantage of affecting the R-R wave interval independently of baroreflex mechanisms (Ismay et al. 1979). This, along with its primary vasoconstrictive mechanism, obliterates any useful index of baroactivation.

11. For better pressure symmetry between conditions, a variable-length atmospheric pressure pulse can separate the suction and positive pressure pulses (Rau et al. 1992). However, this requires additional valves, and, in fact, the methods have never been shown to be functionally different.

12. Two years later, in 1868, Hering and Bruer identified receptors in the lung that initiated respiratory reflexes. For a detailed history of the discovery of the baroreceptors, see Heymans and Neil (1958, pp. 18–25).

13. This said, with historical perspective the distinction between classical and operant (or instrumental) paradigms is actually less definite: Although B. F. Skinner (1981) conceived of the operant response as a rigorously random event, in Neal Miller's (1959) reformulation of instrumental learning, response probabilities (which determine the order of the "response hierarchy") became a deterministic function of the motivational (drive) state, which itself is subject to classical conditioning. Especially for physiological regulatory responses, Miller's idea of a response-determining drive (interoceptive stimulus) state fittingly brings together instrumental and drive-dependent (classical) conditioning.

14. In fact, Cannon (1939) described hunger as "a very disagreeable ache or pang or sense of gnawing or pressure which is referred to the epigastrium" (p. 70); thus, whether hunger actually should be considered nonnoxious interoception is at least arguable.

15. Cannon also had a similar conception of thirst. William James anteceded Cannon at Harvard, and in Cannon's time James's ideas about emotion were still influential. Although Cannon doubted the physiological basis of the peripheral emotion theory of James and Carl Lange, his own conception of motivation unquestionably paralleled it.

16. Motivation might also be derived from positive sensations. Students of learning have long debated the differences between the function of positive and negative sensations

in eliciting reflexes and motivating behavior (Miller 1959, 1966; Stellar & Stellar 1985). For example, Pavlov used both weak acid and meat powder to elicit salivation (Pavlov 1897/1910, p. 83). Acid is an obvious irritant, and the bicarbonate secretion of the salivary reflex neutralizes the acid, but is it reasonable to consider meat powder – in a parallel sense – as an irritant also? Probably not: The effects of the meat are more complicated, and this becomes evident when the acid or meat is used as a behavioral reinforcer to modify more general behavior rather than as simple unconditioned stimuli. The reinforcing effects of the two on antecedent behavior are, in fact, opposite. Along related lines, the sensory effects of the intestinal hormone cholecystokinin have been the subject of vigorous debate. Some investigators assert that CCK produces satiety (i.e., simulating the sensory effects of a satisfactory meal; Smith & Gibbs 1994), but others argue that its effects more closely resemble nausea. Although both may have similar unconditioned effects on eating, the potential motivational consequences are likely quite different.

REFERENCES

Àdàm, G. (1967). *Interoception and Behavior: An Experimental Study*. Budapest: Akademiai Kiado.

Àdàm, G. (1998). *Visceral Perception: Understanding Internal Cognition*. New York: Plenum.

Àdàm, G., Preisich, P., et al. (1965). Changes in human cerebral electrical activity in response to mechanical stimulation of the duodenum. *Electroencephalography and Clinical Neurophysiology, 18*, 409–15.

Adrian, E. D. (1926). The impulses produced by sensory nerve endings. Part 1. *Journal of Physiology, 61*, 49–72.

Axelrod, J. (1974). The pineal gland: A neurochemical transducer. *Science, 184*, 1341–8.

Axelrod, J., & Reisine, D. (1984). Stress hormones: Their interaction and regulation. *Science, 224*, 452–9.

Bàrdos, G., Nagy, J., et al. (1980). Thresholds of behavioral reactions evoked by intestinal and skin stimulation in rats. *Physiology and Behavior, 24*, 661–5.

Berntson, G. G., Cacioppo, J. T., et al. (1991). Autonomic determinism: The modes of autonomic control, the doctrine of autonomic space, and the laws of autonomic constraint. *Psychological Review, 98*, 459–87.

Brenner, J., & Jones, J. M. (1974). Interoceptive discrimination in intact humans: Detection of cardiac activity. *Physiology and Behavior, 13*, 763–7.

Brodal, A. (1969). *Neurological Anatomy*. New York: Oxford University Press.

Bronk, D. W., & Stella, G. (1932). Afferent impulses in the carotid sinus nerve. *Journal of Cell and Comparative Physiology, 1*, 113–30.

Bronk, D. W., & Stella, G. (1935). The response to steady pressures of single end organs in the isolated carotid sinus. *American Journal of Physiology, 110*, 708–14.

Browning, E. T., Brostrom, C. O., & Groppi, V. E., Jr. (1976). Altered adenosine cyclic 3', 5'-monophosphaste synthesis and degradation by C-6 astrocytoma cells following prolonged exposure to norepinephrine. *Molecular Pharmacology, 12*, 32–40.

Bykov, K. M. (1942/1957). *The Cerebral Cortex and the Internal Organs*. New York: Chemical.

Bykov, K. M. (Ed.) (1958). *Textbook of Physiology* (Translated from the Russian by S. Belsky & D. Myshne and Edited by D. Myshne). Moscow: Foreign Languages Publishing.

Bykov, K. M., & Kurtsin, I. T. (1949/1966). *The Corticovisceral Theory of the Pathogenesis of Peptic Ulcer* (Translated from the Russian and Edited by S. A. Corson). Oxford, U.K.: Pergamon.

Cannon, W. B. (1939). *The Wisdom of the Body*, 2nd ed. New York: Norton.

Cannon, W. B., & Washburn, A. L. (1912). An explanation of hunger. *American Journal of Physiology, 29*, 441–55.

Chapman, K. M., & Pankhurst, J. H. (1976). Strain sensitivity and directionality in cat atrial mechanoreceptors in vitro. *Journal of Physiology, 259*, 405–26.

Chernigovskiy, V. N. (1967). *Interoceptors*. Washington, DC: American Psychological Association.

Deguchi, T., & Axelrod, J. (1973). Supersensitivity and subsensitivity of the β-adrenergic receptor in pineal gland regulated by catecholamine transmitter. *Proceedings of the National Academy of Sciences U.S.A., 70*, 24411–14.

Dennett, D. C. (1991). *Consciousness Explained*. Boston: Little, Brown.

Ditchburn, R. W., & Ginsborg, B. L. (1952). Vision with a stabilized retinal image. *Nature, 170*, 36–7.

Dworkin, B. (1988). Hypertension as a learned response: The baroreceptor reinforcement hypothesis. In T. Elbert, W. Langosch, A. Steptoe, & D. Vaitl (Eds.), *Behavioral Medicine in Cardiovascular Disorders*, pp. 17–47. Chichester, U.K.: Wiley.

Dworkin, B. R. (1993). *Learning and Physiological Regulation*. University of Chicago Press.

Dworkin, B. R., & Dworkin, S. (1995). Learning of physiological responses: II. Classical conditioning of the baroreflex. *Behavioral Neuroscience, 109*, 1119–36.

Dworkin, B. R., Elbert, T., et al. (1994). Central effects of baroreceptor activation in humans: Attenuation of skeletal reflexes and pain perception. *Proceedings of the National Academy of Sciences U.S.A., 91*, 6329–33.

Dworkin, B. R., Filewich, R. J., et al. (1979). Baroreceptor activation reduces reactivity to noxious stimulation: Implications for hypertension. *Science, 205*, 1299–1301.

Eckberg, D. L. (1976). Temporal response patterns of the human sinus node to brief carotid baroreceptor stimuli. *Journal of Physiology, 258*, 769–82.

Eckberg, D. L., & Sleight, P. (1992). *Human Baroreflexes in Health and Disease*. Oxford, U.K.: Clarendon.

Elbert, T., Lutzenberger, W., et al. (1988). Baroreceptor stimulation increases pain threshold in borderline hypertensives. *Psychophysiology, 25*, 25–9.

Faber, J. E., & Brody, M. J. (1983). Reflex hemodynamic response to superior laryngeal nerve stimulation in the rat. *Journal of the Autonomic Nervous System, 9*, 607–22.

Furedy, J., Rau, H., et al. (1992). Physiological and psychological differentiation of bi-directional baroreceptor carotid manipulation in humans. *Physiology and Behavior, 52*, 953–8.

Gavin, J. R., Rothe, J., Neville, J. D. M., De Meyts, P., & Buell, D. N. (1974). Insulin-dependent regulation of insulin receptor concentrations: A direct demonstration in cell culture. *Proceedings of the National Academy of Sciences U.S.A., 71*, 84–8.

Ghione, S. (1996). Hypertension-associated hypalgesia. *Hypertension, 28*, 494–504.

Gold, P. E. (1984). Memory modulation: Roles of peripheral catecholamines. In L. R. Squire & N. Butters (Eds.), *Neuropsychology of Memory*, pp. 566–78. New York: Guilford.

Gray, J. A. B., & Malcolm, J. L. (1951). The excitation of touch receptors in a frog's skin. *Journal of Physiology, 115*, 1–15.

Gray, J. A. B., & Matthews, P. B. C. (1951). A comparison of the adaptation of the pacinian corpuscle with the accommodation of its own axon. *Journal of Physiology, 114*, 454–64.

Greeley, J., Le, D. A., et al. (1984). Alcohol is an effective cue in the conditional control of tolerance to alcohol. *Psychopharmacology, 83*, 159–62.

Hefferline, R. F., & Perera, T. B. (1963). Proprioceptive discrimination of a covert operant without its observation by the subject. *Science, 13*, 834–5.

Heymans, C., & Neil, E. (1958). *Reflexogenic Areas of the Cardiovascular System*. Boston: Little, Brown.

Hölzl, R., Erasmus, L., et al. (1994). Analysis of visceral hyperalgesia in symptomatic subgroups of the irritable bowel syndrome. Otto-Seltz-Institut, University of Mannheim.

Hölzl, R., Erasmus, L., et al. (1996). Detection, discrimination and sensation of visceral stimuli. *Biological Psychology, 42*, 199–214.

Hunt, J. N. (1961). Osmotic control of gastric emptying. *Gastroenterology, 41*, 49–51.

Hunt, J. N., & Stubbs, D. F. (1975). The volume and energy content of meals as determinants of gastric emptying. *Journal of Physiology (London), 245*, 209–25.

Ismay, M. J. A., Lumbers, E. R., et al. (1979). The action of angiotensin II on the baroreflex response of the conscious ewe and the conscious fetus. *Journal of Physiology, 288*, 467–79.

Jänig, W., & Häbler, H.-J. (1995). Visceral-autonomic integration. In G. F. Gebhart (Ed.), *Visceral Pain* (Progress in Pain Research and Management, vol. 4), pp. 311–48. Seattle: IASP Press.

Jones, G. E. (1994). Perception of visceral sensations: A review of recent findings, methodologies, and future directions. *Advances in Psychophysiology, 5*, 55–192.

Kappagoda, C. T., & Padsha, M. (1980). Transducer properties of atrial receptors in the dog after 60 min of increased atrial pressure. *Canadian Journal of Physiological Pharmacology, 59*, 837–42.

Kezdi, P. (1962). Mechanism of the carotid sinus in experimental hypertension. *Circulation Research, 11*, 145–52.

Koch, E. B. (1932). Die Irradiation der pressorezeptorischen Kreislaufreflexe. *Klinische Wochenschrift, 2*, 225–7.

Koushanpour, E., & Kelso, D. (1972). Partition of the carotid sinus baroreceptor response in dogs between the mechanical properties of the wall and the receptor elements. *Circulation Research, 31*, 831–45.

Koushanpour, E., & Kenfield, K. J. (1981). Partition of carotid sinus baroreceptor response in dogs with chronic renal hypertension. *Circulation Research, 48*, 267–73.

Kreiger, E. M. (1970). Time course of baroreceptor resetting in acute hypertension. *American Journal of Physiology, 218*, 486–90.

Kukorelli, T., & Juhàsz, G. (1976). Electroencephalographic synchronization induced by stimulation of the small intestine and splanchnic nerve in cats. *Electroencephalography and Clinical Neurology, 41*, 491–500.

Kukorelli, T., & Juhàsz, G. (1977). Sleep induced by intestinal stimulation in cats. *Physiology and Behavior, 19,* 355–8.

Landgren, S. (1952). On the excitation mechanism of the carotid baroceptors. *Acta Physiologica Scandinavica, 26,* 1–34.

Lee, M. H. M., Zaretsky, H. H., et al. (1985). The analgesic effects of aspirin and placebo on experimentally induced tooth pulp pain. *Journal of Medicine, 16,* 417–28.

Lowenstein, W. R., & Mendelson, M. (1965). Components of receptor adaptation in a Pacinian corpuscle. *Journal of Physiology, 177,* 377–97.

Lowenstein, W. R., & Skalak, R. (1966). Mechanical transmission in a Pacinian corpuscle: An analysis and a theory. *Journal of Physiology, 182,* 346–78.

Mallorga, P., Tallman, J. F., Henneberry, R. C., Hirata, F., Strittmatter, W. T., & Axelrod, J. (1980). Mepacrine blocks β-adrenergic agonist-induced desensitization of astrocytoma cells. *Proceedings of the National Academy of Sciences U.S.A., 77,* 1341–5.

McCubbin, J. W., Green, J. H., et al. (1956). Baroreceptor function in chronic renal hypertension. *Circulation Research, 4,* 205–10.

McGaugh, J. L. (1966). Time-dependence processes in memory storage. *Science, 153,* 1351–8.

McGaugh, J. L. (1989). Involvement of hormonal and neuromodulatory systems in the regulation of memory storage. *Annual Review of Neuroscience, 12,* 255–87.

McGaugh, J. L., Cahill, L., & Roozendaal, B. (1996). Involvement of the amygdala in memory storage: Interaction with other brain systems. *Proceedings of the National Academy of Sciences U.S.A., 93,* 13508–14.

McHugh, P. R., & Moran, T. H. (1985). The stomach: A conception of its dynamic role in satiety. *Progress in Psychobiology and Physiological Psychology, 2,* 197–232.

Mei, N. (1978). Vagal glucoreceptors in the small intestine of the cat. *Journal of Physiology (London), 282,* 485–506.

Mifflin, S. W., & Kunze, D. L. (1982). Rapid resetting of low pressure vagal receptors in the superior vena cava of the rat. *Circulation Research, 51,* 241–9.

Miller, N. E. (1959). Liberalization of basic S-R concepts; extensions to conflict behavior, motivation and social learning. In *Psychology: A Study of a Science* (vol. 2, study 1), pp. 196–292. New York: McGraw-Hill.

Miller, N. E. (1966). Experiments relevant to learning theory and psychopathology. In W. S. Sahakian (Ed.), *Psychopathology Today: Experimentation, Theory, and Research*, pp. 148–66. Itasca, IL: Peacock.

Mountcastle, V. (1980). *Medical Physiology.* St. Louis: Mosby.

Norgren, R. (1985). Taste and the autonomic nervous system. *Chemical Senses, 10,* 143–61.

Numao, Y., Siato, M., et al. (1985). The aortic nerve-sympathetic reflex in the rat. *Journal of the Autonomic Nervous System, 13,* 65–79.

Ochoa, J., & Torebjork, E. (1983). Sensations evoked by intraneural microstimulation of single mechanoreceptor units innervating the human hand. *Journal of Physiology, 342,* 633–54.

Paintal, A. S. (1972). Cardiovascular receptors. In E. Neil (Ed.), *Handbook of Sensory Physiology.* New York: Springer.

Pavlov, I. P. (1897/1910). *The Work of the Digestive Glands.* London: Griffin.

Pavlov, I. P. (1940). *Complete Collected Works.* Moscow: Academy of Sciences of the USSR.

Randich, A. R. K., et al. (1990). Electrical stimulation of cervical vagal afferents. II. Central relays for behavioral antinociception and arterial blood pressure decreases. *Journal of Neurophysiology, 64,* 1115–24.

Rau, H., Elbert, T., et al. (1992). PRES: The controlled noninvasive stimulation of the carotid baroreceptors in humans. *Psychophysiology 29,* 165–72.

Riggs, L. A., Ratliff, F., et al. (1953). The disappearance of steadily fixated visual test objects. *Journal of the Optical Society of America, 43,* 495–501.

Rockstroh, B., Dworkin, B. R., et al. (1988). The influence of baroreceptor activation on pain perception. In T. Elbert, W. Langosch, A. Steptoe, & D. Vaitl (Eds.), *Behavioral Medicine in Cardiovascular Disorders,* pp. 49–60. Chichester, U.K.: Wiley.

Sagawa, K. (1983). Baroreflex control of systemic arterial pressure and vascular bed. In J. T. Shepherd & F. M. Abboud (Eds.), *Handbook of Physiology* (vol. 3: The Cardiovascular System), pp. 453–96. Bethesda, MD: American Physiological Society.

Sapru, H. N., Gonzalez, E., et al. (1981). Aortic nerve stimulation in the rat: Cardiovascular and respiratory responses. *Brain Research Bulletin, 6,* 393–8.

Schwartz, G. J., & Moran, T. H. (1996). Sub-diaphragmatic vagal afferent integration of meal-related gastrointestinal signals. *Neuroscience and Biobehavioral Reviews, 20,* 47–56.

Siegel, S., Krank, M. D., et al. (1987). Anticipation of pharmacological and nonpharmacological events: Classical conditioning and addictive behavior. *Journal of Drug Issues, 17,* 83–109.

Skinner, B. F. (1981). Selection by consequences. *Science, 213,* 501–4.

Slucki, H., Àdàm, G., et al. (1965). Operant discrimination of an interoceptive stimulus in rhesus monkeys. *Journal of the Experimental Analysis of Behavior, 8,* 405–14.

Smith, G. P., & Gibbs, J. (1994). Satiating effects of cholecystokinin. *Annals of the New York Academy of Sciences, 713,* 236–41.

Smyth, J. S., Sleight, P., et al. (1969). Reflex regulation of arterial pressure during sleep in man: A quantitative method of assessing baroreflex sensitivity. *Circulation Research, 24,* 109–21.

Stellar, J. R., & Stellar, E. (1985). *The Neurobiology of Motivation and Reward.* New York: Springer-Verlag.

Strulovici, B., Cerione, R. A., Kilpatrick, B. F., Caron, M. G., & Lefkowitz, R. J. (1984). Direct demonstration of impaired functionality of a purified desensitized beta-adrenergic receptor in a reconstituted system. *Science, 225,* 837–40.

Terasaki, W. L., Brooker, G., de Vellis, J., Inglish, D., Hsu, C., & Moylan, R. D. (1978). Involvement of cyclic AMP and protein synthesis in catecholamine refractoriness. In W. J. George & L. J. Ignaro (Eds.), *Advances in Cyclic Nucleotide Research,* vol. 9, pp. 33–52. New York: Raven.

Whitehead, W. E., & Schuster, M. M. (1983). Techniques for the assessment of the anorectal mechanism. In R. Hölzl & W. E. Whitehead (Eds.), *Psychophysiology of the Gastrointestinal Tract,* pp. 311–29. New York: Plenum.

Widdicomb, J. G. (1974). Exteroceptors. In J. J. Hubbard (Ed.), *The Peripheral Nervous System,* pp. 455–85. New York: Plenum.

Zamir, N., & Shuber, E. (1980). Altered pain perception in hypertensive humans. *Brain Research, 201,* 471–4.

CHAPTER NINETEEN

MOTOR PREPARATION

C. H. M. BRUNIA & G. J. M. VAN BOXTEL

Prologue

OVERVIEW

Motor preparation is part of anticipatory behavior. It is an expression of a change in the state of the organism aimed at a better adaptation to expected changes in the environment upon which an adequate response must be given. The setting of the organism implies both the perceptual input and the motor output. In this chapter we will argue that it is impossible to exclusively discuss motor processes without taking into account the related perception. After all, much of our behavior is triggered by changes in our environment, which must therefore be monitored continuously. From the available information in our environment, the relevant part has to be selected and processed further in order to provide an appropriate action.

HISTORICAL BACKGROUND

Information processing takes time because it is based upon physical processes in the central nervous system. For us this is so obvious that it is hard to imagine that the best-known physiologist of the first half of the nineteenth century, Johannes Müller, was convinced that the time needed for an excited nerve to produce a muscle contraction was instantaneous, of the order of the speed of light (Donders 1868/1969). Sensory and motor nerves were considered different but passive channels for the animal spirits since the days of Galen. Bell (1811) and Magendie (1822) discovered that the sensory fibers entered the spinal cord via the dorsal roots, whereas the motor fibers left it via the ventral roots. This became the basis for a distinction between sensory and motor processes – between sensation and movement (Boring 1950). In contrast to the opinion of Müller, his pupil Helmholtz demonstrated in 1850 that the

conduction velocity of a motor nerve in the frog was of the order of a hundred feet per second (Donders 1868/1969). In other words, processes preceding the activation of a muscle had become measurable. The minutes of a meeting of the Dutch Royal Academy of Arts and Sciences in 1865 mention that Donders presented experiments (of his student de Jaager and himself) about measuring the speed of mental processes. Some years later, he wrote his first publication, entitled "On the Speed of Mental Processes," which also appeared in a French and German translation (Donders 1868/1969). The kind of experiments he performed became known as "reaction" experiments, a term coined by Exner (1873).

The basic idea was that information processing is based upon a number of constituent processes, such as "discrimination" or "choice," each taking a circumscribed amount of time. Donders distinguished between the well-known A-, B-, and C-type responses. The A-response was found in a simple reaction time (RT) task in which the subject had to repeat the stimulus word "ki" as quickly as possible. In the B-task, five different stimulus words were used, each of which had to be repeated as quickly as possible. The B-response presumably included discriminative attention and a response choice. In the C-task, only one of the five stimulus words had to be repeated; here a discrimination was needed, but no choice. Presuming that the time needed for a complicated response was that of the simple response plus that of the additional central process, subtraction of A from B or C would provide the time needed for the higher process involved. Donders' method was systematically applied in Wundt's laboratory (Wundt 1893). It became clear that the C-response implied a choice, too – that is, between a Go and a No-Go response. Thus the D-response was added, which required two different responses for two different stimuli (Wundt 1893, pp. 386–9). The notion of "attention" was also needed to explain

John T. Cacioppo, Louis G. Tassinary, and Gary G. Berntson (Eds.), *Handbook of Psychophysiology,* 2nd ed. © Cambridge University Press 2000.

the experimental results; it was used by Lange (1888) to describe a difference between sensorial and muscular reactions. If attention was directed to a fast response (muscular reaction), then one had a shorter RT than when attention was directed toward analyzing the stimulus (sensory reaction). Although in later years the method became more and more criticized, it marked the emergence of experimental psychology from a physiological background.

The reaction time method became combined with a technique that stemmed from the philosophical background of psychology – namely, introspection. This was practiced systematically at the Würzburger school. Külpe contributed to the mental chronometry by an important study of bimanual RTs. He demonstrated the facilitation of the hand toward which attention is directed, supporting the attentional theory of RT (Boring 1950). Yet he soon came to the conclusion that the subtraction method was not justified because it could not be maintained that, in different experimental conditions, just one subprocess was changed. Külpe explained the experimental results of Lange (1888) by a difference in predisposition, in what later became called "attitude." A major topic of the Würzburger school was thinking, a function to be analyzed by the introspective method. Thus, Watt (1904) investigated how associations were brought about by asking his subjects to produce a superordinate for a subordinate or a part for a whole. A crucial conception in this line of research became the *Aufgabe*, the instruction given to a subject to start a thinking process. The instruction was supposed to evoke an *Einstellung* – a "set," as we would say (Boring 1950). So the concept of *set* – a preparedness to cope with a future situation – originated from association psychology. It emerged from experiments in which subjects observed and analyzed their own behavior by systematic experimental introspection. Another notion relevant for preparation is the determining tendency in the formation of associations (Ach 1905). If several associations between different items are of equal strength, the response a subject comes up with might be influenced by an earlier *Aufgabe*. If that instruction predetermines a subject so that even a weaker associative tendency is activated instead of one that is normally stronger, then a determining tendency is operating: a tendency to respond.

In the nineteenth century, psychologists talked about "attention" when the effective tendency was fully conscious and about "expectation" when this was less so. Both were supposed to influence perception and (re)action. It was even suggested that reaction time could be diminished to zero if expectation was optimal by always giving a warning signal at a fixed interval prior to the response stimulus (Boring 1950, p. 715). Too fast, as it happens, since Helmholtz discovered that some time is needed for an excited nerve to activate a muscle. Yet the notion that some form of preparation would result in a faster response was in line with the prevailing way of thinking. It is inter-

esting to note that Külpe supposed that expectancy effects upon perception were based upon spirits entering the sensory fibers from the senses to be later reflected to the muscles. It was said, in other words, that anticipatory behavior was characterized by changes in both the sensory and the motor domain.

It would take some decennia before psychologists would try to measure the physiological changes underlying anticipatory behavior. First the days of introspection came to an end, and behaviorism tried to expel notions like attention and consciousness from the field of scientific psychology. Stimulus and response became the crucial variables. Yet it was clear that psychology could not miss attention, attitude, expectancy, hypothesis, intention, vector, need, perseveration, and preoccupation – all of which were considered to be related to set (Gibson 1941). What these notions had in common was the view of behavior as determined by something other than the immediately preceding sensory stimulation. "It does not deny the importance of the immediate stimulus, it does deny that sensory stimulation is everything in behavior" (Hebb 1949). A new interest emerged in the "central process which seems relatively independent of afferent stimuli." In the same year that Hilgard and Marquis (1940) used this characterization, Davis (1940) published his paper on set and muscular tension. These first psychophysiological results showed a systematic increase in electromyographic (EMG) activity in arm muscles preceding a response stimulus. Two decades later, the first direct recordings of anticipatory brain activity took place. Walter and colleagues (1964) discovered the contingent negative variation, and Kornhuber and Deecke (1965) discovered the *Bereitschaftspotential* or readiness potential. Systematic anticipatory changes were demonstrated not only in the electroencephalogram (EEG), they proved to be present in the electrocardiogram (ECG) as well. The deceleration in heart rate prior to the presentation of an imperative stimulus (Lacey & Lacey 1970), together with other changes in autonomic responses, suggested that anticipatory behavior is reflected in a number of response systems.

Physical Context

INTRODUCTION

Any study of overt behavior is based upon the measurement of some form of movement. Movements are either triggered by some kind of external stimuli or stem from within the organism. It is plausible that both types of movement originate from different brain areas (Passingham 1987). However different the origin, the movement itself can only be brought about via the activation of the relevant motoneurons in brainstem and spinal cord. These constitute the starting point for the final common path (Sherrington 1906/1947) for all movements. The execution of a movement is based upon the contraction of muscles following an excitation of the relevant motoneurons that is sufficiently strong to make them fire. A classical opinion holds that the posterior part of the cerebral cortex is involved in perception and the anterior part in motricity (Luria 1973). We will see later on that this distinction cannot be maintained. Certain neurons in the posterior cortex fire only if a movement is to follow a stimulus presentation, and cells in the anterior cortex fire only after a preceding stimulus presentation. This suggests that, even from a functional anatomical point of view, it is not always easy to define an area as stimulus-bound or response-bound. We will further see that the motor system is really a distributed system in which many cortical and subcortical areas of the central nervous system participate.

The final result of all information processing is the execution of some movement. This chapter is aimed at the discussion of motor preparation, that is, the processes preceding the execution of the movement in question. The notion of preparation implies that there is at least prior knowledge about the necessity of a response, although there might be a temporal uncertainty and an event uncertainty. In experimental circumstances, anticipatory behavior starts with the presentation of a warning stimulus, indicating to the subjects that – after a known or unknown time – a stimulus might be presented, which must be responded to and which might or might not ask for a choice between several response alternatives. Although motor preparation is aimed at the processes at the end of this chain of stages, it is always accompanied by an anticipatory attention to instruction stimuli and possible cues that may or may not be present and that may or may not have behavioral significance. In the actual behavior it is rather artificial to insist upon a strict separation between anticipatory attention and preparation of the response. Anticipatory processes become manifest in more efficient behavior. In laboratory tasks, this all adds up to a shorter reaction time than would have been found without any antecedent knowledge of the experimental situation.

There are several ways to manipulate the subject's expectancy of the experimental situation. They involve stimulus–response compatibility, the number of stimulus–response alternatives, or the relative frequency of stimulus–response alternatives (Requin, Brener, & Ring 1991). Expectancy can also be influenced by giving a cue to a subject that indicates which of several possible alternatives may be needed (Rosenbaum 1980). If there is uncertainty about several variables in a movement at the same time (e.g., the distance that must be bridged, the side at which the response must be made, the finger that must be used), then partial advance information ameliorates the chance that a correct response will be made earlier in time than without that information (Rosenbaum 1985). Although the final result is a shorter RT, this effect hides a number of different mechanisms that might be responsible for it. In a strictly behavioral analysis it is certainly possible to separate some

of the underlying processes. Yet their implementation in the central nervous system remains unknown. Psychophysiology can offer techniques that can help unravel these underlying mechanisms and suggest their possible relation to circumscribed brain areas.

In the following text we will see how psychophysiological variables such as event-related potentials (ERPs) or reflexes can be used to improve the behavioral analysis. However helpful, the ERPs themselves are in general a reflection of cortical activity, since the EEG itself is. From animal and clinical work we know that anticipatory behavior cannot exhaustively be described in terms of cortical processes. Rather, we know that behavior in general is based upon the timely activation of a number of different neural structures, many of which are subcortical. Yet with the exception of some clinical studies, we are generally unable to investigate electrophysiological activity in subcortical human brain areas. Brain imaging studies might be helpful here, but animal studies are also still relevant. If we accept that there are many commonalities between the functioning of the human brain and that of the monkey, this gap in our knowledge can be partly bridged by the study of unit recordings in the nonhuman primate. In this chapter we will try to understand motor preparation as a part of anticipatory behavior, which itself can be described from structural and functional points of view. To appreciate the relevance of the unit recordings in nonhuman primates, an implicit knowledge of the functional neuroanatomy of anticipatory behavior is mandatory; hence we will also provide information about the presumed neuroanatomy of anticipatory behavior.

HOW TO UNDERSTAND BEHAVIOR: BOTTOM-UP OR TOP-DOWN?

The most simple involuntary movement is the *reflex:* an innate obligatory response upon an adequate stimulus. A reflex can be elicited by a proprioceptive stimulus, as is the case with the Achilles tendon reflex or the knee jerk, or by an exteroceptive stimulus, as with the flexion reflex or the blink reflex. The underlying wiring is different: the proprioceptive reflex is the most simple, because it is largely monosynaptic; the exteroceptive reflex is polysynaptic. The Achilles tendon reflex and the knee jerk have similar wiring but at a different level of the spinal cord. In both cases the essential stimulus is the stretching of the muscle by the tap on the tendon. This causes the intrafusal fibers of the muscle spindle to stretch as well, and this is the very trigger for the Ia afferents to send action potentials to the motoneurons in the spinal cord. The Ia afferents excite the alpha-motoneurons via their largely monosynaptic connection and cause these neurons to fire. This results in the obligatory contraction of the triceps surae muscles (in the case of the Achilles tendon reflex) or the quadriceps femoris muscle (in the knee jerk).

These reflexes are an example of a segmental organization of the motor system in the spinal cord: both the reflex afferents and efferents arrive at or leave from the same level. The reflex circuitry itself is under supraspinal control, both from the brainstem and the cortical level. Efferent fibers from brainstem and cortex influence the state of activity of the motoneuron pool. That is what makes the reflex modifiable and so enables its use as a tool to study response preparation (Bonnet, Requin, & Semjen 1981; Brunia & Boelhouwer 1988). If the fibers impinging upon the pool are inhibitory, then the membrane potential of the neurons in the pool moves away from the firing threshold. Thus, fewer elements in the pool will be apt to fire if the adequate stimulus is presented and, consequently, the reflex will show a smaller amplitude. From the other side, if the membrane potential of the motoneurons is moved nearer to the threshold by an excitatory supraspinal influence, then a larger number of them will fire if the adequate stimulus is presented, and the amplitude of the reflex becomes larger than in the absence of that influence. The latency of the reflex remains constant; it is mainly determined by the length of the muscle fibers involved in the reflex (e.g., leg length in the case of the Achilles tendon reflex).

The exteroceptive reflexes, which are evoked by skin stimulation, are determined by similar mechanisms. However, their afferents do not reach the agonist motoneurons directly but rather via interneurons. Hence, the exteroceptive reflexes are polysynaptic. They are also organized at different levels of the spinal cord and the brainstem. In contrast to the monosynaptic reflexes, there is a simultaneous activation of different muscles whose motoneurons are at different levels of the spinal cord. If one steps with naked foot on a drawing pin, an immediate flexion of the leg follows. Now neurons of different pools of flexor muscles of the foot, the limb, and the hip are excited, leading to a coordinated movement away from the stimulus. Exteroceptive reflexes are mostly defense responses.

The blink reflex is a brainstem reflex. Its circuitry is more complex and is not restricted to just one level of the brainstem. It is a polysynaptic reflex with a multimodal direct access for auditory, visual, and somatosensory stimuli. This makes it an interesting tool for studying attentional processes in different modalities (Dawson et al. 1997; Graham & Hackley 1991). The blink reflex is part of a defensive response pattern known as the startle reflex (Landis & Hunt 1939); it has therefore become also a tool for the study of emotional and motivational processes (Lang, Bradley, & Cuthbert 1990; Lang, Simons, & Balaban 1997). Finally, motor preparation has been studied also with the electrically evoked blink reflexes (Boelhouwer 1982; Brunia & Boelhouwer 1988).

The very existence of reflexes suggested to Sherrington (1906/1947) that our complete behavior might be built from reflex chains. The response in one reflex might be the trigger for the next, and so on. Thus, chains of reflexes are brought about by feedback to the central nervous system. This is a clear example of a "bottom-up" organization in behavior. Quite early in this century it had already become clear that deafferentation does not prevent the execution of complicated movements. In 1917, Lashley pointed to the behavior of a patient with a gunshot wound in his spinal cord. The lesion caused a complete anaesthesia for movements of the knee joint. Yet the patient was able to control the extent and speed of flexion and extension movements of the knee like normal people (Lashley 1917). Lashley returned to that finding in a famous paper in which he remarked that a competent musician can play a series of keystrokes at rates too fast to allow feedback to the central nervous system (Lashley 1951). Although the details of that argument do not seem to hold any longer, the interest in the "top-down" organization of the motor system was born; with that, the response-chaining hypothesis came to an end.

In Keele's (1968) notion of a motor program, the possibility for feedback to correct a sequence of movements is explicitly denied. He defined a motor program as "a set of muscle commands that are structured before a movement sequence begins, and that allows the entire sequence to be carried out uninfluenced by peripheral feedback" (1968, p. 387). The specification of response parameters like force, duration, and complexity must be implemented before the movement can be executed. Thus, it is no surprise that the reaction time to the first of a series of responses increases with the length of the series even though that first movement remains identical (Henry & Rogers 1960). This result cannot be explained by peripheral control from proprioceptive feedback. Further supporting evidence for the existence of motor programs came from studies in which nonhuman primates, deprived from proprioceptive feedback via a neurosurgical intervention, were still able to carry out skillful reaching movements (Taub & Berman 1968). A similar result was reported for humans (Forget & Lamarre 1987). Although this underlines the importance of central processes for the initiative of an action, we do not deny the significance of feedback for our behavior in general.

In a cognitive psychological approach of motor preparation, our point of departure is the central organization responsible for development of behavior. Most movements serve a goal – for instance, keeping one's equilibrium, bridging a distance in walking or running, plying a tool, aiming at a target in any kind of shooting, handling a ball in a game, pointing, and grasping. In order to reach the goal, some kind of perceptual control is necessary, be it visual, somatosensory, or auditory. So even if the plan to address a specific action is made and results in a series of voluntary movements, we should keep in mind that these movements must be carried out within the constraints of the available environment. Thus, as soon as the plan is developed and translated into the preparation and execution of certain movements, the environment plays its role. In playing a well-known piece of music, violists might close their eyes; they know the music by heart. Putting the fingers of their left hand on the correct place on the string happens under the control of the auditory and somatosensory feedback: the sound, touch, and vibration of the string. We have seen earlier that playing music has been an argument for Lashley (1951) in favor of the existence of motor programs. Rosenbaum (1980) observed that the very existence of anticipatory effects – both in behavioral output and in the concomitant (psycho)physiological phenomena – is a strong argument against the chaining theory and in favor of the existence of motor programs. Accepting a top-down structure as the basis for interpreting behavior, we argue again that anticipation in our behavior determines not only the output of the system but also the input – that is, both perception and action.

THE NEUROANATOMY OF ANTICIPATORY BEHAVIOR

Motor control is in essence the control of the excitatory and inhibitory influences impinging upon the motoneuron cell columns in the spinal cord. Once these cells discharge, there is no way to stop the final response. The efferent volley is transmitted along the motor fibers to the muscles, resulting in some sort of contraction. In contrast to many situations in everyday life, this is not what one aims at when preparing a response in a reaction time task. Here, the final discharge must be produced at the very moment a stimulus is presented. Such experiments are in a certain sense static. The subject is sitting in a chair and waits upon the arrival of an imperative stimulus. There is not much posture control required, and the activation of only some muscles is needed for the crucial timely response. However artificial this situation might look, the analysis of human behavior under these circumstances has implications for all kinds of supervisory tasks in industrial settings. Its ecological validity can be doubted, however, in a number of other situations. Playing tennis is of course a much more dynamic affair and involves the active assessment of one's ability to answer a future attack. Both posture and beginning arm movements are based upon an estimation of the behavior of the opponent. Neither the spot where the ball will arrive, nor the force with which it will be hit, are known. Preparation implies here a setting of posture and movement under active visuomotor control and is much more complicated than in the RT task. Although different in many important ways, the laboratory and real-life situations both involve a coordinated activation of a number of different brain areas. Consequently, the relevant neuroanatomical structures implicated in the organization of a system of descending fibers to the motoneuron cell columns in the spinal cord will now be discussed, albeit in outline form.

We will first describe the general outline of the motor system. Then we will report a number of anatomical structures in which, by any technique, anticipatory phenomena have been recorded. Next we will discuss some aspects of the visual system in order to later discuss visuomotor control in anticipatory behavior. Finally we will address the role of the prefrontal cortex in the executive control of anticipatory behavior. Although our main focus is on discrete hand responses (such as key presses) in the context of RT experiments, much of what follows is applicable to other types of responses and movements as well.

Contractions of muscles take place after an efferent volley from the motoneurons to the muscles. The motoneuron, its axon, and the muscle fibers innervated are together defined as the *motor unit*. Therefore, one could consider the motoneuron "peripheral" in relation to the rest of the motor system. Holstege (1991) divides the motor system in three parts (see Figure 1). The first motor system is formed by the interneuronal projections into the motoneurons (Holstege 1991, p. 89); they are present in the spinal cord, in the caudal brainstem, and in between. The neurons involved receive information from the periphery (via afferent fibers) and from the second and third motor system. The second motor system sends its fibers to a limited extent directly to the motoneurons but largely to the interneurons of the first system. It has a mediolateral organization; that is, it can be divided into a medial and lateral part with different functions (Holstege 1991; Kuypers 1981). The medial part originates from the brainstem and descends in the ventral funiculus of the spinal cord to terminate on the interneurons of the medial motoneuron column. It is involved in eye and neck movements and in axial and proximal body movements. The lateral part descends from the cortex and (to a lesser extent) from the red nucleus to the lateral motoneuron cell column. From here, the distal body muscles are innervated (Holstege 1991; Kuypers 1981). The third motor system has hardly any overlap with the secondary system. Here, too, is a mediolateral division of labor. The medial component originates from the medial hypothalamus and mesencephalon and terminates in the locus coeruleus, the ventral part of the caudal pons, and the medial tegmentum. The latter structures form the final output to the first system. The lateral part originates in the lateral hypothalamus, the central nucleus of the amygdala, and the bed nucleus of the stria terminalis to terminate in the lateral tegmentum (Holstege 1991).

The third system is a rather recent discovery, based upon new tracer techniques in neuroanatomy (Holstege 1991). It is along this system that emotions enter the motor system. This is an interesting example of "discovery" of a system whose existence was taken for granted by clinicians, who knew that emotional influences played a role in the motor system without knowing the crucial pathways (Gellhorn & Loofbourrow 1963). The medial part of the third system has a diffuse influence on the spinal cord via descending

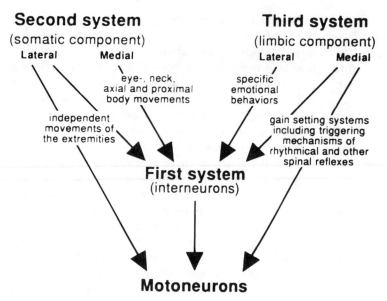

Figure 1. Schematic overview of the three subdivisions of the motor system. Reprinted with permission from Holstege, "Descending motor pathways and the spinal motor system. Limbic and non-limbic components," in Holstege (Ed.), *Role of the Forebrain in Sensation and Behavior* (Progress in Brain Research, vol. 87), pp. 307–421. Copyright 1991 Elsevier Science.

fibers from the locus coeruleus and the raphe nuclei to the motor nuclei and the dorsal horn. The medial part of the third system is activated in the expression of emotions such as laughing or crying; it has the effect of lowering the firing threshold of the motor nuclei of the spinal cord so that their excitation by fibers from the secondary system is facilitated (Holstege 1991). The lateral part of the third motor system projects to the lateral tegmentum, where the interneurons of the primary system are situated. These are involved in rather automatic functions such as respiration, vomiting, swallowing, chewing, and licking.

Structures Involved in Motor Preparation

We will start with a description of relevant cortical structures. The corticalization of the human brain is so impressive that one would be inclined to consider that the prerequisite for any cognitive behavior. This does not imply, however, that we consider behavior to be exclusively a manifestation of cortical processes. Rather, we are convinced of the importance of all kinds of subcortical processes that influence – in a dynamic ongoing gating – the crucial cortical structures. The cortex is certainly involved both in initiating our behavior and in executing all kinds of movements. Yet none of these movements are brought about without the cooperation of the basal ganglia and the cerebellum. These structures handle the information from and to the cortex via different pathways. Both have connections to structures in the brainstem from which the spinal motoneurons are activated.

The Cortex Cerebri. The following parts of the cortex can be considered motor areas (see Figure 2): (1) the precentral gyrus or MI, (2) the premotor cortex, (3) the supplementary motor area, (4) the cingulate motor area, and (5) the frontal eye field.

The precentral gyrus is the motor cortex *sensu strictu*; lying immediately anterior to the central sulcus, it is involved in the execution of voluntary movements. Onset of a movement starts with the discharge of pyramidal tract neurons (Evarts 1968). The firing threshold is lower in the motor cortex than in the premotor or supplementary motor cortex. The activity pattern of a large number of neurons in this area is related to force or speed of a movement. Its cortical sensory input stems for a large part from the adjacent somatosensory areas. Its cortical motor input arrives from the neighboring premotor and supplementary motor areas. Axons of the pyramidal cells descend to the brainstem and spinal motoneurons, either directly or via interneurons. This is the pathway by which discrete skilled movements are realized.

Anterior to the precentral gyrus we find the premotor cortex (PMC), also known as Brodmann's area 6, in which ventral (F4 and F5 in Figure 2) and dorsal (F2 and F7 in Figure 2) parts can be distinguished. The dorsal part of the premotor cortex receives input from the superior parietal lobe, from which sensory information is relayed. A detailed description of the many intricate sensory–motor connections is not possible in this chapter, and the reader is referred to Wise et al. (1997) for more detail. The premotor cortex is better developed in humans than in nonhuman primates. Deiber and associates (1991) asked their subjects to make simple movements with a joystick following the presentation of a tone. In one condition, the movement always had to be made in one direction; in the other condition, a choice had to be made between four possible directions. An increase in regional bloodflow (rCBF), which is an index of increased metabolism, was found in the premotor and supplementary motor cortices in the choice condition, whereas the activity in MI did not differ between the simple and the choice condition. This suggests that the premotor and supplementary motor cortex are involved in response selection. Recording of unit activity in the PMC suggests that this brain area is also responsible for stimulus-guided movements.

Wiesendanger (1993) summarized the possible functions of the supplementary motor area (SMA). Planning of our behavior is attributed to this brain area. Preparation and initialization of movements seem to be organized here, and the SMA is also involved in the translation of motives and intentions in behavior. Timing of our behavior and the control of the sequencing of behavioral elements are possible functions, as are the organization of posture

of certain movements, the environment plays its role. In playing a well-known piece of music, violists might close their eyes; they know the music by heart. Putting the fingers of their left hand on the correct place on the string happens under the control of the auditory and somatosensory feedback: the sound, touch, and vibration of the string. We have seen earlier that playing music has been an argument for Lashley (1951) in favor of the existence of motor programs. Rosenbaum (1980) observed that the very existence of anticipatory effects – both in behavioral output and in the concomitant (psycho)physiological phenomena – is a strong argument against the chaining theory and in favor of the existence of motor programs. Accepting a top-down structure as the basis for interpreting behavior, we argue again that anticipation in our behavior determines not only the output of the system but also the input – that is, both perception and action.

THE NEUROANATOMY OF ANTICIPATORY BEHAVIOR

Motor control is in essence the control of the excitatory and inhibitory influences impinging upon the motoneuron cell columns in the spinal cord. Once these cells discharge, there is no way to stop the final response. The efferent volley is transmitted along the motor fibers to the muscles, resulting in some sort of contraction. In contrast to many situations in everyday life, this is not what one aims at when preparing a response in a reaction time task. Here, the final discharge must be produced at the very moment a stimulus is presented. Such experiments are in a certain sense static. The subject is sitting in a chair and waits upon the arrival of an imperative stimulus. There is not much posture control required, and the activation of only some muscles is needed for the crucial timely response. However artificial this situation might look, the analysis of human behavior under these circumstances has implications for all kinds of supervisory tasks in industrial settings. Its ecological validity can be doubted, however, in a number of other situations. Playing tennis is of course a much more dynamic affair and involves the active assessment of one's ability to answer a future attack. Both posture and beginning arm movements are based upon an estimation of the behavior of the opponent. Neither the spot where the ball will arrive, nor the force with which it will be hit, are known. Preparation implies here a setting of posture and movement under active visuomotor control and is much more complicated than in the RT task. Although different in many important ways, the laboratory and real-life situations both involve a coordinated activation of a number of different brain areas. Consequently, the relevant neuroanatomical structures implicated in the organization of a system of descending fibers to the motoneuron cell columns in the spinal cord will now be discussed, albeit in outline form.

We will first describe the general outline of the motor system. Then we will report a number of anatomical structures in which, by any technique, anticipatory phenomena have been recorded. Next we will discuss some aspects of the visual system in order to later discuss visuomotor control in anticipatory behavior. Finally we will address the role of the prefrontal cortex in the executive control of anticipatory behavior. Although our main focus is on discrete hand responses (such as key presses) in the context of RT experiments, much of what follows is applicable to other types of responses and movements as well.

Contractions of muscles take place after an efferent volley from the motoneurons to the muscles. The motoneuron, its axon, and the muscle fibers innervated are together defined as the *motor unit*. Therefore, one could consider the motoneuron "peripheral" in relation to the rest of the motor system. Holstege (1991) divides the motor system in three parts (see Figure 1). The first motor system is formed by the interneuronal projections into the motoneurons (Holstege 1991, p. 89); they are present in the spinal cord, in the caudal brainstem, and in between. The neurons involved receive information from the periphery (via afferent fibers) and from the second and third motor system. The second motor system sends its fibers to a limited extent directly to the motoneurons but largely to the interneurons of the first system. It has a mediolateral organization; that is, it can be divided into a medial and lateral part with different functions (Holstege 1991; Kuypers 1981). The medial part originates from the brainstem and descends in the ventral funiculus of the spinal cord to terminate on the interneurons of the medial motoneuron column. It is involved in eye and neck movements and in axial and proximal body movements. The lateral part descends from the cortex and (to a lesser extent) from the red nucleus to the lateral motoneuron cell column. From here, the distal body muscles are innervated (Holstege 1991; Kuypers 1981). The third motor system has hardly any overlap with the secondary system. Here, too, is a mediolateral division of labor. The medial component originates from the medial hypothalamus and mesencephalon and terminates in the locus coeruleus, the ventral part of the caudal pons, and the medial tegmentum. The latter structures form the final output to the first system. The lateral part originates in the lateral hypothalamus, the central nucleus of the amygdala, and the bed nucleus of the stria terminalis to terminate in the lateral tegmentum (Holstege 1991).

The third system is a rather recent discovery, based upon new tracer techniques in neuroanatomy (Holstege 1991). It is along this system that emotions enter the motor system. This is an interesting example of "discovery" of a system whose existence was taken for granted by clinicians, who knew that emotional influences played a role in the motor system without knowing the crucial pathways (Gellhorn & Loofbourrow 1963). The medial part of the third system has a diffuse influence on the spinal cord via descending

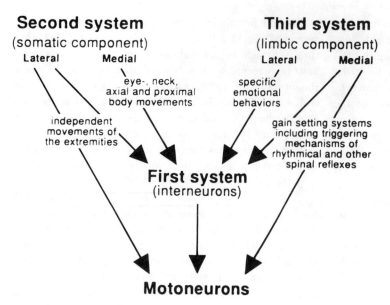

Figure 1. Schematic overview of the three subdivisions of the motor system. Reprinted with permission from Holstege, "Descending motor pathways and the spinal motor system. Limbic and non-limbic components," in Holstege (Ed.), *Role of the Forebrain in Sensation and Behavior* (Progress in Brain Research, vol. 87), pp. 307–421. Copyright 1991 Elsevier Science.

fibers from the locus coeruleus and the raphe nuclei to the motor nuclei and the dorsal horn. The medial part of the third system is activated in the expression of emotions such as laughing or crying; it has the effect of lowering the firing threshold of the motor nuclei of the spinal cord so that their excitation by fibers from the secondary system is facilitated (Holstege 1991). The lateral part of the third motor system projects to the lateral tegmentum, where the interneurons of the primary system are situated. These are involved in rather automatic functions such as respiration, vomiting, swallowing, chewing, and licking.

Structures Involved in Motor Preparation

We will start with a description of relevant cortical structures. The corticalization of the human brain is so impressive that one would be inclined to consider that the prerequisite for any cognitive behavior. This does not imply, however, that we consider behavior to be exclusively a manifestation of cortical processes. Rather, we are convinced of the importance of all kinds of subcortical processes that influence – in a dynamic ongoing gating – the crucial cortical structures. The cortex is certainly involved both in initiating our behavior and in executing all kinds of movements. Yet none of these movements are brought about without the cooperation of the basal ganglia and the cerebellum. These structures handle the information from and to the cortex via different pathways. Both have connections to structures in the brainstem from which the spinal motoneurons are activated.

The Cortex Cerebri. The following parts of the cortex can be considered motor areas (see Figure 2): (1) the precentral gyrus or MI, (2) the premotor cortex, (3) the supplementary motor area, (4) the cingulate motor area, and (5) the frontal eye field.

The precentral gyrus is the motor cortex *sensu strictu*; lying immediately anterior to the central sulcus, it is involved in the execution of voluntary movements. Onset of a movement starts with the discharge of pyramidal tract neurons (Evarts 1968). The firing threshold is lower in the motor cortex than in the premotor or supplementary motor cortex. The activity pattern of a large number of neurons in this area is related to force or speed of a movement. Its cortical sensory input stems for a large part from the adjacent somatosensory areas. Its cortical motor input arrives from the neighboring premotor and supplementary motor areas. Axons of the pyramidal cells descend to the brainstem and spinal motoneurons, either directly or via interneurons. This is the pathway by which discrete skilled movements are realized.

Anterior to the precentral gyrus we find the premotor cortex (PMC), also known as Brodmann's area 6, in which ventral (F4 and F5 in Figure 2) and dorsal (F2 and F7 in Figure 2) parts can be distinguished. The dorsal part of the premotor cortex receives input from the superior parietal lobe, from which sensory information is relayed. A detailed description of the many intricate sensory–motor connections is not possible in this chapter, and the reader is referred to Wise et al. (1997) for more detail. The premotor cortex is better developed in humans than in nonhuman primates. Deiber and associates (1991) asked their subjects to make simple movements with a joystick following the presentation of a tone. In one condition, the movement always had to be made in one direction; in the other condition, a choice had to be made between four possible directions. An increase in regional bloodflow (rCBF), which is an index of increased metabolism, was found in the premotor and supplementary motor cortices in the choice condition, whereas the activity in MI did not differ between the simple and the choice condition. This suggests that the premotor and supplementary motor cortex are involved in response selection. Recording of unit activity in the PMC suggests that this brain area is also responsible for stimulus-guided movements.

Wiesendanger (1993) summarized the possible functions of the supplementary motor area (SMA). Planning of our behavior is attributed to this brain area. Preparation and initialization of movements seem to be organized here, and the SMA is also involved in the translation of motives and intentions in behavior. Timing of our behavior and the control of the sequencing of behavioral elements are possible functions, as are the organization of posture

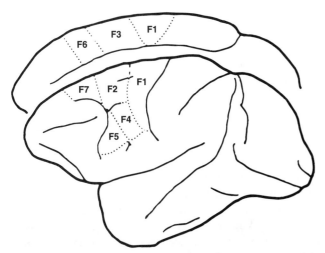

Figure 2. Lateral view of the left hemisphere and medial view of the right hemisphere in the monkey with terminology of Rizzolatti et al. (1996). The primary motor cortex (precentral gyrus, MI, Broadmann's area 4) is designated by F1. The premotor cortex (PMC, Broadmann's area 6) is divided into dorsal (F7 and F2) and ventral (F5 and F4) parts. The supplementary motor area (SMA, Broadman's mesial area 6), is divided in two different areas: F3 (the SMA proper) and F6 (the pre-SMA), with different cytoarchitectonic structures, different subcortical connections, and different functions. Not shown are the frontal eye field (FEF, Broadmann's area 8), situated between F7 and F5, and the cingulate motor areas (Broadmann's areas 23 and 24), situated below the mesial areas F6, F3, and F1. Reprinted (and relabeled) with permission from Rizzolatti, Luppino, & Matelli, "The classic supplementary motor area is formed by two independent areas," in Lüders (Ed.), *Supplementary Sensorimotor Area* (Advances in Neurology, vol. 70), pp. 45–56. Copyright 1996 Lippincott Williams & Wilkins.

during the execution of purposive movements. Furthermore, the control of self-initiated movements is attributed to the SMA. Indeed, the question can be asked whether all this does not point to a supramotor role rather than to a supplementary motor function. It is too early for a definite conclusion, but part of the existing controversy seems to be solved by a paper of Matelli, Luppino, and Rizzolatti (1991; see Figure 2). These authors divide the classic SMA into two parts, the SMA proper (area F3) and, just in front of this, the pre-SMA (area F6). The input to both areas is different: F3 but not F6 is connected to MI. This connection is somatotopically organized (Rizzolatti, Luppino, & Matelli 1996). There are also connections to the dorsal part of the premotor cortex and the cingulate areas. Area F6 is mainly connected to the anterior premotor cortex. It receives an additional input from the prefrontal cortex, which does not hold for F3 (Rizzolatti et al. 1996). The thalamic projections are also different for F3 and F6; F3 gets its major input from the ventrolateral and the posterior ventrolateral nuclei of the thalamus, whereas the input to F6 stems from the dorsomedial and the anterior ventral nucleus of the thalamus.

It is a relatively recent discovery that the cingulate region has a function in motor behavior. As a consequence, this area has not been extensively studied. One of the few

facts known about the cingulate region is that it can be divided in two parts: an anterior and a posterior area, the first of which seems to be related to self-paced motor acts (Rothwell 1995, p. 355).

Area 8 of Brodmann is known as the frontal eye field (FEF). It has strong reciprocal connections to the lateral intraparietal area, situated in the lateral bank of the intraparietal sulcus. Both project to the colliculus superior (Milner & Goodale 1995) and are strongly implicated in the control of saccadic eye movements. The FEF also receives an input from two temporal areas, the medial superior temporal area and the fundus of the superior temporal sulcus (Boussaoud & Wise 1993). These areas seem to be involved in the control of pursuit eye movements (Milner & Goodale 1995). In other words, the control of saccades and of pursuit eye movements seems to be organized into two independent fronto-parietal systems.

The Basal Ganglia. The basal ganglia can be distinguished in the neostriatum. They consist of the caudate nucleus and the putamen, the globus pallidus (pars interna and pars externa), the subthalamic nucleus, and the substantia nigra pars reticulata (Figure 3). Originally, DeLong and Georgopoulos (1981) suggested that there were two loops in which different parts of the basal ganglia are connected to the cortex via different thalamic nuclei: a motor loop and a complex loop. The motor loop directs influences from the sensorimotor and premotor cortices via putamen, pallidum, and thalamus to the premotor cortex. The complex loop connects the association cortex via caudate nucleus, pallidum, and thalamus to the prefrontal cortex. These circuits are independent of each other; they remain segregated, as are the leg and arm representations within the motor loop (DeLong et al. 1984). A couple of years later, Alexander, DeLong, and Strick (1986) suggested the existence of five different circuits between basal ganglia and cortex, all built following the same model. The model itself is discussed further in Alexander and Crutcher (1990) and DeLong (1990), whose description will be followed here. Within the motor loop there are two pathways to the globus pallidus pars interna (GPi) and the substantia nigra pars reticularis (SNr). An indirect pathway passes the globus pallidus pars externa (GPe) and the subthalamic nucleus (STN), and a direct pathway innervates the GPi and SNr monosynaptically. From here is a direct connection to one of the possible thalamic nuclei, which project – depending on which thalamic nucleus was passed – to different cortical areas. The projections from the different cortical areas to the putamen (or the globus pallidus, not depicted here) is excitatory. The direct pathway has an inhibitory connection to the GPe/SNr; in the indirect pathway, two inhibitory connections are followed by one excitatory to the same target (GPe/SNr). From here, there is an inhibitory connection to the thalamus and an excitatory connection to the cortex (Figure 3).

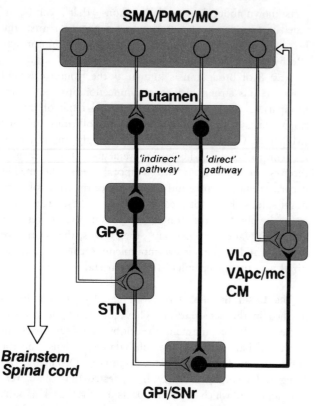

SMA/PMC/MC

Putamen

'indirect' pathway   'direct' pathway

GPe

VLo VApc/mc CM

STN

Brainstem Spinal cord

GPi/SNr

Figure 3. Diagram of the motor circuit in which only the closed loop is depicted. Inhibitory neurons are depicted in black, excitatory neurons in gray. *Key:* CM, center median; GPe, globus pallidus pars externa; GPi, globus pallidus pars interna; MC, primary motor cortex; PMC, premotor cortex; SMA, supplementary motor cortex; SNr, substantia nigra pars reticularis; STN, subthalamic nucleus; VA, nucleus ventralis anterior; VLo, nucleus ventralis pars oralis. Reprinted with permission from Alexander & Crutcher, "Functional architecture of basal ganglia circuits: Neural substrates of parallel processing," *Trends in Neurosciences*, vol. 13, pp. 266–71. Copyright 1990 Elsevier Science.

Although the basal ganglia seem to be involved in different kinds of cognitive functioning, in the present context we will discuss only their role for motor behavior and, more specifically, motor preparation. Schultz and colleagues (1995) provided arguments for this based upon (1) the behavioral effects of lesions in the basal ganglia in animals and humans, (2) the anatomical targets for the output of the basal ganglia (i.e., the motor cortex and the colliculus superior), and (3) the firing of basal ganglia units in relation to force and direction of movements. It is interesting to note that Schultz et al. (1995) found anticipatory firing of units preceding spontaneous and stimulus-triggered movements – and prior to all kind of stimuli that are of relevance for upcoming behavior. This suggests that an almost simultaneous basal ganglia activity is present during all anticipatory EEG activity that we know about in humans (to be discussed later on).

The Cerebellum. The cerebellum receives ascending input from the spinal cord and descending input from senso-

rimotor cortex via the brainstem. Its output to the cortex runs from the dentate nucleus via the thalamus to MI. In line herewith, Thach (1987) reported preparatory activity in dentate nucleus *prior* to that in MI whereas other cerebellar nuclei only fired *after* movement onset; this suggests that the dentate nucleus is involved in motor preparation, with the other nuclei in control of movement execution. Indeed, lesions in the dentate nucleus in nonhuman primates resulted in the absence of a well-known slow wave, the readiness potential, which can normally be recorded prior to voluntary movements. We will discuss this anticipatory slow wave later on, but here we note that subcortical input to MI seems to be obligatory for the emergence of this slow wave. A more general conclusion is that the activity in the motor cortex is based upon an important subcortical input via the thalamus, which enables modulation of the input relevant for sensory processing and for motor processing in a comparable way. In other words, there is a commonality in the organization of anticipatory attention and motor preparation (Brunia 1997).

Structures Involved in Visuomotor Control

Of the three major modalities, the visual system is presumably the best investigated. We will discuss it here in short because many of our movements are in some way or another coupled to what we see. The optic nerve on its way to the cortex passes the lateral geniculate body, considered a "relay" nucleus for visual information. From here, fibers ascend to the visual cortex and participate in a local intracortical circuit, a cortico-cortical circuit, and a thalamo-cortico-thalamic circuit. The first circuit is excitatory, suggesting that a certain input can have an enduring activity in that column (LaBerge 1995). Cortico-cortical pathways are divided into two main streams for visual information, known as the "what" and the "where" systems (Ungerleider & Mishkin 1982). Fibers returning to the thalamus do so to the lateral geniculate body, but also to the pulvinar. The pulvinar is (among others) connected to the parietal cortex, which plays a role in an attentional network (Mesulam 1981; Posner 1994). Yet it should be kept in mind that 50% of the pulvinar cells do not respond to sensory stimulation, so it is doubtful that the only function of the pulvinar is attentional. The same holds for the parietal cortex, with which it has many reciprocal connections. Many parietal neurons are described as responding upon sensory stimulation *only if* a response has to be generated. Moreover, recent studies in patients with certain parietal lesions suggest that their pathology can be described as "not knowing how to act" rather than as a disturbance in the "where" system (Milner & Goodale 1995). These authors noted that picking up an object requires not only a reaching movement but also that hand and fingers be shaped in such a way that size and orientation of the object are anticipated in order to perform a correct grasping movement. Reaching and grasping are temporally coupled under normal circumstances, although they seem to be organized independently (Jeannerod 1997). A combined disturbance can be found in patients with optic ataxia following lesions in the posterior parietal cortex: they not only might fail to reach in the right direction, they also fail to orient their hand and form their grasp appropriately (Milner & Goodale 1995, p. 97). This example clarifies that motor preparation is much more than being ready to press a button. Moreover, it illustrates how the posterior part of the cortex is related not only to perceptual processes but also to the organization of action.

Structures Involved in Executive Control

Anatomically, the prefrontal cortex is defined as the projection area of the dorsomedial nucleus of the thalamus. Apart from that input, the prefrontal cortex also receives fibers from the ventral anterior nucleus and the anterior part of the intralaminar nuclei. According to Fuster (1997), behavior is typified as a hierarchical order of elements that are structured in time. He considers the temporal organization of complex behavior to be the main job of this brain area, and he distinguishes three major functions of the prefrontal cortex: (1) preparation for coming events, (2) memory of recent events, and (3) suppression of interference.

As we argued already in the introduction, preparatory behavior is aimed at the setting of relevant motor structures and also of perceptual systems. Perception can be facilitated by attention, a function that is accomplished by the parietal cortex in collaboration with the pulvinar (LaBerge 1995). The attentional network is under the control of the prefrontal cortex; the same holds for the motor cortex and the dorsomedial nucleus. Elsewhere (Brunia 1997) we have claimed that motor preparation and anticipatory attention are realized via comparable networks in which the reticular nucleus of the thalamus plays a crucial role. The reticular nucleus itself is (among others) under the excitatory influence of the prefrontal cortex. Activation of that pathway results in a relative closing of thalamo-cortical channels. In other words, the thalamo-cortical stream of information – be it in the sensory or in the motor route – can still be modulated just before its entrance into the cortex.

An instruction given to a subject must be kept in a working memory circuit together with other relevant information from comparable situations. Fuster and Alexander (1971) recorded unit activity in the prefrontal cortex that they related to a mnemonic process of retaining a cue. Clinical data also suggest that the prefrontal cortex is involved in holding information that is relevant for only a short time. Neuropsychological research in patients with prefrontal lesions shows that they have a deficient response inhibition. The well-known work of B. Milner (1964) with the Wisconsin card-sorting test demonstrates that patients have difficulties in shifting between response strategies. There is much supporting evidence for the notion that the prefrontal cortex is indeed involved in response inhibition. Fuster (1997) claimed that the medial part of the prefrontal cortex is responsible; Goldman-Rakic (1987) suggested that the function of the prefrontal cortex is initializing, facilitating, or stopping of commands to structures that are involved in motor programming. In other words, the Go–No-Go decision seems to be a function in which the prefrontal cortex participates, as can be concluded from the reports of Sasaki and Gemba (1989; Gemba & Sasaki 1989).

Another function has been suggested by Teuber (1964). In order to distinguish between self-paced movements and externally triggered movements, an organism should be informed about self-initiated movement. Teuber suggested that this is realized via "corollary discharges": a motor command is sent not only to movement-related structures but also to parietal and temporal association areas to inform these areas about the impinging movement. This, too, is an indication of the executive control the prefrontal cortex exerts upon other brain areas. Later on we will see that anticipatory slow waves have a major source in this brain area.

Inferential Context

THE PSYCHOPHYSIOLOGICAL APPROACH TO MOTOR PREPARATION

In the foregoing text we have indicated that, however important the cortex cerebri might be for anticipatory behavior, the role of subcortical structures – the ascending brainstem systems, cerebellum, basal ganglia, and thalamus – must not be forgotten. Much of what happens at the cortical level is, at least partly, a reflection of processes in these structures. As an example we mentioned the well-known anticipatory readiness potential that does not show up if a lesion in the dentate nucleus of the cerebellum is present. This example clarifies the importance of knowledge of subcortical processes for the interpretation of experimental results obtained from the cortex. A real understanding of what happens when a response is prepared and executed must be based upon knowledge of all areas involved. The consequence of this is that we need information from as many different sources as possible.

One psychophysiological approach is to use the EEG (or, more precisely, ERPs) to investigate the relation between behavior and the relevant brain processes. This method can certainly provide results that allow further-reaching conclusions than a strictly behavioral analysis. Yet it should not be forgotten that the EEG and, by implication, most ERPs are a reflection of cortical activity. Changes in this activity that are caused by subcortical processes can certainly be demonstrated in humans, but recordings from subcortical areas can only be obtained in relatively rare clinical cases. Therefore, we also need to know about depth recordings in monkeys under similar experimental conditions to the ones we are interested in. Such recordings concern mostly cell activity. Electromagnetic brain activity reflects changes in postsynaptic membranes of large numbers of cells in the cortex that are activated more or less simultaneously. If the membrane potentials reach the firing threshold, the cells discharge. Thus, the EEG and the unit firing reflect related but different aspects of the same process. There are relatively few studies in which unit firing and slow potentials have been recorded simultaneously (e.g. Arezzo & Vaughan 1980; Fox & Norman 1968). Monkey studies allow the recording of unit firing at both the cortical and subcortical level. If unit recordings at the cortical level in monkeys show commonalities with the ERP recordings in humans, and if subcortical unit activity in monkeys is related to their cortical unit activity, then we are on relatively safe ground when we consider the whole set of data of importance to our understanding of human behavior.

The study of ERPs or event-related fields (ERFs) provides results of high precision in the time domain, but spatial resolution is a problem. The skin, the skull, and the meninges cause a dispersion of the relevant brain activity owing to their different conduction properties. Recently developed techniques of source localization (see Scherg 1990) provide one possible method to overcome this limitation, but the fact remains that we are unable to record subcortical processes directly from the skull.

This problem does not exist with the technique of positron emission tomography (PET), which provides an image of all areas relevant for the execution of a certain task. This advantage goes along with a loss of precision in time, however. Here a better spatial resolution is obtained, and it is possible to record changes in subcortical activation. The newly developed technique of functional magnetic resonance imaging (fMRI) provides a better temporal resolution than the PET studies, so we can expect more fMRI research to take place on the present topic.

Transcranial magnetic stimulation (TMS; Barker, Jalinous, & Freeston 1985) is a technique by which a short magnetic pulse is applied to the motor cortex via the skull, resulting in a short muscle contraction. The pre-existing excitability of the target motoneurons determines the outcome of the stimulation. If a stimulus is applied during the foreperiod of a reaction time task and if an identical stimulus is applied under control conditions, then comparison of both responses provides an insight into the changes in excitability due to the preparation of a response. This is a comparable (yet dissimilar) approach to the use of reflexes as a probe for studying motor preparation.

If an Achilles tendon reflex (or a Hoffmann reflex) is evoked during the foreperiod of a reaction time task, then the amplitude of the reflex is an expression of the number of alpha-motoneurons that fire as a result of the stimulus strength and the pre-existing excitability of the motoneuron pool. Keeping the stimulus strength constant, changes in excitability due to the preparation of the movement can be investigated by comparing the amplitudes of the reflexes evoked during preparation with those evoked under control conditions. The changes in amplitude are a peripheral manifestation of supraspinal preparatory processes.

EVENT-RELATED POTENTIALS

The first electroencephalographic measurement related to a human motor act was reported by Bates (1951), who described a negative potential after movement onset that was interpreted as a reafferent sensory evoked potential. The study of preparatory EEG measurements in humans was initiated by the discovery of the contingent negative variation (CNV) by Walter and his colleagues at the Burden Neurological Institute in Bristol, England (Walter et al. 1964). They recorded a sustained negative potential shift of about -20 μV in the 1-sec interval between a warning stimulus (S1, a single click) and an imperative stimulus (S2, repetitive flashes that could be terminated by a button press). The CNV was discernible in the raw EEG traces but became more evident when noise was reduced by calculating averages of twelve successive trials. The CNV reached its maximum[1] amplitude at the presentation of S2 and returned to the baseline level when the response was made.

At about the same time, Kornhuber and Deecke were studying the brain electrical activity that accompanies voluntary motor actions at the University of Freiburg, Germany. They asked their subjects to press a button at intervals of their own choice and recorded the electrical activity from the scalp on magnetic tape. Backward analysis of the tape recording allowed them to study the brain activity preceding the button press. They found a slowly increasing negative potential shift, starting more than 1 sec before the button press (depending on the rate of responding) and increasing up to the instant of the motor act. This negative shift was labeled *Bereitschaftspotential* or readiness potential (RP; Kornhuber & Deecke 1965).

Kornhuber and Deecke (1965) suggested that the neuronal processes underlying the RP and the CNV were similar. The similarities and differences between these slow brain potentials have been the topic of a considerable amount of research, especially in the 1970s and 1980s. Since the CNV is usually larger than the RP, it was thought that the CNV (i) consisted of an RP associated with the motor response but (ii) was recorded on top of another, presumably nonmotor, negativity. This nonmotor negativity was subsequently isolated and termed stimulus-preceding negativity (Brunia 1988).

An interesting psychophysiological tool that can be applied in the study of motor processes is the lateralized readiness potential (see Coles 1989 for an overview). This measure is based on the observation that the amplitude of the RP becomes greater over the hemisphere contralateral to the responding hand than over the ipsilateral hand.

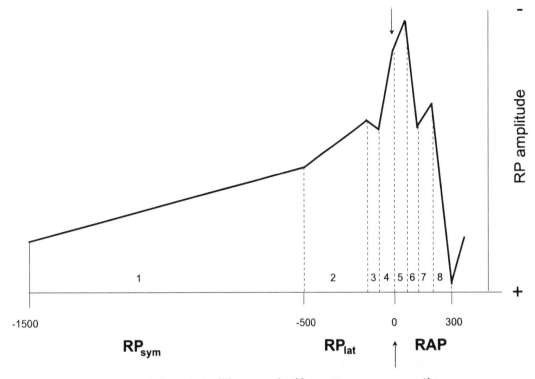

Time in milliseconds (0 = response onset)

Kutas and Donchin (1974) showed that the lateralized portion of the RP could also be measured after an imperative stimulus in a reaction time task if that stimulus indicated the hand with which the response had to be made. The lateralized portion can be isolated by subtracting the ipsilateral from the contralateral potentials, and nonmotor asymmetries in the brain can be removed by subtracting the isolated lateralization for left- and right-hand conditions.

The Readiness Potential

In the original study of Kornhuber and Deecke (1965), four potentials related to the button presses were described: three that occurred before the motor act and one thereafter. By today's standards, one would probably notice that they reported four "components" in the sense of, for instance, Donchin, Ritter, and McCallum (1978). Preceding the button press, Kornhuber and Deecke (1965) distinguished a negative *Bereitschaftspotential,* a premotion positivity, and a negative motor potential. The positive potential complex that followed the button press was designated as a reafferent potential (RAP). In contrast to using names that suggested a functional meaning of these components, other authors preferred to designate the components by polarity and sequence (e.g. Gilden, Vaughan, & Costa 1966) or by polarity and latency (e.g. Shibasaki et al. 1980). Because the number of components studied in various reports has differed somewhat, the naming convention by polarity and sequence has led to some confusion in designating the different components, especially those following the motor act.

Figure 4. Schematic representation of the eight components of the potentials related to motor acts. The terminology used for the various components is given in Table 1. This representation is a theoretical integration of components that were distinguished based on recordings from various electrode positions; a waveform as depicted in this figure cannot be measured at a single electrode.

Brunia (1987) summarized the most common designations that appeared in the literature up to the mid-1980s. Because no new components have been discovered since that time, the survey is still valid. In Figure 4, a systematic representation of the eight known components is presented; the associated nomenclatures are summarized in Table 1. In the present review, which is focused on the components preceding the motor act, we have adhered as much as possible to the original nomenclature of Kornhuber and Deecke (1965) as a tribute to their seminal work. But we do distinguish between the symmetrical and lateralized portions of the RP, designated by RP$_{sym}$ and RP$_{lat}$, respectively. The components following the motor act will be referred to using the polarity–latency convention, which is now the most frequently used. These potentials are not reviewed systematically here.

The RP$_{sym}$ starts between one and two seconds prior to the motor act, depending on factors such as the rate at which the motor acts are issued, their nature and complexity, and the limb with which they are issued. The interval between the start of the RP$_{sym}$ and the motor act is shorter at high rates of successive motor acts (Kornhuber & Deecke 1965). Complex motor acts are usually preceded by an

TABLE 1. Terminology Used to Describe Components of Brain Potentials Related to Motor Acts

1	2	3	4	5	6	7	8	Authors
				N				Bates (1951)
$\leftarrow$ BP $\rightarrow$		PMP	MP		$\leftarrow$	RAP	$\rightarrow$	Kornhuber & Deecke (1965)
$\leftarrow$ N_1 $\rightarrow$		P_1	N_2		P_2			Gilden, Vaughan, & Costa (1966)
$\leftarrow$ N_1 $\rightarrow$		P_1		N_2	P_{2a}		P_{2b}	Gerbrandt, Goff, & Smith (1973)
$\leftarrow$ N_1 $\rightarrow$		P_1	N_2		P_2		P_3	Arezzo & Vaughan (1975)
N_{1a}	N_{1b}	P_1	N_2	N_3	P_{2a}	N_4	P_{2b}	Gerbrandt (1977)
$\leftarrow$ N_1 $\rightarrow$				MCP				Papakostopoulos (1978)
$\leftarrow$ N_1 $\rightarrow$		P_1		P'_1, N_2	P_2		P'_2	Hazemann, Metral, & Lille (1978)
$\leftarrow$ N_1 $\rightarrow$		P_1	N_{2a}	N_{2b}	P_{2a}		$P_{2b}P_3$	Arezzo & Vaughan (1980)
BP	NS	P_{-50}	N_{-10}	N_{+50}	P_{+90}	N_{+160}	P_{+300}	Shibasaki et al. (1980)
RP I	RP II	—						Libet, Wright, & Gleason (1982)
RP_{sym}	RP_{lat}	PMP	MP	N_{50}	P_{90}	N_{160}	P_{300}	This chapter

Note: The sequence numbers of the components refer to Figure 4; arrows indicate the range of the definition relative to the sequential components.

RP_{sym} that starts slightly earlier than when preceding simple motor acts (Lang et al. 1989), and the same is true for foot as opposed to finger movements (Brunia & Van den Bosch 1984). The onset of the RP_{sym} is very consistent within subjects when measured in different recording sessions (Deecke 1987). There are, however, marked differences in onset time between electrode positions. At the vertex electrode (Cz), the RP_{sym} starts as much as 400–500 msec earlier than at precentral or parietal electrode sites (Deecke 1987). The amplitude of the RP_{sym} has a straightforward relation to its onset: it is greater the earlier it starts (Deecke, Grözinger, & Kornhuber 1976). Therefore, the amplitude of the RP_{sym} is also related to the factors influencing its onset, such as response rate, movement complexity, and extremity. In addition, the RP_{sym} has its maximum at the vertex electrode at which the earliest onset was observed.

The early onset and maximum amplitude of the RP_{sym} over the vertex electrode, which is located approximately over the supplementary motor area (SMA), have been used as evidence for the claims that the RP_{sym} is an index of SMA functioning and that SMA activity precedes activity in the primary motor cortex (Deecke 1987). In line with this suggestion, Goldberg (1985) hypothesized that the RP_{sym} is produced by activity in the basal ganglia–dependent loop (see section on basal ganglia), in which input from wide regions of the cortex is gathered and then focused back to restricted premotor regions, especially the SMA. This so-called medial system, as Goldberg referred to it, is schematically represented in Figure 5. Input modulation of this loop is possible at the level of the reticular thalamic nucleus, which overlies the lateral ventral thalamic nucleus and exerts an inhibitory influence on it (Brunia 1993; Skinner & Yingling 1977). It is hypothesized that this loop selects task-relevant features from the environmental context and associates these features with the actions to be executed. Hence, a strategy for future actions is thought to be specified through the activity of this predictive feedforward loop, a process that may be called motor programming.

If it is true that the RP_{sym} is indeed a measure of the functioning of the medial system, then it should be abolished or attenuated in patients with deficiencies in this loop. Indeed, patients with Parkinson's disease seem to have an abnormally small RP_{sym} (Dick et al. 1989). However, generation of the RP_{sym} may not depend only on the medial loop, since Ikeda and co-workers (1994) described a patient with a cerebellar lesion in which the RP_{sym} was completely abolished. Recent attempts to determine the neural generators of the RP_{sym} in healthy subjects using spatiotemporal dipole modeling failed to establish a significant SMA contribution (Böcker, Brunia, & Cluitmans 1994a; Bötzel et al. 1993). However, Praamstra and colleagues (1996b) suggested that this negative finding might be explained by a failure of the previous models to discriminate between SMA and motor cortex contributions to the RP_{sym}; they presented an improved model that included a generator in the SMA. These findings are consistent with intracranial measurements of Ikeda et al. (1992), who recorded an RP_{sym} bilaterally in the SMA. Taken together, the available evidence suggests that the SMA provides a major contribution to the RP_{sym}.

The second component that precedes the motor act is the lateralized portion of the RP, which we termed RP_{lat}. This component, which Shibasaki et al. (1980) referred to as the negative shift (NS'), starts about 500 msec before the motor act, again depending on factors such as the rate with which the actions are issued. Not all researchers recognize the RP_{lat} to be a separate component (see Table 1), but it can be shown to have underlying neural generators that differ from those of the RP_{sym}. We are therefore justified in treating RP_{lat} as a different component. The asymmetry in the RP_{lat} is restricted to central electrode locations, where greater amplitudes can be recorded over the hemisphere contralateral to the hand or finger with which the motor act is performed. Foot movements result in an ipsilaterally greater amplitude of the RP_{lat}; this paradoxical finding was hypothesized by Brunia (1980) to be due to the anatomical organization of the motor cortex. The orientation of the cell columns is such that their activity can be most easily picked up by an electrode over the contralateral hemisphere in the case of hand movements, because the hand area is located in the crown of the gyrus. For foot movements, however, their activity is most easily picked up by an electrode over the ipsilateral hemisphere, since the foot area is located in the mesial wall of the gyrus. This interpretation has been confirmed by spatiotemporal dipole modeling of ERPs (Böcker, Brunia, & Cluitmans 1994b) and magnetoencephalographic (MEG) recordings (Hari et al. 1983).

The foregoing explanation of the paradoxical lateralization for foot movements already suggested that the neuronal sources underlying the RP_{lat} are situated in the primary motor cortex. Indeed, in favor of that view is much evidence based on a variety of different techniques: slow intracortical potential studies in nonhuman primates (Arezzo & Vaughan 1975; Gemba, Sasaki, & Hashimoto 1980; Sasaki et al. 1979); unit studies in nonhuman primates (Requin 1985); MEG measurements in humans (review in Lang et al. 1991); regional cerebral bloodflow studies in humans (Roland et al. 1980), and spatiotemporal dipole modeling of scalp-recorded potentials in humans (Böcker et al. 1994a; Bötzel et al. 1993; Praamstra et al. 1996b). Gemba et al. (1980) recorded a transcranial inversion of the RP not only in the primary motor cortex but also in the premotor and primary somatosensory cortex (of monkeys). Therefore, it is plausible that there are several generators of the RP_{lat}. Although these sources are cortical, it does not mean that the subcortical input is of minor importance. In fact, it seems to be essential since cerebellar hemispherectomy abolished the potentials in all three areas; after a few weeks, recovery in the premotor and somatosensory areas was observed but not in the primary motor cortex (Sasaki et al. 1979). Later on it was demonstrated that the dentate nucleus is essential. Cerebellar outflow runs from the dentate nucleus (via the thalamus) to the motor cortex. In humans, the RP_{lat} depends also on the functioning of this nucleus (Ikeda et al. 1994; Shibasaki et al. 1986).

The finding that the RP_{lat} disappears upon ablation of the dentate nucleus contralateral to the motor cortex in-

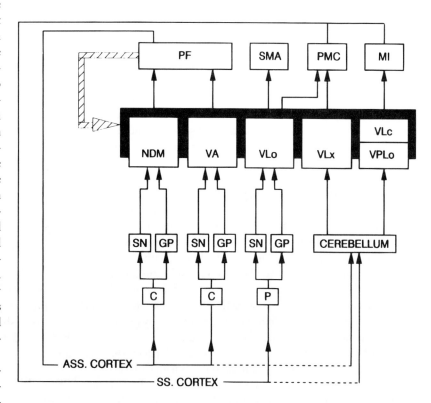

MOTOR PREPARATION

Figure 5. Simplified representation of the different cortical areas connected to caudate nucleus (C), putamen (P), and cerebellum. (Key: MI, primary motor cortex; NDM, dorsomedial nucleus; PF, prefrontal cortex; PMC, premotor cortex; SMA, supplementary motor area; VA, nucleus ventralis anterior; VLc, nucleus ventralis lateralis pars caudalis; VLo, nucleus ventralis lateralis pars oralis; VLx, pars X of the nucleus ventrolateralis; VPLo, nucleus ventralis posterolateralis; black shell, nucleus reticularis thalami, which inhibits locally the underlying relay nuclei.) The major input to the caudate nucleus stems from the association cortex, to the putamen from the somatomotor cortex, and to the cerebellum from the somatomotor cortex but also from the association cortex. The neostriatum outflow runs via the putamen in a motor loop or via the caudate nucleus in different complex loops. Substantia nigra and globus pallidus (externa) are the output channels, which are connected via different thalamic nuclei to different cortical areas. What Goldberg has called the medial and lateral systems are the motor loop via the putamen and the route via the cerebellum, respectively.

volved in the response (hence ipsilateral to the response itself) indicates that the cerebello-thalamo-cortical loop is necessary for the generation of the RP_{lat}. The ipsilateral dentate nucleus of the cerebellum projects to the contralateral thalamus (caudal part of the lateral ventral nucleus) and thence to the contralateral primary motor cortex, while input to the cerebellum is provided by motor and sensory association cortices (Allen & Tsukahara 1974). In the model presented by Goldberg (1985), this loop is called the lateral system (see Figure 5), which is thought to provide context-dependent adjustments of the parameters of the movement strategy selected by the medial system; this loop is therefore a feedback system, in contrast to the medial system (which was thought to operate in a feedforward mode). In patients with Parkinson's disease, the RP_{lat} is greater than in normal age-matched controls (Dick et al. 1989). This finding has been explained by assuming that these patients rely more on the lateral system because their medial system is defective, as indicated by the attenuated RP_{sym}. This explanation is consistent with the clinical observation that patients with Parkinson's disease depend on visual information for the successful initiation and performance of various motor acts (Brooks 1986).

The next component preceding the motor act is the premotion positivity (PMP). The PMP is a widespread bilaterally symmetrical positive wave with a maximum at the midline parietal electrode (Pz). It starts about 50–90 msec before the onset of muscle activity as determined by the EMG. Over central areas, it is more positive over the hemisphere ipsilateral to the response side, probably owing to the overlap with the negative motor potential (which immediately follows the PMP). Deecke and Kornhuber (1977) hypothesized that the PMP corresponds to the actual command for the movement. There are no animal data available related to the possible neuronal generator of the PMP, and spatiotemporal dipole modeling of human scalp potentials have not yielded reliable models of the PMP either (see e.g. Böcker et al. 1994a). It is also possible – as suggested by Neshige, Lüders, and Shibasaki (1988) – that the PMP is merely an epiphenomenon reflecting the transition between two negative waves, the RP_{lat} and the MP, and does not have a real neurophysiological generator. This possibility is supported by the failure to identify the PMP in subdural recordings (Ikeda & Shibasaki 1992).

The motor potential (MP) is the last premovement potential, starting about 10–50 msec prior to the onset of muscle activity. There has been some confusion regarding whether the MP precedes or follows the motor act. Gerbrandt, Goff, and Smith (1973) recorded a negativity after the onset of muscle activity, making its role in initiation of the motor act unlikely. Yet it turned out that the negativity measured by Gerbrandt et al. (1973) was actually part of the reafferent potentials and that the MP indeed occurs preceding the motor act (Gerbrandt 1977; see also Deecke & Kornhuber 1977). The MP is a unilateral negative wave with a maximum over precentral electrode positions contralateral to the responding hand (ipsilateral for foot movements). Combined recording of slow intracortical potentials and unit activity in nonhuman primates (Arezzo & Vaughan 1980) showed that the neuronal source of the MP is located in layer V of the hand area of the primary motor cortex, where a high density of pyramidal tract neurons are known to originate. This location is confirmed by human spatiotemporal dipole models (Böcker et al. 1994a; Bötzel et al. 1993; Praamstra et al. 1996b) and

magnetoencephalographic recordings (Lang et al. 1991). These findings confirm the original interpretation of the MP by Kornhuber and Deecke (1965; see also Deecke & Kornhuber 1977 and Deecke 1987) that the MP reflects the corticospinal outflow initiating the motor act.

In sum, these findings suggest that three processes are involved in the initiation of voluntary, self-paced, motor acts:

1. selecting a motor strategy, presumably an activity of the medial system involving the basal ganglia and the SMA and reflected in the RP_{sym};
2. setting the appropriate parameters for the movement depending on the external context – a function of the lateral system, involving the cerebellum and the primary motor cortex and reflected in the RP_{lat}; and
3. the command to move – involving discharge of pyramidal tract neurons in the primary motor cortex and reflected in the MP.

The independence of the actual motor command from the preparatory processes agrees also with behavioral models of motor preparation and performance, such as Bullock and Grossberg's (1988) vector integration model, in which prepared movements are energized by a separate Go command.

The Contingent Negative Variation

The early work of Walter and his colleagues was aimed not at motor preparation but at the concept of expectancy. Walter et al. (1964) showed that the CNV (a) developed in the 1-sec interval between a click and a series of flashes and (b) was terminated by a button press. The simple pairing of the click and the flashes, without a motor response, did not result in an appreciable potential shift. When S2 (and hence the response) was omitted, the CNV gradually declined; it was restored if the target stimulus was reintroduced. Yet the CNV did not merely depend on the response, because a CNV was found if the subjects had to estimate a time interval *without* producing a response. Walter and co-workers associated the CNV to the probability that a response to S2 was required. Because the attitude of the subjects and the instructions given to them also seemed of importance, the concept of "expectancy" was used, and for some time the CNV was known as the expectancy (E) wave. In subsequent research the CNV was associated with such other constructs as conation (defined as intention to act; Low et al. 1966), motivation (Irwin et al. 1966), and attention (Tecce 1972).

The use of longer intervals between the two successive stimuli showed that the original 1-sec CNV was actually a summation of two separate waves (Loveless & Sanford 1974). The early or O-wave (for orientation) had a frontal maximum and was thought to be a response to the first stimulus because it was shown to be related to such stimulus characteristics as modality, intensity, and duration. The late or E-wave (for expectancy) – sometimes referred

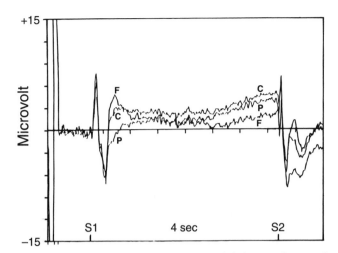

Figure 6. Contingent negative variation recorded during a foreperiod of 4 sec. The early wave after the first stimulus has a frontal maximum decreasing toward more posterior sites. The late wave increases up to the second stimulus and exhibits a central maximum. (Adapted from Brunia & Haagh 1986.)

to as the "terminal" CNV – had a central maximum; it was initially believed to be a sign of the expected occurrence of the second stimulus but was later related to motor programming (see Figure 6). The existence of early and late components with (respectively) frontal and central dominance was demonstrated by McCarthy and Donchin (1978) – using principal components analysis – to constitute the CNV recorded in a short (1-sec) foreperiod. Rohrbaugh, Syndulko, and Lindsley (1976) recorded CNVs in a 4-sec interval between paired stimuli (a tone and a flash, followed by a manual response). They compared the morphology and scalp distribution of the CNV with the potentials elicited by unpaired tones and uncued responses. The early wave of the CNV showed the same morphology and scalp distribution as the potential recorded after the unpaired tone, namely, a frontal maximum and parietal minimum within one second after the tone. The late wave of the CNV had a shape that was similar to the potential elicited by the uncued response and exhibited a central maximum with slightly larger amplitudes over the hemisphere contralateral to the responding hand. Rohrbaugh et al. (1976) concluded that the late CNV is essentially a readiness potential.

In an influential review, Rohrbaugh and Gaillard (1983) reiterated their view that the CNV consisted of an independent early and late wave, of which the late wave was identical to the RP and hence related to motor processes. Their arguments in favor of the motor programming interpretation of the late wave can be summarized as follows.

1. During short foreperiods, the CNV is attenuated when no motor response is required. During longer foreperiods, the late CNV is attenuated (or even absent) when no response to S2 is required or when a delayed instead of an immediate response is required.

2. The amplitude of the late CNV varies as a function of task variables assumed to be related to motor preparation, such as foreperiod duration and foreperiod variability. In addition, it is increased (a) under speed as opposed to accuracy instructions and (b) preceding fast as compared to slow responses within the same series. The late CNV does not vary as a function of sensory manipulations such as stimulus degradation.

3. The late CNV is similar in morphology and scalp distribution to the RP, with a maximum over cortical motor areas. Preceding manual responses, both are dominant over the hemisphere contralateral to the movement side, whereas an ipsilateral dominance is found preceding pedal movements. In addition, the CNV is greater when larger amounts of muscular effort are required for the response to S2, which has also been found for the RP.

Rohrbaugh and Gaillard (1983) also described a number of methodological issues that could bias the interpretation of late CNV findings, such as the length of the foreperiod and the resulting contribution of the early wave as well as the influence of movements (both instructed and non-instructed). In this way, they reinterpreted findings which suggested that the RP and the late CNV were to some extent different phenomena. As a result, the contribution of motor variables to the late CNV is now beyond doubt.

However, there also remain some issues which suggest that the late CNV is more than just an RP. First, the CNV is usually greater than the RP (Brunia & Vingerhoets 1981; van Boxtel & Brunia 1994b), suggesting that additional negativity underlies the CNV. This finding agrees with the clinical observation of Ikeda et al. (1994) that frontal negativity can be measured during the foreperiod of a reaction time task in a patient with a cerebellar lesion that abolished the RP. The additional negativity may be an instance of the stimulus-preceding negativity, which will be briefly discussed in the next section. Second, contralaterally greater amplitudes have been more frequently found for the RP than for the CNV. In part, this may be due to the fact that, in a reaction time task, the lateralized portion of the CNV may be contained in the interval between the second stimulus and the response, and not before S2. However, the more general problem is that the components distinguished in the context of voluntary motor acts, as discussed in the previous section, can not be demonstrated in a CNV paradigm – for instance, by spatiotemporal dipole analysis of scalp-recorded potentials (Böcker 1994). Third, although the late CNV is attenuated when no motor response is given, it can still be recorded when no motor response is required, even when taking into account the methodological pitfalls pointed out by Rohrbaugh and Gaillard (1983; see also Ruchkin et al. 1986).

The RP and the late wave of the CNV are measured in different paradigms in more than one respect. The increased timing constraints induced by the speed instructions in the CNV paradigm may be of special importance. From this perspective, it should come as no surprise that additional waves may be present in the CNV paradigm, contributing to the late wave. For instance, van Boxtel (1994) concluded from a series of precueing studies that at least two nonmotor components contributed to the late wave of the CNV. The first was related to the anticipation of task-relevant stimuli (SPN of second category in next section) and exhibited a bilaterally symmetrical parietal maximum. This component probably reflects the presetting of cortical networks to speed up the imminent processing of stimulus information in these networks. The second nonmotor component was tentatively related to the effortful control over task performance; it showed a bilaterally symmetrical maximum over the frontal cortex. The presence or absence of the various components, motor and nonmotor, depends on the exact task circumstances, instructions to the subjects, their subjective interpretation, and so on. As a consequence, the amplitude and scalp distribution of the CNV late wave is often found to differ from experiment to experiment.

In the more simple CNV tasks, the late wave of the CNV is mainly determined by the level of motor preparation and is therefore at least functionally similar to the RP. The hypothesis that the late wave is mainly determined by activity in the medial (basal ganglia–dependent) system depicted in Figure 5 is supported by two lines of evidence. First, the late wave is attenuated in patients with Parkinson's disease who are thought to have a defective medial system (Praamstra et al. 1996a). Second, CNVs can be recorded in the caudate nucleus of monkeys, although with reversed polarity (Rebert 1977). The presence or absence of the activity in the lateral (cerebellum dependent) system, which produces the contralaterally greater amplitudes, depends on experimental variables that are not yet completely understood. When the side of responding is an important task variable indicated by the second stimulus, then the lateralization can be shown to be present in the reaction time interval (Kutas & Donchin 1974).

The Stimulus-Preceding Negativity

Brunia (1988) hypothesized that the additional negativity distinguishing the CNV from the RP was related to anticipation of the upcoming S2. Motor preparation and stimulus anticipation are necessarily confounded in the foreperiod of a reaction time task. Damen and Brunia (1987) showed that stimulus anticipation without simultaneous motor preparation resulted in a negative wave with a parietal maximum and a right hemisphere preponderance. They termed the negativity stimulus-preceding negativity (SPN); although thought to be exclusively related to nonmotor factors, it frequently contaminates movement-related negativity and it is therefore briefly discussed here. In particular, tasks involving continuous motor output that can

be visually monitored (e.g., tracking tasks) may be susceptible to this contamination. When such tasks are executed with the right hand, the left-hemisphere preponderance of the movement-related potentials is likely to be canceled by the right-hemisphere dominance of the SPN, resulting in a bilaterally symmetrical wave. Whether this is actually the case can be demonstrated by studying responses with the left hand, since right-hemisphere dominance of the SPN is greater for responses with the left than with the right hand (Damen & Brunia 1987).

Van Boxtel (1994) reviewed research into the SPN and concluded that the SPN (a) can be recorded preceding three types of stimuli and (b) probably also has different neural generators in those cases (Figure 7; see also Böcker & van Boxtel 1997).

1. *Stimuli providing knowledge of results about prior performance.* In this case, the SPN has a parietal maximum and a right hemisphere preponderance, especially over anterior electrode positions (Damen & Brunia 1987). This instance of the SPN is probably generated by bilateral parietal sources and a unilateral source in the right fronto-temporal cortex (Böcker 1994).
2. *Stimuli transmitting information about a future task.* In this case the SPN also has a parietal maximum, but it is bilaterally symmetrical and much smaller than the SPN prior to stimuli providing knowledge of results. This instance of the SPN can be recorded preceding all task-relevant stimuli; it contributes to the late wave of the CNV (van Boxtel & Brunia 1994a), although the contribution is small. It probably is generated by a pair of bilateral parietal cortical sources.
3. *Probe stimuli with which the outcome of a previous task must be matched.* Again, a parietal maximum is found in this case, but a left-hemisphere advantage is observed (Chwilla & Brunia 1991). The sources of this instance of the SPN are unknown.

Another negative shift of frontal cortical origin, possibly related to the effortful control over task performance in the forewarned reaction time task, is thought to contribute to the late wave of the CNV (van Boxtel 1994; see also Figure 7). This negativity corresponds to the difference between the RP and the CNV in the cerebellar patient described by Ikeda et al. (1994).

The Lateralized Readiness Potential

The most important development of the last decade in the psychophysiology of motor control is the use of the lateralized readiness potential (LRP). As already indicated, Kutas and Donchin (1974) showed that the lateralized part of the readiness potential (RP_{lat}) can be measured after an imperative stimulus that calls for a response with either the left or the right hand. They suggested that the difference can be used as an on-line index of the degree of motor preparation in reaction time tasks. This idea was

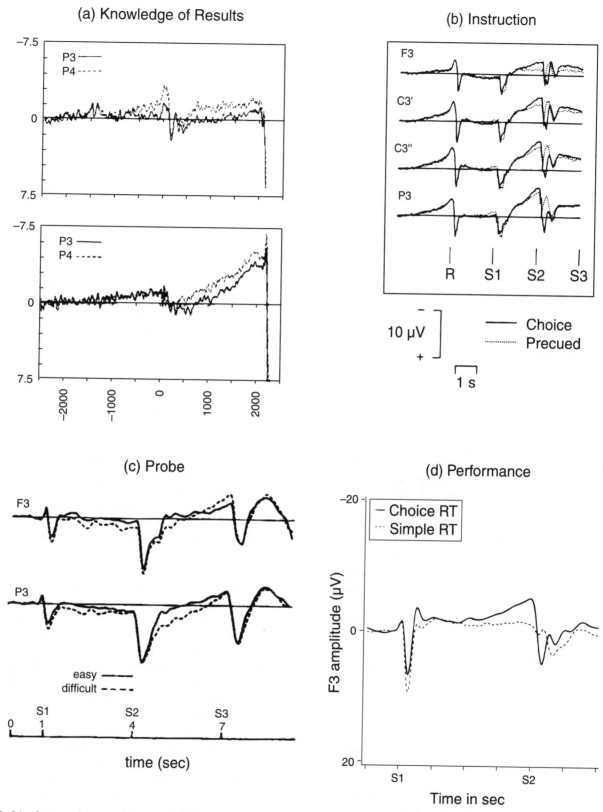

Figure 7. Stimulus-preceding negativity recorded prior to different types of stimuli: (a) preceding a stimulus conveying knowledge of results about prior performance occurring at 2,000 msec after the response (adapted from Damen & Brunia 1987); (b) preceding a stimulus providing an instruction about future performance (S1; adapted from van Boxtel & Brunia 1994b); and (c) preceding a probe stimulus with which the outcome of a previous task has to be matched (S3; adapted from Chwilla & Brunia 1991). Panel (d) shows the frontal negative shift related to the control over task performance (adapted from van Boxtel 1994).

elaborated in the studies of De Jong et al. (1988) and Gratton et al. (1988) and has been frequently used since then to monitor the amount of direction-specific motor preparation (see also Coles 1989). De Jong et al. (1988) termed this measure the "corrected motor asymmetry" in order to avoid any confusion concerning this measure's being obtained in a reaction time task – unlike the RP, which is obtained when movements are self-paced. Nevertheless, the term lateralized readiness potential is used most frequently nowadays, justified by the fact that it is calculated from RP_{lat} even though obtained in a CNV-like paradigm.

Calculation of the LRP is a two-step process. First, the lateralized portion of the signal is isolated by subtracting the ipsilateral potentials from the contralateral potentials, measured over the motor cortex. The next step is to average or subtract the lateralization for left- and right-hand conditions. As a result, asymmetries in the brain that are irrelevant to the direction of the correct response disappear from the signal. Further details about procedures and uses of the LRP in psychological research are outside the scope of this chapter but are discussed elsewhere in this volume (see Chapter 3). We want to emphasize one interesting property of the LRP: around the start of muscle activation, the LRP amplitude is almost constant across conditions (Gratton et al. 1988). Based on this finding, Gratton and colleagues proposed that a fixed level of response activation must be exceeded in order to trigger a response. Cognitive models of response preparation, known as "accumulator" models, similarly assume a gradual accumulation of response-related activity toward a certain threshold. These models account for the observed variability in reaction times by assuming a variable accumulation rate, a variable response threshold, or both. Hanes and Schall (1996) provided support for the fixed-threshold hypothesis with single-cell recordings in the motor areas of monkeys performing specific eye movements. The constancy of the LRP amplitude at muscle activity onset is consistent with that view (Coles 1997).

Whether the amplitude of the LRP at muscle onset provides a reliable index of the response threshold in the motor cortex remains an open question. It can be argued that the threshold is always overestimated in that case, since the neural transmission from the motor cortex to the muscle takes time (estimates range from about 25 msec to 50 msec). De Jong, Coles, and Logan (1995) used the LRP amplitude at 50 msec before response (not muscle) onset as the response threshold. However, it is unknown if the use of that value leads to an underestimation of the response threshold in the motor cortex. This might be the case because, on trials in which no response was issued, the maximum LRP amplitude exceeded the virtual threshold (as determined at 50 msec before response onset) but remained below the amplitude at response onset. Other criteria for the response threshold have been suggested, but to date there does not seem to be a consensus about this matter (Band & van Boxtel 1999). This area will undoubtedly prove to be a fruitful one for future investigations, which will also have to be concerned with the relation of the threshold in the motor cortex and the MP of Kornhuber and Deecke (1965).

REFLEXES

The cortical manifestations of motor preparation discussed so far are a reflection of excitatory postsynaptic changes in the membrane potential of cells in the different motor areas. Firing of these cells excites in turn the cells in brainstem and spinal cord, causing similar changes in their membrane potential. If such changes in membrane potential take place in motoneurons of the spinal cord, they cause a change in that potential toward the firing threshold (but not necessarily so far that the cells discharge). Thus, spinal changes in excitability of motoneurons need not be manifest in the surface EMG. In their survey of a number of monkey studies, Evarts, Shimoda, and Wise (1984) explicitly denied that peripheral anticipatory EMG activity was present; they suggested that a subthreshold activation of motoneurons or interneurons might have taken place. In contrast to Evarts et al. (1984), a small EMG activity was reported in monkeys by Riehle and Requin (1989) – in accord with some EMG studies in humans (Brunia & Vingerhoets 1980; Haagh & Brunia 1984). In the latter study, subjects had to prepare a plantar flexion of the right foot. Apart from a systematic increase in EMG activity in the agonist (the calf muscles), a similar increase was recorded in the antagonist (the anterior tibial muscle) and in several other muscles in the same leg. No such increase in activity was found in the other leg, while a decrease was recorded in the EOG (electro-oculogram) and the mylohyoidius muscle (mouth bottom). So, preparation of a simple foot movement results in a complicated picture. The decrease in facial muscle activity is in line with Obrist's idea that motor preparation goes along with a quieting of irrelevant muscle activity (Obrist 1976), but the rest of the findings do not (Brunia 1984a). The small increase in EMG activity found in a number of leg muscles showed a significant negative correlation with reaction time. However, there was no indication of a stronger correlation for the agonist than for the other muscles. It is therefore doubtful that the slight increase in EMG activity is selectively related to response preparation.

Subthreshold changes in excitability of a motoneuron pool can be investigated with reflexes (Paillard 1955). All other things being equal, an increase in excitability would cause an increase in reflex amplitude and a decrease in excitability would result in a decrease in amplitude. Thus, the size of the reflex amplitude can be considered an estimate of the changes in spinal excitability. Achilles tendon and Hoffmann reflexes have been used to study motor preparation during the foreperiod of a warned reaction time task

(Bonnet et al. 1981; Brunia & Boelhouwer 1988; Requin, Bonnet, & Semjen 1977). These reflexes can be evoked bilaterally in the calf muscles at unpredictable points in time by using a (mechanical or electrical) stimulus while subjects prepare for a unilateral response with the foot or a finger. If a unilateral finger movement is prepared then the calf muscles are not involved in the response, so eventual changes in reflex amplitude cannot be considered to be specifically or selectively related to the preparatory process. If a unilateral plantar flexion is prepared, contralateral calf muscles are likewise not involved in the response. Only changes in amplitude of homolateral reflexes can be considered to be selectively related to the preparatory process. The following picture emerges from our different studies (Brunia, Scheirs, & Haagh 1982; see also Figure 8).

1. The warning stimulus is followed by an increase in reflex amplitude, which is independent from the involvement in the response.
2. In case of unilateral plantar flexion, there is a differential effect present in the second half of the foreperiod. If the calf muscles are uninvolved in the response, the reflex amplitude is larger during the foreperiod than during the intertrial interval. If the calf muscles are involved in the response then the reflex amplitude is slightly larger (or not different) from baseline.
3. Immediately following the imperative stimulus, the differential effect reverses: reflex amplitudes in the involved muscles become larger than in the uninvolved muscles. Both are above baseline.
4. In case of a unilateral finger flexion, both calf muscles are uninvolved. Reflex amplitudes remain larger than baseline.
5. Immediately following the imperative stimulus, a further increase takes place that is comparable to what happens in the contralateral leg with a unilateral plantar flexion.

The changes in reflex amplitude are independent of the length of the foreperiod (Brunia 1983; Brunia et al. 1982). Preceding a unilateral dorsiflexion of the foot, in which the calf muscles are considered uninvolved, reflex amplitudes on both sides remain above baseline (Brunia 1984b).

It is counterintuitive that in none of our experiments was there any sign of increased reflex activity in the agonist, even though indications of an increase in excitability seem to be present when the calf muscles are uninvolved. Although these results might seem puzzling at first, it has been hypothesized (Requin & Paillard 1971) that a presynaptic inhibition of Ia afferents to the agonist motoneuron pool might be the cause of this phenomenon (see also Bonnet et al. 1981; Brunia et al. 1982). We have already discussed the slight increase in surface EMG activity found in the agonist but not in the contralateral calf muscle (Brunia & Vingerhoets 1980; Haagh & Brunia 1985). This points to an increased excitability in the agonist motoneuron pool,

which is stronger than on the uninvolved side. Yet on the uninvolved side there was an increase in reflex amplitudes compared to the control condition, pointing to an increase in excitability on that side, too. The presynaptic inhibition of the Ia afferents from the agonist might be part of the preparatory process, its function being the defense of the motoneuron pool against possibly disturbing influences from the periphery, which might cause a premature response. Thus, the absence of a facilitation of the reflexes evoked via the agonist motoneuron pool might be the result of a balance between an increase in excitability of the cells in the agonist motoneuron pool and the presumed presynaptic inhibition of the Ia afferents from the agonist to that same pool. We therefore consider the reflex findings in the agonist as a lack of facilitation rather than as a sign of inhibition (Brunia 1984b).

This interpretation is at variance with several publications of the Marseille group claiming that reflexes evoked not only in the agonist but also (sometimes) in the uninvolved muscles show a decrease in amplitude (Bonnet et al. 1981; Requin, Lecas, & Bonnet 1984; Requin et al. 1991). Yet in a large series of experiments we have never found a decrease in amplitude below baseline (Brunia 1983, 1984b; Brunia & Vuister 1979; Brunia et al. 1982; Scheirs & Brunia 1982, 1985) – except in one study (Scheirs & Brunia 1986) where the agonist was deliberately contracted. In the latter study a decrease was indeed present. This made us conclude that reflexes are reliable estimators of spinal excitability only when there is no background EMG activity in the agonist. The divergent results between the Marseille group and ours might very well be related to this. Moreover, the decrease in H-reflex amplitude reported by Requin et al. (1977, 1991) is at variance with some of the other studies of the same lab and of others. For example, no such decrement was found during a 1-sec foreperiod (Hayes & Clarke 1978; Sullivan 1980), a 2-sec foreperiod (Semjen & Bonnet 1982), or a 4-sec foreperiod (Brunia & Vuister 1979). Bonnet (1981) did not find a decrease in T-reflex amplitudes below baseline in a 1-sec foreperiod preceding a ballistic movement, and Bonnet and Requin (1982) reported that the M1 response, which is comparable to the T-reflex, remained above baseline as well. Thus, although the results of a large number of experiments do not necessarily point to a rather generalized inhibition, the very existence of the differential effect – that is, the difference in reflex amplitude between muscles involved and uninvolved in the response – is beyond doubt. Still, its predictive value for performance is questioned (Requin et al. 1991) because the size of the effect is not correlated with reaction time. On the contrary, in a Go–No-Go experiment with response probabilities at 80%, 50%, and 20% in blocks, we found only a differential effect in the first condition; in the last condition, reflex amplitudes behaved as uninvolved: they remained above baseline on both sides (Brunia & Boelhouwer 1988).

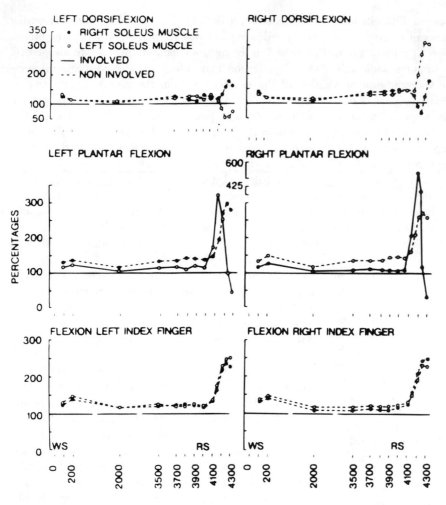

Figure 8. Summary of the results of a number of experiments in which Achilles tendon reflexes were evoked bilaterally in the calf muscles of healthy subjects during the 4-sec foreperiod of a reaction time task. Reflexes evoked during the intertrial interval served as baseline. The responses were: (1) a left or right dorsiflexion of the foot (top); (2) a left or right plantar flexion of the foot (middle); and (3) a button press with the left or right index finger (bottom). Calf muscles are agonist in a plantar flexion. After a phasic increase in amplitude following the warning stimulus, reflex amplitudes in all cases remain above baseline when the muscle is uninvolved in the response (bilateral in 1 and 3 and unilateral in 2). Reflexes evoked in the agonist are not different from baseline. In involved muscles, the differential effect reverses within 100 msec after the imperative stimulus. There is a sharp increase in amplitude in the involved muscles and also (though to a lesser extent) in the uninvolved muscles.

The results of Haagh and Brunia (1984) pointed to an activation of a number of muscles in one and the same leg, rather than to an activation of the agonist alone. This might be related to a stabilizing of the knee and the ankle joint. We have no experimental data to suggest that the afferents from these muscles are also under a presynaptic inhibitory control, although that seems plausible. Taken together, outcomes of the reflex experiments suggest that motor preparation is accompanied by an increase in excitability of agonist motoneurons and of synergist motoneurons, while a presynaptic inhibitory control protects the agonist motoneurons and presumably the synergist motoneurons against a premature firing. There seems to be no reason to think that the preparatory process in the periphery does more than organizing this general response pattern. In other words, most of the preparation is organized at a higher (presumably, cortical) level.

For the analysis of human information processing, investigators mainly studied responses with the upper limb. There is an obvious reason for that, since our hands are pre-eminently the instruments we use to manipulate the world around us. In the studies mentioned before, reflexes were investigated in legs. Although these results may have a degree of ecological validity with respect to automobile driving, it is unclear whether they apply to movements of the upper extremities. The soleus muscle plays a role in the maintenance of posture, while arm and hand are involved in reaching and grasping. Our efforts to start a series of reflex studies in arm muscles failed because it is not possible to evoke sufficiently stable reflexes over the necessary number of trials to permit averaging. However, Bonnet and Requin (1982) were successful in evoking long loop reflexes in arm muscles. If a sudden stretch in a lightly tensed involved muscle is evoked then two responses show up, M1 and M2; M1 is comparable to the monosynaptic reflexes discussed before and M2 is the long loop reflex. The first showed an increase followed by a decrease, while M2 was increased during the whole foreperiod. The authors interpreted the decrease in M1 as due to presynaptic inhibition; the second response was considered a sign of increased excitability of the agonist motoneurons. Up to now, only a few similar studies have been carried out.

Hasbroucq and associates (1997) used transcranial magnetic stimulation to study changes in spinal excitability. This stimulation induces the firing of cortical interneurons that project to the corticofugal pyramidal tract cells. The response obtained in the muscle is the motor-evoked potential (MEP), which has two drawbacks: it is highly variable and it renders impossible any distinction between cortical and spinal contributions. During a short foreperiod, the authors found indications of a decrease in excitability in the agonist motoneurons prior to arrival of the imperative stimulus. How this relates to results obtained with leg reflexes is not clear. It would be interesting to replicate – using this new technique in arm muscles – the series of reflex studies discussed previously.

Epilogue

While a subject is waiting to respond, the arrival of an imperative stimulus is anticipated and the response is prepared. It has been argued here that both processes are based upon a thalamo-cortical stream of information via different thalamic nuclei. Each thalamo-cortical pathway functions as a channel that transmits specific sensory or motor information to the relevant cortical structures. These channels are neither completely open nor completely closed; they can be gated via a control mechanism in which the RN plays a crucial role. This nucleus overlaps the different sensory and motor thalamic relay nuclei and exerts a local, topographically organized, inhibitory influence upon them. The RN itself is open for a generalized inhibition from the reticular formation via the ARAS, as Skinner and Yingling (1977) demonstrated for the sensory nuclei. We claim that the same holds for the motor thalamic nuclei. The generalized inhibition of the locally inhibitory RN cells results in a generalized disinhibition of the thalamic relay nuclei. This process is at the basis of an increase in the state of arousal: all gates are open, both sensory and motor. The RN is also open for an excitatory frontal control mechanism. In contrast to the influence from the reticular formation, this is topographically organized and so allows for a localized activation of the locally active inhibition. The consequence of activity in this system is the closing of a gate. This mechanism is responsible for selection in both the sensory and the motor domain. A gate is open only if the excitation from the frontal cortex does not show up. Neither perception nor movement is possible unless the relevant gates are open. An adequate response to a No-Go or a Stop command could be realized via the immediate closing of the motor gates by frontal excitation of the local inhibitory RN activity.

We have discussed results of ERPs and reflexes. Slow potentials are a manifestation of activity in one or more cortical areas, which are from moment to moment under the influence of subcortical loops (via basal ganglia or cerebellum) and different thalamic nuclei. This subcortical input is a necessary condition for the slow waves to show up.

The results of reflex experiments suggest that, during the fixed foreperiod of reaction time experiments, a general increase in excitability is present that is more pronounced in agonist and synergists but is also present when muscles are not involved in the response. The lack of increase in amplitude in the agonist is thought to be the result of a balance between an increase in excitability of the motoneurons and a simultaneous presynaptic inhibition of the Ia afferents from the muscles. Whether there is really an inhibition during the foreperiod with amplitudes be-

low baseline remains an unsolved problem. We expect that transcranial magnetic stimulation will provide important information in the near future about changes in excitability of motoneurons in arm and hand muscles.

NOTES

G. J. M. van Boxtel is supported by NWO grant 575-63-082B.

1. Consistent with the conventional plotting – with negativity upward – of these kinds of slow potentials, we will use the terms "maximum" and "greater than" to denote "most negative" and "more negative than" (respectively) and the terms "minimum" and "smaller than" to denote "least negative" and "less negative than" (respectively).

REFERENCES

Ach, N. (1905). *Ueber die Willenstätigkeit und das Denken: Eine experimentelle Untersuchung mit einem Anhange über das Hippsche Chronoskop.* Göttingen: VandenHoeck & Ruprecht.

Alexander, G. E., & Crutcher, M. D. (1990). Functional architecture of basal ganglia circuits: Neural substrates of parallel processing. *Trends in Neurosciences, 13,* 266–71.

Alexander, G. E., DeLong, M. R., & Strick, P. L. (1986). Parallel organization of functionally segregated circuits linking basal ganglia and cortex. *Annual Review of Neuroscience, 9,* 357–81.

Allen, G. I., & Tsukahara, N. (1974). Cerebrocerebellar communication systems. *Physiological Reviews, 54,* 957–1006.

Arezzo, J., & Vaughan, H. G., Jr. (1975). Cortical potentials associated with voluntary movements in the monkey. *Brain Research, 88,* 99–104.

Arezzo, J., & Vaughan, H. G., Jr. (1980). Intracortical sources and surface topography of the motor potential and somatosensory evoked potential in the monkey. In H. H. Kornhuber & L. Deecke (Eds.), *Motivation, Motor and Sensory Processes of the Brain* (Progress in Clinical Neurophysiology, vol. 54), pp. 77–83. Amsterdam: Elsevier.

Band, G. P. H., & van Boxtel, G. J. M. (1999). Inhibitory motor control in stop paradigms: Review and reinterpretation of neural mechanisms. *Acta Psychologica, 101,* 179–211.

Barker, A. T., Jalinous, R., & Freeston, I. L. (1985). Noninvasive magnetic stimulation of human motor cortex. *Lancet, 1,* 1106–7.

Bates, J. A. V. (1951). Electrical activity of the cortex accompanying movements. *Journal of Physiology, 113,* 240–57.

Bell, C. (1811). *Idea of a New Anatomy of the Brain: Submitted for the Observations of His Friends.* London: Strahan & Preston. Reprinted 1869 in *Journal of Anatomy and Physiology, 3,* 153–66.

Böcker, K. B. E. (1994). Spatiotemporal dipole models of slow cortical potentials. Doctoral dissertation, Tilburg University, The Netherlands.

Böcker, K. B. E., Brunia, C. H. M., & Cluitmans, P. J. M. (1994a). A spatio-temporal dipole model of the readiness potential in humans. I. Finger movement. *Electroencephalography and Clinical Neurophysiology, 91,* 275–85.

Böcker, K. B. E., Brunia, C. H. M., & Cluitmans, P. J. M. (1994b). A spatio-temporal dipole model of the readiness potential in humans. II. Foot movement. *Electroencephalography and Clinical Neurophysiology, 91,* 286–94.

Böcker, K. B. E., & van Boxtel, G. J. M. (1997). Stimulus-preceding negativity: A class of anticipatory slow potentials. In G. J. M. van Boxtel & K. B. E. Böcker (Eds.), *Brain and Behavior: Past, Present, and Future,* pp. 105–16. Tilburg, The Netherlands: Tilburg University Press.

Boelhouwer, A. J. W. (1982). Blink reflexes and preparation. *Biological Psychology, 14,* 277–85.

Bonnet, M. (1981). Comparison of monosynaptic tendon reflexes during preparation for ballistic or ramp movement. *Electroencephalography and Clinical Neurophysiology, 51,* 353–62.

Bonnet, M., & Requin, J. (1982). Long loop and spinal reflexes in man during preparation for intended directional hand movements. *Journal of Neuroscience, 2,* 90–6.

Bonnet, M., Requin, J., & Semjen, A. (1981). Human reflexology and motor preparation. In D. Miller (Ed.), *Exercise and Sport Science Reviews,* vol. 9, pp. 119–57. Philadelphia: Franklin Institute Press.

Boring, E. G. (1950). *A History of Experimental Psychology.* New York: Appleton-Century-Crofts.

Bötzel, K., Plendl, H., Paulus, W., & Scherg, M. (1993). Bereitschaftspotential: Is there a contribution from the supplementary motor area? *Electroencephalography and Clinical Neurophysiology, 89,* 187–96.

Boussaoud, D., & Wise, S. P. (1993). Primate frontal cortex: Neuronal activity following attentional vs. intentional cues. *Experimental Brain Research, 95,* 15–27.

Brooks, V. B. (1986). *The Neural Basis of Motor Control.* New York: Oxford University Press.

Brunia, C. H. M. (1980). What is wrong with legs in motor preparation? In H. H. Kornhuber & L. Deecke (Eds.), *Motivation, Motor and Sensory Processes of the Brain* (Progress in Clinical Neurophysiology, vol. 54), pp. 232–6. Amsterdam: Elsevier.

Brunia, C. H. M. (1983). Motor preparation: Changes in amplitude of Achilles tendon reflexes during a fixed foreperiod of one second. *Psychophysiology, 20,* 658–64.

Brunia, C. H. M. (1984a). Facilitation and inhibition in the motor system: An interrelationship with cardiac deceleration? In M. G. H. Coles, J. R. Jennings, & J. A. Stern (Eds.), *Psychophysiological Perspectives: Festschrift for Beatrice and John Lacey,* pp. 199–215. New York: Van Nostrand.

Brunia, C. H. M. (1984b). Selective and aselective control of spinal motor structures during preparation for a movement. In S. Kornblum & J. Requin (Eds.), *Preparatory States and Processes,* pp. 285–302. Hillsdale, NJ: Erlbaum.

Brunia, C. H. M. (1987). Brain potentials related to preparation and action. In H. Heuer & A. F. Sanders (Eds.), *Perspectives on Perception and Action,* pp. 105–30. Hillsdale, NJ: Erlbaum.

Brunia, C. H. M. (1988). Movement and stimulus preceding negativity. *Biological Psychology, 26,* 165–78.

Brunia, C. H. M. (1993). Waiting in readiness: Gating in attention and motor preparation. *Psychophysiology, 30,* 327–39.

Brunia, C. H. M. (1997). Gating in readiness. In P. J. Lang, R. F. Simons, & M. T. Balaban (Eds.), *Attention and Orienting: Sensory and Motivational Processes,* pp. 281–306. Mahwah, NJ: Erlbaum.

Brunia, C. H. M., & Boelhouwer, A. J. W. (1988). Reflexes as a tool: A window in the central nervous system. In P. K. Ackles,

J. R. Jennings, & M. G. H. Coles (Eds.), *Advances in Psychophysiology,* vol. 3, pp. 1–67. Greenwich, CT: JAI.

Brunia, C. H. M., & Haagh, S. A. V. M. (1986). Preparation for action: Slow potentials and EMG. In H. Heuer & C. Fromm (Eds.), *Generation and Modulation of Action Patterns* (Experimental Brain Research Series, no. 15), pp. 28–40. Berlin: Springer.

Brunia, C. H. M., Scheirs, J. G. M., & Haagh, S. A. V. M. (1982). Changes of Achilles tendon reflex amplitudes during a fixed foreperiod of reaction time experiments. *Psychophysiology, 19,* 63–70.

Brunia, C. H. M., & Van den Bosch, W. E. J. (1984). Movement-related slow potentials. I. A contrast between finger and foot movements in right-handed subjects. *Electroencephalography and Clinical Neurophysiology, 57,* 515–27.

Brunia, C. H. M., & Vingerhoets, A. J. J. M. (1980). CNV and EMG preceding a plantar flexion of the foot. *Biological Psychology, 11,* 181–91.

Brunia, C. H. M., & Vingerhoets, A. J. J. M. (1981). Opposite hemisphere differences in movement related potentials preceding foot and finger flexions. *Biological Psychology, 13,* 261–9.

Brunia, C. H. M., & Vuister, F. M. (1979). Spinal reflexes as indicator of motor preparation in man. *Physiological Psychology, 7,* 377–80.

Bullock, D., & Grossberg, S. (1988). Neural dynamics of planned arm movements: Emergent invariants and speed accuracy properties during trajectory formation. *Psychological Review, 95,* 49–90.

Chwilla, D. J., & Brunia, C. H. M. (1991). Event-related potential correlates of non-motor anticipation. *Biological Psychology, 32,* 125–41.

Coles, M. G. H. (1989). Modern mind-brain reading: Psychophysiology, physiology, and cognition. *Psychophysiology, 26,* 251–69.

Coles, M. G. H. (1997). Neurons and reaction times. *Science, 275,* 142–3.

Damen, E. J. P., & Brunia, C. H. M. (1987). Changes in heart rate and slow potentials related to motor preparation and stimulus anticipation of a time estimation task. *Psychophysiology 24,* 700–13.

Davis, R. C. (1940). *Set and Muscular Tension* (Science Series, no. 10). Bloomington: Indiana University Press.

Dawson, M. E., Schell, A. M., Swerdlow, N. R., & Filion, D. L. (1997). Cognitive, clinical and neurophysiological implications of startle response modification. In P. J. Lang, R. F. Simons, & M. T. Balaban (Eds.), *Attention and Orienting: Sensory and Motivational Processes,* pp. 281–306. Mahwah, NJ: Erlbaum.

Deecke, L. (1987). Bereitschaftspotential as an indicator of movement preparation in supplementary motor area and motor cortex. In *Motor Areas of the Cerebral Cortex* (Ciba Foundation Symposium, no. 132), pp. 231–50. Chichester, U.K.: Wiley.

Deecke, L., Grözinger, B., & Kornhuber, H. H. (1976). Voluntary finger movement in man: Cerebral potentials and theory. *Biological Cybernetics, 23,* 99–119.

Deecke, L., & Kornhuber, H. H. (1977). Cerebral potentials and the initiation of voluntary movement. In J. E. Desmedt (Ed.), *Attention, Voluntary Contraction and Event-Related Cerebral Potentials* (Progress in Clinical Neurophysiology, vol. 1), pp. 132–50. Basel: Karger.

Deiber, L., Passingham, R. E., Colebatch, J. G., Friston, K. J., Nixon, P. D., & Frackowiak, R. S. J. (1991). Cortical areas and the selection of movement: A study with positron emission tomography. *Experimental Brain Research, 84,* 393–402.

De Jong, R., Coles, M. G. H., & Logan, G. D. (1995). Strategies and mechanisms in nonselective and selective inhibitory motor control. *Journal of Experimental Psychology: Human Perception and Performance, 21,* 498–511.

De Jong, R., Wierda, M., Mulder, G., & Mulder, L. J. M. (1988). Use of partial stimulus information in response processing. *Journal of Experimental Psychology: Human Perception and Performance, 14,* 682–92.

DeLong, M. R. (1990). Primate models of movement disorders of basal ganglia. *Trends in Neurosciences, 13,* 281–5.

DeLong, M. R., & Georgeopoulos, A. R. (1981). Motor function of the basal ganglia. In J. M. Brookhart & V. B. Mountcastle (Eds.), *Handbook of Physiology, I: The Nervous System,* vol. 2 (Motor Control), pp. 1017–61. Bethesda, MD: American Physiological Society.

DeLong, M. R., Georgopoulos, A. P., Crutcher, M. D., Mitchell, S. J., Richardson, R. T., & Alexander, G. E. (1984). Functional organization of the basal ganglia: Contributions of single cell recording studies. In *Functions of the Basal Ganglia* (Ciba Foundation Symposium, no. 107), pp. 64–78. London: Pitman.

Dick, J. P. R., Rothwell, J. C., Day, B. L., Cantello, R., Buruma, O., Gioux, M., Benecke, R., Berardelli, A., Thompson, P. D., & Marsden, C. D. (1989). The Bereitschaftspotential is abnormal in Parkinson's disease. *Brain, 112,* 233–44.

Donchin, E., Ritter, W., & McCallum, W. C. (1978). Cognitive psychophysiology: The endogenous components of the ERP. In E. Callaway, P. Tueting, & S. H. Koslow (Eds.), *Event-Related Brain Potentials in Man,* pp. 349–411. New York: Academic Press.

Donders, F. C. (1868/1969). On the speed of mental processes [Translation by W. G. Koster]. *Acta Psychologica, 30,* 412–31.

Evarts, E. V. (1968). Relation of pyramidal tract activity to force exerted during voluntary movement. *Journal of Neurophysiology, 31,* 14–27.

Evarts, E. V., Shimoda, Y., & Wise, S. P. (1984). *Neurophysiological Approaches to Higher Brain Functions.* New York: Wiley.

Exner, S. (1873). Experimentelle Untersuchung der einfachste psychischen Processe. *Pflügers Archiv, 7,* 601–60.

Forget, R., & Lamarre, Y. (1987). Rapid elbow flexion in the absence of proprioceptive and cutaneous feedback. *Human Neurobiology, 6,* 27–37.

Fox, S. S., & Norman, R. J. (1968). Functional congruence: An index of neural homogeneity and a new measure of brain activity. *Science, 159,* 1257–9.

Fuster, J. M. (1997). *The Prefrontal Cortex,* 3rd ed. Philadelphia: Lippincott-Raven.

Fuster, J. M., & Alexander, G. E. (1971). Neuron activity related to short-term memory. *Science, 173,* 652–4.

Gellhorn, E., & Loofbourrow, G. N. (1963). *Emotions and Emotional Disorders.* New York: Harper & Row.

Gemba, H., & Sasaki, K. (1989). Potential related to no-go reaction of go/no-go hand movement task with color discrimination in human. *Neuroscience Letters, 101,* 263–8.

Gemba, H., Sasaki, K., & Hashimoto, S. (1980). Distribution of premovement slow cortical potentials associated with self-paced hand movements in monkeys. *Neuroscience Letters, 20,* 159–63.

Gerbrandt, L. K. (1977). Analysis of movement potential components. In J. E. Desmedt (Ed.), *Attention, Voluntary Contraction, and Event-Related Cerebral Potentials* (Progress in Clinical Neurophysiology, vol. 1), pp. 174–88. Basel: Karger.

Gerbrandt, L. K., Goff, W. R., & Smith, D. B. (1973). Distribution of the human average movement potential. *Electroencephalography and Clinical Neurophysiology, 34,* 461–74.

Gibson, J. J. (1941). A critical review of the concept of set in contemporary experimental psychology. *Psychological Bulletin, 38,* 781–817.

Gilden, L., Vaughan, H. G., Jr., & Costa, L. D. (1966). Summated human EEG potentials with voluntary movement. *Electroencephalography and Clinical Neurophysiology, 20,* 433–8.

Goldberg, G. (1985). Supplementary motor area structure and function: Review and hypotheses. *Behavioral and Brain Sciences, 8,* 567–616.

Goldman-Rakic, P. S. (1987). Motor control function of the prefrontal cortex. In *Motor Areas of the Cerebral Cortex* (Ciba Foundation Symposium, no. 132), pp. 187–97. Chichester, U.K.: Wiley.

Graham, F. K., & Hackley, S. A. (1991). Passive and active attention to input. In J. R. Jennings & M. G. H. Coles (Eds.), *Handbook of Cognitive Psychophysiology,* pp. 179–251. Chichester, U.K.: Wiley.

Gratton, G., Coles, M. G. H., Sirevaag, E. J., Eriksen, C. W., & Donchin, E. (1988). Pre- and poststimulus activation of response channels: A psychophysiological analysis. *Journal of Experimental Psychology: Human Perception and Performance, 14,* 331–44.

Haagh, S. A. V. M., & Brunia, C. H. M. (1984). Cardiac-somatic coupling during the foreperiod in a simple reaction-time task. *Psychological Research, 46,* 3–13.

Haagh, S. A. V. M., & Brunia, C. H. M. (1985). Anticipatory response-relevant muscle activity, CNV amplitude and simple reaction time. *Electroencephalography and Clinical Neurophysiology, 61,* 30–9.

Hanes, D. P., & Schall, J. D. (1996). Neural control of voluntary movement initiation. *Science, 274,* 427–30.

Hari, R., Antervo, A., Katila, T., Poutanen, T., Seppänen, M., Tuomisto, T., & Varpula, T. (1983). Cerebromagnetic fields associated with voluntary limb movements in man. *Nuovo Cimento, 2D,* 484–95.

Hasbroucq, T., Kaneko, H., Akamatsu, M., & Possamaï, C.-A. (1997). Preparatory inhibition of cortico-spinal excitability: A transcranial magnetic stimulation study in man. *Cognitive Brain Research, 5,* 185–92.

Hayes, K. C., & Clarke, A. M. (1978). Facilitation of late reflexes in humans during the preparatory period of voluntary movements. *Brain Research, 153,* 176–82.

Hazemann, P., Metral, S., & Lille, F. (1978). Influence of force, speed and duration of isometric contraction upon slow cortical potentials in man. In D. A. Otto (Ed.), *Multidisciplinary Perspectives in Event-Related Brain Potential Research,* pp. 107–11. Washington, DC: U.S. Government Printing Office.

Hebb, D. O. (1949). *The Organization of Behavior: A Neuropsychological Theory.* New York: Wiley.

Henry, F. M., & Rogers, D. E. (1960). Increased response latency for complicated movements and a "memory drum" theory of neuromotor reaction. *Research Quarterly, 31,* 448–59.

Hilgard, E. R., & Marquis, D. G. (1940). *Conditioning and Learning.* New York: Appleton-Century.

Holstege, G. (1991). Descending motor pathways and the spinal motor system. Limbic and non-limbic components. In G. Holstege (Ed.), *Role of the Forebrain in Sensation and Behavior* (Progress in Brain Research, vol. 87), pp. 307–421. Amsterdam: Elsevier.

Ikeda, A., Lüders, H. O., Burgess, R. C., & Shibasaki, H. (1992). Movement-related potentials recorded from supplementary motor area and primary motor area. *Brain, 115,* 1017–43.

Ikeda, A., & Shibasaki, H. (1992). Invasive recording of movement-related cortical potentials in humans. *Journal of Clinical Neurophysiology, 9,* 509–20.

Ikeda, A., Shibasaki, H., Nagamine, T., Terada, K., Kaji, R., Fukuyama, H., & Kimura, J. (1994). Dissociation between contingent negative variation and Bereitschaftspotential in a patient with cerebellar efferent lesion. *Electroencephalography and Clinical Neurophysiology, 90,* 359–64.

Irwin, D. A., Knott, J. R., McAdam, D. W., & Rebert, C. S. (1966). The motivational determinants of the "contingent negative variation." *Electroencephalography and Clinical Neurophysiology, 21,* 538–43.

Jeannerod, M. (1997). *The Cognitive Neuroscience of Action.* Oxford, U.K.: Blackwell.

Keele, S. W. (1968). Movement control in skilled motor performance. *Psychological Bulletin, 70,* 387–404.

Kornhuber, H. H., & Deecke, L. (1965). Hirnpotentialänderungen bei Willkürbewegungen und passiven Bewegungen des Menschen: Bereitschaftspotential und reafferente Potentiale. *Pflügers Archiv, 284,* 1–17.

Kutas, M., & Donchin, E. (1974). Studies of squeezing: Handedness, responding hand, response force, and asymmetry of readiness potential. *Science, 186,* 545–8.

Kuypers, H. G. J. M. (1981). Anatomy of the descending pathways. In R. E. Burke (Ed.), *Handbook of Physiology, I: The Nervous System,* vol. 2 (Motor Systems), pp. 597–666. Washington, DC: American Physiological Society.

LaBerge, D. (1995). *Attentional Processing.* Cambridge, MA: Harvard University Press.

Lacey, J. I., & Lacey, B. C. (1970). Some autonomic-central nervous system interrelationships. In P. Black (Ed.), *Physiological Correlates of Emotion,* pp. 205–27. New York: Academic Press.

Landis, C., & Hunt, W. A. (1939). *The Startle Pattern.* New York: Holt, Rinehart & Winston.

Lang, P. J., Bradley, M. M., & Cuthbert, B. N. (1990). Emotion, attention and the startle reflex. *Psychological Review, 97,* 377–95.

Lang, P. J., Simons, R. F., & Balaban, M. T. (1997). *Attention and Orienting: Sensory and Motivational Processes.* Mahwah, NJ: Erlbaum.

Lang, W., Cheyne, D., Kristeva, R., Lindinger, G., & Deecke, L. (1991). Functional localisation of motor processes in the human cortex. In C. H. M. Brunia, G. Mulder, & M. N. Verbaten (Eds.), *Event-Related Brain Research* (Electroencephalography and Clinical Neurophysiology, Suppl. 42), pp. 97–115. Amsterdam: Elsevier.

Lang, W., Zilch, O., Koska, C., Lindinger, G., & Deecke, L. (1989). Negative cortical DC shifts preceding and accompanying simple and complex sequential movements. *Experimental Brain Research, 74,* 99–104.

Lange, L. (1888). Neue Experimente über den Vorgang der einfachen Reaktion auf Sinneseindrücke. *Philisophische Studien, 4,* 479–510.

Lashley, K. S. (1917). The accuracy of movement in the absence of excitation from the moving organ. *American Journal of Physiology, 43,* 169–94.

Lashley, K. S. (1951). The problem of serial order in behavior. In L. A. Jeffress (Ed.), *Cerebral Mechanisms in Behavior,* pp. 112–36. New York: Wiley.

Libet, B., Wright, E. W., Jr., & Gleason, C. A. (1982). Readiness-potentials preceding unrestricted "spontaneous" vs. preplanned voluntary acts. *Electroencephalography and Clinical Neurophysiology, 54,* 322–35.

Loveless, N. E., & Sanford, A. J. (1974). Effects of age on the contingent negative variation and preparatory set in a reaction time task. *Journal of Gerontology, 29,* 52–63.

Low, M. D., Borda, R. P., Frost, J. D., & Kellaway, P. (1966). Surface-negative, slow potential shift associated with conditioning in man. *Neurology, 16,* 771–82.

Luria, A. R. (1973). *The Working Brain.* London: Penguin.

Magendie, F. (1822). Expériences sur les fonctions des racines des nerves rachidiens. *Journal de Physiologie Expérimentale et Pathologie, 2,* 276–9.

Matelli, M., Luppino, G., & Rizzolatti, G. (1991). Architecture of superior and mesial area 6 and of the adjacent cingulate cortex. *Journal of Comparative Neurology, 311,* 445–62.

McCarthy, G., & Donchin, E. (1978). Brain potentials associated with structural and functional visual matching. *Neuropsychologia, 16,* 571–85.

Mesulam, M. M. (1981). A cortical network for directed attention and unilateral neglect. *Annals of Neurology, 10,* 309–25.

Milner, A. D., & Goodale, M. A. (1995). *The Visual Brain in Action.* Oxford University Press.

Milner, B. (1964). Some effects of frontal lobectomy in man. In J. M. Warren & K. Akert (Eds.), *The Frontal Granular Cortex and Behavior,* pp. 313–34. New York: McGraw-Hill.

Neshige, R., Lüders, H., & Shibasaki, H. (1988). Recording of movement-related potentials from scalp and cortex in man. *Brain, 111,* 719–36.

Obrist, P. A. (1976). The cardio-vascular interaction as it appears today. *Psychophysiology, 13,* 95–107.

Paillard, J. (1955). *Réflexes et régulations d'origine proprioceptive chez l'homme.* Paris: Arnette.

Papakostopoulos, D. (1978). Electrical activity of the brain associated with skilled performance. In D. A. Otto (Ed.), *Multidisciplinary Perspectives in Event-Related Brain Potential Research,* pp. 134–7. Washington, DC: U.S. Government Printing Office.

Passingham, R. E. (1987). Two cortical systems for directing movement. In *Motor Areas of the Cerebral Cortex* (Ciba Foundation Symposium, no. 132), pp. 151–61. Chichester, U.K.: Wiley.

Posner, M. (1994). Attention in cognitive neuroscience. An overview. In M. Gazzaniga (Ed.), *The Cognitive Neurosciences,* pp. 615–24. Cambridge, MA: MIT Press.

Praamstra, P., Meyer, A. S., Cools, A. R., Horstink, M. W. I. M., & Stegeman, D. F. (1996a). Movement preparation in Parkinson's disease – Time course and distribution of movement-related potentials in a movement precueing task. *Brain, 119,* 1689–1704.

Praamstra, P., Stegeman, D. F., Horstink, M. W. I. M., & Cools, A. R. (1996b). Dipole source analysis suggests selective modulation of the supplementary motor area contribution to the readiness potential. *Electroencephalography and Clinical Neurophysiology, 98,* 468–77.

Rebert, C. S. (1977). Intracerebral slow potential changes in monkeys during the foreperiod of reaction time. In J. E. Desmedt (Ed.), *Attention, Voluntary Contraction and Event-Related Cerebral Potentials* (Progress in Clinical Neurophysiology, vol. 1), pp. 242–53. Basel: Karger.

Requin, J. (1985). Looking forward to moving soon. Ante factum selective process in motor control. In M. Posner & O. Marin (Eds.), *Attention and Performance,* vol. 11, pp. 147–67. Hillsdale, NJ: Erlbaum.

Requin, J., Bonnet, M., & Semjen, A. (1977). Is there a specificity in the supraspinal control of motor structures during preparation? In S. Dornic (Ed.), *Attention and Performance,* vol. 6, pp. 139–74. Hillsdale, NJ: Erlbaum.

Requin, J., Brener, J., & Ring, C. (1991). Preparation for action. In J. R. Jennings & M. G. H. Coles (Eds.), *Handbook of Cognitive Psychophysiology,* pp. 375–449. Chichester, U.K.: Wiley.

Requin, J., Lecas, J.-C., & Bonnet, M. (1984). Some experimental evidence for a three step model of motor preparation. In S. Kornblum & J. Requin (Eds.), *Preparatory States and Processes,* pp. 259–84. Hillsdale, NJ: Erlbaum.

Requin, J., & Paillard, J. (1971). Depression of spinal monosynaptic reflexes as a specific aspect of motor set in visual reaction time. In *Visual Information Processing and Control of Motor Activity,* pp. 391–6. Sofia: Bulgarian Academy of Sciences.

Riehle, A., & Requin, J. (1989). Monkey primary motor and premotor cortex: Single-cell activity related to prior information about direction and extent of an intended movement. *Journal of Neurophysiology, 61,* 534–49.

Rizzolatti, G., Luppino, G., & Matelli, M. (1996). The classic supplementary motor area is formed by two independent areas. In H. O. Lüders (Ed.), *Supplementary Sensorimotor Area* (Advances in Neurology, vol. 70), pp. 45–56. Philadelphia: Lippincott-Raven.

Rohrbaugh, J. W., & Gaillard, A. W. K. (1983). Sensory and motor aspects of the contingent negative variation. In A. W. K. Gaillard & W. Ritter (Eds.), *Tutorials in Event-Related Potentials Research: Endogenous Components,* pp. 269–310. Amsterdam: North-Holland.

Rohrbaugh, J. W., Syndulko, K., & Lindsley, D. B. (1976). Brain wave components of the contingent negative variation in humans. *Science, 191,* 1055–7.

Roland, P. E., Larsen, B., Lassen, N. A., & Skinhøj, E. (1980). Supplementary motor area and other cortical areas in organization of voluntary movements in man. *Journal of Neurophysiology, 43,* 118–36.

Rosenbaum, D. A. (1980). Human movement initiation: Specification of arm, direction and extent. *Journal of Experimental Psychology: General, 109,* 444–74.

Rosenbaum, D. A. (1985). Motor programming: A review and scheduling theory. In H. Heuer, U. Kleinbeck, & K.-H.

Schmidt (Eds.), *Motor Behavior. Programming, Control and Acquisition,* pp. 1–33. Berlin: Springer.

Rothwell, J. (1995). *Control of Human Voluntary Movement,* 2nd ed. London: Chapman & Hall.

Ruchkin, D. S., Sutton, S., Mahaffey, D., & Glaser, J. (1986). Terminal CNV in the absence of motor response. *Electroencephalography and Clinical Neurophysiology, 63,* 445–63.

Sasaki, K., & Gemba, H. (1989). "No-go potential" in the prefrontal cortex of monkeys. In E. Başar & T. H. Bullock (Eds.), *Brain Dynamics, Progress and Perspective,* pp. 290–301. Heidelberg: Springer.

Sasaki, K., Gemba, H., Hashimoto, S., & Mizuno, N. (1979). Influences of cerebellar hemispherectomy on slow potentials in the motor cortex preceding self-paced hand movements in the monkey. *Neuroscience Letters, 15,* 23–8.

Scheirs, J. G. M., & Brunia, C. H. M. (1982). Effects of stimulus and task factors on Achilles tendon reflexes evoked early during a preparatory period. *Physiology and Behavior, 28,* 681–5.

Scheirs, J. G. M., & Brunia, C. H. M. (1985). Achilles tendon reflexes and surface EMG activity during anticipation of a significant event and preparation for a voluntary movement. *Journal of Motor Behavior, 17,* 96–109.

Scheirs, J. G. M., & Brunia, C. H. M. (1986). Motor preparation and the Achilles tendon reflex: The role of background muscle activity. *Biological Psychology, 23,* 163–78.

Scherg, M. (1990). Fundamentals of dipole source analysis. In F. Grandori, M. Hoke, & G. L. Romani (Eds.), *Auditory Evoked Magnetic Fields and Electric Potentials* (Advances in Audiology, vol. 6), pp. 40–69. Basel: Karger.

Schultz, W., Apicella, P., Romo, R., & Scanati, E. (1995). Context-dependent activity in primate striatum reflecting past and future behavioral events. In J. C. Houk, J. L. Davis, & D. G. Beiser (Eds.), *Models of Information Processing in the Basal Ganglia,* pp. 11–29. Cambridge, MA: MIT Press.

Semjen, A., & Bonnet, M. (1982). Dual effect of response preparation on conditioned H-reflex. *Physiology and Behavior, 28,* 613–17.

Sherrington, C. S. (1906/1947). *The Integrative Action of the Nervous System.* New Haven, CT: Yale University Press.

Shibasaki, H., Barrett, G., Halliday, E., & Halliday, A. M. (1980). Components of the movement-related cortical potential and their scalp topography. *Electroencephalography and Clinical Neurophysiology, 49,* 213–26.

Shibasaki, H., Barrett, G., Neshige, R., Hirata, I., & Tomoda, H. (1986). Volitional movement is not preceded by cortical slow negativity in cerebellar dentate lesion in man. *Brain Research, 368,* 361–5.

Skinner, J. E., & Yingling, C. D. (1977). Reconsideration of the cerebral mechanisms underlying selective attention and slow potential shifts. In J. E. Desmedt (Ed.), *Attention, Voluntary Contraction and Event-Related Cerebral Potentials* (Progress in Clinical Neurophysiology, vol. 1), pp. 30–69. Basel: Karger.

Sullivan, S. J. (1980). Conditioned H-reflexes prior to movement. *Brain Research, 192,* 564–9.

Taub, E., & Berman, A. J. (1968). Movement and learning in the absence of sensory feedback. In S. J. Freeman (Ed.), *The Neuropsychology of Spatially Oriented Behavior,* pp. 173–92. Homewood, NJ: Dorsey.

Tecce, J. J. (1972). Contingent negative variation (CNV) and psychological processes in man. *Psychological Bulletin, 77,* 73–108.

Teuber, H. L. (1964). The riddle of the frontal lobe in man. In J. M. Warren & K. Akert (Eds.), *The Frontal Granular Cortex and Behavior,* pp. 410–44. New York: McGraw-Hill.

Thach, W. T. (1987). Cerebellar inputs to the motor cortex. In *Motor Areas of the Cerebral Cortex* (Ciba Foundation Symposium, no. 132), pp. 201–20. Chichester, U.K.: Wiley.

Ungerleider, L. G., & Mishkin, M. (1982). Two cortical visual systems. In D. J. Ingle, M. A. Goodale, & R. J. W. Mansfield (Eds.), *Analysis of Visual Behavior,* pp. 549–86. Cambridge, MA: MIT Press.

van Boxtel, G. J. M. (1994). *Non-motor components of slow brain potentials.* Doctoral dissertation, Tilburg University, The Netherlands.

van Boxtel, G. J. M., & Brunia, C. H. M. (1994a). Motor and non-motor aspects of slow brain potentials. *Biological Psychology, 38,* 37–51.

van Boxtel, G. J. M., & Brunia, C. H. M. (1994b). Motor and non-motor components of the contingent negative variation. *International Journal of Psychophysiology, 17,* 269–79.

Walter, W. G., Cooper, R., Aldridge, V. J., McCallum, W. C., & Winter, A. L. (1964). Contingent negative variation: An electric sign of sensori-motor association and expectancy in the human brain. *Nature, 203,* 380–4.

Watt, H. J. (1904). *Experimentelle Beiträge zu einer Theorie des Denkens.* Leipzig: Engelmann.

Wiesendanger, M. (1993). The riddle of supplementary motor area function. In N. Mano, I. Hamada, & M. R. DeLong (Eds.), *Role of the Cerebellum and Basal Ganglia in Voluntary Movement,* pp. 253–66. Amsterdam: Elsevier.

Wise, S., Boussaoud, D., Johnson, P. B., & Caminiti, R. (1997). Premotor and parietal cortex: Cortico-cortical connectivity and combinatorial computations. *Annual Review of Neuroscience, 20,* 25–42.

Wundt, W. (1893). *Grundzüge der Physiologischen Psychologie.* Leipzig: Engelmann.

CHAPTER TWENTY

COGNITION AND THE AUTONOMIC NERVOUS SYSTEM
Orienting, Anticipation, and Conditioning

ARNE ÖHMAN, ALFONS HAMM, & KENNETH HUGDAHL

Introduction

EVOLUTIONARY ORIGIN OF MIND–BODY INTEGRATION

The body is not, as folk psychology would have it, a chassis for the mind. The organ of the mind – the brain – is part of the body and is inconceivable without it. Humans, like other organisms, are the product of a biological evolution whose concern has been to perpetuate genetic information across generations rather than to create a mind that is separated from the body. Organisms have evolved to function in their ecological niches by means of intracellular mechanism, efficient metabolism, well-tuned behavioral repertoires, the coordination of societies, or intellectual insights. Psychological functions, like any genetically engineered survival machinery, have been evaluated and approved by natural selection because of their contribution to organismic fitness. In this perspective, there are blurred borders between biological, psychological, social, and cultural levels of discourse. Organisms are undivided, integrated systems designed to exploit their immediate environment in order to promote progeny to flourish in subsequent generations (see e.g. Dawkins 1976; Maynard Smith & Szathmáry 1995; Williams 1997).

Nervous systems play a key role in making organisms integrated systems. Nervous nets coordinate cells and organs to allow nutrition to be located and ingested, dangers to be avoided, and sexual partners to be found. With further evolution, bulbs at the front end of neural tubes developed into machinery for refined control of bodily systems, mechanisms for analyzing external conditions and eliciting appropriate behavior, and eventually to a mind contemplating its location in the universe.

"Mind stuff" (e.g., percepts, memories, thoughts), like all organismic activity, reflects the result of evolutionary processes; unlike bones, however, it is elusive in the paleontological record. Therefore, the evolutionary history of mind stuff must be traced indirectly through studies of bodily design and comparative analyses of modern descendants. Nevertheless, in the evolutionary perspective, mind and body are firmly integrated.

For example, perceiving the world is not a passive process in which energy is simply transferred across separate sensoria. Rather, it utilizes perceptual systems (Gibson 1966) in integrated acts, which are not restricted to the fine-tuning of receptors (eye movements, ear flickering) but include adjustments of the whole body to facilitate sensory analyses. From the neurobiological perspective, sensory information reaching the visual cortex is further analyzed in a ventral and a dorsal stream of cortical information processing. These streams have different evolutionary origins – the former mediating visual experience and the latter visuomotor coordination – yet both cooperate to provide an accurate visual representation of the world (Milner & Goodale 1995). This coordination is obvious in everyday observations. We all recognize the attentive set of a fellow human who is trying to discern the message hidden in a sensory channel: the motionless, tense posture with receptors oriented toward the source of information, the concentrated eye, the frowning brows, hands directed and ready to respond. And if we are good introspectionists we may add the inside story: the "active quiescence," the response readiness, the tuned muscles, and the slowing heart. In effect, psychological events are integrated in a matrix of efferent processes, supporting the view that a primary task of the brain is the organization of efference (Sperry 1952).

THE ROLE OF PSYCHOPHYSIOLOGY

This is where psychophysiology comes in. Through measurements of bodily processes, the data base for analyzing

John T. Cacioppo, Louis G. Tassinary, and Gary G. Berntson (Eds.), *Handbook of Psychophysiology,* 2nd ed. © Cambridge University Press 2000. Printed in the United States of America. ISBN 62634X. All rights reserved.

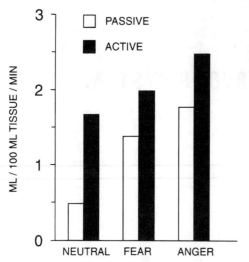

Figure 1. Forearm blood flow (measured by venous occlusion plethysmography) from research participants prompted to imagine personal scripts portraying neutral (resting at a beach), fearful, or angry scenes, involving or not involving motor activity (active and passive, respectively). For example, in the neutral scenes the participants were either resting in a chair at (passive) or slowly jogging along (active) a beach. The active emotional scenes involved aspects of escape (in fear) or attack (in anger). There were significant main effects of both scenes and activity. The subjects imagined each scene for 30 seconds; the graph displays changes from baseline to the imagery period. Note that the mere imagining of motor activity in the neutral scene resulted in significantly enhanced forearm blood flow (Sundin, Melin, & Öhman, unpublished data).

seated position. Thus, the mere thought of using the large musculature induced increased muscular blood flow. Indeed, "the recording of psychophysiological responses may be regarded as a 'window' into the brain and mind" (Hugdahl 1995, p. 3).

Psychophysiological responses have some appealing characteristics for the psychologist looking for handles on otherwise covert psychological processes (e.g. McGuigan 1978). First, unlike verbal reports, they are independent of a folk psychology that embeds observations in a biasing context of presumptions and post hoc interpretations (see e.g. Mandler 1975). Second – and also unlike verbal reports, which must remain retrospective (albeit sometimes with short recall intervals) – physiological measures can track psychological events as they unfold in real time (Beatty 1982). Third, they provide objective, reliable, and easily quantifiable measures that may be related to situational factors and individual characteristics. Fourth, even though the psychophysiological laboratory puts intrusive demands on the comfort of subjects, once they have accepted their predicament it is possible to take measurements unobtrusively that are resilient to voluntary control by the subjects. Fifth, psychophysiological measures provide avenues to psychological processes in nonverbal or barely verbal populations such as animals, infants, the severely retarded, or psychotics. Finally, psychophysiological data invite interpretation in a biological context, promising to bridge the gap between psychology and the biological sciences.

CAVEATS: LIMITATIONS OF THE CONVERGENT INDICATOR PARADIGM

The biological context is important. Psychologists often view physiological measures as *convergent indicators* in efforts to operationally define such concepts as "arousal" or "emotion," and they are then disappointed to discover that various presumed indicators of the concept fail to show reliable correlations (see Lacey 1967). Moreover, dissociations often are found between the physiological indicators, on the one hand, and psychological measures (verbal reports and behavioral observations) of the concept, on the other (Lang 1968).

From psychometric considerations, such dissociations between physiological measures – and between physiological and psychological data domains – are inevitable. A correlation between two measures reflects that a significant proportion of variance in each of them can be attributed to a common source. For example, correlated changes in reaction time and heart rate may be attributed to a common concept labeled "arousal." If both measures exclusively sample this same source of variance, only measurement error prevents the correlation from approaching unity. Such a situation, however, is unlikely when it comes to physiological functions (Berntson, Boysen, & Cacioppo 1992). Heart rate, for example, has more important business to mind

mental activity may be vastly extended. The measurement domains include peripheral nervous activity from both the somatic and the autonomic nervous system (ANS). The responses and response readiness of target muscles can be covertly assessed by electromyographical (EMG) recordings, and because muscular activity invokes demand on the metabolic housekeeping of the organisms, the ANS is invariably recruited, often even in anticipation of overt muscular activity. Thus, as action is contemplated, the heart beats faster and muscular blood flow is adjusted in order to provide a metabolic foundation for the necessary exertion of energy. An example is provided in Figure 1, which shows unpublished forearm blood flow data from an experiment by Sundin, Melin, and Öhman. The subjects, who were comfortably seated, were provided with scripts constructed from personal experience of emotional events as prompts to imagine scenes that differed in emotional content and the muscular activity involved (see Lang 1979). It is obvious that emotional scenes generated larger increases in forearm blood flow than the neutral scenes. This effect was further enhanced when the fear scenes involved aspects of escape behavior and the anger scenes aspects of attack. There was a reliable increase in forearm blood flow even with neutral scenes, as when subjects imagined themselves jogging slowly along a beach when compared to watching the beach scene from a reclined

than informing psychologists about the level of arousal in research participants. In the real world, most measures reflect several sources of variance, and then measures will show appreciable covariation only to the extent that they sample the same sources of variance in approximately the same proportions. Thus, not only will nonshared variance detract from covariation, but even measures that reflect the same variance sources can show low intercorrelation because one of them may be much more affected by variance source A than by source B, for instance, whereas the reverse may be true for the other measure. Hence, in practice there may be severe restriction on the maximum correlation that is possible between, say, physiological and psychological data domains (for a more thorough discussion of this problem, see Öhman 1987, pp. 84–92).

Physiological measures invariably reflect many sources of variance, only a small minority of which will have any psychological relevance. For example, heart rate is determined by mechanical (venous return of blood), hemodynamic (baroreceptor feedback), humoral (circulating catecholamines), neural (sympathetic activation, vagal tone), and central (brainstem, midbrain, cortex) factors. Thus, even though the whole system may be "psychologically driven" in (say) a panic attack, the particular heart rate reached will be determined by a host of factors secondary to or independent of the psychological factors that elicited the response in the first place. Because of this complex causal background, any effort to quantify "anxiety" solely in terms of heart rate is likely to be problematic. To overcome these problems, it is necessary to embed the psychological concept in a biological context that integrates psychological and physiological data and knowledge. For example, panic attacks may be viewed as evolved defense responses promoting escape from suffocation (Klein 1993) that for some reason (including catastrophical interpretations; Clark 1986) are falsely triggered.

Views of the Autonomic Nervous System

THE CLASSICAL VIEW

The classical view of the functional significance of the ANS was formulated by Walter Cannon (1915). Following Claude Bernard's concept of homeostasis – that the body is designed to maintain a constant *milieu interieur* – Cannon regarded the two branches of the ANS (sympathetic and parasympathetic) as opposing reciprocal forces – one anabolic and energy expending, the other catabolic and energy restoring – that in concert maintained the energy balance of the body. In particular, he studied the sympathetic branch, arguing that it serves an emergency function of mobilizing bodily resources to cope with threats through demanding motor output in vigorous attack or escape. For example, sympathetic activation results in increased blood flow to the muscles through elevated heart rate and in-

creased contractile force of the heart beats, resulting in increased arterial pressure, rerouting of blood from intestines to muscles, dilation of lung bronchi to facilitate oxygen uptake, and activation of glucose from the liver to provide energy for muscles and brain.

The sympathetic system, as traditionally conceived, is well designed to serve in emergencies. It has a chain of interconnected ganglia that collect their input from preganglionic fibers originating in the thoracic and lumbar segments of the spinal cord; postganglionic fibers are sent to target organs primarily in the cardiovascular and gastrointestinal systems. Because the ganglia are close to each other with abundant interconnections, activation will spread diffusely across ganglia, resulting in unitary action in virtually all effector systems. This unitary action is further reinforced by sympathetic fibers to the adrenal medulla, which can inject adrenaline into the bloodstream to further stimulate the adrenergic receptors of organs innervated by postganglionic sympathetic fibers.

The notion of the emergency function of the ANS had a strong impact on psychology and psychophysiology. It was incorporated into the concept of stress as a neural hypothalamic-adrenal-medulla axis supplementing the endocrinological pituitary-adrenal-cortex axis described by Selye (1956). It was an important component in notions of energy mobilization (Duffy 1951) and behavioral energetics (Freeman 1948), which – after the discovery of the reticular activation system (Moruzzi & Magoun 1949) – provided the peripheral core of the arousal or "activation" dimension (Lindsley 1951, 1960; Malmo 1959). In turn, this concept could be related to the most influential motivation concept of the time, Hull's (1943) notion of generalized drive (Hebb 1955; Malmo 1959).

At mid-century, it was a widespread belief in psychology that any autonomically innervated effector could serve as an indicator of a unidimensional concept of arousal or activation and so provide compact information about the motivational status of the organism. Soon, however, this notion was subjected to incisive criticism, perhaps most influentially by Lacey (1967). He reviewed the literature to document a degree of statistical independence between behavioral, electrocortical, and autonomic indicators that was hard to reconcile with the notion that a unitary dimension of arousal (or stress) was a major source of variance in each of them.

AUTONOMIC BALANCE

In the tradition shaped by Cannon (1915, 1932), the emphasis was clearly on the sympathetic branch of the ANS as the behaviorally important part of the system. However, other early investigators were interested in the parasympathetic branch and the interaction between the two branches of the ANS. Particular interest was directed toward the vagus, which in evolution predates the sympathetic system

(Campbell, Wood, & McBride 1997). Eppinger and Hess (1915/1976) introduced the notion of "vagotonia" on the basis of pharmacological studies of autonomic effectors, particularly the heart. They argued that "there are individual and varying degrees of tonus of the vagus system in man" (1915/1976, p. 12), as shown, for example, by the varying response to pharmacological agents affecting the vagus, such as atropine and pilocarpine. Eppinger and Hess felt that the concept of vagotonia could help us understand not only general pathology involving the ANS but also various disease pictures, including neuroses. The thesis advanced by Eppinger and Hess had a mixed reception, primarily because of inconsistencies when it came to classifying individuals as vagotonics. However, these inconsistencies could be at least partly accounted for by a methodological problem in testing the effects of pharmacological intervention on autonomic effectors. Wilder (1931/1976) showed that changes in blood pressure and heart rate following injections of atropine, adrenaline, or pilocarpine were determined by the initial value of the physiological parameter: the higher this initial value, the smaller the response. Sometimes even reversals of responses could be seen, so that injections of adrenaline paradoxically resulted in decreases in blood pressure. Hence, this "law of initial values" could explain why an individual could on one occasion be classified as vagotonic and at others as sympathicotonic.

The notion of vagotonia was predicated on an underlying assumption of a general reciprocal relation between the sympathetic and the parasympathetic branches of the ANS; increases in activity of one system were thought to be accompanied, through central integration, by decreases in the other. In this perspective, individuals were expected to differ in a meaningful way in the relative balance between the two systems. This idea was followed up and given a psychometrically sophisticated treatment by Wenger (1941), who used multiple regression techniques to develop an autonomic balance scale on the basis of factor analysis of a large number of psychophysiological measurements. A large database was generated from normal subjects and diverse patient groups (see Wenger & Cullen 1972).

ROLE OF THE VAGUS

Both the notion of an emergency function of the sympathetic branch and the notion of autonomic balance require that ANS function be seen as the interaction between two parallel and relatively unitary systems, reciprocally coupled through central control. However, this notion has been questioned by research showing a fair amount of specificity within the ANS. For example, recordings of neural activity directly in human sympathetic ganglia with microelectrodes often reveal specific responses with little cross-talk between ganglia (Wallin 1981).

Similarly, Porges (1995) argued that the vagal (parasympathetic) system is more diversified than previously

thought. After reviewing the neuroanatomical literature, he suggested that there are two vagal motor systems with different evolutionary origins and distinct locations in the brainstem: one originating in the dorsal motor nucleus, the other in the nucleus ambiguus. In Porges's model, vagal control exerted by the dorsal motor nucleus is associated with reflexive regulation of visceral functions, whereas control by the nucleus ambiguus is associated with cognitive processes, including attention and orienting to changes in the environment. Accordingly, he labeled the branch originating from the dorsal motor nucleus the "vegetative" vagus, whereas the nucleus ambiguus branch (linked to attention and primary emotional affect) was dubbed the "smart" vagus (Porges 1995).

AUTONOMIC SPACE

In traditional terms, the two major divisions of the ANS act as gatekeepers, with the sympathetic branch responding to increased demands for action and the parasympathetic branch responding to decreased demands.

The view that the action of one branch of the ANS is reciprocally related to the other has been questioned by several authors, most influentially by Berntson and Cacioppo and their colleagues (see e.g. Berntson, Cacioppo, & Quigley 1991, 1994b; Berntson et al. 1994a). In their view, the historical doctrine that the two branches of the ANS constitute functionally opposing systems is based on three assumptions: (1) autonomic target organs are innervated by both systems, which allows the sympathetic and parasympathetic branches to exert their opposing effects; (2) the two types of innervations are functionally antagonistic; and (3) the ANS is centrally regulated by reciprocal control.

Berntson and Cacioppo provided several examples of when the sympathetic and parasympathetic branches innervate the same target organ and where they may have similar effects (e.g., the radial and sphincter muscles for bladder function). Another example is the baroreceptor–heart rate reflex, which is controlled by vagal (parasympathetic) activity at high blood pressure but by sympathetic activity at low blood pressure. Berntson and Cacioppo therefore launched an alternative theoretical construct, the "autonomic space," in order to incorporate conditions where the two branches of the ANS obviously do not follow the classic reciprocity principle but may instead be uncoupled or coactive.

Berntson et al. (1991) proposed a multidimensional system to account for autonomic regulation. The multidimensional system may involve both coupled and uncoupled activation modes. A coupled (or coactivation) mode implies that the two ANS branches are activated at the same time; an uncoupled mode means that a change in one branch leaves the other unaffected. A third mode is reciprocal activation, which means that an increase in one branch is paralleled by a decrease in the other branch. Examples of the various modes of autonomic control are seen in Table 1.

The upper left-hand corner of Table 1 indicates a mode of coupled coactivation of both branches of the ANS. This may be seen in fear responses, where signs of sympathetic activity are observed in some target organs (increase in heart rate) while signs of increased parasympathetic activity are observed in other target organs (bladder and bowel functions). One of the branches may act independently of the other in uncoupled control, which may be seen in a moderate increase in heart rate to a physical challenge. Within certain limits, such an increase in heart rate is mediated through vagal (parasympathetic) withdrawal without a reciprocal increase in sympathetic activity.

The different modes of control of the ANS have implications for the directional stability, the dynamic range, and the reactive lability of target–organ responses. For example, the reciprocal mode produces stable, unidirectional responses because both branches operate in the same direction, one actively withdrawing its effect to reinforce the activating effect of the other. The nonreciprocal mode, on the other hand, yields directionally unstable responses because – depending on the relative activation of the two antagonistic branches – the result may be an increase, a decrease, biphasic changes, or no change in target organ activity. This is the case, as we shall see shortly, with heart rate responses to sensory stimuli (see Berntson et al. 1992; Sokolov & Cacioppo 1997). Similarly, the reciprocal mode also results in a larger dynamic range and greater reactivity lability than other modes, owing to the additive effect of the two branches.

The concept of autonomic space liberates thinking about the autonomic nervous system. Rather than expecting rigid reciprocal control of two uniform ANS branches, it gives room for alternative conceptions in which the central neural control of target organs has been evolutionarily tailored for optimal tuning of output depending on circumstances (Porges 1995). Thus, one of the tasks of the psychophysiologist is to disentangle whether a particular effect can be attributed to coupled, uncoupled, or reciprocal interactions between the sympathetic and parasympathetic branches of the ANS. Furthermore, owing to coactivation of the sympathetic and parasympathetic branches, the effects of the two systems may mask each other; this may sometimes produce paradoxical effects that are hard to interpret within more traditional models.

CENTRAL LATERALIZED CONTROL OF AUTONOMIC RESPONSES

Subcortical structures such as the amygdala, hypothalamus, and brainstem have direct effects on autonomic function (Cechetto & Saper 1990; Davis 1992; Mesulam 1985; Smith & DeVito 1984; see also Lane & Jennings 1995). Cortical control of autonomic function involves three main areas: the insular cortex, the infralimbic cortex, and the prelimbic cortex (Cechetto & Saper 1990). Cechetto and Saper (1990) suggested that the insular cortex in the rat, which is located lateral to the basal ganglia, acts as a visceral sensory cortex receiving autonomic afferents. The infralimbic and prelimbic cortices are located anterior and slightly inferior to the anterior section of the corpus callosum. The infralimbic cortex functions as the visceral motor cortex; it is located close to the motor area in the frontal lobe. The infralimbic area has descending projections into the autonomic system. The prelimbic cortex, finally, may be regarded as the visceral premotor area, receiving input from limbic areas and structures but with little motor output of its own.

The psychophysiological interest in autonomic function comes mainly from research on the physiological substrates of emotions. Since there is a large body of empirical evidence showing that both emotional feelings and the expression of emotion are differentially controlled from the two hemispheres of the brain (see Davidson 1995 for an overview), one would expect that autonomic function, at least to some extent, would also be differentially controlled from the left and right hemispheres.

The physiological innervation and control of the heart, or cardiac function, is perhaps the most intensively researched area with regard to asymmetry in the control of autonomic function (for reviews see Hugdahl 1995; Wittling 1997). Whereas cardiologists are aware of anatomical asymmetries – with regard, for example, to vagal innervations of the heart – yet may not give this fact functional significance, most

TABLE 1. Modes of Sympathetic and Parasympathetic Interactions in Autonomic Space

Sympathetic Response	Parasympathetic Response		
	Increase	No Change	Decrease
Increase	Coactivation	Uncoupled sympathetic activation	Reciprocal sympathetic activation
No change	Uncoupled parasympathetic activation	Baseline	Uncoupled parasympathetic withdrawal
Decrease	Reciprocal parasympathetic activation	Uncoupled sympathetic withdrawal	Coinhibition

Source: Adapted from Berntson et al. (1991), with permission from the American Psychological Association and the authors.

psychophysiologists are aware of functional differences yet may be unaware of anatomical differences.

Juxtaposing these perspectives, Lane and Jennings (1995) suggested that sudden cardiac death may be linked to the asymmetrical influences from the brain on heart function. After an extensive review of the literature, they suggested that extreme emotional arousal may trigger ventricular fibrillation (increasing the risk of sudden cardiac death) in a vulnerable individual. In vulnerable individuals, the left hemisphere may be more activated during emotional stress. It has been shown that the left hemisphere is more involved in arrythmogenic activity (Zipes 1991), so an increase in left hemisphere activity may trigger a series of physiological events that lead ultimately to cardiac arrest.

Using a video technique to present films either to the left or the right cerebral hemisphere, Wittling (1990) found that blood pressure increased after right-hemisphere presentations of a sexually arousing film but not after left-hemisphere presentations. It is interesting that Wittling (1990) also found that brain asymmetry in regulating blood pressure (favoring the right hemisphere) was significantly more pronounced in the female subjects.

The asymmetry of function of the autonomic nervous system with regard to cardiac activity has its anatomical counterpart in the asymmetry of parasympathetic innervation of the heart. The right vagus nerve innervates the sinoatrial (SA) node of the heart, which is the main pacemaker for the heart beat. The left branch of the vagus nerve innervates the atrioventricular (AV) node and the AV bundle (Brodal 1981; Schmidt & Thews 1980).

These anatomical observations are further linked to the functional significance of stimulating the right and left sympathetic interganglionic nerve that innervates the SA node. For example, stimulation of the right stellate ganglion resulted in a more pronounced cardiac acceleration than stimulation of the left ganglion (Kamosinska, Nowicki, & Szulczyk 1989; Levy, Ng, & Zieske 1966). It has also been found that deceleration of the heart rate (HR) was greater after right vagus stimulation than after left vagus stimulation (Hageman, Randall, & Armour 1975; see also Wittling 1995 for further details).

Experimental data like these fit quite well with clinical observations of change in HR in brain-lesioned populations. For example, Lane and colleagues (1989) found that epileptic patients tested with the "Wada-test" increased their heart rate after left-hemisphere sodium barbital injections but decreased after right-hemisphere injections. The Wada-test is a preoperative test for localization of language and memory function in epileptic patients undergoing brain surgery. The test consists of injections of sodium barbital (a sedative) that blocks the function of one hemisphere at a time for about 7–10 minutes.

For another autonomic measure often used in psychophysiological laboratories, skin conductance responses (SCRs), data from a large group of patients with well-characterized lesions (Tranel & Damasio 1994) suggested controlling influence from several cortical sites: the dorsolateral and ventromedial frontal cortex, the anterior cingulate, and the inferior parietal cortex. Using positron emission tomography (PET) to correlate cerebral blood flow with number of SCRs emitted during emotional stimulation, Fredrikson and associates (1998) found a positive relation to SCRs for a cluster of voxels comprising the anterior and posterior cingulum and for the primary motor cortex. Negative correlations were reported for clusters incorporating secondary visual and inferior parietal cortices and possibly for the insular cortex. Thus, particularly the cingular and inferior parietal cortices appear to be implicated in the control of SCRs – based on lesion (Tranel & Damasio 1994) and PET (Fredrikson et al. 1998) studies. Lateralized subcortical control of SCRs was suggested by a PET study by Furmark and co-workers (1997), who reported a correlation between activation of the right amygdala and SCRs emitted during aversive visual stimulation.

Attention and the Autonomic Nervous System

INTRODUCTION: A STIMULUS-RICH ENVIRONMENT

The world is replete with events that have more or less direct functional significance for the organism. Evolution has equipped us with perceptual systems that are tuned to particularly informative bandwiths within our "ecology of evolutionary adaptedness" (Tooby & Cosmides 1990). Even within these bandwidths, however, we are constantly exposed to a multitude of environmental events that threaten to overflow our perceptual capacity. Efficient selection of which events to respond to, therefore, is necessary to function adequately in the environment. Evolution has primed organisms to be responsive to stimuli that are more or less directly related to the overall task of promoting one's genes to prosper in subsequent generations. Such stimuli include those related to the survival tasks: finding food, water, "shelters from the storm," and exploitable conspecifics, as well as avoiding and escaping various categories of threats (Öhman, Dimberg, & Öst 1985). They also include stimuli directly associated with reproduction, such as those suggesting sexually accessible mates or offspring to care for. Stimuli of these types are embedded in emotional systems that help regulate behavior within critical functional domains (Tooby & Cosmides 1990). As such, they are not analyzed *in vacuo* by the brain but are immediately connected to output functions, tuning the body for actions that are likely to follow. An important part of the fine-tuning for efficient action concerns the ANS. Thus, any stimulus of even remote functional significance for the organism is likely to elicit ANS responses.

VARIETIES OF ATTENTION

Selecting which stimuli to respond to in a complex array of stimuli is one of the key questions of attention. Following the classical treatment of this topic by James (1890), we shall distinguish between two basic varieties of attention: (i) "passive, reflex, non-voluntary, effortless" attention; and (ii) "active and voluntary" attention (James 1890, p. 416).

Passive attention refers to automatic, reflexive shifts of attention to stimuli that are in some sense interesting: "in *passive immediate sensorial attention* the stimulus is a sense-impression, either very intense, voluminous, or sudden, – in which case it makes no difference what its nature may be, whether sight, sound, smell, blow, or inner pain, – or else it is an *instinctive* stimulus, a perception which, by reason of its nature rather than its mere force, appeals to some one of our normal congenital impulses and has a directly exciting quality" (pp. 416–17; italics in original). In contrast, "*voluntary attention is always derived*" in the sense that "it owes its interest to association with some other immediately interesting thing"; "we never make an *effort* to attend to an object except for the sake of some *remote* interest which the effort will serve" (p. 416; italics in original). Thus, voluntary attention operates in situations where we intentionally exert effort in looking for particular targets among distractor stimuli or when we consciously anticipate that a particular target (e.g., the imperative stimulus in a reaction time task) will occur in a particular time window. In both cases, the effort invested in the attentional process derives from previous instructions, associative learning, or self-generated intentions to locate particular targets in the immediate environment. In passive attention, on the other hand, the power rests with the stimulus itself to capture attention, irrespectively of instructions or intentions. Often this power derives from simple qualities of the stimulus, such as intensity or suddenness of onset, or from its mere novelty. Yet it can also derive from complex but overlearned stimulus information, such as in the power of one's own name to capture one's attention.

Viewed in this way, James's (1890) distinction between passive and active attention overlaps contemporary conceptualizations of attention, such as the distinction between automatic and controlled attentional processes (Schneider, Dumais, & Shiffrin 1984; Shiffrin & Schneider 1977). Automatic processing can occur in parallel across different stimulus attributes; it is involuntary and nonconscious and it does not require effort. Controlled processing, on the other hand, is sequential, voluntary, conscious, and effortful (see Schneider et al. 1984).

Considerable research has been devoted to elucidating psychophysiological responses during passive and active (or automatic and controlled) attention. With regard to passive attention, this work has concentrated on autonomic responses to simple sensory stimuli, and it has typically been performed within the theoretical framework provided by the orienting reflex (OR). Voluntary attentional processes, on the other hand, have typically been studied as anticipatory processes in preparation for speeded response tasks, choice reaction time (RT) tasks, or sensory decisions. These two areas of research will be reviewed in the next sections of this chapter.

The Orienting Reflex

RUSSIAN ORIGINS
One of Pavlov's Discoveries

The *orienting* reflex – or, as he preferred to label it, the "investigatory" or "what-is-it?" reflex – was first described by Pavlov (1927). According to him, the OR was "a very definite motor reaction" (p. 29) by which the animals "immediately orientate their appropriate receptor organ in accordance with the perceptible quality" (p. 12) of the stimulus to allow its full investigation. This reaction was elicited by the "slightest alteration in the environment – even the very slightest sound or faintest odour, or the smallest change in intensity of illumination" (p. 29). He stressed the adaptiveness of the OR, suggesting that without it the life of the animal "would hang at every moment by a thread" (p. 12). Pavlov also continued to speculate that, in humans, the OR provided the primitive origin of epistemic tools culminating in the scientific method.

The Contribution of Sokolov

The OR was forcefully brought to the center of psychophysiological research by the translation into English of the work by E. N. Sokolov (1960, 1963, 1969, 1975), which provided the impetus for extensive research efforts in Europe (including Eastern Europe), Australia, and the United States. This included research by Lynn (1966), Kimmel, van Olst, and Orlebeke (1979), Siddle (1983), Campbell, Hayne, and Richardson (1992), and Lang, Simons, and Balaban (1997b). Sokolov's contributions to the understanding of the OR were manifold, but the treatment in this chapter will focus on two of them. First, Sokolov interpreted the OR within a cognitive context (Sokolov 1960, 1963, 1969), pioneering the idea that elicitation of the OR requires a "comparator" system in the brain (comparing current input to stored representations of past input). Thus, an OR is elicited when there is a discrepancy between current and stored input – that is, when the stimulus is novel or has been changed from previous presentations. Thus, according to Sokolov, the OR is closely related to representations of the world in memory. This aspect of Sokolov's work has been pursued by Öhman (1979) and Siddle (1991), for example. Second, Sokolov (1963) distinguished the OR from other related types of reflexes such as the defense reflex (DR) and specific adaptive reflexes. This line of Sokolov's work was subsequently developed by Graham (e.g. 1979) and Turpin (1986; Cook & Turpin 1997).

For Sokolov (1963), the OR was "the first response of the body to any type of stimulus" (p. 11), and its function was to tune neural systems for sensory analysis "to ensure optimal perception of the stimulus" (p. 11). In addition to the motor component (arrest of ongoing behavior, directing receptors towards the stimulus), Sokolov included autonomic changes (e.g., cardiovascular and skin conductance responses), electrocortical responses (e.g., blocking of the electroencephalographic alpha rhythm), and respiratory changes among the components of the OR.

In Sokolov's (1963) view, the motor and autonomic components of the OR were integrated parts of a centrally coordinated response, the purpose of which was to "establish contact with the stimulus" in order to facilitate its central processing. Indeed, it is easy to see the functionality of eliciting an OR to a novel stimulus in the prevailing context, thus commanding attentional resources to a closer analysis of its nature and possible consequences. As the stimulus, when repeatedly presented, becomes familiar, there is no longer a need for attending to it as long as it is not associated with any significant outcome. Consequently, the OR disappears (i.e., it habituates).

Sokolov (1963) contrasted the OR with the defense reflex (DR). Like the OR, the DR is a generalized response that provides a widespread recruitment of somatic and autonomic activity independently of the sensory modality of the stimulus. Contrary to the OR, however, which *opens* the organism to the environment, the purpose of the DR is to protect the organism from intense and potentially harmful stimuli. Thus, the DR *closes* the organism to the environment by promoting "the breaking away from, or limitation of the activity of the stimulus" (Sokolov 1963, p. 14). In contrast to the habituating OR, the DR remains stable and may even increase across repeated stimulus presentations.

The most convenient index of the OR, often used by Sokolov (1963), is the skin conductance response (SCR) (Öhman 1979; Siddle 1983; see also Chapter 8 of this volume). The SCR is a uniphasic increase in electrical conductivity of the palmar skin elicited by virtually any stimulus; neurally, it reflects exclusive sympathetic control of palmar sweat glands (Wallin 1981). However, a similar (albeit larger) response is elicited also by intense and painful stimuli, which suggests that the SCR is not only an indicator of the OR but is also a component of the DR. Thus, an SCR can be unequivocally identified with an OR only for low to moderate intensities of stimuli, because at high intensities it also reflects the DR.

To distinguish ORs from DRs, Sokolov (1963) measured vasomotor responses from the fingers and the forehead. The theoretical rationale for this measurement channel was that orienting was assumed to be associated with increased – and defense with decreased – cerebral blood flow. These theoretical hunches have more recently been con-

firmed by positron emission tomography (PET) and functional magnetic resonance imaging (fMRI) studies showing increased cerebral blood flow to novel stimuli (Tulving et al. 1994) and decreased blood flow to painful stimuli (Coghill et al. 1994). Assuming that plethysmographically recorded pulse–volume responses in the forehead would to some extent reflect cerebral blood flow, Sokolov expected and observed vasodilatation to orienting stimuli, whereas stimuli eliciting the DR gave a vasoconstrictive forehead response. Both types of stimuli gave vasoconstrictive responses in the finger. This methodology, therefore, differentiated ORs from DRs in terms of qualitatively different cardiovascular response patterns, which provided an important tool in the empirical studies reported by Sokolov (1963). However, these results have proven difficult to replicate in Western laboratories (see Turpin 1983 for an extensive review).

HABITUATION OF THE OR
The Nature of Habituation

Habituation, the waning of a response as its eliciting stimulus is repeated, is a ubiquitous characteristic of organismic life (Thompson & Spencer 1966). Contrary to processes such as sensory adaptation and motor fatigue, it cannot be attributed to peripheral changes in afferent or efferent nerves; rather, it reflects a central process – that is, changes in interneurons at different levels in the central nervous system. Habituation can be observed at many levels of organismic integration, from simple neuronal networks (Kandel 1991) to spinal-level reflexes (Groves & Thompson 1970) to intact organisms (Graham 1973). A

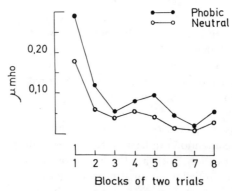

Figure 2. Skin conductance responses (SCRs) to repeated presentations of visual stimuli. One group of nonfearful research participants was exposed to potentially phobic stimuli (snakes) and another group to neutral stimuli (houses). Even though responses in general were larger to the potentially phobic stimuli, the two groups were not significantly different from each other. Note the exponentially decreasing magnitude of SCR with repeated stimulation. Reprinted with permission from Öhman, Eriksson, Fredrikson, Hugdahl, & Olofsson, "Habituation of the electrodermal orienting reaction to potentially phobic and supposedly neutral stimuli in normal human subjects," *Biological Psychology*, vol. 2, pp. 85–93. Copyright 1974 Elsevier Science.

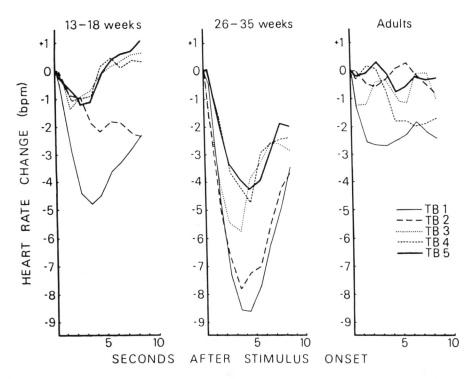

Figure 3. Heart rate in beats per minute (bpm) expressed as change from baseline in young (left panel) and older (middle panel) infants and adults (right panel). Mean baseline heart rates were 149.8, 144.9, and 81.2 (respectively) for the three groups. The graphs show second-by-second changes in heart rate to auditory stimuli for successive trial blocks (TBs) based on two individual trials each. Note the large initial decelerations and the relatively orderly habituation of this response across trial blocks. Note also that habituation is less complete among infants than among adults. Reprinted with permission from Bohlin, Lindhagen, & Hagekull, "Cardiac orienting to pulsed and continuous auditory stimulation: A developmental study," *Psychophysiology*, vol. 18, pp. 440–6. Copyright 1981 Cambridge University Press.

huge literature has accumulated on the topic of habituation (for extensive reviews, see Horn & Hinde 1970; Peeke & Herz 1973a,b; Peeke & Petrinovich 1984; Siddle 1983; Tighe & Leaton 1976).

With regard to the OR, habituation has the status of a defining characteristic – at least when the topic concerns orienting responses to nonsignal stimuli (i.e., stimuli whose significance is limited to their novelty in the context). Thus, both SCR and HR deceleratory components of the OR show rapid habituation over trials, often disappearing within ten presentations of a moderately intense, originally novel stimulus (see e.g. Graham 1973; Siddle, Stephenson, & Spinks 1983). However, even though HR decelerations show a clear-cut decrease in amplitude, they may not disappear altogether; small decelerations may be present even after prolonged stimulus series, particularly in neonates (see Figure 3). Graham (1992) called this habituation-resistant HR deceleration a transient detection response (TDR), postulating that it reflects detection but not necessarily identification of the stimulus. In general, the course of habituation of the OR can be described as an exponential decrease over trials. This is illustrated in Figure 2 for SCRs to auditory and visual stimuli. Figure 3 shows habituation data for heart rate responses in infants and adults.

The data shown in Figures 2 and 3 show actual habituation of specific responses. This response habituation curve may be taken to index an *inferred* central process of habituation. To avoid unnecessary confusion, it is important to distinguish carefully between the observed and the inferred habituation. For example, the common observation that different autonomic responses show different rates of

habituation (see e.g. the review by Graham 1973) does not justify the conclusion that they represent different inferred habituation processes. One might rather claim that they all reflect a common central habituation process (which, however, expresses itself differently in different measures). In other words, the rules of transformation between the central process and the peripheral responses may be different.

Habituation of the OR may be measured in different ways, which do not always provide convergent information. One alternative is to measure the time or the number of trials it takes a subject to reach the state of habituation, typically defined as a sequence of trials (two or three) without any discernible response (Levinson & Edelberg 1984). Alternatively, change in response amplitude can be measured across trials, most simply as the difference in amplitude between early and late trials, or (using all trials) by means of trial × treatment analyses of variance – perhaps supplemented by the analysis of orthogonal trend components. In more sophisticated versions, curve-fitting techniques can be used to derive parameters that reflect rate of change. For example, Lader and Wing (1966) linearized exponential habituation curves by regressing response amplitude on the logarithm of stimulus number; they used the resulting slope coefficient (sometimes with the effect of intercept covaried) as the measure of habituation.

Variables Determining Habituation

Habituation is modulated by a number of independent variables such as stimulus intensity, interstimulus interval, and so forth. These relationships were described as nine parametric relationships of habituation by Thompson and Spencer (1966), who suggested that they collectively provided a complete operational definition of habituation. Even though these characteristics in general are valid for habituation of the OR, complications arise because sometimes the validity depends on the particular measure used. For example, Thompson and Spencer (1966) concluded from the literature that habituation is slower to intense stimuli. Apart from the interpretational complication introduced by the fact that intense stimuli tend to produce DRs rather than ORs, slower habituation (with SCRs as the dependent variable) is observed to more-intense auditory stimuli as long as habituation is measured in terms of number of trials needed to reach a habituation criterion (Graham 1973; Siddle et al. 1983; Turpin & Siddle 1979). However, since more-intense stimuli evoke larger initial SCRs and since the responses in different intensity conditions habituate toward a common asymptote of zero response, the rate of change by necessity becomes larger for intense than for weak stimuli (Jackson 1974).

A further complication in the relationship between stimulus intensity and habituation of the OR comes from Sokolov's (1963) suggestion that threshold level stimuli, because they may be informative but hard to discriminate, tend to elicit large and slowly habituating ORs. This implies that the stimulus intensity–OR habituation relationship may be nonmonotonic, with slow habituation to stimuli of low and high intensities. Such a relationship was, indeed, reported for HR deceleration but not for SCR by Jackson (1974; see Graham 1979 for further discussion).

The interstimulus interval was held to be a primary factor determining rate of habituation by Thompson and Spencer (1966). However, shorter interstimulus intervals necessarily involve more stimuli per unit time, and therefore number of stimuli must be controlled. In general, even though the picture is somewhat complicated (Graham 1973), data indicate that habituation is slower with longer and more variable interstimulus intervals, particularly for the SCR but also for the HR deceleration component of the OR (Gatchel & Lang 1974; see review by Siddle et al. 1983).

Habituation of the OR typically is observed within a session of repeated stimulus presentations. However, the response decrement is ephemeral in the sense that spontaneous recovery of the response can be observed if the stimulus is reintroduced after a resting interval following the habituation session (Thompson & Spencer 1966). Long-term habituation then denotes reduction of the OR across repeated sessions. Such long-term habituation effects have been observed in many response modalities (e.g. Bishop & Kimmel 1969; for reviews see Graham 1973 and Siddle et al. 1983). It is interesting that the effect of interstimulus interval appears to be opposite for short- and long-term habituation. As we have seen, for within-session habituation, response decrement is slower with a long than with a short interstimulus interval. However, if long-term habituation is tested in a subsequent session, better retention of habituation (i.e., smaller ORs in the second session) is observed with longer interstimulus intervals in the training session (Gatchel 1975; see review by Siddle et al. 1983).

Stimulus complexity, the information inherent in the stimulus, was postulated by Sokolov (1969) to be an important determinant of its resistance to habituation. In general, this prediction is borne out by SCR data, particularly when habituation is measured in terms of trials to a criterion of no response (Fredrikson & Öhman 1979; Spinks & Siddle 1976; see Siddle et al. 1983 for a review). However, even though more complex stimuli produce overall more HR deceleration, rate of habituation did not differ for this measure (Fredrikson & Öhman 1979).

ELICITATION OF THE OR
Novelty as the Critical Factor

So far we have bypassed the question of precisely what factors determine the elicitation of the OR and merely presumed that stimuli are in some sense novel to the subject. Most studies have used easily controlled sensory stimuli such as simple tones or geometrical forms. Even though such stimuli are not, strictly speaking, novel to the subjects, at least they are novel within the context of the particular experimental setting. In broad terms, OR habituation could be attributed to the loss of novelty of the stimulus as it is repeated in the experimental context. If the stimulus is reintroduced to the unchanged context – as in tests of spontaneous recovery or in long-term habituation – it is less novel than when presented for the very first time and consequently less orienting will occur, suggesting long-term retention of the first habituation session.

In this perspective, novelty can be more precisely defined in terms of the amount of change a particular stimulus represents in comparison to some standard stimulus that the subject has been exposed to. Such a conceptualization implies that the larger the change, the larger the OR. This is the basic prediction from Sokolov's (1960, 1963) theory of orienting, which suggested that the degree of recovery of the OR on a stimulus change trial should be directly proportional to the difference between the changed test stimulus and the previously presented standard stimulus.

This statement implies that there is generalization of habituation, so that responses to test stimuli are inhibited in an inverse relation to stimulus change (Öhman 1971).

Changes in Simple Sensory Dimensions

In general, the prediction that OR recovers when the stimulus is changed appears to be supported by data (for reviews see Siddle et al. 1983; Siddle & Spinks 1979). This is true for changes in stimulus modality, from auditory to visual stimuli or vice versa (Furedy & Ginsberg 1975; Graham 1973) and for changes in pitch (Graham 1973; Öhman 1971; Siddle & Heron 1976). Because the theory explicitly addresses amount of change rather than direction of change, both increases and decreases in stimulus intensity would be expected to produce OR recovery. However, because of the stimulus intensity dynamism (more intense stimuli producing larger ORs), the effect of decreases in stimulus intensity may be hard to detect. Nevertheless, OR recovery to weaker change trial stimuli has been reported for both the SCR and the HR deceleration component (Siddle & Heron 1977).

Changes in Complex Dimensions

The OR recovery to stimulus change is not restricted to changes in simple physical characteristics of the stimuli. Siddle and colleagues (1979) gave subjects the opportunity to habituate their SCR-ORs to repeatedly presented words. The investigators then examined recovery to test trials involving changes in meaning or in category of words; they reported that SCRs on change trials were larger for participants given both a meaning and a category shift than in participants exposed only to a shift in meaning. Further experiments indicated that recovery was not observed for simple acoustic changes. Even more intriguing, recovery of the OR has been reported for numbers that are presented out of sequence in an otherwise seriatim presentation of numbers (Unger 1964).

Dishabituation of the OR

Recovery of the OR to stimulus change is sometimes confused with dishabituation of the OR. However, whereas OR recovery concerns responses to a changed test stimulus, dishabituation refers to recovery of the OR to the standard stimulus on trials following the changed stimulus. Usually in studies of dishabituation, the changed stimulus interposed in the sequence of standard stimuli is an intense one, which has a generalized arousing effect on the organism. Consequently, dishabituation has been attributed to a separate mechanism of sensitization that enhances responses to all types of stimuli (Groves & Thompson 1970). However, dishabituation can be observed also after nonaversive stimuli (Siddle et al. 1983; Siddle & Lipp 1997), which suggests that at least part of the effect can be attributed to the general change in context produced by the dishabituating stimulus. Thus, the dishabituation stimulus, which is different from previous standard stimuli, may introduce uncertainty as to whether the next stimulus will be a repeated presentation of the dishabituating stimulus or the standard stimulus. Consequently, the standard stimulus after dishabituation is less clearly expected than before dishabituation, and some OR recovery can be expected (Siddle & Lipp 1997).

THEORIES OF HABITUATION: CRITICAL ROLE OF THE COMPARATOR

Theories of OR Habituation

Sokolov (1960, 1963, 1969) presented a two-stage theory of habituation in which ORs were activated by an amplifying system located in the brainstem reticular formation. Whether an OR was elicited or not was determined by a comparator system in the cortex that compared current and stored input. If there was a match between current and stored input then the OR was inhibited, but if there was a mismatch then the OR amplifying system was free to activate the peripheral manifestations of the OR. The memorial representation of the stimulus, the "neuronal model," was assumed to develop into a more and more accurate representation of the stimulus as it was repeatedly encountered. In Sokolov's (1963) version of OR theory, changes in the peripheral response to repeated stimuli therefore reflect processes of perceptual learning and the building of neuronal representations of the environment.

In general, the data on the OR reviewed so far are consistent with Sokolov's (1963) model. However, they are also consistent with the most influential challenger to this model, the dual-process theory of Groves and Thompson (1970; see also Thompson et al. 1973). According to their model, which was developed on the basis of data from habituation of spinal reflexes in cats, overt responses are determined by two independent systems: a specific, phasic stimulus–response (S-R) pathway; and a nonspecific sensitization system, which controls the tonic state of excitation of the organism – that is, its generalized readiness to respond. Habituation is an inferred process that is specific to the S-R pathway and consists of the building up of inhibitory processes, which results in decrements in overt response amplitude. Its characteristics are such that they contribute to explaining the parametric characteristics of habituation described by Thompson and Spencer (1966). Part of the beauty of the dual-process theory is its anchoring in explicit neural systems (Groves & Thompson 1970) and particularly in molecular neural mechanisms (Kandel 1991).

The dual-process theory accounts for response recovery to stimulus change by assuming that similar stimuli share S-R pathways, and more so the more similar they are. For example, habituation to a tone generates inhibition in neural networks that are activated by the tone. Yet other, similar tones activate overlapping networks; thus, when the pitch of the tone is changed, the neural network activated by the new tone is partly inhibited because of shared neurons with the network activated by the standard tone. In this way, more response recovery should be expected the larger the stimulus change. When the neural nets activated by the stimuli no longer overlap, recovery should be complete. Because the dual-process theory appears to account for the data on OR habituation without invoking any comparison between current stimulus input and information stored in memory, it performs as well as Sokolov's (1960, 1963, 1969) theory, but with simpler assumptions about the underlying mechanisms. According to standard scientific canons, it should therefore be preferred. In this perspective, the critical question becomes whether there are data that definitely suggest the need of a comparator process to account for OR data.

Larger Responses on Change Trials than on the First Trial

Graham (1973) raised one critical argument against noncomparator theories such as the dual-process theory. She suggested that cases of larger responses on stimulus change trials than on the first presentation of the standard stimulus are difficult for an overlapping elements model to handle. As we have seen, the dual-process theory would predict total response recovery if there is no overlap between the neural networks activated by two stimuli. However, it is difficult to see why even larger responses sometimes can be produced on the change trial than on the first standard stimulus trial. Such data were reported by Furedy and Ginsburg (1975) when the stimulus change was change in modality of the stimulus, from auditory to visual or vice versa. Another example was provided by Bohlin, Lindhagen, and Hagekull (1981b), who reported HR stimulus change data from infant and adult groups of subjects who were either habituated to a continuous tone and then changed to pulsed tone or vice versa. They found clearly larger HR decelerations on the change trial than on the first trial for the adult group but not for the infant group.

From the comparator type of theory, this result can be understood in terms of the specificity of the memory model. On the first presentation of the standard stimulus, the information available to the subject about the nature of the stimulus is necessarily vague. With repeated stimulus exposures, however, the model becomes a more and more accurate representation of the stimulus. Consequently, when a clearly different stimulus is presented on a change trial, it provides a dramatic mismatch with the model and a very intense OR is elicited, sometimes even larger than the OR shown on the very first trial.

The Effect of Stimulus Omission

Sokolov (1963, 1969) incorporated what he termed the "extrapolating properties of the nervous system" into his model, and he argued that "an orienting reaction develops

at the moment when the stimulus administered ceases to coincide with the 'neuronal model' built up in former applications" (Sokolov 1963, p. 287). This implies that the comparison between memory model and input in effect concerns anticipated and actual stimulation (see Gray 1995 for a similar conception). Thus, Sokolov assumed that the model actively generated expectancies about which stimuli would occur and their characteristics, given the particular context. Such a model can be disconfirmed not only by changes in the anticipated stimulus but also (and perhaps more dramatically) by actual omission of the stimulus. Sokolov (1963) indeed reported ORs to the omission of a stimulus in a regular sequence, but this result has proven elusive in later attempts toward its replication (see review by Siddle et al. 1983).

Siddle (1991; Siddle & Lipp 1997) argued that the omitted stimulus effect provides a decisive way of pitting a comparator theory against a noncomparator model, such as the dual-process theory. In his attempts to provide such a decisive test, he developed a paired stimulus procedure for testing the effect of stimulus omission (Siddle 1985). In this procedure, two stimuli, S1 and S2, are repeatedly presented together. For example, S1 may be a tone of 4-sec duration and S2 an immediately following light of the same duration. After repeated presentations of this stimulus pair, an omission test trial without the S2 is presented, typically followed by a re-presentation trial in which S1 and S2 are again presented together. A control group is given paired presentation of S1 and S2 on all trials. The theoretical assumption is that the subject during training builds up a model of the events, which includes S1 and S2 occurring together. This implies that the occurrence of S2 is anticipated following S1. On the omission trial, this model is violated and an OR occurs to the omitted S2. Data from a large number of experiments (reviewed by Siddle 1991; Siddle & Lipp 1997) showed (a) larger SCR-ORs in experimental groups than control groups on omissions trials and (b) considerably larger responses to the S2 when it was reintroduced on the re-presentation trial. Thus, dishabituation on the following trial is seen as a consequence of the stimulus change provided by the omission of S2. Siddle (1991) argued that this enhanced OR on re-presentation trials was due to the weakening of the S1–S2 expectancy after the omission trial. This was confirmed in experiments directly measuring subjects' expectancies of S2 by requiring them to manipulate a lever to indicate the strength of their expectancy that S2 would occur. The expectancy of S2 to follow S1 developed rapidly over the first few paired presentations and remained at close to a 100% level until the omission trial. The control group (not receiving any omission) remained at that level during the re-presentation trial, but experimental subjects showed conspicuous drops in expectancy – down to about 20%. These data are hard to handle in the dual-process theory; in concert with data showing larger ORs on change than on the first trial, they appear to give decisive support to comparator models such as Sokolov's (1963).

STIMULUS SIGNIFICANCE AND ELICITATION OF THE OR

Theoretical Considerations

So far, our discussion has centered on ORs to stimuli that are in some sense novel. In this perspective, the OR is a means devised by evolution to guarantee that attention and learning resources are focused on unknown events in the environment in order to incorporate them into the brain's representation of the world. However, strong ORs can also be elicited by highly familiar stimuli if they have some degree of significance for the person. Indeed, it is perhaps even more important to respond to stimuli of known significance than to novel ones. Such stimuli were termed "signal stimuli" by Sokolov (1963).

In Sokolov's view, "conditioning" was the general method used to assign signal value to a stimulus (see later sections on conditioning in this chapter). This could be achieved, for example, by having the stimulus followed by another significant event, for which the preceding stimulus then served as signal. However, signal value could also be given to a stimulus simply by instructing the subject of its importance or by requiring some task (such as counting) in response to it. Signal stimuli, therefore, are stimuli with behavioral consequences or stimuli that convey useful information about forthcoming events.

According to Sokolov (1963, pp. 164–6), ORs to signal stimuli are controlled by similar independent variables as ORs to nonsignal stimuli. For example, an orienting response to signal stimuli is curvilinearly related to stimulus intensity, it habituates with repeated stimulation, and it shows recovery with stimulus change. A habituated OR to a nonsignal stimulus reappears if the stimulus is given signal value, and habituation then becomes slower. The functional significance of the signal OR is the same as for the nonsignal OR – to enhance perception of the stimulus (Sokolov 1963, p. 242). These characteristics imply that ORs to signal stimuli are a mixture of characteristics that are shared with ORs to nonsignal stimuli and characteristics that are more unique for signal stimuli.

Because signal stimuli must by definition be familiar, they are represented in well-developed memory models. This is a theoretical problem for stimulus comparator models of orienting, which somehow must account for the fact that both matches *and* mismatches between input and memory model can elicit ORs. One way of approaching this problem is to flip the coin and argue that stimulus significance is the major determinant of the OR, under which novelty (or the related concept of uncertainty) can be subsumed; that is, a novel stimulus will elicit an OR only if it is judged significant (Bernstein 1981; Bernstein & Taylor 1979). In this view, the OR is an attentional response to any significant or potentially significant stimulus, given the current concerns of the organism. Novelty is a powerful elicitor of the OR because novel stimuli may have significant consequences that must be attended to. However, such a theory cannot easily relate to the most appealing aspect of Sokolov's (1963) OR theory, namely, that the OR and its habituation are tied to the development of memorial representations of the world.

Some Data

As we turn to the empirical side, the facts are reasonably clear. Although there is some variability in the results, stimuli that are given signal value tend to elicit larger and more slowly habituating ORs than do nonsignal stimuli (see Siddle et al. 1983 for review). For example, Öhman and Soares (1998, exp. 2) instructed different groups of subjects to try to identify very briefly presented, masked conditioned stimuli, or to estimate probabilities of impending aversive stimuli. The researchers reported overall larger SCRs to the signals in these groups compared to a control group given no extra task. Berggren, Öhman, and Fredrikson (1977) reported slower habituation in groups instructed to press a key at stimulus offset than in groups simply exposed to the stimulus. Orienting responses to signal stimuli are larger than ORs to nonsignal stimuli, but much like the latter, they show habituation across trials and recovery to stimulus change (Öhman 1971).

Significance can be manipulated in other ways than through instructions. Some stimuli have an inherent biological significance ("instinctive" stimuli in the terminology of James 1890). For example, large HR-ORs were elicited in rats exposed to food- and predator-related odors (Campbell et al. 1997); likewise, humans show larger SCRs to biologically relevant threat stimuli such as pictures of snakes and spiders, particularly in an aversive context (Öhman et al. 1974). In a similar vein, Lynn (1966) reviewed Soviet reports of very persistent ORs in rabbits to sounds reminiscent of rustling noises in grass. Furthermore, Boysen and Berntson (1986) examined HR-ORs in chimpanzees to pictures of humans and reported larger decelerations to pictures of the animals' caregiver than to pictures of other humans. Similarly, Tranel, Fowles, and Damasio (1985) reported enhanced SCRs to pictures of the faces of familiar persons interspersed among unfamiliar faces in a stimulus sequence. Finally, Wingard and Maltzman (1980) recruited subjects with exclusive recreational interests (chess, surfing, or fishing) and examined SCR-ORs to pictures related to the different recreational activities as well as to filler slides. They reported specifically enhanced responses to pictures related to an individual's preferred activity; for example, members of a chess club responded more to chess-related pictures than to other pictures.

These data show that significant stimuli are effective in eliciting ORs, but they do not address the question of whether significance is a necessary factor for eliciting

ORs. More recent data and theory, however, clearly indicate that significance and novelty have additive rather than interactive effects on the OR (Ben-Shakhar 1994; Gati & Ben-Shakhar 1990).

Differences between ORs to Signal and Nonsignal Stimuli

Structurally, the ORs to signal and nonsignal stimuli appear to be similar, incorporating components such as HR decelerations (Bohlin & Kjellberg 1979) and SCRs (Öhman 1983). However, they may differ in their functional consequences. The OR to nonsignal stimuli is essentially an alert or alarm reaction mobilizing resources to deal with unknown and potentially dangerous exigencies. Sokolov (1963) talked about "the generalized OR" to capture this aspect of generalized readiness to respond to whatever stimuli might occur. For an OR to a signal stimulus, on the other hand, the situation is quite different. Here the stimulus is a familiar one with well-known consequences, and therefore resources may be specifically directed toward these consequences. To some extent, this is related to Sokolov's (1963) concept of "the localized OR" even though, in his treatment, localized ORs were not restricted to signal stimuli.

These differential effects were illustrated by Bohlin and Graham (1977; Bohlin et al. 1981a; Silverstein, Graham, & Bohlin 1981). When subjects were instructed to focus their attention on a startle probe that followed a signal stimulus, enhanced HR deceleration was seen to the signal, and the startle reflex (SR) to the probe was facilitated (Bohlin & Graham 1977). However, when attention following the signal was directed toward a stimulus presented simultaneously with the startle probe but in another modality (touch), there was still HR deceleration to the signal but now the SR was inhibited (Silverstein et al. 1981). Thus, the signal appeared to direct attention to a particular sensory modality, which resulted in facilitation or inhibition of the SR. However, when on some trials the signal was exchanged for a novel stimulus, large HR decelerations were seen to the novel stimulus but now the SR was facilitated irrespective of the modality of the novel stimulus (Bohlin et al. 1981a). Thus, with a novel stimulus, responses were facilitated regardless of modality; that is, the novel nonsignal stimulus resulted in a generalized increased readiness to respond.

AN INFORMATION-PROCESSING MODEL OF ORIENTING

The Model

Öhman (1979) tried to reconcile the opposing theoretical demands posed by ORs to signal and nonsignal stimuli in an information processing model of orienting. The basic postulate of this model is that the OR reflects the selection of the eliciting stimulus for processing in a channel with limited cognitive resources. Because the limited resource mode of information processing has some important characteristics of consciousness (see Posner & Boies 1971), this notion gives the OR the status of "a gateway to consciousness" (Öhman et al. 1993). Thus, ORs to both signal and nonsignal stimuli have the common cognitive function of promoting limited resource processing of the stimulus.

The model is illustrated in Figure 4. It has two basic assumptions, one pertaining to memory and another to different types of information processing. It is assumed that there are two types of memory systems, one short-term (the STM) and one long-term (the LTM); the former is represented as an activated subset of the latter. Thus, at any moment, memory information that is relevant for the stimulus context and for ongoing activity is in an activated state. It is against this active type of memory information that current input is compared to determine whether new (i.e. mismatching) stimuli are encountered or whether stimuli match memory elements that are primed as in some sense significant.

The other distinction is the one between automatic and controlled information processing (Schneider, Dumais, & Shiffrin 1984; Shiffrin & Schneider 1977). Automatic information processing is fast, effortless, holistic, parallel, nonconscious, and independent of cognitive resources and intentions. Controlled information processing, on the other hand, is slow, effortful, detailed, sequential, often conscious, resource-dependent, and governed by intentions. It is assumed that there are preattentive mechanisms that automatically process input information in relation to the content of the STM. When a significant stimulus – or a stimulus failing to find a match in the STM – is encountered, control over processing must be handed over to the central channel, which works in the controlled processing mode. When control is switched between the two modes of information processing, an OR is elicited and the stimulus enters the focus of attention. The OR was associated with "a call for processing resources" in the central channel. In the original theory, the call and the associated OR were assumed to have a preattentive origin (Öhman 1979). However, this assumption was later modified (Öhman 1992, 1993a) on the basis of data from experiments with masked stimuli, in which masking was used to ensure that stimuli could be processed only at the preattentive level (see the next section). According to the new formulation, only ORs to biologically significant stimuli (e.g., threat-related stimuli such as angry faces; see Dimberg & Öhman 1996) had a preattentive origin, whereas ORs to neutral stimuli (stimuli not implying any degree of biological threat) required central processing for their elicitation.

Tests of the Model

This model incorporates the comparator process of Sokolov's (1963) model but adds the distinction between STM and LTM, which can account for the differences between short- and long-term habituation. By adhering to the distinction between automatic and controlled processes, it places the OR within contemporary attention theory. This is illustrated by the work of Lorch, Anderson, and Weil (1984), who tested some implications of the model using information processing paradigms without any direct measurement of the OR. For example, consistent with the implications of the model, they reported that the opportunity to habituate to irrelevant stimuli – later to be used as distractors in a speeded classification task – reduced the interference effects of the distractors. Furthermore, the distraction effect decreased with training, but the introduction of a novel distractor stimulus disrupted task performance and this effect was smaller if the novel distractor stimulus was similar to stimuli used in initial habituation. Thus, both habituation and larger response recovery with larger stimulus change were demonstrated in disrupted performance.

An important aspect of the model is that it relates the OR to the allocation of cognitive processing resources (see Kahneman 1973). Because it postulates that the OR occurs as the stimulus is selected for limited resource processing, it suggest that further analysis of the stimulus should command processing resources. Stenfert Kroese and Siddle (1983) examined SCR-ORs to distracting tones in subjects engaged in a sustained attention task with two levels of difficulty. Consistent with the assumption of limited processing resources, they reported slower habituation to the tones with a difficult primary task. Furthermore, assum-

ing that the slow habituation to distractor tones with the more difficult attention task would reflect that only limited resources could be allocated to developing a model of the stimulus, they predicted and observed larger recovery to stimulus change during the easier attention task.

The utilization of processing resources can be assessed by assigning subjects a secondary task under the assumption that more processing allocated to the primary task leaves fewer processing resources for the secondary task. Typically, the secondary task involves reaction times (RTs) to occasionally presented probe stimuli (e.g. Posner & Boies 1971). Probes are presented at various stages of processing in the primary task as well as in baseline positions between tasks, and in this way the utilization of processing resources can be traced over time. Dawson and associates (1982) pioneered use of the probe-RT technique in the context of orienting and conditioning. They examined RTs to probes presented during a differential conditioning procedure and reported that stimuli predicting an aversive electric shock (i.e., with signal value) commanded more processing resources than stimuli not followed by shock. Dawson, Filion, and Schell (1989) required their subjects to count longer-than-usual tones presented in one ear and to disregard similar tones presented in the other ear while performing RTs to occasionally presented visual probes. More RT slowing was observed during the presence than in the absence of an orienting stimulus as well as more RT slowing during early than late trials. The researchers also reported a reliable correlation between the SCR-OR and RT slowing to the signal stimulus. Furthermore, when the pitch of the tones were suddenly changed, RT was further slowed. These data were fully replicated by Filion et al. (1991). Similarly, Siddle (1991) reported that signal stimuli gave slower probe RTs than nonsignal stimuli and showed more slowing on early than on late trials for both signal conditions; that is, "habituation" was observed for RT slowing. Furthermore, he confirmed that a stimulus change produced much slower probe RTs than those shown in a control group not exposed to any stimulus change. Indeed, the probe RT on the change trial was significantly slower than probe RTs observed on early trials, thus providing additional evidence consistent with comparator theories as opposed to the dual-process theory (cf. Graham 1973). Siddle and Packer (1987) found significant slowing of probe RTs both during stimulus omissions and during subsequent re-presentation trials, and Packer and Siddle (1989) reported more RT slowing during a miscued than during a correctly cued S2. Thus, consistent with the Öhman (1979) model, stimuli that are in some sense surprising elicit large ORs and also command extra processing resources, as indicated by RT slowing. In general, therefore, the commonalities of

Figure 4. Öhman's (1979) model of elicitation and habituation of the orienting response. Incoming stimuli pass through preattentive mechanisms that automatically compare them to the content in a short-term memory store, understood as an activated subset of long-term memory. Stimuli failing to find a matching memory representation or matching a representation primed as significant are passed on ("call") for processing in a resource-limited central channel, which takes over the analysis of the stimulus as the mode of processing is switched from automatic to controlled. The orienting response is identified with the call for processing resources in the central channel. Redrawn with permission from Öhman, "The orienting response, attention, and learning: An information processing perspective," in Kimmel, van Olst, & Orlebeke (Eds.), *The Orienting Reflex in Humans,* pp. 443–71. Copyright 1979 Lawrence Erlbaum Associates.

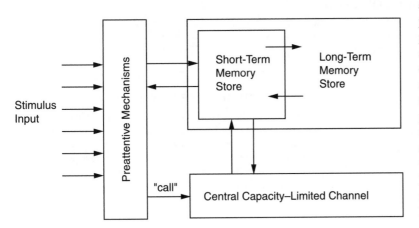

conditions giving rise to SCR-ORs and probe-RT slowing are consistent with the model.

However, some probe-RT observations are more difficult to reconcile with the model. Specifically, Dawson et al. (1989) found a dissociation between SCR-ORs to nonsignal stimuli and RT slowing to probes presented early during these stimuli, particularly when the discrimination between signal and nonsignal stimuli was difficult. Thus, whereas the SCRs were larger to signal than to nonsignal stimuli, RTs were slower to probes presented 150 msec after the onset of the nonsignal stimuli than to probes in this position after signal stimuli. However, a subsequent study (Filion et al. 1991) showed that SC-ORs and RT slowing to nonsignal stimuli exhibited concordant changes – confirming predictions from Öhman's (1979) model – if the signal and nonsignal stimuli were presented in different sensory modalities. Filion et al. (1991) interpreted their data to suggest that RT as an index of the allocation of processing resources was confounded by an "attention switch" to nonsignal stimuli that are similar to signal stimuli. They assumed that preattentive processing identifies a stimulus as task-relevant and calls for processing resources, whereafter resources are allocated to the task associated with the stimulus. When preattentive processing identifies a probable nonsignal stimulus, however, the call elicits a switch of attention (before resources are allocated) in order to confirm that the stimulus is a nonsignal one (rather than allocating resources to task execution). The RT slowing, therefore, is assumed to be due to the disengage–move–engage process of attentional shifts described by Posner (1992) rather than to the allocation of resources to the analysis of orienting stimuli.

Following Wagner (1976), the Öhman (1979) model incorporates priming and associative processes in the explanation of habituation phenomena. Wagner (1976) distinguished between self-generated and retrieval-generated priming of information in STM. Self-generated priming refers to a stimulus priming itself for future presentation. That is, once a stimulus has been presented, its memory model is retrieved from the LTM to the STM, which implies that it will be more available for comparison when the stimulus is presented again and thus a smaller OR will be elicited. Retrieval-generated priming refers to the priming of a memory model because associated stimuli promote the retrieval of the model from the LTM to the STM. For example, in the Siddle (1991) S1–S2 paradigm, S1 retrieves S2 to the STM, thus inhibiting ORs to the S2. However, when the actual S2 is omitted, there is mismatch between OR and the model, and an OR is elicited.

The notion of priming suggests that habituation of the OR should be context-specific. For example, a change in context after the OR has been habituated to a specific stimulus should result in recovery of the OR when the stimulus is presented in the new context. However, this prediction has not been supported by data (Churchill, Remington,

& Siddle 1987; Remington & Churchill 1988; Schaafsma, Packer, & Siddle 1989).

Thus, even though "Öhman's (1979) model may be simplistic" (Wells & Matthews 1994, p. 57), it is consistent with extensive sets of data and has stimulated new research on the role of cognitive processing resources in orienting and habituation. Nevertheless, there are areas in which it does less well, and modifications are called for (see the discussion by Öhman 1992).

THE EFFERENT LINK: PHYSIOLOGICAL MARKERS OF THE OR AND THE DR

Sensory Intake–Rejection and the OR–DR Distinction

In one of the landmark contributions to psychophysiology, Frances Graham and Rachel Clifton (1966) juxtaposed Sokolov's (1963) distinction between the OR and the DR and the Laceys' distinction between sensory intake and rejection. Beatrice and John Lacey (Lacey et al. 1963; Lacey & Lacey 1974) had argued that there is a reciprocal relationship, mediated via the baroreceptor mechanism, between cardiovascular parameters (heart rate and blood pressure) and cortical alertness, so that decreases in blood pressure are associated with increases in cortical alertness and increases in blood pressure with decreases in alertness. This theory was supported by data showing that, in general, tasks requiring sensory intake from the environment produced decreases in heart rate and blood pressure, whereas

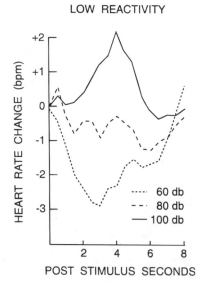

Figure 5. Second-by-second heart rate in beats per minute (bpm) expressed as change from baseline in response to tones of 60, 80, or 100 decibels averaged over twelve research participants. The tones were presented in random order. The graph shows the averaged response over the first three stimulus presentations of each intensity. Note the contrast between the clear deceleration to the lowest stimulus intensity and the acceleration to the highest intensity (unpublished data from an experiment reported by Öhman, Nordby, & d'Elia 1989).

tasks requiring the rejection of sensory information (e.g., painful stimuli, some cognitive tasks) were associated with increased heart rate and blood pressure (Lacey et al. 1963).

Consistent with the conceptual overlap between the intake–rejection and OR–DR distinctions, Graham and Clifton (1966) reviewed the literature to show that what previously had been understood as haphazard directions of heart rate responses (HRRs) to simple sensory stimuli could be interpreted in terms of the distinction between ORs and DRs. Thus, in general, studies using low-intensity stimuli reported decelerating HRRs and those using high intensity stimuli reported accelerating HRRs, particularly if stimulus onset characteristics were uncontrolled. This relationship between the direction of the HRR and stimulus intensity has subsequently been confirmed in a large number of studies (see reviews by Graham 1973, 1979). An example is provided in Figure 5, which shows averaged HRRs for the first three presentations of tone stimuli of 60, 80, and 100 decibels in a group of twelve subjects given the different intensities in random order (data from Öhman, Nordby, & d'Elia 1989).

Autonomic Control of ORs and DRs

From the autonomic space perspective (Berntson et al. 1991, 1992; Sokolov & Cacioppo 1997), it is tempting to surmise that the progression – from a primary decelerative HRR at low stimulus intensity to a bi- or triphasic deceleration–acceleration–deceleration at moderate stimulus intensity to a primarily accelerative response at high stimulus intensity – reflects coactivation of sympathetic and vagal influences on the heart, with the vagal influence dominating at low stimulus intensity and sympathetic dominating at high intensity and with competition between the two branches at moderate intensities (Berntson et al. 1992). In an autonomic blockade study, Quigley and Berntson (1990) examined HRRs to tones of 60 dB and 80 dB intensity in rats injected with saline (control), scopolamine (vagal blockade), and atenolol (sympathetic blockade). Atenolol blocked the accelerative HRR observed in control rats in the high-intensity condition, with little effect of scopolamine, which suggests that acceleration was primarily of sympathetic origin. In the low-intensity condition, however, atenolol enhanced the decelerative response by unleashing the vagus from sympathetic constraints, and scopolamine turned the decelerative response into an accelerative one of apparent sympathetic origin by blocking the vagus. This pattern of data suggests antagonistic coactivation of the two branches in the low-intensity condition. How these data map on to the control of human HRRs, however, remains somewhat unclear. For example, it would be interesting to know whether a still lower stimulus intensity producing uniphasic deceleration (such as the 60-dB condition in Figure 5) would engage an exclusively vagal response. Such vagal effects were reported from rats by Campbell et al. (1997), who concluded that the OR "is produced primarily by centrally driven, vagal stimulation of the heart, occasionally accompanied by sympathetic activation and withdrawal" (p. 58).

Evolutionary Origins of the OR

A rapidly habituating HR deceleration to neutral stimuli has been reported from studies on human adults (see Graham 1973, 1979 for reviews) and infants (reviewed by Graham, Anthony, & Zeigler 1983), on chimpanzees (Berntson & Boysen 1989), and also on rats from as early as 6 days of age and onwards (Richardson, Hayne, & Campbell 1992). Because the behavioral component of the OR involves an arrest of ongoing motor activity (Pavlov 1927; Sokolov 1963), it is possible that the associated quiescence of somatic activity promotes HR deceleration through cardiac–somatic coupling (Obrist 1981). However, whereas somatic activity undoubtedly may affect cardiac orienting (particularly in newborns), in older subjects HR decelerations are readily observed in the absence of somatic changes (Berntson et al. 1992; Richardson et al. 1992).

Campbell et al. (1997) suggested that autonomic ORs to neutral stimuli may have evolved from earlier, more motivationally basic responses, answering the questions "Is it dangerous?" or "Is it food?" rather than the more unspecified "What is it?". Their review of the comparative literature suggests that vagal control of the heart evolved prior to the emergence of sympathetic fibers stimulating the heart, which occurred in amphibians. This neural route supplemented the previously existing endocrinological, catecholaminergic route for exciting the heart. Thus, vagal tone modulating HR by inhibitory control appears to emerge very early in vertebrate evolution, and the dual innervation of the vagus from distinct brainstem nuclei (theoretically exploited by Porges 1995) appears to be present at least in amphibians. Nevertheless, when directly examining HR orienting in reptiles (two species of lizards) and mammals (rats), Campbell et al. (1997) reported no signs of deceleratory HRRs in the lizards either to a neutral stimuli (80-dB pulsating white noise) or to food- and predator-related stimuli (cricket and fox odors, respectively). Rats, however, showed large decelerations to all three types of stimuli. Coupled with reported failures to record deceleratory HR-ORs in avian species (Gabrielsen, Blix, & Ursin 1985), this finding led Campbell et al. (1997) to conclude that "to date there is little evidence that any nonmammalian vertebrate species shows bradycardia to novel, neutral stimuli, suggesting that autonomic orienting responses first appeared somewhere in the course of mammalian evolution" (p. 60).

In contrast, "fear bradycardia," a pronounced HR deceleration to threatening stimuli, is well documented in reptiles such as crocodiles and turtles, as well as in a wide variety of other vertebrate species (Campbell et al. 1997). In aquatic reptilian species, the bradycardia seen during a defensive dive clearly exceeds the bradycardia associated with voluntary dives. Thus, by reducing blood oxygen utilization, fear bradycardia allows longer submergence as a strategy to avoid predators. It is possible that this fear bradycardia associated with diving generalized to terrestrial species as "freezing" responses associated with bradycardia in ecologies where concealment and behavioral immobility served as viable antipredator strategies (Campbell et al. 1997). Although of more ancient evolutionary origin and tied to a more specific stimulus situation, fear bradycardia shows an obvious overlap with the HR-OR. However, it is typically much larger (25%–90% rather than 3%–15% of HR baseline), and even though systematic data are lacking, it appears to habituate much slower (Campbell et al. 1997). In some respects, therefore, fear bradycardia appears related to the DR. Indeed, Sokolov (1963) distinguished between active and passive DRs, the latter one taking "the form of complete immobilization of the animal" (p. 14). In other words, fear bradycardia threatens to undermine the neat distinction between the OR as involving deceleratory and DRs as involving acceleratory HRRs.

The Multiplicity of Responses to Intense Stimuli

The identification of the DR with heart rate acceleration has also stimulated controversy (see Cook & Turpin 1997 for a review). One of the problems with this formulation is that HR acceleration elicited by high-intensity stimuli, contrary to the lack of habituation expected for a DR, shows a clear decrease over trials (Turpin & Siddle 1983). Graham (1979) dealt with the problem of habituating HR accelerations to intense stimuli by arguing that it represented a conglomerate of two reflexes: a slowly or non-habituating DR determined by steady-state characteristics of the stimulus; and a rapidly habituating startle reflex (SR) primarily determined by the onset characteristics of the stimulus. This formulation derived from data reported by Graham and Slaby (1973) demonstrating a very large, short-latency acceleration to an 85-dB white-noise stimulus without controlled gating of onset. This response habituated within five trials. Hatton, Berg, and Graham (1970) directly compared the effect of a short (< 5-μsec) and a long (300-msec) rise time with a 90-dB tone stimulus and found a short-latency acceleration in the former condition and a slower deceleration in the latter. In Graham's (1979, 1992) view, the short-latency HR acceleration is associated with the flexor-contraction component of the rapidly habituating SR and represents a powerful interrupt of motor activity. It is separate from the slowly habituating DR, whose HR acceleratory component has a longer latency and whose function is to provide a general facilitation of motor output.

These conclusions were challenged by Turpin (1986), who suggested that there is a single short-latency acceleratory component of the HRR to intense auditory stimuli that peaks at about 4 sec after stimulus onset, shows habituating, and whose characteristics are determined by overall stimulus energy (onset characteristics, intensity, duration). This response, in his view, is closely related to the blink component of the SR. The DR, on the other hand, was associated with a much slower and larger acceleratory response, peaking about 30 sec after stimulus onset (Eves & Gruzelier 1984; Turpin 1986; Vila, Fernandez, & Godoy 1992). This component may reflect a burst of circulating adrenaline expelled from the adrenal medulla as a response to high-intensity stimuli; according to Turpin (1986), it is more consistent with the timing and characteristics of the active defense reflex described by Sokolov (1963). Thus, even though it is clear that high-intensity stimuli reliably elicit HR accelerations, the exact nature of this response remains somewhat in doubt. Cook and Turpin (1997) suggested that the understanding of this response would profit from considering it in a broader affective perspective than that typically implied in the literature on the OR and the DR. Such a perspective, of course, would also be appropriate for incorporating fear bradycardia into the discussion.

HR Responses to Affective Stimuli

The OR has typically been understood as an affectively neutral response. The terms in the affective lexicon that come to mind are those with a questionable status as labels of emotions: surprise, interest, and curiosity (see e.g. Ortony & Turner 1992). However, the OR has also been identified with the initiation of emotions, as when an emotional stimulus captures attention and becomes the focus of the conscious processing associated with emotional experience (Öhman 1987). In this perspective there is no firm line of demarcation between the presumably affectively neutral OR and emotional responding. For example, as the attention of young males is captured by pictures of attractive female nudes, their HR decelerates (Greenwald, Cook, & Lang 1989; Lang et al. 1993), and it becomes entirely arbitrary which part of this response should be attributed to orienting and which to emotion. Similarly, fear bradycardia may be interpreted as a sequence of events in which an affectively relatively neutral OR in an immobilized organism channels attention to threatening environmental stimuli, promoting an episode of intense anxiety. Research participants exposed to gory pictures of homicide victims and mutilated human bodies show a pronounced HR deceleration (Greenwald et al. 1989; Hamm et al. 1997; Hare et al. 1971; Klorman, Weissberg, & Wiesenfeld 1977; Klorman, Wiesenfeld, & Austin 1975; Lang et al. 1993). In participants reporting high levels of mutilation fear, this deceleratory response is even more pronounced (Hamm et al. 1997; Klorman et al. 1975), even though sometimes preceded by a brief acceleration on early trials (Klorman et al. 1977). In fact, the deceleration of the heart and the associated fall in blood pressure may be so pronounced that the fearful subject actually faints (Öst, Sterner, & Lindahl 1984). These data suggest that deceleratory HRRs to sensory stimuli can occur in contexts of pleasure (erotic pictures) as well as in intensely aversive contexts (pictures of mutilated bodies), where the simple intensity of aversive emotion suggests that it is more appropriate to speak of a DR rather than an OR. Thus, there appears to be a marked discrepancy between the HR deceleration seen in fear bradycardia and to mutilation scenes, on the one hand, and the HR acceleration associated with the DR to intense auditory stimuli, on the other, even though the affective valence of all these situations may be aversive.

There are, however, some circumstances under which HR accelerations can be reliably recorded to affectively aversive stimuli. When subjects who report phobic fear of small animals (e.g., snakes and spiders) are exposed to pictures of their feared creatures, they show a clear HR acceleration, typically peaking within 5 sec after stimulus onset (Fredrikson 1981; Globisch et al. 1999; Hamm et al. 1997; Hare 1973; Hare & Blevings 1975b). Boysen and Berntson (1989) exposed chimpanzees to pictures of other chimpanzees and reported a strong HR acceleration to pictures of individuals that had been aggressive toward the test animal, which contrasted to the primarily decelerative responses shown to pictures of other animals. Assuming that dominant, aggressive animals induce fear in conspecifics (Öhman et al. 1985), this acceleratory HRR – similarly to the response seen in animal phobics – may index fear and a disposition to actively avoid the stimulus. Thus, highly aversive emotion elicited by pictorial stimuli obviously can be accompanied by either HR deceleration or acceleration, even though the phenomenologically obvious emotion in both circumstances appears to be some mixture of fear and disgust.

To some extent, this discrepancy between emotional content and HRRs can be reconciled by recording the eye-blink component of the SR to startle probes presented during visual stimulation. Lang, Bradley, and Cuthbert (1990) postulated that there is a pervasive strategic disposition of approach–avoidance cutting through emotional phenomena, the phenomenological counterpart of which can be described as emotional valence (see Chapter 22 of this volume). Thus, aversive stimuli are associated with avoidance and positive stimuli with approach. These dispositions involve the priming of motor systems, and particularly different types of reflexes, to cope effectively with the situation. An avoidance disposition is associated with the priming of defensive reflex systems, such as the SR (and presumably the DR). Stimuli promoting avoidance (e.g., common fear stimuli such as mutilations and fear-inducing animals) activate defense systems, which would be revealed, for example, by enhanced SRs to startle probes presented during the stimuli. This prediction has been supported by many studies reporting SR data obtained to startle probes presented against a background of aversive, neutral, or positive slides (Globisch et al. 1999; Hamm et al. 1997; Vrana, Spence, & Lang 1988; see Lang,

Bradley, & Cuthbert 1997a for a review). In an intriguing observation, Hamm et al. (1997) reported that, in spite of the widely different HRR patterns seen in mutilation phobics exposed to gory pictures (decelerations) and in spider and snake phobics exposed to pictures of small animals (accelerations), both groups of subjects showed similar enhancements of SRs to probes presented during the pictures. This result suggests that both types of pictures activated an avoidance disposition in both groups of subjects, whereas the HRRs presumably reflected other, more peripheral adjustments to the situation.

Lang et al. (1997a) have further developed a theoretical perspective that may help to reconcile the different types of psychophysiological responses seen to affective and orienting stimuli. They used the concept of a predator imminence continuum (PIC) proposed by Fanselow (1994; Fanselow & Lester 1988) to describe a "defense cascade" of physiological responses to threatening stimuli. This concept is described in Figure 6.

In the first stage, that of pre-encounter with predators, the organism may be unaffected by predators (i.e. dangers) or may take precautionary steps such as avoiding areas where predators have been previously encountered. In this stage, the organism is free to orient to whatever stimulus is novel or of some relevance for current concerns. In the post-encounter stage, a predator (or other danger) has been sighted, the organism becomes aroused, and defensive measures are taken, one of which may be freezing. In Sokolov's (1963) terminology, this corresponds to the passive DR. The deceleration associated with HR orienting to potentially threatening stimuli may now be enhanced into fear bradycardia as attention is focused on the predator and immobility is used as a means of avoiding discovery. However, if the predator approaches (danger is enhanced), the heart may continue to decelerate but startle potentiation begins, even though the organism may still be immobilized and HR may be decelerating. Finally, if the predator attacks (i.e., the danger becomes acute), the circa-strike stage is reached and the flight-or-fight emergency reaction of Cannon (1915) is mobilized, with a pronounced sympathetically dominated response involving HR acceleration and associated strong startle potentiation. This corresponds to the active DR of Sokolov (1963). According to Fanselow (1994), different stages of the PIC are mediated by different brain mechanisms. For example, the responses of the post-encounter stage are primarily mediated by the amygdala, whereas the active defense of the circa-strike stage is primarily mediated by the dorso-lateral gray of the brainstem.

The concept of the PIC puts the distinction between the OR and the DR in a more dynamic ecological context than the simple stimulus intensity dimension advocated by Sokolov (1963) and Graham (1979). Because of the added conceptual richness, this concept may encompass data that provide enigmas for the more traditional approach. For

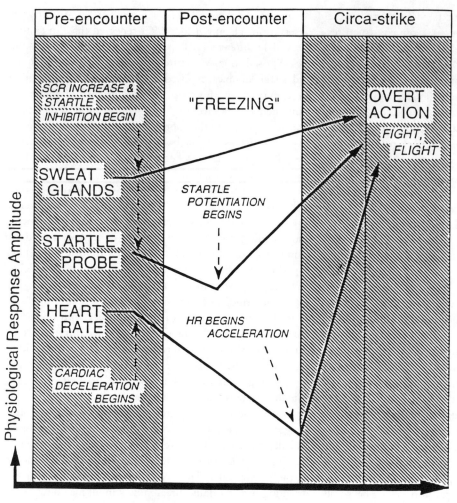

Figure 6. The defense cascade model proposed by Lang et al. (1997a) on the basis of Fanselow's (1994) predatory imminence continuum (PIC). The abscissa shows increasing arousal tracking the intensity of aversive stimulation (closeness of the predator). With little aversive stimulation (no predator present; pre-encounter area of the PIC), increasing level of stimulation produces increases of skin conductance responses (SCRs), startle inhibition, and heart rate deceleration as attention is focused on the stimulus. At moderate levels of aversive stimulation (predator sighted; post-encounter area of the PIC), further attention is invested in the stimulus, with accompanying increase in SCRs and falls in startle modulation and heart rate as the organism is defensively immobilized to avoid discovery. Startle modulation is shifted to enhancement while the heart rate continues dramatically to decrease (fear bradycardia) with increasing arousal. At excessive levels of aversive stimulation (predator attack; circa-strike stage of the PIC), immobility is changed to vigorous action in fight-or-flight responses, recruiting high levels of physiological activity to support emergency action. Reprinted with permission from Lang, Bradley, & Cuthbert, "Motivated attention: Affect, activation, and action," in Lang, Simons, & Balaban (Eds.), *Attention and Orienting: Sensory and Motivational Processes,* pp. 97–136. Copyright 1997 Lawrence Erlbaum Associates.

example, it provides a conceptual bridge between the OR and fear bradycardia, and it explains why some aversive stimuli (mutilations) may promote strong HR decelerations (i.e., fear bradycardia) and startle potentiation whereas others (small animals for animal phobics) may result in HR acceleration and startle potentiation. The implication of this analysis is that mutilation fears are located at the post-encounter stage of the PIC, close to but not crossing the border to the circa-strike stage. The problem for animal phobics, however, is that they automatically are propelled into the circa-strike stage when they encounter

the phobic stimulus even in pictorial form, which should actually motivate only post-encounter defenses.

Voluntary Attention: Anticipation of Impending Stimuli

The OR provides a psychophysiological vehicle for examining a major domain of attention, that of automatic attentional shifts in order to focus on suddenly appearing new or significant stimulation. However, as discussed earlier, attention can also be endogenously driven by voluntarily controlled intentions. We look for predesignated targets or we focus attention in anticipation of a stimulus that is expected to occur at a particular point in time. From an evolutionary perspective, these are critical functions. Efficiently locating the critical target may provide the difference between life and death when the target is a lurking predator, and exact timing of the required response may provide the difference between an empty and a filled stomach for the predator. Thus, this section of the chapter will review research concerned with what might be called "the psychophysiology of anticipation" (Lang, Öhman, & Simons 1978).

THE CONCEPTION OF THE LACEYS

As we saw earlier, Beatrice and John Lacey (Lacey 1967; Lacey & Lacey 1970, 1974) proposed that changes in cardiovascular function may facilitate or inhibit cortical processing. The originality of their argument was that increases or decreases in the intervals between successive heart beats were postulated to have a causal influence on cognitive efficiency. In a way, the Lacey model could be seen as an "attentional" analog to William James's (1884) model of the role of bodily processes in emotional experience. Both the Laceys and James argued that the registration by the brain of a change in a physiological system in the body may be instrumental in shaping further psychological activity.

Specifically, Lacey et al. (1963) suggested that stressful mental activity – such as counting backwards by subtracting numbers – accelerated heart rate, which in turn facilitated the rejection of interfering environmental input. Environmental rejection is a kind of "shut-off" of potentially distracting sensory stimulation through temporary cortical inhibition, caused by increased firing of the baroreceptors in the carotid artery in the neck. As an important component of blood pressure control, the baroreceptors are sensitive to increases and decreases in blood pressure, information on which is fed back to blood pressure regulating nuclei in the medulla for appropriate adjustments. Thus, the baroreceptors increase their firing when blood pressure rises, as in a situation of increased heart rate. The physiological basis of the Lacey hypothesis is provided by findings suggesting that increases in baroreceptor firing are associated with EEG (electroencephalographic) changes indicating that the cortex is de-aroused (Bonvalet, Dell, & Hiebel 1954). The opposite situation would occur if there were a deceleration of heart rate; that is, the cortex would be activated, which (according to the Laceys) would facilitate processing of external stimuli – a situation called sensory intake. The heart rate acceleration seen in a situation of environmental rejection and the deceleration seen in a situation of sensory intake are similar to the cardiovascular response patterns obtained to defensive and orienting stimuli, respectively (cf. Graham & Clifton 1966).

The Lacey hypothesis suggests that cardiovascular responses may be used as tools to modulate cortical activity level in order to deal efficiently with expected stimuli. For example, when a painful stimulus such as the cold pressor test (immersing the hand in ice water) is expected, HR acceleration may attenuate the impact of the stimulus by decreasing cortical sensitivity (Lacey & Lacey 1970). On the other hand, when a stimulus requiring a sensory discrimination or a fast response is anticipated, HR decelerates and so activates the cortex for efficient processing of the expected stimulus and priming of associated responses. Lacey and Lacey (1970) examined this latter hypothesis in a signaled reaction time paradigm, in which the subject released a telegraph key at an imperative stimulus (S2) after a 4-sec anticipation interval following a warning stimulus (S1), which signaled the subject to depress the key. Heart rate invariably decelerated during the successive beats preceding the S2, after an accelerative component following depressing of the key at S1. In agreement with their hypothesis, motivating the subjects to excel in performance (through encouraging instructions and response feedback) elevated the initial acceleratory component to some extent and had a pervasive effect on the deceleration preceding S2. They further reported that omitting the S2 on catch trials resulted in continued deceleration for an additional second or two, as if the subjects continued to anticipate the stimulus. Finally, they reported "a persistent, although modest, correlation" as follows: "the greater the cardiac deceleration, the faster is the reaction time to the imperative stimulus" (Lacey & Lacey 1970, p. 218). Reviewing the literature in search of a relationship between RT and HR deceleration, Bohlin and Kjellberg (1979) supported this conclusion; "there seems to be a tendency for large anticipatory decelerations to covary with fast RT, but the relationship is rather weak and can obviously be attenuated by other influences" (p. 181).

OBRIST AND CARDIAC–SOMATIC COUPLING

Even though he was in general agreement with the Laceys regarding the data, Paul Obrist (a former post-doctoral student with them) challenged their theoretical conclusions. He developed a coherent psychobiological perspective on cardiovascular psychophysiology, stressing the role of the cardiovascular system in providing a metabolic foundation for somatic activity (Obrist 1976, 1981). According to this view, cardiac activity was coupled to somatic outflow at the level of central integration so that, for example, HR tended to mirror the metabolic demands of ongoing somatic activity. Obrist (1976) suggested that the phasic changes in heart rate seen in situations of intake and rejection merely reflected the differences in metabolic needs in these situations. In a situation characterized by sensory intake, the individual typically is quiet and attentive to the outside world, inhibiting task-irrelevant somatic activity in order to focus attention on task-relevant stimuli. Thus, in this perspective, the decrease in heart rate between the S1 and the S2 of a signaled RT task reflects lowered metabolic demands associated with decreased general muscle tonus, rather than the active modulation of cortical activation as posited by the Laceys. In support of this interpretation, Obrist and colleagues (Obrist, Webb, & Sutterer 1969; Obrist et al. 1970) reported that HR decelerations in anticipation of an aversive electric shock or of the imperative stimulus of an RT task were associated with decreases in irrelevant muscle activity, such as spontaneous eye blinks or electromyographic activity from the chin. Similarly, HR acceleration during mental arithmetics – a situation characterized by Lacey as "rejection of the outer world" – may only mean that individuals tense their muscles or show increases in irrelevant muscle activity when trying to solve difficult problems.

According to Obrist's (1981) cardiac–somatic coupling hypothesis, metabolic needs override the emotional impact of the situation. For example, in contrast to predictions from the major theories of emotion and activation of the time (e.g. Lindsley 1960; Malmo 1959), Obrist and co-workers (Obrist, Sutterer, & Howard 1972; Obrist, Wood, & Perez-Reyes 1965) reported that both humans and animals showed heart rate deceleration after the presentation of conditioned stimuli that signaled impending aversive events. In agreement with the cardiac–somatic coupling hypothesis, HR deceleration was accompanied by somatic quieting, as if subjects were passively waiting for the aversive unconditioned stimulus. This was labeled "passive coping" by Obrist (1976), who postulated that it primarily reflected vagal control of the heart. However, when the experimental situation promoted active, effortful responses to cope with aversive stimuli, sympathetic control of the heart could be demonstrated; this was termed "active coping" (Obrist 1976, 1981; Obrist et al. 1974).

EVALUATION OF THE LACEY–OBRIST CONTROVERSY
The Causal Loop from Heart to Brain

In effect, even though the Lacey–Obrist controversy dominated psychophysiology for quite some time, the positions were not as mutually exclusive as implied by their proponents. Both views entailed that the patterned psychophysiological changes occurring during particular experimental situations reflected physiological adjustments promoting optimal transactions with the environment. A prevailing difference is the causal role given by the Laceys to the cardiovascular system in influencing central processing. This is a proposition that is hard to evaluate with human data, but a series of ERP studies by Walker and Sandman (1979, 1982) may shed some light on the causality issue. They recorded event-related potentials (ERPs) to sensory stimuli separately from the left and right hemi-

spheres when their subjects exhibited spontaneous changes in heart rate over time (Walker & Sandman 1979) or at the different blood pressure levels associated with the systolic and diastolic phases of the cardiac cycle (Walker & Sandman 1982). For example, in the latter study, ERPs were triggered during systolic and diastolic phases and averaged across trials. If the baroreceptors mediate between cardiac and behavioral events, then the ERPs recorded at the systolic peak should differ from ERPs recorded at the diastolic peaks. Specifically, Walker and Sandman (1982) hypothesized that the ERPs elicited by stimuli presented during the systole should be smaller than the ERPs to stimuli during the diastolic phase, owing to the inhibitory effects on CNS activity of baroreceptor stimulation. As predicted, the results showed that the P1 peak of the visual ERP was larger at the diastolic phase than at the systolic phase. However, the results also showed that this effect was present only over the right-hemisphere leads, indicating hemisphere differences in CNS–ANS relationships. Hugdahl and associates (1983) reported a similar relationship, although they recorded changes in heart rate when the left and right hemispheres were separately stimulated. In their 1979 paper, Walker and Sandman concluded that "changes in heart rate are reflected more clearly in the right hemisphere than in the left" (p. 727), which later studies also have verified (see Wittling 1995 for review).

Anticipatory HR Deceleration and Expectancy

In an extensive review of the literature on HR changes in S1–S2 paradigms, Bohlin & Kjellberg (1979) concluded that the deceleration preceding S2 was best interpreted as related to an expectancy process whose effect "would be to enhance the perception of the predicted stimulus and to attenuate the reception of stimuli irrelevant to prediction" (p. 192). This is a formulation which retains the relationship between HR deceleration and enhanced capacity for sensory intake postulated by the Laceys (1970, 1974) but which does not make any reference to heart–brain relationships.

Support for an expectancy interpretation can be derived, for example, from studies reporting that the HR deceleration immediately prior to responding to S2 was larger when S2 could be accurately predicted (as seen in comparing fixed and variable S1–S2 intervals; see e.g. van der Molen et al. 1987) and when a response to S2 was highly probable rather than improbable (van der Molen et al. 1989). Furthermore, Bohlin and Graham (1977) reported that the startle reflex was facilitated when the startle probe was heralded by a preceding stimulus that elicited HR deceleration, compared to when the startle stimulus was presented alone with no prior HR deceleration. However, the startle reflex was inhibited when preceded by an HR deceleration elicited by a stimulus directing attention to a tactile stimulus rather than to the auditory startle probe – that is, responses to stimuli that were irrelevant for the task were inhibited (Silverstein et al. 1981).

Further support for an attention–expectancy interpretation of HR deceleration comes from a study by van der Molen, Somsen, and Jennings (1996). They presented monaural tone pips of different pitch to separate ears at a rate (800–1,500 msec) slightly above average intervals between successive heartbeats (interbeat intervals, IBIs). The subjects were instructed to count rare tones of a different pitch in one ear while ignoring pitch changes in the other ear. Rare tones were preceded by 2–12 standard pips. Looking at IBIs preceding rare tones, they found increasing deceleration of the heart with increasing number of standard tones for tones presented in the attended ear but not for those in the nonattended ear. This suggests that the subjects were actively anticipating the rare targets in the attended ear – and more so the longer the sequence of standard tones (up to about eight standard pips, when the effects appeared to level off).

Anticipatory cardiac deceleration appears to be controlled from the right cerebral hemisphere. Using a signaled RT paradigm and patients with lateralized brain lesions as subjects, Yokoyama and colleagues (1987) reported that patients with lesions to the posterior parts of the right hemisphere did not show the expected heart rate deceleration in anticipation of the imperative stimulus.

ANTICIPATORY HR DECELERATION AND MOTOR PROCESSES

Data indicating that the HR deceleration is primarily geared at facilitating stimulus input can be viewed as broadly consistent with the Lacey notion (Lacey & Lacey 1970) that a slowing heart sensitizes central processing of stimulus input. However, the S2 in these experiments typically required an overt motor response. Indeed, Simons, Öhman, and Lang (1979) concluded that the secondary HR deceleration peaking at S2 in an S1–S2 paradigm was uniquely related to response requirement. Thus, when a response was required to S2, the deceleration was larger than when no response was required – even when S2 consisted of highly attractive slides of nude females shown to male undergraduates. Interest value of S2 was reflected in an acceleratory HR component peaking at 3.5 sec after S1 onset, but only when slide duration was controlled by a fast RT to S2 or, in the absence of an overt response requirement, when S2 was of short duration, so that adequate perceptual readiness was a prerequisite for its perception.

The critical role of motor processes for anticipatory HR deceleration has been further documented by Jennings and co-workers (see review by Jennings 1992). Jennings argued that "cardiac deceleration in the foreperiod reflects an aroused state of increased attention but inhibited activity, which gives way to a precisely timed movement and phase-locked heartbeat acceleration" (1992, p. 378) when the S2 is presented. Deceleration, in Jennings's view, is primarily related to inhibition of motor activity. In the S1–S2 interval, the inhibition concerns irrelevant motor activity. The pervasive covariation between motor inhibition and HR deceleration has been documented in RT paradigms involving Go and No-Go contingencies. For example, catch trials in which S2 was omitted resulted in immediate deceleration, particularly when the critical stimulus (i.e., S2 omission) occurred early in an IBI (Jennings et al. 1990). However, on unsuccessful catch trials, when a response was incorrectly emitted, the deceleration was similar to that seen on regular Go trials, when a response was required (and emitted). This suggests that it was the inhibition or emission of the response, rather than the presentation of S2, that was critical for deceleration. Similarly, in a complex choice RT task in which stimuli and responses were related in terms of an arbitrary rule – so that "natural responses" (e.g., press leftmost response key to leftmost stimulus) were inhibited – S2 was associated with clearly prolonged IBIs (Jennings et al. 1991a). Such motor inhibition and HR deceleration contrast with the rapid shift to HR acceleration associated with the correct response to S2. The association here concerns the initiation rather than the completion of the response to S2. For example, the force required for the response to S2 did not affect anticipatory HR deceleration, but more forceful responses prompted earlier and larger HR accelerations when the response was initiated (Jennings et al. 1990).

Following the suggestions by Lacey and Lacey (1978, 1980) that stimuli may have differential effects on HR depending on whether they occur early or late in an HR cycle, Jennings and co-workers systematically presented stimuli at the R-wave of the ECG (electrocardiogram) and at selected delays from the R-wave. For example, Jennings et al. (1991b) reported that sensory stimuli occurring early in a cardiac cycle prolonged that cycle, independently of stimulus intensity and the response requirements of the stimulus. In a study using mathematical modeling techniques to predict the effect of stimuli occurring during that time period within a cardiac cycle when the cardiac pacemaker is maximally sensitive to vagal discharge, Jennings et al. (1992) reported that decelerations were particularly clear to "stop" signals occurring immediately before or during the sensitive period.

The work of Jennings provides a sophisticated contemporary example of how psychophysiological data can be integrated into models of central control of somatic and autonomic activity. In his view, the brain must integrate cognitive activity into such ongoing physiological adjustments as maintaining posture and a regular heart beat. For example, oscillatory activities related to HR must be modulated to allow efficient processing of stimulus input as well as timing of motor output. This mutual dependence between autonomic and motor activity, on the one hand, and the planning and execution of action, on the other, will result in bodily constraints on cognitive activity. The timing of acts will "depend on inhibiting a variety of activities in the interest of resetting oscillators to coordinate phase for new activities. Many of the autonomic responses we observe may be resetting adjustments necessary for new coordinations of behavior. Such resetting adjustments may often occur during what we term emotion, but they are basic as well to the appropriate operation of our information processing system" (Jennings 1992, p. 381).

Pavlovian Conditioning of Autonomic Responses

PAVLOVIAN CONDITIONING, ORIENTING, AND THE NEED FOR CONTROL PROCEDURES

Basic Procedure and Definition of Pavlovian Conditioning

So far, we have encountered S1–S2 paradigms in two different contexts. Siddle (1991) used them to study the effect of stimulus omission on OR recovery, and in the preceding section we made frequent references to S1–S2 paradigms with a motor response required to the S2. These examples illuminate two important effects of S1–S2 paradigms. First, Siddle (1991) claimed that associations are formed if S1 and S2 are repeatedly presented together. This was demonstrated by ORs to S2 omissions, indicating that S1 must have generated an expectancy for S2 to follow. Disconfirmation of this expectancy constituted a surprising event that elicited an OR. Second, when S1 and S2 have occurred together (or if the subject is instructed that S2 will follow S1), S1 allows the subject to prepare for S2. The autonomic correlates of these anticipatory or preparatory processes were extensively discussed in the previous section.

Pavlovian ("classical") conditioning, which is one of psychology's central experimental procedures, is characterized by two salient features: (a) the forming of associations between two paired stimuli, and (b) the use of the first stimulus to prepare for the second. This procedure models a ubiquitous class of adaptive events in the natural environment – the correlations between relatively innocuous and motivationally significant stimuli – which allows the former to be used as predictors of the latter. It takes little reflection to realize that organisms that are able efficiently to utilize such correlations in their behavioral repertoire have an adaptive edge. For example, activating defense responses on the basis of a faint noise associated with predators improves the odds of the prey escaping potentially deadly predator encounters. Thus, one of the evolutionary origins of Pavlovian conditioning is the race between predator agility and prey defense capabilities (Hollis 1982).

In a Pavlovian conditioning arrangement, usually S2 is a stronger stimulus than S1 in the sense that it reliably elicits a response, the so-called unconditioned response (UR). Pavlovian conditioning is understood as the transfer of response-eliciting potential from S2 (the unconditioned stimulus, US) to the originally weaker S1 stimulus (the conditioned stimulus, CS) as the two events are repeatedly presented in a regular temporal relation to each other. As a result, responding to the CS is modified – that is, conditioned responses (CRs) are acquired.

To take fear conditioning as a conventional example, the US is a painful stimulus that induces a conglomerate of defensive responses associated with the circa-strike region of the PIC (Fanselow 1994; cf. Figure 6). As a result of Pavlovian fear conditioning, experimental animals show CRs to the CS; that is, they may be said to "fear" the CS. If blood pressure responses are recorded, for example, animals subjected to fear conditioning procedures show elevated blood pressure responses to the CS after it has been repeatedly paired with an aversive US in the form of foot shocks (LeDoux, Sakaguchi, & Reis 1984).

Because the US has been predicted by the CS on a series of training (or acquisition) trials, aspects of the defensive response may be transferred from the US to the CS. For example, conditioned freezing responses may be acquired as a means of staying in the post-encounter area of the PIC, thus avoiding the potentially lethal circa-strike area. If the context does not allow passive avoidance of threat through freezing, then more active avoidance responses may be conditioned to the CS.

The Role of the OR in Conditioning

Formally, Pavlovian conditioning can be defined as any modification in response to the CS that can be attributed to repeated exposures to contingent presentations of the CS and the US. If this definition is accepted, the OR becomes an important potential confounding factor in many conditioning studies. For example, if the CS elicits an SCR or an HR deceleration, how do we know that these responses are attributable to the CS–US contingency? They may just as well be interpreted as ORs to the CS, if the CS is a novel stimulus, or as a dishabituated OR to the CS, if the OR to the CS was habituated in a series of CS-alone trials before the first presentation of the US, which then acted as a dishabituating stimulus. Furthermore, after conditioning a CS is by definition a signal stimulus, which may be expected to produce augmented and slowly habituating ORs to the signal (i.e., the CS). Finally, if we omit the US to examine whether the CS produces a CR, we know from Siddle's (1991) work that an OR to the omitted stimulus should be expected, and whether this OR also should be regarded as a CR is not immediately clear. Thus, in the cases of ORs to novel CSs and dishabituation of the OR owing to the aversive US, the OR perspective may provide an alternative nonassociative account of findings that the investigator hopes to attribute to the associative process of Pavlovian conditioning (see Badia & Defran 1970).

On the other hand, ORs to signal stimuli or to the omitted US are predicated on the formation of some type of association between the CS and the US, and in this sense they can be attributed to conditioning (Öhman 1983).

However, in other senses such responses do not conform to the characteristics expected of CRs. For example, they would show habituation over trials rather than the growth function expected of a CR, and they would show increasing rather than decreasing generalization gradients with increased stimulus change (see Öhman 1971). However, if one takes the view that conditioning is an associative process that can be indexed by many different measures more or less removed from "the" CR (Rescorla 1980), then ORs may be used to index the underlying associative process regardless of its other characteristics. Thus, autonomic responses attributable to conditioning cannot be unequivocally interpreted as reflecting an acquired CR indexing fear, but may in many instances more parsimoniously be understood in terms of orienting. In this perspective, it is important to define operationally and precisely what we mean when we speak about conditioning.

Control Procedures

In essence, "conditioning" means that a response is attributable to conditioning training, that is, to the repeated contingent presentation of the CS and the US. In order to attribute a putative CR to the CS–US contingency, control procedures are necessary (see Prokasy 1977; Rescorla 1967). To infer that a response results from the history of the eliciting stimulus as a predictor of a US, it is necessary to demonstrate that it is stronger than responses produced by similar stimuli lacking such a history. This can be accomplished either through between-subjects or within-subjects comparisons. In the former case, in a *single-cue* conditioning procedure, an experimental group of subjects is given a sequence of trials in which the CS reliably predicts the occurrence of the US. Responses to the CS from this group are then compared with responses to the CS from a control group given noncontingent (unpaired or random) presentation of the CS and the US during the training trials. Only if responding is reliably larger in the experimental than in the control group can the response legitimately be regarded as CRs elicited by the CS. In a within-subjects control procedure, a *differential* conditioning design may be used in which subjects are exposed to two different CSs that initially do not induce different responses. One stimulus (the CS+) is then followed by the US, whereas the other stimulus (the CS−) serves as a control stimulus never presented with the US. If, as training proceeds, subjects start to show larger responses to the CS+ than to the CS−, differential Pavlovian conditioning has been demonstrated. A more thorough discussion of control procedures is given by Öhman (1983) and Rescorla (1967).

CONDITIONING OF AUTONOMIC RESPONSES
Responses to CS Onset

Using these control procedures, reliable conditioning of autonomic responses can be observed, for example, with

aversive USs (for extensive reviews see Davey 1992a; Dawson & Schell 1985; Öhman 1983). Because of the slow recruitment of autonomic responses, it is preferable to use CS–US intervals that permit the separation of responses to CS onset from responses anticipating the US as well as the UR. With CS–US intervals of a second or less, responses to the CS and the US merge into one response, which means that test trials omitting the US must be used in order to assess CRs to the CS. Because US omission constitutes a surprising event, ORs to the omission may be expected (Siddle 1991; Siddle & Lipp 1997), which leads to interpretational hazards (see Öhman 1983).

Autonomic responses early in the CS–US interval may be interpreted as reflecting orienting to the CS as a signal stimulus. It is well documented that SCRs to CS onset reflect conditioning in the sense that they are larger to stimuli that have been associated with USs than to control stimuli. This is particularly clear in data from differential conditioning paradigms using electric shocks or aversive noise as the US, in which responses invariably are larger to CSs+ than to CSs− (Baer & Fuhrer 1968; Furedy 1970; Maltzman et al. 1977; Öhman et al. 1976b; see Öhman 1983 for a review). When conditioning is assessed with a between-subjects control procedure, on the other hand, the results are more variable (cf. Öhman 1971 and Öhman 1974). However, even though SCRs to CS onset are sensitive to the CS–US contingency, they still retain characteristics of an OR. For example, they habituate over trials rather than showing the gradual response acquisition expected for a CR (see Öhman 1983 for review). Furthermore, they show response recovery with stimulus change – and more so the larger the stimulus change – as would be expected for an OR (Öhman 1971). Thus, SCRs to CS onset show the mixed characteristics of ORs to signal and nonsignal stimuli that should be expected from Sokolov's (1963) description.

A similar conclusion has been reached for the early HR deceleration peaking at about 2 sec after CS onset (Bohlin & Kjellberg 1979). Thus, it is clear that modified orienting is an important effect of Pavlovian contingencies (Öhman 1983).

Responses Anticipating the US

If the CS–US interval is extended, multiple autonomic responses can be observed. For example, with a CS–US interval of 6–10 sec, a distinct response to CS onset is often followed by a second (or sometimes third) response later on in the interval, immediately anticipating the US (Prokasy & Ebel 1967). For SCRs, these responses are uniphasic increases in conductance, but with HR responses there is a sequence of deceleration–acceleration–deceleration, exactly as in the interval between a warning and an imperative stimulus of a signaled RT task (Lacey & Lacey 1970; Obrist et al. 1965, 1969).

With SCRs, the response to CS onset and the second-interval anticipatory responses (SARs) are statistically independent (Öhman 1972; Prokasy & Ebel 1967), which suggests that they reflect different processes. The SAR can be attributed reliably to the CS–US contingency both in differential and single-cue paradigms (see review by Öhman 1983). It appears primarily to reflect forward-directed processes that are determined by characteristics not of the CS but rather of the US. Thus, it can be interpreted as a correlate to a separate process of expectancy learning (Öhman 1979, 1983).

Heart rate changes late in the CS–US interval are differentiated into a mid-interval acceleration and a pronounced late deceleration. It is the late deceleration that most clearly differentiates between CSs followed and not followed by the US (Öhman 1983). Bohlin and Kjellberg (1979) concluded that most experimental manipulations shown to affect the accelerative component can be subsumed under the heading of CS significance. On the other hand, the late deceleration appears, as in signaled RT tasks, primarily to reflect an expectancy for the US to occur at the end of the CS–US interval. There are both human (Obrist et al. 1965) and animal (Iwata & LeDoux 1988) pharmacological blockade studies suggesting that the complex sequence of changes of HR in the CS–US interval reflects competing coactivation of chronotropic sympathetic and vagal innervations of the heart.

CONSCIOUS COGNITION AND CONDITIONING
Verbal Awareness of the CS–US Contingency

The repeated presentation of a CS–US contingency has a multitude of effects in different response domains. One of the effects in humans is that research participants become aware of, and thus able to report verbally on, the contingency. Typically, they quickly pick up that the CS predicts the US and develop an expectancy that can be verbally formulated. However, Pavlovian conditioning can be demonstrated in primitive organisms such as earthworms (see Razran 1971 for review). Furthermore, in mammals, fear conditioning does not require that the sensory cortex analyzing the CS be intact, which demonstrates that such conditioning can be achieved by subcortical circuitry (LeDoux 1996). In general, therefore, it is clear that a highly advanced cognitive apparatus incorporating conscious awareness is not required for Pavlovian conditioning in mammals. In an evolutionary perspective, one would expect that verbal awareness of the CS–US contingency is a consequence of, rather than a prerequisite for, human Pavlovian conditioning. But from the perspective of OR theory (Sokolov 1963) one would expect, first, that responses to CS onset would be related to verbal awareness of the CS–US contingency because it is the very awareness that defines the CS as a signal stimulus. Second, one would expect that the conscious discovery of the CS predicting the US would lead immediately to enhanced responding, because it is exactly at this point

that the CS becomes a signal stimulus for the impending US.

It is well documented that reliable effects on the SCR of contingent CS–US presentations occur only in aware subjects (Dawson & Schell 1985). To take one particularly ingenious example, Dawson and colleagues (1979) managed to compare aware and nonaware contingencies on a within-subjects basis. They used compound CSs that included both auditory and visual components in a masking task allegedly designed to measure relationships between the subject's perceptual performance and physiological activity. The shock US was explained as a way of manipulating physiological state, but in order to assess "potential confounding effects of shock expectancy," the participants were asked to continuously monitor their expectancy of shock. One group, the fully informed one, was instructed that shock could be predicted from stimuli in both sensory modalities. Partially informed participants, however, were only instructed that shocks could be predicted from visual stimuli. The validity of the instruction procedure was confirmed in the shock expectancy ratings. After a series of training trials in which the auditory and visual CSs were perfectly correlated, a series of critical test trials were given with the individual visual and auditory components. In agreement with instructions, the partially informed group clearly differentiated the visual CS+ from the CS– in terms of SCRs to CS onsets, whereas they did not differentiate between auditory CSs+ and CSs–. The fully informed subjects, on the other hand, showed reliable differential conditioning to stimuli in both modalities. Similar results were reported for HR data.

Data of the type reported by Dawson et al. (1979) have been taken to justify the conclusion that awareness of the CS–US contingency is a necessary requirement for SCR conditioning (see e.g. Dawson & Furedy 1976; Öhman 1983). However, whether awareness is really a prerequisite for conditioning – or merely indexes an underlying process that determines both expectancy ratings and SCRs – is difficult to decide from the data. According to Öhman's (1979) model, for example, both ORs and expectancy reflect the common mechanism of controlled processing in a resource-limited information processing channel. Furthermore, awareness is not a sufficient condition for conditioning. There are aware subjects that do not show conditioning (Dawson & Biferno 1973; Pendery & Maltzman 1977) and, once the contingency is discovered, the correlation between measures of awareness and differential SCRs is typically low (see review by Dawson & Furedy 1976).

The second prediction from OR theory, that the emergence of differential SCRs to CSs+ and CSs– should coincide in time with the subject's conscious discovery of the CS–US contingency, has also been vindicated by experimental data. Using a task similar to that used by Dawson et al. (1979) in order to conceal the CS+ and

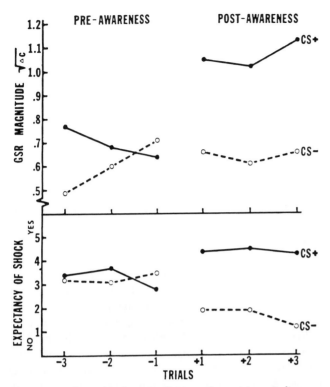

Figure 7. Relationship between (i) research participants' discovery that one conditioned stimulus (the CS+) was consistently followed by the shock unconditioned stimulus (US) whereas another stimulus (the CS−) was not (ratings of "expectancy of shock"; lower panel) and (ii) emergence of differential skin conductance (magnitude of galvanic skin response, GSR; upper panel). As shown in the lower panel, for each research participant, a trial was identified *before* which the subject did not consistently differentiate between the CS+ and the CS− in expectancy but *after* which he did. This shift from nonawareness to awareness of the CS–US contingency was temporally synchronized with the emergence of differential psychophysiological responding. Reprinted with permission from Dawson & Biferno, "Concurrent measurement of awareness and electrodermal classical conditioning," *Journal of Experimental Psychology*, vol. 101, pp. 55–62. Copyright © 1973 by the American Psychological Association.

the CS− and their relationship to the US, Dawson and Biferno (1973) demonstrated that reliable SCR differentiation between the CS+ and the CS− occurred only *after* the trial on which the subjects discovered that the CS+ predicted the US. These results are shown in Figure 7. Similar data were subsequently reported by Öhman, Ellström, and Björkstrand (1976a), Biferno and Dawson (1977), and Pendery and Maltzman (1977). Results of this type have led to the wide acceptance that conscious cognition plays a central part in human conditioning (Davey 1992a; Dawson & Schell 1985; Lovibond 1993; Öhman 1983) and that the data can be understood in terms of OR theory (Dawson & Schell 1985; Öhman 1979, 1983).

Limits of Conscious Cognition

Fear-Relevant CSs. The ubiquitous relationship between conscious cognition and human autonomic conditioning

has been challenged by data on the effects of biologically fear-relevant CSs on human conditioning (reviewed by Öhman 1993b). These data showed that the use of CSs of potentially phobic content – such as snakes and spiders (Öhman et al. 1976b) or angry faces (Öhman & Dimberg 1978; see review by Dimberg & Öhman 1996) – resulted in conditioned SCRs that were much more resistant to extinction (i.e., they persisted even when the US was omitted) than were SCRs conditioned to more neutral stimulus material. This effect was repeatedly reported from Öhman's laboratory (see review by Öhman 1993b) and has subsequently been replicated elsewhere (e.g. Cook, Hodes, & Lang 1986; Davey 1992b; Dawson, Schell, & Banis 1986; Pitman & Orr 1990; Schell, Dawson, & Marinkovic 1991).

A study by Hugdahl and Öhman (1977) (later replicated by Soares & Öhman 1993b) suggested that SCRs conditioned to pictures of snakes and spiders were less related to conscious cognition than were SCRs conditioned to neutral stimuli. Their results suggested that instructing the subjects that no more USs would be presented (verified by the removal of shock electrodes) immediately removed differential SCR responding to neutral stimuli but left conditioned SCRs to potentially phobic CSs virtually unaffected. Thus, it could be argued that subjects conditioned to fear-relevant stimuli showed autonomic responses that were contrary to expectancies.

Again using a complex conditioning paradigm (cf. Dawson & Biferno 1973), Dawson and associates (1986) asked their subjects continuously to rate their US expectancy to potentially phobic and neutral stimuli, some of which predicted the shock US. The researchers reported that the enhanced resistance of extinction of SCRs in subjects conditioned to snakes or spiders was correlated with differences in rated shock expectancies, because shock expectancies were also slower to extinguish to snakes and spiders than to flowers and mushrooms. Furthermore, once the expectancies were extinguished, no more differential SCRs to the CS+ and the CS− were observed. Similarly, Davey (1992b) replicated Hugdahl and Öhman's (1977) finding that SCRs withstood instructions about US omission after conditioning to fear-relevant stimuli. However, Davey (1992b) also reported that the subjects continued to expect the US after the fear-relevant CS+ (according to expectancy ratings), in direct contradiction to the instruction they had received. These two studies (Davey 1992b; Dawson et al. 1986) suggest that conscious cognition as revealed in expectancy ratings is as important in conditioning to fear-relevant stimuli as previously reported for conditioning to neutral stimuli (e.g. Dawson & Schell 1985). However, Schell et al. (1991) later reported continued SCR differential responding after expectancy extinction in subjects conditioned with a shorter CS–US interval (1 sec) than that used in most previous studies (8 sec). Thus, even though the subjects – according to their own expectancy ratings – no longer expected the US after the CS+, they nevertheless showed reliable differential responding between the CS+ and the CS− in their SCRs. Hence there may be one component of the conditioned SCR that reflects a conditioning process distinct from orienting and conscious conditioning.

Masking Studies. Further support for the notion of a conditioned SCR component that cannot be reduced to simple US expectancy comes from conditioning studies using masked stimuli (see Öhman 1996 for review). "Backward masking" is a procedure used to disrupt processing of a target stimulus by an immediately following masking stimulus. When the stimulus–onset asynchrony (SOA) between the target stimulus and the mask is short (about 30 msec), conscious recognition of target facial (Esteves & Öhman 1993) and small animal (snakes and spiders; Öhman & Soares 1993) pictorial stimuli is effectively prevented. See Öhman (1999) for a discussion of the conceptual and methodological implications of perceptual masking.

Öhman and Soares (1993) tested the hypothesis that SCRs conditioned to fear-relevant stimuli (snakes, spiders) could be elicited in response to masked exemplars of the CSs. In support of this hypothesis, they demonstrated that subjects conditioned to the fear-relevant stimuli (i.e., snakes or spiders) showed continued differential responding during the masked extinction trials, whereas no differential responding was observed in subjects conditioned and tested with the masked neutral (i.e., flower and mushroom) stimuli. Thus, in spite of the fact that conscious recognition of the stimuli could be excluded, the subjects nevertheless demonstrated differential SCRs to them as long as their content was fear-relevant. Similar data were reported by Soares and Öhman (1993a,b) and, using angry faces as the fear-relevant stimulus and neutral faces as masks, by Esteves, Dimberg, and Öhman (1994a) and Parra et al. (1997). Furthermore, Öhman and Soares (1994) selected subjects who were fearful of either snakes or spiders and demonstrated differential SCRs to masked presentations of feared and nonfeared stimuli. Thus, stimuli that are emotionally relevant – either through conditioning in the laboratory or because of real-life history – can elicit SCRs even when complete processing is disrupted by masking.

The data so far demonstrate that conditioned autonomic responses can be elicited by masked stimuli. This implies that CRs can be performed without awareness of the eliciting stimulus. However, that they can be nonconsciously performed does not entail that they are nonconsciously learned. To examine whether responses can be conditioned to masked stimuli, Esteves et al. (1994b) exposed normal subjects to effectively masked pictures of angry and happy faces. For some of the subjects, the masked angry face (the CS+) was followed by an electric shock US but a masked happy face (the CS−) was not, whereas other subjects experienced the reversed contingency (i.e., shock following masked happy faces). Different control subjects were given conditioning training to ineffectively masked stimuli, al-

lowing their conscious recognition, or were given random presentation of masked facial stimuli and the shock US. After the masked conditioning (or random presentation of the CS and the US) phase, the masks were removed in an extinction phase and SCRs were measured to nonmasked angry and happy faces. The results showed that conditioning could be obtained to masked stimuli provided that the target stimulus was fear-relevant (i.e., an angry face). Subjects who were conditioned to masked happy faces or were given random presentations of masked faces and the US did not show differential SCRs to angry and happy faces. These data demonstrate that SCRs can be conditioned to fear-relevant stimuli presented outside of awareness, which suggests that conscious awareness of the CS–US contingency is not a necessary requirement for human autonomic conditioning.

Conditioning to masked stimuli was replicated by Öhman and Soares (1998) using snakes and spiders, rather than angry faces, as fear-relevant stimuli. In a second experiment, subjects rated shock as significantly more likely following the masked CS+ than following the masked CS−, even though they were unable to recognize the stimuli. Post hoc analyses revealed that subjects who were unable to differentiate consistently between the CS+ and the CS− in their ratings nevertheless showed reliable differential SCRs. Similarly, when trials were compared in which the subjects expected or did not expect shock, reliable SCR differentiation between the CS+ and the CS− was observed both for trials when shock was expected and when it was not expected. It thus appears that, with masked stimuli, the shock expectancy ratings and the SCRs were essentially orthogonal to each other, which severely discredits any notion that conditioned SCRs were driven by differential expectancies. Thus, we are left with the evidence that there is a component of the conditioned SCR that cannot be reduced to expectancies or understood in terms of orienting. Given that this component is most clearly seen with fear-relevant CSs and aversive USs, it is tempting to conclude that it reflects the conditioning of a genuine fear response. Investigators have just started to delineate the central nervous system mechanisms involved in conditioned fear. Before returning to peripheral conditioned autonomic responses in humans, we digress to the topic of neural mechanisms of conditioned fear as revealed by animal experimentation.

FEAR CONDITIONING AND MODIFICATION OF THE CENTRAL FEAR NEURAL NETWORK

The crucial feature of fear conditioning is the use of aversive, defense-related USs that activate neural pathways in subcortical aversive motivational systems which then prime defensive behavior to the level of primitive reflexes (Konorski 1967; LeDoux 1990). The fact that it signals such an aversive event makes the CS itself aversive, gaining the ability to activate the same affective network as the US. Studying a simple defensive reflex, the startle reflex (SR), Davis and his co-workers elucidated the efferent link of this fear network in the brain (for reviews, see Davis 1992, 1997).

Fear and Potentiated Startle

In its full expression, the SR is a cranial-to-caudal spreading wave of flexor movements along the neural axis that is elicitable by any abruptly occurring sensory stimulus (Landis & Hunt 1939). In contrast to the blink component of the SR typically used in human studies (e.g. Graham 1975; Lang et al. 1997b), the "whole body" startle response – measured as cage floor displacement – is most often used in studies with rodents as subjects (e.g. Brown, Kalish, & Farber 1951; Davis 1984).

In the pioneering study, Brown et al. (1951) used a light–tone compound stimulus as the CS and foot shock as the US. When startle probes (pistol shots) were presented in the presence of the cue that had previously been paired with shock, animals responded with significant potentiation of the whole body SR compared to when SRs were elicited without the CS. This phenomenon has been termed the *fear-potentiated startle effect* and can be routinely demonstrated in animal fear conditioning experiments (e.g. Berg & Davis 1984; Davis & Astrachan 1978; Kurtz & Siegel 1966; see reviews by Davis 1992, 1997).

Pharmacological studies confirm that SR potentiation reflects the acquisition of a central fear state. Substances that have anxiolytic effects in humans (e.g. diazepam; see review by Davis 1992) also reduce fear-induced potentiation of the SR in rats (Berg & Davis 1984; Davis 1979) and humans (Patrick, Berthot, & Moore 1996). In contrast, substances that induce fear in nonanxious persons and that increase symptoms in anxiety patients (e.g. yohimbine) lead to significant SR potentiation in animals (Davis, Redmond, & Baraban 1979). These pharmacological effects are fear-specific because there is no influence on SRs elicited in the absence of a CS. Alcohol, on the other hand, dampens the overall startle reactivity without influencing fear-potentiated SRs (Stritzke, Patrick, & Lang 1995).

Neural Pathways for the Fear-Potentiated Startle

The primary acoustic startle pathway in rodents consists only of three synapses (Davis 1997). When the ear is stimulated by a startle probe, the afferent volley travels to the cochlear root neurons (CRNs), a small group of very large cells embedded in the auditory nerve (Lopez et al. 1993), and then proceeds to the nucleus reticularis pontis caudalis (PnC), the sensorimotor interface in the brainstem. Efferent projections pass from the PnC through the facial motor nucleus (pinna and blink reflex) or spinal cord (whole body startle) to the reflex effectors (Davis 1997). This is the basic obligatory reflex pathway directly driven by the characteristics of the stimulus input (rise time, intensity, frequency, etc.).

The phenomenon of SR potentiation during fear conditioning suggests the existence of an additional, modulatory circuit. Microstimulation of the afferent branch of the obligatory pathway (i.e., prior to the PnC) results in potentiation of the SR during fear (i.e., in the presence of the CS). Electrical stimulation of the efferent branch (i.e., beyond the PnC) does not lead to fear-induced potentiation of the SR (Berg & Davis 1985). The modulating influence of an aversive CS thus appears to be at the PnC. The critical structure of the modulatory circuit is the amygdala, whose central nucleus projects directly to the PnC (Rosen et al. 1991). Accordingly, lesions of the central nucleus of the amygdala, as well as of its efferents to PnC, block the expression of the fear-potentiated SR (Hitchcock & Davis 1991).

Amygdala and the Efferent Organization of Fear

In rabbits, lateral cerebellar lesions (e.g., in the interpositus nucleus) completely block learning and performance of conditioned skeletal responses (e.g., the nictitating membrane response; see review by Thompson 1986) but do not affect the conditioned-fear bradycardia associated with the prototypical behavioral response of rabbits to threat – tonic immobility (Lavond et al. 1984; for an overview see Lavond, Kim, & Thompson 1993). In rats, such lesions do not affect the fear-potentiated SR (Hitchcock & Davis 1986). This points to a dissociation between the brain networks involved in learning and performance of specific motor CRs (see Thompson 1986) and other networks modulating the nonspecific emotional part of fear conditioning, such as startle potentiation and autonomic changes.

The amygdala is the key structure in this latter network. For example, electrical stimulation of the amygdala produces fear-typical behavior (e.g., freezing or passive avoidance) in many animals (Applegate et al. 1983), including humans (Gloor 1992). Furthermore, efferent fibers from the central nucleus of the amygdala project to various regions in the brainstem that are involved in the expression of fear behavior. Thus, electric stimulation of this nucleus produces typical cardiovascular changes (e.g., elevated blood pressure) and increases in SR amplitude (Rosen & Davis 1988).

Lesion experiments have provided evidence that conditioned cardiovascular changes (increase in blood pressure, or bradycardia in rabbits) are regulated in the lateral regions of the hypothalamus that receive projections from the central amygdala (Kapp et al. 1990; LeDoux 1993). It is interesting to note that lesions of the anterior cerebellar vermis, a part of the cerebellum that receives direct projections from the hypothalamus, also disrupted fear bradycardia in rabbits (Supple & Kapp 1993). However, lesions in this region have no influence on somatic components

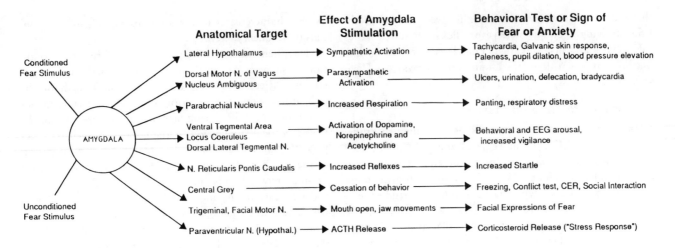

Figure 8. Schematic diagram showing the efferent outflow from the central nucleus of the amygdala to target areas in the midbrain and brainstem. These target areas control physiological systems, the measurable outputs of which are frequently used in animal studies as indicators of fear and anxiety. From Davis, "The role of the amygdala in conditioned fear," in Aggleton (Ed.), *The Amygdala: Neurobiological Aspects of Emotion, Memory, and Mental Dysfunction,* pp. 255–306. Copyright © 1992. Reprinted by permission of Wiley-Liss, Inc., a subsidiary of John Wiley & Sons, Inc.

of the conditioned fear response (freezing). Lesions in another area also receiving fibers from the central nucleus of the amygdala – the ventral central gray of the brainstem – interfere with motor freezing even as conditioned blood pressure responses remain intact (LeDoux et al. 1988). The dorsal gray, on the other hand, is a critical part of the flight-or-fight action circuit (Fanselow 1994). This efferent organization of the fear response is illustrated in Figure 8.

Figure 8 has important implications for the psychophysiologist. It implies that there are hierarchically organized central networks that tie together structures controlling various response outputs. These structures, however, may also have inputs from and output to other networks. For example, cardiovascular responses are recruited by the fear network via nuclei in the lateral hypothalamus and the brainstem. These latter nuclei, however, may also be recruited as parts of other networks and may be susceptible, moreover, to internal constraints of the cardiovascular system (e.g., the baroreceptor control mechanism) working to keep blood pressure within preset limits. Therefore, it is not surprising that the control of cardiovascular responses can be dissociated depending on situational circumstances, only some of which will engage the brain's fear system. Potentiation of the SR, on the other hand, may provide a relatively unequivocal index of amygdala activation.

The Afferent Link of the Central Fear Network

So far we have sketched the downstream organization of the fear response from the central nucleus of the amyg-

dala. But how is the amygdala accessed by fear stimuli, and where is the learning of fear located? LeDoux (1996) proposed answers to these questions in a model of fear learning. His primary data come from a fear conditioning paradigm with auditory CSs and a painful electric shock to the paw as the US, using increases in arterial blood pressure and behavioral freezing as indicators of learned fear. The task LeDoux (1990, 1992, 1996) set himself was to trace the neural circuitry that transferred information from the CS to the CR. By a variety of methods (reviewed by LeDoux 1996), he and his colleagues have been able to specify the afferent pathways of the neural network that encodes emotional information in the amygdala to make contact with the efferent system previously discussed (Figure 8).

Key evidence was provided by the finding that fear CRs to auditory CSs remained intact in spite of complete lesioning of the auditory cortex, which suggested that the amygdala could be activated by only rudimentarily processed CSs. With anatomical tracing techniques, LeDoux and his colleagues discovered that there are direct axonal connections from thalamic regions (the medial geniculate body and the intralaminar nucleus) to the lateral nucleus of the amygdala (LeDoux, Farb, & Ruggiero 1990b; LeDoux, Ruggiero, & Reis 1985). Lesioning of the lateral nucleus of the amygdala led to an immediate loss of fear conditioning (LeDoux et al. 1990a). The lateral nucleus of the amygdala appears to analyze affective characteristics of inputs and to integrate subcortically mediated sensory information with input from the cortex (LeDoux 1992, 1996). Thus, "thalamic inputs to the amygdala allow sensory signals to activate it either before or simultaneous with the arrival of signals at the cortical level, and may therefore play an important role in preconscious and precognitive emotional processing" (LeDoux 1992, p. 192).

From the lateral nucleus, information is conveyed to basolateral nuclei of the amygdala and then on to the central nucleus, which activates neural output indexing fear, such as cardiovascular and skeletal responses (Davis 1992;

LeDoux 1992). The central nucleus of the amygdala also regulates the state of arousal of the neocortex, as revealed by EEG desynchronization (Kapp et al. 1992). This amygdala–cortical link "may allow emotional information processing by the amygdala (particularly by the lateral-basolateral-central connection) to influence perceptual, attentional, memory, and other cognitive processes mediated at the neocortical level" (LeDoux 1992, p. 194). More recent work from LeDoux's laboratory (Rogan, Stäubli, & LeDoux 1997) investigated the cellular mechanisms of fear learning in the amygdala and confirmed the central role of this structure in the learning of fear. The complete LeDoux model is illustrated in Figure 9.

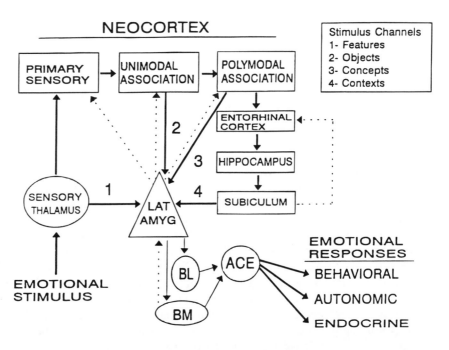

Figure 9. Schematic outline of LeDoux's (1990, 1992, 1995, 1996) fear network emphasizing the central role of the amygdala in fear conditioning. Emotional stimuli are processed through sensory pathways reaching the thalamus, where the sensory information bifurcates. One stream (1) conveys isolated features of the stimulus directly to the lateral nucleus of the amygdala (LAT AMYG), whereas the other stream continues to sensory cortices and then on to association cortices, building representations of objects in relation to concepts and embedded in a specific context. This latter stream sends collateral information to the lateral amygdala at several levels of processing (2, 3, 4). The lateral amygdala tunes these cortical areas on the basis of the already acquired information (dotted arrows). From the lateral nucleus of the amygdala, information is conveyed to the central nucleus of the amygdala (ACE) via the basolateral (BL) and basomedial (BM) nuclei. The central amygdala then activates regions in the midbrain and brainstem controlling emotional output (cf. Figure 8). Reprinted with permission from Gazzaniga (Ed.), *The Cognitive Neurosciences*. Copyright 1995 The MIT Press.

CONDITIONED FEAR IN HUMANS
Role of the Amygdala in Human Fear Conditioning

LeDoux's (1996) work suggests that the learning of fear is accomplished in a neuronal network of the brain, which is centered on the amygdala and can be accessed by sensory stimuli after only minimal processing. This system generates emotional outputs by activating various defense systems with associated autonomic support, and it results in the storage of emotional memories. It is independent of another network, which is centered on the hippocampus and is the substrate of cognitive memories (LeDoux 1996). Thus, if there are similar systems operating in the human brain, one would expect that emotional conditioning is independent of conscious awareness of the stimuli. However, as we have seen in the review of human conditioning studies, conscious cognition appears to play a major role in the conditioning of human autonomic responses, and there is only limited evidence for the conditioning of more primitive emotional responses that could be attributed to the amygdala network.

Nonetheless, support for the critical involvement of the amygdala in human conditioning can be recruited from studies of brain-damaged patients. Bechara et al. (1995) reported that a patient with specific bilateral lesions of the amygdala did not acquire conditioned SCRs in aversive conditioning paradigms even though she did acquire factual knowledge about the conditioning contingency (i.e., she could report the relationship between the various CSs and the US). A patient with bilateral hippocampal damage, on the other hand, failed to provide evidence of learning the contingency at the cognitive level but did acquire con-

ditioned SCRs. Furthermore, LaBar and associates (1995) examined 22 patients who had undergone unilateral removal of the amygdala to control epileptical seizures. They reported impaired SCR conditioning in patients as compared to normal controls, even though patients showed comparable UR magnitudes to those of controls. Furthermore, the overwhelming majority of them were able correctly to report the CS–US contingency. In concert, these two studies support the view that the amygdala is critical for human aversive conditioning.

Nonconscious Fear Conditioning in Humans

If it is assumed that backward masking disrupts cortical processing of visual stimuli at a relatively early stage – before the result is available to consciousness – then LeDoux's (1996) model provides a way of accounting for the masking data reported from Öhman's laboratory (e.g. Öhman 1996).

First, that conditioned SCRs to fear-relevant stimuli (Esteves et al. 1994a; Öhman & Soares 1993) and to fear-related SCRs in fearful subjects (Öhman & Soares 1994) can be elicited by masked stimuli could be explained by collateral neural information to the amygdala from early stages of cortical (and even thalamic) processing of visual stimuli. Thus, even though processing is disrupted before stimuli are consciously recognized, the amygdala – via its access to the result of preliminary analyses – can activate autonomic responses through efference to the lateral hypothalamus and the brainstem.

Second, because fear conditioning is possible in the absence of cortical processing (LeDoux et al. 1984), masked stimuli can serve as effective CSs for aversive USs (Esteves et al. 1994b; Öhman & Soares 1998). Furthermore, the data presented by Öhman and Soares (1998) suggested that nonconscious conditioning was accompanied by some level of awareness of the CS–US contingency as expressed in expectancy ratings. However, SCR conditioning and expectancy learning were orthogonal to each other, as would be expected if they reflected the operation of two different brain systems: one for fear learning and the other for explicit learning of the stimulus contingency.

To directly test whether the amygdala is involved in the generation of conditioned SCRs, Morris, Öhman, and Dolan (1998) used a positron emission tomograph (PET) scanner for measurement of regional cerebral blood flow. They conditioned subjects to one of two angry faces by having it followed by an aversive noise; they then presented extinction trials with these stimuli masked or nonmasked and with the subject placed in the scanner. Contrasts between the CSs+ and the CSs− revealed that the differential brain response to these two stimuli specifically pertained to activation of the amygdala when the CSs+ were presented. The masking factor interacted with laterality. Masked CSs+ specifically activated the right amygdala and nonmasked CSs+ specifically activated the left amygdala. It is striking that the nonmasked stimuli activated the left (verbal) hemisphere whereas the effects of masked CSs were specific to the right (nonverbal) hemisphere. Further support for a role of the amygdala in human fear conditioning was reported by Furmark and colleagues (1997). Using snakes or spiders as CSs and electric shock as the US, they reported a strong correlation between SCRs during presentations of the CS in the PET scanner and conditioned regional cerebral bloodflow in the right amygdala.

The importance of the right hemisphere for human fear conditioning is supported by consistent findings from a series of experiments (Hugdahl & Johnsen 1993; Johnsen & Hugdahl 1991, 1993) using the visual half-field (VHF) technique to assure activation of each hemisphere separately (see McKeever 1986). With this technique, short-duration stimuli are presented either to the left or the right of a fixation point. Because of the incomplete crossing of the visual nerves at the optic chiasma, stimuli falling in the left visual field go initially to the right cerebral hemisphere whereas those in the right visual field go to the left hemisphere. Of most relevance for the present discussion was an experiment by Öhman and co-workers (1988) in which the VHF and masking techniques were combined to present previously conditioned facial stimuli to the left or right hemisphere unbeknown to the participants. Consistent with the PET data reported by Morris et al. (1998), they found reliable differential SCR responses to masked CSs+ and CSs− when the stimuli were presented in the left but not in the right visual half-field – that is, only when the masked CSs were processed by the right hemisphere. The important role of the right hemisphere for human conditioning was further demonstrated in a PET study reported by Hugdahl et al. (1995; see also Hugdahl 1998).

In concert, the neuropsychological, masking, VHF, and PET data present a good case that the amygdala – and particularly the right amygdala – is critically involved in human aversive conditioning, as would be expected from the animal literature. That the masking data on human aversive conditioning were clear-cut only for fear-relevant stimuli (e.g., angry faces or fearsome animals) is consistent with the "preparedness" hypothesis (Seligman 1970, 1971), which suggests that fear conditioning is particularly effective to evolutionarily prepared stimuli. Thus, the hypothesis postulates that stimuli that have provided recurrent survival threats during the evolutionary history of humankind have acquired a genetically based prepotency to enter easily into association with traumatic events. In LeDoux's words, "perhaps neurons in the amygdala that process prepared stimuli have some prewired but normally impotent connections to other cells that control emotional responses. The trauma might only have to mildly massage these pathways rather than create from scratch novel synaptic assemblages between the input and output neurons of the amygdala" (1996, p. 254).

Toward a Two-Level Account of Human Conditioning

Before the wide acceptance of the notion that human autonomic conditioning could be fully accounted for in terms of expectancies (Davey 1992a; Dawson 1973; Dawson & Schell 1985; Lovibond 1993), notions of two levels of learning – one automatic and emotional and the other conscious and cognitive – were quite popular among human autonomic conditioners (Bridger & Mandel 1964; Mandel & Bridger 1973; Razran 1971). For example, Bridger and Mandel (1964) interpreted their findings that instructed extinction was less effective after conditioning to a strong than to a weak US as suggesting that the former condition resulted in a stronger conditioned emotional response resisting the instruction.

Even though notions of expectancy learning have been dominating the field, there have been occasional reports suggesting that more than expectancy is involved in at least some experimental paradigms in which a relatively neutral cue is made contingent on an aversive event. For example, with spider or mutilation slides as USs and subjects selected for fear of spiders and mutilation, Hare and Blevings (1975a) and Klorman and Ryan (1980) found strong accelerative HRRs to tones signaling feared but not to tones signaling neutral material.

An experiment by Hugdahl et al. (1983) suggested that such HR acceleration in anticipation of neutral or emotionally relevant visual stimuli may be controlled from the right cerebral hemisphere. They recorded heart rate change in anticipation of and in response to lateralized visual stimuli presented by a slide projector. The slide stimuli were presented for 200 msec either to the left or right of the fixation point by means of the VHF technique. The fixation point went on 5 sec prior to the slide stimuli. Across three experiments, Hugdahl et al. (1983) reported deceleratory HRRs to the slides, irrespective of which half-field was stimulated. However, HR accelerated in anticipation of stimuli presented in the left visual field (right-hemisphere processing) whereas it decelerated in anticipation of right visual field stimulation (left-hemisphere processing); see Figure 10.

Studying classical conditioning in normal subjects, Cook et al. (1986) reported that pairing fear-relevant stimuli (snakes and spiders) with aversive events (aversive noises or electric shocks) resulted in a reliable conditioned HR acceleration that peaked at about 3 sec after the CS, with the subsequent secondary deceleration hardly reaching below the level achieved by the CS−. This was in marked contrast to conditioning to neutral stimuli, in which the secondary deceleration was the clearly dominant event indexing conditioning. Similar data were reported by Öhman et al. (1985). Finally, Dimberg (1987) found that angry faces paired with shock resulted not only in conditioned SCRs but also in an acceleratory HRR and in a conditioned increase in activity of the corrugator muscle controlling the frowning eyebrow. This pattern clearly suggests the conditioning of a defensive response rather than mere modulation of orienting behavior.

Hodes, Cook, and Lang (1985) used an individual differences approach and examined whether subjects showing HR accelerations before aversive conditioning to snakes and spiders, later to be used as CSs, would also be more prone to show acceleratory conditioned HRRs. This proved to be the case. Furthermore, such subjects showed larger resistance to extinction of the conditioned SCR and also rated the slides as more aversive after conditioning than before. Thus, these subjects appeared to have acquired a defensive response that included a change in the valence of the stimulus. Subjects showing conditioned HR decelerations, on the other hand, showed rapid SCR extinction and no conditioned changes in the valence of the stimuli. Hence, for these subjects, the conditioning contingency appeared to result merely in expectancy changes.

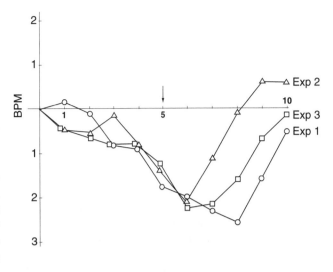

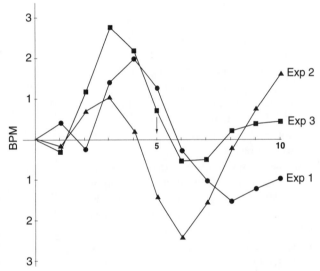

Figure 10. Second-by-second changes in heart rate (in beats per minute, bpm) after the appearance of a fixation point informing the participants that a neutral or emotional slide will be briefly presented (200 msec) after 5 sec (arrow on the abscissa) either to the right (upper panel) or the left (lower panel) visual half-field. Across three independent experiments (Exps 1–3), the participants showed heart rate deceleration in anticipation of slides in the right visual half-field (left-hemisphere processing) and heart rate acceleration in anticipation of slides presented in the left visual field (right-hemisphere processing). Redrawn with permission from Hugdahl, Franzon, Andersson, & Walldebo, "Heart-rate responses (HRR) to lateralized visual stimuli," *Pavlovian Journal of Biological Science*, vol. 18, pp. 186–98. Copyright 1983.

The role of expectancy learning and the patterning of defensive responses during aversive conditioning was further clarified by Hamm and Vaitl (1996). They reported reliable SCR conditioning with both aversive and nonaversive USs (electric shock and a RT task, respectively), with minimal differences as a function of the US condition. Furthermore, with both USs (and consistent with previous findings; see reviews by Dawson & Schell 1985; Öhman 1983), only subjects who were able correctly to identify which stimuli served as the CS+ showed reliable SCR conditioning.

However, in contrast to most previous conditioning studies (but see Hamm et al. 1993; Lipp, Sheridan, & Siddle 1994), Hamm and Vaitl (1996) also measured conditioned modulation of the SR, which (as argued previously) provides a direct index of amygdala involvement in the underlying fear state. Whereas SR magnitudes to probes presented during the CS− did not differ from those presented during the intertrial interval, those to probes presented during the CS+ were clearly enhanced – but only if the US was an aversive event. With the nonaversive RT task US, no startle enhancement was observed. Furthermore, with startle modulation as the dependent variable, there was no relationship between contingency awareness and conditioning. Rather, conditioning was as obvious in subjects failing consciously to pick up the contingency as in those correctly reporting the contingency. These data are shown in Figure 11, which reveals the clear-cut dissociation between the SCR and SR measures.

Finally, Hamm and Vaitl's (1996) data indicated that subjects showing conditioned HR accelerations also showed conditioned modulation of the SR. Those showing conditioned HR decelerations, on the other hand, did not evidence any modulation of the SR to probes presented during the CS+. Thus, from these data it appears that conditioned SR modulation and HR acceleration both index the conditioning of a defensive response, presumably with a neural origin in the amygdala. Conditioned SCRs and HR decelerations, on the other hand, appear to be related to consciously accessible expectancies of the US to follow the CS, with a minimal role for aversiveness and with little modification of the perceived valence of the CS+ (Hodes et al. 1985).

Thus, two types of learning seem to result from the application of a Pavlovian contingency to human subjects. First, they learn that the CS and the US are associated in time. This learning does not require an aversive US (Hamm & Vaitl 1996; Öhman 1974; Siddle 1991); it is consciously mediated (as revealed by verbal reports); and it results in the modification of responses related to the OR, such as SCRs and HR decelerations to signal stimuli. This type of learning can be accounted for in terms of OR theory (Dawson & Schell 1985; Öhman 1979, 1983). Second, an aversive US – particularly if combined with a fear-relevant CS – results in the acquisition of conditioned defense responses involving enhanced SR, HR acceleration, and

Figure 11. Upper panel shows startle responses (standardized mean blink magnitude) to probe stimuli presented during visual stimuli (CS+) predicting the electric shock (aversive) and the imperative stimulus in a reaction time task (nonaversive) unconditioned stimulus (UCS), and to other visual stimuli (CS−) not predicting the UCS, as well as to probes presented during the intertrial intervals (ITI). The lower panel shows skin conductance responses from the same experiment. In both panels the participants have been grouped according to whether or not they could state (in a post-experiment interview) which visual stimulus predicted the UCS (aware and unaware subgroups). Note in the lower panel that skin conductance responses primarily reflect awareness of the CS–UCS relationship; that is, only aware participants showed differential response to the CS+ and the CS−, regardless of the aversiveness of the UCS. According to the upper panel, however, startle response modulation primarily reflects aversiveness of the UCS. That is, startle responses were larger to the CS+ than to the CS− only with the aversive UCS and irrespective of whether or not the participants were aware of the CS–UCS relationship. In other words, the startle response appeared to reflect fear learning and the skin conductance response the cognitive learning of the CS–UCS contingency. Reprinted with permission from Hamm & Vaitl, "Affective learning: Awareness and aversion," *Psychophysiology,* vol. 33, pp. 698–710. Copyright 1996 Cambridge University Press.

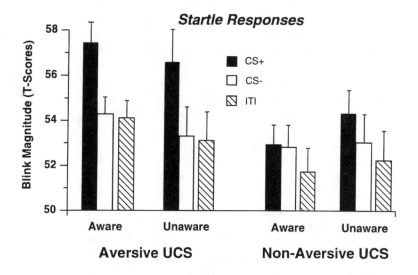

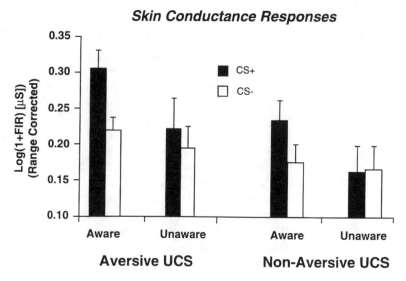

also enhanced SCRs. This conditioned defense response most likely reflects modification of a primitive fear network centered on the amygdala and perhaps lateralized to the right cerebral hemisphere (Hugdahl 1995). It does not require conscious awareness of the CS–US contingency, but it does achieve a modification in the perceived valence of the CS as revealed by ratings (Hodes et al. 1985). Thus, it is appropriate to think of human autonomic conditioning as occurring at two levels: one more primitive and inaccessible to conscious cognition, the other more advanced and cognitively governed.

Concluding Comments

This chapter started with considerations of the evolutionary origin of mind–body integration, and it has taken us through a review of autonomic responses to simple stimuli – in both orienting and conditioning paradigms – to considerations of underlying brain mechanisms. Thus, with evolutionary biology and neural science as cardinal points, this exposé has put psychophysiological data firmly within a biological framework. This is important: Even though psychophysiology has one foot in psychological discourse, it is also embedded among the biological disciplines. In fact, because biology is the science of life, it could be argued that psychology as a whole belongs within the biological sciences. Surely we are trying to understand living creatures. With the advent of evolutionary psychology (e.g. Tooby & Cosmides 1992), there is, indeed, a conceptual framework being developed with the explicit aim of framing psychology in a biological context. Whatever the fate of this larger enterprise, the content of this chapter has shown that the time may be right for more explicitly integrating traditional psychophysiology with the knowledge about the brain generated in contemporary neural science. That we can now understand, for example, important parts of the literature on human fear conditioning in terms of neural systems is a remarkable advance in our understanding. This integration of our discipline with neural science is a promising beginning. Almost certainly, it is a factor that will shape its further destiny.

REFERENCES

Applegate, C. D., Kapp, B. S., Underwood, M. D., & McNall, C. L. (1983). Autonomic and somatomotor effects of the amygdala central n. stimulation in awake rabbits. *Physiology and Behavior, 31,* 353–60.

Badia, P., & Defran, R. H. (1970). Orienting responses and GSR conditioning: A dilemma. *Psychological Review, 77,* 171–81.

Baer, P. E., & Fuhrer, M. J. (1968). Cognitive processes during differential trace and delayed conditioning of the GSR. *Journal of Experimental Psychology, 78,* 81–8.

Beatty, J. (1982). Task-evoked pupillary responses, processing load, and the structure of processing resources. *Psychological Bulletin, 91,* 276–92.

Bechara, A., Tranel, D., Damasio, H., Adolphs, R., Rockland, C., & Damasio, A. R. (1995). Double dissociation of conditioning and declarative knowledge relative to the amygdala and hippocampus in humans. *Science, 269,* 1115–18.

Ben-Shakhar, G. (1994). The roles of stimulus novelty and significance in determining the electrodermal orienting response: Interactive versus additive approaches. *Psychophysiology, 31,* 402–11.

Berg, W. K., & Davis, M. (1984). Diazepam blocks fear-enhanced startle elicited electrically from the brainstem. *Physiology and Behavior, 32,* 333–6.

Berg, W. K., & Davis, M. (1985). Associative learning modifies startle reflexes at the lateral lemniscus. *Behavioral Neuroscience, 99,* 191–9.

Berggren, T., Öhman, A., & Fredrikson, M. (1977). Locus of control and habituation of the electrodermal orienting response to non-signal and signal stimuli. *Journal of Personality and Social Psychology, 35,* 708–16.

Bernstein, A. S. (1981). The orienting response and stimulus significance: Further comments. *Biological Psychology, 12,* 171–85.

Bernstein, A. S., & Taylor, K. W. (1979). The interaction of stimulus information with potential stimulus significance in eliciting the skin conductance orienting response. In Kimmel et al., pp. 499–520.

Berntson, G. G., & Boysen, S. T. (1989). Specificity of the cardiac response to conspecific vocalization in the chimpanzee. *Behavioral Neuroscience, 103,* 235–45.

Berntson, G. G., Boysen, S. T., & Cacioppo, J. T. (1992). Cardiac orienting and defensive responses: Potential origins of autonomic space. In Campbell et al., pp. 163–200.

Berntson, G. G., Cacioppo, J. T., Binkley, P. F., Uchino, B. N., Quigley, K. S., & Fieldstone, A. (1994a). Autonomic cardiac control. III. Psychological stress and cardiac response in autonomic space as revealed by pharmacological blockades. *Psychophysiology, 31,* 599–608.

Berntson, G. G., Cacioppo, J. T., & Quigley, K. S. (1991). Autonomic determinism: The modes of autonomic control, the doctrine of autonomic space, and the laws of autonomic constraint. *Psychological Review, 98,* 459–87.

Berntson, G. G., Cacioppo, J. T., & Quigley, K. S. (1994b). Autonomic cardiac control I. Estimation and validation from pharmacological blockades. *Psychophysiology, 31,* 572–85.

Biferno, M. A., & Dawson, M. E. (1977). The onset of contingency awareness and electrodermal classical conditioning: An analysis of temporal relationships during acquisition and extinction. *Psychophysiology, 14,* 164–71.

Bishop, P. D., & Kimmel, H. D. (1969). Retention of habituation and conditioning. *Journal of Experimental Psychology, 81,* 317–21.

Bohlin, G., & Graham, F. K. (1977). Cardiac deceleration and reflex blink facilitation. *Psychophysiology, 14,* 423–30.

Bohlin, G., Graham, F. K., Silverstein, L. D., & Hackley, S. A. (1981a). Cardiac orienting and startle blink modifications in novel and signal situations. *Psychophysiology, 18,* 603–11.

Bohlin, G., & Kjellberg, A. (1979). Orienting activity in two-stimulus paradigms as reflected in heart rate. In Kimmel et al., pp. 169–97.

Bohlin, G., Lindhagen, K., & Hagekull, B. (1981b). Cardiac orienting to pulsed and continuous auditory stimulation: A developmental study. *Psychophysiology, 18,* 440–6.

Bonvalet, M., Dell, P., & Hiebel, G. (1954). Tonus sympathetique et activité électrique corticale. *Electroencephalography and Clinical Neurophysiology, 6*, 119–44.

Boysen, S. T., & Berntson, G. G. (1986). Cardiac correlates of individual recognition in the chimpanzee (Pan troglodytes). *Journal of Comparative Psychology, 100*, 321–4.

Boysen, S. T., & Berntson, G. G. (1989). Conspecific recognition in the chimpanzee: Cardiac indices of significant others. *Journal of Comparative Psychology, 103*, 215–20.

Bridger, W. H., & Mandel, I. J. (1964). A comparison of GSR fear responses produced by threat and electric shock: *Journal of Psychiatric Research, 2*, 31–40.

Brodal, A. (1981). *Neurological Anatomy in Relation to Clinical Medicine*, 3rd ed. New York: Oxford University Press.

Brown, J. S., Kalish, H. I., & Farber, I. E. (1951). Conditioned fear as revealed by magnitude of startle response to an auditory stimulus. *Journal of Experimental Psychology, 41*, 317–28.

Campbell, B. A., Hayne, H., & Richardson, R. (Eds.) (1992). *Attention and Information Processing in Infants and Adults. Perspectives from Human and Animal Research*. Hillsdale, NJ: Erlbaum.

Campbell, B. A., Wood, G., & McBride, T. (1997). Origins of orienting and defensive responses: An evolutionary perspective. In Lang et al. (1997b), pp. 41–68.

Cannon, W. B. (1915). *Bodily Changes in Pain, Hunger, Fear and Rage*. New York: Appleton.

Cannon, W. B. (1932). *The Wisdom of the Body*. New York: Norton.

Cechetto, D. F., & Saper, C. B. (1990). Role of the cerebral cortex in autonomic functioning. In A. D. Loewy & K. M. Spyer (Eds.), *Central Regulation of Autonomic Functions*, pp. 208–23. New York: Oxford University Press.

Churchill, M., Remington, B., & Siddle, D. A. T. (1987). The effect of context on long-term habituation of the orienting response in humans. *Quarterly Journal of Experimental Psychology, 39B*, 315–38.

Clark, D. M. (1986). A cognitive approach to panic disorder. *Behaviour Research and Therapy, 24*, 461–70.

Coghill, R. C., Talbot, J. D., Evans, A., Meyer, E., Gjedde, A., Bushnell, H. C., & Duncan, G. H. (1994). Distributed processing of pain and vibration by the human brain. *Journal of Neuroscience, 14*, 4095–4108.

Cook, E. W. III, Hodes, R. L., & Lang, P. J. (1986). Preparedness and phobia: Effects of stimulus content on human visceral conditioning. *Journal of Abnormal Psychology, 95*, 280–6.

Cook, E. W. III, & Turpin, G. (1997). Differentiating orienting, startle, and defense responses: The role of affect and its implication for psychopathology. In Lang et al. (1997b), pp. 137–64.

Davey, G. C. L. (1992a). Classical conditioning and the acquisition of human fears and phobias: A review and synthesis of the literature. *Advances of Behaviour Research and Therapy, 14*, 29–66.

Davey, G. C. L. (1992b). An expectancy model of laboratory preparedness effects. *Journal of Experimental Psychology: General, 121*, 24–40.

Davidson, R. J. (1995). Cerebral asymmetry, emotion, and affective style. In R. J. Davidson & K. Hugdahl (Eds.), *Brain Asymmetry*, pp. 361–88. Cambridge, MA: MIT Press.

Davis, M. (1979). Diazepam and flurazepam: Effects on conditioned fear as measured with the potentiated startle paradigm. *Psychopharmacology, 62*, 1–7.

Davis, M. (1984). The mammalian startle response. In R. C. Eaton (Ed.), *Neural Mechanisms of Startle Behavior*, pp. 287–351. New York: Plenum.

Davis, M. (1992). The role of the amygdala in conditioned fear. In J. Aggleton (Ed.), *The Amygdala: Neurobiological Aspects of Emotion, Memory, and Mental Dysfunction*, pp. 255–306. New York: Wiley-Liss.

Davis, M. (1997). The neurophysiological basis of acoustic startle modulation: Research on fear motivation and sensory gating. In Lang et al. (1997b), pp. 69–96.

Davis, M., & Astrachan, D. I. (1978). Conditioned fear and startle magnitude: Effects of different footshock or backshock intensities used in training. *Journal of Experimental Psychology: Animal Behavior Processes, 4*, 95–103.

Davis, M., Redmond, D. E., Jr., & Baraban, J. M. (1979). Noradrenergic agonists and antagonists : Effects on conditioned fear as measured by the potentiated startle paradigm. *Psychopharmacology, 65*, 111–18.

Dawkins, R. (1976). *The Selfish Gene*. Oxford University Press.

Dawson, M. E. (1973). Can classical conditioning occur without contingency learning? A review and evaluation of the evidence. *Psychophysiology, 10*, 82–6.

Dawson, M. E., & Biferno, M. A. (1973). Concurrent measurement of awareness and electrodermal classical conditioning. *Journal of Experimental Psychology, 101*, 55–62.

Dawson, M. E., Catania, J. J., Schell, A. M., & Grings, W. W. (1979). Autonomic classical conditioning as a function of awareness of stimulus contingencies. *Biological Psychology, 9*, 23–40.

Dawson, M. E., Filion, D. L., & Schell, A. M. (1989). Is elicitation of the autonomic orienting response associated with allocation of processing resources? *Psychophysiology, 26*, 560–72.

Dawson, M. E., & Furedy, J. J. (1976). The role of awareness in human differential autonomic classical conditioning: The necessary-gate hypothesis. *Psychophysiology, 13*, 50–3.

Dawson, M. E., & Schell, A. M. (1985). Information processing and human autonomic classical conditioning. *Advances in Psychophysiology, 1*, 89–165.

Dawson, M. E., Schell, A. M., & Banis, H. T. (1986). Greater resistance to extinction of electrodermal responses conditioned to potentially phobic CSs: A noncognitive process. *Psychophysiology, 23*, 552–61.

Dawson, M. E., Schell, A. M., Beers, J. R., & Kelly, A. (1982). Allocation of processing capacity during human autonomic classical conditioning. *Journal of Experimental Psychology: General, 111*, 273–95.

Dimberg, U. (1987). Facial reactions, autonomic activity, and experienced emotion: A three-component model of emotional conditioning. *Biological Psychology, 24*, 105–22.

Dimberg, U., & Öhman, A. (1996). Behold the wrath: Psychophysiological responses to facial stimuli. *Motivation and Emotion, 20*, 149–82.

Duffy, E. (1951). The concept of energy mobilization. *Psychological Review, 58*, 30–40.

Eppinger, H., & Hess, L. (1915/1976). *Vagotonia: A Clinical Study in Vegetative Neurology*. New York: Nervous and Mental

Disease Publishing. Reprinted in S. W. Porges & M. G. H. Coles (Eds.), *Psychophysiology*. Stoudsburg, PA: Dowden, Hutchison & Ross.

Esteves, F., Dimberg, U., & Öhman, A. (1994a). Automatically elicited fear: Conditioned skin conductance responses to masked facial expressions. *Cognition and Emotion, 8*, 393–413.

Esteves, F., Parra, C., Dimberg, U., & Öhman, A. (1994b). Nonconscious associative learning: Pavlovian conditioning of skin conductance responses to masked fear-relevant facial stimuli. *Psychophysiology, 31*, 375–85.

Esteves, F., & Öhman, A. (1993). Masking the face: Recognition of emotional facial expressions as a function of the parameters of backward masking. *Scandinavian Journal of Psychology, 34*, 1–18.

Eves, F. F., & Gruzelier, J. H. (1984). Individual differences in the cardiac response to high intensity auditory stimulation. *Psychophysiology, 21*, 342–52.

Fanselow, M. S. (1994). Neural organization of the defensive behavior system responsible for fear. *Psychonomic Bulletin and Review, 1*, 429–38.

Fanselow, M. S., & Lester, L. S. (1988). A functional behavioristic approach to aversively motivated behavior: Predatory imminence as a determinant of the topography of defensive behavior. In R. C. Bolles & M. D. Beecher (Eds.), *Evolution and Learning*, pp. 185–212. Hillsdale, NJ: Erlbaum.

Filion, D. L., Dawson, M. E., Schell, A. M., & Hazlett, E. A. (1991). The relationship between skin conductance orienting and the allocation of processing resources. *Psychophysiology, 28*, 410–24.

Fredrikson, M. (1981). Orienting and defensive reactions to phobic and conditioned fear stimuli in phobics and normals. *Psychophysiology, 18*, 456–65.

Fredrikson, M., Furmark, T., Olsson, M. T., Fischer, H., Andersson, J., & Långström, B. (1998). Functional neuroanatomical correlates of electrodermal activity: A positron emission tomographic study. *Psychophysiology, 35*, 179–85.

Fredrikson, M., & Öhman, A. (1979). Heart rate and electrodermal orienting responses to visual stimuli differing in complexity. *Scandinavian Journal of Psychology, 20*, 37–41.

Freeman, G. L. (1948). *The Energetics of Human Behavior*. Ithaca, NY: Cornell University Press.

Furedy, J. J. (1970). CS and UCS intervals and orders in human autonomic classical differential trace conditioning. *Canadian Journal of Psychology, 24*, 417–26.

Furedy, J. J., & Ginsberg, S. (1975). Test of an orienting-reaction-recovery account of short-interval autonomic conditioning. *Biological Psychology, 3*, 121–9.

Furmark, T., Fischer, H., Wik, G., Larsson, M., & Fredrikson, M. (1997). The amygdala and individual differences in human fear conditioning. *NeuroReport, 8*, 3957–60.

Gabrielsen, G. W., Blix, A. S., & Ursin, H. (1985). Orienting and freezing responses in incubating ptarmigan hens. *Physiology and Behavior, 34*, 925–34.

Gatchel, R. J. (1975). Effects of interstimulus interval length on short- and long-term habituation of autonomic components of the orienting response. *Physiological Psychology, 3*, 133–6.

Gatchel, R. J., & Lang, P. J. (1974). Effects of interstimulus interval length and variability on habituation of autonomic components of the orienting response. *Journal of Experimental Psychology, 103*, 802–4.

Gati, I., & Ben-Shakhar, G. (1990). Novelty and significance in orientation and habituation: A feature-matching approach. *Journal of Experimental Psychology: General, 119*, 251–63.

Gazzaniga, M. (Ed.) (1994). *The Cognitive Neurosciences*. Cambridge, MA: MIT Press.

Gibson, J. J. (1966). *The Senses Considered as Perceptual Systems*. Boston: Houghton-Mifflin.

Globisch, J., Hamm, A. O., Esteves, F., & Öhman, A. (1999). Fear appears fast: Temporal course of startle reflex potentiation in animal fearful subjects. *Psychophysiology, 36*, 66–75.

Gloor, P. (1992). The role of the amygdala in temporal lobe epilepsy. In J. P. Aggleton (Ed.), *The Amygdala*, pp. 505–38. New York: Wiley-Liss.

Graham, F. K. (1973). Habituation and dishabituation of responses innervated by the autonomic nervous system. In H. S. Peeke & M. J. Hertz (Eds.), *Habituation*, vol. 1 (Behavioral Studies), pp. 163–218. New York: Academic Press.

Graham, F. K. (1975). The more or less startling effects of weak prestimulation. *Psychophysiology, 12*, 238–48.

Graham, F. K. (1979). Distinguishing among orienting, defense, and startle reflexes. In Kimmel et al., pp. 137–67.

Graham, F. K. (1992). Attention: The heartbeat, the blink, and the brain. In Campbell et al., pp. 3–29.

Graham, F. K., Anthony, B. J., & Zeigler, B. L. (1983). The orienting response and developmental processes. In Siddle, pp. 371–430.

Graham, F. K., & Clifton, R. K. (1966). Heart-rate change as a component of the orienting response. *Psychological Bulletin, 65*, 305–20.

Graham, F. K., & Slaby, D. A. (1973). Differential heart rate change to equally intense white noise and tone. *Psychophysiology, 10*, 347–62.

Gray, J. A. (1995). Contents of consciousness: A neuropsychological conjecture. *Behavioral and Brain Sciences, 18*, 659–76.

Greenwald, M. K., Cook, E. W. III, & Lang, P. J. (1989). Affective judgement and psychophysiological response: Dimensional covariation in the evaluation of visual stimuli. *Journal of Psychophysiology, 3*, 347–63.

Groves, P. M., & Thompson, R. F. (1970). Habituation: A dual process theory. *Psychological Review, 77*, 419–50.

Hageman, G. R., Randall, W. C., & Armour, J. A. (1975). Direct and reflex cardiac bradydysrhythmias from small vagal nerve stimulations. *American Heart Journal, 89*, 338–48.

Hamm, A. O., Cuthbert, B. N., Globisch, J., & Vaitl, D. (1997). Fear and the startle reflex: Blink modulation and autonomic response patterns in animal and mutilation fearful subjects. *Psychophysiology, 34*, 97–107.

Hamm, A. O., Greenwald, M. K., Bradley, M. M., & Lang, P. J. (1993). Emotional learning, hedonic change, and the startle probe. *Journal of Abnormal Psychology, 102*, 453–65.

Hamm, A. O., & Vaitl, D. (1996). Affective learning: Awareness and aversion. *Psychophysiology, 33*, 698–710.

Hare, R. D. (1973). Orienting and defensive responses to visual stimuli. *Psychophysiology, 10*, 453–64.

Hare, R. D., & Blevings, G. (1975a). Conditioned orienting and defensive responses. *Psychophysiology, 12*, 289–97.

Hare, R. D., & Blevings, G. (1975b). Defensive responses to phobic stimuli. *Biological Psychology, 3*, 1–13.

Hare, R., Wood, K., Britain, S., & Shadman, J. (1971). Autonomic responses to affective visual stimulation. *Psychophysiology, 7*, 408–17.

Hatton, H. M., Berg, W. K., & Graham, F. K. (1970). Effects of acoustic rise time on heart rate responses. *Psychonomic Science, 19*, 101–3.

Hebb, D. O. (1955). Drives and the C. N. S. (conceptual nervous system). *Psychological Review, 62*, 243–54.

Hitchcock, J. M., & Davis, M. (1986). Lesions of the amygdala but not of the cerebellum or red nucleus block conditioned fear as measured with the potentiated startle paradigm. *Behavioral Neuroscience, 100*, 11–22.

Hitchcock, J. M., & Davis, M. (1991). Efferent pathway of the amygdala involved in conditioned fear as measured with the fear-potentiated startle paradigm. *Behavioral Neuroscience, 105*, 826–42.

Hodes, R. L., Cook, E. W. III, & Lang, P. J. (1985). Individual differences in autonomic response: Conditioned association or conditioned fear? *Psychophysiology, 22*, 545–60.

Hollis, K. L. (1982). Pavlovian conditioning of signal-centered action patterns and autonomic behavior: A biological analysis of function. In J. S. Rosenblatt, R. A. Hinde, C. Beer, & M.-C. Busnell (Eds.), *Advances in the Study of Behavior,* vol. 12. New York: Academic Press.

Horn, G., & Hinde, R. A. (Eds.) (1970). *Short-Term Changes in Neural Activity and Behaviour.* Cambridge University Press.

Hugdahl, K. (1995). *Psychophysiology: The Mind–Body Perspective.* Cambridge, MA: Harvard University Press.

Hugdahl, K. (1998). Cortical control of human classical conditioning: Autonomic and positron emission tomography data. *Psychophysiology, 35*, 170–8.

Hugdahl, K., Berardi, A., Thompson, W. L., Kosslyn, S. M., Macy, R., Baker, D. R., Alpert, N. M., & LeDoux, J. E. (1995). Brain mechanisms in human classical conditioning: A PET blood-flow study. *NeuroReport, 6*, 1723–8.

Hugdahl, K., Franzon, M., Andersson, B., & Walldebo, G. (1983). Heart-rate responses (HRR) to lateralized visual stimuli. *Pavlovian Journal of Biological Science, 18*, 186–98.

Hugdahl, K., & Johnsen, B. H. (1993). Brain asymmetry and autonomic conditioning: Skin conductance responses. In J. C. Roy (Ed.), *Progress in Electrodermal Research*, pp. 271–87. London: Plenum.

Hugdahl, K., & Öhman, A. (1977). Effects of instruction on acquisition and extinction of electrodermal responses to fear relevant stimuli. *Journal of Experimental Psychology: Human Learning and Memory, 3*, 608–18.

Hull, C. L. (1943). *Principles of Behavior.* New York: Appleton-Century-Crofts.

Iwata, J., & LeDoux, J. E. (1988). Dissociation of associative and nonassociative concomitants of classical fear conditioning in the freely behaving rat. *Behavioral Neuroscience, 102*, 66–76.

Jackson, J. C. (1974). Amplitude and habituation of the orienting response as a function of stimulus intensity. *Psychophysiology, 11*, 647–59.

James, W. (1884). What is an emotion? *Mind, 9*, 188–205.

James, W. (1890). *The Principles of Psychology.* New York: Dover.

Jennings, J. R. (1992). Is it important that the mind is in a body? Inhibition and the heart. *Psychophysiology, 29*, 369–83.

Jennings, J. R., van der Molen, M. W., Brock, K., & Somsen, R. J. M. (1991a). Response inhibition initiates cardiac deceleration: Evidence from a sensory-motor compatibility paradigm. *Psychophysiology, 28*, 72–85.

Jennings, J. R., van der Molen, M. W., Brock, K., & Somsen, R. J. M. (1992). On the synchrony of stopping motor responses and delaying heartbeats. *Journal of Experimental Psychology: Human Perception and Performance, 18*, 422–36.

Jennings, J. R., van der Molen, M. W., Somsen, R. J. M., & Brock, K. (1991b). Weak sensory stimuli induce a phase sensitive bradycardia. *Psychophysiology, 28*, 1–10.

Jennings, J. R., van der Molen, M. W., Somsen, R. J. M., & Terezis, C. (1990). On the shift from anticipatory heart rate deceleration to acceleratory recovery: Revisiting the role of response factors. *Psychophysiology, 27*, 383–95.

Johnsen, B. H., & Hugdahl, K. (1991). Hemisphere asymmetry in conditioning to facial emotional expressions. *Psychophysiology, 28*, 154–62.

Johnsen, B. H., & Hugdahl, K. (1993). Right hemisphere representation of autonomic conditioning to facial emotional expressions. *Psychophysiology, 30*, 274–8.

Kahneman, D. (1973). *Attention and Effort.* Englewood Cliffs, NJ: Prentice-Hall.

Kamosinska, B., Nowicki, D., & Szulczyk, P. (1989). Control of the heart rate by sympathetic nerves in the cat. *Journal of the Autonomic Nervous System, 26*, 241–6.

Kandel, E. R. (1991). Cellular mechanisms of learning and the biological basis of individuality. In E. R. Kandel, J. H. Schwartz, & T. M. Jessell (Eds.), *Principles of Neural Science,* 3rd ed., pp. 1009–31. London: Prentice-Hall.

Kapp, B. S., Whalen, P., Supple, W. F., & Pascoe, J. P. (1992). Amygdaloid contributions to conditioned arousal and sensory information processing. In J. P. Aggleton (Ed.), *The Amygdala: Neurobiological Aspects of Emotion, Memory, and Mental Dysfunction,* pp. 229–54. New York: Wiley-Liss.

Kapp, B. S., Wilson, A., Pascoe, J. P., Supple, W., & Whalen, P. J. (1990). A neuroanatomical systems analysis of conditioned bradycardia in the rabbit. In M. Gabriel & J. Moore (Eds.), *Learning and Computational Neuroscience: Foundations of Adaptive Networks,* pp. 53–90. Cambridge, MA: Bradford Books / MIT Press.

Kimmel, H. D., van Olst, E. H., & Orlebeke, J. F. (Eds.) (1979). *The Orienting Reflex in Humans.* Hillsdale, NJ: Erlbaum.

Klein, D. F. (1993). False suffocation alarms, spontaneous panics, and related conditions. *Archives of General Psychiatry, 50*, 306–17.

Klorman, R., & Ryan, R. M. (1980). Heart rate, contingent negative variation, and evoked potentials during anticipation of affective stimulation. *Psychophysiology, 14*, 45–51.

Klorman, R., Weissberg, R. P., & Wiesenfeld, A. R. (1977). Individual differences in fear and autonomic reactions to affective stimulation. *Psychophysiology, 14*, 45–51.

Klorman, R., Wiesenfeld, A. R., & Austin, M. L. (1975). Autonomic responses to affective visual stimuli. *Psychophysiology, 12*, 553–60.

Konorski, J. (1967). *Integrative Activity of the Brain.* University of Chicago Press.

Kurtz, K. H., & Siegel, A. (1966). Conditioned fear and the magnitude of startle response: A replication and extension. *Journal of Comparative and Physiological Psychology, 62*, 8–14.

LaBar, K. S., LeDoux, J. E., Spencer, D., & Phelps, E. (1995). Impaired fear conditioning following unilateral temporal lobectomy in humans. *Journal of Neuroscience, 15,* 6846–55.

Lacey, B. C., & Lacey, J. I. (1974). Studies of heart rate and other bodily processes in sensorimotor behavior. In P. A. Obrist, A. H. Black, J. Brener, & L. V. DiCara (Eds.), *Cardiovascular Psychophysiology,* pp. 538–64. Chicago: Aldine.

Lacey, B. C., & Lacey, J. I. (1978). Two-way communication between the heart and the brain: Significance of time within the cardiac cycle. *American Psychologist, 33,* 99–113.

Lacey, B. C., & Lacey, J. I. (1980). Cognitive modulation of time-dependent bradycardia. *Psychophysiology, 17,* 209–21.

Lacey, J. I. (1967). Somatic response patterning and stress: Some revisions of activation theory. In M. H. Appley & R. Trumbull (Eds.), *Psychological Stress: Issues in Research,* pp. 14–42. New York: Appleton-Century-Crofts.

Lacey, J. I., Kagan, J., Lacey, B. C., & Moss, H. A. (1963). The visceral level: Situational determinants and behavioral correlates of autonomic response patterns. In P. H. Knapp (Ed.), *Expression of Emotion in Man.* New York: International University Press.

Lacey, J. I., & Lacey, B. C. (1970). Some autonomic–central nervous system interrelationships. In P. Black (Ed.), *Physiological Correlates of Emotion,* pp. 205–28. New York: Academic Press.

Lader, M. H., & Wing, L. (1966). *Physiological Measures, Sedative Drugs, and Morbid Anxiety.* London: Oxford University Press.

Landis, C., & Hunt, W. A. (1939). *The Startle Pattern.* New York: Farrar & Rinehart.

Lane, R. D., & Jennings, J. R. (1995). Hemispheric asymmetry, autonomic asymmetry, and the problem of sudden cardiac death. In R. J. Davidson & K. Hugdahl (Eds.), *Brain Asymmetry,* pp. 271–304. Cambridge, MA: MIT Press.

Lane, R. D., Novelly, R., Cornell, C., Zeitlin, S., & Schwartz, G. (1989). Asymmetrical control of heart rate. Paper presented at the Annual Meeting of the Society for Psychophysiological Research (San Francisco, October 1988) and the Annual Meeting of the American Psychiatric Association (San Francisco).

Lang, P. J. (1968). Fear reduction and fear behavior: Problems in treating a construct. In J. M. Shlien (Ed.), *Research in Psychotherapy,* vol. III. Washington, DC: American Psychological Association.

Lang, P. J. (1979). A bio-informational theory of emotional imagery. *Psychophysiology, 16,* 495–512.

Lang, P. J., Bradley, M. M., & Cuthbert, B. N. (1990). Emotion, attention, and the startle reflex. *Psychological Review, 97,* 377–98.

Lang, P. J., Bradley, M. M., & Cuthbert, B. N. (1997a). Motivated attention: Affect, activation, and action. In Lang et al. (1997b), pp. 97–136.

Lang, P. J., Greenwald, M. K., Bradley, M. M., & Hamm, A. O. (1993). Looking at pictures: Affective, facial, visceral, and behavioral reactions. *Psychophysiology, 30,* 261–73.

Lang, P. J., Öhman, A., & Simons, R. F. (1978). The psychophysiology of anticipation. In J. Requin (Ed.), *Attention and Performance,* vol. VII, pp. 469–85. Hillsdale, NJ: Erlbaum.

Lang, P. J., Simons, R. F., & Balaban, M. T. (Eds.) (1997b). *Attention and Orienting: Sensory and Motivational Processes.* Hillsdale, NJ: Erlbaum.

Lavond, D. G., Kim, J. J., & Thompson, R. F. (1993). Mammalian brain substrates of aversive classical conditioning. *Annual Review of Psychology, 44,* 317–42.

Lavond, D. G., Lincoln, J. S., McCormick, D. A., & Thompson, R. F. (1984). Effect of bilateral lesions of the lateral cerebellar nuclei in conditioning of the heart rate and nictitating membrane/eyelid response in rabbit. *Brain Research, 305,* 323–30.

LeDoux, J. E. (1990). Information flow from sensation to emotion: Plasticity in the neural computation of stimulus value. In M. Gabriel & J. Moore (Eds.), *Learning and Computational Neuroscience: Foundations of Adaptive Networks,* pp. 3–51. Cambridge, MA: Bradford Books / MIT Press.

LeDoux, J. E. (1992). Brain mechanisms of emotion and emotional learning. *Current Opinion in Neurobiology, 2,* 191–7.

LeDoux, J. E. (1993). Emotional memory systems in the brain. *Behavioural Brain Research, 58,* 69–79.

LeDoux, J. E. (1995). In search of an emotional system in the brain: Leaping from fear to emotion and consciousness. In M. S. Gazzaniga (Ed.), *The Cognitive Neurosciences,* pp. 1049–61. Cambridge, MA: MIT Press.

LeDoux, J. E. (1996). *The Emotional Brain.* New York: Simon & Schuster.

LeDoux, J. E., Cicchetti, P., Xagoraris, A., & Romanski, L. M. (1990a). The lateral amygdaloid nucleus: Sensory interface of the amygdala in fear conditioning. *Journal of Neuroscience, 10,* 1062–9.

LeDoux, J. E., Farb, C. R., & Ruggiero, D. A. (1990b). Topographic organisation of neurons in the acoustic thalamus that project to the amygdala. *Journal of Neuroscience, 10,* 1043–54.

LeDoux, J. E., Iwata, J., Chicchetti, P., & Reis, D. J. (1988). Different projections of the central amygdaloid nucleus mediate autonomic and behavioral correlates of conditioned fear. *Journal of Neuroscience, 8,* 2517–29.

LeDoux, J. E., Ruggiero, D. A., & Reis, D. J. (1985). Projections to the subcortical forebrain from anatomically defined regions of the medial geniculate body in the rat. *Journal of Comparative Neurology, 242,* 182–213.

LeDoux, J. E., Sakaguchi, A., & Reis, D. J. (1984). Subcortical efferent projections of the medial geniculate nucleus mediate emotional responses conditioned to acoustic stimuli. *Journal of Neuroscience, 3,* 683–98.

Levinson, D. F., & Edelberg, R. (1984). Scoring criteria for response latency and habituation in electrodermal research: A critique. *Psychophysiology, 22,* 417–26.

Levy, M. N., Ng, M. D., & Zieske, H. (1966). Functional distribution of the peripheral cardiac sympathetic pathways. *Circulation Research, 14,* 650–61.

Lindsley, D. B. (1951). Emotion. In S. S. Stevens (Ed.), *Handbook of Experimental Psychology,* pp. 473–516. New York: Wiley.

Lindsley, D. B. (1960). Attention, consciousness, sleep and wakefulness. In J. Field (Ed.), *Handbook of Physiology,* vol. III (Neurophysiology), pp. 1553–93. Washington, DC: American Physiological Society.

Lipp, O. V., Sheridan, J., & Siddle, D. A. T. (1994). Human blink startle during aversive and nonaversive Pavlovian conditioning. *Journal of Experimental Psychology: Animal Behavior Processes, 20,* 380–8.

Lopez, D. E., Merchan, M. A., Bajo, V. M., & Saldana, E. (1993). The cochlear root neurons in the rat, mouse and gerbil. In M.

A. Merchan (Ed.), *The Mammalian Cochlear Nuclei: Organization and Function*, pp. 291–301. New York: Plenum.

Lorch, E. P., Anderson, D. R., & Weil, A. D. (1984). Effects of irrelevant information on speeded classification tasks: Interference is reduced by habituation. *Journal of Experimental Psychology: Human Perception and Performance, 10*, 850–64.

Lovibond, P. F. (1993). Conditioning and cognitive-behaviour therapy. *Behaviour Change, 10*, 119–30.

Lynn, R. (1966). *Attention, Arousal and the Orientation Reaction*. Oxford, U.K.: Pergamon.

Malmo, R. B. (1959). Activation: A neuropsychological dimension. *Psychological Review, 66*, 367–86.

Maltzman, I., Gould, J., Barnett, O. J., Raskin, D. C., & Wolff, C. (1977). Classical conditioned components of the orienting reflex to words using innocuous and noxious unconditioned stimuli under different conditioned stimulus–unconditioned stimulus intervals. *Journal of Experimental Psychology: General, 106*, 185–212.

Mandel, I. J., & Bridger, W. H. (1973). Is there classical conditioning without cognitive expectancy? *Psychophysiology, 10*, 87–90.

Mandler, G. (1975). *Mind and Emotion*. New York: Wiley.

Maynard Smith, J., & Szathmáry, E. (1995). *The Major Transitions in Evolution*. Oxford, U.K.: Freeman.

McGuigan, F. J. (1978). *Cognitive Psychophysiology: Principles of Covert Behavior*. New York: Appleton-Century-Crofts.

McKeever, W. F. (1986). Tachistoscopic methods in neuropsychology. In J. F. Hannay (Ed.), *Experimental Techniques in Human Neuropsychology*. New York: Oxford University Press.

Mesulam, M.-M. (1985). *Principles of Behavioral Neurology*. Philadelpia: Davis.

Milner, A. D., & Goodale, M. A. (1995). *The Visual Brain in Action*. Oxford University Press.

Morris, J., Öhman, A., & Dolan, R. (1998). Modulation of human amygdala activity by emotional learning and conscious awareness. *Nature, 393*, 467–70.

Moruzzi, G., & Magoun, H. W. (1949). Brain stem reticular formation and activation of the EEG. *Electroencephalography and Clinical Neurophysiology, 1*, 455–73.

Obrist, P. A. (1976). The cardiovascular-behavioral interaction – As it appears today. *Psychophysiology, 13*, 95–107.

Obrist, P. A. (1981). *Cardiovascular Psychophysiology: A Perspective*. New York: Plenum.

Obrist, P. A., Lawler, J. E., Howard, J. L., Smithson, K. W., Martin, P. A., & Manning, J. (1974). Sympathetic influences on the heart in humans: Effects on contractility and heart rate of acute stress. *Psychophysiology, 11*, 405–27.

Obrist, P. A., Sutterer, J. R., & Howard, J. L. (1972). Preparatory cardiac changes: A psychobiological approach. In A. H. Black & W. F. Prokasy (Eds.), *Classical Conditioning II: Current Research and Theory*, pp. 312–40. New York: Appleton-Century-Crofts.

Obrist, P. A., Webb, R. A., & Sutterer, J. R. (1969). Heart rate and somatic changes during aversive conditioning and a simple reaction time task. *Psychophysiology, 5*, 696–723.

Obrist, P. A., Webb, R. A., Sutterer, J. R., & Howard, J. L. (1970). The cardiac-somatic relationship: Some reformulations. *Psychophysiology, 6*, 569–87.

Obrist, P. A., Wood, D. M., & Perez-Reyes, M. (1965). Heart rate during conditioning in humans: Effects of UCS intensity, vagal blockade, and adrenergic block of vasomotor activity. *Journal of Experimental Psychology, 70*, 32–42.

Öhman, A. (1971). Differentiation of conditioned and orienting response components in electrodermal conditioning. *Psychophysiology, 8*, 7–22.

Öhman, A. (1972). Factor analytically derived components of orienting, defensive, and conditioned behavior in electrodermal conditioning. *Psychophysiology, 9*, 199–209.

Öhman, A. (1974). Orienting reactions, expectancy learning, and conditioned responses in electrodermal conditioning with different interstimulus intervals. *Biological Psychology, 1*, 189–200.

Öhman, A. (1979). The orienting response, attention, and learning: An information processing perspective. In Kimmel et al., pp. 443–71.

Öhman, A. (1983). The orienting response during Pavlovian conditioning. In Siddle, pp. 315–69.

Öhman, A. (1987). The psychophysiology of emotion: An evolutionary-cognitive perspective. *Advances in Psychophysiology, 2*, 79–127.

Öhman, A. (1992). Orienting and attention: Preferred preattentive processing of potentially phobic stimuli. In Campbell et al., pp. 263–95.

Öhman, A. (1993a). Fear and anxiety as emotional phenomena: Clinical phenomenology, evolutionary perspectives, and information processing mechanisms. In M. Lewis & J. M. Haviland (Eds.), *Handbook of Emotions*, pp. 511–36. New York: Guilford.

Öhman, A. (1993b). Stimulus prepotency and fear learning: Data and theory. In N. Birbaumer & A. Öhman (Eds.), *The Structure of Emotion: Psychophysiological, Cognitive, and Clinical Aspects*, pp. 218–39. Seattle: Hogrefe & Huber.

Öhman, A. (1996). Preferential preattentive processing of threat in anxiety: Preparedness and attentional biases. In R. M. Rapee (Ed.), *Current Controversies in the Anxiety Disorders*, pp. 253–90. New York: Guilford.

Öhman, A. (1999). Distinguishing unconscious from conscious emotional processes: Methodological considerations and theoretical implications. In T. Dalgleish & M. Power (Eds.), *Handbook of Cognition and Emotion*, pp. 321–52. Chichester, U.K.: Wiley.

Öhman, A., & Dimberg, U. (1978). Facial expressions as conditioned stimuli for electrodermal responses: A case of "preparedness"? *Journal of Personality and Social Psychology, 36*, 1251–8.

Öhman, A., Dimberg, U., & Öst, L.-G. (1985). Animal and social phobias: Biological constraints on learned fear responses. In S. Reiss & R. R. Bootzin (Eds.), *Theoretical Issues in Behavior Therapy*, pp. 123–75. New York: Academic Press.

Öhman, A., Ellström, P.-E., & Björkstrand, P.-Å. (1976a). Electrodermal responses and subjective estimates of UCS probability in a long interstimulus interval conditioning paradigm. *Psychophysiology, 13*, 121–7.

Öhman, A., Eriksson, A., Fredrikson, M., Hugdahl, K., & Olofsson, C. (1974). Habituation of the electrodermal orienting reaction to potentially phobic and supposedly neutral stimuli in normal human subjects. *Biological Psychology, 2*, 85–93.

Öhman, A., Esteves, F., Flykt, A., & Soares, J. J. F. (1993). Gateways to consciousness: Emotion, attention, and electrodermal activity. In J.-C. Roy, W. Boucsein, D. C. Fowles, &

J. H. Gruzelier (Eds.), *Progress in Electrodermal Research*, pp. 137–57. New York: Plenum.

Öhman, A., Esteves, F., Parra, C., Soares, J., & Hugdahl, K. (1988). Brain lateralization and preattentive elicitation of conditioned skin conductance responses [Abstract]. *Psychophysiology, 25,* 473.

Öhman, A., Fredrikson, M., Hugdahl, K., & Rimmö, P. A. (1976b). The premise of equipotentiality in human classical conditioning: Conditioned electrodermal responses to potentially phobic stimuli. *Journal of Experimental Psychology: General, 103,* 313–37.

Öhman, A., Nordby, H., & d'Elia, G. (1989). Orienting in schizophrenia: Habituation to auditory stimuli of constant and varying intensity in patients high and low in skin conductance reactivity. *Psychophysiology, 26,* 48–61.

Öhman, A., & Soares, J. J. F. (1993). On the automatic nature of phobic fear: Conditioned electrodermal responses to masked fear-relevant stimuli. *Journal of Abnormal Psychology, 102,* 121–32.

Öhman, A., & Soares, J. J. F. (1994). "Unconscious anxiety": Phobic responses to masked stimuli. *Journal of Abnormal Psychology, 103,* 231–40.

Öhman, A., & Soares, J. J. F. (1998). Emotional conditioning to masked stimuli: Expectancies for aversive outcomes following nonrecognized fear-relevant stimuli. *Journal of Experimental Psychology: General, 127,* 69–82.

Ortony, A., & Turner, T. J. (1992). What's basic about basic emotions? *Psychological Review, 97,* 315–31.

Öst, L.-G., Sterner, U., & Lindahl, B. (1984). Physiological responses in blood phobics. *Behaviour Research and Therapy, 22,* 109–17.

Packer, J., & Siddle, D. A. T. (1989). Stimulus miscuing, electrodermal activity, and the allocation of processing resources. *Psychophysiology, 26,* 192–200.

Parra, C., Esteves, F., Flykt, A., & Öhman, A. (1997). Pavlovian conditioning to social stimuli: Backward masking and the dissociation of implicit and explicit cognitive processes. *European Psychologist, 2,* 106–17.

Patrick, C. J., Berthot, B. D., & Moore, J. D. (1996). Diazepam blocks fear-potentiated startle in humans. *Journal of Abnormal Psychology, 105,* 89–96.

Pavlov, I. P. (1927). *Conditioned Reflexes.* Oxford University Press.

Peeke, H. V. S., & Herz, M. J. (Eds.) (1973a). *Habituation,* vol. 1 (Behavioral Studies). New York: Academic Press.

Peeke, H. V. S., & Herz, M. J. (Eds.) (1973b). *Habituation,* vol. 2 (Physiological Substrates). New York: Academic Press.

Peeke, H. V. S., & Petrinovich, L. (1984). *Habituation, Sensitization, and Behavior.* New York: Academic Press.

Pendery, M., & Maltzman, I. (1977). Instructions and the orienting reflex in "semantic conditioning" of the galvanic skin response in an innocuous situation. *Journal of Experimental Psychology: General, 106,* 120–40.

Pitman, R. K., & Orr, S. P. (1990). Test of the conditioning model of neurosis: Differential aversive conditioning of angry and neutral facial expressions in anxiety disorder patients. *Journal of Abnormal Psychology, 95,* 208–13.

Porges, S. W. (1995). Orienting in a defensive world: Mammalian modifications of our evolutionary heritage. A polyvagal theory. *Psychophysiology, 32,* 301–18.

Posner, M. I. (1992). Attention as a cognitive and neural system. *Current Directions in Psychological Science, 1,* 11–14.

Posner, M. I., & Boies, S. J. (1971). Components of attention. *Psychological Review, 78,* 391–408.

Prokasy, W. F. (1977). First interval skin conductance response: Conditioned or orienting responses? *Psychophysiology, 14,* 360–7.

Prokasy, W. F., & Ebel, H. C. (1967). Three components of the classically conditioned GSR in human subjects. *Journal of Experimental Psychology, 73,* 247–56.

Quigley, K. S., & Berntson, G. G. (1990). Autonomic origins of cardiac responses to nonsignal stimuli in the rat. *Behavioral Neuroscience, 104,* 751–62.

Razran, G. (1971). *Mind in Evolution: An East–West Synthesis of Learned Behavior and Cognition.* New York: Houghton-Mifflin.

Remington, R., & Churchill, M. (1988). Long-term habituation of the orienting response in humans: The effect of intrasession context manipulations. *Journal of Psychophysiology, 2,* 201–12.

Rescorla, R. A. (1967). Pavlovian conditioning and its proper control procedures. *Psychological Review, 74,* 71–80.

Rescorla, R. A. (1980). *Pavlovian Second Order Conditioning. Studies in Associative Learning.* Hillsdale, NJ: Erlbaum.

Richardson, R., Hayne, H., & Campbell, B. A. (1992). The orienting response as a measure of attention and information processing in the developing rat. In Campbell et al., pp. 113–36.

Rogan, M. T., Stäubli, U. V., & LeDoux, J. E. (1997). Fear conditioning induces associative long-term potentiation in the amygdala. *Nature, 390,* 604–7.

Rosen, J. B., & Davis, M. (1988). Enhancement of acoustic startle by electrical stimulation of the amygdala. *Behavioral Neuroscience, 102,* 195–202.

Rosen, J. B., Hitchcock, J. M., Sananes, C. B., Miserendino, M. J. D., & Davis, M. (1991). A direct projection from the central nucleus of the amygdala to the acoustic startle pathway: Anterograde and retrograde tracing studies. *Behavioral Neuroscience, 105,* 817–25.

Schaafsma, M., Packer, J., & Siddle, D. A. T. (1989). The effect of context-change on long-term habituation of the skin conductance response to signal and non-signal stimuli in humans. *Biological Psychology, 29,* 181–91.

Schell, A. M., Dawson, M. E., & Marinkovic, K. (1991). Effects of the use of potentially phobic CSs on retention, reinstatement, and extinction of the conditioned skin conductance response. *Psychophysiology, 28,* 140–53.

Schmidt, R. F., & Thews, G. (1980). *Physiologie des Menschen.* Berlin: Springer-Verlag.

Schneider, W., Dumais, S. T., & Shiffrin, R. M. (1984). Automatic and control processing and attention. In R. Parasuraman & D. R. Davies (Eds.), *Varieties of Attention,* pp. 1–28. Orlando, FL: Academic Press.

Seligman, M. E. P. (1970). On the generality of the laws of learning. *Psychological Review, 77,* 406–18.

Seligman, M. E. P. (1971). Phobias and preparedness. *Behavior Therapy, 2,* 307–21.

Selye, H. (1956). *The Stress of Life.* New York: McGraw-Hill.

Shiffrin, R. M., & Schneider, W. (1977). Controlled and automatic human information processing: II. Perceptual learning, automatic attending, and a general theory. *Psychological Review, 84*, 127–90.

Siddle, D. (Ed.) (1983). *Orienting and Habituation: Perspectives in Human Research*. Chichester, U.K.: Wiley.

Siddle, D. A. T. (1985). Effects of stimulus omission and stimulus change on dishabituation of the skin conductance response. *Journal of Experimental Psychology: Learning, Memory, and Cognition, 11*, 206–16.

Siddle, D. A. T. (1991). Orienting, habituation, and resource allocation: An associative analysis. *Psychophysiology, 28*, 245–59.

Siddle, D. A. T., & Heron, P. A. (1976). Effects of length of training and amount of tone frequency change on amplitude of autonomic components of the orienting response. *Psychophysiology, 13*, 281–7.

Siddle, D. A. T., & Heron, P. A. (1977). Effects of length of training and amount of tone intensity change on amplitude of autonomic components of the orienting response. *Australian Journal of Psychology, 29*, 7–16.

Siddle, D. A. T., Kyriacou, C., Heron, P. A., & Matthews, W. A. (1979). Effects of changes in verbal stimuli on the skin conductance response component of the orienting response. *Psychophysiology, 16*, 34–40.

Siddle, D. A. T., & Lipp, O. V. (1997). Orienting, habituation, and information processing: The effects of omission, the role of expectancy, and the problem of dishabituation. In Lang et al. (1997b), pp. 23–40.

Siddle, D. A. T., & Packer, J. S. (1987). Stimulus omission and dishabituation of the electrodermal orienting response: The allocation of processing resources. *Psychophysiology, 24*, 181–90.

Siddle, D. A. T., & Spinks, J. A. (1979). Orienting response and information processing: Some theoretical and empirical problems. In Kimmel et al., pp. 473–97.

Siddle, D. A. T., Stephenson, D., & Spinks, J. A. (1983). Elicitation and habituation of the orienting response. In Siddle, pp. 109–82.

Silverstein, L. D., Graham, F. K., & Bohlin, G. (1981). Selective attention effects on the reflex blink. *Psychophysiology, 16*, 520–6.

Simons, R. F., Öhman, A., & Lang, P. J. (1979). Anticipation and response set: Cortical, cardiac, and electrodermal correlates. *Psychophysiology, 16*, 222–33.

Smith, O. A., & DeVito, J. L. (1984). Central neural integration for the control of autonomic responses associated with emotions. *Annual Review of Neuroscience, 7*, 43–65.

Soares, J. J. F., & Öhman, A. (1993a). Backward masking and skin conductance responses after conditioning to non-feared but fear-relevant stimuli in fearful subjects. *Psychophysiology, 30*, 460–6.

Soares, J. J. F., & Öhman, A. (1993b). Preattentive processing, preparedness, and phobias: Effects of instruction on conditioned electrodermal responses to masked and non-masked fear-relevant stimuli. *Behaviour Research and Therapy, 31*, 87–95.

Sokolov, E. N. (1960). Neuronal models and the orienting reflex. In M. A. Brazier (Ed.), *The Central Nervous System and Behavior*, pp. 187–276. New York: Joshua Macy Foundation.

Sokolov, E. N. (1963). *Perception and the Conditioned Reflex*. Oxford, U.K.: Pergamon.

Sokolov, E. N. (1969). The modeling properties of the nervous system. In M. Cole & I. Maltzman (Eds.), *A Handbook of Contemporary Soviet Psychology*, pp. 671–704. New York: Basic Books.

Sokolov, E. N. (1975). The neuronal mechanisms of the orienting reflex. In E. N. Sokolov & O. S. Vinogradova (Eds.), *Neuronal Mechanisms of the Orienting Reflex*, pp. 217–35. Hillsdale, NJ: Erlbaum.

Sokolov, E. N., & Cacioppo, J. T. (1997). Orienting and defense reflexes: Vector coding the cardiac response. In Lang et al. (1997b), pp. 1–22.

Sperry, R. W. (1952). Neurology and the mind–brain problem. *American Scientist, 40*, 291–312.

Spinks, J. A., & Siddle, D. A. T. (1976). Effects of stimulus information and stimulus duration on amplitude and habituation of the electrodermal orienting response. *Biological Psychology, 4*, 29–39.

Stenfert Kroese, B., & Siddle, D. A. T. (1983). Effects of an attention-demanding task on amplitude and habituation of the electrodermal orienting response. *Psychophysiology, 20*, 128–35.

Stritzke, W. G. K., Patrick, C. J., & Lang, A. R. (1995). Alcohol and human emotion: A multidimensional analysis incorporating the startle-probe methodology. *Journal of Abnormal Psychology, 104*, 114–22.

Supple, W. F., & Kapp, B. S. (1993). The anterior cerebellar vermis: Essential involvement in classically conditioned bradycardia in the rabbit. *Journal of Neuroscience, 13*, 3705–11.

Thompson, R. F. (1986). The neurobiology of learning and memory. *Science, 233*, 941–7.

Thompson, R. F., Groves, P. M., Teyler, T. J., & Roemer, R. A. (1973). A dual process theory of habituation: Theory and behavior. In H. V. S. Peeke & M. J. Herz (Eds.), *Habituation*, vol. 1 (Behavioral Studies), pp. 239–72. New York: Academic Press.

Thompson, R. F., & Spencer, W. A. (1966). Habituation: A model phenomenon for the study of neuronal substrates of behavior. *Psychological Review, 73*, 16–43.

Tighe, T. J., & Leaton, R. N. (Eds.) (1976). *Habituation: Perspectives from Child Development, Animal Behavior, and Neurophysiology*. Hillsdale, NJ: Erlbaum.

Tooby, J., & Cosmides, L. (1990). The past explains the present: Emotional adaptations and the structure of ancestral environment. *Ethology and Sociobiology, 11*, 375–424.

Tooby, J., & Cosmides, L. (1992). Psychological foundations of culture. In J. H. Barkow, L. Cosmides, & J. Tooby (Eds.), *The Adapted Mind: Evolutionary Psychology and the Generation of Culture*. New York: Oxford University Press.

Tranel, D., & Damasio, H. (1994). Neuroanatomical correlates of electrodermal skin conductance responses. *Psychophysiology, 31*, 427–39.

Tranel, D., Fowles, D. C., & Damasio, A. R. (1985). Electrodermal discrimination of familiar and unfamiliar faces: A methodology. *Psychophysiology, 22*, 403–8.

Tulving, E., Markowitsch, H. J., Kapur, S., Habib, R., & Houle, S. (1994). Novelty encoding networks in the human brain: Positron emission tomography data. *NeuroReport, 5*, 2525–8.

Turpin, G. (1983). Unconditioned reflexes and the autonomic nervous system. In Siddle, pp. 1–70.

Turpin, G. (1986). Effects of stimulus intensity on autonomic responding: The problem of differentiating orienting and defense reflexes. *Psychophysiology, 23*, 1–14.

Turpin, G., & Siddle, D. A. T. (1979). Effects of stimulus intensity on electrodermal activity. *Psychophysiology, 16*, 582–91.

Turpin, G., & Siddle, D. A. T. (1983). Effects of stimulus intensity on cardiovascular activity. *Psychophysiology, 20*, 611–24.

Unger, S. M. (1964). Habituation of the vasoconstrictive orienting reaction. *Journal of Experimental Psychology, 67*, 11–18.

van der Molen, M. W., Boomsma, D. I., Jennings, J. R., & Nieuwboer, R. T. (1989). Does the heart know what the eye sees? A cardiac/pupillometric analysis of motor preparation and response execution. *Psychophysiology, 26*, 70–80.

van der Molen, M. W., Somsen, R. J. M., & Jennings, J. R. (1996). Does the heart know what the ears hear? A heart rate analysis of auditory selective attention. *Psychophysiology, 33*, 547–54.

van der Molen, M. W., Somsen, R. J. M., Jennings, J. R., Nieuwboer, R. T., & Orlebeke, J. F. (1987). A psychophysiological investigation of cognitive-energetic relations in human information processing: A heart rate/additive factors approach. *Acta Psychologica, 66*, 251–89.

Vila, J., Fernandez, M. C., & Godoy, J. (1992). The cardiac defense response in humans: Effects of stimulus modality and gender differences. *Journal of Psychophysiology, 6*, 140–54.

Vrana, S. R., Spence, E. L., & Lang, P. J. (1988). The startle probe response: A new measure of emotion. *Journal of Abnormal Psychology, 97*, 487–91.

Wagner, A. R. (1976). Priming in the STM: An information-processing mechanism for self-generated or retrieval-generated depression of performance. In T. J. Tighe & R. N. Leaton (Eds.), *Habituation: Perspectives from Child Development, Animal Behavior, and Neurophysiology*, pp. 95–128. Hillsdale, NJ: Erlbaum.

Walker, B. B., & Sandman, C. A. (1979). Influences of heart rate on the human visual evoked response. *Journal of Comparative and Physiological Psychology, 93*, 717–29.

Walker, B. B., & Sandman, C. A. (1982). Visual evoked potentials change as heart rate and carotid pressure change. *Psychophysiology, 19*, 520–7.

Wallin, B. G. (1981). Sympathetic nerve activity underlying electrodermal and cardiovascular reactions in man. *Psychophysiology, 18*, 470–6.

Wells, A., & Matthews, G. (1994). *Attention and Emotion: A Clinical Perspective*. Hove, U.K.: Erlbaum.

Wenger, M. A. (1941). The measurement of individual differences in autonomic balance. *Psychosomatic Medicine, 3*, 427–34.

Wenger, M. A., & Cullen, T. D. (1972). Studies of autonomic balance in children and adults. In N. S. Greenfield & R. A. Sternbach (Eds.), *Handbook of Psychophysiology*, pp. 535–69. New York: Holt, Rinehart & Winston.

Wilder, J. (1931/1976). The "law of initial values," a neglected biological law and its significance for research and practice. In S. W. Porges & M. G. H. Coles (Eds.), *Psychophysiology*. Stroudsburg, PA: Dowden, Hutchison & Ross. [Translated from *Zeitschrift für die gesammte Neurologie und Psychiatrie, 37*.]

Williams, G. C. (1997). *Plan and Purpose in Nature*. London: Phoenix.

Wingard, J. A., & Maltzman, I. (1980). Interest as a predeterminer of the GSR index of the orienting reflex. *Acta Psychologica, 46*, 153–60.

Wittling, W. (1990). Psychophysiological correlates of human brain asymmetry: Blood pressure changes during lateralized presentation of an emotionally laden film. *Neuropsychologia, 28*, 457–70.

Wittling, W. (1995). Brain asymmetry in the control of autonomic-physiologic activity. In R. J. Davidson and K. Hugdahl (Eds.), *Brain Asymmetry*, pp. 305–58. Cambridge, MA: MIT Press.

Wittling, W. (1997). Brain asymmetry and autonomic control of the heart. *European Psychologist, 2*, 313–27.

Yokoyama, K., Jennings, J. R., Ackles, P., Hood, P., & Boller, F. (1987). Lack of heart rate changes during an attention-demanding task after right hemisphere lesions. *Neurology, 36*, 624–30.

Zipes, D. P. (1991). The long QT interval syndrome: A Rosetta stone for sympathetic related ventricular tachyarrythmias. *Circulation, 84*, 1414–19.

CHAPTER TWENTY-ONE

LANGUAGE

MARTA KUTAS, KARA D. FEDERMEIER, SEANA COULSON, JONATHAN W. KING,
& THOMAS F. MÜNTE

The Brain – is wider than the sky –
For – put them side by side –
The one the other will contain –
With ease and you beside

The Brain is deeper than the sea –
For – hold them – Blue to Blue –
The one the other will absorb –
As Sponges – Buckets – do

The Brain is just the weight of God –
For – Heft them – Pound for Pound –
And they will differ – if they do –
As Syllable from Sound.

Emily Dickinson (1896/1970)

Historical Context

As Dickinson notes, brains have a remarkable capacity that
differentiates them from other sorts of material substances:
the ability to represent things intentionally. Although we
often take this capacity for granted, it is no small feat that
we are able to entertain the thoughts of a woman who has
long since died. Many consider Dickinson to be a gifted
poet, yet her ability to exploit the representational capacity
afforded by language is shared by all humans. This capacity allows us to communicate with one another across
distances of time and space and to affect one another's
behavior.

Natural language is a species-specific system that enables speakers to evoke cognitive models in listeners via
the systematic combination of vocal sounds or visual signs.
A schematic characterization of the speech event begins
with the speaker's desire to communicate a message and
ends with the listener's apprehension of that message. In
this simplified model of the communicative act, language

mediates between thoughts and motor commands on the
speaker's end, and between acoustic signals and thoughts
on the listener's end. However, the real magic in the system lies in the brains of the speech participants, and it is
to the brain that psychophysiologists turn for answers to
fundamental questions about the nature of language representations and the relationship between language and other
cognitive processes.

Linguists have posited a number of different kinds of
representations to account for language production and
comprehension. These constructs have proven quite useful
for thinking about language processes, but their psychological reality remains a serious question. Much regularity
can be observed in language, but are those regularities due
to the fact that the brain implements linguistic rules? Work
on the psychophysiology of language processing – using
techniques such as ERPs, PET, and fMRI – has attempted
to monitor how the brain changes with manipulations
of particular linguistic representations. The assumption
is that language subprocesses are subserved by different
anatomical and physiological substrates that will generate
distinct patterns of biological activity. These patterns can
then be picked up by methods sensitive to fluctuations in
electromagnetic and hemodynamic activity.

Related to these representational questions has been a
set of issues about the architecture of the language processing system as a whole. Fodor (1983) characterized cognition
as "modular"; that is, as the result of a large number of
autonomous, highly specialized input modules feeding into
a more general-purpose central processor. Input modules
transform particular inputs into representations that can
be handled by the central processor. These input systems
are regarded as "informationally encapsulated" (protected
from influence by other types of information). Additionally, it is argued that the central processor has access
only to the outputs of the input modules and not to any

John T. Cacioppo, Louis G. Tassinary, and Gary G. Berntson (Eds.), *Handbook of Psychophysiology,* 2nd ed. © Cambridge University Press 2000.
Printed in the United States of America. ISBN 62634X. All rights reserved.

intervening representations in the modules themselves. A modular approach to language processing assigns low-level aspects of processing (such as parsing and word recognition) to the input modules while leaving higher-level aspects such as semantics and pragmatics to the central processor. The difference between a modular account of language processing and a nonmodular, or "interactionist," account chiefly concerns the time course of processing. In the modular account, lower levels of processing occur autonomously and are integrated only later by the central processor. By the interactionist account, the lower levels of processing are not independent of higher levels but rather interact continuously with them during the processing of a sentence.

It now seems fairly clear that language processing is neither completely modular nor completely interactionist. However, psycholinguists continue to argue about whether certain language abilities result from dedicated brain regions specialized for specific kinds of linguistic representations, or whether these abilities are more accurately described as resulting from general mechanisms, such as constraint satisfaction as implemented in neural network models. Such models portray language abilities as the outcome of the simultaneous application of general-purpose constraints at many different linguistic levels (MacDonald, Pearlmutter, & Seidenberg 1994).

Psychophysiological studies of language processing are well suited to examine issues of both representation and processing. Techniques with high spatial resolution, such as PET and fMRI, can help pinpoint brain areas important for language processing. Techniques with high temporal resolution, such as ERPs and eye tracking, can help reveal how language processing unfolds over time; they can be used to track the availability of different sorts of linguistic information and the temporal course of their interactions. Additionally, studies of brain-damaged patients, in conjunction with the use of psychophysiological measures, can provide important insights about which brain areas are necessary and/or sufficient for certain types of linguistic processes and about the relationship between language processing and other cognitive abilities. In this chapter, we consider the role of the brain in understanding and producing natural language utterances. We review how psychophysiologists have addressed this issue in the past and consider how these methods might best be employed in the future.

Physical Context

Language production, or speaking, depends on the brain systems that enervate the muscles and coordinate movements of the lungs, vocal cords, jaw, and lips. Language comprehension depends on brain systems which transform the acoustic information that hits the listener's eardrum (or the visual information that hits her eyes, in the case of sign language) into her understanding of what has been said. Language processing thus involves perceptual transformations in auditory and/or visual cortices; motor control processes mediated by the motor cortical areas, basal ganglia, and cerebellum; memory processes – both long-term and working – in hippocampal, medial temporal, and frontal lobe structures; attentional shifts as mediated by the parietal lobe; and so forth. When considering the neural basis of language processing, it is therefore important to appreciate the extent to which the brain as a whole is involved.

Despite the fact that language processing recruits large portions of the brain, some parts of the brain are considered by most to be particularly concerned with the processing of language. An area of the frontal cortex (Brodmann's areas 44 and 45) known as Broca's area is one example. Damage to Broca's area (which usually also includes underlying subcortical tissue and white matter) causes an aphasia characterized by halting, "telegraphic" speech (lacking in function words) but with reasonably good comprehension. In contrast, damage to Wernicke's area (Brodmann area 22) in the parietal cortex produces a "fluent" aphasia (speech has normal rate and rhythm) with impaired comprehension. While Wernicke's aphasics produce speech easily and use function words appropriately, they produce large numbers of paraphasias (incorrect word substitutions) that render their speech nearly incomprehensible. There remain many debates about what Broca's and Wernicke's areas specifically contribute to language processing (e.g., motor vs. sensory, syntax vs. semantics). However, these are two brain areas that are clearly necessary for normal language functions (see Goodglass 1993 for a discussion of other types of aphasia and their neural correlates).

More recently, an area in the basal temporal fusiform gyrus (the basal temporal language area) has been shown to be important for word processing. Stimulation of this area (in epileptic patients undergoing surgery) results in language deficits ranging from anomia to global expressive and receptive aphasias (Luders et al. 1986). The fact that only transient aphasia results from damage to the basal temporal language area suggests that its functions are or can be duplicated by other brain areas. Although not necessary for language function, this area does seem likely to play an important role under normal conditions. In fact, with the advent of noninvasive brain imaging methods (PET, fMRI), a number of areas that seem important (but not necessary) for language functioning have been described. For example, these studies have implicated a left prefrontal area in tasks requiring language production (Petersen & Fiez 1993) or semantic judgments (Kapur et al. 1994); such activations are not observed during the processing of pseudowords, which clearly have many of the phonological and some of the lexical properties of real words but are devoid of meaning.

Imaging studies point consistently to some brain areas as important for language tasks, yet there is considerable diversity in the other areas activated in particular studies (see Fletcher et al. 1995; Petersen et al. 1991; Wise et al. 1991). The precise areas activated in a study depend heavily on the choice of experimental and control tasks and the methods used to process and analyze the data. When drawing conclusions from neuroimaging data, as from all types of psychophysiological data, it is thus important to recognize the inferential leaps required by and the inferential limitations inherent in mappings from physiology to psychology (see Sarter, Berntson, & Cacioppo 1996 and Chapter 1 of this volume).

Social/Cognitive Context

For at least 100,000 years, our species has used language to describe – and construct – the world around us. First, and perhaps most obviously, language provides a medium for the communication of thoughts via a structured stream of sound. Upon hearing language, listeners are somehow able to formulate a mental representation of the speaker's message, which can alter the listener's mental state and affect her subsequent behavior. Language thus provides the primary means of social interaction and enables the coordination of group action. Second, language enables us to transmit cultural knowledge such as customs and values. An integral part of social interaction, it plays an organizing role in social relationships. Like the clothes we wear, the way we talk can reveal much about our cultural heritage. Our accents suggest the place of our upbringing. Our choice of slang words is highly suggestive of group identification. As James Baldwin (1963) noted, "To open your mouth in England is (if I may use Black English) to 'put your business in the street': you have confessed your parents, your youth, your school, your salary, your self-esteem, and, alas, your future." Besides describing the world, language is used to affect and effect it. Language is used to ask questions, make requests, issue warnings; to make promises, enact business contracts, seal marriage vows; to tell stories and lies, crack jokes, and sometimes just to pass the time of day. In short, language is as much a tool for the social construction of reality as a conduit for thoughts and feelings.

The cognitive basis of this complex human skill involves representations and processes at a number of different levels. The study of linguistics is divided into several subdisciplines based on observations of regularities at multiple levels of analysis. Moving from sound to meaning, these disciplines include phonology, the study of linguistic sound; morphology, the study of word formation; grammar (syntax), the study of hierarchical structure in utterances; semantics, the study of context-invariant aspects of meaning; and pragmatics, the study of meaning in use. Although it is unclear how traditional linguistic categories map onto brain structures and functions, it is important to consider the work of linguists as a relevant starting point for exploration of these issues.

Dickinson notes the distinction between syllable, a construct specific to language, and sound, which is more general. Because of naturally occurring anatomical variation in vocal tracts, everyone's voice is different. Factors such as age, sex, health, and size all influence the physical character of speech sounds. Therefore, if we compare the acoustic signal corresponding to the pronunciation of *chowder* by a little girl and an elderly man, the phonetic (i.e., sound) characteristics would differ dramatically. There can even be considerable variation within a given speaker due to factors such as health and mood. Nonetheless, most people would be able to recognize that it was the word *chowder* and not *clams* that was uttered regardless of who says it or how excited the speaker is. This suggests a level of representation of speech that abstracts away from the raw sensory aspects of the acoustic stimulus. These representations are not directly available in the sensory input but rather are constructed in the listener's mind.

Although our intuition is that the fundamental unit of language is the word, linguistic research suggests that words are composed of more fundamental units known as phonemes. For example, the monosyllabic word *cat* is made up of three phonemes /k/, /a/, and /t/, where "phoneme" is defined as the smallest unit of speech input that makes a difference in a word's meaning. So, /k/ and /m/ are both phonemes because we can substitute them for each other in /kat/ and get words with different meanings. Words can also be broken down into "morphemes," which are combinations of phonemes that have their own meaning. As morphemes are the smallest meaning pieces into which a word can be cut, the word *cat* has only one morpheme. In contrast, the word *unsuccessfully* consists of four morphemes, each of which contributes to the meaning of the word as a whole: un-success-ful-ly. This idea of building up meanings by combining representations at different levels is a recurrent one in linguistics because it helps explain how we can express an infinite number of different meanings with a limited repertoire of speech sounds. Thus, phonemes are combined into morphemes, morphemes into lexemes (another word for words), words into phrases, and phrases into sentences.

Just as words are built up out of sounds, sentences are built out of words. The relationship between words and sentences is complex and involves structure at a number of different levels. "Parsing" is the process of analyzing the input into a series of lexical units and then mapping higher-order structures onto those units in a consistent and eventually meaningful way. In addition to what might be called word-level semantics, these include phrase structure, thematic structure, and referential structure, as depicted in Figure 1.

Most students of English grammar have learned that parts of speech can be assigned to words and that certain relationships hold among them (in English, for example, adjectives often precede nouns). Linguists also divide words into different, more abstract, classes and study relationships among them. The study of these relationships is "phrase structure" and is probably what most psychologists would think of as "grammar" or "syntax."

Rules (or regularities) of phrase structure capture our intuitions that, in the following example sentences, the syntax of the phrase *those dogs* is basically similar to that of *those shaggy dogs* and also, perhaps, of *dogs*.

(Dogs) like me.
(Those dogs) like me.
(Those shaggy dogs) like me.

The pronoun *they* may also be interchangeable with the nouns in these examples, when it is known that *they* refers to the dogs in question. English thus has a kind of phrase that contains at least one noun or something acting like one (e.g., a pronoun); these are called "noun phrases" or "NPs." Note that a noun phrase can be used not only as the subject of a sentence, but also as an object: "I want (those dogs)."

The noun phrase thus seems to be a useful description of a variety of word combinations that can be found in different locations in sentences. Note that there are constraints on what can and cannot be found in noun phrases that renders *them want,* which contains a verb, ungrammatical. Likewise, in English, only some word orders are allowed: *shaggy those dogs* is not an acceptable NP.

All these example sentences have the structure [NP V NP] (where V stands for verb). Other types of sentences are possible:

The child slept.
The child slept in the hammock.
The child slept in the afternoon.

These sentences lack an object, ending either with a verb or an optional phrase that indicates where or when the sleeping event took place. Their structure is [NP V location-phrase] or [NP V time-phrase]. The location and time phrases that begin with a preposition are prepositional phrases, or PPs. The sequences [V NP], [V], and [V PP] are all types of "verb phrases" (VPs).

We thus can find structures that have important, stable properties in different sentences and in different parts

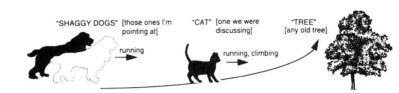

REFERENTIAL

THEMATIC

Caused Motion	*Agent*	causes	*Patient*	to move to	*Goal*
Chase Roles	*Chaser*		*Chasee*		*Chased-to*
Syntax	*Subject*	verb	*Object*		*Oblique*

Those shaggy dogs chased the cat up a tree.

Phonology	Derivational Morphology	Inflectional Morphology	Word Class	
∂oz ʃæg'id agz' (those shaggy dogs)	shag + y ' → shaggy *noun affix adjective*	dog + s ' → dogs *noun affix n. plural*	Open: *shaggy, chased, cat, tree*	Closed: *those, the a, up*

PHRASE STRUCTURE

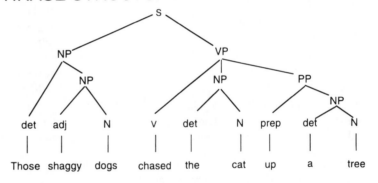

Figure 1. Cartoon view of language processing with illustrations of processes and terms used in this chapter.

of the same sentence. At another level of representation, then, we can characterize sentences (S) as being built up from basic structures like [NP VP]. In turn, NP and VP are built from strings of other categories, which in turn are abstractions for large numbers of individual words. (For more on phrase structure, see e.g. Sells 1985.)

Although the form of the two PP-containing sentences just displayed is the same, there is an obvious difference in meaning between descriptions of location and of time. Locations are interesting linguistically not only because there are so many ways to express the concept but also because there are situations where they must be mentioned in order for a sentence to be grammatical. Consider the following examples.

The shaggy dog put the newspaper into the hammock.
*The shaggy dog put the newspaper.
*The shaggy dog put into the hammock.

Only the first sentence is grammatical. (By convention, ungrammatical sentences are prefixed with an asterisk.) A verb such as *put* requires both an object ("patient") to be placed and a location (or "goal") where it will be placed. In the first sentence, *the newspaper* plays the role of patient while *the hammock* plays the role of goal. *The shaggy dog* is the "agent" who performs the act of putting. Agent, patient, and goal are the three "thematic roles" that are required in a clause where the main verb is *put*; thus, *put* is said to "assign" three thematic roles to the NPs in its clause. In contrast, a verb like *want* assigns only two thematic roles, and *sleep* just one. Information about how many and what thematic roles a verb assigns is referred to as the verb's "argument structure" or "subcategorization requirements" (Sells 1985).

One might assume a hard-wired, one-to-one mapping between a thematic role and particular grammatical category – so that, for example, the agent is mapped to the subject, the patient to the object, and the goal to a prepositional phrase. However, while this might be a canonical mapping, it is not always the case.

John gave the bone to the dog.
subject   object   oblique
agent   patient goal

John gave the dog the bone.
subject   object   object2
agent   goal   patient

The dog was given the bone by John.
subject   object   oblique
goal   patient agent

Thus, for example, a verb like *give* requires that a goal be present, but that goal can be expressed as a subject, an object, or the object of a preposition (here, "oblique" – a term we use loosely for an argument, required by a verb, that is neither subject nor object). In fact, rather than being hard-coded, verb argument structure seems to be sensitive to the existence of form-meaning pairings known as "constructions." For instance, the caused-motion construction described by Goldberg (1995) pairs the [NP V NP PP] structure with a meaning in which the subject (referred to by the first NP) causes the object (referred to in the second NP) to move to the place described in the PP.

He sneezed his napkin off the table.
subject   object   oblique
agent   patient goal

In this example, the man sneezes and causes the napkin to fall off the table. As a so-called intransitive verb, *sneeze* does not normally take a direct object. However, when it participates in the caused-motion construction, it adopts the argument structure of that construction.

The preceding discussion of thematic roles suggested that roles are assigned to the NPs involved. However, they are actually best viewed as mappings from NPs in a sentence to the discourse entities that are the basic units of a "referential" or "message-level" representation. Referential structure is a level of conceptual organization between the situation being described and the linguistic structures that describe it (Langacker 1987). For example, Fauconnier (1994) demonstrated the utility of "mental spaces" as organizational features of referential structure. In Fauconnier's model, a mental space contains a partial representation of the current scenario, including one or more elements and frames that represent relationships among the different discourse entities. Complex scenarios can be represented by positing a number of mental spaces interconnected in various ways.

With all factors taken into consideration, the task of language comprehension involves combining linguistic and nonlinguistic information to construct a message-level representation. Although it is still unclear how much the various aspects of language processing interact, the overall process can be thought of as comprising a number of different subprocesses. The speech stream is decoded into words and other representations (such as morphemes) that can be used in the interpretive process. Parsing involves the assignment of hierarchical structure to the input. Using phonological, morphological, and constructional information, speakers group words into phrases and sentences. Meaning construction is the coordination of linguistic and nonlinguistic information necessary to complete the representation of the discourse event.

Language production involves many of the same computations, albeit in a different order. Here, the speaker's task begins with a message-level representation and ends with the execution of a motor command. Given a message that she would like to evoke, the speaker must choose which words and constructions are most likely to prompt listeners to adopt the desired conceptualization. Moreover, in real time, the speaker must transform these abstract lexical and constructional representations into articulatory commands.

Psychophysiological methods have been used to study language representations and processes at nearly all levels of analysis. Successfully using physiological measures to explore language functions crucially requires that both the right method and the right experimental design be employed to investigate the question of interest. In the remainder of this chapter we describe the types of measures and designs that have been used to study language, as well as the conclusions that have been drawn. We begin with language comprehension, first at the level of the word and then with successively larger units. We then examine language production and studies of brain-damaged individuals. We conclude with a discussion of where psychophysiological approaches to the study of language have brought us – and what remains to be explored.

Inferential Context

FIRST, THERE WAS THE WORD

Until recently, the majority of psychophysiological investigations of language processing have focused on the level of the word. Although there is still considerable debate amongst linguists as to what constitutes a word, we use the term here in its lay sense. Psychophysiological methods have been aimed at better specifying the features of a word, the organization of different kinds of information associated with a word, and the influences on word processing. One proposal is that information about words is represented in a mental dictionary, or "lexicon." This lexicon is thought to contain both low-level phonological and orthographic information and higher-level information such as a word's meaning and its syntactic category. On the standard model, recognizing a word activates the information represented in the lexicon in a process known as "lexical access." This information, in turn, is used to combine the meanings of words into phrases and the meanings of phrases into sentences.

Because information about words is so clearly important for language processing, much psychophysiological research on language has addressed how words are recognized. Event-related potentials provide a continuous, real-time measure of neural processing that is potentially sensitive to qualitatively different kinds of information. Therefore, language researchers have employed this technique to uncover the time at which different types of information about words become available. The first issues we consider are how, where, and when the brain is able to distinguish between sensory input that is treated as language and other sorts of perceptual information. Next, we consider how factors such as global frequency in the language and local frequency in the experimental setting affect the ERPs elicited by words. Finally, we review the literature on the sensitivity of ERPs to linguistic factors such as lexical word class and word meaning.

Lexical versus Perceptual Processing of Word Forms

Does the processing of words differ significantly from the processing of other perceptual forms? If so, when and where in the perceptual stream are recognition processes specific to words first evident? Because, at one level, written words are merely overlearned visual patterns with meaning, we might expect them to be processed similarly to pictures and other kinds of iconic representations. However, at other levels of analysis, words and pictures are quite different and must be differentiated.

Schendan, Ganis, and Kutas (1998) examined the time course of visual classification by comparing the ERPs to objectlike stimuli (real objects, pseudo-objects that were scrambled versions of real objects, and strings of familiar

icons) and wordlike stimuli (words, random letter strings, and a pseudo-font). Regardless of task, at about 95 msec an occipital negativity (N100) distinguished responses to single objectlike stimuli (objects and pseudo-objects) from responses to strings (icon, pseudo-font, random-letter strings, and words). This effect was followed in 10 msec by a further distinction between strings composed of real letters (words and random-letter strings) and nonletters (pseudo-font and icon strings). Thus, in the scalp-recorded ERP, the first sign of specialized processing of letter strings appears at around 105 msec. About 100 msec later, words can be discriminated from random-letter strings; by 250 msec, the ERPs to all stimuli are clearly differentiable from each other (see Figure 2). Overall, the latencies of these ERPs from the human scalp reveal a hierarchy in which visual responses become increasingly selective for classes of visual stimuli over time.

Studies using neuroimaging techniques with high spatial resolution have provided some indications of which brain areas are involved in the processing of words and pictures. As would be predicted from the ERP results, visual areas believed to be early in the visual processing stream show very similar blood flow responses for word and picture stimuli. Differential responses are observed, however, in brain areas further downstream. Left medial extrastriate regions, for example, become active for words and pseudowords but not for nonwords or false fonts (Petersen & Fiez 1993). Further, pictures selectively activate the right middle occipital gyrus, whereas words selectively activate left inferior parietal areas (Vandenberghe et al. 1996).

Similar findings have been reported for the auditory modality. For example, ERPs to meaningful and nonsense words are very similar within the first 150 msec (Novick, Lovrich, & Vaughan 1985), but they begin to diverge by 200–250 msec after stimulus presentation. Findings via PET suggest that activity early in the auditory processing stream – primary auditory cortex and posterior temporal areas – are unlikely to be language-specific. In contrast, responses in and around Wernicke's area seem more specific for words and for tasks requiring phonological processing, such as judging whether two words rhyme (Liotti, Gay, & Fox 1994). Hence, across modalities and methods, observations support the idea that processing of words and other perceptual stimuli diverges within about 200 msec and that this differentiation occurs in secondary perceptual processing areas of the brain.

Frequency, Repetition, and Semantic Variables

Once words have been categorized by the perceptual system, other factors known to play a role in language processing begin to affect the brain's response to them. In fact, around the time that the processing of words and other perceptual stimuli diverges, effects of word frequency are observed. These effects relate to the word's overall

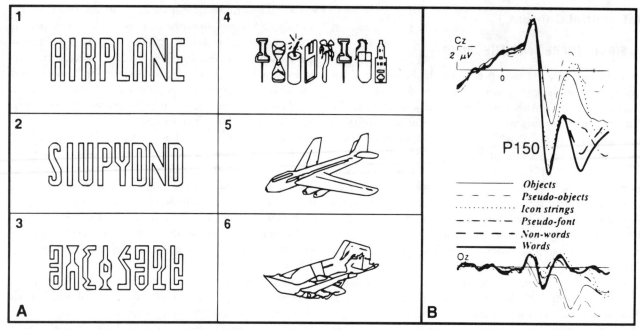

Figure 2. Sample stimuli including words (1), nonwords (2), pseudofont (3), icon strings (4), objects (5), and pseudo-objects (6) and the associated grand average ERPs from a midline central (Cz) and a midline occipital (Oz) electrode site. Note that the P150 is large and equal for words, nonwords and the pseudofont, small and equal for objects and pseudo-objects, and intermediate for icon strings. Negativity is plotted upward on this and all subsequent figures depicting ERPs. Reprinted with permission from Schendan, Ganis, & Kutas, "Neuropsychological evidence for visual perceptual organization of words and faces by 150 ms," *Psychophysiology*, vol. 35, pp. 240–51. Copyright 1998 Cambridge University Press.

frequency in the language as well as the frequency of its occurrence in the experimental situation (i.e. repetition). Between 200 and 400 msec, the ERP to written words shows a sensitivity to the eliciting word's frequency of occurrence in the language (King & Kutas 1998). The highest correlation is shown by the latency of a left anterior negativity, referred to as the lexical processing negativity (LPN); this subsumes the so-called N280 component (Neville, Mills, & Lawson 1992). See Figure 3.

For words occurring in a list rather than in sentences, frequency is also reflected in the amplitude of a negativity with a posterior, slightly right-hemisphere amplitude bias known as N400 (for a review see Kutas & Van Petten 1994). This negativity characterizes the response to any letter string that is orthographically legal and pronounceable. In other words, words and pseudowords elicit an N400 whereas nonwords do not. For real words, the amplitude of the N400 is an inverse function of the word's eliciting frequency, all other factors held constant (Figure 4).

The N400 amplitude is also quite sensitive to repetition (for reviews see Mitchell, Andrews, & Ward 1993; Van Petten et al. 1991). For example, repeating nouns in a list or in text yields a smaller-amplitude N400 on the second as opposed to first presentation – see Figure 4. Such repetition effects occur both within and across the visual and auditory modalities. The N400 repetition effect is also sensitive to the lag between occurrences of the word, the reduction being largest for immediate repetitions.

Another repetition-sensitive component of the ERP is a late positivity (hereafter LPC). In list presentations, the LPC is larger for the second than the first presentation of a word and is specific to low-frequency words (Rugg 1990). There also are some reports of a repetition effect preceding the N400, in the latency range of the P2 (200–250 msec, primarily frontal; Rugg 1987). However, this early effect

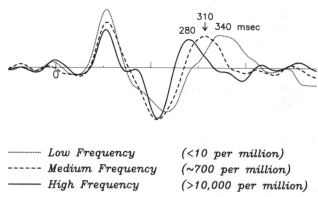

Figure 3. Grand average ERPs from a left anterior site overlying Broca's area in response to words presented one at a time in sentences read for comprehension. Overlapped are three ERPs to words (of both open and closed class) sorted as a function of their frequency of occurrence in the English language and digitally high-pass–filtered at 4 Hz. Note the latency of the negative peak (known as the lexical processing negativity or LPN) is longest for low-frequency words, shortest for high-frequency words, and intermediate in latency for words that are intermediate in frequency.

has been ephemeral – present in some studies but absent in other apparently similar experimental designs, and not always in the same direction (for review, see Van Petten et al. 1991).

During the 200–400-msec time range in which the ERP becomes sensitive to word frequency and repetition, effects of lexical class (open versus closed class) appear. Words with significant semantic content such as nouns and verbs are called "open class" words, while words with more relational content such as determiners and prepositions are called "closed class" or "function" words. Languages tend to have a finite set of closed-class words that remains relatively constant over time; English has had approximately the same 200–300 function words for hundreds of years. In contrast, as knowledge and technology changes, new nouns and verbs are regularly added to the open class (e.g., *motherboard, faxing, camcorder, internet*).

The LPN is sensitive to word frequency, irrespective of word class. Thus, two words with the same frequency in the language elicit LPNs with the same latency even if one is an open-class and the other a closed-class word. In contrast, later components in the ERP are sensitive to lexical class. For example, closed-class words typically elicit much smaller N400s than open-class words, except under particular circumstances where the closed-class word is less expected than usual (King & Kutas 1995; Kluender & Kutas 1993a).

The ERP is also sensitive to further lexical subdivisions within open-class words, such as between nouns and verbs. Koenig and Lehmann (1996) reported ERP laterality differences between nouns and verbs in a list as early as 120 msec, and Brown, Lehmann, and Marsh (1980) likewise noted distributional differences between them beginning about 300 msec after word onset. The latter study used noun–verb homophones (e.g. *fire*), so the processing difference occurred when the same perceptual forms were interpreted either as a noun or as a verb. Differentiations within the category of nouns have also been described. Concrete nouns – those depicting a tangible, often pictureable, entity – elicit larger N400s than do abstract nouns depicting an entity that is not readily pictureable (e.g. *honor*) (Kounios & Holcomb 1994).

The N400 amplitude thus varies with lexical and lexical-semantic factors. As we shall see shortly, N400 amplitude is also sensitive to the semantic relations between words in isolation and within sentences. The results of intracranial recording studies, performed on patients undergoing testing prior to surgery for temporal lobe epilepsy, have suggested that at least some of the activity recorded at the surface in the N400 time window derives from medial temporal lobe structures (Nobre & McCarthy 1995). And PET studies of semantic processing (e.g. Vandenberghe et al. 1996) have described activations in medial temporal lobe

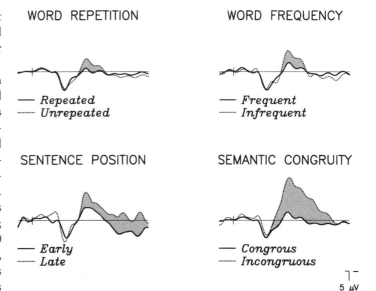

Figure 4. Shown are a sample of N400 effects at a midline parietal recording site averaged across subjects and sentences. *Top left.* Word repetition effect, reflecting the reduction in N400 amplitude with repetition in sentence contexts. *Top right.* Word frequency effect, reflecting the reduction in N400 amplitude with increasing word frequency. *Bottom left.* Sentence position effect, reflecting that – in congruent, declarative sentences – open-class words early in the sentence have larger N400s than those later in the sentence. *Bottom right.* Semantic congruity effect, reflecting the large N400s to semantically incongruous endings.

areas that are consistent with their proposed involvement in lexical and semantic processing.

TWO OF A KIND: PROCESSING OF WORD PAIRS

As previously noted, much language research is predicated on the existence of a mental lexicon and thus is aimed at determining its internal organization. Toward this end, a large number of studies have contrasted the responses to pairs of words that systematically vary along some dimension (orthography, phonology, morphology, semantics) as participants make some decision about them. These studies, only some of which are reviewed here, ask: (1) what features constitute a lexical entry, (2) how words with multiple meanings are represented and accessed (e.g. Van Petten & Kutas 1987); and (3) whether or not it makes sense to talk about an "amodal" representation of the meaning of a concept that can be accessed via written, spoken, and signed words (as well as via pictures).

Phonological and Morphological Relationships in Word Pairs

As interfaces between the perceptual form of a word and its lexical and semantic properties, orthographic and phonological information are important components of most models of the lexicon. Several ERP studies have shown that the influences of these cues can be observed in the N400 time window and beyond. For example, in rhyme judgment tasks, rhyming word pairs elicit a smaller negativity between 250 and 550 msec than do nonrhyming word pairs (Sanquist et al. 1980). When the rhyming pairs are orthographically dissimilar (e.g., *moose–juice*), reduced N400s could be attributed to the phonemic similarity. However, when phonemic and orthographic similarity are crossed, Polich and colleagues (1983) found that both influence the amplitude of the N400, consistent with behavioral reports that orthography cannot be ignored during rhyme judgment (Seidenberg & Tanenhaus 1979). Rugg and Barrett (1987) further demonstrated that orthographic, and not just visual, similarity modulates N400 amplitude.

Morphological influences on word processing also have been observed in the ERP by about 250 msec. Morphological processing involves both the derivation of new words ("derivational morphology") and the marking of case, number, tense, and other word features ("inflectional morphology"). As it happens, for many subsystems of inflectional morphology, regular patterns (e.g., in English past tense: *stretch/stretched*; in English plurals: *friend/friends*) can be contrasted with irregular ones (e.g., *catch/caught*; *woman/women*). A current theoretical debate concerns whether or not the same computational algorithms and/or neural hardware can deal with the analyses of both regular and irregular word forms. Traditionally, our ability to generalize from regularities in the language to novel instances has been taken as evidence that rules of the sort described by linguists are stored in our brains. Proponents of this view contend that there are two distinct mechanisms for dealing with regular and irregular words: (i) a set of rules that are routinely applied to regular forms and to new words, and (ii) a memorized store of a few frequent, irregular forms (e.g. Prince & Pinker 1988). There are those, however, who have argued that a single, domain-general, associative mechanism – as in some connectionist models – can deal with, for instance, past tense formation or plural formation of both regular and irregular words (Plunkett & Marchman 1993). This is a highly controversial area of investigation to which a number of psychophysiological techniques have been summoned.

Because electrophysiological measures reflect subtle processing differences between different classes of stimuli, they are well suited for determining the extent to which regular and irregular word forms are differentially processed. Penke et al. (1997) examined the German past participle system, which is similar to the English past tense in having regular and irregular verbs but different in that all irregular verbs share the same suffix ("-n," with or without a vowel change in the stem). They employed a morphological violation paradigm wherein participants saw both regular and irregular participles with correct and incorrect

suffixes. In three experiments, irregular verbs with the (incorrect) regular inflection elicited a left anterior negativity (LAN); violations of regular verbs showed no such activity. This same pattern of effects was observed for similar comparisons in the German plural system (Weyerts et al. 1997).

Weyerts and co-workers (1995) examined this same issue by comparing ERPs to past participles primed either by themselves (identical repetition) or by their respective infinitive (morphological repetition). For regular verbs, both identical and morphological repetitions showed a similarly sized enhanced positivity from about 250 msec. For irregular verbs, however, the morphological repetition effect was small and delayed relative to identity repetition. In short, various ERP analyses do point to processing differences between regular and irregular morphological forms in adults. Yet it remains an open question exactly how distinct the neural representations of the two are.

Semantic Relations

A number of reaction time and psychophysiological measures indicate that the processing of a single word is facilitated by the prior occurrence of a semantically related word. For instance, the word *cat* is easier to process if it is preceded by a word (such as *dog*) that bears a meaningful relationship to it. This facilitation, known as "semantic priming," is generally interpreted as indicative of the way in which lexical (word) representations are organized in our mental lexicon.

Electrophysiological signs of semantic relations between words have been investigated primarily using two tasks. In the lexical decision task (LDT), participants are asked to decide whether or not a letter string constitutes a real word (Bentin, McCarthy, & Wood 1985; Holcomb 1988). In the category membership verification task, participants indicate whether or not a word is a member of a particular category (Boddy & Weinberg 1981; Fischler et al. 1983; Heinze, Münte, & Kutas 1998; Neville et al. 1986).

In both these tasks, ERPs to semantically primed words are more positive between 200 and 500 msec than are those to unprimed words. The ERP difference is presumably the same N400 component discussed previously in the section on frequency and repetition effects (and to be discussed later with respect to semantic violations in sentences). Very similar effects obtain for written and spoken words – including cross-modally, when one of the words is spoken and the other is written – as well as when priming is by a line drawing, picture, or an environmental sound (Ganis, Kutas, & Sereno 1996; Van Petten & Rheinfelder 1995). The N400 effects in different modalities are similar in consisting of a monophasic negative wave between 200 and 600 msec, but they differ in overall amplitude, onset latency, and scalp distribution. For example, Holcomb and Neville (1990) found that – compared with visual priming – the auditory priming effect was larger, began 50–100 msec earlier, and was more pronounced over frontal and left hemisphere sites. Distributional differences notwithstanding, the reliability with which N400 amplitude is modulated by semantic relations has made it a useful metric for testing various hypotheses about language processing.

Among the more controversial issues in semantic priming literature has been the relative contribution of "automatic" and "attentional" processes to the observed response facilitation (e.g. Den Heyer, Briand, & Dannenbring 1983). This controversy grows out of the larger debate over the modularity of language abilities, with the assumption that modular processes are automatic. Thus, of some interest is the question of whether the N400 component of the ERP indexes automatic lexical (modular) processes or rather nonmodular, controlled effects. Studies examining N400 modulation – by factors such as the proportion of related and unrelated words (Chwilla, Brown, & Hagoort 1995; Holcomb 1988), the stimulus onset asynchrony (SOA) between the prime and target (Anderson & Holcomb 1995), the presence of a mask on the prime or target (Brown & Hagoort 1993; Neville, Pratarelli, & Forster 1989), and subjects' attentional stance with respect to various aspects of the experimental design (Bentin, Kutas, & Hillyard 1995; Gunter et al. 1994; McCarthy & Nobre 1993; Otten, Rugg, & Doyle 1993) – suggest that the N400 in fact indexes processing that is neither completely automatic nor completely controlled.

SENTENCE COMPREHENSION

Even though the psychology of words seems a rich enough field to absorb all of our language research effort for years to come, analyses at the word level alone will not suffice to explain how we derive meaning from language. Many aspects of words themselves are very difficult to understand without appealing to the sentence- or text-level phenomena with which they interact.

Semantic Context in Sentences

Much of the research employing sentences focuses on the response to a particular word that either fits or does not fit with the sentence's meaning or structure. For example, studies using eye movement protocols typically embed words of interest into connected prose and measure eye movement variables on the target word. These variables include the duration of fixation (initial, or total) as well as number of fixations (i.e., if and how often a word is fixated or refixated). Many of these studies test hypotheses about the modularity of language processes such as lexical access. Word forms (either phonological or orthographic) are often associated with more than one meaning (e.g., *bank* – a money-lending institution or the land flanking a river). Controversy surrounds proposals as to how the different meanings for these ambiguous forms are ac-

cessed and the extent to which this lexical access is open to contextual modification.

To address these issues, researchers have compared eye movements to ambiguous and unambiguous words in sentence contexts designed to bias interpretation of the ambiguous word toward one of its several meanings. Ambiguous homographs may be either "biased," where one of the meanings for the word is much more frequent, or "unbiased," where the frequency of occurrence of the multiple meanings is essentially the same. Pacht and Rayner (1993) found in neutral contexts that readers fixated longer on balanced than on biased homographs, suggesting an increased processing load for determining the meaning of an ambiguous word when neither frequency nor context provided clues. However, in biasing contexts (with the bias always toward the subordinate meaning), readers read balanced homographs as quickly as unambiguous controls but fixated on biased homographs for a longer duration. Pacht and Rayner (1993) and subsequently Sereno (1995) suggested that these results from eye movement studies support a "reordered access model" for the processing of ambiguous words in which all meanings of an ambiguous word are accessed independent of context but in an order that is contextually controlled (see Van Petten and Kutas 1987 for an electrophysiological study of homographs).

The processing of words in sentences and their influence by semantic and syntactic constraints has also been extensively studied with ERPs. For instance, Kutas and Hillyard (1980) reported that a semantically anomalous word at the end of a sentence elicits a large negativity peaking around 400 msec (N400) (Figure 4). A similar N400 effect is observed for semantic anomalies in written, spoken, and signed language. Subsequent research has shown that N400 elicitation is not specific to semantic violations and that its amplitude for words in a sentence reflects finer gradations of the semantic constraints placed on that word (for review see Kutas & Van Petten 1994).

In fact, N400 amplitude and the "cloze" probability of a word (i.e., what proportion of subjects will fill in a particular word as being the most likely completion of a sentence fragment; Taylor 1953) are inversely correlated at a level above 90%. In this context, it is important to note the distinction between the cloze probability of a terminal word and the contextual constraint of a sentence fragment per se. For example, "The paint turned out to be the wrong …" is of high contextual constraint in that most people will fill in *color,* whereas "He was soothed by the gentle …" is of low contextual constraint because there are a number of acceptable endings, none of which is clearly preferred over the others (Bloom & Fischler 1980). But both fragments can be completed by words of equal (low) cloze probability, as in, "The paint turned out to be the wrong shade" and "He was soothed by the gentle wind." Crossing several levels of contextual constraint with several levels of cloze probability revealed that N400 amplitude is specifically correlated with the cloze probability of the final word and not with the contextual constraint of the preceding sentence fragment (Kutas & Hillyard 1984; Kutas, Lindamood, & Hillyard 1984). This result was critical in establishing that N400 amplitude does not index the violation of previously established expectancies for a particular word that was not presented; rather, it is sensitive to the degree to which the sentence fragment prepares the way for the word that actually follows.

This effect of contextual constraint on the N400 is also seen in the ERPs to open-class words averaged according to sentence position (Figure 4); the amplitude of the N400 decreases monotonically with a word's ordinal position (Van Petten & Kutas 1991). The observation that this decrement did not occur in random word strings of equal length was taken as evidence that it was due to a sentence-level factor. Semantic context is also capable of eliminating the N400 frequency effect; thus, the effect of larger N400s to low- than high-frequency words observed early in a sentence is absent near the end of a sentence (when N400 amplitudes are equal). This interaction is not apparent in either random word strings or syntactically legal but semantically anomalous sentences, so it seems to be due to semantic factors (Van Petten & Kutas 1990, 1991).

Contrasts of lexical–associative semantic relationships and sentence-level semantic relationships indicate that both independently influence N400 amplitude (Kutas 1993; Van Petten 1995; Van Petten & Kutas 1991; see also Fischler et al. 1985 for a similar conclusion) and interact with comprehension skill (Van Petten et al. 1997). The N400 is thus sensitive to relationships between (i) a word and its immediate sentential context and (ii) a word and other words in the lexicon. Federmeier and Kutas (1999) examined this feature in a study where participants were asked to read pairs of sentences leading to an expectation for a particular item in a particular semantic category.

Ann wanted to treat her foreign guests to an all-American dessert.
So she went out in the back yard and picked some apples.

These sentence pairs were terminated with either the expected item (*apples*), an unexpected item from the expected category (another fruit – e.g. *oranges*), or an unexpected item from a different semantic category (e.g. *carrots*). Both types of unexpected endings elicited an N400 relative to congruent endings. However, even though both kinds of unexpected endings had the same cloze probabilities and were rated as equally implausible, the unexpected item from the expected category had a smaller N400 than did the one from a different category. The extent of this reduction correlated with sentential constraint – that is, how much the expected item was expected. These results suggest that the N400 is sensitive to the organization of background knowledge as well as to the relationship between words and sentence contexts. More generally, the findings

suggest that on-line comprehension processes utilize background semantic knowledge to make sense of sentences.

Syntactic Manipulations

The influence of structural aspects of language is studied in a subfield of psycholinguistics called sentence processing. Psychophysiological approaches to these phenomena have only recently become more common. We begin by describing investigations of subsentence units such as phrases and clauses. We then examine work done at the sentence level, including studies of syntactic violations and ambiguities and argument structure violations.

There has been relatively little work done directly on the psychophysiological correlates of the processing of phrases, especially noun phrases. In fairness, this dearth of research parallels that seen in the behavioral psycholinguistics literature (but see Murphy 1990). (Related, but conceptually distinct, is work in so-called modifier attachment ambiguities, discussed shortly.) Typical of the studies that indirectly address these issues is Neville et al. (1991), where one condition contrasted sentences that had normal phrase structure with those that had the following kind of phrase structure violation.

The scientist criticized Max's proof of the theorem.
*The scientist criticized Max's of proof the theorem.

Loosely speaking, a possessive NP like *Max's* acts like a definite article when it occurs in the context of another NP (here, the expected object of *criticized*). In a typical NP, a definite article is followed by either an adjective or a noun; since *of* is a preposition, this can be viewed as a violation of phrase structure. In this case, this violation was indexed by a brief enhancement of the negativity at left anterior electrode sites followed by a large, widespread positivity that is frequently observed in response to syntactic violations of many kinds.

The Neville et al. (1991) paper illustrates a key difficulty of using the violation approach to investigate phrase structure: generating a phrase structure violation at one point often causes phrase structure violations at other points and very possibly violations of other grammatical principles as well. Thus in the second sentence, *of* should begin a prepositional phrase (PP). The structure of a PP dictates that a preposition be followed by an NP, so *proof* should begin an NP. But this is not the case – one cannot say either "*Max corrected proof" or "*Max corrected proof of the theorem." Similarly, *the theorem* in the second sentence violates the entire VP because the verb *criticized* requires one and only one argument NP and *the theorem* is the second. Neville et al. (1991) focused on "Max's of proof" as an ungrammatical NP and did not discuss what effects these subsequent phrase structure errors had on the recorded ERPs.

Clauses are units larger than phrases. For example, in "The sentences that have been discussed previously

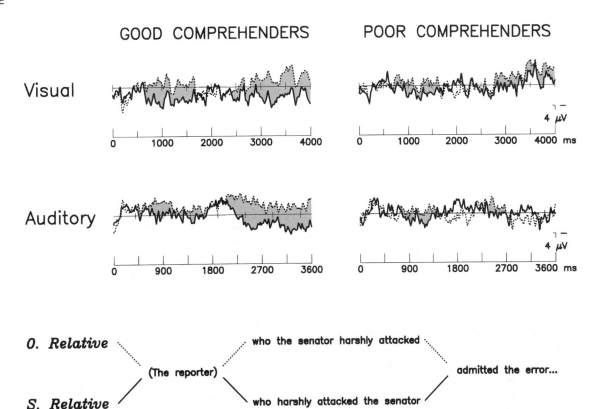

GOOD COMPREHENDERS · POOR COMPREHENDERS

Visual

Auditory

O. *Relative* ····· who the senator harshly attacked ·····
(The reporter) ····· admitted the error...
S. *Relative* ····· who harshly attacked the senator

contained no relative clauses," the subject of the sentence has been modified by a relative clause ("that have been discussed previously"). Conventionally, relative clauses are analyzed as sentences missing one of their NPs – in this case, the object of the verb *discussed*. Since this relative clause is missing its object, it is called an "object relative clause." Sentences like these are known to be more difficult to process than many other sentence types, including others containing relative clauses. Object relatives are particularly difficult to comprehend when the NPs in the main and relative clauses both refer to human, animate actors. Consider the following examples.

Object Relative
The reporter who the senator attacked admitted the error.

Subject Relative
The reporter who attacked the senator admitted the error.

Figuring out who did what to whom is more difficult in an object-relative sentence like the first one than in a so-called subject-relative sentence like the second, whether difficulty is measured using gaze duration (Holmes & O'Regan 1981), word-by-word reading times (King & Just 1991), or pupillary diameter (Just & Carpenter 1993). Based on these measures, the point of greatest difficulty is located at the end of the object-relative clause, when it is necessary to assign thematic roles to the actors involved.

Part of the difficulty involved in parsing these kinds of structures may be related to load they place on working memory (WM). Information provided earlier in the

Figure 5. Comparison of grand average ERPs to subject-relative (solid line) and object-relative (dotted line) sentences from a left anterior site in good and poor comprehenders. The visual sentences were presented one word every 500 msec, whereas the auditory sentences were presented as natural speech. Note that the two sentence types are equivalent both prior to and after the relative clause. The shading represents the area where object-relative sentences are reliably more negative than subject-relative sentences. The visual data are taken from King & Kutas (1995), the auditory data from Mueller, King, & Kutas (1997). Reprinted by permission of the authors.

sentence must be maintained over time in order to determine the identity of the "missing" NP. In fact, the need to maintain information over multiple words is a general property of sentence processing. The earliest emphasis on WM constraints in sentence processing focused on the possibility that limited capacity could lead to parsing failures for otherwise grammatical constructions (Miller & Chomsky 1963). Even when parsing does not fail altogether, however, "subcritical" loads can affect the time course and nature of parsing and interact with reading ability (Just & Carpenter 1992).

Relative clauses provide a controlled way to study working memory and other factors in sentence processing because they differ in complexity despite a close similarity in structure. Moreover, without being ungrammatical, they offer opportunities for making comparisons at multiple time points during processing. Results for English versions of these sentences in both the visual and auditory modality are summarized in Figure 5. These ERPs are the brain responses at a left frontal electrode site elicited by the words throughout relative clauses when read one word at a time (King & Kutas 1995) or heard as natural speech (Mueller, King, & Kutas 1997). As can be seen, the electrophysiological differences are present for good comprehenders and absent for poor comprehenders in both modalities. Although the largest difference between the two sentence types does occur near the end of the relative clause, there is an earlier negativity (left anterior over all scalp sites) that begins as soon as the second NP is encountered in the object-relative clause. This effect has been hypothesized to index the temporary storage of NP-related material in working memory (King & Kutas 1995) and is similar to effects noted in related sentence types by Kluender and Kutas (1993a,b). The later effect in these data may be of similar origin (WM operations required to perform thematic role assignments) or more directly related to the sentence processing task.

Although these relative clause types are unambiguous in English, in German they can be made to be ambiguous until the final word of the clause (Mecklinger et al. 1995). When this is the case, readers appear to expect the more frequent (subject-relative) structure, and a late positivity similar to that seen in response to patently ungrammatical stimuli is elicited by the less frequent object-relative structure. Moreover, if readers are given contextual cues that can be used to generate specific expectancies for a clause type then they appear to do so, as reflected in modulations of the amplitude of the late positivity (Ferstl & Friederici 1997).

Irrespective of clause type, clause boundaries are critical junctures for the study of sentence processing. Eye movement data have revealed that extra processing occurs at these points (Just & Carpenter 1980), while studies using skin conductance responses have suggested that active syntactic processes may be "wrapped up" or relaxed at clause boundaries (Bever, Kirk, & Lackner 1969). There are also clear clause-ending effects in ERP data in both the visual and auditory modalities; these take the form of fronto-central negativities that are larger and more marked over the left than the right hemisphere (Kutas & King 1996; Mueller et al. 1997). These clause-ending negativities (CENs) are different from most of the ERP effects discussed previously in that they do not appear to be just another component of the response to a single word; rather, they are one of several slow brain potential effects that occur during sentence processing.

One brain potential that has played an important role in the study of syntactic and morphosyntactic processing is the P600, sometimes called the syntactic positive shift (SPS). This slow positive shift has been described in several studies (Coulson, King, & Kutas 1998; Hagoort, Brown, & Groothusen 1993; Neville et al. 1991; Osterhout & Holcomb 1992) examining a range of phenomena – including agreement, phrase structure, subcategorization, and subjacency – in three languages (English, German, and Dutch). Although

the nature of the P600 component has not been wholly consistent across studies, it is typically described as beginning around 500 msec and having its midpoint around 600 msec. Its distribution is most often posterior, although anterior effects have also been reported. The P600 component is sometimes preceded by a negativity over left anterior sites.

The P600 has been observed in response to a host of morphosyntactic and syntactic violations, including relatively "local" agreement like subject–verb agreement (Coulson et al. 1998; Hagoort et al. 1993) and pronoun agreement (Coulson et al. 1998). Using Dutch stimuli in which sentential subjects agreed or failed to agree with their verbs, Hagoort and colleagues (1993) observed an SPS (P600), beginning after 500 msec and largest over parietal scalp sites, to the violations. Coulson et al. (1998) likewise observed a P600 to violations of subject–verb agreement ("Every Monday he *mow the lawn) and pronoun agreement ("The plane took *we to paradise and back") in English. However, they found that its amplitude varied with the probability of ungrammatical trials within an experimental block. In fact, the P600 to all improbable trials (collapsed across grammaticality) was indistinguishable from that to all grammatical violations (collapsed across probability) – see Figure 6. These effects of grammaticality and probability were nonadditive, implying overlapping neural generators. Thus, Coulson et al. (1998) argue that the P600 is not a syntactic-specific component but rather a variant of a domain-general component known as P3b, which has been hypothesized to reflect "context updating" (Donchin & Coles 1988).

In addition to indexing local relationships, the P600 has also been observed in response to more global syntactic violations. Both Neville et al. (1991) and Osterhout and

Figure 6. Grand average ERPs to midsentence critical items at a right parietal electrode site. The left half shows a larger late positive wave (P600) to ungrammatical than grammatical continuations of a sentence frame. The right half shows a similar larger late positivity when the continuation, regardless of its grammaticality, was improbable (20%) within that experimental block. Data are from Coulson, King, & Kutas (1998).

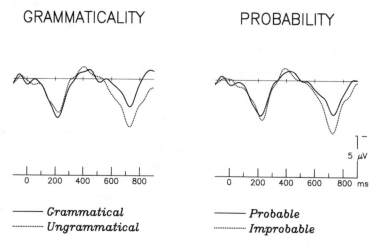

GRAMMATICALITY

——— Grammatical
············ Ungrammatical

PROBABILITY

5 μV

——— Probable
············ Improbable

Holcomb (1992) describe a slow positive shift between 500 and 700 msec to violations of phrase structure in English (e.g., "The broker hoped to sell the stock *was sent to jail"), albeit with different scalp distributions. Hagoort et al. (1993) observed a broadly distributed positivity beginning about 100 msec in response to phrase structure violations in Dutch sentences. Subjacency violations have also been reported to elicit broadly distributed P600 effects beginning after 700 msec (Neville et al. 1991). Finally, Osterhout and Holcomb (1992) reported a posterior P600 effect between 600 and 900 msec to subcategorization violations, an effect that others have failed to observe (Hagoort et al. 1993; Rösler et al. 1993).

In summary, the diversity of the time course and distribution of the ERP potentials labeled P600 or SPS makes it difficult to determine what this component is – if, indeed, it is a single phenomenon. The work by Coulson and colleagues (1998) further suggests that at least the component observed for morphosyntactic violations may not be just a "syntax ERP." However, that a positivity or family of positivities is observed to most syntactic violations at a number of levels provides a convenient tool for testing hypotheses about grammatical processing.

Parsing, as discussed in the introduction, includes the assignment of phrase and argument structure to parts of a sentence. In some cases, however, this assignment can be ambiguous. For example, on hearing "After Joan kicked the ball …" it is unclear whether *ball* is an argument of *kicked* ("After Joan kicked the ball, her brother became angry") or the subject of a new clause ("After Joan kicked, the ball was passed to the other team"). These ambiguities offer an opportunity for examining how different aspects of sentence processing interact (or fail to interact). Can the initial assignment of structure be influenced by semantic context? Or do the assignment of form and the derivation of meaning take place in different modules?

Eye movement studies of reading have suggested that context does not affect a sentence's initial parse. Rather, it appears that a single interpretation is automatically assigned in cases of structural ambiguity. Note that this contrasts with eye movement results for lexical ambiguity, where all possible interpretations seem to be activated. These initial structural assignments, which some have argued are not influenced by linguistic context or world knowledge, may result in misparsings that can be detected by long fixations and/or regressive eye movements at the point in the sentence where the ambiguity is resolved (for a review see Rayner & Morris 1992).

Debate over the influences of context on syntactic processing, however, still looms large. These eye movement results from reading paradigms conflict with those from other paradigms showing that context and/or world knowledge can influence syntactic assignment. Tanenhaus et al. (1995) measured natural eye movements as individuals scanned objects while listening to simple commands. The

assignment of ambiguous prepositions (e.g., whether *on* in "put the red box on the …" modified *red box* or described the location of action) was significantly influenced by the set of items available for manipulation. Furthermore, ERP data suggest that at least some kinds of context can affect parsing during reading.

For example, Garnsey, Tanenhaus, and Chapman (1989) constructed stimulus sentences so that the presence or absence of an ERP violation response would answer the question of whether or not subjects use verb argument preferences as an on-line aid to sentence parsing. They used sentences with embedded questions to determine when subjects would assign a questioned item (i.e. filler) to a possible gap, as follows.

(a) The babysitter didn't know which door the child PUSHED ___ carelessly at the store.
(b) The babysitter didn't know which name the child PUSHED ___ carelessly at the store.
(c) The tour operator wondered which visitor the guide WALKED ___ briskly down the hall.
(d) The tour operator wondered which topic the guide WALKED ___ briskly down the hall.

Because *push* usually takes a direct object, a flexible parsing strategy based on verb argument preferences and an inflexible "first resort" strategy would both assign *door* and *name* to the first possible gap location after the verb. Either strategy would thus result in a semantic incongruity at *pushed* in (b), as indexed by a large N400 relative to the control sentence (a). However, the two strategies predict different outcomes when the verb does not preferentially take an object, as in (c) and (d). Strict adherence to a first-resort strategy would result in a large N400 following the verb *walked* in (d) but not in (c). On the other hand, if the parser were sensitive to verb argument preference then neither (c) nor (d) would be anomalous at the verb and no N400 effect would be observed; this is, indeed, what the results showed. The ERP findings thus suggest that parsing may be more flexible and context-sensitive than eye movement studies have suggested thus far.

The Syntax–Semantics Boundary: Thematic Role Assignment

Thematic role assignments are an integral part of parsing. However, thematic roles also tend to be correlated with semantic properties of words and constructions. This aspect of language processing is thus a good venue for examining the syntax–semantics interface and interactions between these two proposed levels. To date, few psychophysiological studies of thematic role assignment have been conducted.

Weckerly (1995) showed that ERPs are sensitive to the relationship between expected thematic roles and noun animacy. Sentence-initial NPs are likely to be agents in a variety of phrase structure types, and the agent role is usually associated with animate discourse participants. Hence it might be the case that, when an inanimate noun occurs in this position, it will be less expected owing to its mismatch with thematic expectations (even before the verb is encountered) and thus will generate a larger N400 response. This is what Weckerly (1995) observed, among other effects at different locations in object-relative constructions. The fact that readers are sensitive to possible animacy–role conflicts early in the sentence suggests that they are continually monitoring the word input stream for potentially useful information and attempting to construct higher-level structures as quickly as possible – even when lower-level structures are incomplete.

Referential Level Processing

Psychophysiological measures likewise have only rarely been used to study referential effects in sentence processing. However, since pronouns refer directly to discourse participants, the response to a pronoun in context can be used to index the success or failure of referential processing. There are syntactic constraints on the use of pronouns versus reflexive pronouns, and Osterhout and Mobley (1995) have investigated these in English. In an experiment where participants were explicitly judging sentence acceptability, violations of both the number and gender of a reflexive pronoun elicited a P600-like response.

Number Violation
The hungry guests helped themselves to the food.
The hungry guests helped *himself to the food.

Gender Violation
The successful woman congratulated herself on the promotion.
The successful woman congratulated *himself on the promotion.

In another experiment, Osterhout and Mobley (1995) compared the ERPs to pronouns that either matched or mismatched the subject noun in gender.

Matching
The aunt heard that she had won the lottery.

Nonmatching
The aunt heard that *he had won the lottery.

They found that the nonmatching pronouns elicited a larger P600 response, but only for those participants who judged such sentences unacceptable. Of course, these sentences are actually acceptable if no assumption is made that the pronoun refers to the subject NP. For participants who found such sentences acceptable, the ERPs to the nonmatching trials included a larger negativity over Wernicke's area as well as a broadly distributed and bilateral frontal negativity beginning approximately 200 msec after pronoun onset. Note that, in order to make sense of a nonmatching pronoun sentence without any other context,

a reader must hypothesize the existence of an unmentioned discourse participant. The frontal negativity may thus index the processes required to add new elements to the existing message-level representation.

Support for this referential explanation of the frontal negativity comes from King and Kutas (1997), who examined the response to pronouns of both genders in sentence frames where the subject noun was an occupational title that was either more or less likely to be filled by a person of male or female gender.

> The engineer redesigned the circuit because
> he   had detected a flaw.
> ?she

As one might expect, the paucity of female engineers in reality renders the version of this frame with *she* odd at first glance. Readers appear to treat the feminine pronoun here as referring to someone other than the engineer. The ERPs elicited by such "nonstereotypical" pronouns showed a large anterior negativity after about 200 msec (see Figure 7).

Although further work needs to be done using richer contexts, it appears that processes dependent on discourse reference can be systematically studied using on-line ERP data. In the cases just discussed, the recognition that a new discourse participant may have been mentioned forces a reorganization of the referential representation and possibly a shift in the frame or schema guiding comprehension. Coulson (1996) examined the process of frame shifting itself in greater detail using ERPs in a genre where the need for frame shifting is quite pronounced: the one-line joke. For example, in the following joke – "I let my accountant do my taxes because it saves time: Last year it saved me ten years" – the listener begins by setting up a message-level representation structured by a frame in which a busy professional pays an accountant to do his taxes. However, upon encountering *years* this interpretation is no longer tenable, and the reader is forced to map the existing message-level information into a new frame (i.e., to "frame shift"). By reinterpreting the word *time* as jail time, the reader can construct a revised interpretation in which a crooked businessman pays an accountant to conceal illegal financial dealings.

Coulson (1996) recorded ERPs as individuals read sentences that either ended as jokes and required frame shifting or ended with an equally unexpected but nonjoke ending. Although nonjoke endings were low-cloze (equivalent to the joke endings), they were chosen to be consistent with the contextually evoked frame. Jokes elicited greater-amplitude N400 than nonjokes, suggesting that the nonjoke endings were easier to integrate into the established context than were the joke endings. Results thus suggest that frame-based retrieval of background knowledge plays an important role in sentential integration.

Finally, one ERP study to date has examined referential processing in discourse- rather than sentence-level units. St. George, Mannes, and Hoffman (1994) recorded ERPs as participants read paragraphs of text that made sense when presented with a title but – when presented without a title – were quite difficult to comprehend (Bransford & Johnson 1972). They found a much smaller average N400 to words from the titled than untitled paragraphs. These results indicate that the N400 is sensitive to discourse-level as well as to more local, semantic relationships between words.

LANGUAGE PRODUCTION

Language production has been less thoroughly studied with psychophysiological measures than comprehension despite the importance and intricacies of the act of speaking (Levelt 1989). A novel approach to the study of language production was introduced by van Turennout, Hagoort, and Brown (1997). They used Levelt's (1989) model of speech production to derive predictions about the temporal order in which the different types of information become available; then they measured the presence or absence and polarity of the lateralized readiness potential (LRP) to test these predictions. The LRP measure is based on the observation that the brain activity preceding a finger movement is larger over the motor cortex contralateral to the responding hand. After a series of subtractions, this asymmetry can be used as an index of differential motor preparation (Coles, Gratton, & Donchin 1988; Smid, Mulder, & Mulder 1987), even if the prepared response is never actually emitted (as in the No-Go trials of a Go–No-Go task).

According to Levelt's (1989) model, semantic and conceptual information becomes available before phonological information when a person must name a pictured object. To test this hypothesis, van Turennout devised a two-choice Go–No-Go task in which conceptual information (living vs. nonliving) determined the side of the responding hand while phonological information determined whether the participant was to respond; only those pictures whose name ended with a particular phoneme required a response. It was predicted that if semantic information was indeed available before phonological information, then both Go and No-Go trials should be associated with an LRP indicating that the responding hand was prepared (even if the subsequent phonological decision aborted this prepared response on the No-Go trials). The predicted LRP pattern was obtained (see Figure 8). Moreover, instructions were then reversed so that the phonological information determined the responding hand while the conceptual information determined whether or not a response was given; here, no LRP was observed on No-Go trials. These data were

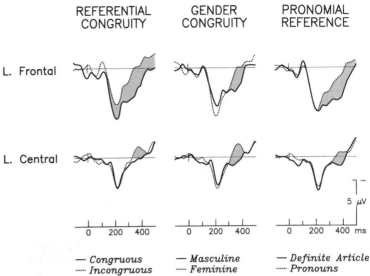

Figure 7. Event-related potential (ERP) effects on pronouns in a sentence context (King & Kutas 1997). Left column shows N400 (at left central site) and anterior negativity (at left frontal site) elicited by pronouns that were of incongruous gender given previous context. Center column shows an overall N400 effect for feminine compared to masculine pronouns, regardless of congruity. Right column shows anterior negativity in responses to pronouns when compared to definite articles; the former require that co-reference be established between the pronoun and referent whereas the latter do not.

offered as support for the temporal order of availability of information for speech in Levelt's (1989) model. In a subsequent study, van Turennout (1997) found that at least some types of syntactic information (the grammatical gender of a noun) also became available prior to phonological information. Most importantly, these studies show how ERPs can be used to investigate the timing of language production.

APPLICATION OF PSYCHOPHYSIOLOGICAL METHODS TO PATIENT POPULATIONS

Many of the initial insights into the relationship between brain areas and language processing came from the study of patients with various kinds of language disorders consequent to brain damage. Their continued study has provided information about the nature of brain–behavior relationships observed in normal individuals (e.g., whether a brain area is necessary for or merely involved in some language process) as well as about the relationship between language processing and other cognitive abilities. In this section we discuss applications of psychophysiological methods to the study of language deficits in Alzheimer's disease, basal ganglia disease, schizophrenia, developmental dyslexia, and aphasia.

Alzheimer's Disease

Alzheimer's disease is a neurodegenerative disease that is defined by a characteristic pattern of neuropathological

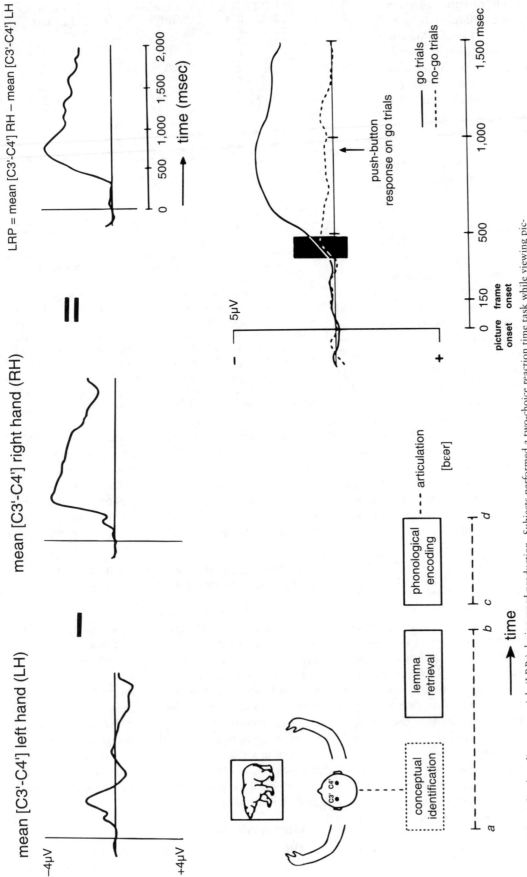

Figure 8. Lateralized readiness potentials (LRPs) during word production. Subjects performed a two-choice reaction time task while viewing pictures of objects and animals in order to name them. The response hand was determined by the living–nonliving distinction; the final phoneme of the word determined whether the response was to be carried out. Preparation of the response hand leads to a lateralized readiness potential that can be differentiated from other lateralized brain activity by a double subtraction (Coles, Gratton, & Donchin 1988; Smid, Mulder, & Mulder 1987), as shown across the top of the figure. As can be seen in the bottom right of the figure, this potential is present even in the No-Go trials, indicating that the semantic (living–nonliving) information was available to the subject before the phonological information. Adapted with permission from van Turennout, Hagoort, & Brown, "Electrophysiological evidence on the time course of semantic and phonological processes in speech production," *Journal of Experimental Psychology: Learning, Memory, and Cognition*, vol. 23, pp. 787–806. Copyright © 1997 by the American Psychological Association.

changes. Among a host of other neuropsychological deficits, patients display language difficulties, primarily naming deficits. Several researchers have found that – like control subjects – patients with probable diagnosis of Alzheimer's disease show reduced N400s to repeated words, despite impairments in their recognition memory (Friedman et al. 1992; Rugg et al. 1994). These results have led to the suggestion that the repetition N400 reflects an intact implicit memory system in Alzheimer's patients.

Smaller and later N400s, however, have been observed in Alzheimer's patients performing more complicated language tasks. Schwartz and co-workers (1996) tested the hypothesis that the hierarchical structure of semantic memory is impaired in Alzheimer's patients so that only broad category memberships are available (Hodges, Salmon, & Butters 1991). They used three levels of categorical abstraction (e.g., living things, plants, flowers) to see if, as predicted from the hierarchical breakdown view, Alzheimer's patients would experience the greatest difficulties with the most specific category members. This was not found to be the case; rather, the congruity effects on reaction times and N400s to the different category levels in patients and controls were similar. However, Alzheimer's patients did have smaller-amplitude N400s at somewhat later latencies than the age-matched controls (see also Iragui, Kutas, & Salmon 1996).

It might prove informative to correlate N400 effects of this type with known neuropathological changes in Alzheimer's disease, including plaques (i.e., aggregates of protein deposited in cortical areas), neurofibrillary tangles, and dramatic decrease in the number of cortical synapses. These changes are most pronounced in the entorhinal cortex and hippocampus, areas that have also been implicated in the generation of the N400 (Nobre & McCarthy 1995). However, the presence of normal N400 word repetition effects in Alzheimer's patients suggests there may be no such significant correlation. Perhaps different neural structures are involved in the generation of the semantic priming (or congruity) N400 effect and the repetition N400 effect.

Basal Ganglia Diseases

Basal ganglia diseases (including Parkinson's disease, Huntington's disease, supranuclear palsy, and others) subsume a set of conditions that – owing to neurodegeneration, predominantly in the basal ganglia – exhibit a complex pattern of hypo- or hyperkinetic movement disorders and associated neurobehavioral symptoms. These symptoms include impairments of executive functions and working memory as well as general slowness of thought processes. These neurobehavioral deficits have been attributed to abnormal functioning of neuronal circuits between the striatum and the cortex, especially frontal regions (Owen et al. 1992).

Disorders of language functioning have also been described in association with basal ganglia diseases. Illes

(1989) noted that spontaneous language production in Huntington's patients was characterized by a reduction in syntactic complexity, semantic paraphasias, and a predominance of closed-class phrases, whereas Parkinson's patients used predominantly open-class phrases. Rosser and Hodges (1994) found that both Huntington's and supranuclear palsy patients performed worse than controls on letter (production of words starting with a given letter) and categorical (production of instances of a category) fluency tasks, suggesting problems with initiation and memory retrieval. In two elegant investigations, Natsopoulos and associates (1991, 1993) showed that basal ganglia patients also experience greater than normal difficulty comprehending relative (especially object-relative) clauses and complement clauses. It is known that working memory plays a crucial role in the comprehension of relative clauses (King & Just 1991). These data therefore imply that – although language functions may be compromised in basal ganglia patients – their difficulties in at least some cases may be a by-product of deficits in more domain-general cognitive functions such as working memory, task initiation, and retrieval from memory.

Schizophrenia

The many symptoms of schizophrenia include several disturbances of language: reduced syntactic complexity (Thomas et al. 1996), the use of novel words (neologism) – including blends of existing words (Rochester & Marin 1979) – and the loosening of semantic associations. It is a matter of debate as to whether these deficits reflect difficulties with language processing per se, abnormal organization of semantic knowledge, or a more pervasive problem with information overload and/or attention (Schwartz 1982). Several groups of electrophysiologists have, with variable success, tested these alternatives using the N400. Smaller N400s have been observed in schizophrenic patients, but generally only when an explicit congruency judgment must be made (Grillon, Ameli, & Glazer 1991; Koyama et al. 1991; Mitchell et al. 1991). Thus it appears that at least part of schizophrenics' language dysfunction may reflect a difficulty in directing attention toward the relationship between words.

Schizophrenic individuals exhibit more than normal numbers of intrusions of semantically related words during spontaneous speech and greater than normal semantic priming effects via behavioral measures (Maher et al. 1987). Andrews and colleagues (1993) used ERPs to assess the abnormal organization of semantic memory that may underlie these phenomena. They employed sentences ending with congruous words, wholly incongruous words, and words that were incongruous but semantically related to the expected endings (e.g., "Father carved the turkey with a spoon"). They expected schizophrenics to show a greater N400 attenuation to semantically related incongruous endings, but both groups generated smaller N400s to related than unrelated endings and did not differ from each other. Thus, electrophysiological evidence for a differential organization of semantic memory in schizophrenia is equivocal. By contrast, however, almost all these studies reported a reliable 40–80-msec delay in the N400 latency. Among the potential explanations for this delay are generally slowed information processing (Grillon et al. 1991), overlap with an abnormal late positive component, and antipsychotic drugs.

Schizophrenic patients have also been investigated with PET and fMRI. These studies have employed verbal fluency tasks, known to pose difficulties for schizophrenic individuals and to activate dorsolateral prefrontal cortex. Frith and associates (1995) did not observe the expected reduced PET activation of the dorsolateral prefrontal cortex in schizophrenic patients, but they did note a greater than normal activation of the superior temporal gyrus. The superior temporal gyrus is presumed to be crucial for word representations, so Frith et al. (1995) attributed the symptomatology of the patients to abnormalities in this region. In a very similar design employing fMRI, Yurgelun-Todd and co-workers (1996) observed both the expected decreased activation in the left dorsolateral prefrontal and the greater activation of the left superior temporal gyrus in schizophrenic individuals.

In summary, the currently available data seem most consistent with the hypothesis that language deficits in schizophrenia are secondary to disturbances in other cognitive mechanisms, although the results are far from consistent. The contradictory findings in the literature undoubtedly stem in part from a lack of appreciation for the well-defined subtypes of schizophrenia, which vary significantly in symptomatology. Directing future research efforts toward the study of homogenous groups of patients may permit a more accurate assessment of the extent of strictly language problems in the most advanced stages of this disease.

Developmental Dyslexia

One of the more frequent learning disabilities, developmental dyslexia has been linked to abnormal development of the magnocellular pathway in the visual system (Lovegrove, Garzia, & Nicholson 1990) and/or reduced asymmetry of the planum temporale (Galaburda et al. 1985). At a psychological level, proposed deficits range from the integration of auditory stimuli (Tallal & Curtiss 1988) to syntactic analysis (Byrne 1981).

Several electrophysiological investigations have been aimed at better defining the psychological deficits involved in developmental dyslexia. Neville and colleagues (1993) found that dyslexic children had enhanced N400 amplitudes to sentence final words and interpreted this as a sign of their greater need to use context to compensate for deficits in visual word recognition. Johannes and co-workers (1995) reported similar findings and conclusions

for adult dyslexics. However, others have reported that dyslexics have smaller than normal N400s in picture-word–priming (Stelmack & Miles 1990) and rhyme-matching (Ackerman, Dykman, & Oglesby 1994) paradigms.

Paulesu and associates (1996) used PET to examine five adult dyslexics as they performed a phonological matching task and a short-term memory task. Broca's area and the temporoparietal areas were activated in both tasks in the normal controls; by contrast, in the dyslexics, Broca's area was active only during phonological matching and the temporoparietal areas were active only during the short-term memory task. These findings were taken as evidence for a functional disconnection between anterior and posterior language areas in dyslexics.

Aphasia

Despite its clinical importance, aphasia has received relatively little attention in psychophysiological investigations. Psychophysiological techniques might be especially revealing, as the language deficits in aphasia often occur without any apparent associated cognitive deficits. Aphasic patients offer an excellent means of determining if there is a direct link between the presence and absence of certain language symptoms (e.g. agrammatism) and certain purportedly linguistic components of the ERP, such as the P600/SPS.

In an elegant series of experiments, Hagoort, Brown, and Swaab (1996) and Swaab, Brown, and Hagoort (1997) investigated semantic analyses in a group of Dutch aphasics, including Wernicke's and Broca's aphasia. In one study, aphasics, nonaphasic right-hemisphere patients, and normal elderly controls heard pairs of words that were either semantically related (*church–villa*), associatively related (*bread–butter*), or unrelated. In normal controls and in those aphasics with mild comprehension deficits, the N400 effects for associative and semantic pairs were of equal size (Hagoort et al. 1996). In contrast, aphasic patients with more pronounced comprehension difficulties showed diminished N400 amplitudes only for the semantically related pairs, fueling speculations about the possible involvement of the right hemisphere in semantic processing (cf. Rodel et al. 1992). Swaab et al. (1997) investigated these same aphasics as they listened to sentences terminated by congruent and incongruent words. The main result was an approximately 100-msec delay of the N400 peak in the aphasic patients with the most profound comprehension deficits. This delay was interpreted as a sign of slower lexical integration, in line with several other reports that aphasics' comprehension difficulties result from a processing rather than a representational deficit (Friederici & Frazier 1992; Haarmann & Kolk 1994). Similar delays in the N400 component have also been observed in closed–head-injury patients who show general cognitive slowing (Münte & Heinze 1994).

Unlike the electrophysiological studies primarily aimed at delineating processing deficits in aphasia, PET studies

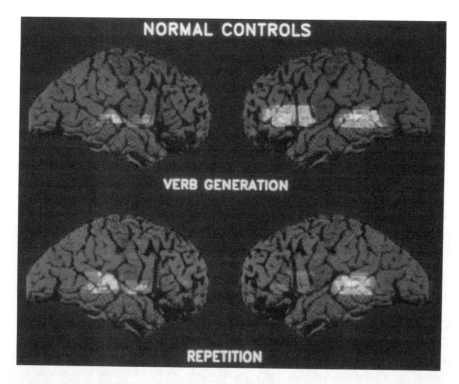

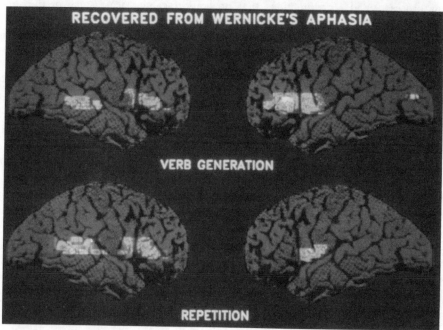

Figure 9. Cerebral regions associated with a verb generation task and a repetition task in six normal volunteers (top) and six patients after recovery from aphasia (bottom), expressed as means for each group based on positron emission tomography (PET). Statistical parametric maps for increases in regional cerebral blood flow during the tasks (compared to rest) rendered onto the lateral surfaces of brains using Talairach and Tournoux coordinates illustrate the distribution of major sites of activation in the right hemisphere. The cutoff for the z-score in the display is 3.09, corresponding to a Bonferroni corrected level of significance of $p < 0.087$. Reprinted with permission from Weiller, Isensee, Rijntjes, Huber, Müller, Bier, Dutschka, Woods, Noth, & Diener, "Recovery from Wernicke's aphasia: A positron emission tomography study," *Annals of Neurology,* vol. 37, pp. 723–32. Copyright © 1995 by the American Neurological Association.

have been focused on the issue of brain plasticity and recovery after language loss. For example, Weiller and colleagues (1995) studied six patients who had recovered from a Wernicke type aphasia. While the expected left hemi-spheric activations were observed in normal controls, the recovered patients showed activation of the homologous right-hemisphere regions (superior temporal gyrus, inferior premotor cortex, lateral prefrontal cortex) – see Figure 9.

These data were interpreted as reflecting a redistribution of language processing within a parallel pre-existing network (see also Ohyama et al. 1996).

Conclusions and Future Directions

Psychophysiological data have converged to build a picture of when and where language processes take place in the brain. In some cases, this information also places constraints on *how* language processing must be occurring.

Perhaps the most striking general conclusion that can be drawn is that language processing is far from a unified phenomenon. Rather, it appears to involve an astonishing array of computational and neurobiological processes that operate on an equally large number of representation types. Much research effort has gone into cataloging and understanding these differences. Both ERP components and fMRI/PET activations have been described that are sensitive to words and no other types of perceptual stimuli. Factors such as word frequency and word class have different ERP signatures. Different ERP indices of semantic and syntactic processing have been proposed.

It is up to future work to piece together the different processes and representations that previous research has defined. That is, while language processing clearly involves a large number of subprocesses, ultimately these must work together to derive meaning from sensory inputs or to instantiate meaning via motor outputs. Understanding language at this level – as an integrated, goal-directed process – will require elucidating the relationships that hold among language subcomponents and between language and other cognitive abilities.

For instance, understanding language utterances necessarily requires that relevant linguistic, contextual, and background knowledge be integrated. Very little is known, however, about the relative importance of immediate context and longer-term background knowledge for meaning construction. The two factors are obviously related: we understand context only because of background knowledge, which in turn is derived (in part) from correspondences we note in various language contexts. How is this relationship instantiated and how are conflicts resolved? We need to design experiments in which both factors are present and to develop measures that can explore their interactions.

It is also important to understand how language representations are built out of both abstract linguistic features and concrete perceptual features. What concrete features allow us to determine that a particular sensory input carries meaning? Do physical features of linguistic stimuli continue to play an important role in language processing beyond the point at which they are classified as words? Do they, for example, help us distinguish nouns from verbs? Does it make sense to talk about a modality-independent language representation at any level of processing?

These questions become especially important when language is taken out of the "white room" – the extremely controlled and fairly artificial setting of the laboratory (Cicourel 1996). In the real world, language processing occurs in a much richer context. Not only are the units of processing larger than those typically studied – discourses, rather than single words or sentences – but there are social and physical cues to guide the language user. In most cases, these cues occur freely interspersed with language; for example, one may point to rather than name an object. In the future we must exploit technological advances to bring more of the world into the laboratory: using tape recorders to study natural conversation, presenting readers with connected texts from natural sources, allowing language users to interact with objects as they process language, and so forth.

Understanding the relationship between aspects of language processing will naturally also entail understanding the role of nonlinguistic factors such as working memory and attention. It is likely that these factors are critical in the integration of more specific language processes, since attentional and working memory capacities may have to be shared across levels of analysis. Furthermore, at least some of the subcomponents of language processing identified thus far may ultimately turn out to be language-specific instantiations of these more general functions. For example, morphosyntactic marking and word order have traditionally been considered purely structural phenomena. However, Langacker (1987) suggested that they – as well as other presumably linguistic phenomena – can be understood more generally as profiling (or attentionally focusing) various aspects of evoked knowledge structures.

This understanding of the relationship between language and other cognitive processes may involve a rethinking of the other processes as well. For example, the exclusive division of cognitive processes into automatic and controlled may not be theoretically useful; rather, one may wish to locate processes on a continuum from automatic to controlled. For example, we briefly reviewed the debate over whether the N400 indexes automatic lexical processing or controlled postlexical processing. Yet the N400 seems in fact to index processes that are automatic in some ways but controlled in others. It has been speculated that semantic priming effects (and associated N400 effects) arise from an obligatory postlexical integrative process (à la Hodgson 1991). This sort of mechanism is neither clearly automatic–modular nor clearly interactive–nonmodular. It resembles modular lexical access in that it is a fast-acting process that acts on every lexical item; in view of large N400 components elicited by pseudowords, it appears moreover to act on every wordlike item. However, it resembles an interactive process in that it is sensitive to high-level inferential information of the sort traditionally associated with attentional processing (as in e.g. Coulson 1996; St. George et al. 1994). By rejecting views of language (or more general) processes that are inflexible and theory-laden, we may derive a more comfortable fit to psychophysiological data and a clearer understanding of language in its cognitive context.

Finally, there is a need to explore connections between language processing and other cognitive feats: the analysis of visual scenes (Sereno 1991), the understanding of diagrams (Hegarty, Carpenter, & Just 1995), and the perception of music (Besson, Faita, & Requin 1994; Besson & Macar 1987). Like language processing, these activities require that meaning be obtained over time from a well-structured source of information. Auditory sentences and music are both inherently structured over time. Diagrammatic processing, like reading, directs attention (and eye movements) from place to place in a surprisingly structured way – in a manner that can be convincingly related to the text that describes them (Hegarty et al. 1995). Visual scenes are less likely to have stereotypical inspection orders, but they are almost as likely to have predictable loci where fixations will occur. By understanding the similarities (and differences) between these types of cognitive processes, we gain insight into the general principles underlying all of cognition as well as an increased understanding of the defining properties of language.

In the future, then, using the various and sundry psychophysiological tools at our disposal, we may yet come to understand how Dickinson used her brain to generate poems … which we use our brains to decipher and appreciate.

NOTE

This work was supported by a postdoctoral fellowship from the McDonnell-Pew Center for Cognitive Neuroscience in Tucson, AZ to S.C., a Predoctoral Fellowship from the Howard Hughes Medical Institute to K.F., a McDonnell-Pew postdoctoral fellowship from the San Diego Center for Cognitive Neuroscience and funds from NIH grant T32 DC00041-01 to J.K., NICHD grant HD22614 and NIA grant AG08313 to M.K., and a grant from the Hermann and Lilly Schilling Foundation, Essen, Germany (TS 013/177/96) to T.M.

REFERENCES

Ackerman, P. T., Dykman, R. A., & Oglesby, D. M. (1994). Visual event-related potentials of dyslexic children to rhyming and nonrhyming stimuli. *J. Clin. Exp. Neuropsychol., 16*, 138–54.

Anderson, J. E., & Holcomb, P. J. (1995). Auditory and visual semantic priming using different stimulus onset asynchronies: An event-related brain potential study. *Psychophysiol., 32*, 177–90.

Andrews, S., Shelley, A. M., Ward, P. B., Fox, A., Catts, S. V., & McConaghy, N. (1993). Event-related potential indices of semantic processing in schizophrenia. *Biol. Psychiatry, 34*, 443–58.

Baldwin, J. (1963). Black man in America: An interview [Sound recording from radio interview with Studs Terkel] (N08P-6396-6397). Cambridge, MA: Credo.

Bentin, S., Kutas, M., & Hillyard, S. A. (1995). Semantic processing and memory for attended and unattended words in dichotic listening: Behavioral and electrophysiological evidence. *J. Exp. Psychol. Hum. Percept. Perf., 21*, 54–67.

Bentin, S., McCarthy, G., & Wood, C. C. (1985). Event-related potentials, lexical decision and semantic priming. *Electroenceph. Clin. Neurophysiol., 60*, 343–55.

Besson, M., Faita, F., & Requin, J. (1994). Brain waves associated with musical incongruities differ for musicians and non-musicians. *Neurosci. Let., 168*, 101–5.

Besson, M., & Macar, F. (1987). An event-related potential analysis of incongruity in music and other non-linguistic contexts. *Psychophysiol., 24*, 14–25.

Bever, T. G., Kirk, R., & Lackner, J. (1969). An autonomic reflection of syntactic structure. *Neuropsychologia, 7*, 23–8.

Bloom, P. A., & Fischler, I. S. (1980). Completion norms for 329 sentence contexts. *Mem. Cogn., 8*, 631–42.

Boddy, J., & Weinberg, H. (1981). Brain potentials, perceptual mechanism and semantic categorization. *Biol. Psychol., 12*, 43–61.

Bransford, J. D., & Johnson, M. K. (1972). Contextual prerequisites for understanding: Some investigations of comprehension and recall. *J. Verb. Learn. Verb. Behav., 11*, 717–26.

Brown, C. M., & Hagoort, P. (1993). The processing nature of the N400: Evidence from masked priming. *J. Cogn. Neurosci., 5*, 34–44.

Brown, W. S., Lehmann, D., & Marsh, J. T. (1980). Linguistic meaning related differences in evoked potential topography: English, Swiss-German, and imagined. *Brain Lang., 11*, 340–53.

Byrne, B. (1981). Deficient syntactic control in poor readers: Is a weak phonetic memory code responsible. *Applied Psycholing., 2*, 201–12.

Chwilla, D. J., Brown, C. M., & Hagoort, P. (1995). The N400 as a function of the level of processing. *Psychophysiol., 32*, 274–85.

Cicourel, A. (1996). Ecological validity and "white room effect": The interaction of cognitive and cultural models in the pragmatic analysis of elicited narratives from children. *Pragmatics Cogn., 4*, 221–64.

Coles, M. G., Gratton, G., & Donchin, E. (1988). Detecting early communication: Using measures of movement-related potentials to illuminate human information processing. *Biol. Psychol., 26*, 69–89.

Coulson, S. (1996). Semantic leaps: Frame-shifting and sentential integration. Ph.D. dissertation, Department of Cognitive Science, University of California, San Diego.

Coulson, S., King, J. W., & Kutas, M. (1998). Expect the unexpected: Event-related brain response to morphosyntactic violations. *Lang. Cogn. Proc., 13*, 21–58.

Den Heyer, K., Briand, K., & Dannenbring, G. L. (1983). Strategic factors in a lexical decision task: Evidence for automatic and attentional-driven processes. *Mem. Cogn., 11*, 374–81.

Dickinson, E. (1896/1970). *Complete Poems of Emily Dickinson* (Edited by T. H. Johnson). London: Faber.

Donchin, E., & Coles, M. G. H. (1988). Is the P300 component a manifestation of context updating? *Behav. Brain Sci., 11*, 357–74.

Fauconnier, G. (1994). *Mental Spaces: Aspects of Meaning Construction in Natural Language.* Cambridge University Press.

Federmeier, K. D., & Kutas, M. (1999). A rose by any other name: Long-term memory structure and sentence processing. *J. Mem. Lang., 41,* 469–95.

Ferstl, E. C., & Friederici, A. D. (1997). Inter-sentential context effects on parsing: A study using event-related potentials. Paper presented at the Tenth Annual CUNY Conference on Human Sentence Processing (Santa Monica, CA).

Fischler, I. S., Bloom, P. A., Childers, D. G., Roucos, S. E., & Perry, N. W. (1983). Brain potentials related to stages of sentence verification. *Psychophysiol., 20,* 400–9.

Fischler, I., Childers, D. G., Achariyapaopan, T., & Perry, N. W., Jr. (1985). Brain potentials during sentence verification: Automatic aspects of comprehension. *Biol. Psychol., 21,* 83–106.

Fletcher, P. C., Frith, C. D., Grasby, P. M., Shallice, T., Frackowiak, R. S., & Dolan, R. J. (1995). Brain systems for encoding and retrieval of auditory-verbal memory. An in vivo study in humans. *Brain, 118,* 401–16.

Fodor, J. A. (1983). *Modularity of Mind: An Essay on Faculty Psychology.* Cambridge, MA: MIT Press.

Friederici, A. D., & Frazier, L. (1992). Thematic analysis in agrammatic comprehension: Syntactic structures and task demands. *Brain Lang., 42,* 1–29.

Friedman, D., Hamberger, M., Stern, Y., & Marder, K. (1992). Event-related potentials (ERPs) during repetition priming in Alzheimer's patients and young and older controls. *J. Clin. Exp. Neuropsychol., 14,* 448–62.

Frith, C. D., Friston, K. J., Herold, S., Silbersweig, D., Fletcher, P., Cahill, C., Dolan, R. J., Frackowiak, R. S., & Liddle, P. F. (1995). Regional brain activity in chronic schizophrenic patients during the performance of a verbal fluency task. *Brit. J. Psychiat., 167,* 343–9.

Galaburda, A. M., Sherman, G. F., Rosen, G. D., Aboitiz, F., & Geschwind, N. (1985). Developmental dyslexia: Four consecutive patients with cortical anomalies. *Ann. Neurol., 18,* 222–33.

Ganis, G., Kutas, M., & Sereno, M. I. (1996). The search for common sense: An electrophysiological study of the comprehension of words and pictures in reading. *J. Cogn. Neurosci., 8,* 89–106.

Garnsey, S. M., Tanenhaus, M. K., & Chapman, R. M. (1989). Evoked potentials and the study of sentence comprehension. *J. Psycholing. Res., 18,* 51–60.

Goldberg, A. E. (1995). *Constructions.* University of Chicago Press.

Goodglass, H. (1993). *Understanding Aphasia.* San Diego: Academic Press.

Grillon, C., Ameli, R., & Glazer, W. M. (1991). N400 and semantic categorization in schizophrenia. *Biol. Psychiat., 29,* 467–80.

Gunter, T. C., Jackson, J. L., Kutas, M., & Mulder, G. (1994). Focusing on the N400: An exploration of selective attention during reading. *Psychophysiol., 31,* 347–58.

Haarmann, H. J., & Kolk, H. H. (1994). On-line sensitivity to subject–verb agreement violations in Broca's aphasics: The role of syntactic complexity and time. *Brain Lang., 46,* 493–516.

Hagoort, P., Brown, C., & Groothusen, J. (1993). The syntactic positive shift (SPS) as an ERP measure of syntactic processing. *Lang. Cogn. Proc., 8,* 439–83.

Hagoort, P., Brown, C. M., & Swaab, T. Y. (1996). Lexical-semantic event-related potential effects in patients with left hemisphere lesions and aphasia, and patients with right hemisphere lesions without aphasia. *Brain, 119,* 627–49.

Hegarty, M., Carpenter, P. A., & Just, M. A. (1995). Diagrams in the comprehension of scientific texts. In R. Barr, M. L. Kamil, P. B. Mosenthal, & P. D. Pearson (Eds.), *Handbook of Reading Research,* vol. 2, pp. 641–68. Mahwah, NJ: Erlbaum.

Heinze, H. J., Münte, T. F., & Kutas, M. (1998). Context effects in a category verification task as assessed by event-related potential (ERP) measures. *Biol. Psychol., 47,* 121–35.

Hodges, J. R., Salmon, D. P., & Butters, N. (1991). The nature of the naming deficit in Alzheimer's and Huntington's disease. *Brain, 114,* 1547–58.

Hodgson, J. M. (1991). Informational constraints on pre-lexical priming. *Lang. Cogn. Proc., 6,* 169–205.

Holcomb, P. J. (1988). Automatic and attentional processing: An event-related brain potential analysis of semantic priming. *Brain Lang., 35,* 66–85.

Holcomb, P. J., & Neville, H. J. (1990). Auditory and visual semantic priming in lexical decision: A comparison using event-related brain potentials. *Lang. Cogn. Proc., 5,* 281–312.

Holmes, V. M., & O'Regan, J. K. (1981). Eye fixation patterns during the reading of relative-clause sentences. *J. Verb. Learn. Verb. Behav., 20,* 417–30.

Illes, J. (1989). Neurolinguistic features of spontaneous language production dissociate three forms of neurodegenerative disease: Alzheimer's, Huntington's, and Parkinson's. *Brain Lang., 37,* 628–42.

Iragui, V., Kutas, M., & Salmon, D. P. (1996). Event-related brain potentials during semantic categorization in normal aging and senile dementia of the Alzheimer's type. *Electroenceph. Clin. Neurophysiol., 100,* 392–406.

Johannes, S., Mangun, G. R., Kussmaul, C. L., & Münte, T. F. (1995). Brain potentials in developmental dyslexia: Differential effects of word frequency in human subjects. *Neurosci. Let., 195,* 183–6.

Just, M. A., & Carpenter, P. A. (1980). A theory of reading: From eye fixations to comprehension. *Psychol. Rev., 87,* 329–54.

Just, M. A., & Carpenter, P. A. (1992). A capacity theory of comprehension: Individual differences in working memory. *Psychol. Rev., 99,* 122–49.

Just, M. A., & Carpenter, P. A. (1993). The intensity dimension of thought: Pupillometric indices of sentence processing. *Canadian J. Exp. Psychol., 47,* 310–39.

Kapur, S., Rose, R., Liddle, P. F., & Zipursky, R. B. (1994). The role of the left prefrontal cortex in verbal processing: Semantic processing or willed action? *Neuroreport, 5,* 2193–6.

King, J., & Just, M. A. (1991). Individual differences in syntactic processing: The role of working memory. *J. Mem. Lang., 30,* 580–602.

King, J. W., & Kutas, M. (1995). Who did what and when? Using word- and clause-related ERPs to monitor working memory usage in reading. *J. Cogn. Neurosci., 7,* 378–97.

King, J. W., & Kutas, M. (1997). Is she an engineer? Brain potentials and anaphora. Poster presentation at the Fourth Annual Meeting of the Cognitive Neuroscience Society (Boston).

King, J. W., & Kutas, M. (1998). Neural plasticity in the dynamics of human visual word recognition. *Neuroscience Letters, 244,* 61–4.

Kluender, R., & Kutas, M. (1993a). Bridging the gap: Evidence from ERPs on the processing of unbounded dependencies. *J. Cogn. Neurosci., 5*, 196–214.

Kluender, R., & Kutas, M. (1993b). Subjacency as a processing phenomenon. *Lang. Cogn. Proc., 8*, 573–633.

Koenig, T., & Lehmann, D. (1996). Microstates in language-related brain potential maps show noun–verb differences. *Brain Lang., 53*, 169–82.

Kounios, J., & Holcomb, P. J. (1994). Concreteness effects in semantic processing: ERP evidence supporting dual-coding theory. *J. Exp. Psychol. Learn. Mem. Cogn., 20*, 804–23.

Koyama, S., Nageishi, Y., Shimokochi, M., Hokama, H., Miyazato, Y., Miyatani, M., & Ogura, C. (1991). The N400 component of event-related potentials in schizophrenic patients: A preliminary study. *Electroenceph. Clin. Neurophysiol., 78*, 124–32.

Kutas, M. (1993). In the company of other words: Electrophysiological evidence for single-word and sentence context effects. *Lang. Cogn. Proc., 8*, 533–72.

Kutas, M., & Hillyard, S. A. (1980). Reading senseless sentences: Brain potentials reflect semantic incongruity. *Science, 207*, 203–5.

Kutas, M., & Hillyard, S. A. (1984). Brain potentials during reading reflect word expectancy and semantic association. *Nature, 307*, 161–3.

Kutas, M., & King, J. W. (1996). The potentials for basic sentence processing: Differentiating integrative processes. In I. Ikeda & J. L. McClelland (Eds.), *Attention and Performance*, vol. 16, pp. 501–46. Cambridge, MA: MIT Press.

Kutas, M., Lindamood, T. E., & Hillyard, S. A. (1984). Word expectancy and event-related brain potentials during sentence processing. In S. Kornblum & J. Requin (Eds.), *Preparatory States and Processes*, pp. 217–37. Mahwah, NJ: Erlbaum.

Kutas, M., & Van Petten, C. K. (1994). Psycholinguistics electrified: Event-related brain potential investigations. In M. A. Gernsbacher (Ed.), *Handbook of Psycholinguistics*, pp. 83–143. San Diego: Academic Press.

Langacker, R. W. (1987). *Foundations of Cognitive Grammar*, vol. 1 (Theoretical Prerequisites). Stanford, CA: Stanford University Press.

Levelt, W. J. M. (1989). *Speaking: From Intention to Articulation*. Cambridge, MA: MIT Press.

Liotti, M., Gay, C. T., & Fox, P. T. (1994). Functional imaging and language: Evidence from positron emission tomography. *J. Clin. Neurophysiol., 11*, 175–90.

Lovegrove, W. J., Garzia, R. P., & Nicholson, S. B. (1990). Experimental evidence for a transient system deficit in specific reading disability. *J. Am. Opt. Ass., 61*, 137–46.

Luders, H., Lesser, R. P., Hahn, J., Dinner, D. S., et al. (1986). Basal temporal language area demonstrated by electrical stimulation. *Neurol., 36*, 505–10.

MacDonald, M. C., Pearlmutter, N. J., & Seidenberg, M. S. (1994). The lexical nature of syntactic ambiguity resolution. *Psychol. Rev., 101*, 676–703.

Maher, N., Manschreck, T. C., Hoover, T. M., & Weisstein, D. D. (1987). Thought disorder and measure features of language production in schizophrenia. In P. Harvey & E. Walker (Eds.), *Positive and Negative Symptoms in Psychosis: Description, Research and Future Directions*, pp. 195–215. Hillsdale, NJ: Erlbaum.

McCarthy, G., & Nobre, A. C. (1993). Modulation of semantic processing by spatial selective attention. *Electroenceph. Clin. Neurophysiol., 88*, 210–19.

Mecklinger, A., Schriefers, H., Steinhauer, K., & Friederici, A. D. (1995). Processing relative clauses varying on syntactic and semantic dimensions: An analysis with event-related potentials. *Mem. Cogn., 23*, 477–94.

Miller, G. A., & Chomsky, N. (1963). Finitary models of language users. In D. Luce, R. Bush, & E. Galanter (Eds.), *Handbook of Mathematical Psychology*, pp. 419–92. New York: Wiley.

Mitchell, P. F., Andrews, S., Fox, A. M., Catts, S. V., Ward, P. B., & McConaghy, N. (1991). Active and passive attention in schizophrenia: An ERP study of information processing in a linguistic task. *Biol. Psychol., 32*, 101–24.

Mitchell, P. F., Andrews, S., & Ward, P. B. (1993). An event-related potential study of semantic congruity and repetition: Effect of content change. *Psychophysiol., 30*, 496–509.

Mueller, H. M., King, J. W., & Kutas, M. (1997). Event-related potentials to relative clause processing in spoken sentences. *Cogn. Brain Res., 5*, 193–203.

Münte, T. F., & Heinze, H. J. (1994). Brain potentials reveal deficits of language processing after closed head injury. *Archives of Neurology, 51*, 482–93.

Murphy, G. L. (1990). Noun phrase interpretation and conceptual combination. *J. Mem. Lang., 29*, 259–88.

Natsopoulos, D., Grouios, G., Bostantzopoulou, S., Mentenopoulos, G., Katsarou, Z., & Logothetis, J. (1993). Algorithmic and heuristic strategies in comprehension of complement clauses by patients with Parkinson's disease. *Neuropsychologia, 31*, 951–64.

Natsopoulos, D., Katsarou, Z., Bostantzopoulou, S., Grouios, G., Mentenopoulos, G., & Logothetis, J. (1991). Strategies in comprehension of relative clauses by Parkinsonian patients. *Cortex, 27*, 255–68.

Neville, H. J., Coffey, S. A., Holcomb, P. J., & Tallal, P. (1993). The neurobiology of sensory and language processing in language-impaired children. *J. Cogn. Neurosci., 5*, 235–53.

Neville, H. J., Kutas, M., Chesney, G., & Schmidt, A. L. (1986). Event-related brain potentials during initial encoding and recognition memory of congruous and incongruous words. *J. Mem. Lang., 25*, 75–92.

Neville, H. J., Mills, D. L., & Lawson, D. S. (1992). Fractionating language: Different neural subsystems with different sensitive periods. *Cerebr. Cort., 2*, 244–58.

Neville, H. J., Nicol, J. L., Barss, A., Forster, K. I., & Garrett, M. F. (1991). Syntactically based sentence processing classes: Evidence from event-related brain potentials. *J. Cogn. Neurosci., 3*, 151–65.

Neville, H. J., Pratarelli, M. E., & Forster, K. A. (1989). Distinct neural systems for lexical and episodic representations of words. *Neuroscience Abstracts, 15*, 246.

Nobre, A. C., & McCarthy, G. (1995). Language-related field potentials in the anterior-medial temporal lobe: II. Effects of word type and semantic priming. *J. Neurosci., 15*, 1090–8.

Novick, B., Lovrich, D., & Vaughan, H. G. (1985). Event-related potentials associated with the discrimination of acoustic and semantic aspects of speech. *Neuropsychologia, 23*, 87–101.

Ohyama, M., Senda, M., Kitamura, S., Ishii, K., Mishina, M., & Terashi, A. (1996). Role of the nondominant hemisphere and undamaged area during word repetition in poststroke aphasics. A PET activation study. *Stroke, 27,* 897–903.

Osterhout, L., & Holcomb, P. (1992). Event-related brain potentials elicited by syntactic anomaly. *J. Mem. Lang., 31,* 785–806.

Osterhout, L., & Mobley, L. A. (1995). Event-related brain potentials elicited by failure to agree. *J. Mem. Lang., 34,* 739–73.

Otten, L. J., Rugg, M. D., & Doyle, M. C. (1993). Modulation of event-related potentials by word repetition: The role of visual selective attention. *Psychophysiol., 30,* 559–71.

Owen, A. M., James, M., Leigh, P. N., Summers, B. A., Marsden, C. D., Quinn, N. P., Lange, K. W., & Robbins, T. W. (1992). Fronto-striatal cognitive deficits at different stages of Parkinson's disease. *Brain, 115,* 1727–51.

Pacht, J. M., & Rayner, K. (1993). The processing of homophonic homographs during reading: Evidence from eye movement studies. *J. Psycholing. Res., 22,* 251–71.

Paulesu, E., Frith, U., Snowling, M., Gallagher, A., Morton, J., Frackowiak, R. S., & Frith, C. D. (1996). Is developmental dyslexia a disconnection syndrome? Evidence from PET scanning. *Brain, 119,* 143–57.

Penke, M., Weyerts, H., Gross, M., Zander-Westphal, E., Münte, T. F., & Clahsen, H. (1997). How the brain processes complex words: An ERP study of German verb inflection. *Cogn. Brain Res., 6,* 37–52.

Petersen, S. E., & Fiez, J. A. (1993). The processing of single words studied with positron emission tomography. *Ann. Rev. Neurosci., 16,* 509–30.

Petersen, S. E., Fox, P. T., Posner, M. I., Mintun, M., & Raichle, M. E. (1991). Positron emission tomographic studies of the processing of single words. *J. Cogn. Neurosci., 1,* 153–70.

Plunkett, K., & Marchman, V. A. (1993). From rote learning to system building: Acquiring verb morphology in children and connectionist nets. *Cognition, 48,* 21–69.

Polich, J., McCarthy, G., Wang, W. S., & Donchin, E. (1983). When words collide: Orthographic and phonological interference during word processing. *Biol. Psychol., 16,* 155–80.

Prince, A., & Pinker, S. (1988). Rules and connections in human language. *Trends Neurosci., 11,* 195–202.

Rayner, K., & Morris, R. K. (1992). Eye movement control in reading: Evidence against semantic preprocessing. *J. Exp. Psychol. Hum. Percept. Perform., 18,* 163–72.

Rochester, S. R., & Marin, J. R. (1979). *Crazy Talk: A Study of the Discourse of Schizophrenic Speakers.* New York: Plenum.

Rodel, M., Cook, N. D., Regard, M., & Landis, T. (1992). Hemispheric dissociation in judging semantic relations: Complementarity for close and distant associates. *Brain Lang., 43,* 448–59.

Rösler, F., Pütz, P., Friederici, A. D., & Hahne, A. (1993). Event-related brain potentials while encountering semantic and syntactic constraint violations. *J. Cogn. Neurosci., 5,* 345–62.

Rosser, A., & Hodges, J. R. (1994). Initial letter and semantic category fluency in Alzheimer's disease, Huntington's disease, and progressive supranuclear palsy. *J. Neurol. Neurosurg. Psychiat., 57,* 1389–94.

Rugg, M. D. (1987). Dissociation of semantic priming, word and nonword repetition by event-related potentials. *Q. J. Exp. Psychol., 39A,* 123–48.

Rugg, M. D. (1990). Event-related brain potentials dissociate repetition effects of high- and low-frequency words. *Mem. Cogn., 18,* 367–79.

Rugg, M. D., & Barrett, S. E. (1987). Event-related potentials and the interaction between orthographic and phonological information in a rhyme-judgement task. *Brain Lang., 32,* 336–61.

Rugg, M. D., Pearl, S., Walker, P., Roberts, R. C., & Holdstock, J. S. (1994). Word repetition effects on event-related potentials in healthy young and old subjects, and in patients with Alzheimer-type dementia. *Neuropsychologia, 32,* 381–98.

St. George, M., Mannes, S., & Hoffman, J. E. (1994). Global semantic expectancy and language comprehension. *J. Cogn. Neurosci., 6,* 70–83.

Sanquist, T. F., Rohrbaugh, J. W., Syndulko, K., & Lindsley, D. B. (1980). Electrocortical signs of levels of processing: Perceptual analysis and recognition memory. *Psychophysiol., 17,* 568–76.

Sarter, M., Berntson, G. G., & Cacioppo, J. T. (1996). Brain imaging and cognitive neuroscience: Toward strong inference in attributing function to structure. *Am. Psychol., 51,* 13–21.

Schendan, H., Ganis, G., & Kutas, M. (1998). Neurophysiological evidence for visual perceptual organization for words and faces by 150 ms. *Psychophysiol., 35,* 240–51.

Schwartz, S. (1982). Is there a schizophrenic language? *Behav. Brain Sci., 5,* 579–626.

Schwartz, T. J., Kutas, M., Butters, N., Paulsen, J. S., & Salmon, D. P. (1996). Electrophysiological insights into the nature of the semantic deficit in Alzheimer's disease. *Neuropsychologia, 34,* 827–41.

Seidenberg, M. S., & Tanenhaus, M. K. (1979). Orthographic effects on rhyme monitoring. *J. Exp. Psychol. Learn. Mem. Cogn., 5,* 546–54.

Sells, P. (1985). *Lectures on Contemporary Syntactic Theories.* Stanford, CA: Center for the Study of Language and Information.

Sereno, M. I. (1991). Language and the primate brain. In *Proceedings, Thirteenth Annual Conference of the Cognitive Science Society,* pp. 79–84. Hillsdale, NJ: Erlbaum.

Sereno, S. C. (1995). Resolution of lexical ambiguity: Evidence from an eye movement priming paradigm. *J. Exp. Psychol. Learn. Mem. Cogn., 21,* 582–95.

Smid, H. G., Mulder, G., & Mulder, L. J. (1987). The continuous flow model revisited: Perceptual and central motor aspects. *Electroenceph. Clin. Neurophysiol., 40,* 270–8.

Stelmack, R. M., & Miles, J. (1990). The effect of picture priming on event-related potentials of normal and disabled readers during a word recognition memory task. *J. Clin. Exp. Neuropsychol., 12,* 887–903.

Swaab, T. Y., Brown, C. M., & Hagoort, P. (1997). Spoken sentence comprehension in aphasia: Event-related potential evidence for a lexical integration deficit. *J. Cogn. Neurosci., 9,* 39–66.

Tallal, P., & Curtiss, S. (1988). From developmental dysphasia to dyslexia: A neurodevelopmental continuum. *J. Clin. Exp. Neuropsychol., 10,* 19.

Tanenhaus, M. K., Spivey-Knowlton, M. J., Eberhard, K. M., & Sedivy, J. C. (1995). Integration of visual and linguistic information in spoken language comprehension. *Science, 268,* 1632–4.

Taylor, W. L. (1953). "Cloze" procedure: A new tool for measuring readability. *Journalism Quarterly, 30,* 415–17.

Thomas, P., Kearney, G., Napier, E., Ellis, E., Leuder, I., & Johnson, M. (1996). Speech and language in first onset psychosis differences between people with schizophrenia, mania, and controls. *Brit. J. Psychiat., 168*, 337–43.

Vandenberghe, R., Price, C., Wise, R., Josephs, O., & Frackowiak, R. S. (1996). Functional anatomy of a common semantic system for words and pictures. *Nature, 383*, 254–6.

Van Petten, C. K. (1995). Words and sentences: Event-related brain potential measures. *Psychophysiol., 32*, 511–25.

Van Petten, C. K., & Kutas, M. (1987). Ambiguous words in context: An event-related potential analysis of the time course of meaning activation. *J. Mem. Lang., 26*, 188–208.

Van Petten, C., & Kutas, M. (1990). Interactions between sentence context and word frequency in event-related brain potentials. *Mem. Cogn., 18*, 380–93.

Van Petten, C., & Kutas, M. (1991). Influences of semantic and syntactic context on open and closed class words. *Mem. Cogn., 19*, 95–112.

Van Petten, C., Kutas, M., Kluender, R., Mitchiner, M., & McIsaac, H. (1991). Fractionating the word repetition effect with event-related potentials. *J. Cogn. Neurosci., 3*, 131–50.

Van Petten, C. K., & Rheinfelder, H. (1995). Conceptual relationships between spoken words and environmental sounds: Event-related brain potential measures. *Neuropsychologia, 33*, 485–508.

Van Petten, C., Weckerly, J., McIsaac, H. K., & Kutas, M. (1997). Working memory capacity dissociates lexical and sentential context effects. *Psychol. Sci., 8*, 238–42.

van Turennout, M. (1997). The electrophysiology of speaking. Doctoral dissertation, Max Planck Institute for Psycholinguistics at Nijmegen, The Netherlands.

van Turennout, M., Hagoort, P., & Brown, C. M. (1997). Electrophysical evidence on the time course of semantic and phonological processes in speech production. *J. Exp. Psychol. Learn. Mem. Cogn., 23*, 787–806.

Weckerly, J. (1995). Object relatives viewed through behavioral, electrophysiological and modeling techniques. Ph.D. dissertation, Department of Cognitive Science, University of California, San Diego.

Weiller, C., Isensee, C., Rijntjes, M., Huber, W., Müller, S., Bier, D., Dutschka, K., Woods, R. P., Noth, J., & Diener, H. C. (1995). Recovery from Wernicke's aphasia: A positron emission tomographic study. *Ann. Neurol., 37*, 723–32.

Weyerts, H., Münte, T. F., Smid, H. G. O. M., & Heinze, H. J. (1995). Mental representation of morphologically complex words: An event-related potential study with adult humans. *Neurosci. Let., 206*, 125–8.

Weyerts, H., Penke, M., Dohrn, U., Clahsen, H., & Münte, T. F. (1997). Brain potentials indicate differences between regular and irregular German noun plurals. *Neuroreport., 8*, 957–62.

Wise, R., Chollet, F., Hadar, U., Friston, K., Hoffner, E., & Frackowiak, R. S. (1991). Distribution of cortical neural networks involved in word comprehension and word retrieval. *Brain, 114*, 1803–17.

Yurgelun-Todd, D. A., Waternaux, C. M., Cohen, B. M., Gruber, S. A., English, C. D., & Renshaw, P. F. (1996). Functional magnetic resonance imaging of schizophrenic patients and comparison subjects during word production. *Am. J. Psychiat., 153*, 200–5.

CHAPTER TWENTY-TWO

EMOTION AND MOTIVATION

MARGARET M. BRADLEY

Prologue

What William James once said about attention could also be said about emotion: "Everyone knows what it is." And, like attention, replacing this intuitive understanding with operational definitions and theoretical constructs – admitting it into the domain of scientific study – is far from a trivial task. Indeed, it sometimes seems that there are as many definitions as there are investigators (see Panksepp 1982 for a representative set). One aspect of emotion that is generally agreed upon, however, is that it is associated with physiological reactions: in emotional situations, the body acts. The heart pounds, flutters, stops, and drops; palms sweat; muscles tense and relax; blood boils; faces blush, flush, frown, and smile. We note these reactions in ourselves, and we make inferences about the emotional life of others based on visible bodily responses.

The link between emotion and bodily action is evident in the derivation of the word "emotion," which stems from the Latin *movere,* meaning to move. In emotional situations, people move: they act and they react. It is informative that the word "motivation" also stems from the same verb; a motive is, literally, "something that moves one." Whereas the term "emotion" is usually reserved for describing stimuli that move people, "motivation" is often used to describe animal behavior. Under conditions of high motivation, animals move: they act and they react. Both emotion and motivation are fundamentally related to action.

Those studying motivated behavior in animal subjects have consistently agreed that action is controlled by two basic parameters of direction and intensity (see e.g. Hebb 1949; Schneirla 1959). That is, even in the simplest organism, stimuli that promote survival (e.g., food, nurturance) elicit approach behaviors, whereas those that threaten the organism prompt withdrawal, escape, or avoidance. All these behaviors can occur with varying strength, speed, and vigor. The motivational parameters of direction (i.e., towards or away) and *intensity* map well onto parameters of hedonic valence (i.e., pleasant or unpleasant) and *arousal* that are recognized as central in emotion. Emotional events can be differentiated on the basis of whether they are good or bad (Arnold 1960), appetitive or aversive (Dickinson & Dearing 1979), agreeable or disagreeable (MacLean 1993), positive or negative (Cacioppo & Berntson 1994), pleasant or unpleasant (Lang, Bradley, & Cuthbert 1990), hospitable or inhospitable (Cacioppo, Bernston, & Crites 1996). These valenced events differ in the degree to which they arouse or engage the individual.

Based on these observations, a number of theorists have advocated a biphasic approach to emotion, which posits that emotion fundamentally stems from varying activation in centrally organized appetitive and defensive motivational systems that have evolved to mediate the wide range of adaptive behaviors necessary for an organism struggling to survive in the physical world (Davidson et al. 1990; Dickinson & Dearing 1979; Konorski 1967; Lang et al. 1990). Neuroscientists have begun to determine how the relationship between stimulus input and behavioral output is mediated through specific, largely subcortical, neural circuits that have evolved to organize and direct adaptive actions (Davis 1989; Fanselow 1994; LeDoux 1987, 1996). A biphasic approach to emotion suggests that its psychophysiological study should assess physiological responses as they vary with systematic variations in hedonic valence and arousal.

Another approach, and one more common thus far in the psychophysiological study of emotion, conceptualizes emotion in terms of a set of discrete states such as fear, anger, sadness, and so forth. Lists of basic emotions have typically varied from theorist to theorist. Descartes (discussed in Panksepp 1982) listed wonder, love, joy, desire,

John T. Cacioppo, Louis G. Tassinary, and Gary G. Berntson (Eds.), *Handbook of Psychophysiology,* 2nd ed. © Cambridge University Press 2000. Printed in the United States of America. ISBN 62634X. All rights reserved.

hate, and sadness as fundamental, and it is interesting that this is the last time positive emotions outrepresented negative and that love was included on the list. Watson (1924), showing allegiance to definitions based on observable behavior, had a short list of fear, rage, and sexual activity. More contemporary lists include surprise, enjoyment, interest, disgust, shame, distress, fear, contempt, and anger (Izard 1972); surprise, acceptance, desire, fear, rage, panic, and disgust (Plutchik 1980); and others. The question of whether specific physiological responses are characteristic of different emotional states has been pursued for almost a century by psychophysiologists, prompted primarily by James's hypothesis regarding the relationship between physiology and specific feelings.

This chapter will begin with a discussion of James's influence on the psychophysiological study of emotion over the course of the last century, reconsidering its implications in light of recent advances in thinking in neuroscience, cognitive psychology, and psychophysiology. A brief review of theory and data relevant to a biphasic approach to emotion will then be presented. Current models of emotional processing at both anatomical and cognitive levels of description will be reviewed, particularly as they describe potential links between stimulus input, motivational activation, and response output. It will then be suggested that three methodological factors loom large when designing or comparing across studies of emotion: (i) the definition of the affective cue, (ii) the determination of the task, and (iii) the description of the response. A brief review of empirical findings in the psychophysiology of emotion will highlight these crucial elements in experimental studies of emotion. It will be suggested that comparisons across studies in which the cues, tasks, or response measures differ have led to a number of difficulties in making sense of the data from psychophysiological inquiries of emotion. Specific issues regarding inter- and intrapersonal differences, conscious experience of emotion, and discrete states will be raised briefly and considered within the context of a biphasic motivational approach to the psychophysiological study of emotion. It will be concluded that inferences about the relationship between emotion and psychophysiological response will be, at first, highly context-dependent.

HISTORICAL BACKGROUND

The psychophysiological study of emotion has been preoccupied for roughly a century with assessing James's hypothesis that physiological responses form the basis of emotional experience. Given the many advances in thinking about the mind and behavior since the time of James, it is not surprising to see that modern viewpoints are somewhat different from those of James, a turn-of-the-century introspectionist whose interest in physiological processes was secondary to his primary goal of explaining feelings – that is, conscious emotional experience. His radical proposal

that feelings *followed* the physiological response elicited by an emotional stimulus represented a nonintuitive reversal of traditional folk wisdom, and provoked the scientific imagination of the psychologist: Is a person afraid because he runs rather than running because he is afraid?

The Jamesian hypothesis defined the central question in the study of emotion as whether specific feeling states were associated with a specific pattern of physiology. To the extent that physiological changes do not uniquely specify different feelings, the Jamesian hypothesis would be disconfirmed. The answer to this question is clearly within the purview of psychophysiologists, who began pursuing answers in investigations spanning the last 100 years using a variety of methods to determine whether specific physiological patterns are associated with specific emotions such as fear and anger (e.g. Ax 1953; Ekman 1971; see Cacioppo et al. 1993 for a review).

Empirical support for the Jamesian hypothesis has not been strong. As noted in a recent review of this literature by Cacioppo et al. (1993), part of the problem stems from inadequate experimental designs in which different studies include different types or numbers of specific emotions than others, do not include appropriate comparison conditions, utilize different dependent measures, or, importantly, investigate emotion in very different experimental contexts. Nonetheless, Cacioppo et al. (1993) selected studies that met a number of important criteria for assessing the question of whether specific physiological patterns accompany specific states of emotional feeling. The data were quite disappointing, with "little evidence for replicable autonomic differences in pairwise comparisons of the emotions on the measures of bodily temperature, systolic blood pressure, facial temperature, respiration, skin conductance level, and cardiac stroke volume" (p. 125). Although heart rate was found to be a relatively effective discriminator, a number of methodological problems led Cacioppo et al. (1993) to conclude that even the meager support provided by this measure was probably an overestimate of actual effect sizes.

In addition to a disappointing lack of empirical confirmation for the Jamesian hypothesis (despite a century of experimentation), there are conceptual difficulties with the question of whether specific emotional states are associated with a specific physiological pattern. These include the facts that (1) physiology varies with specific actions and (2) specific actions can vary both within and across specific emotions. Regarding the link between physiological response and action: it is a truism that most, if not all, peripheral (and, to some degree, central) indices of physiological activity vary as a function of the amount and type of somatic involvement and the accompanying demand for metabolic support. Put bluntly, running will produce a very different configuration of physiological activity than sitting, with activity in one system (e.g. cardiovascular) dependent, to some degree, on activity in another system (e.g. somatic). In addition to these obvious relationships, more subtle interdependencies noted between physiological systems – such as cardiac–somatic coupling (Obrist 1975) and respiratory sinus arrhythmia (Porges 1992) – rule out simple statements about physiology in the absence of specifying a particular action set.

It is also a truism that specific actions can vary in the same emotional state, as well as (more obviously) across different emotional states. For example, both animal and human research indicates that a cue signaling threat can lead to fight, flight, or freezing, as well as a variety of specific idiosyncratic behaviors (see Mackintosh 1983) depending upon available contextual support and the organism's learning history. The physiology of fear in the context of headlong flight will be different from the physiology of fear in the context of freezing, particularly in somatic and cardiovascular systems. Predicting identical physiological patterns in the context of these disparate activities highlights the inappropriateness of the initial question regarding the physiology of fear. At the least, it will be necessary to specify whether the target emotion involves fleeing fear or freezing fear or fighting fear.

Attempts to define emotion's physiology in the absence of information specifying both the context in which it is elicited and the actions it evokes neglect the important context-dependent aspects of emotional actions. To address the role of context in emotion, Lang and his colleagues (1990) distinguished between strategic and tactical aspects of emotion. Whereas *strategies* define the dominant motivational state (i.e., appetitive or defensive), a variety of different *tactics* – diverse, specific, context-bound patterns of action – can be employed in a situation eliciting defense, for example. Thus, a male rat's response to an aversive shock is various: if administered to the rat's feet in a bare chamber, the animal freezes; if delivered by a prod from outside the cage, the rat flees; if suitable material is present, the rat will attempt to bury the shock apparatus; if another male is in the vicinity, a fight ensues (see Mackintosh 1983 for a discussion of these data). This variability in specific emotional behaviors has been a major source of frustration when attempting to extrapolate across instances of the same emotion or to differentiate individual emotions, particularly in terms of assessing their psychophysiological signatures. Tactical variation negates physiological similarity.

Thus, from a modern perspective, the Jamesian question of whether a specific emotion will result in a specific physiological pattern is psychophysiologically naive. For James, however, physiological responses were important only insofar as they provided the ingredients from which conscious experience could be built – he was not explicitly invested in the study of psychophysiological processes per se. Yet Lange, whose ideas are closely linked with James's owing to a similar focus on the role of physiology in emotion, was in fact a physiologist (see Lang 1994b for a thorough discussion of James–Lange theory). For Lange, however, physiological response *was* the emotion – whether a conscious feeling subsequently arose from physiology's activity was not an issue that concerned him. Rather, Lange's goal was simply to characterize similarities and differences in emotion based on empirical patterns of physiological (primarily cardiovascular) response. For psychophysiologists, a shift in emphasis from the study of conscious feelings to the study of physiological patterning redefines the central question from the Jamesian, "Are specific states associated with specific physiology?" to the Langean, "How do physiological patterns vary in different emotional situations?"

Whereas both James and Lange believed that at least some physiological events differentiated among emotions, Cannon (1928) and later Bard (1934) argued that physiological responses, particularly those mediated by the autonomic nervous system, were too general, too diffuse, and too slow to provide a basis for distinguishing different emotional states. Cannon proposed that physiological responses, particularly in aversive contexts, resulted from a general activation of the sympathetic nervous system that he termed the "emergency" reaction. Modern viewpoints again clarify the relevance of the Cannon–Bard theory for current researchers. First, the focus on autonomic responses, particularly those mediated by the sympathetic branch, is quite narrow considering the number and extent of methodologies available to the modern psychophysiologist. In addition, whereas some aspects of autonomic functioning are slow and diffuse, others are more precise and rapid, and the addition of new measures of emotional reactivity in somatic (e.g. reflex), central (e.g., ERP, EEG, fMRI), and neurochemical systems can be profitably employed. Second, the focus on aversiveness renders Cannon's view silent with respect to physiological responses elicited in the context of pleasant, appetitive stimuli.

In this chapter, Lange's empirical approach to the study of emotion is advocated. According to this view, the goal of the psychophysiological study of emotion is the assessment of physiological responses in multiple response systems (unlike Lange's focus on vasomotor) as they vary in well-defined emotional contexts. Perhaps the experimental legacy of the many investigators that pursued the Jamesian hypothesis in the twentieth century will be that these studies highlighted, however indirectly, the context-dependent and tactical nature of emotional response. The data compellingly show that physiological patterns are not the same for a given emotional state, especially if it is prompted in different contexts (Cacioppo et al. 1993; Lacey 1967; Lang et al. 1990).

PLEASURE AND AROUSAL IN EMOTION

James clearly advocated a discrete emotion view, particularly for what he called the "coarse" affects – which included fear, anger, and so on. Because of his influence on psychological research, this theoretical view has received considerable attention in terms of physiological assessment. The simpler dimensional view, however, has not been tested as thoroughly. One benefit of the dimensional view is that it is parsimonious; furthermore, extending back at least to Wundt (1896), there has been agreement among theorists that the basic organizational dimensions of emotion are pleasure and arousal. Moreover, a clear bridge to animal motivation exists, with many scientists equating pleasant events with those that elicit approach behavior and unpleasant events with those eliciting withdrawal or avoidance. For instance, Schneirla (1959) defined the two responses of approach and withdrawal as the only basic patterns "applicable to *all* motivated behavior in *all* organisms." According to his view, approach behaviors (i.e., A-type mechanisms) are elicited in situations such as acquiring food, obtaining shelter, mating, and other activities that promote survival of the individual and the species. Withdrawal (W-type mechanism) behaviors include defense, huddling, flight, and other protective reactions. Schneirla focused on physical intensity as the important parameter eliciting A-type or W-type behaviors, with low-intensity stimuli associated with approach and high-intensity stimuli evoking withdrawal. However, he noted that, for complex organisms such as humans, basic biphasic responses could permute through evolution to provide a basis for more varied types of emotional elicitors (for adult humans, object meaning tends to outweigh stimulus magnitude as the eliciting cue) and emotional activities (e.g., active seeking or avoiding).

Based on a sorting of unconditioned reflexes, Konorski (1967) agreed that a biphasic organization was fundamental, dividing response classes into those that are either protective or defensive. Dickinson and Dearing (1979) developed Konorski's dichotomy into two opponent motivational systems, *aversive* and *attractive,* each activated by a different but equally wide range of unconditioned stimuli. These systems were held to have "reciprocal inhibitory connections" (p. 5) that modulated learned responses and reactions to new, unconditioned input. More recently, Davidson and colleagues (1990; Davidson 1992) and Lang and colleagues (1990) have embraced a biphasic organization, assuming that emotion stems from activation in basic appetitive or defensive motivational systems. In the simplest case, biphasic motivation is defined as a behavioral tendency to approach or withdraw from a stimulus.

There are a number of other factors supporting a simple biphasic organization of emotion. Whereas Schneirla's assertion was based on the behavior of simple creatures such as planaria, Hebb (1949) also concluded – on the basis of studies of higher organisms including rats, cats, dogs, and primates – that a primary parameter of behavior was direction (towards or away). Human developmental data are consistent with the idea that ontogeny recapitulates phylogeny in this sense, as newborns immediately evidence both protective (oral rejection) and appetitive (e.g. sucking) reflexes, indicative of a basic biphasic chassis. Whereas only unconditioned stimuli at first reflexively activate appetitive and defensive systems, experience allows new (conditioned) stimuli to activate these same systems. Thus, infants evidence fear of heights only after they are able to crawl (Campos, Bertenthal, & Kermoian 1992), suggesting that the visual cliff cue activates the defensive system only after experience has forged a connection between it and aversive consequences (i.e., the infant has taken a tumble).

Empirical support for a fundamental biphasic organization of emotion is also clearly seen in studies investigating how adults (as well as children) categorize the world. Osgood's (1969) seminal research demonstrated that, when asked to rate words on attributes that included physical dimensions (heavy–light, thick–thin, hot–cold), psychological descriptors (honest–dishonest, brave–cowardly, kind–cruel), and emotional scales (good–bad, pleasant–unpleasant), factor analyses consistently found that the dimension of hedonic valence was primary in organizing these data and clearly accounted for the most variability in these judgments. A second factor – labeled activation, arousal, or intensity – also accounted for substantial variance. He later found these dimensions were primary for linguistic stimuli in non–English-speaking cultures, as well as in organizing judgments for stimuli ranging from sonar signals to aesthetic paintings (Osgood, Suci, & Tannenbaum 1957). Mehrabian (1970) extended the analysis to nonverbal behavior and again found that hedonic valence and arousal were the basic factors underlying judgments concerning facial expressions, hand and bodily movements, and postural positions.

In short, the world appears to be categorized, fundamentally, in terms of hedonic valence, which can be related to the extent that an event promotes (pleasant) or threatens (unpleasant) life in some way. The fact that human experience, verbal and nonverbal, can consistently be organized in terms of basic appetitive–aversive evaluation provides support for the idea that this dimension is fundamental in human emotion.

Intensity, Arousal, Activation

As just noted, factor analyses of emotional judgments consistently identify a second factor – degree of arousal or activation – as organizing semantic judgments. If, in simple organisms, hedonic valence is directly coupled with behavioral dispositions toward or away from appetitive or aversive stimuli, then its intensity can be measured as the strength or speed of the movement (e.g. Duffy 1962; Hebb 1949; Miller 1959; Schneirla 1959). That is, movement toward or away from a stimulus can be implemented with more or less vigor, energy mobilization, or activation. In simple organisms, behavioral intensity was initially linked to stimulus intensity, with the strength (Miller 1966) or speed (Schneirla 1959) of a withdrawal response varying directly with the degree of shock intensity, for example.

Thus, in its earliest (and simplest) form, intensity characterized the vigor of a response. Subsequently, response vigor was theoretically linked to a central drive state, which was proposed as a primary motivator underlying observed behavior (Hull 1943). The vigor of a response was presumed to directly reflect the intensity of the underlying drive state, allowing response vigor to be used as an index of central motivation. In the Hullian view, stimulus intensity increased motivation (drive), measured in the strength of the resulting (approach or avoidance) behavior. In this view, arousal is conceptualized as a nonspecific, energizing force that intensifies and strengthens either approach or withdrawal.

This nonspecific, activating conception of drive was refined in the late 1950s and early 1960s by a number of theorists who emphasized the activating effects of emotion (Duffy 1962; Lindsley 1951; Malmo 1959). In their view, behavior was conceptualized as varying along a dimension of activity, with coma and death anchoring one end and emotional excitement anchoring the other. Increased activity in cortical, sympathetic, and behavioral systems was predicted as one moved from the calm to excited end of this behavioral dimension, a prediction supported in a number of different studies (see Duffy 1962 for a review).

Activation theory clearly linked increases in arousal to unilateral and monotonic increases in the strength of responding in numerous systems, including cortical (e.g., alpha-band EEG), sympathetic (e.g., heart rate, blood pressure, etc.), and somatic (e.g., muscle tension, motor activity). Lacey (1967) challenged this notion on the basis of data indicating that responses in all systems do not uniformly increase together. For instance, somatic deactivation can be obtained in states of high cortical activation, and pupillary dilatation (a sympathetic response) can occur with cardiac deceleration (a parasympathetic response; Libby, Lacey, & Lacey 1973), effects he termed "directional fractionation." A centerpiece of Lacey's argument was the finding that electrodermal and cardiac responses showed directional fractionation as a function of specific tasks: perception and mentation both result in electrodermal increases, but perception generally involves cardiac deceleration whereas mentation is accompanied by cardiac acceleration.

Modern thinking clarifies different aspects of Lacey's (1967) criticism. First, the notion that cortical activation and somatic or sympathetic activation are necessarily coupled is less reasonable, given current conceptions of the brain. When envisioned as a computational device, it is clear that the brain can be quite busy (i.e. active) when inhibiting somatic or autonomic output, for example, depending upon the goal at hand. Second, the comparison between cardiac responses in different tasks (i.e., percep-

tion and mentation) actually violated Duffy's (1962) caveat that comparisons between differentially arousing contexts could be satisfactorily assessed only with "all other things being equal." That is, tests of arousal theory are more appropriately conducted by varying the level of intensity within the same task context.

Nonetheless, two aspects of activation theory remain untenable today. First is the assumption that increasing arousal uniformly *increases* activity in physiological and behavioral systems. As noted before, behaviors appropriate to a highly arousing, aversive context can include active somatic responses (such as fleeing or fighting) or relatively inactive responses (such as freezing). The degree of somatic activation will depend to a large extent on the specific behavior selected in a particular context. Thus, increases in intensity will not necessarily or uniformly increase somatic and autonomic activation; instead, they will depend upon the response appropriate for the current context and its somatic and metabolic requirements. In this view, arousal amplifies the strength of the associated behavior, which could involve (depending upon the context) decreases rather than increases in activity.

A second unsatisfactory outcome of activation theory is the notion that arousal can be conceptually separated from behavioral direction – that is, the idea that one can consider arousal in the absence of behavior. As noted earlier, arousal was first proposed as a parameter of directed behavior: an organism approached or avoided a stimulus with more or less vigor or strength. The idea that vigor could be removed from the specific behavior, or studied separately, is not a clear corollary of this view. In advocating a unidimensional activation process that energized and amplified all behaviors, regardless of direction, activation theories unwittingly encouraged explorations in which arousal was manipulated (through drugs, motor activity, etc.) in the absence of directed behavior. In fact, Duffy (1962) was quite clear on the centrality of direction (valence) as the main parameter of behavior; her focus on activation was an attempt to deal with the intensive aspects of emotion.

Konorski (1967) clearly advocated activation as a parameter operating within separate appetitive and aversive systems, as did Lang et al. (1990, 1997). In these formulations, arousal is conceived as a hypothetical construct linked with increasing activation in centrally organized appetitive or defensive motivational systems. From this viewpoint, the task of psychophysiologists is to determine how variations in intensity within appetitive and aversive systems affect somatic and autonomic responses in well-defined experimental contexts.

Modes of Biphasic Activation

Assuming that emotion is organized by activity in separable appetitive and aversive systems, one central issue concerns their relationship. An assumption shared by

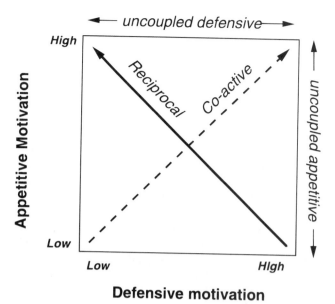

Defensive motivation

Figure 1. Modes of biphasic activation. Activation in hypothetical appetitive and defensive motivation systems can vary from uncoupled activation in each system to coactivation. Adapted with permission from Cacioppo & Berntson, "Relationships between attitudes and evaluative space: A critical review with emphasis on the separability of positive and negative substrates," *Psychological Bulletin,* vol. 115, pp. 401–23. Copyright © 1994 by the American Psychological Association.

many is that these systems are reciprocally inhibited: as activity in one system increases, activity in the other is inhibited (Konorski 1967). Bipolar measures of affective valence reflect this assumption in that a stimulus can be rated as either pleasant or unpleasant, but not both simultaneously. A more flexible conceptualization of biphasic activation was advocated by Cacioppo and Berntson (1994; see also Cacioppo, Gardner, & Berntson 1997), who presented a comprehensive model that allows all possible modes of activation. Figure 1 illustrates this scheme, in which appetitive and defensive activation can vary from being mutually reciprocal to simultaneously active to separably active. Different points in bivariate space identify instances when aversive and appetitive activation are highly coactive to when they reciprocally related.

Defining critical parameters that contribute to reciprocal versus concurrent (or separable) activation of appetitive and aversive systems remains to be worked out. Reciprocal activation is certainly plausible at the stage of actual behavioral output: a specific effector is not always able to respond to two concurrent demands in parallel (i.e., one cannot run both toward and away from a stimulus at the same time). To the extent that one behavior is controlling the organism, it is less likely that another can be simultaneously active. For this reason, Grossman (1967) proposed a central integrator that "decided" which neural system could control behavior at any specific moment. It is also plausible that, at extremely high levels of arousal in either system, the relationship is typically reciprocal – as, for ex-

ample, when the search for food is actively inhibited in a situation involving high threat (see McNaughton 1989).

Conversely, coactivation in both the appetitive and aversive systems may be more probable in moderate or low arousal situations, or in situations that involve multiple independent stimuli or complex unitary (i.e. multifeatured) stimuli that simultaneously activate both the appetitive and defensive systems. Cacioppo and Berntson (1994) originally proposed the bivariate space to deal with attitudes, which are often based on multiple sources of information that have separable appetitive and defensive elements. For instance, when investigating blood or organ donorship, aspects associated with appetitive motivation (e.g., desire to help society) as well as defensive motivation (e.g., fear of pain) are readily elicited from subjects (Cacioppo & Gardner 1993).

A similar instance of coactivation occurs in studies of appetitive behavior, which are often conducted in a context of deprivation (presumably an aversive event) reinforced with food (appetitive motivation). Avoidance learning and active coping paradigms also represent instances of motivational coactivation, since they typically involve an aversive stimulus (e.g. shock) that can be successfully avoided, resulting in a melange of positive and negative cues. Mixed states of appetitive and aversive activation may be the most difficult to understand from the perspective of studying emotion, yet these tasks have been widely used in the study of emotional learning and behavior. To begin with, however, it may be more useful to understand emotional reactions in situations where reciprocal or separable activation is dominant.

System Dominance

A biphasic approach to the study of emotion also raises the issue of whether one or the other system is customarily more dominant or at an advantage in terms of mobilizing the energy and behavioral focus of the organism. When a system is proposed as primary, it is usually the aversive system (Taylor 1991). The adaptive importance of dealing with threats (e.g., defending against a predator) before satisfying appetitive urges lies in the fact that, if the threat is not dealt with, eating may no longer matter: annihilation is a clear bottom line. Therefore, defensive responses seem to take precedence over appetitive.

In a classic situation designed to assess the strength of appetitive and defensive motivation and their relationship to one another, Miller (1966) measured the strength of an animal's approach toward or retreat from a goal box associated with food and/or shock. He found that the slope of the function relating force to distance was steeper for aversive stimuli: as distance to the goal decreased, the strength of withdrawal was greater than approach. Cacioppo and Berntson (1994) characterized this steeper aversive gradient as supporting the idea of an inherent negativity bias in which responding to aversive events has primacy over those that are appetitive. In a recent meta-analysis, Cacioppo and associates (in press) found empirical support for this proposition, with the data demonstrating stronger physiological reactions in the context of negative emotional cues compared with positive ones. We will re-examine this issue later in the chapter.

Physical Context

ANATOMICAL SUBSTRATE

Physiological responses associated with processing appetitive or aversive stimuli in the human psychophysiological laboratory include those in many of the systems discussed in this volume, including electrodermal, cardiovascular, electrocortical, electromyographic, and reflex systems. The reader is encouraged to refer to these chapters for specific information regarding the pertinent anatomical substrates.

NEUROANATOMICAL SUBSTRATE: DEFENSIVE AND APPETITIVE SYSTEMS

In a biphasic approach to the study of emotion, separable motivational systems mediating appetitive and defensive responding are posited. Whether these systems are implemented in the same or different brain structures – and how appetitive and aversive cues come to selectively activate appropriate outputs – are the critical questions when contemplating the neural substrates of emotion. To date, research has tended to focus more on the neural circuitry involved in the defensive motivational system. This is due, at least in part, to the relative ease of presenting intense aversive (compared with appetitive) stimuli in a laboratory setting (but see Ashby, Isen, & Turken 1999; Davidson & Irwin in press).

It is widely agreed that emotion is mediated in subcortical, particularly limbic structures, based mainly on lesion and stimulation studies in animal samples. As LeDoux (1987) noted, "studies of the neural substrates of affective behavior and its autonomic correlates seem always to lead to brain regions traditionally described as components of the limbic system" (p. 425). Knowledge regarding the neural substrates of emotion in humans is still quite cursory, owing to obvious limitations in research investigating the neural circuitry involved. However, new methodologies for studying the human brain in action (e.g., dense electrode arrays, fMRI, PET) promise to greatly accelerate progress in this area.

The Peripheral Nervous System

Because the psychophysiological study of emotion has traditionally focused on autonomic and somatic outputs (e.g., heart rate, blood pressure, electrodermal and muscle tension changes), it is reasonable to start an exploration of its neural substrates from these indices and work backward. Both autonomic and somatic responses are proximally controlled by the peripheral nervous system (see Guyton & Hall 1996 for an overview). In the autonomic system, anatomical and functional distinctions between the parasympathetic and sympathetic branches have been important in the study of emotion. The sympathetic nervous system is characterized by postganglionic fibers, which are quite lengthy and which branch and divide as they make their way to specific target organs. Functionally, this means that a single sympathetic fiber activates a number of different effectors and so provides an anatomical substrate for Cannon's emergency reaction, which proposed a volley of responses – heart rate and blood pressure increases, electrodermal reactions, increase in respiration rate and depth – on the basis of sympathetic activation. Conversely, the postganglionic fibers in the parasympathetic branch are short and hence more likely to target a specific effector.

Most organs are innervated by nerves from both the parasympathetic and sympathetic divisions, which tend to exert opposite effects. Figure 2 lists effects of parasympathetic and sympathetic activation on a variety of different systems typically measured in the study of emotion. The reciprocal effects by these two systems on different organs are mediated by the release of different neurotransmitters at the neuroeffector junction, with acetylcholine released by parasympathetic fibers (cholinergic) and noradrenaline released by sympathetic fibers (adrenergic). Subsequent actions (e.g., increase or decrease in heart rate) are also temporally differentiated by the fact that noradrenaline dissipates slowly whereas acetylcholine dissipates more rapidly. Thus, parasympathetic control will tend to activate specific organs with rapid, phasic effects, whereas sympathetic control is not only more diffuse but also somewhat longer-lasting.

Although sympathetic activity has been associated with mobilization for responding to aversive events, as Cannon originally proposed, some theorists have associated pleasant affect with parasympathetic dominance (Arnold 1960; Gellhorn & Loofbourrow 1963; Schneirla 1959). According to this view, pleasure was presumed to be related to the vegetative, homeostatic controls implemented by the parasympathetic system, because appetitive situations (by definition) do not involve stress and its sympathetic manifestations. Current thinking does not support such a simple relationship. First, rather than simply responding to aversive stimulation, the sympathetic nervous system is more generally designed to prepare and instantiate action, a nonspecific demand. Sympathetic activation clearly occurs in appetitive contexts, such as sexual behavior (Guyton & Hall 1996) and adventure seeking (Zuckerman 1982). To the extent that sympathetic activity is involved in facilitating action, it may play a role in those that subserve either appetitive or aversive motivation.

Organ	Effect of Sympathetic Stimulation	Effect of Parasympathetic Stimulation
Heart Muscle	Increased rate and force of contraction	Decreased rate and force of contraction
Blood Vessels	Most often constricted	Most often little or no effect
Sweat Glands	Copious sweating (cholinergic)	Sweating on palms of hands
Skeletal Muscles	Increased strength & glycogenolysis	None
Apocrine Glands	Thick, odoriferous secretion	None
Pupil of Eye	Dilated	Constricted
Ciliary Eye Muscle	Slight relaxation (far vision)	Constricted (near vision)
Gut (Lumen)	Decreased peristalsis and tone	Increased peristalsis and tone
Gut (Sphincter)	Increased tone (usually)	Relaxed (usually)
Lung Bronchi	Dilated	Constricted
Penis	Ejaculation	Erection
Basal Metabolism	Increased up to 100%	None
Adrenal Medulla	Increased secretion	None

Figure 2. Effects of activity in the sympathetic and parasympathetic branches of the autonomic nervous system on organs often measured in psychophysiological studies of emotion. Adapted with permission from Guyton & Hall, *Textbook of Medical Physiology.* Copyright 1996 W. B. Saunders.

Second, the notion that the aversive system is associated with sympathetic activity and the appetitive with parasympathetic activity suggests a mode of consistent reciprocal activation between the sympathetic and parasympathetic branches that is no longer tenable. This notion has been replaced by the comprehensive view that these systems can be coactive, as illustrated in Figure 3. Berntson, Cacioppo, and Quigley (1991; see also Berntson et al. 1994) proposed a theory of autonomic control in which physiological measures of a dually innervated end organ (e.g. the heart) may differ as a function of the weighting of activation in the parasympathetic and sympathetic systems: systems can be independently active, reciprocally controlled, or coactive. Quigley and Berntson (1990) further demonstrated that heart rate acceleration to an aversive stimulus (in the rat) is larger than to a low-intensity stimulus not because of differential sympathetic activity but because parasympathetic activity decreases with high-intensity stimulation. Similarly, Wenger, Averill, and Smith (1968) concluded

that autonomic responses measured when males processed erotic texts indicated coactivation rather than parasympathetic or sympathetic dominance. This approach suggests that independent measures of sympathetic and parasympathetic autonomic system activation may be essential in understanding peripheral physiological response measured in emotional contexts.

Cortical and Subcortical Controls of Autonomic and Somatic Activity

If activation of the peripheral nervous system is important in modulating the responses in many of the autonomic and somatic systems measured in the psychophysiological study of emotion (e.g., heart, skin, muscles, gut), then

SYMPATHETIC RESPONSE	PARASYMPATHETIC RESPONSE		
	Increase	*No Change*	*Decrease*
Increase	Coactivation	Uncoupled Sympathetic Activation	Reciprocal Sympathetic Activation
No Change	Uncoupled Parasympathetic Activation	Baseline	Uncoupled Parasympathetic Withdrawal
Decrease	Reciprocal Parasympathetic Activation	Uncoupled Sympathetic Withdrawal	Coinhibition

Figure 3. Modes of autonomic control. Activation in the parasympathetic and sympathetic branches of the autonomic nervous system are proposed to vary from coactivation to independent activation. Adapted with permission from Berntson, Cacioppo, & Quigley, "Autonomic determinism: the modes of autonomic control, the doctrine of autonomic space, and the laws of autonomic constraint," *Psychological Review*, vol. 98, pp. 459–87. Copyright © 1991 by the American Psychological Association.

understanding the neural circuits involved in emotion will depend to some degree on determining which brain structures are important in controlling autonomic and somatic activity. Not surprisingly, control systems occur at every level of the central nervous system: from the spinal cord to the brainstem to subcortical and cortical structures (for more extensive discussions see Gellhorn & Loofbourrow 1963; Guyton & Hall 1996; LeDoux 1987). Thus, for instance, mechanisms in the spinal cord can affect the level of activity in sympathetic and parasympathetic fibers in the absence of supraspinal controls.

Among the more important brainstem control structures is the medulla oblongata. Electrical stimulation of the rostral portion of this structure evokes sympathetic reactions throughout the body, including heart rate and blood pressure increases, pupil dilation, inhibition of gastrointestinal activity, secretion of sweat, and so on. Conversely, activation of the vagal nucleus of the medulla oblongata causes a decrease in heart rate and blood pressure and an increase in gastrointestinal activity – reactions associated with parasympathetic activity. Because of its ability to control many elements of autonomic function, the medulla oblongata has been proposed as the final common pathway for autonomic responses associated with defense reactions (LeDoux 1987).

Control of the autonomic as well as the somatic nervous system is clearly tied to activity in brain structures more advanced than either the spinal or brainstem mechanisms. The neural structures proposed to mediate the emotional reactions subserved by the peripheral nervous system continue to evolve as more information becomes available about the brain from both animal and human research. In general, the neural substrates in emotion are not usually discussed with the goal of assessing whether there is evidence for separable appetitive and aversive systems; rather, many theoretical schemes have lumped appetitive and aversive motivation together as involving "emotion" or have implicitly described a system involving aversiveness, since this has proved more amenable to study. Nonetheless, an effort will be made in the following review to highlight research that concerns evidence for or against the notion of separable appetitive and defensive systems. What is clear is how rapidly the views of brain structure in emotion have changed in the last 50 years.

Hypothalamic Focus

Instead of focusing on peripheral physiological changes in emotion, Cannon advocated a more central approach. He maintained that key structures in the brain, particularly the hypothalamus and thalamus, were important in controlling emotional reactions. His view anticipated modern theorizing in that activity in neural circuits was held to affect neurohumoral and neurochemical events that impact on peripheral reactivity. A focus on the hypothalamus as central in emotion was supported by a number of animal studies which demonstrated that electrical stimulation of the hypothalamus produced physiological reactions associated with sympathetic activation – and even full motor sequences indicative of emotion, including freezing, piloerection, hissing, and attack (collectively termed the "defense reaction"; Hess & Burgger 1943) as well as grooming, mating, and feeding or drinking. Lesions of the hypothalamus (Bard 1934) effectively eliminated these reactions.

Many prominent theorists at this time (e.g. Hess 1957; Morgan 1957; Stellar 1954) confidently subscribed to the notion that the hypothalamus was the main structure implicated in emotion, the "hub" of the limbic system (Gellhorn & Loofbourrow 1963), the "driver at the wheel" (MacLean 1954). Stimulation studies suggesting that the anterior and posterior portions of the hypothalamus were differentially associated with parasympathetic and sympathetic reactions (see Grossman 1967 for a review) led some theorists (e.g. Bovard 1962) to suggest that the anterior (and lateral) hypothalamic region was a "positive reward system" whereas the posterior (and medial) region constituted a negative system – a view not widely held today. Despite proposing a much more extensive neural circuit, Papez (1937) also focused on the hypothalamus as a central structure in mediating emotion, particularly bodily responses. In addition to important thalamic-hypothalamic connections, Papez's circuit included the cingulate cortex and hippocampus. This circuit is generally considered incomplete today, mainly because it neglects to include structures currently thought important in emotion (e.g. amygdala) and includes structures (e.g. hippocampus) that are now recognized as more important for memory (LeDoux 1987). Nonetheless, certain key structures in Papez's circuit, such as the thalamus and cingulate cortex, have been implicated in recent neuroimaging explorations of emotional processing (Breiter et al. 1996; George et al. 1995; Lane et al. 1997a,b).

Periacqueductal Central Gray

Grossman (1967) argued that the focus on the hypothalamus was misleading because data showed that hypothalamic lesions are not irreversible and that stimulation or damage to other parts of the limbic system (e.g. amygdala) can affect emotional behaviors as well. His view was that the hypothalamus was part of a larger, more complex system and that the "apparently unique effects of hypothalamic damage or stimulation may be a 'geographic' artifact" (p. 608) due in part to the fact that the "hypothalamus, because of its peculiar anatomical configuration, seems to act as a funnel for most afferent and efferent impulses to the cortex" (p. 612). Support for his view was provided by studies demonstrating that defensive behavior can be elicited by stimulating the central gray, even after the hypothalamus has been lesioned (Hunsberger, cited in LeDoux 1987), and that lesions in the hypothalamus that destroy cell bodies but not fibers of passage do *not* disrupt conditioned emotional behavior (Coyle & Schwarcz 1983) whereas lesions of the central gray do (LeDoux 1987).

A series of studies conducted by Fanselow and his colleagues (1995; Fanselow 1991, 1994) demonstrated that different regions in the periaqueductal central gray of the rat control freezing and active defense, with lesions and stimulation of the ventromedial portion affecting defensive freezing behaviors and those involving the dorsolateral region affecting defensive actions such as attack and escape. It is interesting that distinct actions appear to have anatomical counterparts that are organized longitudinally within the periaqueductal gray region; for example, jumps are elicited by stimulation in caudal regions whereas defensive upright posture and withdrawal are elicited by stimulation in more rostral regions. Based on these and other data, LeDoux (1987) suggested that projections to the central gray may be the important link in the descending *motor* pathway for defensive behavior. Nonetheless, the hypothalamus remains central in mediating many of the *autonomic* responses measured in emotion.

Amygdala

Another limbic structure, the amygdala, has more recently become a focus in neuroanatomical models of emotion – particularly in terms of its role in mediating associations involving motivationally relevant events, positive and negative (Amaral et al. 1992; Gaffen 1992). Not surprisingly, the nature and type of data supporting the role of the amygdala in emotion are very similar to those originally invoked to support the hypothalamus as the center of the emotion system: lesion and stimulation studies have indicated that specific nuclei in this structure mediate specific emotional phenomena, both appetitive and defensive. Stimulation of the amygdala produces rage, attack, and defense reactions similar to those earlier elicited by activation of the hypothalamus. Moreover, bilateral lesions of the amygdala are, in part, responsible for the observance of the Kluver–Bucy syndrome, in which monkeys lose fear behaviors, become hypersexual, and are indiscriminate with respect to mouthing food and nonfood stimuli. Lesions of the amygdala eliminate the fear-potentiated startle response (Davis 1986) and have been implicated in disrupting appetitive behaviors such as mating, food acquisition, and reward learning (Gaffen 1992). An extensive review of research involving effects of amygdala lesion and stimulation is available in the volume edited by Aggleton (1992).

Geschwind (1965) earlier suggested that the amygdala was particularly necessary for associating stimuli with affective or motivational labels. Amaral and co-workers (1992) elaborated on this by suggesting that "the amygdaloid complex might have widespread ... roles ... that might range from facilitating the selection of an appropriate food or mate, to insuring the avoidance of dangerous situations or substances, to facilitating the aesthetic appreciation of art or music" (p. 2). Clearly, this structure is seen as potentially able to mediate a wide range of behaviors relevant in defensive and appetitive motivation.

A primary reason for considering the amygdala a central component in emotion is that, relative to other limbic structures, it includes multiple afferent and efferent connections to cortical, subcortical, and brainstem structures, which allows it to receive inputs from – and control outputs to – many parts of the brain, including those that have

612

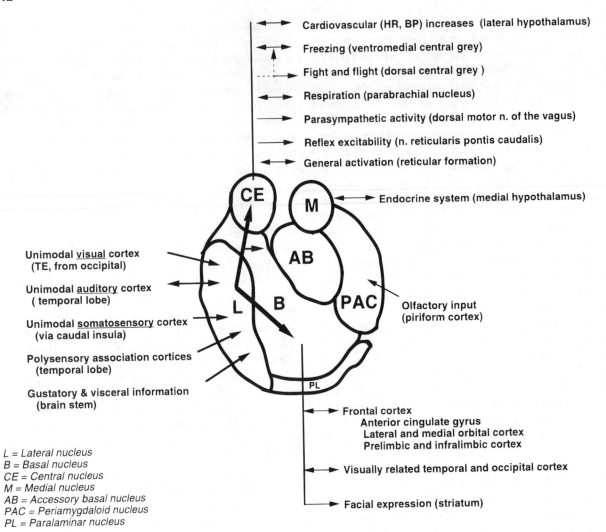

Cardiovascular (HR, BP) increases (lateral hypothalamus)

Freezing (ventromedial central grey)

Fight and flight (dorsal central grey)

Respiration (parabrachial nucleus)

Parasympathetic activity (dorsal motor n. of the vagus)

Reflex excitability (n. reticularis pontis caudalis)

General activation (reticular formation)

Endocrine system (medial hypothalamus)

Unimodal <u>visual</u> cortex
(TE, from occipital)

Unimodal <u>auditory</u> cortex
(temporal lobe)

Unimodal <u>somatosensory</u> cortex
(via caudal insula)

Polysensory association cortices
(temporal lobe)

Gustatory & visceral information
(brain stem)

Olfactory input
(piriform cortex)

CE   M   AB   L   B   PAC   PL

Frontal cortex
  Anterior cingulate gyrus
  Lateral and medial orbital cortex
  Prelimbic and infralimbic cortex

Visually related temporal and occipital cortex

Facial expression (striatum)

L = Lateral nucleus
B = Basal nucleus
CE = Central nucleus
M = Medial nucleus
AB = Accessory basal nucleus
PAC = Periamygdaloid nucleus
PL = Paralaminar nucleus

Figure 4. Inputs, outputs, and intra-amygdala connections illustrate the large variety of sensory and memory inputs to the lateral and basal nuclei of the amygdala as well as various outputs from the central and basal nuclei.

been implicated as important in mediating the autonomic and somatic responses involved in emotional behaviors (Amaral et al. 1992). Thus, the amygdala contains much of the basic architecture necessary for evoking a wide range of behavioral and physiological responses on the basis of multiple types of input cues (i.e., both internal and external). Figure 4 illustrates some of the afferent, efferent, and intra-amygdaloid connections based on a variety of sources, including Amaral et al. (1992), Davis (1989), Fanselow (1994), LeDoux (1987), and Nieuwenhuys, Voogd, and van Huijzen (1988).

A number of general points can be made about the amygdala. First, it is composed of several different nuclei, each of which receives and sends information to a wide variety of different structures. It is no longer tenable to refer to "the amygdala" as having one function or another; rather, different nuclei have both specific inputs

and specific outputs. Whereas some nuclei (e.g. the central nucleus) seem to be predominantly output structures, others (e.g. lateral nucleus) are primarily input structures. Second, the various nuclei within the amygdala are extensively interconnected, with the organization of these connections reflecting the input–output function of different nuclei. Nuclei that primarily serve input functions, such as the lateral and basal nuclei, receive many fewer intra-amygdaloid projections than nuclei that primarily mediate output functions – for example, the central nucleus, which is extensively interconnected with all amygdaloid nuclei (Amaral et al. 1992).

In order to mediate effectively both appetitive and defensive reactions to the variety of potential stimuli encountered in the world, a neural system implementing motivation would need to receive extensive perceptual and memorial information. In fact, inputs to the lateral nucleus of the amygdala (see Figure 4) include those from unimodal cortical sensory areas – including visual, auditory, and somatosensory (via the insula) information – as well as from polysensory association cortex. Olfactory input is relayed to the periamygdaloid (rather than lateral) nucleus, and gustatory information may be relayed to this nucleus via its thalamic input. Information arriving from the senses is in most cases fairly well processed: whereas inputs from primary sensory cortex are few, the presence of multiple unimodal and polymodal inputs suggest the amygdala in general receives information that has received considerable cortical processing. Note especially that inputs representing information on physiological functions are also available to the amygdala, with input from the hypothalamus relayed to the medial nucleus as well as directly to the central nucleus and with visceral information from the brain stem relayed via the thalamus to the lateral nucleus.

The presence of thalamic inputs to the lateral as well as central nuclei indicates that some relatively raw sensory information is probably also available to the amygdala, although this information would presumably be processed only to the level of gross physical features (loud, bright, etc.). As LeDoux (1996) emphasized, these alternative pathways to the amygdala, thalamic and cortical, may play an important role in understanding emotional processing of different sensory stimuli. It is worth emphasizing, however, that (i) complex stimuli (e.g. pictures) that require higher-level perceptual processing for encoding are probably not processed via direct thalamic-amygdaloid input, and (ii) simple unconditioned stimuli are the best candidates for direct activation of the amygdala through thalamic relays.

In the nonhuman primate, the amount of visual information relayed to the amygdala appears to be greater than auditory or somatosensory information (Amaral et al. 1992), which might reflect the fact that, for primates as well as for humans, much behavior is elicited on the basis of visual cues. Consistent with the idea that amygdaloid inputs reflect species-specific perceptual preferences, olfactory-amygdaloid connections are so central in the rodent that Gellhorn and Loofbourrow (1963) concluded the amygdala's role in emotion was only as "a secondary olfactory center."

Outputs from the amygdala are extensive as well, and they include almost all of the structures highlighted as important in emotional processing – with direct connections to the hypothalamus, the central gray, the brainstem, the striatum, and cortical structures including the cingulate gyrus, frontal lobe, visual cortex, and more. Interestingly, a rough division in amygdaloid outputs can be made between the central and basal nuclei. As Figure 4 illustrates, the central nucleus of the amygdala mediates outputs to many of the hypothalamic and brainstem structures involved in emotional responses, whereas outputs from the basal nucleus consist primarily of cortical targets, including visual areas of temporal and occipital lobes as well as frontal, anterior cingulate, and so on. This organization makes it possible for different amygdaloid nuclei to be involved in activating information relevant to physiological response or associative meaning.

An additional output from the basal nucleus is to the nucleus accumbens, which – together with the ventral striatum and other dopaminergically innervated structures – has been implicated as important in modulating appetitive behaviors (Koch & Schnitzler 1997) and in reward learning (see Everitt & Robbins 1992). Activation of both the nucleus accumbens and amygdala have been found in studies investigating the rewarding properties of cocaine use in humans (Breiter et al. 1998), lending support to the notion that the amygdala is a contender as a key component of both appetitive and defensive motivational systems.

Neurohumoral Control

In addition to engaging specific effectors, activation of the sympathetic nervous system has significant implications for release of a number of blood-borne substances that also affect physiological reactivity (for overviews see e.g. Baum, Grunberg, & Singer 1992; Grunberg & Singer 1990). One pathway, emphasized by Cannon, begins with sympathetic activation of the adrenal medulla (in the kidney), which releases catecholamines such as epinephrine and norepinephrine that have the same influence on anatomical structures as direct sympathetic innervation – that is, increasing heart rate, blood pressure, and respiration while redirecting blood flow to active muscles. These sympathetic effects of catecholamines on physiological systems can be longer-lasting than direct sympathetic activation and can also affect organs not directly innervated by sympathetic fibers. A second pathway involves pituitary-adrenocortical activation, a focus of Selye's (1950) work on stress. This path is from the pituitary to the adrenal cortex (also in the kidney), which leads to production of corticosteroids, including the commonly measured substance cortisol. Release of cortisol is stimulated by adrenocorticotropic factor (ACTH) from the brain and functions to increase energy mobilization (see Levine 1986).

Although biochemical measures of catecholamines (e.g., epinephrine, norepinephrine, and cortisol) are common in research investigating both brief and sustained stressors (e.g. Cacioppo et al. 1995), inclusion of these indices of sympathetic activation is less typical in emotion research. Part of the difficulty may lie in obtaining assays (e.g., in blood, urine, or even saliva) at the frequency and rate at which different emotional stimuli are typically presented in emotion research. In addition, early hypotheses (e.g. Ax 1953) that epinephrine and norepinephrine may be differentially associated with fear and anger were disconfirmed, suggesting these biochemical indices could not differentiate among discrete emotions. Rather, catecholamines in particular appeared to be sensitive to the arousing aspects of a situation, increasing in environments that are novel or complex as well as in those that are emotionally arousing (Frankenhaeuser 1975). Such a pattern is clearly informative if the psychophysiological investigation seeks to understand effects of pleasure and arousal on physiological response. Hence, it would be useful to include these measures more routinely in studies of emotion.

Cognitive Models

Neuroanatomical models propose that inputs from a number of different sources converge on subcortical structures such as the amygdala, which controls outputs to the somatic and autonomic nervous system as mediated through various structures, including the central gray and the hypothalamus. This same type of neural network can be described at a cognitive level, where a model of the functional relationship between input and output is provided without identifying specific anatomical structures.

One popular type of cognitive model is instantiated in various forms of "appraisal" theory (Lazarus 1991), in which stored information (appraisals) regarding the stimulus (Arnold 1970) or physiological response (Schacter & Singer 1962) is the critical variable determining the emotionality of an experience. When physiology is the focus of the appraisal process, it is usually conceptualized as involving undifferentiated arousal (Schacter & Singer 1962). Appraisal theories seek to provide a mechanism by which the same stimulus (input) can produce different reports of emotion (output) and by which different situations can produce reports of the same emotion. This is enabled by allowing appraisals – stored interpretations of stimuli and responses – to control emotional experience.

More explicitly information-processing models of emotion propose that emotional representations code multiple types of information, including stimulus characteristics, response features, and stored associations (e.g. Bower 1981; Lang 1979). Lang's bioinformational theory (1979, 1984, 1994a) conceives of emotion as a cognitive network that includes stimulus and response units that are linked by associations (see Figure 5). Lang distinguishes between inputs that are perceptually based (stimulus) and those that are conceptually based (meaning). Whereas "stimulus units" code information regarding sensory and perceptual features (e.g., the visual, acoustic, and tactile features of a snake and the current context), "meaning units" provide semantic information previously learned about the stimulus (e.g., snakes are dangerous). Meaning units are an associationist interpretation of what might typically be termed appraisals (see Lang 1994a). That is, semantic information – previously learned and associated with specific stimulus and response contexts – is part of the memory representation for emotional (and nonemotional) events.

An important feature of Lang's (1979) bioinformational theory is its inclusion of response units in the representation of an emotional stimulus. A number of cognitive models focus almost exclusively on the representation of stimulus and semantic information in memory without considering the coding of relevant behavioral outputs. In bioinformational theory, on the other hand, emotion is instantiated primarily via response units, which code associated actions (e.g. running) and reactions (e.g. heart rate acceleration) that are part of the associative structure of an emotional event. Response information is linked to input cues on the basis of both unconditioned and conditioned associations. Consistent with the use of these terms in the learning literature, unconditioned responses are innate, hard-wired links between stimulus features (e.g. sudden movement) and a particular action (e.g. startle response), whereas conditioned associations reflect links forged through experience.

Network models (e.g. Anderson 1983; Lang 1979) and more recent distributed models of cognition (e.g. McClelland & Rumelhart 1986) view cognitive processing as an iterative process in which information in an input cue initially controls the level of activation in memory. Associated units are activated, and this information is subsequently fed back into the system as a new input cue, allowing different types of information (e.g., stimulus, response, or meaning) to further affect the level of network activation. Thus, whereas physiological responses are often considered outputs of emotional processing, they can also serve as input cues (consistent with James's earlier suggestion). The iterative nature of emotional processing, in which current information regarding both stimulus and response is repeatedly re-entered as input to the processing system, is also highlighted in Cacioppo and colleagues' somatovisceral afference model of emotion (SAME; Cacioppo, Berntson, & Klein 1992a; Cacioppo et al. 1993).

From a methodological perspective, these theories suggest that the nature, quality, type, and amount of information in the input cue is important, since these parameters have implications for the degree of associative activation and physiological output (see e.g. Lang et al. 1980). Because stimulus, response, or meaning information can serve as input that initiates or maintains a processing episode, the bioinformational framework can accommodate theories that identify the primary input to emotion as physiological (e.g., the Jamesian hypothesis or facial feedback theories) as well as more traditional views that focus on sensory stimulation.

All events can be considered as coded and processed in associative structures of the type described here, so what is it that makes a particular cognitive representation "emotional"? Lang (1994b) and LeDoux (1996) agree that it is specific associations to the motivational systems mediating appetitive and defensive behavior (e.g. limbic structures) that are the defining feature of an emotional representation. To the extent that input cues activate these subcortical motivational systems, the resulting cognitive processing can be considered to be emotionally engaging. It is because of associations to these basic biphasic motivational systems (and the resulting activation of relevant autonomic and somatic responses) that physiological activity is a hallmark of emotional processing.

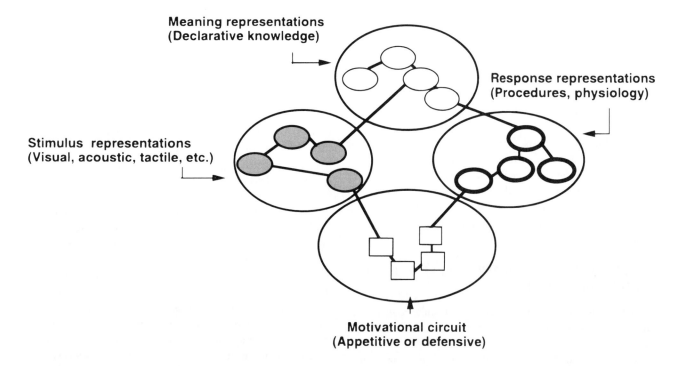

Example: Cognitive representation of a Snake Phobic

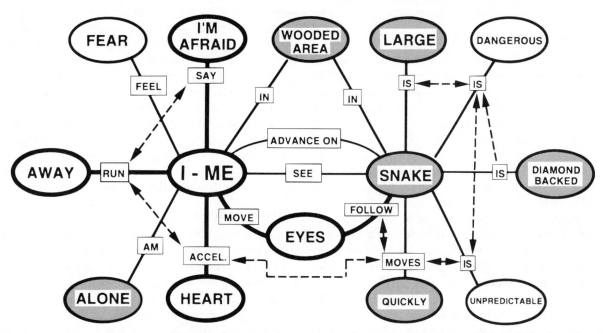

Figure 5. *Top panel*. A cognitive representation of an emotional event includes information relevant to (1) the stimulus and environmental context, (2) learned semantic associates, and (3) appropriate behavioral and physiological responses. Connections to primitive appetitive and defensive motivational systems define an "emotional" event. *Bottom panel*. Example of a cognitive representation coding an encounter with a snake in the woods. Adapted with permission from Lang, "Cognition and emotion: Concept and action," in Izard, Kagan, & Zajonc (Eds.), *Emotion, Cognition and Behavior*. Copyright 1984 Cambridge University Press.

Inferential Context

BIOMETRICS: MENSURATION AND QUANTIFICATION PROCEDURES

Because emotional responses can be measured in many of the physiological systems addressed in this volume, the reader is referred to chapters on specific response systems for information concerning current measurement and quantification techniques. Assessments of changes in electrodermal, somatic, respiratory, reflex, cardiovascular, or cortical activity assessed in the context of emotional (appetitive or aversive) stimulation should be measured, quantified, and mapped to system changes in ways that are consistent with those recommended in this volume.

PSYCHOMETRICS: THE PSYCHOPHYSIOLOGICAL STUDY OF EMOTION

According to the view expressed here, one goal of psychophysiological studies of emotion is to determine the nature of the relationship between inputs (that vary in hedonic valence and arousal) and outputs (measured in a variety of different response systems) as they vary in specific experimental contexts. Making inferences specifically about the psychophysiology of emotion will rely on clearly (1) defining the affective nature of the stimuli, (2) determining the task context, and (3) defining the measured output.

Defining Affective Stimuli

In order to study emotion, it is necessary to manipulate the affective characteristics of experimental stimuli. Research prompted by a biphasic view of emotion suggests that experimental stimuli should systematically vary in terms of pleasure and arousal; a view that sees emotions as discrete, on the other hand, seeks stimuli that vary in terms of eliciting specific emotional states (e.g., fear, anger, sadness). With either paradigm, some type of bootstrapping operation is needed to initially identify stimuli that differ in terms of emotionality.

In human subjects, verbal reports of emotion (e.g., pleasure and arousal ratings; Lang et al. 1990) are often used to classify stimuli a priori. Over the past ten years, our laboratory has developed different sets of experimental stimuli (pictures – Lang, Bradley, & Cuthbert 1998; sounds – Bradley & Lang 1999a; words – Bradley & Lang 1999b) that groups of subjects have rated in terms of both pleasure and arousal. The resulting stimulus collections allow one to select materials that systematically vary in valence and arousal while controlling for other potentially relevant factors (e.g., semantic category). Defining affect in this way allows one to begin to assess the impact of the emotional variables of pleasure and arousal on physiological, behavioral, and subjective report measures.

It is important to include neutral stimuli (i.e., neither highly pleasant nor unpleasant) when investigating emotion in order to assess the physiology associated with the task itself. As discussed more fully in what follows, specific processing tasks can affect the direction of physiological change; the inclusion of neutral stimuli allows one to assess this facet of the experimental procedure. The physiology of the task (imagery, anticipation, etc.) can be determined by assessing each measured response system (cardiovascular, electrodermal, etc.) in the context of processing neutral stimuli. Then, physiological responses associated specifically with emotion will rely on obtaining differences between processing neutral stimuli and those that are affectively engaging.

At the least, then, investigations of emotion should include three groups of affective stimuli, consisting of pleasant (high-arousal), neutral (low-arousal), and unpleasant (high-arousal) stimuli. Use of this minimal affective set allows one to assess effects due to differences in: (i) hedonic valence, where measurable differences are obtained between pleasant and unpleasant stimuli; and (ii) arousal, where significant differences are obtained between arousing (i.e., pleasant or unpleasant) and neutral, calm stimuli. Studies including only two of these three conditions (e.g., aversive–neutral) make it difficult to disassociate effects of stimulus arousal from effects of stimulus valence on physiological and behavioral response.

A more complete experimental design that is consistent with a biphasic view involves manipulating the level of arousal within both pleasant and unpleasant stimulus sets (Cuthbert, Bradley, & Lang 1996); this allows one to assess biphasic reactions at varying levels of intensity. If the goal is further to study whether physiological responses differ in terms of discrete emotions (e.g., fear, anger), it is important to include at least two emotions at each level of valence (e.g., two pleasant emotions; see Cacioppo et al. 1993) – preferably balanced for level of arousal. Otherwise, it is impossible to conclude that obtained differences are due to the physiology associated with the specific emotional state and not simply due to valence or arousal differences.

Determining the Task Context

Comparisons are often made between widely different paradigms of instigation. For example, the physiology during fear has been assessed in contexts as diverse as hearing loud noises, anticipating shock, imagining an intruder in the house, looking at a picture of an amputated leg, viewing a scary film, giving a speech, putting one's hand in cold water ("cold pressor" test), or hearing an anguished scream. Conversely, positive reactions are compared across such diverse contexts as receiving money, listening to joyful music, looking at a picture of puppies, viewing an erotic film, imagining a day on the beach, receiving a good grade, thinking about winning the lottery, or anticipating a vacation.

Making comparisons across very different contexts has led to some confusion when trying to extrapolate effects of emotion on psychophysiological response. For instance, cardiac reactions are often more different when processing affectively similar events in different tasks (e.g., heart rate decelerates during unpleasant picture viewing yet accelerates during unpleasant mental imagery; Lang et al. 1990) than when processing affectively different events in similar tasks (e.g., heart rate accelerates during imagery of pleasant and unpleasant events; Levenson 1992). In this case, the task context of perception or imagination has a strong influence on the direction of heart rate change. Making sense of cardiac patterns as a function of variations in hedonic valence and arousal will require careful consideration of the physiology of the task itself. In addition, whereas both perception and anticipation often produce triphasic cardiac waveforms that include an initial deceleration followed by acceleration and a secondary deceleration, the appearance and weighting of each component can vary with motor requirements (Jennings et al. 1970), ease of stimulus categorization (Bull & Lang 1972), or stimulus familiarity (Bradley, Cuthbert, & Lang 1993a). Thus, individual components of cardiac reactivity can be affected by task variables not particularly relevant to differences in emotion.

The task contexts typically used to induce affective reactions in the laboratory can be roughly sorted into the four categories of perception, anticipation, imagination, and action. In *perception,* the task is to process sensory information that varies in emotion (e.g., hedonic valence and arousal) and that can be presented in various modalities, such as visual (pictures, words, films), acoustic (sounds, music), tactile (shock, cold pressor), olfactory (odors), or gustatory (foods). In *imagination,* the primary task is to generate mentally an emotional stimulus or event. This task relies heavily on the human's ability to internally retrieve and elaborate information relevant to a particular object or event. In *anticipation,* the task is simply to await the presentation of a sensory appetitive or aversive stimulus, usually signaled by a neutral cue (e.g., tone or light). Most classical conditioning paradigms fall into this class. In contexts involving *action,* the task involves a specific overt activity, such as giving a speech or posing facial actions.

Careful attention to the task context should help to terminate comparisons between reactions elicited during presentation of a speech and anticipation of electric shock, for example, on the basis that both may elicit fear or that both are aversive. Rather, the psychophysiological study of emotion will need, at least at first, to restrict comparisons to data obtained in similar contexts. Emotional reactions in perception may differ both quantitatively and qualitatively from emotion in imagination, owing to the requisite physiology of these different tasks as well as to differences in the nature and type of information available in the affective cue. Clearly, the psychophysiology of emotion in action can differ from vigilant anticipation. Parameters

need to be identified, within the context of each task, that have implications for motivational activation – that is, the ease with which hypothetical appetitive and aversive neural systems are activated – as well as for the nature of elicited physiological responses that are related to task but not emotion.

Perception. Perceptual cues can vary in a number of ways that may influence their ability to activate basic motivational systems or the degree of physiological response. Among these are: (1) the sensory modality of the cue (e.g., visual, acoustic, tactile), (2) the degree to which the sensory cue is an unconditioned or conditioned stimulus, (3) the duration of the cue, and (4) whether the information in the cue is static or dynamic.

For instance, cues in different modalities may have differential access to motivational circuits. As noted earlier, visual input to the amygdaloid complex in nonhuman primates is more extensive than auditory input (Amaral et al. 1992), suggesting that modality could be important in activating motivational dispositions. Whether a cue is unconditioned or conditioned reflects the presumed contributions to emotional reactivity of both learning and hard-wired associations. Whereas intense physical stimuli such as painful shocks or loud noises reflexively (and unconditionally) prompt defensive reactions, symbolic stimuli such as the pictures, films, and verbal scripts often used in emotion research rely on learning for motivational activation and may be expected to be more variable.

The importance of stimulus duration in affecting physiological reactions was highlighted in Selye's (1974) general adaptation syndrome, in which a brief stressor was proposed to produce a phasic alarm reaction followed by bodily exhaustion and system collapse after prolonged exposure. More generally, the duration of a specific appetitive or aversive stimulus may control whether sensitization (increased responding) or habituation (decreased responding) is a factor contributing to the pattern of physiological reactivity. Finally, a sensory cue can differ in the amount of information that it provides over time, ranging from a relatively static cue (e.g. a picture) to one that is quite dynamic (a film); see Simons et al. (1999). Physiological systems engaged by novel stimulation (i.e., orienting responses) may contribute substantially to the measured physiology in dynamic processing. Taken together, a keener appreciation of variables that may affect reactivity will help us more clearly interpret effects of emotion on psychophysiological response.

Imagination. Imagery (emotional reliving) paradigms have been used extensively in psychophysiological investigations of emotion. In these tasks, participants are instructed to mentally generate an emotionally evocative event based on either a text cue (i.e., a narrative script) or a perceptual cue (e.g., using a picture or film as an imagery prompt). Important parameters in studies of emotional imagery include: (i) the nature of the information in the imagery cue, (ii) whether the imagined responses are passive or active, and (iii) whether the events imagined have been personally experienced or are fictional.

A number of studies have indicated that the nature of information in the cue affects emotional reactions. Lang and his colleagues (Lang et al. 1980; Miller et al. 1987) have demonstrated that physiological reactions differentiating fearful and neutral imagery are accentuated when response information (e.g., "imagine that your palms are sweaty") is included in the prompt compared to when the imagery cue describes only information related to the stimulus context. Jones and Johnson (1978) demonstrated that imagery cues describing action produced more cardiac reactivity during imagery than cues describing passive scenes. Taken together, these data are consistent with the notion that physiological reactions during imagery reflect activation of response-related information in memory, cued in part by information present in the input prompt. Additionally, when subjects imagine events that they have personally experienced, more appropriate skin conductance and heart rate changes occur than when scripts are imagined that are not personally relevant (Miller et al. 1987), suggesting that motivational and physiological activation is more successful when an existing associative network can be activated. The parameters affecting physiological reactions during emotional imagery are discussed more fully in Cuthbert, Vrana, and Bradley (1991).

Anticipation. Waiting for an unpleasant or pleasant event to occur is the hallmark of classical conditioning studies, in which a neutral cue signals the upcoming occurrence of an unconditioned aversive or appetitive stimulus. Studies of anticipation (and, to some extent, conditioning) focus on physiological reactions during the warning interval – that is, before an emotional stimulus is actually presented. Numerous temporal and associative parameters have been noted as critical in obtaining conditioning effects (Mackintosh 1983; Stern 1972) and are potentially relevant when assessing emotional reactions during anticipation (see Putnam 1990). Critical variables in terms of motivational and physiological activation include: (i) the modality of the warning cue, (ii) whether the warning cue is continuous or discrete, and (iii) whether the warning cue signals a specific (e.g. snake) or nonspecific (e.g. "something bad") target.

The sensory modality of an anticipated perceptual event has been important for theorists such as Graham (1992), who proposed differential modulation of physiological responses (e.g., the acoustic startle reflex) depending upon the modality to which attention is directed. Thus, stimulus modality can affect certain physiological reactions independent of, or in addition to, emotional variables. Whether the warning cue is continuous or discrete has implications for the amount of orienting (perceptual intake) activity

that is occurring concurrent with anticipation, which again can affect the type of physiological reactions during the anticipatory period independent of effects due to affective parameters. Finally, the specificity of the warning cue affects the nature and type of information that can be retrieved or imagined during the anticipatory period, which can affect the pattern of physiological response.

Action. Contexts involving overt action are employed less often in psychophysiological investigations of emotion, and for good reason. Gross motor activity can saturate amplifiers, produce artifact in cardiovascular and electrodermal records, and generally interfere with recording the often smaller physiological effects related to emotional parameters. The main variable in an action context will generally be the required activity: giving a speech will be more physiologically demanding than a simple button press, for example. Assessing changes due to emotional parameters such as pleasure and arousal will be most difficult in contexts that involve considerable activity. Ambulatory monitoring studies, which attempt to study emotional reactions such as panic as they occur in the natural environment, fall within this class of paradigms. These investigators must cope with issues involved in trying to separate the physiology of emotion from the physiology of the ongoing action (see e.g. Turpin 1990; Wilhelm & Roth 1996).

Response Measurement

Most theorists have recognized that the data base of emotion – indices that can be measured and quantified in the laboratory – includes three systems: (1) subjective report, (2) overt action, and (3) physiological response (see e.g. Lang 1968). Subjective reports of affective experience include verbal descriptions (e.g., "I'm afraid"), ratings of emotion (e.g., ratings of fear on a scale of 1 to 10), reports of physiological responses (e.g., identification of bodily responses that occurred), and other methods that elicit reports from subjects regarding their awareness of affective reactions. Overt behaviors – such as running, jumping, fighting, freezing – used extensively in studies of motivated behavior in laboratory animals are somewhat less commonly measured in human studies. Representative overt behaviors in the human laboratory include expressive language (e.g., "I hate you"), vocalization measures (see Scherer 1986), performance measures (e.g., reaction time), and observable facial expressions (Ekman 1971). Physiological responses comprise bodily events that can be assessed using psychophysiological instrumentation and methods yet are not necessarily observable. In emotion research to date, these have included responses in cardiovascular, electrodermal, gastric, somatic, reflex, central, and neurohumoral/neurochemical systems.

There are a number of interesting relationships among three-system measures of emotional responses. First, it is clear that affective reactions can be assessed solely through two measures of overt behavior (e.g. freezing) and physiological (e.g. cardiovascular) response in the absence of verbal reports, as animal studies clearly demonstrate; motivational systems operate independently of a link to a developed language system. Second, when behavior is observable, changes in associated physiological measures will also occur. To the extent a person is overtly smiling, for example, changes will be detected in EMG measures over the appropriate muscles. Thus, behavioral and physiological measures of emotion can be distinguished by whether the response is observable: overt behaviors are visible to an observer, whereas physiological measures can further tap covert, unobservable bodily events. Because of their interdependence, behavioral and physiological measures will not be discordant in the same sense that reports of affective experience and physiology may be. Determining the relationships among three-system responses in specific affective contexts is an important step in the task of understanding human emotional response.

AFFECT, TASK, AND MEASUREMENT: EMPIRICAL FINDINGS

Perceptual information (in some form) is an ingredient in almost all experimental paradigms. Processing a sensory stimulus – as when instructed to look at a picture, listen to a noise, receive a shock, smell an odor, or taste some substance – is here considered to be a prototypical perceptual task. In emotional perception, instructions to simply process sensory stimuli often result in a relatively passive (i.e., physiologically inactive) intake posture.

Earlier investigations exploring emotion in perception assessed autonomic reactions such as vascular changes, electrodermal reactions, and heart rate (Epstein 1971; Roessler, Burch, & Childers 1966; Turpin & Siddle 1983) as a function of differences in stimulus intensity, because this variable was considered critical in eliciting orienting or defense responses. Sensory stimuli of low intensity were held to prompt orienting activity, associated with a pattern of peripheral and cephalic vasoconstriction and heart rate deceleration, whereas intense stimuli prompted a defense response, associated with peripheral vasoconstriction, cephalic vasodilation, and heart rate acceleration (see Graham 1979; Sokolov 1963; Turpin 1986).

Empirical support for a relationship between stimulus intensity (e.g., shock or noise) and predicted patterns of cardiovascular responses was generally good (but see Turpin 1986). Notable exceptions were found, however, particularly when the perceptual stimuli involved pictures. In the picture context, stimulus intensity was generally operationalized as involving variations in hedonic valence, and comparisons were made between pictures that depicted aversive (e.g., car accidents, mutilations) or neutral events. Work by the Laceys (e.g. Libby et al. 1973), Klorman (Klorman, Weissberg, & Austin 1975; Klorman,

Weissbert, & Wiessenfeld 1977), and Hare (e.g. Hare et al. 1971a,b; Hare 1973) consistently found that the heart decelerated when people viewed pictures of unpleasant emotional events, contrary to the notion that such aversive stimuli should prompt defensive heart rate acceleration. Based on these kinds of data, Lacey (1967) introduced the concepts of directional fractionation (i.e., not all physiological responses uniformly increase with increasing arousal) and stimulus specificity (i.e., specific stimuli and tasks are associated with specific patterns of physiological response). That is, although the heart decelerates in a perceptual (sensory intake) context such as picture viewing, increased electrodermal reactions are consistent with sympathetic activation and increasing arousal.

However, pictures differ from the physical stressors (i.e., shock and noise) originally utilized in studies of orienting and defense on a number of the dimensions described earlier. In addition to the obvious modality differences (visual vs. tactile or acoustic), pictures differ from shocks or noises in terms of learning: simple stressors such as painful shock or loud noise are unconditioned stimuli, eliciting defense responses in animals as well as in newborn humans. Pictures, on the other hand, are highly symbolic stimuli whose encoding along affective dimensions requires prior learning as well as cognitive sophistication.

Furthermore, defining stimulus intensity in terms of differences in picture valence (i.e., comparing unpleasant to neutral pictures) confuses the issue of how the intensity of symbolic versus physical stressors affects physiological response. A more systematic approach is to assess how emotional reactions vary with changes in the valence and arousal of picture stimuli. One benefit of using pictures as affective cues is the ease of including pleasant exemplars: when shock serves as an aversive stimulus, for example, it has proven difficult to find an unconditioned tactile stimulus that is as pleasant as shock is unpleasant. Pictures also have the advantage of representing many of the events and stimuli people find affectively engaging in the environment, and these stimuli are experimentally tractable in terms of control and presentation.

Affective Space: Pleasure and Arousal

Recently we collected a set of pictures depicting a wide variety of objects, events, and situations into the International Affective Picture System[1] (IAPS; Lang et al. 1998) with the goal of providing a set of standardized materials for use in studies of emotion. When human subjects are asked to judge the pleasure and arousal of these pictures, an affective space such as that depicted in Figure 6 (top panel) results. In this figure, each symbol represents a picture, plotted as a function of its mean judged pleasure and arousal rating.

The shape of affective space provides support for a fundamental organization of emotion in terms of appetitive and defensive motivation. First, it is clear that stimuli vary in hedonic valence: proceeding vertically in each direction from the center of the space (where neutral events cluster), stimuli are rated as progressively more pleasant or more unpleasant. Second, as ratings of hedonic valence change in either direction, ratings of arousal tend to increase. The boomerang shape of this space is very similar for sets of words or sounds (Bradley & Lang 1999a,b, respectively), instrumental music (van Oyen Witvliet & Vrana 1996), and films (Detenber, Simons, & Bennet 1998), suggesting a common organization for these perceptual stimuli.

The arrows in the top panel of Figure 6 illustrate activation in the hypothetical underlying appetitive and defensive systems. When activation in each system is minimal (neither pleasant or unpleasant), arousal is correspondingly low and events are usually labelled "unemotional" or "neutral." From a motivational perspective, this suggests only a weak tendency to approach or withdraw from the stimulus, with little energy mobilization required for what is essentially a minimal behavioral response. As activation in the defensive system increases (stimuli are rated as increasingly more unpleasant), arousal increases as well, presumably indexing the metabolic requirements required for anticipated and

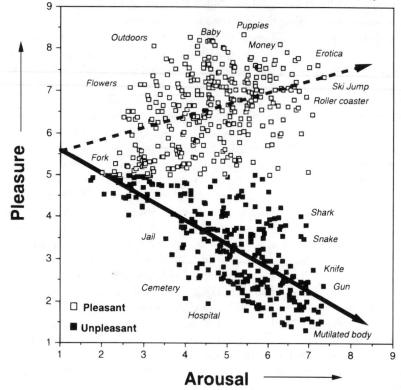

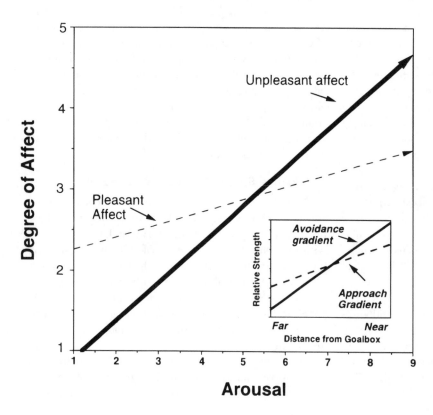

Figure 6. *Top panel.* Pictures from the International Affective Picture System (CSEA 1999) are plotted in a two-dimensional space defined by the mean ratings of judged pleasure and arousal by a large group of subjects. The arrows in the upper and lower portions of affective space indicate varying activation in hypothetical underlying appetitive and defensive motivational systems. *Bottom panel.* The slope of the arousal functions for pleasant and unpleasant pictures (excluding pictures rated in the neutral valence range, i.e., from 4.5 to 5.5 in upper plot), based on subjective reports of pleasure and arousal, closely parallel the approach and avoidance gradients based on direction and intensity of behavior originally noted by Miller (1959; inset) in his classic animal studies. Adapted with permission from Miller, "Liberalization of basic S-R concepts: Extensions to conflict behavior, motivation and social learning," in Koch (Ed.), *Psychology: A Study of a Science,* vol. 2, Study 1. Copyright 1959 The McGraw-Hill Companies.

actual action (e.g., withdrawal, escape, defense). Similarly, increasing activation in the appetitive system is associated with increases in rated arousal, reflecting energy allocated to fueling behaviors involving approach and consummation.

The separate arousal gradients obtained for pleasant and unpleasant pictures in the top panel of Figure 6 are overlaid in the bottom panel of Figure 6. It is striking how well these gradients map onto Miller's classic schematic illustrating differences in approach and avoidance behavior in the rat (inset, bottom panel of Figure 6), since Miller's data were based not on verbal reports but on the strength of the animal's pull toward or away from an appetitive or aversive stimulus. Miller found a prototypical pattern of responding in which withdrawal from an aversive stimulus increased with proximity to it whereas approaching a proximal appetitive stimulus was somewhat less intense. Despite the drastic difference in the measures used to index direction (i.e., withdrawal or approach vs. valence judgments) and degree of activation (behavioral strength vs. arousal judgments), it is clear that reports of arousal for pleasant and unpleasant perceptual stimuli closely parallel Miller's classic motivational gradients. Emotion is fundamentally organized by motivation.

Drawing on data like these, Cacioppo and associates (Berntson, Boysen, & Cacioppo 1993; Cacioppo et al. 1997; Ito, Cacioppo, & Lang 1998) concluded that the positivity offset (i.e., the larger constant for positive motivation) indicates that a weak tendency for activation in the appetitive system exists when neither system is strongly active. They suggest that this tendency to approach, functioning at low levels of motivation, provides a basis for understanding the orienting and exploratory reactions that constitute daily interactions with environmental stimuli that are neither highly threatening nor highly appealing. The negativity bias – the steeper gradient for defensive behaviors – reflects a propensity to respond more strongly to aversive stimulation.

As Figure 6 (top panel) illustrates, the steeper slope for aversive pictures arises from a closer coupling between the degree of (un)pleasantness and arousal: the relationship between valence and arousal ratings for unpleasant pictures is highly linear. For pleasant pictures, on the other hand, reported pleasure and arousal are less tightly coupled – primarily owing to stimuli that are rated as highly pleasant but low in arousal (e.g., clouds, nature scenes). The uncoupling in reports of hedonic valence and action for pleasurable stimuli may reflect the cognitive sophistication underlying aesthetic appreciation.

Physiological Reactions and System Covariation

Stimulus evaluations support the notion that dimensions of pleasure and arousal can be used to organize emotional reactions to picture stimuli. As noted earlier,

however, these judgments are not exhaustive in tapping the subject's affective data base. Using stimuli from the IAPS set, the nature of physiological reactions and their covariation with subjective reports have been assessed in a number of different studies (Greenwald, Cook, & Lang 1989; Lang et al. 1993; for a review see Bradley & Lang in press a). In these experiments, physiological responses such as heart rate, skin conductance, facial EMG activity (e.g., corrugator and zygomatic), blood pressure, respiration, eye movements, and event-related potentials have been measured while subjects simply view emotional and neutral IAPS pictures. Ratings of pleasure and arousal (and, in some cases, of interest, complexity, or familiarity) are obtained after the termination of each picture. Patterns of physiological reactivity as a function of picture valence and arousal have been assessed on the basis of the a priori groupings of pictures (i.e., determined by IAPS norms) as well as by each participant's own reports of pleasure and arousal obtained during the psychophysiological assessment session.

In the latter, covariation method, individuals' reports of experienced pleasure and arousal are related to physiological response by ranking the picture stimuli from lowest to highest on the basis of each subject's own affective judgments. The mean activity in each physiological system is then assessed at each rank, across subjects. This strategy optimizes the opportunity to observe unit changes in physiology coincident with changes in affective judgments, and it provides a meaningful index of affective covariation. The method also allows one to determine whether systematic variations in pleasure or arousal (or their interaction) are associated with systematic changes in physiological response – and, if so, which measures are sensitive to which dimension. On the other hand, if emotion is primarily organized by discrete emotional states then no systematic relationship between variations along these emotional dimensions and physiological response is expected.

Results from these studies are summarized in Figure 7. The left column illustrates the average response pattern for different physiological measures during the time that participants were viewing a 6-sec picture presentation. In each analysis, data were acquired at a 20-Hz sampling rate, reduced off-line into half-second bins, and deviated from a 1-sec baseline just prior to picture onset in order to assess phasic responses to the picture. The center column illustrates the dimensional covariation between physiological responses and affective judgments obtained from a group of subjects and based on the analysis just described. The right column illustrates the size of the dimensional correlation between relevant affective judgments and physiological response for individual male and female subjects. We next discuss these data more fully.

Facial EMG Activity. Facial displays (frowns, grimaces, smiles, etc.) of affective reactions constitute some of the

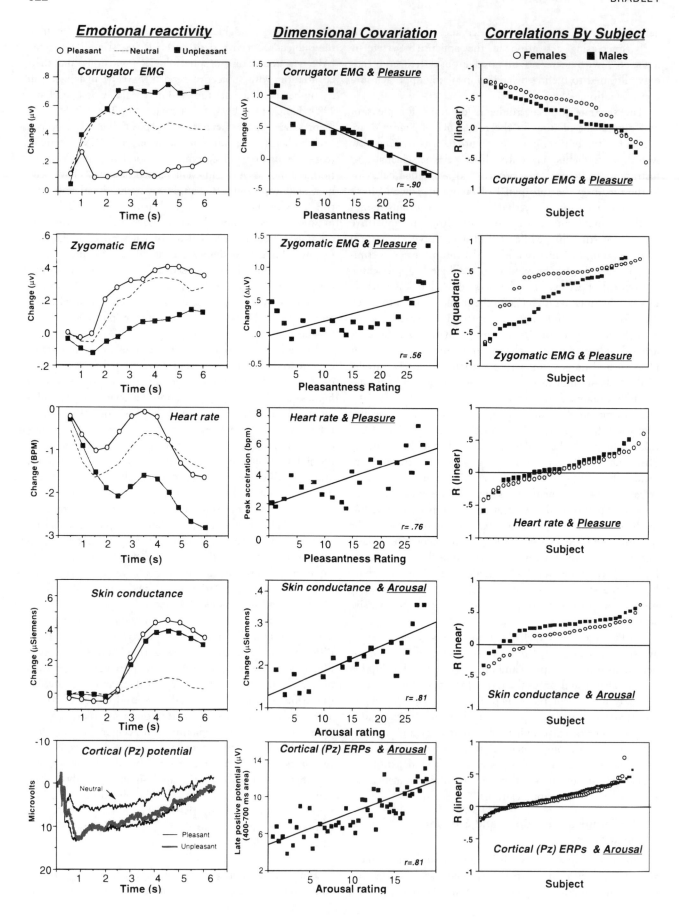

more obvious overt behaviors associated with emotional processing. Whether facial expressions reliably communicate different types of emotion across cultures intrigued even Darwin (1873), and research supports the view that a small set is recognizable pan-culturally (Ekman & Friesen 1986). A number of coding systems have been designed that allow researchers to code facial movement from videotaped displays, which clearly rely on overt expression (e.g., FACS – Ekman & Friesen 1978; MAX – Izard 1979). As Tassinary and Cacioppo (1992) pointed out, electromyographic recordings made using electrodes placed over the relevant muscles further allow measurement of covert facial responses. A number of studies have indicated that emotional processing is associated with significant changes in EMG activity involving different facial muscles (Cacioppo et al. 1986; Dimberg 1990).

A primary issue in this work concerns the extent to which facial EMG activity reflects spontaneous or voluntarily initiated movement, since the strong voluntary control over facial activity poses obvious interpretive problems in studies of emotion (for discussion of these problems, see Tassinary & Cacioppo 1992; Cacioppo, Bush, & Tassinary 1992b). Tassinary, Cacioppo, and Geen (1989) reported that voluntary but not spontaneous facial expressions are associated with the observance of a cortical readiness potential just prior to movement; Ekman, Davidson, and Friesen (1990) suggested that, whereas a spontaneous (Duchenne) smile involves activity in the zygomatic and orbicularis oculi muscles, a posed smile involves only the zygomatic muscle. The fact that facial expressions such as smiling increase when confederates are present in the experimental context (Fridlund 1991) highlights the important role that voluntary control can play in activity of the facial musculature. Interpretation of facial EMG activity in studies of emotion should carefully consider possible demand interpretations of obtained patterns and include, if possible, methods for assessing whether activity was spontaneous or voluntarily initiated and modified.

Corrugator EMG Activity. The corrugator supercilii muscles are responsible for lowering and contraction of the brows. This facial action is held to be an index of distress (see Ekman & Freissen 1986; Fridlund & Izard 1983), and firing of motor units in this muscle region is expected if a stimulus is judged to be unpleasant (even if the degree of unit activity is insufficent to produce visible brow movement). Significant contraction of the corrugator muscle occurs when viewing pictures that are rated as unpleasant

(see Figure 7, left panel). The change in corrugator EMG activity is modest (but still above baseline) when viewing neutral materials, and this muscle often shows relaxation below baseline activity for materials rated as highly pleasant (Figure 7, middle panel).

The dimensional correlation between reports of pleasantness and corrugator EMG activity is quite high. When corrugator EMG activity is averaged over pictures ranked from most to least pleasant for each subject, a strong linear relationship is obtained between valence judgments and corrugator activity (Figure 7, middle panel). As ratings become more unpleasant, activity in the corrugator muscle increases steadily. For the most pleasant materials, activity in the corrugator muscle decreases below baseline. A linear relationship obtained in over 80% of participants in the study by Lang et al. (1993), suggesting that subjective reports of pleasure and corrugator EMG activity are strongly associated in a large proportion of the population (Figure 7, right panel). Activity in the corrugator muscle therefore reflects variations in picture valence, increasing in activity for unpleasant stimuli and decreasing for highly pleasant stimuli.

Zygomatic Major EMG. Activity in this muscle occurs when the cheek is drawn back or tightened (Tassinary et al. 1989); it is involved in facial expressions of smiling. Consistent with this, activity in the zygomatic muscle region increases with increases in hedonic valence and is greatest when viewing pictures judged to be highest in pleasure (see Figure 7, left panel). As Figure 7 (middle panel) illustrates, there is a significant linear correlation between reports of pleasantness and activity in the zygomatic muscle region.

However, for materials rated as most unpleasant – scenes of mutilation and death – there is a tendency for zygomatic EMG activity to again increase. Because of the slight increase in zygomatic EMG activity at the unpleasant end of the valence continuum (and the significant increase at the positive end), there is also usually a reliable quadratic correlation between reports of judged pleasantness and zygomatic EMG activity. Coactivation of zygomatic and corrugator muscles suggests that a facial grimace (involving both lowering of the brow and tightening of the cheek) may accompany perception of some aversive materials.

Roughly two thirds of female subjects show a relationship between zygomatic activity and affective valence, whereas only a quarter of male subjects show this relationship (Figure 7, right panel; Lang et al. 1993). This

---

Figure 7. *Left panel.* Second-by-second changes in facial EMG activity, heart rate, skin conductance, and electrocortieal activity when people view pleasant, neutral, and unpleasant IAPS pictures. *Middle panel.* Facial EMG activity and heart rate change covaries with judgments of rated pleasantness, whereas skin conductance reactions and cortical potentials covary with rated arousal. *Right panel.* Correlations of physiological response with reports of pleasure and arousal are plotted for individual male and female participants. Women show stronger relationships between facial EMG activity and pleasure than men; conversely, men show a stronger relationship between skin conductance change and arousal ratings. Based in part on data from Lang et al. (1993) and Cuthbert et al. (1998).

significant gender difference indicates that women may be more facially expressive than men.

In a recent transfer test, Bradley and Lang (in press b) presented participants with a series of 6-sec sound clips consisting of pleasant, neutral, and unpleasant acoustic events (e.g., rollercoaster, typewriter, bomb), again selected on the basis of normative pleasure and arousal ratings (Bradley and Lang 1999b). Not only were similar patterns of facial EMG changes (i.e., zygomatic and corrugator) obtained when people listened to these affective sounds, the covariation functions and gender distributions were almost identical to those depicted in Figure 7. These data comprise an important next step in emotion research: testing whether patterns obtained with one type of emotional prompt (e.g. pictures) generalize when a specific component of the cue (in this case, sensory modality) is changed.

Patterns of facial EMG activity during mental imagery are also consistent with the notion that activity in the corrugator and zygomatic muscle regions indexes the hedonic valence of the imagined stimulus (Fiorito & Simons 1994; Fridlund, Schwartz, & Fowler 1984; van Oyen Witvliet & Vrana 1995). Schwartz and his colleagues (Schwartz, Ahern, & Brown 1979; Schwartz, Brown, & Ahern 1980) conducted a series of studies which found that corrugator and zygomatic EMG activity primarily differentiated between imagery of negative and positive emotions, whereas EMG activity over the masseter and lateral frontalis muscle regions did not differ. Note also that Schwartz et al. (1980) found women to be more reactive than men, consistent with the gender effects for picture perception. Summarizing the imagery work, Cacioppo et al. (1993) concluded that covert measures of facial EMG activity may reflect "a rudimentary bivalent evaluative disposition or *motivational tendency* rather than discrete emotions" (p. 136).

Whereas facial EMG activity, particularly corrugator, is quite sensitive to hedonic valence in both perception and imagery, these facial muscles are not as reactive in anticipation – particularly when assessed in aversive conditioning studies. For example, Dimberg (1987) did not find reliable conditioning effects in corrugator or zygomatic muscle activity in a differential conditioning design in which faces served as conditioned stimuli and electric shock as the unconditioned stimulus. In a vicarious conditioning paradigm, Vaughan and Lanzetta (1980) showed that, although the reinforced stimulus tended to elicit higher activity in several facial muscles (e.g., masseter, frontalis), findings were not statistically significant or stable across experiments. Hamm and co-workers (1993) similarly did not find differential corrugator EMG activity when subjects were anticipating an aversive shock stimulus as compared to when a cue signaling "safety" was present. A study in which subjects anticipated the presentation of pleasant, neutral, or unpleasant pictures (cued by a light) found no corrugator EMG differences as a function of valence dur-

ing a 6-sec anticipatory interval, even when snake phobics anticipated an upcoming snake picture (Sabatinelli et al. 1996). A number of hypotheses might explain the lack of affective facial EMG changes during anticipation, yet overall these findings still highlight the context-specific nature of emotional reactions in psychophysiological studies, which should encourage analyses in which the task context is specified in drawing inferences about emotion and psychophysiology.

Heart Rate. As noted before, the heart is dually innervated by the parasympathetic and sympathetic nervous systems; hence, a measure such as heart rate can be affected by alteration in the level of activation of either system. When viewing pictures, a classic triphasic pattern of heart rate response (see e.g. Lang & Hnatiow 1962) is obtained that includes an initial deceleration and then an acceleratory response followed by a secondary deceleration. In the picture-viewing context, affective valence contributes primarily to the amount of initial deceleration and subsequent acceleratory activity. As found in earlier studies (Winton, Putnam, & Krauss 1984), unpleasant stimuli produce the greatest initial deceleration. Pleasant pictures, on the other hand, prompt the greatest peak acceleration (see Figure 7, right panel). In fact, the cardiac waveform for unpleasant pictures often shows no clear acceleratory peak but instead a deceleration that is sustained across the picture interval (Bradley, Greenwald, & Hamm 1993b), suggesting that the difference in peak acceleration between pleasant and unpleasant pictures is not due to differential initial deceleration.

Although the averaged cardiac waveform clearly discriminates between pleasant and unpleasant pictures, the dimensional covariation between valence and cardiac rate is relatively more modest than found for facial EMG changes (Figure 7, center panel). On the other hand, a large proportion of participants show a positive correlation between ratings of pleasure and heart rate change, and men and women are equally likely to show a positive relationship (Figure 7, center panel). One important difference between facial EMG reactions and cardiac change is that, whereas the face does not have any other obvious tasks during emotional perception, the primary tasks of the heart are homeostatic and metabolic – that is, basic to the survival of the organism. In addition, factors such as posture, respiration, and physical differences (e.g., body weight, fitness) can conspire to obscure affective covariation in cardiac response.

Significant changes in heart rate also occur purely as a function of motor preparation (Graham 1979; Lacey & Lacey 1970; Obrist 1975), which can affect both the shape of the cardiac waveform in a task and the variations due to emotional parameters. For example, in their picture perception study, Winton et al. (1984) required subjects to press a button at picture offset, which somewhat altered the shape of the heart rate waveform during viewing: both the initial accleratory component and secondary deceleration were accentuated relative to a passive viewing context. Nonetheless, unpleasant pictures led to the greatest initial deceleration and pleasant (erotic) pictures led to the greatest acceleration, as in passive viewing. These data highlight the importance of identifying task variables, such as somatic requirements, that could have a significant impact on physiological measures.

Whereas heart rate during perception of unpleasant pictures results in initial cardiac deceleration, heart rate during unpleasant mental imagery is primarily acceleratory in nature. A number of studies have found that heart rate increases are greater during text-prompted fearful than for neutral imagery (Bauer & Craighead 1979; Cook et al. 1988; Grayson 1982; Grossberg & Wilson 1968; Haney & Euse 1976; Lang et al. 1983; May 1977a,b; Van Egeren, Feather, & Hein 1971) and also greater during unpleasant than pleasant imagery (Fiorito & Simons 1994; van Oyen Witvliet & Vrana 1995). In general, heart rate acceleration during imagery varies most consistently with stimulus arousal – increasing as arousal (either pleasant or unpleasant) of the mental image increases (Cook et al. 1991; Fiorito & Simons 1994; van Oyen Witvliet & Vrana 1995).

In an effort to separate cardiac concomitants of mental imagery from heart rate variance associated with processing text, Schwartz (1971) developed a paradigm in which subjects first memorized emotionally arousing stimuli and then imagined these stimuli in a fixed sequence. Simply imagining arousing stimuli (i.e., without having to process a text prompt) resulted in greater heart rate acceleration than when imagining a neutral sequence (e.g., the letters ABCD). Using tones to cue periods of imagery, May and Johnson (1973) had subjects memorize neutral or arousing words, whereas Vrana, Cuthbert, and Lang (1986) employed sentences describing neutral and unpleasant events. In all cases, heart rate accelerated when imagining arousing compared to neutral events. A follow-up study by May (1977b) found that actively imagining a fearful sentence produced more heart rate acceleration than either thinking the sentence, hearing the sentence, or seeing a picture depicting the same material as described by the sentence.

Lang (1987) has interpreted heart rate acceleration during emotional imagery as "efferent leakage," indicating that – in imagery as in an actual situation – heart rate changes reflect activation of response information associated with appropriate actions. Consistent with this, Jones and Johnson (1978, 1980) obtained faster heart rate during imagery of high-activity sentences (e.g., "I feel happy, and I'm jumping for joy") than during imagery of low-activity, relaxing sentences (e.g., "I feel happy, and I just want to relax"). Miller et al. (1987) demonstrated that, like imagery of fear or anger scenes, imagery of active (neu-

tral) scenes produced greater heart rate acceleration and electrodermal reactivity than neutral scenes involving low activity.

Taken together, the heart rate patterns obtained during emotional perception and imagination are consistent with Lacey's (1967) early observation that deceleration is associated with sensory intake (perception) whereas acceleration is associated with mentation. However, the interpretation that heart rate acceleration in imagery reflects sensory rejection has been refined: rather than focusing on sensory processing (e.g., rejection of perceptual information), a number of theories (see Cuthbert et al. 1991 for a review) now hypothesize that cardiac activity during imagery reflects the activation of somatic activity associated with action in the image (Lang 1979). To the extent that imagining emotional (i.e., pleasant or unpleasant) events involves more activity than neutral events, greater heart rate acceleration during this type of mentation is predicted.

Skin Conductance. Whereas the heart is dually innervated, the electrodermal system is innervated solely by fibers of the sympathetic nervous system, which could make this a useful measure of activation of this autonomic nervous system component. Nonetheless, the mechanism of its action is cholinergic, in contrast to most sympathetic fibers, which are adrenergic. Furthermore, Guyton and Hall (1996) suggested that palmar sweat activity might reflect parasympathetic activity (see Figure 2), as these glands are controlled by the portion of the hypothalamus involved in parasympathetic control.

Usually measured on the palm of the hand, the amount of skin conductance activity increases as the rated arousal of an emotional picture increases, regardless of its emotional valence. Thus, if skin conductance change is plotted as a function of a priori picture valence, a significant quadratic pattern is obtained in which reactivity is generally higher when viewing either pleasant or unpleasant (compared with neutral) materials, as illustrated in Figure 7 (left panel). Winton et al. (1984) also obtained data indicating larger skin conductance responses to slides that were rated as highly pleasant and highly unpleasant. Likewise, Manning and Melchiori (1974) observed this skin conductance pattern when stimuli were words rated as highly pleasant (e.g. "sex") or highly unpleasant (e.g. "violence").

That skin conductance varies consistently with reports of arousal is evident when assessing the dimensional correlation between arousal ratings and skin conductance. A significant linear relationship emerges in which a unit increase in rated arousal (regardless of valence) is associated with an increase in electrodermal reactivity (see Figure 7, center panel). Over 80% of the subjects in Lang et al.'s (1993) study showed a positive correlation between arousal reports and conductance response. A larger proportion of males than females showed a significant correlation, suggesting that – whereas females may be more facially

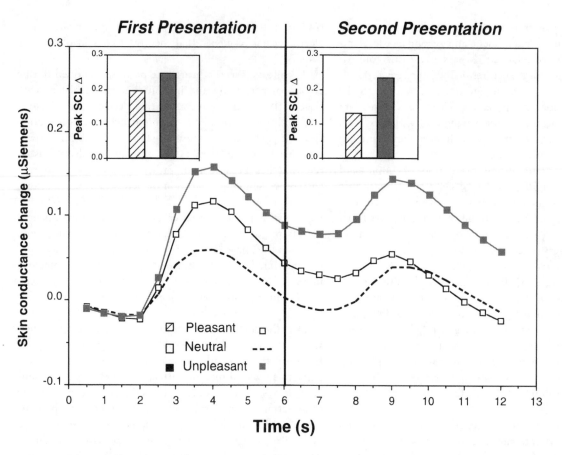

First Presentation   **Second Presentation**

Figure 8. Skin conductance changes when viewing IAPS pictures presented twice in a row indicate a decrease in response magnitude from the first to the second presentation for pleasant but not for unpleasant pictures, suggesting that skin conductance changes for pleasant pictures are mediated in part by novelty.

expressive – males are more reactive in the electrodermal system (Figure 7, right panel).

A similar relationship between skin conductance activity and stimulus arousal is obtained when emotional sounds, rather than pictures, serve as the perceptual stimuli. The covariation functions and gender distributions relating skin conductance response to reports of arousal for sound stimuli were again very similar to those depicted in Figure 7 for pictures (Bradley & Lang in press b).

The magnitude of skin conductance responses has also been found to vary with stimulus arousal in a number of different imagery studies (Cook et al. 1991; Fiorito & Simons 1994; Miller et al. 1987; van Oyen Witvliet & Vrana 1995). Furthermore, a skin conductance increase during anticipation of an aversive electric shock is the prototypical measure of conditioned aversion. That this measure primarily indexes arousal associated with the conditioning procedure – rather than with the aversive stimulus – is supported by findings of significant skin conductance change in appetitive conditioning paradigms (Hamm & Vaitl 1996; Lipp, Sheridan, & Siddle 1994). Significant skin conductance increases were also obtained when subjects

anticipated the presentation of either pleasant or unpleasant pictures as compared with anticipating neutral pictures (Sabatinelli et al. 1996).

Therefore, skin conductance responses appear to be reliably modulated by emotional arousal in perception, anticipation, and imagination. One interpretation is that these effects index sympathetic nervous system reactivity, which is greater for emotionally arousing than for neutral materials. Electrodermal reactions are also quite sensitive to the novelty of both the stimulus and the task: with repeated presentations of the same or different pictures, the size of electrodermal changes rapidly decreases (Bradley, Lang, & Cuthbert 1993c). Effects of novelty suggest that differences in the degree of orienting may underlie some effects of stimulus arousal in this response system. In an effort to separate contributions of stimulus arousal due to novelty from those due to emotion, Bradley et al. (1997) presented unpleasant, pleasant, and neutral pictures twice in a row. The logic was that, during the second presentation, the picture was less novel and so effects due to emotional arousal alone should be accentuated. Figure 8 illustrates the electrodermal data from this experiment. Whereas skin conductance magnitude reached the same level when viewing unpleasant pictures on each of the two presentations, electrodermal reactions to pleasant pictures decreased greatly from the first to second presentation. One interpretation is that electrodermal responses to pleasant pictures may be more related to stimulus novelty than to emotional arousal. More importantly, these data illustrate how one can begin to isolate effects of emotional arousal on physiological response by removing influences due to other factors.

Cortical ERPs and Slow-Wave Activity. When electrocortical (EEG) activity is measured during picture viewing (and subsequently corrected for eye movements), specific event-related potentials and sustained slow-wave activity are observed in response to emotionally arousing picture stimuli, irrespective of affective valence (Crites & Cacioppo 1996; Cuthbert et al. in press; Lifshitz 1966; Palomba, Angrilli, & Mini 1997). As Figure 7 (left panel) illustrates, positive cortical evoked potentials starting at about 400 msec after picture presentation are larger for both pleasant and unpleasant than for neutral materials, and a slow sustained positivity is maintained until picture presentation is terminated.

The dimensional correlation between ratings of arousal and cortical positivity (measured at its maximum, 400–700 msec) is also quite high (see Figure 7, middle panel), indicating that activity measured from the cortical surface primarily indicates whether an emotional (pleasant or unpleasant) or neutral stimulus is the focus of processing. There is evidence from cognitive studies that the positive component occurring around 300 msec after stimulus onset might reflect attentional engagement. For example, if attention is directed toward a stimulus then larger positivity is obtained. On the other hand, the same stimulus that generates a large positivity when associated with a task often does not do so when the stimulus is ignored (see Donchin & Coles 1988). Because emotionally evocative pictures are consistently rated as more interesting and more complex than neutral, low-arousal images (Bradley et al. 1993b; Lang et al. 1990), greater cortical positivity may reflect a variation in attentional engagement that covaries with judged affective arousal.

Crites and Cacioppo (1996) further demonstrated that the local context in which a picture is embedded affects the magnitude of the late positive potential. When a series of pictures of the same valence (say, unpleasant) are presented, the late positive potential for a target that is evaluatively distant (here, pleasant) from the context is greater than for similarly valenced targets. This effect also appears to be larger on the right side of the brain when the task requires an evaluative (but not a semantic) judgment. Cacioppo and his colleagues suggested that these effects index an automatic evaluative process that reflects the distance of a stimulus from the current evaluative set.

Differences in lateralized electrical activity of the brain have also been found when people view pleasant or unpleasant films. Davidson and his colleagues (1990; Wheeler, Davidson, & Tomarken 1993) reported that anterior EEG activity (measured as alpha power) is greater on the left than the right when viewing happy films and vice versa for disgusting films. However, these effects were *not* obtained unless the analysis was constrained to include only epochs containing appropriate facial displays and subjective reports of emotion, suggesting that these cortical effects rely on mobilization of appropriate affective responses in the film-viewing task.

The Startle Reflex: Emotional Priming. The autonomic and somatic physiological responses elicited during picture viewing presumably reflect the engagement of neural structures and pathways, many subcortical, in either the appetitive or defensive motivation systems. Lang and his colleagues (1990, 1997) proposed that, during the period that the subcortical circuitry is active, associations and action programs that are linked to the engaged motivational system are primed and ready to respond. Thus, if the defensive motivational system is dominant (i.e., if the affective state is unpleasant), then other defensive responses are primed. Conversely, responses linked to the nondominant system are inhibited. Because the most fundamental motivational priming is at the level of unconditioned reflexes, a concurrent aversive state should prime defensive reflexes whereas an appetitive state should lead to inhibition of defensive responding.

The startle response has proven to be a defensive reflex that demonstrates this type of priming pattern. Startle is a primitive reflex that serves a protective function, helping to avoid organ injury (as in the eyeblink) and acting as a behavioral interrupt (Graham 1979), clearing processors to deal with possible threat. In studies with human beings, rapid eye closure is one of the most reliable components of the behavioral cascade that constitutes the startle reflex. The magnitude of the blink can be measured by electrodes placed over the orbicularis oculi muscle, just beneath the lower eyelid (see Figure 9). Although intense stimuli in most sensory modalities (e.g., acoustic, visual, tactile) elicit a startle response, the most important feature of a startle-eliciting stimulus is its abruptness; thus, its risetime should ideally be instantaneous (see Anthony 1985 for an overview). The most commonly used startle-eliciting stimulus in human research is a brief (50-msec) burst of white noise at around 95 decibels; this prompts a clear blink response but rarely interferes with ongoing foreground tasks.

When startle probes are administered in the context of affective picture perception, results have consistently conformed to the motivational priming hypothesis. As Figure 10 (top panel) illustrates, a significant linear trend is reliably observed over judged picture valence, with the blink response potentiated when viewing unpleasant pictures and inhibited when viewing pleasant pictures (Lang 1995; Vrana, Spence, & Lang 1988). These effects have proven to be highly replicable (Bradley et al. 1990, 1993c, 1995, in press; Cook et al. 1992; Hamm et al. 1997; Patrick,

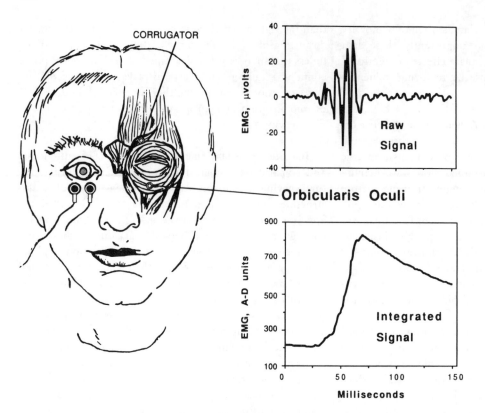

Figure 9. *Left panel.* Illustration of the placement of electrodes for measuring activity over the orbicularis oculi muscle when assessing startle blink responses. *Right panel.* The resulting raw EMG recorded (top) and the rectified, integrated signal from which the magnitude of the blink is scored (bottom). Reprinted with permission from Lang, Bradley, & Cuthbert, "Emotion, attention, and the startle reflex," *Psychological Review,* vol. 97, pp. 377–98. Copyright © 1990 by the American Psychological Association.

Bradley, & Lang 1993; Sutton et al. 1997; Vanman et al. 1996). They also appear relatively early in life: Balaban (1995) found modulation of the startle reflex in 5-month-old infants looking at pictures of angry or happy faces.

The neural circuitry underlying potentiation of the startle response during aversive processing has been extensively investigated by Davis (1986, 1989; Davis, Hitchcock, & Rosen 1987) and others (e.g. Koch & Schnitzler 1997). When stimulated by an abrupt noise, the afferent path of the reflex proceeds from the cochlear nucleus to the reticular formation; from there, efferent connections pass through spinal neurons to the reflex effectors. This is the basic obligatory circuit, driven by the parameters of the input stimulus (e.g., stimulus intensity, frequency, steepness of the onset ramp). Startle modulation by emotion implies that a secondary circuit affects this primary reflex pathway. There is now overwhelming evidence that the amygdala is a critical component of the fear-potentiated startle effect. First, there are direct projections from the amygdala to the reticular site that mediates potentiation (i.e., nucleus reticularis pontis caudalis); second, electrical stimulation of the amygdala enhances startle reflex ampli-

tude; finally, and most important, lesions of the amygdala abolish fear-conditioned startle potentiation.

Affective modulation of the startle reflex does not depend on stimulus novelty. Although there is an overall diminution of the blink reflex with repeated presentation of the startle probe, affective potentiation and inhibition to unpleasant and pleasant pictures remains constant, despite repeated presentation of the same pictures (see Figure 10; Bradley et al. 1993c). Similarly, affective modulation persists when the same (or a different) set of pictures is viewed in separate experimental sessions (Bradley, Gianaros, & Lang 1995).

The startle reflex is modulated by affective valence during picture viewing regardless of whether the startle probe is visual, acoustic, or tactile (Bradley, Cuthbert, & Lang 1990; Hawk & Cook 1997), indicating that modality-specific processes are not central in these modulatory effects. Affective modulation of startle is also not confined to static visual percepts: the startle reflex is also modulated by affective valence when dynamic visual stimuli (e.g. affective films) are presented (Jansen & Frijda 1994) or when the sensory modality involves odors (Erlichman et al. 1995). Furthermore, when the emotional stimuli consist of short, 6-sec sound clips of various affective events (e.g., sounds of love-making, babies crying, bombs bursting) and the startle probe is a visual light flash, the same pattern of affective modulation is obtained (Bradley & Lang in press b). This suggests that its mediation is broadly motivational and thus consistent across affective foregrounds of different stimulus modalities.

The startle reflex has also been used to determine the temporal course of emotional processing. Reflex magnitude is reliably affected by picture valence as early as 500 msec after picture presentation and is maintained throughout a 6-sec viewing interval (Bradley et al. 1993a). The same temporal pattern of modulatory effects occurs regardless of whether the subject ignores or attends to the startle probe (for review see Bradley & Lang in press a), suggesting that reflex modulation is not secondary to modality-driven attentional processes. Interestingly, it is not necessary for the actual picture stimulus to be present: when the picture is removed from view at 500 msec, strong effects of affective valence on reflex modulation are obtained for up to 3 sec, suggesting that the startle stimulus probes the "mind's eye," indexing cognitive and affective processes associated with picture encoding (Codispoti et al. 1999).

If affective priming of the startle reflex is based on motivational variables, then modulatory effects on the startle reflex should increase with greater activation in each motive system. That is, probe startle potentiation should be largest for unpleasant pictures that are highly arousing; conversely, the most arousing *pleasant* pictures should prompt the greatest probe startle *inhibition*. Figure 7 (bottom panel) illustrates reflex modulation for pleasant and unpleasant pictures as they vary in rated arousal (Cuthbert et al. 1996) and supports a motivational priming interpretation: the greatest difference in reflex magnitude is for highly arousing pleasant and unpleasant pictures. For pleasant pictures, startle reflex magnitude decreases progressively with increases in rated arousal. For aversive pictures, an initial reduction in blink magnitude is suggested as arousal begins to increase. Somewhat further along the arousal dimension, however, the direction of reflex modulation is abruptly reversed: startle magnitude begins to increase, peaking for pictures judged unpleasant and highest in arousal.

In many ways, the change in direction of the reflex response that is associated with increasing arousal of unpleasant pictures is reminiscent of Sokolov's (1963) description of the manner in which orienting changes to defense with increasing intensity of physical stimulation after a period of oscillation between the two responses. It is also consistent with Miller's (1959) classic conflict theory (for a more recent assessment, see Cacioppo & Berntson 1994), in which behavior is assumed to be driven by activation along

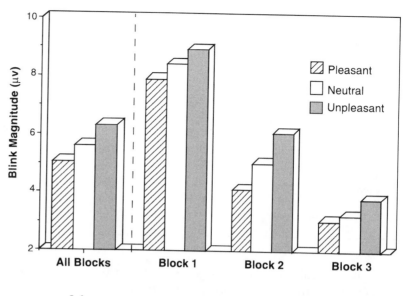

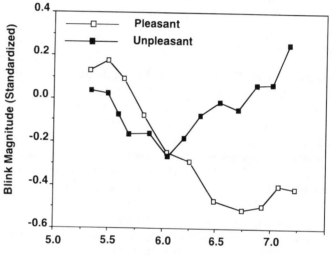

Figure 10. *Top panel.* The startle blink reflex is modulated by affective valence, with blinks potentiated when viewing unpleasant pictures and inhibited when viewing pleasant pictures. Although the obligatory startle reflex habituates with repeated elicitation, affective modulation continues even when the same pictures are repeatedly presented. Reprinted with permission from Bradley, Cuthbert, & Lang, "Pictures as prepulse: Attention and emotion in startle modification," *Psychophysiology,* vol. 30, pp. 541–5. Copyright 1993 Cambridge University Press. *Bottom panel.* The difference in blink magnitude is greatest for pleasant and unpleasant stimuli that are rated as highly arousing, consistent with the notion that affective startle modulation results when appetitive and defensive motivation is intense. Reprinted with permission from Cuthbert, Bradley, & Lang, "Probing picture perception: Activation and emotion," *Psychophysiology,* vol. 33, pp. 103–11. Copyright 1996 Cambridge University Press.

gradients of approach and avoidance. Because aversive pictures are consistently judged to be more "interesting" (Bradley et al. 1993b) than neutral pictures, the initial reflex inhibition to unpleasant stimuli of moderate arousal

TABLE 1. Factor Analysis of Three-System Measures of Emotional Picture Perception

Measure	Factor 1 (Valence)	Factor 2 (Arousal)
Valence ratings	0.86	−0.00
Corrugator muscle	−0.85	0.19
Heart rate	0.79	−0.14
Zygomatic muscle	0.58	0.29
Arousal ratings	0.15	0.83
Interest ratings	0.45	0.77
Viewing time	−0.27	0.76
Skin conductance	−0.37	0.74

may reflect modulation related to orienting, a key feature of appetitive motivation. The abrupt change to increasing startle potentiation reflects the subsequent dominance of defensive motivation as stimuli become more threatening and therefore more arousing.

Summary: Affective Patterns in Physiological Responses.

Taken together, data obtained in the picture perception paradigm are consistent with the hypothesis that motivational variables of affective valence and arousal predominate in organizing physiological and subjective reports of affective reactions. Supporting this, factor analyses conducted on self-report, physiological, and behavioral measures have consistently produced a strong two-factor solution (Lang et al. 1993). As Table 1 illustrates, the first factor involves high loadings for pleasantness ratings, heart rate change, corrugator EMG activity and zygomatic EMG activity, consistent with the interpretation that this is a primary valence factor of appetite or aversion. A second factor involves high loadings for rated experience of arousal, interest ratings, viewing time, skin conductance, and cortical slow waves, all identifiers of an arousal or intensity factor. The cross-loadings for all measures are very low. Thus, affects appear to be built around motivational determinants.

Attention and Emotion: The Defense Cascade

In the picture paradigm, when startle reflex magnitude is considered together with other measures of affective reactivity (e.g., skin conductance, heart rate, facial EMG), it is clear that different response systems change in different ways as activation within each motivational system increases. For instance, specific phobics (like normal subjects) show potentiated startles when viewing unpleasant pictures. However, startle reflexes are even more enhanced when these subjects view pictures of their own phobic objects (Hamm et al. 1997; Sabatinelli et al. 1996). In addition, the typical bradycardia obtained during unpleasant picture viewing does not characterize the response of pho-

bic subjects to pictures of objects they fear (Cook & Turpin 1997; Hamm et al. 1997; Klorman & Ryan 1980; Klorman et al. 1977). Rather, when high-fear subjects view pictures of the phobic object, the sympathetic system dominates and the heart accelerates, in concordance with predictions regarding defense responses in this context. Also, unlike nonphobic subjects, they quickly terminate "looking" in a free-viewing situation. Thus, whereas reflex potentiation to aversive materials characterizes responses to highly arousing unpleasant pictures for both normal and phobic subjects, cardiac and other behavioral measures of attentive orienting are absent when phobics process highly fearful content.

These data suggest that, rather than a single response indicating activation of the defensive motivation system and reflected in a parallel way by all measures, one instead observes a cascade of different response events that change in different ways and at different levels as activation increases. When activation within the defensive system is moderate, a pattern of responding suggestive of oriented attention is obtained: measurable conductance changes, heart deceleration, and inhibited startle reflexes. Thus, attentive orienting is not a response confined solely to neutral or pleasant stimuli. Rather, "natural selective attention" (Lang et al. 1997) is prompted by stimuli that are motivationally relevant – either appetitive or defensive. Consistent with this, Lacey (1958) recognized that, instead of being automatically "rejected," unpleasant events can evoke a physiology consistent with sustained attention. On the other hand, strong aversive motivation is clearly a major factor in initiating defense.

The idea that defense involves stages of responding has been advocated by a number of theorists, including Tinbergen (1951), Blanchard and Blanchard (1989), Fanselow and colleagues (1995; Fanselow & Lester 1988), Masterson and Crawford (1982), and others. For instance, Fanselow (1994) proposed a three-stage model of defensive responding, based on predator imminence, in which defensive responses increased as the threatening stimulus became more proximal. Based on data obtained in the picture perception paradigm, Lang and his colleagues proposed a similar defense cascade that is controlled by increases in motivational activation (as measured by judged arousal) and is considered to be an analog to predator imminence. In Figure 11, the amplitudes of various physiological measures are shown schematically on the ordinate, with increases in arousal on the abscissa. Consistent with Lacey's (1967) rejection of a uniformly increasing response as arousal increases, responses in different systems can initially increase or decrease as the level of arousal increases.

At low to moderate stages of arousal for unpleasant stimuli, a pattern of physiological reactivity consistent with oriented attention is obtained that presumably does not differ fundamentally from appetitive orienting at low levels of activation. This pattern involves:

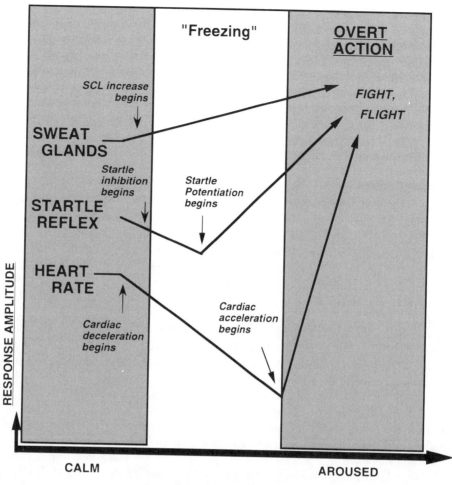

Figure 11. Stages of defensive responding. Different physiological systems change at different rates, based on the intensity of activation in defensive motivation. Reprinted with permission from Lang, Bradley, & Cuthbert, "Motivated attention: Affect, activation and action," in Lang, Simons, & Balaban (Eds.), *Attention and Orienting: Sensory and Motivational Processes.* Copyright 1997 Lawrence Erlbaum Associates.

1. a brief, modest, probably parasympathetically driven heart rate deceleration that occurs in reaction to any stimulus change (this bradycardia becomes larger and more sustained as stimuli are perceived to be more arousing);

2. changes in skin conductance that are small when arousal is low but increase in frequency and amplitude with greater activation; and

3. reflex inhibition to a secondary startle stimulus, consistent with the hypothesis of greater resource allocation to a meaningful foreground.

Defensive responding occurs later in the sequence. Clear evidence that the organism has changed to a defensive posture is first seen in the startle reflex: when defensive activation is high – the threat more imminent – the organism is defensively primed. The startle stimulus acts as a trigger that releases a supranormal reflex reaction. The degree of reflex potentiation increases with greater system activation until the prompting stimulus itself invokes a motivationally relevant action (e.g., fight or flight). Startle potentiation occurs primarily in the context of an increasing attentive focus and a parallel, still increasing and dominant

bradycardia. At the highest activation level, just prior to action, the vagus releases the heart and so enables a sympathetically driven acceleration that is the classic defense response. Thus, for phobic subjects, cardiac acceleration (rather than deceleration) occurs when processing pictures of their feared material because these subjects are further along in the "defense cascade" than normal subjects processing standard unpleasant pictures.

It is interesting to note that incarcerated psychopaths fail to show startle reflex potentiation for aversive pictures; instead, they show reflex inhibition (relative to neutral pictures) when viewing either arousing pleasant *or* arousing unpleasant picture stimuli (Patrick et al. 1993). This finding – quite different from what is seen in the normal population or in specific phobics – is consistent with the hypothesis that unpleasant pictures are relatively less activating for these individuals and that their reflex modulation reflects motivated attention rather than activation of defensive responding. For psychopaths, pictures do not seem to convey the symbolic danger as for normal subjects, nor do they convey an imminent threat that prompts a phobic reaction. These nonempathic individuals remain distanced – and at an early stage in the defense cascade, which might reflect a deficit in defense motivation (Lykken 1957; Patrick 1994).

Social Context

Like most psychophysiological investigations, the study of emotion does not occur in a social vacuum. Perhaps more frequently than in studies of affectless cognition, physiological responses in studies of emotions will vary as a function of important social variables (see Chapter 23 of this volume for further discussion). As noted earlier, for instance, appropriate facial expressions increase in the presence of other people – or even when a subject simply believes another person is observing (Fridlund 1991; Fridlund et al. 1990). More generally, Hatfield, Cacioppo, and Rapson (1993a,b) proposed that people automatically and unintentionally mirror the emotional postures, intonations, and moods of those around them. This phenomenon, termed "emotional contagion," suggests that emotional reactions in the psychophysiology laboratory may depend on variables in the experimental setting that elicit this type of mimicry or modeling.

Individual differences also contribute importantly to the pattern of physiological reactions obtained in studies of emotion, as noted earlier by Duffy (1957). Interpersonal variables particularly relevant to the study of emotion as outlined in this chapter are those relating to (i) individual differences in phasic or tonic activation of appetitive or defensive systems (due e.g. to temperament, gender, cognitive style) and (ii) individual differences in physiological reactivity (e.g., somatic or autonomic).

In terms of differences in motivational activation, current views of personality are converging on the notion that two factors of negative and positive emotionality may underlie temperamental differences in affective reactivity (e.g. Derryberry & Rothbart 1988; Tellegen 1985; Watson, Clark, & Mineka 1994). Empirical evidence that these traits are fundamental in describing personality was provided by Tellegen (1985), who determined (using factor analysis) that a large variety of personality questionnaires share a common variance that is attributable to the existence of two general dimensions of positive and negative affect. Watson et al. (1994) recently conceptualized negative affectivity as a "stable, heritable and a highly general trait dimension" whose affective core comprises "a temperamental sensitivity to negative stimuli" (p. 104). People who are high in negative affect are believed to evidence tonic effects on emotional reactivity (a higher frequency of

negative moods such as anxiety, sadness, and depression) as well as phasic effects, such as greater reactivity to aversive stimuli. Consistent with this, a number of studies have found that highly fearful subjects evidence greater startle potentiation when perceiving (Cook et al. 1991) or imagining (Cook et al. 1992) unpleasant stimuli than do subjects who are low in temperamental fearfulness.

Cognitive style differences, such as imagery ability, also appear to affect physiological mobilization during affective processing, presumably owing to differences in motivational activation. Because experimental cues are often symbolic representations (i.e., pictures, films, textual descriptions) of pleasant or unpleasant stimuli, their ability to activate motivational systems may rely, to some extent, on the subject's ability to elaborate associated information mentally. Differences in retrieval and manipulation of stored information is one facet underlying imagery ability. Lang and his colleagues have consistently found that self-described good imagers respond more during emotional imagery than those reporting poor imagery ability (e.g. Miller et al. 1987; see Cuthbert et al. 1991 for a review). Even more interesting is that imagery ability also affects physiological responsivity when looking at pictures (Lang et al. 1993) or listening to sounds (Bradley & Lang in press b). In both cases, subjects with good imagery ability show a better relationship between their subjective reports of emotion and their physiological responses as well as more reactivity to emotional than to neutral stimulus processing. These data suggest that, when people process degraded stimulus cues (i.e., symbolic representations of objects and events), a cognitive style variable of "good imagery ability" may distinguish those for whom motivational activation and physiological reactivity is more likely to occur.

In addition to individual differences in motivational activation, the notion that people express emotion (especially stress) through different systems (i.e., internal or external) has had a long history in the study of emotion (see Cacioppo et al. 1992c for a review). Early views assumed that some individuals tended to respond in one system (e.g. somatic) rather than in another (e.g. sympathetic), with compensatory effects. Thus, those failing to respond in expressive (somatic) systems were proposed to have greater sympathetic reactivity – along with the long-term damage that accompanies internal stress.

According to PATTERNS, a model of individual differences in physiological function proposed by Cacioppo and colleagues (1992c), these early views were too simplistic. The PATTERNS model assumes that individual reactions result from the operation of different neurophysiological systems that have such operating characteristics as differential response thresholds, onset delays, time constants (recovery periods), and so on. Differences in system gain – the amount of amplification in responding per unit increase in excitation (arousal) – is proposed to be an important individual difference variable in affective reactivity. Individuals with high gain in the sympathetic system ("internalizers") tend to show larger skin conductance reactions with increasing arousal, whereas those with high gain in the somatic system ("externalizers") show greater changes in facial expressivity with increasing arousal. Those with equal gain in both systems ("generalizers") show equivalent changes in electrodermal and facial reactions as arousal increases.

Thus, PATTERNS assumes that, for all neurophysiological systems and all individuals, the greater the neural excitation (e.g., emotional arousal), the greater the output. It is the *amount* of change with increasing arousal that varies with individual differences in system gain. The consistent gender differences obtained in affective perception are consistent with PATTERNS: men tend to be more electrodermally reactive with increasing arousal in emotional perception, whereas women are more facially expressive (Lang et al. 1993); this suggests a higher gain in the sympathetic system for males and a higher gain in expressive reactions for female subjects. It also appears that men and women may differ in ease of activation in different motivational systems. Women tend to be more reactive to unpleasant, arousing perceptual stimuli, whereas men show a bias to respond to pleasant, arousing stimuli (particularly erotic materials). These differences are obtained in subjective reports of pleasure and arousal as well as in autonomic and somatic measures of reactivity. Hence these data suggest differences in the lability of defensive and appetitive reactions as a function of gender.

Epilogue

Emotion and Action

Emotion and motivation have been viewed thus far as processes involving stimuli and events that move an organism toward action. Human emotion, however, differs in some ways from motivated behavior in lower animals. For instance, because of the enormous learning capacity in the human, the range and type of stimuli that come to activate basic subcortical motivational circuits often appear quite distant from those that directly promote or threaten survival. Nonetheless, the mechanisms underlying neural activation can be considered to be similar in both animals and humans. Animal studies have clearly demonstrated that motivational circuits are initially activated by unconditioned stimuli – those that reflexively lead to approach and withdrawal behaviors. New, "conditioned" stimuli come to activate the same circuits, however, through association with these primary appetitive and aversive reinforcers (Halgren 1981). Because humans (as well as animals) learn to respond in adaptive ways to a wide variety of different environmental stimuli and events through this basic learning process, stimuli that activate appetitive and defensive systems through

association can be idiosyncratic, not clearly valenced to bystanders, and not obviously related to basic survival mechanisms.

Second, the close link between emotion and overt action has been loosened in humans, presumably because of the evolution of cortical controls on these fundamental behaviors and development of the ability to mentally process, "off-line," events that are not currently perceptually prompted. Nonetheless, if emotion is intense (e.g., an attacker threatens), then action (e.g. fleeing) is evident, even in humans. However, weaker affective cues (e.g., a movie of the same scene) may elicit only small increases in muscle tension, a mere remnant of the original defensive activity. Thus, emotional reactions in humans often involve primarily a disposition toward or preparation for action (Arnold 1970; Frijda 1986; Lang 1987) rather than clear overt expression. Nonetheless, these can still be considered to be mediated by the same neural circuits originally engaged in activating appropriate approach and defensive behaviors. In this view, motivated behavior can be differentiated from other types of human (and animal) activity primarily in the extent to which this subcortical circuitry is involved during processing (Lang 1994a; Lang et al. 1993; LeDoux 1996).

Conscious Experience of Emotion

If emotion is defined in terms of subjective reports, overt behaviors, and bodily responses, then one might wonder which measure (if any) taps conscious feelings. The issue of the conscious experience of emotion – and how to approach it scientifically – has posed a number of problems in emotion research. As LeDoux (1995) noted, "it is understandable why the field of emotion has had so much trouble in solving the problem of emotion – it has set as its goal the task of understanding consciousness" (p. 1059). Animal theorists, in general, balk at using the term "emotion" in describing motivated behavior in their subjects, mainly because of the added assumption of conscious awareness. The study of motivated behavior, however, does not necessitate taking on the Goliath issue of consciousness – which, in the end, may prove to be more amenable to philosophic than to scientific inquiry.

From a measurement perspective, one solution is to operationally define conscious experience on the basis of subjective reports of emotion. Subjects' reports (verbal or nonverbal) about their emotional experience could be used to index the private, internal state that is usually meant when one speaks of "feelings." Some might argue this is unsatisfactory because of the dependence of personal reports on cultural norms and individual differences in disclosure. In addition, feelings are often held to include the bodily reactions involved in emotional response, such as a racing heart or sweaty palms. A second solution has been to include "conscious awareness" as a fourth type of response system in emotion. The difficulty here is that one needs a reliable operational measure of consciousness and yet, other than three-system measures discussed in this chapter, there are currently no methods for directly measuring an internal feeling state.

To illustrate the problem that conscious feeling states pose in the study of emotion, consider a friend confronted with a fearful cue. If there were neither reports of fear nor overt behaviors associated with fear (e.g., flight, avoidance) nor measurable physiology associated with aversive reactivity (e.g., cardiovascular, somatic, central, neurohumoral), could the individual still be feeling afraid? For some, the answer is a definite Yes: conscious feelings are different from, or more than, the set of empirical responses the scientist can measure. For others, the answer will be No: emotion is solely defined by what can be measured. The concept of internal state also raises more questions than it answers in the study of emotion. That is, it can be invoked not only as a cause (e.g., he ran because he felt afraid) but also as an effect (he saw the snake and so he felt afraid) as well as a mediator between stimuli and response (he saw the snake and felt afraid, so he ran).

Revisiting Discrete States: The Tactics of Emotion

The difference between a biphasic and discrete state view of emotion does not concern whether specific emotional states can be considered appetitive or aversive, since this is clearly possible; rather, it concerns which organization is more fundamental in organizing emotion. Biphasic and discrete state views of emotion are complementary and are not mutually exclusive, as many theorists recognize (see e.g. Mehrabian & Russell 1974). That is, not only can a specific state such as fear be categorized along a dimension of aversiveness, but a particular aversive event can be described as involving fear – assuming a specific definition of this term.

The issue of defining discrete states of emotion is central when distinguishing among specific emotions. Ortony, Clore, and Collins (1988) provided a compelling cognitive analysis detailing the features of situations and stimuli that may differentiate among events that people generally label with different emotional terms. Consistent with a biphasic view, the superordinate division in their scheme is one of hedonic valence, differentiating among desirable and undesirable events. Specific features of environmental events are then proposed to control how different hedonically valenced events are labeled. For instance, "distress" labels the occurrence of an undesirable event and "joy" the occurrence of a desirable event. When there is only a *prospect* of an event occurring, then the situation is labeled "fear" for undesirable events and "hope" for desirable events. The stimulus feature of actual versus prospective maps well onto the distinctions made between perception and anticipation tasks in this chapter. Ortony et al.'s (1988) semantic analysis is consistent with the notion that emotion is fundamentally built on appetitive and defensive motivations, which become increasingly differentiated based on specific stimulus contexts.

Emotional differentiation is based not only on features of the stimulus input, however. As emphasized throughout, emotional reactions are part and parcel of the basic phenomenon. Specific emotions are inferred on the basis of behavioral actions and physiological reactions, and these behaviors also vary depending upon contextual support. As noted earlier, rats engage in a variety of different behaviors in response to electric shock, depending upon their environment (e.g., escaping if there is an exit and attacking if there is a conspecific). If particular emotions were to be distinguished on the basis of behavior, these two contexts might be described as eliciting fear and anger (respectively), despite the similarities in stimulus and motivational activation. The variability of human emotional behavior in a specific context is likewise complex but certainly more creative. This tactical nature of emotional behavior (see Lang et al. 1990) has thwarted the efforts of psychophysiologists to make general inferences regarding the physiology of specific emotional states. Understanding the physiology in situations labeled with discrete emotional states (fear, anger, joy, etc.) will require careful detailing of the elements of behavior elicited (e.g., freezing, fleeing, fighting) as well as the stimulus situation.

Although conscious feeling states are often considered synonymous with a discrete emotion perspective, this is not necessarily the case. Panksepp (1982), for instance, advocates a discrete emotion view in the rat that is based on his hypothesis that four separate neural systems (located mainly in the hypothalamus) of expectancy, rage, fear, and panic underlie motivated behavior. In his view, these emotions stem from systems that have evolved to deal with specific classes of environmental stimuli (i.e., positive incentives, irritation, threat, and loss). The dependence of emotional behavior on specific stimulus contexts is clearly a principal issue in the psychophysiological study of emotion – and one that has been emphasized throughout this chapter. Identifying the critical contextual features in investigations of emotion may help us to understand whether and when there is consistent physiological patterning as a function of contextual similarity.

Arousal and Emotional Intensity

The concept of arousal in the psychophysiological study of emotion has not fared well over the past 30 years, owing in part to Lacey's (1967) observation that physiological responses do not show uniform, parallel increases in direction and strength with increasing arousal (defined as sympathetic activation, metabolic load, or verbal report). This was supported by data from the picture perception paradigm, in which the defense cascade model (Lang et al. 1997), for example, described ways that different physiological systems change at different rates and directions, with increases in some measures (such as startle potentiation) accompanied by decreases in others (e.g., cardiac deceleration). Thus, as Lacey (1967) emphasized, the notion of a parallel increase in all systems as a function of some underlying arousal dimension is not supported by the data.

Nonetheless, emotional arousal – considered as the intensity parameter of the active motive sytem – is a critical factor in organizing the pattern of physiological responses in emotion, as evidenced by factor analyses conducted on an array of evaluative and physiological indices of emotional reactivity (see e.g. Lang et al. 1993). Together, these data redefine the construct of arousal as one that relates to the degree of activation in underlying motivational systems of appetite and defense, rather than a global gain parameter. As noted earlier, high motivational (e.g. defensive) activation can lead to low activity, depending upon contextual constraints. Validating this notion of arousal using the evaluative, physiological, and behavioral indices available in the emotion laboratory remains an important task for the psychophysiologist.

When defining the degree of motivational activation in animals, theorists have relied on a proximity parameter. As discussed previously, Tinbergen (1951) and Fanselow (1994) based their model of defense behavior on "predator imminence" – the distance of a threatening stimulus from the organism – and Miller (1959, 1966) defined activation in both appetitive and defensive systems in terms of the organism's distance from a valent goal. In these conceptions, distance is important because the appropriate action (withdrawal) depends upon where the predator is in the environment; distance clearly covaries with measured behavioral and metabolic indices. When humans encounter motivationally relevant objects in the environment, distance is probably as good an index of motivational activation as it is for animals: As threatening objects come closer, defensive action ensues. In the emotion laboratory, however, the common use of symbolic stimuli (films, pictures, stories, etc.) renders a physical distance metric less informative. Instead, determining the variables that control arousal (i.e., degree of motivational activation) will depend upon systematically exploring how cue and task affect the pattern of evaluative and physiological reactions in studies of emotion.

Conclusion

This chapter has explored the utility of studying emotion's psychophysiology from a biphasic view that posits basic neural systems of defensive and appetitive motivation. Motive systems developed with the brain's evolution, expanding from reflexive approach and withdrawal responses to govern a host of positive incentive and protective behaviors that ensured the survival of our complex species. This motivated visceral and somatic output is parsimoniously described by parameters of hedonic valence and arousal, and both neuroanatomical and cognitive models of emotion have highlighted these organizing dimensions.

Reacting to the James–Cannon debate, psychophysiology began at the forefront of emotion studies, gathering evidence to determine whether physiological patterns are specific to emotional states. Although these efforts were less substantial in result than was hoped, they nevertheless brought into focus the great methodological issues that currently dominate the field of emotion research. It has become increasingly clear that affective cues need to be explicitly defined and somehow standardized and, for example, that the properties of a stimulus such as modality and medium of presentation may have varying physiological impact that can overwhelm indices of affect. Similarly, the importance of determining the experimental task has become clear. That subjects are doing different things – imagining, watching a movie, playing a video game – can lead to very different psychophysiological patterns, despite the experimenter's assumption that a common emotion is evoked. A similar concern encourages better description of the measured responses, underlining the importance of a broad assessment and of analyzing the covariation of evaluative reports with the expressive physiology and behavior.

In summary, emotion research in psychophysiology has matured methodologically. It is beginning to incorporate new techniques of brain imaging, rendering investigators more sensitive to the neural foundations of emotion science. The view that motivation determines emotion and that emotions evolved from survival reflexes has found wide agreement. Although theoretical debate will and should continue, there is an increasing coincidence of method. Standardized stimulus sets are being developed and common experimental paradigms are more widely employed. It is hoped that this evolution in methodology will encourage replication, providing an empirical foundation that is more valuable than isolated results. With a firm foundation, the field may be ready to use shared constructs, which encourages a true cumulative science of emotion.

NOTES

This work was supported in part by National Institute of Mental Health grants MH37757 and MH43975 and by P50-MH52384, an NIMH Behavioral Science grant to the Center for the Study of Emotion and Attention (CSEA), University of Florida, Gainesville.

Many thanks to Peter Lang for his valuable suggestions, discussions, and contributions to this chapter. Thanks also to various members of the NIMH Center for the Study of Emotion and Attention for their assistance, especially Maurizio Codispoti, Dean Sabatinelli, and Thomas Russman.

1. The 1999 International Affective Picture System (IAPS), International Affective Digitized Sounds (IADS), and Affective Norms for English Words (ANEW) are available on CD-ROM; the IAPS is also available as photographic slides. These stimulus sets and technical manuals can be obtained on request from the author at the NIMH Center

for the Study of Emotion and Attention, Box 100165 HSC, University of Florida, Gainesville, FL 32610-0165, USA.

REFERENCES

Aggleton, J. P. (1992). The functional effects of amygdala lesions in humans: A comparison with findings from monkeys. In J. P. Aggleton (Ed.), *The Amygdala: Neurobiological Aspects of Emotion, Memory, and Mental Dysfunction*, pp. 485–503. New York: Wiley-Liss.

Amaral, D. G., Price, J. L., Pitkanen, A., & Carmichael, S. T. (1992). Anatomical organization of the primate amygdaloid complex. In J. P. Aggleton (Ed.), *The Amygdala: Neurobiological Aspects of Emotion, Memory, and Mental Dysfunction*, pp. 1–66. New York: Wiley-Liss.

Anderson, J. R. (1983). *The Architecture of Cognition*. Cambridge, MA: Harvard University Press.

Anthony, B. J. (1985). In the blink of an eye: Implications of reflex modification for information processing. In P. K. Ackles, J. R. Jennings, & M. G. H. Coles (Eds.), *Advances in Psychophysiology*, vol. 1, pp. 167–218. Greenwich, CT: JAI.

Arnold, M. B. (1960). *Emotion and Personality*, vols. I and II. New York: Columbia University Press.

Arnold, M. B. (1970). *Feelings and Emotions*. New York: Academic Press.

Ashby, F. G., Isen, A. M., & Turken, U. (1999). A neuropsychological theory of positive affect and its influence on cognition. *Psychological Review, 106*, 529–50.

Ax, A. F. (1953). The physiological differentiation between fear and anger in humans. *Psychosomatic Medicine, 15*, 433–42.

Balaban, M. T. (1995). Affective influences on startle in five-month-old infants: Reactions to facial expressions of emotion. *Child Development, 66*, 28–36.

Bard, P. (1934). The neurohumoral basis of emotional reactions. In C. Murchinson (Ed.), *Handbook of General Experimental Psychology*. Worcester, MA: Clark University Press.

Bauer, R. M., & Craighead, W. E. (1979). Psychophysiological responses in the imagination of fearful and neutral situations: The effects of imagery instructions. *Behavior Therapy, 10*, 389–403.

Baum, A., Grunberg, N. E., & Singer, J. E. (1992). Biochemical measurements in the study of emotion. *Psychological Science, 3*, 56–60.

Berntson, G. G., Boysen, S. T., & Cacioppo, J. T. (1993). Neurobehavioral organization and the cardinal principle of evaluative bivalence. In F. M. Crinella & J. Yu (Eds.), *Annals of the New York Academy of Sciences*, vol. 702 (Brain Mechanisms: Papers in Memory of Robert Thompson), pp. 75–102. New York Academy of Sciences.

Berntson, G. G., Cacioppo, J. T., & Quigley, K. S. (1991). Autonomic determinism: The modes of autonomic control, the doctrine of autonomic space, and the laws of autonomic constraint. *Psychological Review, 98*, 459–87.

Berntson, G. G., Cacioppo, J. T., Quigley, K. S., & Fabro, V. T. (1994). Autonomic space and psychophysiological response. *Psychophysiology, 31*, 44–61.

Blanchard, R. J., & Blanchard, D. C. (1989). Attack and defense in rodents as ethoexperimental models for the study of emotion. *Progress in Neuro-Psychopharmacology and Biological Psychiatry, 13*, 3–14.

Bovard, E. W. (1962). The balance between negative and positive brain system activity. *Perspectives in Biological Medicine, 6*, 116–27.

Bower, G. H. (1981). Mood and memory. *American Psychologist, 36*, 129–48.

Bradley, M. M., Cuthbert, B. N., & Lang, P. J. (1990). Startle reflex modification: Attention or emotion? *Psychophysiology, 27*, 513–22.

Bradley, M. M., Cuthbert, B. N., & Lang, P. J. (1993a). Pictures as prepulse: Attention and emotion in startle modification. *Psychophysiology, 30*, 541–5.

Bradley, M. M., Cuthbert, B. N., & Lang, P. J. (in press). Affect and the startle reflex. In M. E. Dawson, A. Schell, & A. Boehmelt (Eds.) *Startle Modification: Implications for Neuroscience, Cognitive Science, and Clinical Science*. Cambridge University Press.

Bradley, M. M., Gianaros, P., & Lang, P. J. (1995). As time goes by: Stability of affective startle modulation [Abstract]. *Psychophysiology, 32*, S21.

Bradley, M. M., Greenwald, M. K., & Hamm, A. O. (1993b). Affective picture processing. In N. Birbaumer & A. Ohman (Eds.), *The Structure of Emotion: Psychophysiological, Cognitive, and Clinical Aspects*. Toronto: Hogrefe & Huber.

Bradley, M. M., Kolchakian, M., Cuthbert, B. N., & Lang, P. J. (1997). What's new? What's exciting? Novelty and emotion in perception [Abstract]. *Psychophysiology, 34*, S22.

Bradley, M. M., & Lang, P. J. (1999a). Affective norms for English words (ANEW): Instruction manual and affective ratings. Technical report no. C-1, Center for Research in Psychophysiology, University of Florida, Gainesville.

Bradley, M. M., & Lang, P. J. (1999b). International affective digitized sounds (IADS): Stimuli, instruction manual and affective ratings. Technical report no. B-2, Center for Research in Psychophysiology, University of Florida, Gainesville.

Bradley, M. M., & Lang, P. (in press a). Measuring emotion: Behavior, feeling and physiology. In R. Lane & L. Nadel (Eds.), *Cognitive Neuroscience of Emotion*. Oxford University Press.

Bradley, M. M., & Lang, P. J. (in press b). Affective reactions to acoustic stimuli. *Psychophysiology*.

Bradley, M. M., Lang, P. J., & Cuthbert, B. N. (1993c). Emotion, novelty and the startle reflex: Habituation in humans. *Behavioral Neuroscience, 107*, 970–80.

Breiter, H. C., Gollub, R. L., Weisskoff, R. M., Kennedy, D. N., Makris, N., Berke, J. D., Goodman, J. M., Kantor, H. L., Gastfriend, D. R., Riorden, J. P., Mathew, R. T., Rosen, B. R., & Hyman, S. E. (1996). Acute effects of cocaine on human brain activity and emotion. *Neuron, 19*, 591–611.

Breiter, H., et al. (1998). Cocaine induced brainstem and subcortical activity observed through fMRI with cardiac gating. Paper presented at the annual meeting of the International Society for Magnetic Resonance in Imaging (Sydney).

Bull, K., & Lang, P. J. (1972). Intensity judgments and physiological response amplitude. *Psychophysiology, 9*, 428–36.

Cacioppo, J. T., & Berntson, G. G. (1994). Relationships between attitudes and evaluative space: A critical review with emphasis on the separability of positive and negative substrates. *Psychological Bulletin, 115*, 401–23.

Cacioppo, J. T., Berntson, G. G., & Crites, S. L. (1996). Social neuroscience: Principles of psychophysiological arousal and response. In E. T. Higgins & A. W. Kruglanski (Eds.), *Social Psychology: Handbook of Basic Principles*, pp. 72–101. New York: Guilford.

Cacioppo, J. T., Berntson, G. G., & Klein, D. J. (1992a). What is an emotion? The role of somatovisceral afference, with special emphasis on somatovisceral "illusions." *Review of Personality and Social Psychology, 14,* 63–98.

Cacioppo, J. T., Berntson, G. G., Larsen, J. T., & Poehlmann, K. A. (in press). The psychophysiology of emotion. In R. Lewis & J. M. Haviland (Eds.), *The Handbook of Emotion.* New York: Guilford.

Cacioppo, J. T., Bush, L. K., & Tassinary, L. G. (1992b). Microexpressive facial actions as a function of affective stimuli: Replication and extension. *Personality and Social Psychology Bulletin, 18,* 515–25.

Cacioppo, J. T., & Gardner, W. L. (1993). What is underlying medical donor attitudes and behavior? *Health Psychology, 12,* 269–71.

Cacioppo, J. T., Gardner, W. L., & Berntson, G. G. (1997). Beyond bipolar conceptualizations and measures: The case of attitudes and evaluative space. *Personality and Social Psychology Review, 1,* 3–25.

Cacioppo, J. T., Klein, D. J., Berntson, G. G., & Hatfield, E. (1993). The psychophysiology of emotion. In M. L. & J. M. Haviland (Eds.), *Handbook of Emotions,* pp. 67–83. New York: Guilford.

Cacioppo, J. T., Malarkey, W. B., Kiecolt-Glaser, J. K., Uchino, B. N., Sgoutas-Emch, S. A., Sheridan, J. F., Berntson, G. G., & Glaser, R. G. (1995). Heterogeneity in neuroendocrine and immune responses to brief psychological stressors as a function of autonomic cardiac activation. *Psychosomatic Medicine, 57,* 154–64.

Cacioppo, J. T., Petty, R. E., Losch, M. E., & Kim, H. S. (1986). Electromyographic activity over facial muscle regions can differentiate the valence and intensity of affective reactions. *Journal of Personality and Social Psychology, 50,* 260–8.

Cacioppo, J. T., Uchino, B. N., Crites, S. L., Snydersmith, M. A., Smith, G., Berntson, G. G., & Lang, P. J. (1992c). The relationship between facial expressiveness and sympathetic activation in emotion: A critical review, with emphasis on modeling underlying mechanisms and individual differences. *Journal of Personality and Social Psychology, 62,* 110–28.

Campos, J. J., Bertenthal, B. I., & Kermoian, R. (1992). Early experience and emotional development: The emergence of wariness of heights. *Psychological Science, 3,* 61–4.

Cannon, W. B. (1928). *Bodily Changes in Pain, Hunger, Fear and Rage,* 2nd ed. New York: Appleton-Century-Crofts.

Codispoti, M., Bradley, M. M., Cuthbert, B. N., & Lang, P. J. (1999). Probing the mind's eye: Prepulse inhibition and affective modulation of startle for briefly presented pictures. Manuscript submitted for publication.

Cook, E. W. III, Davis, T. L., Hawk, L. W., Jr., Spence, E. L., & Gautier, C. H. (1992). Fearfulness and startle potentiation during aversive visual stimuli. *Psychophysiology, 29,* 633–45.

Cook, E. W. III, Hawk, L. W., Davis, T. L., & Stevenson, V. E. (1991). Affective individual differences and startle reflex modulation. *Journal of Abnormal Psychology, 100,* 5–13.

Cook, E. W. III, Melamed, B. G., Cuthbert, B. N., McNeil, D. W., & Lang, P. J. (1988). Emotional imagery and the differen-

tial diagnosis of anxiety. *Journal of Consulting and Clinical Psychology, 56,* 734–40.

Cook, E. W. III, & Turpin, G. (1997). Differentiating orienting, startle and defense responses: The role of affect and its implications for psychopathology. In P. J. Lang, R. F. Simons, & M. T. Balaban (Eds.), *Attention and Orienting: Sensory and Motivational Processes.* Hillsdale, NJ: Erlbaum.

Coyle, J. T., & Schwarcz, R. (1983). The use of excitatory amino acids as selective neurotoxins. In A. Björklund & T. Hökfelt (Eds.), *Handbook of Chemical Neuroanatomy. Methods in Chemical Neuroanatomy,* pp. 508–27. Amsterdam: Elsevier.

Crites, S. L., & Cacioppo, J. T. (1996). Electrocortical differentiation of evaluative and nonevaluative categorizations. *Psychological Science, 7,* 318–21.

CSEA [Center for the Study of Emotion and Attention, NIMH] (1999). International affective picture system: Digitized photographs. Center for Research in Psychophysiology, University of Florida, Gainesville.

Cuthbert, B. N., Bradley, M. M., & Lang, P. J. (1996). Probing picture perception: Activation and emotion. *Psychophysiology, 33,* 103–11.

Cuthbert, B. N., Schupp, H. T., Bradley, M. M., Birbaumer, N., & Lang, P. J. (in press). Cortical potentials in emotional perception. *Biological Psychology.*

Cuthbert, B. N., Vrana, S. R., & Bradley, M. M. (1991). Imagery: Function and physiology. In P. K. Ackles, J. R. Jennings, & M. G. H. Coles (Eds.), *Advances in Psychophysiology,* vol. 4, pp. 1–42. Greenwich, CT: JAI.

Darwin, C. (1873). *The Expression of the Emotions in Man and Animals.* New York: Appleton.

Davidson, R. J. (1992). Emotion and affective style: Hemispheric substrates. *Psychological Science, 3,* 39–43.

Davidson, R., Ekman, P., Saron, C. D., Senulis, J. A., & Friesen, W. V. (1990). Approach/withdrawal and cerebral asymmetry: Emotional expression and brain physiology. *Journal of Personality and Social Psychology, 58,* 330–41.

Davidson, R. J., & Irwin, W. (in press). The functional neuroanatomy of emotion and affective style. *Trends in Cognitive Science.*

Davis, M. (1986). Pharmacological and anatomical analysis of fear conditioning using the fear-potentiated startle paradigm. *Behavioral Neuroscience, 100,* 814–24.

Davis, M. (1989). The role of the amygdala and its efferent projections in fear and anxiety. In P. Tyrer (Ed.), *Psychopharmacology of Anxiety,* pp. 52–79. Oxford University Press.

Davis, M., Hitchcock, J., & Rosen, J. (1987). Anxiety and the amygdala: Pharmacological and anatomical analysis of the fear potentiated startle paradigm. In G. H. Bower (Ed.), *Psychology of Learning and Motivation,* vol. 21, pp. 263–305. New York: Academic Press.

Derryberry, D., & Rothbart, M. K. (1988). Arousal, affect and attention as components of temperament. *Journal of Personality and Social Psychology, 55,* 958–66.

Detenber, B. H., Simons, R. F., & Bennett, G. G. (1998). Roll 'em!: The effects of picture motion on emotional responses. *Journal of Broadcasting and Electronic Media, 42,* 113–27.

Dickinson, A., & Dearing, M. F. (1979). Appetitive-aversive interactions and inhibitory processes. In A. Dickinson & R. A. Boakes (Eds.), *Mechanisms of Learning and Motivation,* pp. 203–31. Hillsdale, NJ: Erlbaum.

Dimberg, U. (1987). Facial reactions, autonomic activity and experienced emotion: A three component model of emotional conditioning. *Biological Psychology, 24,* 105–22.

Dimberg, U. (1990). Facial electromyography and emotional reactions. *Psychophysiology, 27,* 481–94.

Donchin, E., & Coles, M. G. (1988). Is the P300 component a manifestation of context updating? *Behavioral and Brain Sciences, 11,* 357–427.

Duffy, E. (1957). The psychological significance of the concept of "arousal" and "activation." *Psychological Review, 64,* 265–75.

Duffy, E. (1962). *Activation and Behavior.* New York: Wiley.

Ekman, P. (1971). Universals and cultural differences in facial expressions of emotion. In J. Cole (Ed.), *Nebraska Symposium on Motivation,* vol. 19, pp. 207–83. Lincoln: University of Nebraska Press.

Ekman, P., Davidson, R. J., & Friesen, W. V. (1990). The Duchenne smile: Emotional expression and brain physiology: II. *Journal of Personality and Social Psychology, 58,* 342–53.

Ekman, P., & Freisen, W. V. (1978). *The Facial Coding System.* Palo Alto, CA: Consulting Psychological Press.

Ekman, P., & Freisen, W. V. (1986). A new pan-cultural facial expression of emotion. *Motivation and Emotion, 10,* 159–68.

Epstein, S. (1971). Heart rate, skin conductance, and intensity ratings during experimentally induced anxiety: Habituation within and among days. *Psychophysiology, 8,* 319–31.

Erlichman, H., Brown, S., Zhu, J., & Warrenburg, S. (1995). Startle reflex modulation during exposure to pleasant and unpleasant odors. *Psychophysiology, 32,* 150–4.

Everitt, B. J., & Robbins, T. W. (1992). Amygdala-ventral striatal interactions and reward related processes. In J. P. Aggleton (Ed.), *The Amygdala: Neurobiological Aspects of Emotions, Memory, and Mental Dysfunction,* pp. 401–29. New York: Wiley-Liss.

Fanselow, M. S. (1991). The midbrain periaqueductal gray as a coordinator of action in response to fear and anxiety. In A. Depaulis & R. Brandler (Eds.), *The Midbrain Periaqueductal Gray Matter,* pp. 151–73. New York: Plenum.

Fanselow, M. S. (1994). Neural organization of the defensive behavior system responsible for fear. *Psychonomic Bulletin and Review, 1,* 429–38.

Fanselow, M. S., DeCola, J. P., De Oca, B. M., & Landeira-Fernandez, J. (1995). Ventral and dorsolateral regions of the midbrain periaqueductal gray (PAG) control different stages of defensive behavior: Dorsolateral PAG lesions enhance the defensive freezing produced by massed and immediate shock. *Aggressive Behavior, 21,* 63–77.

Fanselow, M. S., & Lester, L. S. (1988). A functional behavioristic approach to aversively motivated behavior: Predatory imminence as a determinant of the topography of defensive behavior. In R. C. Bolles & M. D. Beecher (Eds.), *Evolution and Learning,* pp. 185–211. Hillsdale, NJ: Erlbaum.

Fiorito, E. R., & Simons, R. F. (1994). Emotional imagery and physical anhedonia. *Psychophysiology, 31,* 513–21.

Frankenhaeuser, M. (1975). Experimental approaches to the study of catecholamines and emotion. In L. Levi (Ed.), *Emotions – Their Parameters and Measurement,* pp. 209–34. New York: Raven.

Fridlund, A. J. (1991). Sociality of solitary smiling: Potentiation by an implicit audience. *Journal of Personality and Social Psychology, 60,* 229–40.

Fridlund, A. J., & Izard, C. E. (1983). Electromyographic studies of facial expressions of emotion and patterns of emotion. In J. T. Cacioppo & R. E. Petty (Eds.), *Social Psychophysiology,* pp. 243–280. New York: Guilford.

Fridlund, A. J., Sabini, J. P., Hedlund, L. E., & Schaut, J. A. (1990). Audience effects on solitary faces during imagery: Displaying to the people in your head. *Journal of Nonverbal Behavior, 14,* 113–37.

Fridlund, A. J., Schwartz, G. E., & Fowler, S. C. (1984). Pattern recognition of self-reported emotional state from multiple-site facial EMG activity during affective imagery. *Psychophysiology, 21,* 622–37.

Frijda, N. H. (1986). *The Emotions.* Cambridge University Press.

Gaffen, D. (1992). Amygdala and the memory of reward. In J. Aggleton (Ed.), *The Amygdala: Neurobiological Aspects of Emotion, Memory, and Mental Dysfunction,* pp. 471–83. New York: Wiley-Liss.

Gellhorn, E., & Loofbourrow, N. (1963). *Emotions and Emotional Disorders: A Neurophysiological Study.* New York: Harper & Row.

George, M. S., Ketter, T. A., Parekh, B. A., Horowitz, B., Herscovitch, P., & Post, R. M. (1995). Brain activity during transient sadness and happiness in healthy women. *American Journal of Psychiatry, 152,* 341–51.

Geschwind, N. (1965). Disconnection syndromes in animals and man. *Brain, 88,* 237–94.

Graham, F. K. (1979). Distinguishing among orienting, defense, and startle reflexes. In H. D. Kimmel, E. H. van Olst, & J. F. Orlebeke (Eds.), *The Orienting Reflex in Humans* (Conference sponsored by the Scientific Affairs Division of NATO), pp. 137–67. Hillsdale, NJ: Erlbaum.

Graham, F. K. (1992). Attention: The heartbeat, the blink, and the brain. In B. A. Campbell, H. Hayne, & R. Richardson (Eds.), *Attention and Information Processing in Infants and Adults: Perspectives from Human and Animal Research,* pp. 3–29. Hillsdale, NJ: Erlbaum.

Grayson, J. B. (1982). The elicitation and habituation of orienting and defensive responses to phobic imagery and the incremental stimulus intensity effect. *Psychophysiology, 19,* 104–11.

Greenwald, M. K., Cook, E. W. III, & Lang, P. J. (1989). Affective judgement and psychophysiological response: Dimensional covariation in the evaluation of pictorial stimuli. *Journal of Psychophysiology, 3,* 51–64.

Grossberg, J. M., & Wilson, H. K. (1968). Physiological changes accompanying the visualization of fearful and neutral situations. *Journal of Personality and Social Psychology, 10,* 124–33.

Grossman, S. P. (1967). *A Textbook of Physiological Psychology.* New York: Wiley.

Grunberg, N. E., & Singer, J. E. (1990). Biochemical measurement. In J. T. Cacioppo & L. G. Tassinary (Eds.), *Principles of Psychophysiology: Physical, Social, and Inferential Elements,* pp. 149–76. Cambridge University Press.

Guyton, A. C., & Hall, J. E. (1996). *Textbook of Medical Physiology,* rev. ed. Philadelphia: Saunders.

Halgren, E. (1981). The amygdala contribution to emotion and memory: Current studies in humans. In Y. Ben-Ari (Ed.), *The Amygdaloid Complex,* pp. 395–408. Amsterdam: Elsevier.

Hamm, A. O., Globisch, J., Cuthbert, B. N., & Vaitl, D. (1997). Fear and the startle reflex: Blink modulation and autonomic response patterns in animal and mutilation fearful subjects. *Psychophysiology, 34,* 97–107.

Hamm, A. O., Greenwald, M. K., Bradley, M. M., & Lang, P. J. (1993). Emotional learning, hedonic change, and the startle probe. *Journal of Abnormal Psychology, 102,* 453–65.

Hamm, A. O., & Vaitl, D. (1996). Affective learning: Awareness and aversion. *Psychophysiology 33,* 698–710.

Haney, J. N., & Euse, F. J. (1976). Skin conductance and heart rate response to neutral, positive and negative imagery. *Behavior Therapy, 7,* 494–503.

Hare, R. D. (1973). Orienting and defensive responses to visual stimuli. *Psychophysiology, 10,* 453–63.

Hare, R. D., Wood, K., Britain, S., & Frazelle, J. (1971a). Autonomic responses to affective visual stimulation: Sex differences. *Journal of Experimental Research in Personality, 5,* 14–22.

Hare, R. D., Wood, K., Britain, S., & Shadman, J. (1971b). Autonomic responses to affective visual stimulation. *Psychophysiology, 7,* 408–17.

Hatfield, E., Cacioppo, J. T., & Rapson, R. L. (1993a). Emotional contagion. *Psychological Science, 2,* 96–9.

Hatfield, E., Cacioppo, J. T., & Rapson, R. L. (1993b). *Emotional Contagion.* Cambridge University Press.

Hawk, L. W., & Cook, E. W. (1997). Affective modulation of tactile startle. *Psychophysiology, 34,* 23–31.

Hebb, D. O. (1949). *The Organization of Behavior: A Neuropsychological Theory.* New York: Wiley.

Hess, W. R. (1957). *The Functional Organization of the Diencephalon.* New York: Grune & Stratton.

Hess, W. R., & Burgger, M. (1943). The subcortical center for affective defense reactions. *Helvetica Psychologica et Pharmacologica Acta, 1,* 33.

Hull, C. L. (1943). *Principles of Behavior.* New York: Appleton-Century.

Ito, T. A., Cacioppo, J. T., & Lang, P. J. (1998). Eliciting affect using the International Affective Picture System: Trajectories through evaluative space. *Personality and Social Psychology Bulletin, 24,* 855–79.

Izard, C. E. (1972). *Patterns of Emotions.* New York: Academic Press.

Izard, C. E. (1979). The maximally discriminative facial movement coding system (Max). Instructional Technology Center, University of Delaware, Newark.

Jansen, D. M., & Frijda, N. (1994). Modulation of acoustic startle response by film-induced fear and sexual arousal. *Psychophysiology, 31,* 565–71.

Jennings, J. R., Averill, J. R., Opton, E. M., & Lazarus, R. S. (1970). Some parameters of heart rate change: Perceptual versus motor task requirements, noxiousness, and uncertainty. *Psychophysiology, 7,* 194–212.

Jones, G. E., & Johnson, H. J. (1978). Physiological responding during self generated imagery of contextually complete stimuli. *Psychophysiology, 15,* 439–46.

Jones, G. E., & Johnson, H. J. (1980). Heart rate and somatic concomitants of mental imagery. *Psychophysiology, 17,* 339–47.

Klorman, R., & Ryan, R. M. (1980). Heart rate, contingent negative variation, and evoked potentials during anticipation of affective stimulation. *Psychophysiology, 14,* 45–51.

Klorman, R., Weissberg, A. R., & Austin, M. L. (1975). Autonomic responses to affective visual stimuli. *Psychophysiology, 11,* 15–26.

Klorman, R., Weissbert, R. P., & Wiessenfeld, A. R. (1977). Individual differences in fear and autonomic reactions to affective stimulation. *Psychophysiology, 14,* 45–51.

Koch, M., & Schnitzler, H. U. (1997). The acoustic startle response in rats – Circuits mediating evocation, inhibition and potentiation. *Behavioral Brain Research, 89,* 35–49.

Konorski, J. (1967). *Integrative Activity of the Brain: An Interdisciplinary Approach.* University of Chicago Press.

Lacey, J. I. (1958). Psychophysiological approaches to the evaluation of psychotherapeutic process and outcome. In E. A. Rubinstein & M. B. Perloff (Eds.), *Research in Psychotherapy.* Washington, DC: National.

Lacey, J. I. (1967). Somatic response patterning and stress: Some revisions of activation theory. In M. H. Appley & R. Trumbull (Eds.), *Psychological Stress: Issues in Research,* pp. 14–38. New York: Appleton-Century-Crofts.

Lacey, J. I., & Lacey, B. C. (1970). Some autonomic-central nervous system interrelationships. In P. Black (Ed.), *Physiological Correlates of Emotion,* pp. 205–27. New York: Academic Press.

Lane, R. D., Reiman, E. M., Ahern, G. L., Schwartz, G. E., & Davidson, R. J. (1997a). Neuroanatomical correlates of happiness, sadness, and disgust. *American Journal of Psychiatry, 154,* 926–33.

Lane, R. D., Reiman, E. M., Bradley, M. M., Lang, P. J., Ahern, G. L., Davidson, R. J., & Schwartz, G. E. (1997b). Activation of thalamus and medial prefrontal cortex during emotion. *Neuropsychologia, 35,* 1437–44.

Lang, P. J. (1968). Fear reduction and fear behavior: Problems in treating a construct. In J. M. Schlien (Ed.), *Research in Psychotherapy,* vol. 3, pp. 90–103. Washington, DC: American Psychological Association. Reprinted in I. Florin & W. Tunner (Eds.) (1975), *Therapie der Angst: Systematische Desensibilisierung, Forschritte der Klinischen Psychologie, 8.* München: Urban & Schwartzenberg.

Lang, P. J. (1979). A bio-informational theory of emotional imagery. *Psychophysiology, 16,* 495–512.

Lang, P. J. (1984). Cognition in emotion: Concept and action. In C. Izard, J. Kagan, & R. Zajonc (Eds.), *Emotion, Cognition and Behavior.* Cambridge University Press.

Lang, P. J. (1987). Image as action: A reply to Watts and Blackstock. *Cognition and Emotion, 1,* 407–26.

Lang, P. J. (1994a). The motivational organization of emotion: Affect–reflex connections. In S. VanGoozen, N. E. Van de Poll, & J. A. Sergeant (Eds.), *Emotions: Essays on Current Issues in the Field of Emotion Theory,* pp. 61–93. Hillsdale, NJ: Erlbaum.

Lang, P. J. (1994b). The varieties of emotional experience: A meditation on James–Lange theory. *Psychological Review, 101,* 211–21.

Lang, P. J. (1995). The emotion probe: Studies of motivation and attention. *American Psychologist, 50,* 371–85.

Lang, P. J., Bradley, M. M., & Cuthbert, B. N. (1990). Emotion, attention, and the startle reflex. *Psychological Review, 97,* 377–98.

Lang, P. J., Bradley, M. M., & Cuthbert, M. M. (1997). Motivated attention: Affect, activation and action. In P. J. Lang, R. F. Simons, & M. T. Balaban (Eds.), *Attention and Orienting: Sensory and Motivational Processes.* Hillsdale, NJ: Erlbaum.

Lang, P. J., Bradley, M. M., & Cuthbert, B. N. (1998). International affective picture system (IAPS): Technical Manual and

Affective Ratings. Center for Research in Psychophysiology, University of Florida, Gainesville.

Lang, P. J., Greenwald, M. K., Bradley, M. M., & Hamm, A. O. (1993). Looking at pictures: Affective, facial, visceral, and behavioral reactions. *Psychophysiology, 30*, 261–73.

Lang, P. J., & Hnatiow, M. (1962). Stimulus repetition and the heart rate response. *Journal of Comparative and Physiological Psychology, 55*, 781–5.

Lang, P. J., Kozak, M. J., Miller, G. A., Levin, D. N., & McLean, A., Jr. (1980). Emotional imagery: Conceptual structure and pattern of somato-visceral response. *Psychophysiology, 17*, 179–92.

Lang, P. J., Levin, D. N., Miller, G. A., & Kozak, M. J. (1983). Fear imagery and the psychophysiology of emotion: The problem of affective response integration. *Journal of Abnormal Psychology, 92*, 276–306.

Lazarus, R. S. (1991). Cognition and motivation in emotion. *American Psychologist, 46*, 352–67.

LeDoux, J. E. (1987). Emotion. In V. B. Mountcastle, F. Plum, & St. R. Geiger (Eds.), *Handbook of Physiology*, vol. 5 (Section 1: The Nervous System), pp. 419–59. Bethesda, MD: American Physiological Association.

LeDoux, J. E. (1995). In search of an emotional system in the brain: Leaping from fear to emotion and consciousness. In M. S. Gazzaniga (Ed.), *The Cognitive Neurosciences*, pp. 1049–61. Cambridge, MA: MIT Press.

LeDoux, J. E. (1996). *The Emotional Brain: The Mysterious Underpinnings of Emotional Life*. New York: Touchstone / Simon & Schuster.

Levenson, R. W. (1992). Autonomic nervous system differences among emotions. *Psychological Science, 3*, 23–7.

Levine, P. (1986). Stress. In M. G. H. Coles, E. Donchin, & S. W. Porges (Eds.), *Psychophysiology: Systems, Processes, and Applications*, pp. 331–53. New York: Guilford.

Libby, W. L., Jr., Lacey, B. C., & Lacey, J. I. (1973). Pupillary and cardiac activity during visual attention. *Psychophysiology, 10*, 270–94.

Lifshitz, K. (1966). The averaged evoked cortical response to complex visual stimuli. *Psychophysiology, 3*, 55–68.

Lindsley, D. B. (1951). Emotion. In S. S. Stevens (Ed.), *Handbook of Experimental Psychology*. New York: Wiley.

Lipp, O. V., Sheridan, J., & Siddle, D. A. T. (1994). Human blink startle during aversive and nonaversive Pavlovian conditioning. *Journal of Experimental Psychology: Animal Behavior Processes, 20*, 380–9.

Lykken, D. T. (1957). A study of anxiety in the sociopathic personality. *Journal of Abnormal and Social Psychology, 55*, 6–10.

Mackintosh, N. J. (1983). *Conditioning and Associative Learning*. New York: Oxford University Press.

MacLean, P. D. (1954). Studies on limbic system ("visceral brain") and their bearing on psychosomatic problems. In E. D. Wittkower & R. A. Cleghorn (Eds.), *Recent Developments in Psychosomatic Medicine*, pp. 101–25. Philadelphia: Lippincott.

MacLean, P. D. (1993). Cerebral evolution of emotion. In M. L. & J. M. Haviland (Eds.), *Handbook of Emotions*, pp. 67–83. New York: Guilford.

Malmo, R. B. (1959). Activation: A neuropsychological dimension. *Psychological Review, 66*, 367–86.

Manning, S. K., & Melchiori, M. P. (1974). Words that upset urban college students: Measured with GSRs and rating scales. *Journal of Social Psychology, 94*, 305–6.

Masterson, F. A., & Crawford, M. (1982). The defense motivation system: A theory of avoidance behavior. *Behavioral and Brain Sciences, 5*, 661–96.

May, J. R. (1977a). Psychophysiology of self regulated phobic thoughts. *Behavior Therapy, 8*, 150–9.

May, J. R. (1977b). A psychophysiological study of self and externally regulated phobic thoughts. *Behavior Therapy, 8*, 849–61.

May, J. R., & Johnson, H. J. (1973). Physiological activity to internally elicited arousal and inhibitory thoughts. *Journal of Abnormal Psychology, 83*, 239–45.

McClelland, J. L., & Rumelhart, D. E. (1986). *Parallel Distributed Processing: Explorations in the Microstructure of Cognition*, vol. 2 (Psychological and Biological Models). Cambridge, MA: MIT Press.

McNaughton, N. (1989). *Biology and Emotion*. Cambridge University Press.

Mehrabian, A. (1970). A semantic space for nonverbal behavior. *Journal of Consulting and Clinical Psychology, 35*, 248–57.

Mehrabian, A., & Russell, J. A. (1974). *An Approach to Environmental Psychology*. Cambridge, MA: MIT Press.

Miller, G. A., Levin, D. N., Kozak, M. J., Cook, E. W. III, McLean, A., Jr., & Lang, P. J. (1987). Individual differences in imagery and the psychophysiology of emotion. *Cognition and Emotion, 1*, 367–90.

Miller, N. E. (1959). Liberalization of basic S-R concepts: Extensions to conflict behavior, motivation and social learning. In S. Koch (Ed.), *Psychology: A Study of a Science*, vol. 2 (Study 1). New York: McGraw-Hill.

Miller, N. E. (1966). Some animal experiments pertinent to the problem of combining psychotherapy with drug therapy. *Comprehensive Psychiatry, 7*, 1–12.

Morgan, C. T. (1957). Physiological mechanisms of motivation. In M. R. Jones (Ed.), *Nebraska Symposium on Motivation*. Lincoln: University of Nebraska Press.

Nieuwenhuys, R., Voogd, J., & van Huijzen, Chr. (1988). *The Human Central Nervous System: A Synopsis and Atlas*. Berlin: Springer-Verlag.

Obrist, P. A. (1975). The cardiovascular-behavioral interaction – As it appears today. *Psychophysiology, 13*, 95–107.

Ortony, A., Clore, G. L., & Collins, A. (1988). *The Cognitive Structure of Emotions*. Cambridge University Press.

Osgood, C. (1969). The nature and measurement of meaning. In J. G. Snider & C. E. Osgood (Eds.), *Semantic Differential Technique*, pp. 3–41. Chicago: Aldine.

Osgood, C., Suci, G., & Tannenbaum, P. (1957). *The Measurement of Meaning*. Urbana: University of Illinois Press.

Palomba, D., Angrilli, A., & Mini, A. (1997). Visual evoked potentials, heart rate responses, and memory to emotional pictorial stimuli. *International Journal of Psychophysiology, 27*, 55–67.

Panksepp, J. (1982). Toward a general psychobiological theory of emotions. *The Behavioral and Brain Sciences, 5*, 407–67.

Papez, J. W. (1937). A proposed mechanism of emotion. *Archives of Neurology and Psychiatry, 38*, 725–43.

Patrick, C. J. (1994). Emotion and psychopathy: Startling new insights. *Psychophysiology, 31*, 319–30.

Patrick, C. J., Bradley, M. M., & Lang, P. J. (1993). Emotion in the criminal psychopath: Startle reflex modulation. *Journal of Abnormal Psychology, 102*, 82–92.

Plutchik, R. (1980). A general psychoevolutionary theory of emotion. In R. Plutchik & H. Kellerman (Eds.), *Emotion: Theory, Research and Experience*, vol. 1 (Theories of Emotion), pp. 3–31. New York: Academic Press.

Porges, S. W. (1992). Autonomic regulation and attention. In B. A. Campbell, H. Hayne, & R. Richardson (Eds.), *Attention and Information Processing in Infants and Adults*, pp. 201–23. Hillsdale, NJ: Erlbaum.

Putnam, L. E. (1990). Great expectations: Anticipatory responses of the heart and brain. In J. W. Rohrbaugh, R. Parasuraman, & R. Johnson, Jr. (Eds.), *Event-Related Brain Potentials: Basic Issues and Applications*, pp. 109–29. New York: Oxford University Press.

Quigley, K. S., & Berntson, G. G. (1990). Autonomic origins of cardiac responses to nonsignal stimuli in the rat. *Behavioral Neuroscience, 104,* 751–62.

Roessler, R., Burch, N. R., & Childers, H. E. (1966). Personality and arousal correlates of specific galvanic skin responses. *Psychophysiology, 3,* 115–30.

Sabatinelli, D., Bradley, M. M., Cuthbert, B. N., & Lang, P. J. (1996). Wait and see: Aversion and activation in anticipation and perception [Abstract]. *Psychophysiology, 33,* S72.

Schacter, S., & Singer, J. E. (1962). Cognitive, social and physiological determinants of emotional state. *Psychological Review, 69,* 379–99.

Scherer, K. R. (1986). Vocal affect expression: A review and a model for future research. *Psychological Bulletin, 99,* 143–65.

Schneirla, T. (1959). An evolutionary and developmental theory of biphasic processes underlying approach and withdrawal. In M. Jones (Ed.), *Nebraska Symposium on Motivation*, pp. 1–42. Lincoln: University of Nebraska Press.

Schwartz, G. E. (1971). Cardiac responses to self-induced thoughts. *Psychophysiology, 8,* 462–6.

Schwartz, G., Ahern, G., & Bowen, S. (1979). Lateralized facial muscle response to positive and negative emotional stimuli. *Psychophysiology, 16,* 561–71.

Schwartz, G., Brown, S., & Ahern, G. (1980). Facial muscle patterning and subjective experience during affective imagery: Sex differences. *Psychophysiology, 17,* 75–82.

Selye, H. (1950). *The Physiology and Pathology of Exposure to Stress: A Treatise Based on the Concepts of the General Adaptation Syndrome and the Diseases of Adaptation.* Montreal: Acta.

Selye, H. (1974). *Stress without Distress.* Philadelphia: Lippincott.

Simons, R. F., Detenber, B. H., Roedema, T. M., & Reiss, J. E. (1999). Emotion processing in three systems: The medium and the message. *Psychophysiology, 36,* 619–27.

Sokolov, Y. N. (1963). *Perception and the Conditioned Reflex* (Trans. by S. W. Waydenfeld). New York: Macmillan. [Original work published 1958.]

Stellar, E. (1954). The physiology of emotion. *Psychological Review, 61,* 5–22.

Stern, J. A. (1972). Physiological response measures during classical conditioning. In N. S. Greenfield & P. A. Sternbach (Eds.), *Handbook of Psychophysiology*, pp. 197–228. New York: Holt, Rinehart & Winston.

Sutton, S. K., Davidson, R. J., Donzella, B., & Irwin, W. (1997). Manipulating affective state using extended picture presentations. *Psychophysiology, 34,* 217–26.

Tassinary, L. G., & Cacioppo, J. T. (1992). Unobservable facial actions and emotion. *Psychological Sciences, 2,* 28–33.

Tassinary, L. G., Cacioppo, J. T., & Geen, T. R. (1989). Characterizing organismic-environmental transactions: The use of the readiness potential as a marker of voluntary facial behavior. *Psychophysiology, 26,* S60.

Taylor, S. E. (1991). Asymmetrical effects of positive and negative events: The mobilization-minimization hypothesis. *Psychological Bulletin, 110,* 67–85.

Tellegen, A. (1985). Structures of mood and personality and their relevance to assessing anxiety, with an emphasis on self-report. In A. H. Tuma & J. D. Maser (Eds.), *Anxiety and the Anxiety Disorders*, pp. 681–706. Hillsdale, NJ: Erlbaum.

Tinbergen, N. (1951). *The Study of Instincts.* New York: Oxford University Press.

Turpin, G. (1986). Effects of stimulus intensity on autonomic responding: The problem of differentiating orienting and defense reflexes. *Psychophysiology, 23,* 1–14.

Turpin, G. (1990). Ambulatory clinical psychophysiology: An introduction to techniques and methodological issues. *Journal of Psychophysiology, 4,* 299–304.

Turpin, G., & Siddle, D. A. T. (1983). Effects of stimulus intensity on cardiovascular activity. *Psychophysiology, 20,* 611–24.

Van Egeren, L. F., Feather, B. W., & Hein, P. L. (1971). Desensitization of phobias: Some psychophysiological propositions. *Psychophysiology, 8,* 213–28.

Vanman, E. J., Boehmelt, A. H., Dawson, M. E., & Schell, A. M. (1996). The varying time courses of attentional and affective modulation of the startle eyeblink reflex. *Psychophysiology, 33,* 691–7.

van Oyen Witvliet, C., & Vrana, S. R. (1995). Psychophysiological responses as indicators of affective dimensions. *Psychophysiology, 32,* 436–43.

van Oyen Witvliet, C., & Vrana, S. R. (1996). The emotional impact of instrumental music on affect ratings, facial EMG, autonomic measures, and the startle reflex [Abstract]. *Psychophysiology, 33,* S91.

Vaughan, K. B., & Lanzetta, J. T. (1980). Vicarious instigation and conditioning of facial expressive and autonomic responses to a model's expressive display of pain. *Journal of Personality and Social Psychology, 38,* 909–23.

Vrana, S. R., Cuthbert, B. N., & Lang, P. J. (1986). Fear imagery and text processing. *Psychophysiology, 23,* 247–53.

Vrana, S. R., Spence, E. L., & Lang, P. J. (1988). The startle probe response: A new measure of emotion? *Journal of Abnormal Psychology, 97,* 487–91.

Watson, D., Clark, L. A., & Mineka, S. (1994). Temperament, personality, and the mood and anxiety disorders. *Journal of Abnormal Psychology, 103,* 103–16.

Watson, J. (1924). *Behaviorism.* New York: People's Institute.

Wenger, M. A., Averill, J. R., & Smith, D. D. B. (1968). Autonomic activity during sexual arousal. *Psychophysiology, 4,* 408–78.

Wheeler, R. E., Davidson, R. J., & Tomarken, A. J. (1993). Frontal brain asymmetry and emotional reactivity: A biological substrate of affective style. *Psychophysiology, 30,* 82–9.

Wilhem, F. H., & Roth, W. T. (1996). Ambulatory assessment of clinical anxiety. In J. Fahrenberg & M. Myrtek (Eds.), *Ambulatory Assessment: Computer-Assisted Psychological and Psychophysiological Methods in Monitoring and Field Studies.* Göttingen: Hogrefe & Huber.

Winton, W. M., Putnam, L. E., & Krauss, R. M. (1984). Facial and autonomic manifestations of the dimensional structure of emotion. *Journal of Experimental Social Psychology, 20,* 195–216.

Wundt, W. (1896). *Grundriss der Psychologie* [Outlines of Psychology]. Leipzig: Entgelmann.

Zuckerman, M. (1982). Can arousal be pleasurable? *Behavioral and Brain Sciences, 5,* 449.

CHAPTER TWENTY-THREE

INTERPERSONAL PROCESSES

WENDI L. GARDNER, SHIRA GABRIEL, & AMANDA B. DIEKMAN

Introduction

The time: third century B.C. The setting: home of a successful Roman general. Within, the general's teenage son lies stricken by an unknown disease, attended by an array of physicians called to the boy's bedside by his alarmed father. The boy himself says nothing that hints at the possible cause of his illness. He does, however, display a host of discrete physiological symptoms: a racing pulse, a flushed face, and nervous agitation. Only one physician discerns that these symptoms appear most often during the visits of a particularly beautiful woman, his father's new bride. Through careful observation of the co-occurrence of these "symptoms" and the visits of the stepmother, the physician Erasistratos was able to reveal the boy's strange malady to be merely "lovesickness." This diagnosis constituted the first record of using an individual's physiological signs to infer a psychological process of a distinctly interpersonal nature (Mesulam & Perry 1972; cf. Cacioppo 1982).

Erasistratos and the other attending physicians grappled with an obstacle familiar to modern investigators of interpersonal processes: even the most intense or important internal states sometimes go unspoken. The study of social behavior has traditionally relied on observations of interpersonal interaction as well as self-reports of the thoughts and feelings underlying such behavior. Although these methodological mainstays have increased understanding considerably, there are many processes affecting interpersonal behavior that cannot be revealed in this fashion. Whether, as in the case of the unfortunate stepson, the psychological processes are known but not reported because they are somehow socially undesirable (Jones & Sigall 1971) or whether these processes are too fleeting or too complex to be available for conscious reporting (Nisbett & Wilson 1977), those interested in the underpinnings of interpersonal behavior have often needed to go beyond what is overtly communicated in words or actions. For this reason, social psychologists have turned increasingly to psychophysiological paradigms to help delineate the processes underlying interpersonal behavior.

The purpose of this chapter is to illustrate some of the ways in which research and theory in psychophysiology are advancing our understanding of interpersonal processes. A brief history of the field will be presented, after which psychophysiological research conducted within several areas central to the study of interpersonal processes will be reviewed. Obviously, the nature of interpersonal processes may be explored at more than one level of analysis; this chapter will present areas of research at both the individual and group levels of analysis. At the individual level, researchers investigate the intrapersonal processes in which social perception is grounded. The section on individual level analyses will describe advances in the study of both the attitudinal and appraisal processes. Both processes are considered fundamental to an individual's understanding of the social environment and thus play a large role in determining interpersonal interaction. At the group level, the interplay of physiological and social processes present during everyday interpersonal behavior is examined. This interplay will be illustrated by sampling research from the span of interpersonal interaction, ranging from the effects of the mere presence of strangers to the effects of belonging in close relationships and social networks and to the processes underlying intergroup conflict.[1]

History

Although Erasistratos' third-century diagnosis may be heralded as the first foray into "social psychophysiology" (Cacioppo 1982), psychophysiological theory and methods were largely ignored for the first five decades of social

John T. Cacioppo, Louis G. Tassinary, and Gary G. Berntson (Eds.), *Handbook of Psychophysiology*, 2nd ed. © Cambridge University Press 2000. Printed in the United States of America. ISBN 62634X. All rights reserved.

psychological research. Interestingly, the first two authors of textbooks concerning the scientific study of social processes were wildly divergent in their opinions on the utility of a physiological perspective in the study of social behavior. William McDougall (1908) discussed the importance of understanding possible biological influences on interpersonal interaction, although he limited almost all of his discussion of physiology to describing the influence of relatively inflexible instincts. Floyd Allport (1924), on the other hand, dismissed a physiological perspective entirely, focusing instead on the importance of observing the specific overt actions of individuals in the presence of others. Both texts had "social psychology" in their titles, but it was the latter that shaped the field.

Research investigating the physiological concomitants of interpersonal behavior was rare but not altogether absent in the early years of social psychology. For example, Riddle (1925) observed changes in respiration as a marker of interpersonal deception during poker games. Similarly, Lasswell (1936) observed the physiological manifestations of different affective states experienced during an ongoing interpersonal interaction. And Smith (1936), in an ingenious exploration of the intrapersonal processes underlying social conformity, utilized electrodermal responses as an indicator of the anxiety induced by disagreement with the majority opinion.

These early pioneers notwithstanding, the value of a psychophysiological perspective in understanding social processes did not receive much attention until the 1960s. Psychophysiology may have become more attractive to social psychologists at this time for two reasons. First, the concept of "physiological arousal" was at the heart of several influential theories of the decade; for example, cognitive dissonance theory (Festinger 1957), the two-factor theory of emotion (Schacter & Singer 1962), and social facilitation theory (Zajonc 1965) were all highly prominent. Second, physiological measures were becoming recognized as a possible means of collecting data that were less contaminated by social desirability factors (e.g. Rankin & Campbell 1955).

In light of the new advances and research, Shapiro and colleagues (Leiderman & Shapiro 1964; Schwartz & Shapiro 1973; Shapiro & Crider 1969; Shapiro & Schwartz 1970) authored a book and several chapters championing the importance of the interplay between social and physiological processes. These were followed, in the early 1980s, by edited volumes entitled *Social Psychophysiology* (Cacioppo & Petty 1983) and *Sociophysiology* (Waid 1984). As the 1980s drew to a close, Cacioppo, Petty, and Tassinary (1989b) encouraged the field to take "A New Look" at the incorporation of psychophysiological theory and methods into mainstream social psychology, and indeed the 1990s have featured a burgeoning interest in psychophysiological perspectives of interpersonal processes. Since 1986, over 200 studies incorporating physiological variables appeared in mainstream social psychological journals (PsycINFO), and chapters devoted to the interplay between psychophysiological and social processes can now be found in handbooks of the field (e.g. Blascovich 1997; Cacioppo, Berntson, & Crites 1996a).

Given the promise of psychophysiological techniques to illuminate social processes, one might wonder why there was such a delay in the acceptance of the psychophysiological perspective. According to Blascovich (1997), the incorporation of psychophysiological procedures into the study of social processes may have faltered on at least two grounds. First, the technology required for psychophysiological measurement remained inaccessible to many. Second, there was little agreement upon appropriate psychophysiological methodologies and inference techniques among researchers interested in interpersonal processes.

As an example, the construct of "physiological arousal" upon which much of the early work was centered was very generally defined as a nonspecific heightened activation of autonomic and cortical processes. The general nature and function of arousal allowed for application to a broad range of topics, including attitude change (Festinger 1957; Zanna & Cooper 1974), aggression (Christy, Gelfand, & Hartmann 1971; Zillmann 1979), prosocial behavior (Ashton & Severy 1976; Sterling & Gaertner 1984), and interpersonal attraction (Berscheid & Walster 1978; Dutton & Aron 1974), yet this general nature of arousal also had the consequence of leaving the identification of appropriate manipulations and measures unspecified. As a diffuse bodily state, the arousal associated with interpersonal processes was indexed variously by heart rate (Sterling & Gaertner 1984), blood pressure (Zillmann & Cantor 1976), skin conductance (Croyle & Cooper 1983), the facilitation of dominant behavioral responses (Cottrell & Wack 1967; Pallak & Pittman 1972), the moderation of the expected effect by misattribution of arousal to an unrelated but plausible target (Geen, Rakosky, & Pigg 1972; Zanna & Cooper 1974), and by verbal self-reports of "feeling aroused" (Loh & Nuttin 1972).

Given the weak associations that have been found both within and between participants among various autonomic measures of arousal (Lacey & Lacey 1974) – not to mention between autonomic measures and verbal self-reports (Cacioppo et al. 1987) – inconsistencies among the various measures and findings were to be expected (for a discussion see Cacioppo et al. 1996a). However, when such measures contradicted one another, or conflicted with verbal reports of felt arousal, these inconsistencies were often left unresolved. In some cases, the physiological measures of arousal were taken as the valid indices regardless of self-report (Zillmann, Johnson, & Day 1974), whereas in others the verbal reports were taken as veridical and the data provided by the physiological measures were ignored (Breckler 1984; cf. Cacioppo, Petty, & Geen 1989a). Thus, although a focus on "arousal" brought a physiological construct into the mainstream study of interpersonal processes, the vagueness of specification of both the construct itself and the appropriate methods used to quantify it remained problematic (Cacioppo et al. 1996a).

At the opposite extreme, some psychophysiological variables were overspecified; many of the early researchers interested in interpersonal processes expected a physiological measurement to provide a simple one-to-one relationship with the psychological construct of interest. For example, heart rate might be assumed to reflect only emotional arousal, or electrodermal responses utilized as if they unequivocally indexed anxiety. Fortunately, as the epistemological grounds for appropriate inference techniques became better understood (e.g. Cacioppo & Tassinary 1990), the quality and complexity of social psychophysiological research in the field advanced as well (see Blascovich in press for review). Psychophysiological perspectives may now be found in the majority of the mainstream areas of research into interpersonal processes (Baron & Byrne 1997). It is hoped that the sampling of research that follows will serve not only to illustrate how psychophysiological theory and methods have been applied in the field but also to demonstrate the promise of this interplay for furthering our understanding of the processes underlying interpersonal interactions.

Interpersonal Processes at the Level of the Individual

Much of "social reality" can be said to occur in our heads. Indeed, even when alone we remain firmly grounded in the social world – guided in our decisions by concerns about the reactions of others (Baldwin & Holmes 1987) and constrained in our actions by cultural norms (Miller & Prentice 1996). Clearly, the ways in which an individual construes his or her social environment drives that individual's responses, interpersonally and otherwise. Thus, some of the greatest advances in understanding the vagaries of social behavior have been gained by the study of *intrapersonal* processes. Given the importance of an individual's construals of others and the environment to subsequent interpersonal behavior, the current section will review research on the attitudinal and appraisal processes that underlie these construals.

ATTITUDES AND ATTITUDINAL PROCESSES

Perhaps the most central topic in social psychology is the study of attitudes. Simply put, an attitude is an evaluation of an attitude object, or "a psychological tendency that is expressed by evaluating a particular entity with some degree of favor or disfavor" (Eagly & Chaiken 1993, p. 1). These general evaluations are of interest to researchers of interpersonal processes because attitudes are considered central to a wide variety of the psychological

processes that affect social interaction, such as impression formation, interpersonal attraction, self-evaluation and esteem, and stereotyping and prejudice, to name a few.

Throughout the history of attitude research, psychophysiological indexes have been pursued by many as alternatives to self-report measures of attitudes. The accurate measurement of attitudes has always been a vital concern; without reliable and valid measurement, studies of attitudinal process, structure, and function could not be conducted with any assurance of truth. Yet the internal, subjective nature of evaluation presents a challenge when trying to convert individual evaluations into standard attitude scores. The Thurstone (1928) and Guttman (1944) techniques both involve elaborate methods of scaling individuals' responses. Currently, the most commonly used paper-and-pencil measures are Likert-type items and the semantic differential (Likert 1932; Osgood, Suci, & Tannenbaum 1957). Although these measures have the benefit of convenience, any paper-and-pencil measure is obviously subject to an individual's willingness and ability to report his or her attitude. If the attitude object is of a controversial nature, it becomes more challenging to detect individuals' true attitudes, especially if a certain response is socially desirable.

For this reason, then, many researchers explored physiological measurements in the hopes of gaining an index of attitudes that would be less vulnerable to the pressures of social desirability. This exploration proved valuable beyond the realm of mere measurement issues. Psychophysiological investigations in the area of attitudes have provided important insights into the affective and cognitive processes involved in forming, maintaining, and changing attitudes (e.g., Cacioppo & Petty 1981). As such, psychophysiological paradigms have exceeded expectations, not only providing the types of measurements that were hoped for but also allowing fruitful investigations into long-standing questions concerning the nature of attitudinal processing and the functions that attitudes may serve.

Attitude Substrates

Affective Processes. What are the fundamental features of an attitude? One common model of attitudes proposes that attitudes have a tripartite nature, associated with affective reactions to the attitude object, beliefs concerning the positive or negative features of the object, and behaviors performed with respect to the attitude object (Breckler 1984; Katz & Stotland 1959). Early applications of physiological paradigms to attitude assessment were founded upon the belief that they could serve as a type of conduit for purely affective responses, even as "affect" was defined rather broadly. For example, electrodermal (Cooper & Siegel 1956; Rankin & Campbell 1955) and pupillary (Barlow 1969; Hess 1965; Hess & Polt 1960) responses were both initially thought to represent promising alternatives to self-report measures of attitude responses. However, both were subsequently rejected on the grounds that neither psychophysiological measure provided sensitive information concerning the valence of the participant's attitude (Cacioppo & Sandman 1981; Petty & Cacioppo 1983), serving instead as more general indices of attention or orienting (see Chapters 6, 8, and 20 of this volume).

Fortunately, researchers continued to probe the potential of psychophysiological techniques. Although not a conduit to any single attitudinal substrate, facial electromyographic techniques (see Chapter 7), startle responses (Chapter 22), and event-related brain potentials (Chapter 3) all appear to have promise in illuminating both the affective and cognitive underpinnings of attitudes.

Blascovich (1997) highlighted facial electromyography (EMG) and startle probe techniques as two particularly noteworthy paradigms for investigating affective and attitudinal processes. Building on the work of Schwartz and colleagues (1976; Schwartz, Ahern, & Brown 1979) that demonstrated the sensitivity of the zygomatic and corrugator muscles to positive and negative affective states, Cacioppo and colleagues applied facial EMG to the investigation of attitudes (Cacioppo, Bush, & Tassinary 1992; Cacioppo & Petty 1979; Cacioppo et al. 1986, 1988).

The original experiment relating facial EMG to attitudinal responding (Cacioppo & Petty 1979) examined corrugator supercilii (brow) and zygomaticus major (cheek) activity in response to proattitudinal and counterattitudinal messages. Participants were asked to list thoughts that occurred during the message and to give a self-report of their attitude. It was found that EMG activity over the zygomaticus major region varied as a function of the positivity of the affective stimuli and the positivity of affect-laden processing; EMG activity over the corrugator supercilii region was found to vary as a function of the negativity of the affective stimuli and the negativity of affect-laden information processing. Finally, EMG activity over the perioral (e.g., orbicularis oris) region was found to vary as a function of the extent of semantic (e.g., cognitive response) processing. This pattern of facial EMG activity occurred even when participants were neither explicitly advised to collect their thoughts nor warned that they would hear a counterattitudinal message. Thus, facial EMG appeared to hold promise as a method of tapping an individual's spontaneous affective and cognitive responses to an attitude object.

Extensions of this research confirmed the sensitivity of facial EMG as an index of both the valence and intensity of fleeting attitudinal or affective responses that occur in response to the presentation of various positive and negative slides (Cacioppo et al. 1986) or that occur spontaneously during a 30-minute interview (Cacioppo et al. 1988). It is interesting to note that, in both studies, emotional responses that were too subtle and fleeting to be perceived by observers of the participants' overt facial expressions were nonetheless reflected by patterns of facial EMG activity.

Given that the initial interest in physiological indices of attitudes was driven by the potential for measures that were impervious to purposeful distortion, Cacioppo et al. (1992) examined the effects of the intention to communicate one's feelings to others. In this study, participants were instructed to amplify or inhibit facial expressions to an imaginary observer while viewing slides of positive, neutral, or negative valence. This study found that EMG was vulnerable to purposeful distortion, although participants were more successful at moderating zygomatic activity than corrugator activity. Thus, corrugator activity, in contrast with other facial muscle activity, shows potential for the indexing of emotions that are not intended to be communicated.

In light of the communicative value of facial expressions, it is unsurprising that activity of the lower facial musculature should be moderated by conscious intent. In contrast, the reflexive startle blink has received attention as a measure of affect that is thought to be relatively immune to conscious control (Blascovich 1997; see also Chapter 22). To date, this research has been primarily conducted using extreme affective stimuli and may therefore be limited in its application to attitudes that do not entail a strongly emotional basis. However, the reflexive startle blink may still hold promise for increasing the understanding of affective processing that may be similar to, if more extreme than, some types of attitudinal processing.

Lang and Bradley and their colleagues have amassed support for the concept of "synergistic response matching," wherein the reduction or augmentation of any reflex depends on the correspondence between the appetitive or aversive function of that reflex and the ongoing affective state of the individual (Lang, Bradley, & Cuthbert 1990, 1992). Because the startle eye-blink reflex is defensive and therefore negatively toned, the magnitude of the startle eye blink was hypothesized to be enhanced during the experience of negative affect and inhibited during the experience of positive affect. This hypothesis has received support with a wide range of emotional stimuli: the presentation of positive and negatively valenced slides (Bradley, Cuthbert, & Lang 1990; Vrana, Spence, & Lang 1988), the induction of emotional memories and imagery (Vrana & Lang 1990), and conditioned fear (Hamm et al. 1993).[2]

For example, Vrana and co-workers (1988) conducted a study in which the specificity of the startle blink moderation to emotional valence – rather than merely attentional properties – was investigated. Participants were shown positive, neutral, and negative photographic slides that were coupled with an acoustic startle probe. Participants then rated the slides for emotional valence as well as for interest. Besides the "interest" ratings, attention was measured by heart rate and by how long the participant chose to view the slide. Both negative and positive slides drew more attention than neutral slides; however, startle magnitude did not show a similar curvilinear pattern of results. Instead, startle magnitude showed the expected linear increase from pleasant to neutral to unpleasant slides. If positive stimuli simply drew more attention, then attention should show a linear increase from negative to positive stimuli. This discrepancy indicated that attention and emotion did not function in the same way, thus providing support for the emotion hypothesis.

Vrana and Lang (1990) further demonstrated that the moderation of the startle blink reflected internal affective states by having participants engage in pleasant or unpleasant imagery (e.g., imagining a day at the beach versus a visit to the dentist). Startle blinks that were evoked during unpleasant imagery were accentuated, as expected. The extension of this research into the realm of affective conditioning (Hamm et al. 1993) implies that this procedure is sensitive to recently learned changes in valence and thus may be applied to some types of attitude change or persuasion – at least for those attitudes that have a strong emotional basis.

Overall, research examining the affective modulation of the startle response has provided a promising new direction in the psychophysiological study of emotion. Because of their reflexive action, startle responses are not under participants' control and thus can possibly provide the type of unbiased reading of emotional valence that attitude researchers have long been seeking (Blascovich 1997). However, although many attitudes have a strong emotional basis, others may be grounded in belief structures that are less emotionally charged. It is as yet unclear whether the startle blink response could index these types of attitudes.

Cognitive Processes. Whereas the startle responses may provide clues about the affective substrates of attitudes, the use of event-related brain potentials (ERPs) may provide a sensitive measure of attitudes without relying on a strong affective response to the attitude object. The ERP represents an average of electroencephalographic activity in response to repeated time-locked presentations of a stimulus (see Chapter 3). Components within the ERP have traditionally been used as markers of attentional, memorial, motoric, and linguistic processes (Chapters 3, 19, and 21). Cacioppo and associates have applied ERP technology to index attitudinal processing (Cacioppo et al. 1993, 1994; Cacioppo, Crites, & Gardner 1996b; Crites et al. 1995; Crites & Cacioppo 1996; Gardner & Cacioppo in press).

Cacioppo and colleagues (1993) capitalized on the extant research concerning the relationship between a late positive component (the P300 or P3a) and categorization processes (see Chapter 3) to apply ERP techniques to study attitudinal processing. A larger P300 is evoked to categorically inconsistent than consistent information (Donchin 1981; Sutton et al. 1965). Therefore, an attitudinally incon-

sistent object, such as a positive attitude object presented in a context of negative attitude objects, would be expected to evoke a larger P300 than would an attitudinally consistent object, such as a positive attitude object presented in a context of other positive attitude objects. This hypothesis was supported using both idiosyncratically held attitudes (liked and disliked sports teams, celebrities, and foods) and consensually held attitudes (positive and negative personality traits).

Once it was shown that the P300 consistently covaried with attitudinal reports, subsequent research focused upon the utility of the P300 to tap an early stage in the sequence of attitudinal processing. In order to prepare and execute a response to an attitude object, the object must first be categorized as positive or negative. The nature of this early process, termed "evaluative categorization," was somewhat of a mystery – in earlier paradigms (physiologically, behaviorally, or verbally based), this process was thought to depend upon efferent outputs or overt responses. Crites et al. (1995) uncoupled evaluative categorization processes from subsequent response-related processes by instructing participants to misreport their attitudes during half of the attitude sequence. In other words, the output of the evaluative categorization processes and that of the response-related processes were identical for only half the trials; for the other half, output of the evaluative categorization processes was opposite of those of the response-related processes. The P300 remained sensitive to evaluative inconsistency (a positive attitude object in a context of negative objects or vice versa) *regardless* of the veracity of the participants' overt responses. In this way, the utility of the P300 to tap the early stage of evaluative categorization was demonstrated.

The ability to examine this early stage of attitudinal processing separate from downstream processes allowed for insights into the nature of evaluative categorizations. Several debates in the attitudes literature could be addressed. First, the sensitivity of this early process to differences in the extremity of an attitude could be examined. Some researchers believed that the output at early stages of attitudinal processing would be a simple dichotomous "good or bad" evaluation because the primary role of this stage was hypothesized to alert the organism to possible threats in the environment (Chen & Bargh 1999; Fazio 1989). Alternatively, given the importance of assessing the extremity of the positive or negative nature of the attitude object, it had been hypothesized by others that this information, too, would already be reflected in this early stage of the attitudinal processing sequence (Pratto & John 1991; Zajonc 1980a). Research utilizing the P300 paradigm revealed that this ERP technique was sensitive to both the valence and the extremity of an attitude object (Cacioppo et al. 1994) and could even be used to differentiate individuals who possessed different attitudes toward the same object (Gardner & Cacioppo in press). Thus, even at this early stage, the extremity of an attitude object appears to be processed along with its valence.

In addition to illuminating debates concerning the sensitivity of early attitudinal processing, the use of ERPs has been harnessed to answer other fundamental questions about such processing. For example, the general nature of attitudinal processing has been a topic of dispute. Some researchers have postulated that attitudinal processes are "hot" – in other words, that they share features with more rudimentary emotional processes, including the neural substrates proposed to underlie the processing of emotional information (Berntson, Boysen, & Cacioppo 1992; Zajonc 1980a). In contrast, other researchers have conceptualized attitudinal processes as "cold" – to reflect a simple semantic distinction – and thus have refuted the overlap of attitudinal and emotional processes (Millar & Tesser 1992; Zanna & Rempel 1988). New investigations of hemispheric activity in response to attitudinal and nonattitudinal processing may represent an initial step toward resolution of this issue.

Cacioppo et al. (1996b) hypothesized that if different neural generators contributed to attitudinal than to nonattitudinal processes, then these differences would be reflected in a different pattern of electrical activation as measured at the scalp (for reviews see Johnson 1993; Chapter 3 of this volume). Indeed, it was found that in studies in which an attitudinal task was used, the P300s evoked by the target stimuli were right-lateralized (e.g., larger over the right than left hemisphere), whereas in studies in which similar stimuli but a nonattitudinal task was used, the evoked P300s were symmetrically distributed. Further evidence for this effect was provided by Crites and Cacioppo (1996), who showed the right laterality effect could be invoked merely through changing the task instructions. Participants were instructed to categorize different target words (e.g., pear, raspberry, spinach) either as fruits versus vegetables (a nonattitudinal semantic categorization) or as objects that they personally liked versus disliked (an attitudinal categorization). The P300s evoked during the attitudinal task were once again found to be more highly right-lateralized than those evoked to identical stimuli processed in a nonattitudinal fashion.[3]

Although these results support the hypothesis that different neural generators underlie the processing of attitudinal versus nonattitudinal information, neither study entails that these differences arise because of the similarity of attitudinal processes to emotion. However, the role of the right hemisphere in the processing of emotional information is widely held to be important (see Heller 1993 for review); evidence for a right-hemisphere specialization for both the perception (Ross 1981; Spence, Shapiro, & Zaiedel 1996) and the production (Blonder, Bowers, & Heilman 1991; Borod 1993) of emotion has been found in the neuropsychological literature. Clearer evidence for the overlap of emotional and attitudinal processes was provided by

Gardner, Cacioppo, and Berntson (1996); in a study examining the attitudinal processing of photographic slides, they found that slides that were rated as more emotionally intense also evoked more highly right-lateralized P300s than their less emotional counterparts.

It is interesting that the research examining the relationship between emotion, attitudinal processing, and right-hemisphere specialization was foreshadowed by an earlier study that examined EEG (electroencephalograph) measurements in a persuasion context. Cacioppo, Petty, and Quintanar (1982) exposed participants to strong and weak versions of proattitudinal and counterattitudinal messages. A main effect of hemispheric activity on affective polarization demonstrated that individuals who showed relatively more activation in the right hemisphere while listening to the messages also showed a more polarized attitude as indexed by subsequent thought listings. It thus seems highly probable that this study, although utilizing different measures of hemispheric activation, tapped into the same underlying relationship between attitudinal processing and the right hemisphere.

In sum, the use of psychophysiological methodologies to tap attitudinal processes appears to be as fruitful as early researchers had hoped. Facial EMG has been successfully used to assess both spontaneous affective and covert verbal responses to attitude objects. Startle blink responses may someday be used to tap the affective substrates of emotionally based attitudes. Finally, the use of ERP indices has allowed for investigations into the nature of attitudinal processing more generally by providing access to an early stage of evaluative categorization. We turn next to a discussion of another important line of attitudes research, one that focuses not upon how attitudinal information is processed per se but rather upon the reasons why this process is so fundamental – in other words, the very function of attitudes.

Attitude Functions

Why do we hold attitudes? What purpose do they serve? These simple queries represent one of the oldest and most fundamental issues in attitude research (Eagly & Chaiken 1993). As we have seen, psychophysiology has provided new paradigms for the investigation of attitudinal processing, and modern social psychophysiological research has begun to provide interesting answers to even this most basic of questions.

The primary function of attitudes has been hypothesized to be the "knowledge" function (Katz 1960) or the "object appraisal" function (Smith, Bruner, & White 1956). In short, it is thought that holding an attitude toward any person, object, or idea then facilitates any decisions concerning the attitude object, particularly in otherwise demanding situations in which cognitive resources may be low (Fazio 1989). Although intuitively appealing, the ability of attitudes to ease decision making was difficult to address until Blascovich and colleagues (1993; Fazio, Blascovich, & Driscoll 1992) employed autonomic measures to investigate whether holding accessible attitudes results in less physiologically stressful decision making.

Attitude accessibility refers to how quickly and easily the attitude toward any object can be retrieved from memory. Attitudes that are highly accessible have been thought to be those most likely to hold the knowledge or object-appraisal function and thus ease decision making (Fazio 1989). Blascovich and colleagues hypothesized that, were this the case, then highly accessible attitudes should result in lower autonomic indicators of stress than their less accessible counterparts during a decision-making task concerning the attitude objects.

In an initial study, Fazio et al. (1992) demonstrated that attitude rehearsal leads to lower diastolic blood pressure when faced with a decision task involving the attitude. This effect was demonstrated by giving participants an opportunity to form attitudes toward abstract paintings;[4] subsequently, they were shown pairs of the paintings and asked to decide which they preferred. In this pairwise decision task, participants who had been able to rehearse their attitudes displayed lower diastolic blood pressure than participants who were not given an opportunity for attitude rehearsal.

In an extension of this work, Blascovich et al. (1993) used more sensitive measures of autonomic reactivity (e.g., pre-ejection period, stroke volume, cardiac output, pulse transit time) and also employed manipulations that ruled out object familiarity and attitude extremity as possible confounds. The results of two studies provided further support for the functional utility of attitudes; autonomic reactivity, particularly sympathetic arousal, was reduced during a decision-making task when participants held accessible attitudes toward the stimuli. In combination, these studies provide striking psychophysiological evidence that attitude accessibility affects the ease of decision making. Although this function of attitudes has been studied for many years, these studies provide a convincing physiological demonstration that attitudes function to help individuals make decisions easily and effectively.

In conclusion, the incorporation of psychophysiological paradigms and perspectives into the field of attitude research has clearly been fruitful. In the past decade, the psychophysiological perspective has opened new avenues of inquiry by providing both theoretical frameworks and advances in measurement. Thus, although psychophysiological techniques have finally fulfilled the initial promissory note of veridical, nonverbal measures of attitudes, the contribution of psychophysiology exceeds the mere provision of new methodological tools. Instead, a burgeoning interest in the interplay among physiological and attitudinal processes continues to advance the field by enabling new investigations of fundamental questions.

APPRAISALS OF THE SOCIAL ENVIRONMENT: THREAT VERSUS CHALLENGE

A key tenet in the study of interpersonal processes is that the appraisal of an individual's social environment is fundamental to his or her subsequent behavior. Simply put, social behavior does not vary with the objective situation but rather with the individual's appraisal of the situation (for a review see Olson, Roese, & Zanna 1996). Just as an attitude represents an evaluation of a person, object, or idea, an appraisal represents an evaluation of the current situation – or, more specifically, an individual's evaluation of his or her personal ability to cope with the situation at hand (Lazarus 1991). The initiation of behaviors as diverse as applying for a job, asking an acquaintance out for coffee, helping a stranger in distress, or initiating an argument with a spouse are all strongly driven by whether the individual involved views each situation to be a threat (e.g., exceeding one's personal resources or capabilities) or a challenge (e.g., within one's personal ability).

The importance of such appraisal processes for emotional experience and social behavior has been acknowledged since the 1960s (e.g. Arnold 1960; Lazarus & Alfert 1964). Much of the focus of the early appraisal literature emphasized the importance of appraisal processes in moderating emotional and physiological reactions to passive coping situations in which an individual must endure some stressor (e.g., white noise, unpleasant films). For example, Speisman, Lazarus, and Davison (1964) exposed participants to an emotionally stressful film while encouraging participants to view the film in a more or less threatening fashion (some participants heard a narrative that intellectualized the film, decreasing threat appraisals; others heard a narrative that enhanced threat appraisals). Results of this and similar studies (e.g. Lazarus & Alfert 1964) revealed that the reduction of threat appraisals lowered both subjective feelings of stress and physiological reactivity (e.g., skin conductance responses) while viewing the films.

More recent appraisal research has focused upon active as well as passive coping situations. Active coping situations, in which an individual appraises the situation in terms of his or her ability to gain a desired outcome, are more akin to the social stressors faced during interpersonal interactions and are also much more likely to allow for either threat or challenge appraisals (cf. Tomaka et al. 1993). For example, Hu and Romans-Kroll (1995) reported that focusing speech-anxious participants on the challenging but positive features of giving a speech decreased both subjective fear and physiological reactivity during the speech task itself.

Researchers have also added a larger battery of physiological measures that may, in combination, serve as markers of threat or challenge appraisals. Specifically, Blascovich, Tomaka, and colleagues (Blascovich & Tomaka

1996; Tomaka & Blascovich 1994; Tomaka et al. 1993, 1997) reasoned that cardiac performance (as measured by pre-ejection period, stroke volume, and cardiac output; see Chapter 9) would increase in any active coping situation, reflecting increased levels of motivation. For individuals who appraised the situation as a challenge, these increases in cardiac performance would be accompanied by vasodilation (e.g., a decrease in total peripheral resistance), an adaptive pattern associated with increased energy mobilization and performance for coping with the situation. Alternatively, individuals who appraised the situation as a threat would show increased cardiac performance coupled with vasoconstriction, a defensive pattern reflecting perhaps a shielding of resources from attack (Dienstbier 1989) and one that has been linked to cardiovascular disease (Manuck 1994).

In the first study examining autonomic markers of threat and challenge, Tomaka et al. (1993) presented participants with an active coping task (mental arithmetic) and observed both self-reported psychological responses and physiological responses during the task. As expected, those participants who viewed the situation as a challenge showed increased cardiac performance and decreased total peripheral resistance as compared with those who viewed the situation as a threat. Challenged participants also reported feeling less stressed during the task, and they outperformed their threatened counterparts.

The differentiation of threat and challenge allows for more direct examinations of social variables on appraisal processes and responses to stress. For example, it has been argued that individuals who possess a strong belief in a "just world" (e.g., that the world is a fair place and thus people generally get what they deserve) are able to maintain more positive expectancies about the social environment and increased motivation in the face of minor stressors (Lerner 1980). Indeed, Tomaka and Blascovich (1994) demonstrated that individuals with higher just-world beliefs were more likely to exhibit patterns indicating challenge than threat when faced with a minor stressor. Similarly, the importance of mastery versus performance goals for determining adaptive responses to academic situations has been emphasized in modern educational research (see Dweck 1996 for review). Tomaka et al. (1997) manipulated participants' goals via the instructional "set" – stressing either effort (mastery) or accuracy (performance) before the task. Results revealed that participants who had been given instructions stressing mastery responded both psychologically and physiologically as challenged, whereas those who had been given performance goals responded as threatened.

Overall, studies examining intrapersonal appraisal processes have illustrated the importance of the subjective construals of the environment on affective responding and subsequent social behavior. Research has begun to delineate the probable physiological functions (mobilization of energy versus defensive protection of resources) underlying challenge versus threat responses as well as the possible health consequences of such appraisals. A growing body of research has linked the prevalence of positive expectancies to better physical well-being. This relationship holds equally well for dispositional positive expectancies or optimism (Antoni & Goodkin 1988; Scheier & Carver 1985; see Scheier & Carver 1992 for review) and situationally specific positive expectancies concerning a particular health challenge such as heart transplantation (Leedham et al. 1995). The mechanisms underlying this relationship remain unclear, but certainly one possibility is that positive expectations lead to treating stressors as challenges rather than threats, rendering the autonomic consequences of stress less physically damaging. By differentiating patterns of autonomic responding evoked by threat versus challenge appraisals during active coping tasks, other research programs – in addition to illuminating the possible health implications of expectancies – have allowed for investigations of variables (e.g., belief in a just world, mastery versus performance goals) that are clearly relevant to social responding. The importance of such appraisal processes for interpersonal interaction will be seen in the next section.

Interpersonal Processes at the Level of the Group

Human beings are social creatures; much of daily life is spent navigating a sea of interpersonal exchanges with colleagues, strangers, friends, and family. Thus, although one focus within the study of interpersonal processes is the perceptions of social reality that occur within an individual, it is equally important to study the individual within the social environment. This social environment can be defined rather broadly; for example, as simple a social stimulus as the mere presence of a stranger has been shown to affect behavior. Additionally, the quality of our interactions with close others has been a focus of much research, as has the importance of being embedded within a social network. Finally, intergroup interaction – in which the individual becomes part of the larger whole defined by group membership (e.g., racial, national, religious) and acting primarily for the group interest – has become an increasingly important topic. All of these varieties of interpersonal interaction take place (for most of us) on a daily basis, and the current section will illustrate some of the research in each area.

MERE PRESENCE

The first empirical study of interpersonal processes (Triplett 1898) concerned the effects of the presence or absence of a social environment on individual performance. An avid bicyclist, Triplett observed that the presence of another rider on the track improved riding speed as compared to the speed of the same individual when riding the track alone. Triplett's initial interpretation was nonpsychological in nature; he studied the patterns of wind resistance, believing the presence of a second rider shielded the individual from wind that would otherwise decrease the rider's speed. It was only when this physical hypothesis was disconfirmed by careful testing that he began to focus on the social psychological aspects of the situation. In an ingenious experiment, Triplett observed children as they reeled in a length of fishing wire as fast as possible; half of the children were randomly assigned to perform the task alone and half were assigned to perform the task in pairs. Triplett found that the children assigned to perform the task in pairs were faster than those who performed the task alone, and thus social facilitation – the first empirically tested theory in interpersonal psychology – was born.

In the ensuing years, both facilitory and inhibitory effects of the presence of others were observed, yet it was not until almost 70 years later that Zajonc (1965) integrated these disparate findings and postulated a common physiological mechanism. Zajonc's explanation of the effects of observation contained two postulates: (1) the mere presence of others, as spectators or co-actors, elevates nonspecific physiological arousal; and (2) this physiological arousal facilitates "dominant" responses, which enhance the performance of simple or well-learned tasks but inhibit the performance of difficult or novel tasks (Zajonc 1965, 1980b). The effect of conspecifics on arousal and performance was not limited to humans and was assumed to occur across species. Indeed, Latane and Cappell (1972) found that the mere presence of other rats caused an increase in physiological arousal as measured by heart rate, and Zajonc (1980b) reported facilitation and inhibition of the behavioral performance in cockroaches when they ran an easy or difficult maze either alone or "observed" by conspecifics.

The second postulate of social facilitation theory – that an increase in arousal results in the facilitation of dominant responses – has rarely been questioned (Graydon & Murphy 1995). However, the first postulate – that the mere presence of others is sufficient to induce these arousal differences – has been a topic of controversy (see Kent 1994 for review). The proposed psychological mediators of this effect have generally fallen into one of three frameworks: (i) anxiety induced by self-presentational concerns (Bond 1982; Bond & Titus 1983); (ii) distraction induced by the presence of others (Baron 1986); and (iii) an increase in energy expenditure and task engagement when performance is public rather than private (Musante & Anker 1972; Obrist 1981). Each of these three explanations has received varying levels of support moderated by the nature of the audience, the nature of the task, and the physiological indices of arousal employed. For example, electrodermal reactivity consistently increases under observed conditions, but heart rate and EMG have not been as consistently af-

fected (Bond & Titus 1983; Evans 1979; Geen & Gange 1977; Moore & Baron 1983). One reason for the inconsistencies was undoubtedly the aforementioned treatment of "arousal" as generalized nonspecific activation, thought to affect not only autonomic indices but skeletal musculature and electroencephalographic activity as well. This perspective of arousal as nondifferentiated, together with a focus upon single psychological mediators, led to a wide array of physiological measures of arousal across many different paradigms – and, not surprisingly, to contradictory findings (see Cacioppo et al. 1996a). A reconsideration of each of the underlying physiological systems and their response sensitivities was necessary to illuminate and organize the various findings supportive of the different models of social facilitation.

In Cacioppo and Petty's (1986) review of the mere-presence literature, two discrete psychological processing stages were proposed, each of which could be expressed through different physiological systems. First, the presence of others was hypothesized to cause psychological stress and an increased sensitivity to possible threats in the environment. Second, such appraisals were hypothesized to affect energy mobilization or effortful striving on the part of the individual. This two-stage analysis was based, in part, upon the pattern of physiological response in the social facilitation literature. The sensitivity of electrodermal but not heart rate or skeletomuscular responses to the potentially supportive or threatening aspects of the audience shares similarities with the pattern of response to potentially threatening stimuli (Fowles 1980). Thus, the effect of mere presence may be interpreted to first moderate the appraisals of the threatening aspects of failure and then, on that basis, to motivate increased effort on the task. This two-stage analysis has received more attention in the past decade, and it seems to organize much of the past literature.

Cacioppo and co-workers (1990) found mere presence insufficient to increase basal electrodermal arousal but sufficient to increase the physiological responses to an environmental change. These findings are thus consistent with the notion that the presence of others increases the likelihood of the perception of punitive consequences of environmental change. Of course, human associates may have stress-buffering as well as stress-inducing effects. Most studies have investigated the effects of the mere presence of strangers, in which it may be assumed that failure would be seen poorly. Indeed, the expectancies of positive or negative evaluation from an unknown audience interacts with social facilitation effects (Sanna & Shotland 1990). Further, research that has varied the relationship of an observer (friend versus stranger) has provided additional support for an initial appraisal stage that results in an increase in arousal for situations in which the presence of another is perceived as threatening but a decrease when the presence is perceived as supportive. Kissel (1965) found that electrodermal activity was higher for individuals who performed an anagram task in the presence of a stranger than a friend. Similarly, Snydersmith and Cacioppo (1992) and Edens, Larkin, and Abel (1992) demonstrated that cardiovascular reactivity increased during difficult laboratory tasks with observation by strangers as compared to friends. Finally, Allen and associates (1991) reported the stress-buffering effects of pets: participants showed lowered physiological reactivity during the performance of a stressful task when near their pets than they did in the presence of a human friend or when performing the task alone.

The second stage of effortful striving has also received support. Dienstbier (1989) proposed that brief periods of cardiovascular reactivity reflect energy mobilization to perceived challenges. Wright and colleagues (1995) demonstrated that social evaluation spurred cardiovascular reactivity if a behavioral challenge was unfixed and thus required enhanced effort to succeed, but not when the task was fixed and relatively easy to meet without enhanced effort. When participants perceived failure on the task to be unlikely, no increased output (as assessed by cardiovascular measures) was found. Note that cardiovascular reactivity had not been shown to vary as a function of factors increasing anxiety or threat appraisal in the first stage of social facilitation. As further support, Chapman (1973, 1974) reported that electromyographic indicators of task engagement increase as a function of the presence or absence of an audience and the nature of the task, but not as a function of anxiety.

It therefore appears that prior studies that depended upon electrodermal responses may have been sensitive only to the anxiety components of the presence of others, whereas studies using other autonomic and electromyographic indices may have been primarily sensitive to task engagement. Recall that, across studies, the moderation of performance by the presence or absence of others could (and did) reflect an enhancement or disruption of either stage. Additionally, the treatment of all physiological response systems as identical initially obfuscated the separability of the stages of social facilitation. Thus, a social-psychophysiological analysis – one that considers the psychological states aroused by the presence of others (e.g., socially induced anxiety and increased task engagement) as well as the discrete physiological response systems involved in the expression of those states – illuminates a controversial effect roughly a century after its first observation.

CLOSE RELATIONSHIPS AND SOCIAL NETWORKS

Studies investigating the effects of observation have, with few exceptions, investigated the impact of the presence of strangers. Of course, many of our daily social interactions are not with strangers but rather with close associates, friends, and family. Indeed, it is these interactions that are expected to have the greatest effects and so to carry the largest potential for reward or punishment. It is to these effects that we now turn.

Humans have been hypothesized to possess a fundamental "need to belong" (Baumeister & Leary 1995; Gardner, Pickett, & Brewer in press), and data from current national surveys certainly appear to provide supportive evidence of the beneficial effects of affiliation with others. When asked "What is necessary for happiness?", the majority of respondents rate relationships with family and friends as most important (Berscheid 1985). Likewise, in a large study conducted by the National Opinion Research Center (Burt 1986), participants who reported having contact with five or more intimate friends in the prior six months were 60% more likely (than those who did not report such contact) to report that their lives were "very happy." In fact, close social ties are important across the lifespan. Studies conducted with children (Newcomb & Bagwell 1995), young adults (Manning & Fullerton 1988; Perkins 1991), and the elderly (Gupta & Korte 1994) all demonstrate a significant link between high-quality social relationships and mental well-being.

The beneficial impact of satisfying close relationships is not limited to psychological well-being. House, Landis, and Umberson (1988) reviewed evidence that linked social isolation with high mortality rates; in fact, across six studies, isolation from others emerged as a risk factor that was every bit as powerful as smoking or hypertension. Meta-analyses conducted in the 1990s have further underscored the importance of social relationships to physical well-being. Reifman (1995) reported the beneficial effects of social relationships (particularly marital relationships) on recovery from myocardial infarction. Smith and coworkers (1994) and Uchino, Cacioppo, and Kiecolt-Glaser (1996) provided more general reviews linking social support – the perception of emotional, instrumental, or informational resources that are provided by an individual's social network – to a wide variety of health outcomes. These meta-analyses have revealed that the relationship between social isolation and physical well-being appears to generalize across age groups (Hansell 1985; Seeman et al. 1994; Uchino et al. 1995), gender (Bland et al. 1991; Kaufmann & Beehr 1986), and culture (Dressler 1983; Janes 1990). In short, individuals with a higher level of social support appear to suffer fewer physical symptoms of illness and to show increased recovery from cancer, lower cardiovascular reactivity, and heightened endocrine and immune function.

The effect of satisfactory close relationships on physical and mental well-being is therefore fairly clear. However, the social and physiological mechanisms underlying this effect are still being explored (see Uchino et al. 1996 for review). A predominant view in the literature is that perceptions of social support may "buffer" the individual from the harmful effects of psychological stress (Cohen & McKay 1984).

The experience of acute psychological stress in the laboratory has been shown to increase cardiovascular reactivity, which in turn has been shown to affect endocrine (e.g., plasma cortisol levels) and immune (e.g., natural killer cell activity) functioning (Kamarck et al. 1992; Manuck 1994; Sgoutas-Emch et al. 1994; Uchino et al. 1995). Perceptions of social support appear to moderate these stress-induced physiological changes. Tardy, Thompson, and Allen (1989), Boyce and Chesterman (1990), and Knox (1993) all demonstrated that individuals higher in perceived social support demonstrated lower levels of cardiovascular reactivity during the experience of psychological stress in the laboratory. Studies examining short-term naturalistic stressors provide additional evidence of the beneficial effect of perceived social support. For example, medical students undergoing exams show stress-induced decrements in immune functioning that are particularly pronounced for those students who report being lonely (Glaser et al. 1992; Kiecolt-Glaser et al. 1984).

Social support may be particularly important in times of chronic stress. Uchino, Kiecolt-Glaser, and Cacioppo (1992) examined stress-induced cardiovascular reactivity in spousal caregivers of patients with Alzheimer's disease. Caregivers low in social support showed age-related increases in heart rate reactivity in response to two acute laboratory stressors, whereas caregivers high in social support showed age-related decreases in heart rate reactivity. Immune measures taken from the same sample of caregivers showed that low social support was also associated with greater declines in immune function over the course of a year (Kiecolt-Glaser et al. 1991). Similarly, Baron and associates (1990) examined the immune responses of spouses of cancer patients and found that lower immune functioning was associated with lower perceptions of social support.

How do close relationships buffer stress? What functions do close others serve? Social support is a multidimensional construct that encompasses perceptions of both tangible and emotional resources (Cohen & McKay 1984), and the match between the type of stressor and type of support may be an important factor (Cutrona & Russell 1990). However, it generally appears that the emotional more so than the tangible support provided by others is key in buffering effects of the majority of stressors.

One dimension of emotional support is appraisal support: the perception that there are others with whom the individual can discuss problems (Cohen & McKay 1984). Results of a survey of 1,000 respondents conducted by Reis and Franks (1994) stressed the importance of appraisal support as well as feelings of intimacy with others in the prediction of physical and psychological well-being. Additionally, Uchino et al. (1995) found that appraisal support was an important moderator of age-related differences in cardiovascular functioning. The mediators of this effect are unclear. One possibility is that the mere knowledge that there are others with whom an individual can discuss a stressor serves to change appraisals of that stressor and thus cardiovascular response (Tomaka et al. 1997) and subsequent immune function. Another possibility is that this type of social support promotes health because of the actual effects of confiding in others (Pennebaker 1989).

Over the past decade, Pennebaker and colleagues have conducted an impressive series of studies illustrating the benefits of having someone with whom to discuss problems (see Pennebaker 1989 for a review). For example, Pennebaker and Beall (1986) randomly assigned individuals a "daily diary" task in which they were encouraged either to write about past emotional stressors or about more superficial events. Those individuals who had been provided an outlet for expressing problems were found to have suffered fewer illnesses requiring visits to a physician in the subsequent 14 months (see also Pennebaker & Francis 1996). Further, individuals who have been encouraged to disclose emotional traumas have shown healthier levels of immune function, including heightened immune response to mitogens (Pennebaker, Kiecolt-Glaser, & Glaser 1988), moderation of Epstein–Barr virus reactivation (Esterling et al. 1994), and better responses to a hepatitis vaccination (Petrie et al. 1995). Given that individuals who are high in appraisal support are more likely to be provided with a sympathetic ear in times of stress, these beneficial effects of disclosure may therefore provide an alternative mediator of the protective association between positive social relationships and health.

Nowhere is the impact of the quality of close relationships more greatly revealed than in the research examining the physiological effects of marriage. The spouse is often the central figure in an individual's support network, and indeed the quality of the marital relationship contributes more to overall life satisfaction for married individuals than does any other variable (Glenn & Weaver 1981). Not surprisingly, most married individuals characterize their spouse as the principal source of emotional comfort (Antonucci & Jackson 1987). The relationship between marital status and health serves to illustrate both the positive and negative aspects of such high levels of emotional interdependence. Such intimacy with a spouse is likely to make an individual more resilient to disease and more likely to recover after a health crisis (Case, Moss, & Case 1992; Williams, Barefoot, & Califf 1992), and the loss of this relationship – whether through divorce (Kiecolt-Glaser et al. 1988) or bereavement (Irwin et al. 1987) – compromises health for the individual who is newly alone.

Further, marriage is not always a "safe harbor" of social and emotional support and – because the marriage is most often the primary emotional relationship – unhappiness with a spouse can have particularly deleterious outcomes. Marital conflict has been shown to invoke cardiovascular (Gottman & Levenson 1992), endocrine (Kiecolt-Glaser et al. 1996) and immune (Glaser & Kiecolt-Glaser 1994;

Kiecolt-Glaser et al. 1993) responses that leave the individual more vulnerable to disease. This is particularly true for dissatisfied couples, who are likely to engage in higher levels of negative communication (Markman 1991) and negative reciprocity (Sher & Weiss 1991) than their more satisfied counterparts. Indeed, research in which couples are brought into the laboratory to discuss areas of conflict revealed that the subsequent endocrine and immune responses were more severe for those couples engaging in hostile behavior during the discussion (for a review see Kiecolt-Glaser et al. 1994).

Heightened physiological reactivity during conflict has even been examined as a barometer of marital quality. Levenson, Gottman, and colleagues have found that heightened cardiovascular reactivity during arguments is related to current marital dissatisfaction (Levenson & Gottman 1983) and is also a strong predictor of continued decreases in marital satisfaction over a three-year period (Levenson & Gottman 1985). These associations held even for couples who had been married for decades (Levenson, Carstenson, & Gottman 1994). Additionally, heightened cardiovascular reactivity during marital conflict has been shown to be an independent and significant predictor of future marital dissolution (Gottman & Levenson 1992).

The finding that physiological reactivity during the discussion of marital problems has predictive power above and beyond current reports of marital dissatisfaction may at first seem surprising. However, it is likely that heightened reactivity may serve as a marker for hostile attributional processes, which are known to precede declines in marital satisfaction and to predict marital dissolution (Fincham & Bradbury 1992; Fincham & O'Leary 1983). In fact, the particular pattern of physiological reactivity reported by Gottman and Levenson (1992) – namely, increased heart rate coupled with vasoconstriction – is strikingly similar to the cardiovascular concomitants of threat appraisal (Tomaka et al. 1997). Recall that an appraisal of threat is one in which the individual judges the situation to be beyond his or her personal capabilities or control. It is well known that individuals in distressed marriages often view a spouse's negative behaviors to arise from immutable dispositional deficiencies rather than changeable situational pressures (Kayser 1993). The biased attributional processes that have been shown to accompany marital dissatisfaction might thus be expected to be associated with physiological markers of threat.

In sum, close interpersonal relationships are "double-edged swords" for psychological and physical well-being. Those closest to us provide many resources: feelings of intimacy, tangible and emotional succor, and sympathetic outlets when we undergo problems. All of those resources may protect the individual in times of stress. However, these same social relationships may themselves be a source of stress or conflict, and the individual may become more vulnerable to psychological or physical disease when close emotional ties are lost or threatened. The physiological mechanisms underlying the association between interpersonal relationships and health have just begun to be systematically explored, but a perspective that takes both social and physiological factors into account is clearly necessary to understand both the benefit and harm conferred by our intimate ties with others.

SOCIAL IDENTITY AND INTERGROUP CONFLICT

In addition to the influence of close others, the social groups of which we are members contribute heavily to our perceptions, emotions, and interpersonal behavior. All individuals name important group memberships (e.g. ethnic, religious, or social groups) as self-defining at least some of the time (Brewer & Gardner 1996; Gardner, Gabriel, & Lee 1999). Likewise, the evaluation of a group's standing relative to other groups, as well as the evaluation of one's own suitability as a group member, play a large role in individual self-esteem (Luhtanen & Crocker 1992).

Such linkage of the group with the self represents the heart of social identity theory (Tajfel & Turner 1986). Both perception and behavior change radically on the basis of whether a social interaction is seen as interpersonal (the individuals involved are representing themselves) or intergroup (the individuals involved are representing their groups) in nature (Hoyle, Pinkley, & Insko 1989; Sherif 1966). Because individuals strive to maintain positive social identities, they are often biased in their perceptions of groups in which they share membership (in-groups) versus groups in which they do not share membership (out-groups). These biased perceptions lead to in-group favoritism and out-group derogation, prejudicial tendencies that (if left unchecked) can result in social and economic discrimination or even genocide. Indeed, much of the past four decades of research in intergroup relations was spurred by the atrocities of the Second World War – in the hope of defusing future intergroup conflict (see e.g. Baron & Byrne 1997).

The broad conceptualization of what constitutes a social group has given social psychologists the latitude to study a variety of different groups in their attempts to understand the basic processes and motivations that underlie intergroup conflict. A great deal of this work has focused on the function, structure, and pervasiveness of stereotypes of all kinds (Hamilton & Sherman 1994). At their most basic, stereotypes represent specific descriptive beliefs, positive or negative, that are attributed on the basis of membership in a particular group (Bodenhausen, Macrae, & Garst 1997). Stereotypes are posited to be activated automatically upon encounter with an out-group (Devine 1989) and, once activated, to affect the retrieval and processing of social information (see Hilton & von Hippel 1996 for a review).

Because it is often considered socially unacceptable to express negative stereotypes or prejudicial feelings toward an out-group member, valid assessment of intergroup attitudes has often been problematic. Traditionally, experimental social psychologists have studied intergroup prejudice using self-report data, such as questionnaires (e.g. Devine 1989; McConahay 1986). However, doubts have been raised about the validity of some of these measures (Fazio et al. 1995). At the core of this controversy is the lack of correspondence between the levels of prejudice that are verbally expressed versus actual behavior (Crosby, Bromly, & Saxe 1980; Weitz 1972). Crosby et al.'s (1980) review of the relationship between self-reported racial attitudes and actual behavior of Caucasians toward African-American targets found a striking disparity; similar disparities have been found in studies of attitudes toward the disabled (see Archer 1985 for a review).

The lack of correspondence between stated prejudice and actual behavior can be explained several ways. A simple explanation is that individuals are simply dishonest on self-report measures (McConahay 1986). Alternatively, people may not be consciously aware of their prejudices (Gaertner & Dovidio 1986). Regardless of the underlying reasons, the disparity between expressed prejudice and prejudicial behavior has caused quite a bit of consternation for those researchers wishing to study prejudice. Researchers hoped that, as with other attitudes, physiological measures would prove useful in revealing prejudicial attitudes that individuals were unwilling or unable to report.

The goal of nonverbal measurement of prejudice spurred the earliest work in intergroup processes and physiology. Rankin and Campbell (1955) examined the effects of incidental contact by African-American and Caucasian experimenters on electrodermal responses. Forty Caucasian male students participated in what they thought was a word association test; during the course of the experiment two male experimenters, one African-American and one Caucasian, made adjustments to the dummy apparatus attached to the participant's left hand while the apparatus attached to the right hand remained operational. Participants showed increased electrodermal responding when in contact with the African-American experimenter as compared to the Caucasian experimenter. Rankin and Campbell (1955) interpreted these electrodermal differences as reflections of racial prejudice. This interpretation was supported by a replication attempt of Porier and Lott (1967), who found that electrodermal responses to an African-American experimenter in this paradigm were indeed correlated with the California "e scale," a measure of prejudice.

Given the aforementioned difficulties in using electrodermal responses as an indicator of attitudes, researchers have turned to alternative physiological means, such as facial EMG (Vanman et al. 1990; Vanman, Kaplan, & Miller 1991) and ERPs (Osterhout, Bersick, & McLaughlin 1997), to assess stereotypes and prejudice. For example, Van-

man et al. (1990) asked Caucasian participants to imagine working in a number of situations with either another Caucasian or with an African-American. Meanwhile, facial EMGs were recorded on their cheeks, brows, and lips. This EMG activity varied as a function of race of the target (increased corrugator and decreased zygomaticus with African-American targets). Although self-reports of feelings about the interaction did not correlate with EMG activity, it is plausible that participants were disguising their true feelings about a cross-race interaction. A second experiment seems to support this hypothesis: Vanman et al. (1991) replicated the EMG findings with in-groups and out-groups in which there were fewer social desirability concerns for the expression of dislike. In this study, students who were not involved in the Greek (fraternity/sorority) system were exposed to slides and bogus information about in-groups (non-Greeks and other students from the same university) and out-groups (Greeks in addition to students from a rival university). In this case, EMG activity varied in the predicted fashion as a function of group membership of target (increased corrugator and decreased zygomaticus for out-group targets as compared to in-group targets), and self-reports of liking for the targets did correlate with EMG activity.

Taken together, the results from these two experiments are intriguing. The first experiment used racial groups concerning which there is a strong social norm that makes expressing prejudicial feelings unacceptable. The second used Greek and university affiliations, memberships that may have strong meaning for the individuals involved in them but with fewer societal ramifications and demands of social desirability. The two experiments reported similar EMG activity for out-group targets and in-group targets; only the self-reports of prejudicial feelings differed. These results suggest that a subject may be unwilling rather than unable to report negative feelings evoked by an out-group, and they aptly illustrate the use of facial EMG to tap feelings of intergroup prejudice – whether or not verbally reported.

Although racial stereotypes are often accompanied by negative prejudicial feelings, gender stereotypes are thought to be rooted in beliefs concerning appropriate roles for men and women (Eagly & Steffen 1984). Because of the lack of generalized affective negativity directed toward women, ERPs rather than facial EMGs have been used to tap these stereotypes. Osterhout et al. (1997) used the N400 component of the ERP to examine expectancy violations that had been generated by placing women in high-status occupations. The N400 has been shown to be a sensitive marker of semantic expectancy (see Chapter 21). Thus, it was predicted that a female name paired with a high-status occupation would evoke larger N400s than a male name placed with the same occupation. In fact, the N400 evoked by the violation of such semantic expectancies as the target sentence "Sally is a waiter" (as compared to "waitress") was only slightly larger than those sentences that violated societal expectancies, such as "Sally is a surgeon" (as compared to "nurse"). This ingenious study thus provides evidence that physiological measures may be used to reveal even those stereotypes that do not have a strongly affective basis.

Measurement issues aside, physiological paradigms have also been applied to the examination of the motivational and cognitive processes underlying intergroup discrimination and conflict. Van Egeren (1979) reported increased cardiovascular arousal any time an individual was placed in a competition or conflict situation. Given the increases in competitive threat perceived when two groups (not simply two individuals) are in conflict (Hoyle et al. 1989; Rehm, Steinleitner, & Lilli 1987), the arousal induced by intergroup conflict should be even greater than that of individual competition. Indeed, Branscombe and Wann (1992) hypothesized that merely observing a competition between two individuals (e.g., a boxing match between an American and a Russian) would lead to increased cardiovascular activity for those who were highly nationally identified and thus for whom the match represented a threat to a valued social identity. This hypothesis was supported; those participants for whom national identity was important exhibited increased diastolic and systolic blood pressure in response to the boxing match. Further, the highly identified participants were more likely to derogate the out-group (Russians), and the level of arousal evoked by the match was correlated with the amount of out-group derogation.

Although Branscombe and Wann (1992) found that physiological arousal correlated with out-group derogation, it is unclear whether arousal contributed to the increased negativity expressed toward the out-group or merely coincided with it. However, a separate body of literature has emerged that examines the causal power of arousal in evoking stereotyping and prejudice. This research focuses primarily on physiological arousal as a determinant of cognitive capacity, for one prevailing conceptualization of the function of stereotypes is that they serve as judgmental heuristics that can be used to simplify social perception (see e.g. Bodenhausen & Wyer 1985). If this is the case, then any variable that moderates cognitive capacity would be likely to modify the reliance on stereotypes and the resultant prejudicial perceptions as well. Because the relationship between physiological arousal and cognitive capacity is hypothesized to be quadratic (perhaps best described as an inverted U in which cognitive capacity is decreased at both extremely low and extremely high levels of arousal), investigations of the effects of arousal levels on stereotyping have taken place at both extremes.

Bodenhausen (1990) relied upon individuals' own peaks and valleys in circadian arousal to examine the impact of arousal on stereotyping. In two studies, participants classified as either "morning" or "night" people were assigned to participate in an experiment at either their most or least optimal time. The first experiment examined the effects of arousal on the likelihood to commit the "conjunction fallacy" (Tversky & Kahneman 1988), the erroneous belief that the probability of two events both being true is greater than the probability of either event being true. The conjunction fallacy is a common error when individuals are asked to estimate the probabilities of a stereotyped element existing in conjunction with a neutral element as opposed to a neutral element existing alone (Gilovich 1991). For example, people are more likely to believe that a woman described in terms representative of the stereotypical librarian (e.g., quiet, likes to read, wears glasses) is "a librarian who plays jazz as a hobby" than simply "someone who plays jazz for a hobby." As expected, Bodenhausen (1990) found that participants operating at nonoptimal, low-arousal times of day were more likely to commit the conjunction fallacy than participants operating at optimal times. A second experiment illustrated the relationship between nonoptimally low arousal and discrimination: participants tested at nonoptimal times were more likely to utilize their racial stereotypes in evaluating the guilt or innocence of a minority target accused of a crime. The results of both studies were interpreted as evidence of the influence of cognitive capacity limitations on the use of stereotypes.

Of course, cognitive capacity can also be decreased by a level of arousal that is too high. Several studies have examined the effects of exercise-induced physiological arousal upon intergroup perceptions and behavior. Consistent with the cognitive capacity model, high levels of arousal have been found to decrease perceived complexity and increase stereotypes of out-groups for people highly identified with their group (Wann & Branscombe 1995). Additionally, Kim and Baron (1988) found that high levels of arousal (as measured by changes in heart rate and blood pressure after exercise) increased the occurrence of the illusory correlation, another common bias that contributes to the formation and maintenance of negative stereotypes concerning out-group members (see Hamilton & Rose 1980).

Finally, several studies have investigated emotion as a moderator of arousal and subsequent intergroup judgments (see Mackie & Hamilton 1993 for review) and have found the arousal properties of an emotion to be an important determinant of its consequences on judgments of out-group members. Individuals show more evidence of stereotype persistence when they have been highly aroused through the experimental induction of emotions such as anxiety or anger (Bodenhausen, Sheppard, & Kramer 1994; Stroessner & Mackie 1992; Wilder & Shapiro 1989), again thought to result from a reduction in cognitive capacity. Given that anger and anxiety constitute the two most common emotional responses to initial intergroup contact (Jackson & Sullivan 1989; Vanman & Miller 1993), it is perhaps no surprise that stereotypes about out-groups persist even after contact with nonstereotypic out-group members.

Taken as a whole, examination of intergroup relations with physiological procedures reveals a vicious cycle among out-group biases, physiological arousal, and the persistence of prejudicial beliefs. First, whenever a social identity is threatened, intergroup contact results in increased negative affect coupled with high physiological arousal. Second, high physiological arousal is sufficient to decrease cognitive capacity and thus compromises social perception and judgment through increasing stereotype usage. Finally, increased stereotypically driven thinking maintains or even strengthens the original prejudice felt toward the out-group as well as the superiority of the individual's own social identity.

The area of physiology and intergroup conflict is relatively young, yet it appears to have great potential for growth. The feasibility of physiological measures of prejudice, an area fraught with previous difficulty in measurement, is certainly promising. Moreover, it is hoped that a physiological perspective may help clarify the processes underlying intergroup conflict by providing new methodologies as well as new ideas with which to explore the interplay between affect, cognition, and intergroup relations.

Concluding Thoughts

The psychophysiological perspective appears to be finally coming of age in the study of interpersonal processes. The field of social psychophysiology – which could be characterized (until the past two decades) as consisting primarily of the search for nonverbal measures of psychological processes – has, in the 1980s and 1990s, seen an explosion of new research in which psychophysiological procedures are used to delineate the processes underlying basic social behavior. Throughout this chapter, we have tried to illustrate both the historical and theoretical progress of psychophysiology within given areas.

We have reviewed literature concerning the intrapersonal psychological processes upon which social perceptions are based and also the interpersonal processes that become invoked by interactions with others. In many ways this is a false dichotomy, for intrapersonal and interpersonal processes coexist in a state of dynamic co-dependence. For example, individually held attitudes toward social groups foster biased perceptions and interactions during instances of intergroup contact. Likewise, the intrapersonal appraisal processes of each spouse in a marital interaction determine, in large part, the interpersonal behaviors exhibited during conflict. In each case, knowledge about the attendant physiological responses has added much to the understanding of these fundamentally important interpersonal interactions.

In sum, this chapter has attempted to illustrate how psychophysiological perspectives and paradigms have increased our understanding of interpersonal processes at all levels of analysis. The past few decades have seen a burgeoning number of researchers pursuing basic questions in the field with increasingly sophisticated social psychophysiological paradigms. The field of interpersonal psychology appears at last to be bringing Erasistratos' centuries-old insight to fruition: when interested in interpersonal relations, sometimes listening to the body will best communicate the mind.

NOTES

1. This chapter does not seek to provide an exhaustive review of the literature; the areas reviewed illustrate only some of the ways in which psychophysiological theory and methods have been incorporated into the study of interpersonal processes. The absence of many areas – such as interpersonal attraction, aggression, prosocial behavior, and intragroup dynamics – should not be taken as an indication that psychophysiological perspectives have been ignored in these areas.

2. Not all reflexes are useful indices of affective state. For example, some reflexes, such as the spinal tendinous reflex, have been related to arousal but not emotional valence of a stimulus and thus lack directionality as a measure of attitude (Bonnet et al. 1995).

3. Two pieces of evidence suggest that the right laterality reported here is a different phenomenon than the hemispheric asymmetries in response to affective state reported by Davidson and colleagues (e.g. Davidson 1995). First, the right lateralization was not moderated by the valence of the stimuli but rather was found equally for both positive and negative attitude objects. Second, largest foci of activity were in the centroparietal rather than frontal regions. Thus, the right lateralization in response to attitudinal processing in general most likely reflects a different (but possibly related) psychophysiological process.

4. Because the accessibility of attitudes can be temporarily manipulated through attitude rehearsal (Fazio et al. 1982), it was possible to test the stress reduction hypothesis of attitudes without having to rely on pre-existing idiosyncratic attitudes, which may have raised concerns of likely confounds with attitude extremity or importance.

REFERENCES

Allen, K. M., Blascovich, J., Tomaka, J., & Kelsey, R. M. (1991). Presence of human friends and pet dogs as moderators of autonomic responses to stress in women. *Journal of Personality and Social Psychology*, 61, 582–9.

Allport, F. H. (1924). *Social Psychology*. Boston: Houghton-Mifflin.

Antoni, M. H., & Goodkin, K. (1988). Host moderator variables in the promotion of cervical neoplasia: I. Personality facets. *Journal of Psychosomatic Research*, 32, 327–38.

Antonucci, T. C., & Jackson, J. S. (1987). Social support, interpersonal efficacy, and health: A life course perspective. In L. L. Carstensen & B. A. Edelstein (Eds.), *Handbook of Clinical Gerontology*, pp. 291–311. New York: Pergamon.

Archer, D. (1985). Social deviance. In G. Lindzey & E. Aronson (Eds.), *Handbook of Social Psychology*, 3rd ed., vol. 2, pp. 743–804. New York: Random House.

Arnold, M. B. (1960). *Emotion and Personality*. New York: Columbia University Press.

Ashton, N. L., & Severy, L. J. (1976). Arousal and costs in bystander intervention. *Personality and Social Psychology Bulletin, 2*, 268–72.

Baldwin, M. W., & Holmes, J. G. (1987). Salient private audiences and awareness of the self. *Journal of Personality and Social Psychology, 52*, 1087–98.

Barlow, J. D. (1969). Pupillary size as an index of preference in political candidates. *Perceptual and Motor Skills, 28*, 587–90.

Baron, R. A., & Byrne, D. (1997). *Social Psychology*. Needham Heights, MA: Allyn & Bacon.

Baron, R. S. (1986). Distraction-conflict theory: Progress and problems. In L. Berkowitz (Ed.), *Advances in Experimental Social Psychology*. Orlando, FL: Academic Press.

Baron, R. W., Cutrona, C. E., Hicklin, D., Russell, D. W., & Lubaroff, D. M. (1990). Social support and immune function among spouses of cancer patients. *Journal of Personality and Social Psychology, 59*, 344–52.

Baumeister, R. F., & Leary, M. R. (1995). The need to belong: Desire for interpersonal attachment as a fundamental human motivation. *Psychological Bulletin, 117*, 497–529.

Berntson, G. G., Boysen, S. T., & Cacioppo, J. T. (1992). Neurobehavioral organization and the cardinal principle of evaluative bivalence. In F. M. Crinella & J. Yu (Eds.), *Brain Mechanisms: Papers in Memory of Robert Thompson*, pp. 75–102. New York: Annals of the New York Academy of Sciences.

Berscheid, E. (1985). Interpersonal attraction. In G. Lindzey & E. Aronson (Eds.), *The Handbook of Social Psychology*. New York: Random House.

Berscheid, E., & Walster, G. W. (1978). *Interpersonal Attraction*, 2nd ed. Reading, MA: Addison-Wesley.

Bland, S. H., Krigh, V., Winkelstein, W., & Trevisan, M. (1991). Social network and blood pressure: A population study. *Psychosomatic Medicine, 53*, 598–607.

Blascovich, J. (in press). Using physiological indexes of psychological processes in social psychological research. In C. M. Judd & H. Reis (Eds.), *Handbook of Advanced Research Methods in Social Psychology*. London: Cambridge University Press.

Blascovich, J., Ernst, J. M., Tomaka, J., Kelsey, R. M., Salomon, K. A., & Fazio, R. H. (1993). Attitude as a moderator of autonomic reactivity. *Journal of Personality and Social Psychology, 64*, 165–76.

Blascovich, J., & Tomaka, J. (1996). The biopsychosocial model of arousal regulation. In M. Zanna (Ed.), *Advances in Experimental Social Psychology*, vol. 28, pp. 1–51. New York: Academic Press.

Blonder, L. X., Bowers, D., & Heilman, K. M. (1991). The role of the right hemisphere in emotional communication. *Brain, 114*, 1115–27.

Bodenhausen, G. V. (1990). Stereotypes as judgmental heuristics: Evidence of circadian variations in discrimination. *Psychological Science, 1*, 319–22.

Bodenhausen, G. V., Macrae, C. N., & Garst J. (1997). Stereotypes in thought and deed: Social-cognitive origins of intergroup discrimination. In C. Sedikides, J. Schopler, & C. A.

Insko (Eds.), *Intergroup Cognition and Intergroup Behavior*. Mahwah, NJ: Erlbaum.

Bodenhausen, G. V., Sheppard, L. A., & Kramer, G. P. (1994). Negative affect and social judgment: The differential impact of anger and sadness. *European Journal of Social Psychology, 24*, 45–62.

Bodenhausen, G. V., & Wyer, R. S., Jr. (1985). Effects of stereotypes on decision making and information processing strategies. *Journal of Personality and Social Psychology, 48*, 262–82.

Bond, C. F. (1982). Social facilitation: A self-presentational view. *Journal of Personality and Social Psychology, 42*, 1042–50.

Bond, C. F., & Titus, L. J. (1983). Social facilitation: A meta-analysis of 241 studies. *Psychological Bulletin, 94*, 265–92.

Bonnet, M., Bradley, M. M., Lang, P. J., & Requin, J. (1995). Modulation of spinal reflexes: Arousal, pleasure, action. *Psychophysiology, 32*, 367–72.

Borod, J. C. (1993). Cerebral mechanisms underlying facial, prosodic, and lexical emotional expression: A review of neuropsychological studies and methodological issues. Special Section: Neuropsychological perspectives on components of emotional processing. *Neuropsychology, 7*, 445–63.

Boyce, T. W., & Chesterman, E. (1990). Life events, social support, and cardiovascular reactivity in adolescence. *Developmental and Behavioral Pediatrics, 11*, 105–11.

Bradley, M. M., Cuthbert, B. N., & Lang, P. J. (1990). Startle reflex modification: Attention or emotion? *Psychophysiology, 27*, 513–22.

Branscombe, N. L., & Wann, D. L. (1992). Physiological arousal and reactions to outgroup members during competitions that implicate an important social identity. *Aggressive Behavior, 18*, 85–93.

Breckler, S. J. (1984). Empirical validation of affect, behavior and cognition as distinct components of attitude. *Journal of Personality and Social Psychology, 47*, 1191–1205.

Brewer, M. B., & Gardner, W. L. (1996). Who is this "we"? Levels of collective identity and self representations. *Journal of Personality and Social Psychology, 71*, 83–93.

Burt, R. S. (1986). Strangers, friends, and happiness. GSS Technical report no. 72, National Opinion Research Center, University of Chicago.

Cacioppo, J. T. (1982). Social psychophysiology: A classic perspective and contemporary approach. *Psychophysiology, 19*, 241–51.

Cacioppo, J. T., Berntson, G. G., & Crites, S. L. (1996a). Social neuroscience: Principles of psychophysiological arousal and response. In E. T. Higgins & A. W. Kruglanski (Eds.), *Social Psychology: Handbook of Basic Principles*. New York: Guilford.

Cacioppo, J. T., Bush, L. K., & Tassinary, L. G. (1992). Microexpressive facial actions as a function of affective stimuli: Replication and extension. *Personality and Social Psychology Bulletin, 18*, 515–26.

Cacioppo, J. T., Crites, S. L., Berntson, G. G., & Coles, M. G. H. (1993). If attitudes affect how stimuli are processed, should they not affect the event-related brain potential? *Psychological Science, 4*, 108–12.

Cacioppo, J. T., Crites, S. L., Jr., & Gardner, W. L. (1996b). Attitudes to the right: Evaluative processing is associated with lateralized late positive event-related brain potentials. *Personality and Social Psychology Bulletin, 22*, 1205–19.

Cacioppo, J. T., Crites, S. L., Gardner, W. L., & Berntson, G. G. (1994). Bioelectrical echoes from evaluative categorization: I. A late positive brain potential that varies as a function of trait negativity and extremity. *Journal of Personality and Social Psychology, 67,* 115–25.

Cacioppo, J. T., Martzke, J. S., Petty, R. E., & Tassinary, L. G. (1988). Specific forms of facial EMG response index emotions during an interview: From Darwin to the continuous flow hypothesis of affect-laden information processing. *Journal of Personality and Social Psychology, 54,* 592–609.

Cacioppo, J. T., & Petty, R. E. (1979). Attitudes and cognitive response: An electrophysiological approach. *Journal of Personality and Social Psychology, 37,* 2181–99.

Cacioppo, J. T., & Petty, R. E. (1981). Electromyograms as measures of extent and affectivity of information processing. *American Psychologist, 36,* 441–56.

Cacioppo, J. T., & Petty, R. E. (Eds.) (1983). *Social Psychophysiology: A Sourcebook.* New York: Guilford.

Cacioppo, J. T., & Petty, R. E. (1986). Social processes. In G. H. Coles, E. Donchin, & S. Porges (Eds.), *Psychophysiology: Systems, Processes, and Applications,* pp. 646–82. New York: Guilford.

Cacioppo, J. T., Petty, R. E., & Geen, T. R. (1989a). Attitude structure and function: From the tripartite to the homeostasis model of attitudes. In A. Pratkanis, S. Breckler, & A. Greenwald (Eds.), *Attitude Structure and Function,* pp. 275–309. Hillsdale, NJ: Erlbaum.

Cacioppo, J. T., Petty, R. E., Losch, M. E., & Kim, H. (1986). Electromyographic activity over facial muscle regions can differentiate the valence and intensity of affective reactions. *Journal of Personality and Social Psychology, 50,* 260–8.

Cacioppo, J. T., Petty, R. E., & Quintanar, L. R. (1982). Individual differences in relative hemispheric alpha abundance and cognitive responses to persuasive communications. *Journal of Personality and Social Psychology, 43,* 623–36.

Cacioppo, J. T., Petty, R. E., & Tassinary, L. G. (1989b). Social psychophysiology: A new look. *Advances of Experimental Social Psychology, 22,* 39–91.

Cacioppo, J. T., Rourke, P. A., Marshall-Goodell, B. S., Tassinary, L. G., & Baron, R. S. (1990). Rudimentary physiological effects of mere observation. *Psychophysiology, 27,* 177–86.

Cacioppo, J. T., & Sandman, C. A. (1981). Psychophysiological functioning, cognitive responding, and attitudes. In R. Petty, T. Ostrom, & T. Brock (Eds.), *Cognitive Responses in Persuasion,* pp. 81–103. Hillsdale, NJ: Erlbaum.

Cacioppo, J. T., & Tassinary, L. G. (1990). Inferring psychological significance from physiological signals. *American Psychologist, 45,* 16–28.

Cacioppo, J. T., Tassinary, L. G., Stonebraker, T. B., & Petty, R. E. (1987). Self-report and cardiovascular measures of arousal: Fractionation during residual arousal. *Biological Psychology, 25,* 135–51.

Case, R. B., Moss, A. J., & Case, N. (1992). Living alone after myocardial infarction. *Journal of the American Medical Association, 267,* 515–19.

Chapman, A. J. (1973). An electromyographic study of apprehension about evaluation. *Psychological Reports, 33,* 811–14.

Chapman, A. J. (1974). An electromyographic study of social facilitation: A test of the "mere presence" hypothesis. *British Journal of Psychology, 65,* 123–8.

Chen, M., & Bargh, J. A. (1999). Consequences of automatic evaluation: Immediate behavioral predispositions to approach or avoid the stimulus. *Personality and Social Psychology Bulletin, 25,* 215–24.

Christy, P. R., Gelfand, D. M., & Hartmann, D. P. (1971). Effects of competition-induced frustration on two classes of modeled behavior. *Developmental Psychology, 5,* 104–11.

Cohen, S., & McKay, G. (1984). Social support, stress, and the buffering hypothesis: A theoretical analysis. In A. Baum, S. E. Taylor, & J. E. Singer (Eds.), *Handbook of Psychology and Health,* pp. 253–67. Hillsdale, NJ: Erlbaum.

Cooper, J. B., & Siegel, H. E. (1956). The galvanic skin response as a measure of emotion in prejudice. *Journal of Psychology, 42,* 149–55.

Cottrell, N. B., & Wack, D. L. (1967). Energizing effects of cognitive dissonance upon dominant and subordinate responses. *Journal of Personality and Social Psychology, 6,* 132–8.

Crites, S. L., & Cacioppo, J. T. (1996). Electrocortical differentiation of evaluative and non-evaluative categorizations. *Psychological Science, 7,* 318–21.

Crites, S. L., Cacioppo, J. T., Gardner, W. L., & Berntson, G. G. (1995). Bioelectrical echoes from evaluative categorization: II. A late positive brain potential that varies as a function of attitude registration rather than attitude report. *Journal of Personality and Social Psychology, 68,* 997–1013.

Crosby, F., Bromly, S., & Saxe, L. (1980). Recent unobtrusive studies of black and white discrimination and prejudice: A literature review. *Psychological Bulletin, 87,* 546–63.

Croyle, R., & Cooper, J. (1983). Dissonance arousal: Physiological evidence. *Journal of Personality and Social Psychology, 45,* 782–91.

Cutrona, C. E., & Russell, D. W. (1990). Type of support and specific stress: Toward a theory of optimal matching. In B. R. Sarason, I. G. Sarason, & G. R. Pierce (Eds.), *Social Support: An Interactional View,* pp. 319–66. New York: Wiley.

Davidson, R. J. (1995). Cerebral asymmetry, emotion, and affective style. In R. J. Davidson & K. Hugdahl (Eds.), *Brain Asymmetry,* pp. 361–87. Cambridge, MA: MIT Press.

Devine, P. G. (1989). Stereotypes and prejudice: Their automatic and controlled components. *Journal of Personality and Social Psychology, 56,* 5–18.

Dienstbier, R. A. (1989). Arousal and physiological toughness: Implications for mental and physical health. *Psychological Review, 96,* 84–100.

Donchin, E. (1981). Surprise! ... surprise? *Psychophysiology, 8,* 493–513.

Dressler, W. (1983). Blood pressure, relative weight, and psychosocial resources. *Psychosomatic Medicine, 53,* 608–20.

Dutton, D. G., & Aron, A. P. (1974). Some evidence for heightened sexual attraction under conditions of high anxiety. *Journal of Personality and Social Psychology, 30,* 510–17.

Dweck, C. S. (1996). Implicit theories as organizers of goals and behavior. In P. M. Gollwitzer & J. A. Bargh (Eds.), *The Psychology of Action: Linking Cognition and Motivation to Behavior,* pp. 69–90. New York: Guilford.

Eagly, A. H., & Chaiken, S. (1993). *The Psychology of Attitudes.* San Diego: Harcourt Brace Jovanovich.

Eagly, A. H., & Steffen, V. J. (1984). Gender stereotypes stem from the distribution of women and men into social roles. *Journal of Personality and Social Psychology, 46,* 735–54.

Edens, J. L., Larkin, K. T., & Abel, J. L. (1992). The effects of social support and physical touch on cardiovascular reactions to mental stress. *Journal of Psychosomatic Research, 36*, 371–82.

Esterling, B. A., Antoni, M. H., Fletcher, M. A., Margulies, S., & Schneiderman, N. (1994). Emotional disclosure through writing or speaking modulates latent Epstein–Barr virus reactivation. *Journal of Consulting and Clinical Psychology, 62*, 130–40.

Evans, G. W. (1979). Behavioral and physiological consequences of crowding in humans. *Journal of Applied Social Psychology, 9*, 27–46.

Fazio, R. H. (1989). On the power and functionality of attitudes: The role of attitude accessibility. In A. R. Pratkanis & S. J. Breckler (Eds.), *Attitude Structure and Function*, pp. 153–79. Hillsdale, NJ: Erlbaum.

Fazio, R. H., Blascovich, J., & Driscoll, D. M. (1992). On the functional value of attitudes: The influence of accessible attitudes upon the ease and quality of decision making. *Personality and Social Psychology Bulletin, 18*, 388–401.

Fazio, R. H., Chen, J., McDonel, E. C., & Sherman, S. J. (1982). Attitude accessibility, attitude-behavior consistency, and the strength of the object-evaluation association. *Journal of Experimental Social Psychology, 18*, 339–57.

Fazio, R. H., Jackson, J. R., Dunton, B. C., & Williams, C. J. (1995). Variability in automatic activation as an unobtrusive measure of racial attitudes: A bona fide pipeline? *Journal of Personality and Social Psychology, 69*, 1013–27.

Festinger, L. (1957). *A Theory of Cognitive Dissonance.* Evanston, IL: Row, Peterson.

Fincham, F. D., & Bradbury, T. N. (1992). Assessing attributions in marriage: The Relationship Attribution Measure. *Journal of Personality and Social Psychology, 62*, 457–68.

Fincham, F. D., & O'Leary, K. D. (1983). Causal inferences for spouse behavior in maritally distressed and nondistressed couples. *Journal of Social and Clinical Psychology, 1*, 42–57.

Fowles, D. C. (1980). The three arousal model: Implications of Gray's two factor learning theory for heart rate, electrodermal activity, and psychopathy. *Psychophysiology, 17*, 87–104.

Gaertner, S. L., & Dovidio, J. F. (1986). The aversive form of racism. In J. F. Dovidio & S. L. Gaertner (Eds.), *Prejudice, Discrimination, and Racism*, pp. 61–89. San Diego: Academic Press.

Gardner, W. L., & Cacioppo, J. T. (in press). A brain based index of evaluative processing: A late positive brain potential reflects individual differences in the extremity of a negative evaluation. *Social Cognition.*

Gardner, W. L., Cacioppo, J. T., & Berntson, G. G. (1996). Right lateralized P300s in response to emotional stimuli. *Psychophysiology, 33*, S55.

Gardner, W. L., Gabriel, S., & Lee, A. Y. (1999). "I" value freedom, but "we" value relationships: Self-construal priming mirrors cultural differences in judgment. *Psychological Science, 10*, 321–6.

Gardner, W. L., Pickett, C. A., & Brewer, M. B. (in press). Social exclusion and selective memory: How the need to belong biases processing of social information. *Personality and Social Psychology Bulletin.*

Geen, R. G., & Gange, J. J. (1977). Drive theory of social facilitation: Twelve years of theory and research. *Psychological Bulletin, 84*, 1267–88.

Geen, R. G., Rakosky, J. J., & Pigg, R. (1972). Awareness of arousal and its relation to aggression. *British Journal of Social and Clinical Psychology, 11*, 115–21.

Gilovich, T. (1991). *How We Know What Isn't So: The Fallibility of Human Reason in Everyday Life.* New York: Free Press.

Glaser, R., & Kiecolt-Glaser, J. K. (1994). Stress-associated immune modulation and its implications for reactivation of latent herpes viruses. In R. Glaser & J. Jones (Eds.), *Human Herpes Virus Infections*, pp. 245–70. New York: Dekker.

Glaser, R., Kiecolt-Glaser, J. K., Bonneau, R., Malarkey, W., & Hughes, J. (1992). Stress-induced modulation of the immune response to recombinant hepatitis B vaccine. *Psychosomatic Medicine, 54*, 22–9.

Glenn, N. D., & Weaver, C. N. (1981). The contribution of marital happiness to global happiness. *Journal of Marriage and Family, 43*, 161–8.

Gottman, J. M., & Levenson, R. W. (1992). Marital processes predictive of later dissolution: Behavior, physiology, and health. *Journal of Personality and Social Psychology, 63*, 221–33.

Graydon, J., & Murphy, T. (1995). The effect of personality on social facilitation whilst performing a sports related task. *Personality and Individual Differences, 19*, 265–7.

Gupta, V., & Korte, C. (1994). The effects of a confidant and a peer group on the well-being of single elders. *International Journal of Aging and Human Development, 39*, 293–302.

Guttman, L. A. (1944). A basis for scaling qualitative data. *American Sociological Review, 9*, 139–50.

Hamilton, D. L., & Rose, T. L. (1980). Illusory correlation and the maintenance of stereotypic beliefs. *Journal of Personality and Social Psychology, 39*, 832–45.

Hamilton, D. L., & Sherman, J. W. (1994). Stereotypes. In R. S. Wyer, Jr. & T. K. Srull (Eds.), *Handbook of Social Cognition*, vol. 2, pp. 1–68. Hillsdale, NJ: Erlbaum.

Hamm, A. O., Greenwald, M. K., Bradley, M. M., & Lang, P. J. (1993). Emotional learning, hedonic change, and the startle probe. *Journal of Abnormal Psychology, 102*, 453–65.

Hansell, S. (1985). Adolescent networks and distress at school. *Social Forces, 63*, 698–715.

Heller, W. (1993). Neuropsychological mechanisms of individual differences in emotion, personality, and arousal. Special Section: Neuropsychological perspectives on components of emotional processing. *Neuropsychology, 7*, 476–89.

Hess, E. H. (1965). Attitude and pupil size. *Scientific American, 212*, 46–54.

Hess, E. H., & Polt, J. M. (1960). Pupil size as related to the interest value of visual stimuli. *Science, 132*, 349–50.

Hilton, J. L., & von Hippel, W. (1996). Stereotypes. *Annual Review of Psychology, 47*, 237–71.

House, J. S., Landis, K. R., & Umberson, D. (1988). Social relationships and health. *Science, 241*, 540–5.

Hoyle, R. H., Pinkley, R. L., & Insko, C. A. (1989). Perceptions of social behavior: Evidence for different expectations for interpersonal and intergroup interaction. *Personality and Social Psychology Bulletin, 15*, 365–76.

Hu, S., & Romans-Kroll, J. (1995). Effects of positive attitude toward giving a speech on cardiovascular and subjective fear responses during speech in anxious subjects. *Perceptual and Motor Skills, 81,* 609–10.

Irwin, M., Daniels, M., Smith, T. L., Bloom, E., & Weiner, H. (1987). Impaired natural killer cell activity during bereavement. *Brain, Behavior, and Immunity, 1,* 98–104.

Jackson, L. A., & Sullivan, L. A. (1989). Cognition and affect in evalutions of stereotypes by group members. *Journal of Social Psychology, 129,* 659–72.

Janes, C. R. (1990). Migration, changing gender roles, and stress: The Samoan case. *Medical Anthropology, 12,* 217–48.

Johnson, R. (1993). On the neural generators of the P300 component of the event-related potential. *Psychophysiology, 30,* 90–7.

Jones, E. E., & Sigall, H. (1971). The bogus pipeline: A new paradigm for measuring affect and attitude. *Psychological Bulletin, 76,* 349–64.

Kamarck, T. W., Jennings, R. J., Debski, T. T., Glickman-Weiss, E., Johnson, P. S., Eddy, M. J., & Manuck, S. B. (1992). Reliable measures of behaviorally invoked cardiovascular reactivity form a PC based test battery: Results from student and community samples. *Psychophysiology, 29,* 17–28.

Katz, D. (1960). The functional approach to the study of attitudes. *Public Opinion Quarterly, 24,* 163–204.

Katz, D., & Stotland, E. (1959). A preliminary statement to a theory of attitude structure and change. In S. Koch (Ed.), *Psychology: A Study of a Science,* vol. III (Formulations of the Person in the Social Context). New York: McGraw-Hill.

Kaufmann, G. M., & Beehr, T. A. (1986). Interactions between job stressors and social support: Some counterintuitive results. *Journal of Applied Psychology, 71,* 522–6.

Kayser, K. (1993). *When Love Dies: The Process of Marital Disaffection.* New York: Guilford.

Kent, M. V. (1994). The presence of others. In A. Hare, H. Blumberg, M. Davies, & M. Kent (Eds.), *Small Group Research: A Handbook,* pp. 81–105. Norwood, NJ: Ablex.

Kiecolt-Glaser, J. K., Dura, J. R., Speicher, C. E., Trask, O. J., & Glaser, R. (1991). Spousal caregivers of dementia victims: Longitudinal changes in immunity and health. *Psychosomatic Medicine, 53,* 345–62.

Kiecolt-Glaser, J. K., Garner, W., Speicher, C. E., Penn, G., & Glaser, R. (1984). Psychosocial modifiers of immunocompetence in medical students. *Psychosomatic Medicine, 46,* 7–14.

Kiecolt-Glaser, J. K., Kennedy, S., Malkoff, S., Fisher, L., Speicher, C. E., & Glaser, R. (1988). Marital discord and immunity in males. *Psychosomatic Medicine, 55,* 395–409.

Kiecolt-Glaser, J. K., Malarkey, W., Cacioppo, J. T., & Glaser, R. (1994). Stressful personal relationships: Immune and endocrine function. In R. Glaser & J. K. Kiecolt-Glaser (Eds.), *Handbook of Human Stress and Immunity,* pp. 321–39. San Diego: Academic Press.

Kiecolt-Glaser, J. K., Malarkey, W., Chee, M., Newton, T., Cacioppo, J. T., Mao, H., & Glaser, R. (1993). Negative behavior during marital conflict is associated with immunological down-regulation. *Psychosomatic Medicine, 55,* 395–409.

Kiecolt-Glaser, J. K., Newton, T., Cacioppo, J. T., MacCallum, R., Glaser, R., & Malarkey, W. (1996). Marital conflict and endocrine function: Are men really more physiologically affected than women? *Journal of Consulting and Clinical Psychology, 64,* 324–32.

Kim, H. S., & Baron, R. S. (1988). Exercise and the illusory correlation: Does arousal heighten stereotypic processing? *Journal of Experimental Social Psychology, 24,* 366–80.

Kissel, S. (1965). Stress reducing properties of social stimuli. *Journal of Personality and Social Psychology, 2,* 378–84.

Knox, S. S. (1993). Perception of social support and blood pressure in young men. *Perceptual and Motor Skills, 77,* 132–4.

Lacey, J. I., & Lacey, B. C. (1974). On heart rate responses and behavior: A reply to Elliott. *Journal of Personality and Social Psychology, 30,* 1–18.

Lang, P. J., Bradley, M. M., & Cuthbert, B. N. (1990). Emotion, attention, and the startle reflex. *Psychological Review, 97,* 377–95.

Lang, P. J., Bradley, M. M., & Cuthbert, B. N. (1992). A motivational analysis of emotion: Reflex-cortex connections. *Psychological Science, 3,* 44–9.

Lasswell, H. D. (1936). Certain changes during trial (psychoanalytic) interviews. *Psychoanalytic Review, 23,* 241–7.

Latane, B., & Cappell, H. (1972). The effects of togetherness on heart rate in rats. *Psychonomic Science, 29,* 177–9.

Lazarus, R. S. (1991). Progress on a cognitive-motivational-relational theory of emotion. *American Psychologist, 46,* 819–34.

Lazarus, R. S., & Alfert, E. (1964). Short-circuiting of threat by experimentally altering cognitive appraisal. *Journal of Abnormal and Social Psychology, 69,* 195–205.

Leedham, B., Meyerowitz, B., Muirhead, J., & Frist, W. (1995). Positive expectations predict health after heart transplantation. *Health Psychology, 14,* 74–9.

Leiderman, P. H., & Shapiro, D. (1964). *Psychobiological Approaches to Social Behavior.* Stanford, CA: Stanford University Press.

Lerner, M. J. (1980). *The Belief in a Just World: A Fundamental Delusion.* New York: Plenum.

Levenson, R. W., Carstenson, L. L., & Gottman, J. M. (1994). The influence of age and gender on affect, physiology, and their interrelations: A study of long term marriage. *Journal of Personality and Social Psychology, 67,* 56–68.

Levenson, R. W., & Gottman, J. M. (1983). Marital interaction: Physiological linkage and affective exchange. *Journal of Personality and Social Psychology, 45,* 587–97.

Levenson, R. W., & Gottman, J. M. (1985). Physiological and affective predictors of change in relationship satisfaction. *Journal of Personality and Social Psychology, 49,* 85–94.

Likert, R. A. (1932). A technique for measurement of attitudes. *Archives of Psychology, 140,* 1–55.

Loh, W. D., & Nuttin, J. M. (1972). Effects of interethnic-group comparisons and attitudes on task performance. *Journal of Personality and Social Psychology, 24,* 291–300.

Luhtanen, R., & Crocker, J. (1992). A collective self-esteem scale: Self-evaluation of one's social identity. *Personality and Social Psychology Bulletin, 18,* 302–18.

Mackie, D. M., & Hamilton, D. L. (1993). *Affect, Cognition, and Stereotyping: Interactive Processes in Group Perception.* San Diego: Academic Press.

Manning, F. J., & Fullerton, T. D. (1988). Health and well-being in highly cohesive units of the U.S. Army. *Journal of Applied Social Psychology, 18,* 503–19.

Manuck, S. B. (1994). Cardiovascular reactivity in cardiovascular disease: Once more into the breach. *International Journal of Behavioral Medicine, 1,* 4–31.

Markman, H. (1991). Constructive marital conflict is *not* an oxymoron. *Behavioral Assessment, 13,* 83–96.

McConahay, J. B. (1986). Modern racism, ambivalence, and the modern racism scale. In J. F. Dovidio & S. L. Gaertner (Eds.), *Prejudice, Discrimination, and Racism,* pp. 91–125. Orlando, FL: Academic Press.

McDougall, W. (1908). *An Introduction to Social Psychology.* London: Methuen.

Mesulam, M., & Perry, J. (1972). The diagnosis of lovesickness: Experimental psychophysiology without the polygraph. *Psychophysiology, 9,* 546–51.

Millar, M. G., & Tesser, A. (1992). The role of beliefs and feelings in guiding behavior: The mismatch model. In L. L. Martin & A. Tesser (Eds.), *The Construction of Social Judgments,* pp. 277–300. Hillsdale, NJ: Erlbaum.

Miller, D. T., & Prentice, D. (1996). The construction of social norms and standards. In E. T. Higgins & A. W. Kruglanski (Eds.), *Social Psychology: Handbook of Basic Principles,* pp. 799–829. New York: Guilford.

Moore, D. L., & Baron, R. S. (1983). Social facilitation: A social psychophysiological approach. In J. T. Cacioppo & R. E. Petty (Eds.), *Social Psychophysiology: A Sourcebook.* New York: Guilford.

Musante, G., & Anker, J. M. (1972). Experimenter's presence: Effects on subjects' performance. *Psychological Reports, 30,* 903–4.

Newcomb, A. F., & Bagwell, C. (1995). Children's friendship relations: A meta-analytic review. *Psychological Bulletin, 117,* 306–47.

Nisbett, R. E., & Wilson, T. D. (1977). Telling more than we can know: Verbal responses on mental processes. *Psychological Review, 84,* 231–59.

Obrist, P. A. (1981). *Cardiovascular Psychophysiology: A Perspective.* New York: Plenum.

Olson, J. M., Roese, N. J., & Zanna, M. P. (1996). Expectancies. In E. T. Higgins & A. Kruglanski (Eds.), *Social Psychology: Handbook of Basic Principles,* pp. 211–38. New York: Guilford.

Osgood, C. E., Suci, G. J., & Tannenbaum, P. H. (1957). *The Measurement of Meaning.* Urbana: University of Illinois Press.

Osterhout, L., Bersick, M., & McLaughlin, J. (1997). Brain potentials reflect violations of gender stereotypes. *Memory and Cognition, 25,* 273–85.

Pallak, M. S., & Pittman, E. S. (1972). General motivational effects of dissonance arousal. *Journal of Personality and Social Psychology, 21,* 349–58.

Pennebaker, J. W. (1989). Confession, inhibition, and disease. *Advances in Experimental Social Psychology, 22,* 211–44.

Pennebaker, J. W., & Beall, S. K. (1986). Confronting a traumatic event: Toward an understanding of inhibition and disease. *Journal of Abnormal Psychology, 95,* 274–81.

Pennebaker, J. W., & Francis, M. E. (1996). Cognitive, emotional, and language processes in disclosure: Physical health and adjustment. *Cognition and Emotion, 10,* 601–26.

Pennebaker, J. W., Kiecolt-Glaser, J. K., & Glaser, R. (1988). Disclosure of traumas and immune function: Health implications for psychotherapy. *Journal of Consulting and Clinical Psychology, 56,* 239–45.

Perkins, H. W. (1991). Religious commitment, "yuppie" values, and well-being in post collegiate life. *Review of Religious Research, 32,* 244–51.

Petrie, K. J., Booth, R. J., Pennebaker, J. W., Davison, K. P., & Thomas, M. G. (1995). Disclosure of trauma and immune response to a hepatitis B vaccination program. *Journal of Consulting and Clinical Psychology, 63,* 787–92.

Petty, R. E., & Cacioppo, J. T. (1983). The role of bodily responses in attitude measurement and change. In J. T. Cacioppo & R. E. Petty (Eds.), *Social Psychophysiology: A Sourcebook.* New York: Guilford.

Porier, G. W., & Lott, A. J. (1967). Galvanic skin responses and prejudice. *Journal of Personality and Social Psychology, 5,* 253–9.

Pratto, F., & John, O. P. (1991). Automatic vigilance: The attention-grabbing power of negative social information. *Journal of Personality and Social Psychology, 61,* 380–91.

Rankin, R. E., & Campbell, D. T. (1955). Galvanic skin responses to Negro and white experimenters. *Journal of Abnormal and Social Psychology, 51,* 30–3.

Rehm, J., Steinleitner, J., & Lilli, W. (1987). Wearing uniforms and aggression: A field experiment. *European Journal of Social Psychology, 17,* 357–60.

Reifman, A. (1995). Social relationships, recovery from illness, and survival: A literature review. *Annals of Behavioral Medicine, 17,* 124–31.

Reis, H. T., & Franks, P. (1994). The role of intimacy and social support in health outcomes: Two processes or one? *Personal Relationships, 1,* 185–97.

Riddle, E. M. (1925). Aggressive behavior in a small social group. *Archives of Psychology, 78,* 111–21.

Ross, E. D. (1981). The aprosodias: Functional-anatomical organization of the affective components of language in the right hemisphere. *Archives of Neurology, 38,* 561–9.

Sanna, L. J., & Shotland, R. L. (1990). Valence of anticipated evaluation and social facilitation. *Journal of Experimental Social Psychology, 26,* 82–92.

Schacter, S., & Singer, J. E. (1962). Cognitive, social, and physiological determinants of affective state. *Psychological Review, 69,* 379–99.

Scheier, M. F., & Carver, C. S. (1985). Optimism, coping, and health: Assessment and implications of general outcome expectancies. *Health Psychology, 4,* 219–47.

Scheier, M. F., & Carver, C. S. (1992). Effects of optimism on psychological and physical well-being: Theoretical overview and empirical update. *Cognitive Therapy and Research, 16,* 201–28.

Schwartz, G. E., Ahern, G. L., & Brown, S.-L. (1979). Lateralized facial muscle response to positive and negative emotional stimuli. *Psychophysiology, 16,* 561–71.

Schwartz, G. E., Fair, P. L., Salt, P., Mandel, M. R., & Klerman, G. L. (1976). Facial muscle patterning to affective imagery in depressed and nondepressed subjects. *Science, 192,* 489–91.

Schwartz, G. E., & Shapiro, D. (1973). Social psychophysiology. In W. F. Prokasky & D. C. Raskin (Eds.), *Electrodermal Activity in Psychological Research.* New York: Academic Press.

Seeman, T. E., Berkman, L. F., Blazer, D., & Rowe, J. W. (1994). Social ties and support and neuroendocrine function: The MacArthur studies of successful aging. *Annals of Behavioral Medicine, 16,* 95–106.

Sgoutas-Emch, S. A., Cacioppo, J. T., Uchino, B. N., Malarkey, W., Pearl, D., Kiecolt-Glaser, J. K., & Glaser, R. (1994). The effects of an acute psychological stressor on cardiovascular, endocrine, and cellular immune response: A prospective study of individuals high and low in heart rate reactivity. *Psychophysiology, 31,* 264–71.

Shapiro, D., & Crider, A. (1969). Psychophysiological approaches in social psychology. In G. Lindzey & E. Aronson (Eds.), *Handbook of Social Psychology,* vol. 3, pp. 1–49. Reading, MA: Addison-Wesley.

Shapiro, D., & Schwartz, G. E. (1970). Psychophysiological contributions to social psychology. *Annual Review of Psychology, 21,* 87–112.

Sher, T. G., & Weiss, R. L. (1991). Negativity in marital communication: Where's the beef? *Behavioral Assessment, 13,* 1–5.

Sherif, M. (1966). *Group Conflict and Co-operation: Their Social Psychology.* London: Routledge & Kegan Paul.

Smith, C. (1936). The autonomic excitation resulting from the interaction of individual opinion and group opinion. *Journal of Abnormal and Social Psychology, 30,* 138–64.

Smith, C., Fernengal, K., Holcroft, C., Gerald, K., & Marien, L. (1994). Meta-analysis of the associations between social support and health outcomes. *Annals of Behavioral Medicine, 16,* 352–62.

Smith, M. B., Bruner, J. S., & White, R. W. (1956). *Opinions and Personality.* New York: Wiley.

Snydersmith, M. A., & Cacioppo, J. T. (1992). Parsing complex social factors to determine component effects: I. Autonomic activity and reactivity as a function of human association. *Journal of Social and Clinical Psychology, 11,* 263–78.

Speisman, J. C., Lazarus, R. S., & Davison, L. (1964). Experimental analysis of a film used as a threatening stimulus. *Journal of Consulting Psychology, 28,* 23–33.

Spence, S., Shapiro, D., & Zaidel, E. (1996). The role of the right hemisphere in the physiological and cognitive components of emotional processing. *Psychophysiology, 33,* 112–22.

Sterling, B., & Gaertner, S. L. (1984). The attribution of arousal and emergency helping: A bidirectional process. *Journal of Experimental Social Psychology, 20,* 586–96.

Stroessner, S. J., & Mackie, D. L. (1992). The impact of induced affect on the perception of variability in social groups. *Personality and Social Psychology Bulletin, 18,* 546–54.

Sutton, S., Braren, M., Zubin, S., & John, E. R. (1965). Information delivery and the sensory evoked potential. *Science, 155,* 1436–9.

Tajfel, H., & Turner, J. (1986). The social identity theory of intergroup behavior. In S. Worchel & W. G. Austin (Eds.), *Psychology of Intergroup Relations,* pp. 7–24. Chicago, IL: Nelson.

Tardy, C. H., Thompson, W. R., & Allen, M. T. (1989). Cardiovascular responses during speech: Does social support mediate the effects of talking on blood pressure? *Journal of Language and Social Psychology, 8,* 271–85.

Thurstone, L. L. (1928). Attitudes can be measured. *American Journal of Sociology, 33,* 529–44.

Tomaka, J., & Blascovich, J. (1994). Effects of justice beliefs on cognitive appraisal of subjective, physiological, and behavioral responses to potential stress. *Journal of Personality and Social Psychology, 67,* 732–40.

Tomaka, J., Blascovich, J., Kelsey, R. M., & Leitten, C. L. (1993). Subjective, physiological, and behavioral effects of threat and challenge appraisal. *Journal of Personality and Social Psychology, 65,* 248–60.

Tomaka, J., Blascovich, J., Kibler, J., & Ernst, J. M. (1997). Cognitive and physiological antecedents of threat and challenge appraisal. *Journal of Personality and Social Psychology, 73,* 63–72.

Triplett, N. (1898). The dynamogenic factors in pacemaking and competition. *American Journal of Psychology, 9,* 507–33.

Tversky, A., & Kahneman, D. (1988). Extensional versus intuitive reasoning: The conjunction fallacy in probability judgment. In A. M. Collins & E. E. Smith (Eds.), *Readings in Cognitive Science: A Perspective from Psychology and Artificial Intelligence,* pp. 440–51. San Mateo, CA: Morgan Kaufmann.

Uchino, B. N., Cacioppo, J. T., & Kiecolt-Glaser, J. K. (1996). The relationship between social support and physiological process: A review with emphasis on underlying mechanisms and implications for health. *Psychological Bulletin, 119,* 488–531.

Uchino, B. N., Cacioppo, J. T., Malarkey, W., Glaser, R., & Kiecolt-Glaser, J. K. (1995). Appraisal support predicts age-related differences in cardiovascular function in women. *Health Psychology, 14,* 556–62.

Uchino, B. N., Kiecolt-Glaser, J. K., & Cacioppo, J. T. (1992). Age-related changes in cardiovascular response as a function of a chronic stressor and social support. *Journal of Personality and Social Psychology, 63,* 839–46.

Van Egeren, L. F. (1979). Cardiovascular changes during social competition in a mixed-motive game. *Journal of Personality and Social Psychology, 37,* 858–64.

Vanman, E. J., Kaplan, D. L., & Miller, N. (1991). Facial EMG activity and bias between social groups: A replication and extension. *Psychophysiology, 28,* S59.

Vanman, E. J., & Miller, N. (1993). Applications of emotion research theory and research to stereotyping and intergroup relations. In D. M. Mackie & D. L. Hamilton (Eds.), *Affect, Cognition, and Stereotyping: Interactive Processes in Group Perception,* pp. 213–38. New York: Academic Press.

Vanman, E. J., Paul, B. Y., Kaplan, D. L., & Miller, N. (1990). Facial electromyography differentiates racial bias in imagined cooperative settings. *Psychophysiology, 27,* S63.

Vrana, S. R., & Lang, P. J. (1990). Fear imagery and the startle-probe reflex. *Journal of Abnormal Psychology, 99,* 181–9.

Vrana, S. R., Spence, E. L., & Lang, P. J. (1988). The startle probe response: A new measure of emotion? *Journal of Abnormal Psychology, 97,* 487–91.

Waid, W. M. (1984). *Sociophysiology.* New York: Springer-Verlag.

Wann, D. L., & Branscombe, N. R. (1995). Influence of identification with a group and physiological arousal on perceived intergroup complexity. *British Journal of Social Psychology, 34,* 223–35.

Weitz, S. (1972). Attitude, voice and behavior: A repressed affect model of interracial interactions. *Journal of Personality and Social Psychology, 24,* 14–21.

Wilder, D. A., & Shapiro, P. (1989). Role of competition-induced anxiety on limiting the beneficial impact of positive behavior by an out-group member. *Journal of Personality and Social Psychology, 56,* 60–9.

Williams, R. B., Barefoot, J. C., & Califf, R. M. (1992). Prognostic importance of social and economic resources among medically treated patients with angiographically documented coronary artery disease. *Journal of the American Medical Association, 267,* 520–4.

Wright, R. A., Tunstall, A. M., Williams, B. J., Goodwin, S. J., & Harmon-Jones, E. (1995). Social evaluation and cardiovascular response: An active coping approach. *Journal of Personality and Social Psychology, 69,* 530–43.

Zajonc, R. (1965). Social facilitation. *Science, 149,* 269–74.

Zajonc, R. (1980a). Feeling and thinking: Preferences need no inferences. *American Psychologist, 35,* 151–75.

Zajonc, R. (1980b). Compresence. In P. B. Paulus (Ed.), *Psychology of Group Influence.* Hillsdale, NJ: Erlbaum.

Zanna, M., & Cooper, J. (1974). Dissonance and the pill: An attribution approach to studying the arousal properties of dissonance. *Journal of Personality and Social Psychology, 29,* 703–9.

Zanna, M., & Rempel, J. (1988). Attitudes: A new look at an old concept. In D. Bar-Tal & A. Kruglanzkie (Eds.), *The Social Psychology of Knowledge,* pp. 315–34. Cambridge University Press.

Zillmann, D. (1979). *Hostility and Aggression.* Hillsdale, NJ: Erlbaum.

Zillmann, D., & Cantor, J. R. (1976). Effect of timing of information about mitigating circumstances on emotional responses to provocation and retaliatory behavior. *Journal of Experimental Social Psychology, 12,* 38–55.

Zillmann, D., Johnson, R. C., & Day, K. D. (1974). Provoked and unprovoked aggressiveness in athletes. *Journal of Research in Personality, 8,* 139–52.

CHAPTER TWENTY-FOUR

DEVELOPMENTAL PSYCHOPHYSIOLOGY
Conceptual and Methodological Perspectives

NATHAN A. FOX, LOUIS A. SCHMIDT, & HEATHER A. HENDERSON

Historical Introduction

Developmental psychophysiology is the study of behavior–physiology relations in infants and young children. Issues commonly studied by psychophysiologists with adult populations – such as cognitive processing, emotion–cognition interactions, or responses to stress – may be examined in populations of young children as well. Using age-appropriate paradigms, interested researchers have investigated infant visual attention through the measurement of cardiac orienting (Field 1979; Sameroff, Cashmore, & Dykes 1973); others have examined infant discrimination of human faces by recording event-related potentials (de Haan & Nelson 1997; Nelson & Collins 1991, 1992). Such research has been quite valuable in revealing the links between physiological response and behavior in infants and children of different ages. When multiple ages are utilized, such studies have also revealed age differences in physiology–behavior linkages (Richards 1985, 1989).

Developmental psychophysiology, however, may offer the greater promise of revealing the processes by which both physiology and behavior change over time. Such an approach necessitates a three-tier investigation. First, there must be a description of age-related changes in behavioral performance and physiological response. Second, there must be an attempt to describe how the physiological system itself is developing and changing over time, often as a function of the stimuli that are being studied. Third, there should be some attempt at integration of physiology and behavior. An example of this approach may be seen in the study of infant memory for faces. Such research has used event-related potentials (ERPs) to examine multiple age groups (Nelson & Collins 1991, 1992). These studies found decreasing latency and increasing amplitude of particular components of the ERP with age (see Neslon 1994 for a review). Decreasing latency and increasing ampli-

tude of the ERP have further been linked with increased memory performance across childhood (Howard & Polich 1985). Together these results suggest that with age there is an increasing speed in processing stimuli, including faces.

These findings are an important first step, but the developmental psychophysiologist should ask the next set of questions. Specifically, in the study of systems that change over time, it is critical to understand what system parameters may be contributing to the response being measured. In the case of the increasing amplitude and decreasing frequency of the ERP, we need to know what physical and physiological changes have occurred over developmental time that may contribute to these changes in the ERP. For example, it is possible that changes in myelination of brain areas putatively involved in the behavior may affect the latency of the response. There may be changes in skull thickness or cortico-cortical connections that affect the pattern of the response. And there are clearly certain cognitive processes involved in the development of face recognition and discrimination that contribute to the behavioral response. Finally, although direct comparisons between adult and child behaviors may not be appropriate (i.e., each group may solve a particular problem with different strategies and perhaps with different underlying neural mechanisms), similarities in performance between these groups or deficits in one group may be useful for raising hypotheses about the underlying bases of the behavior.

For example, Schacter, Kagan, and Leichtman (1995) reviewed studies of adult clinical populations who showed patterns of amnesia for episodic memory or confabulatory behaviors. Many of these adult subjects had injury to areas of the prefrontal region. Indeed, the clinical data on brain-damaged adults suggest that injury to certain areas of the prefrontal cortex may be associated with source memory deficits. Schacter et al. (1995) drew a comparison between the responses of adult brain-damaged patients and the behaviors that young children exhibit when tested for episodic or source memory. Although not suggesting that the processes responsible for adult or child errors were similar, the researchers did raise interesting hypotheses regarding the role of the prefrontal region in episodic memory.

Thus, developmental psychophysiology has the opportunity to study changes in response systems over age as well as the processes underlying this change. Change in the response system must not only be measured; it must, moreover, be understood as a function of the physical and psychological maturation of the organism under study. These added elements of developmental change create a new level of complexity (Emde & Walker 1976; Richards 1989; Snidman et al. 1995), in contrast to the psychophysiological study of adult populations.

MODELS OF DEVELOPMENT

Developmental change has been modeled in many different ways. The model one adopts as well as the processes one examines will determine the questions that are asked. There are a number of different models of development, each with a different emphasis on the roles of environment and biology in influencing behavior. Application of one of these models to a particular study will influence the manner in which questions are asked and variables are measured.

Biologically Determined Model of Development

This model postulates that development is a function of the unfolding of predetermined biological processes. The underlying structures of the brain develop and hook up with one another via predetermined processes that have a great deal to do with the action and expression of certain genes (Edelman 1987). Thus, neuroblasts migrate and generate particular layers of cortical and subcortical structures during embryonic development similarly for all individuals – in the absence of toxic environments (e.g., in utero exposure to drugs, alcohol, or radiation) (Huttenlocher 1979; Sidman & Rakic 1973). Likewise, the formation of the nuclei responsible for cardio-respiratory control and vagal innervation of the heart occur on a standard developmental timetable except in the presence of toxic environmental effects. Of course, even with well-programmed neural development there are individual differences in growth outcomes that may result from differences in intrauterine environments or the timing of particular stressors (Huttenlocher 1979). Such differences reflect a critical variable that any developmental model must take into account. The timing with which certain environmental events impact upon preprogrammed biological growth is a critical area of study. Ultimately, though, the timing of neural development is presumed – in biological models of development – to be preprogrammed and to occur in an orderly fashion in the absence of negative environmental events.

Critical Period Model of Development

A second model of development is one that takes into account environmental input and emphasizes the criticality of the timing at which this input is presented. This model is best thought of as reflecting the concept of a critical period. The idea of a critical period is that there is a window of opportunity through which particular environmental input will have a major influence on the organization of behavior (Hubel & Wiesel 1970). For example, there is some evidence that exposure to language during the early years of life is critical for the adequate formation of appropriate language ability (Lenneberg 1967; Petitto 1993). Such a notion implies that exposure prior to or after this window of opportunity will not have the same effect upon the neural organization underlying this behavior (but see Mills, Coffey-Corina, & Neville 1994). In addition, it implies that appropriate exposure during the critical period will lead to the organization of structures in such a way that they will henceforth underlie the more mature behavioral pattern. The critical period model of development is akin to an "innoculation" model in that appropriate development necessitates input at a particular time. Neural reorganization occurs as a function of this input, which then underlies subsequent behavior. This reorganization of behavior is a second process that plays an important role in our understanding of behavioral change. After receiving the appropriate environmental input, the infant is protected (innoculated) from other competing environmental inputs.

Stage Model of Development

A third model is one in which development is explained as a series of different periods of reorganization of both physiology and behavior (Case 1992; Fischer 1983, 1987; Thatcher 1991, 1994). Such a model is derivative of Piaget's view of development. He viewed an organism's development as consisting of a continuous process of accommodating and assimilating environmental information. At particular points in development, a subject's interpretation of the information changes qualitatively – moving, for example, from a sensorimotor view to a more concrete operational one. At these transition moments, there are behavioral and accompanying physiological reorganizations that reflect changes in the manner in which the child operates on the world. There is interesting, though indirect, psychophysiological evidence to support this view. Thatcher, Walker, and Giudice (1987) examined changes in intra- and interhemispheric coherence of the EEG (electroencephalograph) across multiple ages. They found what they described as lawful patterns of reorganization of coherence both within and between the left and right hemispheres. The ages at which these changes occurred seemed to correspond to periods of cognitive reorganization proposed by Piaget.

A number of "stage" or reorganization models describe the transformation of existing behavioral/cognitive structures at particular periods of time into more sophisticated structures for the purpose of assimilating new and more complex information (Case 1992; Fischer 1980). Further, behavioral/cognitive reorganization is supposedly mimicked at the neural level (Fischer 1987; Fischer & Rose 1994). For example, in a re-analysis of longitudinal EEG data collected by Matousek and Petersén (1973), John (1977) described distinct periods of reorganization of power in anterior to posterior scalp locations that coincided with age periods thought to represent times of cognitive change. In a more discrete study of brain–behavior relations, Bell and Fox (1992) reported on changes in EEG power recorded from the frontal scalp leads in infants who had and had not mastered an object permanence ("A not B") task, which is thought to involve the activity of the dorsolateral frontal cortex (Diamond & Goldman-Rakic 1983, 1986, 1989). The timing of changes in behavior and EEG for successful infants was tightly locked, so that reorganization of behavior and EEG (reflected not only in power but also coherence) were similar in scope.

Interactionist Model of Development

A fourth approach to the study of development is one that views the process as involving a continuous interaction between (a) the genetic and biological disposition of the individual and (b) environmental factors impinging upon that individual (Gottlieb 1976). The goal of research is to understand the processes involved in this interaction. In order to do so, one must assess not only the biological and physiological status of the organism but also the manner in which various types of environmental contexts affect that status. Such an approach involves the study of individual differences and the role of the environment in affecting these differences.

The study of individual differences is, in fact, a major topic in psychophysiology. Researchers have for some time recognized that individuals differ in their initial or baseline pattern of physiology and have attempted to take these differences into account when understanding subject response to stimulation (see Zahn 1986 for a review). Indeed, a number of investigators have given specific emphasis to the psychological meaning of these individual differences in physiology. For example, Davidson and colleagues argued that the resting pattern of frontal EEG activation reflects a disposition for individuals to respond in a particular hedonic manner (Davidson 1984a,b, 1995). Adults with resting right frontal EEG asymmetry are more likely to respond with a negative hedonic valence than are adults exhibiting left frontal activation. Within the domain of autonomic activity, Porges (1992) argued that individual levels of heart

rate variability or vagal tone will affect the subject's response to a stimulus or to a mild stressor. Individuals with low vagal tone are less likely than those with higher levels to display significant cardiac orienting. Porges' work is unique in that he extended these findings from adult to infant and child populations.

Fox and colleagues extended Davidson's model to examine temperamental differences among infants and young children. In a series of studies, they showed that infants with right frontal baseline EEG asymmetry are more likely than those with left frontal asymmetry to display distress and negative affect to unfamiliar stimuli (Calkins, Fox, & Marshall 1996; Fox, Bell, & Jones 1992). They also showed that children displaying this pattern of right frontal asymmetry are more likely to show social withdrawal and reticence in a social situation with unfamiliar peers (Fox et al. 1995).

Although most developmental psychologists subscribe to the interactionist model to describe developmental processes, few studies actually capture the interactional component of the model. Most studies and researchers of individual differences are able to characterize the individual, and often the environment, but are less likely to describe the manner in which these factors mutually influence one another. Any understanding of development, however, must ultimately take into account such interaction. Such a model necessitates the integration of timing and reorganization of physiology as a function of experience; it must take into account when exposure to certain events occurs and how this affects the organization of physiology and behavior.

Each of the four models just described provides important insight into developmental processes. There are clearly some changes that are under greater genetic control than others (e.g., migration of nerve cells in the embryological development of the brain), other changes that necessitate environmental input at a particular moment if they are to function properly (e.g., the need for visual stimulation in the organization of the visual system), and still other changes that show transformations over time as a function of interaction with the environment (e.g., means–end ability). The choice of a model may be a function of the processes under study. At a macro level, there must be some integration of these frameworks for understanding the complex manner in which development occurs in the central nervous system (CNS).

Physical Context: Systems in Developmental Psychophysiology

In this section, we review two major psychophysiological systems (electrocortical and cardiovascular) for which the four models discussed previously have been used in the study of biology–behavior relations during development.

We describe the historical precedents for each of these systems and review studies focusing on developmental issues.

THE ELECTROCORTICAL SYSTEM: EEG AND ERP

Overview

As with any system undergoing change, there are dramatic differences in activity of the EEG during the first two years of life. Changes in power and frequency of the EEG during this time period may be a function of certain developmental changes in specific brain parameters. For example, it is possible that changes in myelination of axons, changes in dendritic branching, and the sculpting of neuronal patterns (both in terms of cell proliferation and cell death) all affect the pattern of electrical energy recorded off the scalp. We know, however, precious little about the development of any of these physical parameters. The data on myelination of brain areas comes from studies such as those conducted by Benes and co-workers (1994) and Gilles, Shankle, and Dooling (1983). The data on dendritic changes and sculpting comes from studies by Huttenlocher and colleagues (e.g. Huttenlocher 1984; Huttenlocher & de Courten 1987; Huttenlocher et al. 1982). None of these studies has directly linked anatomical changes to behavior.

The paucity of information regarding growth and development of the systems under study obviously makes interpretation of the pattern of responses being measured from these systems somewhat problematic. For example, adult alpha, recorded over the occipital cortex, is defined as comprising the frequency band of 8–13 Hz. This frequency band seems to respond reliably to changes in visual attention (eyes open vs. eyes closed produces alpha suppression). There is, however, little power in the 8–13-Hz frequency band through late childhood. On the other hand, there is a reliable rhythm recorded over the occipital cortex that is responsive in similar ways to visual input in the first year of life. This rhythm has a frequency centered at 4 Hz with a band defined around 3–5 Hz. Later in the second year of life, the rhythm has a frequency centered at 7 Hz with a band defined around 6–8 Hz. The change in this frequency band may be of significance for understanding not only basic neural development but also the relation between EEG and behavioral changes. That is, the increase in frequency of the infant's alpha-like rhythm may tell us something about the development of the underlying neural generators in the thalamus that are purportedly responsible for generating adult alpha rhythm (Nunez 1981).

Developmental changes in psychophysiological measures may also reflect functional changes in the way the brain processes information. It is possible that certain brain structures are present early on but do not come "on line" until later in development. Changes in psychophysiological responses may thus result from the appearance of new functional operations rather than from the physical maturation of any structures. For instance, some patterns of electrical activity are less a result of anatomical variations and more a reflection of functional changes. One example is the pattern of frontal EEG asymmetry reported in infant and adult studies. Individuals may show a predominant asymmetry pattern at rest (either left or right frontal EEG asymmetry). But there are also clear shifts in these same individuals as a function of affective state or cognitive activity. For example, individuals with a pattern of resting left frontal EEG asymmetry may display right frontal EEG asymmetry in response to an aversive film clip (Jones & Fox 1992; Tomarken, Davidson, & Henriques 1990). These shifts seem to suggest that the pattern of changes in EEG asymmetry reflect functional changes in brain activation rather than anatomical differences. There may, of course, be developmental changes in the degree to which these functional differences emerge and are utilized. Nevertheless, individual differences in psychophysiological measures such as EEG asymmetry may reflect important functional rather than structural differences.

Historical Background

Berger (1929, 1932a,b) was the first to use the electroencephalogram to assess human brain development. Berger found little brain electrical activity before 1 month of age, after which time EEG frequency and amplitude increased in the occipital region. Following Berger's important work, a number of longitudinal studies on EEG development were conducted with full-term and premature infants and with a focus on distinguishing between sleep and wake states. Overall, the early studies found that EEG frequency and amplitude increased during the first year of life in the full-term infant, whereas brain electrical activity of the premature infant was similar to the in utero infant (Dreyfus-Brisac & Monod 1975). More recent studies have also noted reduced EEG amplitude in pre-term compared with full-term infants (Duffy, Als, & McAnulty 1990).

The early EEG studies were, however, limited on several fronts (Berger 1932a,b; Smith 1938a,b,c, 1939). First, most of the studies were largely descriptive. They attempted to detail the development of various components of the EEG in the absence of any information regarding the physical development of the nervous system. Second, attempts at quantification of EEG frequency and amplitude were done by hand with a ruler, possibly limiting the precision of calculations; many of the early studies predated the use of computers and frequency analyzers. Third, adult parameters (such as sleep staging) were used to index EEG development in the infant. Fourth, there were a limited number of sites from which EEG recordings were made. A majority of studies recorded from only one or two scalp sites, possibly precluding the contribution of brain maturation in other regions relative to the sites collected.

The EEG has been used by both clinicians and basic researchers as an instrument to understand complex brain–behavior relations. Traditionally, the EEG has been used in clinical settings to diagnose neuropathology. In this setting, the neurologist primarily uses qualitative interpretation of the EEG signal to understand brain anomalies such as seizures or tumor. More recently, quantitative EEG (qEEG) has been used in basic research settings by investigators interested in understanding issues related to normal as well as atypical brain development. For example, some researchers have examined changes in EEG frequency (Hagne 1968, 1972) and coherence (Thatcher, Krause, & Hrybyk 1986) in relation to brain maturation. Still others have related regional EEG activation to the emergence of particular functions in the developing brain. For example, patterns of frontal EEG activation have been examined in relation to emotional (Dawson et al. 1992b; Fox et al. 1992; see also Fox 1991, 1994) and cognitive (Bell & Fox 1994) development during infancy as well as the development of maladaptive social behavior during early childhood (Fox et al. 1996).

With the advent of new computer technologies, the collecting of ongoing EEG at a high rate of speed is now a reality. Such advances allow for reliable temporal resolution between underlying neurophysiology and psychological processes. Furthermore, unlike more intrusive brain imaging procedures such as positron emission tomography (PET) and functional magnetic resonance imaging (fMRI), the EEG is a relatively noninvasive neuroimaging procedure, making it more tractable with pediatric populations. These methodological improvements and considerations, in combination with recent theoretical advances in the neurosciences, provide an exciting atmosphere for researchers interested in using the EEG to understand the developing human brain. However, the use of EEG in understanding human brain development has been limited because there have been relatively few longitudinal studies in which quantitative EEG has been used to assess brain maturation. In addition, the EEG suffers from poor spatial resolution. Neuroimaging techniques such as PET and fMRI have superior spatial resolution. On the other hand, EEG is superior to these neuroimaging techniques in that it provides temporal information about brain processes.

Studies Relating EEG to Early Brain Development

A number of longitudinal studies have been directed toward examining EEG frequency development during the first two years of life. Most of these studies examined posterior EEG frequency development and noted that a dominant EEG frequency emerged between 3–5 Hz during the first 6 months of life and between 6–8 Hz by the end of the first year. Smith (1938a,b,c, 1939) was one of the first researchers to examine EEG frequency development in the developing brain. Smith (1938b) noted that, by age 3–4 months, a characteristic alpha-like rhythm appeared in the occipital region in the human infant. The occipital rhythm increased to 6–7 Hz by age 12 months (1938b, 1939, 1941).

Smith (1938b) suggested that the onset of occipital activity at 3–4 months was linked to maturation of visual systems. Smith (1939, 1941) also noted a 7-Hz alpha-like frequency at age 3–4 months in the central region that increased in frequency after 10 months. Smith (1941) speculated that this shift in pattern was linked to the emergence of reaching behavior in the infant. Lindsley (1939) also noted the development of an alpha-like rhythm between 3 Hz and 5 Hz in the occipital region at age 3–4 months, which increased to 6 Hz by age 12 months. Lindsley (1939) postulated that the development of this rhythm was related to the ontogeny of visual perception. Henry (1944) reported a 3–4-Hz rhythm in the occipital region at 3–4 months that increased to 7 Hz by age 12 months.

Following this early work, longitudinal studies of EEG frequency development waned for nearly three decades until the work of Hagne and her colleagues (Hagne 1968, 1972; Hagne et al. 1973). Hagne's work is of particular importance for at least three reasons. First, unlike earlier studies that calculated frequency data by hand, she performed frequency analyses using a fast Fourier transform. Second, Hagne recorded from multiple sites representing anterior and posterior regions of the brain. Third, Hagne was interested in relative power and peak frequency. Hagne (1968, 1972) reported that the delta (1.5–3.5-Hz) to theta (3.5–7.5-Hz) frequency ratio changed between 8 and 12 months, with increases in theta and decreases in delta. This pattern of change was a function of electrode location: theta activity decreased in P3 and O1 between 8 and 10 months and increased between 10 and 12 months, while theta activity in C3 and Cz increased between 8 and 12 months. Still others (Mizuno et al. 1970) examined relative power in the right occipital area using a quotient of alpha (7.17–10.3 Hz) over delta (2.4–3.46 Hz). Mizuno et al. (1970) found that this quotient increased from 1 to 12 months of age, with increases in alpha activity and corresponding decreases in the delta band.

Another measure used in the study of brain development is EEG coherence, a measure of the phase relation of two processes at a specific frequency band. Coherence values range from 0 (there is no phase relation) to 1 (the two signals are either completely in or out of phase with each other). A number of researchers have speculated on the interpretation of changes in EEG coherence. Nunez (1981) suggested that coherence between two EEG electrode locations may reflect the activity of axonal connections between two regions. Others have postulated that coherence values may be related to the activity of short- and long-fiber networks of the axons (Thatcher et al. 1986, 1987). Thatcher postulated that development in the cortex involves processes of increasing communication between regionally distinct locations as well as increased differentiation of regions across the cortex. Thatcher used a ratio score of long- to short-distance coherence to demonstrate this model. By examining the coherence of long-distance sites (assuming increases to reflect increased long-distance communication) and also of short-distance sites (assuming decreases to reflect regional specialization), Thatcher et al. (1987) were able to model the growth of the cerebral hemispheres across the first ten years of life. The researchers reported that periods of major change in short- and long-distance coherence coincided with what appear to be major stage transitions in cognitive growth. Thatcher argued that this is an indirect confirmation of his model of neural change as reflected in the EEG measure of coherence.

If coherence does reflect the connectivity between different regions, then it may change as a function of the degree to which that connectivity increases or decreases. Studies of both human (Huttenlocher 1979; Huttenlocher et al. 1982) and nonhuman (Greenough & Volkmar 1973) primate cortical development have reported that, during early development, there is an overpopulation of neurons in the cortex that seem also to be selectively pruned. Bell and Fox (1996) wondered if these processes were reflected in measures of EEG coherence and took as their model the timing of self-produced locomotion during the first year of life. They recorded EEG from four groups of 8-month-old infants who varied in the degree of experience they had with self-produced locomotion (one group was not yet crawling; a second group crawled for one to two weeks; a third group from three to six weeks; and a fourth group had been crawling for more than seven weeks). Bell and Fox argued that coherence measures should differ as a function of the degree of experience that infants had with crawling. This model of experience-dependent changes in neural patterning was first proposed by Greenough (Greenough & Black 1992; Greenough, Black, & Wallace 1987), who predicted an inverted U-shaped function in the number of connections (with an increase at the onset of particular expected experiences and a decrease as pruning occurred once a particular competency had been mastered). Bell and Fox (1996) found this same inverted U-shaped function for intrahemispheric coherence in the EEG among the four groups. Infants with no experience in crawling showed less coherence than those with only a short period of crawling experience. By seven weeks of experience, the level of coherence had again dropped.

Studies Relating ERP Morphology to Early Brain Development

Developmentalists who subscribe to early critical periods are interested in (a) how environmental input can affect brain development and (b) the emergence of particular competencies during development. One such example is the acquisition of language. There seem to be critical periods around which particular components of language emerge. During the first half of the first year of life, all infants are capable of discriminating across lexical boundaries the sounds of any language. Thus, infants raised in an English-speaking environment in the United States are capable of discriminating across certain boundaries of Chinese or Japanese (Best 1993). After six to eight months, this ability to discriminate any boundary seems to disappear, and children are able to make these discriminations only for their native language – the language to which they have been exposed. These changes clearly suggest the reorganization of neural centers as a function of language input and the critical period during which this reorganization is said to occur. However, not all neural reorganization for language necessitates the input of oral communication.

In a series of studies, Neville and her colleagues showed that congenitally deaf subjects differ from hearing subjects in the pattern of their ERP responses to language (Neville, Kutas, & Schmidt 1982a,b). Whereas hearing subjects displayed a prototypical left-hemisphere distribution of the ERP in response to language stimuli, deaf subjects showed the opposite pattern (right-hemisphere distribution). Neville reports that this pattern of right-hemisphere activity in the ERP of deaf subjects may be a function of the type of language input they receive. Whereas hearing subjects receive oral auditory input, deaf subjects were more likely to receive visual-spatial input as communication. The type of language communication therefore reorganized the patterns of hemisphereic dominance, which were reflected in the asymmetry of the ERP.

THE CARDIOVASCULAR SYSTEM: HEART PERIOD AND HEART RATE VARIABILITY
Overview

The cardiovascular system is relatively well developed at birth, and recording of the ECG (electrocardiogram) is relatively easy even during the newborn period, thus providing researchers and clinicians with a useful and noninvasive means for assessing the developmental status of infants. Measures of heart period (the time interval between successive heart cycles, or the interbeat interval) and heart rate variability (a general term used to refer to beat-to-beat changes in heart rate or heart period) serve as indices of autonomic nervous system (ANS) regulatory activities and have been related to individual differences in attention, cognition, and emotion in both child and adult populations. The interpretation of the autonomic origins of cardiovascular response patterns, whether in the context of intraindividual responses to discrete stimuli or interindividual differences in baseline cardiovascular patterns, is complicated by the fact that the heart is dually innervated by the parasympathetic and sympathetic branches of the ANS. Yet methodological advances, such as the incorporation of spectral analytic techniques into the analysis of heart rate variability data, allow for the isolation and quantification of particular sources of heart rate variability (Mezzacappa et al. 1994).

The ability to empirically link basic cardiovascular measures such as heart period to higher-order processes such as attention and information processing has been particularly useful in the field of child development, where researchers are faced with the difficulty of gathering information from infants who have yet to acquire language or complex motor behaviors. Thus, cardiovascular measures have become a useful tool for the study and assessment of sensory, perceptual, and cognitive development in infants. Conversely, infant development provides a useful means for studying the development of autonomic functioning and its role in psychological processes.

Beyond infancy, cardiovascular functioning has been related to the development of emotional and behavioral disorders in childhood and adolescence. The cardiovascular system has been related to problem behaviors based on the theoretical assumption that cardiovascular functioning is related to higher-order cognitive processes such as information processing. In older children and adults, information processing expands beyond simply attending to stimuli in the environment to allocating attention between internal (i.e. self-focused) and external (other-focused) events.

Historical Background

There are excellent reviews of the historical development of the use of cardiovascular measures in psychological research on adult populations (see e.g. Hassett & Danforth 1982). Cardiovascular measures were originally used as an index of general arousal or emotion. Darrow (1929) first documented adults' physiologically distinct responses to classes of stimuli differing in the extent to which they were psychologically arousing. Specifically, when adults were presented with disturbing or arousing words, Darrow recorded a rise in blood pressure along with increases in heart rate. In contrast, there was little elevation (and sometimes very slight drops) in blood pressure in response to benign sensory stimuli. In addition, Darrow found that heart rate and respiration were more tightly associated during psychologically arousing than in more benign conditions. Together, Darrow's findings demonstrated that stimuli with distinct characteristics and psychological meanings evoked physiologically unique responses. In addition, increased respiratory-cardiac coupling under psychologically arousing conditions was attributed to increased autonomic arousal.

Ax (1953) extended Darrow's findings by demonstrating that specific emotions were associated with distinct physiological reaction patterns. During anger provocation in the laboratory, Ax found that adults responded with increased diastolic blood pressure and decreased heart rate. In contrast, there were fewer consistent reaction patterns during the induction of fear. Further, Ax noted that there was a greater association between physiological measures during anger induction. Ax interpreted these differences in the concordance of physiological measures as reflecting greater integration or organization during anger versus fear. From an evolutionary perspective, Ax related the increased phys-

iological integration during anger reactions to a complete mobilization of resources, in contrast to a relative lack of integration or paralysis of bodily functions during fear reactions.

Lacey (1967) provided compelling ideas as well as empirical evidence to argue against general activation theories of emotion. Lacey argued that physiological activation could not simply be conceptualized as a unidimensional continuum in which the degree of physiological activation directly maps onto the intensity of emotion or behavior. Rather, Lacey proposed that activation is multidimensional and that physiological reaction patterns reflect not only the intensity but also the intended goal or aim of an emotion or behavior. In a series of experiments, Lacey reported that the direction of cardiovascular response was telling of a subject's intention (e.g., approach vs. avoidance or withdrawal) toward external stimuli. Through directional reactions, the cardiovascular system serves to meet the varying metabolic demands of the body. Cardiac decelerations in response to arousing stimuli were thought to reflect stimulus detection and active intake from the environment; cardiac accelerations were thought to reflect active mental work, an internal focus, and the active filtering of irrelevant external stimuli.

The application of spectral analytic techniques to the study of both intra- and interindividual differences in heart rate variability has allowed for more precise interpretations regarding the autonomic origins of these differences. Using power spectral analysis, heart rate signals are decomposed into a series of component frequencies, with each component contributing to the total variance in the signal. The distribution of the total variance across the frequency range studied is associated with particular sources of the heart rate variability and the related parasympathetic and sympathetic nervous system mediators (Akselrod et al. 1981, 1985).

In adults, the majority of heart rate variability is contained within the frequency range of 0.0–0.5 Hz, with the 0.15–0.5-Hz components referred to as high-frequency (HF) and the 0.04–0.15-Hz components referred to as low-frequency (LF). The HF band marks the component of heart rate variability associated with respiratory sinus arrhythmia (RSA; Hirsch & Bishop 1981). However, developmental changes in respiratory rate will affect the boundaries of this band. The influences of respiration on heart rate variability are mediated primarily by changes in parasympathetic control over the heart via the vagus nerve (Katona & Jih 1975). Thus, spectral power in the HF band has been used as a measure of the magnitude of RSA, which in turn has been used as an index of vagal control over the heart. However, the predictive relations between RSA and cardiac vagal control are reduced by nonrespiratory parasympathetic contributions to heart rate variability and by within-subject changes in respiratory parameters, making RSA an imperfect estimate of vagal cardiac control (see Berntson et al. 1997 for a review). Despite these limitations, RSA remains among the most selective noninvasive indices of parasympathetic cardiac control (Berntson, Cacioppo, & Quigley 1993).

The neural origins of LF variability are more diffuse, since they are mediated by both the parasympathetic and sympathetic branches of the autonomic nervous system. Low-frequency power varies with sympathetic control, but only under limited and very specific conditions (Berntson et al. 1997). Measures of the LF/HF ratio have been used to index the balance between sympathetic and vagal cardiac control (Malliani, Pagani, & Lombardi 1994). But for several reasons – including the fact that the sympathetic and the parasympathetic nervous systems are not always reciprocally controlled – this method of estimating sympathovagal balance remains controversial (Berntson et al. 1997). Further, measurement of LF power requires heart period data to be collected over several minutes, with minimal motor movement and regular respiration (Snidman et al. 1995). These constraints are particularly challenging to overcome in work with infants and young children.

Sympathetic cardiac control has also been evaluated by measuring the duration of pre-ejection period (PEP; Cacioppo et al. 1994). The PEP is the period over which the left ventricle generates force, or the interval from the onset of ventricular depolarization to the beginning of ejection; it is inversely related to sympathetic inotropy (Binkley & Boudoulas 1986). Systolic time intervals such as PEP can be derived from information provided by impedance cardiography or from a combination of concurrent electrocardiographic, phonocardiographic, and pulse measurements. Again, application of this method of assessing sympathetic cardiac control may be problematic in studies of infants and children.

In summary, advances in measurement techniques provide researchers with a means for empirically evaluating the specific relations between parasympathetic and sympathetic influences and a variety of cognitive, emotional, and behavioral measures (Mezzacappa et al. 1997). Owing to the relative ease of isolating the parasympathetic influences on cardiac control, there have been more empirical studies relating psychological indices to vagal influences over the heart. Methods for noninvasively estimating sympathetic influences over the heart continue to be refined, but as of yet there is no agreed-upon measure (Berntson et al. 1997). Further, pragmatic constraints limit the extent to which methods for assessing sympathetic cardiac control can be applied to studies of infants and young children.

Cardiovascular psychophysiology is based, in part, on the premise that both the direction and magnitude of cardiovascular responses are sensitive to stimulus characteristics and reflect not only the intensity of one's reaction but the intention as well. Cardiovascular measures can also serve as markers of individual differences in these reaction tendencies. The demonstration and articulation of these properties of the cardiovascular response system has triggered growing interest by developmental psychologists in cardiovascular development and in the development of ANS–CNS integration. Moreover, developmental psychologists have used cardiovascular measures and psychophysiological paradigms to index perceptual and cognitive processing abilities and risk status in preverbal infants. Finally, a good deal of developmental work has been completed on cardiovascular markers of individual differences in response tendencies within both cognitive and social domains.

Social-Psychological Context

EEG AND COGNITIVE DEVELOPMENT: THE CASE OF THE FRONTAL LOBES

There is a good deal of interest in the study of relations between maturation of specific brain areas and the development of cognitive processes (Bell & Fox 1994; Diamond & Goldman-Rakic 1989; Fox & Bell 1990; Thatcher 1994). The frontal region is one brain area that has held interest both for those interested in individual differences and for those interested in cognitive–brain relations. The dorsolateral area of the frontal region is known to play a critical role in processes associated with working memory. Goldman-Rakic (1987a,b; Goldman-Rakic et al. 1983) and Diamond (Diamond & Goldman-Rakic 1983, 1986, 1989; Diamond, Zola-Morgan, & Squire 1989) demonstrated how maturation of this area is critical in the performance of certain cognitive tasks that develop in the first and second years of life in the human infant. More recently, Diamond and colleagues (1997) showed how variations in infant diet could affect infants with PKU (phenylketonuria) and ultimately compromise their frontal functioning. There is also a good deal of speculation on the role that the frontal lobes might play in inhibition, planning, and executive function behaviors (Chelune et al. 1986; Dennis 1991; Welsh, Pennington, & Groisser 1991). The frontal cortex is also directly involved in multiple behavioral components associated with emotion, such as the motor facilitation of emotion expression, the organization and integration of cognitive processes underlying emotion, and the ability to regulate emotions (Dawson 1994; Fox 1994).

Although a large corpus of evidence exists on EEG frequency development in posterior regions, there has been little research directed toward frontal EEG development. Much of the hesitation in examining frontal EEG stemmed from the belief that the frontal lobes did not develop until later childhood. However, recent neuroimaging studies suggest otherwise. Chugani and Phelps (1986) found an increase in glucose metabolism in the frontal cortex in human infants between 8 and 12 months, providing evidence for changes in frontal activity during the first year of life.

Developmental research with nonclinical populations utilizing measures of brain electrical activity (whether via

EEG or ERP) has examined changes in frontal lobe activity over the first years of life (Bell & Fox 1994, 1996). There are also studies that have used measures of EEG or ERP as dependent variables, examining frontal response as a function of cognitive challenge (Nelson 1994). Some studies have attempted to link these measures to known developmental changes in specific brain structures and the behaviors purportedly subsumed by those structures.

One example of this linkage may be found in the sequence of studies by Diamond and Goldman-Rakic (1989) and Bell and Fox (1992, 1994). Diamond and Goldman-Rakic studied infant nonhuman primates and were able to show (by ablation of specific regions of frontal cortex) that performance on paradigms such as the delayed response task or Piaget's A-not-B task involved maturation and integrity of the dorsolateral frontal cortex. Bell and Fox (1992) followed up on this work, recording EEG monthly from infants aged 6 to 12 months. At each session, infants were assessed on the A-not-B task. Bell and Fox (1992) found a correlation between EEG recorded over the frontal region and performance on the A-not-B task in human infants. They suggested that the EEG recordings reflected activity generated from the dorsolateral frontal cortex. Such studies are suggestive of the manner in which EEG may inform knowledge of cognitive development.

Fox (Fox & Bell 1990; Fox et al. 1992) explored frontal lobe maturation during the latter half of the first year of life using frontal EEG frequency measures. The EEG was recorded from left and right frontal, parietal, and occipital scalp locations monthly in a group of 13 healthy full-term infants from 7 until 12 months of age. A measure of relative power for each region was computed using the ratio of 6–9-Hz to 1–4-Hz power at each age. The data revealed an increase in 6–9-Hz power in the frontal region over age, suggesting an increase in EEG power from the frontal region in the second half of the first year of life. These EEG data, in combination with the neuroimaging findings mentioned earlier, suggest that the frontal lobes are active and developing during the latter half of the first year of life. Changes in EEG power in the frontal region during the latter half of the first year of life might reflect frontal lobe maturation.

Bell and Fox (1994) also examined EEG coherence values between anterior and posterior electrode locations in the sample just described. They found stronger coherence between the frontal and occipital sites across age compared with the frontal and parietal sites. This pattern of long- versus short-distance coherence suggests the maturation of anterior and posterior connections over the second half of the first year of life – connections that are necessary for the sequencing of complex behavior (Pribram 1973).

EEG AND THE DEVELOPMENT OF EMOTIONS

Based upon a series of adult studies indicating that the frontal region is involved in certain aspects of emotional behavior (Schwartz, Davidson, & Maer 1975; Schwartz et al. 1976), Fox and Davidson completed a series of papers in which they examined the relation between EEG asymmetry and the expression of emotion in human infants. Their first study (Davidson & Fox 1982) investigated EEG in 10-month-old infants who viewed a videotape of an actress while the actress was smiling or crying. In two independent studies, Davidson and Fox found that infants exhibited greater left frontal EEG asymmetry when viewing the smiling face than when viewing the crying face. Fox and Davidson (1984) interpreted these results as suggesting that the frontal region was specialized for the control of the expression of behaviors involved in approach and withdrawal. Emotions constitute a class of behaviors that can be parsed into those associated with approach (such as joy or interest) or withdrawal (disgust, fear, distress) (see Fox 1991).

In a subsequent test of this model, Fox and Davidson (1986a) presented 1- and 2-day-old infants with different liquid tastes (sugar water, citric acid, and plain water). They recorded EEG in response to the presentation of the tastes and found differences in asymmetry along the approach–withdrawal dimension. Further studies with 10-month-old infants who were responding to the approach of an unfamiliar adult (Fox & Davidson 1987) or maternal separation (Fox & Davidson 1988) confirmed the role of behaviors associated with either approach or withdrawal as being associated with left or right frontal EEG asymmetry.

Subsequently, both Davidson (1995; Wheeler, Davidson, & Tomarken 1993) and Fox (1991) found that the pattern of resting or baseline frontal EEG asymmetry was itself a marker for the disposition of the subject to express affects associated with either approach or withdrawal. For example, Davidson and Fox (1989) reported that differences in tonic frontal EEG arousal predicted infants' emotional responses. Infants who displayed a pattern of greater relative right frontal EEG activation exhibited a shorter latency to cry in response to maternal separation at age 10 months compared with infants who displayed left frontal asymmetry. Individual differences in frontal EEG were also shown to predict affective style and personality in young adults. Adults who displayed a pattern of greater relative right frontal EEG asymmetry rated film clips more negatively (Tomarken et al. 1990) and were less sociable in a dyadic interaction (Schmidt & Fox 1994) than subjects exhibiting left frontal EEG asymmetry. Together, these studies suggest that stable individual differences in frontal EEG (e.g. Fox et al. 1992) may reflect individual differences in temperamental characteristics of the individual. Additional work from Fox's laboratory with behaviorally inhibited toddlers and preschool children seems to confirm this notion (Fox et al. 1995).

Behavioral inhibition reflects a tendency to display fear and wariness in response to novel stimuli (Kagan, Reznick, & Snidman 1987). Behaviorally inhibited children display long latencies before approaching novel stimuli, exhibit a high frequency of negative affect, and remain in close proximity to their mothers in response to the presentation of novel stimuli. Children who display this pattern of behavior toward novel social stimuli have been characterized as shy and timid. In addition, children who remain inhibited during the first few years of life are at risk for anxiety disorders in later childhood (Hirshfeld et al. 1992).

Calkins et al. (1996) examined frontal lobe development in a group of infants selected for temperamental constellations thought to predict behavioral inhibition and shyness in early childhood. Eighty-one healthy infants were selected at 4 months of age from a larger sample of 207 using procedures similar to those reported by Kagan and Snidman (1991). Infants were observed in their homes at 4 months of age and videotaped as they responded to novel auditory and visual stimuli. The 81 infants were selected based upon their frequency of motor activity and their degree of positive and negative affect displayed in response to these novel stimuli. Three groups were formed on the basis of behavior at age 4 months. The Negative group comprised infants who responded to the stimuli with high motor activity, high negative affect, and low positive affect. Kagan and Snidman (1991) found that this temperamental group of infants was behaviorally inhibited at 14 months of age. The Positive group consisted of infants who responded with high amounts of both motor activity and positive affect but low amounts of negative affect. The third group of infants – referred to as the Low responders – were characterized by their low levels of activity, including motor activity and both positive and negative affect.

The infants were seen again at 9, 14, and 24 months, at which times their EEGs were recorded. At 14 months, each infant was observed interacting during a free play situation and with a series of unfamiliar stimuli designed to elicit his or her response to novelty. The data revealed that infants who were easily distressed by novelty at 4 months of age exhibited greater relative right frontal EEG activation asymmetry at 9 months (as well as at 24 months) than infants in the other two groups. These same infants likewise displayed a greater number of behaviors reflecting inhibition at both 14 and 24 months of age. It is also important to note that infants who displayed a pattern of stable right frontal EEG across the first two years tended to be more inhibited at both 14 and 24 months compared with infants who exhibited a pattern of stable left frontal EEG during this time (Fox, Calkins, & Bell 1994).

These data suggest that greater activity in the right versus left frontal region may serve as a marker for infants' temperamental wariness in response to novelty. Infants who display a pattern of right frontal EEG activation appear less able to successfully regulate the arousal of negative affect, and this may serve as a marker of subsequent behavioral inhibition in toddlers.

The pattern of frontal EEG asymmetry and inhibition is critical for understanding the development of social withdrawal in the school years. The preschool years coincide with the development of social skills and peer interactions, both of which are determinants of the child's subsequent social development. Children who are shy and socially reticent often fail to develop such skills and hence are at risk for social withdrawal, social anxiety, and internalizing problems during the early school years (Rubin, Stewart, & Coplan 1995). Conversely, children who are aggressive and intrusive with other children often fail to develop social skills and peer relationships. This group of children may be at risk for externalizing problems during the early school years. The origins of both forms of maladaptive social behavior may be linked to emotion regulatory problems and frontal dysfunction.

In an attempt to examine this issue, Fox et al. (1995) observed 48 4-year-old children during play in groups of four. These groups consisted of children who were unfamiliar to one another but were of the same age and sex. The play session was divided into five parts: (1) unstructured free play, (2) clean-up, (3) birthday speeches, (4) cooperation task, and (5) unstructured free play. The children were unobtrusively observed during this time, and their social behaviors were subsequently coded for measures of social participation.

A composite measure of social reticence was computed from behaviors displayed during the play session. This composite included the following standardized measures: (1) proportion of anxious behavior, latency to first spontaneous utterance, and proportion of reticent behavior (unoccupied and onlooking behavior) during freeplay; (2) proportion of unoccupied behavior during clean-up and cooperation task; (3) the inverse of speech episode duration and the inverse of total time talking during the speech episode.

Each child was seen individually some two weeks after the group visit, at which time EEG was recorded for three minutes while the child was seated and attending to a visual stimulus. The data revealed that children who displayed a high proportion of anxious behavior and wariness in response to their peers during the play session exhibited greater relative right frontal EEG activation – a function of less power (more activation) in the right than the left frontal site – compared with their more sociable and less anxious peers.

In a second study, Fox et al. (1996) observed an additional 48 4-year-olds using the same procedures. This study examined whether the interaction of resting frontal EEG asymmetry and social behavior during peer play was related to the occurrence of maladaptive behavior in preschoolers. The data suggested that highly sociable children who were "right frontal" were more likely to exhibit externalizing problems than sociable children who were "left frontal." In addition, shy children who displayed right frontal EEG asymmetry were more likely to exhibit internalizing problems than shy children who displayed left frontal EEG asymmetry. These findings suggest that individual differences in frontal EEG activation may play an important role in the development of maladaptive social behavior during the preschool years. Children who display greater right frontal EEG activation may not have such competencies as verbal mediation skills and analytic abilities – thought to be subserved by the left frontal region – which are necessary to successfully regulate affective arousal. Children who display a pattern of right frontal EEG activation and extreme social reticence or sociability may be at risk for subsequent affective and behavioral problems. Indeed, frontal dysregulation has been implicated in conduct disorders by others (Moffit & Henry 1989).

EEG AND THE DEVELOPMENT OF BEHAVIOR PROBLEMS IN OLDER CHILDREN AND ADULTS

Psychophysiologists have long been interested in psychopathology. There is a long history of research investigating CNS responses (via EEG and ERPs) of clinical populations, including patients diagnosed with schizophrenia, depression, and psychosis (Lahmeyer et al. 1989; Miller & Lesser 1988; Niznikiewicz et al. 1997; Pollock & Schneider 1990; Pritchard 1986). There have also been a number of studies of CNS responding with children who have been diagnosed with specific psychiatric disorders, such as hyperactivity, attention deficit disorder, and conduct disorder (Chelune et al. 1986; Raine & Venables 1987; Raine, Venables, & Williams 1990a). These studies have, by and large, attempted to outline the physiological mechanisms that are associated with the cognitive or affective deficits seen in these child clinical populations.

Over the past ten years there has been an increased interest in processes associated with the development of psychopathology in children, along with a rethinking of the manner in which these issues ought to be approached. In particular, questions arise about the origins and factors (including environmental) that predispose some children to certain conditions and, more generally, about the nature of the interaction between dispositions and environments that may be the ultimate cause of certain types of psychopathology in children (Cicchetti 1993). Researchers have recognized that certain forms of child psychopathology (particularly internalizing or externalizing disorders) do not arise *de novo* but rather are the end product of multiple factors – including infant or child temperament, parenting style, and certain environmental correlates (see e.g. Cicchetti & Richters 1993). Such an approach is analogous to the interactionist model detailed earlier, and it necessitates (for the psychophysiologist) an analysis at the level of individual differences in child or infant disposition that incorporates the effects of environment (or parenting) on these initial dispositions.

One example of this approach is the work on the effects of maternal depression on infant physiology and ultimately on child behavioral outcomes. Such studies have examined the effects of maternal depression on infant physiology (Dawson et al. 1992a; Field et al. 1995). It is widely known that adults who are depressed display less positive affect and more anxiousness than their nondepressed counterparts. Depressed adults are also known to exhibit reduced left frontal EEG activation (Henriques & Davidson 1991) and greater right frontal EEG activation (Henriques & Davidson 1990; Schaffer, Davidson, & Saron 1983) than nondepressed adults. Women who are depressed are known to display less positive affect and reduced levels of stimulation when interacting with their infants (Cohn et al. 1986; Cohn & Tronick 1989; Field 1986; Field et al. 1988). Infants of depressed mothers display less positive affect and increased irritability (Cohn et al. 1986; Field 1986; Field et al. 1985) as well as greater frontal EEG activation than infants of nonsymptomatic mothers (Dawson et al. 1992a). The findings reported by Dawson and her colleagues were for infants who ranged in age from 11 to 17 months. A similar pattern of frontal EEG asymmetry was documented in infants as early as the first six months of life (Field et al. 1995).

Field et al. (1995) recorded baseline EEG in infants of depressed and nondepressed adolescent mothers. Infants ranged in age from 3 to 6 months, and the EEG was recorded during an alert state of attention. Infants of depressed mothers exhibited greater right frontal activation than infants of nondepressed mothers. Collectively, these studies suggest that maternal depression may affect infant physiology in the first two years of life. The fact that maternal depression affects brain electrical activity is consistent with an interactionist approach to development. It is also possible that the pattern of frontal EEG asymmetry in infants of depressed mothers may reflect a heritable component of the mothers' depression. There have been relatively few studies conducted on the possible genetic basis of EEG patterns. Further, it remains unknown whether the patterns of EEG asymmetry observed in infancy remain stable over time (given certain types of parenting and environments) or whether children who display these EEG patterns as infants exhibit behavioral difficulties as they become older. However, answers to these questions will require longitudinal studies that operationalize and assess the interactive processes involved in development.

CARDIOVASCULAR MEASURES AND THE STUDY OF COGNITIVE DEVELOPMENT

Berg and Berg (1979) emphasized the utility of cardiovascular and other autonomic measures in the study of developmental psychology because these systems are relatively well developed at birth and during infancy. For example, the heart begins to beat by the fourth week after conception, and with the development of central control mechanisms the heart becomes responsive to state changes (Groome et al. 1997). By 30 weeks after conception, heart rate changes are reliably associated with changes in internal states such as sleep cycles.

As with adults, infants demonstrate directional cardiac responses to external stimuli. The direction of change is directly related to the development of neural control over the heart. In both humans and rats, Porges (1983) reported monotonic increases in the extent of vagal control over the heart across gestational age (see also Porges, McCabe, & Yongue 1982). At birth, infants show reliable heart rate accelerations in response to stimulation (airstreams); however, by 2.5 months of age, infants show consistent heart rate decelerations in response to the same stimulus (Berg & Berg 1979). Others have noted significant shifts in baseline levels of heart rate variability at around 2–4 months of age (Attuel et al. 1986; Lewis et al. 1970). These shifts in baseline and reactive cardiac patterns may reflect a general physiological reorganization of the CNS related to increasing cortical control. By 3–4 months of age, infants show consistent heart rate decelerations in response to stimulation regardless of modality (i.e., visual, acoustic, or tactile). These decelerative responses are interpreted as reflecting infants' active processing of sensory events.

Infants do not simply respond indiscriminately to the environment; rather, their orienting responses are sensitive to stimulus parameters. Even newborns show visual preferences for horizontal versus vertical gratings, curved versus straight contours, and novel versus repeated stimuli (Slater & Morison 1991). These visual preferences are accompanied by larger and longer decelerative heart rate responses (Lewis et al. 1966; McCall & Kagan 1967). That infants can discriminate among such stimuli and that these discriminations are reflected in different patterns of heart rate change gave rise to important developments in experimental paradigms for work with infants. For example, the habituation–dishabituation paradigm (Graham & Clifton 1966) provides a means for indexing fundamental cognitive processes such as attention, memory, and responsiveness to novelty, and it is still used as an index of basic sensory capacities. Specifically, with repeated exposure to the same stimulus, behaviors (i.e., visual attention) and physiological responses (i.e., heart rate decelerations) become habituated or less pronounced, reflecting an infant's waning attention. During dishabituation trials, a novel stimulus is presented and stimulus detection is marked by restored responding such as renewed visual attention or cardiac decelerations.

Differences in tonic and reactive cardiac responses can also serve as markers of individual differences in physical and/or cognitive status. For example, differences in parasympathetic tone have been related to levels of infant attentiveness and reactivity (Richards 1987). Perinatal events (e.g., physical stress and recovery from maternal medication) have been reported to temporarily block the decelerative response (Adkinson & Berg 1976), and more enduring conditions such as malnourishment have longer-term effects on cardiac reactivity (Lester 1975). Thus, cardiovascular responses can serve as a means for studying development within particular domains of psychology (including cognitive, sensory, and perceptual development) as well as a means of assessing individual differences in the neurally mediated capacity to respond within these domains.

In order to serve as a marker of enduring individual differences, as opposed to simply differences in state, cardiac measures must show stability over time and over shifts in development and maturation (Porges et al. 1994b). Individual differences in cardiovascular measures, including heart period and heart rate variability, show little stability from birth until at least 3 months of age (Fracasso et al. 1994; Snidman et al. 1995; Stifter & Fox 1990). For example, Stifter and Fox (1990) found little stability from birth to 5 months of age on measures of heart period, heart rate variance, and vagal tone, but moderate stability from 5 to 14 months of age. Similarly, Fracasso et al. (1994) assessed vagal tone and mean heart period during baseline and following the presentation of emotion-eliciting stimuli at four time points between 5 and 13 months of age. These measures were significantly related at all ages, with the magnitude of the correlations increasing with age.

With older children, Fox and Field (1989) reported moderate stability in vagal tone and heart rate variability across a six-month period in a sample of preschool-aged children. Longer-term stabilities, from infancy into early childhood, were reported by Porges et al. (1994b) for both heart period and vagal tone. From 9 months until 3 years of age, heart period and vagal tone increased across the entire group, but children maintained their rankings relative to the group across the same time interval. Porges et al. (1994b) further reported that the stability of heart period and vagal tone was similar in magnitude to the stability of maternal reports of temperament over the same time period.

CARDIOVASCULAR MEASURES AS INDICES OF RISK STATUS

Premature neonates demonstrate different patterns of both tonic and reactive cardiovascular activity than do full-term newborns. For example, premature infants – both those who are healthy and those who are at greater risk due to various medical complications – tend to have higher heart rates (Krafchuk, Tronick, & Clifton 1983) and greater heart rate variability than full-term infants. Premature infants also demonstrate patterns of cardiovascular responding to environmental stimuli that are markedly different than those of full-term infants. Rose, Schmidt, and Bridger (1976) reported that sleeping preterm infants exhibited depressed cardiac responses to various tactile stimuli in comparison with full-term infants. Further, Krafchuk et al.

(1983) found that, compared to full-term infants, high-risk premature infants showed slower and smaller magnitude cardiac changes in response to auditory stimuli and in response to a dishabituation trial (in which the head end of the infant's bassinet was raised 2–3 inches and then released). However, once the high-risk group reacted to the stimuli, particularly the dishabituation stimulus, they took longer to habituate their cardiac response. The mix of hypo- and hyperresponsiveness was interpreted as reflecting the relative immaturity of the CNS. This pattern of reacting provides an infant with less control and flexibility with which to regulate his or her responses to the environment.

Global cardiac measures such as heart period and heart period variability have been used as a means for detecting gross dysfunction (i.e., severe brain damage) among neonates with a variety of clinical pathologies. For instance, Porges (1983) used vagal tone, thought to provide a more sensitive index of CNS functioning, to classify a group of neonates along a continuum reflecting the severity of neuropathology. Higher vagal tone was associated with lower risk status. Higher vagal tone has also been associated with better cognitive outcomes by the end of the first year of life. For example, infants with higher vagal tone at birth had higher Bayley MDI scores at both 8 and 12 months than did infants with lower vagal tone (Fox & Porges 1985). Although children in the extremes of the distribution of vagal tone had consistent outcomes, there was not a perfect linear relationship. That is, not all children with low vagal tone performed poorly on the Bayley MDI. These findings raise the more general issue of how different patterns of early reactivity, as reflected in cardiovascular measures, affect (and are affected by) the nature of interactions with environment and caregivers in promoting development.

CARDIOVASCULAR MEASURES AND EMOTIONAL DEVELOPMENT

In general, greater heart rate variability during the first year of life is associated with greater reactivity, both cardiovascular and behavioral, to environmental stimulation. These differences apply not only to sensory stimuli but also to social stimuli, which for young infants consists primarily of interactions with caregivers. Work by Fox (1989) suggests that these differences in global reactivity are associated with differences in self-regulation and the development of particular social behaviors.

In infants, differences in heart period variability have been associated with differences in facial expressivity. Specifically, 3-month-old infants with greater heart rate variability displayed interest expressions of longer duration in face-to-face interactions with their mothers (Fox & Gelles 1984). Stifter and Fox (1990) found that, at 5 months of age, infants with greater heart rate variability displayed

more negative expressions in response to an arm restraint procedure used to elicit distress or anger in the laboratory. Stifter, Fox, and Porges (1989) further reported that 5-month-olds with higher levels of heart rate variability expressed a greater number of positive emotional expressions, especially in response to an approaching stranger. Thus, heart rate variability appears to be related to global reactivity or responsivity (both positive and negative) in early infancy.

Heart rate variability is also associated with infants' capacities to flexibly regulate their own reactions. Infants with greater heart rate variability at birth displayed more self-regulatory behaviors in response to an arm restraint procedure at 5 months of age (Fox 1989). Behaviors such as looks to mother, looks at self in the mirror, arm and leg thrusts, and vocalizations were coded as self-regulatory. Heart rate variability is likely related to self-regulatory behaviors via the common relations with infants' capacities to flexibly implement strategies for managing interactions with the environment. By the second year of life, differences in reactivity and regulation are apparent in children's behaviors in social contexts. At 14 months of age, children with high vagal tone approached an adult stranger more readily and spent less time in close proximity to mother during a laboratory visit. Vagal tone measured at 14 months of age related to the same infants' reactions and use of self-regulatory behaviors during their 5-month visit. Specifically, children with high vagal tone at 14 months of age expressed more negative affect during the 5-month visit and were more likely to have cried during the arm restraint procedure (at 5 months) than children with low vagal tone.

Cardiovascular measures, as assessed during infancy, have concurrent relations to temperament and also predictive relations to temperament at later ages. For example, Porges et al. (1994b) found that high vagal tone was related to maternal reports of difficult temperament at 9 months of age. It is interesting that – although no concurrent relations were found between vagal tone and temperament ratings at the 3-year assessment – higher vagal tone as assessed at 9 months of age was predictive of maternal reports of less difficult temperament when the same children were 3 years old. Nine-month vagal tone predicted 3-year temperament reports independently of any relations between the 9-month and 3-year temperament reports.

This apparent switch in the direction of relation between vagal tone and temperament is probably best explained by considering the influences of early temperament on infants' interactions with their environment, particularly their interactions with caregivers. High vagal tone during early infancy appears to be associated with greater global reactivity, which is likely to be interpreted by caregivers as "difficult." However, vagal tone is also related to infants' abilities to self-regulate their reactions. Thus, the capacity to self-regulate at 3 years of age is likely interpreted by caregivers as reflecting a relatively easy temperament. It may be that infants who are reactive to their environments from birth, in a sense, create more opportunities for learning how to flexibly regulate their own arousal. Reactivity likely leads to more contact with caregivers, leading to more socialization experiences related to issues of regulating reactivity. In contrast, less reactive infants may have fewer learning experiences related to issues of self-regulation. However, hypotheses regarding the ways in which reactivity, regulation, and socialization experiences interact to promote development have yet to be empirically examined.

CARDIOVASCULAR MEASURES AND THE DEVELOPMENT OF BEHAVIOR PROBLEMS IN OLDER CHILDREN AND ADOLESCENTS

Individual differences in the tonic level of activation and in the degree of reactivity of the ANS have been related to the development of specific behavior problems. There have been mixed results relating tonic levels of autonomic activity to behavior problems. For example, in a prospective study of criminal behavior, Raine et al. (1990a) found that lower resting heart rate and fewer nonspecific skin conductance responses assessed in a sample of 15-year-old boys were associated with an increased likelihood of criminal behavior at 24 years of age. These findings suggest that ANS underarousal may be associated – perhaps even causally – with criminal behavior. This global pattern of underarousal may lead individuals to seek out stimulation, for example, by engaging in antisocial or criminal behaviors. In the studies by Raine and his colleagues, ANS underarousal has been hypothesized to be attibutable to both reduced sympathetic modulation (Raine et al. 1990a,b) and enhanced vagal modulation (Raine & Jones 1987; Raine & Venables 1984). In contrast, Zahn and Kruesi (1993) concluded that there were no consistent differences in tonic levels of arousal or generalized ANS activity between boys with behavior disorders and their same-aged peers. Indeed, in a review of studies, Raine (1993) reported on the inconsistencies of the findings relating global underarousal to antisocial behaviors.

Using spectral analytic techniques, Mezzacappa et al. (1997) examined more directly the relations between adolescent boys' self-reports of antisocial behavior and autonomic regulatory influences over the heart. Mezzacappa and co-workers analyzed the transfer of respiratory variability to heart rate variability. This transfer can essentially be thought of as the heart rate response to quantified changes in respiration, with individual differences in the transfer dynamics implying differences in the central processing of cardiorespiratory interactions. Using this logic, the findings indicated that the central processing of respiratory–heart rate relations was disrupted in antisocial individuals, which would support the literature relating

parasympathetic control to the integrity of regulatory processes (Porges, Doussard-Roosevelt, & Maiti 1994a).

In addition to tonic levels of autonomic arousal, antisocial behaviors have been related to unique patterns of autonomic reactions to various environmental stimuli. Autonomic reactivity has been related to the development of behavior problems through their common relations to orienting responses and orienting deficits. Cardiovascular reactivity can serve as an index of the orienting reflex, which assesses the extent to which a subject attends to and processes an eliciting stimulus. Raine et al. (1990b) found that criminal behavior at 24 years of age was predicted by hyporeactive heart rate responses to auditory stimuli as assessed at 15 years of age. This pattern of hyporesponsivity was predictive over and above the predictive effects of tonic heart rate, suggesting that the response deficit was not simply a function of lower overall physiological arousal and that it may be a risk factor for later criminal behavior.

More recently, Raine and his colleagues expanded their work to explore patterns of psychophysiological responding that may serve to protect antisocial adolescents from going on to commit crimes in early adulthood. Specifically, they hypothesized that adolescents who engage in antisocial behavior but who do *not* go on to commit crimes in adulthood may have distinctly hyperreactive patterns of physiological responding in comparison to normal individuals and to those antisocial adolescents who do go on to commit crimes in early adulthood (Raine, Venables, & Williams 1995). Such a model goes against previous theories in which "adolescent-limited" antisocial individuals are seen as falling between their more resistant antisocial peers and their normal peers on a continuum of antisocial behavior. Indeed, Raine et al. (1995) reported that adolescent-limited antisocial individuals had higher resting heart rates and greater electrodermal orienting responses than their resistant antisocial peers. Raine et al. (1995) further reported that the adolescent-limited antisocial individuals had higher heart rates and greater electrodermal orienting responses when compared also with a sample of normal adolescents; however, these differences did not reach statistical significance. It is therefore difficult to deduce whether this pattern of greater autonomic arousal indeed reflects a unique protective mechanism against committing crime or whether the adolescent-limited antisocial individuals simply respond autonomically like their non-antisocial peers. Regardless, the work of Raine and his colleagues highlights the relation between both tonic and reactive patterns of autonomic responding and antisocial behaviors.

The direction of heart rate change in response to environmental stimuli has further been interpreted in the context of social information processing. Cardiac decelerations, as in work with infants, are interpreted as reflecting the active intake of information from the environment. This style of responding may serve as a marker of such other-oriented focused attention as the experiences of empathy and sympathy. In contrast, cardiac accelerations are interpreted as reflecting the rejection of environmental inputs and may serve as a marker of a person's attempt to actively cope with personal distress or anxiety (Zahn-Waxler et al. 1995). For example, preschoolers who responded with cardiac decelerations to a videotape designed to induce sadness were observed displaying more prosocial behavior and greater empathic concern in response to others' distress when compared to children who responded with little or no cardiac deceleration. In contrast, children with lower tonic heart rates while viewing the sadness induction tape were observed demonstrating more avoidance and joy reactions during others' distress.

In contrast to the findings linking cardiac hypoactivation to conduct problems, cardiac hyperactivation may be related to behavior problems of an internalizing nature. Children who expressed few emotions while viewing a mood induction tape were found to have higher, more stable heart rates, lower vagal tone, and less change in heart rate (from baseline) in response to the mood induction tape (Cole et al. 1996). This pattern of cardiovascular responding was interpreted as reflecting a resistance to external input and an increased focus on internal state. The pattern of high, stable heart rate is similar to that reported by Kagan and his colleagues relating cardiovascular measures to behavioral inhibition in children (Kagan, Reznick, & Snidman 1987, 1988). In an examination of the changes in the frequency components of heart rate variability during cognitive challenge, Kagan et al. (1987, 1988) found that behaviorally inhibited children displayed greater shifts in the distribution of heart rate variability toward the LF band of the distribution. Kagan and colleagues interpreted this shift as reflecting an increase in sympathetic influences over the heart during the cognitive challenge. In a more direct examination of the associations between anxiety and sympathetic cardiac influences, Mezzacappa et al. (1997) used the change in LF heart rate variability with postural manipulations (supine to standing) as an indicator of sympathetic cardiac influences on heart rate. Sympathetic influences were positively correlated with adolescent boys' self-reports of anxiety.

Inferential Context: Methodological Issues in the Psychophysiological Study of Infants and Children

There are obvious methodological issues involved in the recording of EEG, ERPs, or ECG in adult populations. These have been discussed in detail elsewhere, and there are published recommendations regarding standards of methods for each measure (Berntson et al. 1997; Pivik et al. 1993; Task Force 1996). Additionally, there are unique methodological problems when using these measures with infants and young children. These include movement and

muscle artifact, placement of electrodes, state changes of the infant or young child, definition of a baseline, and the need to link physiology to behavioral response. It should be noted that these methodological issues are not specific to acquiring EEG, ERP, or ECG response measures but in fact are common to the recording of all psychophysiological responses.

Movement and Muscle Artifact. Obviously, one cannot instruct infants or young children to sit still so as to record resting levels of physiology. And, when presenting either auditory or visual stimuli, it is not possible with infants or young children to issue instructions to pay attention to the stimulus or not to move. Therefore, recording of either autonomic or brain electrical activity is fraught with the possibility of confounding by unwarranted movement artifact. Researchers have attempted to design studies that capture the young subject's attention for long enough periods of time so as to provide data for analysis. Further, developmental psychophysiologists have usually designed systems that allow them the ability and flexibility to edit their physiological records for periods of artifact. Nevertheless, the problem is a critical one for investigators wishing to study these populations. Studies that do not report how they edited or artifact-scored the data or that do not report the ratio of artifact-rejected to "good" data may be including points that are unwarranted.

Electrode Placement. Prior to the advent of neuroimaging techniques such as MRI, the placement of electrodes was accomplished by the examination of brain geometry and topography via autopsy, and these findings were generalized to create a set of standard placement sites (Jasper 1958). Jasper mapped what became accepted as an international set of placements of 20 electrodes over the scalp, reflecting the major cortical divisions as well as the various sulci of the cortex. A unique set of problems arise in the application of the 10–20 system for use with infants and young children. In the Jasper system, the placement of electrodes relies on a ratio of distances between anterior and posterior sites. It is unclear whether this same ratio exists across development or whether different regions of the brain mature (physically) at different rates, leading to differences in the relation between anterior to posterior growth. A number of researchers (e.g. Myslobodsky et al. 1990) have examined this problem, primarily again through autopsy, and have found that the 10–20 system does an adequate job in defining placement of electrodes across key cortical regions. With the advent of MRI, a number of studies have begun to examine the accuracy of electrode placement with respect to actual physical landmarks of cortical topography (Lagerlund et al. 1993). Overall, these studies have found that, by and large, the 10–20 system does a good job in defining the location of electrodes over significant cortical landmarks in adult populations. Less is known, however, about the adequacy of this system for use with infants and children.

State Change. A third methodological issue involves the need to attend to the state of the subject, particularly when they are infants or young children. Again, it is not possible to issue instructions regarding level of task attention to these populations, nor is it always possible to time laboratory visits so that they are optimal for the level of attention necessary for the task. These issues are particularly salient for infants whose ability to maintain a particular state of attention may be fragile. Often researchers working with infants will time their assessments with the sleep-wake-eating cycle of the child. Subjects are often seen prior to a feeding, when they are awake and alert – or after a feeding and a sleep cycle. Aside from concern regarding the timing of the assessment, it is incumbent upon the researcher to monitor behavioral state so as to ensure that the physiological responses recorded across subjects are done so consistently with respect to their states.

Definition of a Baseline. Very often psychophysiologists are interested in the change in response of a measure from a "resting baseline" to some other state that has been elicited as a function of cognitive or affective challenge. Alternatively, researchers may be interested in individual differences in the level of resting state of a group of individuals (for measures of EEG, blood pressure, or heart rate). In all instances, the assumption underlying measurement of a resting baseline or a prechallenge condition is that subjects are all in the same affective and cognitive state. It is not always clear that this assumption is being met with adult populations, and it is even more difficult with infant and child populations. It is sometimes impossible to instruct subjects to remain in a particular state for a period of time, and state variability is great for very young infants. Researchers have met this challenge by presenting infants with certain types of stimuli that have a general appeal and create conditions of quiet attention across large groups of subjects. So, for example, Fox and colleagues present infants with a rotating bingo wheel that contains multicolored bingo balls. This display captivates most infants' attention, and EEG can be collected during these times because it remains relatively free of movement artifact. However, this event and the state it elicits from infants is one of focused attention, which is obviously different from the "resting baseline" collected in some adult studies. State control and equivalence of baseline are thus critical issues as you go up the developmental ladder.

Linking Physiological Responses to Behavior. Monitoring behavior during the experiment leads to another critical methodological issue for studies with infant and young child populations. In the absence of self-report, it is necessary that infant or young child psychophysiological responses be anchored to behavior. If the researcher does not have this anchor, then it will be difficult to interpret the physiological response being recorded. For example, in studies of infant face discrimination, Nelson and colleagues (e.g. Nelson & Collins 1992) routinely tested infants in behavioral paradigms to ensure they are able to make the types of discriminations being presented in the ERP study. The coordination of behavioral testing and ERP testing lends support to any interpretation these workers may have about neural processing of face discrimination. Fox argued that inference about physiological correlates of emotion response should be made only in the presence of observable behavioral measures such as facial or vocal expressions (Fox 1994; Fox & Davidson 1986b). In his work there is a link between report of EEG activity during the expression of certain emotions and behavioral signs of these emotions. Obviously, as children develop and are able to provide self-report measures or appropriate motor responses, these should be used in linking physiology to behavior. In general, however, physiological reactivity should be reported in infants or young children only in the presence of observable behavioral response.

Signal Localization. Aside from these unique methodological problems, recording EEG and ERPs from infants and young children poses additional issues to researchers interested in the localization of these signals. In a sense, these issues go beyond the very real concerns about localization that researchers have for the signals recorded from adults. The morphological changes that occur over development during the first years of life may influence the localization of electrical activity emanating from the brain. These changes include myelination of certain brain areas as well as dendritic arborization (Greenough et al. 1987; Greenough & Volkmar 1973). The little we know about neural development compounds the problem of accurate localization of source activity in the young infant. In addition, the fontanelle does not close in most infants until the second half of the first year of life. The fontanelle may actually create an electrical "sink hole" around which current will not flow; obviously, this could change the nature of the signals being transduced off the scalp.

THOUGHTS ON THE STUDY OF DEVELOPMENTAL PSYCHOPHYSIOLOGY

Psychophysiology has lagged behind other branches of psychology in integrating knowledge of developmental processes into its approach to research. A survey of papers or posters presented over the past ten years at psychophysiology conferences finds only a handful of presentations in which children are studied and fewer yet in which developmental questions are asked. Too often, when infants or children are studied, their responses are treated similarly to adult data. These populations have often been approached as if they were "little adults," with the measurements and interpretations of their responses viewed against a background of group differences (infant, child, adult) attributed to age. To some extent, the lack of interest in developmental processes is changing within the psychophysiological community. There is increased interest within cognitive neuroscience in the development of processes, such as memory or attention, that have been studied intensively within psychophysiology. This renewed interest has developed alongside improved technology that makes the psychophysiological study of developmental populations more accessible.

Through the integration of research in the areas of developmental psychology and psychophysiology, advances have been made in understanding the structural and functional developments of the autonomic and central nervous systems in infancy and childhood. Substantial progress has been made toward unraveling the intricate processes underlying development in these systems and the relations these developments have to changes in cognition and behavior during childhood. That children and adults differ in the organization of physiological systems highlights the need to investigate the development of these systems in detail. The better these systems are understood as they exist and develop in children, the more they contribute both conceptually and methodologically to our understanding of the development of basic psychological processes, including cognition, perception, and emotion. Further, stable individual differences in the activity and reactivity of these systems provide insight into the basic processes involved in the development of both normal and problem behaviors.

REFERENCES

Adkinson, C. D., & Berg, W. K. (1976). Cardiac deceleration in newborns: Habituation, dishabituation, and offset responses. *Journal of Experimental Child Psychology, 21,* 46–60.

Akselrod, S., Gordon, D., Madwed, J. B., Snidman, N. C., Shannon, D. C., & Cohen, R. J. (1985). Hemodynamic regulation: Investigation by spectral analysis. *American Journal of Physiology, 249,* H867–H875.

Akselrod, S., Gordon, D., Ubel, R. A., Shannon, D. C., Barger, A. C., & Cohen, R. J. (1981). Power spectrum analysis of heart rate fluctuation: A quantitative probe of beat-to-beat cardiovascular control. *Science, 213,* 220–2.

Attuel, P., Leporho, M. A., Ruta, J., Lucet, V., Steinberg, C., Azancot, A., & Coumel, P. (1986). The evolution of the sinus heart rate and variability as a function of age from birth to 16 years. In E. F. Doyle (Ed.), *Pediatric Cardiology: Proceedings of the Second World Congress 1985.* New York: Springer-Verlag.

Ax, A. F. (1953). The physiological differentiation between fear and anger in humans. *Psychosomatic Medicine, 15,* 433–42.

Bell, M. A., & Fox, N. A. (1992). The relations between frontal brain electrical activity and cognitive development during infancy. *Child Development, 63,* 1142–63.

Bell, M. A., & Fox, N. A. (1994). Brain development over the first year of life. Relations between electroencephalographic frequency and coherence and cognitive and affective behaviors. In G. Dawson & K. W. Fischer (Eds.), *Human Behavior and the Developing Brain,* pp. 314–45. New York: Guilford.

Bell, M. A., & Fox, N. A. (1996). Crawling experience is related to changes in cortical organization during infancy: Evidence from EEG coherence. *Developmental Psychobiology, 29,* 551–61.

Benes, F. M., Turtle, M., Khan, Y., & Farol, P. (1994). Myelination of a key relay zone in the hippocampal formation occurs in human brain during childhood, adolescence and adulthood. *Archives of General Psychiatry, 51,* 477–84.

Berg, W. K., & Berg, K. M. (1979). Psychophysiological development in infancy: State, sensory function and attention. In J. D. Osofsky (Ed.), *Handbook of Infant Development,* pp. 283–343. New York: Wiley.

Berger, H. (1929). Über das Elektrenkephalogramm des Menschen: I. *Archiv für Psychiatri und Nervenkrankheiten, 87,* 527–70.

Berger, H. (1932a). Über das Elektrenkephalogramm des Menschen: IV. *Archiv für Psychiatri und Nervenkrankheiten, 97,* 6–26.

Berger, H. (1932b). Über das Elektrenkephalogramm des Menschen: V. *Archiv für Psychiatri und Nervenkrankheiten, 98,* 231–54.

Berntson, G. G., Bigger, J. T., Eckberg, D. L., Grossman, P., Kaufman, P. G., Malik, M., Nagaraja, H. N., Porges, S. W., Saul, J. P., Stone, P. H., & van der Molen, M. W. (1997). Heart rate variability: Origins, methods, and interpretive caveats. *Psychophysiology, 34,* 623–48.

Berntson, G. G., Cacioppo, J. T., & Quigley, K. S. (1993). Respiratory sinus arrhythmia: Autonomic origins, physiological mechanisms, and psychophysiological implications. *Psychophysiology, 30,* 183–96.

Best, C. T. (1993). Emergence of language-specific constraints in perception of non-native speech: A window on early phonological development. In B. de Boysson-Bardies, S. de Schonen, P. Jusczyk, P. MacNeilage, & J. Morton (Eds.), *Developmental Neurocognition: Speech and Face Processing in the First Year of Life,* pp. 289–304. Boston: Kluwer.

Binkley, P. F., & Boudoulas, H. (1986). Measurement of myocardial inotropy. In C. V. Leier (Ed.), *Cardiotonic Drugs: A Clinical Survey,* pp. 5–48. New York: Dekker.

Cacioppo, J. T., Berntson, G. G., Binkley, P. F., Quigley, K. S., Uchino, B. N., & Fieldstone, A. (1994). Autonomic cardiac control. II. Basal response, noninvasive indices, and autonomic space as revealed by autonomic blockades. *Psychophysiology, 31,* 586–98.

Calkins, S. D., Fox, N. A., & Marshall, T. R. (1996). Behavioral and physiological antecedents of inhibited and uninhibited behavior. *Child Development, 67,* 523–40.

Case, R. (1992). The role of the frontal lobes in the regulation of cognitive development. Special Issue: The role of frontal lobe maturation in cognitive and social development. *Brain and Cognition, 20,* 51–73.

Chelune, G. J., Ferguson, W., Koon, R., & Dickey, T. O. (1986). Frontal lobe disinhibition in attention deficit disorder. *Child Psychiatry and Human Development, 16,* 221–34.

Chugani, H. T., & Phelps, M. E. (1986). Maturational changes in cerebral function in infants determined by 18FDG positron emission tomography. *Science, 231,* 840–3.

Cicchetti, D. (1993). Developmental psychopathology: Reactions, reflections, projections. Special Issue: Setting a path for the coming decade – Some goals and challenges. *Developmental Review, 14,* 471–502.

Cicchetti, D., & Richters, J. E. (1993). Developmental considerations in the investigation of conduct disorder. Special Issue: Toward a developmental perspective on conduct disorder. *Development and Psychopathology, 5,* 331–44.

Cohn, J. F., Matias, R., Tronick, E. Z., Connell, D., & Lyons-Ruth, D. (1986). Face-to-face interactions of depressed mothers and their infants. In E. Z. Tronick & T. Field (Eds.), *Maternal Depression and Infant Disturbance,* pp. 31–45. San Francisco: Jossey-Bass.

Cohn, J. F., & Tronick, E. Z. (1989). Specificity of infants' response to mothers' affective behavior. *Journal of the American Academy of Child and Adolescent Psychiatry, 28,* 242–8.

Cole, P. M., Zahn-Waxler, C., Fox, N. A., Usher, B. A., & Welsh, J. D. (1996). Individual differences in emotion regulation and behavior problems in preschool children. *Journal of Abnormal Psychology, 105,* 518–29.

Darrow, C. W. (1929). Electrical and circulatory responses to brief sensory and ideational stimuli. *Journal of Experimental Psychology, 12,* 267–300.

Davidson, R. J. (1984a). Affect, cognition and hemispheric specialization. In C. E. Izard, J. Kagan, & R. B. Zajonc (Eds.), *Emotions, Cognition and Behavior,* pp. 320–65. Cambridge University Press.

Davidson, R. J. (1984b). Hemispheric asymmetry and emotions. In K. R. Scherer & P. Ekman (Eds.), *Approaches to Emotion,* pp. 39–57. Hillsdale, NJ: Erlbaum.

Davidson, R. J. (1995). Cerebral asymmetry, emotion, and affective style. In R. J. Davidson & K. Hugdahl (Eds.), *Brain Asymmetry,* pp. 361–87. Cambridge, MA: MIT Press.

Davidson, R. J., & Fox, N. A. (1982). Asymmetrical brain activity discriminates between positive versus negative stimuli in human infants. *Science, 218,* 1235–7.

Davidson, R. J., & Fox, N. A. (1989). The relation between tonic EEG asymmetry and ten month old emotional response to separation. *Journal of Abnormal Psychology, 98,* 127–31.

Dawson, G. (1994). Development of emotional expression and emotion regulation in infancy: Contributions of the frontal lobe. In G. Dawson & K. W. Fischer (Eds.), *Human Behavior and the Developing Brain,* pp. 346–79. New York: Guilford.

Dawson, G., Grofer Klinger, L., Panagiotides, H., Hill, D., & Spieker, S. (1992a). Frontal lobe activity and affective behavior in infants of mothers with depressive symptoms. *Child Development, 63,* 725–37.

Dawson, G., Panagiotides, H., Grofer Klinger, L., & Hill, D. (1992b). The role of frontal lobe functioning in the development of self-regulatory behavior in infancy. *Brain and Cognition, 20,* 152–75.

de Haan, M., & Nelson, C. A. (1997). Recognition of the mother's face by six-month-old infants: A neurobehavioral study. *Child Development, 68,* 187–210.

Dennis, M. (1991). Frontal lobe function in childhood and adolescence: A heuristic for assessing attention regulation, executive control, and the intentional states important for social discourse. *Developmental Neuropsychology, 7,* 327–58.

Diamond, A., & Goldman-Rakic, P. S. (1983). Comparison of performance on a Piagetian object permanence task in human infants and rhesus monkeys: Evidence for involvement of prefrontal cortex. *Society for Neuroscience Abstracts, 9,* 641.

Diamond, A., & Goldman-Rakic, P. S. (1986). Comparative development in human infants and infant rhesus monkeys of cognitive functions that depend on prefrontal cortex. *Neuroscience Abstracts, 12,* 742.

Diamond, A., & Goldman-Rakic, P. S. (1989). Comparison of human infants and rhesus monkeys on Piaget's AB task: Evidence for dependence on dorsolateral prefrontal cortex. *Experimental Brain Research, 74,* 24–40.

Diamond, A., Prevor, M. B., Callender, G., & Druin, D. P. (1997). *Prefrontal Cortex Cognitive Deficits in Children Treated Early and Continuously for PKU* (Monographs of the Society for Research in Child Development, vol. 62/4, serial no. 252). University of Chicago Press.

Diamond, A., Zola-Morgan, S., & Squire, L. R. (1989). Successful performance by monkeys with lesions of the hippocampal formation on A-not-B and object retrieval, two tasks that mark developmental changes in human infants. *Behavioral Neuroscience, 103,* 526–37.

Dreyfus-Brisac, C., & Monod, N. (1975). The electroencephalogram of full term newborns and premature infants. In G. C. Lairy (Ed.), *Handbook of Electroencephalography and Clinical Neurophysiology,* vol. 6 (The Normal EEG throughout Life), pp. 6B-6–6B-30. Amsterdam: Elsevier.

Duffy, F. H., Als, H., & McAnulty, G. B. (1990). Behavioral and electrophysiological evidence for gestational age effects in healthy preterm and fullterm infants studied two weeks after expected due date. *Child Development, 61,* 1271–86.

Edelman, G. M. (1987). *Neural Darwinism: The Theory of Neuronal Group Selection.* New York: Basic Books.

Emde, R. N., & Walker, S. (1976). Longitudinal study of infant sleep: Results of 14 subjects studied at monthly intervals. *Psychophysiology, 13,* 456–61.

Field, T. M. (1979). Visual and cardiac responses to animate and inanimate faces by young term and preterm infants. *Child Development, 50,* 188–94.

Field, T. (1986). Models for reactive and chronic depression in infancy. In E. Z. Tronick & T. Field (Eds.), *Maternal Depression and Infant Disturbance,* pp. 47–60. San Francisco: Jossey-Bass.

Field, T., Fox, N. A., Pickens, J., & Nawrocki, T. (1995). Relative right frontal EEG activation in 3- to 6-month-old infants of "depressed" mothers. *Developmental Psychology, 31,* 358–63.

Field, T., Healy, B., Goldstein, S., Perry, S., Bendall, D., Schanberg, S., Zimmerman, E., & Kuhn, C. (1988). Infants of depressed mothers show "depressed" behavior even with nondepressed adults. *Child Development, 59,* 1569–79.

Field, T., Sandberg, D., Garcia, R., Vega-Lahr, N., Goldstein, S., & Guy, L. (1985). Prenatal problems, postpartum depression, and early mother-infant interaction. *Developmental Psychology, 12,* 1152–6.

Fischer, K. W. (1980). A theory of cognitive development: The control and construction of hierarchies of skills. *Psychological Review, 87,* 477–531.

Fischer, K. W. (1983). Developmental levels as periods of discontinuity. *New Directions for Child Development, 21,* 5–20.

Fischer, K. W. (1987). Relations between brain and cognitive development. *Child Development, 58,* 623–32.

Fischer, K. W., & Rose, S. P. (1994). Dynamic development of coordination of components in brain and behavior: A framework for theory and research. In G. Dawson & K. Fischer (Eds.), *Human Behavior and the Developing Brain,* pp. 3–66. New York: Guilford.

Fox, N. A. (1989). Heart-rate variability and behavioral reactivity: Individual differences in autonomic patterning and their relation to infant and child temperament. In J. S. Reznick (Ed.), *Perspectives on Behavioral Inhibition.* University of Chicago Press.

Fox, N. A. (1991). If it's not left, it's right: Electroencephalogram asymmetry and the development of emotion. *American Psychologist, 46,* 863–72.

Fox, N. A. (1994). Dynamic cerebral processes underlying emotion regulation. In N. A. Fox (Ed.), *The Development of Emotion Regulation: Behavioral and Biological Considerations* (Monographs of the Society for Research in Child Development, vol. 59/2–3, serial no. 240), pp. 152–66. University of Chicago Press.

Fox, N. A., & Bell, M. A. (1990). Electrophysiological indices of frontal lobe development: Relations to cognitive and affective behavior in human infants over the first year of life. *Annals of the New York Academy of Sciences, 608,* 677–98.

Fox, N. A., Bell, M. A., & Jones, N. A. (1992). Individual differences in response to stress and cerebral asymmetry. *Developmental Neuropsychology, 8,* 161–84.

Fox, N. A., Calkins, S. D., & Bell, M. A. (1994). Neural plasticity and development in the first two years of life: Evidence from cognitive and socioemotional domains of research. *Development and Psychopathology, 6,* 677–96.

Fox, N. A., & Davidson, R. J. (1984). Hemispheric substrates of affect: A developmental model. In N. A. Fox & R. J. Davidson (Eds.), *The Psychobiology of Affective Development,* pp. 353–81. Hillsdale, NJ: Erlbaum.

Fox, N. A., & Davidson, R. J. (1986a). Taste-elicited changes in facial signs of emotion and the asymmetry of brain electrical activity in human newborns. *Neuropsychologia, 24,* 417–22.

Fox, N. A., & Davidson, R. J. (1986b). Psychophysiological measures of emotion: New directions in developmental research. In C. E. Izard & P. Read (Eds.), *Measuring Emotions in Infants and Children,* vol. II, pp. 13–47. Cambridge University Press.

Fox, N. A., & Davidson, R. J. (1987). EEG asymmetry in ten month old infants in response to approach of a stranger and maternal separation. *Developmental Psychology, 23,* 233–40.

Fox, N. A., & Davidson, R. J. (1988). Patterns of brain electrical activity during the expression of discrete emotions in ten month old infants. *Developmental Psychology, 24,* 230–6.

Fox, N. A., & Field, T. (1989). Young children's responses to entry into preschool: Psychophysiological and behavioral finding. *Journal of Applied Developmental Psychology, 10,* 527–40.

Fox, N. A., & Gelles, M. (1984). Face-to-face interaction in term and preterm infants. *Infant Mental Health Journal, 5,* 192–205.

Fox, N. A., & Porges, S. W. (1985). The relation between neonatal heart period patterns and developmental outcome. *Child Development, 56,* 28–37.

Fox, N. A., Rubin, K. H., Calkins, S. D., Marshall, T. R., Coplan, R. J., Porges, S. W., Long, J. M., & Stewart, S. (1995). Frontal activation asymmetry and social competence at four years of age. *Child Development, 66,* 1770–84.

Fox, N. A., Schmidt, L. A., Calkins, S. D., Rubin, K. H., & Coplan, R. J. (1996). The role of frontal activation in the regulation and dysregulation of social behavior during the preschool years. *Development and Psychopathology, 8,* 89–102.

Fracasso, M. P., Porges, S. W., Lamb, M. E., & Rosenberg, A. A. (1994). Cardiac activity in infancy: Reliability and stability of individual differences. *Infant Behavior and Development, 17,* 277–84.

Gilles, F. H., Shankle, W., & Dooling, E. C. (1983). Myelinated tracts: Growth patterns. In F. H. Gilles, A. Leviton, & E. C. Dooling (Eds.), *The Developing Human Brain: Growth and Epidemiologic Neuropathology,* pp. 117–83. Boston: John Wright / PSG.

Goldman-Rakic, P. S. (1987a). Development of cortical circuitry and cognitive function. *Child Development, 58,* 601–22.

Goldman-Rakic, P. S. (1987b). Circuitry of the prefrontal cortex and the regulation of behavior by representational knowledge. In F. Plum & V. Mountcastle (Eds.), *Handbook of Physiology,* vol. 5, pp. 373–417. Bethesda, MD: American Physiological Society.

Goldman-Rakic, P. S., Isseroff, A., Schwartz, M., & Bugbee, N. (1983). The neurobiology of cognitive development. In M. M. Haith & J. J. Campos (Eds.), *Handbook of Child Psychology,* vol. II (Infancy and Developmental Psychobiology), pp. 281–344. New York: Wiley.

Gottlieb, G. (1976). The role of experience in the development of behavior and the nervous system. In G. Gottlieb (Ed.), *Neural and Behavioral Specificity: Studies on the Development of Behavior and the Nervous System,* vol. 3, pp. 25–54. New York: Academic Press.

Graham, F. K., & Clifton, R. K. (1966). Heart-rate changes as a component of the orienting response. *Psychological Bulletin, 65,* 305–20.

Greenough, W. T., & Black, J. E. (1992). Induction of brain structure by experience: Substrates for cognitive development. In M. R. Gunnar & C. A. Nelson (Eds.), *Minnesota Symposia on Child Psychology,* vol. 24 (Developmental Behavioral Neuroscience), pp. 155–200. Hillsdale, NJ: Erlbaum.

Greenough, W. T., Black, J., & Wallace, C. (1987). Effects of experience on brain development. *Child Development, 58,* 540–59.

Greenough, W. T., & Volkmar, F. R. (1973). Pattern of dendritic branching in the occipital cortex of rats reared in complex environments. *Experimental Neurology, 40,* 491–504.

Groome, L. J., Swiber, M. J., Atterbury, J. L., Bentz, L. S., & Holland, S. B. (1997). Similarities and differences in behavioral state organization during sleep periods in the perinatal infant before and after birth. *Child Development, 68,* 1–11.

Hagne, I. (1968). Development of the waking EEG in normal infants during the first year of life. In P. Kellaway & I. Petersén (Eds.), *Clinical Electroencephalography of Children,* pp. 97–118. New York: Grune & Stratton.

Hagne, I. (1972). Development of the EEG in normal infants during the first year of life. *Acta Pediatrica Scandinavica (Suppl. 232),* 25–32.

Hagne, I., Persson, J., Magnusson, R., & Petersén, I. (1973). Spectral analysis via fast Fourier transform of waking EEG in normal infants. In P. Kellaway & I. Petersén (Eds.), *Automation of Clinical EEG*, pp. 103–43. New York: Raven.

Hassett, J., & Danforth, D. (1982). An introduction to the cardiovascular system. In J. T. Cacioppo & R. E. Petty (Eds.), *Perspectives in Cardiovascular Psychophysiology*, pp. 4–18. New York: Guilford.

Henriques, J. B., & Davidson, R. J. (1990). Regional brain electrical asymmetries discriminate between previously depressed subjects and healthy controls. *Journal of Abnormal Psychology, 99*, 22–31.

Henriques, J. B., & Davidson, R. J. (1991). Left frontal hypoactivation in depression. *Journal of Abnormal Psychology, 100*, 535–45.

Henry, J. R. (1944). *Electroencephalograms of Normal Children* (Monographs of the Society for Research in Child Development, vol. 9/3, serial no. 39). University of Chicago Press.

Hirsch, J. A., & Bishop, B. (1981). Respiratory sinus arrhythmia in humans: How breathing pattern modulates heart rate. *American Journal of Physiology, 241*, H620–H629.

Hirshfeld, D. R., Rosenbaum, J. F., Biederman, J., Bolduc, E. A., Faraone, S. V., Snidman, N., Reznick, J. S., & Kagan, J. (1992). Stable behavioral inhibition and its association with anxiety disorder. *Journal of the American Academy of Child and Adolescent Psychiatry, 31*, 103–11.

Howard, L., & Polich, J. (1985). P300 latency and memory span development. *Developmental Psychology, 21*, 283–9.

Hubel, D. H., & Wiesel, T. N. (1970). The period of susceptibility to the physiological effects of unilateral eye closure in kittens. *Journal of Physiology (London), 206*, 419–36.

Huttenlocher, P. R. (1979). Synaptic density in human frontal cortex: Developmental changes and effects of aging. *Brain Research, 163*, 195–205.

Huttenlocher, P. R. (1984). Synapse elimination and plasticity in developing human cerebral cortex. *American Journal of Mental Deficiency, 88*, 488–96.

Huttenlocher, P. R., & de Courten, C. (1987). The development of synapses in striate cortex of man. *Human Neurobiology, 6*, 1–9.

Huttenlocher, P. R., de Courten, C., Garey, L. J., & Van der Loos, H. (1982). Synaptogenesis in human visual cortex: Evidence for synapse elimination during normal development. *Neuroscience Letters, 33*, 247–52.

Jasper, H. H. (1958). The ten-twenty electrode system of the International Federation. *Electroencephalography and Clinical Neurophysiology, 10*, 371–5.

John, E. R. (1977). *Functional Neuroscience*, vol. 2 (Neurometrics). Hillsdale, NJ: Erlbaum.

Jones, N. A., & Fox, N. A. (1992). Electroencephalogram asymmetry during emotionally evocative films and its relation to positive and negative affectivity. *Brain and Cognition, 20*, 280–99.

Kagan, J., Reznick, J. S., & Snidman, N. (1987). The physiology and psychology of behavioral inhibition. *Child Development, 58*, 1459–73.

Kagan, J., Reznick, J. S., & Snidman, N. (1988). Biological bases of childhood shyness. *Science, 240*, 167–71.

Kagan, J., & Snidman, N. (1991). Infant predictors of inhibited and uninhibited profiles. *Psychological Science, 2*, 40–4.

Katona, P. G., & Jih, F. (1975). Respiratory sinus arrhythmia: A noninvasive measure of parasympathetic cardiac control. *Journal of Applied Physiology, 39*, 801–5.

Krafchuk, E. E., Tronick, E. Z., & Clifton, R. K. (1983). Behavioral and cardiac responses to sound in preterm neonates varying in risk status: A hypothesis of their paradoxical reactivity. In T. M. Field & A. Sostek (Eds.), *Infants Born at Risk: Physiological and Perceptual Processes*, pp. 99–128. New York: Grune & Stratton.

Lacey, J. I. (1967). Somatic response patterning and stress: Some revisions of activation theory. In M. H. Apley & R. Trumbull (Eds.), *Psychological Stress*, pp. 14–42. New York: Appleton-Century-Crofts.

Lagerlund, T. D., Sharbrough, F. W., Rack, C. R., Erickson, B., Strelow, D. C., Cicora, M., & Busacker, N. E. (1993). Determination of 10–20 system electrode locations using magnetic resonance image scanning with markers. *Electroencephalography and Clinical Neurophysiology, 86*, 7–14.

Lahmeyer, H. W., Reynolds, C. F., Kupfer, D. J., & King, R. (1989). Biologic markers in borderline personality disorder: A review. *Journal of Clinical Psychiatry, 50*, 217–25.

Lenneberg, E. (1967). *Biological Foundations of Language*. New York: Wiley.

Lester, B. M. (1975). Cardiac habituation of the orienting response to an auditory signal in infants of varying nutritional status. *Developmental Psychology, 11*, 432–42.

Lewis, M., Kagan, J., Campbell, H., & Kalafat, J. (1966). The cardiac response as a correlate of attention in infants. *Child Development, 37*, 63–71.

Lewis, M., Wilson, C. D., Ban, P., & Baumel, M. H. (1970). An exploratory study of resting cardiac rate and variability from the trimester of prenatal life through the first year of postnatal life. *Child Development, 41*, 799–812.

Lindsley, D. B. (1939). A longitudinal study of the occipital alpha rhythm in normal children: Frequency and amplitude standards. *Journal of Genetic Psychology, 55*, 197–213.

Malliani, A., Pagani, M., & Lombardi, F. (1994). Physiology and clinical implications of variability of cardiovascular parameters with focus on heart rate and blood pressure. *American Journal of Cardiology, 73*, 3C–9C.

Matousek, M., & Petersén, I. (1973). Frequency analysis of the EEG in normal children and adolescents. In P. Kellaway & I. Petersén (Eds.), *Automation of Clinical Electroencephalography*, pp. 75–102. New York: Raven.

McCall, R. B., & Kagan, J. (1967). Attention in the infant: Effects of complexity, contour, perimeter, and familiarity. *Child Development, 38*, 939–52.

Mezzacappa, E., Kindlon, D., Earls, F., & Saul, J. P. (1994). The utility of spectral analytic techniques in the study of the autonomic regulation of beat-to-beat heart rate variability. *International Journal of Methods in Psychiatric Research, 4*, 29–44.

Mezzacappa, E., Tremblay, R. E., Kindlon, D., Saul, J. P., Arseneault, L., Seguin, J., Pihl, R. O., & Earls, F. (1997). Anxiety, antisocial behavior, and heart rate regulation in adolescent males. *Journal of Child Psychology and Psychiatry, 38*, 457–69.

Miller, B. L., & Lesser, I. M. (1988). Late-life psychosis and modern neuroimaging. *Psychiatric Clinics of North America, 11*, 33–46.

Mills, D. L., Coffey-Corina, S. A., & Neville, H. J. (1994). Variability in cerebral organization during primary language acquisition. In G. Dawson & K. Fischer (Eds.), *Human Behavior and the Developing Brain*, pp. 427–55. New York: Guilford.

Mizuno, T., Yamauchi, N., Watanabe, A., Komatsushiro, M., Takagi, T., Iinuma, K., & Arakawa, T. (1970). Maturation of patterns of EEG: Basic waves of healthy infants under 12 months of age. *Tohoku Journal of Experimental Medicine, 102,* 91–8.

Moffit, T. E., & Henry, B. (1989). Neuropsychological assessment of executive functions in self-reported delinquents. *Development and Psychopathology, 1,* 105–18.

Myslobodsky, M. S., Coppola, R., Bar-Ziv, J., & Weinberger, D. R. (1990). Adequacy of the international 10–20 electrode system for computed neurophysiologic topography. *Journal of Clinical Neurophysiology, 7,* 507–18.

Nelson, C. A. (1994). Neural correlates of recognition memory in the first postnatal year. In G. Dawson & K. W. Fischer (Eds.), *Human Behavior and the Developing Brain*, pp. 269–313. New York: Guilford.

Nelson, C. A., & Collins, P. F. (1991). Event-related potential and looking time analysis of infants' responses to familiar and novel events: Implications for visual recognition memory. *Developmental Psychology, 27,* 50–8.

Nelson, C. A., & Collins, P. F. (1992). Neural and behavioral correlates of visual recognition memory in 3- and 8-month-old infants. *Brain and Cognition, 19,* 105–21.

Neville, H. J., Kutas, M., & Schmidt, A. (1982a). Event-related potential studies of cerebral specialization during reading: II. Studies of congenitally deaf adults. *Brain and Cognition, 16,* 316–37.

Neville, H. J., Kutas, M., & Schmidt, A. (1982b). Event-related potential studies of cerebral specialization during reading: I. Studies of normal adults. *Brain and Cognition, 16,* 300–15.

Niznikiewicz, M. A., O'Donnell, B. F., Nestor, P. G., Smith, L., Law, S., Karapelou, M., Shenton, M. E., & McCarley, R. W. (1997). ERP assessment of visual and auditory language processing in schizophrenia. *Journal of Abnormal Psychology, 106,* 85–94.

Nunez, P. (1981). *Electric Fields of the Brain*. New York: Oxford University Press.

Petitto, L. A. (1993). On the ontogenetic requirements for early language acquisition. In B. de Boysson-Bardies, S. Schonen, P. Jusczyk, P. F. MacNeilage, & J. Morton (Eds.), *Developmental Neurocognition: Speech and Face Processing in the First Year of Life*, pp. 365–83. Dordrecht: Kluwer.

Pivik, R. T., Broughton, R. J., Coppola, R., Davidson, R. J., Fox, N., & Nuwer, M. R. (1993). Guidelines for the recording and quantitative analysis of electroencephalographic activity in research contexts. *Psychophysiology, 30,* 547–58.

Pollock, V. E., & Schneider, L. S. (1990). Quantitative, waking EEG research on depression. *Biological Psychiatry, 27,* 757–80.

Porges, S. W. (1983). Heart rate patterns in neonates: A potential diagnostic window to the brain. In T. Field & A. Sostek (Eds.), *Infants Born at Risk: Physiological and Perceptual Processes*, pp. 3–22. New York: Grune & Stratton.

Porges, S. W. (1992). Vagal tone: A physiologic marker of stress vulnerability. *Pediatrics, 90,* 498–504.

Porges, S. W., Doussard-Roosevelt, J. A., & Maiti, A. K. (1994a). Vagal tone and the physiological regulation of emotion. In N. A. Fox (Ed.), *The Development of Emotion Regulation: Biological and Behavioral Considerations* (Monographs of the Society for Research in Child Development, vol. 59/2–3, serial no. 240), pp. 167–88. University of Chicago Press.

Porges, S. W., Doussard-Roosevelt, J. A., Portales, A. L., & Suess, P. E. (1994b). Cardiac vagal tone: Stability and relation to difficulties in infants and 3-year-olds. *Developmental Psychobiology, 27,* 289–300.

Porges, S. W., McCabe, P. M., & Yongue, B. G. (1982). Respiratory-heart rate interactions: Physiological implications for pathophysiology and behavior. In J. Cacioppo & R. Petty (Eds.), *Perspectives in Cardiovascular Psychophysiology*, pp. 223–64. New York: Guilford.

Pribram, K. H. (1973). The primate frontal cortex: Executive of the brain. In K. H. Pribram & A. R. Luria (Eds.), *Psychophysiology of the Frontal Lobes*, pp. 293–314. New York: Academic Press.

Pritchard, W. S. (1986). Cognitive event-related potential correlates of schizophrenia. *Psychological Bulletin, 100,* 43–66.

Raine, A. (1993). *The Psychopathology of Crime: Criminal Behavior as a Clinical Disorder*. San Diego: Academic Press.

Raine, A., & Jones, F. (1987). Attention, autonomic arousal, and personality in behaviorally disordered children. *Journal of Abnormal Child Psychology, 15,* 583–99.

Raine, A., & Venables, P. H. (1984). Tonic heart rate level, social class, and antisocial behavior in adolescents. *Biological Psychology, 18,* 123–32.

Raine, A., & Venables, P. H. (1987). Contingent negative variation, P3 evoked potentials, and antisocial behavior. *Psychophysiology, 24,* 191–9.

Raine, A., Venables, P. H., & Williams, M. (1990a). Relationships between central and autonomic measures of arousal at age 15 years and criminality at age 24 years. *Archives of General Psychiatry, 47,* 1003–7.

Raine, A., Venables, P. H., & Williams, M. (1990b). Autonomic orienting responses in 15-year-old male subjects and criminal behavior at age 24. *American Journal of Psychiatry, 147,* 933–7.

Raine, A., Venables, P. H., & Williams, M. (1995). High autonomic arousal and electrodermal orienting at age 15 years as protective factors against criminal behavior at age 29 years. *American Journal of Psychiatry, 152,* 1595–1600.

Richards, J. E. (1985). The development of sustained visual attention in infants from 14 to 26 weeks of age. *Psychophysiology, 22,* 409–16.

Richards, J. E. (1987). Infant visual sustained attention and respiratory sinus arrhythmia. *Child Development, 58,* 488–96.

Richards, J. E. (1989). Development and stability in visual sustained attention in 14, 20, and 26 week old infants. *Psychophysiology, 26,* 422–30.

Rose, S., Schmidt, K., & Bridger, W. H. (1976). Cardiac and behavioral responsivity to tactile stimulation in premature and fullterm infants. *Developmental Psychology, 12,* 311–20.

Rubin, K. H., Stewart, S. L., & Coplan, R. J. (1995). Social withdrawal in childhood: Conceptual and empirical perspectives. In T. Ollendick & R. Prinz (Eds.), *Advances in Clinical Child Psychology*, vol. 17, pp. 157–96. New York: Plenum.

Sameroff, A. J., Cashmore, T. F., & Dykes, A. C. (1973). Heart rate decelerations during visual fixation in human newborns. *Developmental Psychology, 8,* 117–99.

Schacter, D. L., Kagan, J., & Leichtman, M. (1995). True and false memories in children and adults: A cognitive neuroscience perspective. *Psychology, Public Policy and Law, 2,* 411–28.

Schaffer, C. E., Davidson, R. J., & Saron, C. (1983). Frontal and parietal electroencephalogram asymmetry in depressed and nondepressed subjects. *Biological Psychiatry, 18,* 753–62.

Schmidt, L. A., & Fox, N. A. (1994). Patterns of cortical electrophysiology and autonomic activity in adults' shyness and sociability. *Biological Psychology, 38,* 183–98.

Schwartz, G. E., Davidson, R. J., & Maer, F. (1975). Right hemisphere lateralization for emotion in the human brain: Interaction with cognition. *Science, 190,* 286–8.

Schwartz, G. E., Fair, P. L., Salt, P., Mandel, M., & Klerman, G. L. (1976). Facial muscle patterning to affective imagery in depressed and nondepressed subjects. *Science, 192,* 489–91.

Sidman, R. L., & Rakic, P. (1973). Neuronal migration with special reference to developing human brain: A review. *Brain Research, 62,* 1–35.

Slater, A., & Morison, V. (1991). Visual attention and memory at birth. In M. J. Weiss & P. R. Zelazo (Eds.), *Newborn Attention: Biological Constraints and the Influence of Experience,* pp. 256–77. Norwood, NJ: Ablex.

Smith, J. R. (1938a). The electroencephalogram during normal infancy and childhood: I. Rhythmic activities present in the neonate and their subsequent development. *Journal of Genetic Psychology, 53,* 431–53.

Smith, J. R. (1938b). The electroencephalogram during normal infancy and childhood: II. The nature and growth of alpha waves. *Journal of Genetic Psychology, 53,* 455–69.

Smith, J. R. (1938c). The electroencephalogram during normal infancy and childhood: III. Preliminary observations on the pattern sequence during sleep. *Journal of Genetic Psychology, 53,* 471–82.

Smith, J. R. (1939). The "occipital" and "pre-central" alpha rhythms during the first two years. *Journal of Psychology, 7,* 223–6.

Smith, J. R. (1941). The frequency and growth of the human alpha rhythms during infancy and childhood. *Journal of Psychology, 11,* 177–98.

Snidman, N., Kagan, J., Riordan, L., & Shannon, D. C. (1995). Cardiac function and behavioral reactivity during infancy. *Psychophysiology, 32,* 199–207.

Stifter, C. A., & Fox, N. A. (1990). Infant reactivity and regulation: Physiological correlates of newborn and five-month temperament. *Developmental Psychology, 26,* 582–8.

Stifter, C. A., Fox, N. A., & Porges, S. W. (1989). Facial expressivity and heart rate variability in five- and ten-month-old infants. *Infant Behavior and Development, 12,* 127–37.

Task Force of the European Society of Cardiology and the North American Society of Pacing and Electrophysiology (1996). Heart rate variability: Standards of measurement, physiological interpretation, and clinical use. *Circulation, 93,* 1043–65.

Thatcher, R. W. (1991). Maturation of the human frontal lobes: Physiological evidence for staging. Special Issue: Developmental consequences of early frontal lobe damage. *Developmental Neuropsychology, 7,* 397–419.

Thatcher, R. W. (1994). Psychopathology of early frontal lobe damage: Dependence on cycles of development. Special Issue: Neural plasticity, sensitive periods, and psychopathology. *Development and Psychopathology, 6,* 565–96.

Thatcher, R. W., Krause, P., & Hrybyk, M. (1986). Corticocortical association fibers and EEG coherence: A two compartmental model. *Electroencephalography and Clinical Neurophysiology, 64,* 123–43.

Thatcher, R. W., Walker, R. A., & Giudice, S. (1987). Human cerebral hemispheres develop at different rates and ages. *Science, 236,* 1110–12.

Tomarken, A. J., Davidson, R. J., & Henriques, J. B. (1990). Resting frontal brain asymmetry predicts affective responses to films. *Journal of Personality and Social Psychology, 59,* 791–801.

Welsh, M. C., Pennington, B. F., & Groisser, D. B. (1991). A normative-developmental study of executive function: A window on prefrontal function in children. *Developmental Neuropsychology, 7,* 131–49.

Wheeler, R. E., Davidson, R. J., & Tomarken, A. J. (1993). Frontal brain asymmetry and emotional reactivity: A biological substrate of affective style. *Psychophysiology, 30,* 82–9.

Zahn, T. P. (1986). Psychophysiological approaches to psychophysiology. In M. G. H. Coles, E. Donchin, & S. W. Porges (Eds.), *Psychophysiology: Systems, Processes, and Applications,* pp. 508–610. New York: Guilford.

Zahn, T. P., & Kruesi, M. J. P. (1993). Autonomic activity in boys with disruptive behavior disorders. *Psychophysiology, 30,* 605–14.

Zahn-Waxler, C., Cole, P. M., Darby Welsh, J., & Fox, N. A. (1995). Psychophysiological correlates of empathy and prosocial behaviors in preschool children with behavior problems. *Development and Psychopathology, 7,* 27–48.

CHAPTER TWENTY-FIVE

SLEEP AND DREAMING

R. T. PIVIK

Introduction

The majority of our behavioral and cognitive lives are spent in the waking state – a time during which activities viewed as essential to personal existence and continuation of the species are accomplished. It is therefore to be expected that for many the waking state is likely to be considered "the sole portion of ... existence that 'counts' in any way, sleep appearing as 'time out' from the game of living" (Kleitman 1963, p. 3). However, although sleep may appear to constitute an interruption of the critical activities of wakefulness, it is indisputable that the alternation between sleep and wakefulness is essential to "normal" existence in all higher life forms. The importance of sleep to normal waking activities can be immediately appreciated when the well-documented adverse effects of sleep reduction on waking behavioral and psychological functions are considered – effects extending from decreased alertness and impaired performance (Gillberg & Åkerstedt 1994; Monk 1991) to death (Bentivoglio & Grassi-Zucconi 1997; Everson 1995; Horne 1988). Clearly, these two states interact in a complementary and synergistic relationship to maintain and extend life. Although the precise nature of this co-dependence has, to a great extent, been obscured by a lack of detailed knowledge regarding the physiology and psychology of sleep, recent advances in these areas have provided significant insights into these puzzling within- and between-state variations and relationships.

It is at the same time surprising and revealing that sleep should support any form of cognitive activity – surprising since at first glance it is difficult to imagine the purpose of mental activity during such sustained periods of disengagement from the environment, and revealing because of the unexpected psychophysiological relationships the presence of such activity implies. Still, if concepts subscribing to the interaction or psychophysiological parallelism of mind–body relationships are even closely approximated, then it would be expected that the marked behavioral and physiological sleep–wakefulness differences would be reflected in equally marked differences in the characteristics of associated cognitive activity. In this instance, state-dependent expectations are apparently reinforced: unlike the generally more organized, rational, self-directed nature of waking cognition, cognitive activity during sleep is seemingly disorganized, distorted, and subject to little volitional control. This distinctive cognitive behavior – not associated with an abnormal state or condition, yet so apparently different from waking mental activity – has been provided with an appropriately distinctive name: dreaming.

Historical Background

The relative inaccessibility of processes underlying sleep and dreaming fostered wide-ranging speculation regarding the nature and function of these activities. Early theories attributed sleep to various changes in the distribution, temperature, or constitution of blood, and many considered the difference between sleep and death simply a matter of degree (Kleitman 1963; Nitz 1993). Later concepts extending into the early twentieth century localized sleep to the brain and ascribed many functions to this state, including enhancing digestion, creating new "animal spirits" required for waking behavior, and eliminating potentially harmful "humors" from the body (Wittern 1989). Paralleling these notions were beliefs that dreams contained messages foretelling the future, revealed cures for illnesses, or provided unique access to the unconscious (Kramer 1994; Webb 1993). These various conceptualizations had in common a view of sleep as a unimodal state and dreams as sporadic, relatively rare events.

Although sleep and dreaming have long been sources of fascination and speculation, scientific interest in these

John T. Cacioppo, Louis G. Tassinary, and Gary G. Berntson (Eds.), *Handbook of Psychophysiology*, 2nd ed. © Cambridge University Press 2000. Printed in the United States of America. ISBN 62634X. All rights reserved.

behaviors significantly intensified in the twentieth century. In the second edition of his classic text summarizing information regarding sleep and wakefulness, Kleitman (1963) listed over 4,000 references, of which less than 2% referred to publications before the twentieth century. However, the most marked acceleration of experimental studies into the nature of sleep physiology and psychology can be traced to the mid-twentieth century, when Eugene Aserinsky, a physiology doctoral student at the University of Chicago, observed episodes of eye movement activity during sleep in what were the first whole-night polygraphic recordings of such activities (Aserinsky 1953). Although he observed they were slower than waking eye movements of comparable amplitude and was more impressed with their "jerkiness" than their velocity, Aserinsky nevertheless elected to characterize this as "rapid eye movement" or REM activity, in large part to avoid "the anticipated taunts relative to the popular slang meaning of 'jerk'" (Aserinsky 1996, p. 218).

This observation – utilizing a newly emerging technology that made possible long-term recordings of electrophysiological activities – led to a series of publications that revolutionized and redirected thinking regarding both the nature of sleep and the occurrence of dreaming (Aserinsky & Kleitman 1953, 1955; Dement 1955; Dement & Kleitman 1957a,b; Dement & Wolpert 1958a,b). The finding of recurring episodes of physiological activation embedded within sleep that were unlike either wakefulness or the remainder of sleep flew in the face of existing concepts of sleep as a unitary, passive state. So unique were these rapid eye movement periods that they prompted investigators to consider REM sleep as a third state of existence (Dement 1969; Snyder 1966; Steriade & McCarley 1990). Not only did these REM periods deviate in their physiological characteristics from other normal states, but upon awakening from these episodes subjects commonly reported dreaming, suggesting that an objective index had been identified for determining "the incidence and duration of periods of dreaming" (Aserinsky & Kleitman 1953, p. 274).

Although electrographic recordings of brain wave and oculomotor activities assisted in the discovery of REM sleep and its association with dreaming, these observations did not require such technological assistance. Determination of whether an individual is asleep can be made subjectively with reasonable reliability, and movements of the eyes are readily apparent from associated displacements of the corneal bulge under the eyelids. Furthermore, because of the prominence of visual images in dream reports, it had long been speculated that dreams would be accompanied by eye movements (Griesinger 1868; Ladd 1892). Given such considerations, why hadn't these remarkable periods of physiological and cognitive activation – which occur nightly, are distributed across the night, and which may last 20 minutes or longer – been previously discovered? In a publication in which he chronicled the discovery of REM sleep, Aserinsky (1996) considered this question as follows:

the obvious answer must lie in human behavior. Since the first REM period is not obvious during the first couple of hours of sleep, and cyclicity would require a still longer period of observation, the discovery of REM would have required an obsessive, highly motivated individual to peer continually for hours at a sleeper's eyes. This would explain the failure of the layman to discover REM, but what about scientists who are infamous for both obsessiveness and motivation, and thus should have looked for the eye movements? My guess is that no one was sufficiently driven to spend an inordinate amount of time to fill in the gaps of sleep studies in which the position of the eyes was noted by occasional lifting of the sleeper's eyes. (pp. 226–7)

The technological capability of recording physiological measures over long periods of time may not have been required for the discovery of REM sleep, but it was essential for the subsequent exploration and detailing of the general physiology of sleep. Although Aserinsky (1996) considered the relationship of rapid eye movements in sleep to dreaming as "almost incidental with respect to its import in understanding brain function" (p. 226), it was the linkage of sleep-state physiology to sleep-state cognitive activity that provided the major impetus for the next two decades of sleep and dream research and established the foundation for what could be considered the "new sleep research." Furthermore, this focus on psychophysiological relationships during sleep presented an opportunity to determine if such relationships are maintained across states and, consequently, to provide a broader understanding of mind–body relationships. Even before specific physiological sleep–wakefulness differences were determined, it was apparent that these states differed along significant dimensions, among which was the profound change in level of consciousness. Relative to wakefulness, there is a dramatic decrease in awareness of both the external and internal physical environments during sleep, as reflected by increased sensory thresholds to external and internal stimulation as well as by an absence of appreciation of significant physiological variations, such as galvanic skin response activation during slow-wave sleep or breathing cessation associated with sleep apnea (Guilleminault 1994; Johnson 1973). With few exceptions (e.g. lucid dreaming), this decrease in awareness is accompanied by a general loss of volitional control over physiological and psychological processes. The relative inaccessibility of sleep processes, together with the associated greatly diminished awareness and control, created both real and apparent obstacles to the scientific study of these behaviors. Still, the very factors that complicated the study of these processes also removed or attenuated potentially confounding variables commonly associated with investigations during wakefulness – for example, stress, expectations, and undefined variations in level of arousal – raising the possibility that relationships either obscured by or absent during wakefulness would be unmasked during sleep.

Physical Context

Questions concerning why and how wakefulness–sleep state alternations occur have motivated speculation and inquiry into the mechanisms of these variations. Early views of sleep – as the passive behavioral default that results when wakefulness-maintaining activities from specific sensory (Bremer 1937, 1938) or nonspecific brainstem reticular pathways (Moruzzi & Magoun 1949) were withdrawn – had to be modified to incorporate evidence of active sleep-promoting processes. This evidence was provided by brainstem and cortical stimulation and lesion studies (reviewed in Jones 1994; Steriade & McCarley 1990) as well as by indications of active control processes effecting and modulating sleep, such as recurring periods of activated (REM) sleep and predictable sleep pattern variations across the night (i.e., the sleep cycle). The separation of sleep-promoting mechanisms into passive and active categories provided a conceptual framework within which studies could be formulated and interpreted. However, technological advances permitting more discerning anatomical and neurophysiological evaluations of systems and processes underlying sleep and waking behavior made it apparent that the passive–active dichotomy was too simplistic, and that sleep initiation and maintenance most likely involved cascading effects and interactions resulting from both the passive effects of functional deafferentation and the activation of structures with hypnogenic properties. The search for specific brain regions or centers whose activation might be essential to the occurrence or promotion of sleep identified several candidates: the solitary tract nucleus in the medulla, the preoptic basal forebrain area, the anterior hypothalamus, and the brain stem raphe nuclei for non–rapid eye movement (NREM) sleep; and the pons for REM sleep (see Jones 1994; Steriade & McCarley 1990).

Paralleling and complementing these studies were those capitalizing on developments in the detection and localization of biochemicals in the peripheral and central nervous systems and exploring how these compounds were related to state determination. Although the notion of a chemical hypnogenic factor had been hypothesized early in the twentieth century (Pieron 1913), the technology necessary to effectively pursue this line of inquiry was not available until the 1950s and 1960s; since that time, this technology has become increasingly sensitive and sophisticated. Studies using these techniques have implicated interactions among a wide range of chemicals that exert sleep- or wakefulness-promoting influences and have reinforced those focused on anatomical or neurophysiological aspects of sleep in demonstrating the complexity of systems involved in determining states of sleep and wakefulness. These compounds – produced centrally and peripherally and acting as neurotransmitters, neuromodulators, or neurohormones – have been variously localized to neurons, cerebrospinal fluid, and blood (for reviews see Jones 1994; Krueger & Karnovsky 1995; Steriade & McCarley 1990). These quests for sleep centers and chemical sleep factors have proven to be highly informative and heuristically beneficial, and the outcomes of these studies have been summarized as follows: "no sleep or wake state *in toto* can be said to have a center and ... few, if any, components of waking–sleep states have 'a center'" (Steriade & McCarley 1990, p. 21); and "no single chemical neurotransmitter, neuromodulator, or neurohormone has been identified that is necessary or sufficient for the generation and maintenance of sleep or waking. Instead, multiple factors and systems are involved in the onset and maintenance of these states" (Jones 1994, p. 157). The idea of distributed and interacting systems is being increasingly utilized in theoretical formulations integrating neuronal and neurochemical processes that attempt to explain state determination (Krueger et al. 1995; McCarley & Hobson 1975). Ultimately, understanding the mechanisms responsible for state determination and the relationship of these mechanisms to behavior will provide insights into the function of sleep – an enigma that continues to elude resolution (Rechtschaffen 1998).

Social Context

It requires little reflection to appreciate that the results of scientific investigations may be unintentionally influenced by such aspects of the experimental process as the laboratory environment, measurement apparatus, experimental demands, and the presence of investigators. These factors may exert what have been termed "reactive measurement effects" (Campbell 1957) on study outcome measures. Recognizing that the sleeping environment, sleep behavior, and associated personal thoughts (dreams) of individuals are usually considered among the most private of behavioral domains, attempts to study these behaviors would seem to require obtrusive intervention and present multiple opportunities for reactive measurement effects. In attempts to control for or at least minimize such effects, investigators have applied several techniques or procedures. For example, in addition to assuring subject confidentiality with respect to study results, it has proven helpful to introduce subjects to the laboratory environment, procedures, and personnel prior to undertaking sleep recordings. Still, in view of the apparent intrusiveness of procedures necessary to evaluate sleep physiology, statements referring to such procedures as "noninvasive" and "minimally sleep disturbing" would seem to underestimate the sleep disturbance expected under these conditions. However, studies of sleep in populations across the pediatric to geriatric age range during the past 45 years have clearly established that most subjects can, and do, sleep well under these circumstances. Commonly, the initial nights in the laboratory are accompanied by sleep disturbance in the form of increased latencies to sleep onset, more body movements, and fragmentation of sleep patterns. Since sleep patterns normally stabilize subsequent to this initial period, these variations have been considered to be transient responses to the novel sleeping environment and instrumentation. This adaptation phenomenon has been termed the "first night effect" (Agnew, Webb, & Williams 1966). Once adaptation has occurred, the night-to-night stability of many sleep measures is remarkable. This consistency is expressed across several variables, including the amounts and cyclic characteristics of sleep stages (see Figure 3 in the next section), autonomic measures (heart rate and variability – Pivik et al. 1996; see Figures 5 and 6), and specific electrographic events (K-complexes – Johnson 1973; ponto-geniculo-occipital spike activity – Jouvet 1972). The development of portable instrumentation to record physiological parameters necessary for sleep–wakefulness differentiation and sleep staging has allowed the comparison of results from recordings made in subjects' home environments with those obtained from the same subjects studied in the laboratory. That such comparisons have revealed minimal between-condition differences (Sewitch & Kupfer 1985) attests to the general robustness of sleep processes and the adaptability of subjects.

Concerns regarding the influence of experimental factors on sleep mentation reports have focused on (i) possible confabulation by subjects in the interest of pleasing the investigator and (ii) the extent to which the laboratory environment may directly affect the content in these reports. The potential for experimental confounds due to confabulation is always of concern in situations where other procedures (e.g., physiological or performance indices) cannot be used as corroborative measures. This issue, of long-standing concern to investigators studying sleep mentation, was effectively addressed by Rechtschaffen (1967) in a series of logical considerations to be used as guidelines for evaluating the acceptance of such reports as true representations of sleep experiences. These guidelines are briefly summarized as follows (Pivik 1986, p. 393).

1. *Parsimony* – interpretations requiring the fewest assumptions are favored.
2. *Prevalence* – phenomena known to occur most frequently are favored over those of rare occurrence. For example, in the absence of indications of impaired memory in the recall processes in wakefulness, the subject's postarousal report is accepted as a valid representation of his or her experience, rather than questioned on the grounds of cognitive impairment.
3. *Plausibility* – an extension of the prevalence guideline, which, however, "gives special emphasis to frequency and occurrence in given situations" (Rechtschaffen 1967, p. 7). For example, although it could be assumed that

subjects are lying when questioned about the presence and details of dream experiences, on the basis of current understanding of the motivational factors promoting lying, one would consider it unlikely that subjects would lie so consistently about dream reports.
4. *Private experience* – in the absence of objective indices, there is a strong tendency to accept the existence of phenomena if they have been part of one's own experience.

As might be expected, elements of the experimental environment or procedures may be incorporated into dream reports (Domhoff & Kamiya 1964; Okuma, Fukuma, & Kobayashi 1976). Although some content differences may exist between dreams collected at home and those collected in the laboratory (Lloyd & Cartwright 1995; Weisz & Foulkes 1970), these differences are minor. A more significant issue relates to whether dreams collected in the laboratory are so influenced by the experimental conditions that they provide an unfaithful representation of the subject's dream life – depicting it as more mundane, realistically oriented, or coherent than it may be (Dorus, Dorus, & Rechtschaffen 1971; Snyder 1970). The studies just cited indicating content similarities between home and laboratory dreams (when collected under similar sampling conditions) suggest that reports collected in the laboratory do not provide an unrepresentative view of dream content and processes. Furthermore, it has been argued (Foulkes & Cavallero 1993) that spontaneous recall of dreams in the home environment may, in fact, present an atypical view of dream content because laboratory dreams are better sampled and home dreams that are remembered may be so because of bizarre, emotional, or vivid characteristics.

Inferential Context

Every area of scientific endeavor is confronted with unique methodological challenges, but for sleep research the usual challenges – such as satisfying criteria fundamental to the reliable and valid measurement of physiological and cognitive processes – are compounded by the need to obtain these measures from the sleeping organism while maintaining state integrity and continuity. This state maintenance is, and continues to be, critical to the recognition of physiological indices that may be used as more discrete and objective correlates of sleep behaviors and also to the valid assignment of behaviors to their proper state domain.

In this regard, it is instructive to consider how demand characteristics differ between studies conducted during wakefulness and sleep, the methodological challenges these differences create, and how some of these challenges have been resolved. During waking investigations, which generally extend for a few minutes up to perhaps two hours, subjects are aware of transducers attached to their bodies and can comply with instructions to avoid or minimize behaviors (such as body movements and eye

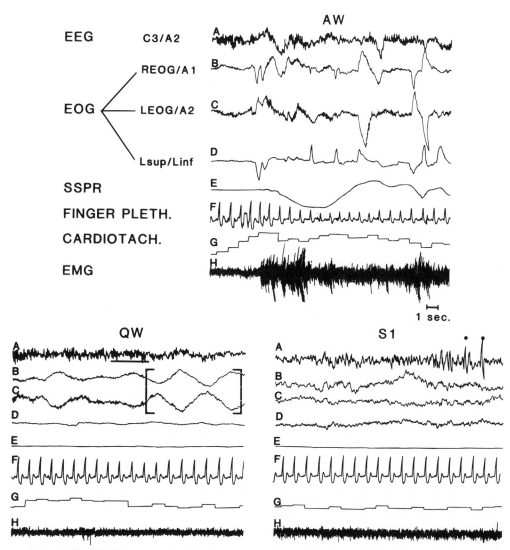

EEG   C3/A2

EOG   REOG/A1

      LEOG/A2

      Lsup/Linf

SSPR

FINGER PLETH.

CARDIOTACH.

EMG

Figure 1. Polygraphic tracings of physiological measures associated with sleep–wakefulness state variations. Eight channels of activity (A–H) are depicted during active and quiet wakefulness (AW and QW, respectively) and the first stage of sleep (NREM stage 1, or S1). The recorded variables include the electroencephalogram (EEG; C3/A2, channel A); the electro-oculogram (EOG; horizontal right and left outer canthi and vertical placements superior and inferior to right eye orbit, channels B, C, and D, respectively); autonomic activity (spontaneous skin potential response, SSPR; channel E); finger plethysmogram (channel F); cardiotachometer recordings (channel G); and the facial (orbicularis oris) electromyogram (EMG; channel H). In these examples, the passive decrease in EMG activity that commonly occurs at sleep onset (S1) does not become evident until slow-wave sleep (Figure 2, S3 and S4). Electrophysiological features of note: alpha activity (underscored, channel A) and slow rolling eye movements (channels B and C) preceding sleep onset in QW; vertex sharp waves in stage 1 (see dots, channel A). See text for discussion of sleep stage definitions and electrophysiological composition. Reprinted with permission from Pivik 1986, © The Guilford Press.

blinks) that might compromise the quality of the recordings. By comparison, sleep recordings normally last at least 6–8 hours, and sleeping subjects do not have volitional control over biological sources of artifact, such as the frequent adjustments in body position that take place during the course of a normal night of sleep (Altshuler & Brebbia 1967; DeKoninck, Lorrain, & Gagnon 1992; Kleitman 1963). Accordingly, it was necessary to develop procedures to more securely attach transducers for reliable recordings over these extended periods of time, and it has often been necessary to design special devices or techniques to access measures of interest while minimizing

sleep disturbance. For example, electrodes used to record the electro-oculogram (EOG) also detect brain waves or electroencephalographic (EEG) signals (see Figures 1 and 2, S1–S4), and to obtain eye movement recordings not contaminated by these signals required transducers that could be applied to the eyelids to register mechanical movements of the eye (Baldridge, Whitman, & Kramer 1963; Gross, Byrne, & Fisher 1965). Although such cross-talk is diminished when low-amplitude, fast-frequency EEG activity predominates (e.g., during waking and REM sleep) and does not generally compromise state identification, even at these times EEG events may influence EOG recordings

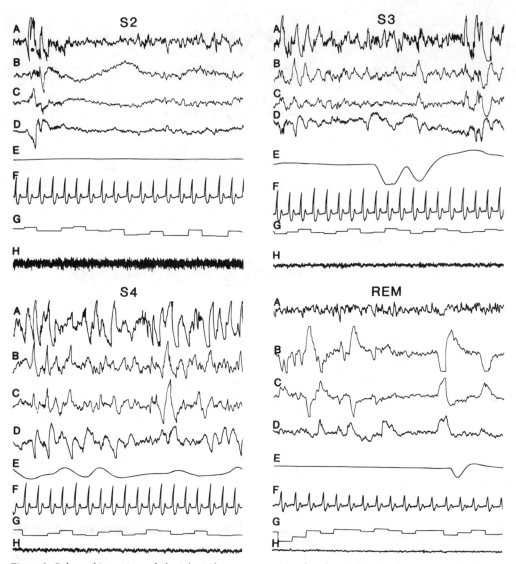

Figure 2. Polygraphic tracings of physiological measures associated with variations in sleep stages – NREM stages 2–4 (S2–S4) and REM. For explanation of channels A–H, see Figure 1. Of note is the occurrence of stage-2 K-complexes (see dot, channel A). See text for discussion of sleep stage definitions and electrophysiological composition. Reprinted with permission from Pivik 1986, © The Guilford Press.

(Iacono & Lykken 1981) and EOG events may influence EEG recordings (see Chapters 2 and 3 of this volume). In order to investigate variations in spinal monosynaptic reflex activity recorded from leg musculature, a method of leg restraint was devised that maintains the positions of stimulating and recording electrodes without altering reflex responses or disturbing sleep as a result of excessive restraint (Mercier & Pivik 1983; Pivik 1971; Pivik & Dement 1970). A variety of devices that can be comfortably inserted into the external auditory canal have been developed for: controlling stimulus delivery in sleep auditory arousal threshold (Busby, Mercier, & Pivik 1994) or evoked potential (Campbell & Bartoli 1986) studies; providing measures of middle ear muscle activity by converting changes in sound pressure level to variations in impedance (Pessah & Roffwarg 1972); and measuring core body temperature by

means of a thermistor positioned near the eardrum (Palca, Walker, & Berger 1981). In addition to these examples, the field of sleep disorders medicine has developed many novel approaches to assess physiological functioning during sleep (see Kryger, Roth, & Dement 1994).

The amount of data collected in even the most fundamental of sleep studies using electrographic techniques is formidable. Over an 8-hr period, a single channel of EEG recording (at the recommended paper speed of 10 mm/sec) will trace a trail on paper extending 0.2 miles or, if digitized, will require approximately 25 megabytes of computer storage space. When it is considered that multiple channels of physiological information are commonly recorded for 2–5 nights, the magnitude of the associated information acquisition, processing, and storage requirements can be appreciated. Increasingly, sleep investigations are utilizing new developments in computer technology that make these challenges more manageable and greatly facilitate associated data analysis (Armitage 1995a; Kubicki & Herrmann 1996). Examples of the application of computerized methods of analysis to an autonomic measure (heart rate) and EEG are presented in the next section in Figures 4–6 and 7–8, respectively.

The organizing principle which imposed meaning on these extensive data (and which was key to the recognition of REM sleep as a discrete entity) involved discerning and clustering patterns of activity into larger blocks of behavior termed "states and stages." These concepts, often loosely applied, are important to distinguish because of the significantly different implications they carry for the conceptualization and understanding of behavior. In the physical world the difference between states is often quite distinct; for example, the defining state characteristics of H_2O when it exists in a liquid, frozen, or gaseous form are clearly evident. In living organisms, however, where behaviors are based on complex interactions among a variety of systems, state definition is often more equivocal and more judgmental. Still, as indicated by the following definitions, even under these more complex conditions there is common agreement regarding criteria for state determination. For instance, a state may be defined as: "a cluster of attributes whose simultaneous and repeated occurrence is highly unique" (Dement & Mitler 1974, p. 278); "a recurring temporally enduring constellation of values of a set of indicator variables of the organism" (Steriade & McCarley 1990, p. 8); or "constellations of functional patterns and physiological variables which may be relatively stable and which seem to repeat themselves" (Prechtl et al. 1968, p. 200). According to these criteria, existence in mammals generally may be partitioned into three states – namely, wakefulness, REM sleep and NREM sleep.

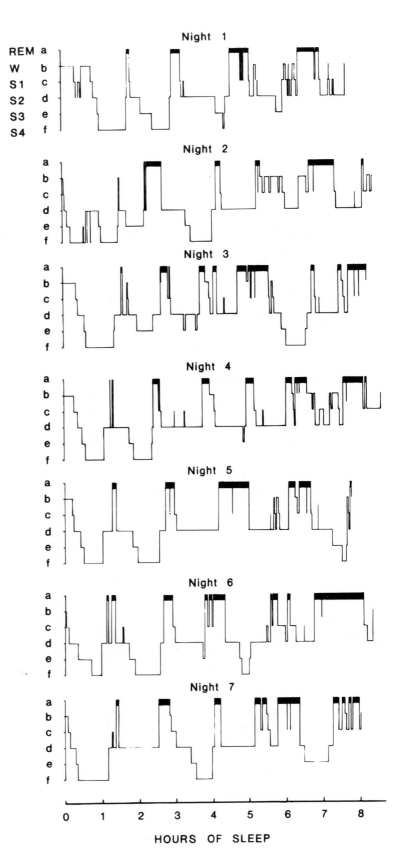

Figure 3. Sleep profiles depicting variations in sleep stages (ordinate) as a function of time asleep (abscissa). These profiles, based on seven consecutive nights of baseline sleep in a young adult, illustrate the stability of sleep patterns across nights, the presence of patterned oscillations between REM (darkened rectangles) and NREM sleep (i.e., sleep cycle), and the decrease in stage-4 and increase in REM sleep as a function of sleep time within a given night. Reprinted with permission from Pivik 1986, © The Guilford Press.

If a *state* may be likened to the gestalt that emerges from associated, defining attributes, then a *stage* represents the identification of progressive within-state changes in these attributes. These component stages are defined by relatively precise but nevertheless arbitrary criteria. Referring again to the different states H_2O may assume, it is possible to define stages of transition bridging these states as a function, for example, of precise temperature and pressure variations. By analogy, the NREM sleep state in humans has been divided into four stages based on EEG criteria. Although REM sleep has been differentially examined on the basis of the presence or absence of various activities (e.g., eye movements or autonomic activation), further fragmentation of REM sleep into stages has not been proposed.

To arrive at valid and enduring state and stage criteria necessitates the development of an adequate and reliable descriptive database from which such criteria can be derived. The initial set of such criteria for sleep states and stages was proposed within five years of the discovery of REM sleep and the use of all-night polygraphic recordings of sleep electrophysiology (Dement & Kleitman 1957a), but it would be more than another decade before standardized scoring manuals would be developed. These manuals defined criteria for the reliable scoring and interpretation of electrophysiological sleep recordings based on the evaluation of 20–30-sec epochs (Anders, Emde, & Parmelee 1971; Rechtschaffen & Kales 1968), and they provided a reasonable solution for managing the large data sets associated with such studies. The choice of the specific scoring epochs for chunking sleep behavior was not specifically rationalized and did not reflect a validated 20- or 30-second behavioral sleep unit. Instead, it was most likely based on several practical factors, including discriminability of recordings, reduction of an extensive database to more manageable dimensions, and providing the best fit between physiological data and technical parameters of recording instrumentation. It is of historical interest in this regard that the early electrographic recordings of human sleep were conducted using a recorder that every 20 or 30 seconds cut a moving strip of paper on which variations in brain potentials were traced (Loomis, Harvey, & Hobart 1938). A caveat to the use of such relatively long scoring epochs is the resultant smoothing of the dynamic flux of physiological changes that occurs within briefer time intervals, giving the impression that sleep states are played out in a very stable and continuous manner and that state and stage transitions are relatively abrupt.

The extent to which the duration of the scoring epoch contributes to this impression was underscored in an investigation in which 24-hour recordings of sleep in the cat were analyzed using a 3-sec scoring interval (Ferguson et al. 1969). With this procedure it was found that uninterrupted intervals of either wakefulness or NREM sleep were quite brief, about one or two minutes. Briefer scoring intervals have also been applied in humans to provide more precise assessments of variations in normal (Ogilvie & Wilkinson 1984; Pivik, Busby, & Brown 1993) or disruptive physiological processes during sleep (ASDA 1992). However, obtaining information of such temporal precision presents additional data processing and conceptual demands. For example, in terms of data processing, using 3-sec scoring intervals in the 24-hr animal recordings increases the number of individual data samples to be analyzed tenfold (i.e., from 2,880 to 28,800). Focusing on ever briefer intervals also requires valid and reliable scoring criteria for these intervals and, most importantly, raises the question of what is the smallest meaningful unit of sleep behavior that can be practically determined. The feasibility of analyzing extended data sets using more discrete time intervals has been significantly facilitated by computer technology. However, when such technology has been applied to studies of sleep, the convention of reporting computerized results based on 20–30-sec (or longer) intervals has been generally maintained (Armitage 1995b; Itil 1969, 1970; Sussman et al. 1979).

Microepoch analyses of physiological variables during sleep provide a more faithful representation of the actions and interactions of these variables; moreover, the resulting enhanced microstructural view of sleep variables may help resolve questions relating to sleep–wakefulness interactions that remain unanswered. For example, the basis for what constitutes a "refreshing" night of sleep remains undetermined, but there is growing emphasis on sleep continuity as an important contributing factor (Carskadon, Brown, & Dement 1982; Stepanski et al. 1984). In this regard, it has been shown that discrete interruptions of sleep, either spontaneously occurring or resulting from external stimulation, can be associated with enhanced daytime sleepiness and reports of significantly reduced sleep quality, even though these disturbances may not effect a significant reduction in total sleep time (Roehrs et al. 1994; Stepanski et al. 1987).

As new methods of data acquisition and analysis have developed, the descriptive picture of sleep physiology has become increasingly detailed and has provided information relevant to the study of psychophysiological relationships during sleep. Still, accounts of thought processes can be directly accessed or confirmed only by means of verbal communication. Although verbalization may occur during both REM and NREM sleep, intelligent dialog with a sleeping subject has not been initiated or maintained, and attempts to provide subjects with posthypnotic suggestions to relate ongoing mentation without awakening have been unsuccessful (Arkin 1978; Arkin et al. 1970). Inferences can be made about thought processes from nonverbal measures – for example, motor responses (Berger & Oswald 1962b; Dement & Wolpert 1958b; Shimizu & Inoue 1986; see also Chapter 3) or autonomic responses (Hobson, Goldfrank, & Snyder 1965; Laberge, Greenleaf,

& Kedzierski 1983; see Chapters 6, 8–10, and 20 of this volume). But such inferences are most reliably determined during wakefulness in the context of a controlled experiment and not during sleep, when directional control over subjects' behavior and associated thought processes is minimal if not absent. Furthermore, although some variation in state can be said to occur when subjects are required to provide a verbal report of immediately preceding experiences, this shift is much greater for the reporting of sleep mentation where a major between-state change must occur (sleep to wakefulness) as compared to the relatively minor within-state change associated with wakeful reports of waking experiences. The more extreme nature of the state change required to access reports of sleep cognition distinguishes studies of sleep mentation from others, which do not feature such marked disparity between the conditions of experience and reporting.

The inability to more directly and immediately access cognitive activity in the sleeping subject, coupled with aspects of sleep physiology that differ remarkably from those commonly associated with cognitive activity during wakefulness, prompted skepticism regarding whether postawakening reports reflected cognitive activity occurring during sleep. Alternative explanations considered included suggestions that the reports reflected hypnopompic experiences generated in the process of waking up (Goblot 1896) or were intentionally contrived in the interest of pleasing the experimenter. Experimental data addressing these concerns will be presented once fundamental attributes of sleep physiology and psychology have been considered.

Sleep Physiology and Psychology: Descriptive Aspects

Nearly two decades before the discovery of REM sleep, Loomis, Harvey, and Hobart (1937, 1938) recorded EEG activity in sleeping subjects and described five sequential brain potential patterns, which they referred to as "stages or states of sleep" (Loomis et al. 1938, p. 421). These patterns (designated A, B, C, D, and E), generally similar across subjects and occurring reliably across recording sessions in the same subjects, were characterized as follows: A, intermittent alpha activity; B, low-voltage potentials (theta); C, the occurrence of 14-Hz spindles; D, spindles in conjunction with 1-Hz delta waves; and E, increased delta activity with less conspicuous spindling (Loomis et al. 1938). It was noted that "during the night of sleep a sleeper continually shifts back and forth from one state to another, either spontaneously or as the result of stimuli" (p. 422). These investigators did not comment on the remarkable implication of their findings that sleep was not the unitary phenomenon it had been traditionally considered to be. It was to be another two decades before a more comprehensive differentiation of EEG patterns during sleep – using numbers instead of letters to designate stage

and including the newly discovered state of REM sleep – was presented (Dement & Kleitman 1957a). It was also in the late 1950s that a second fundamental characteristic of sleep was recognized: sleep stage pattern variations across the night are largely predictable from night to night, indicating the existence of a sleep cycle (Dement & Kleitman 1957a; see also Figure 3).

The discovery of REM sleep and the sleep cycle had far-reaching implications for both biological and psychological processes during sleep. Physiologically, in contrast to previous thinking that sleep occurred passively in response to the absence of wakefulness, these findings indicated that sleep was governed by active mechanisms. Furthermore, since the extended time intervals involved in stage and cycle variations could not be explained by short-term neurophysiological processes, it was necessary to invoke neurochemical mechanisms with longer time constants. In terms of concepts of sleep cognition, these discoveries had equally dramatic effects. Now that dreaming could be associated with a physiological state that recurred predictably each night and that (in the adult) normally accounted for one quarter of each night of sleep, beliefs that dreams occurred only sporadically and under special conditions had to be rejected.

Although the scoring criteria in the Dement and Kleitman (1957a) publication provided descriptions of EEG frequency, amplitude, and waveform characteristics associated with sleep stages, an interlaboratory scoring reliability study conducted by Monroe (1969) revealed an unacceptable level of scoring differences across laboratories. Preliminary reports of Monroe's findings were instrumental in the development of a *Manual of Standardized Terminology, Techniques and Scoring for Sleep Stages of Human Subjects* (Rechtschaffen & Kales 1968), which presented more precise definitions of sleep states and stages and provided the standardized criteria since used for the recording and reliable analysis of adult human sleep. Figures 1 and 2 provide examples of physiological variations characteristic of sleep and wakefulness as well as within-sleep stage differentiations described in that manual. These figures illustrate not only basic measures required for sleep evaluation (EEG, EOG, and EMG; channels A, B, C, and H) but also include optional measures, such as recordings of vertical eye movements (channel D) and autonomic activity (channels E, F, and G). In these tracings, wakefulness (AW and W) is associated with a low-voltage, mixed-frequency EEG that may contain varying amounts of alpha (8–12-Hz) activity. Wakefulness is also usually associated with blinking, rapid eye movements, and variations in the levels of tonic facial EMG activity.

As accurately described 30 years previously (Davis et al. 1938), alpha activity is attenuated in the transition from wakefulness to sleep. There is a concurrent slowing of EEG activity, with an increase in 4–7-Hz theta activity coupled with the sporadic occurrence of vertex sharp

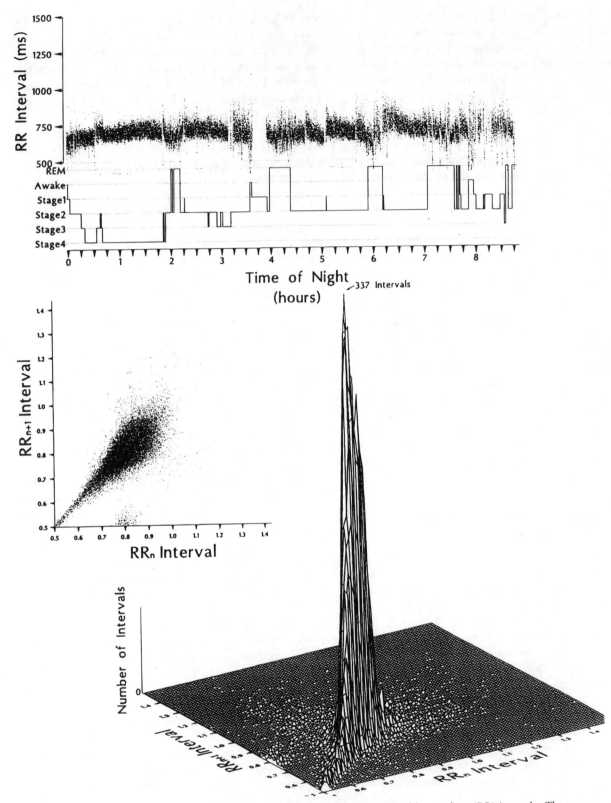

Figure 4. Analyses of heart rate across a night of sleep based on computer-determined beat-to-beat (RR) intervals. The upper graph depicts a sleep histogram with associated RR interval plots. In the middle graph, each RR interval (RR_n) is plotted against the subsequent interval (RR_{n+1}) to produce a graph known as a Poincaré plot, reflecting the beat-to-beat dispersion for specific heart rate intervals as well as interbeat interval variability as heart rate changes. Expanding the two-dimensional Poincaré plot into three dimensions (lower figure) more clearly illustrates the density distribution of graphed values. In this Poincaré plot and those in Figures 5 and 6, RR interval values (both axes) extend from 0 to 1.4 sec in 100 msec intervals.

waves (see Figure 1, S1). The transition from wakefulness to stage 1 is also accompanied by slow horizontal eye movements, and facial muscle tonus is usually decreased relative to that of relaxed wakefulness (Figure 1). Stage 2 is characterized by the intermittent occurrence of K-complexes and 12–14-Hz spindle activity against a relatively low-amplitude, mixed-frequency background (Figure 2). Stages 3 and 4, which together constitute "slow-wave sleep," differ from stage 2 and from each other in the amount of delta (0.5–4-Hz) activity present in each scoring epoch. Stage 3 epochs must contain 20%–50% – and stage-4 epochs more than 50% – of this activity. Defining characteristics of REM sleep include a relatively low-voltage, mixed-frequency EEG without K-complexes or spindles, the sporadic occurrence of eye movements, and reduced levels of submental and facial EEG activity (Figure 2). Although not required for REM sleep determination, other distinctive EEG features that may be present include bursts of theta activity (sawtooth waves) preceding clusters of eye movements (Berger, Olley, & Oswald 1962), and alpha activity 1–2 Hz slower than the subject's waking alpha frequency (Johnson et al. 1967).

These criteria underscore the emphasis on EEG activity for discriminating state and stages – an emphasis which for NREM sleep is absolute and which for REM sleep includes also a requirement of relatively reduced EMG activity. Paradoxically, REM sleep can occur in the relative (i.e., epochs within REM periods without eye movement) or absolute (as in the congenitally blind; Berger et al. 1962) absence of the very parameter for which the state was initially named.

The following quotation (Pivik 1986, p. 384) places the Rechtschaffen and Kales scoring criteria in a broader physiological context and notes fundamental ways in which these criteria describe the difference between sleep and wakefulness.

1. The presence of waveforms unique to sleep – for example, endogenously determined K-complexes, 12 to 14 Hz spindle activity, vertex sharp waves, and frontal sawtooth waves.
2. The prevalence and concentration of activities – for example, the enhancement of slower EEG frequencies (delta and theta), and the concentration of these and other activities, such as eye movements or galvanic skin responses (GSRs), at specific times of the night. With respect to EEG activity, computerized analyses have shown that in only rare instances is the EEG composed of a single frequency; even in the desynchronized low-

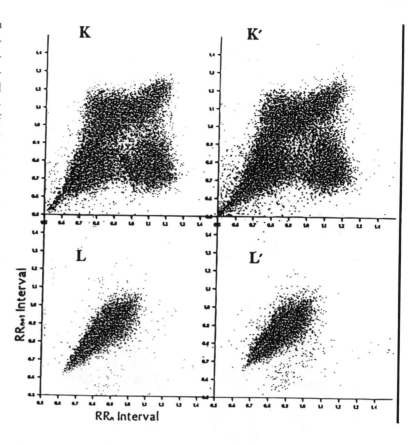

Figure 5. Whole-night Poincaré plots for two subjects (K and L) on two consecutive baseline nights (night 3, left column; night 4, right column). In these graphs, the within-subject consistency and between-subject variability across nights are notable. Reprinted with permission from Pivik, Busby, Gill, Hunter, & Nevins, "Heart rate variations during sleep in preadolescents," *Sleep*, vol. 19, pp. 117–35. Copyright 1996 American Sleep Disorders Association and Sleep Research Society.

voltage EEG of wakefulness in normal individuals, there is a small but nonetheless real component of delta activity present (Lubin, Johnson, & Austin 1969; Hoffman et al. 1979). The shift away from the higher frequencies associated with arousal during wakefulness and the concentration on slower activities are what make sleep unique.

3. The predictable constellations of physiological patterns that occur – for example, concentrations of delta activity are associated with high GSR activation during slow-wave sleep, and indices of cortical, ocular-motor, and autonomic arousal are associated with sustained muscular inhibition during REM sleep.

Sleep profiles (Figure 3) are useful for representing such general sleep characteristics as latencies, cyclicity, stage distribution, and relative amounts of sleep disturbance. However, these graphs do not communicate more rapid physiological variations that occur as sleep patterns play out across the night and that are often most frequent during shifts between states and stages. These transitional

698

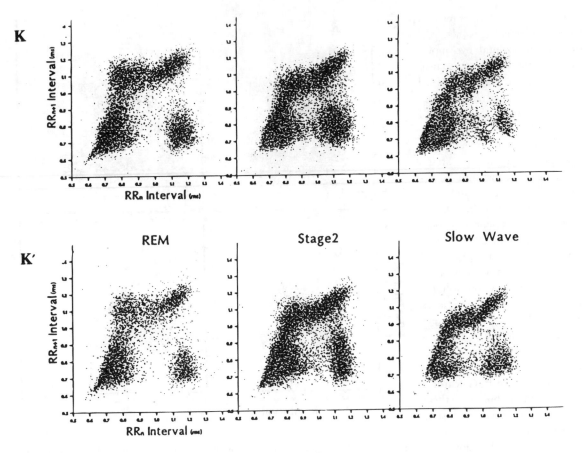

Figure 6. Sleep-stage Poincaré plots illustrating night-to-night similarities for two subjects, M and K (upper and lower plots derived, respectively, from whole-night plots). Reprinted with permission from Pivik, Busby, Gill, Hunter, & Nevins, "Heart rate variations during sleep in preadolescents," *Sleep*, vol. 19, pp. 117–35. Copyright 1996 American Sleep Disorders Association and Sleep Research Society.

periods reflect shifting physiological priorities, the determinants of which are not well understood. Among these state transitions, one that has been the focus of great interest is the sleep onset period. Although most investigators identify sleep onset with the presence of stage-1 EEG patterns, others (Agnew & Webb 1972; Johnson 1973; Ogilvie, Wilkinson, & Allison 1989) – because of inconsistencies in the covariation of psychological and behavioral measures with EEG criteria for sleep – have argued for considering initial stage 2 as sleep onset. It is clear that the EEG changes that take place at sleep onset (Figures 1, 7, and 8) do not occur in physiological isolation. For example, several measures – including oculomotor activity in the form of slow horizontal eye movements (Foulkes & Vogel 1965; Rechtschaffen & Kales 1968), variations in skin potential (Hori 1982), decreased ventilation (Naifeh & Kamiya 1981; Trinder et al. 1992), and decreased heart rate (Pivik & Busby 1996; Zemaityte, Varoneckas, & Sokolov 1984) – may anticipate stage-1 EEG changes by several seconds. Such systematic and coordinated changes across systems are consistent with concepts of physiological state. How-

ever, the relationship between these physiological changes and the point of perceptual disengagement from the waking environment is imperfect, as indicated both by studies of sleep onset mentation (Foulkes & Vogel 1965; Vogel, Foulkes, & Trosman 1966) and by researchers' ability to elicit behavioral responses to external stimulation (in some individuals) in stage 1 and, to a lesser extent, in the initial moments of stage 2 (Ogilvie & Wilkinson 1984; Ogilvie et al. 1989). Another indication that transitions between states or stages are commonly not achieved abruptly is reflected in the practice of many investigators not to accept a single epoch of stage 1 or stage 2 as the time of sleep onset but rather to require several consecutive epochs of these stages for this determination (Born, Muth, & Fehm 1988; Mercier, Pivik, & Busby 1993; Reynolds et al. 1983).

Associated with global patterns of state change across the night are predictable variations in the presence and distribution of physiological activity within sleep stages. For example, stage 4 occurs predominantly in the first third of the night and REM sleep in the last third (Williams, Agnew, & Webb 1964, 1966; see Figure 3) – observations reflected in the exponential decrease in delta activity across the night as determined from more recent computerized analyses of EEG sleep data (Feinberg et al. 1978; Feinberg, Fein, & Floyd 1980). Other notable stage-related physiological variations include: increases in body movements and K-complexes just prior to REM periods (Dement &

Kleitman 1957a; Halasz et al. 1977; Pivik & Dement 1968); reduced incidence of K-complexes and increased spindle activity in the few minutes subsequent to REM periods (Azumi, Shirakawa, & Takahashi 1975; Pivik & Dement 1968); the relative difficulty in engaging REM mechanisms early in the night, as indicated by the brevity or even omission of a REM period within the first two hours of sleep (Berger & Oswald 1962a; Dement & Kleitman 1957a; Roffwarg, Muzio, & Dement 1966); and increased density of eye movements as a function of time both within individual REM periods and within REM periods across the night (Aserinsky 1969, 1971).

It might be expected that state and stage distinctions made in the 1950s would undergo significant modification when subjected to the scrutiny of intense investigation over several decades. However, those definitions have been preserved, and the ensuing research has detailed characteristics of physiological measures that, although not integral to stage determination, have nevertheless served to reinforce and extend our understanding of state physiology. Prominent among these observations is the presence of generalized physiological activation during REM sleep, including increases in the rate and irregularity of respiratory (Aserinsky 1965; Snyder et al. 1964) and cardiovascular (Pivik et al. 1996; Snyder, Hobson, & Goldfrank 1963; Snyder et al. 1964) activities. Electrodermal activity in REM sleep is limited in incidence and is more similar in form to responses of this system during wakefulness (Broughton, Poire, & Tassinari 1965; Hauri & Van de Castle 1973b). These variations occur against a background of centrally mediated inhibition of facial and submental musculature and spinal monosynaptic reflexes (Berger 1961; Hodes & Dement 1964; Jacobson et al. 1964; Jouvet & Michel 1959; Pompeiano 1966, 1967).

Compared with REM sleep, physiological activation in the majority of NREM sleep is unremarkable. Exceptions to this generalization are the unusual levels of autonomic, hormonal and motor activation present during slow-wave sleep, particularly stage 4. During stage 4, there is commonly a dramatic increase in electrodermal activity (Broughton et al. 1965; Johnson & Lubin 1966; see Figure 2), which, in its extreme, has been referred to as "GSR storms" (Burch 1965). Normally, electrodermal activation of this intensity would suggest an enhanced level of

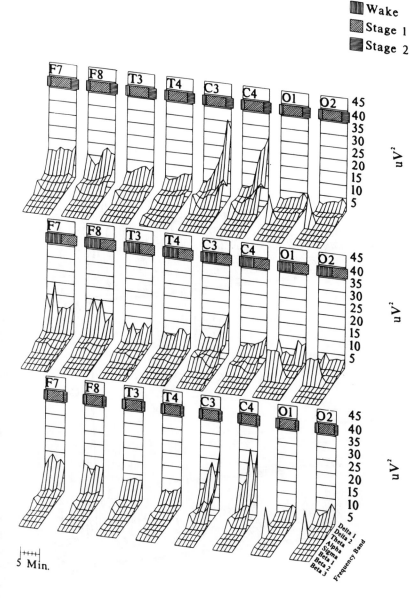

Figure 7. Variations in sleep onset EEG and as reflected in computerized analysis of activity from eight homologous scalp placements (frontal, F; temporal, T; central, C; occipital, O) across three nights in the same subject. The graphs display these data in absolute (μV^2) values following fast Fourier transform and power spectral analysis. These figures show within-subject differences as a function of recording site and night. Reproduced with permission from Pivik, "The several qualities of sleepiness: Psychophysiological considerations," in Monk (Ed.), *Sleep, Sleepiness and Performance.* Copyright 1991 John Wiley & Sons Limited.

arousal, yet arousal threshold during stage 4 is the highest of all sleep stages (Bonnet & Moore 1982; Busby et al. 1994; Goodenough et al. 1965; Lammers & Badia 1991). Consequently, the excessive electrodermal activity during stage 4 has been considered to result from the release of subcortical brain areas involved in the production of these responses from inhibition by higher centers and *not* to index

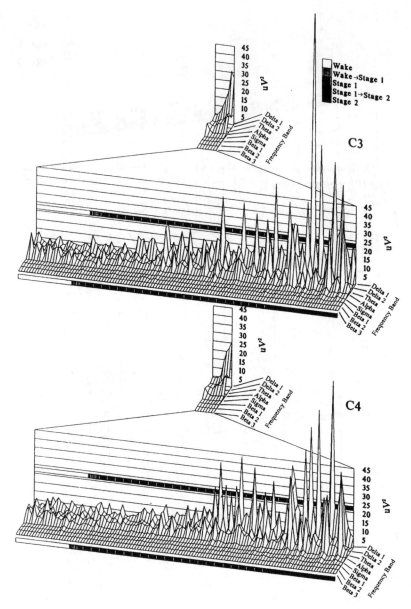

Figure 8. These illustrations expand the 8-min time base charted for bilateral central recordings depicted in the upper and middle panels in Figure 7 and present absolute power data in 4-sec bins. Using modified Rechtschaffen and Kales (1968) criteria, each 4-sec bin was classified into state categories as indicated in the legend. These figures demonstrate the complexities in EEG variations across hemispheres and nights in a single subject during the transition from wakefulness to sleep. Reproduced with permission from Pivik, "The several qualities of sleepiness: Psychophysiological considerations," in Monk (Ed.), *Sleep, Sleepiness and Performance.* Copyright 1991 John Wiley & Sons Limited.

enhanced physiological arousal (Johnson 1973; Johnson & Lubin 1966; see also Chapter 8). Slow-wave sleep is also the time when approximately 80% of the total daily secretion of growth hormone is released (Born et al. 1988; Sassin et al. 1969; Takahashi, Kipnis, & Daughaday 1968) and during which a variety of arousal disorders, termed "para-

somnias," occur (Roffwarg 1979). These disorders are characterized by varying degrees of motor and autonomic activity and include such behaviors as sleep walking, sleep talking, enuresis, night terrors, and confusional arousals. For more detailed consideration of the nosology, description, and treatment of these and other sleep-related disorders, the interested reader is referred to the *International Classification of Sleep Disorders Diagnostic and Coding Manual* (DCSC 1990) or to the text entitled *Principles and Practice of Sleep Medicine* (Kryger et al. 1994).

The initial wave of psychophysiological studies of sleep that followed the discovery of REM sleep were driven by the emphatic physiological distinctions between REM and NREM sleep and were essentially studies of state relationships. They were significantly influenced by the belief that REM sleep provided an objective measure of dreaming and that dreaming occurred only during these periods. For the most part, these studies reported a high incidence (approximately 80%) of recall following arousals from REM sleep – although subsequent investigations also detected subjects who typically fail to recall dreams (Goodenough 1978; Goodenough et al. 1959) – and a relative mental void in NREM sleep (less than 10% recall). However, reports suggesting that mental activity was present during NREM sleep (Goodenough et al. 1959) continued to accumulate, so that by 1967 data were available from nine studies reporting NREM recall values ranging from 23% to 74% (reviewed in Foulkes 1967). To some extent, the apparent discrepancy between the early and later studies regarding the presence of NREM mentation can be attributed to differences in what investigators were willing to accept as a dream. The early studies relied on an intuitive and implicit understanding of the nature of dreaming and consequently did not provide an operational definition of this variable. The first study to provide some clarification in this regard was published in 1957 and entitled "The Relation of Eye Movements during Sleep to Dream Activity: An Objective Method to the Study of Dreaming" (Dement & Kleitman 1957b). In this study, subjects were queried upon awakening as to "whether or not they had been dreaming"; only those reports that related a "coherent, fairly detailed description" (p. 341) of the sleep mental experience qualified as dreams. Reports of having dreamed "without recall of content, or vague fragmentary impressions of content" (p. 341) were considered negative and disregarded. Based on these criteria, observations conformed to the commonly reported REM–NREM recall differentiation (80% recall in REM and 7% in NREM). These early studies, restrictive as they were with respect to dream definition, nevertheless provided an important insight into the nature of the dreaming process – namely, that in most individuals this process occurs with its greatest intensity during REM sleep.

It became obvious that a systematic and effective evaluation of mental activity during sleep would require a more detailed operational definition of what would be accepted as a dream, and many such definitions have been advanced. For example, the dream has been variously characterized as a "verbal report describing an occurrence involving multisensory images and sensations, frequently of a bizarre and unreal nature and involving the narrator himself" (Berger 1967, p. 16); "the presence of any sensory imagery with development and progression of mental activity" (Kales et al. 1967, p. 556); "any occurrences with visual, auditory or kinesthetic imagery" (Foulkes 1962, p. 17); a "multidimensional conglomerate of a hallucinatory belief in the actual occurrence of an imagined experience which, in turn, tends to be an extended visual, sometimes bizarre, drama" (Antrobus et al. 1978b, p. 40); or simply "thinking" (Foulkes 1978, p. 3).

The range of definitions represented by these examples places various constraints on which reports would be accepted into the "dreaming" data set, consequently tailoring the perception of the general nature of cognitive activity during sleep and more profoundly affecting the incidence of acceptable reports of dreaming occurring outside the confines of REM sleep. However, when reports elicited from arousals during sleep were examined using more permissive criteria that allow more fragmentary and less perceptual reports to be accepted as data, the presence of a much more extensive mental life during sleep was revealed. Lifting these definitional restrictions primarily affected the amounts of recall from NREM sleep arousals, with observations of more than 50% recall not being uncommon (Foulkes 1962; Goodenough et al. 1959; Herman, Ellman, & Roffwarg 1978; Molinari & Foulkes 1969; Pivik & Foulkes 1968; Zimmerman 1970). As suggested by the substantial increase in amounts of NREM recall that became apparent once a more relaxed definition of sleep mentation was used, there are qualitative distinctions that differentiate REM and NREM reports. The major differences that have been repeatedly observed (Antrobus 1983; Foulkes & Rechtschaffen 1964; Pivik 1971; Rechtschaffen, Verdone, & Wheaton 1963a) may be summarized as follows:

reports obtained in periods of REM activity showed more organismic involvement in affective, visual and muscular dimensions and were more highly elaborated than non-REMP reports. REMP reports showed less correspondence to the waking life of the subjects than did reports from spindle and delta sleep. The relatively frequent occurrence of thinking and memory processes in spindle and delta sleep was an especially striking result. (Foulkes 1962, pp. 24–5)

Distinctions between REM and NREM amounts of recall and associated qualitative report characteristics seemed to imply a fundamental difference in cognitive activity during these states, with more complex, vivid, and bizarre "dreaming" during REM sleep and less developed, more mundane "thinking" during NREM sleep. However, NREM reports of dreaming have been observed to be as common (Goodenough et al. 1965) or more common (Bosinelli et al. 1968; Foulkes 1960, 1962; Pivik 1971; Pivik & Foulkes 1968; Rechtschaffen, Vogel, & Shaikun 1963b; Zimmerman 1968) than NREM thinking reports. Still, when reports from the two kinds of sleep are contrasted directly via paired comparison, judges are generally able to reliably discriminate REM from NREM reports (Bosinelli et al. 1968; Monroe et al. 1965). An exception to this discriminability is the NREM mentation elicited following arousals during sleep onset. Reports of mental activity at this time share many features with REM sleep reports that make it difficult to discriminate between them, including incidence, hallucinatory dramatic quality, and report length (Foulkes, Spear, & Symonds 1966; Foulkes & Vogel 1965; Vogel 1978; Vogel et al. 1966) as well as perceptual and emotional qualities (Vogel, Barrowclough, & Giesler 1972). Two implications of the recognition that dreamlike mentation occurred outside REM sleep were (i) REM sleep deprivation could not be equated with dream deprivation (Dement 1960) and (ii) REM sleep dreams were not vital to psychological normality during wakefulness (Sampson 1965, 1966; Vogel 1975; Vogel et al. 1975).

Subsequent research has confirmed the characteristics of NREM mentation outlined in cognitive sleep studies conducted during the initial 15 years following the discovery of REM sleep. Yet, despite the weight and persistence of such evidence, there was substantial reluctance to acknowledge the validity of mental activity during sleep occurring outside REM sleep. Although it was necessary to consider other plausible explanations for reports of NREM mentation – such as viewing them as artifacts of arousal generated in the process of waking up, or confabulated in an effort to please the investigators, or reflecting recall of mental activity from previous REM periods – skepticism remained even when such possibilities had been effectively countered. Foulkes (1967, p. 31) offered several probable reasons for this unwillingness to accept the authenticity of NREM mentation despite convincing arguments to the contrary:

(a) while the low-voltage random EEG of REM sleep is compatible with the existence of ongoing thought processes, the high-voltage, low-frequency EEG of NREM is not;

(b) a report of a mental experience is not credible unless supported by public behavioral or physiological observation; and,

(c) REM sleep is so vastly different physiologically from NREM sleep that there must also be a vast psychological difference between the two, such as vivid dreaming vs. little or no mental activity.

This quotation is consistent with the emphasis on physiological correlates as validating indices of psychological experience. Although they provide useful guidelines, a dependence on such physiological correlates can, in the extreme, command an unsupportable degree of mind–body isomorphism. The points outlined by Foulkes serve to illustrate the extent to which prevailing theoretical thinking can promote expectations that interfere with scientific objectivity. The concept of NREM mentation was no more iconoclastic than that of recurrent phases of physiological activation occurring during sleep, yet the latter reports were not met with the same degree of skepticism as reports of NREM mentation. Even though the association between REM sleep and dreaming dramatically altered existing views regarding the nature of dreaming, dreaming was already accepted as a sleep-related cognitive event. Furthermore, because visual experiences are perhaps the most common and compelling components of dreams, the finding that the experience of dreaming appeared to be associated with these periods of rapid eye movements simply confirmed prior expectations. Aserinsky (1996) explicitly refers to this situation when he notes that "the prospect that these eye movements may be associated with dreaming did not arise as a lightning stroke of insight" (p. 217) since the notion of "an association of the eyes with dreaming is deeply engrained in the unscientific literature and can be categorized as common knowledge" (p. 218).

Although not extensive, there was evidence of the kind of linkage between NREM reports and preawakening events that provided precisely the kind of "public evidence" demanded to validate NREM mentation. These preawakening events took the form of either spontaneously occurring activity, such as sleep talking (Arkin et al. 1970; Rechtschaffen, Goodenough, & Shapiro 1962) or experimentally induced incorporations of external stimuli (Foulkes 1967; Foulkes & Rechtschaffen 1964; Rechtschaffen et al. 1963a).

It is likely that a detailed search for observable physiological events to be correlated with, validate, and perhaps explain psychological activity during sleep would have occurred regardless of the REM–NREM mentation controversy. However, if the presence of cognitive activity during NREM sleep had been dismissed then these studies would have focused exclusively on REM sleep, and our appreciation of the physiological conditions and requirements underlying cognitive activity would have been significantly diminished. In this search for psychophysiological measures that might best predict the presence of mental activity during sleep, it is not surprising that EEG activity – despite limitations in understanding the precise nature and origin of such activity (Niedermeyer & Lopes da Silva 1993) – would be a primary focus.

The similarity between EEG activity during waking and REM sleep has been previously noted, and Dement and Kleitman (1957a) suggested that generally this pattern was a better correlate of dreaming than were eye movements. Subsequent research has supported this impression. As EEG activity becomes more desynchronized, there is greater recall and the reports obtained contain more vivid and bizarre dreamlike material. Accordingly, arousals from sleep where the background EEG activity consists of low-voltage, mixed-frequency patterns (stage 1 and REM) produced the highest incidence of recall as well as recall of the most vivid, bizarre, and emotional nature (Dement 1955; Dement & Kleitman 1957b; Foulkes & Vogel 1965; Vogel et al. 1966) as compared to recall obtained from arousals where the sleep EEG is characterized by slower and higher-amplitude patterns (Armitage 1980; Pivik 1971; Pivik & Foulkes 1968). The positive relationship between levels of EEG activation and the quantity and quality of recall is consistent with findings of increased recall of more dreamlike material across the night (Foulkes 1960; Goodenough et al. 1959; Pivik & Foulkes 1968; Shapiro, Goodenough, & Gryler 1963; Verdone 1963, 1965), since there is marked reduction in slower EEG activity and a greater presence of faster frequencies in the second half of the night. As indicated in Figure 3, these variations reflect a concentration of slow-wave sleep early in the night and more stage-2 and REM sleep later.

This confounding of sleep stage and time of night frustrates attempts to determine independent relationships between these variables and aspects of sleep cognition. One approach to circumventing this confound has been to focus on stage 2, which is more prevalent later in the night yet normally occurs throughout the night. When stage-2 mentation is sampled across the night, increases in both recall and dreamlike quality in reports elicited later in the night have been observed (Arkin et al. 1978b; Pivik & Foulkes 1968). Although these findings suggest a time-of-night rather than background EEG influence on sleep mentation, computer analyses of all-night sleep EEG recordings have shown a covariation between EEG activity and time of night – that is, linear decreases across the night in alpha (Harman & Pivik 1996) and delta (Feinberg et al. 1980) bands, indicating that stage 2 early in the night contains greater amounts of slow EEG activity than later in the night. These observations underscore the importance of supplementing, where possible, standard analyses with procedures that may provide additional information. In this case, computer analysis more precisely quantifies the above-threshold delta activity (scoring criteria for stage 2 allow up to 20% per epoch of ≥ 75-μV delta activity) as well as activity occurring below the criterion level, thereby providing a more faithful representation of the amount of this activity within each epoch (Armitage 1995b).

Attention has also been drawn to the occurrence of synchronized fast EEG rhythms (20–40 Hz) during both wakefulness and sleep in animals and humans (Franken et al. 1994; Llinas & Ribary 1993; Steriade, Amzica, & Contreras 1996). These rhythms are most prevalent during wakefulness and REM sleep but have been detected during NREM sleep as well. The cognitive correlates of this activity are only beginning to be studied, and whether (or how) this activity might be implicated in aspects of consciousness and cognition remains to be determined (Kahn, Pace-Schott, & Hobson 1997).

The global time-of-night–EEG–sleep mentation relationships noted here indicate variations in mental activity over relatively long periods of time, but short-term temporal relationships between recall and physiological events have also been reported. For example, recall of REM sleep mentation is reduced if awakenings are made soon after a gross body movement (Dement & Wolpert 1958b; Wolpert & Trosman 1958). Other investigations have shown that duration of time in a sleep stage prior to arousal may influence the amount and quality of recalled material. Arousals made early in REM periods produce fewer reports and reports of less dreamlike quality relative to those obtained from arousals later in REM (Foulkes 1962; Kramer, Roth, & Czaya 1975; Whitman 1969). Although arousals from stage 4 generally produce less recall and recall that is less dreamlike than that from other sleep stages, such differences between stage 4 and stage 2 are minimized when the amount of within-stage time prior to awakening is controlled (Tracy & Tracy 1974). Furthermore, recall rates between REM and slow-wave sleep (SWS) are not as widely discrepant (89% versus 65%, respectively) when temporal factors such as time of night and time into stage are regulated (Cavallero et al. 1992).

The general differences in incidence and qualitative aspects of REM and NREM mentation favor the more "awake-like" stage-1 pattern as a reasonable predictor of dreamlike cognitive activity, but the fact that NREM sleep stages with quite different EEG patterns also support an extensive amount of cognitive activity – often dreamlike – forces the conclusion that these tonic background patterns are at best only global correlates of mental activity during sleep. This conclusion is further affirmed by observations of within-state variations and between-state similarities in the frequency and characteristics of recalled material. Clearly, the psychophysiological relationship between sleep cognition and EEG activity is imperfect.

The characterizations that developed from early studies in sleep cognition – REM sleep mentation as visual, bizarre experiences and NREM mentation as more thoughtlike and mundane – seemed to fit well with an extensive and developing literature in waking subjects that indicated cortical hemispheric specialization for different features of cognitive activity. Neurophysiological and psychophysiological studies in waking subjects assigned linguistic and analyt-ical processes to the left hemisphere and visuospatial and holistic processes to the right hemisphere (Geschwind & Galaburda 1987). The electrophysiological measure that came to be accepted as a primary index of differential hemispheric EEG activation was the amount of alpha activity, since increases in this activity have been related to decreases in attention or effort. For example, higher alpha amplitude has been noted over the right hemisphere during performance on verbal tasks and over the left hemisphere on spatial tasks (Doyle, Ornstein, & Galin 1974; Galin & Ornstein 1972). Accordingly, global REM–NREM variations suggested differential cerebral hemispheric involvement, with the visuomotor loading of REM sleep dreams suggesting greater right-hemisphere involvement during REM sleep (Broughton 1975; Goldstein, Stolzfus, & Gardocki 1972). Close visual examination of EEG recordings may reveal interhemispheric differences in such activity across homologous sites, but quantification of such differences has relied almost exclusively on electronic processing of EEG recordings.

Although it is specifically formulated with respect to the amount of alpha activity, the concept of greater amplitude (or power) of EEG activity as an index of decreased cortical activation – and hence of reduced hemispheric involvement – has been generalized across EEG frequency bands and applied as well to total EEG power measures. At a strictly electrophysiological level, findings with respect to REM–NREM hemispheric activation have been inconsistent in supporting the right-hemispheric nature of REM sleep (Antrobus, Ehrlichman, & Wiener 1978a; Armitage, Hoffman, & Moffitt 1992; Bertini & Violani 1992; Doricchi & Violani 1992). The few studies that have specifically documented the extent of EEG lateralization in conjunction with concomitant sleep mentation have, with few exceptions (e.g. Angeleri, Scarpino, & Signorino 1984), *not* supported the postulated dichotomy between right-hemisphere REM and left-hemisphere NREM (Armitage et al. 1992; Cohen 1977; Guevara et al. 1995; Moffitt et al. 1982; Pivik et al. 1982). It should be emphasized, however, that interpretation of interhemispheric EEG sleep data is complicated by variations in subject characteristics, scalp recording sites, EEG frequency bands considered, and analytical procedures used (Armitage et al. 1992; Pivik et al. 1982; see also Chapter 2), and it may vary dynamically with specific features of ongoing mentation (Bertini & Violani 1992; Doricchi & Violani 1992).

In addition to EEG variables, efforts to determine physiological correlates of mental activity during sleep have also examined autonomic and motor variables. Among autonomic measures investigated in this respect are heart and respiratory rates, electrodermal activity, and penile erections. In general, robust relationships between tonic levels of autonomic activity and either the incidence or qualitative aspects of recalled mentation have not been observed. Furthermore, when positive correlations have been observed, they have often been in association with transient changes in these measures (for reviews see Pivik 1991a; Rechtschaffen 1973).

Perhaps most remarkable are the apparent dissociations between certain autonomic measures and cognitive activity during sleep. Prominent in this regard is the stormlike occurrence of electrodermal activity during stages 3 and 4 (Burch 1965). It would be expected that these high rates of electrodermal activity would have some impact on associated mental activity in terms of enhanced recall or qualitative aspects of recalled mentation, but such relationships have not been observed (Hauri & Rechtschaffen 1963; Pivik 1971; Tracy & Tracy 1974). Similarly, the increased blood flow to the genitalia during REM sleep, resulting in penile erections (Fisher, Gross, & Zuch 1965; Karacan et al. 1966) or clitoral engorgement (Cohen & Shapiro 1970), would suggest that the great majority of REM reports would contain overt sexual content. However, with the exception of lucid dreaming (LaBerge 1985; LaBerge et al. 1983), REM reports with manifest sexual features are relatively uncommon (Fisher 1966; Hall & Van de Castle 1966). It is interesting that lucid dreams containing sexual activity are associated with expected variations in some (respiration and skin conductance) but not all (heart rate) autonomic measures (LaBerge 1985, 1992).

With the exception of occasional twitches and body movements, sleep would appear to the casual observer to be a state of general motor quiescence – an impression physiologically documented for trunk and limb musculature (Jacobson et al. 1964). Not apparent to the observer would be the previously noted tonic inhibition of face and neck muscles that accompanies (and may slightly anticipate the onset of) REM sleep (Berger 1961; Jacobson et al. 1964). Because tonically reduced EMG activity is a defining characteristic of REM sleep, it is not possible to determine the relationship between this variable and ongoing mentation independent of that in other systems (such as those measured by EEG) that are also tonically active at this time. However, because of the variability in the timing of EMG inhibition and EEG desynchronization signaling REM sleep onset, it has been possible to systematically examine characteristics of NREM sleep mentation (generally in stage 2) immediately preceding REM sleep as a function of the presence or absence of tonic EMG inhibition. It was expected that the pre-REM decrease in facial and submental muscle activity might signal a shift to more REM-like mental activity, but instead these low-EMG pre-REM periods yielded fewer reports as well as reports that were less dreamlike than those from awakenings at high-EMG levels (Larson & Foulkes 1969; Pivik 1971).

Tonic–Phasic Distinctions

As indicated by the foregoing review and commented upon by others (Antrobus & Bertini 1992), the relationship between tonic physiological activation and cognitive activity is complex, with the strongest psychophysiological association to emerge being that between the presence of a stage-1 EEG pattern and recall of dreamlike mentation. Although the psychophysiological sleep studies conducted during the decade and a half following the discovery of REM sleep emphasized general state relationships, it had been apparent that – even though sleep stages were defined primarily in terms of tonic physiological criteria – the stages were nevertheless characterized by transient variations in these measures. In fact, a closer psychophysiological correspondence was generally obtained when reports were elicited following such abrupt variations. This improved relationship was reflected in increased recall and/or qualitative variations in recalled material and was observed across EEG, autonomic, and motor systems (Pivik 1986, 1991a). Among such phasically occurring physiological activity, the relationship of one type of discrete motor activity

Figure 9. An example of the correspondence between eye movements and dream content. Immediately following a series of horizontal nystagmoid eye movements (designated by dots) during REM sleep, the subject was awakened (vertical line, lower channels) and related a dream experience (viewing parallel parking lines while riding by in a car) that provided the precise perceptual conditions required to elicit optokinetic nystagmus. In this example, the EMG recordings contain ECG (electrocardiograph) artifact made more prominent by the tonic EMG inhibition during REM sleep. However, this artifact does not interfere with the general purpose of EMG recordings during sleep (i.e., stage differentiation). Reprinted with permission from Pivik 1986, © The Guilford Press.

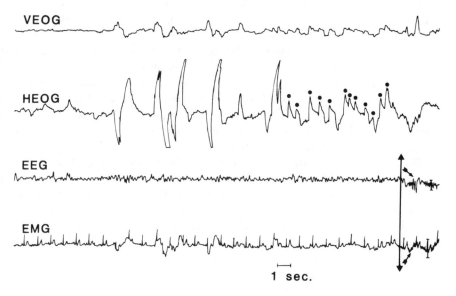

VEOG

HEOG

EEG

EMG

1 sec.

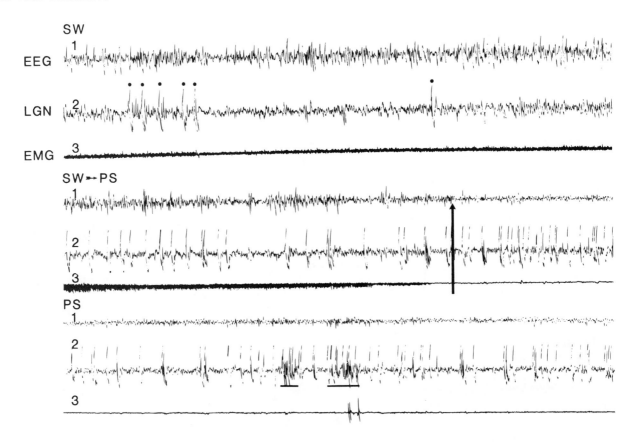

Figure 10. Electrographic variations during the transition between slow-wave (SW) and paradoxical sleep (PS) in the cat. Spontaneous PGO spike activity recorded from electrodes implanted in the lateral geniculate nucleus (LGN) occur in isolated fashion (dots in the upper SW tracings) preceding PS onset (vertical arrow SW → PS tracings) and singly and in clusters during PS (underscored in lower tracings). Reprinted with permission from Pivik 1986, © The Guilford Press.

(eye movements) to REM sleep mentation has been most intensively investigated. These studies have evaluated this relationship not only in terms of general associations but also in trying to determine if a strict relationship existed between eye movements and dream images. In terms of the more nonspecific approach, although increased eye movement activity is commonly associated with enhanced recall, the magnitude of this relationship is not particularly remarkable (Pivik 1991a). Likewise, reports obtained in association with increased eye movement are often, but not consistently, more vivid and emotional (Ellman et al. 1974; Hobson et al. 1965). It is interesting to note that increased eye movement may not always be a good predictor of the amount of activity reported in the dream (Berger & Oswald 1962a; Firth & Oswald 1975; Hauri & Van de Castle 1973a; Pivik & Foulkes 1968).

The discovery of the association between REM sleep and dreaming confirmed the expectation that visual dreams would be accompanied by eye movements. It also suggested the corollary hypothesis that these eye movements were not random but were functioning as they would during wakefulness – to view the perceived images (in this case, dream images). This precise relationship between eye movements and dream imagery of REM sleep has come to be known as the "scanning" hypothesis (Roffwarg et al. 1962). Although intuitively appealing and appearing to provide an ideal opportunity for demonstrating the extent to which psychophysiological isomorphy can occur during sleep, at-

tempts to substantiate this relationship have met with mixed success. Although examples of highly specific correspondence have been noted (Figure 9), demonstrating this relationship as a general feature of REM sleep has been largely unsuccessful (reviewed in Pivik 1991a; Rechtschaffen 1973). However, interpretation of these generally negative results needs to be tempered with an appreciation of the experimental demands inherent in such studies. These include (i) investigators highly skilled in interviewing procedures and techniques, with a detailed understanding of head–eye movement relationships, and (ii) highly motivated subjects who can awaken quickly and provide high-quality detailed recall of dream imagery and associated gaze shifts.

Insight into the difficulty of determining whether (or the extent to which) eye movements during REM sleep are scanning dream images was provided by an investigation conducted during wakefulness in which eye movements were recorded and subjects were periodically interviewed and requested to detail their eye movements in the few seconds prior to the interview (Bussel, Dement, & Pivik 1972). These reports were then correlated with the associated eye

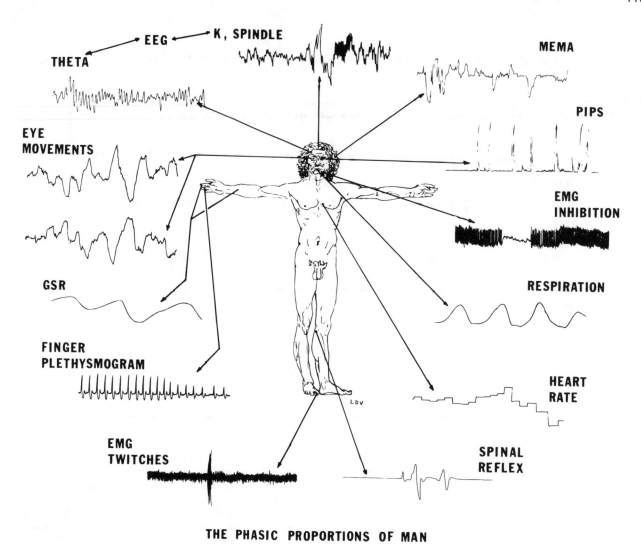

THETA EEG K, SPINDLE

MEMA

PIPS

EYE MOVEMENTS

EMG INHIBITION

GSR

RESPIRATION

FINGER PLETHYSMOGRAM

HEART RATE

EMG TWITCHES

SPINAL REFLEX

THE PHASIC PROPORTIONS OF MAN

Figure 11. Illustrations of various phasically occurring electrophysiological measures that have been investigated in the context of psychophysiological studies of sleep. These variables, with approximate designations of anatomical areas from which they are recorded, include the following: EEG measures (K-complex, spindle, and theta activity); expressions of muscle activity from auditory (middle ear muscle activity, MEMA), visual (eye movements and periorbital integrated potentials, PIPS), and skeletal musculature (facial EMG inhibition, spinal reflexes, and EMG twitches) systems; and autonomic activity (galvanic skin response, finger plethysmogram, respiration, and heart rate). Reprinted with permission from Pivik 1986, © The Guilford Press.

movement recordings. It was observed that subjects' reports during wakefulness could not be related to polygraphically recorded eye movement activity with any greater reliability than has been possible in the REM dream–eye movement studies. There has been a resurgence of interest in this relationship, with indications of more positive associations between eye movement and imagery in lucid dreams (LaBerge 1992) as well as indirect support from studies using imaging technology indicating involvement of the same cortical areas in the control of both waking and REM

sleep eye movements (Hong et al. 1995) and from studies using more nonspecific, correlational techniques associating numbers of eye movements with the amount of visual imagery in dream reports (Hong et al. 1997).

Interest in the association between more discrete variations in physiological activity during sleep and associated mentation – exemplified by the eye movement–REM dream imagery relationship – became part of a more general shift in focus from state to event relationships that significantly affected both physiological and psychophysiological sleep studies. The critical differentiation focused on the duration and temporal clustering of events: sustained or tonic activities lasting several seconds or minutes (e.g., background EEG and EMG stage correlates) were contrasted with sporadic or phasic activities lasting less than a second (e.g., muscle twitches, rapid eye movements, or K-complexes) or, at most, a few seconds (e.g., isolated transient autonomic variations). Initially based on such events during REM sleep in the cat (Moruzzi 1963), this reconceptualization was soon extended to NREM sleep events as well (Grosser & Siegal 1971). Notable influences of this tonic–phasic distinction on psychophysiological studies of sleep included: (1) providing a structured physiological framework within which to consider these studies; (2) suggesting that REM–NREM physiological differences were quantitative and not absolute; and (3) providing what came to be considered a prototypic phasic event that served as a model in the search for the human analog of such activity – namely, the PGO spike. This event, named for the brain regions from which it was most readily recorded (i.e., the Pons, lateral Geniculate bodies, and Occipital cortex), acquired psychophysiological prominence in part because of the anatomical and sleep stage distribution of this activity. Consistent with both the visual emphasis in dreams and the high incidence of dream reports from REM sleep, PGO spikes were most prominent in the visual system during REM sleep (Brooks 1967, 1968; Jouvet 1972; see Figure 10). Furthermore, the occurrence of PGO spikes during NREM sleep – most intensely just prior to REM onset and less frequently at other times in the NREM cycle – held out promise that this activity might provide a physiologic correlate of NREM mentation.

The tonic–phasic distinction provided the theoretical orientation which dominated the field for many years and which continues to influence psychophysiological sleep studies (Antrobus & Bertini 1992; Pivik 1978, 1991a; Rechtschaffen 1973). This model prompted increasing numbers of studies comparing reports obtained from awakenings following episodes of tonic or phasic physiological activation during sleep, stimulated the search for physiological measures that might reflect activity of the phasic event system proposed by Moruzzi (1963; see Figure 11 for examples of the range of events examined in these studies), and led to the formulation of new proposals regarding the relationship between phasic events and sleep mentation (Hobson 1992; Hobson & McCarley 1977).

These investigations provided new insights into sleep physiology and psychophysiology, but they failed to indicate either that phasic events were a prerequisite for the presence of cognitive activity during sleep or that these events could be reliably related to specific qualitative measures of sleep mentation, such as the degree of cognitive processing of dream experiences (Foulkes & Pope 1973; Molinari & Foulkes 1969) or the presence of discontinuity and bizarreness within reports (Foulkes & Pope 1973; Ogilvie et al. 1982; Reinsel, Antrobus, & Wollman 1985; Watson 1972). Furthermore, there are unusual features differentiating sleep from waking cognitive activity that have received little attention in terms of either general or tonic–phasic physiological sleep correlates. Among these are what has been termed the "single-mindedness" and "nonreflectiveness" of dreams. Single-mindedness refers to "the strong tendency for a single train of related thoughts and images to persist over extended periods without disruption or competition from other simultaneous thoughts and images" (Rechtschaffen 1978, p. 97). It has been suggested that this attribute is a reflection of a combination of increased sensory thresholds and cortical activation during sleep (Reinsel, Antrobus, & Wollman 1992). Nonreflectiveness refers to the attenuation or arrest of judgmental processes during dreaming (Kleitman 1967; Rechtschaffen 1978) – that is, the general acceptance of events or images during dreaming without the critical evaluation that normally takes place during waking. This characteristic may reflect the possibility that an inherent feature of dreaming is the absence of the need for "a constant regulating function of self-evaluation" (Meier 1993, p. 64). The apparent limited use of evaluative information from waking cognitive experiences in this context implies either restricted access to such information during sleep or a discontinuity between selective waking and sleeping cognitive processes (Foulkes 1993).

Sleep Cognition: Reconceptualizations

For the first 25 years following the discovery of the relationship between REM sleep and dreaming, investigations into the psychology of sleep were largely physiologically driven. Nevertheless, there were concurrent lines of research that provided information regarding more general issues concerning both the circumstances under which dreaming occurs and the nature of dreams – research from which is emerging a significantly modified view of dreaming. In the process of documenting the apparent pervasiveness of mental activity across sleep stages, investigators provided insights into what may generally be considered the necessary and sufficient conditions for dreaming to occur. Studies of variations in mental activity during the transition from waking to sleep were particularly revealing in this regard. Early investigations identified four stages of EEG–EOG patterns occurring sequentially during this sleep onset period and studied the variations in mental activity associated with these stages, defined as:

1) alpha EEG, generally continuous with one or more REMs a few seconds prior to the "awakening"; 2) alpha EEG often discontinuous, with pronounced SEMs [slow eye movements] covering at least the 20–30 secs. of the record prior to the experimenter's call; 3) descending Stage 1 EEG (almost always, but not necessarily, accompanied by SEMs); and, 4) descending Stage 2 EEG of at least 30 secs. but not more than 2.5 mins. duration (usually, but not necessarily accompanied by SEMs). (Foulkes & Vogel 1965, p. 233)

Mental activity – much of it dreamlike – was reported on 90%–98% of arousals from these stages.

The similarities between these reports and those from REM sleep were emphasized in subsequent studies (Foulkes et al. 1966; Vogel et al. 1972). Furthermore, reports of mental activity changed in a systematic way as subjects progressed from the alpha REM stage to stage 2. These variations began with subjects initially relinquishing control over the course of mental activity, then becoming unaware of the environment, and finally losing reality orientation and having hallucinatory experiences (Vogel et al. 1966). These results suggested that reduced sensory input and subsequent abrogation of voluntary ideational control are essential for dream production. It is notable that when these conditions have been established in waking subjects – either in the context of classic sensory deprivation studies (e.g. Freedman, Grunebaum, & Greenblatt 1971) or under more benign conditions – dreamlike, bizarre, hallucinatory experiences have occurred (Foulkes & Fleisher 1975; Foulkes & Scott 1973; Reinsel et al. 1992; Singer 1978). These observations, coupled with accumulating evidence that REM and NREM reports were not so qualitatively dissimilar (Antrobus 1983; Cavallero et al. 1992; Foulkes & Schmidt 1983), led to the proposition of a single dream system or process that functions across states at different levels of activation (Cavallero & Cicogna 1993; Foulkes & Cavallero 1993). This conceptualization identifies REM sleep as one condition among many that would be expected to be accompanied by dreaming and thereby minimizes the expectation that REM sleep physiology will provide an explanation for dreaming (Foulkes & Cavallero 1993).

However, just as brain injury may affect the characteristics of cognitive activity during both wakefulness and sleep (Kerr 1993), so too must characteristics of sleep cognition be influenced by alterations of the functional architecture of the sleeping relative to the waking brain. Brain imaging studies in humans (Braun et al. 1997, 1998; Hong et al. 1995; Maquet et al. 1996) are beginning to document similarities and differences in cortical and subcortical activation between the waking and sleeping brain that may offer new possibilities for understanding specific dream characteristics. For example, the reported deactivation during REM sleep of areas of the frontal cortex known to be involved in integration of sensory information during wakefulness (Braun et al. 1997) may be consistent with the absence of reflectiveness characteristic of REM dream reports.

In addition to the findings indicating qualitative similarities between REM and NREM mentation, some reports have contradicted the generally accepted view of dreams as characteristically bizarre, unusual, and dramatic experiences that differ significantly from waking thought (Dorus et al. 1971; Foulkes et al. 1967; Snyder 1970). On the basis of these reports and others that compare, for example, the nature of dreams collected in home versus laboratory environments, Foulkes (1996) concluded that "representatively sampled dream experiences, in both content and form, have a texture not so vastly different from, or unfamiliar to, waking experience" (p. 615). These observations effectively demystify the dreaming process and, while acknowledging variations that occur as a consequence of state differences, nevertheless suggest fundamental cross-state similarities between waking and sleeping cognitive systems. Support for

this commonality has been provided by studies indicating that individuals with waking cognitive or sensory defects (e.g., resulting from brain damage) show deficits consistent with these impairments in dream experiences (Doricchi & Violani 1992; Kerr 1993).

Another source of support comes from developmental studies of dreaming. These are particularly relevant not only because of their normative nature but also because features of the ontogeny of physiological aspects of sleep offer unusual opportunities to investigate the development of dreaming. Many of the physiological characteristics of sleep in the adult are not present in the newborn, but perhaps the most dramatic difference is the predominance of REM sleep at this time (40%–70% of total sleep time), with an approximation of adult levels of REM sleep not occurring until after the first year (Louis et al. 1997; Pivik 1983; Roffwarg et al. 1966). The presence of large amounts of this state at a time in development when neuronal processes underlying central nervous system (CNS) maturation are highly active prompted Roffwarg et al. (1966) to suggest that REM-associated activity provided a source of endogenous stimulation important for aspects of normal CNS development. This hypothesis, which is consistent with the influence of activity-dependent factors on neural development, has received support from animal studies demonstrating that interruption of REM sleep phasic influences early in the postnatal period – either by REM sleep deprivation or suppression of PGO spike activity – impaired the course of visual system development (Marks et al. 1995; Oksenberg et al. 1996). However, to expect that the REM sleep–dreaming association so prominent in adults would be present in early development, when waking sensory and cognitive skills are only beginning to form, would require ascribing extraordinary psychological functions to the REM state. At what point does the REM sleep–dreaming relationship become evident, and with what implications for distinguishing cognitive processes during wakefulness versus sleep? Given the research emphasis on adult sleep physiology and psychology soon after the discovery of associations between dreams and REM sleep, it is not surprising that answers to these questions were not immediately forthcoming. When the results of studies of dreaming in early childhood were presented (Foulkes 1982; Foulkes et al. 1990, 1991), they revealed that (i) reports of REM dreams with formal properties of adult dreams did not become evident until the age of 8 or 9 and (ii) the processes required for imagery during waking and sleep develop in parallel. It was concluded that dreaming "is a symbolic process with strong cognitive prerequisites and with a developmental history much like that of waking symbolic thought [and waking consciousness]" (Foulkes 1996, p. 619). Consistent with this parallelism between waking and sleeping cognitive processes is the observation that visual imagery is absent in the dreams of the congenitally blind or those blinded before the age of 5 (i.e., before dreaming can be demonstrated) but present in those blinded at or after this time, when dreaming with properties essentially similar to those in adults occurs (Foulkes 1993; Kerr 1993).

Conclusions, Unanswered Questions, and Future Directions

Overviews of research fields too often emphasize unresolved issues or areas of contention and neglect to emphasize accomplishments. In little more than one generation, research into the related topics of sleep and dreaming has produced remarkable achievements and revelations. These areas, once almost exclusively the topic of anecdotal and speculative discussion, have been redefined by the application of rigorous scientific investigation – with resulting significant empirical revelations regarding the physiological and psychological nature of these ubiquitous human experiences. At the physiological level, enough has been discovered about sleep mechanisms, influences on these mechanisms, and normative aspects of sleep (McGinty et al. 1985; Montplaisir & Godbout 1990; Steriade & McCarley 1990) to permit the extensive differentiation of a variety of sleep abnormalities, many of which can now be effectively treated (DCSC 1990; Kryger et al. 1994). Nevertheless, questions remain regarding the processes underlying virtually every aspect of sleep control: the initiation, maintenance, and termination of sleep as a state as well as between- and within-sleep stage variations. These are truly complex questions, but the coupling of new molecular and genetic methods with those of anatomy, neurophysiology, and biochemistry (Cirelli, Pompeiano, & Tononi 1996; Pack & Mackiewicz 1996; Thakkar 1996) to address these issues offers real promise that they may be resolved.

In terms of the psychology of sleep, studies of sleep cognition have produced results that are no less remarkable. These investigations have broadened our understanding of the organization and formal characteristics of dreams, and they have demonstrated that dreaming is a pervasive behavior not restricted to a particular sleep stage or even to sleep (Antrobus & Bertini 1992; Cavallero & Foulkes 1993; Ellman & Antrobus 1991; Foulkes 1985). Furthermore, the evidence showing that this behavior requires cognitive abilities that normally are not developed until well into the first decade of life (Foulkes 1982, 1993) indicates that dreaming is not an automatic and inevitable consequence of REM sleep. The many empirical accomplishments resulting from years of research into sleep cognition have significantly informed us regarding many aspects of dreams and the dreaming process, but they have also raised new questions (e.g., what features and processes are common to, or distinguish between, cognitive activity during wakefulness and sleep?) and left us still contemplating fundamental questions, such as why dreams are so readily forgotten and whether dreaming has an adaptive function.

Dreaming is still most likely to be reported from the REM sleep state, yet – except for the general association between REM sleep physiology and dreaming – attempts to determine reliable links between sleep physiology and sleep cognition have been largely unsuccessful. Perhaps, as suggested by Rosenlicht and Feinberg (1997) for REM sleep (and as may apply to any situation where dreaming occurs), this apparent "gross psychophysiological *mismatch*" may reflect an inherent dissociation during dreaming that relates to physiological and/or psychological state function at that time. If, as Foulkes suggests for "minds capable of conscious representational and self-representational intelligence" (1997, p. 4), "dreaming is the form assumed by consciousness whenever there is residual but somewhat dissociated cognitive/cerebral activation in the relative absence of direction either from the person's environment or from voluntary self-control" (p. 3), then perhaps these dissociations may be better understood in terms of the functional activation of various brain areas and systems at the time of the dream relative to that observed during nondream experiences. Promising indications that such understanding may not be beyond our reach can be found in the application of functional imaging technology to the study of physiological and cognitive processes during sleep (Braun et al. 1997, 1998; Hong et al. 1995; Maquet et al. 1996), in the refinement of instruments to evaluate features of these cognitive experiences such as "bizarreness" (Reinsel et al. 1992) and sensory qualities (Antrobus et al. 1987; Rechtschaffen & Buchignani 1992), and in the development of heuristic theoretical models that integrate these complex data (Antrobus 1993; Kahn et al. 1997). The continuing development of such technological and methodological procedures and their combined application in the same subjects at times associated with the occurrence of dreamlike mentation – as well as during wakefulness under conditions where levels of perceptual processing and symbolic cognition are controlled – will facilitate the identification of similarities and differences in cross-state processes. Such studies will most likely reveal that the sleep–wakefulness state barrier is more permeable than once thought and that the biological and cognitive processes defining these states are more meaningfully related than many previously imagined.

NOTE

The author gratefully acknowledges the assistance of Ralph Nevins and Jane Buttrum in the preparation of figures, Drs. K. Busby and K. Harman for helpful comments on early drafts of the manuscript, and Jane Buttrum for secretarial support.

REFERENCES

Agnew, H. W., Jr., and Webb, W. B. (1972). Measurement of sleep onset by EEG criteria. *Am. J. EEG Technol.*, 12, 127–34.

Agnew, H. W., Jr., Webb, W. B., & Williams, R. L. (1966). The first night effect: An EEG study of sleep. *Psychophysiology, 2,* 263–6.

Altshuler, K. Z., & Brebbia, D. R. (1967). Body movement artifact as a contaminant in psychophysiological studies of sleep. *Psychophysiology, 3,* 86–91.

Anders, T., Emde, R., & Parmelee, A. (Eds.) (1971). *A Manual of Standardized Terminology, Techniques and Criteria for Scoring of States of Sleep and Wakefulness in Newborn Infants.* Los Angeles: UCLA Brain Information, NIMDS Neurological Information Network.

Angeleri, F., Scarpino, O., & Signorino, M. (1984). Information processing and hemispheric specialization: Electrophysiological study during wakefulness, stage 2 and stage REM sleep. *Res. Commun. Psychol., Psychiatry, Behav., 9,* 121–38.

Antrobus, J. S. (1983). REM and NREM sleep reports: Comparison of word frequencies by cognitive classes. *Psychophysiology, 20,* 562–8.

Antrobus, J. S. (1993). The dreaming mind/brain: Understanding its processes with connectionist models. In Cavallero & Foulkes, pp. 77–92.

Antrobus, J. S., & Bertini, M. (Eds.) (1992). *The Neuropsychology of Sleep and Dreaming.* Hillsdale, NJ: Erlbaum.

Antrobus, J., Ehrlichman, H., & Wiener, M. (1978a). EEG asymmetry during REM and NREM: Failure to replicate [Abstract]. *Sleep Res., 7,* 24.

Antrobus, J. S., Fein, G., Jordan, L., Ellman, S. J., & Arkin, A. M. (1978b). Measurement and design in research on sleep reports. In Arkin et al. (1978a), pp. 19–55.

Antrobus, J., Hartwig, P., Rosa, D., Reinsel, R., & Fein, G. (1987). Brightness and clarity of REM and NREM imagery: Photo response scale. *Sleep Res., 16,* 240.

Arkin, A. M. (1978). Sleeptalking. In Arkin et al. (1978a), pp. 513–32.

Arkin, A. M., Antrobus, J. S., & Ellman, S. J. (Eds.) (1978a). *The Mind in Sleep.* Hillsdale, NJ: Erlbaum.

Arkin, A. M., Antrobus, J. S., Ellman, S. J., & Farber, J. (1978b). Sleep mentation as affected by REMP deprivation. In Arkin et al. (1978a), pp. 459–84.

Arkin, A. M., Toth, M., Baker, J., & Hastey, J. M. (1970). The frequency of sleep-talking in the laboratory among chronic sleep-talkers and good dream recallers. *J. Nerv. Ment. Dis., 151,* 369–74.

Armitage, R. (1980). Changes in dream content as a function of time of night, stage of awakening and frequency of recall. Master's thesis, Carleton University, Ottawa.

Armitage, R. (1995a). Microarchitectural findings in sleep EEG in depression: Diagnostic implications. *Biol. Psychiatry, 37,* 72–84.

Armitage, R. (1995b). The distribution of EEG frequencies in REM and NREM sleep stages in healthy young adults. *Sleep, 18,* 334–41.

Armitage, R., Hoffmann, R., & Moffitt, A. (1992). Interhemispheric EEG activity in sleep and wakefulness: Individual differences in the basic rest–activity cycle (BRAC). In Antrobus & Bertini, pp. 17–45.

ASDA [American Sleep Disorders Association and Sleep Research Society] (1992). Atlas Task Force Report. EEG arousals: Scoring rules and examples. *Sleep, 15,* 173–84.

Aserinsky, E. (1953). Ocular motility during sleep and its application to the study of rest–activity cycles and dreaming. Thesis, University of Chicago.

Aserinsky, E. (1965). Periodic respiratory pattern occurring in conjunction with eye movements during sleep. *Science, 150,* 763–6.

Aserinsky, E. (1969). The maximal capacity for sleep: Rapid eye movement density as an index of sleep satiety. *Biol. Psychiatry, 1,* 147–59.

Aserinsky, E. (1971). Rapid eye movement density and pattern in the sleep of normal young adults. *Psychophysiology, 8,* 361–75.

Aserinsky, E. (1996). The discovery of REM sleep. *J. Hist. Neurosci., 5,* 213–27.

Aserinsky, E., & Kleitman, N. (1953). Regularly occurring periods of eye motility and concomitant phenomena during sleep. *Science, 118,* 273–5.

Aserinsky, E., & Kleitman, N. (1955). Two types of ocular motility occurring during sleep. *J. Appl. Physiol., 8,* 1–10.

Azumi, K., Shirakawa, S., & Takahashi, S. (1975). Periodicity of sleep spindle appearance in normal adults [Abstract]. *Sleep Res., 4,* 263.

Baldridge, B. J., Whitman, R. M., & Kramer, M. (1963). A simplified method for detecting eye movements during dreaming. *Psychosomatic Med., 25,* 78–82.

Bentivoglio, M., & Grassi-Zucconi, G. (1997). The pioneering experimental studies on sleep deprivation. *Sleep, 20,* 570–6.

Berger, R. J. (1961). Tonus of extrinsic laryngeal muscles during sleep and dreaming. *Science, 134,* 840.

Berger, R. J. (1967). When is a dream is a dream is a dream? *Exp. Neurol., 19,* 15–28.

Berger, R. J., Olley, P., & Oswald, L. (1962). The EEG, eye movements, and dreams of the blind. *Quarterly J. Exp. Psychol., 14,* 183–6.

Berger, R. J., & Oswald, I. (1962a). Effects of sleep deprivation on behavior, subsequent sleep, and dreaming. *J. Ment. Sci., 108,* 457–65.

Berger, R. J., & Oswald, I. (1962b). Eye movements during active and passive dreams. *Science, 137,* 601.

Bertini, M., & Violani, C. (1992). The postawakening testing technique in the investigation of cognitive asymmetries during sleep. In Antrobus & Bertini, pp. 47–62.

Bonnet, M. H., & Moore, S. E. (1982). The threshold of sleep: Perception of sleep as a function of time asleep and auditory threshold. *Sleep, 5,* 267–76.

Born, J., Muth, S., & Fehm, H. L. (1988). The significance of sleep onset and slow wave sleep for nocturnal release of growth hormone (GH) and cortisol. *Psychoneuroendocrinology, 13,* 233–43.

Bosinelli, M., Molinari, S., Bagnaresi, G., & Salzarulo, P. (1968). Caratteristiche dell attiva psicofisiologica durante il sonno: Un contributo alle techniche di valutazion. *Riv. Speriment. Freiatria, 92,* 128–50.

Braun, A. R., Balkin, T. J., Wesensten, N. L., Carson, R. E., Varga, M., Baldwin, P. S., Selbie, J., Belenky, G., & Herscovitch, P. (1997). Regional cerebral blood flow throughout the sleep–wake cycle: An H$_2$^{15}O PET study. *Brain, 120,* 1173–97.

Braun, A. R., Balkin, T. J., Wesensten, N. L., Carson, R. E., Varga, M., Baldwin, P. S., Selbie, J., Belenky, G., & Herscovitch, P. (1998). Dissociated pattern of activity in visual cortices and their projections during human rapid eye movement sleep. *Science, 279,* 91–5.

Bremer, F. (1937). L'activité cérébrale au cours du sommeil et de la narcose. Contribution a l'étude du mécanisme du sommeil. *Bull. Acad. R. Med. Belg.*, *4*, 68–86.

Bremer, F. (1938). L'activité électrique de l'écorce cérébrale et le probleme physiologique du sommeil. *Boll. Soc. Ital. Biol. Sper.*, *13*, 271–90.

Brooks, D. C. (1967). Localization of the lateral geniculate nucleus monophasic waves associated with eye movements in the cat. *Electroencephalogr. Clin. Neurophysiol.*, *23*, 123–33.

Brooks, D. C. (1968). Localization and characteristics of the cortical waves associated with eye movements in the cat. *Exp. Biol.*, *22*, 603–13.

Broughton, R. J. (1975). Biorhythmic variations in consciousness and psychological function. *Can. Psychological Rev.*, *16*, 217–39.

Broughton, R. J., Poire, R., & Tassinari, C. A. (1965). The electrodermogram (Tarchanoff effect) during sleep. *Electroencephalogr. Clin. Neurophysiol.*, *18*, 691–708.

Burch, N. (1965). Data processing of psychophysiological recordings. In L. D. Proctor & W. R. Adey (Eds.), *Symposium on the Analysis of Central Nervous System and Cardiovascular Data Using Computer Methods*, pp. 165–180. Washington, DC: National Aeronautics and Space Administration.

Busby, K. A., Mercier, L., & Pivik, R. T. (1994). Ontogenetic variations in auditory arousal threshold during sleep. *Psychophysiology*, *31*, 182–8.

Bussell, J., Dement, W., & Pivik, R. T. (1972). The eye movement–imagery relationship in REM sleep and waking [Abstract]. *Sleep Res.*, *1*, 100.

Campbell, D. T. (1957). Factors relevant to the validity of experiments in social settings. *Psych. Bull.*, *54*, 297–312.

Campbell, K., & Bartoli, E. (1986). Human auditory evoked potentials during natural sleep: The early components. *Electroencephal. Clin. Neurophysiol.*, *65*, 142–9.

Carskadon, M. A., Brown, E. D., & Dement, W. C. (1982). Sleep fragmentation in the elderly: Relationship to daytime sleep tendency. *Neurobiology of Aging*, *3*, 321–7.

Cavallero, C., & Cicogna, P. (1993). Memory and dreaming. In Cavallero & Foulkes, pp. 38–57.

Cavallero, C., Cicogna, P., Natale, V., Occhionero, M., & Zito, A. (1992). Slow wave sleep dreaming. *Sleep*, *15*, 562–6.

Cavallero, C., & Foulkes, D. (Eds.) (1993). *Dreaming as Cognition*. New York: Harvester Wheatsheaf.

Cirelli, C., Pompeiano, M., & Tononi, G. (1996). New perspectives on sleep and gene expression. *SRS Bull.*, *2*, 12–17.

Cohen, D. B. (1977). Changes in REM dream content during the night: Implications for a hypothesis about changes in cerebral dominance across REM periods. *Percept. Mot. Skills*, *44*, 1267–77.

Cohen, H. D., & Shapiro, A. (1970). Vaginal blood flow during sleep [Abstract]. *Psychophysiology*, *1*, 338.

Davis, H., Davis, P. A., Loomis, A. L., Harvey, E. N., & Hobart, G. (1938). Human brain potentials during the onset of sleep. *J. Neurophysiol.*, *1*, 24–38.

DCSC [Diagnostic Classification Steering Committee] (1990). *International Classification of Sleep Disorders: Diagnostic and Coding Manual*. Rochester, MN: American Sleep Disorders Association.

DeKoninck, J., Lorrain, D., & Gagnon, P. (1992). Sleep positions and position shifts in five age groups: An ontogenetic picture. *Sleep*, *15*, 143–9.

Dement, W. C. (1955). Dream recall and eye movement during sleep in schizophrenics and normals. *J. Nerv. Ment. Dis.*, *122*, 263–9.

Dement, W. C. (1960). The effect of dream deprivation. *Science*, *131*, 1705–7.

Dement, W. C. (1969). A new look at the third state of existence. *Stanford Medical Alumni Association*, *8*, 2–8.

Dement, W. C., & Kleitman, N. (1957a). Cyclic variations in EEG during sleep and their relation to eye movements, bodily motility and dreaming. *Electroencephalogr. Clin. Neurophysiol.*, *9*, 673–90.

Dement, W. C., & Kleitman, N. (1957b). The relation of eye movements during sleep to dream activity: An objective method for the study of dreaming. *J. Exp. Psychol.*, *53*, 339–46.

Dement, W. C., & Mitler, M. M. (1974). An introduction to sleep. In O. Petre-Quadens & J. D. Schlag (Eds.), *Basic Sleep Mechanisms*, pp. 271–96. New York: Academic Press.

Dement, W., & Wolpert, E. (1958a). Interrelations in the manifest content of dreams occurring on the same night. *J. Nerv. Ment. Dis.*, *126*, 568–78.

Dement, W., & Wolpert, E. (1958b). The relation of eye movements, body motility, and external stimuli to dream content. *J. Exp. Psychol.*, *55*, 543–54.

Domhoff, G. W., & Kamiya, J. (1964). Problems in dream content study with objective indicators: 1. A comparison of home and laboratory dream reports. *Arch. Gen. Psychiatry*, *11*, 519–24.

Doricchi, F., & Violani, C. (1992). Dream recall in brain-damaged patients: A contribution to the neuropsychology of dreaming through a review of the literature. In Antrobus & Bertini, pp. 99–140.

Dorus, E., Dorus, W., & Rechtschaffen, A. (1971). The incidence of novelty in dreams. *Arch. Gen. Psychiatry*, *25*, 364–8.

Doyle, J. C., Ornstein, R., & Galin, D. (1974). Lateral specialization of cognitive mode: EEG frequency analysis. *Psychophysiology*, *11*, 567–78.

Ellman, S. J., & Antrobus, J. S. (Eds.) (1991). *The Mind in Sleep*, 2nd ed. New York: Wiley.

Ellman, S. J., Antrobus, J. S., Arkin, A. M., Farber, J., Luck, D., Bodnar, R., Sanders, K., & Nelson, W. J., Jr. (1974). Sleep mentation in relation to phasic and tonic events – REMP and NREM [Abstract]. *Sleep Res.*, *3*, 115.

Everson, C. A. (1995). Functional consequences of sustained sleep deprivation in the rat. *Behav. Brain Res.*, *69*, 43–54.

Feinberg, I., Fein, G., & Floyd, T. C. (1980). Period and amplitude analysis of NREM EEG in sleep: Repeatability of results in young adults. *Electroencephalogr. Clin. Neurophysiol.*, *48*, 212–21.

Feinberg, I., March, J. D., Fein, G., Floyd, T. C., Walker, J. M., & Price, L. (1978). Period of amplitude analysis of 0.5–3 c/sec activity in NREM sleep of young adults. *Electroencephalogr. Clin. Neurophysiol.*, *44*, 202–13.

Ferguson, J., Cohen, H., Barchas, J., & Dement, W. (1969). Sleep and wakefulness: A closer look. Paper presented at a meeting of the Federation of American Society for Experimental Biology's Symposium on Neurohumoral Aspects of Sleep and Wakefulness (Atlantic City, NJ).

Firth, H., & Oswald, I. (1975). Eye movements and visually active dreams. *Psychophysiology*, *12*, 602–5.

Fisher, C. (1966). Dreaming and sexuality. In R. Lowenstein, L. Newman, M. Shur, & A. Solnit (Eds.), *Psychoanalysis: A General Psychology*. New York: International Universities Press.

Fisher, C., Gross, J., & Zuch, J. (1965). Cycles of penile erection synchronous with dreaming (REM) sleep. *Arch. Gen. Psychiatry, 12*, 29–45.

Foulkes, D. (1960). Dream reports from different stages of sleep. Doctoral dissertation, University of Chicago.

Foulkes, D. (1962). Dream reports from different stages of sleep. *J. Abn. Soc. Psychol., 65*, 14–25.

Foulkes, D. (1967). Nonrapid eye movement mentation. *Exp. Neurol., 19*, 28–38.

Foulkes, D. (1978). *A Grammar of Dreams*. New York: Basic Books.

Foulkes, D. (1982). *Children's Dreams: Longitudinal Studies*. New York: Wiley.

Foulkes, D. (1985). *Dreaming: A Cognitive-Psychological Analysis*. Hillsdale, NJ: Erlbaum.

Foulkes, D. (1993). Children's dreaming. In Cavallero & Foulkes, pp. 114–32.

Foulkes, D. (1996). Dream research: 1953–1993. *Sleep, 19*, 609–24.

Foulkes, D. (1997). A contemporary neurobiology of dreaming. *SRS Bull., 3*, 2–4.

Foulkes, D., & Cavallero, C. (1993). Introduction. In Cavallero & Foulkes, pp. 1–17.

Foulkes, D., & Fleisher, S. (1975). Mental activity in relaxed wakefulness. *J. Abnorm. Psychol., 84*, 66–75.

Foulkes, D., Hollifield, M., Bradley, L., Terry, R., & Sullivan, B. (1991). Waking self-understanding, REM-dream self representation, and cognitive ability variables at ages 5–8. *Dreaming, 1*, 41–51.

Foulkes, D., Hollifield, M., Sullivan, B., Bradley, L., & Terry, R. (1990). REM dreaming and cognitive skill at ages 5–8: A cross-sectional study. *Int. J. Behav. Devel., 13*, 447–65.

Foulkes, D., Pivik, T., Steadman, H. S., Spear, P. S., & Symonds, J. D. (1967). Dreams of the male child: An EEG study. *J. Abn. Psychology, 72*, 457–67.

Foulkes, D., & Pope, R. (1973). Primary visual experience and secondary cognitive elaboration in stage REM: A modest confirmation and an extension. *Percept. Mot. Skills, 37*, 107–18.

Foulkes, D., & Rechtschaffen, A. (1964). Presleep determinants of dream content: Effects of two films. *Percept. Mot. Skills, 19*, 983–1005.

Foulkes, D., & Schmidt, M. (1983). Temporal sequence and unit composition in dream reports from different stages of sleep. *Sleep, 6*, 265–80.

Foulkes, D., & Scott, E. (1973). An above-zero waking baseline for the incidence of momentarily hallucinatory mentation [Abstract]. *Sleep Res., 2*, 108.

Foulkes, D., Spear, P. S., & Symonds, J. (1966). Individual differences in mental activity at sleep onset. *J. Abnorm. Psychol., 71*, 280–6.

Foulkes, D., & Vogel, G. (1965). Mental activity at sleep onset. *J. Abnorm. Psychol., 70*, 231–43.

Franken, P., Dijk, D. J., Tobler, I., & Borbely, A. A. (1994). High-frequency components of the rat electrocorticogram are modulated by the vigilance states. *Neurosci. Lett., 167*, 89–92.

Freedman, S. J., Grunebaum, H. U., & Greenblatt, M. (1971). Perceptual and cognitive changes in sensory deprivation. In P. Solomon, P. E. Kubzansky, P. H. Leiderman, J. H. Mendelson, R. Trumbull, & D. Wexler (Eds.), *Sensory Deprivation*

(A Symposium Held at Harvard Medical School), pp. 58–71. Cambridge, MA: Harvard University Press.

Galin, D., & Ornstein, R. (1972). Lateral specialization of cognitive mode: An EEG study. *Psychophysiology, 9*, 412–18.

Geschwind, N., & Galaburda, A. M. (Eds.) (1987). *Cerebral Lateralization: Biological Mechanisms, Associations, and Pathology*. Cambridge, MA: MIT Press.

Gillberg, M., & Åkerstedt, T. (1994). Sleep restriction and SWS-suppression: Effects on daytime alertness and night-time recovery. *J. Sleep Res., 3*, 144–51.

Goblot, E. (1896). Sur le souvenir des rêves. *Revue Philosophique, 42*, 288.

Goldstein, L., Stolzfus, N., & Gardocki, J. (1972). Changes in interhemispheric amplitude relations in EEG during sleep. *Physiological Behav., 8*, 811–15.

Goodenough, D. R. (1978). Dream recall: History and current status of the field. In Arkin et al. (1978a), pp. 113–40.

Goodenough, D. R., Lewis, H. B., Shapiro, A., & Sleser, I. (1965). Some correlates of dream reporting following laboratory awakenings. *J. Nerv. Ment. Dis., 140*, 365–73.

Goodenough, D. R., Shapiro, A., Holden, M., & Steinschriber, L. (1959). A comparison of "dreamers" and "nondreamers": Eye movements, electroencephalograms and the recall of dreams. *J. Abnorm. Psychol., 59*, 295–302.

Griesinger, X. X. (1868). Physio-psychologische Selbstbeobachtungen. *Arch. Psychiatr. Nervenkr., 1*, 200–4.

Gross, J., Byrne, J., & Fisher, C. (1965). Eye movements during emergent stage I EEG in subjects with life-long blindness. *J. Nerv. Ment. Dis., 141*, 365–70.

Grosser, G., & Siegal, A. (1971). Emergence of a tonic–phasic model for sleep and dreaming: Behavioral and physiological observations. *Psychol. Bull., 75*, 60–72.

Guevara, M. A., Lorenzo, I., Arce, C., Ramos, M., & Corsi-Cabrera, M. (1995). Inter- and intrahemispheric EEG correlation during sleep and wakefulness. *Sleep, 18*, 257–65.

Guilleminault, C. (1994). Clinical features and evaluation of obstructive sleep apnea. In M. H. Kryger, T. Roth, & W. C. Dement (Eds.), *Principles and Practice of Sleep Medicine*, 2nd ed., pp. 667–77. Philadelphia: Saunders.

Halasz, P., Rajna, P., Pal, I., Kundra, O., Vargha, A., Balogh, A., & Kemeny, A. (1977). K-complexes and micro-arousals as functions of the sleep process. In W. P. Koella & P. Levin (Eds.), *Sleep 1976*, pp. 292–4. Basel: Karger.

Hall, C., & Van de Castle, R. L. (1966). *The Content Analysis of Dreams*. New York: Appleton-Century-Crofts.

Harman, K., & Pivik, R. T. (1996). Site-specific variations in alpha activity across sleep cycles in normal adults [Abstract]. *Sleep Res., 25*, 127.

Hauri, P., & Rechtschaffen, A. (1963). An unsuccessful attempt to find physiological correlates of NREM recall. Paper presented at the meeting of the Association for the Psychophysiological Study of Sleep (New York).

Hauri, P., & Van de Castle, R. L. (1973a). Psychophysiological parallelism in dreams. *Psychosomatic Med., 35*, 297–308.

Hauri, P., & Van de Castle, R. L. (1973b). Psychophysiological parallels in dreams. In U. J. Jovanovic (Ed.), *The Nature of Sleep*, pp. 140–2. Stuttgart: Fischer.

Herman, J. H., Ellman, S. J., & Roffwarg, H. P. (1978). The problem of NREM dream recall re-examined. In Arkin et al. (1978a), pp. 59–92.

Hobson, J. A. (1992). A new model of brain–mind state: Activation level, input source, and mode of processing (AIM). In Antrobus & Bertini, pp. 227–45.

Hobson, J. A., Goldfrank, F., & Snyder, F. (1965). Respiration and mental activity in sleep. *J. Psychiatric Res., 3,* 79–90.

Hobson, J. A., & McCarley, R. W. (1977). The brain as a dream state generator: An activation-synthesis hypothesis of the dream process. *Am. J. Psychiatry, 134,* 1335–48.

Hodes, R., & Dement, W. C. (1964). Depression of electrically induced reflexes ("H"-reflexes) in man during low voltage EEG "sleep." *Electroencephalogr. Clin. Neurophysiol., 17,* 617–29.

Hoffman, R. F., Moffitt, A. R., Shearer, J. C., Sussman, P. S., & Wells, R. B. (1979). Conceptual and methodological considerations towards the development of computer-controlled research on the electro-physiology of sleep. *Waking and Sleeping, 3,* 1–16.

Hong, C. C.-H., Gillin, J. C., Dow, B. M., Wu, J., & Buchsbaum, M. S. (1995). Localized and lateralized cerebral glucose metabolism associated with eye movements during REM sleep and wakefulness: A positron emission tomography (PET) study. *Sleep, 18,* 570–80.

Hong, C. C.-H., Potkin, S. G., Antrobus, J. S., Dow, B. M., Callaghan, G. J., & Gillin, J. C. (1997). REM sleep eye movement counts correlate with visual imagery in dreaming: A pilot study. *Psychophysiology, 34,* 377–81.

Hori, T. (1982). Electrodermal and electro-oculographic activity in a hypnagogic state. *Psychophysiology, 19,* 668–72.

Horne, J. (1988). *Why We Sleep. The Functions of Sleep in Humans and Other Mammals.* Oxford University Press.

Iacono, W. G., & Lykken, D. T. (1981). Two-year retest stability of eye tracking performance and a comparison of electro-oculographic and infrared recording techniques: Evidence of EEG in the electro-oculogram. *Psychophysiology, 18,* 49–55.

Itil, T. (1969). Digital computer "sleep prints" and psychopharmacology. *Biol. Psychiatry, 1,* 91–5.

Itil, T. (1970). Digital computer analysis of the electroencephalogram during eye movement sleep state in man. *J. Nerv. Ment. Dis., 150,* 201–8.

Jacobson, A., Kales, A., Lehmann, D., & Hoedemaker, F. S. (1964). Muscle tonus in human subjects during sleep and dreaming. *Exp. Neurol., 10,* 418–24.

Johnson, L. C. (1973). Are stages of sleep related to waking behavior? *Am. Scientist, 61,* 326–38.

Johnson, L. C., & Lubin, A. (1966). Spontaneous electrodermal activity during waking and sleeping. *Psychophysiology, 3,* 8–17.

Johnson, L. C., Nute, C., Austin, M. J., & Lubin, A. (1967). Spectral analysis of the EEG during waking and sleeping. *Electroencephalogr. Clin. Neurophysiol., 23,* 80.

Jones, B. E. (1994). Basic mechanisms of sleep–wake states. In M. H. Kryger, T. Roth, & W. C. Dement (Eds.), *Principles and Practice of Sleep Medicine,* 2nd ed., pp. 145–62. Philadelphia: Saunders.

Jouvet, M. (1972). The role of monoamines and acetylcholine-containing neurons in the regulation of the sleep–waking cycle. *Ergeb. Physiol., 64,* 166–307.

Jouvet, M., & Michel, F. (1959). Correlations electromyographiques du sommeil chez le chat decortique et mesencephalique chronique. *Compte Rendu Sociologie et Biologie (Paris), 153,* 422–5.

Kahn, D., Pace-Schott, E. F., & Hobson, J. A. (1997). Consciousness in waking and dreaming: The roles of neuronal oscillation and neuromodulation in determining similarities and differences. *Neuroscience, 78,* 13–38.

Kales, A., Hoedemaker, F., Jacobson, A., Kales, J., Pawlson, M., & Wilson, T. (1967). Mentation during sleep: REM and NREM recall reports. *Percept. Mot. Skills, 24,* 556–60.

Karacan, I., Goodenough, D. R., Shapiro, A., & Starker, S. (1966). Erection cycle during sleep in relation to dream anxiety. *Arch. Gen. Psychiatry, 15,* 183–9.

Kerr, N. H. (1993). Mental imagery, dreams and perception. In Cavallero & Foulkes, pp. 18–37.

Kleitman, N. (1963). *Sleep and Wakefulness,* 2nd ed. University of Chicago Press.

Kleitman, N. (1967). The basic rest–activity cycle and physiological correlates of dreaming. *Exp. Neurol., 19,* 2–4.

Kramer, M. (1994). The scientific study of dreaming. In M. H. Kryger, T. Roth, & W. C. Dement (Eds.), *Principles and Practice of Sleep Medicine,* 2nd ed., pp. 394–9. Philadelphia: Saunders.

Kramer, M., Roth, T., & Czaya, J. (1975). Dream development within a REM period. In P. Levin & W. P. Koella (Eds.), *Sleep,* pp. 406–9. Basel: Karger.

Krueger, J. M., & Karnovsky, M. L. (1995). Sleep as a neuroimmune phenomenon: A brief historical perspective. *Adv. Neuroimmunol., 5,* 5–12.

Kryger, M. H., Roth, T., & Dement, W. C. (Eds.) (1994). *Principles and Practice of Sleep Medicine,* 2nd ed. Philadelphia: Saunders.

Kubicki, S., & Herrmann, W. M. (1996). The future of computer-assisted investigation of the polysomnogram: Sleep microstructure. *J. Clin. Neurophysiol., 13,* 285–94.

LaBerge, S. (1985). *Lucid Dreaming.* Los Angeles: Tarcher.

LaBerge, S. (1992). The postawakening testing technique in the investigation of cognitive asymmetries during sleep. In Antrobus & Bertini, pp. 289–303.

LaBerge, S., Greenleaf, W., & Kedzierski, B. (1983). Physiological responses to dreamed sexual activity during lucid REM sleep. *Psychophysiology, 20,* 454–5.

Ladd, G. T. (1892). Contributions to the psychology of visual dreams. *Mind, 1 (N.S.),* 299–304.

Lammers, W. J., & Badia, P. (1991). Motor responsiveness to stimuli presented during sleep: The influence of time-of-testing on sleep stage analyses. *Physiology and Behavior, 50,* 867–8.

Larson, J. D., & Foulkes, D. (1969). Electromyogram suppression during sleep, dream recall and orientation time. *Psychophysiology, 5,* 548–55.

Llinás, R., & Ribary, U. (1993). Coherent 40-Hz oscillation characterized dream state in humans. *Proc. Natl. Acad. Sci. USA, 90,* 2078–81.

Lloyd, S. R., & Cartwright, R. D. (1995). The collection of home and laboratory dreams by means of an instrumental response technique. *Dreaming: J. Assoc. Study Dreams, 5,* 63–73.

Loomis, A. L., Harvey, E. N., & Hobart, G. A. (1937). Cerebral states during sleep as studied by human brain potentials. *J. Exp. Psychol., 21,* 127–44.

Loomis, A. L., Harvey, E. N., & Hobart, G. A. III (1938). Distribution of disturbance-patterns in the human electroencephalogram, with special reference to sleep. *J. Neurophysiol., 1,* 413–30.

Louis, J., Cannard, C., Bastuji, H., & Challamel, M.-J. (1997). Sleep ontogenesis revisited: A longitudinal 24-hour home polygraphic study on 15 normal infants during the first two years of life. *Sleep, 20,* 323–33.

Lubin, A., Johnson, L. C., & Austin, M. J. (1969). Discrimination among states of consciousness using EEG spectra. *Psychophysiology, 6,* 122–32.

Maquet, P., Péters, J.-M., Aerts, J., Delfiore, G., Degueldre, C., Luxen, A., & Granck, G. (1996). Functional neuroanatomy of human rapid-eye-movement sleep and dreaming. *Nature, 383,* 163–6.

Marks, G. A., Shaffery, J. P., Oksenberg, A., Speciale, S. G., & Roffwarg, H. P. (1995). A functional role for REM sleep in brain maturation. *Behav. Brain Res., 69,* 1–11.

McCarley, R. W., & Hobson, J. A. (1975). Neuronal excitability modulation over the sleep cycle: A structural and mathematical model. *Science, 189,* 58–60.

McGinty, D. J., Drucker-Colín, R., Morrison, A., & Parmeggiani, P. L. (Eds.) (1985). *Brain Mechanisms of Sleep.* New York: Raven.

Meier, B. (1993). Speech and thinking in dreams. In Cavallero & Foulkes, pp. 58–76.

Mercier, L., & Pivik, R. T. (1983). Spinal motoneuronal excitability during wakefulness and non-REM sleep in hyperkinesis. *J. Clin. Neurophysiology, 5,* 321–36.

Mercier, L., Pivik, R. T., & Busby, K. (1993). Sleep patterns in reading disabled children. *Sleep, 16,* 207–15.

Moffitt, A., Hoffmann, R., Wells, R., Armitage, R., Pigeau, R., & Shearer, J. (1982). Individual differences among pre- and post-awakening EEG correlates of dream reports following arousals from different stages of sleep. *Psych. J. Univ. Ottawa, 7,* 111–25.

Molinari, S., & Foulkes, D. (1969). Tonic and phasic events during sleep: Psychological correlates and implications. *Percept. Mot. Skills, 29,* 343–68.

Monk, T. H. (Ed.) (1991). *Sleep, Sleepiness and Performance.* Chichester, U.K.: Wiley.

Monroe, L. J. (1969). Inter-rater reliability and the role of experience in scoring EEG sleep records: Phase I. *Psychophysiology, 5,* 376–84.

Monroe, L. J., Rechtschaffen, A., Foulkes, D., & Jensen, J. (1965). Discriminability of REM and NREM reports. *J. Pers. Soc. Psychol., 2,* 456–60.

Montplaisir, J., & Godbout, R. (Eds.) (1990). *Sleep and Biological Rhythms.* New York: Oxford University Press.

Moruzzi, G. (1963). Active processes in the brain stem during sleep. *Harvey Lecture Series, 58,* 233–97.

Moruzzi, G., & Magoun, H. W. (1949). Brain stem reticular formation and activation of the EEG. *Electroencephalogr. Clin. Neurophysiol., 1,* 455–73.

Naifeh, K. H., & Kamiya, J. (1981). The nature of respiratory changes associated with sleep onset. *Sleep, 4,* 49–59.

Niedermeyer, E., & Lopes da Silva, F. (Eds.) (1993). *Electroencephalography: Basic Principles, Clinical Applications, and Related Fields,* 3rd ed. Baltimore: Williams & Wilkins.

Nitz, D. (1993). Early sleep theories. In M. A. Carskadon (Ed.), *Encyclopedia of Sleep and Dreaming,* pp. 200–1. New York: Macmillan.

Ogilvie, R. D., Hunt, H. T., Sawicki, C., & Samahalskyi, J. (1982). Psychological correlates of spontaneous middle-ear muscle activity during sleep. *Sleep, 5,* 11–27.

Ogilvie, R. D., & Wilkinson, R. T. (1984). The detection of sleep onset: Behavioral and physiological convergence. *Psychophysiology, 21,* 510–20.

Ogilvie, R. D., Wilkinson, R. T., & Allison, S. (1989). The detection of sleep onset: Behavioral, physiological, and subjective convergence. *Sleep, 12,* 458–74.

Oksenberg, A., Shaffery, J. P., Marks, G. A., Speciale, S. G., Mihailoff, G., & Roffwarg, H. P. (1996). Rapid eye movement sleep deprivation in kittens amplifies LGN cell-size disparity induced by monocular deprivation. *Dev. Brain Res., 97,* 51–61.

Okuma, T., Fukuma, E., & Kobayashi, K. (1976). "Dream detector" and comparison of laboratory and home dreams collected by REMP-awakening technique. *Adv. Sleep Res., 2,* 223–31.

Pack, A. I., & Mackiewicz, M. (1996). Potential molecular biological approaches to the study of sleep. *SRS Bull., 2,* 2–7.

Palca, J. W., Walker, J. M., & Berger, R. J. (1981). Tympanic temperature and REM sleep in cold exposed humans. *Acta Universitatis Carolinae – Biologica 1979,* 225–7.

Pessah, M., & Roffwarg, H. (1972). Spontaneous middle ear muscle activity in man: A rapid eye movement phenomenon. *Science, 178,* 773–6.

Pieron, H. (1913). *Le problème physiologique du sommeil.* Paris: Masson.

Pivik, R. T. (1971). Mental activity and phasic events during sleep. Doctoral dissertation, Stanford University, Stanford, CA.

Pivik, R. T. (1978). Tonic states and phasic events in relation to sleep mentation. In Arkin et al. (1978a), pp. 245–71.

Pivik, R. T. (1983). Order and disorder during sleep ontogeny: A selective review. In P. Firestone, P. J. McGrath, & W. Feldman (Eds.), *Advances in Behavioral Medicine for Children and Adolescents,* pp. 75–102. Hillsdale, NJ: Erlbaum.

Pivik, R. T. (1986). Sleep: Physiology and psychophysiology. In G. H. Coles, E. Donchin, & S. W. Porges (Eds.), *Psychophysiology,* pp. 378–406. New York: Guilford.

Pivik, R. T. (1991a). Tonic states and phasic events in relation to sleep mentation. In S. J. Ellman & J. S. Antrobus (Eds.), *The Mind in Sleep,* 2nd ed., pp. 214–47. New York: Wiley.

Pivik, R. T. (1991b). The several qualities of sleepiness: Psychophysiological considerations. In T. H. Monk (Ed.), *Sleep, Sleepiness and Performance,* pp. 3–37. Chichester, U.K.: Wiley.

Pivik, R. T., & Busby, K. (1996). Heart rate associated with sleep onset in preadolescents. *J. Sleep Res., 5,* 33–6.

Pivik, R. T., Busby, K., & Brown, M. (1993). Characteristics of sleep onset in adolescents: Temporal relationships among cardiovascular and EEG power spectral measures. Paper presented at the Conference on Sleep Onset Mechanisms: Normal and Abnormal Processes (Niagara-on-the-Lake, Ontario, Canada).

Pivik, R. T., Busby, K. A., Gill, E., Hunter, P., & Nevins, R. (1996). Heart rate variations during sleep in preadolescents. *Sleep, 19,* 117–35.

Pivik, R. T., Bylsma, F., Busby, K., & Sawyer, S. (1982). Interhemispheric EEG changes: Relationship to sleep and dreams in gifted adolescents. *Psychiat. J. Univ. Ottawa, 7,* 56–76.

Pivik, T., & Dement, W. (1968). Amphetamine, REM deprivation and K-complexes [Abstract]. *Psychophysiology, 5,* 241.

Pivik, T., & Dement, W. C. (1970). Phasic changes in muscular and reflex activity during non-REM sleep. *Exp. Neurol., 27,* 115–24.

Pivik, T., & Foulkes, D. (1968). NREM mentation: Relation to personality, orientation time, and time of night. *J. Consult. Clin. Psychol., 37*, 144–51.

Pompeiano, O. (1966). Muscular afferents and motor control during sleep. In R. Granit (Ed.), *Muscular Afferents and Motor Control*, pp. 415–36. Stockholm: Almqvist & Wiksell.

Pompeiano, O. (1967). The neurophysiological mechanism of the postural and motor events during desynchronized sleep. In S. S. Kety, E. V. Evarts, & H. L. Williams (Eds.), *Sleep and Altered States of Consciousness*. Baltimore: Williams & Wilkins.

Prechtl, H. F. R., Akiyama, Y., Zinkin, P., & Grant, D. K. (1968). Polygraphic studies of the full-term newborn. 1. Technical aspects and qualitative analysis. In M. C. Bax & R. C. MacKeith (Eds.), *Studies in Infancy*, pp. 1–21. London: Heinemann.

Rechtschaffen, A. (1967). Dream reports and dream experiences. *Exp. Neurol., 19 (Suppl. 4)*, 4–15.

Rechtschaffen, A. (1973). The psychophysiology of mental activity during sleep. In F. J. McGuigan & R. A. Schoonover (Eds.), *The Psychophysiology of Thinking*, pp. 153–205. New York: Academic Press.

Rechtschaffen, A. (1978). The single-mindedness and isolation of dreams. *Sleep 1*, 97–109.

Rechtschaffen, A. (1998). Current perspectives on the function of sleep. *Perspect. Biol. Med., 41*, 359–90.

Rechtschaffen, A., & Buchignani, C. (1992). The visual appearance of dreams. In Antrobus & Bertini, pp. 143–55.

Rechtschaffen, A., Goodenough, D., & Shapiro, A. (1962). Patterns of sleep talking. *Arch. Gen. Psychiatry, 7*, 418–26.

Rechtschaffen, A., & Kales, A. (Eds.) (1968). *A Manual of Standardized Terminology, Techniques and Scoring System for Sleep Stages of Human Subjects* (NIM Publication no. 204). Washington, DC: U.S. Government Printing Office.

Rechtschaffen, A., Verdone, P., & Wheaton, J. (1963a). Reports of mental activity during sleep. *Can. Psychiat. Assoc. J., 8*, 409–14.

Rechtschaffen, A., Vogel, G., & Shaikun, G. (1963b). Interrelatedness of mental activity during sleep. *Arch. Gen. Psychiatry, 9*, 536–47.

Reinsel, R., Antrobus, J., & Wollman, M. (1985). The phasic–tonic difference and the time-of-night effect. *Sleep Res., 14*, 115.

Reinsel, R., Antrobus, J., & Wollman, M. (1992). Bizarreness in sleep and waking mentation. In Antrobus & Bertini, pp. 157–86.

Reynolds, C. F., Taska, L. S., Jarrett, D. B., Coble, P. A., & Kupfer, D. J. (1983). REM latency in depression: Is there one best definition? *Biol. Psychiatry, 18*, 849–63.

Roehrs, T., Merlotti, L., Petrucelli, N., Stepanski, E., & Roth, T. (1994). Experimental sleep fragmentation. *Sleep, 17*, 438–43.

Roffwarg, H. P. (1979). Diagnostic classification of sleep and arousal disorders. *Sleep, 2*, 1–137.

Roffwarg, H., Dement, W., Muzio, J., & Fisher, C. (1962). Dream imagery: Relationship to rapid eye movements of sleep. *Arch. Gen. Psychiatry, 7*, 235–58.

Roffwarg, H., Muzio, J. N., & Dement, W. C. (1966). Ontogenetic development of the human sleep–dream cycle. *Science, 152*, 604–19.

Rosenlicht, N., & Feinberg, I. (1997). REM sleep = dreaming: only a dream. *SRS Bull., 3*, 10–12.

Sampson, H. (1965). Deprivation of dreaming sleep by two methods: 1. Compensatory REM time. *Arch. Gen. Psychiatry, 13*, 79–86.

Sampson, H. (1966). Psychological effects of deprivation of dreaming sleep. *J. Nerv. Ment. Dis., 143*, 305–17.

Sassin, J. F., Parker, D. C., Mace, J. W., Gotlin, R. W., Johnson, L. C., & Rossman, L. G. (1969). Human growth hormone release: Relation to slow-wave sleep and sleep-waking cycles. *Science, 165*, 513–15.

Sewitch, D. E., & Kupfer, D. J. (1985). A comparison of the Telediagnostic and Medilog systems for recording normal sleep in the home environment. *Psychophysiol., 22*, 718–26.

Shapiro, A., Goodenough, D. R., & Gryler, R. B. (1963). Dream recall as a function of method of awakening. *Psychosom. Med., 25*, 174–80.

Shimizu, A., & Inoue, T. (1986). Dreamed speech and speech muscle activity. *Psychophysiology, 23*, 210–14.

Singer, J. L. (1978). Experimental studies of daydreaming and the stream of thought. In K. S. Pope & J. L. Singer (Eds.), *The Stream of Consciousness*, pp. 187–223. New York: Plenum.

Snyder, F. (1966). Toward an evolutionary theory of dreaming. *Am. J. Psychiatry, 123*, 121–42.

Snyder, F. (1970). The phenomenology of dreaming. In H. Madow & L. H. Snow (Eds.), *The Psychodynamic Implications of the Physiological Studies on Dreams*, pp. 124–51. Springfield, IL: Thomas.

Snyder, F., Hobson, J., & Goldfrank, F. (1963). Blood pressure changes during human sleep. *Science, 142*, 1313–14.

Snyder, F., Hobson, J., Morrison, D., & Goldfrank, F. (1964). Changes in respiration, heart rate, and systolic blood pressure in human sleep. *J. Appl. Physiol., 19*, 417–22.

Stepanski, E., Lamphere, J., Badia, P., Zorick, F., & Roth, T. (1984). Sleep fragmentation and daytime sleepiness. *Sleep, 7*, 18–26.

Stepanski, E., Lamphere, J., Roehrs, T., Zorick, F., & Roth, T. (1987). Experimental sleep fragmentation in normal subjects. *Intern. J. Neuroscience, 33*, 207–14.

Steriade, M., Amzica, F., & Contreras, D. (1996). Synchronization of fast (30–40 Hz) spontaneous cortical rhythms during brain activation. *J. Neurosci., 16*, 392–417.

Steriade, M., & McCarley, R. W. (1990). *Brainstem Control of Wakefulness and Sleep*. New York: Plenum.

Sussman, P., Moffitt, A., Hoffman, R., Wells, R., & Shearer, J. (1979). The description of structural and temporal characteristics of tonic electrophysiological activity during sleep. *Waking and Sleeping, 3*, 279–90.

Takahashi, Y., Kipnis, D. M., & Daughaday, W. H. (1968). Growth hormone secretion during sleep. *J. Clin. Investigations, 47*, 2079–90.

Thakkar, M. (1996). REM sleep: A biochemical perspective. *SRS Bull., 2*, 22–8.

Tracy, R. L., & Tracy, L. N. (1974). Reports of mental activity from sleep stages 2 and 4. *Percept. Motor Skills, 38*, 647–8.

Trinder, J., Whitworth, F., Kay, A., & Wilkin, P. (1992). Respiratory instability during sleep onset. *J. Appl. Physiol., 73*, 2462–9.

Verdone, P. (1963). Variables related to the temporal reference of manifest dream content. Doctoral dissertation, University of Chicago.

Verdone, P. (1965). Temporal reference of manifest dream content. *Percept. Mot. Skills, 20*, 1253–68.

Vogel, G. W. (1975). Review of REM sleep deprivation. *Arch. Gen. Psychiatry, 32,* 749–61.

Vogel, G. W. (1978). Sleep-onset mentation. In Arkin et al. (1978a), pp. 97–108.

Vogel, G. W., Barrowclough, B., & Giesler, D. (1972). Limited discriminability of REM and sleep onset reports and its psychiatric implications. *Arch. Gen. Psychiatry, 26,* 449–55.

Vogel, G. W., Foulkes, D., & Trosman, H. (1966). Ego functions and dreaming during sleep onset. *Arch. Gen. Psychiatry, 14,* 238–48.

Vogel, G. W., Thurmond, A., Gibbons, P., Sloan, K., Boyd, M., & Walker, M. (1975). REM sleep reduction effects on depression syndromes. *Arch. Gen. Psychiatry, 32,* 765–77.

Watson, R. K. (1972). Mental correlates of periorbital potentials during REM sleep. Doctoral dissertation, University of Chicago.

Webb, W. B. (1993). Dream theories of the ancient world. In M. A. Carskadon (Ed.), *Encyclopedia of Sleep and Dreaming,* pp. 192–4. New York: Macmillan.

Weisz, R., & Foulkes, D. (1970). Home and laboratory dreams collected under uniform sampling conditions. *Psychophysiology, 6,* 588–96.

Whitman, R. (1969). A summary. In M. Kramer (Ed.), *Dream Psychology and the New Biology of Sleep,* pp. 405–42. Springfield, IL: Thomas.

Williams, R. L., Agnew, H. W., Jr., & Webb, W. B. (1964). Sleep patterns in young adults: An EEG study. *Electroencephalogr. Clin. Neurophysiol., 17,* 376–81.

Williams, R. L., Agnew, H. W., Jr., & Webb, W. B. (1966). Sleep patterns in the young adult female: An EEG study. *Electroencephalogr. Clin. Neurophysiol., 20,* 264–6.

Wittern, R. (1989). Sleep theories in antiquity and the Renaissance. In J. A. Horne (Ed.), *Sleep '88,* pp. 11–22. Stuttgart: Fischer-Verlag.

Wolpert, E. A., & Trosman, H. (1958). Studies in psychophysiology of dreams. I: Experimental evocation of sequential dream episodes. *Am. Assoc. Arch. Neurol. Psychiatry, 79,* 603–6.

Zemaityte, D., Varoneckas, G., & Sokolov, E. (1984). Heart rhythm control during sleep. *Psychophysiology, 21,* 279–89.

Zimmerman, W. B. (1968). Psychological and physiological differences between "light" and "deep" sleepers [Abstract]. *Psychophysiology, 4,* 387.

Zimmerman, W. B. (1970). Sleep mentation and auditory awakening thresholds. *Psychophysiology, 6,* 540–9.

PART FOUR

APPLICATIONS

CHAPTER TWENTY-SIX

PSYCHOPHYSIOLOGY IN THE STUDY OF PSYCHOPATHOLOGY

JENNIFER KELLER, BLAIR D. HICKS, & GREGORY A. MILLER

Introduction

The application of psychophysiological measures to the study of psychopathology has resulted in many findings about variations in processing during the course of mental disorder. Psychophysiological measures provide an alternate and sometimes unique view of an individual's functioning. Psychophysiological findings can corroborate (or contradict) findings from more traditional psychological measures of functioning, including self-report scales, behavioral performance, informant data, and diagnostic interviews. Psychophysiological findings are also useful in monitoring the time course of mental processes involved in task performance, in measuring mental processes that the individual does not report, and in assessing behavior when the production of an overt response is undesired or unavailable (Coles 1989). A number of excellent reviews, including a remarkably comprehensive chapter by Zahn (1986), have examined applications of psychophysiological measures to the study of psychopathology. A variety of more specialized reviews are also available, including those by Braff (in press), Bruder (1995), Dawson, Schell, and Böhmelt (1999), Dawson et al. (1995), Depue and Iacono (1989), Fernandes and Miller (1995), Ford, Pfefferbaum, and Roth (1992), Holzman (1987), McCarley et al. (1996), Miller and Yee (1994), Pritchard (1986), Raine, Lencz, and Benishay (1995), Sponheim, Allen, and Iacono (1995), Taitano and Miller (1998), Turpin (1989a), and Yee (1995).

A goal of this chapter is to review how theories about psychopathology guide the application of psychophysiological measures and provide a context within which to interpret results. Turpin (1989b) distinguished between theory-driven applications of psychophysiological measures and the isolated use of psychophysiological techniques as correlates of a psychological or physiological process. In

the former, separate theories about the physiological and psychological *processes* (as opposed to *measures*) involved in a task are integrated. The subsequent selection of psychophysiological measure(s) is driven by the theories about the processes. In contrast, the latter approach is typified by assessment of an isolated psychological *or* physiological process using a physiological measure. In many cases there is a theoretical basis for either the psychological or physiological phenomena under study, but there is no integration between theories about the psychological and physiological phenomena. Although this chapter will follow Turpin's advice to focus on integrative approaches, it should be clear that the two constitute different points on a spectrum and not qualitatively different approaches. Where theory about psychological and physiological processes is well advanced, psychophysiological approaches can integrate those theories. Where strong theory is lacking, even the isolated use of psychophysiological techniques may aid in the eventual development of strong theories. Ultimately, the usefulness of psychophysiological approaches depends more on the availability of strong theories about psychological and physiological processes and their role in psychopathology than on the choice of which psychophysiological variable to investigate.

The boundaries and utility of psychophysiological measures in the study of psychopathology are much in debate for reasons we shall discuss but not resolve within a single chapter. Instead, this chapter will consider how best to study psychopathology with psychophysiological measures. When studying psychophysiology in psychopathology, either domain can be the independent or dependent variable. Often the researcher's predilections determine what is manipulated and what is measured, but sometimes a particularly rich paradigm will be more tractable with a particular configuration of independent and dependent variables.

John T. Cacioppo, Louis G. Tassinary, and Gary G. Berntson (Eds.), *Handbook of Psychophysiology,* 2nd ed. © Cambridge University Press 2000. Printed in the United States of America. ISBN 62634X. All rights reserved.

PSYCHOPATHOLOGY FOR THE PSYCHOPHYSIOLOGIST

For the researcher interested in studying general mental processes using psychophysiological variables, research on psychopathology provides information that may enhance models of normal mental functioning. Psychopathology research may suggest the existence of a mental process not previously recognized. Studies of psychopathology may also indicate which processes are susceptible to disturbance and which remain intact. Information about the relative vulnerability of specific mental processes may reveal information about how mental processes are organized. Although studies of psychopathology can provide much information about normal mental functioning, the usefulness of such research is limited by how well the disrupted mental process is understood. Thus, theories about normal mental processing and about psychopathology benefit to the extent that they share information.

Comprehensive theories of mental functioning must be able to account for the types of disturbances associated with mental disorders. Theories that are unable to do so not only ignore an important source of potential validation but also fail to address the heterogeneity inherent in how individuals approach a task. An important question to be addressed when proposing models of mental functioning is the prevalence of a particular mental strategy. Whereas some processes are believed to be ubiquitous, others are merely potential strategies among which individuals choose. Theories that are sufficiently developed to address this heterogeneity will be better able to account for the alternative strategies used by individuals with psychopathology.

PSYCHOPHYSIOLOGY FOR THE PSYCHOPATHOLOGIST

For researchers interested in studying psychopathology, psychophysiological approaches can be especially enticing. Electrophysiological measures offer a noninvasive method for monitoring physiological activity with excellent temporal resolution. However, when used to monitor the physiological activity from inside the skull, these measures are limited in the amount of spatial resolution that they can provide. Magnetoencephalographic measures are noninvasive, provide excellent temporal resolution, and are better suited for studying neural events in that they avoid interference from bone and tissue separating the sensor from the neuronal activity. Hemodynamic methods (based on blood flow, blood oxygenation, etc.) offer only indirect information about the timing of events. A subset of hemodynamic approaches (e.g., PET, fMRI) can be used to monitor intracranial physiology but are far more expensive and less widely available than electrophysiological measures. Whenever possible, psychophysiological approaches that combine several of these different types of measures can provide a

rich view of the gross physiological activity associated with psychopathology. Particularly promising is the ability of psychophysiology to define the endophenotype (Klein & Anderson 1995; Shields, Heston, & Gottesman 1975), the manifestation of a disorder via anomalies not observable by diagnostic interview or observation of overt behavior. This may prove to be crucial, for example, for identifying affected individuals in genetic linkage studies (Iacono 1998).

Two comments are in order regarding the potential appeal of psychophysiological measures to psychopathology. First, these measures are valuable in that they reflect the operation of mental processes associated with symptoms of psychopathology. Similar disturbances in mental processing can lead to different symptoms, just as disturbances of different mental processes can lead to similar symptoms. By studying mental processes as opposed to symptoms alone, it is possible to determine the effects of the disease process on different aspects of cognitive and emotional functioning. Thus, an exclusive focus on behavioral symptoms can be a frustrating basis for determination of the mental processes of which symptoms are a manifestation. Second, although the present chapter reflects the historical emphasis on psychological processes in psychophysiology, the psychophysiological approach is equally valuable for research questions emphasizing physiological processes (Miller & Ebert 1988). Thus, for example, psychopathology is by definition a disorder of psychological and not of biological functioning, but the value of understanding the neurobiology of normal and abnormal psychological functioning is now widely appreciated. Because of its noninvasive technology and its sophistication in psychological theory and experimental design, psychophysiology remains at the forefront of the increasingly biological agenda in psychopathology research.

Although psychophysiological measures can provide the psychopathologist with an additional realm of valuable information, there is substantial disagreement about the perceived utility of these methods. One common objection is that psychophysiological measures are sometimes part of an attempt to explain psychopathology entirely at the level of biology. However, this objection is a misunderstanding of the application of psychophysiological measures. Psychophysiology provides information that may not be obtainable with verbal or overt behavioral measures, but this information should not be considered more accurate, more representative, or sufficient for characterizing an individual's mental status or functioning (Lang 1968). As we argue throughout this chapter, psychophysiology is best utilized in conjunction with verbal and behavioral measures – not in place of those measures. In any case it should be clear that biological reductionism of psychopathology is not feasible (Miller 1996).

Some concerns about psychophysiological measures are based on appropriate conceptualizations of their role. One concern is about the often considerable amount of technical expertise required – an amount that is frequently underestimated. Another concern pertains to the generalizability of information obtained during situations in which subjects know that their physiology is being monitored. Other concerns arise from the expense of psychophysiological equipment relative to the cost of diagnostic interviews or psychometric tests. However, recent innovations in available psychophysiological equipment have addressed these concerns to some degree. Integrated physiological data collection systems, low-cost computing, and ambulatory monitoring techniques have all combined to lower the costs and increase the feasibility of psychophysiological measures in clinical contexts, although no foreseeable technical advance can lessen the methodological expertise required.

HISTORICAL CONTEXT OF THE PSYCHOPHYSIOLOGICAL STUDY OF PSYCHOPATHOLOGY

Theories of psychopathology often encompass physiological systems, and psychophysiology has been a useful tool for the investigation of clinical phenomena. Historically as well as presently, much of the best psychophysiological work on psychopathology was driven by prevailing theories of psychopathology. In order to gain insight into the history of psychophysiological investigation of psychopathology, it is important to consider the work in the context of the predominant theoretical concepts of the time (see Alexander 1972).

The concept of nonspecific physiological reactivity was an early influence on the study of psychopathology using psychophysiological measures. Clinically, patients with schizophrenia and depression were often noted to appear withdrawn and to exhibit blunted affect. Much early work attempted to account for this behavioral hyporeactivity by looking for physiological hyporeactivity. This was consistent with the James–Lange theory of emotion, which described emotions directly in terms of physiological change. In an attempt to explain emotional abnormalities in psychopathology, researchers studied abnormal physiology (e.g. Malmo & Shagass 1949).

Landis (1932) conducted an extensive review of electrodermal studies looking for a consistent pattern of abnormal physiology in schizophrenia, but none was found. Later, Cohen and Patterson (1937) found that changes in pulse rate tended to be larger in patients than controls. Malmo and Shagass (1949, 1952) examined the responsivity of multiple ANS (autonomic nervous system) measures – including heart rate, electrodermal responses, respiration, and blood pressure – in acute and chronic schizophrenia. First-episode schizophrenia patients showed greater reactivity to stressors than either chronic patients or controls; the latter two groups demonstrated similar levels of reactivity. Such findings were used to argue against the notion that behavioral hyporesponsiveness can be attributed to physiological hyporesponsiveness.

Lang and Buss (1968) reviewed the literature of physiological responsivity and found evidence that some individuals with psychopathology were physiologically hyporesponsive to particular stressors. The fact that the hyporesponsiveness was limited to certain types of stressors suggests that a generalized deficit in physiological responsivity cannot account for the pervasive deficits seen in psychopathology. Overall, early studies of physiological reactivity in psychopathology suggested that hyporeactivity is more prevalent in more chronic individuals but that generally patients will react normally under higher levels of stimulus intensity. Historically, many studies examining reactivity did not provide important methodological information, such as adequate description of the patient sample or the stimuli. Furthermore, comparing physiological reactions is problematic in that differences in basal levels can complicate interpretation of the response (Lacey 1956; Wilder 1950).

Over time, the concept of nonspecific physiological reactivity proved not to be broadly viable. Lacey (1967), Lang (1968), and others (see Miller & Kozak 1993) argued convincingly that different response systems too often diverge for such a concept to be of general use. Unfortunately, the overwhelming evidence for that conclusion is not widely appreciated, and vague concepts of generalized arousal are still invoked all too often in studies of psychopathology and psychophysiology. This usage should be distinguished from arousal concepts applied more defensibly in narrower domains, as in self-report measurement of the dimensions of emotion (e.g. Lang, Bradley, & Cuthbert 1990) or theories of region-specific brain activity in emotion and psychopathology (to be reviewed shortly).

Another theoretical concept guiding research was physiological activation. Clinical observations suggested that certain psychiatric groups may be distinguished from controls by their baseline level of physiological activity, as opposed to their responses to specific stressors. Muscle tension was a common measure of activation, with the general finding that some patients demonstrate greater skeletal tension than controls (Duffy 1962). Another method used to assess activation was electroencephalography (EEG), which assumes that brain activity is monotonically related to EEG frequency: activity in the 8–13-Hz (alpha) range is presumed to indicate relatively little brain activation, with activity at higher frequencies indicating greater activation. In a study with an exceptionally large sample size, Davis and Davis (1939) found that patients demonstrated significantly less alpha than did control subjects. Other studies found that anxious subjects demonstrated less resting alpha and more activity in higher and lower bands (Ulett et al. 1953; see Duffy 1962 for a review of EEG findings in psychopathology). Although finding group differences in EEG is not uncommon, the functional significance of such differences is typically unclear. Global EEG activity as a measure of resting nonspecific activation has not proven very useful in psychopathology research. More recent work on region-specific alpha (discussed later) renders the non-specific activation concept obsolete.

A third concept that has received substantial psycho-physiological attention is defective physiological regulation in psychopathology. This work investigated not only how physiological patterns were disrupted but also the circumstances that could influence their regulation. Buck, Car-scallen, and Hobbs (1950, 1951) reported that schizophrenic individuals demonstrated significantly lower body tempera-ture than controls and that their range of temperatures over a 24-hour period was smaller than the range demonstrated by controls. Ax (1962) analyzed physiological regulation in schizophrenia and suggested that dysregulation was best observed when comparing multiple systems that typically operate together (such as heart rate, HR, and respiration). The dysregulation that he observed appeared between mul-tiple systems that were not coordinating properly, rather than within a single system. Because respiration affects HR by means of proprioceptive signals from the chest, diaphragm, and lungs, Ax (1962) suggested that such sig-nals are impaired in schizophrenia. More recent theories of schizophrenia have suggested that an impairment of proprioceptive information may also be involved with the development of positive symptoms (Frith 1992). The find-ings on dysregulation reinforce the approach of examining multiple physiology systems. This theme is repeated in the review of current studies of psychopathology presented in this chapter. Although the study of physiological regula-tion offers important information about psychopathology, there have been relatively few empirical studies investigat-ing this phenomenon. However, as theories are developed that specify testable hypotheses about what role physiolog-ical dysregulation may have in psychopathology, the allure of such studies will attract an increased amount of empiri-cal research.

SOME PROBLEMS WITH COMMON THEORETICAL ASSUMPTIONS

The potential of psychophysiology to contribute to the study of psychopathology has been undermined histori-cally by two common, problematic assumptions. First, naively reductionistic conceptualizations of the relation-ship between psychological and physiological phenomena have been a recurring embarrassment in psychopathology research for decades. Approaches that aim to identify either the biological or the psychological phenomena "underly-ing" psychopathology fail to recognize that psychopathol-ogy must be understood in terms of both biological and psychological factors. The most subtle manifestation of the problem is when overly narrow or reductionistic conceptu-alizations guide research but are not clearly stated. When a particular relationship is explicitly proposed, it is open to validation or disconfirmation through critical analysis

and empirical research. Attempts to avoid such scrutiny by assuming rather than articulating such a relationship need to be avoided (see Miller 1996 for further discussion).

The second problematic assumption is primarily in the psychological realm, but it has implications for the selec-tion and interpretation of biological measures. Phenomena of interest in psychopathology, and psychology in general, are often dichotomized into emotional and cognitive pro-cessing. In psychophysiology, this dichotomy is frequently expressed as an implicit assumption that central nervous system measures are appropriate for the study of cogni-tion, whereas peripheral nervous system measures are better suited to the study of emotion. Yet there is very little theo-retical basis or empirical support for dichotomizing mental processing into cognitive or emotional processing or for limiting the type of events for which physiological measures are appropriate (see Miller 1996 for further discussion).

Much empirical work has been overlooked or misinter-preted because of these problematic assumptions. A multi-level approach is essential, one in which the utility of each level of explanation is respected. This synergistic approach has been developed elsewhere (Cacioppo & Berntson 1992; Lang 1968, 1978, 1984; Miller & Kozak 1993; see also Chapter 1 of this volume). No level is inherently privi-leged. Thus, although psychophysiology will be empha-sized, this chapter will attempt to integrate measures of these components to develop a better understanding of the processes involved in psychopathology.

The preceding introductory comments have addressed a variety of issues relevant to psychopathology research. In particular, it has been argued that naive or haphazard approaches have diluted the contributions of some empir-ical research, including those utilizing psychophysiological measures. The following sections will focus on integrat-ing psychophysiological research to demonstrate how it has advanced the study of psychopathology. These sections are organized around three types of psychopathology – anx-iety, mood, and schizophrenia spectrum disorders. There is an ongoing debate in the psychopathology literature about whether to view psychological disorders as discrete categories or within a dimensional framework (see Clark, Watson, & Reynolds 1995; Millon 1991), but the bulk of psychophysiological research has assumed a categori-cal approach. Further, the framework will be used to demonstrate how different levels of description (i.e., not just diagnoses) can be used to better interpret many of the current findings and to guide future psychophysiological investigations of psychopathology.

Psychophysiology Applied to the Study of Psychopathology: Physical and Social Contexts

No review of the study of psychopathology can hope to be comprehensive. Even when limiting our focus to only those studies that have employed psychophysiological measures, the amount of material to be covered is entirely too broad. The *Diagnostic and Statistical Manual of Mental Disorders,* fourth edition (DSM-IV; APA 1994) lists seventeen separate classifications of mental disorders. Most, if not all, of those classifications have been assessed using psychophysiological techniques. The focus herein upon the three classifications that have received the most attention from psychophysiological studies should not be considered an endorsement of the categorical approach or a judgment that these classifications are most appropriate for psychophysiological study. As discussed earlier, psychopathology is a concept that encompasses biological, psychological, and environmental factors. Trying to pull these factors apart in order to consider the physical context of psychopathology separate from its social context is simply not viable. Indeed, the strongest reason for using psychophysiology to study psychopathology is that psychophysiology is uniquely suited to simultaneously examine both the physical and the social contexts of psychopathology.

ANXIETY DISORDERS

There are twelve superficially distinct anxiety disorders listed in DSM-IV. That list does not include additional subtypes of anxiety suggested in the literature (e.g. Barlow 1988, 1991; Heller et al. 1997) or subclinical forms or degrees of anxiety studied in the personality literature and probably of great clinical relevance. As noted before, there is some debate about whether mental disorders should be seen as discrete categories or as points on a continuum of behavior. This debate is prominent in the anxiety literature, where it is unclear whether subclinical anxiety and the various anxiety disorders are best conceptualized in terms of one or more dimensions or as qualitatively distinct phenomena. Even if healthy and pathological anxiety represent distinct phenomena, there may be some overlap between them, including their physiology. It is valuable to study nonclinical individuals under stressful and anxiety-provoking conditions as well as individuals with pathological anxiety. Psychophysiological correlates of stress have been reviewed elsewhere (see Chapter 13) and will not be covered here. Cuthbert & Lang (1989), Hugdahl (1989), Öst (1989), Sartory (1989), and Yeudall et al. (1983) have reviewed various aspects of the psychophysiology of anxiety. The present section will focus on the fit between available theoretical models of anxiety and available empirical studies using psychophysiological measures.

When studying psychopathology with psychophysiological measures, one issue is whether the focus of study is the psychopathology itself or the consequences of the psychopathology. Physiological differences are often discussed as if they are *due to* anxiety rather than being *part of* anxiety. Such a view may misrepresent the role of physiology in anxiety or in any emotion. Lang (1968, 1978) addressed the

study of emotions by proposing the "three-systems" model. He suggested that emotions are expressed in three systems: verbal, physiological, and behavioral activity. Emotion potentially entails all three of these components, meaning that a complete picture of normal and pathological emotion requires assessment of all three. Lang suggested that the activity of all three systems is part of anxiety and not due to anxiety (see Miller & Kozak 1993 for discussion). For example, elevated heart rate or lateralized EEG patterns are not responses to an anxious state but rather part of what it means to be in an anxious state; such physiological events are not responses to fearful imagery but part of the process of imagery.

Regional Brain Activity Associated with Anxiety

Psychophysiological approaches to anxiety historically focused on autonomic measures (see Zahn 1986). More recently, interest has grown in modulation of the startle reflex (see Chapters 20 and 22) and in brain regions (see Chapters 2 and 36) that become more or less active during periods of anxious mood. Although some studies have found no relationship between anxiety and cerebral metabolism (Buchsbaum et al. 1985; Giordani et al. 1990), most have suggested that one hemisphere is more active during anxiety than the other. There is, however, considerable variance in which hemisphere has been implicated (for review see Heller et al. 1997). For example, Tucker and colleagues (1978; Tyler & Tucker 1982) found anxiety to be associated with left-hemisphere hyperactivity, as indicated by behavioral tasks associated with left-hemisphere function. Greater left-hemisphere activity has also been suggested by EEG (Carter, Johnson, & Borkovec 1986) and cerebral blood flow (rCBF) studies (e.g. Baxter et al. 1987; Fredrikson et al. 1993; Swedo et al. 1989). However, other studies using behavioral and psychophysiological measures have found anxiety to be associated with greater right-hemisphere activity, specifically in panic disorder patients (e.g. Reiman et al. 1984), highly anxious individuals (Reivich, Gur, & Alavi 1983) identified by the State-Trait Anxiety Inventory (Spielberger 1968), generalized anxiety disorder patients (Buchsbaum et al. 1987; Wu et al. 1991), controls taking antianxiety medication (Mathew, Wilson, & Daniel 1985), and social phobics (Davidson et al. 1997).

In light of these inconsistencies, Gruzelier (1989) and Heller and colleagues (Heller, Etienne, & Miller 1995; Heller et al. 1997) suggested that anxiety may favor either hemisphere, the direction being dependent on the severity and subtype of anxiety. They suggested that the left hemisphere is more involved when there are strong cognitive components such as ruminations and obsessional thoughts (Gruzelier 1989) or anxious apprehension (e.g. worry; Heller et al. 1997), whereas the right hemisphere is more involved when activity in the sympathetic nervous system is heightened, such as in generalized anxiety

(Gruzelier 1989) or anxious arousal (e.g. panic; Heller et al. 1997). These subtypings have been based primarily on lateralized EEG findings and behavioral data from lateralized tasks, although evidence using autonomic measures also suggests that subtypes of anxiety can be dissociated (see Zahn 1986). Beyond Heller et al. (1997), this distinction between anxious apprehension and anxious arousal has not yet been systematically assessed. Approaches that investigate both central and autonomic measures associated with anxiety will be necessary in order to develop a more complete theory of these subtypes.

Post-Traumatic Stress Disorder

Diagnostic categories of anxiety are distinguished in part by whether the anxiety is in response to a specific event. Research on anxiety disorders in which specific stressors or circumstances are found to elicit anxiety – such as simple phobias (e.g. snake phobia), social phobia, and post-traumatic stress disorder (PTSD) – have found a number of psychophysiological changes during exposure to the anxiety-eliciting stimuli. When anxiety has a specific prompt, the individual generally responds with increased autonomic activity (see Hugdahl 1989 and Öst 1989 for reviews on simple phobias and on panic disorder, agoraphobia, and social phobia, respectively).

Whereas research on generalized anxiety has used central nervous system (CNS) measures such as EEG and rCBF, the vast majority of research on stimulus-specific anxiety disorders has employed only autonomic measures. This emphasis on autonomic measures in the study of emotion probably reflects two arguable assumptions. The first assumption is that anxiety is an *emotional* disorder as opposed to a disorder of *cognition*. As discussed earlier, it is unnecessary to assume that a given psychological phenomenon should be understood in exclusively emotional or exclusively cognitive terms. The second problematic assumption is that, if anxiety is a disorder of emotion, then it is appropriate to study it using physiological measures historically associated with emotion rather than those typically associated with cognition. Yet theories about anxiety disorders make assertions about mental events that can be investigated equally well with central and peripheral measures.

To illustrate the utility of employing both central and peripheral measures when researching anxiety disorders, we will review here the psychophysiological findings for PTSD. Post-traumatic stress disorder warrants attention for several reasons. Although it is a rapidly growing research area, there have been few broad reviews of psychophysiological studies on PTSD (Orr & Kaloupek 1997; Prins, Kaloupek, & Keane 1995; see also Lating & Everly 1995; Orr 1994; Pitman 1997), and many important questions have yet to be addressed adequately. Research on PTSD can be particularly challenging owing to diagnostic comorbidity issues discussed later in this chapter. Nevertheless,

many of the issues arising in the assessment of PTSD are equally applicable to other anxiety disorders.

Historically viewed as a disorder that afflicts war veterans, the diagnosis of PTSD has broadened to include victims of other types of trauma (e.g., rape, motor vehicle accidents; Helzer, Robins, & McEvoy 1987). Symptoms of PTSD include re-experiencing the event (e.g., nightmares, flashbacks), avoidance of stimuli associated with the event, general numbing of responsiveness (e.g., poor recall, feeling detached), and hyperarousal (e.g., insomnia, exaggerated startle response). Several theories have suggested that the physiological symptoms of PTSD, such as exaggerated startle, are a result of classical conditioning (Keane, Zimering, & Caddell 1985; Kolb 1984). These theories of PTSD suggest that unconditioned expressive, experiential, and physiological responses to traumatic events become conditioned to otherwise neutral stimuli, which then elicit a "fight or flight" response. Other theories have presented information processing models of PTSD (Foa & Kozak 1986; Foa & Riggs 1993). More recently, Brewin, Dalgleish, and Joseph (1996) outlined an information processing model of PTSD that offers specific predictions about memory and attentional biases. Nadel and Jacobs (in press) proposed that some symptoms of PTSD reflect hippocampal damage secondary to stress-related steroid exposure (see also the review chapters in Friedman, Charney, & Deutch 1995).

As indicated earlier, most psychophysiological research on PTSD has been confined to autonomic measures. Patients with PTSD are consistently found to react to trauma-related stimuli with elevated autonomic activity compared with a variety of groups, including non-PTSD trauma victims, nonpsychiatric controls, and other anxiety-disordered patients. This finding has been reported across a variety of experimental contexts, including paradigms using auditory and visual traumatic stimuli and script-driven imagery (Orr et al. 1993; Pitman et al. 1987; see also Prins et al. 1995).

A few studies have used central measures to examine responses to trauma-related stimuli. McCaffrey et al. (1993) found increased relative left-hemisphere alpha activity in PTSD veterans to one specific trauma-related odor compared to veterans with adjustment-related but non-PTSD problems. However, the study did not sufficiently explain why that particular trauma-related odor was associated with increased alpha whereas others were not. Patients with PTSD were found to have rCBF increases during trauma-related scripts relative to nontrauma scripts. These increases were seen in a variety of brain regions, including right-hemisphere limbic and paralimbic structures believed to be involved in intense emotion (Rauch et al. 1996). However, because this study lacked a control group, it is unclear whether these findings are specific to PTSD.

With PTSD patients clearly hyperresponsive to trauma-related stimuli, it is of interest whether the hyperresponsiveness is *limited* to trauma-related stimuli. Some studies have found that PTSD patients are not hyperresponsive to nontrauma, neutral stimuli such as mental arithmetic (Blanchard et al. 1996; Gerardi, Blanchard, & Kolb 1989; Pallmeyer, Blanchard, & Kolb 1986), whereas others have found an exaggerated startle response to neutral auditory stimuli (Prins et al. 1995).

Findings on startle responses in PTSD vary depending on how the startle response is measured. To date, startle paradigms using skin conductance and heart rate responses have consistently found an exaggerated startle response, whereas paradigms using electro-oculogram (EOG) have not. Stimulus intensity has varied across studies, with louder tones more likely to elicit an exaggerated startle response. It is possible that louder tones are more reminiscent of some traumas (e.g. gunfire) and more likely to elicit exaggerated startle for that reason (Prins et al. 1995). Butler et al. (1990) reported a larger startle response in PTSD combat veterans than in controls for acoustic stimuli but not for tactile stimuli. It is interesting to note that Morgan et al. (1995) found that stressful task conditions mediated the startle response. When paired with shock, PTSD patients exhibited a larger startle response (fear-potentiated startle) than did controls. This difference was not present in nonstress (no-shock) conditions. The authors concluded that enhanced startle is specific to trauma-related or trauma-reminiscent stimuli.

Other studies have examined PTSD patients' responses to nontrauma stimuli and found differences in various event-related brain potential (ERP) components. Perhaps the most commonly studied ERP component is the P300, which is a positive voltage shift in the EEG time-locked to an infrequent stimulus event. Charles et al. (1995) examined P300 in a standard "oddball" paradigm and found smaller P300 for PTSD patients than for non-PTSD trauma victims. However, because they reported difference scores without reporting separate amplitude scores for rare and frequent tones, it is unclear what aspect of P300 carried the effect (e.g., overall reduction vs. lack of target–rare effect vs. exaggerated nontarget–frequent response). McFarlane, Weber, and Clark (1993) examined midline ERPs in a three-tone auditory oddball task. For the PTSD group, the N200 (a negative-going ERP component that typically occurs following the recognition of a change in the present stimuli) occurred later, and P300 amplitude was smaller and did not distinguish the infrequent tones. In contrast, controls demonstrated larger P300 to targets than to distractors. McFarlane et al. (1993) suggested that the patients spent more time on stimulus discrimination (reflected in N200 latency) and had fewer resources available for subsequent processing, as evidenced by decreased P300 amplitude.

Paige et al. (1990) examined ERPs using tones of four different intensities. Based on slope changes in P200 amplitude, they characterized most control subjects as "augmenters" (P200 amplitude and stimulus intensity positively correlated) and most PTSD subjects as "reducers" (P200 amplitude and stimulus intensity negatively correlated). The P200 ERP is considered to be a response to an exogenous event, and it can be enhanced by focusing attention upon exogenous events. The study also examined heart rate in the same subjects but not simultaneously or under the same task conditions. Heart rate increased twice as much in PTSD patients as in controls. The P200 findings have recently been replicated using magnetoencephalographic (MEG) recordings (Lewine et al. 1997). These findings merit follow-up to determine, for example, if the reduction reflects a compensatory mechanism driven by the exaggerated responsiveness observed in some peripheral measures.

Distinct from research on reactivity in PTSD, several studies have investigated whether PTSD patients are chronically hyperaroused. Blanchard (1990) reviewed baseline studies and concluded that PTSD veterans have an increased resting heart rate and blood pressure. However, more recent studies have not found these differences (McFall, Veith, & Murburg 1992; Pitman et al. 1990). As McFall et al. (1992) and Prins et al. (1995) discussed, some of the disparate findings may be an artifact of baseline length. Baseline differences are generally found in studies using shorter baselines, suggesting an acute reaction to the experimental context rather than a true tonic elevation.

The inability to recall important aspects of the trauma is a symptom of PTSD, and the hippocampus is involved in memory function. However, there are as yet few psychophysiological studies of specific cognitive dysfunction in PTSD. Bremner et al. (1995) used MRI (magnetic resonance imaging) to examine hippocampal volume in PTSD patients. They found less right hippocampal volume in PTSD participants than in controls, consistent with a hypothesis of memory problems. These PTSD patients also were found to have lower scores on the Weschler Memory Scale (WMS) for both immediate and delayed verbal recall relative to controls, with no differences found in visual memory. Similarly, Gurvits et al. (1996) found reduced hippocampal volume in PTSD patients compared to non-PTSD combat veterans and nonveteran controls. They also found that hippocampal volume was negatively correlated with the amount of combat exposure, suggesting that repeated traumatic stress may damage the hippocampus. Further, Semple et al. (1993) reported decreased blood flow to the hippocampal area, although another group failed to replicate this finding (Rauch et al. 1996). These findings suggest that PTSD may be associated with hippocampal attrition. As noted previously, Nadel and Jacobs (in press) proposed a mechanism for this attrition. Yehuda (1997) also proposed a mechanism for this attrition – one that implicates the hypothalamic-pituitary-adrenal (HPA) axis, which is involved in coordinating the body's response to stress.

The few studies that have used central measures in PTSD have tended to be problematic, such as lacking a control group or relying on nonstandard data analytic methods. Brewin et al.'s (1996) theory suggests that exposure to traumatic memories should be effective at extinguishing emotional reactions experienced during the trauma itself but not secondary reactions arising from subsequent cognitive appraisal of the situation. Based on this theory, it would be interesting to investigate habituation to a suitable range of trauma-related stimuli using central and autonomic measures simultaneously. More elaborate paradigms using such stimuli may shed light on the impact of PTSD-related anxiety on associated cognitive deficits.

Post-traumatic stress disorder has been shown to have a high rate of comorbid diagnoses, including major depression, other anxiety disorders, and substance abuse (Green et al. 1989; Helzer et al. 1987; Keane & Wolfe 1990). It has been hypothesized that comorbidity with other disorders accounts for some of the discrepant PTSD findings. Successful investigations of PTSD will need to deal with comorbidity issues. Heller and Nitschke (1998) and Mineka, Watson, and Clark (1998) discussed this issue for anxiety and related disorders more generally.

Summary

Complementing the long tradition of autonomic studies of anxiety, more recent psychophysiological research has found that different subtypes of anxiety are associated with distinct regional patterns of brain activity. Failure to consider such differences may account for a considerable portion of the discrepant central and peripheral findings reported to date. The functional significance of this regional differentiation remains to be determined, although Davidson (1984, 1992) and Heller (1993; Heller & Nitschke 1998) have provided some proposals. Autonomic measures have been the predominant psychophysiological tool in anxiety research, but it is becoming clear that central measures provide valuable information about the nature of anxiety. For example, Brewin et al.'s (1996) theory of PTSD provides a useful framework for guiding psychophysiological investigations of anxiety. Conceptualizations that focus on the integral role of physiological activity *in* anxiety, rather than as a response *to* anxiety, are also promising.

MOOD DISORDERS

Research on mood disorders and research on anxiety disorders share a few key elements (see Heller & Nitschke 1998). One element is the specificity of each disorder. Mood and anxiety are both broad constructs, and even diagnostic criteria designed to provide discrete boundaries for each disorder may leave much ambiguity. In the case of depression, DSM-IV recognizes several mood disorders, including major depression, dysthymia, and bipolar disorder, as well as several subtypes, such as depression with atypical or melancholic features. Additional categorizations of depression have been utilized, including endogenous–

exogenous and agitated–retarded as well as a depressive personality subtype (Klein 1990; Klein & Miller 1993, 1997; Klein & Shih 1998). This range of depressive syndromes can complicate the interpretation of findings from studies on depression. A second issue is the problem of comorbidity and symptom overlap with other disorders. Depression often co-occurs with anxiety, substance abuse, and other disorders. Additionally, isolated or subsyndromal symptoms of depression and anxiety are found in other psychological disorders, and symptoms of other disorders may occur in individuals whose primary disorder is depression or anxiety. Research based on well-defined theoretical models and well-characterized subject groups can help address these issues, but for the most part there is not enough research available to permit much integration. This appears to be an area especially in need of the improved delimitation of homogeneous endophenotypes that psychophysiology may foster, as discussed earlier.

Although depressed mood is by far the most commonly encountered mood symptom (Zahn 1986), elevated, expansive, and irritable mood are also associated with mood disorders. Psychophysiological studies of mood have most often focused on depression, perhaps in part owing to the difficulty of working with manic patients. Because manic patients often share certain symptoms with schizophrenic patients, they are often used as a comparison group for studies into potential vulnerability markers, such as eye tracking deficits and changes in the P300 component of the ERP (Adler et al. 1990; Souza et al. 1995). Blackwood et al. (1996) examined the prevalence of changes in P300 latency and eye tracking in families of bipolar probands. They found neither strong evidence for an increase in these physiological vulnerability factors among affected families nor any evidence for diagnostic specificity of the physiological factors. Impairment of smooth pursuit eye movements has been reported but was originally suspected of being a consequence of lithium treatment (Holzman, O'Brian, & Waternaux 1991). However, Gooding and associates (1993) were unable to find any effect of lithium treatment on eye tracking ability. Because bipolar disorder may constitute a mix of mood and psychotic features, this group may be useful in bridging the gap in our understanding between specific mental processes and psychophysiology in mood and psychotic disorders.

Cyclothymia is a disorder that is similar to but less severe than bipolar disorder. Virtually no studies have examined physiology in this group. Lenhart and Katkin (1986; Lenhart 1985) studied a mixed group of dysthymics and cyclothymics and reported eye movement abnormalities and reduced skin conductance responding. The latter finding is consistent with reports on patients with severe mood disorder (reviewed by Zahn 1986). Fernandes et al. (1999) found that cyclothymics were very similar to dysthymics in seeming to process recurrent stimuli as if novel – this inferred from N200 responses. The very limited psychophysiological literature on these groups warrants expansion and linkage to theoretical work on more traditional mood disorders.

Depression is often associated with disturbances of cognition, perhaps stemming from the same mental dysfunction (Tariot & Weingartner 1986). Reviews of psychophysiological findings in mood disorder include Bruder (1995), Sponheim et al. (1995), and Yee (1995). Reflecting the abundance of empirical research on depression relative to other mood disorders, the present section will focus on the use of psychophysiology to address questions about depression.

Regional Brain Activity Associated with Depression

One emphasis that has received increasing attention in psychophysiological research is the relationship between specific brain regions and affect. Valence is a dimension of affect that has been found to vary systematically with activity in specific brain regions. Davidson (1984, 1992) and Heller (1990, 1993) suggested that pleasant valence is associated with greater left than right anterior activity and that unpleasant valence is associated with greater right than left anterior activity. Consistent with this suggestion, Gainotti and colleagues (Gainotti 1972; Gainotti, Caltagirone, & Zoccolotti 1993) found that the left frontal region is involved in the experience of positive mood and that damage to (or inactivation of) that region results in depressed mood. Hemodynamic and EEG studies of depression have also reported decreased left anterior brain activity (Baxter et al. 1985; Bench et al. 1993; see also Henriques & Davidson 1989). Although most studies find greater relative left frontal *alpha* activity during depression, it is unclear whether this is due to an increase in right frontal activation, a decrease in left frontal activation, or some combination of both. However, other studies have reported increased activity (i.e., less alpha) in left prefrontal regions in depression (Drevets et al. 1992), and still others have found no effects for depression (Tomarken & Davidson 1994) or for positive or negative affect (Sutton & Davidson 1997).

Heller (1993) further suggested that autonomic activity related to emotion is modulated by right posterior brain activity. Reduced right posterior activity is associated with depressed mood; increased right posterior activity is associated with anxiety characterized by autonomic hyperarousal. Support for this hypothesis comes from studies showing that depressed individuals have a selective deficit on right-hemisphere tasks (Rubinow & Post 1992; Silberman, Weingartner, & Post 1983). Depressed individuals have also shown right-hemisphere deficits in paradigms using lateralized presentation of stimuli (Bruder 1995). This abnormal lateralization has been linked to clinical features of depression, including subtype and treatment outcome. Furthermore, depressed subjects have been reported to show reduced attentional bias in favor of the right hemisphere (Heller et al. 1995; Jaeger, Borod, & Peselow 1987; Keller et al. in press) on the Chimeric Faces Task, a free-vision facial processing test (Levy et al. 1983).

Right-parietal involvement in depression has also been supported by EEG studies that report decreased brain activity near right posterior areas in depressed patients during tasks of dichotic listening (Bruder et al. 1995), nonlateralized emotional face presentation (Deldin et al. in press), language processing (Keller et al. 1995), and verbal memory (Henriques & Davidson 1995). Decreased right posterior activity has also been found in remitted depressed patients (Henriques & Davidson 1990), suggesting a relationship between brain activity patterns and trait characteristics of depression. Blood flow studies have reported similar findings (Flor-Henry 1979; Post et al. 1987; Uytdenhoef et al. 1983) but with some exceptions (see Davidson & Tomarken 1989). In order to confirm this relationship between right posterior activity and depression and anxiety, future studies need to deal with their considerable comorbidity.

Information Processing in Depression

Several theories of depression have discussed abnormal information processing in mood disorders. Ellis and Ashbrook (1988) suggested that depression depletes the amount of processing that an individual can complete within a fixed time. Thus, depressed individuals are more likely than nondepressed individuals to be impaired on tasks requiring sustained and controlled processing. Hertel and colleagues (Hertel & Hardin 1990; Hertel & Rude 1991) suggested that deficits in depression are a result of a lack of cognitive initiative or motivation. Depressed individuals will appear impaired on high-demand tasks as predicted by Ellis and Ashbrook (1988), but the impairment may reflect a failure to engage in controlled processing rather than a reduced amount of available processing resources. This notion is similar to an effortful or controlled processing account of attention (e.g. Hasher & Zacks 1979; Posner & Snyder 1975). Based on psychophysiological and neuropsychological data, Heller and Nitschke (1997) furthered Hertel's position and suggested that depressed patients' fundamental deficits were in initiative and in strategic use of information.

The foregoing theories suggest a variety of anomalies in depressed individuals, such as deficits on tasks that require sustained attention, larger amounts of cognitive capacity, or frontal lobe function. Some of the behavioral findings are consistent with the theories, suggesting a deficit in controlled rather than automatic processing. In several studies, depressed inpatients demonstrated a significant impairment in effortful cognitive tasks (requiring sustained concentration or attention or larger amounts of cognitive capacity) compared with nondepressed subjects (Roy-Byrne et al. 1986; Weingartner & Silberman 1982). However, in less effortful, more automatic tasks, depressed patients performed as well as nondepressed subjects. Tancer et al. (1990) compared depressed inpatients to nondepressed inpatients on more or less effortful tasks. Depressed individuals remembered significantly fewer words at free recall than did nondepressives, but they did not differ from non-depressives on less effortful tasks. In addition, providing problem-solving strategies for depressed individuals leads to improved performance (Silberman et al. 1983); when these strategies are not provided, depressed people utilize less of the available information (Conway & Giannopoulos 1993).

Available psychophysiological findings are largely consistent with theories suggesting that less effortful mental processes are intact in depression. Early ERP components, which are thought to reflect basic sensory processing and attention, are relatively intact in depressed patients (Bruder et al. 1995; Katsanis, Iacono, & Beiser 1996), although there are some exceptions (Roth et al. 1981; Shagass 1981; Yee, Deldin, & Miller 1992). One early component that may be reduced in depression (Ogura et al. 1993) is mismatch negativity (MMN), a subcomponent of N200; however, Fernandes et al. (1999) observed MMN to be intact.

Other physiological measures such as longer-latency ERPs and autonomic orienting – which reflect higher-order mental processes such as stimulus evaluation and working memory – have received more attention in depression. As suggested by theories of depression, these higher-order processes are more likely to be disrupted in depression. In an extensive review of the P300 literature, Roth et al. (1986) found that half of the studies found significant reduction in P300 amplitude. However, most of the studies reviewed examined P300 in a simple auditory oddball task. Roth et al. (1986) argued for the need to go beyond the oddball paradigm and to assess ERPs during more cognitively challenging tasks. They further suggested that tasks should be developed from theories about specified dysfunction in depression. Using a very demanding dual-task paradigm, Yee and Miller (1994) examined individuals who reported moderate levels of chronic depression and were at risk for developing major depressive disorder. This dysthymic sample demonstrated both smaller P300s overall and a lack of modulation of P300 as a function of task demands, suggesting problems in both resource amount and resource allocation. More recently, Hicks and co-workers (1998) studied college students who had met DSM-IV criteria for past or present major depression or bipolar disorder. By using more homogeneous groups and more stringent analytic procedures, they determined that the P300 differences between controls and mood-disordered subjects reflected differences in resource allocation.

Studies examining another N200 subcomponent, N2b, provide some evidence of abnormal short-term memory in depression. The N2b appears sensitive to whether an incoming stimulus matches a cognitive template in short-term memory (Näätänen 1990; Pritchard, Shappell, & Brandt 1991; Ritter & Ruchkin 1992). El Massioui and Lesèvre (1988) observed a smaller N2b and a larger late frontal negativity in depression. This combination of results suggests that depressed individuals rely on later, more effortful processing strategies to perform the task. This is consistent with behavioral data suggesting that depressed people have some difficulty in tasks that require sustained attention and controlled processing. Giese-Davis, Miller, and Knight (1993) and Fernandes et al. (1999) reported exaggerated N2bs in nonpatient dysthymics. Fernandes et al. further found that a subset of subjects meeting criteria for DSM-III major depression showed the same pattern. These subjects were college students functioning relatively well, whereas patients in the El Massioui and Lesèvre (1988) study, which found decreased N2b, were severely depressed inpatients. There are a number of possible explanations for this discrepancy. As Fernandes, Hicks, and Miller (1995) suggested, the difference may reflect severity of the depression and extent of cognitive difficulties. They suggested that the enhanced N2b in depressed nonpatients may reflect a compensatory mechanism that deteriorates with increased psychopathology. Another possibility is that differences in the tasks could account for the inconsistencies. For example, the probability of the target tone and difficulty of the tone discrimination task differed between these two studies and may influence ERP responses.

Further evidence that depressed individuals have difficulty maintaining attention to relevant stimuli comes from measures of the orienting response. Orienting appears to reflect the allocation of attentional resources to the processing of a novel stimulus (Dawson, Filion, & Schell 1989; Öhman 1979). The contingent negative variation (CNV) is a scalp-negative voltage shift typically observed after presentation of a warning stimulus and resolving after presentation of an imperative stimulus in a fixed-foreperiod, warned reaction time paradigm (Pritchard 1986). Within the foreperiod, CNV appears initially to reflect orienting to the warning stimulus and then begins to index anticipation of the imperative stimulus (Simons, Öhman, & Lang 1979). The amplitude of the CNV appears to be proportional to the level of sustained attention focused on the detection of the imperative stimulus (Näätänen & Michie 1979). Depressed and dysthymic individuals' decreased CNV amplitude (see Sponheim et al. 1995) suggests that they are less able to stay focused on an anticipated event. Reductions in CNV have been shown to be related to the severity of depression, normalizing when the depression remits (Ashton et al. 1988), and are associated with longer reaction times.

A variety of autonomic measures have been used to assess aspects of information processing such as orienting and attention in depression. Results have been inconsistent across different measures. Orienting involves directing attention and extracting information from the environment (Sokolov 1990). Research on orienting has primarily been measured via electrodermal activity (EDA; see Henriques & Davidson 1989 for a review). It has been suggested that different aspects of skin responses are associated with different psychological functions: the phasic skin conductance orienting responses (SCOR) are associated with attention and information processing, whereas tonic skin conductance level (SCL) and nonspecific skin conductance responses (NS-SCORs) have been said to reflect general states of activation and arousal (Boucsein 1992; Dawson, Schell, & Filion 1990), although – as discussed before – the latter are no longer particularly viable constructs.

Depressed patients and dysthymics have consistently been found to have fewer and smaller SCORs (Bernstein et al. 1988; Dawson & Nuechterlein 1984; Ford et al. 1992; Iacono, Ficken, & Beiser 1993; Iacono et al. 1983; Öhman, Nordby, & d'Elia 1986; Simons 1981; Ward, Doerr, & Storrie 1983; Yee 1995; Yee & Miller 1988) and lower SCL (Ward & Doerr 1986), indicating hyporeactivity (Zahn 1986). This electrodermal hypoactivity appears to be a trait difference and not a state difference, since it has been observed following remission of depressive episodes. Lower electrodermal levels have been correlated with more severe depression (see Sponheim et al. 1995). Some other physiological measures that are less well researched have also been found to be diminished in depression: heart rate orienting (Dawson et al. 1985), forearm blood flow (Williams, Iacono, & Remick 1985), and salivary response (Noble & Lader 1971). Furthermore, some putative ERP measures of orienting (e.g., CNV and N200) are diminished in patient depressives (Ashton et al. 1988; Ogura et al. 1993), suggesting dysfunctional orienting. The primarily electrodermal hyporesponsiveness of depressed individuals has often been interpreted as evidence for an overall orienting deficit, but other measures of orienting do not always suggest a general deficit. For example, Bernstein et al. (1988) found that depressed subjects had normal finger pulse volume (FPV) response despite reduced SCOR, and Steinhauer and Zubin (1982) reported normal levels of pupillary dilation response in depressed subjects.

We have discussed how much research has shown that physiological response systems do not necessarily move in concert, yet it would be beneficial to understand why certain systems appear intact and others are disrupted in depression. A number of authors have suggested that particular neurotransmitter systems are involved in specific physiological systems. For example, Bernstein et al. (1988) suggested that the pattern of autonomic results (decreased SCOR and normal FPV and pupillary dilation response) in depression reflect a cholinergic deficit and not a general orienting deficit. Timsit-Berthier et al. (1987) suggested that catecholaminergic dysfunction, particularly dopaminergic functioning, results in CNV amplitude reductions during depression. Investigation of the relationships among depression, various physiological measures, and particular neurotransmitter systems is still in its infancy, and further research is warranted to understand the discordance of various systems.

Language processing, which requires both sustained attention and working memory (Docherty et al. 1996), has received little attention in depression. The N400, a negative voltage shift in the EEG, is enhanced when a terminal word in a sentence is incongruent with the text preceding it (Kutas & Van Petten 1994). It is elicited without a behavioral response and can be used as an index of semantic processing. Because sustained attention is impaired in depression, they may show N400 abnormalities. Keller et al. (1995) found that, unlike nonpsychiatric controls, depressed inpatients' N400s failed to distinguish semantically congruent and incongruent sentence endings. However, Deldin, Casas, and Best (1998) found that depressed individuals' N400s differentiated congruent and incongruent sentence endings and that they did not differ from controls. In each study, subjects were also exposed to sentence endings that were emotionally congruent or incongruent with the subject's mood state. Neither group found that depressed individuals' N400s differentiated positive or negative sentence endings. However, Chung et al. (1996) found that N400 responses differentiated positive and negative words in nonpatient subjects in whom a sad mood had been induced. Although the very limited available data show some inconsistencies, this research on cognitive and emotional processing in mood disorders is a potentially exciting area that has potential to integrate theories of depression and psychophysiology.

Summary

In the past decade, there has been an increasing focus on the role of attentional resources and on whether resource allocation is deficient in depression. However, it is unclear whether the psychological deficits seen in depression are due to reduced initiative or motivation or whether depression depletes resources so that adequate processing of the material cannot be completed. Research in depression has benefitted from the use of both central and peripheral measures, although very few studies have used these measures together. Findings for depression and dysthymia have been quite consistent across some autonomic measures. The inconsistencies in N2b and P300 components of the ERP suggest that major depression is accompanied by the failure of a compensatory strategy operative in dysthymia, with samples in various studies differing in the particular features of depression represented. A conclusive determination about orienting and higher-level processing awaits further research.

SCHIZOPHRENIA SPECTRUM DISORDERS

Schizophrenia is thought of as primarily a disorder of cognition, although a variety of other symptoms are frequently present also. A large body of psychophysiological research is available for schizophrenia (see Blackwood et al. 1996; Friedman & Squires-Wheeler 1994; Holzman 1987; Pritchard 1986; Shajahan et al. 1997; Turetsky, Colbath, & Gur 1998a,b; Zahn 1986), and research is growing for "spectrum" disorders in which subjects have only a subset of symptoms or are simply at risk for schizophrenia (Dawson et al. 1995; Hicks et al. 1998; Trestman et al. 1996). Studies of cognitive deficits in schizophrenia spectrum disorders point to several broad areas of disturbance, including attention (Gold & Harvey 1993; Knight 1992), working memory (Cohen et al. 1994; Goldman-Rakic 1991), language (Andreasen 1979), and emotional processing (Kring & Neale 1996). Reflecting the general similarity of psychophysiological findings across this spectrum, this section will consider the schizophrenia spectrum as a whole rather than distinguishing schizophrenia, schizotypal, psychotic, or relevant at-risk groups. Occasions where findings for the groups are divergent or where only one group was investigated will be noted. Given the wealth of literature, the discussion will be particularly selective and is organized around issues in attention, working memory, language, and emotion.

Attention

It has long been established that individuals with schizophrenia spectrum disorders demonstrate impairments in selective and sustained attention (McGhie & Chapman 1961; Venables 1964). The impairment in selective attention reflects an apparent tendency for all incoming information to be treated as important, whereas impairment in sustained attention reflects a reduction in the processing of stimuli presented in attended channels (Oltmanns 1978). The combined effect of these attentional deficits is an inefficient allocation of processing capacity, resulting in a failure to process important information adequately and in time wasted processing irrelevant information. Several theories have proposed that some schizophrenic symptoms, such as hallucinations and ideas of reference, may be a consequence of an impaired attentional filter (Braff 1993; McGhie & Chapman 1961; Silverman 1964). The purpose of such a filter is to protect limited-capacity systems from being overloaded with too much incoming information (Broadbent 1982). An impaired filter would lead to the inability to process adequately the most important information as well as to a tendency to attribute special or inappropriate significance to other information.

Disturbance in attentional filtering has been studied extensively in recent years through the use of startle or prepulse modulation paradigms. Presentation of loud, fast-onset tones evokes a startle reflex that can be measured several ways, including magnitude of eye blinks and skin conductance responses. The startle reflex is modulated when a low-intensity stimulus (prepulse) is presented shortly before the onset of the startle stimulus (Anthony 1985). If the interval between the prepulse and startle stimulus is relatively short (e.g., 30–300 msec), there is a

reduction in the magnitude of the startle reflex. The reflex inhibition is believed to reflect the operation of an attentional filter that blocks out environmental information occurring during the initial phases of processing of the prepulse stimulus (Braff & Geyer 1990). Longer intervals between the prepulse and startle stimuli (e.g., greater than 1,000 msec) lead to an enhanced startle reflex. The facilitation of the startle reflex appears to be due to the focusing of attention on the prepulse stimulus occurring in the same channel as the startle stimulus.

Prepulse inhibition occurs regardless of whether stimuli are task-relevant. It is an automatic process (Braff & Geyer 1990; Graham 1975), which makes this paradigm especially appropriate for working with clinical populations who may have problems understanding or adhering to task instructions. Numerous studies have found that prepulse inhibition is reduced in schizophrenia (Braff et al. 1978; Braff, Grillon, & Geyer 1992; Dawson et al. 1993; Grillon et al. 1992; Hazlett et al. 1998) and in nonpatients putatively at risk for schizotypy (Cadenhead, Geyer, & Braff 1993; Cadenhead, Kumar, & Braff 1996; Dawson et al. 1995; Schell et al. 1995; Simons & Giardina 1992). The lack of inhibition of the startle reflex suggests that schizophrenia spectrum individuals fail to block out incoming information during the period in which they should be processing the prepulse stimulus. In addition, schizophrenic patients fail to show the expected enhancement of the startle reflex following longer interstimulus intervals (Dawson et al. 1993; Hazlett et al. 1998), reflecting a failure to sustain attention in the channel in which the startle stimulus occurs. Although prepulse inhibition is an automatic process, it can be modified if the subject attends to the prepulse stimulus (Filion, Dawson, & Schell 1993): when controlled attentional processing is focused on the prepulse stimulus, the inhibition of the startle reflex is even greater. As with automatic prepulse inhibition, schizophrenia spectrum individuals appear to be deficient in the ability to modulate prepulse inhibition by focusing their attention on the prepulse stimulus (Dawson et al. 1993; Schell et al. 1995). Results from positron emission tomography (PET; Hazlett et al. 1998) and dopamine receptor (Ellenbroek, Budde, & Cools 1996) studies implicate medial prefrontal cortex as being involved in the modulation of prepulse inhibition. As we shall discuss, this region is implicated in other physiological measures that are attenuated in schizophrenia.

Conceptually related to attentional filtering is the study of sensory gating deficits in schizophrenia spectrum disorders. Paired-stimulus paradigms reliably find that there is a smaller P50 ERP component to the second stimulus than to the first stimulus of the pair. The reduction is often quantified as the ratio of the two P50 amplitudes. Schizophrenic individuals show larger S2/S1 P50 ratios (implying less filtering) than controls (Adler et al. 1982; Freedman et al. 1983; Smith, Boutros, & Schwarzkopf 1994a). Larger ratios have been observed in nonmedicated schizophrenic individuals (Freedman et al. 1983), first-degree relatives of schizophrenia patients (Clementz, Geyer, & Braff 1997b), and bipolar patients (Franks et al. 1983).

Serious methodological problems and inconsistencies have undermined the P50 suppression literature, including the frequently poor reliability of the P50 ratio measure itself (Smith et al. 1994). After the initial report of reduced suppression in schizophrenia, nearly a decade elapsed before the first attempts at replication in other laboratories appeared, each differing significantly in methodology. Sufficient replications now exist that the basic phenomenon can be considered to be well established (Boutros, Overall, & Zouridakis 1991; Light & Braff 1998), but some uncertainty remains as to the relationship of P50 amplitude and suppression to diagnostic subtypes, task demands, and experimental conditions (for reviews see White & Yee 1997, 1998; Yee & White 1998). Issues such as posture of the subject during recording and selection of valid trials have yet to be resolved. It is unclear whether P50 is a single positive shift or if it is a subcomponent of a larger response – specifically, a change in gamma activity in the EEG (Clementz, Blumenfeld, & Cobb 1997a). Temporal factors also appear to have a significant impact on the nature of the observed ratio. Clementz et al. (1997b) found that P50 suppression was more pronounced during trials presented early in the study (see White & Yee 1998). In an analysis of P50 at the single-trial level, Jin et al. (1998) found that the P50 ratio difference was a result of greater trial-to-trial latency variability in responses to the first stimulus in schizophrenia patients than in controls. Accurate measurement of P50 can be compromised by the fact that several components (e.g., P30, N40, N100, Nd) occur during or adjacent to P50. Some of these are sensitive to attention and have been shown to differentiate schizophrenia patients and controls, complicating the interpretation of observed differences in P50 suppression.

There are also a number of problems pertaining to the theoretical understanding of P50 suppression. Although interest in P50 suppression in schizophrenia is based on the assumption that sensory gating deficits are related to the clinical phenomena of perceptual abnormalities, Jin et al. (1998) found that patients reporting perceptual abnormalities demonstrated P50 ratios consistent with normal controls. Moreover, patients not reporting perceptual abnormalities demonstrated abnormal P50 ratios. There is also some evidence that P50 is subject to attentional and stress manipulations as well as to diagnostic subtype (Boutros et al. 1993; Cullum et al. 1993; Guterman, Josiassen, & Bashore 1992; White, Yee, & Nuechterlein 1997; Yee, White, & Nuechterlein 1996; but see Jerger, Biggins, & Fein 1992 and White & Yee 1997 for failures to find an attention effect). Further study of these issues is needed before the nature of P50 suppression and its suitability as a measure of disturbed filtering in schizophrenia spectrum disorders can be fully determined.

Another ERP component that is sensitive to selective attention has been called negative difference (Nd; Hansen & Hillyard 1980) or processing negativity (PN; Näätänen, Gaillard, & Mantysalo 1978). Interpretation of this effect is complicated because Nd is usually scored by subtracting activity in the unattended channel from activity in the attended channel. In controls, the expected finding is larger negativity following stimuli presented in the attended channel. If there is an attentional filter deficit in schizophrenia spectrum disorders, then negativity in the unattended channel should be as large as negativity in the attended channel. If, instead, the deficit is related to individuals being unable to sustain attention in a specific channel, then negativity in the attended channel should be as small as negativity in the unattended channel. Schizophrenic individuals (Iwanami et al. 1998; Ward et al. 1991) and their children (Schreiber et al. 1992) demonstrated a smaller Nd to the stimuli in the attended channel than did controls. This difference is the result of attended-channel responses being as small as unattended-channel responses, suggesting that abnormalities may involve a failure to attend to relevant stimuli and not an inability to filter irrelevant information. Such a conclusion must be offered very cautiously, however, because a given task may be more suited for evaluating one aspect of processing than another. In addition, the pattern of Nd differences distinguishes paranoid from nonparanoid schizophrenic individuals (Oades, Zerbin, & Eggers 1994; Oades et al. 1997), demonstrating the importance of adequate diagnostic screening.

A different approach to investigating selective attention deficits in schizophrenia spectrum disorders is to examine patterns of brain activity during selective attention tasks. The left temporal lobe, especially the region around the left superior temporal gyrus (STG), has been identified as key in cerebral lateralization deficits in schizophrenia across physiological measures (Crow 1990; McCarley et al. 1993; O'Leary et al. 1996). Volume measures of the left STG and surrounding areas have indicated that this region is especially reduced in schizophrenia (Crow 1990). Several MRI studies have found a negative correlation between left STG volume and positive symptoms such as auditory hallucinations (Barta et al. 1990; Menon et al. 1995) and thought disorder (Shenton et al. 1992). The size of the left STG has also been found to be negatively correlated with P300 amplitude measured over left temporal (T3) and central (C3) sites (McCarley et al. 1993). Also, P300 reductions have been consistently reported in nonpatient anhedonics (Fernandes & Miller 1995) for whom there is evidence of elevated risk for schizophrenia (Erlenmeyer-Kimling et al. 1993; Freedman et al. 1998), with several studies reporting that the amplitude difference between schizophrenia spectrum individuals and controls is greatest over the left hemisphere (Bruder et al. 1992; McCarley et al. 1991; Salisbury et al. 1996). Activity in the STG has also been studied by rCBF during a dichotic listening task (O'Leary et al.

1996). Control subjects demonstrated an increase in activity in the STG contralateral to the attended ear and a decrease in activity in the STG ipsilateral to the attended ear. Schizophrenic patients demonstrated greater activity in the left STG regardless of the direction of attention. Taken together, these studies suggest that in schizophrenia the left STG is smaller and is associated with smaller P300s over the left scalp, yet it receives more blood flow. This somewhat complex relationship suggests that, although schizophrenic individuals have structural deficits in the left STG, they persist in trying to activate that region.

The ability to focus attention over time in preparation for a stimulus is referred to as sustained attention (Nuechterlein et al. 1986). In paradigms where a cue indicates the location of an imminent target stimulus, the ability of schizophrenic patients to benefit from that cue declines as the time interval between cue and target increases (Fukushima et al. 1990; Sereno & Holzman 1996). Assuming there are no distracting stimuli, the decline suggests an impairment in sustained attention. Further evidence that schizophrenic individuals have difficulty maintaining attention to relevant stimuli comes from CNV studies. Reduced CNV is observed in many, though not all, schizophrenic patients (Pritchard 1986; Rockstroh et al. 1989), and CNV reduction in acute schizophrenia is more prevalent when the patient exhibits more positive than negative symptoms (Abraham & McCallum 1977; Bachneff & Engelsmann 1980; McCallum & Abraham 1973; Wagner et al. 1996). Further, there is some evidence that CNV tends to normalize when acute patients remit (Pritchard 1986). Patients with a more chronic course of schizophrenia demonstrate more robust CNV reductions (Rizzo et al. 1983).

Other evidence suggests that the observed attentional deficit in schizophrenia spectrum subjects is dependent on controlled processing. Reduced CNV has been observed in college students with high scores on the Revised Physical Anhedonia Scale (Chapman, Chapman, & Raulin 1976) when high-interest nude slides are used as stimuli (Miller, Simons, & Lang 1984). However, the CNV attenuation in anhedonics was not found when other, nonsexual stimuli were used (Miller & Yee 1985), suggesting that differences between anhedonics and controls arise only when controls are highly engaged in focusing attention on the incoming stimulus or when the anticipated stimulus has strong appetitive value. Although CNV attenuation in nonpatient anhedonics is apparently not as severe as in schizophrenic patients, it suggests that attentional impairments involving controlled processing develop before the onset of diagnosable psychopathology.

A deficit in sustained attention can underlie an apparent selective attention deficit if the individual fails to engage a stimulus to the point that subsequent stimuli need to be filtered out. In a similar manner, a selective attention deficit can interfere with sustained attention if the subject fails to filter out even trivial stimulation that may then disrupt the subject's ability to sustain attention. Thus, an ambiguity about the attentional findings reviewed here is whether there is a primary deficit in either selective or sustained attention alone or whether there are deficits in each not solely due to the other. Knight (1993) reviewed a number of studies of attention in schizophrenia and suggested that the reported deficits in attention may be associated with a deficit in short-term memory – a deficit in what the subject does with the stimulus after it has been perceived, rather than what the subject does in preparation for the stimulus. Patients with schizophrenia appear capable of filtering out information that clearly has no meaning (Knight 1992). Their selective attention deficit shows up when an "irrelevant" stimulus appears to contain meaningful information. Knight (1993) hypothesized that schizophrenic individuals fail to focus adequately on task-relevant information and therefore allow new information to distract them. Although such a pattern could result from a failure to prioritize task-relevant above task-irrelevant information or an inability to inhibit task-irrelevant information, schizophrenic patients' ability to inhibit random noise stimuli favors the former explanation. They are able to filter meaningless information, but meaningful information – whether it is task-relevant or task-irrelevant – may be unavoidably processed.

Working Memory

The distinction between what happens before and after the occurrence of a stimulus implies a separation between attentional and memory processes. Knight's hypothesis illustrates the difficulty of formally separating the two stages of processing on the basis of performance scores. Investigations utilizing psychophysiological measures may be more successful in distinguishing between these stages of processing. Like attention, memory has also been subdivided into different types, including sensory or iconic store, short-term memory, working memory, and long-term memory. This section will focus on working memory, which has been shown to be particularly deficient in schizophrenia spectrum disorders.

Information in working memory is preserved by means of conscious memory routines, such as rehearsal, which can extend the duration of storage indefinitely (Atkinson & Shiffrin 1968). Working memory is often conceptualized as more than merely storage; it involves integration of information from a range of sources, which allows the individual to guide his or her behavior on the basis of internalized representations of the outside world, including ideas and thoughts, as opposed to external stimulation exclusively (Goldman-Rakic 1994). Tasks that require individuals to maintain an elaborated or rehearsed representation of a stimulus over a span of several seconds in the *absence* of any external representation of the stimulus are well suited for testing working memory. A commonly used example of this type of task is the Wisconsin Card Sorting Test (WCST). Schizophrenic individuals have been shown to be particularly deficient on this test (Weinberger, Berman, & Zec 1986), often performing at a level equivalent to individuals with prefrontal lesions. The poor performance of schizophrenic patients on this test appears to be due primarily to deficits in working memory and not to other features of the test, such as abstract reasoning and problem solving (Goldberg et al. 1993).

Studies on working memory have linked poor performance to hypofunction in both prefrontal cortex and temporal lobe structures (see Velakoulis & Pantelis 1996). Activity in these two regions has been shown to be correlated during working memory tasks (Cohen et al. 1994; Friedman, Janas, & Goldman-Rakic 1990). The relationship between these two regions may be specific to working memory tasks, since it has not been observed during performance on the Raven's Progressive Matrices – another abstract reasoning–problem solving task that does not involve a working memory component (Berman et al. 1993; Obiols et al. 1993). As discussed earlier, reduced activity in the prefrontal cortex has also been linked to deficits in attentional filtering. Filtering deficits may in turn disrupt working memory. A disruption in the prefrontal–temporal link in schizophrenia, as indicated by prefrontal or temporal abnormalities, may contribute to working memory difficulties in this disorder (Weinberger et al. 1994).

Evidence about the brain regions involved in the generation of N200 and P300 suggests that those components are closely tied to regions associated with long-term and working memory (Egan et al. 1994; Nielsen-Bohlman & Knight 1994). In schizophrenic populations, MMN and N200 reductions have been linked to auditory sensory and working memory impairments (Catts et al. 1995; Javitt et al. 1995; O'Donnell et al. 1993). However, N2b enhancement has been reported in nonpatient anhedonics (Fernandes et al. 1999; Giese-Davis et al. 1993). The enhancement appears to reflect both an excessive response to incoming stimuli and a tendency to treat familiar stimuli as novel, consistent with a memory impairment. The enhancement in at-risk individuals may be associated with an attempt to compensate for incipient memory problems. This compensatory effort may be terminated at the onset of schizophrenia, resulting in the N200 reduction observed in patients. The P300 reflects activity in prefrontal as well as temporoparietal cortex (Knight et al. 1989; Neshige & Luders 1992; Simson, Vaughan, & Ritter 1976). Decreased P300 amplitude is one of the most reliable psychophysiological findings in schizophrenia (Ford et al. 1994b; McCarley et al. 1996; Pritchard 1986; Turetsky et al. 1998a). As noted previously, reduced P300 is consistently found in schizophrenia spectrum individuals even in the absence of performance differences (Fernandes & Miller 1995). These findings suggest that ERPs may provide a particularly sensitive tool for determining which memory processes are impaired in schizophrenia as well as when such memory impairments develop.

Habituation of orienting involves a decrease in response with repeated presentations of a stimulus. If, as suggested by Öhman (1979, 1986), orienting involves the initiation of controlled processing in order to handle novel incoming stimuli, then habituation reflects a reduced need for or call on controlled processing. The reduction in controlled processing is believed to reflect the successful establishment of an internalized template for the presented stimulus (Siddle 1991). Because this template must last throughout the interval between stimulus presentations (often up to 60 sec in common autonomic orienting paradigms), it is probable that the template resides in working memory rather than a short-term iconic store.

Schizophrenia patients have been shown to demonstrate a wide range of abnormalities in the SCOR – predominantly hyporesponsiveness, either not responding at all or habituating quickly (Bernstein et al. 1982; Dawson & Nuechterlein 1984; Öhman 1981). Attenuated SCOR has also been reported for nonpatient anhedonics (Simons 1981). More recent studies have suggested that SCOR habituation failures are not consistent with a pervasive failure of habituation in schizophrenia patients (Braff et al. 1992). Some studies have found a bimodality in schizophrenia, with both hyporesponsive (nonresponding) and hyperresponsive (slow to habituate) patients (Bernstein et al. 1982; Dawson et al. 1989). Other studies have not found differences in responsiveness between schizophrenic individuals and controls (Braff et al. 1992; Iacono et al. 1993). Distinct from anomalies in the SCOR to incoming stimuli, schizophrenia is also associated with elevated skin conductance level. Particularly promising is preliminary evidence that a short-term increase in skin conductance level reliably precedes symptom exacerbation in (previously improved) schizophrenia outpatients (Hazlett et al. 1997).

A possible explanation for the complex and inconsistent findings for habituation in schizophrenia is that habituation may vary over time. Thus, studies that average orienting data across trials are unlikely to detect fluctuations in habituation. Raine et al. (1997) found abnormal SCOR habituation in schizotypal subjects. The nature of the habituation abnormalities suggests that schizotypals took longer to develop a cognitive template for the incoming stimulus; once the template was established, however, schizotypals demonstrated appropriate habituation. This points to deficits in the *establishment* rather than *maintenance* of material within working memory in schizotypal personality disorder. Delayed development of cardiac orienting was similarly observed in a sample of nonpatient anhedonics putatively at risk for schizophrenia (Ebert 1987). Further exploration of the time course of orienting template development in schizophrenia spectrum individuals is warranted by the important implications for memory function.

Dysfunction of prefrontal and temporal cortex during working memory tasks is consistent with the possibility that schizophrenic patients rely on long-term memory systems involving limbic regions to compensate for their compromised working memory (which is dependent on neocortical function). In a study of monozygotic twins discordant for schizophrenia, Berman et al. (1993) found the expected hypoactivity in dorsal prefrontal cortex in affected twins during WCST performance. It is interesting that, although the affected twins showed less frontal activity, they showed greater hippocampal activity. This pattern suggests that schizophrenic patients did not employ working memory to complete the task but instead attempted to rely on mental processes typically associated with long-term memory (Weinberger et al. 1994). This compensatory route may rely on the early selection of incoming information as requiring processing for long-term storage in the limbic region. The enhanced N2b found in at-risk individuals who have not developed schizophrenia may thus reflect successful selection of incoming information. As the schizophrenia disease process develops, this compensatory process may be disrupted. Such a disruption could account for reduced N200 amplitude and poorer working memory skills in schizophrenic individuals.

Language Disturbances

Clinical studies of schizophrenia have noted several abnormal language patterns in schizophrenia (Andreasen 1979), and a number of different approaches have been suggested for studying these language difficulties. Patterson (1987) suggested that language disturbance in schizophrenia might be related to a failure to generate appropriate linguistic expectancies. Others have studied these language difficulties using models of lexical memory (Anderson 1983; Morton 1969) that suggest that the presence of one word can prime recall for similar words in an associative network. Several studies have suggested that schizophrenic patients have more widespread priming than do controls (Kwapil et al. 1990; Manschreck et al. 1988; Spitzer et al. 1994), resulting in increased semantic interference. However, Barch et al. (1996) pointed out a number of methodological problems with these studies and reported normal semantic priming in schizophrenia. Barch and Berenbaum (1996) proposed instead that various language production processes were differentially related to subtypes of thought disorder.

These language disturbances in schizophrenia have been investigated with psychophysiological techniques. As noted before, N400 has been shown to be sensitive to various aspects of linguistic processing. Consistent with models of lexical memory, N400 is believed to be influenced by an automatic process of spreading activation throughout semantic networks (Fischler & Raney 1989; Kutas & Hillyard 1989). Additionally, N400 is sensitive to semantic expectancies. Its magnitude is inversely related to the amount of semantic priming of and expectancy for a particular word (Kutas & Hillyard 1984). As an index of semantic pro-

cessing, N400 can be used to indicate whether the amount of priming in schizophrenia spectrum individuals is greater (decreased N400 amplitude) or if the process of semantic priming takes longer or occurs later in schizophrenia spectrum individuals (delayed or prolonged N400 latency). The N400 can also be used to indicate whether schizophrenic patients' language disturbance might be related to a failure to generate appropriate linguistic expectancies (increased N400).

Studies of semantic priming and semantically incongruous sentences in schizophrenia have had variable results. Some researchers have found reduced N400 amplitude and longer latency for some but not all schizophrenic subjects (Adams et al. 1993; Grillion, Ameli, & Glazer 1991), whereas others have found increased N400 amplitude and longer N400 latency in schizophrenic subjects (Niznikiewicz et al. 1997). Still others have found no N400 amplitude anomalies in schizophrenia (Andrews et al. 1989). As noted earlier, these language tasks require sustained attention, which has been found to be deficient in schizophrenia. It is unclear to what extent these N400 anomalies are due to specific language deficits or to more general attentional deficits. Anomalous N400 in schizophrenia is not surprising in that language abilities have been linked with the left posterior temporal lobe, a region described as being important in the etiology of schizophrenia (Crow 1990). Additionally, McCarthy and colleagues (1995; Nobre & McCarthy 1995) reported a negative polarity field potential (peak latency, 400–500 msec) within the anterior-medial temporal lobe that was consistently elicited by anomalous sentence endings and unprimed words. If this area is important in the generation of N400 then an abnormal N400 would be expected, since this temporal region has been implicated in schizophrenic illness. Further work with N400 and perhaps other language-sensitive ERP components (Kutas 1997) is warranted to build on these initial processing studies aimed at understanding language deficits in schizophrenia.

Emotion

Working memory and attentional deficits potentially explain many of the psychological dysfunctions seen in schizophrenia spectrum disorders. However, it is not obvious how these deficits could explain the notable affective disturbances seen in these individuals. Affective disturbance in schizophrenia spectrum disorders has been noted in numerous reports on the clinical characteristics of the disorder. Although affective disturbance takes many forms in schizophrenia, flattened affect is a common observation. It is often associated with chronic course (Knight et al. 1979) and is usually indicative of poor prognosis (Carpenter et al. 1978; Fenton & McGlashan 1991). Several studies have assessed emotional expression concurrently in self-report and overt behavioral domains (e.g. Berenbaum & Oltmanns 1992; Dworkin et al. 1993; Krause et al. 1989).

The consistent finding has been that schizophrenic patients *demonstrate* less emotional expression than do controls (e.g., based on observers' ratings of facial emotion) but *report* equivalent levels of emotional experience. This discordance among two of Lang's three systems (verbal, physiological, and overt behavioral domains) is intriguing, given the absence of a "gold standard" for emotion (Miller 1996). Although schizophrenic patients are commonly medicated, this seems unable to account for this emotional discordance (for a review of medication confounds in schizophrenia research, see Blanchard & Neale 1992).

Studies of affect in schizophrenia that employ psychophysiological along with overt behavioral and verbal measures may thus be crucial in evaluating apparent emotional deficits. Kring and Neale (1996) examined skin conductance responses in schizophrenic patients and controls during presentation of emotional film clips. Consistent with previous work, schizophrenic individuals demonstrated less overt emotion (based on facial ratings quantified using the Facial Expression Coding System, FACES) while reporting equal emotional experience. However, in that study schizophrenic patients produced more nonspecific skin conductance responses than did controls. Intense emotional experience is typically associated with greater physiological reactivity (Lang 1995). However, schizophrenic individuals demonstrated more skin conductance responses across the board – during emotionally neutral, positive, and negative film clips. Thus, the heightened activity was not limited to putatively emotional contexts. Sison et al. (1996) measured heart rate and facial EMG (electromyographic) activity during emotional imagery. Schizophrenic patients were found to have reduced emotional expression behaviorally (facial EMG) but normal verbal and physiological activity. Additional psychophysiological evaluation could productively investigate the physiological and psychological components of emotional expressivity in schizophrenia. Psychophysiological evaluation of emotion in nonpatients potentially at risk for schizophrenia has been more extensive and suggests a breakdown of the coherence of different emotional response channels (for reviews see Fernandes & Miller 1995; Miller & Yee 1994; Simons, Fitzgibbons, & Fiorito 1993).

Summary

Psychophysiological research has suggested that certain mental functions are abnormal in schizophrenia spectrum disorders. Specifically, sustained attention and working memory deficits may contribute to problems in these individuals. Working memory is perhaps receiving the greatest emphasis in recent psychophysiological research on schizophrenia and may underlie some aspects of filtering and sustained attention problems. Psychophysiological measures have very recently been used to explore deficits in language and affective processing.

Psychophysiological Study of Psychopathology: Inferential Context

SOME PROBLEMS IN COMPARING POPULATIONS

The study of psychopathology often involves the comparison of groups of individuals in an attempt to understand what is specific to one or more populations. This comparison introduces a host of problems related to the interpretation of group differences. Because the groups typically differ prior to the experiment, it is difficult to determine whether measured differences are the result of experimental manipulations or attributable to pre-existing differences. For example, the law of initial values indicates that the level of physiological response to experimental manipulations is related to the pre-experimental level of the physiological measure (Benjamin 1967; Jin 1992; Wilder 1957). Since psychopathological studies cannot rely on random assignment to avoid such differences, alternative approaches must be considered.

Two approaches that may appear useful – but have been shown to be ineffective as general solutions – are matching samples and analysis of covariance. Many researchers have attempted to match patient and control groups on the basis of pre-experimental scores on various measures, such as intelligence or physiological responsiveness. A major problem with matching samples on some measure is that, if the populations from which the samples are drawn do in fact differ on the measure, then matching subjects will result in high scorers from one group being paired with low scorers from the second group. Neither sample is representative of its respective population. Furthermore, such matching can lead to situations in which high scorers will tend to perform less well under retest conditions (regress to the mean), just as the low scorers will tend to perform better (Chapman & Chapman 1973). In addition, matching subjects on one variable tends to unmatch the groups systematically on other variables.

The second approach involves the use of analysis of covariance in hopes of removing the effect of score differences on one test from scores on a second test. Unfortunately, this is not generally a valid use of analysis of covariance when the question at hand involves group differences. Score differences may reflect real, substantive differences between groups. No statistical technique can "correct" for a real difference between groups (Benjamin 1967; Chapman & Chapman 1973; Fleiss & Tanur 1973; Miller, Chapman, & Isaacks 1998); to "correct for" group differences is not even an appropriate goal. For example, confining an analysis to fast-responding depressed patients and slow-responding nonpatients, so that the two samples have comparable reaction times, does not control for the fact that depressed individuals tend to show long reaction times. When a potential covariate is related to the grouping variable, removing variance associated with the covariate necessarily distorts the grouping variable. Analysis of covariance (ANCOVA) is designed for removing noise variance, not systematic variance. Studies of psychopathology that examine group differences are typically inappropriate for analysis of covariance.

There are several ways to compare groups – methods that deal more appropriately with pre-existing differences. One way is to employ *multiple measures* of performance on the *same task*. Performance measures are carefully selected in order to tap distinct subsets of the mental operations involved in task performance. Evaluation of the pattern of results obtained from the different measures may isolate specific mental operations that are demonstrably affected or unaffected by psychopathology. Psychophysiological approaches are particularly well suited for this type of approach, as they provide an additional measure of aspects of task performance. Measurement of physiological responses during a task can often provide sufficient resolution to allow discrete mental operations to be observed (Coles 1989).

A second approach involves the use of the *same or similar measures* across *several tasks* in order to determine to what extent a deficit on one task may exceed a deficit on another task. Measures are considered similar based on their being matched on administration format, difficulty, and reliability. Using this approach, individuals with psychopathology may score below normal controls across all tasks measured. However, the difference between the groups on one task may be substantially larger than the difference on another task. Such a pattern would suggest that the larger deficit involves mental processes that are especially deficient in one group (Chapman & Chapman 1973). The challenge is finding tasks and measures that are equated in terms of difficulty and reliability across groups. Differences in difficulty or reliability can produce artifactual findings that misrepresent the importance of a specific deficit. Davidson and colleagues (1990) discussed these issues and provided a rare example of a study that handled them explicitly.

A third way to address pre-existing differences is to manipulate task difficulty so that each group performs an equally difficult task. The standard implementation of this approach is to adjust task difficulty until each group attains accuracy scores approximating 50% (Chapman & Chapman 1989). A more sophisticated version of this approach – only recently developed and not yet applied in psychophysiological research – is to employ a task in which each group's performance is equally distant from 50% (Miller et al. 1995). In some ways, titration of task difficulty is similar to adjusting stimulus intensity in accordance with each subject's threshold detection level. The drawback of this approach is that tasks of interest are not always readily adjustable.

A fourth approach to addressing pre-existing differences is related to ANCOVA but does not require that the groups be comparable on the covariate. Rather than treating the apparently tangential variable on which the groups differ as a covariate, the analysis can incorporate it and attempt to understand its substantive role. Procedurally, this can be accomplished (in a standard hierarchical regression analysis) by treating the variable as another predictor of interest – especially if its interaction with other variables of interest is included in the analysis. Leutner and Rammsayer (1995) discussed this approach in a personality–self-report context, and their examples generalize well to psychopathology and psychophysiology.

A final approach attempts to sidestep the problem of group differences by using groups whose members exhibit characteristics of psychopathology but are sufficiently well functioning that their performance is substantially equal to that of controls. One way to accomplish this is to study individuals who may be likely (or more likely than the general population) to develop psychopathology yet who are still fully functional (Edell 1995; Klein & Anderson 1995). Such at-risk individuals may include relatives of patients, demographically similar individuals, or individuals exhibiting subthreshold or few symptoms. In some cases, at-risk individuals have earned that designation on the basis of their having disturbances of the same psychological or biological processes as individuals with more severe psychopathology. Because onset of psychopathology is presumably determined by a multitude of factors, it is not necessary for at-risk individuals to develop psychopathology in order for research into their cognition to be useful. They provide the opportunity to study disturbed mental processes that are important in psychopathology while avoiding many of the complications that result from more severe psychopathology.

PROBLEMS IN STUDYING AFFECTED POPULATIONS

The range of dysfunction in psychopathology research is quite broad, from "normal" controls or relatives of patients to acute inpatients. Different issues may arise when conducting psychophysiological research at different levels of severity. In general, the greater the severity, the more concerns exist that need to be addressed.

One difficulty when working with more severely affected individuals is treatment with psychotropic medications (Blanchard & Neale 1992). Conflicting findings have made it difficult to draw firm conclusions about the effects of medications on various physiological measures (see e.g. Buschbaum et al. 1988; Ford et al. 1994a; Matsuoka et al. 1996; Scrimali et al. 1990). Even with individuals not receiving prescription medication, self-medication (i.e., tobacco, alcohol, illicit drugs) can have an effect. Much more research is needed in this area. Another concern is the ability to provide informed consent for participation in clinical research. Individuals with psychopathology will vary in their ability to understand the research, its risks, and its implications (for discussion of the ethics of informed consent with patients, see Zaubler, Viederman, & Fins 1996). This topic is receiving increasing attention and more systematic empirical research. There are also a number of important practical issues in conducting research with hospitalized patients, including the relationship with the clinical staff and obtaining approval from hospital administration. Yet another set of issues arises in research with at-risk individuals, as discussed by Edell (1995).

Despite serious difficulties in working with psychiatric populations, there are ways to address many of these problems. Although medication is often not under the control of the research team and random assignment is not normally possible, researchers can obtain information about the medication of the participants and consider this information when analyzing the data. Research-specific diagnostic screening is especially important to ensure adequate characterization and appropriate group assignment of patients, especially since treatment and research staff may use diagnoses for different purposes. Careful screening procedures may also address such problems as substance abuse and comorbidity (see discussion in next section). These issues must be considered when designing or evaluating research.

Another challenge in studying psychopathology is identifying appropriate control or comparison groups. Depending on the research question posed, other patient groups or nonpatient controls may be most appropriate. Patient groups offer a population that is perhaps comparably medicated and hospitalized, factors that may influence the phenomena of interest. Nonpsychiatric groups provide a basis for comparison to nonpsychopathology research but can be difficult to find given the high rate of subthreshold and undiagnosed disorders in the general population (Schechter et al. 1994). Although under ideal circumstances researchers could recruit both psychiatric and nonpsychiatric control groups, this is often not feasible. Ultimately, researchers need to choose comparison groups based on their experimental questions.

An alternative to working with patients is to work with nonpatients who are at risk for developing diagnosable psychopathology or who already show certain symptoms. As noted earlier, there are several advantages to using at-risk groups to examine psychopathology (see Edell 1995; Klein & Anderson 1995; Mednick & McNeill 1968). First, the use of at-risk groups can avoid problems associated with patient status, such as medication effects, informed consent, and tolerance for research protocols. Second, if a deficit in a particular mental function is fundamental to the development of a disorder, then indications of that deficit should be manifest prior to the actual onset of the disorder. Third, it may be advantageous to examine problems before rather than after onset of the disorder. This would allow researchers to identify possible compensatory mechanisms that at-risk individuals could employ to de-

lay the onset of more severe psychopathology. Information gained from such at-risk studies would be useful both in understanding the process of the disorder and in developing preventive or ameliorative interventions.

PROBLEMS OF COMORBIDITY

Different patterns of symptoms can be associated with the same mental disorder, as reflected in the flexibility of the diagnostic criteria in the DSM-IV. This heterogeneity can be problematic in drawing conclusions in psychopathology research. For psychophysiological research, it is important to consider the prevalence and theoretical significance of particular physiological symptoms in order to select appropriate measures for study. Psychopathology may involve verbal, physiological, and behavioral symptoms (Lang 1968). Because traditional diagnostic categories rely predominantly on verbal and behavioral symptoms, they typically fail to consider the role of physiological symptoms or nonsymptomatic physiological manifestations of relevant processes.

Another problem that complicates psychopathological research is comorbidity, the co-occurrence of different mental disorders in the same individual (Heller & Nitschke 1998; Mineka et al. 1998). Because each diagnosis is associated with somewhat different clusters of verbal, physiological, and behavioral symptoms, comorbidity becomes problematic when co-occurring disorders have divergent effects on the same measure. For example, if depression and anxiety have divergent effects on a physiological symptom (e.g., EEG alpha suppression), then the co-occurrence of these disorders will confound measurement of this physiological variable. This problem occurs more subtly when an individual meets criteria for one diagnosis and is subthreshold for another diagnosis.

Both heterogeneity within a diagnosis and comorbidity between diagnoses can affect the prevalence of the verbal, physiological, and behavioral symptoms within a sample. These factors may differ between studies or research sites and may undermine replicability. Potential physiological measures are almost always ignored by traditional diagnostic screening procedures and so variability in this domain is unknown. One way to address this issue would be to employ psychophysiological screening procedures as part of group selection in research. For example, Blanchard et al. (1996) screened PTSD patients for baseline physiological responsiveness before an experimental task. However, the relevance of the physiological measure must have been established beforehand. Further, as noted previously, initial differences between groups can complicate interpretation of changes in the psychophysiological variable following experimental manipulation. Despite these complications, good experimental design can enhance psychopathological study via the use of psychophysiological variables as independent and dependent variables.

Researchers need to make decisions about whether heterogeneity and comorbidity are problematic in their study. Investigators have a choice of describing psychopathology in terms of a diagnosis (e.g., schizophrenia), a symptom (e.g., disorganized speech, depressed mood, exaggerated startle response), or an inferred mental process (e.g., working memory). Although not themselves constituting psychopathology, genetic and other biological phenomena may be a focus of research on psychopathology. These levels of description may be differentially affected by the issues of heterogeneity and comorbidity. The investigator's choice depends on many things, including the level of resolution needed to answer the research question (Cacioppo & Berntson 1992), which in turn is dependent on (usually implicit) value judgements about what is most important or most promising. In many areas, psychophysiological investigations have been applied at these different levels haphazardly, causing the literature to be spread rather thinly with little conclusive evidence at any level. In other areas, the choice has been more consistent and the data are clear.

Suggestions for Future Research on Psychopathology

This chapter has attempted to examine some key findings and trends in psychopathology research that employs psychophysiological techniques. We have argued that findings that are particularly meaningful share a common feature: the integration of good psychological with good physiological theory. However, much of what is reported does not involve such integration. The modal report is simply one more empirical demonstration that individuals with psychopathology differ from controls. We should ask more of our field.

We have also emphasized the importance of a number of issues that arise in psychopathology research, issues that are crucial though not specific to psychophysiological measurement. For example, thorough and reliable diagnostic screening is essential for clear characterization of subject samples. Consideration of the rates of diagnostic comorbidity – as well as delineation and evaluation of relevant subtypes – is also necessary.

Current theories of psychopathology do not provide a justification for examining only one measurement domain (e.g., physiology) or, within a domain, only one variable (e.g., regional cerebral blood flow). Lang's three-systems approach to anxiety and Bernstein's studies of orienting in depression are examples of contexts in which multiple-system assessment is essential to understanding the phenomenon. Such multidomain and multivariable approaches have long been recommended in both psychophysiological and nonpsychophysiological literatures (Campbell & Fiske 1959; Lang 1968). However, we have noted that even psychophysiological research is often parochial in typically confining its measurement of emotion, for example, to autonomic measures. The issue is not that having more data is better, since in most cases there is no agreed-upon standard for an observable manifestation of some theoretical construct. Multiple measures of the construct are needed in order to improve the construct validity of the research.

Psychophysiological research on psychopathology tends to rely on a traditional subset of measures to examine a given type of psychopathology. Yet when research on a specific psychological disorder is limited to a narrow subset of measures, crucial information about response patterns may be overlooked. Indeed, this bias limits direct comparison of findings across psychological disorders and thus may reify a categorical approach to psychological disorder when a dimensional approach might well be more fruitful. Future investigators should consider a broader range of measures as potentially informative about the constructs of interest.

In particular, they can explore measures traditionally used to study one psychological disorder to study other types. For example, startle paradigms have contributed significantly to the schizophrenia and anxiety literature, although few studies have systematically assessed startle in depression. Those studies that have looked at startle reflex in depression using affective stimuli have found inconsistent results (see Cook 1999). Prominent psychological models of depression suggest that depressed individuals respond differently to positive and negative information (Beck 1976; Bower 1981). Prominent physiological models of the startle reflex (e.g. Braff & Geyer 1990; Davis 1986; Davis et al. 1995) could be integrated with models of depression, especially given the growing literature on startle modulation by emotional valence (Lang 1995; Lang et al. 1990; Simons & Zelson 1985). Another example is the literature on regional brain activity in emotion, which has predominantly been used in the study of anxiety and depression (Heller & Nitschke 1998). In schizophrenia research, regional brain activity is usually examined in relation to cognitive processing differences. Given the growing interest in the role of emotional processing in schizophrenia, research that examines how emotion may be reflected in brain activity could be valuable for clarifying patterns of regional activity in schizophrenia and also for evaluating whether and how they are distinct from those in depression.

A research agenda that encompasses multiple measures across multiple domains is ambitious. For the most part, it is probably not feasible to conduct experiments that can individually account for a reasonable set of measures across multiple domains. Instead, most research is necessarily incremental, each step testing a subset of the variables of interest. The expectation is that further research will extend the relevant findings and contribute to the process of developing a representative picture of the phenomena of interest. In order to accomplish this, it is necessary to develop systematic research on the basis of phenomena that can be consistently and operationally defined and thus are testable under a variety of conditions.

Knight and Silverstein (1998) outlined such an approach for the study of schizophrenia, and it applies as well to other forms of psychopathology. Rather than relying on broad constructs such as "working memory," the goal is to identify more specific processes believed to produce the behaviors of interest. These relevant processes can be assessed using a full range of measures from the verbal, physiological, and behavioral domains. For example, amplitude reductions in P300 have consistently been observed in schizophrenia. Long after this was established, however, it was still not clear what processes contribute to the P300 reduction. It was comparatively recently that Ford et al. (1994b) finally determined the reduction to be the result of a multitude of factors (fewer P300s on a single-trial basis, smaller P300s when they do occur, etc.). Other robust findings should similarly be decomposed in order to understand their nature and particularly their relationship to clinical manifestations of psychopathology.

ADVANCING PSYCHOPHYSIOLOGICAL RESEARCH ON PSYCHOPATHOLOGY

Psychophysiological research on psychopathology can address a wide range of questions. Here are a few we deem particularly worthy of attention in future research.

What are the psychological and physiological causes of the psychophysiological difference? More useful than knowing that there is a difference in psychopathological groups is to understand the basis of the psychophysiological difference. Theories about what the mind is doing must be compatible with measures of what the brain is doing. To illustrate, there are many potential physiological bases for P300 reduction in psychopathology: less tissue in or near the hippocampus or left temporal lobe, different orientation of the neurons that generate P300, fewer neurons firing, fewer neurons synchronized, and so on. Further, there are numerous psychological explanations for P300 reduction: poor working memory, dearth of resources, attentional deficits, lack of motivation, and so on. A major goal of psychophysiological research in psychopathology should be to develop and test theories that integrate the psychological and physiological domains of explanation.

At what stage in processing do individuals with psychopathology begin to diverge from controls? We need not assume that individuals with psychopathology engage in entirely unique strategies to process information. Instead, such individuals may share processing strategies with nonpsychiatric controls, especially in early stages of processing. As processing continues, individuals with psychopathology diverge from controls in how they handle incoming or retrieved information. It is not clear, however, when this divergence occurs or on what it depends. Alternative to an information processing structure that assumes discrete steps, both functions and dysfunctions may be modeled in terms of reciprocal circuits (Robertson &

Powers 1990). Either way, similarities as well as differences in information processing – and strengths as well as deficits – warrant study. This type of analysis can also reveal whether the locus of a difference changes with the progression and remission of the disorder, which will be a central issue in sophisticated psychopathology research.

Under what conditions are individuals with psychopathology able to mimic controls in their performance of mental operations? In some cases, individuals with psychopathology may perform as well as controls in a specific domain but perform differently in another domain. Understanding the disparities in these domains may highlight the dysfunctional processes. For example, Hertel and Hardin (1990) found that depressed individuals performed as well as controls on a memory retrieval task when given an explicit strategy but exhibited significant memory deficits in unstructured recall conditions. This finding suggests that depressed people are capable of adequate information recall but that the conditions in which they will do so are limited. Similar approaches for examining other psychopathological deficits not only highlight which dysfunctional processes are the most crucial but also suggest strategies for treatment. This issue has received relatively little attention in psychophysiological studies.

Do the processing differences reflect a deficit or a compensatory tactic? It is often unclear whether anomalous processing is due to a deficit to be avoided or treated (the usual assumption) or, instead, reflective of an effort at compensation or another form of protective factor that perhaps should be encouraged or taught to others with the disorder (or at risk for it). This issue is largely uncharted territory for biologically oriented approaches to psychopathology, although it is well established in the psychology literature. Psychophysiology may make a substantial contribution.

Psychophysiology as an innovative tradition and as a powerful set of tools can provide valuable information in understanding psychopathology. A number of important considerations have been outlined that influence the significance and utility of psychophysiological research on psychopathology. Research in this area will be most beneficial when strong theories of the fundamental psychological disturbance are integrated with solid theories of related physiological processes.

NOTE

The writing of this chapter was supported by NIMH grant MH39628 to Gregory A. Miller and by the University of Illinois Departments of Psychology and Psychiatry and Beckman Institute. Jennifer Keller was supported by NIMH Institutional National Research Service Award MH19554 and Individual Research Service Award MH11758. We gratefully acknowledge the comments of Rebecca Compton, Wendy Heller, Brandy Isaacks, Jack Nitschke, Patrick Palmieri, and Keolani Taitano on an earlier draft.

REFERENCES

Abraham, P., & McCallum, W. C. (1977). A permanent change in the EEG (CNV) of schizophrenics. *Electroencephalography and Clinical Neurophysiology, 43*, 533.

Adams, J., Faux, S. F., Nestor, P. G., Shenton, M., Marcy, B., Smith, S., & McCarley, R. W. (1993). ERP abnormalities during semantic processing in schizophrenia. *Schizophrenia Research, 10*, 247–57.

Adler, L. E., Gerhardt, G. A., Franks, R., Baker, N., Nagamoto, H., Drebing, C., & Freedman, R. (1990). Sensory physiology and catecholamines in schizophrenia and mania. *Psychiatry Research, 31*, 297–309.

Adler, L. E., Pachtman, E., Franks, R. D., Pecevich, M., Waldo, M. C., & Freedman, R. (1982). Neurophysiological evidence for a defect in neuronal mechanisms involved in sensory gating in schizophrenia. *Biological Psychiatry, 17*, 639–54.

Alexander, A. A. (1972). Psychophysiological concepts of psychopathology. In N. S. Greenfield & R. A. Sternbach (Eds.), *Handbook of Psychophysiology*, pp. 925–66. New York: Holt, Rinehart & Winston.

APA [American Psychiatric Association] (1994). *Diagnostic and Statistical Manual of Mental Disorders*, 4th ed. Washington, DC: American Psychiatric Association.

Anderson, J. R. (1983). A spreading activation theory of memory. *Journal of Verbal Behavior, 22*, 261–95.

Andreasen, N. C. (1979). Thought, language, and communication disorders. I. Clinical assessment, definition of terms, and evaluation of their reliability. *Archives of General Psychiatry, 36*, 1315–21.

Andrews, S., Shelley, A., Ward, P. B., Fox, A., Catts, S. V., & McConaghy, N. (1993). Event-related potential indices of semantic processing in schizophrenia. *Biological Psychiatry, 34*, 443–58.

Anthony, B. J. (1985). In the blink of an eye: Implications of reflex modification for information processing. In P. K. Ackles, J. R. Jennings, & M. G. H. Coles (Eds.), *Advances in Psychophysiology*, vol. 1, pp. 167–218. Greenwich, CT: JAI.

Ashton, H., Golding, J. F., Marsh, V. R., Thompson, J. W., Hassanyeh, F., & Tyrer, S. P. (1988). Cortical evoked potentials and clinical rating scales as measures of depressive illness. *Psychological Medicine, 18*, 305–17.

Atkinson, R. F., & Shiffrin, R. M. (1968). Human memory: A proposed system and its control processes. In K. W. Spence & J. T. Spence (Eds.), *The Psychology of Learning and Motivation: Advances in Research and Theory*, vol. 2, pp. 89–195. New York: Academic Press.

Ax, A. F. (1962). Psychophysiological methodology for the study of schizophrenia. In R. Roessler & N. S. Greenfield (Eds.), *Physiological Correlates of Psychological Disorder*. Madison: University of Wisconsin Press.

Bachneff, S. A., & Engelsmann, F. (1980). Contingent negative variation, postimperative negative variation, and psychopathology. *Biological Psychiatry, 15*, 323–8.

Barch, D. M., & Berenbaum, H. (1996). Language production and thought disorder in schizophrenia. *Journal of Abnormal Psychology, 105*, 81–8.

Barch, D. M., Cohen, J. D., Servan-Schreiber, D., Steingard, S., Steinhauer, S. S., & van Kammen, D. P. (1996). Semantic priming in schizophrenia: An examination of spreading acti-

vation using word pronunciation and multiple SOAs. *Journal of Abnormal Psychology, 105*, 592–601.

Barlow, D. H. (1988). *Anxiety and Its Disorders: The Nature and Treatments of Anxiety and Panic*. New York: Guilford.

Barlow, D. H. (1991). Disorders of emotion. *Psychological Inquiry, 2*, 58–71.

Barta, P. E., Pearlson, G. D., Powers, R. E., Richards, S. S., & Tune, L. E. (1990). Auditory hallucinations and smaller superior temporal gyral volume in schizophrenia. *American Journal of Psychiatry, 147*, 1457–62.

Baxter, L. R., Phelps, M. E., Mazziotta, J. C., Guze, B. H., Schwartz, J. M., & Selin, C. E. (1987). Local cerebral glucose metabolic rates in obsessive-compulsive disorder. *Archives of General Psychiatry, 44*, 211–18.

Baxter, L. R., Phelps, M. E., Mazziotta, J. C., Schwartz, J. M., Berner, R. H., Selin, C. E., & Sumida, R. M. (1985). Cerebral metabolic rates for glucose in mood disorders: Studies with positron emission tomography and fluorodeoxyglucose F 18. *Archives of General Psychiatry, 42*, 441–7.

Beck, A. T. (1976). *Cognitive Therapy and the Emotional Disorders*. New York: International University Press.

Bench, C. J., Friston, K. J., Brown, R. G., Frackowiak, R. S. J., & Dolan, R. J. (1993). Regional cerebral blood flow in depression measured by positron emission tomography: The relationship with clinical dimensions. *Psychological Medicine, 23*, 579–90.

Benjamin, L. S. (1967). Facts and artifacts in using analysis of covariance to "undo" the law of initial values. *Psychophysiology, 4*, 187–206.

Berenbaum, H., & Oltmanns, T. F. (1992). Emotional experience and expression in schizophrenia and depression. *Journal of Abnormal Psychology, 101*, 37–44.

Berman, K. F., Ostrem, J. L., Van Horn, J. D., Mattay, V. S., Esposito, G., & Weinberger, D. R. (1993). A comparison between normal monozygotic and dizygotic twins studied during cognition with positron emission tomography abstract. *Society for Neuroscience Abstracts, 19*, 792.

Bernstein, A. S., Frith, C. D., Gruzelier, J. H., Patterson, T., Straube, E. R., Venables, P. H., & Zahn, T. P. (1982). An analysis of the skin conductance orienting response in samples of American, British, and German schizophrenics. *Biological Psychology, 14*, 155–211.

Bernstein, A. S., Riedel, J. A., Graae, F., Seidman, D., Steele, H., Connolly, J., & Lubowsky, J. (1988). Schizophrenia is associated with altered orienting activity: Depression with electrodermal (cholinergic?) deficit and normal orienting response. *Journal of Abnormal Psychology, 97*, 3–12.

Blackwood, D. H., Sharp, C. W., Walker, M. T., Doody, G. A., Glabus, M. F., & Muir, W. J. (1996). Implications of comorbidity for genetic studies of bipolar disorder: P300 and eye tracking as biological markers for illness. *British Journal of Psychiatry, 30*, 85–92.

Blanchard, E. B. (1990). Elevated basal levels of cardiovascular responses in Vietnam veterans with PTSD: A health problem in the making? *Journal of Anxiety Disorders, 4*, 233–7.

Blanchard, E. B., Kickling, E. J., Bucklye, T. C., Taylor, A. E., Vollmer, A., & Loos, W. R. (1996). Psychophysiology of posttraumatic stress disorder related to motor vehicle accidents: Replication and extension. *Journal of Consulting and Clinical Psychology, 64*, 742–51.

Blanchard, J. J., & Neale, J. M. (1992). Medication effects: Conceptual and methodological issues in schizophrenia research. *Clinical Psychology Review, 12,* 345–61.

Boucsein, W. (1992). *Electrodermal Activity.* New York: Plenum.

Boutros, N. N., Overall, J., & Zouridakis, G. (1991). Test–retest reliability of the P50 mid-latency auditory evoked response. *Psychiatry Research, 39,* 181–92.

Boutros, N., Zouridakis, G., Rustin, T., Peabody, C., & Warder, D. (1993). The P50 component of the auditory evoked potential and subtypes of schizophrenia. *Psychiatry Research, 47,* 243–54.

Bower, G. H. (1981). Mood and memory. *American Psychologist, 36,* 129–48.

Braff, D. L. (1993). Information processing and attention dysfunctions in schizophrenia. *Schizophrenia Bulletin, 19,* 233–59.

Braff, D. L. (in press). Psychophysiological and information processing approaches to schizophrenia. In D. S. Charney, E. Nestler, & B. S. Bunney (Eds.), *Neurobiological Foundations of Mental Illness.* New York: Oxford University Press.

Braff, D. L., & Geyer, M. A. (1990). Sensorimotor gating and schizophrenia: Human and animal model studies. *Archives of General Psychiatry, 47,* 181–8.

Braff, D. L., Grillon, C., & Geyer, M. A. (1992). Gating and habituation of the startle reflex in schizophrenia. *Archives of General Psychiatry, 49,* 206–15.

Braff, D. L., Stone, C., Callaway, E., Geyer, M., Glick, I., & Bali, L. (1978). Pre-stimulus effects on human startle reflex in normals and schizophrenics. *Psychophysiology, 14,* 339–43.

Bremner, J. D., Randall, P., Scott, T. M., Bronen, R. A., Seibyl, J. P., Southwick, S. M., Delaney, R. C., McCarthy, G., Charney, D. S., & Innis, R. B. (1995). MRI-based measurement of hippocampal volume in patients with combat-related posttraumatic stress disorder. *American Journal of Psychiatry, 152,* 973–81.

Brewin, C. R., Dalgleish, T., & Joseph, S. (1996). A dual representation theory of posttraumatic stress disorder. *Psychological Review, 103,* 670–86.

Broadbent, D. E. (1982). Task combination and selective intake of information. *Acta Psychologica, 50,* 253–90.

Bruder, G. E. (1995). Cerebral laterality and psychopathology: Perceptual and event-related potential asymmetries in affective and schizophrenic disorders. In K. W. Spence & J. T. Spence (Eds.), *Brain Asymmetry,* pp. 661–91. Cambridge, MA: MIT Press.

Bruder, G. E., Stewart, J. W., Towey, J. P., Friedman, D., Tenke, C. E., Voglmaier, M. M., Leite, P., Cohen, P., & Quitkin, F. M. (1992). Abnormal cerebral laterality in bipolar depression: Convergence of behavioral and brain event-related potential findings. *Biological Psychiatry, 32,* 33–47.

Bruder, G. E., Tenke, C. E., Stewart, J. W., Towey, J. P., Leite, P., Voglmaier, M. M., & Quitkin, F. M. (1995). Brain event-related potentials to complex tones in depressed patients: Relation to perceptual asymmetry and clinical features. *Psychophysiology, 32,* 373–81.

Buchsbaum, M. S., DeLisi, L., Holcomb, H. H., Hazlett, E., & Kessler, R. (1985). In T. Greitz, D. H. Ingvar, & L. Widen (Eds.), *The Metabolism of the Human Brain Studied with Positron Emission Tomography,* pp. 471–84. New York: Raven.

Buchsbaum, M. S., Lee, S., Haier, R., Wu, J. C., Green, M., & Tang, S. W. (1988). Effects of Amoxapine and Imipramine on

evoked potentials in the continuous performance test in patients with affective disorder. *Neuropsychobiology, 20,* 15–22.

Buchsbaum, M. S., Wu, J., Haier, R., Hazlett, E., Ball, R., Katz, M., Sokolski, K., Lagunas-Solar, M., & Langer, D. (1987). Positron emission tomography assessment of effects of benzodiazepines on regional glucose metabolic rate in patients with anxiety disorder. *Life Science, 20,* 2392–2400.

Buck, C. W., Carscallen, H. B., & Hobbs, G. E. (1950). Temperature regulation in schizophrenia: I. Comparison of schizophrenic and normal subjects. II. Analysis of duration of psychosis. *Archives of Neurology and Psychiatry, 64,* 828–42.

Buck, C. W., Carscallen, H. B., & Hobbs, G. E. (1951). Effect of prefrontal lobotomy on temperature regulation in schizophrenic patients. *Archives of Neurology and Psychiatry, 65,* 197–205.

Butler, R. W., Braff, D. L., Rausch, J. L., Jenkins, M. A., Sprock, J., & Geyer, M. A. (1990). Physiological evidence of exaggerated startle response in a subgroup of Vietnam veterans with combat related PTSD. *American Journal of Psychiatry, 147,* 1308–12.

Cacioppo, J. T., & Berntson, G. G. (1992). Social psychological contributions to the Decade of the Brain: Doctrine of multilevel analysis. *American Psychologist, 47,* 1019–28.

Cadenhead, K. S., Geyer, M. A., & Braff, D. L. (1993). Impaired startle prepulse inhibition and habituation in patients with schizotypal personality disorder. *American Journal of Psychiatry, 150,* 1862–7.

Cadenhead, K. S., Kumar, C., & Braff, D. L. (1996). Clinical and experimental characteristics of "hypothetically psychosis prone" college students. *Journal of Psychiatric Research, 30,* 331–40.

Campbell, D. T., & Fiske, D. W. (1959). Convergent and discriminant validation by the multirating-multimethod matrix. *Psychological Bulletin, 56,* 81–105.

Carpenter, W. T., Bartko, J. J., Strauss, J. S., & Hawk, A. B. (1978). Signs and symptoms as predictors of outcome: A report from the International Pilot Study of Schizophrenia. *American Journal of Psychiatry, 135,* 940–5.

Carter, W. R., Johnson, M. C., & Borkovec, T. D. (1986). Worry: An electrocortical analysis. *Advances in Behavioral Research and Therapy, 8,* 193–204.

Catts, S. V., Shelley, A. M., Ward, P. B., Liebert, B., McConaghy, N., Andrews, S., & Michie, P. T. (1995). Brain potential evidence for an auditory sensory memory deficit in schizophrenia. *American Journal of Psychiatry, 152,* 213–19.

Chapman, L. J., & Chapman, J. P. (1973). Problems in the measurement of cognitive deficit. *Psychological Bulletin, 79,* 380–5.

Chapman, L. J., & Chapman, J. P. (1989). Strategies for resolving the heterogeneity of schizophrenics and their relatives using cognitive measures. *Journal of Abnormal Psychology, 98,* 357–66.

Chapman, L. J., Chapman, J. P., & Raulin, M. L. (1976). Scales for physical and social anhedonia. *Journal of Abnormal Psychology, 85,* 374–82.

Charles, G., Hansenne, M., Anssea, M., Pitchot, W., Machowski, R., Schittecatte, M., & Wilmotte, J. (1995). P300 in posttraumatic stress disorder. *Neuropsychobiology, 32,* 72–4.

Chung, G., Tucker, D. M., West, P., Potts, G. F., Liotti, M., Luu, P., & Hartry, A. L. (1996). Emotional expectancy: Brain electrical activity associated with an emotional bias in interpreting life events. *Psychophysiology, 33,* 218–33.

Clark, L. A., Watson, D., & Reynolds, S. (1995). Diagnosis and classification of psychopathology: Challenges to the current system and future directions. *Annual Review of Psychology, 46,* 121–53.

Clementz, B. A., Blumenfeld, L. D., & Cobb, S. (1997a). The gamma band response may account for poor P50 suppression in schizophrenia. *Neuroreport, 8,* 3889–93.

Clementz, B. A., Geyer, M. A., & Braff, D. L. (1997b). P50 suppression among schizophrenia and normal comparison subjects: A methodological analysis. *Biological Psychiatry, 41,* 1035–44.

Clementz, B. A., Geyer, M. A., & Braff, D. L. (1998). Poor P50 suppression among schizophrenia patients and their first-degree biological relatives. *American Journal of Psychiatry, 155,* 1691–4.

Cohen, J. D., Forman, S. D., Braver, T. S., Casey, B. J., Servan-Schreiber, D., & Noll, D. C. (1994). Activation of prefrontal cortex in a nonspatial working memory task with functional MRI. *Human Brain Mapping, 1,* 293–304.

Cohen, L. H., & Patterson, M. (1937). Effect of pain on the heart rate of normal and schizophrenic individuals. *Journal of General Psychology, 17,* 273–89.

Coles, M. G. H. (1989). Modern mind–brain reading: Psychophysiology, physiology, and cognition. *Psychophysiology, 26,* 251–69.

Conway, M., & Giannopoulos, C. (1993). Dysphoria and decision making: Limited information use in the evaluation of multiattribute targets. *Journal of Personality and Social Psychology, 64,* 613–23.

Cook, E. W. (1999). Affective individual differences, psychopathology, and startle reflex modification. In M. E. Dawson, A. M. Schell, & A. H. Böhmelt (Eds.), *Startle Modification: Implications for Neuroscience, Cognitive Science, and Clinical Sciences,* pp. 187–208. Cambridge University Press.

Crow, T. J. (1990). Temporal lobe asymmetries as the key to the etiology of schizophrenia. *Schizophrenia Bulletin, 16,* 433–43.

Cullum, C. M., Harris, J. G., Waldo, M. C., Smernoff, E., Madison, A., Nagamoto, H. T., Griffith, J., Adler, L. E., & Freedman, R. (1993). Neurophysiological and neuropsychological evidence for attentional dysfunction in schizophrenia. *Schizophrenia Research, 10,* 131–41.

Cuthbert, B. N., & Lang, P. J. (1989). Imagery, memory and emotion: A psychophysiological analysis of clinical anxiety. In G. Turpin (Ed.), *Handbook of Clinical Psychophysiology,* pp. 105–34. New York: Wiley.

Davidson, R. J. (1984). Affect, cognition and hemispheric specialization. In C. E. Izard, J. Kagan, & R. Zajonc (Eds.), *Emotion, Cognition and Behavior,* pp. 320–65. Cambridge University Press.

Davidson, R. J. (1992). Anterior cerebral asymmetry and the nature of emotion. *Brain and Cognition, 20,* 125–51.

Davidson, R. J., Chapman, J. P., Chapman, L. J., & Henriques, J. B. (1990). Asymmetrical brain electrical activity discriminates between psychometrically matched verbal and spatial cognitive tasks. *Psychophysiology, 27,* 528–43.

Davidson, R. J., Marshall, J. R., Tomarken, A. J., & Henriques, J. B. (1997). While a phobic waits: Regional brain electrical and autonomic activity predict anxiety in social phobics during anticipation of public speaking. Manuscript submitted for publication.

Davidson, R. J., & Tomarken, A. J. (1989). Laterality and emotion: An electrophysiological approach. In F. Boller & J. Grafman (Eds.), *Handbook of Neuropsychology,* pp. 419–41. Amsterdam: Elsevier.

Davis, M. (1986). Pharmacological and anatomical analysis of fear conditioning using the fear-potentiated startle paradigm. *Behavioral Neuroscience, 100,* 814–24.

Davis, M., Campeau, S., Kim, M., & Falls, W. A. (1995). Neural systems of emotion: The amygdala's role in fear and anxiety. In J. L. McGaugh, N. M. Weinberger, & G. Lynch (Eds.), *Brain and Memory: Modulation and Mediation of Neuroplasticity,* pp. 3–40. New York: Oxford University Press.

Davis, P. A., & Davis, H. (1939). The electroencephalograms of psychotic patients. *American Journal of Psychiatry, 95,* 1007–25.

Dawson, M. E., Filion, D. L., & Schell, A. M. (1989). Is elicitation of the autonomic orienting response associated with allocation of processing resources? *Psychophysiology, 26,* 560–72.

Dawson, M. E., Hazlett, E. A., Filion, D. L., Nuechterlein, K. H., & Schell, A. M. (1993). Attention and schizophrenia: Impaired modification of the startle reflex. *Journal of Abnormal Psychology, 102,* 633–41.

Dawson, M. E., & Nuechterlein, K. H. (1984). Psychophysiological dysfunctions in the developmental course of schizophrenic disorders. *Schizophrenia Bulletin, 10,* 204–32.

Dawson, M. E., Schell, A. M., & Böhmelt, A. H. (Eds.) (1999). *Startle Modification: Implications for Neuroscience, Cognitive Science, and Clinical Science.* Cambridge University Press.

Dawson, M. E., Schell, A. M., Braaten, J. R., & Catania, J. J. (1985). Diagnostic utility of autonomic measures for major depressive disorders. *Psychiatry Research, 15,* 261–70.

Dawson, M. E., Schell, A. M., & Filion, D. L. (1990). The electrodermal system. In J. T. Cacioppo & L. G. Tassinary (Eds.), *Principles of Psychophysiology: Physical, Social, and Inferential Elements,* pp. 295–324. Cambridge University Press.

Dawson, M. E., Schell, A. M., Hazlett, E. A., Filion, D. L., & Nuechterlein, K. H. (1995). Attention, startle eye-blink modification, and psychosis proneness. In A. Raine, T. Lencz, & S. A. Mednick (Eds.), *Schizotypal Personality,* pp. 250–71. Cambridge University Press.

Deldin, P. J., Casas, B., & Best, J. (1998). Semantic and emotional expectancy in major depression and dysthymia. Paper presented at the annual meeting of the Society for Psychophysiological Research (Denver).

Deldin, P. J., Keller, J., Gergen, J. A., & Miller, G. A. (in press). N200 right parieto-temporal reductions in major depression. *Journal of Abnormal Psychology.*

Depue, R. A., & Iacono, W. G. (1989). Neurobehavioral aspects of affective disorders. *Annual Review of Psychology, 40,* 457–92.

Docherty, N. M., Hawkins, K. A., Hoffman, R. E., Quinlan, D. M., Rakfeldt, J., & Sledge, W. H. (1996). Working memory, attention, and communication disturbances in schizophrenia. *Journal of Abnormal Psychology, 105,* 212–19.

Drevets, W. C., Videen, T. O., Preskorn, S. H., Price, J. L., Carmichael, S. T., & Raichle, M. E. (1992). A functional anatomical study of unipolar depression. *Journal of Neuroscience, 12,* 3628–41.

Duffy, E. (1962). *Activation and Behavior.* New York: Wiley.

Dworkin, R. H., Cornblatt, B. A., Friedmann, R., Kaplansky, L. M., Lewis, J. A., Rinaldi, A., Shilliday, C., & Erlenmeyer-Kimling, L. (1993). Childhood precursors of affective vs. social deficits in adolescents at risk for schizophrenia. *Schizophrenia Bulletin, 19,* 563–77.

Ebert, L. (1987). Orienting and habituation in anhedonic and dysthymic college students. Master's thesis, University of Illinois, Urbana.

Edell, W. S. (1995). The psychometric measurement of schizotypy using the Wisconsin scales of psychosis proneness. In G. A. Miller (Ed.), *The Behavioral High-Risk Paradigm in Psychopathology,* pp. 3–46. New York: Springer-Verlag.

Egan, M. F., Duncan, C. C., Suddath, R. L., Kirch, D. G., Mirsky, A. F., & Wyatt, R. J. (1994). Event-related potential abnormalities correlate with structural brain alterations and clinical features in patients with chronic schizophrenia. *Schizophrenia Research, 11,* 259–71.

Ellenbroek, B. A., Budde, S., & Cools, A. R. (1996). Prepulse inhibition and latent inhibition: The role of dopamine in the medial prefrontal cortex. *Neuroscience, 75,* 535–42.

Ellis, H. C., & Ashbrook, P. A. (1988). Resource allocation model of the effects of depressed mood states on memory. In K. Fiedler & J. Forgas (Eds.), *Affect, Cognition, and Social Behavior,* pp. 25–43. Toronto: Hogreff.

El Massioui, F., & Lesèvre, N. (1988). Attention impairment and psychomotor retardation in depressed patients: An event-related potential study. *Electroencephalography and Clinical Neurophysiology, 70,* 46–55.

Erlenmeyer-Kimling, L., Cornblatt, B. A., Rock, D., Roberts, S., Bell, M., & West, A. (1993). The New York High-Risk Project: Anhedonia, attentional deviance, and psychopathology. *Schizophrenia Bulletin, 19,* 141–53.

Fenton, W. S., & McGlashan, T. H. (1991). Natural history of schizophrenia subtypes: II. Positive and negative symptoms and long-term course. *Archives of General Psychiatry, 48,* 978–86.

Fernandes, L. O. F., Hicks, B. D., & Miller, G. A. (1995). Psychophysiology of schizotypic features: Cognitive and emotional anomalies associated with the Chapman Scales. Paper presented at the annual meeting of the Society for Psychophysiological Research (October, Toronto).

Fernandes, L. O. F., Keller, J., Giese-Davis, J. E., Hicks, B. D., Klein, D. N., & Miller, G. A. (1999). Converging evidence for a cognitive anomaly in early psychopathology. *Psychophysiology, 36,* 511–21.

Fernandes, L. O. L., & Miller, G. A. (1995). Compromised performance and abnormal psychophysiology associated with the Wisconsin Psychosis-Proneness Scales. In G. A. Miller (Ed.), *The Behavioral High-Risk Paradigm in Psychopathology,* pp. 47–87. New York: Springer-Verlag.

Filion, D. L., Dawson, M. E., & Schell, A. M. (1993). Modification of the acoustic startle-reflex eyeblink: A tool for investigating early and late attentional processes. *Biological Psychology, 35,* 185–200.

Fischler, I., & Raney, G. E. (1989). Language by eye: Behavioral, autonomic and cortical approaches to reading. In J. R. Jennings & M. G. H. Coles (Eds.), *Handbook of Cognitive Psychology: Central and Autonomic Nervous System,* pp. 511–77. New York: Wiley.

Fleiss, J. L., & Tanur, J. M. (1973). The analysis of covariance in psychopathology. In M. Hammer, K. Salzinger, & S. Sutton (Eds.), *Psychopathology: Contributions from the Social, Behavioral, and Biological Sciences,* pp. 509–27. New York: Wiley.

Flor-Henry, P. (1979). On certain aspects of the localization of the cerebral systems regulating and determining emotion. *Biological Psychiatry, 14,* 677–98.

Foa, E. B., & Kozak, M. J. (1986). Emotional processing of fear: Exposure to corrective information. *Psychological Bulletin, 99,* 20–35.

Foa, E. B., & Riggs, D. S. (1993). Posttraumatic stress disorder and rape. In R. Pynoos (Ed.), *Posttraumatic Stress Disorder: A Clinical Review,* pp. 133–63. Lutherville, MD: Sidron.

Ford, J. M., Pfefferbaum, A., & Roth, W. (1992). P3 and schizophrenia. In D. Friedman & G. E. Bruder (Eds.), *Psychophysiology and Experimental Psychopathology: A Tribute to Samuel Sutton* (Annals of the New York Academy of Sciences, vol. 658), pp. 146–62. New York Academy of Sciences.

Ford, J. M., White, P. M., Csernansky, J. G., Faustman, W. O., Roth, W. T., & Pfefferbaum, A. (1994a). ERPs in schizophrenia: Effects of antipsychotic medication. *Biological Psychiatry, 36,* 153–70.

Ford, J. M., White, P., Lim, K. O., & Pfefferbaum, A. (1994b). Schizophrenics have fewer and smaller P300s: A single-trial analysis. *Biological Psychiatry, 35,* 96–103.

Franks, R. D., Adler, L. E., Waldo, M. C., Alpert, J., & Freedman, R. (1983). Neurophysiological studies of sensory gating in mania: Comparison with schizophrenia. *Biological Psychiatry, 18,* 989–1005.

Fredrikson, M., Gustav, W., Greitz, T., Eriksson, L., Stonee-Elander, S., Ericson, K., & Sedvall, G. (1993). Regional cerebral blood flow during experimental phobic fear. *Psychophysiology, 30,* 126–30.

Freedman, L. R., Rock, D., Roberts, S. A., Cornblatt, B. A., & Erlenmeyer-Kimling, L. (1998). The New York High-Risk project: Attention, anhedonia and social outcome. *Schizophrenia Research, 30,* 1–9.

Freedman, R., Adler, L. E., Waldo, M. D., Pachtman, E., & Franks, R. D. (1983). Neurophysiological evidence for a defect in inhibitory pathways in schizophrenia: Comparison of medicated and drug-free patients. *Biological Psychiatry, 18,* 537–52.

Friedman, D., & Squires-Wheeler, E. (1994). Event-related potentials (ERPs) as indicators of risk for schizophrenia. *Schizophrenia Bulletin, 20,* 63–74.

Friedman, H. R., Janas, J. D., & Goldman-Rakic, P. S. (1990). Enhancement of metabolic activity in the diencephalon of monkeys performing working memory tasks: A 2-deoxyglucose study in behaving rhesus monkeys. *Journal of Cognitive Neuroscience, 2,* 18–31.

Friedman, M. J., Charney, D. S., & Deutch, A. Y. (Eds.) (1995). *Neurobiological and Clinical Consequences of Stress: From Normal Adaption of PTSD.* New York: Raven.

Frith, C. D. (1992). *The Cognitive Neuropsychology of Schizophrenia.* Hove, U.K.: Erlbaum.

Fukushima, J., Fukushima, K., Morita, N., & Yamashita, I. (1990). Further analysis of the control of voluntary saccadic eye movements in schizophrenic patients. *Biological Psychiatry, 28,* 943–58.

Gainotti, G. (1972). Emotional behavior and hemisphere side of lesion. *Cortex, 8,* 41–55.

Gainotti, G., Caltagirone, C., & Zoccolotti, P. (1993). Left/right and cortical/subcortical dichotomies in the neuropsychology of emotion. *Cognition and Emotion, 7,* 71–93.

Gerardi, R. J., Blanchard, E. B., & Kolb, L. C. (1989). Ability of Vietnam veterans to dissimulate a psychophysiological assessment for post-traumatic stress disorder. *Behavior Therapy, 20,* 229–43.

Giese-Davis, J. E., Miller, G. A., & Knight, R. A. (1993). Memory template comparison processes in anhedonia and dysthymia. *Psychophysiology, 30,* 646–56.

Giordani, B., Boibin, M. J., Berent, S., Betley, A. T., Kieppe, R. A., Rothley, J. M., Modell, J. G., Hichwa, R. D., & Kuhl, D. E. (1990). Anxiety and cerebral cortical metabolism in normal persons. *Psychiatry Research: Neuroimaging, 35,* 49–60.

Gold, J. M., & Harvey, P. D. (1993). Cognitive deficits in schizophrenia. *Schizophrenia, 162,* 295–312.

Goldberg, T. E., Greenberg, R. D., Griffin, S. J., Gold, J. M., Kleinman, J. E., Pickar, D., Schulz, S. C., & Weinberger, D. R. (1993). Impact of clozapine on cognitive impairment and clinical symptoms in patients with schizophrenia. *British Journal of Psychiatry, 162,* 43–8.

Goldman-Rakic, P. S. (1991). Prefrontal cortical dysfunction in schizophrenia: The relevance of working memory. In B. Carroll (Ed.), *Psychopathology and the Brain,* pp. 1–23. New York: Raven.

Goldman-Rakic, P. S. (1994). Working memory dysfunction in schizophrenia. *The Journal of Neuropsychiatry and Clinical Neurosciences, 6,* 348–57.

Gooding, D. C., Iacono, W. G., Katsanis, J., Beiser, M., & Grove, W. M. (1993). The association between lithium carbonate and smooth pursuit eye tracking among first-episode patients with psychotic affective disorders. *Psychophysiology, 30,* 3–9.

Graham, F. K. (1975). The more or less startling effects of weak prestimuli. *Psychophysiology, 12,* 219–30.

Green, B. L., Lindy, J. D., Grace, M. C., & Glesser, G. C. (1989). Multiple diagnosis in posttraumatic stress disorder: The role of war stressors. *Journal of Nervous and Mental Disease, 177,* 329–35.

Grillon, C., Ameli, R., Charney, D. S., Kristal, J., & Braff, D. L. (1992). Startle gating deficits occur across prepulse intensities in schizophrenic patients. *Biological Psychiatry, 32,* 939–43.

Grillon, C., Ameli, R., & Glazer, W. M. (1991). N400 and semantic categorization in schizophrenia. *Biological Psychiatry, 29,* 467–80.

Gruzelier, J. H. (1989). Lateralization and central mechanisms in clinical psychophysiology. In G. Turpin (Ed.), *Handbook of Clinical Psychophysiology,* pp. 135–74. New York: Wiley.

Gurvits, T. V., Shenton, M. E., Hokama, H., & Ohta, H. (1996). Magnetic resonance imaging study of hippocampal volume in chronic, combat-related posttraumatic stress disorder. *Biological Psychiatry, 40,* 1091–9.

Guterman, Y., Josiassen, R. C., & Bashore, T. R. (1992). Attentional influence on the P50 component of the auditory event-related potential. *International Journal of Psychophysiology, 12,* 197–209.

Hansen, J., & Hillyard, S. (1980). Endogenous brain potentials associated with selective auditory attention. *Electroencephalography and Clinical Neurophysiology, 54,* 311–21.

Hasher, L., & Zacks, R. T. (1979). Automatic and effortful processes in memory. *Journal of Experimental Psychology: General, 108,* 356–88.

Hazlett, E. A., Buchsbaum, M. S., Haznedar, M. M., Singer, M. B., Germans, M. K., Schnur, D. B., Jimenez, E. A., Buchsbaum, B. R., & Troyer, B. T. (1998). Prefrontal cortex glucose metabolism and startle eyeblink modification abnormalities in unmedicated schizophrenic patients. *Psychophysiology, 35,* 186–98.

Hazlett, H., Dawson, M. E., Schell, A. M., & Nuechterlein, K. H. (1997). Electrodermal activity as a prodromal sign in schizophrenia. *Biological Psychiatry, 41,* 111–13.

Heller, W. (1990). The neuropsychology of emotion: Developmental patterns and implications for psychopathology. In N. Stein, B. L. Leventhal, & T. Trabasso (Eds.), *Psychological and Biological Approaches to Emotion,* pp. 167–211. Hillsdale, NJ: Erlbaum.

Heller, W. (1993). Neuropsychological mechanisms of individual differences in emotion, personality, and arousal. *Neuropsychology, 7,* 476–89.

Heller, W., Etienne, M. A., & Miller, G. A. (1995). Patterns of perceptual asymmetry in depression and anxiety: Implications for neuropsychological models of emotion. *Journal of Abnormal Psychology, 104,* 327–33.

Heller, W., & Nitschke, J. B. (1997). The puzzle of regional brain activity in depression and anxiety: The importance of subtypes and comorbidity. *Cognition and Emotion, 12,* 421–8.

Heller, W., & Nitschke, J. B. (1998). Regional brain activity in emotion: A framework for understanding cognition in depression. *Cognition and Emotion, 11,* 637–61.

Heller, W., Nitschke, J. B., Etienne, M. A., & Miller, G. A. (1997). Patterns of regional brain activity differentiate anxiety subtypes. *Journal of Abnormal Psychology, 106,* 375–85.

Helzer, J. E., Robins, L. N., & McEvoy, L. (1987). Post-traumatic stress disorder in the general population: Findings of the Epidemiologic Catchment Area Survey. *New England Journal of Medicine, 317,* 1630–4.

Henriques, J. B., & Davidson, R. J. (1989). Affective disorders. In G. Turpin (Ed.), *Handbook of Clinical Psychophysiology,* pp. 357–92. New York: Wiley.

Henriques, J. B., & Davidson, R. J. (1990). Regional brain electrical asymmetries discriminate between previously depressed and healthy control subjects. *Journal of Abnormal Psychology, 99,* 22–31.

Henriques, J. B., & Davidson, R. J. (1995). Event related potential asymmetries differentiate between depressed and control participants. Poster presented at the annual meeting of the Society for Psychophysiological Research (October, Toronto).

Hertel, P. T., & Hardin, T. S. (1990). Remembering with and without awareness in a depressed mood: Evidence for deficits in initiative. *Journal of Experimental Psychology: General, 119,* 45–59.

Hertel, P. T., & Rude, S. S. (1991). Depressive deficits in memory: Focusing attention improves subsequent recall. *Journal of Experimental Psychology: General, 120,* 301–9.

Hicks, B. D., Yee, C. M., Isaacks, B. G., Klein, D. N., & Miller, G. A. (1998). Problems in resource allocation, not resource availability, in schizotypy. Manuscript submitted for publication.

Holzman, P. S. (1987). Recent studies of psychophysiology in schizophrenia. *Schizophrenia Bulletin, 13,* 49–75.

Holzman, P. S., O'Brian, C., & Waternaux, C. (1991). Effects of lithium treatment on eye movements. *Biological Psychiatry, 29,* 1001–15.

Hugdahl, K. (1989). Simple phobias. In G. Turpin (Ed.), *Handbook of Clinical Psychophysiology,* pp. 283–308. New York: Wiley.

Iacono, W. G. (1998). Identifying risk for psychopathology. *Psychophysiology, 35,* 621–37.

Iacono, W. G., Ficken, J. W., & Beiser, M. (1993). Family studies of electrodermal habituation and psychopathology. In J. C. Roy, W. Boucsein, D. C. Fowles, & J. Gruzelier (Eds.), *Progress in Electrodermal Research,* pp. 239–50. New York: Plenum.

Iacono, W., Lykken, D., Peloquin, L., Lumry, A., Valentine, R., & Tuason, V. (1983). Electrodermal activity in euthymic unipolar and bipolar affective disorders. *Archives of General Psychiatry, 40,* 557–68.

Iwanami, A., Isono, H., Okajima, Y., Noda, Y., & Kamijima, K. (1998). Event-related potentials during a selective attention task with short interstimulus intervals in patients with schizophrenia. *Journal of Psychiatry and Neuroscience, 23,* 45–50.

Jaeger, J., Borod, J. C., & Peselow, E. (1987). Depressed patients have atypical hemispace biases in the perception of emotional chimeric faces. *Journal of Abnormal Psychology, 96,* 321–4.

Javitt, D. C., Doneshka, P., Grochowski, S., & Ritter, W. (1995). Impaired mismatch negativity generation reflects widespread dysfunction of working memory in schizophrenia. *Archives of General Psychiatry, 52,* 550–8.

Jerger, K., Biggins, C., & Fein, G. (1992). P50 suppression is not affected by attentional manipulations. *Biological Psychiatry, 31,* 365–77.

Jin, P. (1992). Toward a reconceptualization of the law of initial value. *Psychological Bulletin, 111,* 176–84.

Jin, Y., Bunney, W. E., Jr., Sandman, C. A., Patterson, J. V., Fleming, K., Moenter, J. R., Kalali, A. H., Hetrick, W. P., & Potkin, S. G. (1998). Is P50 suppression a measure of sensory gating in schizophrenia? *Biological Psychiatry, 43,* 873–8.

Katsanis, J., Iacono, W. G., & Beiser, M. (1996). Visual event-related potentials in first-episode psychotic patients and their relatives. *Psychophysiology, 33,* 207–17.

Keane, T. M., & Wolfe, J. (1990). Comorbidity in post-traumatic stress disorder: An analysis of community and clinical studies. *Journal of Applied Social Psychology, 20,* 1776–88.

Keane, T. M., Zimering, R. T., & Caddell, J. N. (1985). A behavioral formulation of post-traumatic stress disorder in Vietnam veterans. *The Behavior Therapist, 8,* 9–12.

Keller, J., Deldin, P. J., Gergen, J. A., & Miller, G. A. (1995). Evidence for a semantic processing deficit in depression. Paper presented at the annual meeting of the Society for Psychophysiological Research (October, Toronto).

Keller, J., Nitschke, J. B., Bhargava, T., Deldin, P. J., Heller, W., Gergen, J. A., & Miller, G. A. (in press). Neuropsychological differentiation of depression and anxiety. *Journal of Abnormal Psychology.*

Klein, D. N. (1990). Depressive personality: Reliability, validity, and relation to dysthymia. *Journal of Abnormal Psychology, 99,* 412–21.

Klein, D. N., & Anderson, R. L. (1995). The behavioral high-risk paradigm in the mood disorders. In G. A. Miller (Ed.), *The Behavioral High-Risk Paradigm in Psychopathology,* pp. 199–221. New York: Springer-Verlag.

Klein, D. N., & Miller, G. A. (1993). Depressive personality in non-clinical subjects. *American Journal of Psychiatry, 150,* 1718–24.

Klein, D. N., & Miller, G. A. (1997). Depressive personality: Relationship to dysthymia and major depression. In H. S. Akiskal & G. B. Cassano (Eds.), *Dysthymia and the Spectrum of Chronic Depressions,* pp. 85–93. New York: Guilford.

Klein, D. N., & Shih, J. H. (1998). Depressive personality: Associations with DSM-III-R mood and personality disorders and negative and positive affectivity, 30-month stability, and prediction of course of Axis I depressive disorders. *Journal of Abnormal Psychology, 107,* 319–27.

Knight, R. A. (1992). Specifying cognitive deficiencies in poor premorbid schizophrenics. In E. F. Walker, R. Dworkin, & B. Cornblatt (Eds.), *Progress in Experimental Psychology and Psychopathology Research,* vol. 15, pp. 252–89. New York: Springer.

Knight, R. A. (1993). Comparing cognitive models of schizophrenics' input dysfunction. In R. L. Cromwell & C. R. Snyder (Eds.), *Schizophrenia: Origins, Processes, Treatment and Outcome,* pp. 151–75. Oxford University Press.

Knight, R. A., Roff, J. D., Barnett, J., & Moss, J. L. (1979). Concurrent and predictive validity of thought disorder and affectivity: A 22-year follow-up of acute schizophrenics. *Journal of Abnormal Psychology, 88,* 1–12.

Knight, R. T., Scabini, D., Woods, D. L., & Clayworth, C. C. (1989). Contributions of the temporo-parietal junction to the human auditory P3. *Brain Research, 502,* 109–16.

Knight, R. A., & Silverstein, S. M. (1998). The role of cognitive psychology in guiding research on cognitive deficits in schizophrenia: A process-oriented approach. In M. F. Lenzenweger & R. H. Dworkin (Eds.), *Origins and Development of Schizophrenia: Advances in Experimental Psychopathology,* pp. 247–95. Washington, DC: American Psychological Association.

Kolb, L. C. (1984). The post-traumatic stress disorders of combat: A subgroup with conditioned emotional response. *Military Medicine, 149,* 237–43.

Krause, R., Steimer, E., Sanger, A. C., & Wagner, G. (1989). Facial expression of schizophrenic patients and their interaction partners. *Psychiatry, 52,* 1–12.

Kring, A. M., & Neale, J. M. (1996). Do schizophrenic patients show a disjunctive relationship among expressive, experiential, and psychophysiological components of emotion? *Journal of Abnormal Psychology, 105,* 249–57.

Kutas, M. (1997). Views on how the electrical activity that the brain generates reflects the functions of different language structures. *Psychophysiology, 34,* 383–98.

Kutas, M., & Hillyard, S. A. (1984). Brain potentials during reading reflect word expectancy and semantic association. *Nature, 307,* 161–3.

Kutas, M., & Hillyard, S. A. (1989). An electrophysiological probe of incidental semantic association. *Journal of Cognitive Science, 1,* 38–49.

Kutas, M., & Van Petten, C. (1994). Psycholinguistics electrified: Event-related brain potential investigations. In M. A. Gernsbacher (Ed.), *Handbook of Psycholinguistics,* pp. 83–143. New York: Academic Press.

Kwapil, T. R., Hegley, D. C., Chapman, L. J., & Chapman, J. P. (1990). Facilitation of word recognition by semantic priming in schizophrenia. *Journal of Abnormal Psychology, 99,* 215-21.

Lacey, J. I. (1956). The evaluation of autonomic responses: Toward a general solution. *Annals of the New York Academy of Sciences, 67,* 123–64.

Lacey, J. I. (1967). Somatic response patterning and stress: Some revisions of activation theory. In M. H. Appley & R. Trumbull (Eds.), *Psychological Stress: Issues in Research,* pp. 14–38. New York: Appleton-Century-Crofts.

Landis, C. (1932). Electrical phenomena of the skin. *Psychological Bulletin, 29,* 693–752.

Lang, P. J. (1968). Fear reduction and fear behavior: Problems in treating a construct. In J. M. Shlien (Ed.), *Research in Psychotherapy,* vol. 3, pp. 90–102. Washington, DC: American Psychological Association.

Lang, P. J. (1978). Anxiety: Toward a psychophysiological definition. In H. S. Akiskal & W. L. Webb (Eds.), *Psychiatric Diagnosis: Exploration of Biological Criteria,* pp. 265–389. New York: Spectrum.

Lang, P. J. (1984). Cognition in emotion: Concept and action. In C. E. Izard, J. Kagan, & R. B. Zajonc (Eds.), *Emotion, Cognition and Behavior,* pp. 192–228. Cambridge University Press.

Lang, P. J. (1995). The emotion probe: Studies of motivation and attention. *American Psychologist, 50,* 372–85.

Lang, P. J., Bradley, M. M., & Cuthbert, B. N. (1990). Emotion, attention, and the startle reflex. *Psychological Review, 97,* 377–95.

Lang, P. J., & Buss, A. H. (1968). Psychological deficit in schizophrenia: II. Interference and activation. In D. S. Holmes (Ed.), *Reviews of Research in Behavior Pathology,* pp. 400–52. New York: Wiley.

Lating, J. M., & Everly, G. S., Jr. (1995). Psychophysiological assessment of PTSD. In G. S. Everly, Jr. & J. M. Lating (Eds.), *Psychotraumatology,* pp. 129–45. New York: Plenum.

Lenhart, R. E. (1985). Lowered skin conductance in a subsyndromal high-risk depressive sample: Response amplitudes versus tonic levels. *Journal of Abnormal Psychology, 94,* 649–52.

Lenhart, R. E., & Katkin, E. S. (1986). Psychophysiological evidence for cerebral laterality effects in a high-risk sample of students with subsyndromal bipolar depressive disorder. *American Journal of Psychiatry, 143,* 602–7.

Leutner, D., & Rammsayer, T. (1995). Complex trait-treatment-interaction analysis: A powerful approach for analysing individual differences in experimental designs. *Personality and Individual Differences, 19,* 493–511.

Levy, J., Heller, W., Banich, M. T., & Burton, L. A. (1983). Asymmetry of perception in free viewing of chimeric faces. *Brain and Cognition, 2,* 404–19.

Lewine, J. D., Cañive, J. M., Orrison, W. W., Jr., Edgar, C. J., Provencal, S. L., Davis, J. T., Paulson, K., Graeber, D., Roberts, B., Escalona, P. R., & Calais, L. (1997). Electrophysiological abnormalities in PTSD. In R. Yehuda & D. McFarlane (Eds.), *Psychobiology of Post-Traumatic Stress Disorder,* pp. 508–11. New York Academy of Sciences.

Light, G. A., & Braff, D. L. (1998). The "incredible shrinking" P50 event-related potential. *Biological Psychiatry, 43,* 918–20.

Malmo, R. B., & Shagass, C. (1949). Physiological studies of reaction to stress in anxiety states and early schizophrenia. *Psychosomatic Medicine, 11,* 9–24.

Malmo, R. B., & Shagass, C. (1952). Studies of blood pressure in psychiatric patients under stress. *Psychosomatic Medicine, 14,* 82–93.

Manschreck, T. C., Maher, B. A., Milavetz, J. J., Ames, D., Weisstein, C. C., & Schneyer, M. L. (1988). Semantic priming in thought disordered schizophrenic patients. *Schizophrenia Research, 1,* 61–6.

Mathew, R. J., Wilson, W. H., & Daniel, D. G. (1985). The effect of nonsedative doses of Diazepam on regional cerebral blood flow. *Biological Psychiatry, 20,* 1109–16.

Matsuoka, H., Saito, H., Ueno, T., & Sato, M. (1996). Altered endogenous negativities of the event-related potential in remitted schizophrenia. *Electroencephalography and Clinical Neurophysiology, 100,* 18–24.

McCaffrey, R. J., Lorig, T. S., Pendrey, D. L., McCutcheon, N. B., & Garrett, J. C. (1993). Odor-induced EEG changes in PTSD Vietnam veterans. *Journal of Traumatic Stress, 6,* 213–24.

McCallum, W. C., & Abraham, P. (1973). The contingent negative variation in psychosis. *Electroencephalography and Clinical Neurophysiology (Suppl.), 53,* 329–35.

McCarley, R. W., Faux, S., Shenton, M., Nestor, P., & Adams, J. (1991). Event-related potentials in schizophrenia: Their biological and clinical correlates and a new model of schizophrenic pathophysiology. *Schizophrenia Research, 4,* 209–31.

McCarley, R. W., Hsiao, J. K., Freedman, R., Pfefferbaum, A., & Donchin, E. (1996). Neuroimaging and the cognitive neuroscience of schizophrenia. *Schizophrenia Bulletin, 22,* 703–25.

McCarley, R. W., Shenton, M. E., O'Donnell, B. F., & Nestor, P. G. (1993). Uniting Kraepelin and Bleuler: The psychology of schizophrenia and the biology of temporal lobe abnormalities. *Harvard Review of Psychiatry, 1,* 36–56.

McCarthy, G., Nobre, A. C., Bentin, S., & Spencer, D. D. (1995). Language-related field potentials in the anterior-medial temporal lobe: I. Intracranial distribution and neural generators. *The Journal of Neuroscience, 15,* 1080–9.

McFall, M. E., Veith, R. C., & Murburg, M. M. (1992). Basal sympathoadrenal function in posttraumatic stress disorder. *Biological Psychiatry, 31,* 1050–6.

McFarlane, A. C., Weber, D. L., & Clark, C. R. (1993). Abnormal stimulus processing in posttraumatic stress disorder. *Biological Psychiatry, 34,* 311–20.

McGhie, A., & Chapman, J. (1961). Disorders of attention and perception in early schizophrenia. *British Journal of Medical Psychology, 34,* 103–16.

Mednick, S. A., & McNeill, T. (1968). Current methodology in research on the etiology of schizophrenia. *Psychological Bulletin, 70,* 681–93.

Menon, R. R., Barta, P. E., Aylward, E. H., Richards, S. S., Vaughn, D. D., Tien, A. Y., Harris, G. J., & Pearlson, G. D. (1995). Posterior superior temporal gyrus in schizophrenia: Grey matter changes and clinical correlates. *Schizophrenia Research, 16,* 127–35.

Miller, G. A. (1996). Presidential address: How we think about cognition, emotion, and biology in psychopathology. *Psychophysiology, 33,* 615–28.

Miller, G. A., Chapman, J. P., & Isaacks, B. G. (1998). Misunderstanding analysis of covariance. Manuscript submitted for publication.

Miller, G. A., & Ebert, L. (1988). Conceptual boundaries in psychophysiology. *Journal of Psychophysiology, 2,* 13–16.

Miller, G. A., & Kozak, M. J. (1993). Three-system assessment and the construct of emotion. In N. Birbaumer & A. Öhman (Eds.), *The Structure of Emotion: Psychophysiological, Cognitive and Clinical Aspects*, pp. 31–47. Seattle: Hogrefe & Huber.

Miller, G. A., Simons, R. F., & Lang, P. J. (1984). Electrocortical measures of information processing deficit in anhedonia. *Annals of the New York Academy of Sciences, 425*, 598–602.

Miller, G. A., & Yee, C. M. (1985). Affective responsiveness in anhedonia and dysthymia. Paper presented at the meeting of the Society for Psychophysiological Research (October, Houston, TX).

Miller, G. A., & Yee, C. M. (1994). Risk for severe psychopathology: Psychometric screening and psychophysiological assessment. In P. K. Ackles, J. R. Jennings, & M. G. H. Coles (Eds.), *Advances in Psychophysiology*, vol. 5, pp. 1–54. London: Jessica Kingsley.

Miller, M. B., Chapman, J. P., Chapman, L. J., & Collins, J. (1995). Task difficulty and cognitive deficits in schizophrenia. *Journal of Abnormal Psychology, 104*, 251–8.

Millon, T. (1991). Classification in psychopathology: Rationale, alternatives, and standards. *Journal of Abnormal Psychology, 100*, 245–61.

Mineka, S., Watson, D., & Clark, L. A. (1998). Comorbidity of anxiety and unipolar mood disorders. *Annual Review of Psychology, 49*, 377–412.

Morgan, C. A., Grillon, C., Southwick, S. M., Davis, M., & Charney, D. S. (1995). Fear-potentiated startle in posttraumatic stress disorder. *Biological Psychiatry, 38*, 378–85.

Morton, J. (1969). Interaction of information processing in word recognition. *Psychological Review, 76*, 163–78.

Näätänen, R. (1990). The role of attention in auditory information processing as revealed by event-related potentials and other brain measures of cognitive function. *Behavioral and Brain Sciences, 13*, 201–28.

Näätänen, R., Gaillard, A. W. K., & Mantysalo, S. (1978). The N2 effect of selective attention reinterpreted. *Acta Psychologica, 42*, 313–29.

Näätänen, R., & Michie, P. T. (1979). Early selective attention effects on the evoked potential. A critical review and reinterpretation. *Biological Psychology, 8*, 81–136.

Nadel, L., & Jacobs, W. J. (in press). The role of the hippocampus in PTSD, panic and phobia. In N. Kato (Ed.), *Hippocampus: Functions and Clinical Relevance*. Amsterdam: Elsevier.

Neshige, R., & Luders, H. (1992). Recording of the event-related potentials (P300) from human cortex. *Journal of Clinical Neurophysiology, 9*, 294–8.

Nielsen-Bohlman, L., & Knight, R. T. (1994). Electrophysiological dissociation of rapid memory mechanisms in humans. *Neuroreport, 5*, 1517–21.

Niznikiewicz, M. A., O'Donnell, B. F., Nestor, P. G., Smith, L., Law, S., Karapelou, M., Shenton, M. E., & McCarley, R. W. (1997). ERP assessment of visual and auditory language processing in schizophrenia. *Journal of Abnormal Psychology, 106*, 85–94.

Noble, P., & Lader, M. (1971). Depressive illness, pulse rate, and forearm blood flow. *British Journal of Psychiatry, 119*, 261–6.

Nobre, A. C., & McCarthy, G. (1995). Language-related field potentials in the anterior-medial temporal lobe: II. Effects of word type and semantic priming. *The Journal of Neuroscience, 15*, 1090–8.

Nuechterlein, K. H., Edell, W. S., Norris, M., & Dawson, M. E. (1986). Attentional vulnerability indicators, thought disorder, and negative symptoms. *Schizophrenia Bulletin, 12*, 408–26.

Oades, R. D., Dittmann-Balcar, A., Zerbin, D., & Grzella, I. (1997). Impaired attention-dependent augmentation of MMN in nonparanoid vs paranoid schizophrenic patients: A comparison with obsessive-compulsive disorder and healthy subjects. *Biological Psychiatry, 41*, 1196–1210.

Oades, R. D., Zerbin, D., & Eggers, C. (1994). Negative difference (Nd), an ERP marker of stimulus relevance: Different lateral asymmetries for paranoid and nonparanoid schizophrenics. *Pharmacopsychiatry, 27*, 65–7.

Obiols, J. E., Garcia-Domingo, M., de Trincheria, I., & Domenech, E. (1993). Psychometric schizotypy and sustained attention in young males. *Personality and Individual Differences, 14*, 381–4.

O'Donnell, B. F., Shenton, M. E., McCarley, R. W., Faux, S. F., Smith, R. S., Salisbury, D. F., Nestor, P. G., Pollak, S. D., Kikinis, R., & Jolesz, F. A. (1993). The auditory N2 component in schizophrenia: Relationship to MRI temporal lobe gray matter and to other ERP abnormalities. *Biological Psychiatry, 34*, 26–40.

Ogura, C., Nageishi, Y., Omura, F., Kozo, F., Ohta, H., Kishimoto, A., & Matsubayshi, M. (1993). N200 component of event-related potentials in depression. *Biological Psychiatry, 33*, 720–6.

Öhman, A. (1979). The orienting response, attention, and learning: An information processing perspective. In H. Kimmel, E. van Olst, & J. Orlebeke (Eds.), *The Orienting Reflex in Humans*, pp. 443–71. Hillsdale, NJ: Erlbaum.

Öhman, A. (1981). Electrodermal activity and vulnerability to schizophrenia: A review. *Biological Psychology, 12*, 87–145.

Öhman, A. (1986). Face the beast and fear the face: Animal and social fears as prototypes for evolutionary analyses of emotion. *Psychophysiology, 23*, 123–45.

Öhman, A., Nordby, H., & d'Elia, G. (1986). Orienting and schizophrenia: Stimulus significance, attention, and distraction in a signalled reaction time task. *Journal of Abnormal Psychology, 95*, 326–34.

O'Leary, D. S., Andreasen, N. C., Hurtig, R. R., Kesler, M. L., Rogers, M., Arndt, S., Cizadlo, T., Watkins, G. L., Ponto, L. L. B., Kirchner, P. T., & Hichwa, R. D. (1996). Auditory attentional deficits in patients with schizophrenia: A positron emission tomography study. *Archives of General Psychiatry, 53*, 633–41.

Oltmanns, T. F. (1978). Selective attention in schizophrenia and manic psychoses: The effects of distraction on information processing. *Journal of Abnormal Psychology, 87*, 212–25.

Orr, S. P. (1994). An overview of psychophysiological studies of PTSD. *PTSD Research Quarterly, Winter*, 1–3.

Orr, S. P., & Kaloupek, D. G. (1997). Psychophysiological assessment of posttraumatic stress disorder. In J. P. Wilson & T. M. Keane (Eds.), *Assessing Psychological Trauma and PTSD*, pp. 69–97. New York: Guilford.

Orr, S. P., Pitman, R. K., Lasko, N. R., & Herz, L. R. (1993). Psychophysiological assessment of posttraumatic stress disorder imagery in World War II and Korean combat veterans. *Journal of Abnormal Psychology, 10*, 152–9.

Öst, L. (1989). Panic disorder, agoraphobia, and social phobia. In G. Turpin (Ed.), *Handbook of Clinical Psychophysiology*, pp. 309–28. New York: Wiley.

Paige, S. R., Reid, G. M., Allen, M. G., & Newton, J. E. O. (1990). Psychophysiological correlates of posttraumatic stress disorder in Vietnam veterans. *Biological Psychiatry, 27,* 419–30.

Pallmeyer, T., Blanchard, E., & Kolb, L. (1986). The psychophysiology of combat induced post-traumatic stress disorder in Vietnam veterans. *Behaviour Research and Therapy, 24,* 645–52.

Patterson, T. (1987). Studies toward the subcortical pathogenesis of schizophrenia. *Schizophrenia Bulletin, 13,* 555–76.

Pitman, R. K. (1997). Overview of biological themes in PTSD. In R. Yehuda & D. McFarlane (Eds.), *Psychobiology of Post-Traumatic Stress Disorder,* pp. 1–9. New York Academy of Sciences.

Pitman, R. K., Orr, S. P., Forgue, D. F., Altman, B., de Jong, J. B., & Herz, L. R. (1990). Psychophysiologic responses to combat imagery of Vietnam veterans with posttraumatic stress disorder versus other anxiety disorder. *Journal of Abnormal Psychology, 99,* 49–54.

Pitman, R. K., Orr, S. P., Forgue, D. F., de Jong, J., & Claiborn, J. (1987). Psychophysiologic assessment of posttraumatic stress disorder imagery in Vietnam combat veterans. *Archives of General Psychiatry, 44,* 970–5.

Posner, M. I., & Synder, C. R. R. (1975). Attention and cognitive control. In R. L. Sloso (Ed.), *Information Processing and Cognition: The Loyola Symposium,* pp. 55–85. Hillsdale, NJ: Erlbaum.

Post, R. M., DeLisi, L. E., Holcomb, H. H., Uhde, T. W., Cohen, R., & Buchsbaum, M. (1987). Glucose utilization in the temporal cortex of affectively ill patients: Positron emission tomography. *Biological Psychiatry, 22,* 545–53.

Prins, A., Kaloupek, D. G., & Keane, T. M. (1995). Psychophysiological evidence for autonomic arousal and startle in traumatized adult populations. In M. J. Friedman, D. S. Charney, & A. Y. Deutch (Eds.), *Neurobiological and Clinical Consequences of Stress: From Normal Adaption of PTSD,* pp. 291–314. New York: Raven.

Pritchard, W. S. (1986). Cognitive event-related potential correlates of schizophrenia. *Psychological Bulletin, 100,* 43–66.

Pritchard, W. S., Shappell, S. A., & Brandt, M. E. (1991). Psychophysiology of N200/N400: A review and classification scheme. In J. R. Jennings, P. K. Ackles, & M. G. H. Coles (Eds.), *Advances in Psychophysiology,* vol. 4, pp. 43–106. London: Jessica Kingsley.

Raine, A., Benishay, D., Lencz, T., & Scarpa, A. (1997). Abnormal orienting in schizotypal personality disorder. *Schizophrenia Bulletin, 23,* 75–82.

Raine, A., Lencz, T., & Benishay, D. S. (1995). Schizotypal personality and skin conductance orienting. In A. Raine, T. Lencz, & S. A. Mednick (Eds.), *Schizotypal Personality,* pp. 219–49. Cambridge University Press.

Rauch, S. L., van der Kolk, B. A., Fisler, R. E., Alpert, N., Orr, S. P., Savage, C. R., Fischman, A. J., Jenkie, M. A., & Pittman, R. K. (1996). A symptom provocation study of posttraumatic stress disorder using positron emission tomography and script-driven imagery. *Archives of General Psychiatry, 53,* 380–7.

Reiman, E. M., Raichle, M. E., Butler, F. K., Herscovitch, P., & Robins, E. (1984). A focal brain abnormality in panic disorder, a severe form of anxiety. *Nature, 310,* 683–5.

Reivich, M., Gur, R., & Alavi, A. (1983). Positron emission tomographic studies of sensory stimuli cognitive processes and anxiety. *Human Neurobiology, 2,* 25–33.

Ritter, W., & Ruchkin, D. S. (1992). A review of event-related potentials discovered in the context of studying P3. In D. Friedman & G. Bruder (Eds.), *Psychophysiology and Experimental Psychopathology* (Annals of the New York Academy of Sciences, vol. 658), pp. 1–32. New York Academy of Sciences.

Rizzo, P. A., Albani, G. F., Spadaro, M., & Morocutti, C. (1983). Brain slow potentials CNV, prolactin, and schizophrenia. *Biological Psychiatry, 18,* 175–83.

Robertson, R. J., & Powers, W. T. (1990). *Brain Slow Potentials (CNV), Prolactin, and Schizophrenia.* Gravel Switch, KY: Control Systems Groups.

Rockstroh, B., Elbert, T., Canavan, A., Lutzenberger, W., & Birbaumer, N. (1989). *Slow Cortical Potentials and Behavior,* pp. 177–205. Munich: Urban & Schwarzenberg.

Roth, W. T., Duncan, C. C., Pfefferbaum, A., & Timsit-Berthier, M. (1986). Applications of cognitive ERPs in psychiatric patients. In W. C. McCallum, R. Zappoli, & F. Denoth (Eds.), *Cerebral Psychophysiology: Studies in Event-Related Potentials EEG* (Suppl. 38), pp. 419–38. Amsterdam: Elsevier.

Roth, W. T., Pfefferbaum, A., Kelly, A. F., Berger, P. A., & Kopell, B. S. (1981). Auditory event-related potentials in schizophrenia and depression. *Psychiatry Research, 4,* 199–212.

Roy-Byrne, P. P., Weingartner, H., Bierer, L. M., Thompson, K., & Post, R. M. (1986). Effortful and automatic cognitive processes in depression. *Archives of General Psychiatry, 43,* 265–7.

Rubinow, D. R., & Post, R. M. (1992). Impaired recognition of affect in facial expression in depressed patients. *Biological Psychiatry, 31,* 947–53.

Salisbury, D. F., Voglmaier, M. M., Seidman, L. J., & McCarley, R. W. (1996). Topographic abnormalities of P3 in schizotypal personality disorder. *Biological Psychiatry, 40,* 165–72.

Sartory, G. (1989). Obsessional-compulsive disorder. In G. Turpin (Ed.), *Handbook of Clinical Psychophysiology,* pp. 329–56. New York: Wiley.

Schechter, D., Strasser, T. J., Santangelo, C., Kim, E., & Endicott, J. (1994). "Normal" control subjects are hard to find: A model for centralized recruitment. *Psychiatry Research, 53,* 301–11.

Schell, A. M., Dawson, M. E., Hazlett, E. A., & Filion, D. L. (1995). Attentional modulation of startle in psychosis-prone college students. *Psychophysiology, 32,* 266–73.

Schreiber, H., Stolz-Born, G., Kornhuber, H. H., & Born, J. (1992). Event-related potential correlates of impaired selective attention in children at high risk for schizophrenia. *Biological Psychiatry, 32,* 634–51.

Scrimali, T., Grasso, F., Franciforti, M., Gilotta, S., Saraceno, C., Zerbo, S., & Paoletti, C. (1990). Multi-factorial evaluation of the pharmacodynamic action and therapeutic profile of a new serotoninergic antidepressant: Fluoxetine. *New Trends in Experimental and Clinical Psychiatry, 6,* 91–7.

Semple, W. E., Goyer, P., McCormick, R., Morris, E., Compton, B., Muswick, G., Nelson, D., Donovan, B., Leisure, G.,

Berridge, M., Miraldi, F., & Schultz, S. C. (1993). Preliminary report: Brain blood flow using PET in patients with posttraumatic stress disorder and substance-abuse histories. *Biological Psychiatry, 34,* 115–18.

Sereno, A. B., & Holzman, P. S. (1996). Spatial selective attention in schizophrenic, affective disorder, and normal subjects. *Schizophrenia Research, 11,* 33–50.

Shagass, C. (1981). Neurophysiological evidence for different types of depression. *Journal of Behavior Therapy and Experimental Psychiatry, 12,* 99–111.

Shajahan, P. M., O'Carroll, R. E., Glabus, M. F., Ebmeier, K. P., & Blackwood, D. H. (1997). Correlation of auditory "oddball" P300 with verbal memory deficits in schizophrenia. *Psychological Medicine, 27,* 579–86.

Shenton, M. E., Kikinis, R., Jolesz, F. A., Pollak, S. D., LeMay, M., Wible, C. G., Hokama, H., Martin, J., Metcalf, D., Coleman, M., & McCarley, R. W. (1992). Abnormalities of the left temporal lobe and thought disorder in schizophrenia: A quantitative magnetic resonance imaging study. *New England Journal of Medicine, 327,* 604–12.

Shields, J., Heston, L. L., & Gottesman, I. I. (1975). Schizophrenia and the schizoid: The problem for genetic analysis. In R. R. Fieve, D. Rosenthal, & H. Brill (Eds.), *Genetic Research in Psychiatry,* pp. 167–97. Baltimore: Johns Hopkins University Press.

Siddle, D. A. T. (1991). Orienting, habituation, and resource allocation: An associative analysis. *Psychophysiology, 28,* 245–60.

Silberman, E. K., Weingartner, H., & Post, R. M. (1983). Thinking disorder in depression: Logic and strategy in an abstract reasoning task. *Archives of General Psychiatry, 40,* 775–80.

Silverman, J. (1964). The problem of attention in research and theory in schizophrenia. *Psychological Review, 71,* 352–79.

Simons, R. F. (1981). Electrodermal and cardiac orienting in psychometrically defined high risk subjects. *Psychiatry Research, 4,* 347–56.

Simons, R. F., Fitzgibbons, L., & Fiorito, E. (1993). Emotion-processing in anhedonia. In N. Birbaumer & A. Öhman (Eds.), *The Organization of Emotion,* pp. 288–306. Toronto: Hogrefe & Huber.

Simons, R. F., & Giardina, B. D. (1992). Reflex modification in psychosis-prone young adults. *Psychophysiology, 29,* 8–16.

Simons, R. F., Öhman, A., & Lang, P. J. (1979). Anticipation and response set: Cortical, cardiac, and electrodermal correlates. *Psychophysiology, 16,* 222–33.

Simons, R. F., & Zelson, M. F. (1985). Engaging visual stimuli and reflex blink modification. *Psychophysiology, 22,* 44–9.

Simson, R., Vaughan, H., & Ritter, W. (1976). The scalp topography of potentials associated with missing auditory or visual stimuli. *Electroencephalography and Clinical Neurophysiology, 62,* 25–31.

Sison, C. E., Alpert, M., Fudge, R., & Stern, R. M. (1996). Constricted expressiveness and psychophysiological reactivity in schizophrenia. *Journal of Nervous and Mental Disease, 184,* 589–97.

Smith, D. A., Boutros, N. N., & Schwarzkopf, S. B. (1994). Reliability of P50 auditory event-related potential indices of sensory gating. *Psychophysiology, 31,* 495–502.

Sokolov, E. N. (1990). The orienting response, and future directions of its development. *Pavlovian Journal of Biological Science, 25,* 142–50.

Souza, V. B., Muir, W. J., Walker, M. T., Glabus, M. F., Roxborough, H. M., Sharp, C. W., Dunan, J. R., & Blackwood, D. H. (1995). Auditory P300 event-related potentials and neuropsychological performance in schizophrenia and bipolar affective disorder. *Biological Psychiatry, 37,* 300–10.

Spielberger, C. D. (1968). Self-evaluation questionnaire. STAI Form X-2. Palo Alto, CA: Consulting Psychologists Press.

Spitzer, M., Weisker, I., Winter, M., Maier, S., Hermle, L., & Maher, B. A. (1994). Semantic and phonological priming in schizophrenia. *Journal of Abnormal Psychology, 103,* 485–94.

Sponheim, S. R., Allen, J. J., & Iacono, W. G. (1995). Psychophysiological measures in depression: The significance of electrodermal activity, electroencephalographic asymmetries, and contingent negative variation to behavioral and neurobiological aspects of depression. In G. A. Miller (Ed.), *The Behavioral High-Risk Paradigm in Psychopathology,* pp. 222–49. New York: Springer-Verlag.

Steinhauer, S., & Zubin, J. (1982). Vulnerability to schizophrenia: Information processing in the pupilla and event-related potential. In E. Usdin & I. Hanin (Eds.), *Biological Markers in Psychiatry and Neurology,* pp. 371–85. Oxford, U.K.: Pergamon.

Sutton, S. K., & Davidson, R. J. (1997). Prefrontal brain asymmetry: A biological substrate of the behavioral approach and inhibition systems. *Psychological Science, 8,* 204–10.

Swedo, S. E., Schapiro, M. B., Grady, C. L., Cheslow, D. L., Leonard, H. L., Kumar, A., Friedland, R., Rapoport, S. L., & Rapoport, J. L. (1989). Cerebral glucose metabolism in childhood-onset obsessive compulsive disorder. *Archives of General Psychiatry, 46,* 518–23.

Taitano, K., & Miller, G. A. (1998). Neuroscience perspectives on emotion in psychopathology. In W. Flack & J. Laird (Eds.), *Emotion in Psychopathology: Theory and Research,* pp. 20–44. New York: Oxford University Press.

Tancer, M. E., Brown, T., Evans, D., Ekstrom, D., Haggerty, J., Pedersen, C., & Golden, R. (1990). Impaired effortful cognition in depression. *Psychiatric Research, 31,* 161–8.

Tariot, P. N., & Weingartner, H. (1986). A psychobiologic analysis of cognitive failures: Structure and mechanisms. *Archives of General Psychiatry, 43,* 1183–8.

Timsit-Berthier, M., Mantanus, H., Ansseau, M., Devoitille, J. M., Dal Mas, A., & Legros, J. J. (1987). Contingent negative variation in major depressive patients. *Electroencephalography and Clinical Neurophysiology (Suppl.), 40,* 762–71.

Tomarken, A. J., & Davidson, R. J. (1994). Frontal brain activation in repressors and nonrepressors. *Journal of Abnormal Psychology, 103,* 339–49.

Trestman, R. L., Horvath, T., Kalus, O., Peterson, A. E., Coccaro, E., Mitropoulou, V., Apter, S., Davidson, M., & Siever, L. J. (1996). Event-related potentials in schizotypal personality disorder. *Journal of Neuropsychiatry and Clinical Neuroscience, 8,* 33–40.

Tucker, D. M., Antes, J. R., Stenslie, C. E., & Barnhardt, T. M. (1978). Right hemisphere activation during stress. *Neuropsychologia, 15,* 697–700.

Turetsky, B. I., Colbath, E. A., & Gur, R. E. (1998a). P300 subcomponent abnormalities in schizophrenia: I. Physiological evidence for gender and subtype specific differences in regional pathology. *Biological Psychiatry, 43,* 84–96.

Turetsky, B. I., Colbath, E. A., & Gur, R. E. (1998b). P300 subcomponent abnormalities in schizophrenia: II. Longitudinal stability and relationship to symptom change. *Biological Psychiatry, 43,* 31–9.

Turpin, G. (1989a). *Handbook of Clinical Psychophysiology.* New York: Wiley.

Turpin, G. (1989b). An overview of clinical psychophysiological techniques: Tools or theories? In G. Turpin (Ed.), *Handbook of Clinical Psychophysiology,* pp. 3–44. New York: Wiley.

Tyler, S. K., & Tucker, D. M. (1982). Anxiety and perceptual structure: Individual differences in neuropsychological function. *Journal of Abnormal Psychology, 91,* 210–20.

Ulett, G. A., Gleser, G., Winokur, G., & Lawler, A. (1953). The EEG and reaction to photic stimulation as an index of anxiety-proneness. *Electroencephalography and Clinical Neurophysiology, 5,* 23–32.

Uytdenhoef, P., Portelange, P., Jacquy, J., Charles, G., Linkowshi, P., & Mendlewicz, J. (1983). Regional cerebral blood flow and lateralized hemispheric dysfunction in depression. *British Journal of Psychiatry, 143,* 128–32.

Velakoulis, D., & Pantelis, C. (1996). What have we learned from functional imaging studies in schizophrenia? The role of frontal, striatal and temporal areas. *Australian and New Zealand Journal of Psychiatry, 30,* 195–209.

Venables, P. H. (1964). Input dysfunction in schizophrenia. In B. A. Maher (Ed.), *Progress in Experimental Personality Research.* New York: Academic Press.

Wagner, M., Rendtorff, N., Kathmann, N., & Engle, R. R. (1996). CNV, PINV and probe-evoked potentials in schizophrenics. *Electroencephalography and Clinical Neurophysiology, 98,* 130–43.

Ward, N. G., & Doerr, H. O. (1986). Skin conductance: A potentially sensitive and specific marker for depression. *Journal of Nervous and Mental Disease, 174,* 553–9.

Ward, N. G., Doerr, H. O., & Storrie, M. (1983). Skin conductance: A potentially sensitive test for depression. *Psychiatry Research, 10,* 295–302.

Ward, P. B., Catts, S. V., Fox, A. M., Michie, P. T., & McConaghy, N. (1991). Auditory selective attention and event-related potentials in schizophrenia. *British Journal of Psychiatry, 158,* 534–9.

Weinberger, D. R., Aloia, M. S., Goldberg, T. E., & Berman, K. F. (1994). The frontal lobes and schizophrenia. *Journal of Neuropsychiatry and Clinical Neurosciences, 6,* 419–27.

Weinberger, D. R., Berman, K. F., & Zec, R. F. (1986). Physiologic dysfunction of dorsolateral prefrontal cortex in schizophrenics. I. Regional cerebral blood flow evidence. *Archives of General Psychology, 43,* 114–24.

Weingartner, H., & Silberman, E. (1982). Models of cognitive impairment: Cognitive changes in depression. *Psychopharmacological Bulletin, 18,* 27–42.

White, P. M., & Yee, C. M. (1997). Effects of attentional and stressor manipulations on the P50 gating response. *Psychophysiology, 34,* 703–11.

White, P. M., & Yee, C. M. (1998). P50 sensitivity to physical and psychological influences. Manuscript submitted for publication.

White, P. M., Yee, C. M., & Nuechterlein, K. H. (1997). The post-auricular reflex in schizophrenia: A potential measure of impaired suppression. Paper presented at the annual meeting of the Society for Psychophysiological Research (October, Cape Cod, MA).

Wilder, J. (1950). The law of initial values. *Psychosomatic Medicine, 12,* 392–401.

Wilder, J. (1957). The law of initial values in neurology and psychiatry. *Journal of Nervous and Mental Disease, 125,* 73–86.

Williams, K. M., Iacono, W. G., & Remick, R. A. (1985). Electrodermal activity among subtypes of depression. *Biological Psychiatry, 20,* 158–62.

Wu, J. C., Buchsbaum, M. S., Hershey, T. G., Hazlett, E., Sicotte, N., & Johnson, J. C. (1991). PET in generalized anxiety disorder. *Biological Psychiatry, 29,* 1181–99.

Yee, C. M. (1995). Implications of the resource allocation model for mood disorders. In G. A. Miller (Ed.), *The Behavioral High-Risk Paradigm in Psychopathology,* pp. 271–88. New York: Springer-Verlag.

Yee, C. M., Deldin, P. J., & Miller, G. A. (1992). Stimulus intensity effects in dysthymia and anhedonia. *Journal of Abnormal Psychology, 101,* 230–3.

Yee, C. M., & Miller, G. A. (1988). Emotional information processing: Modulation of fear in normal and dysthymic subjects. *Journal of Abnormal Psychology, 97,* 54–63.

Yee, C. M., & Miller, G. A. (1994). A dual-task analysis of resource allocation in dysthymia and anhedonia. *Journal of Abnormal Psychology, 103,* 625–36.

Yee, C. M., & White, P. M. (1998). Experimental modification of P50 suppression. Manuscript submitted for publication.

Yee, C. M., White, P. M., & Nuechterlein, K. H. (1996). Effects of attention on P50 gating in schizophrenia. Paper presented at the annual meeting of the Society for Psychophysiological Research (October, Vancouver, CA).

Yehuda, R. (1997). Sensitization of the hypothalamic-pituitary-adrenal axis in posttraumatic stress disorder. *Annals of the New York Academy of Sciences, 821,* 57–75.

Yeudall, L. T., Schopflocher, D., Sussman, P. S., Barabash, W., Warneke, I. B., Gill, D., Otto, W., Howarth, B., & Termansen, P. E. (1983). Panic attack syndrome with and without agoraphobia: Neuropsychological and evoked potential correlates. In P. Flor-Henry & J. Gruzelier (Eds.), *Laterality and Psychopathology,* pp. 195–216. New York: Elsevier.

Zahn, T. P. (1986). Psychophysiological approaches to psychopathology. In M. G. H. Coles, E. Donchin, & S. W. Porges (Eds.), *Psychophysiology: Systems, Processes, and Applications,* pp. 508–610. New York: Guilford.

Zaubler, T. S., Viederman, M., & Fins, J. J. (1996). Ethical, legal, and psychiatric issues in capacity, competency, and informed consent: An annotated bibliography. *General Hospital Psychiatry, 18,* 155–72.

CHAPTER TWENTY-SEVEN

PSYCHOPHYSIOLOGICAL APPLICATIONS IN CLINICAL HEALTH PSYCHOLOGY

CATHERINE M. STONEY & LISA MANZI LENTINO

Introduction

Health psychology has experienced substantial growth over the last 20 years, both in the number of members affiliating with the field as well as in the diversity and scope of the research and clinical services subsumed under the field. At the crux of the discipline is the belief that there is an inherent interaction between psychological and physiological processes. This holistic view of mind–body interactions is primarily an outgrowth of the early psychosomatic movement. Although this movement was somewhat limited – by methodological flaws in research, by the restrictive nature of the questions addressed by early pioneers of the field, and by a general unwillingness to accept factors such as genetic predisposition, environmental stressors, and cognitions as important contributions to health and illness (Engel 1980; Schwartz 1982) – many of these limitations have resulted in important strengths of health psychology today. For example, rigorous training in research methodology and design, as well as the broad nature and range of health conditions and issues addressed in health psychology, are hallmarks of the field and are likely consequences of perceived deficiencies within the psychosomatic movement. Other, more recent societal influences have also contributed to the emergence of health psychology, including the predominance of chronic illnesses as the leading causes of mortality. These social influences have necessitated taking a lifespan approach – and the consequent consideration of behavioral, psychological, and preventive factors – when investigating etiologic influences and treatment options.

Perhaps the most substantial contribution of the psychosomatic movement to the development and emergence of health psychology is the commitment to the biopsychosocial model of health and illness. This model posits that health and illness are best conceptualized by using a systems-based approach that incorporates biological, psychological, and social factors. In many ways, this model is a reaction to the traditional biomedical model, which is reductionistic in nature, adheres to the philosophy of mind–body dualism, and holds that a single primary principle can elicit a complex phenomenon. In contrast, the biopsychosocial model proposes that health is best understood by examining the interaction of a variety of variables across a variety of levels. Inherent in the biopsychosocial model is the need for an interdisciplinary approach for addressing both empirical and clinical issues. Because of their natural commonalities, health psychology and psychophysiology often become intertwined in the process of resolving research and clinical questions.

In this chapter, we demonstrate how the collaborative relationship between health psychology and psychophysiology has made substantial contributions to both clinical and basic research issues in health and illness. Psychophysiological techniques and approaches have been used by health psychologists in the assessment, etiology, and treatment of a diverse range of disorders and conditions, including diseases of the cardiovascular and neuromuscular systems, disorders of respiration, and sleep disturbances (see Table 1). While psychophysiological investigations of disorders within some systems have concentrated primarily on issues regarding assessment, others have focused more on treatment approaches. For example, investigations of electroencephalography (EEG) and electrodermal activity for the diagnosis of schizophrenia are well-represented (Öhman 1981; Venables 1983; Zahn 1986; see also Chapter 26 of this volume), yet there is a dearth of similar studies for chronic pain. Conversely, a plethora of psychophysiologically based interventions for the treatment of various types of chronic pain (Cox, Freundlich, & Meyer 1975; Holroyd, Andrasik, & Noble 1980) are evident, whereas essentially no comparable investigations are available for schizophrenia. Although decisions regarding whether or not to utilize

John T. Cacioppo, Louis G. Tassinary, and Gary G. Berntson (Eds.), *Handbook of Psychophysiology*, 2nd ed. © Cambridge University Press 2000. Printed in the United States of America. ISBN 62634X. All rights reserved.

TABLE 1. Examples of Psychophysiological Applications for the Assessment and Treatment of a Range of Conditions

Conditions	Psychophysiological Assessment and Etiologic Approaches	Psychophysiologic Treatment Approaches
Hypertension	Blood pressure control Blood pressure reactivity Stress hormones	Blood pressure biofeedback Heart rate biofeedback EMG biofeedback Relaxation
Rheumatoid arthritis	—	EMG biofeedback Skin temperature biofeedback Relaxation
Headache pain	Vascular reactivity Cerebrovasoconstriction EMG activity	TENS Skin temperature biofeedback EMG biofeedback Relaxation
Temporomandibular disorder	EMG activity EMG reactivity	TENS EMG biofeedback Nocturnal EMG biofeedback Relaxation
Insomnia	EEG activity Polysomnographic studies	EMG biofeedback EEG biofeedback Relaxation

Key: EEG, electroencephalogram; EMG, electromyogram; TENS, transelectrical nerve stimulation.

these techniques – in general and in regard to the specific systems chosen for investigation – could be theoretically based, often they are not. In this chapter we will thus refer not only to what is known but also to that which is yet unexamined.

We have organized coverage of these topics by first providing a brief description of the nature and prevalence of the relevant disorder or condition, followed by a characterization of the underlying psychophysiological principles involved in the assessment or etiology of the disorder, and finally a consideration of the psychophysiological treatments utilized for each disorder. The issues covered are by no means meant to be an exhaustive account of how psychophysiologically based paradigms have been applied to issues in health psychology. Rather, they were selected to highlight representative approaches to disparate systems and disorders.

Psychophysiological Paradigms in Etiology and Assessment

The use of psychophysiological techniques in the assessment and etiology of various disorders is nearly always limited by the complexity of the systems being monitored, the technical aspects of the measurement and analytic strategies, and the frequent presence of confounding variables. For example, pharmacotherapy (including neuroleptics, antidepressants, and anxiolytics) for the treatment of sleep disorders, hypertension, and psychopathology will alter physiological and psychological functioning and can impede our ability to understand the very relationships being investigated (Iacono 1991; Turpin 1991). The choice of system to be measured can be made on both theoretical and practical grounds; this choice involves consideration of the basis for the presumed association, the time course of interest, the resources available, and the technical expertise of the clinical researcher.

Perhaps the most common use of psychophysiologically based paradigms in the clinical research literature is in the assessment and diagnosis of psychopathologies, including anxiety disorders, schizophrenia, and phobias. Although there are few clinicians who routinely use psychophysiological techniques for assessment or diagnosis, these strategies hold promise for assisting in the differential diagnoses of certain disorders. For example, psychophysiological techniques can potentially clarify some of the pervasive difficulties with the DSM-IV (*Diagnostic and Statistical Manual of Mental Disorders,* fourth edition), such as overlap among diagnostic categories and questionable validity of some disorders. By subclassing individuals according to their psychophysiological responses, clinicians can identify subtypes of disorders that differ significantly with regard to etiology or treatment response (Iacono 1991).

In addition to differential diagnosis, there are several other contributions that could be made by psychophysiology to the understanding of a variety of disorders. Because psychophysiological measures often have both state and trait properties, they may be more sensitive to temporal fluctuations in states of a disorder than traditionally used measures (Iacono 1991). Psychophysiological measures can also serve as important indicators of risk and thus assist in the design of preventive measures. Psychophysiological assessment techniques have the advantage of being independent of self-report and are consequently useful with uncooperative individuals or those with poor communication skills or children (Iacono 1991). More importantly, discordance between physiological markers and self-report of symptoms has assisted in diagnosis – as, for example, with a series of studies on panic disorder (Margraf et al. 1987). Finally, advances in ambulatory monitoring devices (Turpin 1990) have created the possibility of assessing individuals' responses throughout their daily lives as well as during treatment (Margraf et al. 1987).

Psychophysiological Paradigms in Treatment

The utility of psychophysiologically based paradigms in the treatment of various disorders has focused on three main techniques. Perhaps the most widely studied in the empirical literature is biofeedback, which has been applied in the treatment of cardiovascular, neuromuscular, sleep, respiratory, and sexual disorders (Table 2). Second, relax-

TABLE 2. Representative Physiological Systems Used in Biofeedback Treatment Paradigms for Various Pathophysiological and Psychopathological Conditions

Measure	Condition
Blood pressure	Anxiety disorders, panic Hypertension
Bronchoconstriction	Asthma
EEG	Epilepsy Sleep disorders, insomnia
EMG	Chronic back pain Rheumatoid arthritis Sleep disorders, insomnia Tension and migraine headache TMD
Heart rate	Anxiety disorders, panic Neurocardiogenic syncope Sinus tachycardia
Respiration	Asthma Hyperventilation Panic disorder
Skin temperature (thermal)	Hypertension Migraine headache Rheumatoid arthritis

Key: EEG, electroencephalogram; EMG, electromyogram; TMD, temporomandibular joint disorder.

ation techniques (with or without biofeedback) are used clinically in the treatment of the same list of disorders. Although many different relaxation techniques are available and widely practiced, they all share the common behavioral features of deep breathing and the repetitive subvocalization of a sound or word, for the ultimate purpose of attention deployment. Finally, the utility of transdermal electrical nerve stimulation (TENS) in the treatment of a host of pain conditions has shown promise and represents a psychophysiological technique with direct clinical applicability.

BIOFEEDBACK AND RELAXATION

Biofeedback for the clinical treatment of a large number of disorders, including cardiovascular diseases, has been used with varying degrees of success since the 1960s. The general premise of the biofeedback technique is that measurement and display of a particular physiological system (using visual, auditory, or tactile information) and subsequent presentation of those electrophysiological signals will provide exteroceptive feedback to subjects and so enable them to alter what might otherwise be considered an involuntary physiological system. Clear instructions regarding the direction and time course of change desired are important determinants of biofeedback efficacy in both laboratory and clinical settings. However, the actual presentation of information appears to be less important. For example, individuals who are simply given instructions to reduce heart rate (in the absence of actual feedback) are somewhat successful at doing so, particularly early in training (Cuthbert et al. 1981; Stoney et al. 1986), although individuals receiving biofeedback become more adept with increased training (Lo & Johnston 1984). In addition, increasing the amount of information presented to subjects in a biofeedback task does little to improve performance (Blanchard et al. 1974). Thus, the specific elements that enhance the efficacy of these techniques are still elusive.

In research settings, biofeedback has been shown to enable the direct modification of a host of physiological parameters, such as heart rate, blood pressure, rate pressure product, and pulse transit time (see Table 2). By far the most common cardiovascular parameter studied in biofeedback has been heart rate, largely because of its measurement accessibility and range. Thus, much of our understanding of the conceptual basis for voluntary control of autonomic functioning is derived from biofeedback studies of heart rate. In contrast, biofeedback in the clinical setting is more typically used in conjunction with relaxation or meditation procedures to facilitate the relaxation response. In this latter case, information regarding muscle tension, skin temperature, or skin conductance might be used, since changes in these parameters are expected to occur during relaxation.

Clinically, several issues regarding the mechanisms and efficacy of biofeedback-assisted relaxation have dominated the field. First, the utility of identifying in advance those individuals who will exhibit the greatest success with the technique is obvious. Second, understanding the specificity of the response has implications not only for the theoretical understanding of the technique but also for its clinical utility. For example, the degree to which the response is generalizable will dictate the availability of the systems that can be tapped. Finally, the duration of treatment effectiveness has clear implications for clinical utility. Many of these issues have been examined in psychophysiological investigations.

Individual difference factors that predict success at control of autonomic functioning might be likely to serve an important clinical role. Large between-subject variability in ability to control autonomic functioning has led to the investigation of those factors predisposing some individuals to greater control. The most consistent finding is that greater physiological reductions are noted in subjects who have elevated basal levels than in those who have normal or low resting physiological levels. This difference in individual efficacy may be due to an initial values effect, and it has led to the assertion that control of visceral systems cannot supercede the biological constraints of that system (Schwartz 1975). The implication is that biofeedback may be especially successful among those clinical populations who already have elevated basal levels of autonomic activation.

In fact, this hypothesis has been tested and shown to be partly true. That is, normal subjects with high resting heart rate or high heart rate variability are most successful in heart rate biofeedback paradigms (Stoney et al. 1986). In addition, those presenting with exercise-induced (Lo & Johnston 1984; Perski & Engel 1980), stress-induced (Steptoe & Ross 1982; Stoney et al. 1987), or task-induced (Riley & Furedy 1981) elevations in heart rate or pulse transit time are most successful at accomplishing heart rate deceleration during heart rate biofeedback. More important is the question of whether biofeedback of autonomic functioning is effective in patient populations, many of whom may have sustained elevations in parameters that have been shown to be modifiable by biofeedback. These latter studies have focused on the use of biofeedback as a treatment for hypertension, sinus tachycardia, neurocardiogenic syncope, and other cardiac disorders (Engel & Bleecker 1979; Fredrikson & Engel 1992; Patel 1977). In general, moderate effects for treatment have been noted (Kaufmann et al. 1988), with some important exceptions (Jacob et al. 1991). In addition to predicting response on the basis of initial levels of autonomic activity, other investigations have examined additional potential predictors. For example, anxiety and other psychological factors, social and environmental factors, and demographic variables have all been tested as possible predictors of treatment response; to date, none have been found to be as powerful predictors of success at biofeedback as psychophysiological predictors (McGrady 1996).

Despite the earlier studies of Miller and colleagues (e.g. Miller & DiCara 1967) demonstrating (in curarized animals) that operant and bidirectional control of heart rate could be obtained in the absence of somatic mediation, there is still controversy regarding the specificity of the response to biofeedback (Brener, Phillips, & Connally 1980; Manuck 1976). Nonetheless, most researchers today would agree that the control of most autonomic parameters is in part mediated by respiratory and somatomotor influences. For example, heart rate biofeedback has been shown to be most successful when respiratory and gross somatic parameters are unconstrained (Obrist 1981). Under conditions of severe constraint, some voluntary control over heart rate can still be achieved, but the magnitude of the changes demonstrated are appreciably smaller than when biofeedback procedures are presented to unrestrained participants (Obrist 1976). When monitoring respiratory and somatomotor changes during heart rate biofeedback, generally some changes in respiratory functioning occur concomitant with alterations in heart rate or blood pressure (Stoney et al. 1986). Thus, although some amount of cardiac specificity has been noted (Manuck 1976; Stoney et al. 1986), the effects are not totally independent of alterations in respiratory or somatic activity. These findings are consonant with the hypothesis that voluntary heart rate changes that occur with biofeedback covary in a consistent and positive manner with somatic-metabolic activity.

In addition to understanding the specificity of the response, the duration of the clinical effects of biofeedback and relaxation training provide additional indication of the clinical efficacy of the techniques. Several factors are important in determining success of direct biofeedback therapy or biofeedback-assisted relaxation on control of autonomic functioning. For example, sufficient trials of learning must be presented in order to effect adequate response duration to the training. This dose–response phenomenon is also apparent when comparing studies that instructed patients to self-monitor and practice the techniques at home with those that only incorporated a few clinic-based sessions. Dosage may be additionally important in determining duration of the response. There is some evidence that biofeedback in combination with relaxation is more effective than either therapy alone – dating from the pioneering studies in this area (Benson et al. 1971; Patel 1973) to more recent investigations (McGrady, Olson, & Kroon 1995). Finally, as with most other types of therapies, adherence to treatment is essential for a successful outcome.

TRANSDERMAL ELECTRICAL NERVE STIMULATION

Biofeedback and relaxation techniques are widely used in the treatment of a variety of pathologies, but other psychophysiological techniques are more specifically applied to

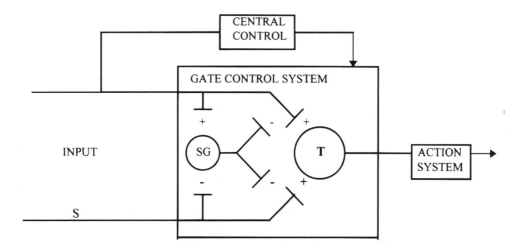

Figure 1. Schematic diagram of the gate control theory of pain. L, large-diameter fibers; S, small-diameter fibers; T, first central transmission cells; SG, substantia gelatinosa; −, inhibition; +, excitation. The L fibers increase and the S fibers decrease the SG inhibition on the afferent fiber terminals. Reprinted with permission from Melzack & Wall, "Pain mechanisms: A new theory," *Science,* vol. 150, pp. 971–9. Copyright 1965 American Association for the Advancement of Science.

particular conditions. One such example that has shown clinical promise is the use of transcutaneous electrical nerve stimulation (TENS) in the treatment of chronic pain conditions. TENS is a noninvasive, self-administered technique which involves electrical stimulation of the peripheral nervous system and which has proven to be an effective adjunct in the global treatment of pain conditions (Long 1991). For example, TENS has been found to be effective in reducing migraine headaches (Annal et al. 1992); in treating low back pain (Bourke 1994); in the treatment of acute oro-facial and various other forms of chronic and transient pain (Choudhury & Ffoulkes-Crabbe 1988); and for the relief of anginal pain (Mannheimer et al. 1986). TENS has been shown to reduce pain perception and also to increase pain thresholds (Johnson et al. 1991a; Johnson, Ashton, & Thompson 1991b). Although TENS probably contains a placebo component (Marchand et al. 1993), the procedure is more effective than placebo (Bourke 1994; Marchand et al. 1993) and no less effective than aspirin (Lundeberg 1984) in reducing pain.

The precise mechanism behind the effectiveness of the TENS procedure is still uncertain. However, the most probable explanation is one based on the "gate" theory of pain (Melzack & Wall 1965). This theory posits that portions of the CNS are uniquely involved in the experience of pain by operating a gatelike mechanism in the dorsal horn of the spinal column, which in turn modifies the sensation of pain. Nonpainful stimuli carried in large-diameter myelinated nerve fibers excite inhibitory interneurons in the substantia gelatinosa; these interneurons inhibit pain impulses by controlling the gate mechanism. Stimulation of small-diameter nociceptive afferents inhibits the afferent fiber terminals in the substantia gelatinosa, opens the gate, and allows the experience of pain (see Figure 1 for a schematic diagram). Thus, this central control mechanism is able to either facilitate or inhibit the flow of neural transmissions based on appraisals of the potentially painful experience. TENS selectively stimulates large afferent fibers using low-intensity, high-frequency stimula-

tion, thereby reducing the experience of pain (Wang, Mao, & Han 1992). The pain-reducing effects of TENS are not reversed by opiate antagonists, so the mechanism of action is not opiate-dependent (Freeman, Campbell, & Long 1983; Sjoland & Erikson 1979).

Although TENS has been found to be effective in reducing pain symptoms in various disorders, the level of obtained analgesic response is highly variable (Johnson et al. 1991b). For example, approximately one third of patients using TENS receive no benefits from the procedure or quickly become tolerant. Among those who initially respond, only one third continue to experience pain relief after two years (Bates & Nathan 1980). The mechanism by which patients become tolerant to TENS may be related to adaptation of the nervous system to the repetitive stimulation of TENS, ultimately decreasing the efficacy of the procedure (Pomeranz & Niznick 1987).

To increase both the number of those who benefit from TENS as well as the duration of benefits, several variations of the technique have been introduced. In addition to the conventional technique just described, an acupuncture-like variation and a brief, intense TENS procedure have been utilized, with variation primarily in the stimulation parameters used (Mannheimer & Lampe 1984; Ottoson & Lundeberg 1988). Brief, intense TENS consists of high-frequency stimulation applied for a short duration (Lander & Fowler-Kerry 1993), while acupuncture-like TENS consists of high-intensity, low-frequency pulses. Both variations on the conventional TENS technique have been found to be occasionally more efficacious (Eriksson, Sjolund, & Nielzen 1979). Some clinicians have chosen to use different patterns of pulse delivery or electrode sizes to help increase the efficacy of the TENS procedure. For example, increasing electrode size activates a larger number of large-diameter afferents, which in turn leads to a greater inhibition of nociceptive information from small-diameter afferents in the spinal cord and ultimately enhances the analgesic effects of TENS (Johnson et al. 1991b).

Clinically speaking, there are several types of TENS equipment on the market (Solomon & Guglielmo 1985) and several variations in TENS techniques (Hansson & Akblom 1983; Mannheimer & Carlsson 1979). Those patients who do not respond to a particular variation of TENS, or who develop tolerance to the procedure, may find that alternative frequencies and modes of stimulation are more effective (Johnson et al. 1991b). Because the effects of TENS are additive over time, patients should be instructed to use TENS repetitively over a short period of time to enhance its analgesic effects. Finally, although TENS is an effective pain-reducing procedure, efficacy is enhanced when it is included as one component of a more complete multidisciplinary pain management program (Marchand et al. 1993).

Disorders

HYPERTENSION

Hypertension refers to a sustained elevation in systolic and diastolic blood pressure, although the exact blood pressure level that should be considered to signify hypertension is somewhat arbitrary. In fact, the cardiovascular risks associated with blood pressure rise progressively over the range of pressure, with no clear precipitous rise at a given pressure. In addition, blood pressure varies widely with different activity levels, stress, posture, and dietary influences, and during sleep. In many cases, these elevations serve a homeostatic or adaptive role and thus do not have pathophysiological consequences, as in the case of acute bouts of exercise. However, in other cases the upward adjustments in blood pressure do not serve an apparent metabolic role and can therefore be considered excessive, relative to the needs of the organism. A diagnosis of hypertension is therefore dependent not only upon how the disease is defined but also on how well-controlled are a number of behavioral, environmental, and individual difference factors.

For a small percentage of those affected, hypertension is developed secondary to renal, endocrine, or congenital disorders. In otherwise healthy young women, secondary hypertension may also develop with the use of estrogen-containing oral contraceptives and during pregnancy. However, in over 90% of cases of hypertension in the United States, the origin of the disease is unknown; in such cases, the term "essential" hypertension is applied. The prevalence of the disease is widespread, with conservative estimates of about 50 million (15%) of Americans affected.

Hypertension is a progressive and self-accelerating disease; if untreated, it contributes significantly to the development of coronary heart disease, stroke, heart failure, and target organ damage and thus is a major factor contributing to cardiovascular pathology. For psychophysiologists and health psychologists, the relevance of hypertension lies in the abundant evidence showing that social, psychological, and behavioral factors likely affect the initiation, progression, and course of the disorder (Lawler & Cox 1985; Pickering & Gerin 1990).

Etiology and Assessment

Essential hypertension is one of the most well-researched disorders in all of psychophysiology. An extensive literature is replete with psychological and behavioral variables that (i) influence the blood pressure of both normotensives and hypertensives, (ii) may contribute to the initiation of hypertension, and (iii) can affect the progression of the pathophysiology of hypertension. Very early psychophysiological studies examined the impact of environmental stimuli, emotional states, and cognition on blood pressure control mechanisms. In fact, the first investigations in the arena of health psychology involved application of the basic psychophysiological principles to understanding blood pressure control in hypertension.

There are three major and overlapping goals of health psychology when applying psychophysiological principles to the study of hypertension and blood pressure control. The first goal is to index the pattern of physiological and behavioral responses to various stimuli (among healthy normotensives and hypertensives) for the identification of *markers* or *risk factors* for sustained essential hypertension. From a clinical standpoint, these studies are concerned with early identification of those who display particular response patterns; this will presumably aid in the early treatment of the disorder. Second, there has been a substantial effort to record physiologic patterns to various environmental stimuli – among hypertensives and those at risk for hypertension – in order to identify the *mechanisms* by which these influences are implicated in the development and progress of the disease. These investigations have also aided in the enhanced understanding of the role of social, emotional, and gross behavioral influences on blood pressure control. Third, investigations abound of the impact of various environmental stimuli on blood pressure among both normotensives and hypertensives, and these should help develop behavioral approaches to the *treatment* of the disorder. The first two of these goals are covered in the following section; biobehavioral treatment approaches are discussed in a subsequent section.

The diagnosis of essential hypertension is (by definition) a diagnosis of exclusion, as the origin of the disease is not known. In part for this reason, the group of individuals for whom such a diagnosis has been made is generally heterogeneous with respect to mechanisms related to the initiation of the disease, effective treatment of the disorder, and development of compensatory adjustments that occur as a consequence of sustained high blood pressure. In fact, individual differences in these compensatory adjustments (in the later stages of the disease) are what make understanding the mechanisms responsible for initiation of (early) hypertension difficult. Thus, there is considerable utility in studying the very earliest stages of hypertension, particularly with regard to psychological influences on disease progression.

Many investigations have employed the technique of monitoring blood pressure reactivity among apparently healthy individuals who are at elevated risk for future development of hypertension. For example, numerous investigations of normotensive offspring of hypertensive parents show that these healthy normotensive individuals show generally higher blood pressure and heart rate reactivity to stress when compared with normotensive offspring of normotensive parents (Fredikson & Matthews 1990). Other presumably high-risk groups – such as those with a family history of cardiovascular disease, borderline hypertensives, and healthy young people with mildly elevated blood pressure – have been shown to have exaggerated cardiovascular and/or neuroendocrine reactivity to acute psychological stress (Stoney & Matthews 1988). In some cases, exaggerated blood pressure responsivity to alpha-adrenergically mediated stimuli among healthy individuals predicted subsequent development of sustained hypertension. Because hyperreactivity among high-risk or borderline hypertensives is often reduced or eliminated after pretreatment with adrenergic blockade, the early phase of hypertension is frequently considered to be characterized by increased sympathetic contributions to cardiac response (Langer et al. 1985). However, a more circumscribed literature, including both pharmacological manipulation and behavioral studies, has specifically examined parasympathetic contributions to the hyperkinetic state characterizing some borderline hypertensive patients. These studies indicated diminished cardiac parasympathetic tone among borderline and essential hypertensives, due either to impaired vagal tone alone or to dysfunctional cardiac sympathetic–vagal interactions (Grossman, Brinkman, & de Vries 1992). Taken together, these disparate findings suggest that the early phase of hypertension cannot be uniformly characterized; it may be a function of exaggerated sympathetic nervous reactivity, impaired vagal tone, or dysfunction in central nervous system integration of autonomic outflow.

Although the mechanisms related to the development of essential hypertension are not yet clear, psychophysiological investigations such as these have identified several pathophysiological candidates. These include numerous investigations of various stress hormones and neurotransmitters, particularly the opioid peptides. For example, endogenous opiates have hypotensive actions, are known to modulate cardiovascular responses to physical and psychological stress, and assist in baroreflex control of blood pressure (McCubbin, Surwit, & Williams 1985). Moreover, the relaxation-induced attenuated blood pressure reactivity to stress among borderline hypertensive men is mediated in part by endogenous opioid mechanisms (McCubbin et al. 1996). These and related data further advance the notion that opioid mechanisms are under some degree of behavioral control and thus may be of substantial clinical utility in addressing stress-associated disorders of the cardiovascular system.

Treatment

Many of the behavioral treatment modalities for hypertension focus on altering the patterns of sympathetic nervous system activation, either at rest or in response to behavioral stimuli. Although the specifics of these treatments vary with regard to implementation, clinical utility, and ease of use, they all share the common goal of altering (either directly or indirectly) the typical physiological responses to stimuli in order to diminish blood pressure. The implicit assumption is that clinically improved control of blood pressure regulatory mechanisms will carry over into less structured environments and so lessen the likelihood of further pathophysiology.

The success of relaxation techniques for the treatment of hypertension has been somewhat variable, which is due at least in part to the different patient populations examined and the generally diverse methods used. The most recent reports are generally equivocal regarding evidence for the efficacy of these behavioral treatments in hypertension. In a longitudinal, randomized clinical trial designed to test the efficacy of nonpharmacologic treatment of mild diastolic hypertension, a stress management arm was included in the intervention (Group 1992). Stress management therapy included a combination of relaxation, mental imagery, and managing perceptions of stress. In general, little success was found for these stress management techniques in reducing either systolic or diastolic blood pressure, although adherence to the training was not assessed and the amount of training was probably suboptimal. Two recent reviews concluded that very limited support is available for the notion that standard relaxation therapy results in clinically significant declines in blood pressure among hypertensive patients (Jacob et al. 1991; Linden & Chambers 1994).

The success of direct biofeedback or biofeedback-assisted relaxation has shown somewhat more promise as a therapeutic technique in treating hypertension. In general, both biofeedback and biofeedback-assisted relaxation training over the course of several sessions results in initial reductions in diastolic (but not systolic) blood pressure among hypertensive patients, and it may increase baroreceptor sensitivity (Steptoe & Sawada 1989). However, many fewer investigations have been able to demonstrate sustained control of blood pressure. There are exceptions:

among mildly hypertensive patients, sustained reductions in stress-induced systolic and diastolic blood pressure were apparent six months after training (Paran, Amir, & Yaniv 1996). Thermal biofeedback to increase hand or foot warming had some initial success among hypertensives, but this was not sustained in subsequent follow-up studies among this investigative team (Blanchard et al. 1996).

In addition to strategies designed to reduce physiological arousal, a number of cognitive coping strategies have been experimentally employed to alter subjects' appraisals of potentially threatening situations. Although these strategies have typically measured only heart rate responses to stress and have generally been employed in healthy, normotensive individuals, they have been instructive in increasing our awareness of the role of cognition on blood pressure control mechanisms. In one set of studies, participants were taught the strategy of redefining an aversive stimulus. For example, Holmes and Houston (1974) showed that thinking about a potential shock threat as a "different" rather than a "painful" sensation resulted in lower heart rate reactivity to that threat. These data are similar to studies that have demonstrated that diverting one's attention from potentially painful stimuli enhances coping with the threat, increases pain tolerance, and also diminishes heart rate responsivity to that threat (Bloom et al. 1977; Grimm & Kanfer 1976). Other strategies – such as increased availability of social support, various cognitive belief systems, and teaching the use of positive self-statements, stress denial, and detachment – have also been tested in experimental models (Ahles, Blanchard, & Leventhal 1983; Kamarck, Manuck, & Jennings 1990; Tomaka & Blascovich 1994; Uchino, Cacioppo, & Kiecolt-Glaser 1996). Each has found clinical utility as an effective coping strategy for stress management and many have also been shown to reduce cardiovascular (primarily heart rate) reactivity to stress. For hypertensive individuals, however, the efficacy of these cognitive coping strategies in reducing blood pressure responses to situational stressors is less well investigated.

PAIN

Pain accounts for more than 80% of all physician visits, affects over 50 million Americans, and costs over $70 billion in health care costs and lost productivity annually in the United States alone (Gatchel & Turk 1996). Chronic pain often leads not only to substantial physical and economic costs but to emotional and psychological costs as well. Feelings of helplessness, hopelessness, despair, and depression are commonly experienced by chronic pain sufferers – and also by those who care for the pain patient.

Because persistent pain is not solely a physical phenomenon but also a psychological, emotional, interpersonal, and financial one, the traditional biomedical model of pain is insufficient for either assessing intractable pain or designing effective treatment strategies. Biological and physical factors cannot completely account for reported symptoms of pain. For example, there is frequent discordance between physical pathology or damage and the experience of pain (Melzack & Wall 1965). Despite this, traditional medicine continues to adhere to this unidimensional construct of pain by focusing solely on correcting the biological dysfunction or abnormality (Turk 1996).

In response to the unidimensional biomedical model of pain, Melzack and Wall (1965) developed the *gate control* theory of pain (described previously). This theory represents the first attempt to integrate both psychological and physiological factors in understanding pain. By establishing the role of a central nervous system mechanism in nociceptive processing and perception, this theory provides a physiological basis for the role of psychological factors in chronic pain. It also integrates sensory, affective, cognitive, and ultimately behavioral components into a model explaining the experience of pain (Turk 1996). Although there have been challenges and criticisms (Nathan 1976), the gate control theory has proven to be remarkably resilient and has demonstrated the importance of viewing pain more broadly than is possible under the biomedical model. Therefore, the evidence suggests that, in order to gain a more comprehensive understanding of pain, we must examine the phenomenon from a biopsychosocial perspective.

Despite the potential benefits that gate control theory may have for advancing our knowledge and understanding of chronic pain, much of the existing psychophysiological research on chronic pain has failed to fully incorporate psychological, behavioral, or social factors in their investigations (see Flor & Turk 1989). This lack of attention to current theoretical models and consequent methodological flaws has inevitably hindered progress in conceptualizing the psychophysiology of chronic pain.

Early psychophysiological research relied upon general activation models such as Selye's general adaptation syndrome. However, these theories fail to explain why specific body sites or systems are affected or why there exist individual differences in psychophysiological responding. This has led to the development of specificity models – including individual response specificity, stimulus response specificity, symptom specificity, and motivational response specificity (Ax 1964; Flor & Turk 1989; Lacey & Lacey 1958; Malmo & Shagass 1949) – in attempts to explain idiosyncratic psychophysiological responses and the development of different psychophysiological disorders, including chronic pain. For example, Flor and her colleagues (Flor & Turk 1989) have elegantly developed and applied the work of Malmo (1975) to understanding patterns of chronic pain. Her model is based on the essential notion that individuals with chronic localized musculoskeletal pain have significantly greater stress-induced muscle tension and pain severity ratings at the site of injury but not at other sites (Burns et al. 1997; Flor & Turk 1989). Even though other models of response pattern specificity could be considered when conducting psychophysiological research into such a complex phenomenon as chronic pain, in practice most psychophysiological clinical research has not taken such a comprehensive approach to examining pain conditions.

Three common chronic pain conditions (rheumatoid arthritis, tension and migraine headaches, and temporomandibular joint disorder) will be described next. Again, the discussion of these conditions is not meant to represent an exhaustive account of psychophysiology in the assessment and treatment of pain but is designed rather to highlight representative issues in pain conditions that are particularly relevant to health psychology. Methodological and theoretical limitations on the psychological and physiological factors involved in chronic pain conditions are apparent throughout the research in this area. For example, the chronicity of pain engenders antecedent psychological consequences that make causal inferences difficult. A more rigorous examination of the psychophysiological antecedents and consequences of chronic pain would assist in elucidating the physiological patterns involved in chronic pain conditions.

RHEUMATOID ARTHRITIS

Rheumatoid arthritis (RA) is a chronic systemic inflammatory disorder that is marked by pain (often debilitating) and deterioration of peripheral joints. The most commonly affected joints are those of the feet, hands, and wrist – typically in a bilateral and symmetric manner. However, the effects of rheumatoid arthritis are not restricted to the joints; they can be manifest through other systemic and nonspecific changes. For example, disfiguring rheumatoid nodules occur in 10%–15% of patients, as do inflammatory responses in vascular, cardiac, pulmonary, muscular, and ocular tissue. Additional symptoms accompanying rheumatoid arthritis may include fever, fatigue, and sleep disturbances (Young 1993).

Approximately 1% of the general population is affected with rheumatoid arthritis, with women being three times more likely than men to contract this disorder. The disease most commonly develops between the ages of 20 and 50; those at the older end of this age range are at greater risk for developing rheumatoid arthritis than those at the younger end (Young 1993). The impact of this disorder is felt not only physically but emotionally, interpersonally, and economically as well. For example, 60% of those with the disorder become unable to work and earn substantially less income than those without arthritis (Mitchell, Burkhauser, & Pincus 1988).

Etiology and Assessment

The precise etiological mechanism behind rheumatoid arthritis is still unknown. Because the RA lesions consist of cellular components of the immune system, such as macrophages and T-cells, it is thought that the disorder may result from a foreign antigen that targets the synovia and ultimately results in a chronic immune response (Liao & Haynes 1995). Much of the current research focuses on genetic aspects of the disease and on understanding which cytokines and inflammatory mediators are produced at the disease site (Goronzy & Weyand 1995). It is now recognized that the migration of inflammatory cells into the tissue has etiological significance. Therefore, it is likely that rheumatoid arthritis is an antigen-driven and thus a T-cell–mediated disease (Harris 1990; Weyand & Goronzy 1997). However, nonimmune tissues and mechanisms should also be taken into consideration when trying to understand this complex disorder, owing to the (limited) evidence that they may also play a role in the etiology of rheumatoid arthritis. Furthermore, there is compelling evidence to suggest that there may be a genetic link behind this disease (Weyand & Goronzy 1997). Despite promising models (using arthritis-susceptible rats) that suggest some common central nervous system pathways for inflammatory and emotional responsivity (Sternberg 1995), quite limited psychophysiologically based research on humans has targeted the assessment and etiology of rheumatoid arthritis as a research focus.

Treatment

Because the exact etiological mechanism of rheumatoid arthritis is still uncertain, medical interventions are predominantly palliative in nature, emphasizing pain relief or pain management. Some of the most common psychophysiological techniques used in the treatment of rheumatoid arthritis are relaxation techniques (progressive muscle relaxation, controlled breathing, visual imagery) and both electromyographic and thermal biofeedback, which have proven to be effective in reducing pain symptoms in rheumatoid arthritis patients. For example, relaxation and temperature biofeedback have been reported to reliably decrease pain, improve joint functional ability, and improve sleep (Achterberg, McGraw, & Lawlis 1981). In a treatment program incorporating imagery and temperature biofeedback, patients experienced significantly decreased pain and stiffness and improved overall condition (Mitchell 1986). In another example incorporating relaxation, temperature biofeedback, and cognitive-behavioral treatment techniques, Bradley et al. (1987) found decreased pain, pain behaviors, anxiety, and objective and subjective ratings of disease activity. These responses are not specific to rheumatoid arthritis and are typical of the general relaxation response. More specific understanding of the process involved in the development of rheumatoid arthritis will result in more effective psychophysiologic treatment strategies.

HEADACHE

Headache is one of the most common ailments reported today, with over 90% of the United States population reporting the experience of headache at least once per year. Based on telephone survey data, 57.1% of males and 76.5% of females reported experiencing a headache during the four weeks prior to interview (Linet et al. 1989). Lifetime prevalence rates for episodic or chronic tension headache have been estimated at 88% for women, 69% for men, and an overall 78% when both sexes are combined (Rasmussen et al. 1991). Migraine headaches are experienced more frequently by women than by men; a survey of over 20,000 men and women in the United States (Stewart et al. 1992) showed that 17.6% of women and 5.7% of men experience one or more migraine headaches per year, with those between the ages of 35 and 45 the most frequently and seriously affected.

Variability in both the type and severity of headache is substantial. For example, the International Headache Society (IHS 1988) has described over 100 different types of headaches that vary with regard to etiology, symptomatology, and progression. The two most common types of headaches are migraine (with and without aura) and tension headaches.

Migraine headaches without aura are idiopathic, recurring disorders that may last up to three days and involve pulsating, unilateral pain of moderate to severe intensity. This type of headache is often aggravated or precipitated by physical activity, stress, and certain environmental influences (IHS 1988). Migraine without aura may or may not be associated with nausea, photophobia, and phonophobia. In contrast, migraine headache with aura may occasionally occur without pain (IHS 1988). This latter disorder, typically with nausea and photophobia, usually follows neurological aura symptoms that have been found to be localized over the cerebral cortex or brainstem.

Tension headaches are recurrent headaches that can last for as little as a few minutes to as long as a few days. The pain is typically described as pressing or tightening in quality, bilateral in location, and not exacerbated by physical activity, with varying degrees of intensity reported. Unlike with migraine, nausea is absent, although the pain may worsen with exposure to light and/or noise (IHS 1988).

Headache severity can vary greatly among those afflicted, ranging from mild (managed by over-the-counter analgesics) to totally disabling. Over 11 million individuals in the United States experience some level of disability due to headache (Stewart et al. 1992); for some unfortunate individuals, headaches become totally disabling. Despite the significant number of individuals affected by headaches and despite the physical, psychological, and economic costs associated with them, conclusive clarification regarding the psychophysiological mechanisms behind headache has been elusive.

Etiology and Assessment

The prime mechanism underlying migraine headache has traditionally been thought to be vascular in nature; specifically, abnormal vascular activity of the cranial arteries has been proposed (Wolff 1963). Several early psychophysiological studies provided some support for this hypothesis. For example, when migraine sufferers were administered a vasoconstrictor during a migraine attack, they subsequently experienced a decrease in blood volume pulse and a concurrent decrease in subjective headache intensity (Wolff 1963). However, research examining the validity of this hypothesized vascular mechanism has yielded inconsistent and inconclusive findings. For example, whereas some studies have discovered abnormalities of temporal blood flow (Morley 1985), higher heart rate (Drummond 1982), and elevated diastolic blood pressure (Drummond 1982) among individuals suffering from migraines relative to healthy controls, other studies have failed to find such differences in these cardiovascular measures (Arena 1985; Thompson & Adams 1984).

Such inconsistencies have also been found in studies that have examined individuals during active headache versus headache-free periods (Thompson & Adams 1984) and those that induced stress experimentally and examined the subsequent recovery period (Andrasik 1982; Gannon et al. 1981). Amongst these studies, some investigators found cerebrovasoconstriction (as measured by blood volume pulse recordings) to be associated with migraine (Gannon et al. 1981); others found no differences in cerebral blood flow activity among migraine, muscle contraction, and normal subjects (Andrasik 1982; Thompson & Adams 1984). Similarly, some investigators (Bakal & Kaganov 1977; Kroner-Herwig et al. 1988) found no differences in blood volume pulse patterns between migraine and muscle contraction subjects, whereas others (Arena 1985; Gannon et al. 1981), who found no differences while at rest, did find elevated blood volume pulse during recovery.

Some investigators have outwardly challenged the role of vasodilation as the primary cause of pain in migraine patients (Olesen et al. 1990). These investigators found changes in cerebral blood flow to be independent of subjects' experience of pain. This observation led to the conclusion that increased cerebral blood flow and migraine pain are not directly related, although there is considerable debate regarding this conclusion (McGrady et al. 1994).

Migraine and tension headaches frequently become altered during the experience of the pain, and it is not uncommon for migraine pain to become more like tension headache pain and vice versa. Olesen (1991) proposed a model suggesting that the experience of all types of headache pain is the result of the summed effects of perivascular, supraspinal, and myofascial inputs. With migraine headaches, the primary nociception is vascular, whereas in tension headaches it is most commonly myofascial. However, the importance of the three inputs (perivascular, supraspinal, and myofascial) may vary between patients and even within the same individual over time. Much of the complexity of migraine and tension headaches can be accommodated with this relatively new model.

A novel approach to studying the specific vascular aspect of headaches was reported by Martins and colleagues (1993). Patients who have undergone intracranial endovascular procedures for the treatment of arteriovenous malformations or aneurism often developed headaches that are well defined and describe consistent patterns. During such procedures, segmental vascular stimulation is accomplished using either a balloon inflation technique or the injection of embolic material (Nichols et al. 1990). The headaches occurred suddenly but were of short duration; they were nonthrobbing, with a unilateral focal localization. Martins et al. (1993) concluded that these headaches were most likely directly attributable to the stimulation of the arterial wall at the site of the arterial occlusion. Thus, although irritation of the vascular wall was apparently responsible for producing the headaches, the resulting headaches were quite different in symptomatology from migraine headaches, which are thought to have at least a partly vascular origin. Even in migraine patients who underwent the procedure, the resulting headaches did not resemble migraines. The authors suggest that these results provide evidence against a purely vascular origin of migraine attacks. Research incorporating more migraineurs will be necessary for a more comprehensive understanding of the complex vascular aspects of migraine headaches.

Etiological processes for tension headaches are typically thought to differ from those for migraine headaches. For example, it has traditionally been asserted that tension headaches are related to sustained contraction in cranial and neck muscles (Bakal 1975; Haynes 1981). However, as in the case of migraine headache, the psychophysiological mechanisms behind tension headache are elusive. For example, investigations have compared muscle tension differences between tension headache sufferers, migraine patients, and controls during rest. Although some studies have found support for the sustained contraction hypothesis in the form of elevated frontal electromyographic muscle tension (Murphy & Lehrer 1990; Poziak-Patweica 1976; Vaughn, Pall, & Haynes 1977), others have failed to find differences in electromyographic frontal muscle activity among tension, vascular, or headache-free subjects (Flor & Turk 1989; Gannon et al. 1981; Martin & Mathews 1978). During stress, however, there is somewhat more consistent evidence that tension headache sufferers exhibit exaggerated electromyographic increases (Flor & Turk 1989). Support for this hypothesis comes from several studies finding greater frontalis and temporal electromyogram increases in response to a personally relevant stressor among headache sufferers. However, some research has failed to find differences in electromyogram response to stress between tension headache and nonheadache subjects (Martin & Mathews 1978). Thus, there is not clear universal support for the symptom specificity model for headache pain.

Another hypothesized mechanism of tension headache postulates a vascular etiology. Tunis and Wolff (1953, 1954) found that tension headache subjects had greater levels of vasoconstriction than normal subjects, and that these elevated levels coincided with headache-active and not headache-free periods. These investigators used this observation as a basis for the hypothesis that prolonged muscle contraction led to restricted blood supply to the muscles. Other investigations (Ostfeld, Reis, & Wolff 1957; Wolff 1963) yielded similar results, while still others have suggested that tension headaches may be associated with localized cephalic vasodilation rather than vasoconstriction (Martin & Mathews 1978; Onel, Friedman, & Grossman 1961). Generally, abnormal blood flow patterns in the cerebral vessels of tension headache sufferers are apparent, implicating an intracranial vascular mechanism (Wallasch 1992).

Further support for the role of vascular factors in tension headache is provided by evidence that headache subjects – whether tension, migraine, or mixed – have distended temporal arteries between pressure pulses (relative to controls) that appear to be driven by blood pressure (Martin, Marie, & Nathan 1992). Between pulses, the temporal arteries of headache sufferers did not return to the same diameter as those of the nonheadache controls, and active headache subjects had consistently dilated arteries between pressure pulses when compared with headache-free controls.

Some cite practical methodological considerations – such as sample characteristics or the reliability and validity of psychophysiological measurements (Blanchard & Andrasik 1982) – as reasons why some research supports a vascular mechanism while other research supports a muscular component, but the inconsistencies in the literature on tension headache may more substantially reflect the complexity of the headache phenomenon. Headache has proven to be an especially difficult ailment to assess and diagnose. Such limitations have undoubtedly hindered the ability of researchers to obtain clear answers regarding the etiological mechanisms behind headaches. With such great variation in type and severity, our diagnostic category of "tension headache" may actually include a rather heterogenous collection of headaches. Therefore, results that fail to support the role of muscular mechanisms (or that appear to support the role of vascular mechanisms) behind tension headaches may reflect the variation in headache type or severity rather than the relative validity of the proposed mechanisms. For example, in less complex muscular disorders such as temporomandibular disorder and chronic low back pain, there is greater support for the symptom-specificity hypothesis (Flor et al. 1991). Therefore, there may be a subset of tension headache sufferers who tend to demonstrate exaggerated electromyographic responses to stress and still another subset whose members usually exhibit atypical vascular responses. Or perhaps, as suggested by the myofascial-supraspinal-vascular model of tension headaches proposed by Olesen et al. (1990), muscular and vascular components may both be involved in tension headaches or at least in a subset of them.

Practical considerations of methodology, such as adequate acclimation periods and appropriate control groups (Blanchard & Andrasik 1982), may help lead to conclusive findings. However, more conceptual issues – such as the diagnostic complexity of headache and decisions as to which muscle beds to assess or which psychophysiological systems to monitor – must first be addressed. For example, some researchers have suggested that the neck muscles may be more appropriate for assessing electromyographic responses than the typically used frontalis region (Gannon et al. 1987). It has also been suggested that an idiographic approach, which analyzes the specific antecedent and enduring facets of headache and designs specific treatment strategies that meet the needs of each individual, may be a more effective approach to diagnosing and treating headache than the nomothetic approaches typically used (Biondi & Portuesi 1994). Another methodological issue involves the ability to accurately establish cause–effect directionality with regard to muscular and vascular activity or changes. Although it is tempting to view such muscular or vascular activity as etiological factors in headache, the possibility remains that a third mediating variable or variables, such as headache state, may actually *cause* differences in psychophysiological variables (Haynes 1983). Haynes and colleagues proposed that causal pathways can only be established through longitudinal studies that accurately assess psychophysiological indices prior to, during, and after a headache.

Treatment

The most common psychophysiological treatment approaches for migraine headaches involve a combination of thermal biofeedback and relaxation training (Arena & Blanchard 1996). These techniques have proven effective in helping approximately 50% of individuals reach significant clinical improvement in headache activity (Blanchard et al. 1985, 1990). Thermal biofeedback as a treatment strategy for migraine headache has been employed for the past 25 years (Sargent, Green, & Walters 1972). During this technique, patients are instructed to warm their fingers through digital vasodilation while receiving relatively immediate sensory feedback (Arena & Blanchard 1996). Like the case of electromyographic (EMG) biofeedback in the treatment of tension headache, the precise mechanism that makes thermal biofeedback an effective treatment for migraine headaches is unclear (Hatch 1993). The exact nature of the relationship between vasodilation of the blood vessels in the periphery and the reduction of migraine pain warrants further investigation. Some have speculated that the treatment effects associated with thermal biofeedback may be due to a subsequent reduction in sympathetic activity, the induction of a global relaxation response, or nonspecific effects on other biochemical processes that may contribute to the development of headache (Arena & Blanchard 1996; Hatch 1993).

As with migraine headache, EMG biofeedback and relaxation training (or a combination of the two) are typically used in the treatment of tension headache, with about the same level of efficacy. For example, results of several studies have shown these techniques to be more effective than placebo control, with efficacy estimates for both EMG biofeedback and relaxation training showing approximately 50% of patients clinically improved (Andrasik & Blanchard 1987; Blanchard 1992; Holroyd & Penzien 1986).

The more controversial issue regarding the treatment methods of biofeedback and relaxation training is not if they work but rather *how* they work. In theory, these techniques work by making patients aware of muscle tension and teaching them how to relax painful muscles; however, as our discussion has indicated, the role of muscle hyperactivity in tension headaches is certainly debatable (Hatch 1993). Inconsistent associations between muscle activity and headache pain raise further doubt that muscle tension is the precise mechanism through which biofeedback and relaxation training alleviate tension headache pain (Nuechterlein & Holroyd 1980). Furthermore, the effectiveness of electromyographic biofeedback and relaxation therapy in treating tension headaches appears to involve a large cognitive component (Blanchard et al. 1993), because some studies find that significant improvement in symptoms is more a function of verbal feedback from the experimenter regarding success at the biofeedback or relaxation strategies and less a function of the subject's actual success at mastering the techniques.

TEMPOROMANDIBULAR JOINT DISORDER

Temporomandibular joint disorder (TMD) is a common psychophysiological disorder of the neuromuscular system. Those who suffer from TMD often experience a dull, muscular ache in the jaw region that worsens with extended use of those muscles. Pain can also be felt at the base of the skull, the temporomandibular joint (TMJ), and the masseter and temporalis muscles (McNeill et al. 1990). Individuals with TMD often have trouble opening or closing their jaw, and such action is often accompanied by a "click" or popping sound in the TMJ (Griffiths 1983). In addition, patients sometimes report that their bite feels out of alignment. The pain associated with TMD is often dispersed and can affect the ear canal, neck, supraorbital area, temporal areas, occiputs, sinuses, or teeth. It can also cause a range of problems such as headache, other fascial pains, earache, dizziness, ringing in the ears, or pain in the neck, shoulder, and upper and lower back (Chase, Hendler, & Kraus 1988; Glaros & Glass 1993). The pain associated with TMD is typically experienced in a cyclic nature, with pain coinciding with flare-ups in the masticatory muscles (Dworkin et al. 1994).

Estimates of the prevalence of TMD vary widely owing to differences in how this disorder is specifically defined and how estimates are collected. For example, median prevalence rates of TMD diagnosis among population-based studies have been as high as 50%–60% (Gale 1992; Glaros & Glass 1993; Okeson 1989). However, the median prevalence rate drops to about 32% (with a range of 16%–59%) when reported symptoms of TMD are used as the criterion (Glaros & Glass 1993). When incapacitating pain or dysfunction are the diagnostic criteria used, prevalence rates drop to between 3% and 5% (De Kanter et al. 1992; Dworkin et al. 1990; Glaros & Glass 1993; Schiffman et al. 1990). Hence, there is compelling evidence that many individuals in the general population who meet clinical criteria for TMD are coping with their symptoms without the assistance of health-care professionals. TMD is reported in women about three to four times as often as in men. This gender difference may be a function of reporting bias rather than biological influences (Bush et al. 1993), because women with the disorder are more apt than men to seek treatment (Chase et al. 1988). Alternatively, the gender difference may be a function of differences in circulating estrogens; the prevalence of TMD is highest in premenopausal women, in women taking oral contraceptives, and in postmenopausal women using estrogen replacement therapy (Stohler 1997).

Etiology and Assessment

Research examining the physical components of TMD has revealed that TMD can be subclassified into muscle disorders, intracapsular derangements, and degenerative arthritic changes of the TMJ (Dworkin & LeResche 1992; Maixner et al. 1995). Although some patients may report symptoms that suggest the pain is originating predominantly from either the joint (i.e. arthralgia) or the muscles (i.e. myalgia), most patients report a combination of these symptoms (Dworkin & LeResche 1992). Schiffman and colleagues (1990) report that approximately 23% of TMD patients have muscle disorders, 19% have either internal derangements or degenerative changes in the TMJ, and 27% have combined muscle–joint disorder. In addition to degenerative or arthritic changes in the TMJ, several other factors – such as infectious processes; hormonal, nutritional, and metabolic conditions; and vascular problems – can predispose an individual to TMD (Glaros & Glass 1993).

According to the psychophysiological model of TMD (Laskin 1969), the pain associated with this disorder is primarily due to masticatory muscle spasms that result from muscle fatigue. This muscle fatigue is thought to be typically and primarily caused by maladaptive tension-relieving behaviors such as clenching. Theoretically, chronic muscle fatigue eventually leads to organic changes such as occlusal disharmonies (poor alignment within the jaw), degenerative arthritis, and contracture (abnormal shortening of the muscle or tendon). These organic changes may subsequently perpetuate the TMD.

Consistent with this model is the principle of response stereotypy (Lacey & Lacey 1958; Malmo & Shagass 1949), which would predict that individuals tend to demonstrate a consistent physiological response pattern to stress over time. Those who experience particularly strong muscular reactions (specifically in their head, neck, and jaw regions) are those most likely to develop TMD. In fact, several studies have demonstrated elevated baseline and enhanced EMG responses to various environmental stressors in TMD patients relative to controls (Dahlstrom et al. 1985; Kapel, Glaros, & McGlynn 1989). For example, in support of the principle of physiological response stereotypy in TMD patients, Flor and colleagues (1991) found that TMD subjects showed significant increases in right masseter electromyogram levels, as well as trends for significant increases in left masseter electromyogram levels, during both neutral and stressful images when compared with healthy subjects and those with chronic low back pain. In another example, individuals with myofascial pain and dysfunction had higher resting electromyogram levels and showed lower heart rate and higher frontalis EMG responses to stressors than did controls (Kapel et al. 1989).

However, not all studies have found results that are consistent with this principle of response stereotypy. For example, some studies have found no differences between TMD individuals and healthy controls with regard to EMG levels either at baseline or in response to experimentally induced stressors (Intrieri, Jones, & Alcorn 1994; Katz et al. 1989). Such discrepancies in the literature may be due to different diagnostic criteria used when selecting subjects, the types of stressors used, and other methodological and statistical considerations (Intrieri et al. 1994).

More recent research has suggested that TMD patients are more sensitive to noxious stimuli than healthy controls (Maixner et al. 1995). These researchers used a submaximal effort tourniquet procedure to produce ischemic muscle pain. Results demonstrated that TMD patients had significantly lower thermal pain threshold, ischemic pain threshold, and ischemic pain tolerance values. (It should be noted that this pain sensitivity was observed at a site other than the head and neck region.) These results were used as support for the position that TMD is a psychophysiological disorder that involves central nervous system (CNS) pain regulatory systems, which consequently leads to maladaptive emotional, physiological, and neuroendocrine responses to emotional and physical stressors. As further evidence for this view, Maixner and colleagues (1995) cited findings that 70%–80% of TMD patients suffer from other psychophysiological disorders such as ulcers, migraine headaches, lower back pain, asthma, or dermatitis (Laskin 1969; Rugh & Solberg 1976). Other researchers have also found TMD individuals to have lower finger pressure and lower electric pain thresholds than control subjects (Malow, Grimm, & Olsson 1980).

The enhanced pain sensitivity found in TMD patients may be indicative of alterations in how the CNS processes nociceptive information (Maixner et al. 1995). Although the specific CNS regions involved in these alterations have not been identified, it has been proposed that the ascending reticular activation system may be involved. The reticular activation system is involved in the regulation of sensory perception, emotional responses, arousal, endocrine responses, somatomotor output, and autonomic reactivity to environmental stimuli (Steriade & Llinas 1988; Whitsel et al. 1990). Disinhibition of this system could lead to the enhanced pain sensitivity and the maladaptive psychological, sensory, motor, autonomic, and neuroendocrine changes found in TMD patients. Such disinhibition may occur as a function of baroreflex or opioid malfunctioning or of impaired regulation of nociception (Maixner et al. 1995; Olson 1980). Although highly speculative, the focus of pain in the head and neck regions of TMD patients may reflect the high density of sensory input to the somatosensory system found in the head and neck relative to other areas of the body (Maixner et al. 1995). More research is needed to determine the exact nature of the relationship between individuals' pain sensitivity and their susceptibility to developing TMD and other related disorders.

Treatment

Individuals with TMD often engage in parafunctional behaviors such as clenching and grinding of their teeth, which can either exacerbate or initiate TMD symptoms (Katz et al. 1989). Psychophysiological monitoring devices, which make the individual aware of these behaviors, have been used to help reduce their occurrence. Although the devices presently available for ambulatory EMG monitoring have not yet reached adequate levels of sensitivity or specificity, some devices have been used to detect nocturnal bouts of clenching and grinding. When these devices detect EMG activity reflective of clenching or grinding, the individual is awoken by an alarm. Although such devices have been shown to be effective in reducing incidents of clenching or grinding, further refinements and careful documentation of their effectiveness are needed (Cassisi, McGlynn, & Belles 1987).

The most common psychophysiological approaches used in the treatment of TMD are EMG biofeedback, relaxation training, or a combination of these two techniques. Electromyogram biofeedback is typically focused around the masseter, temporalis, or frontalis muscular regions. Results of several studies indicate that EMG biofeedback is an effective treatment technique for TMD (Dahlstrom et al. 1985; Dalen et al. 1986). Such biofeedback has been shown to be as effective as dental splints, which are used to decrease parafunctional behaviors such as clenching or

grinding (Crockett et al. 1986; Dahlstrom, Carlsson, & Carlsson 1982). There is also some evidence that the treatment gains following EMG biofeedback are maintained after one year following treatment (Dahlstrom & Carlsson 1984).

As with EMG biofeedback treatment of tension headaches, the precise mechanism by which biofeedback alleviates TMD symptoms is not clearly understood. One hypothesized mechanism is that biofeedback effectively reduces EMG activity in the facial or jaw muscles, which subsequently leads to a reduction in pain sensation (Glaros & Glass 1993). However, there is some evidence demonstrating that there is not always a direct correspondence between EMG activity and a subject's experience of pain (Burdette & Gale 1988; Dahlstrom & Carlsson 1984).

Such findings have prompted alternative explanations for the effectiveness of EMG biofeedback. One such explanation is that this technique instructs individuals in the use of general relaxation and/or adaptive coping skills (Glaros & Glass 1993). It has also been proposed that biofeedback may simply increase an individual's awareness of elevated tension levels and maladaptive parafunctional behaviors such as clenching. Such awareness may be sufficient to enable the individual to cease such behavior and potentially alleviate the TMD symptoms (Dalen et al. 1986).

INSOMNIA

Insomnia is the most common sleep disorder experienced in this and most Westernized countries, with one-year prevalence estimates for chronic insomnia of 15%–20% and lifetime prevalence rates for transient insomnia as high as 40%. Insomnia is essentially a subjective assessment of disturbed sleep; it can include difficulty in falling asleep, inability to maintain sleep because of frequent awakenings, and assessment of poor sleep quality. Because insomnia is defined by subjective experiences of sleep difficulty, the consequences are usually pervasive and affect most aspects of daily living, leading to irritability, exhaustion, anxiety, and somatic complaints.

Assessment and Etiology

Insomnia may result from specific organic disease, psychiatric disorders, environmental factors, and drug use or abuse. However, roughly one quarter of all cases of insomnia have no identified etiology and may be clinically referred to as psychophysiological insomnia. In general, assessment of insomnia is difficult because clinicians typically rely on reports of subjective experiences and because the disorder is often multifaceted. The diagnosis of insomnia is made after extensive psychiatric and medical interviews to identify known causes of insomnia. For those cases with no known etiology, a clinical diagnosis of psychophysiological insomnia is made after polysomnographic sleep efficiency studies (Kales & Kales 1984). These studies

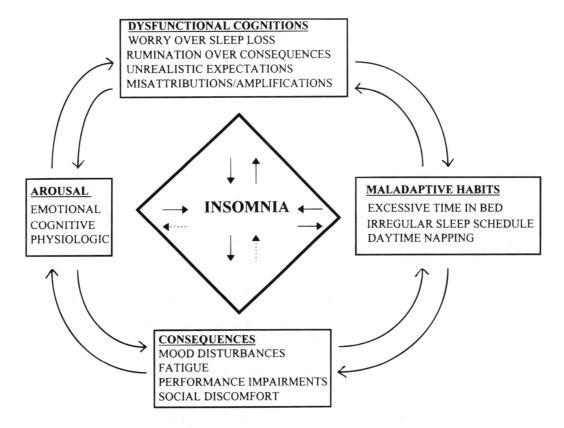

Figure 2. A microanalytic model of insomnia. Reprinted with permission from Morin, *Insomnia*. Copyright 1993 The Guilford Press.

show less total and delta sleep, lower sleep efficiency, longer sleep latency, and more intermittent waking time. A great deal of recent research has focused on the magnocellular regions of the basal forebrain in the regulation of the sleep–wake cycle and has identified GABAergic projection neurons as important components (Szymusiak 1995). However, virtually no research has examined changes in the basal forebrain during behavioral intervention for insomnia. Thus, the electrophysiological documentation has proven useful for the clinical assessment and diagnosis of insomnia, but it has not yet advanced our understanding of the disorder's etiology.

Treatment

Nonpharmacologic approaches to the treatment of insomnia have been advocated because of the significant iatrogenic and paradoxical effects of most hypnotic agents. This has led to the clinical application of a variety of behavioral treatments for chronic insomnia, including relaxation techniques, biofeedback, cognitive-behavioral therapy, stimulus control, sleep restriction, and paradoxical intention. For example, biofeedback based on the EMG (Budzynski 1973) or to enhance theta or sensorimotor rhythm activity (Hauri et al. 1982) diminishes insomnia symptoms in patients presenting with complaints. Although others of these behavioral techniques do not involve direct psychophysiological measurements, all are thought to operate (at least partially) by decreasing physiological arousal and thus effecting shorter sleep onset latency and decreased awak-

enings. For example, Figure 2 shows a cognitive-behavioral model for insomnia that incorporates physiological arousal as both a consequence and a precipitant of insomnia. In addition, the emotional and cognitive impairments that can occur coincident with insomnia may also affect the maladaptive arousal. Treatments for either the direct or indirect reduction of sympathetic arousal may be expected to alter these cycles and alleviate some of the symptoms of insomnia. In addition, relaxation and biofeedback approaches may enhance parasympathetic activity and further diminish autonomic tone.

The efficacy of behavioral treatments has been tested in several quantitative reviews comparing various relaxation strategies with other cognitive and behavioral therapies for insomnia (Lacks & Morin 1992; Murtagh & Greenwood 1995). Overall, behavioral treatments for insomnia are generally highly effective in reducing sleep onset latency and improving quality of sleep, are clinically durable, and perform significantly better than placebo control conditions. However, no strategy is generally found to be more efficacious than another, and the mechanisms of action by which these strategies operate to reduce the subjective and objective experiences of insomnia are still unclear. Although some have suggested that relaxation treatments are superior in terms of enhancing the quality of sleep (Espie et al. 1989), others have found relaxation to be most effective for promoting total sleep time (Murtagh & Greenwood 1995). Comparison of behavioral interventions to pharmacotherapy has provided mixed data, with most studies showing the efficacy of drug in comparison to nondrug interventions to be highly dependent on the specific characteristics of insomnia examined.

Conclusions

From the foregoing discussion, it is apparent that a range of psychophysiological paradigms have been widely used in the broad field of health psychology. Although not offering a comprehensive assessment of all physical and psychological conditions where psychophysiological techniques have been applied, we have presented a representative sample of clinical and basic science studies to illustrate the diverse nature of these paradigms.

Investigations regarding the etiology, diagnosis, and assessment of both pathophysiological and psychopathological conditions are increasingly present in the literature, reflecting greater appreciation of the combined and complementary roles of behavior, cognition, and physiological processes. The pervasive failure of early clinical psychophysiological investigations to acknowledge the role of cognition is being replaced by a new perspective, which is largely a contribution of health psychology. This integration will become more ubiquitous as more and more health psychologists become rigorously trained in both psychology and physiology fundamentals, and the conceptual and practical value of applying psychophysiological paradigms to clinical conditions will then be even more apparent.

NOTE

The authors are grateful to Tilmer O. Engebretson for his insightful comments on an earlier version of this chapter. Preparation of this chapter was supported in part by NHLBI grants HL48363 and HL44847 to C. M. Stoney.

REFERENCES

Achterberg, J., McGraw, P., & Lawlis, G. F. (1981). Rheumatoid arthritis: A study of the relaxation and temperature biofeedback training as an adjunctive therapy. *Biofeedback and Self-Regulation, 6,* 207–33.

Ahles, T. A., Blanchard, E. B., & Leventhal, H. (1983). Cognitive control of pain: Attention to the sensory aspects of the cold pressor stimulus. *Cognitive Therapy and Research, 7,* 159–78.

Andrasik, F. (1982). Psychophysiology of recurrent headache: Methodological issues and new empirical findings. *Behavior Therapy, 13,* 407–29.

Andrasik, F., & Blanchard, E. B. (1987). Biofeedback treatment of muscle contraction headache. In J. P. Hatch, J. G. Fisher, & J. D. Rugh (Eds.), *Biofeedback: Studies in Clinical Efficacy,* pp. 281–315. New York: Plenum.

Annal, N., Soundappan, S. V., Subbu Palaniappan, K. M., & Chandrasekar, S. (1992). Introduction of transcutaneous, low-voltage, non-pulsatile direct current (DC) therapy for migraine and chronic headaches: A comparison with transcutaneous electrical nerve stimulation (TENS). *Headache Quarterly, 3,* 434–42.

Arena, J. G. (1985). Psychophysiological comparisons of three kinds of headache subjects during and between headache states: Analysis of post-stress adaptation periods. *Journal of Psychosomatic Research, 29,* 427–41.

Arena, J. G., & Blanchard, E. B. (1996). Biofeedback and relaxation therapy. In R. J. Gatchel & D. C. Turk (Eds.), *Psychological Approaches to Pain Management: A Practitioner's Handbook,* pp. 179–230. New York: Guilford.

Ax, A. F. (1964). Goals and methods of psychophysiology. *Psychophysiology, 1,* 8–25.

Bakal, D. A. (1975). Headache: A biopsychological perspective. *Psychological Bulletin, 82,* 369–82.

Bakal, D. A., & Kaganov, J. A. (1977). Muscle contraction and migraine headache: Psychophysiological comparison. *Headache, 17,* 208–15.

Bates, J. A. V., & Nathan, P. W. (1980). Transcutaneous electrical nerve stimulation for chronic pain. *Anaesthesia, 35,* 817–22.

Benson, H., Shapiro, D., Tursky, B., & Schwartz, G. E. (1971). Decreased systolic blood pressure through operant conditioning techniques in patients with essential hypertension. *Science, 173,* 740–2.

Biondi, M., & Portuesi, G. (1994). Tension-type headache: Psychosomatic clinical assessment and treatment. *Psychotherapy and Psychosomatics, 61,* 41–64.

Blanchard, E. B. (1992). Psychological treatment of benign headache disorder. Special Issue: Behavioral medicine: An update for the 1990s. *Journal of Consulting and Clinical Psychology, 60,* 537–51.

Blanchard, E. B., & Andrasik, F. (1982). Psychological assessment and treatment of headache: Recent developments and emerging issues. *Journal of Consulting and Clinical Psychology, 50,* 859–79.

Blanchard, E. B., Andrasik, F., Appelbaum, K. A., Evans, D. D., Burish, S. E., Teders, S. J., Rodichok, L. D., & Barron, K. D. (1985). The efficacy and cost-effectiveness of minimal-therapist-contact, non-drug treatments of chronic migraine and tension headache. *Headache, 25,* 214–20.

Blanchard, E. B., Appelbaum, K. A., Nicholson, N. L., Radnitz, C. L., Morrill, B., Michultka, D., Kirsch, C., Hillhouse, J., & Dentinger, M. P. (1990). A controlled evaluation of the addition of cognitive therapy to a home-based biofeedback and relaxation treatment of vascular headache. *Headache, 30,* 371–6.

Blanchard, E. B., Eisele, G., Vollmer, A., Payne, A., Gordon, M., Cornish, P., & Gilmore, L. (1996). Controlled evaluation of thermal biofeedback in treatment of elevated blood pressure in unmedicated mild hypertension. *Biofeedback and Self-Regulation, 21,* 167–90.

Blanchard, E. B., Kim, M., Hermann, C., & Steffek, B. D. (1993). Preliminary results of the effects on headache relief of perception of success among tension headache patients receiving relaxation. *Headache Quarterly, 4,* 249–53.

Blanchard, E. B., Scott, R. W., Young, L. D., & Haynes, M. R. (1974). The effects of feedback signal information content on the long-term self-control of heart rate. *Journal of General Psychology, 91,* 175–87.

Bloom, L. R., Houston, B. K., Holmes, D. S., & Burish, T. G. (1977). The effectiveness of attentional diversion and situation redefinition for reducing stress due to an ambiguous threat. *Journal of Research in Personality, 11,* 83–94.

Bourke, D. L. (1994). TENS vs. placebo. *Pain, 56,* 122–3.

Bradley, L. A., Young, L. D., Andersen, K. O., Turner, R. A., Agudelo, C. A., McDaniel, L. K., Pisko, E. J., Semble, E. L., & Morgan, T. M. (1987). Effects of psychological therapy on pain behavior of rheumatoid arthritis patients: Treatment outcome and six-month follow-up. *Arthritis and Rheumatism, 30,* 1105–14.

Brener, J., Phillips, K., & Connally, S. (1980). Energy expenditure, heart rate, and ambulation during shock-avoidance conditioning of heart rate increases and ambulation in freely-moving rats. *Psychophysiology, 17,* 64–74.

Budzynski, T. H. (1973). Biofeedback procedures in the clinic. *Seminars in Psychiatry, 5,* 537–47.

Burdette, B. H., & Gale, E. N. (1988). The effects of treatment of masticatory muscle activity and mandibular posture in myofascial pain-dysfunction patients. *Journal of Dental Research, 67,* 1126–30.

Burns, J. W., Wiegner, S., Derleth, M., Kiselica, K., & Pawl, R. (1997). Linking symptom-specific physiological reactivity to pain severity in chronic low back pain patients: A test of mediation and moderation models. *Health Psychology, 16,* 319–26.

Bush, F. M., Harkins, S. W., Harrington, W. G., & Price, D. D. (1993). Analysis of gender effects on pain perception and symptom presentation in temporomandibular pain. *Pain, 53,* 73–80.

Cassisi, J. E., McGlynn, F. D., & Belles, D. R. (1987). EMG-activated feedback alarms for the treatment of nocturnal bruxism: Current status and future directions. *Biofeedback and Self-Regulation, 12,* 13–30.

Chase, D. C., Hendler, B. H., & Kraus, S. L. (1988). A commonsense approach to TMJ pain. *Patient Care, 22,* 57–68.

Choudhury, K. J., & Ffoulkes-Crabbe, D. J. (1988). Experience with transcutaneous electrical nerve stimulation (TENS) for relief of pain. *Pain Clinic, 2,* 91–5.

Cox, D. J., Freundlich, A., & Meyer, R. G. (1975). Differential effectiveness of electromyographic feedback, verbal relaxation, and medication placebo with tension headaches. *Journal of Consulting and Clinical Psychology, 43,* 892–8.

Crockett, D. J., Foreman, M. E., Alden, L., & Blasberg, B. (1986). A comparison of treatment modes in the management of myofascial pain dysfunction syndrome. *Biofeedback and Self-Regulation, 11,* 279–91.

Cuthbert, B., Kristeller, J., Simons, R., Hodes, R., & Lang, P. J. (1981). Strategies of arousal control: Biofeedback, meditation, and motivation. *Journal of Experimental Psychology: General, 110,* 518–46.

Dahlstrom, L., Carlsson, G. E., & Carlsson, S. G. (1982). Comparison of effects of electromyographic biofeedback and occlusal splint therapy on mandibular dysfunction. *Scandinavian Journal of Dental Research, 90,* 151–6.

Dahlstrom, L., & Carlsson, S. G. (1984). Treatment of mandibular dysfunction: The clinical usefulness of biofeedback in relation to splint therapy. *Journal of Oral Rehabilitation, 11,* 277–84.

Dahlstrom, L., Carlsson, S. G., Gale, E. N., & Jansson, T. G. (1985). Stress-induced activity in mandibular dysfunction: Effects of biofeedback training. *Journal of Behavioral Medicine, 8,* 191–9.

Dalen, K., Ellertsen, B., Espelid, I., & Gronningsaeter, A. G. (1986). EMG feedback in the treatment of myofascial pain dysfunction syndrome. *Acta Odontologica Scandinavica, 44,* 279–84.

De Kanter, R. J. A. M., Kayser, A. F., Battistuzzi, P. G. F. C. M., Truin, G. J., & Van 't Hof, M. A. (1992). Demand and need for treatment of craniomandibular dysfunction in the Dutch adult population. *Journal of Dental Research, 71,* 1607–12.

Drummond, P. D. (1982). Extracranial and cardiovascular reactivity in migrainous subjects. *Journal of Psychosomatic Research, 28,* 133–8.

Dworkin, S. F., Huggins, K. H., LeResche, L., Von Korff, M., Howard, J., Truelove, E., & Sommers, E. (1990). Epidemiology of signs and symptoms in temporomandibular disorders: I. Clinical signs in cases and controls. *Journal of the American Dental Association, 120,* 273–81.

Dworkin, S. F., & LeResche, L. (1992). Research diagnostic criteria for temporomandibular disorders: Review, criteria, examinations and specifications, critique. *Journal of Craniomandibular Disorders: Facial and Oral Pain, 6,* 301–55.

Dworkin, S. F., Turner, J. A., Wilson, L., & Massoth, D. (1994). Brief group cognitive-behavioral intervention for temporomandibular disorder. *Pain, 59,* 175–87.

Engel, B. T., & Bleecker, E. R. (1979). Application of operant conditioning techniques to the control of the cardiac arrhythmias. In A. H. B. P. A. Obrist, J. Brener, & L. V. DiCara (Eds.), *Cardiovascular Psychophysiology: Current Issues in Response Mechanisms, Biofeedback and Methodology,* pp. 456–76. Chicago: Aldine.

Engel, G. L. (1980). The clinical application of the biopsychosocial model. *American Journal of Psychiatry, 137,* 535–44.

Eriksson, M. B. E., Sjolund, B. H., & Nielzen, S. (1979). Long term results of peripheral conditioning stimulation as an analgesic measure in chronic pain. *Pain, 6,* 335–47.

Espie, A., Linday, W. R., Brooks, D. M., Hood, E. M., & Turvey, T. (1989). A controlled comparative investigation of psychological treatments for chronic sleep-onset insomnia. *Behavioral Research Therapy, 27,* 79–88.

Flor, H., Birbaumer, N., Schulte, W., & Roos, R. (1991). Stress-related electromyographic responses in patients with chronic temporomandibular pain. *Pain, 46,* 145–52.

Flor, H., & Turk, D. C. (1989). Psychophysiology of chronic pain: Do chronic pain patients exhibit symptom-specific psychophysiological responses? *Psychological Bulletin, 105,* 215–59.

Fredrikson, M., & Engel, B. T. (1992). Learned control of heart rate during exercise in patients with borderline hypertension. *European Journal of Applied Physiology and Occupational Physiology, 54,* 315–20.

Fredrikson, M., & Matthews, K. A. (1990). Cardiovascular responses to behavioral stress and hypertension: A meta-analytic review. *Annals of Behavioral Medicine, 12,* 30–9.

Freeman, T. B., Campbell, J. N., & Long, D. M. (1983). Naloxone does not affect pain relief induced by electrical stimulation in man. *Pain, 17,* 189–95.

Gale, E. N. (1992). Epidemiology. In B. G. Sarnat & D. M. Laskin (Eds.), *The Temporomandibular Joint: A Biological Basis for Clinical Practice,* 4th ed., pp. 237–48. Philadelphia: Saunders.

Gannon, L. R., Haynes, S. N., Cuevas, J., & Chavez, R. (1987). Psychophysiological correlates of induced headaches. *Journal of Behavioral Medicine, 10,* 411–23.

Gannon, L. R., Haynes, S. N., Safranek, R., & Hamilton, J. A. (1981). A psychophysiological investigation of muscle contraction and migraine headache. *Journal of Psychosomatic Research, 25,* 271–80.

Gatchel, R. J., & Turk, D. C. (Eds.) (1996). *Psychological Approaches to Pain Management: A Practitioner's Handbook.* New York: Guilford.

Glaros, A. G., & Glass, E. G. (1993). Temporomandibular disorders. In R. J. Gatchel & E. B. Blanchard (Eds.), *Psychophysiological Disorders: Research and Clinical Applications,* pp. 299–356. Washington, DC: American Psychological Association.

Goronzy, J. J., & Weyand, C. M. (1995). T and B cell-dependent pathways in rheumatoid arthritis. *Current Opinion in Rheumatology, 7,* 214–21.

Griffiths, R. H. (1983). Report of the President's conference on the examination and management of temporomandibular disorders. *Journal of the American Dental Association, 166,* 75–7.

Grimm, L., & Kanfer, F. H. (1976). Tolerance of aversive stimulation. *Behavior Therapy, 7,* 593–601.

Grossman, P., Brinkman, A., & de Vries, J. (1992). Cardiac autonomic mechanisms associated with borderline hypertension under varying behavioral demands: Evidence for attenuated parasympathetic tone but not for enhanced beta-adrenergic activity. *Psychophysiology, 29,* 698–711.

Group [The Trials of Hypertension Prevention Collaborative Research Group] (1992). The effects of nonpharmacologic interventions on blood pressure of persons with high normal levels. *Journal of the American Medical Association, 267,* 1213–20.

Hansson, P., & Akblom, A. (1983). Transcutaneous electrical nerve stimulation (TENS) as compared to placebo TENS for the relief of acute oro-facial pain. *Pain, 15,* 157–65.

Harris, E. D. J. (1990). Rheumatoid arthritis: Pathophysiology and implications for therapy. *New England Journal of Medicine, 322,* 1277–89.

Hatch, J. P. (1993). Headache. In R. J. Gatchel & E. B. Blanchard (Eds.), *Psychophysiological Disorders: Research and Clinical Applications,* pp. 111–49. Washington, DC: American Psychological Association.

Hauri, P. J., Pery, L., Hellekson, C., Hartmann, E., & Russ, D. (1982). The treatment of psychophysiologic insomnia with biofeedback: A replication study. *Biofeedback and Self-Regulation, 7,* 223–35.

Haynes, S. N. (1981). Muscle contraction headache – A psychophysiological perspective. In S. N. Haynes & L. R. Gannon (Eds.), *Psychosomatic Disorders: A Psychophysiological Approach to Etiology and Treatment.* New York: Praeger.

Haynes, S. N. (1983). The psychophysiological assessment of muscle-contraction headache subjects during headache and nonheadache conditions. *Psychophysiology, 20,* 393–9.

Holmes, D. S., & Houston, B. K. (1974). Effectiveness of situation redefinition and affective isolation in coping with stress. *Journal of Personality and Social Psychology, 29,* 212–18.

Holroyd, K. A., Andrasik, F., & Noble, J. (1980). Comparison of EMG biofeedback and credible pseudotherapy in treating tension headache. *Journal of Behavioral Medicine, 3,* 29–39.

Holroyd, K. A., & Penzien, D. B. (1986). Client variables and the behavioral treatment of recurrent tension headache: A meta-analytic review. *Journal of Behavioral Medicine, 9,* 515–36.

Iacono, W. G. (1991). Psychophysiological assessment of psychopathology. *Psychological Assessment, 3,* 309–20.

IHS [International Headache Society] (1988). Classification and diagnostic criteria for headache disorders, cranial neuralgias and fascial pain. *Cephalalgia, 8,* 1–96.

Intrieri, R. C., Jones, G. E., & Alcorn, J. D. (1994). Masseter muscle hyperactivity and myofascial pain dysfunction syndrome: A relationship under stress. *Journal of Behavioral Medicine, 17,* 479–500.

Jacob, R. G., Chesney, M. A., Williams, D. M., Ding, Y., & Shapiro, A. P. (1991). Relaxation therapy for hypertension: Design effects and treatment effects. *Annals of Behavioral Medicine, 13,* 5–17.

Johnson, M. I., Ashton, C. H., Bousfield, D. R., & Thomson, J. W. (1991a). Analgesic effects of different pulse patterns of transcutaneous electrical nerve stimulation on cold-induced pain in normal subjects. *Journal of Psychosomatic Research, 35,* 313–21.

Johnson, M. I., Ashton, C. H., & Thompson, J. W. (1991b). The consistency of pulse frequencies and pulse patterns of transcutaneous electrical nerve stimulation (TENS) used by chronic pain patients. *Pain, 44,* 231–4.

Kales, A., & Kales, J. D. (1984). *Evaluation and Treatment of Insomnia.* New York: Oxford University Press.

Kamarck, T. W., Manuck, S. B., & Jennings, J. R. (1990). Social support reduces cardiovascular reactivity to psychological challenge: A laboratory model. *Psychosomatic Medicine, 52,* 42–58.

Kapel, L., Glaros, A. G., & McGlynn, F. D. (1989). Psychophysiological responses to stress in patients with myofascial pain-dysfunction syndrome. *Journal of Behavioral Medicine, 12,* 397–406.

Katz, J. O., Rugh, J. P., Hatch, J. P., Langlais, R. P., Terezhalmay, G. T., & Borcherding, S. H. (1989). Effect of experimental stress on masseter and temporalis muscle activity in human subjects with temporomandibular disorders. *Archives of Oral Biology, 34,* 393–8.

Kaufmann, P. G., Jacob, R. G., Ewart, C. K., Chesney, M. A., Muenz, L. R., Doub, N., & Mercer, W. (1988). Hypertension Intervention Pooling Project. *Health Psychology, 7 (Suppl.),* 209–24.

Kroner-Herwig, B., Diergarten, D., Diergarten, D., & Seeger-Siewart, R. (1988). Psychophysiological reactivity of migraine sufferers in conditions of stress and relaxation. *Journal of Psychosomatic Research, 32,* 483–92.

Lacey, J. I., & Lacey, B. C. (1958). Verification and extension of the principle of autonomic response stereotypy. *American Journal of Psychology, 71,* 50–73.

Lacks, P., & Morin, C. M. (1992). Recent advances in the assessment and treatment of insomnia. *Journal of Consulting and Clinical Psychology, 60,* 586–94.

Lander, J., & Fowler-Kerry, S. (1993). TENS for children's procedural pain. *Pain, 52,* 209–16.

Langer, A. W., McCubbin, J. A., Stoney, C. M., Hutcheson, J. S., Charlton, J. D., & Obrist, P. A. (1985). Cardiopulmonary adjustments during exercise and an aversive reaction time task: Effects of beta-adrenoceptor blockade. *Psychophysiology, 22,* 59–68.

Laskin, D. M. (1969). Etiology of the pain–dysfunction syndrome. *Journal of the American Dental Association, 79,* 147–53.

Lawler, J. E., & Cox, R. H. (1985). The borderline hypertensive rat (BHR): A new model for the study of environmental factors in the development of hypertension. *Pavlovian Journal of Biological Sciences, 30,* 101–15.

Liao, H.-X., & Haynes, B. F. (1995). Role of adhesion molecules in the pathogenesis of rheumatoid arthritis. *Rheumatic Diseases Clinics of North America, 21,* 715–40.

Linden, W., & Chambers, L. (1994). Clinical effectiveness of non-drug treatment for hypertension: A meta-analysis. *Annals of Behavioral Medicine, 16,* 35–45.

Linet, M. G., Stewart, W. F., Celentano, D. D., Ziegler, D., & Sprecher, M. (1989). An epidemiologic study of headache among adolescents and young adults. *Journal of the American Medical Association, 261,* 2211–16.

Lo, C. R., & Johnston, D. W. (1984). Cardiovascular feedback during dynamic exercise. *Psychophysiology, 21,* 199–206.

Long, D. M. (1991). Fifteen years of transcutaneous electrical stimulation for pain control. *Stereotactic and Functional Neurosurgery, 56,* 2–19.

Lundeberg, T. (1984). The pain suppressive effect of vibratory stimulation and transcutaneous electrical nerve stimulation (TENS) as compared to aspirin. *Brain Research, 294,* 201–9.

Maixner, W., Fillingim, R., Booker, D., & Sigurdsson, A. (1995). Sensitivity of patients with painful temporomandibular disorders to experimentally evoked pain. *Pain, 63,* 341–51.

Malmo, R. B. (1975). *On Emotions, Needs, and Our Archaic Brain.* New York: Holt, Rinehart & Winston.

Malmo, R. B., & Shagass, C. (1949). Physiologic study of symptom mechanism in psychiatric patients under stress. *Psychosomatic Medicine, 11,* 25–9.

Malow, R. M., Grimm, L., & Olsson, R. E. (1980). Differences in pain perception between myofascial pain dysfunction patients and normal subjects: A signal detection analysis. *Journal of Psychosomatic Research, 24,* 303–9.

Mannheimer, C., & Carlsson, C. (1979). The analgesic effect of transcutaneous electrical nerve stimulation (TENS) in patients with rheumatoid arthritis. A comparative study of different pulse patterns. *Pain, 6,* 329–34.

Mannheimer, C., Carlsson, C., Vedin, A., & Wilhemsson, C. (1986). Transcutaneous electrical nerve stimulation. *Acta Anaesth. Scand., 22,* 589–92.

Mannheimer, C., & Lampe, G. (1984). *Clinical Transcutaneous Electrical Nerve Stimulation.* Philadelphia: Davis.

Manuck, S. B. (1976). The voluntary control of heart rate under differential somatic restraint. *Biofeedback and Self-Regulation, 1,* 273–84.

Marchand, S., Charest, J., Li, J., Chenard, J., Lavignolle, B., & Laurencelle, L. (1993). Is TENS purely a placebo effect? A controlled study on chronic pain. *Pain, 54,* 99–106.

Margraf, J., Taylor, C. B., Ehlers, A., Roth, W. T., & Agras, W. S. (1987). Panic attacks in the natural environment. *Journal of Nervous and Mental Disease, 175,* 558–65.

Martin, P. R., Marie, G. V., & Nathan, P. R. (1992). Psychophysiological mechanisms of chronic headaches: Investigation using pain induction and pain reduction procedures. *Journal of Psychosomatic Research, 36,* 137–48.

Martin, P. R., & Mathews, A. (1978). Tension headaches: Psychophysiological investigation and treatment. *Journal of Psychosomatic Research, 22,* 389–99.

Martins, L. P., Baeta, E., Paiva, T., & Campos, J. (1993). Headaches during intracranial endovascular procedures: A possible model of vascular headache. *Headache, 33,* 227–33.

McCubbin, J. A., Surwit, R. S., & Williams, R. B., Jr. (1985). Endogenous opiate peptides, stress reactivity, and risk for hypertension. *Hypertension, 7,* 808–11.

McCubbin, J. A., Wilson, J. F., Bruehl, S., Ibarra, P., Carlson, C. R., Norton, J. A., & Colclough, G. W. (1996). Relaxation training and opioid inhibition of blood pressure response to stress. *Journal of Consulting and Clinical Psychology, 64,* 593–601.

McGrady, A. (1996). Good news – bad news: Applied psychophysiology in cardiovascular disorders. *Biofeedback and Self-Regulation, 21,* 335–47.

McGrady, A., Olson, R. P., & Kroon, J. S. (1995). Biobehavioral treatment of essential hypertension. In M. S. Schwartz (Ed.), *Biofeedback – A Practitioner's Guide,* 2nd ed., pp. 445–67. New York: Guilford.

McGrady, A., Wayquier, A., McNeil, A., & Gerard, G. (1994). Effect of biofeedback-assisted relaxation on migraine headache and changes in cerebral blood flow velocity in the middle cerebral artery. *Headache, 34,* 424–8.

McNeill, C., Mohl, N. D., Rugh, J. D., & Tanaka, T. T. (1990). Temporomandibular disorders: Diagnosis, management, education, and research. *Journal of the American Dental Association, 120,* 253–63.

Melzack, R., & Wall, P. D. (1965). Pain mechanisms: A new theory. *Science, 150,* 971–9.

Miller, N. E., & DiCara, L. (1967). Instrumental learning of heart rate changes in curarized rats: Shaping, and specificity to discriminative stimulus. *Journal of Comparative and Physiological Psychology, 63,* 12–19.

Mitchell, J., Burkhauser, R., & Pincus, T. (1988). The importance of age, education, and comorbidity in the substantial earnings losses of individuals with symmetric polyarthritis. *Arthritis and Rheumatism, 31,* 348–57.

Mitchell, K. R. (1986). Peripheral temperature autoregulation and its effect on the symptoms of rheumatoid arthritis. *Scandinavian Journal of Behavioral Therapy, 15,* 55–64.

Morin, C. M. (1993). *Insomnia.* New York: Guilford.

Morley, S. (1985). Migraine: A generalized vasomotor dysfunction? A critical review of evidence. *Headache, 17,* 71–4.

Murphy, A. I., & Lehrer, P. M. (1990). Headache versus non-headache state: A study of electrophysiological and affective changes during muscle contraction headaches. *Behavioral Medicine, 16,* 23–30.

Murtagh, D. R. R., & Greenwood, K. M. (1995). Identifying effective psychological treatments for insomnia: A meta-analysis. *Journal of Consulting and Clinical Psychology, 63,* 79–89.

Nathan, P. W. (1976). The gate control theory of pain: A critical review. *Brain, 99,* 123–58.

Nichols, F. T. III, Mawad, M., Mohr, J. P., Stein, B., Hilal, S., & Michelsen, W. J. (1990). Focal headache during balloon inflation in the internal carotid and middle cerebral arteries. *Stroke, 21,* 555–9.

Nuechterlein, K. H., & Holroyd, J. C. (1980). Biofeedback in the treatment of tension headache. *Archives of General Psychiatry, 37,* 866–73.

Obrist, P. A. (1976). The cardiovascular-behavioral interaction as it appears today. *Psychophysiology, 13,* 95–107.

Obrist, P. A. (1981). *Cardiovascular Psychophysiology: A Perspective.* New York: Plenum.

Öhman, A. (1981). Electrodermal activity and vulnerability to schizophrenia: A review. *Biological Psychology, 12,* 87–145.

Okeson, J. P. (1989). *Management of Temporomandibular Disorders and Occlusion,* 2nd ed. St. Louis: Mosby.

Olesen, J. (1991). Clinical and pathophysiological observations in migraine and tension-type headache explained by integration of vascular, supraspinal and myofascial inputs. *Pain, 46,* 125–32.

Olesen, J., Friberg, L., Olsen, T. S., Iverson, H. K., Lassen, N. A., Anderson, A. R., & Karle, A. (1990). Timing and topography of cerebral blood flow, aura, and headache during migraine attacks. *Annals of Neurology, 28,* 791–8.

Olson, R. E. (1980). Myofascial pain-dysfunction syndrome: Psychological aspects. In B. G. Sarnet & D. M. Laskin (Eds.), *The Temporomandibular Joint: A Biological Basis for Clinical Practice,* vol. 3, pp. 300–14. Springfield IL: Thomas.

Onel, Y., Friedman, A. P., & Grossman, J. (1961). Muscle blood flow studies in muscle-contraction headaches. *Neurology, 11,* 935–9.

Ostfeld, A. M., Reis, D. J., & Wolff, H. G. (1957). Studies on headache: Bulbar conjunctival ischemia and muscle contraction headache. *Arch. Neurol. Psych., 77,* 113–19.

Ottoson, D., & Lundeberg, T. (1988). *Pain Treatment by TENS.* Berlin: Springer.

Paran, E., Amir, M., & Yaniv, N. (1996). Evaluating the response of mild hypertensives to biofeedback-assisted relaxation using a mental stress test. *Journal of Behavior Therapy and Experimental Psychiatry, 27,* 157–67.

Patel, C. H. (1973). Yoga and biofeedback in the management of hypertension. *Lancet, 2,* 1053–5.

Patel, C. H. (1977). Biofeedback-aided relaxation and meditation in the management of hypertension. *Biofeedback and Self-Regulation, 2,* 1–41.

Perski, A., & Engel, B. T. (1980). The role of behavioral conditioning in the cardiovascular adjustment to exercise. *Biofeedback and Self-Regulation, 5,* 91–104.

Pickering, T. G., & Gerin, W. (1990). Cardiovascular reactivity in the laboratory and the role of behavioral factors in hypertension: A critical review. *Annals of Behavioral Medicine, 12,* 3–16.

Pomeranz, B., & Niznick, G. (1987). Codetron: A new electrotherapy device overcomes the habituation problems of conventional TENS devices. *American Journal of Electromedicine, 1,* 22–6.

Poziak-Patweica, E. (1976). Cephalic spasm of the head and neck muscles. *Headache, 14,* 261–9.

Rasmussen, B. K., Jensen, R., Schroll, M., & Olesen, J. (1991). Epidemiology of headache in a general population: A prevalence study. *Journal of Clinical Epidemiology, 44,* 1147–57.

Riley, D. M., & Furedy, J. J. (1981). Effects of instructions and contingency of reinforcement on the operant conditioning of human phasic heart rate change. *Psychophysiology, 18,* 75–81.

Rugh, J. D., & Solberg, W. K. (1976). Psychological implications of temporomandibular pain and dysfunction. *Oral Science Review, 7,* 3–30.

Sargent, J. H., Green, E. E., & Walters, E. D. (1972). The use of autogenic feedback training in a pilot study of migraine and tension headaches. *Headache, 12,* 120–4.

Schiffman, E. L., Fricton, J. R., Haley, D. P., & Shapiro, B. L. (1990). The prevalence and treatment needs of subjects with temporomandibular disorders. *Journal of the American Dental Association, 120,* 295–303.

Schwartz, G. E. (1975). Biofeedback, self-regulation, and the patterning of physiological processes. *American Scientist, 63,* 314–24.

Schwartz, G. E. (1982). Testing the biopsychosocial model: The ultimate challenge facing behavioral medicine? *Journal of Consulting and Clinical Psychology, 50,* 1040–53.

Sjoland, B. H., & Erikson, M. B. E. (1979). The influence of naloxone on analgesia produced by peripheral conditioning stimulation. *Brain Research, 173,* 295–301.

Solomon, S., & Guglielmo, K. M. (1985). Treatment of headache by transcutaneous electrical stimulation. *Headache, 25,* 12–15.

Steptoe, A., & Ross, A. (1982). Voluntary control of cardiovascular reactions to demanding tasks. *Biofeedback and Self-Regulation, 7,* 149–66.

Steptoe, A., & Sawada, Y. (1989). Assessment of baroreceptor reflex function during mental stress and relaxation. *Psychophysiology, 26,* 140–7.

Steriade, M., & Llinas, R. R. (1988). The functional states of the thalamus and the associated neuronal interplay. *Physiological Review, 68,* 649–742.

Sternberg, E. M. (1995). Neuroendocrine factors in susceptibility to inflammatory disease: Focus on the hypothalamic-pituitary-adrenal axis. *Hormone Research, 43,* 159–61.

Stewart, W. F., Lipton, R. B., Celentano, D. D., & Reed, M. L. (1992). Prevalence of migraine headache in the United States. Relation to age, income, race and other sociodemographic factors. *Journal of the American Medical Association, 267,* 84–9.

Stohler, C. S. (1997). Masticatory myalgias. *Pain Forum, 6,* 176–80.

Stoney, C. M., Langer, A. W., Sutterer, J. R., & Gelling, P. D. (1986). Biofeedback-assisted heart rate deceleration: Specificity of cardiovascular and metabolic effects in normal and high risk subjects. In P. Grossman, K. H. L. Janssen, & D. Vaitl (Eds.), *Cardiorespiratory and Cardiosomatic Psychophysiology.* New York: Plenum.

Stoney, C. M., Langer, A. W., Sutterer, J. R., & Gelling, P. D. (1987). A comparison of biofeedback-assisted cardiodeceleration in type A and B men: Modification of stress-associated cardiopulmonary and hemodynamic adjustments. *Psychosomatic Medicine, 49,* 79–87.

Stoney, C. M., & Matthews, K. A. (1988). Parental history of hypertension and myocardial infarction predicts cardiovascular responses to behavioral stressors in middle-aged men and women. *Psychophysiology, 25,* 269–77.

Szymusiak, R. (1995). Magnocellular nuclei of the basal forebrain: Substrates of sleep and arousal regulation. *Sleep, 18,* 478–500.

Thompson, K. J., & Adams, H. E. (1984). Psychophysiological characteristics of headache patients. *Pain, 18,* 41–52.

Tomaka, J., & Blascovich, J. (1994). Effects of justice beliefs on cognitive appraisal of and subjective, physiological, and behavioral responses to potential stress. *Journal of Personality and Social Psychology, 67,* 732–40.

Tunis, H., & Wolff, H. (1953). Studies on headache: Long-term observations of the reactivity of the cranial arteries in subjects with vascular headache of the migraine type. *Archives of Neurology Psychiatry, 70*, 551–7.

Tunis, H., & Wolff, H. (1954). Studies on headache: Cranial artery vasoconstriction and muscle contraction headache. *Archives of Neurology Psychiatry, 71*, 425–34.

Turk, D. C. (1996). Biopsychosocial perspective on chronic pain. In R. J. Gatchel & D. C. Turk (Eds.), *Psychological Approaches to Pain Management: A Practitioner's Handbook*. New York: Guilford.

Turpin, G. (1990). Ambulatory clinical psychophysiological monitoring: Proceedings of a symposium held at the World Congress of Behavior Therapy, Edinburgh, Scotland, September 1988. *Journal of Psychophysiology, 4*, 297–304.

Turpin, G. (1991). The psychophysiological assessment of anxiety disorders: Three-systems measurement and beyond. *Psychological Assessment, 3*, 366–75.

Uchino, B. N., Cacioppo, J. T., & Kiecolt-Glaser, J. K. (1996). The relationship between social support and physiological processes: A review with emphasis on underlying mechanisms and implications for health. *Psychological Bulletin, 119*, 488–531.

Vaughn, R., Pall, M. L., & Haynes, S. N. (1977). Frontalis EMG responses to stress in subjects with frequent muscle contraction headaches. *Headache, 16*, 313–17.

Venables, P. H. (1983). Some problems and controversies in the psychophysiological investigation of schizophrenia. In A. G. J. A. Edwards (Ed.), *Physiological Correlates of Human Behavior*, pp. 207–32. London: Academic Press.

Wallasch, T. M. (1992). Transcranial doppler ultrasonic features in episodic tension-type headache. *Cephalalgia, 12*, 293–6.

Wang, J. Q., Mao, L., & Han, J. (1992). Comparison of the antinociceptive effects induced by electroacupuncture and transcutaneous electrical nerve stimulation in the rat. *International Journal of Neuroscience, 65*, 117–29.

Weyand, C. M., & Goronzy, J. J. (1997). Pathogenesis of rheumatoid arthritis. *Medical Clinics of North America, 81*, 29–55.

Whitsel, B. L., Favorov, O. V., Kelly, D. G., & Tommerdahl, M. (1990). Mechanisms of dynamic peri- and intra-columnar interactions in somatosensory cortex: Stimulus-specific contrast enhancement by NMDA receptor activation. In O. Franzen & J. Westman (Eds.), *Information Processing in the Somatosensory System*. London: Macmillan.

Wolff, H. G. (1963). *Headache and Other Head Pain*. New York: Oxford University Press.

Young, L. D. (1993). Rheumatoid arthritis. In R. J. Gatchel & E. B. Blanchard (Eds.), *Psychophysiological Disorders: Research and Clinical Applications*, pp. 269–98. Washington DC: American Psychological Association.

Zahn, T. P. (1986). Psychophysiological approaches to psychopathology. In M. G. H. Coles, E. Donchin, & S. W. Porges (Eds.), *Psychophysiology: Systems, Processes, and Applications*, pp. 508–610. New York: Guilford.

CHAPTER TWENTY-EIGHT

THE DETECTION OF DECEPTION

WILLIAM G. IACONO

Deception is common in human interchange. The consequences of deception, being deceived, or being detected can be substantial, leading to ruined relationships, lawsuits, and even world war. Psychology has not ignored this important aspect of human behavior (e.g. Ben-Shakar & Furedy 1990; Depaulo 1992; Ekman 1991; see also edited volumes by Giacalone & Rosenfeld 1989; Memon, Vrij, & Bull 1998; Rogers 1997; Yuille 1989). However, given the widespread nature of deception and the premium placed on honesty, it is somewhat surprising that greater effort has not been devoted to developing a scientific basis for understanding deception and its detection. In their review, Bashore and Rapp (1993) noted the continuing need to develop psychological theory and approaches to understanding deception and its detection. Empirical study is needed to better delineate the components of deception, which obviously involve much more than lying when asked a question. Studies are also needed that build on psychological knowledge about cognitive processes and emotion in order to develop theories related to deception and its detection.

It is against this backdrop of a relative dearth of theory and research on deception that polygraph testing has evolved over the last 75 years, becoming the most prevalent application of a psychophysiological technique and emerging as one of few psychological tests that can have life-altering consequences for those who take it. Despite the obvious need to evaluate applied polygraphy, few scientists have been actively engaged in research on this topic. As a result, basic questions pertaining to the accuracy of commonly applied lie detection procedures remain unanswered and there are no generally accepted theories regarding the psychophysiological detection of deception. The facts that

1. there is no consensus among scientists that there exists an adequate foundation for the application of polygraph tests,

2. the profession of polygraphy operates outside the purview of any scientific organization and is practiced mostly by law enforcement officials trained at free-standing polygraph schools, and

3. polygraph tests can have a profound effect on individuals subjected to them

all combine to make polygraph testing highly controversial.

In this chapter, I will review the existing research on deception detection, focusing especially on the recent literature. In the process, I hope to offer some insights into why controversy persists in this field and why the state of knowledge remains primitive – even though polygraph testing has been with us for most of the last century.

Historical Context

OVERVIEW OF MODERN POLYGRAPHY

Although the Employee Polygraph Protection Act of 1988 (Public Law 100-347) eliminated most private sector uses of polygraph tests, federal national security and law enforcement agencies (as well as state and local police departments) still rely on polygraph tests to determine employee honesty, screen the integrity of prospective new employees, and help close out criminal investigations. Honts (1991) noted that government figures reveal the use of polygraph tests is increasing substantially each year. Horvath (1993), in a survey of law enforcement agencies' use of screening tests, noted that more than 67,000 police job applicants take these tests each year, with 22% rejected because they appear deceptive to one or more of the issues covered by the tests.

Polygraph test results are sometimes presented to the court in criminal as well as civil proceedings, and they are used in a wide variety of commercial contexts where verifying someone's truthfulness is important (e.g., many fishing

John T. Cacioppo, Louis G. Tassinary, and Gary G. Berntson (Eds.), *Handbook of Psychophysiology,* 2nd ed. © Cambridge University Press 2000. Printed in the United States of America. ISBN 62634X. All rights reserved.

tournaments use them to verify that a prospective winner actually caught the fish on the designated lake on the day of the tournament; insurance companies "polygraph" policy holders with suspicious claims). Various government agencies (e.g., the CIA, FBI, NSA) have research programs focused on the use of lie detection techniques, the most ambitious of which is based at the Department of Defense Polygraph Institute in Alabama. These agencies have intramural research programs and they also let contracts to both individuals and organizations to answer specific research questions of interest to the government.

ORIGINS OF POLYGRAPHY

The origins of the psychophysiological detection of deception can be traced to the Greek physician Erasistratus who, almost two millennia ago, was asked to treat ailing Antiochus, the son of one of Alexander the Great's generals who ruled over Syria. During his examination of Antiochus, Erasistratus found occasion to palpate the young man's pulse while discussing the virtues of his father's beautiful new wife. Detecting a "tumultuous rhythm," Erasistratus concluded Antiochus was feeling guilty over his love for his stepmother, a hypothesis subsequently supported by the accused pair's having a daughter together.

Technology was apparently first used to detect lying by Lombroso, who in 1895 monitored cardiovascular activity while criminal suspects were interrogated. However, the birth of modern applications to detect lying can be traced to William M. Marston (1917), a Harvard psychologist who was also trained as a lawyer. Marston was a student of another Harvard professor, Hugo Munsterberg, one of the first psychologists to advocate that principles of psychological science could be used to benefit forensic investigation (Munsterberg 1908). Marston (1938) took seriously the teachings of his mentor, eventually introducing a "lie detector" test in which blood pressure was monitored when a subject denied wrongdoing. Marston's conviction in the validity of his invention was brought out in a now famous case in which James Frye, accused of murder, tried to have introduced as evidence the results of Marston's blood pressure lie test showing that he did not commit the crime. In *Frye v. United States* (293 F.1013 1924), the U.S. Supreme Court ruled against Mr. Frye and used the opportunity to articulate standards for what constitutes acceptable scientific evidence of any kind. Many state courts still use the *Frye* rules to determine the acceptability of scientific evidence, and current federal court standards (*Daubert v. Merrell Dow Pharmaceuticals,* 113 C. Ct. 2786 1993; see Faigman 1995) continue to show the influence of *Frye*.[1] In 1998, in *United States v. Scheffer* (118 S. Ct. 1261, 140 L. Ed. 2d 413; see Faigman et al. 1999), the Supreme Court addressed the rules of admissibility as they apply specifically to a defendant's right to introduce the results of a passed polygraph test as evidence in military court. The Court ruled that a defendant does not have the right to admit such evidence.

RELEVANT/IRRELEVANT TEST

Marston (1938) was a firm believer in the notion that there was a specific lie response – a unique psychophysiological reaction associated with lying. Yet those who followed his lead greeted his claim with skepticism (e.g. Larson 1932, 1938); they understood that there was an obvious advantage to comparing physiological reactions to different kinds of questions, at least one of which was relevant to the issue at hand. The first polygraph technique to include comparison questions, the relevant/irrelevant test (RIT), was introduced into the scientific literature by Larson (1921).

As its name implies, the RIT includes two types of questions. The relevant or "did you do it" question addresses the suspect's involvement in the alleged misdeed. In criminal investigations (or any situation where a specific incident is alleged to have occurred), this question deals with a single issue and takes the form of an accusation. In the case of a murder or an arson, for instance, respective relevant questions might be phrased "Did you shoot Clem Fisbee?" or "Did you light the fire that burned your house down?" Interposed among such relevant questions are queries that deal with irrelevant issues, such as "Is your name William?" or "Are you now in Minneapolis?" The subject is expected to answer these items truthfully. They are intended to provide an index of physiological reactivity against which the responses to the relevant questions can be compared. If the relevant questions elicit larger responses than the irrelevant comparison items, the individual is deemed to be deceptive. Responses of equivalent size to the two types of questions indicate truthfulness.

The RIT is most often used today as an employee screening tool to evaluate the character of employees and determine if they follow employer regulations. Although some commercial businesses (e.g., pharmaceutical companies and security firms) are allowed by the Employee Polygraph Protection Act to use the RIT this way, it is the federal government (which exempted itself from coverage by this Act) that most commonly employs the RIT for employee screening. Although this variant of the RIT still includes relevant and irrelevant questions, the form of the relevant questions and the purpose of the irrelevant questions are different from those in the criminal case.

Because it is unclear that an employee has necessarily done anything wrong, relevant questions cannot deal with a specific incident. Instead, they cover the likelihood, in general, that an employee (or prospective hire) has done something the employer would like to know about. Hence, relevant questions might deal with topics such as whether the subject has lied or omitted information on an employment application, taken anything of value from a prior employer, come to work while under the influence of a drug, left a classified file unattended, divulged secret information to foreign nationals, and so forth. Irrelevant questions, rather than serving a comparison purpose, are designed to provide a respite in what otherwise would be a long series of emotionally laden questions.

The interpretation of this test depends more on how responses to the different relevant questions may identify an area of special sensitivity. For instance, if the employee shows more physiological reactivity to drug and alcohol questions than to questions dealing with employee dishonesty, the examiner may focus on the area of substance use, ultimately failing the subject if strong reactions to such questions continue and the employee has no reasonable explanation for this apparent excessive sensitivity. Employees who are socially skilled and able to convincingly "explain away" their reactions are thus likely to avoid incrimination. Thurber (1981) found that, among applicants for police officer jobs, those who scored highest on a measure of impression management were most likely to pass a polygraph screening test.

"CONTROL" QUESTION TEST

The obvious problem with the specific-incident version of the RIT is that the irrelevant questions do not provide an adequate control for the emotional impact of being asked the accusatory relevant questions. Even an innocent person can reasonably be expected to show more physiological disturbance to "Did you fondle your daughter's genitals when you gave her a bath?" than to "Is today Tuesday?" In 1947, John Reid described a different procedure, one requiring that responses to relevant questions be evaluated against the response to comparison questions that were themselves designed to elicit emotional reactions. These "control" questions were supposed to deal with an issue thematically related to the matter under investigation, involving some misdeed that presumably everyone has been guilty of at some time in their lives.[2] In a case of theft or murder, for example, the control question might take the form "Have you ever taken something from someone who trusted you?" or "Have you ever deliberately hurt someone to get revenge?" The assumption is that everyone has done these sorts of things – or, if they have not, they are nevertheless concerned about the truthfulness of their answer to the control question.

The CQT (control question test) theory assumes that guilty people will be more concerned about their lie to the relevant question than by their denial to the innocuous control question. Consequently, their nervous systems should react more strongly to relevant than control questions. Innocent people, by contrast, should be unconcerned about their responses to the relevant question because they are not, after all, guilty. Because they are supposed to be more worried about their response to the control question,

they are expected to respond more strongly to it than to the relevant question. The CQT theory predicts this result because innocent individuals are led to believe that lying to this question is also cause for failing the test. How it is that they should reach this conclusion is explained (for a case of theft) as follows:

"Since this is a matter of a theft, I need to ask you some general questions about yourself in order to assess your basic honesty and trustworthiness. I need to make sure that you have never done anything of a similar nature in the past and that you are not the type of person who would do something like stealing that ring and then would lie about it.... So if I ask you, 'Before the age of 23, did you ever lie to get out of trouble ...?' you could answer that no, couldn't you?" Most subjects initially answer no to the control questions. If the subject answers yes, the examiner asks for an explanation ... [and] leads the subject to believe that admissions will cause the examiner to form the opinion that the subject is dishonest and therefore guilty. This discourages admissions and maximizes the likelihood that the negative answer is untruthful. However, the manner of introducing and explaining the control questions also causes the subject to believe that deceptive answers to them will result in strong physiological reactions during the test and will lead the examiner to conclude that the subject was deceptive with respect to the relevant issues concerning the theft. In fact, the converse is true. Stronger reactions to the control questions will be interpreted as indicating that the subject's denials to the relevant questions are truthful. (Raskin 1989, pp. 254–5)

Perhaps the most significant development for the CQT since Reid introduced it was Backster's (1962) modifications. Prior to Backster, the autonomic tracings generated during polygraph examinations were largely evaluated subjectively. This subjective evaluation, which subsequently has been referred to as "global scoring," was based in part on examination of the polygraph charts but also on other possible indications of guilt uncovered by the examiner, such as inconsistencies in the subject's account of the alleged incident or aspects of an individual's demeanor (e.g., failure to maintain eye contact) that might suggest guilt (Reid & Inbau 1977). A student of Reid, Backster introduced a semiobjective "numerical" scoring procedure to quantify the outcome of the examination (to be described shortly).

The CQT is more appropriately considered a collection of related techniques than a single technique. In this family of procedures, the number of questions and charts, the phrasing, content, and positioning of questions, the nature of "filler" questions, global and numerical scoring procedures, and the autonomic measures employed may all differ across examiners, especially those trained in different schools or working in different settings.

One variant in procedure involves the use of a "stimulation" or "stim" test, introduced by Keeler (1930, 1939).

The purpose of this procedure is to convince examinees that their psychophysiological reactions will indeed give them away if they lie. There are many variations on how a stim test is carried out, but one approach involves having subjects pick a card from a deck, concealing it from the examiner. The examiner then asks a series of questions ("Was it a club?", "Was it a face card?", etc.) having the subject respond No to each item until the card can be identified through inspection of the examinee's physiological responses. Because it is possible that the examiner will make a mistake, which would achieve the opposite of the intended effect, some examiners use marked decks so they know which card was chosen. Others will have the subject place the card face up so both can see it, ask the same questions, and then announce that it is obvious the subject's lying will be detectable. To further convince the subject, if necessary, the examiner may show the subject the recording of his or her physiological reactions while pointing out that the largest response seems to be associated with the correct answer. Sometimes examiners alter amplifier settings to artificially augment the response when the key question is asked so it will be clear to the examinee that he or she is detectable.

When the stim test is introduced to the subject, if at all, is a matter of examiner choice. Some examiners conduct the stim test before asking the CQT questions. Others first ask the CQT questions and then introduce the stim test, followed by one or more repetitions of the CQT items. Still others will use their discretion to decide where to place the stim test. For example, they may elect not to use it at all if, after the first run through the CQT questions, the response pattern seems clear (i.e., there may be no perceived need to "stimulate" the subject to obtain a definitive polygraph verdict).

Perhaps the variation of the CQT that is most unlike the others in this class is the directed lie test (DLT). With this recent innovation, the subject is "directed" to answer the control questions deceptively. An example would be "Have you ever told even one lie?" or "Have you ever broken even one rule?", to which subjects are told to answer No. Subjects are also instructed to think about a particular time they told a lie or broke a rule when they are asked these questions. Directed lie questions are explained to the subject by the examiner as follows (Raskin 1989, p. 271): "I need to have questions to which you and I both know you are lying. That way, I can be sure that you continue to respond appropriately when you are lying and that you remain a suitable subject throughout this test." As with the conventional CQT, guilty subjects are expected to give stronger reactions to the relevant questions. However, subjects who respond truthfully to the relevant questions should be worried about whether their directed lie responses will demonstrate that their reactions are different when they are truthful. According to Raskin (1989), this concern should enhance their reactions to the directed lie controls, making them stronger than reactions to the relevant questions.

PEAK OF TENSION TEST AND GUILTY KNOWLEDGE TEST

The forerunner of the guilty knowledge test (GKT) is the peak of tension test (POTT; Keeler 1939). Keeler introduced the notion that one could present to a suspect a question along with multiple possible answers, with only the guilty and law enforcement authorities aware of the correct answer. In a bank robbery, for instance, if the amount stolen was not divulged to the public then only the police and the robber would know that the amount stolen was $20,000. Attached to a polygraph, the suspect could be asked "Was the amount taken from the bank ... $5,000 ... $10,000 ... $15,000 ... $20,000 ... $25,000?" The suspect's "psychological tension" as well as his or her autonomic reaction would be expected to build to a "peak" at $20,000 and subsequently decline, thus revealing knowledge and likely involvement in the crime.

The "searching" peak of tension test differs from the standard POTT in that the examiner does not know the answer to the question. Instead, the subject's maximum response is used to discover what the answer is. An example of an application of this procedure might involve the bank robber, who has hidden the money, being asked if it is located at any of various numbered locations indicated on a map. As the suspect is asked to look at each numbered location, the examiner endeavors to determine the location associated with the greatest physiological arousal, presumably revealing where the money was hidden.

The GKT, developed by David Lykken (1959, 1960), is a refinement of the POTT in which a series of multiple choice questions, all dealing with facts with which only those knowledgeable about the crime would be familiar. The GKT assumes that the guilty individual's recognition of the correct multiple choice alternative (the "key") will lead to stronger physiological responses to this than to the other alternatives for a given question. The incorrect alternatives indicate what the response to the correct alternative should look like if the subject is innocent, unaware of which answer conveys guilty knowledge. Unlike the other deception detection techniques, the GKT and the POTT are seldom used in forensic applications.

Physical Context

There is no unique physiological response associated with lying, and there is no known physical substrate underlying what these tests measure. In fact, it is not clear what psychological processes are tapped by the techniques employed in applied polygraphy – or even how important deception per se is to their outcome (Furedy & Ben-Shakar 1991; Furedy, Davis, & Gurevich 1988; Saxe 1991).

Poiygraph operators are taught that their procedures most likely depend on a subject's fear of the consequences of being detected. However, little research has been directed at this issue; it remains possible that other psychological constructs, such as the guilt and anxiety associated with lying or belief that the test works, are important. Because the psychological underpinnings of applied polygraphy are so poorly understood, it should be no surprise that the physical substrate underlying these techniques has received virtually no attention beyond the level of identifying useful peripheral measures. Given this background, this section will characterize the psychophysiological measurements associated with polygraph testing.

INSTRUMENTATION

Regardless of the type of test they give, polygraphers typically rely on a portable field polygraph, often no larger than a brief case, to monitor autonomic reactions to the test questions. Recorded activity includes electrodermal responsivity (either skin resistance or conductance), monitored from stainless steel electrodes attached to the fingertips; respiration, recorded from pneumatic belts positioned around the upper chest and abdomen; and a "cardio" channel in which relative changes in blood pressure are determined by observing pressure oscillations obtained from a standard, partially inflated sphygmomanometer cuff placed on the subject's arm. In addition, some examiners add a channel in which digital vasomotor activity is recorded using a plethysmograph.

For older field polygraphs, respiration and blood pressure were mechanically recorded. Changes in air pressure in the pneumatic belts used to record respiration and in the blood pressure cuff caused bellows in the polygraph to expand and collapse. By attaching the polygraph pens to these bellows, a record of pressure changes can be recorded on the chart paper. Some polygraphers, especially those trained to use this type of equipment, prefer to make recordings using these mechanically coupled devices even though more sensitive electronic modules are available. Patrick and Iacono (1991a) compared the recordings obtained from a typical field polygraph that used both mechanical and electronic recording modules to those simultaneously monitored by a quality laboratory polygraph and showed that the two instruments produced similar recordings that, when numerically scored, yielded almost identical results.

The most obvious change in field polygraphy during the last decade has been the computerization of the recordings. Computers and software are available that digitize and store the analog recordings, which can be edited off-line and inspected on computer monitors or plotted out. In addition, software is available to score records and even interpret them, at least for CQT polygraphy. Some scoring programs provide a statement of the probability that an individual was truthful in response to the relevant questions. Because this software is proprietary, nothing is known about the algorithms and data base used to support such decisions, and little is known about their validity.

SCORING

Although global evaluation of polygraph tests used to be common and is still important for employee screening, semiobjective numerical approaches are now typically applied to the CQT. In the variant of numerical scoring that is now most prevalent, control and relevant questions (which are usually presented to the subject one after the other) are scored in pairs. For each physiological channel, a determination is made regarding whether the control question or the relevant question paired with it elicited the larger response. If the control question produces the larger response, a number from 1 to 3 is assigned for that channel depending on how much larger the response to the control question is. If the relevant question generates the larger reaction, scores from −1 to −3 are assigned, as appropriate. Typically, there are three pairs of control and relevant questions per "chart" (a chart is the physiological record generated by a single run through all the questions). There are three charts, each generated by the same question list (usually about ten questions are asked, including some irrelevant items that do not figure in the scoring), with the questions presented in a different order each time. By summing these scores over each of the three channels (electrodermal, respiration, and cardio) and each chart, a total score is obtained. Scores of 6 or higher indicate truthfulness; scores from 5 to −5 are considered inconclusive; −6 or lower indicates deception.

Social Context

Many psychological tests are individually administered (e.g., the Wechsler family of intelligence tests), requiring a trained examiner to interact with an examinee in order to obtain a valid test administration. Although these tests are thus partially dependent on the quality of the social interaction between two people, they are actually constructed and administered in such a way as to minimize the likelihood that the outcome is dependent on the examiner. This result is accomplished in part by having standardized test stimuli administered to each test subject in the same manner. Polygraph tests are also individually administered, but they are not standardized: an individual tested by two different examiners might be asked quite different questions, presented in different formats, with or without a "stim" test, and so on. In fact, there is virtual unanimity among practicing polygraphers that the behavior of the examiner and the quality of his or her interaction with the subject is critical to the outcome of any particular polygraph test.

For instance, the examiner must:

1. use the information collected during the pretest interview to develop questions using a vocabulary the examinee can understand;
2. review those questions with the examinee to be certain their meaning is clear;
3. convince the examinee that failing the control questions will lead to a deceptive test outcome (i.e., so that the previously quoted result described by Raskin 1989 is achieved); and
4. decide whether and when to use a stim test to boost the examinee's confidence in the procedure.

Failure to achieve these objectives, all of which depend in part on the quality of the social interaction between examiner and examinee, would serve to invalidate a given test administration.

Because of the importance of interpersonal factors to polygraph test outcome, in this section I will describe how social context is important to the practice of polygraphy and how the format of the test, which is built in part around the examiner's ability to interact effectively with examinees, leads polygraphers to the unwarranted conclusion that the techniques they employ are highly accurate. In the process, I hope to make apparent that a polygraph test can more appropriately be considered an interview *cum* interrogation assisted by the recording of psychophysiological data than a conventional, objective psychological test (see also Ben-Shakar & Furedy 1990 for an evaluation of the degree to which polygraph techniques constitute tests).

COMPONENTS OF A FIELD POLYGRAPH TEST

Polygraph tests, especially the CQT, have three components. The first is the pretest interview, during which the examiner collects information from the subject such as medical and psychological history, attitudes about the importance of one's character and integrity, and the subject's account of the crime. This information is then used to formulate the relevant and control questions, which are subsequently reviewed with the subject to make certain each question can be answered Yes or No. During the pretest interview, the polygrapher is also likely to review the subject's views about polygraphy, including whether the subject has taken prior tests, and attempt to reassure the subject that the test is highly accurate. The second stage of the examination consists of asking the test questions while recording physiological responses; it also involves evaluating the physiological data and making a diagnosis. If the verdict is truthful, the subject is free to leave. If it is inconclusive, arrangements might be made to resolve the matter by scheduling another test session. But if it is deceptive, the examiner will interrogate the subject, using the failed test plus the information collected during the pretest interview to attempt to elicit a confession. Being told that one has

failed the lie detector, that "this impartial, scientific instrument tells me that you are not telling the truth about this," can be a powerful inducer of confessions from guilty (and sometimes even from innocent) suspects. This posttest interrogation thus becomes the third and final component of the examination.

It is not generally recognized that specific-incident polygraph tests are typically administered after a thorough investigation has uncovered ambiguous evidentiary data that are unlikely to be resolved through further investigation (Patrick & Iacono 1991b). The test represents an opportunity to close the case, one that is best realized if suspects who fail the test confess to wrongdoing. Hence, one of the chief aims of test administration is to resolve the case by obtaining further evidence in the form of admissions or a confession from those subjected to the stress of interrogation. That a small but substantial fraction of those failing the test make such admissions speaks to the utility of polygraph testing as a forensic investigative tool. Although this phenomenon does not directly address the issue of validity, the fact that failing the test leads to confessions helps to convince examiners that their tests are infallible.

WHY POLYGRAPHERS BELIEVE IN THEIR TECHNIQUES: THE IMPORTANCE OF CONFESSIONS

The problem with reasoning that the test must be accurate – because many who fail then confess – is that it does not account for the biased manner in which polygraphers are likely to obtain feedback regarding the accuracy of their decisions. Because these tests are typically administered when the facts are ambiguous, there is little likelihood that an adequate criterion for what constitutes "ground truth" will ever become apparent. It is unlikely that these cases will go to trial; if the facts were clear enough for a legal resolution, there would have been no need to conduct the polygraph test. Moreover, if the case were to be resolved by trial and the outcome was at variance with the polygrapher's diagnosis, the trial verdict can be easily dismissed as an error, stemming perhaps from the requirement that the accused must be seen as guilty beyond a reasonable doubt, from court rules that render some incriminating evidence inadmissible (e.g., the polygraph test results!), or from jury error.

What the polygrapher actually becomes aware of, then, is whatever can be derived from a general absence of follow-up information regarding ground truth. More explicitly, if a person passes a polygraph test then that person will not be asked to confess, and the polygrapher will most likely never know if this was an instance where a guilty person generated a false negative outcome. Likewise, if the person fails but does not confess, the examiner will never know if this was a case of an innocent person producing a "false positive" error. In fact, the only time the examiner is likely to get any feedback is if an individual confesses following a failed test. Thus, the examiner has no realistic opportunity ever to be made aware of errors, and the only feedback likely to be received will always confirm the test outcome. It is for this reason that examiners can honestly make claims asserting that they have given thousands of tests but have never been shown to be wrong – there is really little likelihood they would ever uncover unambiguous evidence of guilt or innocence that could be used to substantiate an error.

FRIENDLY VERSUS ADVERSARIAL TESTS

Martin Orne (1975) was first to draw attention to the possibility that polygraph tests might yield different verdicts depending on the circumstances of test administration. "Adversarial" tests are those administered by law enforcement officials. The results of these tests are likely to be known to the prosecution and may affect the likelihood that the police will intensify their investigation of an individual if the test is failed. A "friendly" test is one arranged by a suspect's attorney; its outcome is protected by attorney–client privilege. The results of friendly tests are likely to become public only if the suspect passes the test, in which case the result will be used to argue the innocence of the suspect. Friendly tests have been criticized as likely to be more easily passed than adversarial tests because less is at stake with a friendly administration. Besides the examinee having less to fear regarding the consequences of being found deceptive, there is greater likelihood with a friendly test that the test will be subtly influenced by the belief that the suspect, who is paying the polygrapher's fee in hopes of a nondeceptive outcome, is innocent.

Currently there are no empirical data that bear directly on the differential validity of tests administered under these two different sets of circumstances. All field studies conducted to assess the accuracy of polygraph tests have used subjects tested in adversarial cases. Thus, little is known about the accuracy of friendly tests per se. This is a serious shortcoming of the existing literature, because it is the results of friendly tests that are most often presented in court.

DO POLYGRAPHERS ALLOW SUBJECTIVE EVALUATION TO AFFECT THEIR DECISIONS?

Although polygraph testing clearly has many subjective elements, empirical data are needed to address the possibility that the nature of the dyadic interaction can affect the outcome of the test. Such data are available from a study of Royal Canadian Mounted Police (RCMP) polygraph practices that was conducted by Patrick and Iacono (1991b). The RCMP, Canada's national police force, is recognized as having among the best trained polygraph examiners in the world – examiners who use state-of-the-art

techniques, who receive continuing education training, and whose work is reviewed periodically to ensure its quality. There is thus no reason to suppose the work of these examiners represents anything less than the finest that professional polygraphy has to offer.

In their field study, Patrick and Iacono (1991b) identified RCMP criminal investigations involving a polygraph test and examined the complete set of cases for a specified region of British Columbia over a five-year period. The police officers who administered the control question polygraph tests were trained to numerically score the autonomic data. Their personal disdain for the global approach to scoring was reinforced by their training, which emphasized that their decisions were not to be based on their subjective evaluation of case information or suspect characteristics.

To determine if their decisions were in fact based entirely on chart data, we compared the verdicts announced in their written reports for each case with their own numerical scores as well as with numerical scores obtained by having other examiners blindly rescore their charts ($n = 276$). Of the 73 tests the original examiners scored as truthful, all but one generated a written verdict indicating nondeception. For the 132 tests that were originally scored deceptive, only 82% of the suspects were diagnosed deceptive. In effect, the examiner overruled the conclusion that should have been dictated by his own numerical score, deciding that 18% of the individuals with deceptive numerical scores were truthful or that the situation was inconclusive. Another 69 cases fell into the numerically inconclusive zone; 45% of these were interpreted as truthful and 4% as deceptive.

These findings indicate that examiners disregard their own evaluations of the physiological data, relying instead on extrapolygraphic cues to render their verdicts. However, there is an obvious lack of symmetry in how they make these adjustments: of the 59 times examiners contradicted their own numerical scoring, 93% of the time they offered opinions that favored the truthfulness of the suspect by rendering inconclusive or truthful verdicts when the physiological scoring indicated deception or truthful diagnoses when inconclusive scores were obtained.

Inspection of the blind rescore data showed that the original examiners also tended to adjust their numerical scores to favor truthfulness. For example, 72 suspects received numerical scores indicating truthfulness from the original examiner, but only 51 (29% fewer) of the blindly rescored charts indicated truthfulness. This result obtained not merely because the blind examiners were more cautious in their numerical scoring and therefore more likely to arrive at inconclusive scores. Of all the charts that were originally numerically scored as other than inconclusive, 40% fell in the truthful range. For the blindly rescored charts that yielded non-inconclusive scores, only 32% were truthful. Hence, the original examiners were more likely to generate numerically truthful scores than the blind scorers, further suggesting that their original scores also reflected their tendency to believe many of the suspects were innocent.

The final interesting observation related to these data was the finding that the original examiners were more accurate with their written verdicts for truthfulness than in their numerical scoring or than the numerical scoring of the blind examiners. For subjects who met the ground truth criteria for innocence (they were cleared by the confession of another implicated individual), the original examiners were correct 90% of the time. By contrast, the accuracy of their numerical chart scores was 70%, and the accuracy of the blind scorers' numerical evaluations was only 55%.

These data suggest the following important conclusions.

1. Even though numerical scoring was supposed to dictate the verdicts of the examiners, they relied on information not contained in the polygraph charts to make their diagnoses.
2. These extrapolygraphic data also affected the decisions they made when they numerically scored their charts.
3. Both their opinions and their numerical scores were adjusted to favor the likelihood that suspects were innocent.
4. Their behavior actually led to more accurate decisions than would have obtained had their decisions been made from a strict evaluation of the charts.
5. In order to determine the validity of the psychophysiological test (i.e., what the decision would be if only the psychophysiological data were used), it is necessary to have the charts blindly scored by someone who knows nothing about the case.

A major criticism of the CQT, forcefully advanced by Lykken (1974), is that it is biased against innocent people because even innocent individuals are likely to be more disturbed by the threatening accusations contained in the relevant questions than by the comparatively innocuous nature of the material covered by the control questions. These RCMP data would seem to suggest that, on some level, the examiners were aware of this bias. To avoid misclassifying innocent individuals, they look for case and suspect data that convinces them to override the physiological data if it does not gibe with the extrapolygraphic information.

THE BOGUS PIPELINE

Saxe (1991) noted that the social context of the testing situation is likely to influence physiological responding. In particular, he draws attention to the possibility that the CQT may work in part because people believe it works. I have already noted why polygraphers come to believe that their techniques are virtually infallible, and that an important aspect of the procedure is to convey this conviction to suspects. Is the effectiveness of polygraph tests determined in part by a type of "placebo response" governed by the polygrapher's ability to convince the subject of the efficacy of polygraphy?

It was this type of possibility that was explored with the "bogus pipeline" paradigm of Jones and Sigall (1971). Concerned that people were not reporting racial attitudes honestly, Jones and Sigall examined the effect that hooking subjects up to a phony lie detector machine had on their reporting of racial prejudice. Those who thought they were being polygraphed (and thus were detectable if they lied) revealed more negative racial attitudes than those who were not connected to the lie detecting equipment. This bogus pipeline effect may account for why suspects make damaging admissions and even confess under the duress of polygraphic interrogation. If they are convinced the test works, then they are likely to believe either that they (a) will be detected, in which case they might as well admit their wrongdoing before the test is finished, or (b) have been detected by a procedure that is recognized as accurate, so they may as well confess during the posttest interrogation that follows a failed test.

It is because of this effect that polygraph tests have often been used by sex offender treatment programs to verify the good behavior of and encourage full reporting from clients (Abrams 1989). For example, Emerick and Dutton (1993) examined the effects of polygraph testing on the disclosures adolescent sex offenders made about their deviant sexual behavior when referred for treatment intake assessments. Sexual histories were obtained by both clinical interview and a "confirmation polygraph" interrogation that was designed in part to verify the truthfulness of the sexual behavior reported during the interview. Although in the absence of ground truth the validity of any elicited information is unknown, it is nevertheless interesting that the polygraph test generated substantially more admissions (often two to three times as many) than the interview regarding the number of child victims, frequency of assaults, use of force, and prior exposure to pornographic material. Abrams (1989, pp. 176–7), in discussing this application of polygraph testing, expresses the concern that if subjects pass these types of tests then they may come to believe they have beaten the polygraph, because a pass implies truthfulness on the control questions that "almost definitely" involve lies. Abrams warns that this can create a "placebo effect," giving the subject confidence that he can mislead the examiner on the relevant questions, leading to a false negative finding on subsequent tests. To combat this possibility, the examiner should draw attention to the control questions, indicate that the subject has shown signs of deception, and seek at least a "minor" admission. Abrams concludes, "In no case should the subject be allowed to leave believing that he has beaten the test." As noted previously, applications like these speak to the utility of polygraph testing and help explain why there is so much support for their continued use.

Saxe (1994) extended the bogus pipeline concept by arguing that an examinee who believes that a test is accurate is likely to show more physiological disturbance when responding deceptively and to feel reassured or less reactive when responding truthfully. Those with little confidence in the test are hypothesized to be less aroused by answering questions with lies and highly anxious when answering honestly. Lykken (1974, 1975) offered similar speculation regarding the effect confidence in the procedure can be expected to have on a subject's autonomic reactivity. Saxe (1991) reported the results of a mock crime study from his laboratory that were consistent with such reasoning. Guilty subjects were told they could keep money they "stole" if they could pass a CQT. Both innocent and guilty subjects were told either that the test was essentially infallible or that it had questionable validity. A stim test was also used, but in the latter condition the demonstration of its effectiveness failed. Guilty subjects were detectable only when they believed the test was accurate. In fact, none of the guilty subjects were detected when they did not believe in the efficacy of the CQT.

Inferential Context

RELIABILITY
Test–Retest Reliability

Almost nothing is known about polygraph test–retest reliability. This is unfortunate for several reasons. First, given the lack of standardization of applied polygraph tests and the extent to which subjective factors influence examiner opinion, it is of considerable interest whether different examiners would reach the same conclusion when testing the same subject. Second, in real life, situations often arise where the value of testing a subject a second time is raised. A second test may be proposed if the first produced an inconclusive result. Second tests are also often proposed when the defense and prosecution stipulate to the admissibility of polygraph results at trial and in advance of a test being taken. Often, the prosecution will suggest dropping the charges if a defendant passes a test. If the test is failed, the defendant is then asked to take a retest. If that test is passed then charges are dismissed, but if it too is failed then the results of both tests will be used as evidence to prosecute the suspect. Third, in real life, often the first test a suspect takes is a friendly test arranged by the defense. An issue that frequently arises focuses on the pros and cons of that suspect taking a second test administered by the police. Fourth, sometimes defendants pass two tests and wish the court to consider the possibility that it is thus especially unlikely that the defendant is guilty. It is not known to what extent having passed one test influences the likelihood of passing a second. For instance, would it necessarily be the case that guilty suspects who pass a first test could be expected to fail a second

test? Fifth, the role of habituation on the outcome of the second test is potentially important to consider. Iacono, Boisvenu, and Fleming (1984) showed that habituation can be pronounced over the course of a question sequence. Also, because the control questions are more likely than the relevant questions to vary substantially from one testing to the next, habituation may have a more pronounced effect on the relevant questions and thereby increase the likelihood of passing a second test. The effect of differential habituation to the two types of questions over multiple occasions needs to be addressed.

Interscorer Reliability

There is no debate in the literature about interscorer reliability, which has been shown to be uniformly high across a wide variety of studies. For instance, among field studies that draw subjects from real-life cases, Horvath (1977) found that blind evaluators trained to score charts globally consistently scored them as the original examiners did (average $r = 0.87$). Both Patrick and Iacono (1991b) and Honts (1996) reported the reliability of blind chart evaluation of numerically scored charts to be over 0.90. Patrick and Iacono (1991b) reported high reliabilities for each of the three channels of autonomic data when blindly rescored, with the highest reliability associated with electrodermal recording ($r > 0.90$) and the lowest with respiration ($r < 0.80$).

VALIDITY
The Difficulty of Determining Validity

There are two types of studies that one can examine to assess validity. *Laboratory studies* require volunteer subjects to act out a mock crime and then to lie about it on a polygraph test. *Field studies* use criminal suspects who have taken a test and for whom evidence of ground truth exists. Both types of investigation have serious limitations that undermine their value for estimating validity under real-life circumstances (e.g. Abrams 1989; Ben-Shakar & Furedy 1990; Furedy & Heslegrave 1988; Iacono & Patrick 1987, 1988, 1997, 1999; Lykken 1981; Raskin 1986).

Laboratory Studies. Since it is the relative emotional impact of the relevant and control questions that determines the outcome of the test, it is reasonable to ask whether the emotional impacts experienced in the laboratory can be considered similar to those produced in the interrogation of criminal suspects in real life. One might suppose that the embarrassing nature of the control questions is reasonably comparable in both situations. However, for innocent subjects in a laboratory study, these questions are the only ones they are asked that deal with potentially sensitive subject matter, a fact that is likely to make innocent laboratory subjects relatively more responsive (than innocent subjects in real life) to control than relevant questions. Were this to be the case, laboratory studies would overestimate the accuracy of polygraph tests for innocent individuals.

However, it is the emotional impact of the relevant questions that differs substantially from laboratory to real-life settings. This would be the case for both innocent and guilty subjects, both of whom would reasonably be expected to be more worried about their responses to relevant questions when their futures are perceived to hang on how those responses are evaluated by the polygrapher. Moreover, the emotional impact of giving a false answer on instruction (as with directed lie control questions) cannot be assumed to be comparable to giving a false answer by one's own choice in the hope of evading detection for a real crime of which one is guilty. Another difference between laboratory and field settings is that laboratory tests are carried out as part of a standardized experimental procedure. Field tests are likely to vary substantially across examiners and suspects, even for suspects accused of fairly similar crimes. Given all these differences between laboratory and field situations, one cannot safely extrapolate to real-life criminal investigation from simulations where noncriminal subjects are merely following instructions and where neither "guilty" nor "innocent" subjects have anything to fear should the polygrapher conclude that they are lying (for an elaboration of these arguments, see e.g. Barland & Raskin 1973; Iacono & Patrick 1987; Kugelmass & Lieblich 1966).

This conclusion is supported by two laboratory studies that attempted to achieve greater verisimilitude, both of which obtained higher rates of error than typical laboratory studies cited by CQT proponents (see Kircher, Horowitz, & Raskin 1988 for a review). Patrick and Iacono (1989) used prison inmates who were led to believe that failing the polygraph might put them at risk of reprisals from their fellow inmates, who also participated in the same study. Forman and McCauley (1986) permitted their subjects to privately choose whether to be "innocent" or, to win a larger money bonus if they passed the CQT, to be "guilty" – thus increasing the sense of personal involvement both in the mock crime and in the decision to lie during the CQT. In these two studies, the average CQT accuracy was 73% – considerably lower than that for many laboratory studies without such manipulations, whose average accuracy is 88% (Kircher et al. 1988).

Field Studies. The standard design for a field study of polygraph validity is to select polygraph charts obtained in actual criminal investigations in which the suspect tested was later proved through a confession either to be deceptive or truthful. These verified charts are then rescored blindly by another examiner who is unacquainted with the suspect and with the case facts. In this way one can be sure that the diagnostic decision is based solely on the charts and not on information irrelevant to the psychophysiological determination of guilt, such as the case facts and information the polygrapher obtains interviewing the suspect.

The difficulty in conducting an adequate field study lies in obtaining a sufficient sample of cases in which the suspect tested was later proved to be either guilty or innocent by a method that is independent of the outcome of the polygraph test (Patrick & Iacono 1991b). As noted previously, polygraphers seldom learn the final outcome of cases in which they are involved. Virtually the only credible evidence a forensic polygrapher ever receives pertaining to the accuracy of his or her diagnoses arises when a suspect confesses at the conclusion of a failed polygraph examination. In cases where there are multiple suspects, the confession of one may verify that alternative suspects previously tested were truthful during their CQTs. Field studies of CQT accuracy have employed these polygraph-induced confessions, which identify the guilty and exonerate co-suspects, as their criterion of ground truth.

Polygraph tests that yield confessions are invariably confirmed by those confessions to be accurate because suspects do not confess unless they are interrogated and they will not be interrogated unless the examiner concludes, after evaluating the charts, that they have been deceptive. Half of all guilty suspects would fail even if the test outcome were to be actually determined by a coin toss. Believing in the "scientifically validated" polygraph procedure, some of these persons will confess. The verification of these selected charts thus tells us nothing about the actual validity of the CQT; that is, some unknown proportion of guilty suspects will have passed the test while some equally unknown proportion of innocent suspects will have failed but refused to confess.[3]

Those charts confirmed as truthful by the confessions of alternative suspects also are not representative of the charts of truthful suspects generally. The reason for this is that polygraphers, believing in the accuracy of their procedures, will not ordinarily proceed to test an alternative suspect once one suspect has failed and thus (in their view) has been shown to be the culprit sought. This means that, as a rule, the only charts verified as truthful will be those of suspects who have been previously diagnosed as truthful by the original examiner – who then proceeded to test an alternative suspect who failed and confessed.

Because the evaluation of polygraph charts is highly reliable, having confession-verified charts blindly rescored will of course tend to confirm the scoring of the original examiner, forcing the agreement between the blindly scored data and the confession criterion. These studies thus inform more about the reliability of chart scoring than about validity. Iacono (1991) illustrated that, if polygraph testing had exactly chance accuracy, then research based on confessions derived from tests conducted following the typical field and research practices outlined here would misleadingly imply that polygraph testing was essentially infallible.

Thus, existing field studies that have employed polygraph-induced confessions as criteria of ground truth have relied on a selection of charts that systematically excludes potentially invalid ones – both deceptive suspects who were classified as truthful and truthful suspects classified as liars. Such studies therefore inevitably result in estimates of validity, including *sensitivity* (the success with which the guilty are identified) as well as *specificity* (the degree to which the innocent are recognized as truthful), that are inflated to some unknown extent.

It turns out that the original examiners in these studies permit their knowledge of the case facts or their subjective impressions of the suspects tested to override the indications provided by the charts (cf. previous discussion of RCMP examiners; see also Patrick & Iacono 1991b). Most often this results in their concluding that a suspect may be innocent even though he or she received a failing or inconclusive result when the charts were scored by the standard rules. Sometimes this has led the original examiners to proceed to test an alternative suspect who also failed, was interrogated, and confessed, thus confirming their subjective belief in the first suspect's innocence. When these verified-truthful charts are included in the selection of charts to be rescored as part of a field study, those few truthful charts are likely to be scored as deceptive, thus reducing the overestimate of the CQT's specificity. The conclusion suggested by these considerations is that the existing field studies of CQT validity must overestimate its sensitivity and also (though to a lesser extent) the ability of the CQT to detect truthful responding.

Conclusions Concerning Validity

The great difficulty that exists evaluating the accuracy of polygraph tests, coupled with their widespread use, has served to fuel much of the controversy surrounding these applications. At one end are the professional polygraph community and psychologists who have been trained in polygraphy and practice as polygraph operators, all of whom believe that the existing evidence – despite any perceived limitations – supports their use of a forensic tool that has proven utility (if not validity). At the other end are social scientists, with no background in professional polygraphy, who believe that compelling evidence of validity should be in place before techniques are adopted that can have such profound consequences on our judicial system and the civil liberties of those tested. The result is a highly polarized field in which it is easier to point to areas of disagreement than to areas of agreement. In this section, I will highlight some key aspects of this controversy by drawing from reviews of the field over the last decade (Abrams 1989; Bashore & Rapp 1993; Ben-Shakar & Furedy 1990; Furedy & Heslegrave 1988; Honts & Quick 1996; Honts, Raskin, & Kircher 1997; Iacono & Lykken 1997a,b,c, 1999; Iacono & Patrick 1997, 1999; Lykken 1998; Raskin 1989; Raskin, Honts, & Kircher 1997a,b; Saxe 1991, 1994). Although all of these reviews are pertinent, the reader wishing to consider more thoroughly how I arrived at these conclusions can find all the arguments and ap-

propriate references in the exchanges between Iacono and Lykken (1997a,b,c) and Raskin et al. (1997a,b; Honts et al. 1997).

Status of the Relevant/Irrelevant Test. There is little advocacy for the use of the RIT in criminal or any type of specific incident investigation. The RIT is almost universally considered to be strongly biased against innocent individuals, an opinion that was reinforced by a recent mock crime study indicating over a 70% error rate among innocent research participants subjected to this technique (Horowitz et al. 1997).

Little is known about the accuracy of the employee screening version of the RIT. However, in one study carried out at the Department of Defense Polygraph Institute, only 34% of subjects who participated in an act of mock espionage were detected by federally certified polygraph examiners whose main duty was to conduct these types of examinations (Barland, Honts, & Barger 1989; Honts 1994). Data supplied by the Department of Defense to Congress on its use of counterintelligence polygraphs indicate that few individuals actually fail these tests. In one report, of 12,306 tests, only 23 (0.2%) were failed, and eight of these individuals received their security clearance anyway (Iacono 1994). Findings such as these led Honts (1994) to conclude that because examiners expect to find few "spies" working for the government, they adjust their decision rules to pass almost everyone. Such an interpretation helps explain why only 34% of the guilty in the mock espionage study were detected. The examiners, not knowing that the base rate of guilt in this study approached 50% and accustomed to a base rate under 1%, maintained their habit of tending to pass most of those tested. Although it is possible that periodic screening of government employees deters possible misbehavior, findings such as these provide insight into how the notorious CIA spy Aldrich Ames was able to pass two polygraph tests. They also raise serious questions about the effectiveness of the government's counterintelligence polygraph screening program.

CQT. Because most of the research on polygraphy has been directed toward the CQT, more is known about this procedure than any of the others. The CQT debate revolves around the following points of contention.

Accuracy with Innocent Subjects. One of the most serious criticisms against the CQT is that, because the control questions do not control for the accusatory impact of being asked the relevant question, even innocent subjects are likely to fail this test. Skeptics argue that the research literature indicates that it is unlikely the CQT has much more than 50% (or chance) accuracy with innocent subjects. In stark contrast, advocates argue from the same studies that the existing research supports the conclusion that the accuracy with innocent persons exceeds 90%.

Accuracy with Guilty Subjects. Proponents argue that the accuracy of the CQT with guilty subjects exceeds 95% and that it is very difficult for guilty individuals to learn how to appear nondeceptive by relying on countermeasures to defeat the test. Citing studies by Honts and associates (Honts, Hodes, & Raskin 1985; Honts, Raskin, & Kircher 1994), critics note that mock crime subjects seem to be unable to determine on their own how to effectively beat the CQT by using countermeasures. Instead, they need specific instructions on how to recognize relevant and control questions coupled with advice on how to unobtrusively augment their responses to control questions. Proponents also believe there are no important differences between friendly and adversarial tests, and draw attention to the fact that there are no studies indicating that the outcomes of the two types of test differ. In contrast, skeptics argue that the accuracy with guilty subjects is probably closer to 75%, provided they do not use countermeasures, and decidedly less if they do use countermeasures. Citing the same studies of Honts et al. (1985, 1994), proponents note that the subjects in these studies easily learned to use countermeasures such as biting their tongues or silently performing serial subtraction when control questions were presented. The total instruction time in CQT theory and how to implement countermeasures was less than 30 minutes, and subjects were able to effectively learn to use their countermeasures (i.e., they not only beat the test, their use of countermeasures went undetected by experienced examiners) despite never being hooked up to a polygraph and thus never receiving feedback or coaching on how they might best manipulate their physiological responses. Anyone who reads the method sections of the reports of Honts and colleagues or turns to other sources of information about polygraph testing (e.g., Lykken's 1981 or 1998 books or the web page [www.polygraph.com] of D. Williams on "How to Sting the Polygraph") may learn how to employ countermeasures. Critics note that the differences between friendly and adversarial tests seem substantial, especially given the commonly held notion that the effectiveness of the CQT for detecting deception derives from the fear of being detected. The results of existing field studies derive from adversarial tests and therefore should not be generalized to friendly tests. The burden of proof rests with those who wish to rely on friendly tests to show they are equal to adversarial tests in their validity.

Acceptable Data for Deriving Accuracy Estimates. Reviewers of the literature are able to reach such different estimates of accuracy because they use different criteria to evaluate the adequacy of studies. Thus, the studies they consider to support their respective conclusions overlap little. Even when they rely on the same studies, they often reach quite different conclusions.

To enable the reader to gain some insight into the quality of arguments that have led to this polarization of views, it is illustrative to consider how one study, that of Patrick

and Iacono (1991b), has been interpreted. In their RCMP field study, Patrick and Iacono (1991; Iacono & Patrick 1988) followed the standard field study procedure of using confessions following failed tests to identify the guilty and exonerate the innocent. As noted previously, when confessions are used this way, it is extremely likely that the blindly rescored charts – especially from confirmed guilty subjects – will be "corroborated" by the confession, because chart scoring is very reliable and the original examiner's decision that the subject had tested positive always preceded obtaining the confession. Thus it should be a surprise to no one that, for confession-confirmed guilty subjects, Patrick and Iacono (1991b) reported that the original examiners' scoring of the charts was 100% accurate and that the blind evaluators were 98% accurate.

Despite the virtual certainty of obtaining such results under the circumstances – and despite Patrick and Iacono's arguments regarding why they could *not* be used to estimate validity – when Abrams (1989) reported the results of this study, he cited it as showing 98% accuracy for guilty subjects. Honts and Quick (1996) and Raskin et al. (1997a) cited the same data as supporting the high accuracy of the CQT with guilty suspects. Because none of these three reviews offered specific counterarguments to Patrick and Iacono's admonishment against relying on confession-confirmed charts for appraising validity, it is not possible to determine why they believe it appropriate to rely on them or on the results of other field studies, all of which are vulnerable to this same confession confound. Both Honts and Quick (1996) and Raskin et al. (1997b) further argued that blind scoring should not be used to assess the accuracy of the original examiner because the blind scorer rarely testifies in court. They argue that "the true figure of merit for the CQT in legal settings is the accuracy of the original examiners, whose decisions would be the evidence actually presented in court" (p. 627). They go on to claim that the proper figure to use from Patrick and Iacono (1991b) for estimating the accuracy of the CQT with guilty subjects is 100%. Of course, this figure does not tell us anything at all about the accuracy of the original examiner. It only indicates that, for the subset of suspects who fail the original examiner's CQT and confess, the "deception indicated" opinion of the original examiner matches the confession in every instance.

What was unique about the Patrick and Iacono investigation was their attempt to circumvent the confession confound by searching for ground truth evidence that was not dependent on the outcome of the CQT. They did this by searching the police files of all the subjects (from 402 cases, many of which involved more than one subject) who received polygraph tests to uncover ground truth data that was not dependent on an individual's having failed the CQT (e.g., a confession that arose outside the context of the polygraph examination). In what turned out to be an interesting revelation about police practices, independent evidence of ground truth was found for only one guilty individual. This situation arose because the investigating officers who referred suspects for polygraph evaluations essentially closed their cases to additional investigation once a suspect failed the test. From these officers' point of view, this was a reasonable practice. Their investigation was already at a dead end when they made the case referral. The failed polygraph confirmed their suspicions but, absent a posttest confession, provided no new evidence that could be used to prosecute the suspect. Believing they "had their man," the Mounties closed the case file.

A rather different scenario was associated with nondeceptive polygraph outcomes. In these cases, the referring officer assumed that the suspect was innocent and that someone else must have committed the crime. Hence, case files tended to be left open for further investigation. For 24 subjects, continued investigation uncovered evidence that they were in fact innocent – either because someone else confessed to the crime or because it was evident that no crime was committed (e.g., an item reported stolen was subsequently found to have been misplaced by the owner). When the polygraph tests from these innocent individuals were blindly evaluated, 57% of the conclusive verdicts indicated truthfulness.

The Patrick and Iacono (1991b) study is the only one to date to offer validity data that are not contaminated by polygraph test-induced confessions. It showed that the psychophysiological test had only slightly better than chance accuracy for innocent people.

GKT. There is no controversy regarding the accuracy of the GKT in laboratory investigations. Repeatedly, reviews of the relevant literature have shown that in the laboratory, the GKT is often 100% accurate with innocent subjects and accurate about 85%–90% of the time with guilty research participants (Ben-Shakar & Furedy 1990; Iacono 1985; Iacono & Patrick 1988, 1999; Lykken 1988; Raskin et al. 1997a). It is of interest to note that proponents of the GKT are those most critical of CQT polygraphy, while critics of the GKT tend to be advocates for the CQT. One area about which there is agreement concerns the theoretical foundation of the GKT. There is no dispute that the GKT has a sound scientific foundation. The one other area of agreement concerns the conclusion that false positives are less of a problem for the GKT than false negatives. The areas of disagreement concern the following points.

Real-Life Applicability. For the GKT to have real-life applicability, several conditions must be satisfied. The crime under investigation must yield factual evidence that can be developed into GKT items. Robberies, burglaries, arsons, sex crimes, and many homicides leave trails of evidence suitable for this purpose, but some crimes (e.g., random acts of violence or sex crimes where the only issue is consent) do not lend themselves to the GKT format. The information from these crimes that is used to develop

GKT items must be known to both the police and the perpetrator but not to innocent suspects (although innocent subjects aware of crime facts may be distinguishable from both innocent but uninformed and guilty subjects; Bradley & Rettinger 1992). Facts that are too obscure to be remembered will not make good items.

Critics argue that it is too difficult to find crimes that satisfy these requirements. For instance, Podlesny (1993; Podlesny, Nimmich, & Budowle 1995) reviewed FBI case files to determine if they contained evidence that could be used to develop GKT items and concluded that perhaps no more than 15% of the case files could be used for this purpose. Proponents argue that what is needed are carefully conducted field studies using investigators who are trained to identify evidence suitable for GKT items. With regard to the Podlesny findings, much of what characterizes a crime scene may make excellent material for GKT items (e.g., characterization of specific aspects of the decor in a burglarized home) yet not be useful as evidence and are therefore not contained in an investigative file.

Interpretation of Existing Field Studies. There are now two published studies, both from the Israeli police, evaluating the performance of the GKT in actual criminal cases (Elaad 1990; Elaad, Ginton, & Jungman 1992). These studies showed hit rates above 95% for innocent suspects but somewhat high false negative rates (47%–58%) for guilty suspects. Although these results are disappointing, they are unlikely to be definitive to GKT advocates because the Elaad studies used an average of fewer than two items per GKT. Because the power of the GKT to detect the guilty increases exponentially with the number of items asked, it remains an open question how well GKTs based on longer question lists might fare.

Effectiveness of Countermeasures. Only two investigations of GKT susceptibility to countermeasures exist. Although Lykken (1960) showed that it is difficult to defeat a GKT, a more recent study by Honts and co-workers (1996) indicated that most mock crime guilty subjects could be trained to use countermeasures and so appear as though they did not possess guilty knowledge. Although the Honts et al. (1996) study is limited in several important respects (Iacono & Patrick 1999), it may be that a GKT based on autonomic measures is vulnerable to the countermeasure training of Honts et al. (1996). Were this shown to be the case, basing the GKT on cerebral measures such as the event related potential (ERP) might not only increase the effectiveness of the GKT but also substantially reduce the likelihood that these types of countermeasures can easily be used to defeat it (Bashore & Rapp 1993).

For instance, Allen, Iacono, and Danielson (1992) developed an ERP variant of the GKT that they evaluated by having study participants learn two word lists (from seven possible choices), one of which was known to the experimenter and the other of which was unknown or hidden from the experimenter (representing the equivalent of guilty knowledge). Words from these lists were mixed with novel words that participants had not seen before. Because both the known and hidden word lists had special significance to the subjects and were presented infrequently compared to the novel words, they elicited larger P3 brainwave voltages than the novel words. This situation would be analogous to showing criminal suspects pictures of a crime scene that the guilty should recognize intermixed with pictures of unfamiliar crime scenes, one subset of which was previewed in detail with the suspect.

In Allen et al. (1992), the subject's task was to prevent the experimenter from identifying the hidden word list while pressing a response key to indicate whether the word was novel or learned after each word was presented. In order to succeed in the task, the subject had to "lie" by using the response key to indicate that the hidden words were novel. This response requirement served as a check to ensure that subjects were actually paying attention to the stimuli. To determine the nature of the subject's "guilty knowledge," the ERPs to the seven word lists were averaged separately. The word list that generated an averaged ERP that was most similar to that generated by the learned list was assumed to be the hidden list. Using this procedure, the hidden list was identified accurately about 95% of the time. Because each subject served as his or her own control in this study, beating this test requires subjects to somehow generate an ERP to the hidden list that looks more like the ERP to the novel than learned words while consistently generating behavioral responses indicating correct classification of all the hidden and novel words as novel and the learned words as learned. Note that both "errors" – a hidden word misclassified as learned, or relatively longer response latencies to hidden than novel words – would be incriminating. It may be possible to train someone to beat such a test, but it is not obvious how this might be accomplished. Moreover, it would appear to be substantially more difficult to manipulate ERPs and manual response behavior (which is accurately measured to the nearest thousandth of a second) in this context than it would be to augment autonomic reactions in a typical GKT.

SCIENTIFIC OPINION

The opinions of scientists regarding polygraphy are important for two reasons. First, given the extreme unlikelihood that any line of research will yield findings that resolve concerns about accuracy, there is considerable value in a broad-based sampling of the opinions of scientists with sufficient background and expertise to evaluate polygraph tests. In fact, given how polarized the field is, there is obvious value in tapping the opinions of those with such expertise who are *not* considered to be the "experts" involved in the controversies about validity, since a poll of such experts would amount to little more than a head

count of those aligned with one viewpoint or the other. Second, the U.S. Supreme Court, in *Frye* and again in *Daubert* and *Scheffer,* has made the views of the scientific community about the general acceptance of a technique important to the determination of whether it can be used to develop evidence (see Faigman et al. 1997b, 1999 regarding the legal status of polygraph evidence in light of these and other court rulings). Hence, the legal community has a legitimate interest in prevailing scientific opinion about the theory and accuracy of polygraph tests.

Members of the Society for Psychophysiological Research (SPR) have been surveyed three times regarding their views on polygraphy (Amato 1993; Gallup Organization 1984; Iacono & Lykken 1997d). Polygraphy proponents (Murphy & Murphy 1997; Raskin et al. 1997a) as well as critics (Iacono & Lykken 1997a) have noted that polling SPR members is relevant to determining whether there exists a consensus among scientists about the validity of polygraph tests. The three surveys have in common the question presented in Table 1. Raskin, Honts, and their colleagues (Amato & Honts 1993; Honts & Quick 1996; Raskin et al. 1997a) have drawn attention to the fact that about 60% of respondents in the two earlier surveys endorsed alternative "B," indicating that polygraph interpretation "is a useful diagnostic tool." This finding led Amato and Honts (1993) to conclude that the membership of SPR consider polygraph tests "useful for legal proceedings" (p. S22), even though the question does not ask for an opinion about the use of polygraph tests in court. This question is ambiguous in other ways as well: it could be interpreted to deal with utility rather than validity, and it does not make clear what type of test is to be considered.

This lack of clarity led Iacono and Lykken (1997d) to conduct their own survey, asking this same question (so the three surveys would have this one feature in common) but also expanding the question list to include many other items in order to more fully flesh out the opinions of SPR members. A second group, the Fellows of the American Psychological Association's (APA) Division of General Psychology, was also polled (APA psychologists have also been recognized as having expertise appropriate to the evaluation of polygraphy; Murphy & Murphy 1997). Because it is the psychological and psychometric properties of polygraph tests that make them controversial, it seemed appropriate to survey this distinguished group of psychologists to supplement the views of the SPR membership and determine the extent to which common opinions are shared widely among psychologists. Because the psychological aspects of polygraph testing span many areas of psychology (e.g., experimental, social, clinical, physiological, measurement), the polling of general psychologists seems especially pertinent to the evaluation of polygraph testing.

In the Iacono and Lykken (1997d) surveys, only SPR members were asked the question reproduced in Table 1. As the table reveals, they obtained a pattern of responses

---

TABLE 1. SPR Member Opinions Regarding Usefulness of Polygraphy in Three Surveys

	Percent Who Agree		
	Gallup (1984) $N = 152$	**Amato (1993)** $N = 135$	**Iacono & Lykken (1997d)** $N = 183$
A. "A sufficiently reliable method to be the sole determinant"	1	1	0
B. "A useful diagnostic tool when considered with other available information"	62	60	44
"Between B and C"	2	—	2
C. "Of questionable usefulness, entitled to little weight against other available information"	33	37	53
D. "Of no usefulness"	3	2	2

Notes: Members of the Society for Psychophysiological Research were asked the following question: "Which one of these four statements best describes your own opinion of polygraph test interpretations by those who have received systematic training in the technique, when they are called upon to interpret whether a subject is or is not telling the truth?"

Although not offered as an option, in two of the surveys respondents indicated a choice that fell between alternatives B and C.

---

that differed significantly from that of the two earlier surveys. In particular, more individuals in the Iacono and Lykken survey thought polygraph tests were of "questionable usefulness" and fewer thought they were a "useful diagnostic tool." The reasons for these discrepant results are not clear but may derive from two factors. First, in the Iacono and Lykken survey only, respondents were specifically told that the focus of the survey was the CQT, and

they were also given a description of the CQT to reduce ambiguity concerning what it was. Because many members of SPR are likely to be as familiar with the GKT as with the CQT, their response to this question in the two earlier surveys may have been influenced by their greater confidence in the GKT coupled with their inclusion of the GKT among the techniques covered by the question. Second, the response rate to this question among the random group of

---

TABLE 2. Responses to Questions Asked of SPR and APA Members

Questionnaire Item	**Percent Who Agree**	
	SPR	APA
1. "Would you say that [the CQT, GKT, DLT] is based on scientifically sound psychological principles or theory?"		
a. CQT	36	30
b. DLT	NA	22
c. GKT	77	72
2. "Would you advocate that courts admit into evidence the outcome of control question polygraph tests, that is, permit the polygraph examiner to testify before a jury that in his/her opinion, the defendant was [deceptive or truthful] when denying guilt?"		
a. deceptive	24	20
b. truthful	27	24
3. Is it reasonable to conclude that an individual who fails 8 out of 10 GKT items has guilty knowledge?	72	75

Key: APA, American Psychological Association's Division of General Psychology; CQT, control question test; DLT, directed lie test; GKT, guilty knowledge test; NA, question not asked; SPR, Society for Physiological Research.

SPR members surveyed was over 85% for the Iacono and Lykken poll but only 30% for that of Amato. No information was provided about the Gallup survey's success in eliciting participation from the total sample of those contacted for their poll. It is possible that the earlier surveys drew samples generally favorable to polygraphy. Because Iacono and Lykken's sample was composed of the vast majority of those surveyed, it is unlikely to have drawn disproportionately from any subgroups within SPR (such as individuals with specialized training in polygraphy) and thus can be considered to be more broadly representative of the views of the SPR membership.

Table 2 presents the findings for questions asked in common to the membership of both organizations. The results are remarkably consistent, and they indicate that the CQT is viewed as neither scientifically sound nor suitable as scientific evidence. The Amato (1993) survey also failed to uncover much support for the CQT from SPR members. Respondents were asked to rate the accuracy of the CQT on a 5-point scale, with 1 reflecting chance and 5 indicating 100% accuracy. Means near the scale midpoint were obtained for accuracy with both innocent ($M = 2.7$) and guilty ($M = 3.1$) suspects. Likewise, APA fellows were unimpressed with the foundation for the DLT. Members of both groups saw the GKT as having a solid psychological basis. The contrast in the regard with which the CQT and GKT are held by scientists is important because it indicates that respondents are not generally against detection of deception techniques but are specifically skeptical about the CQT and its variant, the DLT. The similarity in responses of the members of these two organizations suggests that it is reasonable to assume agreement on the questions that were unique to each group.

Table 3 summarizes responses, grouped by topic, to several of the key questions that were unique to each organization. The first question listed was designed to determine if respondents believed the CQT to be correct at least 85% of the time. As indicated previously, proponents actually argue that the accuracy of the CQT is over 90% for innocent and 95% for guilty people. Obviously, the scientists polled are dubious of such claims and – as the responses to items 2 and 3 indicate – would require considerably better or more convincing evidence, ideally from field studies, to alleviate such doubts. The last two items

TABLE 3. SPR and APR Member Opinions about Polygraphy

Questionnaire Item (Group Asked)	Percent Who Agree
Psychometrics	
1. CQT is at least 85% accurate. (SPR)	
a. in tests of guilty suspects	27
b. in tests of innocent suspects	22
2. Strong empirical evidence is required before accuracy claims of proponents are believed. (APA)	93
3. It is reasonable for courts to give "substantial weight" to results of laboratory studies to estimate CQT validity in real life. (SPR)	17
4. The CQT can "accurately be called a standardized procedure." (APA)	20
5. The CQT is "relatively independent of differences among examiners in skill and subjective judgment." (APA)	10
Friendly Tests	
6. "Friendly" CQTs are more likely to be passed than those taken under adversarial conditions. (SPR)	75
7. If guilty, would take a "friendly" CQT. (APA)	72
8. If innocent, would take an "adversarial" CQT. (APA)	35
Countermeasures	
9. "CQT can be beaten by augmenting one's response to the control questions." (SPR)	99
10. Criminals and spies are likely to beat a CQT. (APA)	92
11. Confident could personally learn how to defeat a CQT. (APA)	75

Key: See Table 2.

in this category reveal that APA fellows believed that the CQT was neither a standardized nor objective procedure. The remaining data summarized in Table 3 points to the following conclusions: scientists believe that friendly tests are easier to pass than adversarial tests and that countermeasures can be used effectively to defeat a CQT.

With regard to the question in Table 1, in order to determine if opinions about polygraph testing varied as a function of how informed respondents were, all three studies divided respondents into those who were more or less informed about polygraphy based on their self-rated knowledge of the field. In the Iacono and Lykken survey, respondents were asked to report how many articles they had read or presentations they had attended dealing with polygraph test validity. The response to this question correlated 0.87 with self-rated knowledge, indicating that respondents tended to rate how informed they were based on how familiar they were with scientific research and presentations. For the three surveys, 30%–33% of respondents were considered to be "more informed" than the rest, based on their self-rated knowledge. Only the Amato survey reported a difference in how respondents answered the question in Table 1, with about 81% of those who considered themselves more informed selecting option B. In the Gallup and the Iacono and Lykken surveys, 60% and 48% (respectively) of the more informed endorsed this option. In these two surveys, endorsement rates were very similar to those observed for the respondents taken as a whole. To determine if respondents who were even more informed differed from the group as a whole, it was possible to identify from the Iacono and Lykken survey a "very informed" subgroup representing about 21% of the entire sample. Of this group, 48% picked option B, a result that did not differ from that obtained when the larger group of "more informed" individuals was considered. Iacono and Lykken (1997d) also examined the 44% of the sample who selected option B to see if they (as concluded by Amato and Honts 1993) would favor the use of the CQT in legal proceedings as indicated by their response to question 2 in Table 2. Only about half of those who thought the CQT to be a "useful diagnostic tool" favored its use in court. In addition, over 60% thought the CQT was less than 85% accurate in their response to item 1 in Table 3.

Taken in the aggregate, the responses of the SPR members and APA Fellows indicate substantial skepticism about the CQT and the claims made by CQT proponents. It is apparent from the Iacono and Lykken data that CQT polygraphy is not "generally accepted" by the majority of scientists polled. This impression is shared by J. K. Murphy, Chief of Polygraph for the Federal Bureau of Investigation (Murphy & Murphy 1997) as well as by writers of introductory textbooks in psychology. In a review of 37 texts published between 1987 and 1994 (Devitt, Honts, & Vondergeest 1997), only four of the books were judged to contain any citations favorable toward polygraph testing, and neither of two psychophysiologists reviewing the material on polygraphy in these texts judged even one of them as presenting a positive impression of polygraphy.

Epilogue

UNANSWERED QUESTIONS

A number of important issues concerning this area of applied psychophysiology deserve further attention. These issues are outlined next, together with some comments highlighting their complexity and the hurdles that must be overcome to resolve them.

RIT

Even though little is known about the accuracy of the RIT – because it is seldom used in specific-incident investigations and receives little advocacy for this purpose – little is to be gained by further research designed to evaluate its use in this context. In contrast, the employment screening variant of the RIT warrants considerably greater research. The validity and utility of this application are essentially unknown. Agencies that rely on employment screening polygraph tests assume that they deter undesirable applicants for jobs, reduce misconduct and employee turnover, are cheaper and more effective than conventional background investigations, encourage greater honesty, and lead to a higher-quality work force (Horvath 1993). If employee polygraph screening actually produces such results then it is no wonder that employers wish to use them. However, there has been little empirical evaluation of these purported benefits and no serious consideration of the possibly deleterious effects of screening. At issue are the civil rights of employees and employee prospects who fail tests and are denied employment; false positive errors and the self-removal of employees from consideration for jobs that require them to undergo a procedure they believe to be objectionable or invalid, both of which limit the employer's ability to hire the most talented individuals for a job; and false negative errors that allow undesirable employees, who now know they have "gotten away" with something and are unlikely to be suspected of wrongdoing should they engage in dishonest behavior, to hold secure jobs.

CQT

The central issue confronting CQT polygraphy is whether a research paradigm can be developed that would provide an unbiased test of the field accuracy of this technique. As noted repeatedly in this review and elsewhere (e.g., Iacono & Lykken 1997a), current field practices make it almost impossible to collect criterion ground truth data that is independent of someone having failed a polygraph test. Although confessions are themselves problematic as the standard for ground truth (e.g., only a select subgroup of those failing CQTs confess, and some confessions may be false), the serious problem with confessions is that they necessarily confirm the original examiner's polygraph verdict. The RCMP investigation of Patrick and Iacono (1991b) indicated that, although it may be possible to circumvent this problem to assess CQT validity for innocent people, it will not be possible to do so with guilty people. Raskin et al. (1988) required that ground truth in their field study be established both by a confession and the recovery of confirmatory evidence. Although the additional requirement of confession-corroborating information should eliminate false confessions, it does not deal with the confession confound because the additional evidence would not have been obtained had the suspect not failed the CQT, confessed, and led investigators to the evidence.

Other approaches to establishing ground truth are also problematic. Judicial outcomes are dependent on legal maneuvering and procedures, some of which are likely to have been influenced by the existence of polygraph data. This confound, coupled with the fact that the judicial outcome may not reflect the "truth," renders the use of judicial proceedings undesirable for the purpose of making a precise estimate of field polygraph accuracy. Another approach is to rely on an "expert panel" to review the case facts without concern about the admissibility of evidence or legal issues. This approach has been used in two field studies (Barland & Raskin 1976; Bersh 1969). Unfortunately, in both studies, the evidence presented to the panels included confessions from those who failed polygraph tests, thus undermining the independence of the panel.[4] Also, it was difficult for the panels in both studies to reach consensus on the guilt of those who took CQTs, and questions have been raised by the authors of one of the studies regarding the adequacy of data that panels had available for this purpose (Barland 1982; Barland & Raskin 1976; Raskin 1986).

To determine if the panel approach could be improved and to assess the validity of panel decisions themselves, Dohm and Iacono (1993) carried out an investigation in which panels of lay persons, police investigators, and attorneys reviewed multiple-suspect, specific-incident military criminal investigative files that ultimately led to the suspects taking CQTs. Twenty-seven cases were used for this purpose. In all these cases, one of the suspects who took a polygraph test confessed. However, this confession – rather than being presented as evidence to the panel – was withheld and served as the criterion against which to evaluate the panel's ability to decide who committed the crime. The panel was also not given the results of any of the polygraph tests. Prior to beginning the study, two judges reached consensus that, for the cases chosen, the confessions clearly confirmed the accusations against suspects that were contained in the CQT relevant questions. The reliability with which the panels made their determinations differed little across the three six-member panels and, although reasonable for social science research (average $r = 0.75$), was less than the interscorer reliability of the CQT. Ideally, these reliabilities would have to be above 0.9 to avoid the criticism that a mismatch between the polygraph and examiner verdicts was not attributable to panel decision-making inconsistency. Turning to the validity of panel decision making, panels had difficulty identifying the guilty: the overall hit rate was under 25%. Although these results are disappointing and indicate that panels are unlikely to be useful in the determination of ground truth, they are not surprising. As noted previously, had it been easy to decide from the case evidence who was guilty then the criminal investigation would probably have led to an indictment rather than to a polygraph test. The Dohm and Iacono findings also indicate that field studies, such as that of Honts (1996), in which polygraph case file evidence is reviewed to reach ground truth determinations cannot be accepted at face value unless evidence is presented about the likely validity of such determinations.

To solve the confession bias problem, a different approach to collecting CQT and ground truth information is needed. To eliminate the contamination that arises when confessions are used to establish ground truth, an adequate field study would require that some large police agency (e.g., a federal agency or a large city police department) administer polygraph tests to all criminal suspects brought in for questioning but without posttest interrogation of the suspects and without scoring the charts or communicating the test results to anyone; the charts would then be sealed and stored awaiting resolution of the case. At the time a case is to be closed, an independent panel would consider the case-related questions – the CQT relevant questions – put to each suspect and evaluate the available case material to decide the truthfulness of that suspect's answers. In this manner, the ground truth criterion, which could still be confession-based (because now whatever confession arose would have been independent of the results of the sealed polygraph exam), would be obtained independently of the outcome of the CQT. When sufficient cases have been closed to yield, say, 100 unanimous panel decisions each of "deceptive" and "truthful," the 200 polygraph charts associated with these ground-truth assessments would be independently scored and compared with the criterion judgments. If the results were sufficiently encouraging, then one would want to replicate this field study with a different police agency and different examiners. Practical concerns, such as those focused on suspects' rights and the likelihood of getting subjects and/or their attorneys to agree to such a study, make it unlikely that it would ever be executed. Moreover, since police polygraphers are already convinced that the CQT has near-perfect validity and since there is no indication that the use of polygraphy by law enforcement agencies will be restricted owing to concerns about validity, police agencies are likely to have no interest in cooperating with such a project. However, as long as no such study exists, it will not be possible to determine the field accuracy of the CQT.

GKT

An adequate field study of the GKT must deal with the same concerns just outlined for the CQT. Elaad (1990; Elaad et al. 1992) was able to lessen the confession confound problem in his studies because the GKT always followed a CQT, which presumably provided the primary basis for the polygrapher to interrogate a suspect in order to obtain a confession. The confession confound could have been lessened further by having the GKT administered by a different examiner who was blind to the outcome of the CQT. Then the first examiner, following standard procedure but unaware of the GKT results, could interrogate those who failed the CQT. The resulting confessions, when they occurred, would have been independent of the GKT outcome and thus could serve as a reasonable criterion of ground truth for the GKT. However, the issue of how the GKT's always following the CQT might affect the outcome of the GKT would still have to be addressed (see Iacono & Patrick 1999).

A good GKT field study would require the GKT items to be developed by criminalists or other investigators who were on the crime scene. In the Eland field studies, the polygrapher was faced with the burden of developing GKT items, a task rendered difficult by the fact that polygraphers do not visit the crime scene. Moreover, those at the crime scene, not anticipating the GKT, were not primed to examine the appropriateness of the evidence for the development of GKT items. Finally, there is no reason for such evidence to find its way into the police file that polygraphers review for background before testing a subject. With all these factors working against the polygrapher, it is little wonder that practicing polygraphers find the application of the GKT fraught with logistical problems. A GKT field study could overcome many of them by training criminalists to identify good GKT material and having them develop the questions for the polygraph test. Lykken (1981) provided an excellent example of how a criminal case might be investigated to optimize the development of a GKT.

The strength of the GKT has typically been hailed as deriving from its low false positive rate or high specificity. With enough questions, it is difficult to see how a competently administered GKT could be failed by an innocent person. However, this is not a selling point for law enforcement agents, who are more worried about guilty persons going free and the GKT's false negative rate. To increase the interest of law enforcement in the GKT, much more must be made of its positive predictive power or the likelihood that a failed test correctly identifies a guilty person. A competently administered test that is failed provides compelling evidence of guilt, a feature of the GKT easily recognized by the scientific community (see the survey results for item 3 in Table 2). As I have already pointed out, the Elaad investigations do not fully tap the potential of the GKT, and it is arguable that the GKT can only be used in a small fraction of cases as Podlesny (1993; Podlesny et al. 1995) has asserted. Like other kinds of evidence that are not available for all crimes (e.g., fingerprint and ballistics test results), GKT evidence would be highly incriminating when present.

Both laboratory and field studies indicate that the GKT's specificity (proportion of innocent classified as innocent) is very high. Ben-Shakar and Furedy (1990) reviewed ten GKT laboratory studies published between 1959 and 1987. The median and modal specificity for these studies was 100%; the weighted average specificity was 94%. In the Elaad field studies (Elaad 1990; Elaad et al. 1992), the average specificity was 98%. Figure 1 illustrates the positive predictive value of a test, as a function of its sensitivity and specificity, for the average specificities of 0.94 and 0.98 reported in the laboratory and field work and also for lower specificities of 0.86 and 0.90. A glance at the figure illustrates that, with specificities as high as these, only moderate sensitivity is needed to achieve high predictive value. For instance, consider the predictive power obtained when the sensitivity is only 0.48, as it was in the pooled data from the Elaad reports. Under these circumstances,

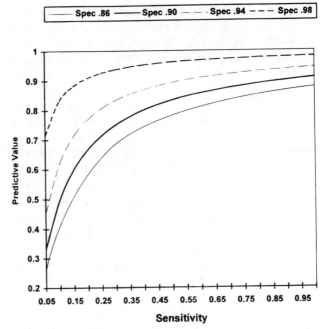

Figure 1. Positive predictive value of the guilty knowledge test as a function of sensitivity for four different estimates of test specificity.

the likelihood that a failed GKT comes from a guilty person is well above 0.7 even if the GKT were to have an (unlikely) specificity as low as 0.86. At the specificity of 0.98 evident in the Elaad studies, the graph reveals a predictive value of 0.96; this indicates that, 96% of the time, a failed GKT would come from a guilty person.

Because most people can easily grasp the sound logic of the GKT, evidence from a failed GKT (e.g., "the defendant's largest response was to the guilty knowledge alternative in nine of the ten questions asked") can be presented in a simple, straightforward manner to a court and jury. The jury does not need to be told, as is the case with the CQT, that the person has "failed" or be asked to resolve complex issues such as whether the relevant and control questions achieved their intended effect; they need only know the number of items indicating guilty knowledge. Assuming that the defendant has no explanation for the possession of guilty knowledge (it would have to be denied when reviewing the items for the GKT or there would be no reason to administer the test), that the test was administered in such a manner as to minimize examiner influence (e.g., the examiner was blind regarding the correct answers[5]), and that ten known innocent individuals were given the same test and none failed more than four items, wouldn't the test results seem to have compelling evidentiary value?

FUTURE DIRECTIONS

There are no psychological tests that have more profound consequences for those who take them than the employee screening RIT and the CQT. Yet few academic and applied psychologists pay much attention to this important area of applied psychology. The result of this indifference and neglect is a lack of systematic and edifying research, leading to the current sad state of scientific knowledge regarding the validity of these techniques. Unlike other areas of applied psychology, with polygraphy the applied techniques were developed in the absence of the basic research needed to support their use and yet have flourished nonetheless. Consequently, scientific psychology has spent the last several decades playing "catch-up," focusing on their validity with the hope that empirical research could be used to legitimize, modify, or stop their use. It is perhaps time to face the possibility that this goal will never be realized. Polygraphy has been with us for most of this century. The CQT, undergoing little more than cosmetic change, has passed its fiftieth birthday. The practice of polygraphy is unlikely to go away or change substantially any time soon, no matter what new research initiatives are launched.

I agree with the recommendations of Bashore and Rapp (1993), who argued in part that psychophysiologists can best contribute to this field by moving away from research focused on conventional polygraph procedures and methods and toward developing a *science* of deception detection. As Bashore and Rapp (1993) noted, event-related potential research using P300 "oddball" and N400 semantic incongruity paradigms represents one welcome step in this direction (see e.g. Allen & Iacono 1997; Boaz et al. 1991; Farwell & Donchin 1991; Rosenfeld et al. 1991). Other methodologies, such as those based on facial electromyography and pupillography, may also have much to offer in such an enterprise.

NOTES

1. For a more thorough review of the early history of lie detection, the interested reader is referred to Abrams (1989), Ben-Shakar & Furedy (1990), Lykken (1981, 1998), and especially Trovillo (1939a,b).
2. These control questions are not controls in the scientific sense, since they are not comparable to the relevant question in their significance to the subject. Because of this, this test might be more appropriately labeled the *comparison* question test (Ben-Shakar & Furedy 1990).
3. Note that false confessions given by innocent individuals who confess after failing a polygraph test also would go undetected as errors. The inclusion of such data in the cases chosen for a field study would serve to inflate accuracy estimates.
4. The Bersh (1969) study was also flawed by providing the panelists with the results of the polygraph tests.
5. Elaad (1997) obtained the somewhat surprising finding that examiner awareness of the guilty knowledge alternative led to the subject producing smaller responses to this item. This finding implies that examiners without such awareness are likely to be better able to detect guilty individuals.

REFERENCES

Abrams, S. (1989). *The Complete Polygraph Handbook*. Lexington, MA: Lexington Books.

Allen, J. J. B., & Iacono, W. G. (1997). A comparison of methods for the analysis of event-related potentials in deception detection. *Psychophysiology, 34*, 234–40.

Allen, J. J., Iacono, W. G., & Danielson, K. D. (1992). The identification of concealed memories using the event-related potential and implicit behavioral measures: A methodology for prediction in the face of individual differences. *Psychophysiology, 29*, 504–22.

Amato, S. L. (1993). A survey of the Society for Psychophysiological Research regarding the polygraph: Opinions and interpretations. Master's thesis, University of North Dakota, Grand Forks.

Amato, S. L., & Honts, C. R. (1993). What do psychophysiologists think about polygraph tests? A survey of the membership of SPR [Abstract]. *Psychophysiology, 31*, S22.

Backster, C. (1962). Methods of strengthening our polygraph technique. *Police, 6*, 61–8.

Barland, G. H. (1982). On the accuracy of the polygraph: An evaluative review of Lykken's *Tremor in the Blood. Polygraph, 11*, 258–72.

Barland, G. H., Honts, C. R., & Barger, S. D. (1989). *Studies of the Accuracy of Security Screening Polygraph Examinations*. Ft. McClellan, AL: Department of Defense Polygraph Institute.

Barland, G. H., & Raskin, D. C. (1973). The use of electrodermal activity in the detection of deception. In W. F. Prokasy & D. C. Raskin (Eds.), *Electrodermal Activity in Psychological Research*. New York: Academic Press.

Barland, G. H., & Raskin, D. C. (1976). Validity and reliability of polygraph examinations of criminal suspects. Report no. 76-1 (Contract no. N1-99-0001). National Institute of Justice, Department of Justice, Washington, DC.

Bashore, T. R., & Rapp, P. E. (1993). Are there alternatives to traditional polygraph procedures? *Psychological Bulletin, 113*, 3–22.

Ben-Shakar, G., & Furedy, J. J. (1990). *Theories and Applications in the Detection of Deception*. New York: Springer-Verlag.

Bersh, P. J. (1969). A validation study of polygraph examiner judgments. *Journal of Applied Psychology, 53*, 393–403.

Boaz, T. L., Perry, N. W., Raney, G., Fischler, I. S., & Shuman, D. (1991). Detection of guilty knowledge with event related potentials. *Journal of Applied Psychology, 76*, 788–95.

Bradley, M. T., & Rettinger, J. (1992). Awareness of crime-relevant information and the guilty knowledge test. *Journal of Applied Psychology, 77*, 55–9.

DePaulo, B. M. (1992). Nonverbal behavior and self-presentation. *Psychological Bulletin, 111*, 203–43.

Devitt, M. K., Honts, C. R., & Vondergeest, L. (1997). Truth or just bias: The treatment of the psychophysiological detection of deception in introductory psychology textbooks. *Journal of Credibility Assessment and Witness Psychology, 1*, 9–32.

Dohm, T. E., & Iacono, W. G. (1993). Design and pilot of a polygraph field validation study. Technical report no. 227, Personnel Decisions Research Institute, Minneapolis, MN.

Ekman, P. (1991). *Telling Lies: Clues to Deceit in the Marketplace, Politics, and Marriage*. New York: Norton.

Elaad, E. (1990). Detection of guilty knowledge in real-life criminal applications. *Journal of Applied Psychology, 75,* 521–9.

Elaad, E. (1997). Polygraph examiner awareness of crime-relevant information and the guilty knowledge test. *Law and Human Behavior, 21,* 107–20.

Elaad, E., Ginton, A., & Jungman, N. (1992). Detection measures in real-life criminal guilty knowledge tests. *Journal of Applied Psychology, 77,* 757–67.

Emerick, R. L., & Dutton, W. A. (1993). The effect of polygraphy on the self-report of adolescent sex offenders: Implications for risk assessment. Paper presented at the Annual Conference on the Assessment and Treatment of Sexual Abusers (Portland, OR).

Faigman, D. L. (1995). The evidentiary status of social science under *Daubert*: Is it "scientific," "technical," or "other" knowledge? *Psychology, Public Policy, and Law, 1,* 960–79.

Faigman, D. L., Kaye, D. H., Saks, M. J., & Sanders, J. (1997a). *Modern Scientific Evidence: The Law and Science of Expert Testimony.* St. Paul, MN: West Publishing.

Faigman, D. L., Kaye, D. H., Saks, M. J., & Sanders, J. (1997b). The legal relevance of scientific research on polygraph tests. In Faigman et al. (1997a), pp. 554–64.

Faigman, D. L., Kaye, D. H., Saks, M. J., & Sanders, J. (1999). The legal relevance of scientific research on polygraph tests. In D. L. Faigman, D. Kaye, M. J. Saks, & J. Sanders (Eds.), *Modern Scientific Evidence: The Law and Science of Expert Testimony* (Pocket Part., vol. 1), pp. 156–60. St. Paul, MN: West Publishing.

Farwell, L. A., & Donchin, E. (1991). The truth will out: Interrogative polygraphy ("lie detection") with event related brain potentials. *Psychophysiology, 28,* 531–47.

Forman, R. F., & McCauley, C. (1986). Validity of the positive control test using the field practice model. *Journal of Applied Psychology, 71,* 691–8.

Furedy, J. J., & Ben-Shakar, G. (1991). The roles of deception, intention to deceive, and motivation to avoid detection in the psychophysiological detection of guilty knowledge. *Psychophysiology, 28,* 163–71.

Furedy, J. J., Davis, C., & Gurevich, M. (1988). Differentiation of deception as a psychological process: A psychophysiological approach. *Psychophysiology, 25,* 683–8.

Furedy, J. J., & Heslegrave, R. J. (1988). Validity of the lie detector: A psychophysiological perspective. *Criminal Justice and Behavior, 15,* 219–46.

Gallup Organization (1984). Survey of members of the American Society for Psychophysiological Research concerning their opinion of polygraph test interpretation. *Polygraph, 13,* 153–65.

Giacolone, R. A., & Rosenfeld, P. (Eds.) (1989). *Impression Management in the Organization.* Hillsdale, NJ: Erlbaum.

Honts, C. R. (1991). The emperor's new clothes: Application of polygraph tests in the American workplace. *Forensic Reports, 4,* 91–116.

Honts, C. R. (1994). Psychophysiological detection of deception. *Current Directions, 3,* 77–82.

Honts, C. R. (1996). Criterion development and validity of the CQT in field application. *Journal of General Psychology, 123,* 309–24.

Honts, C. R., Devitt, M. K., Winbush, M., & Kircher, J. C. (1996). Mental and physical countermeasures reduce the accuracy of the concealed knowledge test. *Psychophysiology, 33,* 84–92.

Honts, C. R., Hodes, R. L., & Raskin, D. (1985). Effects of physical countermeasures on the physiological detection of deception. *Journal of Applied Psychology, 70,* 177–87.

Honts, C. R., & Quick, B. D. (1996). The polygraph in 1995: Progress in science and the law. *North Dakota Law Review, 71,* 987–1020.

Honts, C. R., Raskin, D., & Kircher, J. (1994). Mental and physical countermeasures reduce the accuracy of polygraph tests. *Journal of Applied Psychology, 79,* 252–9.

Honts, C. R., Raskin, D. C., & Kircher, J. C. (1997). A rejoinder to Iacono and Lykken. In Faigman et al. (1997a), pp. 629–31.

Horowitz, S. W., Kircher, J. C., Honts, C. R., & Raskin, D. C. (1997). The role of comparison questions in physiological detection of deception. *Psychophysiology, 34,* 108–15.

Horvath, F. (1977). The effect of selected variables on the interpretation of polygraph records. *Journal of Applied Psychology, 62,* 127–36.

Horvath, F. (1993). Polygraph screening of candidates for police work in large police agencies in the United States: A survey of practices, policies, and evaluative comments. *American Journal of Police, 12,* 67–86.

Iacono, W. G. (1985). Guilty knowledge. *Society, 22,* 52–4.

Iacono, W. G. (1991). Can we determine the accuracy of polygraph tests? In J. R. Jennings, P. K. Ackles, & M. G. H. Coles (Eds.), *Advances in Psychophysiology,* vol. 4, pp. 201–7. London: Jessica Kingsley.

Iacono, W. G. (1994). Government makes mistakes in relying on lie detectors. *Star Tribune,* April 5, p. 9A.

Iacono, W. G., Boisvenu, G. A., & Fleming, J. A. (1984). The effects of diazepam and methylphenidate on the electrodermal detection of guilty knowledge. *Journal of Applied Psychology, 69,* 289–99.

Iacono, W. G., & Lykken, D. T. (1997a). A rejoinder to Raskin, Honts, and Kircher. In Faigman et al. (1997a), pp. 631–3.

Iacono, W. G., & Lykken, D. T. (1997b). A response to professors Raskin, Honts, and Kircher. In Faigman et al. (1997a), pp. 627–9.

Iacono, W. G., & Lykken, D. T. (1997c). The scientific status of research on polygraph techniques: The case against polygraph tests. In Faigman et al. (1997a), pp. 582–618.

Iacono, W. G., & Lykken, D. T. (1997d). The validity of the lie detector: Two surveys of scientific opinion. *Journal of Applied Psychology, 82,* 426–33.

Iacono, W. G., & Lykken, D. T. (1999). Update: The scientific status of research on polygraph techniques: The case against polygraph tests. In D. L. Faigman, D. Kaye, M. J. Saks, & J. Sanders (Eds.), *Modern Scientific Evidence: The Law and Science of Expert Testimony* (Pocket Part., vol. 1), pp. 174–84. St. Paul, MN: West Publishing.

Iacono, W. G., & Patrick, C. J. (1987). What psychologists should know about lie detection. In A. K. Hess & I. B. Weiner (Eds.), *Handbook of Forensic Psychology.* New York: Wiley.

Iacono, W. G., & Patrick, C. J. (1988). Polygraph techniques. In R. Rogers (Ed.), *Clinical Assessment of Malingering and Deception.* New York: Guilford.

Iacono, W. G., & Patrick, C. J. (1997). Polygraphy and integrity testing. In R. Rogers (Ed.), *Clinical Assessment of Malingering and Deception,* 2nd ed., pp. 252–81. New York: Guilford.

Iacono, W. G., & Patrick, C. J. (1999). Polygraph ("lie detector") testing: The state of the art. In A. K. Hess & I. B. Weiner

(Eds.), *The Handbook of Forensic Psychology*, 2nd ed., pp. 440–73. New York: Wiley.

Jones, E. E., & Sigall, H. (1971). The bogus pipeline: A new paradigm for measuring affect and attitude. *Psychological Bulletin, 76*, 349–64.

Keeler, L. (1930). A method for detecting deception. *American Journal of Police Science, 1*, 38–52.

Keeler, L. (1939). Problems in the use of the "lie detector." *Police Year Book 1938–1939*, pp. 136–42. Washington, DC: International Association of Chiefs of Police.

Kircher, J. C., Horowitz, S. W., & Raskin, D. C. (1988). Meta-analysis of mock crime studies of the control question polygraph technique. *Law and Human Behavior, 12*, 79–90.

Kugelmass, S., & Lieblich, I. (1966). The effects of realistic stress and procedural interference in experimental lie detection. *Journal of Applied Psychology, 50*, 211–16.

Larson, J. A. (1921). Modification of the Marston deception test. *Journal of the American Institute of Criminal Law and Criminology, 12*, 391–9.

Larson, J. A. (1932). *Lying and Its Detection: A Study of Deception and Deception Tests*. University of Chicago Press.

Larson, J. A. (1938). The lie detector polygraph: Its history and development. *Journal of the Michigan State Medical Society, 37*, 893–7.

Lombroso, C. (1895). *L'homme criminel*. Paris: Felix Alcan.

Lykken, D. T. (1959). The GSR in the detection of guilt. *Journal of Applied Psychology, 43*, 385–8.

Lykken, D. T. (1960). The validity of the guilty knowledge technique: The effects of faking. *Journal of Applied Psychology, 44*, 258–62.

Lykken, D. T. (1974). Psychology and the lie detector industry. *American Psychologist, 29*, 725–39.

Lykken, D. T. (1975). The right way to use a lie detector. *Psychology Today, 8*, 56–60.

Lykken, D. T. (1981). *A Tremor in the Blood: Uses and Abuses of the Lie Detector*. New York: McGraw-Hill.

Lykken, D. T. (1988). Detection of guilty knowledge: A comment on Forman and McCauley. *Journal of Applied Psychology, 73*, 303–4.

Lykken, D. T. (1998). *A Tremor in the Blood: Uses and Abuses of the Lie Detector*, 2nd ed. New York: Plenum.

Marston, W. M. (1917). Systolic blood pressure changes in deception. *Journal of Experimental Psychology, 2*, 143–63.

Marston, W. M. (1938). *The Lie Detector Test*. New York: R. R. Smith.

Memon, A., Vrij, A., & Bull, R. (1998). *Accuracy and Perceived Credibility of Victims, Witnesses, and Suspects*. Chichester, U.K.: Wiley.

Munsterberg, H. (1908). *On the Witness Stand*. New York: Doubleday.

Murphy, C. A., & Murphy, J. K. (1997). Polygraph admissibility. *Update, 10*, nos. 1/2.

Orne, M. T. (1975). Implications of laboratory research for the detection of deception. *Polygraph, 2*, 169–99.

Patrick, C. J., & Iacono, W. G. (1989). Psychopathy, threat, and polygraph test accuracy. *Journal of Applied Psychology, 74*, 347–55.

Patrick, C. J., & Iacono, W. G. (1991a). A comparison of field and laboratory polygraphs in the detection of deception. *Psychophysiology, 28*, 632–8.

Patrick, C. J., & Iacono, W. G. (1991b). Validity of the control question polygraph test: The problem of sampling bias. *Journal of Applied Psychology, 76*, 229–38.

Podlesny, J. A. (1993). Is the guilty knowledge polygraph technique applicable in criminal investigations? A review of FBI case records. *Crime Laboratory Digest, 20*, 57–61.

Podlesny, J. A., Nimmich, K. W., & Budowle, B. (1995). A lack of case facts restricts applicability of the guilty knowledge deception detection method in FBI criminal investigations. Technical report, FBI Forensic Research and Training Center, Quantico, VA.

Raskin, D. (1986). The polygraph in 1986: Scientific, professional and legal issues surrounding applications and acceptance of polygraph evidence. *Utah Law Review, 1*, 29–74.

Raskin, D. (1989). Polygraph techniques for the detection of deception. In D. Raskin (Ed.), *Psychological Methods in Criminal Investigation and Evidence*, pp. 247–96. New York: Springer.

Raskin, D. C., Honts, C. R., & Kircher, J. C. (1997a). The scientific status of research on polygraph techniques: The case for polygraph tests. In Faigman et al. (1997a), pp. 565–82.

Raskin, D. C., Honts, C. R., & Kircher, J. C. (1997b). A response to professors Iacono and Lykken. In Faigman et al. (1997a), pp. 619–27.

Raskin, D. C., Kircher, J. C., Honts, C. R., & Horowitz, S. W. (1988). A study of the validity of polygraph examinations in criminal investigation (Final Report to the National Institute of Justice). Department of Psychology, University of Utah, Salt Lake City.

Reid, J. E. (1947). A revised questioning technique in lie-detection tests. *Journal of Criminal Law and Criminology, 37*, 542–7.

Reid, J. E., & Inbau, F. E. (1977). *Truth and Deception: The Polygraph ("Lie Detector") Technique*, 2nd ed. Baltimore: Williams & Wilkins.

Rogers, R. (Ed.) (1997). *Clinical Assessment of Malingering and Deception*, 2nd ed. New York: Guilford.

Rosenfeld, J. P., Angell, A., Johnson, M., & Qian, J. (1991). An ERP-based, control-question lie detector analog: Algorithms for discriminating effects within individuals' average waveforms. *Psychophysiology, 38*, 319–35.

Saxe, L. (1991). Science and the CQT polygraph: A theoretical critique. *Integrative Physiological and Behavioral Science, 26*, 223–31.

Saxe, L. (1994). Detection of deception: Polygraph and integrity tests. *Current Directions, 3*, 69–73.

Thurber, S. (1981). CPI variables in relationship to the polygraph performance of police officer candidates. *Journal of Social Psychology, 113*, 145–6.

Trovillo, P. V. (1939a). A history of lie detection. *American Journal of Police Science, 29*, 848–81.

Trovillo, P. V. (1939b). A history of lie detection. *Journal of Criminal Law and Criminology, 30*, 104–19.

Yuille, J. (Ed.) (1989). *Credibility Assessment*. Norwell, MA: Kluwer.

CHAPTER TWENTY-NINE

APPLICATIONS OF PSYCHOPHYSIOLOGY TO HUMAN FACTORS

ARTHUR F. KRAMER & TIMOTHY WEBER

The main goal of this chapter is to illustrate how psychophysiological techniques – as well as scientific theories that integrate behavioral and psychophysiological levels of description – can be used to address problems and concerns in the field of human factors. In order to accomplish this goal we will begin with a brief discussion of human factors and describe a limited but important subset of current issues. Next we will describe some of the criteria that must be met for psychophysiological measures to serve a useful function in assisting human factors researchers and practitioners in enhancing the functionality, efficiency, and safety of current and future human–machine systems. We will then briefly describe a few illustrative examples of human factors issues that are addressed with a series of converging operations, which include psychophysiological measures and models. More specifically, we will focus on the topics of the evaluation of vigilance decrements (lapses in alertness), the assessment of mental workload, and the development of adaptive automated systems. However, it is important to note that we have chosen to focus on these three application domains because psychophysiology has already made inroads – in both the laboratory and applied settings – in these research areas and not because we believe that they provide the only potential applications. There are clearly a number of additional human factors issues and concerns that are ripe for psychophysiological application. These include the assessment of operator training and skill development (Hoffman 1990; Strayer & Kramer 1990), the assessment of multimodal displays (Yagi 1997), and the examination and prediction of errors and error compensation strategies in complex systems (Gehring et al. 1993; Reason 1990; Scheffers et al. 1996).

In recent years there have been a number of reviews of applications of psychophysiology topics related to human factors, most notably mental workload assessment (Gevins et al. 1995; Kramer 1991; Kramer & Spinks 1991; Parasur-

aman 1990; Wickens 1990; Wilson & Eggemeier 1991) and adaptive automation (Byrne & Parasuraman 1996; Kramer, Trejo, & Humphrey 1994). Given that these authors have provided extensive historical reviews of this literature, we will mainly focus our discussion on relevant research within the past decade (but see the section entitled "A Brief History" for a review of earlier work). We will also attempt, whenever possible, to focus on empirical studies that have evaluated the major topics of interest in extralaboratory environments – that is, in simulators and operational environments. Finally, given that other chapters in this volume provide an extensive treatment of the physiological mechanisms underlying the psychophysiological measures that we discuss, our discussion will focus on the utility of these measures as indices of psychological constructs pertaining to system design, system evaluation, and operator training.

A Brief Introduction to Human Factors

Human factors has been defined as the study of human capabilities and limitations that affect the design of human–machine systems (Wickens 1992). However, the field of human factors extends beyond the theoretical and empirical study of human behavior and cognition in complex systems to the formulation of guidelines, principles, and models that can be used to design systems that accommodate human users and operators (Meister 1989). In other words, human factors is neither a domain that resides solely in the laboratory nor one that focuses solely on the engineering of new (or the retrofitting of old) human–machine systems. That is, the field of human factors endeavors moreover to provide a bridge between (i) the study of human behavior and cognition in laboratory and simulated environments and (ii) the design and evaluation of human–machine systems. These systems range from (purportedly) simple consumer products such as TVs and

John T. Cacioppo, Louis G. Tassinary, and Gary G. Berntson (Eds.), *Handbook of Psychophysiology*, 2nd ed. © Cambridge University Press 2000. Printed in the United States of America. ISBN 62634X. All rights reserved.

VCRs to large and complex systems such as automobiles, aircraft, process control plants, and the World Wide Web.

Over the years, the core topics of interest within the human factors community have changed with the development of technology – more specifically, technologies that have reduced the need for humans to serve as manual laborers and controllers and shifted the role of humans to system managers and supervisors. Although such developments in technology have generally been advantageous for the humans who have participated in the operation of complex systems and products, there have also been a number of costs associated with the transition of humans from the role of manual controller to that of supervisor (and occasionally more active participant) in semiautomated and automated systems.

For example, one recurrent problem has been referred to as automation-induced complacency. This occurs when human operators are expected to perform a series of manual tasks while also monitoring automated systems. Under such conditions, monitoring performance often decreases precipitously rather quickly, often within 30 minutes. However, such performance decrements occur less often when the human operator's only task is to monitor the automated systems (Parasuraman, Molloy, & Singh 1993; Parasuraman, Mouloua, & Molloy 1994). Thus, if human operators are expected to perform multiple tasks, some of which require active intervention and manual control, then the monitoring of automated systems may suffer. Of course, one solution to such a problem might be to also automate the manual tasks and thereby unburden the operator from the dual tasks of manual control and supervisory management. However, such a change is often technically impractical and may also overwhelm the human operator with excessive monitoring demands. Even when highly automated systems are a practical alternative, operators have been shown to overestimate the automated systems' reliability and succumb thereby to automation-induced complacency even in the absence of manual control demands (Lee & Moray 1992; Riley 1994).

Another problem associated with highly automated systems has been referred to as out-of-the-loop unfamiliarity or, more generally, as a lack of situation awareness (Endsley 1994; Wickens 1992). This occurs when human operators must suddenly, and often without warning, get back into the control loop and either perform manual control duties and/or detect and diagnose problems with automated systems. In such cases the human operators are both slower and more error-prone in carrying out these duties than if they had been an active participant in the operation of the system rather than a passive system monitor. Important questions with regard to this problem include how to keep the operator continuously aware of the state of important systems and how best to monitor (human) operator readiness to take over important duties should automation fail (Scerbo 1994).

There is still another set of important issues arising in the context of complex semiautomated and automated systems. How should the often overwhelming amounts of multimodal information be presented to human operators, and how should we assess whether mission-critical information has been adequately extracted and retained by the operators? These general issues include questions of both a sensory and perceptual nature. Is critical information sufficiently distinct from background information? Is critical information displayed long enough for operators to note and extract task-critical components? There are also important cognitive concerns. Is the information presented to the operator in a format that is consistent with his or her mental representation of the system? Do the working memory requirements exceed operator capacity? Given the rapid development of "virtual reality" technology for operator training and system control, the sensory, perceptual, and cognitive issues associated with information presentation and multimodal integration have become more than an academic exercise. These issues are now on the verge of becoming a serious bottleneck for the effective use of this technology.

The issues raised here (and many others) have been and continue to be addressed through the application of a variety of traditional human factors methodologies. For example, the question of when to automate system functions has been addressed with several different methods, including (1) the use of models of human performance and cognition to predict the situations in which human performance is likely to degrade and (2) the continuous assessment of human performance via measurement of overt actions and responses. Indeed, the model-based and assessment-based procedures have also been combined into a hybrid approach to enhance the efficiency of adaptively automated systems (Byrne & Parasuraman 1996). Similar techniques have been employed to evaluate new display concepts and to ensure that information is presented in formats consistent with the perceptual capabilities and cognitive representations of human operators.

Role of Psychophysiology in Human Factors

Given that there are a multitude of techniques available to address human factors problems and issues, one must ask what role psychophysiology might play in human factors research and application. Certainly, to the extent that information gained through psychophysiological measurement is redundant with that obtained from other measures and models employed by the human factors community, psychophysiological measures will be unlikely to gain wide acceptance. This is likely to be the case for the foreseeable future in light of the relatively high cost of (and substantial amount of expertise required for) collecting, analyzing, and interpreting psychophysiological measures when compared with the subjective rating and performance-based measurement techniques traditionally employed by human factors practitioners and researchers.

Thus, for psychophysiological measurement techniques to gain acceptance in the human factors community, these measures must:

1. prove to be more valid or reliable indices of relevant psychological (or, in some cases, physiological) constructs than traditional behavioral and subjective measures; or
2. enable the measurement of constructs that are difficult or impossible to measure with traditional measures; or
3. enable the measurement of relevant constructs in situations where other types of measures are unavailable.

Indeed, there is evidence (to be discussed shortly) that each of these three criteria has been or can be met within a human factors context and with measures obtained via psychophysiologically inspired models.

Another important consideration is the temporal sensitivity of psychophysiological measures. In many human factors contexts – such as the evaluation of new display concepts, the examination of the effects of different environmental conditions (e.g., differences in ambient temperature, humidity) on human performance and information processing, the evaluation of training proficiency, and the assessment of fitness for duty – data can be collected and then analyzed and interpreted off-line (i.e., at a later time that might, depending on circumstances, range from minutes to days). In such situations, enough effort can be devoted to deal adequately with potential artifacts in the psychophysiological data and enough data can usually be collected to ensure adequate signal-to-noise ratios. On the other hand, there are also a number of human factors contexts that demand almost instantaneous data processing and interpretation. For example, given the increasing trend toward adaptive automation in systems such as aircraft and process control, it has become important to develop measures that can both describe and predict changes in psychological constructs such as mental workload, alertness, and information processing strategies – in real time or near-real time. Such information could then serve – along with inferences about human information processing capacities extracted from dynamic models of the interaction between humans, tasks, and environment – as input to algorithms that determine the dynamic task allocation policy between humans and automated systems. Of course, such situations pose technical problems for psychophysiological measures that are not encountered in off-line contexts, such as rapid data collection, processing, artifact rejection, and interpretation. Additionally, the bandwidth of some systems (e.g. high-performance aircraft) may be high enough to preclude collecting sufficient amounts of (at least some types of) psychophysiological data to ensure adequate reliability or signal-to-noise ratios.

One additional issue that merits some discussion is the applicability of psychophysiological measurement techniques to extralaboratory environments. Most psychophysiological research has focused on explicating the functional significance of different measures and components with relatively simple tasks in well-controlled laboratory environments. Even so, a great deal of effort has been expended on the elimination of potential artifacts (e.g., from ambient electrical fields, contamination from other physiological signals that may mask the signal of interest, individual differences in baselines, or a measure's morphology or topography). When such artifacts are difficult or impossible to eliminate during data recording, the focus has been on adjusting the physiological measures in order to minimize the impact of artifacts on data interpretation. Given the diversity and magnitude of the artifacts encountered in such well-controlled settings, is it a reasonable expectation to collect valid and reliable psychophysiological data in less well-controlled environments such as high-fidelity (and sometimes motion-based) simulators or operational environments? Although collecting psychophysiological data in such environments clearly provides a considerable technical challenge, there have been a number of promising developments in the design of miniaturized recording equipment that can withstand the rigors of operational environments (Caldwell 1995; Miller 1995; Sterman & Mann 1995). There have also been developments in pattern recognition and signal analysis techniques that enhance the detection of some physiological signals in noise (Trejo & Shensa 1993; Westerkamp & Williams 1995), as well as development of automated artifact rejection procedures (Du, Leong, & Gevins 1994). For example, Gevins et al. (1995) reported the development of a "smart helmet" system, which incorporates a combination of 32 EEG and EOG electrodes along with miniaturized preamplifiers into a flight helmet. Barring technological roadblocks, such developments should continue to increase the potential for recording psychophysiological signals in a number of complex environments.

In summary, each of the issues discussed so far needs to be carefully considered when psychophysiological measures are to be used in addressing human factors problems and concerns. Indeed, it is likely that some types of psychophysiological measures will be appropriate for only a subset of situations in which human factors issues are examined, whereas other measures may be more widely applicable. In an effort to make some of these considerations more concrete, we now turn to a critical review of current applications of psychophysiological measurement issues in the human factors field.

Psychophysiology and Human Factors: A Brief History

Human factors developed as a unique discipline in response to human performance questions that arose around the time of World War II. For the first time, systems such as military aircraft, ships, and ground vehicles were becoming sufficiently complex that more numerous (and sometimes catastrophic) errors were observed – even though the systems were functioning as designed from a mechanical standpoint. That is, human operators either could not execute their assigned functions as expected or they did not have sufficient training to do so. As a consequence of these system problems and the well-founded suspicion that systems were not being designed to ensure adequate human performance, experimental psychologists were called upon to evaluate the human–machine interface and training regimes, to diagnose the problems (and potential problems not yet observed), and to suggest system improvements and training modifications to ensure safe and efficient system operation (Fitts & Jones 1947; Mackworth 1948).

It is interesting that psychophysiological measures, principally measures of gaze direction, played an important role in the examination of human performance in complex systems during the early years of human factors. Fitts and colleagues (Fitts, Jones, & Milton 1950; Jones, Milton, & Fitts 1950; see also Gainer & Obermayer 1964) used measures of gaze direction, gaze duration, and the sequence of eye movements to examine the information extraction strategies employed by novice and experienced aircraft pilots during instrument flight. Data acquired from these studies were used to reconfigure instrument panels to optimize the speed and accuracy with which pilots could locate and extract flight-relevant information. Eye scan measures continue to be used today, in conjunction with measures of pilot performance, to assess pilot strategies for extracting information as well as mental workload and skill acquisition in military and civilian flight (Bellenkes, Wickens, & Kramer 1997; Fox et al. 1996; Kotulak & Morse 1995).

The use of other psychophysiological measures to examine issues of interest to the human factors community soon followed the pioneering research of Fitts and co-workers. For example, Sem-Jacobsen and colleagues (Sem-Jacobsen 1959, 1960, 1961; Sem-Jacobsen et al. 1959; Sem-Jacobsen & Sem-Jacobsen 1963) recorded electroencephalographic (EEG) activity from pilots as they flew missions of varying difficulty in simulated and actual flight in an effort to examine the utility of this psychophysiological measure for assessing the deleterious effects of high-G environments and mental and emotional workload. It was also speculated that psychophysiological measures, and in particular measures of the EEG, would prove useful for the selection and evaluation of pilots for high-performance aircraft and for adaptively automated systems (see also Gomer 1981). Although Sem-Jacobsen's visions for applications have not yet been realized, our review of the current literature will indicate that at least some of these applications are soon to be realized.

Finally, measures of heart rate and heart rate variability have long been used to provide a continuous record of the cardio-respiratory function and mental workload of operators in complex simulated and real-world systems. Heart rate measures have been recorded as aircraft pilots execute a number of maneuvers in simulated and actual aircraft such as landing (Ruffel-Smith 1967), refueling during long-haul flights (Brown et al. 1969), performing steep descents (Roscoe 1975), and flying combat missions (Roman, Older, & Jones 1967). Such measures continue to be used today, often in the context of other psychophysiological measures and along with a more sophisticated appreciation for the underlying physiology.

In summary, although the application of psychophysiological techniques to issues of human factors has a relatively recent history, these measures provide useful insights into human performance and cognition in extralaboratory environments. We turn now to a discussion of recent applications of psychophysiological measures to three different topics of interest to the human factors community: assessment and prediction of vigilance decrements, assessment of mental workload, and potential psychophysiological inputs to adaptively automated systems.

Assessment and Prediction of Vigilance Decrements

Interest in the human factors community in the detection and prediction of vigilance decrements – and especially in operator performance, which is crucial to mission success – has been expressed since at least the 1950s (Broadbent 1971; Broadbent & Gregory 1965; Davies & Parasuraman 1980). Indeed, early interest in vigilance decrements focused on two aspects of the phenomenon: (i) the characterization of behavioral and information processing changes that accompany reduced vigilance, often through the utilization of signal detection theory (i.e., examining the influence of vigilance changes on the sensitivity and response criteria of human observers); and (ii) changes in physiological indices of arousal (Hockey 1984; Parasuraman 1984). However, it soon became clear that arousal could not be treated as a unitary concept but instead was multidimensional in nature (Gopher & Sanders 1984; Pribram & McGuinness 1975).

A good deal of laboratory and applied research in recent years has focused on explicating the multiple interacting mechanisms that underlie the maintenance of alertness (or, conversely, the onset of sleep – Akerstedt & Folkard 1996; Lavie & Zvulini 1992). Much of this research has concentrated on work environments, such as long-haul truck driving, train driving, and transoceanic flight. In these environments, irregular hours of sleep and activity are the norm and work often occurs during the evening or nighttime hours (Boucsein & Ottmann 1996; Kecklund & Akerstedt 1993; Miller 1995).

The measurement of EEG has been the "gold standard" against which alertness has been verified in much of this work. This measure has long served as the method of choice for the categorization of stages of sleep (Goeller & Sinton 1989; Loomis, Harvey, & Hobart 1937). Also, changes in EEG, particularly in the alpha and theta bands, have been found to be predictive of performance changes in sleep-deprived individuals (Beatty et al. 1974; Smulders et al. 1997; Townsend & Johnson 1979). Other measures – such as EOG (electro-oculogram), pupil diameter, slow eye movements, respiration, electrodermal activity, and ERPs (event-related potentials) – have also demonstrated some success in tracking the onset of sleep (Harsh et al. 1993; Miller 1995; Torsvall & Akerstedt 1987, 1988; Yamamoto & Isshiki 1992). However, within the human factors community, the interest is not in categorizing sleep stages but rather in identifying and predicting when loss of alertness or increased sleepiness will detrimentally influence performance.

In recent years, there have been a number of attempts to employ psychophysiological markers of alertness to predict vigilance decrements in laboratory and extralaboratory settings. In some cases, the identification and prediction of changes in alertness resulting in performance decrements have taken place off-line. In other studies, the focus has been on using psychophysiological measures to develop on-line, closed-loop systems to predict (and sometimes reduce) performance decrements. For example, Morris and Miller (1996) recorded EOG as ten sleep-deprived military pilots flew an extended series of instrument maneuvers in a moving-base flight simulator. The investigators were able to account for 61% of the variance in a composite measure of flight performance. The composite measure included three EOG measures, blink amplitude (i.e., the extent of eyelid movement), long closure rate (i.e., the number of closures longer than 500 msec), and blink duration. Similar relationships between eye blink measures and performance in sleep-deprived individuals have been reported in both laboratory and automobile simulator studies (Stern, Boyer, & Schroeder 1994; Wierwille 1994). Such results, when considered along with the underlying neuronal substrates, have led these researchers to suggest that endogenous blinks may be a useful index of tonic activation of the rostral central nervous system – that portion of the nervous system responsible for the maintenance of alertness.

Other researchers have examined the usefulness of ERPs and EEG in tracking performance decrements that accompany decreases in alertness. Humphrey, Kramer, and Stanny (1994) examined the changes in ERPs – more specifically, the amplitude and latency of the P300 component – as sleep-deprived subjects performed memory and visual search tasks throughout the night and into the morning. Reaction times (RTs) and lapses increased, accuracy decreased, P300 latencies increased, and P300 amplitudes decreased with increasing time on task. Indeed, the magnitude of the changes in P300 latency and RT were quite similar as a function of time on task. Given that the P300 appears to be sensitive to stimulus evaluation processes while being relatively insensitive to motor processes, it would appear that decrements in performance were due, in large part, to reduced efficiency of perceptual processes (see also Koelega et al. 1992).

Two research groups have focused on developing EEG-based closed-loop systems for the prediction of vigilance decrements. Pope, Bogart, and Bartolome (1995) had participants perform a multitask consisting of monitoring, tracking, communication, and resource management subtasks, each of which could be performed manually or automatically. The EEG was recorded continuously during performance of these tasks and was used to adjust the level of automation (i.e., the number of subtasks that were performed automatically) on the basis of changes in alertness or task engagement as inferred from a number of different EEG-based metrics. The EEG-based detection algorithms were tested in two different control modes, as both a negative and positive feedback system. In the case of the negative feedback system, the objective was to detect a decrease in task engagement and then require that a subtask be performed manually. This, in turn, would result in an EEG-based indication of increased task engagement (alertness). For the positive feedback system, the objective was to increase the discrepancy between the EEG-based indication of alertness at time n and time $n+1$ by further reducing manual control requirements when reduced alertness was detected. Thus, within this control theory approach, an effective EEG-based index of alertness or task engagement would be expected to produce relatively rapid and stable oscillatory behavior with the negative feedback system. On the other hand, a slow and less stable oscillation would be expected with the positive feedback system. Several of the EEG derivations produced such behavior. However, the derivation that was most successful was beta power divided by the sum of alpha power and theta power. This is most likely due to the fact that the other derivations included either high-frequency EEG or EMG (electromyographic) components, neither of which has been reported to be sensitive to changes in alertness.

Makeig and colleagues (1990; Makeig & Inlow 1993; Makeig & Jung 1996) have investigated the efficacy of EEG-based alertness detection systems for the prediction of missed responses during simulated sonar tasks using U.S. Navy sonar operators. In their studies, sonar operators attempted to detect 300-msec noise-burst targets embedded in a white noise background. In some of the studies, particularly those in which ERPs were of interest, brief task-irrelevant tones were also occasionally presented. Operator-specific EEG algorithms were derived by employing several different frequencies in the delta, theta, and alpha bands to predict vigilance decrements. These multiple regression–based algorithms were quite successful. The algorithms developed on data from one experimental session were capable of accounting for between 75% and 85% of the variance in error rates (i.e., response omissions or lapses) obtained in a second experimental session. Other results suggested that on-line algorithms, which detected changes in theta and gamma (> 35 Hz) activity, were capable of predicting missed target detection responses up to ten seconds in advance of the occurrence of a target. Finally, ERP components (more specifically, N200 amplitude and latency and P100/N100 amplitude difference) elicited by task-irrelevant auditory probes did a reasonable job of predicting changes in error rates within a 32-sec moving window.

The results from the Pope et al. and Makeig et al. studies suggest that it is now possible, in simulated real-world tasks, to detect and predict changes in alertness or task engagement that have important implications for system performance. One wonders, however, whether physiologically based alertness detection and prediction systems could be further improved by incorporating a number of psychophysiological measures, rather than a single measure as in the Pope et al. and Makeig et al. studies. Indeed, a number of studies suggest that this may be the case. For example, Torsvall and Akerstedt (1988) reported that changes in the alpha and theta bands of the EEG, along with slow eye movements detected in the EOG, could reliably predict that a target would be missed a full minute in the future. Varri et al. (1992) reported the development of a computerized system for predicting the onset of sleepiness that incorporated measures based on EOG, EEG, and EMG. Preliminary tests of the system showed promise when compared against the scoring of the physiological data by sleep experts. Thus, it would appear that a promising area of future research is the incorporation of a number of different physiological measures into alertness detection systems. Clearly, another important direction is the transition of psychophysiologically based alertness detection systems out of the laboratory and into operational environments. This is a particularly important step, because many of the vigilance decrements observed in laboratory research have not been reported in the field. This is likely due to the differential incentives to maintain adequate performance in these two settings (Wickens 1992).

Assessment of Mental Workload

THEORY

Although there is, at present, no commonly agreed-upon definition of the construct of mental workload, it has often been conceptualized as the processing costs incurred by a human operator in the performance of a single or multiple tasks (Kramer 1991; Wickens 1992). These costs have been associated with the effort or resources required to maintain an acceptable level of performance in the face of varying environmental and task conditions.

Early models of mental workload assumed that a single capacity or undifferentiated resource was sufficient to ac-

count for performance decrements observed with changes in task difficulty or variations in external (e.g., temperature, humidity, barometric pressure, noise, lighting) or internal (e.g., fatigue, illness) stressors (Moray 1967). In these unitary capacity models, it is assumed that a single pool of capacity is available and that the requirement to perform additional tasks (or increases in task difficulty) will require the allocation of resources. As task demands continue to increase, the supply of resources is diminished and performance declines. It is interesting to note that, within some of these early models, there was a degree of elasticity in the supply of resources available for task performance. For example, in Kahneman's (1973) model, the supply of resources could be expanded to a limited extent with increases in arousal. Thus, in a sense, humans could self-regulate the quality of their performance (at least within circumscribed limits) by varying their level of arousal.

However, this self-regulation of performance through the expansion of processing resources soon became viewed as a two-edged sword. That is, while the conceptualization of resources as a somewhat elastic commodity – driven by variations in effort, arousal, and motivation – was seen as an important method of compensating for variations in task difficulty as well as internal and external stressors, it also rendered it difficult to predict patterns of task interactions in multitask environments. Thus, an important interest in the 1970s and 1980s was the description of processing resource trade-offs between concurrently performed tasks and their implications for task performance (Norman & Bobrow 1975; Sperling & Melcher 1978). In such a context, it was important to fix the total amount of resources, so that allocating x resources to one task left $1 - x$ resources available for the performance of other tasks (Navon & Gopher 1979). Without such a restriction on the notion of resources or processing capacity, it would be difficult to map resource consumption to performance quality in any meaningful way – especially in the absence of a detailed knowledge of how and when other factors (e.g., arousal, effort, and motivation) influenced the quantity of available resources.

A number of data visualization tools were developed within this fixed-resource framework as an aid to the qualitative and quantitative conceptualization of the relationship between performance and resource allocation policy. For example, a performance operating characteristic (POC) is illustrated in Figure 1: performance on two concurrently performed tasks is cross-plotted to indicate the extent to which the two tasks require resources to be adequately performed. In deriving a POC, participants are asked to vary their priority, across blocks of trials, on two tasks. For example, in one block of dual-task trials, participants might be instructed to perform as best as possible on task A and devote any spare capacity to task B. In another block of trials, participants would be instructed to treat the tasks

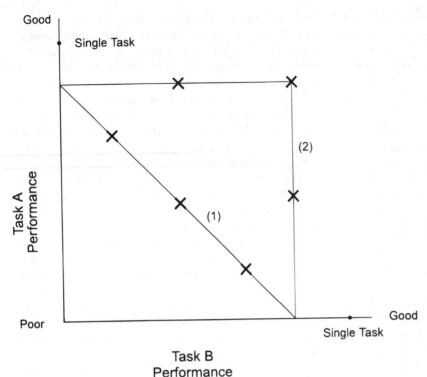

Figure 1. Illustration of a performance operating characteristic (POC). Curve 1 illustrates a situation in which the performance of one task is dependent on the performance of the other task. In such cases it is assumed that the two tasks require the same variety of processing resources or capacity. Curve 2 illustrates a situation in which the performance of one task is insensitive to the performance of the other, concurrent task. In such cases it is assumed that either the two tasks require few resources for performance (i.e., they can be performed automatically) or that the tasks require different processing resources.

where performance is resource-limited: performance improves in a monotonic fashion with the investment of additional resources. Such a function would be likely to underlie the performance relationship illustrated in curve 1 of Figure 1. On the other hand, curve 2 in Figure 2 indicates that task performance is data-limited; that is, the investment of additional resources beyond an initial (and minimal) allocation will have little additional influence on performance. Such a performance/resource relationship could arise for several reasons. First, the task could be very difficult, as when a human operator is required to maintain twenty unrelated pieces of information in working memory. Because such a task is obviously beyond the capabilities of most of us, investing additional resources would have little or no beneficial effect on performance. Second, a PRF function like that illustrated in curve 2 could indicate that performance on a task had been sufficiently automated that few resources are needed to achieve optimal performance – for example, the manual control of an automobile on a straight highway by an experienced driver. Curve 2 in the PRF function would likely underlie the performance relationship illustrated in curve 2 of Figure 1, where changes in the performance on one task had little influence on the performance of the other task (i.e., assuming the two tasks were data-limited).

A number of psychophysiological studies have been conducted to examine the predictions of the resource models

with equal priority. Finally, in a third block consisting of dual-task trials, participants would be asked to favor task B. Single-task conditions, in which participants perform one of the two tasks and completely ignore the other, are also included to provide anchors for the POC.

Curve 1 illustrates a situation in which there is a 1:1 trade-off between two concurrently performed tasks; that is, performance on one task declines with increases in the performance of the other. In contrast, curve 2 illustrates a situation in which performance of one task is insensitive to the level of performance on the other, concurrent task. Although the POC illustrates only the relationship between the performance of two concurrently performed tasks, the relationship between the hypothetical construct of resources and performance can be inferred from the shape of the function in the POC. This relationship can be further illustrated in a performance resource function (PRF), which plots performance against resources.

Figure 2 illustrates the resource/performance relation that would be expected to underlie the performance functions plotted in Figure 1. Curve 1 in Figure 2 depicts the case

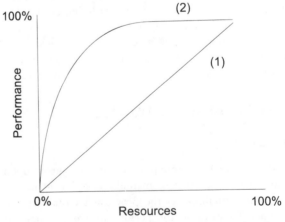

Figure 2. Illustration of a performance resource function (PRF). Curve 1 illustrates a situation in which the investment of additional processing resources results in a corresponding improvement in performance. Curve 2 represents a situation in which optimal performance is achieved after the investment of minimal resources, with the additional investment of resources having little or no effect on the quality of performance.

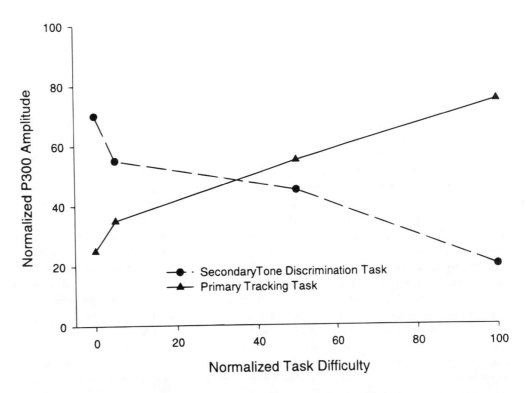

Figure 3. Illustration of a P300 reciprocity effect, where P300s elicited by events in a tracking task increase with the difficulty of the tracking task while P300s elicited by tones in a secondary tone discrimination task decrease in amplitude with increases in the difficulty of the tracking task. The performance and P300 measures were normalized (i.e., by subtracting the minimum score in each task from each condition and dividing these products by the differences between the minimum and maximum score in each task) to facilitate comparisons across the primary and secondary tasks.

of mental workload. Studies examining the P300 and N100 components of the ERP have confirmed a number of predictions of resource models of mental workload. One important prediction of resource models is that resource-limited tasks should entail a monotonic relationship between resources and performance. Kramer, Wickens, and Donchin (1985) confirmed this prediction when they found that increasing the difficulty of a tracking task systematically decreased the amplitude of the P300 component of the ERP elicited by a secondary visual discrimination task. Thus, it would appear that the P300 might provide an index of the allocation of resources: increased resource demands by the primary task would lead to diminished resources for the secondary task, which in turn would be reflected by decreases in the P300 amplitude. Indeed, this relationship between P300 and task difficulty under dual-task conditions was confirmed in a variety of studies that used tasks such as visual search, memory search, visual and auditory discrimination, and tracking (Hoffman et al. 1985; Kramer & Strayer 1988; McCallum, Cooper, & Pocock 1987; Natani & Gomer 1981; Strayer & Kramer 1990).

However, if ERPs and more specifically P300s reflect resource allocation, then we would expect a reciprocity in P300s elicited by two concurrently performed tasks. That is, fixed-capacity models (Navon & Gopher 1979; Norman & Bobrow 1975) argue that, as one task becomes more difficult or more important, additional resources will be allocated for the performance of that task, leaving fewer resources for the concurrently performed task. If P300s reflect such a process then we would expect a reciprocity in P300 amplitude, so that increases in the amplitude of

P300s elicited by events in one task should be accompanied by decreases in the amplitude of P300s elicited in another, concurrent task. Indeed, such an effect has been reported. Sirevaag et al. (1987; see also Wickens et al. 1983) found that P300s elicited by changes in target position in a tracking task increased in amplitude with increases in the difficulty of the task. Correspondingly, the amplitude of P300s elicited by events in a task of lesser importance (an auditory discrimination task) decreased with increases in the difficulty of the primary (tracking) task. The results from this study are illustrated in Figure 3. Thus, it would appear that changes in P300 amplitude in dual-task studies mimic the resource reciprocity effects predicted by fixed-capacity models.

The P300 reciprocity effects are important for several reasons. First, they provide converging support for the notion of resource trade-offs among tasks, support that is independent of the performance effects traditionally used to define resource allocation policies. Second, the P300 data can be obtained in the absence of overt responses, thus enabling the assessment of resource allocation policies in situations where actual behavior occurs infrequently (e.g., a quality control inspector monitoring a visual display, a pilot monitoring the status of the aircraft while flying on autopilot). Finally, as we review next, reciprocity effects have been found for components of the ERP other than the P300, suggesting the potential of resource trade-offs for different processing operations.

Similar reciprocity effects have been reported for other components of the ERP, such as the P100, N100, and P200 (Mangun & Hillyard 1990; Parasuraman 1985). Note, however, that in the study of Mangun and Hillyard (1990), the P100 and N100 components showed reciprocity patterns like that illustrated in curve 1 of Figure 1 (or similar to that shown in Figure 3), reflecting a trade-off in the processes underlying these components between locations in a spatial attention task (e.g., attend to the left or the right to detect an infrequent target), whereas P300s and performance measures displayed a pattern more like that illustrated in curve 2 of Figure 1. The authors explained this apparent dissociation between reciprocity patterns for the earlier ERP components (P100 and N100) and the later ERP component and performance measures by suggesting that, "as attention was increasingly withdrawn from one visual field and allocated to the other, higher perceptual processes were still able to extract and analyze the information from the progressively diminishing sensory signal" (Mangun & Hillyard 1990, p. 548). In other words, more than a single variety of processing resources or capacity can underlie performance in a divided attention task.

The suggestion that a single resource or capacity is insufficient to account for the pattern of performance and processing interactions in dual-task situations has been supported by a variety of behavioral and electrophysiological studies. For example, there have been a number of reports of failures to find performance trade-offs between two resource-limited tasks (North 1977; Shaffer 1975; Wickens 1992). There have also been reports that some psychophysiological measures such as the P300 and heart rate variability (HRV) are sensitive to only a limited subset of processing demands. For example, P300 appears to be sensitive to central processing but not motor demands (Isreal et al. 1980); P100 and N100 appear to reflect early selective attention processes and more specifically the distribution of attentional resources in visual space (Mangun & Hillyard 1990). The 0.10-Hz component of HRV appears to be sensitive to working memory demands but insensitive to response or motor demands (Aasman, Mulder, & Mulder

1987; Jorna 1992). As a result of findings like these and others, a number of theorists have proposed that mental workload should be conceptualized as a multidimensional rather than a unidimensional construct, so that two concurrently performed tasks will show trade-offs only when the tasks require the same types of processing resources or capacity (Polson & Freidman 1988; Wickens 1992).

It is interesting that some psychophysiological measures appear to be diagnostic of particular varieties of processing resources whereas other measures are less diagnostic and appear instead to reflect general or undifferentiated processing demands imposed upon the human. Psychophysiological measures that fall into this latter category include respiration, heart rate (HR), eye blinks, electrodermal activity, and some components of electroencephalographic activity (Fogarty & Stern 1993; Kramer 1991; Wilson & Eggemeier 1991). The sensitivity of these measures to general or undifferentiated processing demands can have advantages and disadvantages both. On the positive side, such measures could be used in a wide variety of settings and across a number of different systems to provide a general indication of the mental workload experienced by the human operator. In many cases, such information can be extremely valuable to system designers who are interested in the overall magnitude of processing demands imposed upon the human operator. However, if more specific information concerning the type of processing demands is needed – for example, to discern whether

---

TABLE 1. Assessment Measures Mapped to Workload Components

Physiological Measure	Psychological Constructs	
	Primary	**Additional**
P300 component of the ERP	Perceptual/central processing resources	Memory updating
P100/N100 components of the ERP	Spatial attention	
EEG – alpha activity	General processing demands	Alertness
EEG – theta activity	General processing demands	Alertness
Heart rate	General processing demands	Physical and emotional workload
Heart rate variability (0.10-Hz component)	Working memory demands	Problem-solving demands
Eye scan pattern	Visual information extraction strategies	
Blink rate	Visual demands	Alertness
Blink duration	Visual demands	Alertness

Note: Listed are psychophysiological measures that have been employed in the assessment of the multidimensional construct of mental workload in applied settings, along with a hypothesized mapping between measures and mental workload components.

the response demands of a new control system or the perceptual demands of a new display configuration are responsible for increased mental workload – then more diagnostic measures will be necessary. A summary of the inferred relationship between different psychophysiological measures and different aspects or components of mental workload is presented in Table 1.

APPLICATIONS

We have provided a brief description of the theoretical framework in which psychophysiological measures of mental workload have been explored. Now we turn to a discussion of extralaboratory applications of physiological measurement of mental workload in simulator and operational environments. Aircraft flight is the context in which, by far, the most extralaboratory research has been pursued. Indeed, early applications of psychophysiological measurement of workload and other psychological constructs date back to the late 1940s. At that time, Paul Fitts and his colleagues (Fitts et al. 1950; Jones et al. 1950) employed measures of eye gaze direction to determine the manner in which pilots extracted information from instrument panels. The results of these studies led to the development of aircraft instrument panels that configured instruments on the basis of importance (defined in terms of the number and duration of eye fixations) and sequential scan strategies.

In the past decade, a number of studies have been conducted to evaluate the utility of different psychophysiological measures as metrics of mental workload in simulator and operational environments. For example, Kramer, Sirevaag, and Braune (1987) examined whether the inverse relationship between P300s elicited by secondary task events and the difficulty of a primary task, which had previously been reported in laboratory studies, would be obtained in an aircraft simulator. Seven student pilots flew an instrument flight plan with a single-engine aircraft simulator while concurrently counting one of two tones that were presented via earphones. The P300s elicited by the secondary task tones decreased in amplitude with increases in the difficulty of the flight task, which was produced by increasing turbulence and subsystem failures. Similar effects were reported for P300 amplitude and latency (Fowler 1994) and P200 amplitude (Wilson, Fullenkamp, & Davis 1994) for simulated visual flight (i.e., flight in which the pilot flies with reference only to the ground) and actual flight in military aircraft, respectively. It is important to note that, in each of these studies, ERPs were elicited by tones from an "oddball" task in which the pilots were required to either covertly count or manually respond to the relevant tones.

Even though this "relevant probe" technique appears to produce relatively consistent data in simulator and operational environments, there is an important drawback to using this method for eliciting ERPs in nonlaboratory en-

vironments. Namely, it is conceivable that the requirement to count or overtly respond to auditory (or visual) probes will increase workload in already demanding environments. Furthermore, safety concerns will likely preclude the imposition of additional task demands on operators in many real-world environments. Therefore, although the relevant probe technique would appear appropriate for the assessment for mental workload in laboratory and simulator environments, it is unlikely to see wide application in operational contexts.

Given these potential limitations of the relevant probe technique, what other psychophysiological measures might be used to examine mental workload in simulator and operational environments? There are at least three possibilities. First, an "irrelevant probe" technique has been used to elicit ERPs in aircraft simulators. In this technique, additional stimuli (e.g. tones) are presented but participants are not required to count or overtly respond to them (Papanicolaou & Johnstone 1984). Thus, at the very least, the irrelevant probe technique minimizes response or motor interference with the task of interest. Sirevaag et al. (1993) employed this technique to assess the mental workload experienced by senior helicopter pilots using a variety of different communication systems. The P300s elicited by irrelevant probes decreased in amplitude with increases in the communication load in different phases of low-level high-speed flight in a high-fidelity helicopter simulator. Thus, like the P300 effects obtained with secondary task-relevant probes, it would appear that the P300 provides an index of the residual processing resources that remain after performing the primary task (in both cases, flight control). However, there are also cases in which P300s elicited by irrelevant probes have not proven sensitive to the mental workload experienced in simulators. Kramer, Trejo, and Humphrey (1995) had ten highly trained U.S. Navy radar operators perform a simulated radar task that was varied in difficulty by manipulating the number of targets to be tracked in a limited period of time; ERPs were elicited by auditory irrelevant probes. Although the amplitude of the P300 decreased when the tone task alone was compared to the radar task with the irrelevant tones, no further decrease in P300 amplitude was observed with increases in the difficulty of the radar task.

An important question is why the irrelevant probe task was sensitive to levels of mental workload in the Sirevaag et al. (1993) study but not in the Kramer et al. (1995) experiment. Although there are a number of differences in these two studies, including the type of system being simulated, one intriguing possibility concerns the nature of the operators' tasks. In the Sirevaag et al. (1993) study, the pilots were constantly communicating with air traffic control, ground controllers, and other aircraft. That is, they were monitoring auditory messages presented via headphones. In contrast, verbal communication was quite infrequent for the radar operators in the Kramer et al.

(1995) study. Therefore, it seems conceivable that the P300 elicited by the irrelevant auditory probes reflected variations in mental workload in the Sirevaag et al. study because the auditory channel was being actively monitored and attended, whereas the auditory channel was not very important in the radar monitoring task examined in Kramer at al. (1995). In other words, it may be that P300s elicited by irrelevant probes reflect mental workload only if they occur within an attended modality or source of information. This hypothesis is consistent with the findings of Verbaten, Huyben, and Kemner (1997) and Makeig et al. (1990). These researchers found that ERPs elicited by task-irrelevant probes were sensitive to variations in mental workload in cases where the irrelevant probes were presented in the same modality as the task of interest. In any event, additional research is warranted before the irrelevant probe technique will be ready for application in simulator and operational settings.

Another alternative to the relevant probe technique for the assessment of mental workload in simulator and operational environments has been referred to as the "primary task" technique (Kramer et al. 1985). In this technique, psychophysiological measures (in particular, ERPs) are elicited by relevant events in the task of interest. For example, in the Sirevaag et al. (1993) study, P300s elicited by changes in the position of the target in the tracking task increased in amplitude with increases in the difficulty of tracking. A clear advantage of this technique is that the mental workload (as well as other processing operations) can be assessed with respect to specific events that occur within the operator's task(s). Furthermore, unlike the relevant or irrelevant probe techniques, no additional stimuli need be introduced into the task, thereby negating concerns regarding performance disruption and operator safety. Thus, within aircraft simulators and during actual flight, psychophysiological measures could be recorded based on radio communications, the presentation of navigational fixes on multifunction displays, and the occurrence of various warning indicators in the cockpit. However, there are also several drawbacks associated with the primary task technique with regard to psychophysiological measurement. First, the technique requires that relevant discrete events be found in the tasks of interest and that the simulators (or operational systems) be modified so that these events can be used as triggers for the psychophysiological measures. However, modification of complex systems – particularly operational systems – is usually quite difficult, if not impossible. Second, given the low signal-to-noise ratio of many ERP components (i.e., those psychophysiological measures that are triggered by discrete events), there must be a sufficient number of discrete events within the task of interest in order for the technique to be feasible. Given these constraints, there are limited opportunities for the use of the primary task technique in simulator and operational environments.

Nonetheless, psychophysiological measures that do not require the imposition of additional stimuli might still be employed. Indeed, the great majority of psychophysiological measures that have been used to assess mental workload in simulator and operational environments fall into this category. These measures include eye movements, blinks, heart rate, heart rate variability, respiration, electrodermal measures, hormonal measures, and EEG activity. The only potential drawback of these measures is that they are not, in general, diagnostic with regard to the varieties of mental workload that are experienced by the human operator. However, these techniques have been used successfully in a number of applied contexts to track changes in mental workload with variations in task and environmental demands.

For example, measures of HR and HRV have proven sensitive to variations in the difficulty of flight maneuvers and phases of flight (e.g., straight and level, takeoffs, landings) in both fixed-wing and rotary-wing military and commercial aviation (Boer & Veltman 1997; Roscoe 1993; Veltman & Gaillard 1996; Wilson & Fisher 1995), automobile driving (Brookhuis & de Waard 1993), air traffic control (Brookings, Wilson, & Swain 1996), and electroenergy process control (Rau 1996). In each of these cases, heart rate measures have served as a relatively continuous index of mental workload in simulated or operational environments.

It is important to note, however, that changes in heart rate and components of heart rate variability do not always produce the same pattern of effects with regard to their sensitivity to mental workload and task difficulty (Jorna 1992; Mulder 1992; Porges & Byrne 1992; Wilson 1992). This is likely due, in large part, to the fact that these measures are influenced by different physiological systems responsible for maintaining homeostasis. Thus, we wish to underscore that, although it may be relatively easy to record heart rate measures in applied situations (but see Wilson 1992 and Jorna 1992 for in-depth discussion of potential artifacts in applied settings), changes in these measures are multiply determined by different physiological systems and therefore are likely to be influenced by different physical and psychological phenomena (Berntson, Cacioppo, & Quigley 1993; Cacioppo et al. 1994). In fact, spectral analysis of heart rate is traditionally differentiated into three functionally distinct bands as follows.

1. A low-frequency band ranges from 0.02 to 0.06 Hz and appears to reflect the regulation of body temperature.
2. A mid-frequency band ranges from 0.07 to 0.14 Hz and is apparently related to the short-term regulation of blood pressure.
3. A high-frequency band ranges from 0.15 to 0.50 Hz and appears to reflect momentary respiratory influences (i.e. respiratory sinus arrhythmia, RSA) on heart rate.

The relative sensitivity of HR and HRV measures to changes in mental workload has been examined in a number of applied studies. Tattersall and Hockey (1995) analyzed HR and HRV measures recorded during a three-hour cockpit training study of eleven novice flight engineers. They reported that (i) HRV in the mid-frequency band was reduced during demanding problem-solving activities during straight and level flight and (ii) HR was higher during the take-off and landing phases of flight. The authors speculated that HR provides a sensitive index of the higher arousal or stress experienced by the flight engineers during takeoff and landing phases of flight, whereas HRV in the mid-frequency band reflects the mental effort expended during difficult problem-solving operations. Wilson (1993) recorded HR from aircraft pilots and weapon systems officers as they flew a variety of maneuvers in an F4 Phantom aircraft. For the pilots, HR increased from ground-based operations to flight as well as during a number of different flight segments (i.e., takeoff and landing, low-level flight, target acquisition). The HRs were generally lower for the weapon systems officer than for the pilot, with one important exception: weapon systems officer HRs were higher than pilot HRs during the one flight segment in which the weapon systems officers flew the aircraft.

In general, HRV was less sensitive to changes in workload than HR. For the pilot, HRV decreased from preflight to flight segments, but this pattern was reversed for the weapon systems officers. Wilson speculated that the different HRV patterns for the pilot and weapon systems officer might be attributable to different patterns of respiration. Indeed, Veltman and Gaillard (1996; see also Sirevaag et al. 1993) reported a confound between HRV in the mid-frequency band and respiration in a simulated flight task. However, when they deconfounded HRV and respiration by scaling HRV with blood pressure variability (BPV) – essentially removing the influence of respiration on the derived measure – they found that the derived HRV measure did discriminate among preflight and different flight segments. Thus, although there are important concerns with regard to respiratory confounds on mid-frequency HRV measures, there also appear to be procedures that can be used to address such concerns (see also Mulder 1992). Therefore, as suggested by our preceding discussion as well as by the mapping of psychophysiological measures to cognitive constructs (Table 1), the choice of whether HR or a component of HRV is to be employed in any particular setting should be predicated upon (i) the potential artifacts that might be encountered as well as (ii) the mental workload aspect(s) of interest to the researcher or human factors practitioner.

In addition to HR and HRV, a number of other measures have been used to assess mental workload in applied settings without requiring additional task requirements (e.g., the probe techniques necessary for elicitation of ERPs). Electro-oculographic measures – including blink rate, blink amplitude, blink duration, and saccade length and velocity – have been employed to assess mental workload in simulator and operational environments. Consistent with laboratory studies, blink rate has been found to reflect changes in mental workload in applied settings, although these changes are in visual workload rather than mental workload in general (Sirevaag et al. 1993; Wilson 1994; Wilson et al. 1994). For example, Veltman and Gaillard (1996) found that blink rate discriminated between flight conditions and landing (with lower blink rates during landing) yet was insensitive to different levels of task demands during flight. Likewise, Brookings et al. (1996) reported that blink rate discriminated among a number of different aircraft density conditions during a simulated air traffic control task (with reduced blink rates while monitoring an increasing number of aircraft) yet did not discriminate among scenarios characterized by different levels of complexity (i.e., as defined by increasing the heterogeneity of aircraft types to be controlled). These results led the researchers to conclude that – although blink rate distinguishes among different levels of *visual* load, with decreasing blink rates while extracting more information from the visual environment – blink rates are evidently insensitive to cognitive load in applied settings.

These findings and conclusions are somewhat perplexing when viewed in the context of laboratory-based research that has found blink rate to be sensitive to both visual and cognitive workload (Kramer 1991; Stern, Walrath, & Goldstein 1984). For example, Bauer, Goldstein, and Stern (1987) reported that blink rate reflected the memory processes necessary to maintain either few or many items in memory for a brief period of time, a situation in which cognitive but not visual load varied. Given such a pattern of results, why then does blink rate appear to be insensitive to cognitive load in applied settings? One possible explanation concerns the relative sensitivity of blink rate to visual and cognitive load. It is conceivable that blink rate is not sufficiently sensitive to relatively fine distinctions between high levels of cognitive load that are experienced in applied settings (e.g., the distinction between straight and level flight versus landing). That is, unlike laboratory conditions in which gradual increases in task demands are implemented, comparisons between task conditions in applied settings are often between very low-demand situations (e.g. resting baselines) and a variety of what are often high-demand task conditions. Blink measures may just not be sensitive to cognitive load differences in high-demand situations.

Blink duration measures – that is, the amount of time the eyelids are closed during a blink – have produced more variable results than have blink rate measures in applied settings. Sirevaag et al. (1993) reported decreases in blink duration with increases in communication load during rotary wing flight, regardless of whether communication was carried out visually (by reading messages from a multifunction display and responding manually) or orally. However, other researchers have either found blink duration to discriminate between the same conditions as blink rate measures (Veltman & Gaillard 1996) or to be less sensitive to visual load conditions than blink rate (Wilson 1994; Wilson et al. 1994). Thus, clearly more research is needed to discern the relative sensitivity of different blink measures to mental workload as well as to examine the range of sensitivity of electro-oculographic measures to cognitive aspects of mental workload in applied settings.

Unlike ERPs, which require the presentation of a discrete event for their elicitation, electroencephalographic measures can be recorded independently of ongoing stimulus and response activity. Indeed, EEG measures in the form of the traditional frequency bands (see Chapter 2 of this volume for an in-depth discussion of the spectral decomposition of EEG activity) have been used in a limited number of applied settings (aircraft flight and automobile driving) as indices of mental workload. Measures of EEG have more frequently been employed in the assessment of low levels of arousal in vigilance situations and as input for closed-loop adaptive systems to monitor alertness in real time or near-real time. These applications will be discussed next.

Sterman and colleagues (1994; Sterman & Mann 1995; Sterman, Mann, & Kaiser 1992) examined EEG changes in the 8–12-Hz (alpha) band during a series of simulated and operational military flights. For example, Sterman et al. (1992) reported a systematic decrease in the power of 8–12-Hz EEG activity as control responsiveness was degraded in a T4 aircraft. Furthermore, these spectral changes were sensitive to the time course of the variations in task difficulty within the flights. Sterman and Mann (1995) likewise reported graded decreases in this alpha power as U.S. Air Force pilots flew progressively more difficult in-flight refueling missions in a B2 aircraft simulator. As in their previous study, alpha suppression varied within each flight according to momentary demands of the tasks and mission. Brookings et al. (1996) reported changes in both theta (4–8-Hz) and alpha (8–12-Hz) power as a number of experienced air traffic controllers performed a series of control tasks varying in task complexity and aircraft density. Alpha power decreased with increases in the heterogeneity of the aircraft types to be controlled, whereas theta power increased with the absolute number of aircraft to be controlled. Brookhuis and de Waard (1993) reported that a derived EEG measure – (alpha + theta)/beta – reflected the difficulty of an automobile driving task, decreasing in power as driving difficulty increased.

Thus, the EEG measures, particularly in the alpha and theta bands, have proven sensitive to variations of mental workload in applied settings. Furthermore, these measures have the potential to track momentary fluctuations in mental workload that result from relatively rapid changes in task demands. However, it still remains to be determined whether changes in these components of the EEG reflect general variations in the arousal or preparatory state of the organism or instead more specific cognitive operations or processes. Topographic analyses of spectral changes across the scalp are likely to provide insight into this issue (Andrew & Pfurtscheller 1996; Gevins et al. 1995; Sterman & Mann 1995).

In summary, a number of psychophysiological recording techniques that have been developed in the laboratory have been successfully implemented in extralaboratory contexts such as simulators and operational environments. Although the psychophysiological measures discussed here have proven useful in the assessment of mental workload in applied contexts, there is clearly a need for the development of additional and more efficacious procedures for signal extraction, pattern recognition, and artifact detection and compensation if psychophysiological measures are to become more widely used in the human factors context.

In addition to the need for further development of technology and methodology, there is also a need for a reconsideration of the theoretical framework in which mental workload has been examined in applied contexts. As described earlier in this section, the modal view of mental workload has been the fixed (unitary or multidimensional) resource or capacity view. Although this conceptualization has provided a reasonable starting point for the examination of performance trade-offs between concurrently performed tasks in applied settings, it is unnecessarily restrictive when complex task performance is considered within the context of the stresses (e.g., sleep loss, fatigue, illness, variations in motivation) of everyday life. That is, the fixed-capacity view does not permit the compensatory and often strategic control of performance that is needed to cope with the common stressors encountered in most jobs and tasks. Indeed, theorists such as Hockey (1997; see also Gaillard 1993; Gopher & Sanders 1984; Pribram & McGuinness 1975) have argued the need for multiple-level compensatory control mechanisms. According to this view, performance is monitored, and if it is found to be deficient then either of two solutions is available. In one solution, additional resources are recruited to improve performance – with the assumption of concomitant expenses in subjective effort and behavioral and physiological cost (both short- and potentially long-term costs in the form of psychosomatic illnesses). In the second solution, performance goals are revised and performance strategies are modified. Of course, the examination of mental workload within such a theoretical framework, although much more inclusive in terms of the important factors such as stress effects, also requires a more detailed understanding of the interaction among physiological, behavioral, and subjective factors that influence performance in applied contexts. Yet such a level of complexity is clearly necessary to develop an adequate understanding of human performance and information processing in extralaboratory environments.

The fixed-resource notion has also come under attack in recent years by researchers who have suggested that, rather than conceptualizing multitask performance in terms of graded capacity sharing, additional consideration should be given to all-or-none performance trade-offs and strategic modifications of processing strategies under difficult dual-task conditions (Allport 1987; Meyer & Kieras 1997; Navon & Miller 1987). Indeed, Pashler (1994) provided relatively strong empirical evidence in favor of bottleneck models (cf. Broadbent 1958). According to these models, the availability of a processing operation is restricted to a single task at a time. Therefore, multitask decrements can be attributed to the delay in the availability of the processing mechanisms rather than a lack of capacity or resources.

The important question, however, is what implications these theoretical considerations have for the psychophysiological assessment of mental workload in applied settings. At the very least, such considerations suggest a broader role for psychophysiological measures. For example, the concern for compensatory regulation of behavior suggests that psychophysiological measures may serve a role in assessing and predicting short- and long-term physiological or health costs as well as in assessing momentary fluctuations in mental workload. Indeed, psychophysiological measures have played an increasingly important role in the investigation of the efficacy of different coping styles in the workplace (Gaillard & Kramer in press). Similarly, the concern with changes in information processing strategies with variations in mental workload could be addressed with psychophysiological measures that have not been traditionally used in workload assessment. For example, ERP components have been identified and characterized that would provide additional insights concerning: the monitoring and detection of errors (the error related negativity – Gehring et al. 1993; Scheffers et al. 1996); the programming and execution of overt actions (the lateralized readiness potential – Coles, Scheffers, & Fournier 1995; Osman, Moore, & Ulrich 1995); the updating of working memory (the slow-wave component – Rosler, Heil, & Roder 1997); and the detection of semantically incongruent information (the N400 – Kutas & Van Petten 1994). Thus, psychophysiology could play an important role in the examination of a broadened conceptualization of mental workload in applied settings.

Psychophysiological Inputs to Adaptively Automated Systems

In a previous section (Assessment and Prediction of Vigilance Decrements), we briefly described two alertness detection systems (Makeig & Inlow 1993; Pope et al. 1995) that, in essence, provide the possibility for the allocation of tasks between humans and machines on the basis of an assessment of the human operator's level of alertness or task engagement. In many ways, the application of psychophysiology to the on-line detection and prediction of

vigilance decrements is well on its way to implementation in operational systems, at least in those systems where operator movements and physical activity are somewhat constrained (e.g., automobile driving, train driving, piloting, quality control inspection, process control). This is due in large part to the fairly well-developed concept of alertness at both a physiological and a psychological level of description. Additionally, there is a substantial body of empirical research both in the laboratory and in simulators that suggests physiological measures can indeed be successfully employed to detect and predict vigilance decrements, particularly in terms of response omissions or lapses.

However, can we expect on-line applications of psychophysiological measures to other issues of concern to human factors professionals, such as the assessment of changes in mental workload or the direction of attention? In many ways, the detection and prediction of behavioral implications of variations in mental workload and attention are harder than assessing performance implications of lapses in alertness. This follows because in many cases the major concern in alertness detection is whether behavior is present or absent – that is, whether the human operator is awake and performing or asleep. Although this is certainly somewhat of an oversimplification of the vigilance or alertness problem(s), just being able to make the binary decision that the operator will be awake or asleep during critical task periods would be a major contribution to the field. However, the assessment of mental workload and attention goes beyond simply making a binary decision (although in many cases even this would be a great improvement in our knowledge about the psychological state of the human operator). Instead, it often involves the assessment of graded changes in performance quality and oftentimes changes in information processing and performance strategies. Thus, these areas of application of psychophysiology demand much greater precision of measurement than does alertness detection.

Given these situational constraints, several important questions must be answered before psychophysiological measures can be employed in real-time adaptive systems. One question, which has been addressed (in part) by research discussed in the previous section on the assessment of mental workload, is the sensitivity of different psychophysiological measures to levels and types of processing demand or mental workload. As discussed earlier, some psychophysiological measures (e.g., ERP components) are quite diagnostic with regard to the nature of processing demands. Other measures, however, are sensitive to changes in a host of psychological and sometimes physical constructs (e.g., respiration, eye blinks, electrodermal activity) but are not diagnostic of specific types of demands. Clearly, the decision of which measure to employ depends upon the nature of the question, particularly in terms of the system performance implications for detecting and predicting general or specific changes in psychological processes. Another related question – which has received much less attention but is no less important in the context of real-world systems – is whether particular psychophysiological measures are sensitive to the entire range or only a limited range of the psychological construct of interest (e.g., mental workload, attention, alertness).

A number of studies have examined the extent to which EEG can be used to distinguish among the types of processing required to perform different tasks as a starting point for the development of psychophysiologically based communication systems. For example, Wilson and Fisher (1995) examined the extent to which EEG data could be used to classify which of 14 different tasks (e.g., simple auditory and visual RT, spatial processing, memory search, visual monitoring) a subject was performing. A principal components analysis (PCA) was used to determine the EEG frequency bands, which were then submitted to a stepwise discriminant analysis procedure. This was done to classify the EEG according to which of the different tasks was being performed during the recording (see also Mecklinger, Kramer, & Strayer 1992 for further discussion of the PCA technique applied to EEG frequency band determination). An average classification accuracy of 86% (with a range of 61%–95%) was achieved across seven participants. However, the frequencies above 30 Hz at lateral recording sites were heavily represented in the classifier. Thus, it is conceivable that the high classification accuracy might to some extent be due to muscle activity of the neck and scalp rather than to electrical activity of the brain. Kerin and Aunon (1990) performed a similar study in an effort to determine whether EEG frequency band asymmetry ratios (the ratio of power in the traditional frequency bands across homologous sites on the right and left side of the scalp) obtained from 2-sec data samples could be used to discriminate among the performance of a variety of different tasks (mental rotation, mental multiplication, mental composition of a letter, visual imagery) under ten different experimental conditions. In this case, however, the investigators ensured that the EEG effects were not contaminated by muscle artifacts. The classification accuracies (percentages) ranged from the mid-80s to 90s, which were similar to those reported by Wilson and Fisher (1995). Unfortunately, however, it is difficult to directly compare the findings of the Kerin and Aunon (1990) and Wilson and Fisher (1995) studies owing to their use of different classification procedures and tasks. Nonetheless, the data from the two studies are promising and suggest that the varieties of processing associated with different types of tasks can be distinguished by an on-line analysis of relatively short samples of EEG. Clearly, however, additional studies are needed that systematically compare the efficacy of different classification algorithms with a large corpus of perceptual, cognitive, and psychomotor tasks.

Other researchers have demonstrated that on-line analysis of EEG and ERPs can be used to communicate at least two-state information to a computer. Farwell and Donchin (1988) developed an ERP (P300-based) communication system in which participants attended to 1 of 36 cells in a 6×6 matrix of letters and symbols. The rows and columns of the matrix were randomly flashed and ERPs were elicited by the flashes. Discriminant analysis algorithms were developed to capitalize on differences in amplitude in the P300 and slow wave, which discriminated between attended and unattended elements in the matrix. The system was able to communicate, with 95% accuracy, approximately 2.3 letters per minute. Although this communication rate was quite slow, the system was far from optimized in that only a portion of the ERP waveform was used from a single scalp site for classification. Indeed, Humphrey and Kramer (1994) demonstrated classification accuracies above 95% between conditions of high versus low workload. They used dual tasks with average ERPs consisting of 10 sec of data (i.e., ten 1-sec ERPs) and combined the ERP data from several electrodes (see also Trejo, Kramer, & Arnold 1995).

Other researchers (Pfurtscheller et al. 1996; Wolpaw & McFarland 1994) have trained participants to utilize their EEG to move cursors around a computer screen. Wolpaw et al. (1991) trained participants, over the course of five one-hour sessions, to modify the amplitude of their 8–12-Hz mu rhythm to move a cursor into a target. The target was randomly positioned at the top or the bottom of a computer screen. Participants learned to modify their mu rhythm, which was recorded over the motor cortex, by thinking about performing either a physical activity such as lifting weights (which increased the amplitude of the mu rhythm) or relaxing (which decreased the amplitude of the mu rhythm). The investigators persuasively ruled out contamination of the mu rhythm by eye blinks or by other potential activity that might increase local EMG activity.

In terms of assessing the direction of attention, particularly in the visual domain, another promising technology is eye tracking. In recent years eye trackers have evolved from cumbersome devices that require constraining the observer with a chin rest and bite bar – which, of course, precluded speaking and many other complex actions – to relatively light, head-mounted devices or (in some cases) completely unobtrusive recording devices. Although there are certainly still constraints on the conditions under which eye movements can be reliably recorded (e.g., the observer must be relatively nonambulatory and, in the case of nonobtrusive eye trackers, facing the tracker), it is now possible to record the position of the eyes – with relatively high temporal and spatial precision – in a laboratory, a simulator, and a number of operational environments. Indeed, given the research suggesting visual attention and eye position are often closely coupled (Deubel & Schneider 1996; Kowler et al. 1995; Zelinsky & Sheinberg 1997; but see Fox et al. 1996), eye trackers can be used to dynamically track the allocation of attention to different regions of the visual field.

Such information can be extremely valuable in the context of on-line monitoring of operator information extraction strategies. This ensures that critical information has been noted and that operators are sampling information with sufficient frequency to ensure an up-to-date mental model of the task and environment.

In summary, although the application of psychophysiology to on-line assessment is still in its infancy, the laboratory and simulator research that has been conducted thus far has made a promising start toward the development of physiologically based on-line assessment of alertness, attention, and mental workload. Clearly, continued progress will depend on the integration of multiple psychophysiological measures with other measures of the constructs of interest. It depends, as well, on the continued development of signal detection and pattern recognition techniques that can hasten the extraction of the measures from the background noise experienced in simulator and operational settings.

Psychophysiological Inference in Human Factors

Human factors researchers and practitioners have used psychophysiological measures in at least two different ways to make inferences about important psychological processes in applied settings. At the most fundamental level, human factors researchers have used psychophysiological measures as an index of whether two conditions, systems, or individuals differ. In such a case, the main interest is often whether a particular display, control device, or novel design produces a general difference in brain function (e.g., via measures of EEG or ERPs) or autonomic nervous system responsivity (via measures of heart rate, heart rate variability, or respiration). The psychophysiological information obtained in these studies, often along with behavioral and subjective assessments, is then used to decide whether the modified system produces equivalent human responses as compared to a baseline system (especially when additional functions or features are added to the system and the question is whether the human operator can still adequately perform the requisite tasks) or perhaps whether the modified system has led to an enhancement in human responses.

However, the ability to discern whether two systems result in a difference in the physiological responsivity of human operators is not always sufficient. In many cases, the human factors researcher is interested in discerning the nature of the psychological difference engendered by two or more tasks or systems. Only with such information can the proposed tasks or systems be further refined or modified to best accommodate the human operator. For example, in order to reduce mental workload it is often important to know whether high levels of workload are the result of excessive perceptual, memory, or motor de-

mands (or some combination of these different types of processing demands). Such knowledge can then enable system modifications that are targeted to the specific nature of processing demands, thereby reducing the time and cost necessary for system improvements. Indeed, as has been illustrated in previous discussions and the hypothesized mapping in Table 1, psychophysiological measures have been used to indicate whether specific types (and magnitudes) of processing demands differ across systems, settings, and individuals in applied contexts such as piloting, air traffic control, sonar and radar monitoring, and automobile and truck driving. However, although such inferences are routinely made, it is important to keep in mind that the mapping between physiological measures and psychological constructs is rarely one-to-one (Cacioppo & Tassinary 1990). That is, as illustrated in Table 1, the great majority of psychophysiological measures are related in a one-to-many fashion with psychological constructs, so there clearly is a need for the use of converging operations (and measures – including physiological, behavioral, and subjective) to isolate the influence of system changes on psychological processes.

Conclusions

In this chapter we have provided a brief synopsis of several current issues in the field of human factors that would likely benefit from the application of psychophysiological techniques and psychophysiologically inspired models and theories. In discussing each of these potential application areas, we have endeavored, whenever possible, to describe studies in which psychophysiological measures have been used to address issues of concern to the human factors community in applied settings – that is, in complex simulators and in operational environments. Indeed, if psychophysiology is to make a lasting contribution to the field of human factors, it is important that we "transition" our measurement techniques from the relatively sterile yet well-controlled environment of the laboratory to the much richer but less controlled operational settings. Clearly, as evidenced by our critical review of the literature, such transitions are beginning to take place.

In each of the research and application domains that we discussed – the assessment of mental workload, the detection and prediction of lapses in alertness, and the on-line assessment of information processing activities and strategies – there have been demonstrations of successful applications of psychophysiology. In these cases, psychophysiological measurement has either (a) provided converging support, along with performance and subjective measures, of important changes in information processing strategies, alertness, or attention, or (b) provided insights that were not available with other measures – for example, by providing information concerning physiological coping strategies with implications for short- and long-term psychological and physical health, by indicating changes in resource allocation strategies with implications for multitask performance, and by predicting when vigilance decrements will be observed. Clearly, given the continued development of semiautomated and automated systems in which human operators monitor rather than actively control system functions, there will be numerous additional opportunities for the use of psychophysiological measures to provide insights into the covert processes of the mind.

However, in each of the research domains that we have discussed, there remain a number of important challenges for psychophysiological measurement. These challenges include:

1. the development and further refinement of signal extraction, pattern recognition, and artifact rejection and compensation algorithms that can be employed in relatively noisy environments;
2. the continued development of physiological and psychological models of psychophysiological measures; and
3. the mapping of these models and measures to models developed by other research domains, such as cognitive science and neuroscience.

Indeed, there appears to be activity on each of these fronts and in particular on the integration of psychophysiological, neuroscience, cognition, and emotion in the development of macro models of human psychological function.

NOTE

The preparation of this chapter was supported by the U.S. Army Research Laboratory under a cooperative research agreement (DAAL01-96-2-0003) and by a grant from the Office of Naval Research N00014-93-1-0253.

REFERENCES

Aasman, J., Mulder, G., & Mulder, L. (1987). Operator effort and the measurement of heart-rate variability. *Human Factors, 29*, 161–70.

Akerstedt, T., & Folkard, S. (1996). Predicting sleep latency from the three-process model of alertness. *Psychophysiology, 33*, 385–9.

Allport, A. (1987). Selection for action: Some behavioral and neurophysiological considerations of attention and action. In H. Heuer & A. Sanders (Eds.), *Perspectives on Perception and Action*, pp. 395–418. Hillsdale, NJ: Erlbaum.

Andrew, C., & Pfurtscheller, G. (1996). Event-related coherence as a tool for studying dynamic interactions of brain regions. *Electroencephalography and Clinical Neurophysiology, 98*, 144–8.

Bauer, L. O., Goldstein, R., & Stern, J. A. (1987). Effects of information processing demands on physiological response patterns. *Human Factors, 29*, 213–34.

Beatty, J., Greenberg, A., Deibler, W., & O'Hanlon, J. (1974). Operant control of occipital theta rhythm affects performance in a radar monitoring task. *Science, 183*, 871–3.

Bellenkes, A. H., Wickens, C. D., & Kramer, A. F. (1997). Visual scanning and pilot expertise: The role of attentional flexibility and mental model development. *Aviation, Space and Environmental Medicine, 68*, 869–79.

Berntson, G. G., Cacioppo, J. T., & Quigley, K. S. (1993). Respiratory sinus arrhythmia: Autonomic origins, physiological mechanisms, and psychophysiological implications. *Psychophysiology, 30*, 183–96.

Boer, L. C., & Veltman, J. A. (1997). From workload assessment to system improvement. Paper presented at the NATO Workshop on Technologies in Human Engineering Testing and Evaluation (June 24–26, Brussels).

Boucsein, W., & Ottmann, W. (1996). Psychophysiological stress effects from the combination of night-shift work and noise. *Biological Psychology, 42*, 301–32.

Broadbent, D. (1958). *Perception and Communication.* London: Pergamon.

Broadbent, D. (1971). *Decision and Stress.* New York: Academic Press.

Broadbent, D., & Gregory, M. (1965). Effects of noise and signal rate upon vigilance as analyzed by means of decision theory. *Human Factors, 7*, 155–62.

Brookhuis, K. A., & de Waard, D. (1993). The use of psychophysiology to assess driver status. *Ergonomics, 36*, 1099–1110.

Brookings, J., Wilson, G. F., & Swain, C. R. (1996). Psychophysiological responses to changes in workload during simulated air traffic control. *Biological Psychology, 42*, 361–77.

Brown, W. K., Rogge, J. F., Buckley, C. J., & Brown, C. A. (1969). Aeromedical aspects of the first non-stop transatlantic helicopter flight: II. Heart rate and ECG changes. *Aerospace Medicine, 40*, 714–17.

Byrne, E. A., & Parasuraman, R. (1996). Psychophysiology and adaptive automation. *Biological Psychology, 42*, 249–68.

Cacioppo, J. T., Berntson, G. G., Binkley, P. F., Quigley, K. S., Uchino, B. N., & Fieldstone, A. (1994). Autonomic cardiac control. II. Noninvasive indices and basal response as revealed by autonomic blockades. *Psychophysiology, 31*, 586–98.

Cacioppo, J. T., & Tassinary, L. G. (1990). Psychophysiology and psychophysiological inference. In J. T. Cacioppo & L. G. Tassinary (Eds.), *Principles of Psychophysiology: Physical, Social and Inferential Aspects,* pp. 3–33. Cambridge University Press.

Caldwell, J. (1995). Assessing the impact of stressors on performance: Observations on levels of analysis. *Biological Psychology, 40*, 197–208.

Coles, M. G. H., Scheffers, M., & Fournier, L. (1995). Where did you go wrong? Errors, partial errors, and the nature of human information processing. *Acta Psychologica, 90*, 129–44.

Davies, D. R., & Parasuraman, R. (1980). *The Psychology of Vigilance.* London: Academic Press.

Deubel, H., & Schneider, W. (1996). Saccade target selection and object recognition: Evidence for a common attentional mechanism. *Vision Research, 36*, 1827–37.

Du, W., Leong, H., & Gevins, A. (1994). Ocular artifact rejection by adaptive filtering. Paper presented at the 7th IEEE SP Workshop on Statistical Signal and Array Processing (Quebec City, CA).

Endsley, M. R. (1994). Automation and situation awareness. In M. Mouloua & R. Parasuraman (Eds.), *Human Performance in Automated Systems: Current Research and Trends,* pp. 163–81. Hillsdale, NJ: Erlbaum.

Farwell, L., & Donchin, E. (1988). Talking off the top of your head: Toward a mental prosthesis utilizing event-related brain potentials. *Electroencephalography and Clinical Neurophysiology, 70,* 510–23.

Fitts, P., & Jones, R. (1947). Analysis of factors contributing to 460 "pilot error" experiences in operating aircraft controls. Memorandum report no. TSEA 4-694-12, Harry Armstrong Aerospace Medical Research Laboratory, Wright-Patterson AFB, Ohio.

Fitts, P., Jones, R., & Milton, J. (1950). Eye fixations of aircraft pilots III: Frequency, duration and sequence of fixations while flying Air Force Ground Controlled Approach System (GCA). Air Material Command Technical report no. USAF TR-5967.

Fogarty, C., & Stern, J. (1993). Eye movements and blinks: Their relationship to higher cognitive processes. *International Journal of Psychophysiology, 8,* 35–42.

Fowler, B. (1994). P300 as a measure of workload during a simulated aircraft landing task. *Human Factors, 36,* 670–83.

Fox, J., Merwin, D., Marsh, R., McConkie, G., & Kramer, A. (1996). Information extraction during instrument flight: An evaluation of the validity of the eye–mind hypothesis. Proceedings of the Human Factors Society, 40th Annual Meeting (Philadelphia).

Gaillard, A. W. K. (1993). Comparing the concepts of mental load and stress. *Ergonomics, 36,* 991–1005.

Gaillard, A. W. K., & Kramer, A. F. (in press). Theoretical and methodological considerations in psychophysiological research. In R. Backs (Ed.), *Engineering Psychophysiology.* Hillsdale, NJ: Erlbaum.

Gainer C. A., & Obermayer, R. W. (1964). Pilot eye fixations while flying selected maneuvers using two instrument panels. *Human Factors, 6,* 485–501.

Gehring, W., Goss, B., Coles, M. G. H., Meyer, D., & Donchin, E. (1993). A neural system for error detection and compensation. *Psychological Science, 4,* 385–90.

Gevins, A., Leong, H., Du, R., Smith, M., Le, J., DuRousseau, D., Zhang, J., & Libove, J. (1995). Towards measurement of brain function in operational environments. *Biological Psychology, 40,* 169–86.

Goeller, C., & Sinton, C. (1989). A microcomputer-based sleep stage analyzer. *Computer Methods and Programs in Biomedicine, 29,* 31–6.

Gomer, F. E. (1981). Physiological monitoring and the concept of adaptive systems. In J. Morel & K. F. Kraiss (Eds.), *Manned Systems Design,* pp. 271–87. New York: Plenum.

Gopher, D., & Sanders, A. F. (1984). S-Oh-R: Oh stages! Oh resources! In W. Printz & A. F. Sanders (Eds.), *Cognition and Motor Processes.* Berlin: Springer-Verlag.

Harsh, J., Voss, U., Hull, J., Schrepfer, S., & Badia, P. (1993). ERP and behavioral changes during the wake/sleep transition. *Psychophysiology, 31,* 244–52.

Hockey, G. R. J. (1984). Varieties of attentional state: The effects of environment. In R. Parasuraman & D. R. Davies (Eds.), *Varieties of Attention,* pp. 449–84. New York: Academic Press.

Hockey, G. R. J. (1997). Compensatory control in the regulation of human performance under stress and high workload: A cognitive energetical framework. *Biological Psychology, 45,* 73–94.

Hoffman, J. (1990). Event-related potentials and automatic and controlled processes. In J. Rohrbaugh, R. Parasuraman, & R. Johnson (Eds.), *Event-Related Brain Potentials: Basic Issues and Applications,* pp. 145–57. New York: Oxford University Press.

Hoffman, J., Houck, M., MacMillian, F., Simons, R., & Oatman, L. (1985). Event related potentials elicited by automatic targets: A dual-task analysis. *Journal of Experimental Psychology: Human Perception and Performance, 11,* 50–61.

Humphrey, D., & Kramer, A. (1994). Towards a psychophysiological assessment of dynamic changes in mental workload. *Human Factors, 36,* 3–26.

Humphrey, D., Kramer, A. F., & Stanny, R. (1994). Influence of extended-wakefulness on automatic and non-automatic processing. *Human Factors, 36,* 652–69.

Isreal, J., Chesney, G., Wickens, C., & Donchin, E. (1980). P300 and tracking difficulty: Evidence for multiple resources in dual-task performance. *Psychophysiology, 17,* 259–73.

Jones, R., Milton, J., & Fitts, P. (1950). Eye fixations of aircraft pilots IV: Frequency, duration and sequence of fixations during routine instrument flight. Technical report no. 5795, Wright-Patterson AFB, Ohio.

Jorna, P. G. A. M. (1992). Spectral analysis of heart rate and psychological state: A review of its validity as a workload index. *Biological Psychology, 34,* 237–57.

Kahneman, D. (1973). *Attention and Effort.* Englewood Cliffs, NJ: Prentice-Hall.

Kecklund, G., & Akerstedt, T. (1993). Sleepiness in long distance truck driving: An ambulatory EEG study of night driving. *Ergonomics, 36,* 1007–17.

Kerin, Z., & Aunon, J. (1990). Man–machine communications through brain processing. *IEEE Engineering in Medicine and Biology, 90,* 55–7.

Koelega, H. S., Verbaten, M. N., van Leeuwen, T. H., Kenemans, J. L., Kemner, C., & Sjouw, W. (1992). Time effects on event-related brain potentials and vigilance performance. *Biological Psychology, 34,* 59–86.

Kotulak, J. C., & Morse, S. E. (1995). Oculomotor responses with aviator helmet-mounted displays and their relation to in-flight symptoms. *Human Factors, 37,* 699–710.

Kowler, E., Anderson, E., Dosher, B., & Blaser, E. (1995). The role of attention in the programming of saccades. *Vision Research, 35,* 1897–1916.

Kramer, A. F. (1991). Physiological metrics of mental workload: A review of recent progress. In D. Damos (Ed.), *Multiple Task Performance,* pp. 279–328. London: Taylor & Francis.

Kramer, A. F., Sirevaag, E., & Braune, R. (1987). A psychophysiological assessment of operator workload during simulated flight missions. *Human Factors, 29,* 145–60.

Kramer, A. F., & Spinks, J. (1991). Capacity views of information processing. In R. Jennings & M. Coles (Eds.), *Psychophysiology of Human Information Processing: An Integration of Central and Autonomic Nervous System Approaches,* pp. 179–250. New York: Wiley.

Kramer, A. F., & Strayer, D. (1988). Assessing the development of automatic processing: An application of dual-task and event-related brain potential methodologies. *Biological Psychology, 26,* 231–68.

Kramer, A. F., Trejo, L., & Humphrey, D. (1994). Psychophysiological measures of workload: Potential applications to adaptively automated systems. In M. Mouloua & R. Parasuraman (Eds.), *Human Performance in Automated Systems: Current Research and Trends,* pp. 137–62. Hillsdale, NJ: Erlbaum.

Kramer, A. F., Trejo, L., & Humphrey, D. (1995). Assessment of mental workload with task-irrelevant auditory probes. *Biological Psychology, 40,* 83–100.

Kramer, A. F., Wickens, C. D., & Donchin, E. (1985). The processing of stimulus properties: Evidence for dual task integrality. *Journal of Experimental Psychology: Human Perception and Performance, 11,* 393–408.

Kutas, M., & Van Petten, C. (1994). Psycholinguistics electrified: Event-related brain potential investigations. In M. Gernsbacher (Ed.), *Handbook of Psycholinguistics,* pp. 83–144. San Diego: Academic Press.

Lavie, P., & Zvulini, A. (1992). The 24 hour sleep propensity function: Experimental bases for somnotypology. *Psychophysiology, 29,* 566–75.

Lee, J., & Moray, N. (1992). Trust, control strategies and allocation of function in human–machine systems. *Ergonomics, 35,* 1243–70.

Loomis, A. L., Harvey, E., & Hobart, G. A. (1937). Cerebral states during sleep as studied by brain potentials. *Journal of Experimental Psychology, 21,* 127–44.

Mackworth, N. H. (1948). The breakdown of vigilance during prolonged visual search. *Quarterly Journal of Experimental Psychology, 1,* 5–61.

Makeig, S., Elliot, F. S., Inlow, M., & Kobus, D. A. (1990). Predicting lapses in vigilance using brain evoked responses to irrelevant auditory probes. Unpublished manuscript.

Makeig, S., & Inlow, M. (1993). Lapses in alertness: Coherence of fluctuations in performance and EEG spectrum. *Electroencephalography and Clinical Neurophysiology, 86,* 23–35.

Makeig, S., & Jung, T. P. (1996). Tonic, phasic and transient EEG correlates of auditory awareness in drowsiness. *Cognitive Brain Research, 4,* 15–25.

Mangun, G. R., & Hillyard, S. A. (1990). Allocation of visual attention to spatial locations: Tradeoff functions for event-related brain potentials and detection performance. *Perception and Psychophysics, 47,* 532–50.

McCallum, C., Cooper, R., & Pocock, P. (1987). Event-related and steady state changes in the brain related to workload during tracking. In K. Jensen (Ed.), *Electric and Magnetic Activity of the Central Nervous System: Research and Clinical Applications in Aerospace Medicine.* France: NATO AGARD.

Mecklinger, A., Kramer, A. F., & Strayer, D. L. (1992). Event related potentials and EEG components in a semantic memory search task. *Psychophysiology, 29,* 104–19.

Meister, D. (1989). *Conceptual Aspects of Human Factors.* Baltimore: Johns Hopkins University Press.

Meyer, D. E., & Kieras, D. E. (1997). A computational theory of executive control processes and multiple-task performance: Part I. Basic Mechanisms. *Psychological Review, 104,* 3–65.

Miller, J. C. (1995). Batch processing of 10,000 hours of truck driver EEG data. *Biological Psychology, 40,* 209–22.

Moray, N. (1967). Where is capacity limited? A survey and a model. *Acta Psychologica, 27,* 84–92.

Morris, T. L., & Miller, J. C. (1996). Electro-oculographic and performance indices of fatigue during simulated flight. *Biological Psychology, 42,* 343–60.

Mulder, L. J. M. (1992). Measurement and analysis methods of heart rate and respiration for use in applied environments. *Biological Psychology, 34,* 205–36.

Natani, K., & Gomer, F. (1981). Electrocortical activity and operator workload: A comparison of changes in the electroencephalogram and event-related potentials. Technical report no. MDC E2427, McDonnel Douglas Corporation, St. Louis.

Navon, D., & Gopher, D. (1979). On the economy of the human processing system. *Psychological Review, 86,* 214–55.

Navon, D., & Miller, J. (1987). The role of outcome conflict in dual-task interference. *Journal of Experimental Psychology: Human Perception and Performance, 13,* 435–48.

Norman, D., & Bobrow, D. (1975). On data-limited and resource-limited processes. *Cognitive Psychology, 7,* 44–64.

North, R. (1977). Task functional demands as factors in dual-task performance. In *Proceedings of the 21st Annual Meeting of the Human Factors Society.* San Francisco: Human Factors Society.

Osman, A., Moore, C., & Ulrich, R. (1995). Bisecting RT with lateralized readiness potentials: Precue effects after LRP onset. *Acta Psychologica, 90,* 111–27.

Papanicolaou, A. C., & Johnstone, J. (1984). Probe evoked potentials: Theory, method and applications. *International Journal of Neuroscience, 24,* 107–31.

Parasuraman, R. (1984). Sustained attention in detection and discrimination. In R. Parasuraman & D. R. Davies (Eds.), *Varieties of Attention,* pp. 243–72. New York: Academic Press.

Parasuraman, R. (1985). Event related brain potentials and intermodal divided attention. *Proceedings of the Human Factors Society, 29,* 971–5.

Parasuraman, R. (1990). Event-related brain potentials and human factors research. In J. Rohrbaugh, R. Parasuraman, & R. Johnson (Eds.), *Event-Related Brain Potentials: Basic Issues and Applications,* pp. 279–300. New York: Oxford University Press.

Parasuraman, R., Molloy, R., & Singh, I. L. (1993). Performance consequences of automation induced complacency. *International Journal of Aviation Psychology, 3,* 1–23.

Parasuraman, R., Mouloua, M., & Molloy, R. (1994). Monitoring automation failures in human machine systems. In M. Mouloua & R. Parasuraman (Eds.), *Human Performance in Automated Systems: Current Research and Trends,* pp. 45–9. Hillsdale, NJ: Erlbaum.

Pashler, H. (1994). Dual-task interference in simple tasks: Data and theory. *Psychological Bulletin, 116,* 220–44.

Pfurtscheller, G., Kalcher, J., Neuper, C., Flotzinger, D., & Pregenzer, M. (1996). On-line EEG classification during externally-paced hand movements using a neural network-based classifier. *Electroencephalography and Clinical Neurophysiology, 99,* 416–25.

Polson, M., & Freidman, A. (1988). Task sharing within and between hemispheres: A multiple resource approach. *Human Factors, 30,* 633–43.

Pope, A., Bogart, E., & Bartolome, D. (1995). Biocybernetic system evaluates indices of operator engagement in automated task. *Biological Psychology, 40,* 187–95.

Porges, S. W., & Byrne, E. A. (1992). Research methods for the measurement of heart rate and respiration. *Biological Psychology, 34,* 93–130.

Pribram, K. H., & McGuinness, D. (1975). Arousal, activation and effort in the control of attention. *Psychological Review, 27,* 131–42.

Rau, R. (1996). Psychophysiological assessment of human reliability in a simulated complex system. *Biological Psychology, 42,* 287–300.

Reason, J. (1990). *Human Error*. Cambridge University Press.

Riley, V. (1994). A theory of operator reliance in automation. In M. Mouloua & R. Parasuraman (Eds.), *Human Performance in Automated Systems: Current Research and Trends*, pp. 8–14. Hillsdale, NJ: Erlbaum.

Roman, J., Older, H., & Jones, W. L. (1967). Flight research program. VII: Medical monitoring of Navy carrier pilots in combat. *Aerospace Medicine, 38*, 133–9.

Roscoe, A. H. (1975). Heart rate monitoring of pilots during steep gradient approaches. *Aviation, Space and Environmental Medicine, 46*, 1410–15.

Roscoe, A. H. (1993). Heart rate as a psychological measure for in-flight workload assessment. *Ergonomics, 36*, 1055–62.

Rosler, F., Heil, M., & Roder, B. (1997). Slow negative brain potentials as reflections of specific modular resources of cognition. *Biological Psychology, 45*, 109–42.

Ruffel-Smith, H. P. (1967). Heart rate of pilots flying aircraft on scheduled airline routes. *Aerospace Medicine, 38*, 1117–19.

Scerbo, M. (1994). Theoretical perspectives on adaptive automation. In M. Mouloua & R. Parasuraman (Eds.), *Human Performance in Automated Systems: Current Research and Trends*, pp. 37–64. Hillsdale, NJ: Erlbaum.

Scheffers, M., Coles, M. G. H., Bernstein, P., Gehring, W., & Donchin, E. (1996). Event-related brain potentials and error related processing: An analysis of incorrect responses to go and no-go stimuli. *Psychophysiology, 33*, 42–53.

Sem-Jacobsen, C. W. (1959). Electroencephalographic study of pilot stress. *Aerospace Medicine, 30*, 797–803.

Sem-Jacobsen, C. W. (1960). Recording of in-flight stress in jet fighter planes. *Aerospace Medicine, 31*, 320–35.

Sem-Jacobsen, C. W. (1961). Black-out and unconsciousness revealed by airborne testing of fighter pilots. *Aerospace Medicine, 32*, 247–53.

Sem-Jacobsen, C. W., Nilseng, O., Patten, C., and Eriksen, O. (1959). Electroencephalographic recording in simulated flight in a jet fighter plane. *Journal of Electroencephalography and Clinical Neurophysiology, 11*, 22–9.

Sem-Jacobsen, C. W., & Sem-Jacobsen, J. E. (1963). Selection and evaluation of pilots for high performance aircraft and spacecraft by in-flight EEG study of stress tolerance. *Aerospace Medicine, 34*, 605–9.

Shaffer, L. (1975). Multiple attention in continuous tasks. In P. Rabbitt & S. Dornic (Eds.), *Attention and Performance*. London: Academic Press.

Sirevaag, E., Kramer, A., Coles, M., & Donchin, E. (1987). Resource reciprocity: An event-related brain potentials analysis. *Acta Psychologica, 70*, 77–90.

Sirevaag, E., Kramer, A., Wickens, C., Reisweber, M., Strayer, D., & Grenell, J. (1993). Assessment of pilot performance and workload in rotary wing helicopters. *Ergonomics, 9*, 1121–40.

Smulders, F., Kenemans, J., Jonkman, L., & Kok, A. (1997). The effects of sleep loss on task performance and the electroencephalogram in young and elderly subjects. *Biological Psychology, 45*, 217–39.

Sperling, G., & Melcher, M. (1978). The attention operating characteristic: Examples from visual search. *Science, 20*, 315–18.

Sterman, B., & Mann, C. (1995). Concepts and applications of EEG analysis in aviation performance evaluation. *Biological Psychology, 40*, 115–30.

Sterman, B., Mann, C., & Kaiser, D. (1992). Quantitative EEG patterns of in-flight workload. In *1992 Space Operations Applications and Research Proceedings*, pp. 466–73. Houston, TX: Johnson Space Center.

Sterman, B., Mann, C., Kaiser, D., & Suyenobu, B. (1994). Multiband topographic EEG analysis of a simulated visuo-motor aviation task. *International Journal of Psychophysiology, 16*, 49–56.

Stern, J. A., Boyer, D., & Schroeder, D. (1994). Blink rate: a possible measure of fatigue. *Human Factors, 36*, 285–97.

Stern, J., Walrath, L. C., & Goldstein, R. (1984). The endogenous eyeblink. *Psychophysiology, 21*, 22–33.

Strayer, D., & Kramer, A. F. (1990). Attentional requirements of automatic and controlled processes. *Journal of Experimental Psychology: Learning, Memory and Cognition, 16*, 67–82.

Tattersall, A. J., & Hockey, G. R. (1995). Level of operator control and changes in heart rate variability during simulated flight maintenance. *Human Factors, 37*, 682–98.

Torsvall, L., & Akerstedt, T. (1987). Sleepiness on the job: Continuously measured EEG changes in train drivers. *Electroencephalography and Clinical Neurophysiology, 66*, 502–11.

Torsvall, L., & Akerstedt, T. (1988). Extreme sleepiness: Quantification of EOG and spectral EEG parameters. *International Journal of Neuroscience, 38*, 435–41.

Townsend, R. E., & Johnson, L. C. (1979). Relation of frequency analyzed EEG to monitoring behavior. *Electroencephalography and Clinical Neurophysiology, 47*, 272–9.

Trejo, L., Kramer, A. F., & Arnold, J. (1995). Event-related potentials as indices of display monitoring performance. *Biological Psychology, 40*, 33–72.

Trejo, L. J., & Shensa, M. J. (1993). Linear and neural network models for predicting human signal detection performance from event-related potentials: A comparison of wavelet transforms with other feature extraction methods. *Proceedings of the International Simulation Conference* (November 7–10). San Diego: Society for Computer Simulation.

Varri, A., Hirvonen, K., Hasan, J., Loula, P., & Hakkinen, V. (1992). A computerized analysis system for vigilance studies. *Computer Methods and Programs in Biomedicine, 39*, 113–24.

Veltman, J. A., & Gaillard, A. W. K. (1996). Physiological indices of workload in a simulated flight task. *Biological Psychology, 42*, 323–42.

Verbaten, M. N., Huyben, M. A., & Kemner, C. (1997). Processing capacity and the frontal P3. *International Journal of Psychophysiology, 25*, 37–48.

Westerkamp, J., & Williams, R. (1995). Adaptive estimation of single response evoked potentials. *Biological Psychology, 40*, 161–8.

Wickens, C. D. (1990). Applications of event-related potential research to problems in human factors. In J. Rohrbaugh, R. Parasuraman, & R. Johnson (Eds.), *Event-Related Brain Potentials: Basic Issues and Applications*, pp. 301–9. New York: Oxford University Press.

Wickens, C. D. (1992). *Engineering Psychology and Human Performance*. New York: Harper-Collins.

Wickens, C. D., Kramer, A. F., Vanesse, L., & Donchin, E. (1983). The performance of concurrent tasks: A psychophysiological analysis of the reciprocity of information processing resources. *Science, 221*, 1080–2.

Wierwille, W. W. (1994). Overview of research on driver drowsiness definition and driver drowsiness detection. Paper presented at the 14th Annual Technical Conference on the Enhanced Safety of Vehicles (ESV) (May, Munich).

Wilson, G. F. (1992). Applied use of cardiac and respiration measures: Practical considerations and precautions. *Biological Psychology, 34,* 163–78.

Wilson, G. F. (1993). Air-to-ground training missions: A psychophysiological workload analysis. *Ergonomics, 36,* 1071–87.

Wilson, G. F. (1994). Workload assessment monitor (WAM). In *Proceedings of the Human Factors and Ergonomics Society,* pp. 944–8. Santa Monica, CA: Human Factors Press.

Wilson, G. F., & Eggemeier, F. T. (1991). Psychophysiological assessment of workload in multi-task environments. In D. Damos (Ed.), *Multiple Task Performance,* pp. 329–60. London: Taylor & Francis.

Wilson, G. F., & Fisher, F. (1995). Cognitive task classification based on topographic EEG data. *Biological Psychology, 40,* 239–50.

Wilson, G. F., Fullenkamp, P., & Davis, I. (1994). Evoked potential, cardiac, blink and respiration measures of pilot workload in air to ground missions. *Aviation, Space and Environmental Medicine, 65,* 100–5.

Wolpaw, J. R., & McFarland, D. J. (1994). Multichannel EEG-based brain computer communication. *Electroencephalography and Clinical Neurophysiology, 90,* 444–9.

Wolpaw, J. R., McFarland, D. J., Neat, G. W., & Forneris, C. A. (1991). An EEG-based brain computer interface for cursor control. *Electroencephalography and Clinical Neurophysiology, 78,* 252–9.

Yagi, A. (1997). Application of saccade evoked cortical models to display evaluation. Paper presented at the Workshop on Applied Psychophysiology (June, Helsinki).

Yamamoto, Y., & Isshiki, H. (1992). Instrument for controlling drowsiness using galvanic skin reflex. *Medical and Biological Engineering, 30,* 562–4.

Zelinsky, G. J., & Sheinberg, D. L. (1997). Eye movements during parallel-serial visual search. *Journal of Experimental Psychology: Human Perception and Performance, 23,* 244–62.

CHAPTER THIRTY

ENVIRONMENTAL PSYCHOPHYSIOLOGY

RUSS PARSONS & TERRY HARTIG

Every scientific psychology must take into account whole situations, i.e., the state of both person and environment. (Lewin 1936, p. 12)

Introduction

Physical environments are not typically manipulated by research psychologists, though aspects of the physical environment are often held constant in psychological research. The physical world we experience on a daily basis, however, is not held constant. We are active participants in continuously ongoing transactions, and thus we are continuously experiencing change in our environments. Change in the physical environment is the stuff of human perceptions, cognitions, emotions, memories, development – in short, the stuff of our basic psychological processes. That psychologists take care to control physical environments in their research reflects their appreciation of the power of changing physical contexts to influence human behavior. Because physical environments ordinarily coincide with and lend structure to social environments, often in particular ways and toward particular ends, they are central to the study of social psychological processes as well. This dynamic conception of person-and-environment has been periodically expressed by psychologists and philosophers over the past 60 years (see Altman & Rogoff 1987), though it has had relatively little impact in psychophysiology. Although the amount of psychophysiological research on the physical environment is not small in an absolute sense, manifold possibilities for the systematic study of physical environments have yet to be seriously explored. In this chapter we examine how psychophysiological constructs and methods can be used to understand human transactions with the physical environment.

Despite the inchoate nature of this work, we believe that the existing body of literature can be characterized

as a distinct field of inquiry, environmental psychophysiology. We follow Tassinary (1995) in defining the field as "the study of relationships between organism–place transactions and physiological events." The conceptualization of environment and methodological approaches used in environmental psychophysiology derive largely from three disciplines within the life sciences: *environmental psychology,* in which relationships between human behavior and well-being and sociophysical environments are studied (Stokols & Altman 1987); *psychophysiology,* in which psychological phenomena related to and revealed through physiological principles and events are studied (Cacioppo & Tassinary 1990b); and *environmental physiology,* which involves the study of animal–environment relationships with particular attention paid to the biological effects of changes in the geophysical environment (Tassinary 1995). Environmental psychophysiology can also be distinguished from the related subdisciplines of cognitive psychophysiology and social psychophysiology; the former is concerned with intra-organismic information processing whereas the latter focuses on inter-organismic information processing (see Chapter 1 of this volume).[1] This fairly broad disciplinary heritage implies an extensive purview for this new field. However, we will limit the scope of our coverage of environmental psychophysiology in this chapter to minimize overlap with other chapters in this volume, especially those in Part Three (Processes). The focus of this chapter will be the physical aspects of environments ordinarily encountered, and the level of analysis will emphasize the psychological import of the physical environments of daily life.

The research in environmental psychophysiology so defined and delimited has three noteworthy characteristics. First, research interest has focused on relatively *discrete* physical environmental dimensions and features, especially those features that can be conceived of as environmental stressors. Although some studies have considered whole

John T. Cacioppo, Louis G. Tassinary, and Gary G. Berntson (Eds.), *Handbook of Psychophysiology,* 2nd ed. © Cambridge University Press 2000. Printed in the United States of America. ISBN 62634X. All rights reserved.

environments or situations, most have examined particular environmental dimensions, such as light or sound. This follows in part from a desire to understand the effects of different environmental stressors, but some research has also been motivated to discover information that can inform the design and management of environments in which we live, work, and relax. This is the second noteworthy characteristic of the research to be reviewed: its *applied* orientation. From examinations of traffic congestion to the design of lighting for work environments and the effects of overflight noise in elementary school districts, research in environmental psychophysiology has generated information of direct relevance for policy and decision makers who can influence the design and management of everyday environments. Finally, it is noteworthy as well that much of the research in environmental psychophysiology is *interdisciplinary* in nature. Research in the field has often been conducted by nonpsychologists or by researchers trained in psychology and psychophysiological methods but who have primary institutional affiliations with design-oriented colleges, departments, and other applied institutes. Although this interdisciplinary character may mean that the research to be reviewed is in some instances less technically sophisticated than that found in "mainstream" psychophysiology, this work has the virtue of suggesting interesting new possibilities for the application of psychophysiological methods and constructs.

Because of the applied character of environmental psychophysiology, the organization of this chapter diverges somewhat from that of chapters in the previous parts of this volume. In the pages that follow, we examine work in three broad areas: environmental stress, restorative environments, and topographic cognition. We have chosen these areas both to exemplify existing work and to suggest the broad potential for the application of psychophysiological constructs and methods to the study of human transactions with the physical environment. The research we discuss ranges from commonly encountered psychophysiological applications in environmental stress, through more recent applications of similar constructs and methods to examine the restorative potential of large-scale outdoor environments, to the emerging use of functional brain imaging techniques to draw inferences about the neural substrates of "wayfinding" and related spatial behaviors. In keeping with the major themes of this volume, we provide an appropriate historical context for the material covered in each of these sections, as well as discussions of relevant biological (anatomic/neural/hormonal substrates) and experimental (e.g., research setting, individual differences) contexts.

Environmental Stress: Human Transactions with Noise

The term "environmental stress" is typically construed broadly to include both social and physical environmental stressors, though socially oriented daily life events are often of primary interest.[2] Here, however, we examine what is perhaps the quintessential physical environmental stressor – noise. We consider stress to be a psychophysiological state arising from one of two general types of suboptimal person–environment transactions: (1) the environment presents demands that a person is ill-prepared to meet; or (2) environmental opportunities for goal attainment are either absent or thwarted. Along with most other environmental psychologists (see Evans & Cohen 1987), we advocate a relational concept of stress wherein appraisal of the fit between the environment (demands and opportunities) and oneself (capacities and goals) is central to the stress that is experienced and the coping that is engaged. Despite this interactive or relational perspective, we acknowledge the possibility of normative environmental stressors, such as noisome odors or nociceptive sounds, that are widely experienced as noxious (see Moos & Swindle 1990). We acknowledge as well the possibility that chronic environmental stressors may go largely unnoticed and yet contribute to the stress that is experienced over the course of a day. What these and other limitations of the relational perspective suggest is that there is more to the stressor-appraisal-coping process than can be learned from self-reports of daily life events. Thus, knowledge of individual differences, psychophysiological assessments of situational experience, and objective measurements of physical conditions can all help to understand a process that is unlikely to be either completely available to or accurately represented by conscious recollection.

NOISE

Noise, n. A stench in the ear. Undomesticated music. The chief product and authenticating sign of civilization. (Bierce 1911/1993, p. 85)

In antiquity there was only silence. In the nineteenth century, with the invention of the machine, Noise was born. Today, Noise triumphs and reigns supreme over the sensibility of men. (Russolo 1913/1971, p. 166)

As these epigrams suggest, noise has long been regarded as an Industrial Age phenomenon with untoward psychological consequences. Much of the early research on the effects of noise, however, focused on establishing dose–response curves for potential hearing loss as a function of stimulus intensity and duration of exposure (see Kryter 1994 for a review). Our primary concern here will be with the *nonauditory* effects of noise, which are all those effects not directly related to hearing loss (DeJoy 1984). The modal definition of noise in this literature is "unwanted sound" (Evans & Cohen 1987; Kryter 1994; McLean & Tarnopolsky 1977; Ward & Suedfeld 1973), a definition that clearly implies the importance of cognitive interpretations and the psychological meaning of sound independent

817

of its physical characteristics. In particular, the controllability and predictability of sound are critically important to understanding the nonauditory effects of noise. And, as we shall see, personality and other individual differences also can be used to predict psychophysiological responsiveness and the performance effects of noise, as can nonauditory situational attributes (e.g. effort) of transactions with the sociophysical environment. We begin with brief overviews of epidemiological, animal, and human laboratory work on the nonauditory effects of noise, highlighting inferential issues pertinent to the conduct of field research. We then examine two areas of field research (noise in sleep and school environments) that exemplify the application of psychophysiological constructs and methods to human transactions with the physical environment.

EPIDEMIOLOGICAL AND ANIMAL RESEARCH

Extensive research on the nonauditory effects of noise is a relatively recent phenomenon, arising 20–30 years ago out of public concern for possible health effects of noise pollution in industrial and other workplace environments (DeJoy 1984). Reviewers of the epidemiological research on industrial noise exposure have generally concluded that the strongest evidence for potential health effects is from long-term (3–5 years) exposure to noise at or above 85 dBA (Stansfeld & Haines 1997; Welch 1979). Under these conditions, cardiovascular effects are typically reported (e.g. Parvizpoor 1976; Zhao et al. 1993), with peripheral vasoconstriction (Jansen 1969) and elevated blood pressure (Anticaglia & Cohen 1970) being the symptoms most commonly associated with occupational noise (for reviews see DeJoy 1984; McLean & Tarnopolsky 1977; Smith 1991; Thompson 1996). Occupational noise has also been associated with higher rates of cardiovascular disease (Knipschild 1977, 1980) and myocardial infarction (Ising et al. 1996). However, it is difficult to draw conclusions about health effects based on this work because (i) not all of the epidemiological studies suggest that there are deleterious effects (see e.g. Cohen, Taylor, & Tubbs 1980a; Lees, Romeril, & Wetherall 1980; Van Dijk, Verbeek, & De Vries 1987) and (ii) other studies indicate that harmful effects accrue only after very long exposures on the job (≥ 25 years; Lang, Fouriaud, & Jacquinet-Salord 1992). Moreover, many of the studies that do show effects have not included adequate control groups. Thus, causal inferences based on this literature are unwarranted, because there are usually numerous confounds associated with industrial noise exposure, including the presence of other physical environmental stressors (e.g., heat, dangerous machinery). Throughout this work, the presumed mechanism of the nonauditory health effects of noise is that noise is a stressor, and the complementary laboratory and quasi-experimental research on the nonauditory effects of noise has emphasized measurement of the physiological concomitants of stress and coping.

Early laboratory work with mice and rats suggests that noise-related arousal effects can include increased activation of the cardiovascular system (Smookler & Buckley 1969, hypertension in rats), the sympathetic adrenomedullary system (Ogle & Lockett 1968, increased urinary epinephrine), and the hypothalamic-pituitary-adrenocortical system (Henkin & Knigge 1963, increased plasma hydroxycorticosteroids). Recent work with these species has also indicated cellular immune system effects (e.g. Freire-Garabal et al. 1995, reduced NK cell activity). Generalizations are not straightforward from this research to humans, however, as there are significant structural and functional differences between rodent and human auditory systems (DeJoy 1984). In particular, the rodent auditory system is most sensitive to frequencies in the 15–40-kHz range, while the comparable range of sensitivity for humans is 1–4 kHz (McLean & Tarnopolsky 1977). There is greater similarity among human and nonhuman primate auditory systems and hearing capacities, and work with various monkey species has indicated that noise exposures can produce cardiovascular (Peterson et al. 1984) and endocrine (Hanson, Larson, & Snowdon 1976; Kalin et al. 1985) effects similar to those reported in the rodent literature. For instance, in an oft-cited study by Peterson and his colleagues (1981), rhesus monkeys were exposed to a complex series of environmental sounds, ranging from 30–102 dBA (L_{eq24} = 85 dBA),[3] 24 hours per day for nine months while heart rate and blood pressure (BP) were monitored continuously (see Table 1). Relative to both their own pre-exposure BP and the BP of control animals during the exposure period, the experimental animals showed elevated mean arterial BP throughout the 9-month exposure as well as throughout the day on a daily basis. Pre- and post-exposure tests of auditory sensitivity suggest that these BP changes were not a function of hearing loss. It is interesting to note that BP also remained elevated in the experimental animals throughout the 27-day post-exposure monitoring period. Although one can find methodological weaknesses in this study,[4] these basic findings have been replicated in subsequent work with a related species (*Macaca fascicularis*; Peterson et al. 1984), and they represent some of the strongest results to date from the animal literature regarding the cardiovascular effects of environmental noise.

HUMAN LABORATORY RESEARCH

With the exception of the effects of noise on sleep (summarized in the next section), much of the human laboratory research on the nonauditory effects of noise has emphasized effects on the performance of cognitive and psychomotor tasks. Very often, complete factorial designs (i.e., those including noise-only conditions) are not used, and thus it becomes difficult to assess the physiological effects of noise independent of the physiological activation required to perform the task. Those laboratory studies

TABLE 1. Schedule of Daily Sounds Presented to Rhesus Monkeys by Peterson et al. (1981)

Time	Contents	L$_{eq}$	Range of Measures (dBA)
0700–0730	*Morning Household Noise* Alarm TV on and channel change, "Today Show" Shower with radio and shower doors sliding Hair dryer, shaver, water running, throat clear, toilet flush, gargle (with radio)	81 dBA, fast	51–94
0730–0800	*Transportation Noise (Automobile)* Eight conditions: Windows up or down Speed fast or slow Radio on or off	78 dBA, fast	54–92
0800–1200	*Work Noise (Noisy Industry)* Pile-driver impact noise Bulldozer and diesel generator operation (Background)	82 dBA, fast (0.861 on) 97 dBA, peak (0.139 on)	58–92 92–102
1200–1300	*Cafeteria Noise*	71 dBA, fast	56–82
1300–1700	*Work Noise (repeat)*		
1700–1730	*Transportation Noise (repeat)*		
1730–2230	*Evening Household Noise* Football game on TV	63 dBA, fast	30–75
2230–0700	*Night Noise Intrusions* Heavy vehicle passbys, flyovers, birds chirping (A/C on in background)	48 dBA, fast	30–74
		L$_{eq24}$ = 85 dBA	

that have examined the effects of noise independent of task performance have generally found mild cardiovascular effects, including peripheral vasoconstriction (Kryter & Poza 1980), increased diastolic BP, decreased systolic BP, and sinus arrhythmia (Mosskov & Ettema 1977a,b), and a reduction in cardiac output (Andren et al. 1979, 1980). Many of these same cardiovascular effects emerge under task performance, and they are exacerbated when task performance is accompanied by noise (Carter & Beh 1989; Conrad 1973; Kryter & Poza 1980; Millar & Steels 1990; Mosskov & Ettema 1977a,b). Some sympathoadrenal and adrenocortical endocrine effects associated with task performance and noise have been found as well, including increased epinephrine (Frankenhaeuser & Lundberg 1974, aftereffects only) and elevated cortisol responding (Brandenberger et al. 1980; Follenius et al. 1980), but the effects for these systems are much less consistent.

Although laboratory research on the nonauditory effects of noise on humans has emphasized the ergonomics of performance, some of the findings from this work can be used to help interpret field studies of noise exposure, where the emphasis has been on the potential health effects of environmental noise. There are several reasons for this. First, laboratory work focusing on transient exposures to noise in the context of cognitive performance can offer a reasonable model for the effects of environmental noise in school and occupational settings. Though the tasks used in laboratory noise research typically do not have direct analogs in school and occupational settings, the generalizability of these findings is not necessarily restricted accordingly. What we would expect to generalize from the laboratory to nonlaboratory settings is not the effects of noise on the particular cognitive tasks used in the laboratory but rather the effects of noise on more general psychological processes, such as attention and short-term memory, which are central to performance of those tasks (see Anderson & Bushman 1997 for a fuller exposition of this point). These same psychological processes are likely central to the performance of many tasks found in school and occupational settings as well, and thus the laboratory findings can be relevant for those settings. The focus on *transient* noise in laboratory research is also relevant to nonlaboratory settings, because much of the noise experienced in school, occupational, and other nonlaboratory settings is transient in nature (e.g., oscillating traffic volumes, airplane overflights, aperiodic neighborhood noise).

Laboratory research can also be used to isolate different aspects of human–environment transactions that can mediate the effects of environmental stressors. For instance, experimental work indicates that task performance and psychophysiological responding can be influenced by the perceived predictability and controllability of the stimulus source. Though many laboratory studies have failed to find performance effects of noise exposures (e.g. Conrad 1973; Millar & Steels 1990), careful reviews of this varied and complex body of work have repeatedly concluded that noise can have definite effects on performance that depend upon both the nature of the noise and the nature of the task (for reviews see Broadbent 1979; Kjellberg 1990; Smith 1991). To the extent that environmental noise is uncontrollable, aperiodic, or experienced for extended periods – as may well be the case in many occupational and school settings – tasks requiring concentration and sustained attention are likely to suffer. Several classic physiological studies have found that autonomic responsiveness to noise is decreased when participants are given control over the noise, even when control is not exercised (Glass, Singer, & Friedman 1969). Lundberg and Frankenhaeuser (1978), for instance, reported significantly elevated heart rates for students performing math under uncontrollable noise relative to those who could set noise levels. Breier and colleagues (1987) found significant increases in skin conductance during uncontrollable noise relative to controllable noise, as well as increased levels of epinephrine and adrenocorticotropic hormone during performance of a postnoise anagram task among those who had experienced uncontrollable noise. Thus, there is evidence that the actual and perceived stimulus characteristics of noise that influence task performance also influence stress-related psychophysiological responding.

Other laboratory work suggests that an understanding of situational characteristics could be critical to the interpretation of potential health and other effects of environmental noise exposures in the field. Several studies relying on self-report measures indicate that exposure to noise can elicit negative changes in mood when noise interferes with ongoing activities (Aniansson, Pettersson, & Peterson 1983; Jones & Broadbent 1979; Öhrström & Rylander 1982). In a rare study that used psychophysiological measures and constructs to examine affective consequences of noise, Dimberg (1990) monitored facial EMG (electromyographic) activation during exposures to loud (95-dBA) and moderate (75-dBA) 1,000-Hz tones. He found that activity recorded from *corrugator supercilii* and *zygomaticus major* muscle regions was congruent with the negative and positive emotional responses that participants reported for the loud and soft tones, respectively. In both the short term and the long term, noise-induced changes in mood could have deleterious health effects (Stone et al. 1987, 1994). Such changes could also have important implications in school and occupational settings, where changes in mood could in-

fluence self-imposed performance standards (Cervone et al. 1994) and possibly increase the stress of maintaining performance standards in challenging working conditions. A recent study by Tafalla and Evans (1997), which examined an "adaptive costs" model of physiological activation and performance under stress, highlights this possibility.

The autonomic effects of noise (and other stressors) in the laboratory, coupled with reports of minimal negative performance effects for many tasks, have prompted several research groups to propose the "adaptive costs" model of stress to account for both sets of findings (Cohen et al. 1980b, 1986; Frankenhaeuser 1980; Glass & Singer 1972). According to this model, adequate or superior performance levels are maintained under noise through dint of increased effort, which is reflected in increased autonomic responding. Thus, though performance may be maintained in the face of environmental noise, health costs are ultimately thought to accrue through repeated or sustained increases in autonomic activation, such as sustained increases in cardiovascular responding (Krantz et al. 1988). Consistent with the adaptive costs hypothesis, there is good evidence in the psychophysiological literature that cardiovascular activation, for instance, is greatest when effort and active coping are high (Lovallo et al. 1985; Obrist et al. 1978). Coping and sustained effort to perform in the face of noise in particular have been shown to elicit sustained increases in heart rate, blood pressure (Carter & Beh 1989), and peripheral vasoconstriction (Millar & Steels 1990).

Building on work by Frankenhaeuser and her colleagues (Frankenhaeuser & Lundberg 1977; Lundberg & Frankenhaeuser 1978) suggesting that there may be a trade-off between performance under noise and psychophysiological responding, Tafalla and Evans (1997) explicitly manipulated effort and environmental noise while participants performed mental arithmetic. The presence of uncontrollable noise did not impair performance when increased effort was encouraged, but these conditions did elicit increases in heart rate, norepinephrine, and cortisol. Conversely, when increased effort was not induced, performance declined under uncontrollable noise but cardiovascular and neuroendocrine responding did not change from levels observed during task performance in quiet surroundings. These findings have direct implications for those occupational settings where workers are exposed to uncontrollable noise and yet have strong incentives to maintain performance levels (e.g., exacting quality standards or high productivity requirements). Such conditions may obtain in a wide range of occupations from blue-collar industrial workers to white-collar office employees, and they may also occur in urban school settings where various kinds of transportation noise are often unavoidable. An appropriate assessment of human–environment transactions in noisy (and other stressful) environments should therefore include an examination of sociophysical aspects of environments, such as controllability of potential physical stressors and psychosocial incentives to perform (see Evans, Johansson, & Carrère 1994).

Apart from stimulus properties, situational characteristics, and state-dependent individual responding, state-independent individual characteristics have also been examined in the laboratory. Perhaps the most obviously pertinent state-independent individual characteristic is sensitivity to noise, though the evidence for sensitivity as a stable trait that accounts for variability in performance and physiological responding is checkered (see Kjellberg 1990). Anxiety and neuroticism have been popularly linked to noise sensitivity, and a classic study by Bennett (1945) indicated that questions regarding annoyance with noise were useful in discriminating normal individuals from those diagnosed as neurotic. More recent evidence, however, has been mixed. Several studies suggest that there is no relationship between self-reported sensitivity to noise and scores on the Eysenck Personality Inventory (EPI), Cattell's 16 PF, or the Minnesota Multiple Phasic Inventory (MMPI) (see Griffiths & Delauzun 1977; Moreira & Bryan 1972). Conversely, introverts have been found to prefer lower environmental noise levels (Standing, Lynn, & Moxness 1990) and lower laboratory noise stimulation levels (Hockey 1972), findings that hold when scores for neuroticism are controlled (Geen 1984). Geen (1984) also reported greater cardiovascular and electrodermal reactivity among introverts compared to extroverts at moderate noise exposure levels (55–75 dBA); in a second experiment, however, cardiovascular responding did not differ at very low (40-dBA) or very high (85-dBA) noise levels. It is interesting that there was no difference in physiological reactivity between introverts and extroverts when participants from each group were exposed to *preferred* noise stimulation levels (55 dBA and 72 dBA, respectively), regardless of whether exposure levels were chosen or assigned.

Several researchers have suggested that inconsistencies in the evidence for noise sensitivity as a stable trait reflect the fact that putative measures of noise sensitivity may actually measure general annoyance with environmental stimuli (Kjellberg 1990; Weinstein 1980). Consistent with this, Thomas and Jones (1982) reported that 35% of the variability in noise annoyance scores can be accounted for by responses to a general annoyance questionnaire. However, though discomfort thresholds for noise, light, heat, and cold are moderately related (pairwise r values range from 0.25 to 0.52), sensitivity to noise below the discomfort threshold seems to be unrelated to sensitivities to these other physical environmental stimuli (Öhrström, Björkman, & Rylander 1988). This finding would not be predicted if noise sensitivity were simply an indication of a more general underlying sensitivity to environmental conditions. Thus, researchers have yet to conclusively determine the extent to which noise sensitivity and general environmental sensitivity overlap, or even whether either type of sensitivity constitutes a stable individual characteristic.

FIELD RESEARCH

Except for epidemiological research on the effects of noise in occupational settings (summarized previously), much of the field research on noise has examined effects in sleep environments and the deleterious effects of noise on children in school and home environments. We will consider each of these broad areas in turn. Sleep environment research is conducted both in field and laboratory settings, with reasonably good evidence suggesting that laboratory methods and findings can generalize to non-laboratory environments (Coates et al. 1979; Johns 1977). Although noise-induced *awakenings* tend to be more likely in laboratory studies (see review by Pearsons, Barber, & Tabachnick 1990), various sleep *disturbances* have been found in both field and laboratory settings. These disturbances often take the form of increases in cortical arousal or changes in sleep stage that do not lead to awakenings. For instance, early laboratory research suggested that relatively loud aircraft flyovers (peak intensities of 65–80 dBA) reliably elicit increases in cortical arousal (LeVere & Davis 1977) and are associated with performance decrements on reaction time (RT) tasks administered upon awakening, despite the absence of noise-induced awakenings during the night (LeVere, Bartus, & Hart 1972). These results parallel findings in the field, which indicate that body movements (Öhrström & Björkman 1983), transient electroencephalographic (EEG) fluctuations (Vallet et al. 1983a), shifts to lighter sleep levels (Stevenson & McKellar 1988; Vallet et al. 1983a), and phasic cardiovascular responding (Tulen, Kumar, & Jurriëns 1986; Vallet et al. 1983a,b) are linearly related to decibel levels of noise events. Such linear relationships are often established by recording all instances of a particular class of outdoor noise event (e.g., automobile passbys or airplane overflights) and correlating peak SPLs (sound pressure levels) for these events with various physiological measures. Apart from correlational analyses, these data sets lend themselves to more detailed examinations of transient physiological responding to nocturnal noise events. Heart rates of sleeping field participants, for example, tend to increase momentarily when cars or airplanes pass by, followed by a deceleration that mimics the receding noise level of the sound source (Muzet & Ehrhart 1980).

In part because there are difficulties associating specific noise events with specific sleep disturbances (e.g., when there are multiple, simultaneous automobile passbys), many researchers have examined the *quality* of sleep in noisy versus quiet field settings. Sleep quality is typically inferred from sleep stage analyses based on EEG and electro-oculogram (EOG) recordings in which the duration, distribution, and latency-to-onset of sleep stages are examined. Studies using quasi-experimental designs to manipulate noise exposure provide the strongest evidence for deleterious effects of noise on sleep quality. Manipulations of noise exposures in the field include the introduction of double-glazed windows (Öhrström & Björkman 1983; Tulen et al. 1986; Wilkinson & Campbell 1984), the use of sound-dampening insulation on single-glazed windows (Eberhardt & Akselsson 1987), open versus closed windows (Griefahn & Gros 1986; Tulen et al. 1986), earplugs versus none (Griefahn & Gros 1986), and moving participants' sleep locations from noisy to quiet parts of their dwellings (Vallet et al. 1983a). Two prominent findings emerge from this work, indicating that both slow-wave sleep (stages 3 and 4 – Bergamasco, Benna, & Gilli 1976; Eberhardt & Akselsson 1987; Griefahn & Gros 1986; Wilkinson & Campbell 1984) and rapid eye movement (REM) sleep (Jurriëns 1981; Vallet et al. 1983a) can be adversely affected by noise. Researchers have repeatedly found that latency-to-onset increases and that duration decreases for both slow-wave sleep and REM sleep as peak SPLs increase. Yet these effects of noise are rarely observed for both types of sleep in the same study, an occurrence that Eberhardt and Akselsson (1987) attributed to the inhibition that each sleep stage exerts on the other. They suggested that the particular deleterious effects observed in any given study are a result of the distribution of peak noise events relative to the occurrence of sleep stages. If peak noise events happen to cluster toward the beginning of the sleep period, for instance, then the latency and duration of slow-wave sleep are more apt to be influenced. This is because slow-wave sleep stages predominate in the early hours of sleep whereas the longer periods of REM occur toward the end of the sleep period (Lukas 1976).

Several researchers have reported that peak characteristics of nocturnal noise events are more closely related to sleep quality (Eberhardt & Akselsson 1987; Tulen et al. 1986) and transient sleep disturbances (Vallet et al. 1983a) than measures that integrate acoustic energy over protracted periods (e.g., L_{eq8}). Among researchers who report peak SPLs, there is some consistency in suggesting that noise events producing indoor peak SPLs of 45–55 dBA and above are more likely to cause transient disturbances and/or influence sleep stage parameters than noise events with lower peak SPLs (Eberhardt & Akselsson 1987; Öhrström & Björkman 1983; Vallet et al. 1983a). Despite some consensus regarding peak thresholds of noise that will cause disturbances, other peak characteristics have been much less carefully studied in field settings. Both the rise time (Tulen et al. 1986) and the duration (Lukas 1976; Tulen et al. 1986) of peak noise events have been suggested as important stimulus parameters, though neither is reported with sufficient regularity to warrant a reasonable assessment of their respective contributions to sleep disturbances. There is some evidence regarding certain situational characteristics of peak noise events that may also influence the likelihood and nature of sleep disturbances. For instance, the likelihood that a given peak SPL will elicit a sleep disturbance depends in part upon the background noise level (Vallet et al. 1983a; Vallet, Gagneux, &

Simonnet 1980). Thus, although there may be difficulties in obtaining data regarding the specific characteristics of each noise event over the course of a night's sleep, information such as time of occurrence and relative magnitude may well be critical to understanding the potential deleterious effects of nighttime noise.

This conclusion is underscored by research concerning habituation to environmental noise after years of exposure. Sleep researchers have repeatedly found that the sleep quality of those who have slept in noisy environments for one or more years improves significantly when changes are introduced (sound insulation, double-glazed windows) to reduce indoor peak SPLs (Eberhardt & Akselsson 1987; Griefahn & Gros 1986; Vallet et al. 1983a; Wilkinson & Campbell 1984). Laboratory and field research indicate that although behavioral habituation to nocturnal noise events does occur (e.g., number of awakenings; Thiessen & Lapointe 1978), EEG arousals (Townsend, Johnson, & Muzet 1973), shifts in sleep level (Thiessen & Lapointe 1978), and phasic cardiovascular responding (Vallet et al. 1983b) are much less resistant to extinction. These findings are consistent with animal research, which suggests that cells in the dorsal raphe nuclei are responsible for regulating ultradian sleep cycles (e.g. Lydic, McCarley, & Hobson 1987; Shima, Nakahama, & Yamamoto 1986), and that these cells do not habituate to auditory and visual stimuli during sleep while other cells in the classical reticular formation do (Heym, Trulson, & Jacobs 1982). It may be unlikely, then, that complete adaptation to nocturnal noise events ordinarily occurs in field settings, highlighting the need to characterize carefully the potential health effects of chronic exposure to noise in sleep environments.

The effects of chronic exposure to noise have also been the focus of research on children in home and school environments. Unlike research in sleep environments, there have been few quasi-experimental studies of children's noise exposure in which noise levels have been manipulated by the investigators. Occasionally, however, researchers have been able to capitalize on nonexperimental changes or differences in existing noise levels. In an early classic study, noise levels in apartment buildings that spanned a busy highway were associated with impaired auditory discrimination and reading abilities of children who lived in the apartments (Cohen, Glass, & Singer 1973). Several researchers have highlighted cardiovascular and other stress-related physiological responding to examine the potential health effects of chronic noise exposure on school-age children (Cohen et al. 1980b, 1981; Evans, Bullinger, & Hygge 1998; Evans, Hygge, & Bullinger 1995; Regecová & Kellerová 1995). Early work examining aircraft (Karogodina 1969) and traffic (Karsdorf & Klappach 1968) noise suggested that children in noisy schools had higher resting blood pressure than their counterparts in quiet schools, a finding that has generally been confirmed by more recent studies (see review by Evans & Lepore 1993). For instance,

Cohen and his colleagues (1980b) reported cross-sectional data from an oft-cited study of children attending noisy schools underneath busy air corridors (one flight every 2.5 min) surrounding Los Angeles International airport. Compared to children from quiet schools (matched for grade level, ethnic and racial distribution of children, and parents' occupations and education levels), children from schools under the noisy air corridors had higher resting SBP and DBP (systolic and diastolic blood pressure) when measured in a quiet environment. Subsequent longitudinal data did not support habituation of these effects over time (Cohen et al. 1981).

This early evidence for nonhabituation of cardiovascular responding among school children exposed to noise is consistent with a large-scale study ($n = 1{,}542$), conducted in Bratislava, comparing children who were exposed to different levels of traffic noise (Regecová & Kellerová 1995). Children attending schools in noisy urban areas (> 60 dBA L_{eq24}) showed elevated resting SBP and DBP relative to that of children attending schools in quiet urban areas (< 60 dBA L_{eq24}) after relevant physical (height and weight), demographic, and socioeconomic variables were controlled. This study was also consistent with the Los Angeles air corridor study with respect to differences noted between noisy and quiet home environments versus noisy and quiet school environments. In Bratislava, noise levels obtained from the streets where the children lived were not as closely related to cardiovascular responding as noise levels for the schools. This mirrors cardiovascular and cognitive performance data from the Los Angeles study, where no differences were found between students *living* in quiet versus noisy overflight areas (Cohen et al. 1980b). One interpretation of data from these two studies suggesting greater physiological impacts of noise in school than in home environments follows from the laboratory research mentioned previously regarding increased negative affect when noise interferes with cognitive processing. Noise may have greater negative consequences in school environments to the extent that children are more likely to be cognitively challenged in school than at home.

Regecová and Kellerová (1995) also reported lower resting heart rates (HRs) for children attending schools in noisy areas of Bratislava. In light of the elevated resting BP for these children, they attributed the lower HRs to inhibition of sympathetic nervous system (SNS) activation by baroreceptor reflex responses. They did not measure SNS activity, however; nor did they present evidence regarding the implied permanent modulation of heart rate by repeated baroreceptor reflex response inhibition of SNS activation. Unfortunately, though BP is commonly measured, most other studies of children's exposure to environmental noise have neither reported HR nor measured SNS activity (see Evans & Lepore 1993), and thus the generalizability of this finding is uncertain. In particular, the causal attribution of lower HRs to baroreceptor-mediated SNS in-

hibition is not as straightforward as it seems. Evidence for a dissociation between baroreceptor reflex responses and SNS inhibition under stressful conditions (e.g. Anderson, Sinkey, & Mark 1987) suggests that alternative explanations for lower HRs among the noisy-school children must be considered, especially given the typical conceptualization of environmental noise as a stressor. As Johnson and Anderson (1990) suggested, it is difficult to draw inferences about regulated physiological endpoints (e.g., HR and BP) without knowledge of the activity of the controlling mechanisms (e.g., SNS activation).

Two studies by Evans and his colleagues (1995, 1998) on the effects of overflight noise on school children can be used to illustrate important methodological considerations for conducting psychophysiological research in situ. In both studies, they explicitly included endocrine measures to help interpret anticipated cardiovascular differences between children from noisy and quiet environments. In the first study, compared to control children living in quiet urban neighborhoods (matched for socioeconomic status, family size, and parental education and occupations), children from noisy communities near Munich International Airport had marginally higher SBP ($p = 0.08$) and significantly higher overnight urinary epinephrine and norepinephrine levels (Evans et al. 1995). Children from the noisy communities also exhibited lower SBP reactivity when challenged with a reading task under noisy conditions. Their long-term memory for the reading material was significantly worse, they were less persistent in their attempts to solve an insoluble puzzle, and their performance on a standardized reading test suffered relative to that of children from quiet neighborhoods. Although the weight of these converging lines of evidence militates in favor of a clear difference between children from noisy and quiet communities, neither the stressful nature of that difference nor the attribution of the difference to chronic noise exposure is unambiguous. First, although the overnight endocrine measures may suggest differences in chronic stress levels, their help in interpreting phasic cardiovascular responding (lowered SBP reactivity) to the noisy reading task is limited. A concomitant phasic measure of SNS activation would have been more informative (e.g., skin conductance – a minimally invasive and easily collected measure well suited for work with children). This is especially important given that the resting cardiovascular measures showed no significant differences between groups.

Second, from the information reported, it is difficult to assess noise exposure for the two groups. The sound measure used was L_{eq24}, but it is not clear whether decibel levels were measured in home environments, school environments, or both. If noise exposure was not essentially the same in both school and home environments, and if measurements were made in one environment or the other, then the L_{eq24} measure would be misleading because it integrates acoustic energy over 24 hours. Children would have been absent for a signifi-cant proportion of the time over which measurements were averaged if measurements were made in one environ-ment or the other. Another potential problem with the L_{eq} measure as reported is the extent to which a single neighborhood or community-level L_{eq} accurately represents noise exposures at individual residences. Noise exposure levels within the noisy and quiet com-munity groups were unlikely to have been uniform across households, and thus within-group variability could be masking more and/or stronger effects than those reported. One way to ad-dress this concern is to densely monitor overflight noise, either on a residence-by-residence basis or by using a noise-and-number index (NNI; Tarnopolsky, Watkins, & Hand 1980) to establish contour lines around a point source for noise pollution, such as an airport. More densely recorded noise exposure levels could then be used to de-velop dose–response curves for noise exposure and each of the dependent variables. The added information that multiple exposure levels would yield is critically important in those situations where nonmonotonic dose–response (or time–response) relationships are suspected (Miller 1985), as has been suggested for children chronically exposed to environmental noise (Cohen et al. 1980b).[5] Figure 1 sug-gests how pairwise comparisons among groups exposed to different noise levels can be misleading when the dose–response relationship is nonmonotonic. For instance, the lower SBP reactivity for the high-noise group in the Evans et al. (1995) study could emerge from the relationship de-picted in Figure 1 if groups exposed to noise levels 1 and 2 were compared, but no difference would have emerged if slightly higher noise levels had been found for the noisy neighborhoods (level 1 and 3 comparison), and *greater* SBP reactivity would have been observed with still higher noise levels (any level compared with level 4).

Evans et al. (1998) capitalized on the construction of a new airport outside Munich to collect prospective data on the effects of overflight noise in a study that illustrates the importance of collecting multiple data points over time (to properly characterize environmental exposures) as well as some of the difficulties in interpreting field studies. Resting SBP and overnight catecholamine levels of noise-exposed children showed greater increases over two years (spanning 6 months prior to and 18 months after the airport open-ing) than those of children from quiet communities. It is important to note that quality-of-life indicators that were initially at odds with the physiological data (*increasing* for the noise-exposed children in the first 6 months after open-ing) ultimately showed a sharp decline among the noise-

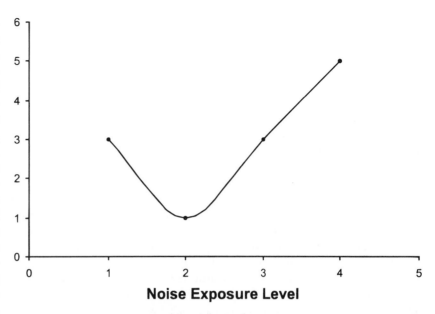

Figure 1. Illustration of a potential nonmonotonic dose–response re-lationship between noise and cardiovascular responding. Pairwise comparison between groups exposed to any two noise levels can be misleading.

exposed children relative to the quality of life reported for those in quiet communities. However, attribution of these effects to overflight noise alone was not possible because of the concomitant increases in road traffic, land develop-ment, and other sociophysical environmental changes that accompanied the new airport. Even so, when considered in light of the laboratory and cross-sectional field research reviewed previously, these complementary prospective data represent a significant contribution to the mounting evi-dence for deleterious effects of chronic noise exposure.

We turn now from our examination of this quintessen-tial environmental stressor to a review of more positively toned transactions with the physical environment: those that are thought to reduce psychological stress.

Restorative Environments

If we analyze the operation of scenes of beauty upon the mind, and consider the intimate relation of the mind upon the nervous system and the whole physical economy, the ac-tion and reaction which constantly occur between bodily and mental conditions, the reinvigoration which results from such scenes is readily comprehended.

[T]he enjoyment of scenery employs the mind without fatigue and yet exercises it; tranquilizes it and yet enlivens it; and thus, through the influence of the mind over the body, gives the effect of refreshing rest and reinvigoration to the whole system. (F. L. Olmsted, 1865)

Frederick Law Olmsted was instrumental in the inception of urban parks throughout the United States in the period

1857–96 (Fein 1972), most notably Central Park in New York. Moreover, according to one biographer, Olmsted articulated "a philosophic base for the creation of state and national parks" in a report on the Yosemite Valley area, the first public lands in the United States to be set aside by Congress as a scenic reserve (see Olmsted 1865/1952, p. 13). Olmsted's professional activities built on an appreciation of the psychological demands of urban life and anticipated current views on biopsychosocial mechanisms mediating environmental effects on health (see also Olmsted 1870).

With related interests in environmental design and management applications in the service of health promotion, a small but growing number of environment–behavior researchers have over recent decades been casting light onto Olmsted's early notions. This work has joined inquiry related to stress with research on psychologically beneficial experiences in natural environments (Hartig 1993; Parsons 1991a). Studies of noise and other stressors, such as crowding and commuting (e.g. Baum & Paulus 1987; Evans & Cohen 1987; Singer, Lundberg, & Frankenhaeuser 1978), have been concerned with correcting deleterious conditions in those places where people and their activities are concentrated. Together with psychological analyses of urban life (Milgram 1970), they point to reasons why urban settings might hinder recovery from or exacerbate the effects of role and task demands faced in one's work and home environments. Through discussions of the effects of overload and chronically elevated arousal, the stress literature informs us about sociophysical environmental conditions that prompt a need for restoration.

Instead of specifying deleterious environmental conditions that might be corrected, restoration research has provided a basis for efforts to protect and promote psychologically positive values of natural environments that would otherwise be lost to urbanization and resource-intensive land management practices (Hartig & Evans 1993; Pitt & Zube 1987; Saegert 1976). The study of restorative environments has its roots in several areas concerned with nature experience. Surveys of outdoor recreationists have consistently shown that stress reduction is a desired benefit motivating visits to natural areas (Knopf 1983). Aside from stress reduction, various other personal, interpersonal, and social benefits have been identified in studies of wilderness users and evaluations of various outdoor programs (Driver, Nash, & Haas 1987; Kaplan & Kaplan 1989; Knopf 1987). In addition, environmental evaluation research has revealed the properties of scenes that contribute to visual preferences and aesthetic responding (Daniel & Vining 1983; Kaplan & Kaplan 1989; Ulrich 1983). Studies in this area have consistently documented a preference for scenes dominated by natural elements such as vegetation and water (Hartig 1993; Knopf 1987).

In specifying negative conditions that lead people to seek recovery, restorative environments theories have incorporated or reacted to environmental stress research. Much of the theory and research on environmental stressors, however, presumes that recovery from a stressor takes place in its absence. Although this is a reasonable assumption, it is likely that a more complex state of affairs awaits further consideration (Hartig et al. 1996). This is not to say that studies of recovery are absent in the stress literature; they are present in various forms, including those studies that focus on the importance of individual differences, variability in social situations, and task characteristics of stressors. For example, psychophysiological stress recovery has been treated as an interindividual difference variable related to personality dimensions such as neuroticism (Johansson & Frankenhaeuser 1973), and it has been used to understand the relationship between stress and ill health (Gannon et al. 1989; O'Brien, Haynes, & Mumby 1998; see review by Haynes et al. 1991). There is evidence as well that the rate of recovery or "unwinding" following stress may be affected by one's sensitivity to hassles on the job (Johansson et al. 1996). Associations between the character of tasks giving rise to psychophysiological stress and the time course of subsequent recovery also have been documented, both in laboratory experimentation (Lundberg et al. 1993) and in occupational studies (Melin & Lundberg 1997). In short, recovery has been recognized by some as a variable that, like reactivity, reflects individual differences, situational parameters, and characteristics of stressors. As such, it can contribute to the explanation of stress-related health outcomes (see also Turner 1994). Yet the positive, recovery-promoting qualities of sociophysical environments (i.e., rather than the mere absence of particular stressors) have largely been neglected in the stress literature.

In the following we briefly overview two theories that have guided research on restorative environments. Although these theories are products of inquiry into the experience of natural environments, their applicability extends beyond such experiences to those of human environments more generally. We then selectively review studies that have a bearing on restorative environments theories. Among these are some studies not concerned with restorative environments per se but which nonetheless inform us about the restorative valences of environments. We close this section with a discussion of how psychophysiological methods and constructs may be used to help clarify pertinent conceptual issues in the study of environmental restoration.

RESTORATIVE ENVIRONMENTS THEORY

A cognitive theory concerned with recovery from directed attention fatigue (e.g. Kaplan & Kaplan 1989) and a theory focused on psychophysiological stress recovery (e.g. Ulrich 1983) provide conceptual tools for better understanding restoration and restorative environments. Both theories posit an evolutionary adaptiveness for environmental evaluation and restoration, and both build on assumptions about the adaptiveness of human psychological and physiological response capabilities to conditions that were likely to have held in natural environments of pre-urban history. These assumptions support statements about the relative restorative potentials of natural and contemporary built environments. A number of differences between the theories stem from their specifications of the negative antecedent conditions from which people will be restored and the mechanisms for their restoration. The stress recovery approach emphasizes variables associated with emotional and psychophysiological restoration from stress, which is conceived of as a process of responding to a situation that challenges or threatens well-being (Ulrich et al. 1991). Among the corollaries of stress specified are self-reports of negative emotions and short-term changes in physiological systems (i.e., cardiovascular, neuroendocrine, musculoskeletal) indicative of heightened arousal and negative affect (Ulrich et al. 1991; see also Parsons 1991a).

According to this theory, restoration from stress is one of several potential affectively oriented and aesthetically mediated consequences of passive visual encounters with environments (Ulrich 1983). The experience of visually pleasant physical surroundings is thought to reduce stress by eliciting positive emotions, sustaining nonvigilant attention, restricting negative thoughts, and returning physiological arousal to more moderate levels (see also Ulrich et al. 1991). Such aesthetic and restorative responding is thought to be evoked by qualities of the visual stimulus array such as moderate depth, moderate complexity, the presence of a focal point, and the presence of natural contents such as vegetation or water. In specifying collative properties such as complexity, the theory's emphasis on stress-related affect and arousal constructs in characterizing antecedent conditions is complemented by an acknowledgment of the importance of cognitively oriented assessments in restorative person–environment transactions. This latter acknowledgment is largely derived from Berlyne's (1960, 1971) work on experimental aesthetics (see Ulrich 1981, 1983). Perceptual evaluations leading to restoration are assumed to occur very rapidly, and empirical investigations based on this theory have emphasized methods that assess relatively short-term emotional and physiological changes, though implications have been examined for more slowly developing outcomes such as the postoperative use of strong painkillers (Ulrich 1984). The emphasis on short-term change in this work is also premised on the understanding that many encounters with aesthetic (natural) environments are brief and are made in passing.

"Attention restoration" theorists (e.g. Kaplan 1995) have emphasized the negative consequences of directed attention fatigue – especially its effects on human performance. Directed attention fatigue is thought to stem from depletion of a central inhibitory capacity. This capacity is depleted in the effort to exclude stimuli that compete for attention with a focal undertaking. When this capacity is overdrawn, the resultant fatigue may manifest in irritability and other negative affects, inability to plan, diminished helping behavior, failure to recognize interpersonal cues, and increased likelihood of error in performance.

A cognitive mechanism thought to support recovery from directed attention fatigue was discerned in William James's (1892) description of involuntary attention, which refers to attention driven by interest rather than force of will (Kaplan 1978; Kaplan & Kaplan 1982). This form of attention, renamed *fascination,* is assumed to be effortless and without capacity limitations. It can be engaged by objects and events as well as by exploring and making sense of some physical or conceptual environment. If a given situation permits reliance on fascination then directed attention can be rested, and one's limited supply of this cognitive resource can be replenished. Though fascination is necessary to restore directed attention, it is not sufficient. Three other factors that may characterize person–environment transactions are central to attention restoration theory: being away from usual routines and goals that lack interest; the coherence and scope perceived in a potentially restorative environment; and compatibility among one's behavioral inclinations, limitations, and opportunities for action in the environment (Kaplan 1983). To the extent that these factors operate, restoration can take place. Over extended periods, the restorative process may encourage reflection – an activity with a variety of proactive implications, such as changes in life perspectives (Kaplan & Talbot 1983) and adherence to medical treatment regimens (Cimprich 1993).

As these synopses indicate, attention restoration theory emphasizes cognitive aspects of restorative experience and does not attempt to account for possible psychophysiological restoration. Conversely, stress restoration theory emphasizes affective and arousal components of restoration but considers less fully the potential cognitive antecedents and sequelae of restorative experiences. Despite this difference in emphasis, there is considerable conceptual overlap between these accounts of restoration, and it is appropriate to ask how psychophysiological constructs and methods might be used to clarify distinctions between these theoretical positions (cf. Hartig & Evans 1993). Before exploring this point in a discussion of conceptual issues, we selectively review empirical work pertinent to these theories.

EMPIRICAL RESEARCH ON RESTORATIVE ENVIRONMENTS

There is a small but growing body of evidence that differences in sociophysical environments are reflected in patterns of psychophysiological stress recovery. Of particular interest here are studies in which there was both (1) an initial stress induction manipulation or an assessment of naturalistically occurring stress, providing the opportunity to assess recovery, and (2) between-subjects variation in sociophysical aspects of the environment subsequently available for recovery.

In an initial test of the nature restoration hypothesis, students who had just completed a stressful course examination provided emotion self-reports before and after experiencing an 18-min photographic simulation of outdoor environments (Ulrich 1979). Those participants who viewed slides of natural scenes showed declines in sadness and anger and an increase in positive affects from pre- to posttest, whereas the opposite pattern held for participants who viewed urban slides. However, psychophysiological methods were not used to assess the expected change in arousal. In a subsequent study (Ulrich et al. 1991), the relative effects of natural and urban visual environments on recovery were examined for participants who viewed a stressful industrial accident film followed by a 10-min videotape of nature, urban traffic, or an outdoor pedestrian mall setting. Poststressor recovery trajectories for continuously monitored frontalis muscle tension (via EMG), skin conductance (SC), and pulse transit time (PTT) differed as a function of the environment viewed, with nature scenes promoting the fastest returns toward baseline and the lowest overall levels. Skin conductance responses declined most quickly, with the nature scenes eliciting greater decline in spontaneous fluctuations within the first 4 min of viewing. The natural and urban videos showed divergent levels of PTT and EMG within 5–7 min of viewing. Stressor offset to postenvironment changes in self-reported fear, anger/aggression, and positive affect echoed those seen in the 1979 study and also implicated the greater restorative potency of the nature videos.

Several conceptual replications of the Ulrich et al. (1991) research have appeared in both laboratory and field studies. As with Ulrich et al. (1991), Parsons (1991b) showed participants brief videotaped stressors followed by videotaped natural and urban environments while psychological and physiological indicators of arousal and emotion were monitored. Apart from their natural versus urban character, the environments also differed with respect to the presence or absence of water (i.e., a river). A distinction between water and nonwater environments is consistent with theoretically predicted and empirically verified findings in environmental preference research showing water to be a very powerful variable, often accounting for most of the explained variance when used as a predictor (Dearinger 1979; Pomeroy, Fitzgibbon, & Green 1989; Shafer, Hamilton, & Schmidt 1969; Zube, Pitt, & Anderson 1975). Evidence from autonomic arousal measures (SC and respiration rate) indicated that the nature-dominated environments and those with water facilitated recovery to a greater extent than either the urban or nonwater environments. Facial EMG measures indicative of negative affective responding (corrugator supercilii and medial frontalis placements) suggested that a nonwater natural environment (i.e., a meadow) was less likely to elicit negative emotions than were the other environments. One notable implication of these findings was that sufficiently pleasant urban surroundings (e.g., interesting architecture and a water feature) can have restorative effects similar to those reported for nature-dominated environments. Recently, Parsons and colleagues (1998) used video simulations of drives through areas with different roadside environments to test the hypothesis that a nature-dominated drive will facilitate quicker and more complete recovery from stress. Stress was induced with either a 10-min industrial accident film (passive stressor) or mental arithmetic (active stressor) immediately prior to a 10-min video of a drive through predominantly forested or rural areas, urban settings, residential areas with golf courses, or mixed residential and commercial areas. A second stressor was presented after the environment video to test the hypothesis that environments might not only facilitate recovery but also ameliorate the negative consequences of a future stressor. Facial muscle activity, heart rate, blood pressure, electro-oculograms, and skin conductance were monitored continuously to assess autonomic and somatic activity. The findings indicated that, relative to transactions with urban roadsides, even superficial transactions with nature-dominated roadside environments (the drive videos primarily depicted the road ahead) were sufficient to positively impact sympathetic arousal in both recovery and immunization contexts.

Hartig and his colleagues (submitted; see also Hartig 1993) have examined these same issues in multiple field settings, most recently using ambulatory blood pressure monitoring. In this experiment, young adults were seated in a windowless room or in a room with a view out onto trees for ten minutes. Just prior to the 10-min period with or without a window view, half of the participants in each condition had completed 60 min of rapid-paced, attentionally demanding tasks (Stroop, binary classification) intended to be both stressful and attentionally fatiguing. The remaining participants had just completed a drive to the field site. During the post-stressor period with or without window views, linear DBP recovery trajectories were steeper for those with the window view. After the initial ten minutes poststressor, the participants walked for 50 min in either a nature reserve or an area of medium-density urban development. Ambulatory blood pressure readings obtained at regular intervals during the walk also indicated a stronger stress dampening effect of the contact with nature (Hartig et al. submitted), with the mean SBP trajectory of the nature participants declining during the initial 20 min in contrast to the rise seen in the mean trajectory of urban participants. In an earlier field experiment, Hartig, Mang, and Evans (1991) found that participants who walked in a regional wilderness park after 40 min of fast-paced, attentionally demanding tasks (Stroop, binary classification) had higher posttest levels of self-reported positive affect, less anger and aggression, and better proofreading performance than those who either walked in an urban area or sat in a laboratory reading magazines and listening to music. However, there were no differences in postwalk BP or heart rate, which might be due to the time required to reinstrument the participants after the walk. In contrast, using the ambulatory measurement protocol, Hartig et al. (submitted) did find that posttest DBP was, relative to baseline, lower after the walk in the nature reserve as compared to the urban area. In both of the field studies, research assistants led the subjects at a slow pace (saunter) along pre-established routes on gentle terrain, so the different outcomes cannot be attributed to differences in physical exertion.

Other studies that have not been explicitly concerned with restorative environments nonetheless inform us about the restorative valences of different environments or the utility of the theories overviewed here. A report by Fredrickson and Levenson (1998) is informative in both senses. Noting that positive emotions have presented problems to theories of emotion that have been oriented toward associating specific action tendencies with given emotions, Fredrickson and Levenson propose that, rather than initiating specific actions, one function of positive emotions may be to "undo" elevated autonomic arousal brought on by negative emotions. They suggest that "the positive emotions of contentment and amusement act in the service of homeostasis, restoring quiescence; as such, a switch from a negative emotion to one of these positive emotions may in effect rid individuals of the psychological and physiological sequelae of action readiness, allowing them to pursue a wider variety of actions or experiences" (p. 193). In essence, their "undoing hypothesis" view of the recovery process is similar to Ulrich's (1983), but without specific reference to aesthetic environments as a source of positive emotions.

Fredrickson and Levenson (1998, study 1) do, however, report results that bear on the restorative power of a natural environment. Participants who viewed a brief (83-sec) film clip of a man in danger of falling from a ledge were randomly assigned to one of four 100-sec secondary film conditions. The secondary films were intended to induce a predominating sense of contentment (waves breaking on a beach), amusement (a puppy playing with a flower), sadness (a boy crying as he watches his father die), or a more neutral state (a growing pile of colored sticks). Participants provided real-time ratings of positive–negative affectivity and measures of heart period (HP), finger pulse amplitude (FPA), and pulse transmission time to both an ear (PTE) and a finger (PTF). The recovery index used was *reactivity duration*, which was defined as "the time elapsed after the offset of the initial fear film until cardiovascular levels returned to within an individual's own confidence interval and remained within this confidence interval for at least five of six consecutive seconds" (p. 200). As hypothesized, duration of reactivity to the fear film varied as a function of the secondary film valence. The shortest mean dura-

tion – and so fastest recovery – was seen for participants who watched the positively toned films. For each of these, reactivity duration was significantly shorter ($\sim$ 20 sec) than that observed for the neutral ($\sim$ 40 sec) and sad ($\sim$ 60 sec) films. The contentment (breaking waves) and amusement (puppy) films produced similarly speedy recovery.

The study by Fredrickson and Levenson (1998) is interesting for several reasons. Aside from independent substantiation of an affective mechanism that works to accelerate recovery from psychophysiological stress, it provides a bit of additional evidence that the passive visual experience of a physical environment (i.e., a beach with breaking waves) can facilitate cardiovascular recovery following an emotionally negative antecedent. It also documents comparably accelerated cardiovascular recovery with a simulation that encompasses a large-scale environment and one that focuses on relatively small, discrete aspects of an environment (puppy and flower). Manipulations in experimental research on restorative environments have involved large-scale environments, natural and urban in particular, though it is understood that attention will often be engaged by discrete features of those environments. Further, the study shows cardiovascular recovery differentials emerging within a much briefer period than those reported in previous studies explicitly concerned with rapid environmental facilitation of stress recovery; compare the $\sim$ 20-sec recovery period recorded by Fredrickson and Levenson with the 5–7 min documented by Ulrich et al. (1991) for PTT and the 10-min period of Hartig et al. (submitted) for BP. This finding should aid efforts to estimate the temporal parameters of restoration along the given recovery dimensions represented in Fredrickson and Levenson's aggregate reactivity duration index.

Final mention here goes to a study by Frankenhaeuser et al. (1989), which reminds us that under naturalistic circumstances the restorativeness of an environment may be contingent upon individual and situational characteristics. In a study of the effects of gender and occupational status on stress and "unwinding" in white-collar workers, Frankenhaeuser et al. reported that women in managerial positions had greater conflict between demands from their paid job and demands from other duties than did male managers and both female and male clerical workers. The female managers also had higher competitiveness scores, which were derived from a structured interview assessing type-A behavior pattern. Further, the female managers had masculinity scores as high as those of male managers and clerical workers *and* femininity scores as high as those of the female clerical workers. Finally, the after-work SBP and epinephrine levels of the female managers distinguished them from their male counterparts as well, with the former measure remaining elevated after work and the latter increasing. The characterization that emerges from these data is one of the female managers struggling to resolve conflicts between work and family life.

These are select results from a large set of cardiovascular, neuroendocrine, and self-report measures obtained during and after work. It is noteworthy that "after work" did in fact mean "at home," which was expected to be a place where women and men alike could unwind. Indeed, the pattern of measures obtained at home on a work-free day indicate lower arousal, greater relaxation, and more positive mood (although here too the female managers distinguish themselves with relatively high norepinephrine levels). However, the results regarding unwinding in the home after work suggest that the restorative potential of the home, which many would implicitly assume is substantial, varies as a function of situational conditions and individual differences (see also Frankenhaeuser 1991). These results encourage consideration of cultural expectations regarding the circumstances under which people might seek and find restoration. The home was the primary workplace for most women not so long ago, and the responsibility for housework and child rearing still is borne mainly by women. In the case of the female managers, Frankenhaeuser et al.'s (1989) findings highlight the role of individual, situational, and sociocultural factors as additional determinants of the restorativeness of a given place at a given time.

CONCEPTUAL AND METHODOLOGICAL ISSUES

There are a number of interrelated conceptual and methodological issues in the foregoing overview of theory and research, some of which we briefly sketch here. We start by considering whether a distinction can be made between stress recovery and directed attention restoration, an issue with implications for choices regarding the selection, frequency, and timing of measures in studies of environmental restorativeness. As we suggested earlier, there is a fair degree of conceptual overlap between these models. Ulrich et al. (1991), for instance, suggested that the directed attention fatigue (DAF) construct can be accommodated by such existing models of environmental stress as information overload (e.g. Cohen 1978; Cohen & Spacapan 1978). Kaplan and Kaplan (1982), however, maintain that DAF can be experienced independently of stressful conditions, and that consequently it represents a distinct psychological state. Though several operationalizations of DAF have appeared in the literature (e.g. Cimprich 1993; Hartig et al. submitted), they have not been adequately distinguished from stress manipulations (Kaplan 1995), so the construct validity of DAF has yet to be empirically verified. As we have described, psychophysiological constructs and methods have been central to the development of the stress recovery model and only incidental to the directed attention restoration model. However, we see an opportunity for these psychophysiological tools to help determine the relative utility of DAF as a construct and, by extension, the ultimate heuristic value of distinguishing between stress

recovery and directed attention restoration (cf. Hartig & Evans 1993).

As an example, consider the problem of determining whether DAF can be experienced independently of stress. Directed attention fatigue is thought to occur through prolonged bouts of focal attention, and it has been operationalized in terms of performance on tasks that require vigilance. The experience of stress is typically described as resulting from a perception of threat or harm, and it is often operationalized in terms of autonomic reactivity, such as changes in blood pressure, skin conductance, and so forth. Thus, to determine whether procedures thought to produce DAF were also stressful, we might monitor a measure such as skin conductance during administration of vigilance tasks. This approach is problematic, however, to the extent that our measure of stress is also responsive to manipulations of attention, which is the case for many autonomic measures, including skin conductance (Strube 1990, p. 49). Clearly what is needed is a pair of measures, one that indexes stress but is relatively nonresponsive to focal attention, and one that indexes focal attention but is relatively nonresponsive to stress. Tasks that lead to increases in the latter and quiescence (or decreases) in the former would be likely candidates for DAF procedures.

Though we are not aware of ideal measures that uniquely index stress and focal attention, psychophysiological measures that might be used to assess the suitability of DAF tasks can be found among the growing number of components identified in event-related brain potentials (ERPs). Over the last 30 years, extensive evidence in the psychophysiological literature has established that the amplitude of negative ERPs occurring 100–150 msec (N100) after a target stimulus is related to selective attention (see Coles, Gratton, & Fabiani 1990 for a review). Attended stimuli elicit larger (more negative) N100s relative to nonattended stimuli. Because the onset latency of a variant of the N100, *processing negativity*, has been associated with the allocation of attentional resources (see Coles et al. 1990; Hansen & Hillyard 1983), this class of ERP may well be useful in tracking deteriorating attentional capacity – DAF. A more recently identified ERP component, the P50 (positive deflection, ~ 50-msec peak latency) has been shown to be insensitive to changes in directed attention under certain circumstances, yet it is influenced by stress manipulations (White & Yee 1997). Thus, examination of these ERP components during the performance of tasks that putatively require directed attention yet are thought to be nonstressful may help to determine the construct validity of DAF and, more broadly, the relative utility of a distinction between the stress recovery and directed attention restoration models of environmental restorativeness.

A set of issues related to the conceptualization of DAF (i.e., its stressful versus nonstressful character) concern operationalizations of restoration, which have been inadequately addressed in the literature on restorative environments. Restoration has not been consistently defined in the environmental literature, nor has recovery been consistently defined in the stress recovery literature. Haynes et al. (1991) defined recovery from stress as "changes in stressor-induced responses following stressor termination" (p. 356). This broad definition incorporates both nonlinear and bidirectional changes in variables following stressor offset, allowing for "recovery" that does not necessarily reflect a return to prestressor response levels. In particular, however, if the word "stimulus" is used in place of "stressor" in this definition, then the simple notion of "changes following stimulus offset" is broad enough to capture the presumed depletion–replenishment cycle of DAF and restored attentional capacity as well as the experience of stress and the return to autonomic equanimity. "Stress recovery" would no longer be appropriate for the term being defined, though "restoration" is suitable, as it could be applied both to the replenishment of a capacity and to the return to physiological homeostasis.

Under this conceptualization, then, if restoration can involve the replenishment of a capacity, then the operationalization of restoration does not necessarily imply the measurement of autonomic (and other) stress-related variables. For instance, just as the N100 ERP component may prove useful in determining the construct validity of DAF, the onset latency of processing negativity also may be useful in assessing the restoration of directed attentional capacity. The onset latency of processing negativity increases as the difficulty in discriminating between attended and unattended channels increases. Presumably, the difficulty of a given attentional discrimination is related to the available directed attentional capacity; as this capacity is depleted, attentional discriminations become more difficult. Thus, the onset latency of processing negativity might be expected to increase as directed attentional capacity is depleted – that is, as DAF increases, discriminations among attended and unattended channels should be more difficult. Conversely, as directed attentional capacity is restored, the onset latency of processing negativity might be expected to decrease, as attentional discriminations should become easier.

Even if DAF is eventually resolved to be a stressful psychological state, it may still be useful to distinguish it from other stressors – in part because of the complex nature of physiological mechanisms that underlie stress responses and stress recovery. As typically conceived (Kaplan 1995) and induced (Hartig et al. submitted), DAF unfolds over a protracted period of focused cognitive activity. The slowly developing nature of DAF has direct implications for the stress-related physiological mechanisms that may be engaged by this psychological state and, ultimately, for any health-related consequences that may be inferred (which has been a prime concern in the restorative environments literature; see Parsons 1991a). As Haynes et al. (1991) noted, the duration of a stressor has important influences on patterns of physiological responding. Relatively brief, acute stressors (such as the math tasks, extemporaneous speeches, and iced appendages that abound in the stress literature) engage the sympathetic adrenomedullary system, which quickly leads to increased levels of immune activity and circulating epinephrine and norepinephrine. More long-lived stressors engage the hypothalamic-pituitary-adrenocortical system, leading to the release of cortisol and its attendant immunosuppressive effects. Thus, the physiological parameters that may be useful in assessing DAF and the associated restoration of directed attention (ERPs, corticosteroids, and immunocompetence) differ from the primarily cardiovascular and sympathetically mediated (e.g. SCR) measures that have characterized empirical investigations of the stress recovery model of environmental restorativeness.

To close this section, we mention in passing several methodological issues related to environmental sampling and representativeness that have also been inadequately addressed in this relatively young field. Environmental psychologists have often been concerned with the representativeness of the environments under study. For our purposes here, this concern refers not only to the sampling of environments across the effective range of the physical variables of interest but also to the restorative implications of sociophysical changes in environments over time, as suggested by the Frankenhaeuser et al. (1989) study described ealier. In the empirical examinations of restorative environments thus far, environmental classes such as "natural" or "urban" have too often been represented by very small numbers of exemplars, leaving the interpretation of results open to attributions to particular environmental instantiations rather than to the environmental classes or variables of interest. Although this particular problem in environmental sampling can be easily resolved (at least conceptually), others are less tractable, such as the selection of appropriate comparison or "control" conditions. Because people are never encountered outside of an environment, the concept of a "no-environment" control condition has no meaning (see Fredrickson & Levenson 1998). Finally, we raise the difficult issue of the ecological validity of environmental surrogates. Psychophysiological research on environmental restorativeness is more conveniently conducted in the laboratory than in the field, and thus a reliance on environmental surrogates is a primary concern. If the restorative qualities of environments can be adequately represented visually, then high-quality photography and videography may well produce adequate surrogates. However, to the extent that the environmental qualities of interest (restorative or otherwise) are not well represented by visually oriented technologies, then the adequacy of environmental surrogates is called into question. This issue, in the guise of adequately represented movement through space, receives more careful consideration in the following section.

Topographic Cognition

Don't know where I am and got no mother to guide me home. (Chariton 1990, p. 141)

One can define spatial cognition broadly as any aspect of an organism's behavior that involves space and is informed by cerebral activity (Kritchevsky 1988). Topographic cognition refers to a subset of these behaviors wherein cerebral activity guides an organism's movement through the molar environment. For purposes of this discussion, and as is typically conceived in studies of topographic cognition (e.g. Aguirre, Zarahn, & D'Esposito 1998; Allen 1985; Kuipers 1982; Maguire 1997), the molar environment is large in scale and/or visually occluded so that it cannot be completely perceived from a single vantage point. Thus, walking a maze in a laboratory room, navigating a building, or exploring a city all constitute transactions with molar environments that engage topographic cognition.

Though we do it every day, mostly without thinking about it, finding our way through the world is both a critically important and quite complex behavior. Common animal behaviors that are crucial to survival – such as gathering food, finding mates or shelter, hunting prey, avoiding predators, and cacheing of young – all depend on an organism's ability to understand and navigate its physical surroundings (Spencer, Blades, & Morsley 1989). Although few of us still rely on our hunting skills for survival, case study evidence from clinical neuropsychology suggests that topographic disorientation can nevertheless be quite devastating (Cammalleri et al. 1996; Habib & Sirigu 1987; Landis et al. 1986; Whiteley & Warrington 1978). Wayfinding is a complex behavior as well; it requires the coordination of spatial perception, memory, and attention, and it often involves dynamic spatial processes, such as mental rotation and the construction of spatial imagery (Kritchevsky 1988). In the last section of this chapter, we examine the contributions that psychophysiology can make to our understanding of these processes. We briefly review historical and recent work in clinical neuropsychology, psychobiology, and cognitive psychology that suggests the importance of multimodal integration of perceptual information for topographic cognition. We then highlight some very interesting work that exploits recent advances in functional brain imaging techniques to investigate wayfinding. The reliance on transactions with environmental surrogates in this research prompts a discussion of how representations of large-scale environments can be assessed in psychophysiology, which is still largely a laboratory science.

ORIGINS AND RECENT RESEARCH ON TOPOGRAPHIC COGNITION

The origins of our current understanding of topographic cognition can be traced to fin de siécle Europe, when clinical reports of spatial disorders associated with topographic disorientation began appearing in the medical literature. There were reports of impaired wayfinding in familiar environments (Badal 1888/1982; Jackson 1876/1958) and inability to recognize familiar places (Meyer 1900/1996) as well as reports of retained spatial knowledge accompanied by the inability to apply it (Wilbrand 1892/1982). Although most researchers during this period distinguished these spatial deficits from more common aphasias, they typically did not acknowledge a commonality among reports – that many of these problems were associated with posterior lesions in the right hemisphere (Morrow & Ratcliff 1988). In an influential series of papers, Zangwill and his colleagues (Ettlinger, Warrington, & Zangwill 1957; McFie, Piercy, & Zangwill 1950; Paterson & Zangwill 1944, 1945) documented the importance of the posterior right hemisphere for spatial behavior (DeRenzi 1982); in particular, Paterson and Zangwill (1945) identified a key distinction between two visuospatial deficits (topographic agnosia and amnesia) that continues to inform the bulk of latter-day theory and research on topographic cognition. Topographic agnosics have difficulty recognizing familiar buildings and landmarks, while topographic amnesics cannot readily specify routes within or draw maps of familiar territory.

Echoing these neuropsychological findings, complementary strands of research in psychobiology and cognitive and environmental psychology have developed similar distinctions between topographic recognition and memory abilities. Early Hullian stimulus–response accounts of spatial behavior and learning in nonhuman animals have been supplanted by "cognitive mapping" explanations (Tolman 1948), which assume that animals use allocentric[6] representations of the spatial relationships among environmental features to navigate their surroundings (see Allen 1985, 1987; Schacter & Nadel 1991). In particular, work with animals suggests a clear maturational distinction between landmark learning ability (early onset) and map learning ability (later onset; see Schacter & Nadel 1991), and neural localization studies with animals (primarily the rat) have also been important in isolating the hippocampal formation as central to cognitive mapping functions (see O'Keefe & Nadel 1978 for a review and seminal theoretical account of this work). Cognitive and environmental psychologists have devoted much of their research efforts to identifying and understanding types of topographic knowledge. Following Shemyakin's (1962) early theoretical account, researchers have generally identified three types of topographic knowledge: landmark knowledge, route knowledge, and configural or survey knowledge (Allen 1985; Golledge & Stimson 1997; Schacter & Nadel 1991; Siegel & White 1975; Thorndyke 1981). Landmark knowledge confers the ability to recognize previously encountered, distinctive environmental features and to use them as reference points for locomotion through the environment. Route knowledge comprises spatiotemporal relations among sequentially ordered environmental features coordinated with motor actions required to traverse set paths through an environment. And possession of the most complex form of topographic knowledge, configural or survey knowledge, implies the ability to infer spatial relations among multiply interconnected environmental features from an allocentric frame of reference (for variations on these basic definitions, see Allen 1987; Schacter & Nadel 1991; Thorndyke 1981). More colloquially, configural knowledge refers to the possession of a "cognitive" or "mental" map, which allows one to interact flexibly with the environment to recognize short-cuts, generate new routes when existing ones are blocked, judge distance to and direction of occluded elements, and so forth.

Although most researchers acknowledge these three basic types of topographic knowledge and regard both the microgenetic acquisition and the ontogenetic development of landmark, route, and configural knowledge and abilities to be sequential (Allen 1985; Golledge 1987; Siegel & White 1975), the consensus is not absolute (see Golledge & Stimson 1997, chap. 5; Spencer et al. 1989, chap. 1). Some have questioned the evidentiary basis of configural knowledge (e.g. Pick 1993) or suggested that true configural knowledge cannot develop independently of exposure to symbolic representations of the environment (Moeser 1988), and others have questioned the *sequential* microgenetic acquisition of topographic knowledge types (Montello 1998). What these questions suggest is that the simple description of an orderly development of topographic knowledge and abilities is likely overly simple and perhaps wrong in several respects, as others have noted (Magliano et al. 1995; Mandler 1988; Montello 1998; Pick 1993; Spencer et al. 1989). In particular, two distinctions regarding the manner in which topographic information is acquired have important implications for the brain imaging research described in the next section. First, topographic information about the environment can be gained through direct experience with the world or through interaction with symbolic representations of the environment, such as maps or verbal descriptions of routes. Presson and Hazelrigg (1984) labeled the former *primary* and the latter *secondary* spatial learning, and many researchers have found that performance on topographic tasks can depend upon this distinction (Evans & Pezdek 1980; Howard & Kerst 1981; Scholl 1987; Thorndyke & Hayes-Roth 1982). Evans and Pezdek (1980), for example, reported that latencies to judge the accuracy of spatial relations among triads of buildings are linearly related to rotational disparity from typical Cartesian presentation (i.e., $0° =$ north) for students who learned the building locations from a map, though latencies are unrelated to Cartesian coordinates for those who learned the locations in situ.

Second, evidence suggests that a distinction between *passive* and *active* primary spatial learning may be impor-

tant (see Cohen & Cohen 1985 for a review). In general, active engagement with the environment is thought to produce more flexible cognitive maps (Cohen & Cohen 1985; Siegel & White 1975), whereas passive interactions tend to produce orientation-specific representations (e.g. Hintzman, O'Dell, & Arndt 1981). This distinction is supported by both correlational (Acredolo 1988; Appleyard 1970; Beck & Wood 1976; Golledge & Spector 1978) and experimental (Cohen & Weatherford 1980, 1981; Klatzky et al. 1998; Simons & Wang 1998) work, and the importance of active engagement seems not to lie with movement through the environment per se but rather with the opportunity to monitor the environment that movement affords (Acredolo, Adams, & Goodwyn 1984; Böök & Gärling 1980a,b, 1981). Many researchers have suggested that the integration of perceptual information during locomotion is central to maintaining orientation in and constructing representations of environments (Evans & Pezdek 1980; Gärling, Böök, & Lindberg 1985; Montello 1998; Spencer et al. 1989). Although some researchers have emphasized the importance of integrating multiple visual perceptions over time (Heft 1983), others have suggested that periodic attention to retinal flow information in the environment can be used to calibrate orientation estimates gleaned from biomechanical and proprioceptive afferents (Pick 1993).[7] Rieser and his colleagues (1995) showed that the accuracy of biomechanical estimates of distance (i.e., walking to a target with eyes closed) can be manipulated when prior biomechanical and visual feedback regarding rate of travel are mismatched. Rieser et al. (1995) observed similar inaccuracies for orientation judgments after participants experienced a rotational visual–biomechanical discontinuity, and scene recognition also suffers following a change in perspective that disrupts vestibular and proprioceptive feedback (Simons & Wang 1998). These findings suggest that biomechanical actions (and associated kinesthetic afferents) performed during self-locomotion are important sources of information regarding course and distance knowledge, and that the accuracy of this knowledge is periodically updated by the opportunity to integrate visual and nonvisual information sources.

In sum, it seems clear that movement through the environment has the potential to influence the manner in which topographic information is acquired and used. As we shall see next, this has implications for the use of functional brain imaging techniques to study topographic cognition.

TOPOGRAPHIC COGNITION, FUNCTIONAL BRAIN IMAGING, AND VIRTUAL REALITY

To date, researchers have used two functional brain imaging techniques to study topographic cognition in humans: functional magnetic resonance imaging (fMRI) and positron emission tomography (PET). In both techniques, inferences about areas of brain activation are made based on evidence for regional cerebral blood flow (rCBF), in the former provided by magnetic echoes and in the latter by regional concentrations of blood-borne radioisotopes (see Chapter 4). Because of the restrictive nature of brain imaging equipment, research participants' transactions with environments are limited to either recollections of actual environments or perceptions of environmental surrogates, with the latter approach predominating. Environmental surrogates have included videotaped "walk-throughs" (Maguire, Frakowiak, & Frith 1996) and modified versions of commercially available computer games that allow participants to control apparent movement through maze-like or townlike environments (Aguirre & D'Esposito 1997; Aguirre et al. 1996; Maguire et al. 1998a,b). Topographic tasks have included imagined point-to-point (PTP) traversals of previously learned actual environments (Ghaem et al. 1997; Maguire, Frakowiak, & Frith 1997), exploration of novel computer-represented environments (Aguirre et al. 1996; Maguire et al. 1998b), learning of videotaped environments (Maguire et al. 1996), and traversals and directional judgments in previously learned computer environments (Aguirre et al. 1996; Aguirre & D'Esposito 1997; Maguire et al. 1998a). Despite these differences in environmental representations and tasks – as well as differences in specific research questions – the primary focus among investigators using functional brain imaging to study topographic cognition has been to localize neural substrates involved in the learning and retrieval of topographic information. They have found that learning and retrieval of topographic information activate many of the same structures in the medial temporal, posterior parietal, and occipitotemporal regions, including the hippocampus, parahippocampus, posterior cingulate (retrosplenial) cortex, fusiform and lingual gyri, precuneus, and the inferior and superior parietal lobules (see summary in Table 2).

In particular, activations of the hippocampus, parahippocampus, posterior cingulate, and precuneus have consistently been associated with more complex topographic tasks, including those putatively requiring allocentric representations of the environment. Activation of these structures for complex topographic behavior is consistent with animal models of navigation, which suggest that egocentric (head- and body-centered) reference coordinates (based in part on externally acquired landmark information) are integrated with an internally generated sense of direction (based on vestibular, proprioceptive, and motor afferents) to produce allocentric reference coordinates used to navigate complex environments (McNaughton, Knierim, & Wilson 1995; Taube et al. 1996). Evidence suggests that posterior parietal regions, including the precuneus, are important for generating egocentric coordinates (Anderson et al. 1993), whereas several models have focused on the hippocampal formation for processing of idiothetic (internally generated) heading information used to produce allocentric coordinates (Burgess, Recce, & O'Keefe 1994;

McNaughton, Chen, & Markus 1991). The contribution of the posterior cingulate to this process has been represented as the starting point for the transformation of coordinates from egocentric to allocentric (Vogt, Finch, & Olson 1992) or, alternatively, as processing parietal coordinate information to update idiothetic position signals, which tend to drift independent of external verification (McNaughton et al. 1991, 1995).

This broad consistency between structures implicated in topographic cognition of intact humans with those structures being delineated as integral to navigational neural circuits in animals is encouraging. However, several important caveats must be raised regarding interpretation of the brain imaging work, and these caveats in turn have important implications for the ulimate utility of brain imaging methods for the study of human topographic cognition. We will briefly mention three issues that are common inferential concerns in functional brain imaging research, regardless of the psychological phenomena of interest; we will then concentrate on a fourth issue that has specific import for those studying topographic cognition. First, with respect to fMRIs and PET scans, there are issues associated with the functional significance of neural activation inferred from rCBF. Although increased blood flow to a particular region may be associated with increased neural activity, the functional significance of that activity is difficult to determine in the absence of any information regarding the specific nature (e.g., excitatory vs. inhibitory) or patterns of neuronal firing (for discussion of similar concerns, see Posner & Raichle 1994; Sarter, Berntson, & Cacioppo 1996).

Second, though recent advances in brain imaging techniques have dramatically improved the spatial resolution of both PET and fMRI scans, the temporal resolution of these techniques is still rather limited (Brodal 1998). In the brain imaging work outlined here, data from brain scans during the performance of topographic tasks were integrated over anywhere from 45 sec to 90 sec, a long period of time during which participants may engage in both task-focused and off-task processing. Researchers may assume that off-task processing is randomly distributed among experimental conditions, though it is not clear how one could convincingly test this assumption. But when cerebral localization of cognitive functioning is the primary purpose of the research, attempts should be made to limit the likelihood of off-task processing. Participants may also engage in unexpected task-focused processing, which may also limit the attribution of functional significance to particular brain regions when data from rCBF are intergrated over long epochs. Aguirre and D'Esposito (1997), for example, trained participants to a 90% accuracy criterion for topographic knowledge of a computer-simulated town; subjects were then given prescanning practice on two tasks that putatively discriminated landmark cognitive processing from survey (allocentric) cognitive processing. Note that these

TABLE 2. Summary of Reviewed Neuroimaging Studies

Study	Subject Gender (F/M)	Scan Technique	Encoding Stimuli	Retrieval Task	Control Task(s)	Observed Activations
Maguire et al. 1996	0/8	PET	2 videotaped walks (scanned during 2nd walk)	N/A	1. Stationary video 2. Random colors	*ES–CT1* R – hippocampus B – parahippocampus – precuneus
Aguirre et al. 1996	0/9	fMRI	VR maze (Wolf 3D), with 3 intersections, 5 cul-de-sacs, and 2–4 learning trials (scanned)	PTP navigation	Movement through looping VR corridor	*ES–CT (Ret–CT same)* B – posterior parietal B – posterior cingulate B – lingual gyrus B – parahippocampus
Aguirre & D'Esposito 1997	1/3	fMRI	VR town (Marathon2), with 16 places, 4×4 grid, and 2–3 hr training	1. ID place image 2. PTP navigation	Scrambled VR pixels, nonsense labels	*Ret1–Ret2* R – fusiform gyrus R – parahippocampus L – lingual gyrus R – occip./mid-occip. gyri *Ret2–Ret1* R – inf. parietal lobule L – precuneus L – sup. parietal lobule L – sup. frontal gyrus L – premotor cortex
Ghaem et al. 1997	0/5	PET	800-m suburban walk, actual environment, 3 trials	1. Mental route simulation 2. Imagine landmarks	Rest	*Ret1–Ret2* L – med. hippocampal region L – precuneus L – insula
Maguire et al. 1997	0/11		Experienced London taxi drivers	1. PTP route descrip. 2. Landmark descrip. 3. Retell film plots 4. Describe film frames	Number repetition	*Ret1–Ret2* – medial parietal cortex – posterior cingulate R – hippocampus
Maguire et al. 1998a	0/10	PET	VR town (DukeNukem 3D), with 4 streets, buildings, shops, and access to rooms in buildings	1. PTP navigation 2. PTP navigation and detours 3. Route following	Static scenes from town	*(Ret1 & Ret2)–Ret3* R – hippocampus L – occipital cortex L – sup. frontal gyrus
Maguire et al. 1998b	0/11	PET	1. VR room maze with objects (DoomII) 2. VR room maze without objects (both tasks scanned)	N/A	1. Random color/ texture images 2. Single empty room	*ES1–CT1* B – precuneus B – occipitotemporal B – cerebellum R – parahippocampus *ES2–CT2* B – precuneus B – occipitotemporal B – cerebellum

Key: fMRI, functional magnetic resonance imaging; PET, positron emission tomography; VR, virtual reality; PTP, point-to-point; ID, identify. *Note:* Listed activations include those that addressed the central research questions of each study, listed according to the hemispheric activations (Left, Right, or Bilateral) that remained after the indicated subtractions were made. ES, encoding stimuli; CT, control task; Ret, retrieval task. If no hemisphere is indicated then it was not specified in the report.

tasks were administered within subjects and were self-paced during (separate) 60-sec scanning blocks. Given the prior training to a knowledge criterion (i.e., acquisition of *both* landmark and survey knowledge), exposure to both tasks beforehand, and the time to implement any desired strategies during scanned task performance, participants may well have used both types of knowledge for both tasks, regardless of the instructions and the presumed task requirements. The authors did find an expected dorsal–ventral split in activated brain regions when activation during the two topographic tasks was directly compared; however, when each of the topographic tasks was compared to a nontopographic control, a broad swath of posterior dorsal and ventral stuctures was found to be activated for *both* topographic tasks. Thus, a specific mapping of function to structure was likely limited (in part) by the temporal integration of neural activity over long epochs relative to the time required to perform the tasks.

This example also helps to illustrate the third general caveat to the interpretation of brain imaging research: there are limitations associated with the "subtractive logic" routinely used to draw inferences about the functional significance of regional neural activity. In a continuously active system such as the human brain, observed activations at a particular period of time under a given set of conditions are only meaningful relative to activations observed under a comparison set of conditions. When observed activations associated with comparison conditions are subtracted from those associated with the experimental conditions of interest, the remaining activations are assumed to be functionally significant – that is, selectively associated with the cognitive processes engaged by the experimental conditions. For a number of reasons (see Sarter et al. 1996), however, when such subtractions are made it is possible that information is lost regarding the neural substrates subserving the functions of interest. For example, regions that are active to a similar extent for both experimental and control tasks may be active for different reasons (i.e., they subserve different functions), and thus experimentally relevant and interpretable activations would be lost to subtraction. Andersen et al. (1993), for instance, reported evidence for posterior parietal cell assemblies that contribute to the representation of space in both head-centered and body-centered coordinates, depending upon the conditions under which activation is elicited. In a situation where activations associated with both sets of conditions were directly compared, the subtractive logic of imaging techniques could well lead to a discounted role for this parietal region in both functions.

Given these concerns, it is important that brain imaging evidence for the localization of cognitive functions be interpreted in light of pertinent evidence from related disciplines, such as psychobiological work with animals and neuropsychological research with impaired human populations. Inferences for the localization of cognitive function

to candidate neural structures based on brain imaging data become much stronger if it can also be shown that lesions of the same structures in animals and humans lead to deficits in behaviors that (putatively) require the function in question. To their credit, the researchers pioneering funcional brain imaging of topographic cognition have assiduously marshalled psychobiological and neuropsychological evidence to support the neural localization inferences they have made. However, we believe that there is another set of concerns specific to the study of topographic cognition that require further interpretational caution and that may suggest a modification of typical experimental procedures. This fourth set of concerns is related to a critical assumption that is made when environmental surrogates are paired with brain imaging techniques to study topographic cognition – namely, assuming that participants' interactions with environmental surrogates engage the same cognitive processes that encounters with actual environments engage (Aguirre et al. 1998). To illustrate the nature of these concerns, we will focus on conflicting evidence from recent brain imaging work regarding the relative contribution of the hippocampus to human topographic cognition.

As briefly mentioned in the preceding review, there is good evidence from the animal literature that the hippocampus is central to processing that requires allocentric spatial representations. Much of this evidence comes from work with rodents (for reviews see McNaughton et al. 1995; O'Keefe & Nadel 1978), though research with avian species also supports the importance of the hippocampus for complex spatial behavior (Bingman & Jones 1994; Sherry, Jacobs, & Gaulin 1992). There has been some work with nonhuman primates that is supportive as well (Feigenbaum & Rolls 1991; Rolls, Robertson, & Georges-François 1995), though the issue of topographic cognition has been less intensively explored with these animals than with rodents. Finally, the evidence from clinical neuropsychology has been much less clear-cut, in large part because focal damage to the hippocampus proper is a relatively rare event.[8] There has been some neuropsychological evidence, however, that *parahippocampal* damage can lead to topographic disorientation (with primarily spatial location deficits rather than landmark agnosia; see Habib & Sirigu 1987). Aguirre et al. (1998) cited this evidence of parahippocampal involvement in topographic cognition to support findings in their brain imaging work that also implicate the parahippocampus. They suggest that neural substrates for allocentric representations of space may differ in primates and rats, with the parahippocampus being more important in the former and the hippocampus in the latter. In two recent studies, they collected fMRI data while participants explored either a computer-simulated maze (Aguirre et al. 1996) or a computer-simulated town (Aguirre & D'Esposito 1997). Although the specific research questions were slightly different in these two studies (acquisition vs. retrieval of topographic information in one, place identity vs. topographic location in the other), activations in the medial temporal regions implicated the parahippocampus in both studies; the hippocampus proper was not recruited in either study.

In contrast, Maguire and her colleagues have reported three PET scan studies in which the right hippocampus was activated for both learning (Maguire et al. 1996) and retrieval (Maguire et al. 1997, 1998a) of complex topographic information relative to activations observed for less complex topographic and nontopographic tasks. Considering possible reasons for this conflicting evidence regarding the contribution of the hippocampus proper to complex topographic cognition, we can quickly dispatch two possibilities by referring to a fourth study by Maguire and her colleagues. Although separate laboratories using different brain imaging techniques have reported this conflicting evidence (Aguirre et al. using fMRI; Maguire et al. using PET), Maguire et al. (1998b) found that medial temporal activation for topographic tasks was limited to the right parahippocampal gyrus. Thus, the cross-study differences in implicated neural substrates do not appear to be attributable to differences in laboratories or imaging techniques per se, because Maguire et al. (1998b) again used PET but this time failed to find activation of the hippocampus proper. We suggest that a more likely explanation for the conflicting evidence across studies (regarding the contribution of the hippocampus to topographic cognition) lies in the specific nature of the participants' environmental transactions. The three studies that failed to find hippocampal activation for complex topographic cognition all used relatively simple computer simulations of either mazes (Aguirre et al. 1996; Maguire et al. 1998b) or a town with distinctly mazelike characteristics (Aguirre & D'Esposito 1997).[9] On the other hand, the three studies in which the hippocampus *was* implicated in complex topographic cognition all relied on much more complex environmental transactions. Maguire et al. (1997) scanned participants while they described routes through London based on their intimate first-hand knowledge of the city from years of driving taxis; Maguire et al. (1996) scanned participants while they viewed information-rich videotaped urban "walks"; and although Maguire et al. (1998a) did use a computer-simulated town, the published depictions and verbal descriptions of the town suggest that it was substantially more sophisticated than previously used simulations. The town comprised four streets with shops, bars, a cinema, church, bank, train station and a video-game arcade, and the buildings were accessible and navigable, lending considerable complexity to environmental transactions.

Whether these differences in environmental transactions can account for the differential activation of the hippocampus across imaging studies is difficult to determine. At the very least, given the evidence from these initial imaging studies, it is probably premature to assume that all simulated environmental transactions engage the same cognitive processes (or engage them to the same degree) as those engaged for transactions with actual environments. Although the environmental transactions in all three studies that elicited hippocampal activation differed from the simple computer-simulated transactions in those that did not, the nature of those differences was not uniform. In one case we might focus on the visual complexity of videotaped environments (Maguire et al. 1996), in another on the visual and interactive richness of a recalled, familiar actual environment (Maguire et al. 1997), and in the third on a visually and navigationally complex perceptual interaction with a computer-simulated environment (Maguire et al. 1998a). However, the common thread among these environmental transactions is not obvious, other than a vague notion that each is more compelling or complex than transactions with computer-simulated mazes.

One possibility for why a more compelling environmental transaction would be more likely to recruit hippocampal activation concerns the depiction of movement through the environment. As we have seen in the studies reviewed here, active engagement with the environment may well influence the way people represent space and perform spatial tasks; in particular, the opportunity to integrate visual and kinesthetic inputs when people move through space may play a key role in the cognitive processing of topographic information. Prominent animal models of hippocampal involvement in navigation have also identified movement through the environment as being requisite for the generation of allocentric referents and the calibration of an idiothetic sense of direction (Burgess et al. 1994; McNaughton et al. 1991, 1995). It is noteworthy that these models were developed based on research with freely moving animals. This research has provided abundant evidence, such as hippocampal "place" cells,[10] for the involvement of the hippocampus in the performance of complex navigational tasks (see O'Keefe 1991). Recent work with animals indicates that the firing rate of hippocampal place cells is linked to the speed and direction of an animal's movement (Wiener, Paul, & Eichenbaum 1989). It is interesting that hippocampal place cells cease firing almost completely when animals are passively restrained (Foster, Castro, & McNaughton 1989). Thus, to the extent that the environmental simulations used in the topographic brain imaging studies convincingly mimicked the perceptual experiences of movement, they may have been more apt to engage cognitive processes that recruit hippocampal activation. Also, the data from recent animal work suggests that the physical restraint required by brain imaging techniques likely has a direct bearing on any inferences made regarding the neural substrates of human topographic cognition. However, because "wearable" brain scanning devices have yet to be developed, environmental simulations are likely to play an important role in brain imaging investigations of topographic cognition for the foreseeable future, as well as in other environmentally oriented psychophysiological work.

Thus, we see a critical need for a conceptual framework that specifies criteria by which researchers can discriminate stronger from weaker environmental simulations, especially with respect to the simulation of movement. We sketch one here that borrows heavily from concepts in the communications literature.

In developing a definition of virtual reality (VR), Steuer (1992) proposed a set of criteria for assessing the "telepresence" of VR systems. Telepresence refers to a feeling of being in a physical environment that is spatially and/or temporally removed from one's immediate physical surroundings; this feeling is produced by *mediated* rather than direct perceptual experience. In Steuer's model, mediation is through any indirect form of communication, so even relatively simple technologies (letters, telephones) can function as VR systems. This expansive potential for VR is felicitous for examining the simulated environmental transactions used in brain imaging research, as it allows us to assess such media as videotape and sophisticated three-dimensional computer animations within the same conceptual framework. The criteria Steuer presents are similar in content to those developed by others in the communications field (e.g. Zeltzer 1992) and focus on two dimensions of presentation media that are presumed to elicit a feeling of telepresence: vividness and interactivity. *Vividness* refers to the representational richness of a simulated environment and can be judged in terms of the breadth and depth of the sensory information presented. "Breadth" refers here to the range of perceptual systems simultaneously addressed by a presentation medium. Redundant information contained in multimodal sensory presentations is thought to eliminate competing perceptual interpretations and thereby enhance a given perceptual experience. "Depth" is determined individually for each sensory channel and is gauged according to its resolution, or density of data. The second media dimension determining telepresence, *interactivity*, is the extent to which users can manipulate the content and form of a simulated environment. Interactivity can be assessed in terms of the speed (real-time or slower) and range of available manipulations, as well as the fidelity of actions required to manipulate simulated environments (often referred to as "mapping"). Using a steering wheel to control simulated driving, for instance, constitutes a more veridical VR interaction than would button presses or keypad-controlled motion.

We want to emphasize that we sketch this model for illustrative purposes only. To our knowledge, the dimensions and underlying variables of telepresence have not been empirically verified, nor are these dimensions and variables likely to be the only relevant factors (see Biocca & Levy 1995; Cutting 1996, 1997). However, this model does give us a vocabulary and initial conceptual framework within which the simulated environmental transactions used in brain imaging research can be evaluated. For example, video game systems routinely trade off visual depth, and thereby vividness, to retain real-time motion in the service of interactivity. If we compare Maguire et al.'s (1996) videotaped environmental simulation, which did activate the hippocampus, and the two simulated maze-environments used by Aguirre and colleagues (Aguirre et al. 1996; Aguirre & D'Esposito 1997), which did not, we may reach the tentative conclusion that visually vivid simulations are more apt to recruit hippocampal involvement than are more visually impoverished (albeit) interactive simulations. Comparing Maguire et al.'s (1998a) more complex VR town with Aguirre's and D'Esposito's (1997) mazelike VR town, we can begin to parse the differences in complexity in terms of the former simulation's (apparently) greater visual depth *and* broader range of interactivity (provided by building accessibility and functioning doors). Comparisons with the remaining PET study eliciting hippocampal activation (Maguire et al. 1997) are problematic within this conceptual framework because the taxi drivers' environmental transactions were with recalled actual environments. This presents two problems. First, the definition of telepresence specifies a mediated perception of being in a physical environment other than one's immediate spatiotemporal surroundings, but recalled (and imagined) environments are internally generated, not perceived. Thus, we need a term (and definition) similar to telepresence yet broad enough to incorporate recalled and imagined source stimuli for simulated environmental transactions. We suggest *immersion,* which refers to a perceptual, mnestic, or imaginal feeling of being in a physical environment that is spatially and/or temporally removed from one's immediate physical surroundings. This definition is essentially the same as that for telepresence, yet it allows for mediated perception rather than requiring it and is expanded to include internally generated environmental transactions.

A second problem presented by a conceptual framework that must accommodate both internally and externally generated source stimuli for simulated environmental transactions is the need for person-centered assessment dimensions to complement vividness and interactivity, which are technology- or medium-centered. As an example, we consider one such dimension here, "familiarity," which we suggest can take at least two forms. *Specific familiarity* refers to one's personal knowledge of the environments to be simulated. Given the behavioral evidence described earlier regarding the microgenetic and ontogenetic development of topographic knowledge and abilities, we might expect a shift in the cognitive processes used to perform spatial tasks as one's familiarity with a particular environment increases, a shift that may be reflected in patterns of recruited neural activation. There is minimal evidence of this in the topographic brain imaging research conducted thus far. Aguirre et al. (1996) did report greater parahippocampal activation for maze-environment acquisition relative to retrieval, but the issue has not been addressed with complex environments that are difficult to learn. Specific familiarity with environments is an area that deserves careful study, however, as there are important opportunities to address the methodological concerns of using functional brain imaging to study topographic cognition. For example, one approach to examining the critical assumption that transactions with computer-simulated environments engage the same cognitive processes as transactions with actual environments would be to simulate existing environments. Heretofore, the computer simulations used in brain imaging studies of topographic cognition have depicted nonexistent environments. Simulations of existing environments would allow researchers to directly compare the behavior and neural activity of individuals who had acquired topographic information in actual environments versus those acquiring the same information through simulations. Similar regional patterns of neural activations across groups under these circumstances – during a topographic recall task, for instance – would help to support the assumption of similar engagement of cognitive processes for simulated and real-world transactions.

We might also expect the cognitive processes engaged by topographic behavior to differ as a function of one's *general familiarity* with the means of environmental simulation. With respect to internally generated source stimuli, individual differences in experience generating environmental imagery, route information, relative spatial locations, and so forth may lead people to develop different ways of processing topographic information. Cab drivers, for instance, routinely generate complex point-to-point route information, whereas bus drivers (with well-learned, set routes) would likely have less experience generating novel route information, as would those who are not professional drivers. With respect to externally generated source stimuli, there may be perceptual learning curves associated with the emergent technologies used to create and display environmental simulations, and individual differences in familiarity with such technologies could influence the cognitive processes they engage. Over the past 200 years, one psychologically interesting by-product of industrialization has been the continual creation of novel sensory phenomena, the perceptual mastery of which has occasionally been physically unpleasant for members of our species (Schivelbusch 1986). To use an example cited by Cutting et al. (1992), the advent of widespread train travel in the mid-nineteenth century was accompanied by clinical reports of eye fatigue, back strain, and overall body stress. The eye fatigue was presumably due to novice train travelers' inexperience in engaging the visual environment at previously unknown speeds.[11] More recently, reports of "side effects" associated with immersive VR environments include dizziness, headaches, eyestrain, and nausea (Regan & Price 1994), symptoms that can be reduced with the prior administration of anti–motion-sickess drugs (e.g. scopolamine hydrobromide; Regan & Ramsey 1996). Although it is not yet clear whether symptoms such as these

would subside with increasing VR experience, their relatively common occurrence (upwards of 60% of participants experiencing at least one symptom; Regan & Price 1994) represents prima facie evidence that VR environmental simulations may not engage the same cognitive processes as those engaged by actual environments. Indeed, one reason why videotaped environmental simulations elicit increased hippocampal activations while computer simulations do not may be broad familiarity with the former medium relative to the latter, especially with respect to the perception of motion.

In sum, the brain imaging studies reviewed here represent a promising initial psychophysiological foray into the investigation of human topographic cognition. Serious concerns regarding the interpretation of neural substrates recruited during topographic behavior have been met with felicitous reference to pertinent theory and converging lines of evidence from neuropsychology, psychobiology, and cognitive and environmental psychology. Inferential concerns regarding the comparability of cognitive processing engaged by transactions with simulated versus actual environments, however, have been less well met. The importance of these concerns is thrown into sharp relief by the research described here regarding the distinction between primary and secondary acquisition of topographic information, the importance of active relative to passive engagement with environments, and the emerging reports of perceptual maladies associated with immersive VR environments. Because brain imaging techniques have the potential to make important contributions to our understanding of human topographic cognition, the assumption regarding transactional comparability between simulated and actual environments deserves careful scrutiny, and we have outlined a conceptual framework that can facilitate comparisons among simulated environmental transactions. Additional psychophysiological measures might also be used, however, to examine comparability among environmental simulations. If some simulations are substantially better than others – for instance, at depicting self-locomotion through the environment – then EMG recordings from muscle groups involved in locomotion may reveal increased activations associated with those more immersive simulations.

Beyond examinations of the comparability among simulations, there are other techniques (as well as constructs and research) within psychophysiology that can be brought to bear on the inferential issues raised by the use of brain imaging to investigate topographic cognition. For example, interpretation of the localization of neural substrates associated with the performance of various topographic tasks could benefit from an analysis of task-related activations in terms of both cortical and autonomic arousal. Some of the structures activated by topographic tasks in these brain imaging studies (and interpreted solely in terms of the cognitive processes engaged) have also been implicated in the production of skin conductance responses elicited by nontopographic tasks (Tranel & Damasio 1994). Thus, increased activation in the right inferior parietal region may reflect cognitive processes associated with a survey-oriented relative to a landmark-oriented task (Aguirre & D'Esposito 1997), but it may also reflect the relative difficulty of the tasks independent of the specific cognitive processes engaged. To date, only one of the reviewed brain imaging studies (Ghaem et al. 1997) has measured autonomic or other psychophysiological concomitants of rCBF during topographic cognition. Thus, it seems there are broad opportunities here for the application of psychophysiological methods and constructs that could help brain imaging researchers address some of the inferential concerns inherent in laboratory studies of topographic cognition.

Concluding Remarks

As stated at the beginning of this chapter, environmental psychophysiology is not a field as such. However, we believe that the existing work regarding the significant effects that ordinary transactions with the physical environment can have argue strongly for the psychophysiological study of human–environment transactions. As our reviews of environmental noise, restorative environments, and topographic cognition indicate, psychophysiological constructs and methods have already been used profitably in this regard over a wide range of transactions. There are other areas as well, not reviewed here, where psychophysiology has contributed to our knowledge of how people engage the physical environment. These include: other areas of environmental stress, such as thermal extremes and crowding (Baum & Paulus 1987; Taylor, Allsopp, & Parkes 1995); less obviously oppressive environmental transactions, including chronobiological and other effects of light (Küller & Laike 1998; Küller & Mikellides 1993); as well as emerging fields of investigation regarding the effects of environmental elements such as negative air ions and olfactory stimuli (Morton & Kershner 1987; Miltner et al. 1994).

Although considerable work has been done in environmental psychophysiology as we have described it, more explicit recognition of this subdiscipline may well have advantages. The coordinated development and use of shared methodological approaches, for instance, would arguably be more easily accomplished with the institutional infrastructure (e.g., conferences, journal outlets) of a more formal discipline. In particular, given the repeated references in this chapter to the ecological validity of simulating large-scale environmental conditions in the laboratory, further development of lightweight, affordable ambulatory psychophysiological recording systems is a prime concern. Institutional imprimatur of this fledgling field could also facilitate the acquisition of research support and help to set research agendas that are responsive to needs in the field. For instance, as indicated in the section on to-

pographic cognition, some psychophysiological methods (such as brain imaging techniques) that are ill-suited to field research must rely on environmental simulations; thus, research questions regarding human transactions with various kinds of simulations will have to be addressed (e.g., why do immersive VR systems elicit nausea?).

Thus, we present the material in this chapter in part to exemplify the application of psychophysiology to human transactions with the physical environment but also to foster the recognition and nurture the development of environmental psychophysiology as a subdiscipline.

NOTES

For their helpful comments and assistance with technical literature, we thank Phyllis Sanchez, Psychiatry and Behavioral Sciences, Harborview Medical Center, Seattle; Staffan Hygge, Igor Knez, and Hans Allan Löfberg of the Laboratory of Applied Psychology, Centre for Built Environment, Swedish Royal Institute of Technology; Rikard Küller, Jans Janssens, and Thorbjörn Laike of the Environmental Psychology Unit, School of Architecture, Lund Institute of Technology. The first author also gratefully acknowledges several travel grants that supported our collaboration on this project as provided by the Institute for Housing Research, Uppsala University, and the College of Fine and Applied Arts and the Department of Landscape Architecture, University of Illinois, Urbana-Champaign.

1. Readers familiar with Andreassi's (1995) psychophysiology text will recognize that "environmental psychophysiology" is not being minted here. Andreassi's use of the term, however, is somewhat more restricted than ours, though his definition obscures the fact. He maintains that environmental psychophysiology refers to "the effects of physical environments on the physiology of a behaving person" (Andreassi 1995, p. 360). This seemingly broad consideration of potential effects belies the narrowly focused content of his environmental psychophysiology chapter. The physical environment of interest is the *internal* physical environment, primarily as it is influenced by changing hormone levels, the ingestion of drugs, and exposure to neurotoxic chemicals. As indicated in the introduction, our understanding of the physical environment is much more broadly conceived, in keeping with Lewin's and other psychologists' long-standing admonitions to consider "whole situations."

2. This is especially true of the clinical literature. See, for instance, the "Environmental Perspective" section of a recent book on measuring stress (Cohen, Kessler, & Gordon 1995), in which all four chapters are heavily slanted toward measuring socially oriented life events, such as problems on the job and marital conflicts.

3. L_{eq} is the multiple-event sound equivalent level (in decibels), a measure of exposure that is proportional to the sum of sound energy in 1-sec SPLs averaged over a specified period (see Kryter 1994, p. 7). In this instance, the L_{eq24} indicates the average over a 24-hour period.

4. For instance, as Table 1 indicates, the series of environmental sounds (suggested by the Environmental Protection Agency; see Peterson et al. 1980) presented to the monkeys has reasonable face validity for urban human populations, but it is unclear how such sounds are interpreted by nonhuman species. These stimuli may well be more threatening to a rhesus monkey than to humans, and the reported sound–no-sound differences in cardiovascular responding may be inflated accordingly.

5. See Cohen et al.'s (1980b, p. 239) discussion of children's distractibility as a function of school noise level and duration of exposure. Children from noisy schools initially performed better than those from quiet schools (i.e., were less distractible). With longer exposure in the noisy school environment, their performance was maintained or improved slightly, though with the longest exposures (more than 4 years) their performance dropped precipitously, falling well below that of children with similar tenure in quiet schools.

6. The terms "allocentric" and "egocentric" are used in the general literature on spatial cognition to refer to reference frames: environment-centered and person-centered, respectively. Egocentric frames of reference include retinocentric, craniocentric, and somatocentric, whereas allocentric frames of reference may include any (usually stable) element or set of elements in the environment other than the self. Developmentally, egocentric frames of reference emerge first, followed by simple allocentric reference frames focusing on proximal elements in the environment, progressing through allocentric frames focused on more distal elements (including those beyond the immediate perceptual horizon).

7. Pick (1993, p. 36) actually used the term "optical flow," though the context suggests that the intended meaning was retinal flow. Retinal flow is motion as it is presented to the retina, and it comprises both rotational flow and optical flow. The former is due to motion produced by eye movements, while the latter is produced by movement of the observer through the environment (see Cutting et al. 1992).

8. We note, however, that Morris and his colleagues (1996) have recently published a short report on the spatial abilities of temporal lobe resection (TLR) patients suffering from focal temporal lobe epilepsy. Resections, which were confined to the amygdala and the anterior two thirds of the hippocampus, impaired both egocentric and allocentric spatial performance of right TLR patients relative to left TLR patients and controls.

9. The town is laid out in a 4×4 grid of named places, and though the presence of a background skyline suggests the possibility of using distal features for orientation within the immediate environment, the authors claimed that this was not possible (Aguirre & D'Esposito 1997, p. 2513, fig. 2). In other respects, the published map and first-person views of the environment are strongly suggestive of a maze.

10. These are hippocampal cells selectively tuned for an animal's location in space, regardless of its orientation (i.e., its egocentric perspective).

11. Scanning patterns that are appropriate at pedestrian speeds – roughly equal numbers of fixations on proximal and distal cues – are extremely difficult to maintain at high speeds, and attempts to do so will probably lead to eye strain.

REFERENCES

Acredolo, L. P. (1988). Infant mobility and spatial development. In Stiles-Davis et al., pp. 157–66.

Acredolo, L. P., Adams, A., & Goodwyn, S. W. (1984). The role of self-produced movement and visual tracking in infant spatial orientation. *Journal of Experimental Child Psychology, 38*, 312–27.

Aguirre, G. K., & D'Esposito, M. (1997). Environmental knowledge is subserved by separable dorsal/ventral neural areas. *Journal of Neuroscience, 17*, 2512–18.

Aguirre, G. K., Detre, J. A., Alsop, D. C., & D'Esposito, M. (1996). The parahippocampus subserves topographic learning in man. *Cerebral Cortex, 6*, 823–9.

Aguirre, G. K., Zarahn, E., & D'Esposito, M. (1998). Neural components of topographical representation. *Proceedings of the National Academy of Sciences U.S.A., 95*, 839–46.

Allen, G. L. (1985). Strengthening weak links in the study of the development of macrospatial cognition. In R. Cohen (Ed.), *The Development of Spatial Cognition*, pp. 301–22. Hillsdale, NJ: Erlbaum.

Allen, G. L. (1987). Cognitive influences on the acquisition of route knowledge in children and adults. In P. Ellen & C. Thinus-Blanc (Eds.), *Cognitive Processes and Spatial Orientation in Animal and Man*, pp. 274–83. Boston: Nijhoff.

Altman, I., & Rogoff, B. (1987). World views in psychology: Trait, interactional, organismic and transactional perspectives. In Stokols & Altman, pp. 7–40.

Altman, I., & Wohlwill, J. F. (Eds.) (1983). *Human Behavior and Environment: Advances in Theory and Research*. New York: Plenum.

Andersen, R. A., Snyder, L. H., Li, C. S., & Stricanne, B. (1993). Coordinate transformations in the representation of spatial information. *Current Opinion in Neurobiology, 3*, 171–6.

Anderson, C. A., & Bushman, B. J. (1997). External validity of "trivial" experiments: The case of laboratory aggression. *Review of General Psychology, 1*, 19–41.

Anderson, E. A., Sinkey, C. A., & Mark, A. L. (1987). Mental stress increases sympathetic nerve activity and arterial pressure despite stimulation of arterial baroreceptors. *Circulation Monograph, 9*, IV-347.

Andreassi, J. L. (1995). *Psychophysiology: Human Behavior and Physiological Response*, 3rd ed. Hillsdale, NJ: Erlbaum.

Andren, L., Hansson, L., Bjorkman, M., & Jonsson, A. (1980). Noise as a contributory factor in the development of elevated arterial pressure. *Acta Medica Scandinavica, 207*, 493–8.

Andren, L., Hansson, L., Bjorkman, M., Jonsson, A., & Borg, K. O. (1979). Haemodynamic and hormonal changes induced by noise. *Acta Medica Scandinavica, 625 (Supp.)*, 13–18.

Aniansson, G., Pettersson, K., & Peterson, Y. (1983). Traffic noise annoyance and noise sensitivity in persons with normal and impaired hearing. *Journal of Sound and Vibration, 88*, 85–97.

Anticaglia, J. R., & Cohen, A. (1970). Extra-auditory effects of noise as a health hazard. *American Industrial Hygiene Association Journal, 31,* 277–81.

Appleyard, D. (1970). Styles and methods of structuring a city. *Environment and Behavior, 2,* 100–17.

Badal, J. (1888/1982). Contribution a l'étude des cécités psychiques. Alexie, agraphie, hémianopsie inférieure, trouble du sens d'l'espace. *Arch. Ophthalmol., 140,* 97–117. [As cited in DeRenzi 1982, chap. 1.]

Baum, A., & Paulus, P. (1987). Crowding. In Stokols & Altman, pp. 533–70.

Beck, R. J., & Wood, D. (1976). Cognitive transformation of information from urban geographic fields to mental maps. *Environment and Behavior, 8,* 199–238.

Bennett, E. (1945). Some tests for the discrimination of neurotic from normal subjects. *British Journal of Medical Psychology, 20,* 271–7.

Bergamasco, B., Benna, P., & Gilli, M. (1976). Human sleep modifications induced by urban traffic noise. *Acta Oto-Laryngology, 339 (Supp.),* 33–6.

Berlyne, D. E. (1960). *Conflict, Arousal, and Curiosity.* New York: McGraw-Hill.

Berlyne, D. E. (1971). *Aesthetics and Psychobiology.* New York: Appleton-Century-Crofts.

Bierce, A. (1911/1993). *The Devil's Dictionary.* Toronto: Dover Publications. [Original work published as vol. VII of *The Collected Works of Ambrose Bierce* (New York: Neale Publishing).]

Bingman, V. P., & Jones, T. J. (1994). Sun compass–based spatial learning impaired in homing pigeons with hippocampal lesions. *Journal of Neuroscience, 14,* 6687–94.

Biocca, F., & Levy, M. R. (Eds.) (1995). *Communication in the Age of Virtual Reality.* Hillsdale, NJ: Erlbaum.

Böök, A., & Gärling, T. (1980a). Processing of information about location during locomotion: Effects of a concurrent task and locomotion patterns. *Scandinavian Journal of Psychology, 21,* 185–92.

Böök, A., & Gärling, T. (1980b). Processing of information about location during locomotion: Effects of amount of visual information about the locomotion pattern. *Perceptual and Motor Skills, 51,* 231–8.

Böök, A., & Gärling, T. (1981). Maintenance of orientation during locomotion in unfamiliar environments. *Journal of Experimental Psychology: Human Perception and Performance, 7,* 995–1006.

Brandenberger, G., Follenius, M., Wittersheim, G., Salame, P., Siméoni, M., & Reinhardt, B. (1980). Plasma catecholamines and pituitary adrenal hormones related to mental task demand under quiet and noise conditions. *Biological Psychology, 10,* 239–52.

Breier, A., Albus, M., Pickar, D., Zahn, T. P., Wolkowitz, O. M., & Paul, S. M. (1987). Controllable and uncontrollable stress in humans: Alterations in mood, neuroendocrine and psychophysiological function. *American Journal of Psychiatry, 144,* 1419–25.

Broadbent, D. E. (1979). Human performance and noise. In C. S. Harris (Ed.), *Handbook of Noise Control,* pp. 2066–85. New York: McGraw-Hill.

Brodal, P. (1998). *The Central Nervous System: Structure and Function.* New York: Oxford University Press.

Burgess, N., Recce, M., & O'Keefe, J. (1994). A model of hippocampal function. *Neural Networks, 7,* 1065–81.

Cacioppo, J. T., & Tassinary, L. G. (Eds.) (1990a). *Principles of Psychophysiology: Physical, Social, and Inferential Elements.* Cambridge University Press.

Cacioppo, J. T., & Tassinary, L. G. (1990b). Psychophysiology and psychophysiological principles. In Cacioppo & Tassinary (1990a), pp. 3–33.

Cammalleri, R., Gangitano, M., D'Amelio, M., Raieli, V., Raimondo, D., & Camarda, R. (1996). Transient topographical amnesia and cingulate cortex damage: A case report. *Neuropsychologia, 34,* 321–6.

Carter, N. L., & Beh, H. C. (1989). The effect of intermittent noise on cardiovascular functioning during vigilance task performance. *Psychophysiology, 26,* 548–59.

Cervone, D., Kopp, D. A., Schaumann, L., & Scott, W. D. (1994). Mood, self-efficacy and performance standards: Lower moods induce higher standards of performance. *Journal of Personality and Social Psychology, 67,* 499–512.

Chariton, W. O. (1990). *This Dog'll Hunt: An Entertaining Texas Dictionary.* Plano, TX: Wordware.

Cimprich, B. (1993). Development of an intervention to restore attention in cancer patients. *Cancer Nursing, 16,* 83–92.

Coates, T. J., Rosekind, M. R., Strossen, R. J., Thoresen, C. E., & Kirmil-Gray, K. (1979). Sleep recordings in the laboratory and home: A comparative analysis. *Psychophysiology, 16,* 339–46.

Cohen, A., Taylor, W., & Tubbs, R. (1980a). Occupational exposures to noise, hearing loss and blood pressure. In Tobias et al., pp. 322–6.

Cohen, R., & Weatherford, D. L. (1980). Effects of route traveled on the distance estimates of children and adults. *Journal of Experimental Child Psychology, 29,* 403–12.

Cohen, R., & Weatherford, D. L. (1981). The effect of barriers on spatial representations. *Child Development, 52,* 1087–90.

Cohen, S. (1978). Environmental load and the allocation of attention. In A. Baum, J. E. Singer, & S. Valins (Eds.), *Advances in Environmental Psychology,* vol. 1, pp. 1–29. Hillsdale, NJ: Erlbaum.

Cohen, S. L., & Cohen, R. (1985). The role of activity in spatial cognition. In R. Cohen (Ed.), *The Development of Spatial Cognition,* pp. 199–223. Hillsdale, NJ: Erlbaum.

Cohen, S., Evans, G. W., Krantz, D. S., & Stokols, D. (1980b). Physiological, motivational and cognitive effects of noise on children: Moving from the laboratory to the field. *American Psychologist, 35,* 231–43.

Cohen, S., Evans, G. W., Krantz, D. S., Stokols, D., & Kelly, S. (1981). Aircraft noise and children: Longitudinal and cross-sectional evidence on adaptation to noise and the effectiveness of noise abatement. *Journal of Personality and Social Psychology, 40,* 331–45.

Cohen, S., Evans, G. W., Stokols, D., & Krantz, D. S. (1986). *Behavior, Health and Environmental Stress.* New York: Plenum Press.

Cohen, S., Glass, D. C., & Singer, J. E. (1973). Apartment noise, auditory discrimination, and reading ability in children. *Journal of Experimental Social Psychology, 9,* 407–22.

Cohen, S., Kessler, R. C., & Gordon, L. U. (1995). *Measuring Stress: A Guide for Health and Social Scientists.* New York: Oxford University Press.

Cohen, S., & Spacapan, S. (1978). The aftereffects of stress: An attentional interpretation. *Environmental Psychology and Nonverbal Behavior, 3,* 43–59.

Coles, M. G. H., Gratton, G., & Fabiani, M. (1990). Event-related brain potentials. In Cacioppo & Tassinary (1990a), pp. 413–55.

Conrad, D. W. (1973). The effects of intermittent noise on human serial decoding performance and physiological response. *Ergonomics, 16,* 739–47.

Cutting, J. E. (1996). Wayfinding from multiple sources of local information in retinal flow. *Journal of Experimental Psychology: Human Perception and Performance, 22,* 1299–1313.

Cutting, J. E. (1997). How the eye measures reality and virtual reality. *Behavior Research Methods, Instruments and Computers, 29,* 27–36.

Cutting, J. E., Springer, K., Braren, P. A., & Johnson, S. H. (1992). Wayfinding on foot from information in retinal, not optical, flow. *Journal of Experimental Psychology: General, 121,* 41–72.

Daniel, T. C., & Vining, J. (1983). Methodological issues in the assessment of landscape quality. In Altman & Wohlwill, pp. 39–84.

Dearinger, J. A. (1979). Measuring preferences for natural landscapes. *Journal of the Urban Planning and Development Division, 105,* 63–80.

DeJoy, D. M. (1984). The nonauditory effects of noise: Review and perspectives for research. *Journal of Auditory Research, 24,* 123–50.

DeRenzi, E. (1982). *Disorders of Space Exploration and Cognition.* New York: Wiley.

Dimberg, U. (1990). Facial electromyographic reactions and autonomic activity to auditory stimuli. *Biological Psychology, 31,* 137–47.

Driver, B. L., Nash, R., & Haas, G. (1987). Wilderness benefits: A state-of-knowledge review. In R. C. Lucas (Ed.), *Proceedings – National Wilderness Research Conference: Issues, State of Knowledge, Future Directions* (USDA Forest Service General Technical report no. INT-220), pp. 294–319. Ogden, UT: USDA Forest Service Intermountain Research Station.

Eberhardt, J. L., & Akselsson, K. R. (1987). The disturbance by road traffic noise of the sleep of young male adults as recorded in the home. *Journal of Sound and Vibration, 114,* 417–34.

Ettlinger, G., Warrington, E. K., & Zangwill, O. L. (1957). A further study of visual-spatial agnosia. *Brain, 80,* 335–61.

Evans, G. W., Bullinger, M., & Hygge, S. (1998). Chronic noise exposure and physiological response: A prospective study of children living under environmental stress. *Psychological Science, 9,* 75–7.

Evans, G. W., & Cohen, S. (1987). Environmental stress. In Stokols & Altman, pp. 571–610.

Evans, G. W., Hygge, S., & Bullinger, M. (1995). Chronic noise and psychological stress. *Psychological Science, 6,* 333–8.

Evans, G. W., Johansson, G., & Carrère, S. (1994). Psychosocial factors and the physical environment: Inter-relations in the workplace. In C. L. Cooper & I. T. Robertson (Eds.), *International Review of Industrial and Organizational Psychology,* vol. 9, pp. 1–29. Chichester, U.K.: Wiley.

Evans, G. W., & Lepore, S. J. (1993). Nonauditory effects of noise on children: A critical review. *Children's Environments, 10,* 31–51.

Evans, G. W., & Pezdek, K. (1980). Cognitive mapping: Knowledge of real world distance and location information. *Journal of Experimental Psychology: Human Learning and Memory, 6,* 13–24.

Feigenbaum, J., & Rolls, E. T. (1991). Allocentric and egocentric spatial information processing in the hippocampal formation of the behaving primate. *Psychobiology, 19,* 21–40.

Fein, A. (1972). *Frederick Law Olmsted and the American Environmental Tradition.* New York: Braziller.

Follenius, M., Brandenberger, G., Lecornu, C., Simeoni, M., & Reinhardt, B. (1980). Plasma catecholamines and pituitary adrenal hormones in response to noise exposure. *European Journal of Applied Physiology, 43,* 253–61.

Foster, T. C., Castro, C. A., & McNaughton, B. L. (1989). Spatial selectivity of rat hippocampal neurons is dependent upon preparedness for movement. *Science, 244,* 1580–2.

Frankenhaeuser, M. (1980). Psychoneuroendocrine approaches to the study of person–environment transactions. In H. Selye (Ed.), *Selye's Guide to Stress Research,* vol. 1, pp. 46–70. New York: Van Nostrand Reinhold.

Frankenhaeuser, M. (1991). The psychophysiology of sex differences as related to occupational status. In M. Frankenhaeuser, U. Lundberg, & M. A. Chesney (Eds.), *Women, Work, and Health,* pp. 39–61. New York: Plenum.

Frankenhaeuser, M., & Lundberg, U. (1974). Immediate and delayed effects of noise on performance and arousal. *Biological Psychology, 2,* 127–33.

Frankenhaeuser, M., & Lundberg, U. (1977). The influence of cognitive set on performance and arousal under different noise loads. *Motivation and Emotion, 1,* 139–49.

Frankenhaeuser, M., Lundberg, U., Fredrikson, M., Melin, B., Tuomisto, M., Myrsten, A.-L., Hedman, M., Bergman-Losman, B., & Wallin, L. (1989). Stress on and off the job as related to sex and occupational status in white-collar workers. *Journal of Organizational Behavior, 10,* 321–46.

Fredrickson, B. L., & Levenson, R. W. (1998). Positive emotions speed recovery from the cardiovascular sequelae of negative emotions. *Cognition and Emotion, 12,* 191–220.

Freire-Garabal, M., Núñez-Iglesias, M. J., Balboa, J. L., Fernández-Rial, J. C., & Rey-Mendéz, M. (1995). Effects of buspirone on the immune response to stress in mice. *Pharmacology, Biochemistry and Behavior, 51,* 821–5.

Gannon, L., Banks, J., Shelton, D., & Luchetta, T. (1989). The mediating effects of psychophysiological reactivity and recovery on the relationship between environmental stress and illness. *Journal of Psychosomatic Research, 33,* 167–75.

Gärling, T., Böök, A., & Lindberg, E. (1985). Adults' memory representations of the spatial properties of their everyday physical environment. In R. Cohen (Ed.), *The Development of Spatial Cognition.* Hillsdale, NJ: Erlbaum.

Geen, R. (1984). Preferred stimulation levels in introverts and extroverts: Effects on arousal and performance. *Journal of Personality and Social Psychology, 46,* 1303–12.

Ghaem, O., Mellet, E., Crivello, F., Tzourio, N., Mazoyer, B., Berthoz, A., & Denis, M. (1997). Mental navigation along memorized routes activates the hippocampus, precuneus and insula. *Neuroreport, 8,* 739–44.

Glass, D. C., & Singer, J. E. (1972). *Urban Stress: Experiments in Noise and Social Stressors.* New York: Academic Press.

Glass, D. C., Singer, J. E., & Friedman, L. N. (1969). Psychic cost of adaptation to an environmental stressor. *Journal of Personality and Social Psychology, 12,* 200–10.

Golledge, R. G. (1987). Environmental cognition. In Stokols & Altman, pp. 131–74.

Golledge, R. G., & Spector, A. N. (1978). Comprehending the urban environment: Theory and practice. *Geographical Analysis, 10,* 401–26.

Golledge, R. G., & Stimson, R. J. (1997). *Spatial Behavior: A Geographical Perspective.* New York: Guilford.

Griefahn, B., & Gros, E. (1986). Noise and sleep at home: A field study on primary and after-effects. *Journal of Sound and Vibration, 105,* 373–83.

Griffiths, I. D., & Delauzun, F. R. (1977). Individual differences in sensitivity to traffic noise: An empirical study. *Journal of Sound and Vibration, 55,* 93–107.

Habib, M., & Sirigu, A. (1987). Pure topographical disorientation: A definition and anatomical basis. *Cortex, 23,* 73–85.

Hansen, J. C., & Hillyard, S. A. (1983). Selective attention to multidimensional auditory stimuli in man. *Journal of Experimental Psychology: Human Perception and Performance, 9,* 1–19.

Hanson, J. D., Larson, M. E., & Snowdon, C. T. (1976). The effects of control over high intensity noise on plasma cortisol levels in rhesus monkeys. *Behavioral Biology, 16,* 333–40.

Hartig, T. (1993). Nature experience in transactional perspective. *Landscape and Urban Planning, 25,* 17–36.

Hartig, T., Böök, A., Garvill, J., Olsson, T., & Gärling, T. (1996). Environmental influences on psychological restoration. *Scandinavian Journal of Psychology, 37,* 378–93.

Hartig, T., & Evans, G. W. (1993). Psychological foundations of nature experience. In T. Gärling & R. G. Golledge (Eds.), *Behavior and Environment,* pp. 427–57. Amsterdam: Elsevier.

Hartig, T., Evans, G. W., Jamner, L. D., Davis, D., & Gärling, T. (submitted). Stress recovery enhanced by natural environment experiences.

Hartig, T., Mang, M., & Evans, G. W. (1991). Restorative effects of natural environment experiences. *Environment and Behavior, 23,* 3–26.

Haynes, S. N., Gannon, L. R., Orimoto, L., O'Brien, W. H., & Brandt, M. (1991). Psychophysiological assessment of post-stress recovery. *Psychological Assessment, 3,* 356–65.

Heft, H. (1983). Way-finding as the perception of information over time. *Population and Environment: Behavioral and Social Issues, 6,* 133–50.

Henkin, R. I., & Knigge, K. M. (1963). Effects of sound on the hypothalamic-pituitary-adrenal axis. *American Journal of Physiology, 204,* 710–14.

Heym, J., Trulson, M. E., & Jacobs, B. L. (1982). Raphe unit activity in freely moving cats: Effects of phasic auditory and visual stimuli. *Brain Research, 232,* 29–39.

Hintzman, D. L., O'Dell, C. S., & Arndt, D. R. (1981). Orientation in cognitive maps. *Cognitive Psychology, 13,* 149–206.

Hockey, G. R. J. (1972). Effects of noise on human efficiency and some individual differences. *Journal of Sound and Vibration, 20,* 299–304.

Howard, J. H., & Kerst, S. M. (1981). Memory and perception of cartographic information for familiar and unfamiliar environments. *Human Factors, 23,* 495–504.

Ising, H., Babisch, W., Kruppa, B., Lindthammer, A., & Wiens, D. (1996). Subjective work noise – A major risk factor in myocardial infarction. In *Proceedings of the International Congress on Noise Control Engineering,* vol. 4, pp. 2159–64. St. Albans, U.K.: Institute of Acoustics.

Jackson, J. H. (1876/1958). Case of large cerebral tumor without optic neuritis and with left hemiplegia and imperception. Reprinted in J. Taylor (Ed.), *Selected Writings of John Hughlings Jackson,* pp. 146–52. New York: Basic Books.

James, W. (1892). *Psychology: The Briefer Course.* New York: Holt.

Jansen, G. (1969). Effects of noise on physiological state. In W. D. Ward & J. E. Fricke (Eds.), *Noise as a Public Health Problem,* pp. 89–98. Washington, D.C.: American Speech and Hearing Association.

Johansson, G., Evans, G. W., Rydstedt, L., & Carrère, S. (1996). Job hassles and cardiovascular reaction patterns among urban bus drivers. Report no. 823, Department of Psychology, Stockholm University.

Johansson, G., & Frankenhaeuser, M. (1973). Temporal factors in sympatho-medullary activity following acute behavioral activation. *Biological Psychology, 1,* 63–73.

Johns, M. W. (1977). Validity of subjective reports of sleep latency in normal subjects. *Ergonomics, 20,* 683–90.

Johnson, A. K., & Anderson, E. A. (1990). Stress and arousal. In Cacioppo & Tassinary (1990a), pp. 216–52.

Jones, D., & Broadbent, D. E. (1979). Side-effects of interference with speech by noise. *Ergonomics, 22,* 1073–81.

Jurriëns, A. A. (1981). Noise and sleep in the home: Effects on sleep stages. In W. P. Koella (Ed.), *Sleep 1980: Fifth European Congress on Sleep Research,* pp. 217–20. Basel: Karger.

Kalin, N. H., Gibbs, D. M., Barksdale, C. M., Shelton, S. E., & Carnes, M. (1985). Behavioral stress decreases plasma oxytocin concentrations in primates. *Life Sciences, 36,* 1275–80.

Kaplan, R., & Kaplan, S. (1989). *The Experience of Nature: A Psychological Perspective.* Cambridge University Press.

Kaplan, S. (1978). Attention and fascination: The search for cognitive clarity. In S. Kaplan & R. Kaplan (Eds.), *Humanscape,* pp. 84–90. Ann Arbor, MI: Ulrich's Books.

Kaplan, S. (1983). A model of person–environment compatibility. *Environment and Behavior, 15,* 311–32.

Kaplan, S. (1995). The restorative benefits of nature: Toward an integrative framework. *Journal of Environmental Psychology, 15,* 169–82.

Kaplan, S., & Kaplan, R. (1982). *Cognition and Environment: Functioning in an Uncertain World.* New York: Praeger.

Kaplan, S., & Talbot, J. F. (1983). Psychological benefits of a wilderness experience. In Altman & Wohlwill, pp. 163–203.

Karogodina, I. L. (1969). Effect of aircraft noise on population near airports. *Hygiene and Sanitation, 34,* 182–7.

Karsdorf, G., & Klappach, H. (1968). The influence of traffic noise on the health and performance of secondary school students in a large city (Transl. by Literature Research Company). [Original work published in *Zeitschrifte für die Gesammte Hygiene, 14,* 52–4; as cited in Evans & Lepore 1993.]

Kjellberg, A. (1990). Subjective, behavioral and psychophysiological effects of noise. *Scandinavian Journal of Work Environments and Health, 16 (Suppl.),* 29–38.

Klatzky, R. L., Loomis, J. M., Beall, A. C., Chance, S. S., & Golledge, R. G. (1998). Spatial updating of self-position and orientation during real, imagined and virtual locomotion. *Psychological Science, 9,* 293–8.

Knipschild, P. (1977). Medical effects of aircraft noise: Community cardiovascular survey. *International Archives of Occupational and Environmental Health, 40,* 185–90.

Knipschild, P. (1980). Aircraft noise and hypertension. In Tobias et al., pp. 283–7.

Knopf, R. C. (1983). Recreational needs and behavior in natural settings. In Altman & Wohlwill, pp. 205–40.

Knopf, R. C. (1987). Human behavior, cognition, and affect in the natural environment. In Stokols & Altman, pp. 783–825.

Krantz, D. S., Contrada, R. J., Hill, D., & Friedler, E. (1988). Environmental stress and biobehavioral antecedents of coronary heart disease. *Journal of Consulting and Clinical Psychology, 56*, 333–41.

Kritchevsky, M. (1988). The elementary spatial functions of the brain. In Stiles-Davis et al., pp. 111–40.

Kryter, K. D. (1994). *The Handbook of Hearing and the Effects of Noise: Physiology, Psychology and Public Health.* San Diego: Academic Press.

Kryter, K. D., & Poza, F. (1980). Effects of noise on some autonomic system activities. *Journal of the Acoustical Society of America, 67*, 2036–44.

Kuipers, B. (1982). The "map in the head" metaphor. *Environment and Behavior, 14*, 202–20.

Küller, R., & Laike, T. (1998). The impact of flicker from fluorescent lighting on well-being, performance, and physiological arousal. *Ergonomics, 41*, 433–47.

Küller, R., & Mikellides, B. (1993). Simulated studies of color, arousal, and comfort. In R. W. Marans & D. Stokols (Eds.), *Environmental Simulation,* pp. 163–90. New York: Plenum.

Landis, T., Cummings, J. L., Benson, F., & Palmer, P. (1986). Loss of topographic familiarity: An environmental agnosia. *Archives of Neurology, 43*, 132–6.

Lang, T., Fouriaud, C., & Jacquinet-Salord, M. C. (1992). Length of occupational noise exposure and blood pressure. *International Archives of Occupational and Environmental Health, 63*, 369–72.

Lees, R. E. M., Romeril, C. S., & Wetherall, L. D. (1980). A study of stress indicators in workers exposed to industrial noise. *Canadian Journal of Public Health, 71*, 261–5.

LeVere, T. E., Bartus, R. T., & Hart, F. D. (1972). Electroencephalographic and behavioral effects of nocturnally occurring jet aircraft sounds. *Aerospace Medicine, 43*, 384–9.

LeVere, T. E., & Davis, N. (1977). Arousal from sleep: The physiological and subjective effects of a 15 dB(A) reduction in aircraft flyover noise. *Aviation, Space and Environmental Medicine, 48*, 607–11.

Lewin, K. (1936). *Principles of Topological Psychology* (Transl. by F. Heider & G. M. Heider). New York: McGraw-Hill.

Lovallo, W. R., Wilson, M. F., Pincomb, G. A., Edwards, G. L., Tompkins, P., & Brackett, D. J. (1985). Activation patterns to aversive stimulation in man: Passive exposure versus effort to control. *Psychophysiology, 22*, 283–91.

Lukas, J. S. (1976). Noise and sleep: A literature review and a proposed criterion for assessing effect. *Journal of the Acoustical Society of America, 58*, 1232–42.

Lundberg, U., & Frankenhaeuser, M. (1978). Psychophysiological reactions to noise as modified by personal control over noise intensity. *Biological Psychology, 6*, 51–9.

Lundberg, U., Melin, B., Evans, G. W., & Holmberg, L. (1993). Physiological deactivation after two contrasting tasks at a video display terminal: Learning vs. repetitive data entry. *Ergonomics, 36*, 601–11.

Lydic, R., McCarley, R. W., & Hobson, J. A. (1987). Serotonin neurons and sleep: II. Time course of dorsal raphe discharge, PGO waves, and behavioral states. *Archives Italiennes de Biologie, 126*, 1–28.

Magliano, J. P., Cohen, R., Allen, G. L., & Rodrigue, J. R. (1995). The impact of a wayfinder's goal on learning a new environment: Different types of spatial knowledge as goals. *Journal of Environmental Psychology, 15*, 65–75.

Maguire, E. A. (1997). Hippocampal involvement in human topographical memory: Evidence from functional imaging. *Philosophical Transactions of the Royal Society of London, Ser. B, 352*, 1475–80.

Maguire, E. A., Burgess, N., Donnett, J. G., Frakowiak, R. S. J., Frith, C. D., & O'Keefe, J. (1998a). Knowing where and getting there: A human navigation network. *Science, 280*, 921–4.

Maguire, E. A., Frakowiak, R. S. J., & Frith, C. D. (1996). Learning to find your way: A role for the human hippocampal formation. *Proceedings of the Royal Society of London, Ser. B, 263*, 1745–50.

Maguire, E. A., Frakowiak, R. S. J., & Frith, C. D. (1997). Recalling routes around London: Activation of the right hippocampus in taxi drivers. *Journal of Neuroscience, 17*, 7103–10.

Maguire, E. A., Frith, C. D., Burgess, N., Donnett, J. G., & O'Keefe, J. (1998b). Knowing where things are: Parahippocampal involvement in encoding object locations in virtual large-scale space. *Journal of Cognitive Neuroscience, 10*, 61–76.

Mandler, J. M. (1988). The development of spatial cognition: On topological and Euclidean representation. In Stiles-Davis et al., pp. 423–32.

McFie, J., Piercy, M. F., & Zangwill, O. L. (1950). Visual-spatial agnosia associated with lesions of the right cerebral hemisphere. *Brain, 73*, 167–90.

McLean, E. K., & Tarnopolsky, A. (1977). Noise, discomfort and mental health: A review of the socio-medical implications of disturbance by noise. *Psychological Medicine, 7*, 19–62.

McNaughton, B. L., Chen, L. L., & Markus, E. J. (1991). "Dead reckoning," landmark learning and sense of direction: A neurophysiological and computational hypothesis. *Journal of Cognitive Neuroscience, 3*, 190–202.

McNaughton, B. L., Knierim, J. J., & Wilson, M. A. (1995). Vector encoding and vestibular foundations of spatial cognition: Neurophysiological and computational mechanisms. In M. S. Gazzaniga (Ed.), *The Cognitive Neurosciences,* pp. 585–95. Cambridge, MA: MIT Press.

Melin, B., & Lundberg, U. (1997). A biopsychosocial approach to work-stress and musculoskeletal disorders. *Journal of Psychophysiology, 11*, 238–47.

Meyer, O. (1900/1996). Ein- und doppelseitige homonyme Hemianopsie mit Orientirrungsstören. *Monatsschrift für Psychiatrie und Neurologie, 8*, 440–56.

Milgram, S. (1970). The experience of living in cities. *Science, 167*, 1461–8.

Millar, K., & Steels, M. J. (1990). Sustained peripheral vasoconstriction while working in continuous intense noise. *Aviation, Space and Environmental Medicine, 61*, 695–8.

Miller, N. E. (1985). Effects of emotional stress on the immune system. *Pavlovian Journal of Biological Science, 20*, 47–52.

Miltner, W., Matjak, M., Braun, C., Diekmann, H., & Brody, S. (1994). Emotional qualities of odors and their influence on the startle reflex in humans. *Psychophysiology, 31*, 107–10.

Moeser, S. D. (1988). Cognitive mapping in a complex building. *Environment and Behavior, 20*, 21–49.

Montello, D. R. (1998). A new framework for understanding the acquisition of spatial knowledge in large-scale environments. In M. J. Egenhofer & R. G. Golledge (Eds.), *Spatial and Temporal Reasoning in Geographic Information Systems*, pp. 143–54. New York: Oxford University Press.

Moos, R. H., & Swindle, R. W. (1990). Person-environment transactions and the stressor-appraisal-coping process. *Psychological Inquiry, 1*, 30–2.

Moreira, N. M., & Bryan, M. E. (1972). Noise annoyance susceptibility. *Journal of Sound and Vibration, 21*, 449–62.

Morris, R. G., Pickering, A., Abrahams, S., & Feigenbaum, J. D. (1996). Space and the hippocampal formation in humans. *Brain Research Bulletin, 40*, 487–90.

Morrow, L., & Ratcliff, G. (1988). The neuropsychology of spatial cognition. In Stiles-Davis et al., pp. 5–32.

Morton, L. L., & Kershner, J. R. (1987). Negative ion effects on hemispheric processing and selective attention in the mentally retarded. *Journal of Mental Deficiency Research, 31*, 169–80.

Mosskov, J. I., & Ettema, J. H. (1977a). Extra-auditory effects in short-term exposure to aircraft and traffic noise. II. *International Archives of Occupational and Environmental Health, 40*, 165–73.

Mosskov, J. I., & Ettema, J. H. (1977b). Extra-auditory effects in short-term exposure to aircraft and traffic noise. IV. *International Archives of Occupational and Environmental Health, 40*, 177–84.

Muzet, A., & Ehrhart, J. (1980). Habituation of heart rate and finger pulse responses to noise in sleep. In Tobias et al., pp. 401–4.

O'Brien, W. H., Haynes, S. N., & Mumby, P. B. (1998). Differences in cardiovascular recovery among healthy young adults with and without a parental history of hypertension. *Journal of Psychophysiology, 12*, 17–28.

Obrist, P. A., Gaebelein, C. J., Teller, E. S., Langer, A. W., Grignolo, A., Light, K., & McCubbin, J. A. (1978). The relationship among heart rate, carotid dP/dt, and blood pressure in humans as a function of the type of stress. *Psychophysiology, 15*, 102–15.

Ogle, C. W., & Lockett, M. F. (1968). The urinary changes induced in rats by high-pitched sound. *Journal of Endocrinology, 42*, 253–60.

Öhrström, E., & Björkman, M. (1983). Sleep disturbance before and after traffic noise attentuation in an apartment building. *Journal of the Acoustical Society of America, 73*, 877–9.

Öhrström, E., Björkman, M., & Rylander, R. (1988). Noise annoyance with regard to neurophysiological sensitivity, subjective noise sensitivity and personality variables. *Psychological Medicine, 18*, 605–13.

Öhrström, E., & Rylander, R. (1982). Sleep disturbance effects of noise – A laboratory study on after effects. *Journal of Sound and Vibration, 84*, 87–103.

O'Keefe, J. (1991). The hippocampal cognitive map and navigational strategies. In J. Paillard (Ed.), *Brain and Space*, pp. 273–95. Oxford University Press.

O'Keefe, J., & Nadel, L. (1978). *The Hippocampus as a Cognitive Map*. Oxford, U.K.: Clarendon.

Olmsted, F. L. (1865/1952). The Yosemite Valley and the Mariposa big trees: A preliminary report. Reprinted [with an introductory note by L. W. Roper] in *Landscape Architecture, 43*, 12.

Olmsted, F. L. (1870). *Public Parks and the Enlargement of Towns*. Cambridge, MA: Riverside.

Parsons, R. (1991a). The potential influences of environmental perception on health. *Journal of Environmental Psychology, 11*, 1–23.

Parsons, R. (1991b). Recovery from stress during exposure to videotaped outdoor environments. Doctoral dissertation, Department of Psychology, University of Arizona, Tucson.

Parsons, R., Tassinary, L. G., Ulrich, R. S., Hebl, M. R., & Grossman-Alexander, M. (1998). The view from the road: Implications for stress recovery and immunization. *Journal of Environmental Psychology, 18*, 113–40.

Parvizpoor, D. (1976). Noise exposure and prevalence of high blood pressure among weavers in Iran. *Journal of Occupational Medicine, 18*, 730–1.

Paterson, A., & Zangwill, O. L. (1944). Disorders of visual space perception associated with lesions of the right cerebral hemisphere. *Brain, 67*, 331–58.

Paterson, A., & Zangwill, O. L. (1945). A case of topographical disorientation associated with unilateral cerebral lesion. *Brain, 68*, 188–211.

Pearsons, K. S., Barber, D. S., & Tabachnick, B. G. (1990). Analyses of the predictability of noise-induced sleep disturbance. Report no. HSD-TR-89-029. Wright-Patterson AFB, Ohio.

Peterson, E. A., Augenstein, J. S., Hazelton, C. L., Hetrick, D., Levene, R. M., & Tanis, D. C. (1984). Some cardiovascular effects of noise. *Journal of Auditory Research, 24*, 35–62.

Peterson, E. A., Augenstein, J. S., Tanis, D. C., & Augenstein, D. G. (1981). Noise raises blood pressure without impairing auditory sensitivity. *Science, 211*, 1450–2.

Peterson, E. A., Tanis, D. C., Augenstein, J. S., Seifert, R. A., & Bromley, H. R. (1980). Noise and cardiovascular function in rhesus monkeys II. In Tobias et al., pp. 246–53.

Pick, H. L. (1993). Organization of spatial knowledge in children. In N. Eilan, R. McCarthy, & B. Brewer (Eds.), *Spatial Representation*, pp. 31–42. Cambridge, MA: Blackwell.

Pitt, D., & Zube, E. (1987). Management of natural environments. In Stokols & Altman, pp. 1009–42.

Pomeroy, J. W., Fitzgibbon, J. E., & Green, M. B. (1989). The use of personal construct theory in evaluating landscape aesthetics. In P. Dearden & B. Sadler (Eds.), *Landscape Evaluation*. Victoria, BC: University of Victoria.

Posner, M. I., & Raichle, M. E. (1994). *Images of Mind*. New York: Freeman.

Presson, C. C., & Hazelrigg, M. D. (1984). Building spatial representations through primary and secondary learning. *Journal of Experimental Psychology: Learning, Memory and Cognition, 10*, 716–22.

Regan, E. C., & Price, K. R. (1994). The frequency of occurrence and severity of side-effects of immersion virtual reality. *Aviation Space and Environmental Medicine, 65*, 527–30.

Regan, E. C., & Ramsey, A. D. (1996). The efficacy of hyoscine hydrobromide in reducing side-effects during immersion in virtual reality. *Aviation Space and Environmental Medicine, 67*, 222–6.

Regecová, V., & Kellerová, E. (1995). Effects of urban noise pollution on blood pressure and heart rate in preschool children. *Journal of Hypertension, 13*, 405–12.

Rieser, J. J., Pick, H. L., Ashmead, D. H., & Garing, A. E. (1995). Calibration of human locomotion and models of perceptual-motor organization. *Journal of Experimental Psychology: Human Perception and Performance, 21*, 480–97.

Rolls, E. T., Robertson, R. G., & Georges-François, P. (1995). The representation of space in the primate hippocampus. *Society for Neuroscience Abstracts, 21*, 1492.

Russolo, L. (1913/1971). *The Art of Noise* (Futurist Manifesto). [Translated and reprinted in M. Kirby, *Futurist Performance* (New York: Dutton).]

Saegert, S. (1976). Stress-inducing and reducing qualities of environments. In H. M. Proshansky, W. H. Ittelson, & L. Rivlin (Eds.), *Environmental Psychology*, 2nd ed., pp. 218–23. New York: Holt, Rinehart & Winston.

Sarter, M., Berntson, G., & Cacioppo, J. T. (1996). Brain imaging and cognitive neuroscience: Toward strong inference in attributing function to structure. *American Psychologist, 51*, 13–21.

Schacter, D. L., & Nadel, L. (1991). Varieties of spatial memory: A problem for cognitive neuroscience. In R. G. Lister & H. J. Weingartner (Eds.), *Perspectives on Cognitive Neuroscience*. New York: Oxford University Press.

Schivelbusch, W. (1986). *The Railway Journey*. Berkeley: University of California Press.

Scholl, M. J. (1987). Cognitive maps as orienting schemata. *Journal of Experimental Psychology: Learning, Memory and Cognition, 13*, 615–28.

Shafer, E. L., Hamilton, J. F., & Schmidt, E. A. (1969). Natural landscapes preferences: A predictive model. *Journal of Leisure Research, 1*, 1–19.

Shemyakin, F. N. (1962). General problems of orientation in space and space representations. In B. G. Anan'yev, et al. (Eds.), *Psychological Science in the USSR*, vol. 1, pp. 184–225. NTIS Report no. TT62-11083, Office of Technical Services, Washington, DC. [As cited in Golledge & Stimson 1997.]

Sherry, D. F., Jacobs, L. F., & Gaulin, S. J. (1992). Spatial memory and adaptive specialization of the hippocampus. *Trends in Neuroscience, 15*, 298–303.

Shima, K., Nakahama, H., & Yamamoto, M. (1986). Firing properties of two types of nucleus raphe dorsalis neurons during the sleep–waking cycle and their responses to sensory stimuli. *Brain Research, 399*, 317–26.

Siegel, A. W., & White, S. H. (1975). The development of spatial representation of large-scale environments. In H. W. Reese (Ed.), *Advances in Child Development and Behavior*, vol. 10, pp. 9–55. New York: Academic Press.

Simons, D. J., & Wang, R. F. (1998). Perceiving real-world viewpoint changes. *Psychological Science, 9*, 315–20.

Singer, J. E., Lundberg, U., & Frankenhaeuser, M. (1978). Stress on the train: A study of urban commuting. In A. Baum, J. E. Singer, & S. Valins (Eds.), *Advances in Environmental Psychology*, vol. 1, pp. 41–56. Hillsdale, NJ: Erlbaum.

Smith, A. (1991). A review of the nonauditory effects of noise on health. *Work and Stress, 5*, 49–62.

Smookler, H. H., & Buckley, J. P. (1969). Relationships between brain catecholamine synthesis, pituitary adrenal function and the production of hypertension during prolonged exposure to environmental stress. *International Journal of Neuropharmacology, 8*, 33–41.

Spencer, C., Blades, M., & Morsley, K. (1989). *The Child in the Physical Environment: The Development of Spatial Knowledge and Cognition*. New York: Wiley.

Standing, L., Lynn, D., & Moxness, K. (1990). Effects of noise upon introverts and extroverts. *Bulletin of the Psychonomic Society, 28*, 138–40.

Stansfeld, S. A., & Haines, M. (1997). Environmental noise and health: A review of nonauditory effects. Report, Department of Health, London.

Steuer, J. (1992). Defining virtual reality: Dimensions determining telepresence. *Journal of Communications, 42*, 73–93.

Stevenson, D. C., & McKellar, N. R. (1988). The effect of traffic noise on sleep of young adults in their home. *Journal of the Acoustical Society of America, 85*, 768–71.

Stiles-Davis, J., Kritchevsky, M., & Bellugi, U. (Eds.) (1988). *Spatial Cognition: Brain Bases and Development*. Hillsdale, NJ: Erlbaum.

Stokols, D., & Altman, I. (Eds.) (1987). *Handbook of Environmental Psychology*. New York: Wiley.

Stone, A. A., Cox, D. S., Valdimarsdottir, H., Jandorf, L., & Neale, J. M. (1987). Secretory IgA as a measure of immunocompetence. *Journal of Human Stress, 13*, 136–40.

Stone, A. A., Neale, J. M., Cox, D. S., Napoli, A., Valdimarsdottir, H., & Kennedy-Moore, E. (1994). Daily events are associated with a secretory immune response to an oral antigen in men. *Health Psychology, 13*, 440–6.

Strube, M. J. (1990). Psychometric principles: From physiological data to psychological constructs. In Cacioppo & Tassinary (1990a), pp. 34–57.

Tafalla, R. J., & Evans, G. W. (1997). Noise, physiology and human performance: The potential role of effort. *Journal of Occupational Health Psychology, 2*, 148–55.

Tarnopolsky, A., Watkins, G., & Hand, D. J. (1980). Aircraft noise and mental health: I. Prevalence of individual symptoms. *Psychological Medicine, 10*, 683–98.

Tassinary, L. G. (1995). Unpublished lecture notes.

Taube, J. S., Goodridge, J. P., Golob, E. J., Dudchenko, P. A., & Stackman, R. W. (1996). Processing the head direction cell signal: A review and commentary. *Brain Research Bulletin, 40*, 477–86.

Taylor, N. A. S., Allsopp, N. K., & Parkes, D. G. (1995). Preferred room temperature of young vs. aged males: The influence of thermal sensation, thermal comfort and affect. *Journal of Gerontology: Medical Sciences, 50A*, M216–M221.

Thiessen, G. J., & Lapointe, A. C. (1978). Effect of intermittent truck noise on percentage of deep sleep. *Journal of the Acoustical Society of America, 64*, 1078–80.

Thomas, J. R., & Jones, D. M. (1982). Individual differences in noise annoyance and the uncomfortable loudness level. *Journal of Sound and Vibration, 82*, 289–304.

Thompson, S. (1996). Non-auditory health effects of noise: An updated review. In *Proceedings of the International Congress on Noise Control Engineering*, vol. 4, pp. 2177–82. St. Albans, U.K.: Institute of Acoustics.

Thorndyke, P. W. (1981). Spatial cognition and reasoning. In J. H. Harvey (Ed.), *Cognition, Social Behavior and the Environment*, pp. 137–49. Hillsdale, NJ: Erlbaum.

Thorndyke, P. W., & Hayes-Roth, B. (1982). Differences in spatial knowledge acquired from maps and navigation. *Cognitive Psychology, 14*, 560–89.

Tobias, J. V., Jansen, G., & Ward, W. D. (Eds.) (1980). *Noise as a Public Health Problem: Proceedings of the 3rd International Congress* (ASHA Reports, no. 10). Rockville, MD: American Speech-Language-Hearing Association.

Tolman, E. C. (1948). Cognitive maps in rats and men. *Psychological Review, 55,* 189–208.

Townsend, R. E., Johnson, L. C., & Muzet, A. (1973). Effects of the long term exposure to tone pulse noise on human sleep. *Psychophysiology, 10,* 369–76.

Tranel, D., & Damasio, H. (1994). Neuroanatomical correlates of electrodermal skin conductance responses. *Psychophysiology, 31,* 427–38.

Tulen, J. H. M., Kumar, A., & Jurriëns, A. A. (1986). Psychophysiological acoustics of indoor sound due to traffic noise during sleep. *Journal of Sound and Vibration, 110,* 129–41.

Turner, J. R. (1994). *Cardiovascular Reactivity and Stress: Patterns of Physiological Response.* New York: Plenum.

Ulrich, R. S. (1979). Visual landscapes and psychological well-being. *Landscape Research, 4,* 17–23.

Ulrich, R. S. (1981). Natural vs. urban scenes: Some psychophysiological effects. *Environment and Behavior, 13,* 523–56.

Ulrich, R. S. (1983). Aesthetic and affective response to natural environment. In Altman & Wohlwill, pp. 85–125.

Ulrich, R. S. (1984). View through a window may influence recovery from surgery. *Science, 224,* 420–1.

Ulrich, R. S., Simons, R., Losito, B. D., Fiorito, E., Miles, M. A., & Zelson, M. (1991). Stress recovery during exposure to natural and urban environments. *Journal of Environmental Psychology, 11,* 201–30.

Vallet, M., Gagneux, J. M., Blanchet, V., Favre, B., & Labiale, G. (1983a). Long-term sleep disturbance due to traffic noise. *Journal of Sound and Vibration, 90,* 173–91.

Vallet, M., Gagneux, J. M., Clairet, J. M., Laurens, J. F., & Letisserand, D. (1983b). Heart rate reactivity to aircraft noise after a longterm exposure. In *The 4th International Congress on Noise as a Public Health Problem,* pp. 965–71. Milan: Centro Richerche E Studi Amplifon.

Vallet, M., Gagneux, J. M., & Simonnet, F. (1980). Effects of aircraft noise on sleep: An *in situ* experience. In Tobias et al., pp. 391–6.

Van Dijk, F. J. H., Verbeek, J. H. A. M., & De Vries, F. F. (1987). Nonauditory effects of noise in industry, V: A field study in a shipyard. *International Archives of Occupational and Environmental Health, 59,* 55–62.

Vogt, B. A., Finch, D. M., & Olson, C. R. (1992). Functional heterogeneity in cingulate cortex: The anterior executive and posterior evaluative regions. *Cerebral Cortex, 2,* 435–43.

Ward, L. M., & Suedfeld, P. (1973). Human responses to highway noise. *Environmental Research, 6,* 306–26.

Weinstein, N. D. (1980). Individual differences in critical tendencies and noise annoyance. *Journal of Sound and Vibration, 68,* 241–8.

Welch, B. L. (1979). Extra-auditory health effects of industrial noise: Survey of foreign literature. Aerospace Medical Research Laboratory Technical report no. AMRL-TR-79-41. Wright-Patterson AFB, Ohio.

White, P. M., & Yee, C. M. (1997). Effects of attentional and stressor manipulations on the P50 gating response. *Psychophysiology, 34,* 703–11.

Whiteley, A. M., & Warrington, E. K. (1978). Selective impairment of topographic memory: A single case study. *Journal of Neurology, Neurosurgery and Psychiatry, 41,* 575–8.

Wiener, S. I., Paul, C. A., & Eichenbaum, H. (1989). Spatial and behavioral correlates of hippocampal neuronal activity. *Journal of Neuroscience, 9,* 2737–63.

Wilbrand, H. (1892/1982). Ein Fall von Seelenblindheit und Hemianopsie mit Sections-befund. *Deutsch. Z. Nervenheilk., 2,* 361–87. [As cited in DeRenzi 1982, chap. 8.]

Wilkinson, R. T., & Campbell, K. B. (1984). Effects of traffic noise on quality of sleep: Assessment by EEG, subjective report, or performance the next day. *Journal of the Acoustical Society of America, 75,* 468–75.

Zeltzer, D. (1992). Autonomy, interaction and presence. *Presence: Teleoperators and Virtual Environments, 1,* 127–32.

Zhao, Y., Zhang, S., Selvin, S., & Spear, R. (1993). A dose–response relationship between cumulative noise exposure and hypertension among female textile workers without hearing protection. In M. Vallet (Ed.), *Noise as a Public Health Problem: Proceedings of the 6th International Congress,* vol. 3, pp. 274–9. Arcuil Cedex, France: l'INRETS.

Zube, E., Pitt, D. G., & Anderson, W. T. (1975). Perception and prediction of scenic resource values in the Northeast. In E. Zube, R. Brush, & J. Fabos (Eds.), *Landscape Assessment.* Stroudsberg, PA: Dowden, Hutchinson & Ross.

PART FIVE

METHODOLOGY

CHAPTER THIRTY-ONE

PSYCHOMETRICS

MICHAEL J STRUBE

All scientists must grapple with the limitations of faulty observations. Rarely are the concepts that are embedded in theories easily revealed or conveniently available with little error. This is particularly the case in psychophysiology, where an attempt is made to link physical processes to psychological constructs. The ability to make those linkages rests on attention to important psychometric principles. After all, physiological measurement, like all other forms of measurement, is the replicable assignment of numbers to represent properties (cf. Campbell 1957). Accordingly, basic psychometric principles are as relevant to psychophysiological assessment as they are to the measurement of intelligence, the assessment of job performance, or the self-report of emotion. The purpose of this chapter is to provide a guide to the issues requiring attention when inferences about psychological constructs are based on the collection of physiological data. In the discussion that follows, the core psychometric issues relevant to measurement in any area will be outlined, but with an emphasis on their psychophysiological application.

A topic as broad as psychometrics cannot possibly be covered comprehensively in a single chapter. It ranges widely and includes topics and issues that overlap with research design and statistics.[1] There is a danger that a chapter attempting to summarize such a broad topic will devolve into a selective listing of formulas and facts. To avoid that problem, I will attempt to emphasize and illustrate a very simple theme that has wide-reaching implications: Science is essentially an error-correcting enterprise. The ability to uncover "truth" hinges on the ability to identify, estimate, and remove error from fallible observations. I will show how this theme underlies traditional psychometric principles and why psychophysiologists should be concerned about these principles. The emphasis will be on general principles to the exclusion of problems specific to particular modes of physiological measurement. The num-

ber of physiological systems now measured is so numerous and the technological advances are so rapid (see e.g. Cacioppo & Tassinary 1990b; Coles, Donchin, & Porges 1986; Druckman & Lacey 1989) that an attempt to discuss particular measurement problems would be highly selective and not particularly educational. Other chapters in this volume amply document the measurement nuances and idiosyncrasies for particular problem areas. It is worth emphasizing, however, that inadequate technical knowledge and inadequate statistical representation can hinder inferences for particular physiological measures, a point made persuasively by Cacioppo and Tassinary (1990a; see also Sarter, Berntson, & Cacioppo 1996). This chapter will focus instead on principles that are general to all psychophysiological measurement.

THE BASIC INFERENTIAL TASK

The behavioral sciences encompass a staggering number of topics, and even narrowing the focus to psychophysiology does not do much to reduce the impression of amazing diversity. Fortunately, all scientists attempt to solve the same basic problem depicted in Figure 1. The basic task of science is to make inferences about *hypothetical constructs* (e.g., stress, compliance, reactivity, attention, memory) that cannot be observed directly. This task requires operationalizing those constructs so that numbers can be attached to them in a meaningful way that can be replicated by others.[2] This allows the logic and power of research design and statistics to be brought to bear on the problem. It is this operationalization stage that also makes necessary the careful attention to psychometric principles, because the quality of the inferences about constructs and construct relations will depend on the quality of the measurements that will stand for or represent those constructs. The ability to make accurate and complete descriptive statements about the

John T. Cacioppo, Louis G. Tassinary, and Gary G. Berntson (Eds.), *Handbook of Psychophysiology,* 2nd ed. © Cambridge University Press 2000. Printed in the United States of America. ISBN 62634X. All rights reserved.

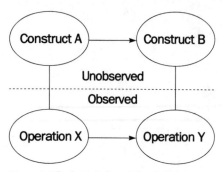

Figure 1. The basic inferential task in science.

constructs (e.g., how much stress a sample is experiencing) and the ability to make logically justified inferences about construct relations (e.g., stress is caused by control loss) rests on the extent to which the observations that represent those constructs possess desirable psychometric qualities.

The problem is illustrated by the simple example shown in Figure 2. Suppose that a researcher posed the hypothesis that control loss is stressful. This implies a causal relation between two constructs. This hypothesis would presumably be derived from some carefully developed conceptual model. These constructs, however, cannot be observed directly. Instead, clear, specific, and measurable operational definitions must be established that will "stand for" or represent the underlying constructs. Control loss, for example, might be operationally defined as the number of daily frustrations from a list of 40 possible frustrations that a person claims to have experienced on a given day. Stress might be defined by a physiological measure of reactivity such as systolic blood pressure. Two inferential problems are immediately obvious. First, under what conditions can we safely infer that a causal relation exists between number of daily frustrations and systolic blood pressure? Second, given that such an empirical inference is warranted, under what conditions can we make the more important inference that control loss is causally antecedent to the experience of stress? The answers to both questions rely on relatively error-free operational definitions. Psychometric principles guide the development of operational definitions that are (relatively) free of error.

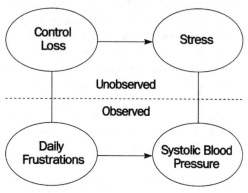

Figure 2. An example of the basic inferential task.

Before proceeding, it is important to emphasize another feature embedded in Figures 1 and 2 and assumed throughout this chapter: Scientific progress is guided by clear and carefully derived statements about constructs and construct relations. The ability to plan quality research and the ability to make clear inferences from that research depend on the clarity of the guiding conceptual model. The most conscientious attention to the psychometric principles discussed here will be wasted if those principles are applied to poorly defined conceptual hypotheses. Psychometric principles, then, are aids to – but not replacements for – creative thought and logical analysis.

With this basic view of the scientific inference process in mind, we can now turn to a discussion of the psychometric principles that guide the identification, estimation, and control of error in measurement.

Reliability

The ability to make inferences about constructs depends upon the ability to "see" those constructs clearly, that is, to have relatively error-free representations of them. Estimating and controlling error in measurement requires a theory about measurement that defines the nature of error in operational definitions. In the sections that follow, two measurement theories will be described. The first, known as *classical theory,* is very simple and provides a convenient vehicle for introducing some important ideas about measurement. It also is the view of measurement upon which many common reliability estimates are based. The classical view of reliability, however, has two important limitations: it views error as (i) entirely random and (ii) a unitary entity. A more complex and more realistic view of measurement, called *generalizability theory,* overcomes these limitations and provides a very general and far-reaching approach to measurement.

THE CLASSICAL THEORY OF RELIABILITY

The classical theory of reliability[3] assumes that an observation (x) is composed of a *true score* (t) and an *error score* (e), which are related in a very simple way:

$$x = t + e. \tag{1}$$

The true score is assumed to represent the standing of a given individual (or other object of measurement) on the construct of interest – that is, the score that would be obtained under ideal (error-free) conditions. The observed score deviates from the true score due to the influence of error, which in the classical view of reliability is assumed to be random. Random error is the noise against which the signal of the true score is detected; large amounts of random error obscure the scientist's ability to "see" the true score clearly.

According to the classical view, if an obtained score is composed of a true score and random error, then the variability of a sample of obtained scores (symbolized as σ_x^2) will likewise be composed of true score variance (σ_t^2) and error variance (σ_e^2):

$$\sigma_x^2 = \sigma_t^2 + \sigma_e^2. \tag{2}$$

This view of obtained score variability provides the basis for the classical definition of reliability. A relatively error-free measure will produce scores that vary because they contain more true score variance than error variance. In other words, the obtained scores will vary because the objects of measurement are truly different in terms of the construct being measured and not because of random differences. An intuitively appealing way to represent this idea is the proportion of obtained score variance that is due to true score variance,

$$\text{reliability} = \frac{\sigma_t^2}{\sigma_t^2 + \sigma_e^2}. \tag{3}$$

This ratio is, in fact, the classical definition of reliability, symbolized r_{xx} (see e.g. Nunnally & Bernstein 1994). The square root of the reliability coefficient estimates the correlation of obtained scores with true scores,

$$r_{xt} = \sqrt{r_{xx}}, \tag{4}$$

and emphasizes quite clearly that, as reliability increases, obtained scores become better estimates of true scores. This definition also makes clear why the reliability of a measure is often described with such terms as *consistency, repeatability,* and *dependability.* If a measure is reliable, then similar obtained score distributions should emerge on different measurement occasions because the true score component is assumed not to change over those measurement occasions.

Classical theory also allows a more formal statement of the way random error can obscure the ability to detect relationships between two operational definitions and thus thwart the goal of identifying causal relations (see Figures 1 and 2):

$$r_{xy} = \rho_{xy}\sqrt{r_{xx}r_{yy}}. \tag{5}$$

Here r_{xy} is the obtained correlation between two different operational definitions (x and y), ρ_{xy} is their correlation under conditions of perfect measurement, and r_{xx} and r_{yy} are the reliabilities associated with the measurement of x and y, respectively. Equation (5) makes one point quite clear: low reliability in *either* measure can impair the ability to detect relationships.[4]

Because classical theory assumes that error is random, it provides a convenient way to estimate reliability: the correlation between "parallel" measures over different measurement occasions. The logic is simple. If two measures of the same true score are correlated, then that correlation

can only be due to their shared true score variability; the random error components by definition cannot correlate with anything. By definition, a correlation is equal to a covariance between two measures divided by the standard deviations of those measures:

$$r_{xy} = \frac{\sigma_{xy}}{\sigma_x \sigma_y}. \tag{6}$$

If x and y are in deviation score form and are measures of the same true score (i.e., parallel forms), then their covariance takes on a familiar form:

$$
\begin{aligned}
\sigma_{xy} &= \frac{1}{n}\sum_1^n (t_i + e_{x_i})(t_i + e_{y_i}) \\
&= \frac{\sum_1^n t_i^2}{n} + \frac{\sum_1^n t_i e_{x_i}}{n} + \frac{\sum_1^n t_i e_{y_i}}{n} + \frac{\sum_1^n e_{x_i} e_{y_i}}{n} \\
&= \frac{\sum_1^n t_i^2}{n} = \sigma_t^2,
\end{aligned}
\tag{7}
$$

because true scores cannot correlate with the random error components nor can different random error components (e_{x_i} and e_{y_i}) correlate with each other. Furthermore, because the two measures are assumed to be parallel measures, σ_x and σ_y are assumed to be equal (at least in the population) and so the denominator of equation (6) can be assumed to equal the variance of either measure. Accordingly, the correlation between two measures of the same true score is equal to true score variance divided by obtained score variance – the classical definition of reliability. Thus, if two parallel measures are correlated then those measures must each be composed of shared true score variance; the higher the correlation, the more true score variance (relative to error variance) they contain. This idea gives rise to three popular reliability estimates: test–retest reliability, alternative forms reliability, and internal consistency.

Test–retest reliability is simply the correlation between the same measure on two different occasions. *Alternative forms reliability* is the correlation between two different measures, each assumed to measure the same true score, administered on different occasions. *Internal consistency* is based on the correlations among multiple items of one test or measure. In each case, the different measurement "occasions" (different times, different forms, different items) are assumed to differ only in their random components, so that the correlation between occasions reveals the relative amounts of true score variance that the measures contain. Of course, if the true score has changed between measurement occasions (i.e., the construct is unstable), then the reliability estimate is ambiguous as an indicator of measurement error.

In addition to providing a means of estimating reliability, the classical theory also suggests an important way to reduce error and make measures more reliable: *aggregation.* If multiple observed scores of the same construct are combined, the random sources of error that contaminate each observed score have a chance to cancel out and leave standing a better estimate of the true score. If a measure of a construct is based on a single observation, then the obtained score for a given individual will be biased up or down to some extent because of the random error. If we had a second observation that was also a measure of the same true score, it would also have an error component, but the direction in which this error influenced the obtained score would likely be different than for the first item (because error is random in the classical view). If we averaged the two observations, that average might provide a better measure because the two error components might partly cancel each other out. They will not completely cancel each other out unless their influences are directly opposite, but if we average more and more observations – each with its own random error source but measuring the same true score – then the odds of the error canceling out keep improving. This is a fundamental idea in measurement. Aggregating items or observations that measure the same true score will allow the random error components to cancel and provide a more reliable measure. In fact, the well-known Spearman–Brown prophesy formula is based on this idea (see Nunnally & Bernstein 1994).

Although we have emphasized r_{xx} as a measure of reliability, there is another way to view it. We could just as easily think about reliability of measures in terms of the amount of error those measures contain (σ_e^2). The square root of this variance, the *standard error of measure* (σ_{meas}), gauges the uncertainty inherent in an obtained score by providing an estimate of how much obtained scores would be expected to vary on subsequent measurement occasions even though the true score remained constant:

$$\sigma_{\text{meas}} = \sigma_x \sqrt{1 - r_{xx}}. \qquad (8)$$

The σ_{meas} communicates reliability in terms of the original scale of measurement, which can be quite revealing.

Although the classical view is very popular and widely used, it suffers from an important flaw: it views error as a unitary entity. This flaw may be shown by considering closely the different ways that reliability can be estimated. Each defines error in slightly different ways and thus the different estimates need not reach the same conclusions about reliability. For example, the internal consistency approach to reliability construes error as random fluctuations that vary across responses to multiple items given at the same time. Sources of error that might change from one day to another do not have any opportunity to show up as error. Indeed, on any one measurement occasion, such sources masquerade as true score because they impose a constant influence on the observed scores for all items for a particular individual. For example, a bad headache would impair my concentration and influence my responses to all items on a cognitive abilities test. I would not get the score

I truly deserve. On a different day, my headache might be better and so too would my performance, but not because of any change in my underlying cognitive abilities. Yet for any given measurement occasion, my health is not variable and so does not have an opportunity to emerge as a source of error. Instead, its constant status makes it act like true score. In contrast, test–retest reliability *would* show as error the health changes and other changes for individuals over time. The major point here is that a source of error only "counts" in classical theory if it can show variability for a particular individual across measurement occasions. Clearly, then, error is multidimensional, and a means of capturing this multidimensionality would provide a more powerful approach to estimating and controlling error.

GENERALIZABILITY THEORY

The major advantage of generalizability theory (Brennan 1992; Cronbach et al. 1972; Shavelson & Webb 1991; Shavelson, Webb, & Rowley 1989) over the traditional classical approach is its ability to specify and estimate more precisely the multiple sources of error that can contaminate obtained scores. This is accomplished by specifying carefully the conditions of measurement and estimating the influence of those conditions of measurement as sources of error variance in the obtained scores. In generalizability theory, the conditions of measurement are known as *facets*. A facet is simply a clearly defined way that measurement occasions can vary and so represents a potential source of influence on obtained scores in addition to true score variance. Different days on which a measure could be collected, for example, are a facet of measurement. Measures collected on one day could vary systematically from those collected on another day (an overall effect for everyone), or the relative standing of participants might differ across days. In either case, scores could vary by day so that any one obtained score would not necessarily provide a dependable indication of a person's real standing on the construct being measured. Multiple items on a test, multiple recordings on the same day, and multiple judges of the same behavior are all examples of measurement conditions that could introduce variability into obtained scores and so obscure the ability to detect true score differences. The list of possible measurement facets is very long and depends on the specific measurement problem. Accordingly, a key problem in generalizability theory is the identification of important measurement facets.

Generalizability theory gets its name from the idea that the ability to generalize obtained scores across conditions of measurement requires explicitly specifying and testing the conditions of measurement that might affect obtained score variability. Generalizability theory thus bounds conclusions about reliability to well-defined measurement facets. Collectively, these measurement facets define the *universe of admissible observations,* the boundaries within which the investigator considers observations potentially to be interchangeable. That exchangeability, however, is an empirical question. Thus, according to generalizability theory, there is no one reliability for a measure. Reliability depends on the conditions of measurement, and there are potentially as many reliabilities for a measure as there are unique uses or conditions of measurement.

Generalizability theory essentially defines true score and error more carefully than the traditional classical view. The somewhat nebulous idea of a true score is replaced in generalizability theory with the *universe score,* the average of all observations in the universe of admissible observations. Although this too is a hypothetical value, it is at least bounded by well-specified measurement conditions. The unitary error score of the classical view is replaced by several error scores, again defined by the conditions of measurement. Generalizability theory is designed to estimate these multiple components of obtained score variability and to use those components to explore the consequences of different sources of measurement error.

The variance estimation part of generalizability theory is known as a *generalizability study,* or *G-study* for short. G-studies can take several forms, defined by the design used to collect the measurements. For example, suppose that a researcher wished to explore the reliability of systolic blood pressure (SBP) measurement, perhaps because SBP is to be used in research on the cardiovascular effects of cognitive and physical challenges. The ability to detect changes in SBP relies on knowing a person's "true" blood pressure, but that true value might be obscured by several kinds of error (see e.g. Llabre et al. 1988). Hence, the G-study must be designed to include facets of measurement that could create variability in blood pressure readings so those sources of variability can be estimated separately. One source of variability will be characteristics of the participants in the study. In generalizability theory, this facet of measurement is known as the *object of measurement.* Variability for this facet is desirable and corresponds to true score variance in classical theory. This is referred to as the *p* facet for *persons* or *participants.* Another source of error might be called observer (*o*) and represents fluctuations that depend on the person recording the blood pressure (e.g., some variant of "white-coat syndrome"). Variability in the obtained scores due to ob-

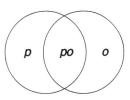

Figure 4. Sources of variance for a person (*p*) × observer (*o*) G-study.

server differences would be an undesirable source because it obscures the underlying universe score. If we have each observer collect the blood pressures from each person, the G-study is a *crossed design.* If we have two observers record blood pressures from five people, the data collection design would look like that depicted in Figure 3. In practice, of course, many more people would be sampled and more observers would be desirable so that sources of variance are estimated with higher precision.

Figure 4 displays a Venn diagram depicting the unique sources of variance in this *po* design. The sources indicate an expanded view of obtained score variability:

$$\sigma_x^2 = \sigma_p^2 + \sigma_o^2 + \sigma_{po}^2. \tag{9}$$

The variance estimates in a G-study are estimated from the mean squares provided by *analysis of variance,* which in this case yields three distinct sources of variance: person (*p*), observers (*o*), and person × observers (*po*) (for details on variance component estimation, see Cronbach et al. 1972; Shavelson & Webb 1991). With one exception, the mean squares in analysis of variance are not themselves pure variance component estimates. For the simple *po* design, the mean squares have the expected values

$$\text{EMS}(p) = \sigma_{po}^2 + n_o\sigma_p^2, \tag{10}$$

$$\text{EMS}(o) = \sigma_{po}^2 + n_p\sigma_o^2, \tag{11}$$

$$\text{EMS}(po) = \sigma_{po}^2, \tag{12}$$

which allows the following algebraic manipulation of mean squares to obtain variance component estimates:

$$\hat{\sigma}_p^2 = [\text{MS}_p - \text{MS}_{po}]/n_o, \tag{13}$$

$$\hat{\sigma}_o^2 = [\text{MS}_o - \text{MS}_{po}]/n_p, \tag{14}$$

$$\hat{\sigma}_{po}^2 = \text{MS}_{po}. \tag{15}$$

Rules for generating variance components from more complicated designs are described by Cronbach et al. (1972), Shavelson and Webb (1991), and Brennan (1992).

The person (*p*) component represents real differences in the systolic blood pressures of the participants. It is interpreted like any other variance, but in this case it refers to the variance of universe scores representing the average of all recordings in the universe of admissible observations. The observer (*o*) component represents systematic differences between the observers. For example, if readings were

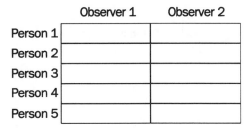

	Observer 1	Observer 2
Person 1		
Person 2		
Person 3		
Person 4		
Person 5		

Figure 3. Data collection design for a simple person × observer G-study.

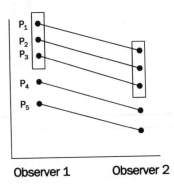

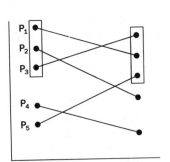

Figure 5. Sources of error for a relative decision.

systematically lower for one observer, perhaps due to that person's calmer demeanor, then this would show up in the *o* component of variance and would affect scores for all individuals equally. The person × observer (*po*) component reflects differences in the relative standing of participants for the two observers, plus any unaccounted for random sources of variability. The person × observer interaction might represent, for example, systematically different ways that particular individuals react to particular observers. These effects, however, cannot be separated from the random errors of measurement in this design.[5]

It should be clear by now that classical theory and generalizability theory view error in fundamentally different ways. In the classical view, random error is the only source of error. In generalizability theory, random error is a default category that represents error that could not be defined by conditions of measurement. Conditions of measurement reflect systematic ways in which obtained scores can vary that have nothing to do with the universe score variability, that is, systematic error. Stated more strongly: in generalizability theory, the presence of random error signals a relatively poor understanding of how measurement conditions affect obtained score variability.

The *o* and *po* components both represent sources of error, but their impact is different and depends on how objects of measurement will be distinguished. There are two kinds of distinctions that can be made. The first, known as a *relative decision*, reflects only the relative standing of the objects of measurement. The second, known as an *absolute decision*, takes the absolute value of the scores

into account as well. Figures 5 and 6 display the nature of these two decisions and the influence of different error components on them.

The top panel of Figure 5 shows that the two observers provide the same relative rank ordering for the participants. If we wanted to identify the participants with the three highest blood pressures, we would get the same answer from either observer. This occurs despite the fact that all recordings are systematically lower for the second observer. This reflects an observer effect (i.e., the *o* component would be large), but this source of error does not affect the relative decision. The bottom panel of Figure 5 depicts a different pattern. In this case, the relative standing of the participants is different for the two observers. This person × observer interaction obscures our ability to identify the three people with the highest blood pressures. The *po* component *is*, then, a source of error for a relative decision. More generally, any interaction that involves the object of measurement will be a source of error for relative decisions. Such interactions indicate that the differences between the objects of measurement shift in magnitude across facet levels, making it difficult to consistently identify their relative standing.

Figure 6 displays the same two data patterns but now with reference to a criterion score. This criterion might represent an established cut-off score for defining high blood pressure. In other words, rather than defining high blood pressure as the three highest scores, an external criterion is used. Now the absolute values of the recordings are important and not just their relative standing. As the

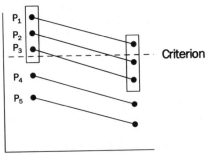

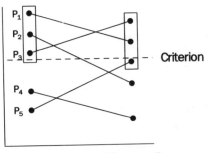

Figure 6. Sources of error for an absolute decision.

top panel indicates, the overall observer differences (i.e., the o component) influence whether a given participant exceeds the criterion. The bottom panel indicates that interactions involving the object of measure affect absolute decisions as well. Absolute decisions are influenced by any source of variance that influences the value of the obtained score. That means that all sources other than the object of measurement will be a source of error for absolute decisions.

The simple person × observer design could be expanded to include other facets. For example, we might include day of examination as an additional condition of measurement. On any given day, a person's blood pressure might be depressed or elevated for idiosyncratic reasons (e.g., attending a yoga class, drinking an extra cup of coffee). Those influences could obscure the detection of the person's true or typical blood pressure. The influence would be constant for a particular person on that day and so would be confused as true score; from the standpoint of identifying typical blood pressure, this person would not get the value he or she deserves. The only way to separate out this source of error is to include it explicitly in the measurement design. Adding a day (d) component to the design and crossing it with the other facets produces a completely crossed person × observer × day design. Figure 7 shows the sources of variance that can be estimated from this design. As before, the person (p) component is desirable variance. The remaining variance sources are error, and their influence depends on the type of decision that will be made. For relative decisions, the po, pd, and pod sources all make it difficult to know with confidence the relative standing of participants. The pd component reflects changes in the relative standing of the participants between the different days on which recordings are made. The pod component reflects changes in relative blood pressure that vary simultaneously by observer and day; this component also contains other random sources of error. All of the variance sources other than p would contaminate absolute decisions.

An example will help illustrate some of the points just made. Assume that a completely crossed random effects G-study with two observers and four days was conducted. The analysis of variance for that design produces seven sources of variation that are estimated by mean squares,

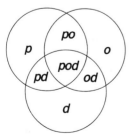

Figure 7. Sources of variance for a person (p) × observer (o) × day (d) G-study.

TABLE 1. Expected Mean Squares and Variance Component Estimation for a Completely Crossed Design (Persons × Observers × Days)

Expected Mean Squares

$$\mathrm{EMS}(p) = \sigma_{pod}^2 + n_o\sigma_{pd}^2 + n_d\sigma_{po}^2 + n_o n_d\sigma_p^2$$
$$\mathrm{EMS}(o) = \sigma_{pod}^2 + n_p\sigma_{od}^2 + n_d\sigma_{po}^2 + n_p n_d\sigma_o^2$$
$$\mathrm{EMS}(d) = \sigma_{pod}^2 + n_p\sigma_{od}^2 + n_o\sigma_{pd}^2 + n_p n_o\sigma_d^2$$
$$\mathrm{EMS}(po) = \sigma_{pod}^2 + n_d\sigma_{po}^2$$
$$\mathrm{EMS}(pd) = \sigma_{pod}^2 + n_o\sigma_{pd}^2$$
$$\mathrm{EMS}(od) = \sigma_{pod}^2 + n_p\sigma_{od}^2$$
$$\mathrm{EMS}(pod) = \sigma_{pod}^2$$

Estimated Variance Components

$$\hat{\sigma}_p^2 = (\mathrm{MS}_p - n_o\hat{\sigma}_{pd}^2 - n_d\hat{\sigma}_{po}^2 - \hat{\sigma}_{pod}^2)/(n_o n_d)$$
$$\hat{\sigma}_o^2 = (\mathrm{MS}_o - n_p\hat{\sigma}_{od}^2 - n_d\hat{\sigma}_{po}^2 - \hat{\sigma}_{pod}^2)/(n_p n_d)$$
$$\hat{\sigma}_d^2 = (\mathrm{MS}_d - n_p\hat{\sigma}_{od}^2 - n_o\hat{\sigma}_{pd}^2 - \hat{\sigma}_{pod}^2)/(n_p n_o)$$
$$\hat{\sigma}_{po}^2 = (\mathrm{MS}_{po} - \hat{\sigma}_{pod}^2)/n_d$$
$$\hat{\sigma}_{pd}^2 = (\mathrm{MS}_{pd} - \hat{\sigma}_{pod}^2)/n_o$$
$$\hat{\sigma}_{od}^2 = (\mathrm{MS}_{od} - \hat{\sigma}_{pod}^2)/n_p$$
$$\hat{\sigma}_{pod}^2 = \mathrm{MS}_{pod}$$

---

whose expected values are listed in Table 1. As can be seen, each mean square (with one exception) is a linear combination of variance components. Accordingly, some simple algebraic manipulation can isolate each variance component for the generalizability theory analysis. Some hypothetical variance components are listed in Table 2, which also lists the proportions of the total variance (the sum of all the variance components) accounted for by each component so that their relative size can be gauged more easily. The largest source of variance is universe score variability (p), indicating that much of the total variability is due to real differences in systolic blood pressure – at least as defined within this universe of admissible observations. The remaining sources of variability are error, and some of them are relatively large. For example, the person × day (pd) component accounts for 17% of the variance in total

TABLE 2. Hypothetical Variance Components for a Completely Crossed G-Study of Systolic Blood Pressure Measurement

Source of Variance	Component of Variance	Proportion of Total Variance
Person (p)	180	0.40
Observer (o)	25	0.06
Day (d)	15	0.03
po	40	0.09
pd	75	0.17
od	10	0.02
pod	105	0.23

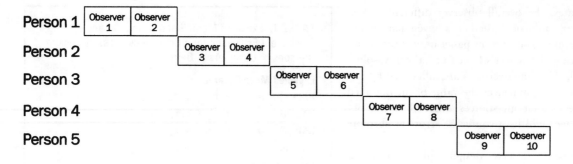

Figure 8. Data collection design with observers (*o*) nested within persons (*p*).

variability. This component reflects a shift in the relative differences of individuals over days and makes all decisions – relative and absolute – less reliable. By contrast, the modest *o* effect (only 6% of the variance) would hinder only absolute decisions.

There is one other design variation that arises frequently in generalizability studies: *nested designs.* In the simple design with observers as the only condition of measurement, it might not be possible to have the same observers test each participant. Instead, a different pair of observers might test each participant (perhaps this would occur if participants were patients being seen in different physicians' offices). In this case, observers are no longer crossed with persons; rather, they are nested within persons. The data collection design is shown in Figure 8 and is sometimes symbolized as *o : p* to indicate that observers (*o*) are nested (:) within persons (*p*). The major consequence of nesting is that some variance components that can be estimated separately in a crossed design are confounded in a nested design. As the Venn diagram in Figure 9 shows, the person × observer (*po*) interaction cannot be separated from the observer (*o*) effect. The overlap of the observer component and the person component (which defines the interaction *po*) is completely contained in the observer (*o*) component. Only two components of variance can be estimated in this design: a *p* component and a combined component that contains both the *o* source of variance and the *po* source of variance.

Designs can have both crossed and nested features. For example, the person × observer × day design might not be feasible. Although it might be possible to assess all participants on each day (person and day are crossed), it might not be possible for each observer to record the blood pressures of all participants. This creates a partially nested design (see Figure 10). With observers nested within persons, the observer (*o*) source of variance is confounded with the person × observer (*po*) interaction. As Figure 10 indicates, the *od* and *pod* sources of variance are also confounded. Consequently, only five sources of variance can be estimated from this design.

Generalizability theory makes one additional important distinction: random versus fixed effects. An effect is *random* if the facet levels are considered exchangeable with any other facet levels.[6] By contrast, an effect is *fixed* if the levels used are the only ones of interest. When an effect is fixed, there is no intent to generalize to some larger population, either because there is no larger population (all facet levels are included) or because the ones included in the study are the only ones that the researcher cares about. This distinction between fixed and random effects is important for appropriate estimation of variance components. Two approaches have been recommended (see Shavelson & Webb 1991). First, separate generalizability analyses can be carried out at each level of the fixed effect. This makes sense if each level of the fixed effect was selected because there was particular interest in that level. Second, if a researcher wants an overall average of the generalizability of the measure, then averaging across the fixed effects is another option (Cronbach et al. 1972; Shavelson & Webb 1991). However, large variance components for the fixed effect

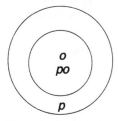

Figure 9. Sources of variance for a design with observers (*o*) nested within persons (*p*).

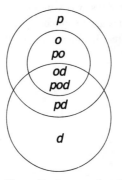

Figure 10. Sources of variance for a partially nested design in which observers (*o*) are nested within persons (*p*) and both are crossed with days (*d*).

would dictate caution in using the averaging approach, because it obscures an important source of variance.

Just like classical theory, generalizability theory also provides coefficients that gauge the reliability of measures. These coefficients, however, are calculated differently depending on the kind of decision that will be made about the objects of measurement. Reliability estimates for relative decisions, called *generalizability coefficients,* represent the proportion of obtained score variance that is due to universe score variance:

$$E\rho^2 = \frac{\sigma_p^2}{\sigma_p^2 + \sigma_\delta^2}. \tag{16}$$

The term σ_δ^2 refers to the error variance for a relative decision and varies according to the type of design used in the G-study. For the examples described previously, the error terms would be:

$$po: \sigma_\delta^2 = \frac{\sigma_{po}^2}{n_o}, \tag{17}$$

$$pod: \sigma_\delta^2 = \frac{\sigma_{po}^2}{n_o} + \frac{\sigma_{pd}^2}{n_d} + \frac{\sigma_{pod}^2}{n_o n_d}, \tag{18}$$

$$d(o:p): \sigma_\delta^2 = \frac{\sigma_{o,po}^2}{n_o} + \frac{\sigma_{pd}^2}{n_d} + \frac{\sigma_{od,pod}^2}{n_o n_d}, \tag{19}$$

where n_o and n_d refer to the number of facet levels for observers and days, respectively. The first term and the last term in (19) reflect the fact that some variance components cannot be estimated separately in nested designs. For the example in Table 2, the generalizability coefficient is

$$E\rho^2 = \frac{\sigma_p^2}{\sigma_p^2 + \dfrac{\sigma_{po}^2}{n_o} + \dfrac{\sigma_{pd}^2}{n_d} + \dfrac{\sigma_{pod}^2}{n_o n_d}}$$

$$= \frac{0.40}{0.40 + \dfrac{0.09}{2} + \dfrac{0.17}{4} + \dfrac{0.23}{2(4)}} = 0.77. \tag{20}$$

For absolute decisions, the reliability coefficient is called the *index of dependability* (symbolized as ϕ; Brennan & Kane 1977) and is defined as follows:

$$\phi = \frac{\sigma_p^2}{\sigma_p^2 + \sigma_\Delta^2}. \tag{21}$$

The term σ_Δ^2 refers to the error variance for absolute decisions. For the designs described previously, those error terms are

$$po: \sigma_\Delta^2 = \frac{\sigma_o^2}{n_o} + \frac{\sigma_{po}^2}{n_o}, \tag{22}$$

$$pod: \sigma_\Delta^2 = \frac{\sigma_o^2}{n_o} + \frac{\sigma_d^2}{n_d} + \frac{\sigma_{od}^2}{n_o n_d}$$
$$+ \frac{\sigma_{po}^2}{n_o} + \frac{\sigma_{pd}^2}{n_d} + \frac{\sigma_{pod}^2}{n_o n_d}, \tag{23}$$

$$d(o:p): \sigma_\Delta^2 = \frac{\sigma_d^2}{n_d} + \frac{\sigma_{o,po}^2}{n_o} + \frac{\sigma_{pd}^2}{n_d} + \frac{\sigma_{od,pod}^2}{n_o n_d}. \tag{24}$$

Using equation (23), the example in Table 2 yields an index of dependability of 0.72, smaller than the generalizability coefficient because of the additional sources of error that hinder absolute decisions.

Several aspects of the reliability estimates provided by generalizability theory are clear from equations (16)–(24). First, reliability estimates are design dependent. Second, reliability depends on the number of facet levels (i.e., the aggregation principle). Third, reliability depends on the type of decision that will be made. Finally, reliability depends as much on the universe score variance (σ_p^2) as it does on error variance. This is a key point. Inadequate sampling of the objects of measurement can distort reliability estimates. This can occur because a restricted sample does not fairly capture the natural variation in the objects of measurement or because intentional sampling inflates the apparent variability of the objects of measurement. A fair sample represents a random sample from the population to which inferences will be made. All of these points underscore a comment made earlier that there are as many reliabilities for a measure as there are conditions of measurement. In other words, there is an external validity to reliability estimation that is quite explicitly modeled by generalizability theory.

Generalizability theory clearly provides a powerful way to determine the multiple sources of error in a measure. It provides an equally powerful way to estimate the consequences of those error sources so that future measurement efforts can be planned carefully. In generalizability theory, these forecasting and planning efforts are known as *decision studies,* or D-studies for short. A D-study uses the variance components from the G-study to pose "what if" questions about future possible ways to collect data. Different D-studies can estimate the consequences of changing the number of facet levels (i.e., the aggregation principle) and the consequences of changing the data collection and decision design (i.e., the definition of error).

The essential difference between a G-study and a D-study is that data are collected and variance components are estimated in a G-study; those variance components are then used in D-studies to pose questions about alternative data collection options. The different data collection options (facets and facet levels) define the *universe of admissible generalization,* the D-study parallel to the universe of admissible observations in the G-study. In a D-study, the number of facet levels and their arrangements are modified to determine how reliability changes with different

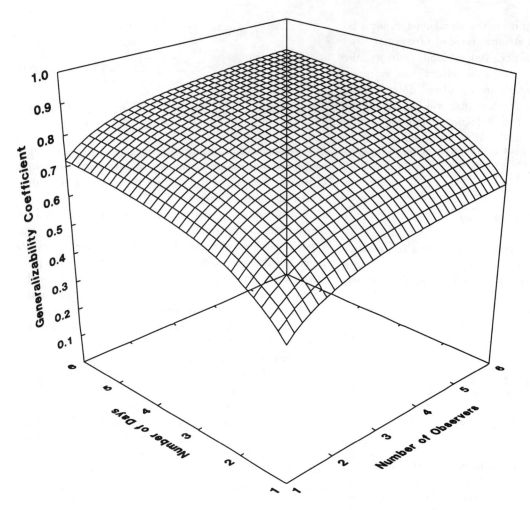

Figure 11. D-study results for a completely crossed design using variance components from Table 2.

kinds of designs. For example, the D-study generalizability coefficient for a person × observer × day design would be defined as

$$E\rho^2 = \frac{\sigma_p^2}{\sigma_p^2 + \dfrac{\sigma_{po}^2}{n_o'} + \dfrac{\sigma_{pd}^2}{n_d'} + \dfrac{\sigma_{pod}^2}{n_o'n_d'}}, \qquad (25)$$

where the primes indicate that, rather than being a constant as in the G-study, the number of facet levels is free to vary in the D-study.[7]

Using the variance components from Table 2, Figure 11 illustrates the impact on the generalizability coefficient for a crossed design of varying the numbers of observers and days of observation. As expected, reliability increases as the number of observers and days increases, but the rate of increase is different for the two facets; increasing the number of days has a larger influence. This could have been anticipated from Table 2 in which the *pd* component is the largest source of error; hence that component will show the largest effect of aggregation. Nonetheless,

Figure 11 also shows that aggregation over both days and observers will be necessary to achieve a modest reliability (with modest cost).

Figure 12 represents the same information as Figure 11 but with reference to the standard error of measure (i.e., the square root of the error variance). The same conclusions would be drawn from this figure, but it represents reliability in the metric of the measure that will be used. This allows a better sense of the uncertainty we will have about a person's systolic blood pressure for different combinations of observers and days of observation.[8] For example, with two observers and two days of observation, the standard error for a relative decision will be 9.15. Using this to set confidence intervals reveals that the same universe score would be consistent with obtained scores that differ by as much as 37 points (with 95% confidence; see Feldt & Brennan 1989 or Nunnally & Bernstein 1994). This might be quite sobering and more informative to a researcher or practitioner than knowing that the generalizability coefficient under these conditions is 0.68.

The design is free to vary, too, provided the appropriate variance components are available from the G-study. For example, the G-study might have been a completely crossed design, but different D-studies could explore partially

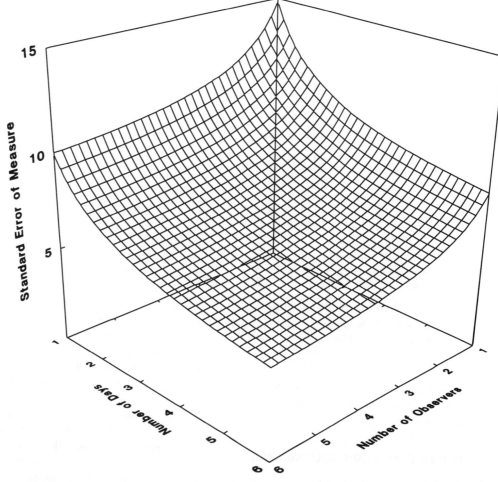

Figure 12. Projected standard errors of measure for a completely crossed design using variance components from Table 2.

nested (e.g., $d(o : p)$) or completely nested (e.g., $o : d : p$) options. Each D-study, then, defines a different universe of admissible generalization. This allows careful planning that can optimize reliability while taking design cost into account (Marcoulides & Goldstein 1990). If two designs produce essentially the same reliability then the researcher can choose the one that is easier or is less costly to conduct. Alternatively, for a fixed cost a researcher can identify the design that maximizes reliability.

A D-study can be used to ask "trade-off" questions as well. We can ask, for example, what numbers of observers and days of observation will produce a reliability or standard error of a given amount. Figure 13 displays the results of asking this question for a completely crossed design and a generalizability coefficient of 0.80, a common reliability benchmark. Clearly more than one day of observation will be necessary, and the trade-off to limiting the number of days is a larger number of observers. Depending on the costs of training observers and collecting data over multiple days, a sensible combination of observers and days can be determined. If no combination will produce the desired reliability at a reasonable cost, then efforts must be made to reduce error in other ways (e.g. standardization) or through inclusion of additional measurement facets. However, any

change in the measurement protocol must be accompanied by a new G-study to estimate new variance components.

The results in Figures 11, 12, and 13 assume that a relative decision will be made using a completely crossed design, yet D-studies can determine the consequences for other designs and other decisions. If the blood pressure readings will be used to identify at-risk individuals, then an external criterion will be used; the decision is absolute and subject to more sources of error. If the crossed design is unrealistic, then D-studies can be used to explore the consequences of nesting. Note that D-studies are limited only by the design of the original G-study: they cannot address questions about measurement facets that were not included in the original G-study, nor can they estimate the consequences of different designs if the variance components are not available from the G-study. Had the G-study been a partially nested day × (observer within person) design, then separate estimates of the o, po, od, and pod components of variance would not be available – they would be contained in confounded variance components. Consequently, it would not be possible to conduct D-studies for designs

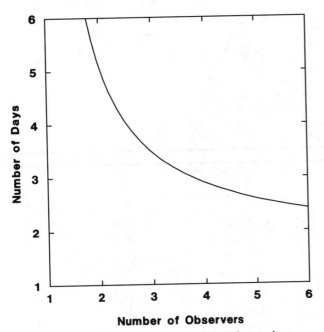

Figure 13. Combinations of observers and days that produce a generalizability coefficient of 0.80 (based on variance components from Table 2).

requiring separate variance components for these effects. The widest range of D-study questions can be posed if the G-study is completely crossed.[9]

IDENTIFYING AND CONTROLLING ERROR

Generalizability theory emphasizes the estimation of separate error components, but that estimation hinges on correctly identifying those error components in the first place. Incorrect identification of error sources can lead to faulty interpretations (see Schmidt & Hunter 1996 for an excellent discussion of the general problem of error identification and correction). One common problem is to ignore "hidden" facets. For example, a researcher might administer multiple items to a group of respondents on one occasion and forget that, although occasion is a constant in the study, it likely will be a source of variability and thus should be considered as error in application. The problem is that occasion variance (what Schmidt & Hunter 1996 call transient error) acts like a constant for each individual on a given occasion and so is counted as true score or universe score for each individual. It may be idiosyncratic for each object of measurement or it may be constant for all objects of measurement. Either way, its effect will be indistinguishable from universe score variance. For example, the systolic blood pressure of participants could be temporarily elevated or depressed on any given occasion in ways that are idiosyncratic (e.g., one person meditated that day, another person nearly had a traffic accident) or constant for all (e.g., the fire alarm was activated in the building on the day of examination). These sources exert

a systematic effect that cannot be distinguished from the universe score on a single measurement occasion. Their status as error is only revealed through their variability over multiple measurement occasions. The effect of transient error can only be estimated if multiple occasions are included in the measurement design.

Similarly, error specific to a particular test condition or mode of measurement (what Schmidt & Hunter 1996 refer to as specific error) can masquerade as universe score variance unless test condition or measurement mode is explicitly included in the measurement design and its contribution to error is estimated (see e.g. Llabre et al. 1988, 1991). The G-study in our example could be expanded to include a standard mercury sphygmomanometer, a Dynamap automatic blood pressure monitor, and an ambulatory blood pressure monitor (Llabre et al. 1988). Variability due to measurement mode could then be estimated (although in this example it might be argued that measurement mode is a fixed effect). The general principle here is simple: Universe score variability and error variability depend on the conditions of measurement and the conditions of application. Careful attention must be given to what should count as error, and the measurement design must then be constructed such that all sources of error can emerge and be estimated correctly.

There is, of course, another option for the control of error. Rather than letting an error source be free to vary and harnessing that error through aggregation, the error source could also be controlled effectively through standardization. Standardization is simply the attempt to control the measurement conditions carefully so that no extraneous sources of error are allowed to influence scores. For example, the same instructions delivered in the same way should precede a measure. Otherwise, individuals' obtained scores might vary slightly in response to differences in instructions, and that would be an additional source of error that obscures our ability to detect the true score. Similarly, environmental conditions should be the same for all respondents; otherwise, respondents' scores could vary depending on temperature, humidity, or ambient noise. The important point about standardization is that when measurement conditions are standardized, potential sources of variance become constants and so cannot influence the variability of obtained scores. When is an error source a constant and when is it a hidden facet? That depends on the intended application. Conditions that will be free to vary in an application must be free to vary – and their influence estimated – in a generalizability study.

Three additional points about error are pertinent. First, reliability of measurement does not ensure sensitivity of measurement. A poor choice of measurement instrument may preclude detecting the phenomenon of interest even though what is detected is done so reliably. The distinction here is between a measure's reliability and its sensitivity. For example, verbal reports of physical symptoms may be quite reliable, but they are notoriously insensitive to specific visceral reactions (Pennebaker 1982). Second, reliable measurement alone will not ensure a correct causal inference. Reliability increases the maximum possible correlation that can be detected between two operational definitions (equation (5)), but this does not imply that a causal relation exists between those operational definitions. Additional requirements for inferring causality must be considered (i.e., internal validity; see Cook & Campbell 1979). In fact, reliable measures may fail to reveal associations between variables because other statistical assumptions are not met (i.e., statistical conclusion validity; see Cook & Campbell 1979). Finally, standards of reliability should be recognized as arbitrary and crude benchmarks for the control of error in measurement. To be sure, with reliability, higher is better. But attempting to achieve a particular reliability value may provide only a crude approximation to the real goal of keeping measurement error at a known level or achieving an acceptably sensitive test for an effect of known size. Accordingly, concerns about statistical power (see e.g. Bollen 1989; Fleiss & Shrout 1977; Humphreys & Drasgow 1989; Kopriva & Shaw 1991; Williams & Zimmerman 1989; Zimmerman & Williams 1986) and the setting of confidence intervals should guide the choice of a reliability value to achieve.

Validity

Validity is traditionally defined as the extent to which a measure assesses what it purports to measure. Perhaps a better way to think about validity is the appropriateness of the label that is applied to a given application for a measure (Messick 1989). This reminds us that, as with reliability, there are as many validities for a measure as there are applications for it.

The basic problem of *in*validity can be viewed as an extension of our previous discussion of reliability. In classical theory an obtained score is conceptualized as being composed of a true score plus a random error score. In generalizability theory, this idea was expanded to include multiple error sources, some of them systematic. That is, in generalizability theory, there may be some components of variance that exert a predictable influence on the scores of individuals even though those components have nothing to do with the true or universe score. If those variance sources (e.g. observers) influence the obtained variability to a great extent then the labeling of the measure as an indication of stress could be inappropriate, especially if the universe score variability is quite small. In this sense, generalizability theory is appropriately described as blending the concepts of reliability and validity (Shavelson & Webb 1991). It suggests as well that the two concerns of psychometrics – reliability and validity – each address aspects of measurement error. Invalidity represents the erroneous labeling of what an operational definition means.

More generically, the conceptualization of an obtained score can be displayed simply as

$$x = t_1 + t_2 + e, \qquad (26)$$

where t_1 represents the true score of primary interest, t_2 represents the true score for another construct, and e (as before) represents random error. If the variability in x due to t_1 is substantial, then the label applied to x is appropriate – it is valid. If, however, the variability in x is due primarily to t_2, then a label based on t_1 would be invalid. For example, heart rate would be a relatively poor measure of sympathetic nervous system influence because it is affected by both sympathetic (t_1) and parasympathetic (t_2) systems.

Strictly speaking, then, a measure is not validated; rather, the interpretation or purpose for which the measure will be used is validated. Accordingly, the number of validities for a measure can vary considerably (see e.g. Fahrenberg et al. 1986). The ways that measures can be validated can likewise vary widely. Indeed, it would be accurate to say that most of science is a process of validation. There are several well-defined approaches to validation, and our review will emphasize some useful points.

CONTENT VALIDATION

Content validation is a consensual approach that relies on expert agreement about the content universe or domain, the degree to which a given indicator or item represents that domain, and the degree to which a collection of indicators adequately represents all facets of the domain. Representation here might include issues about the appropriate measurement circumstances and the particular profile or patterning of responses over time or situation (Cacioppo & Tassinary 1990a). The question is essentially whether a given operational definition is a good proxy for the underlying construct – that is, the extent to which most experts agree that it "stands for" the construct. Broadly speaking, content validity refers to consensus on the universe of admissible observations.

There are two distinct types of content validation. The first and more common approach is to assess expert agreement about representativeness after the measure has been developed. For example, if our intent were to assess cardiovascular function, then we could propose a set of indicators (e.g., systolic blood pressure, diastolic blood pressure, pulse transit time, forearm blood volume, heart rate) and measure expert agreement concerning the suitability of each indicator and the representativeness of any set of indicators. This might be accomplished by (i) having a group of experts rate each indicator, indicator profile, and measurement circumstance (e.g., on a seven-point scale) according to their appropriateness given the construct definition and then (ii) assessing expert agreement using generalizability theory (see e.g. Crocker, Llabre, & Miller 1988).[10]

A second and more preferred approach is to use expert opinion in the measurement development phase. Each expert would generate indicators or measurement conditions believed to be appropriate given the construct definition. Those indicators or measurement conditions generated by a sizable majority of the experts would be selected for inclusion (e.g., parallel panels approach; Ghiselli, Campbell, & Zedeck 1981). For example, experts could be queried about the times of day, testing conditions, and other situational influences that should be covered to ensure adequate sampling of the blood pressure domain (cf. Pickering et al. 1982). These facets of measurement can affect the obtained scores and potentially challenge the preferred labeling of those obtained scores. Similarly, expert opinion can be sought about the appropriate response dimensions to use (e.g., amplitude, frequency), the correct profile to construct, or the appropriate ways to represent a measure statistically. Accordingly, it is more appropriate to speak of content-oriented measurement development than of content validation (Guion 1978).

Not surprisingly, content validation is easiest when constructs are simple and well-defined. In this case the body of content is clear and there is a greater likelihood of agreement among experts. But even for relatively concrete constructs, the content validation approach is not without problems. One crucial decision is selection of experts. They should possess technical competence, have adequate knowledge of the field, and be unbiased in their research and theoretical orientations. An aggressive attempt should be made to prevent the kind of confirmatory bias that can so easily enter into validation attempts as a function of the critical choices made in structuring the research setting (Greenwald 1975; Greenwald et al. 1986).

Content validation is easiest when the "distance" from the construct to the operation is fairly short. When the construct is more abstract, the identification of an adequate sample of operational definitions is more difficult. In this case, the content validation approach can be thought of as an initial quality check on the operational definitions with the need for additional construct validation.

CRITERION-RELATED VALIDATION

A second approach to validation – the criterion-related approach – is essentially based on the desire for a measure that can substitute for the criterion. In other words, there is an agreed-upon "gold standard" but (a) the criterion is too difficult or costly to assess, (b) the criterion has not yet occurred but a measure that can predict its likely occurrence is desired, or (c) the criterion has occurred in the past but is no longer directly accessible. These three are referred to respectively as *concurrent* validity, *predictive* validity, and *postdictive* validity. An example of concurrent validity is the substitution of X-rays for the more costly but more accurate surgical detection of tumors. An

example of predictive validity is the search for cardiovascular markers of future hypertension and coronary disease. An example of postdictive validation is the use of electrocardiography to determine past occurrence of myocardial infarction.

Criterion-related validation is common in psychophysiology owing to the cost, invasiveness, and difficulty of measuring physiological variables for certain samples or under specific conditions. Examples include the substitution of self-reported sleep for physiologically documented sleep (Hoch et al. 1987), development of an efficient measure of sleep parameters for use in the home (Helfand, Lavie, & Hobson 1986), investigation of an indirect measure of beat-to-beat change in blood pressure (Shapiro et al. 1981), and development of a measure of neonate blood pressure (Hall et al. 1982).

In choosing the criterion-related approach to validation, researchers need to be aware of some potential dangers. First, selection of a criterion may be quite arbitrary and no more representative of the construct than the proposed predictor. The criterion is ideally the most appropriate operational definition from a theoretical standpoint that has itself been validated rigorously. Accordingly, the criterion-related approach should not become a mindlessly empirical effort in which, in order to find a suitable substitute, any measure is correlated with the criterion but without regard for the theoretical appropriateness or meaning of the predictor. To be sure, for some applied problems there is often little interest in the nature of the predictor so long as it provides a statistically reliable means of assessing the past, current, or future presence of the criterion. This is not necessarily inappropriate if one's interests are purely functional. More care is necessary, however, if advances in conceptual understanding are to be gained. Note as well that a purely empirical search for predictors places one at the mercy of correlations that are either inflated owing to chance or dependent on unknown moderator variables.

A second danger is the assumption of an isomorphic relation between the criterion and the proxy. Their consistent and perhaps high association does not necessarily warrant the conclusion that they have a one-to-one relation (see Cacioppo & Tassinary 1990a). Although a proxy variable might be highly associated with a criterion, the proxy could well have a different pattern of relations with other constructs that could alter the meaning of the proxy. This problem highlights that linking a measure to an existing criterion is a valuable validation tool yet is *not* a complete validation exercise. Additional evidence is needed to establish firmly the correct label for a measure.

The practical utility of the criterion-related approach is limited in that it presupposes that a carefully validated and reliable criterion has already been established (Cole, Howard, & Maxwell 1981). In one sense, then, the criterion-related approach to validation represents a somewhat later phase in a complete validation program: (a) an

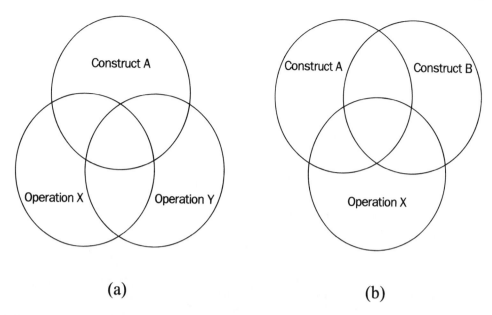

(a)   (b)

Figure 14. Two problems with operational definitions: (a) underrepresentativeness; (b) overrepresentativeness.

important construct is identified and defined, (b) an operational definition of that construct is developed (perhaps via content validation), (c) the link between construct and operational definition is validated (via construct validation), and (d) a decision is made to find additional operational definitions that are easier to obtain than the original and that can be used in future theory-based and applied research. The validity of these additional operational definitions is examined via the criterion-related approach with the original operational definition as the criterion (see Ghiselli et al. 1981 for a discussion of additional statistical issues that can arise with the criterion-related approach), and the validity of that criterion-based label is further verified via construct validation. A good example of a criterion-related substitute measure is the use of glycosylated hemoglobin (HbA_1) as an indicator of recent compliance with a blood glucose control regimen (Bunn 1981; Kennedy & Merimee 1981). (For comments about the validity of a biochemical index of smoking behavior, see Bliss & O'Connell 1984.)

CONSTRUCT VALIDATION

Although content validation and criterion-related validation are important parts of the measurement labeling process, more convincing evidence for an operational definition's interpretation derives from *construct* validation. The hallmark of the construct validation process is the placement of a construct within a network of logically and theoretically justified constructs and construct relations along with specifications as to how these translate into observable operational definitions (i.e., a nomological network – Cronbach & Meehl 1955; Messick 1981). The validation of a construct then entails validating the multiple operation-level relations that are derived. The network or theory surrounding the constructs informs and guides

the researcher as to the operational definitions that should and should not be related and also to the direction and magnitude of those relations. For example, if we were attempting to validate systolic blood pressure as a measure of stress, our theory might dictate that stress occurs in response to control loss (see Figure 2). Accordingly, establishing an empirical relation between control loss and systolic blood pressure provides *partial* validation of systolic blood pressure as a measure of stress. Other empirical relations (e.g., correlations with other validated measures of stress) would add to or detract from our confidence in this interpretation, depending on their magnitude and the conditions under which they are obtained. So too would relations with non–stress-related measures; these relations would challenge the appropriateness of the label.

Demonstrating construct validity is typically hampered by two common characteristics of operational definitions: (i) any one operational definition may capture only part of the underlying construct, and (ii) operational definitions are multidimensional and may represent two or more constructs. These relations are depicted in Figure 14 (see also Cook & Campbell 1979; Fiske 1987). Note that the claim that a construct is either underrepresented or overrepresented at the operation level assumes that the construct is clearly defined in the first place. Consequently, construct invalidity can be seen to arise from problems with methods or operations (this point is argued in a very compelling fashion by Fiske 1987).

The dangers of incomplete representation are twofold. First, it is possible that a particularly crucial aspect of the construct has been missed. For example, the full range of a construct may not be included in an experimental manipulation. Failure to find an empirical relation between the operational definitions might then lead to the inference that the constructs are not related when in fact an adequate test has not been performed. In psychophysiology, exclusive use of verbal reports to measure stress or emotion may lead to the conclusion that a stimulus has no long-lasting effects on behavior. But this may be incorrect, as Zillmann (1978) demonstrated in his work on excitation transfer. Zillmann found that residual arousal from a prior stimulus (e.g. physical exercise) can influence later behavior (e.g. aggression), despite reports by participants that they are no longer aroused. Second, if only part of the construct has been tested and an empirical relation is found, there is no guarantee that the results generalize to the more complete construct. Additional work may, in fact, suggest the need for a narrower construct (Fiske 1987).

Operational definitions may also represent more than one construct (Figure 14). This situation often reflects the actual state of affairs: most behaviors are multiply determined and can be expected to be influenced by more than one source of variance. Indeed, the ease with which researchers can come up with alternative explanations for internally valid empirical relations speaks to the complex and multiple constructs tapped to varying degrees by incomplete or inaccurate operational definitions. An example is the skin conductance response, which has long been recognized as being affected by widely varying stimulus conditions and across sense modalities, with interpretations that include an index of specific emotions, a measure of motivation, a measure of attention, and a personality index. A less obvious danger to overrepresentation is the assumption that obtained relations between operational definitions imply an isomorphic relation, a point to which I return later.

The underrepresentation and overrepresentation problems indicate that (i) reliance on any one operation could lead to seriously distorted conclusions and (ii) the validity of any one operational definition depends on convergent and discriminant evidence. The solution to both problems is *multiple operationism* – that is, to specify a set of correspondence rules that serve to associate a single concept with multiple operations. Only when empirical relations replicate across multiple operations can any confidence in construct relations be attained and the proper interpretation of an operational definition be made confidently. The logic of multiple operationism, depicted in Figure 15, is based on the simultaneous collection of convergent and discriminant validation evidence. Each hypothetical study in Figure 15 tests the same conceptual hypothesis: A → B. In each study, however, a different set of operations is used, each of which is overrepresented and underrepresented. Across studies, the "excess" representation varies, whereas the relation between constructs A and B is constant. Likewise, across studies, the incomplete construct coverage in any one study is compensated for by differ-

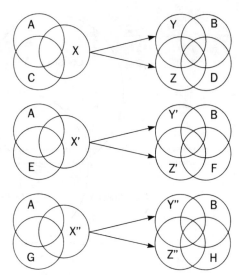

Figure 15. The consequences of multiple operationism.

ent coverage in other studies. Based on supportive and consistent empirical relations, the most parsimonious explanation for the entire set of results is that construct A is causally related to construct B. Although it is not possible to rule out entirely the conclusion that, for example, construct C caused construct D in study 1, construct E caused construct F in study 2, and construct G caused construct H in study 3, such a complex model is less parsimonious and becomes less plausible as additional supportive studies are added. Ordinarily, of course, many more such conceptual replications are necessary in order to establish firmly the appropriate label for a measure.

Multiple operationism actually refers to two distinct tasks. First, any one construct will give rise to many possible operational definitions (e.g., the many ways that arousal can be operationalized physiologically). The relations among these operations must be examined for their internal consistency. This *monoconstruct* multiple operationism provides information about the validity of interpreting any given operation as representing the construct. Second, relations among constructs must be tested by examining the interrelatedness of different sets of operations. For example, if we were to investigate the hypothesis that arousal increases vigilance, we would want to examine relations between multiple measures of arousal (e.g., heart rate and skin conductance) and multiple measures of vigilance (e.g., reaction time and event-related potentials). This *multiconstruct* multiple operationism speaks to the validity of the proposed construct linkages. Both validation tasks are crucial to model testing and both are represented in Figure 15, in which monoconstruct multiple operationism is represented within each study for dependent variables and multiconstruct multiple operationism occurs across studies.

An additional word of caution regarding multiple operationism is in order. The power of using multiple operations is greatest when they diverge substantially from each other. There is little to be gained from using two self-report measures or two nearly identical modes of physiological assessment. Any correlation between the operations might reflect their similarity in method rather than any common underlying construct. Stated differently, a construct should not be method-bound, unless one is taking a particularly narrow view of a construct. The only way to demonstrate the independence of method and construct is through multiple operationism. The importance of avoiding method artifact has led to the development of the multiattribute–multimethod matrix procedure (Campbell & Fiske 1959; Fiske 1987; Hammond, Hamm, & Grassia 1986), a technique for identifying the degree to which operational relations are contaminated by method variance.

An example might make some of the preceding discussion clearer. Expanding the previous example in Figure 2, we might propose that the following conditions are representative of *control loss* and will bring about an increase in *stress:* (a) failing a driving test, (b) unexpectedly losing a job, (c) getting caught in a traffic jam, (d) having someone cut in line just as you near the ticket counter, and (e) getting caught in the rain without an umbrella. In successive investigations, we could devise operational definitions and examine their relation to our operational definition of stress: systolic blood pressure (perhaps measured using an ambulatory monitor). We could also include in each study additional measures of stress. Taken together, this type of evidence would provide convergent validation that systolic blood pressure measures stress. On the other hand, our model might also predict that stress is not related to (f) simple physical exertion or (g) chemical stimulation. Accordingly we would not predict empirical relations between operational definitions of these variables (e.g., treadmill test, ingestion of caffeine) and systolic blood pressure. That these relations would most assuredly be found would indicate a lack of discriminant validity.

In our previous discussion of reliability we noted that aggregation is an important principle for the suppression of error. Over repeated measurement occasions, random errors have an increasing chance of canceling out and leaving the true score more apparent. A similar aggregation principle operates for validation via multiple operationism. Over repeated studies using multiple operations, errors due to construct mislabeling have a chance to be corrected because systematic (but idiosyncratic) errors have a chance to cancel – assuming those errors do not have a constant bias in all studies.

THE PROCESS OF CONSTRUCT VALIDATION

As might be clear by now, construct validation is an iterative, evolving, programmatic process. This can be highlighted by examining more closely the logic involved in making inferences based on data-level relations (see also Nunnally & Bernstein 1994). Consider again the original diagram of the basic inferential task (Figure 1). All that we have to base our inferences on is a relation between operational definitions X and Y; perhaps this is a causal relation, $X \rightarrow Y$. Any inference that we make, however, involves three other relations: (i) the extent to which X is a valid representation of construct A, (ii) the extent to which Y is a valid representation of construct B, and (iii) the extent to which A is causally related to B. In any one study we cannot simultaneously make inferences about all three of these relations. Rather, we must first assume two of them to be true, and then allow the empirical relation $X \rightarrow Y$ to inform us about the plausibility of the remaining relation. For example, if our intent were to make inferences about $A \rightarrow B$, then we must assume that X and Y are valid representations of constructs A and B, respectively. In other words, if we wish to make inferences about construct relations, then we must assume that the operational definitions have construct validity. Likewise, if we wish to make inferences about the construct validity of Y, then we must assume that A and B are causally linked and that X is a valid representation of A. Our assumptions about the truth of the relations in our conceptual model are based on research (our own or previous research conducted by others). If our ultimate goal is making causal inferences, then we must proceed by first generating empirical evidence for the construct validity of our measures. This is a necessary first step because we must assume construct validity is present when causal hypotheses are tested; without such evidence, lack of empirical support for the causal hypothesis is uninterpretable. Furthermore, past research must be able to support considerable confidence in such assumptions because the appropriate interpretation of positive or negative empirical results hinges on the validity of those assumptions. An incorrect assumption can alter the direction of subsequent research and make the construct validation process inefficient if not completely misleading. This incremental view of construct validation returns us to a point made at the beginning of this chapter: research must be guided by a very clear view of what one intends to infer from the data.

Several final comments about construct validation are in order. First, the construct validity of *both* the independent and dependent variables require careful attention. Psychophysiological research tends to emphasize the construct validity of physiological signals as dependent measures. But the construct validity of the eliciting conditions for those signals is equally important. For example, work on the physiological markers of stress has used a wide variety of stressors (e.g., physically demanding tasks, mental arithmetic, cold pressor task). The conceptual equivalence of those tasks is an important consideration that influences the labeling of the physiological signal. Second, conceptual models should be responsive to empirical findings. A conceptual hypothesis is only an educated guess about how things work. If the evidence indicates a need for revision, it behooves researchers to let their models evolve rather than fall prey to confirmatory bias (although it may be obvious, it is important that model revisions be tested on new samples). In a similar fashion, researchers should test their models aggressively – that is, provide empirical tests of hypotheses that are not immune to falsification. Researchers should assume that their measures and models contain errors and then set out aggressively to find and correct those errors (rather than assuming measures and models are true and finding ways to protect that fragile perception). Finally, researchers should realize that construct validation is a slow, methodical process. The building of a conceptual model should be taken one sure-footed step at a time.

PSYCHOLOGICAL LABELS FOR PHYSIOLOGICAL SIGNALS

Whenever labels are attached to numbers, there is a danger of assuming an isomorphic relation between the measures on which the labeling is based. This is particularly a problem in psychophysiology, where the "label" attached to a physiological signal is quite frequently a psychological state or process (Cacioppo & Tassinary 1990a; Sarter et al. 1996). As Cacioppo and Tassinary point out, an important goal of psychophysiological research is to specify the functional relation between elements in the psychological domain (Ψ) and elements in the physiological domain (Θ): $\Psi = f(\Theta)$. Often this functional relation is investigated by manipulating some element in the psychological domain and measuring the consequent response in the physiological domain. It is tempting to conclude that corresponding signal differences can be labeled with the psychological element that produced them. As Cacioppo and Tassinary (1990a) remind us, however, "simply knowing that manipulating a particular psychological element such as emotional arousal leads to a particular physiological response such as electrodermal activation does not logically enable inferences about the former based on observations of the latter" (p. 24). The problem here is that the relations between elements in the psychological domain and elements in the physiological domain may not be one-to-one. Consequently, the probability of a physiological response given a psychological event, $P(\Theta \mid \Psi)$, is not necessarily equal to the probability of the psychological event given the physiological signal, $P(\Psi \mid \Theta)$. More than one distinct psychological event could produce the same physiological signal, for example (what Cacioppo and Tassinary call a many-to-one relation; see also Chapter 1 of this volume). The problem is perhaps clearest in cognitive neuroscience (Sarter et al. 1996). Cognitive operations are manipulated (e.g., using memory tasks or naming tasks) to determine the effect on brain images in order to isolate the brain structures that *may* be responsible for the psychological process. Finding such associations

(i.e., $P[\Theta \mid \Psi] > 0$) does not justify labeling the structure a particular cognitive center in the brain and inferring that a change in that structure would produce the psychological event (i.e., $P[\Psi \mid \Theta] > 0$), and it certainly does not justify the isomorphic inference that $P(\Psi \mid \Theta) = P(\Theta \mid \Psi)$. Such invariant relations are a noble goal, but they require more evidence than is usually gathered in any single investigation.

The lessons to be learned from the inferential pitfalls identified by Cacioppo and Tassinary (1990a) and Sarter et al. (1996) are that (i) strong inferences should not be assumed when the empirical relations do not justify them, and (ii) one's research strategy should be planned to achieve strong inference when possible. The latter goal can be achieved through careful attempts to transform many-to-one, one-to-many, and many-to-many relations between the psychological and physiological domains into one-to-one relations. This may require thinking of the "elements" in those domains as sets or profiles of responses that may have a temporal nature to them and may require restricting the circumstances under which they are measured. This brings us back to a theme that has been emphasized throughout this chapter: the characteristics of operations (e.g., reliability, validity, and relations) are not ordinarily invariant. They depend on the circumstances of measurement, broadly defined. Striving for such invariance requires increasing specification that might seem to limit the utility of the measures and defeat the goal of broad generalizability. Yet such striving is actually in the spirit of error reduction that has been emphasized throughout this chapter.

Conclusion

The psychometric principles discussed in this chapter lie at the very heart of scientific progress. Although most researchers have a rudimentary understanding of these principles, their importance and specific application are often ignored. This arises, perhaps, because psychometric principles are most often associated with the classic psychometric traditions of intelligence, ability, and personality assessment. Nonetheless, as emphasized throughout this chapter, attention to psychometric principles is crucial no matter what form measurement takes. Whether one is attempting to map the physiological structure of mood, to identify stable physiological markers of future disease risk, to develop procedures for determining the physiological concomitants of cognitive function, or to demonstrate the practical utility of physiologically based lie detection, psychometric principles provide essential "rules of evidence" that are used to judge the adequacy of our conceptual and applied conclusions.

Science is aptly described as a truth-seeking enterprise, but it may be more accurately described as an error-correction enterprise. After all, scientists rarely find the truth staring them in the face. Instead, it emerges grudgingly after careful trimming and winnowing of the numerous error sources that obscure the view. Careful attention to psychometric principles can make that winnowing process more efficient and effective.

NOTES

1. This chapter will not attempt to provide a comprehensive coverage of psychometric principles; that task is ably accomplished in numerous book-length treatments (e.g. Ghiselli et al. 1981; Nunnally & Bernstein 1994). Instead, the discussion will focus on key issues and their application. Similarly, discussion of closely related issues in research design and statistics can be found in numerous sources (e.g. Cohen & Cohen 1983; Cook & Campbell 1979; Maxwell & Delaney 1990; Myers & Well 1991; Whitley 1996; Winer 1971).

2. To be sure, the "distance" from constructs to operations varies considerably and for some topics the leap is not all that great. For most areas in the behavioral sciences, however, the constructs are not isomorphic with their measurements, requiring careful attention to psychometric principles to avoid leaps of faith.

3. There are actually several classical views of reliability that make slightly different assumptions. Those differences are not important here but are described in detail elsewhere (see e.g. Feldt & Brennan 1989; Ghiselli et al. 1981; Nunnally & Bernstein 1994). Furthermore, the classical view is only one way to conceptualize measurement, albeit a very popular one. Another increasingly popular view – with some advantages over the classical view – is *item response theory* (Hambleton, Swaminathan, & Rogers 1991).

4. Another point is more subtle but also important. One of the variables in equation (5) could be a manipulated independent variable in an experiment. It is easy to imagine that this variable will have perfect reliability. After all, everyone in a particular experimental condition gets the same "score." But the crucial question is whether everyone in an experimental condition is brought to the same psychological state (Strube 1989). For example, an experiment that uses mental arithmetic to examine the physiological consequence of a cognitive challenge assumes that the experimental manipulation is equally challenging to all participants in that condition. This may not be true, however. Subtle variations in the delivery of the challenge act like random variability because all participants in a condition get the same score but not necessarily the score they "deserve."

5. In general, the highest-order effect is confounded with random error.

6. Ideally, they would be randomly sampled from the population of possible levels. In theory this population would be infinite, but in practice it is usually just very large. Furthermore, the levels actually used in a generalizability study may not be truly random samples; it is sufficient to assume that they are if there is no particular interest in the levels used and any other levels would work equally well.

7. D-studies forecast expected results but are limited by the precision of the variance components from the G-study. Confidence intervals can be placed around variance components (and around other parameter estimates) to provide an appropriate level of caution (Brennan 1992; Cronbach et al. 1972). Sampling variability can be reduced by increasing the number of subjects and facet levels.

8. Generalizability theory, like classical theory, provides a single standard error of measure that applies to all objects of measurement regardless of their universe score. Measurement error may not be equivalent for all score levels, however. Recent work has attempted to overcome this problem (e.g. Brennan 1996; Feldt & Qualls 1996; Kolen, Hanson, & Brennan 1992).

9. There are additional features of generalizability theory that cannot be described in detail here but which expand its potential range of application. For example, any facet can take on the role of objects of measurement (Cardinet, Tourneur, & Allal 1976, 1981). A familiar example makes this clear. In a typical experimental design, persons are nested within groups ($p : g$) and groups are the objects of measurement. That is, decisions will be made about groups (e.g., are they different?). The generalizability coefficient then refers to the reliability of group means (Brennan 1995), and the standard error of measure is the familiar standard error of the mean. Another example is the use of within-person correlations, such as between physiological measures collected over multiple tasks or eliciting conditions. In this case, tasks would be the object of measurement and variability in the within-person correlations would emerge as a sizable task × person interaction. There is also a multivariate extension of generalizability theory that allows examining the influence of measurement conditions on the covariances between multiple outcome measures (Brennan, Gao, & Colton 1995; Cronbach et al. 1972; Marcoulides 1994; Nussbaum 1984; Webb & Shavelson 1981; Webb, Shavelson, & Maddahian 1983).

10. Agreement in categorical judgments would be assessed using Cohen's kappa to guard against capitalization on change agreement (see Cohen 1960, 1968; Conger 1980; Fleiss 1971; Kraemer 1980; Uebersax 1982, 1987, 1988).

REFERENCES

Bliss, R. E., & O'Connell, K. A. (1984). Problems with thiocyanate as an index of smoking status: A critical review with suggestions for improving the usefulness of biochemical measures in smoking cessation research. *Health Psychology, 3,* 563–81.

Bollen, K. A. (1989). *Structural Equations with Latent Variables.* New York: Wiley.

Brennan, R. L. (1992). *Elements of Generalizability Theory,* rev. ed. Iowa City, IA: American College Testing.

Brennan, R. L. (1995). The conventional wisdom about group mean scores. *Journal of Educational Measurement, 32,* 385–96.

Brennan, R. L. (1996). Conditional standard errors of measurement in generalizability theory. ITP Occasional paper no. 40. Iowa Testing Programs, University of Iowa, Iowa City.

Brennan, R. L., Gao, X., & Colton, D. A. (1995). Generalizability analyses of work keys listening and writing tests. *Educational and Psychological Measurement, 55,* 157–76.

Brennan, R. L., & Kane, M. T. (1977). An index of dependability for mastery tests. *Journal of Educational Measurement, 14,* 277–89.

Bunn, H. F. (1981). Evaluation of glycosylated hemoglobin in diabetic patients. *Diabetes, 30,* 613–17.

Cacioppo, J. T., & Tassinary, L. G. (1990a). Inferring psychological significance from physiological signals. *American Psychologist, 45,* 16–28.

Cacioppo, J. T., & Tassinary, L. G. (Eds.) (1990b). *Principles of Psychophysiology. Physical, Social, and Inferential Elements.* Cambridge University Press.

Campbell, D. T., & Fiske, D. W. (1959). Convergent and discriminant validation by the multitrait–multimethod matrix. *Psychological Bulletin, 56,* 81–105.

Campbell, N. R. (1957). *Foundations of Science; The Philosophy of Theory and Experiment.* New York: Dover.

Cardinet, J., Tourneur, Y., & Allal, L. (1976). The symmetry of generalizability theory: Applications to educational measurement. *Journal of Educational Measurement, 13,* 119–35.

Cardinet, J., Tourneur, Y., & Allal, L. (1981). Extension of generalizability theory and its applications in educational measurement. *Journal of Educational Measurement, 18,* 183–204.

Cohen, J. (1960). A coefficient of agreement for nominal scales. *Educational and Psychological Measurement, 20,* 37–46.

Cohen, J. (1968). Weighted kappa: Nominal scale agreement with provision for scaled disagreement or partial credit. *Psychological Bulletin, 70,* 213–20.

Cohen, J., & Cohen, P. (1983). *Applied Multiple Regression/ Correlation Analysis for the Behavioral Sciences.* Hillsdale, NJ: Erlbaum.

Cole, D. A., Howard, G. S., & Maxwell, S. E. (1981). Effects of mono- versus multiple-operationalization in construct validation efforts. *Journal of Consulting and Clinical Psychology, 49,* 395–405.

Coles, M. G. H., Donchin, E., & Porges, S. W. (1986). *Psychophysiology: Systems, Processes, and Applications.* New York: Guilford.

Conger, A. J. (1980). Integration and generalization of kappa for multiple raters. *Psychological Bulletin, 88,* 322–8.

Cook, T. D., & Campbell, D. T. (1979). *Quasi-Experimentation: Design and Analysis Issues for Field Settings.* Chicago: Rand-McNally.

Crocker, L., Llabre, M., & Miller, M. D. (1988). The generalizability of content validity ratings. *Journal of Educational Measurement, 25,* 287–99.

Cronbach, L. J., Gleser, G. C., Nanda, H., & Rajaratnam, N. (1972). *The Dependability of Behavioral Measurements: Theory of Generalizability for Scores and Profiles.* New York: Wiley.

Cronbach, L. J., & Meehl, P. E. (1955). Construct validity in psychological tests. *Psychological Bulletin, 52,* 281–302.

Druckman, D., & Lacey, J. I. (1989). *Brain and Cognition.* Washington, DC: National Academy Press.

Fahrenberg, J., Foerster, F., Schneider, H. J., Müller, W., & Myrtek, M. (1986). Predictability of individual differences in activation processes in a field setting based on laboratory measures. *Psychophysiology, 23,* 323–33.

Feldt, L. S., & Brennan, R. L. (1989). Reliability. In R. L. Linn (Ed.), *Educational Measurement,* 3rd ed., pp. 105–46. New York: Macmillan.

Feldt, L. S., & Qualls, A. L. (1996). Estimation of measurement error variance at specific score levels. *Journal of Educational Measurement, 33,* 141–56.

Fiske, D. W. (1987). Construct invalidity comes from method effects. *Educational and Psychological Measurement, 47,* 285–307.

Fleiss, J. L. (1971). Measuring nominal scale agreement among many raters. *Psychological Bulletin, 76,* 378–82.

Fleiss, J. L., & Shrout, P. E. (1977). The effects of measurement errors on some multivariate procedures. *American Journal of Public Health, 67,* 1188–91.

Ghiselli, E. E., Campbell, J. P., & Zedeck, S. (1981). *Measurement Theory for the Behavioral Sciences.* New York: Freeman.

Greenwald, A. (1975). Consequences of prejudice against the null hypothesis. *Psychological Bulletin, 82,* 1–20.

Greenwald, A., Pratkanis, A. R., Leippe, M. R., & Baumgardner, M. H. (1986). Under what conditions does theory obstruct research progress? *Psychological Review, 93,* 216–29.

Guion, R. M. (1978). Scoring of content domain samples: The problem of fairness. *Journal of Applied Psychology, 63,* 499–506.

Hall, P. S., Thomas, S. A., Friedman, E., & Lynch, J. J. (1982). Measurement of neonatal blood pressure: A new method. *Psychophysiology, 19,* 231–6.

Hambleton, R. K., Swaminathan, H., & Rogers, H. J. (1991). *Fundamentals of Item Response Theory.* Newbury Park, CA: Sage.

Hammond, K. R., Hamm, R. M., & Grassia, J. (1986). Generalizing over conditions by combining the multitrait–multimethod matrix and the representative design of experiments. *Psychological Bulletin, 100,* 257–69.

Helfand, R., Lavie, P., & Hobson, J. A. (1986). REM/NREM discrimination via ocular and limb movement monitoring: Correlation with polygraphic data and development of a REM state algorithm. *Psychophysiology, 23,* 334–9.

Hoch, C. C., Reynolds, C. F. III, Kupfer, D. J., Berman, S. R., Houck, P. R., & Stack, J. A. (1987). Empirical note: Self-report versus recorded sleep in healthy seniors. *Psychophysiology, 24,* 293–9.

Humphreys, L. G., & Drasgow, F. (1989). Some comments on the relation between reliability and statistical power. *Applied Psychological Measurement, 13,* 419–25.

Kennedy, A. L., & Merimee, T. J. (1981). Glycosylated serum protein and hemoglobin A_1 levels to measure control of glycemia. *Annals of Internal Medicine, 95,* 56–8.

Kolen, M. J., Hanson, B. A., & Brennan, R. L. (1992). Conditional standard errors of measurement for scale scores. *Journal of Educational Measurement, 29,* 285–307.

Kopriva, R. J., & Shaw, D. G. (1991). Power estimates: The effect of dependent variable reliability on the power of one-factor ANOVAs. *Educational and Psychological Measurement, 51,* 585–95.

Kraemer, H. C. (1980). Extension of the kappa coefficient. *Biometrics, 36,* 207–16.

Llabre, M. M., Ironson, G. H., Spitzer, S. B., Gellman, M. D., Weidler, D. J., & Schneiderman, N. (1988). How many blood pressure measurements are enough? An application of generalizability theory to the study of blood pressure reliability. *Psychophysiology, 25*, 97–106.

Llabre, M. M., Spitzer, S. B., Saab, P. G., Ironson, G. H., & Schneiderman, N. (1991). The reliability and specificity of delta versus residualized change as measures of cardiovascular reactivity to behavioral challenges. *Psychophysiology, 28*, 701–11.

Marcoulides, G. A. (1994). Selecting weighting schemes in multivariate generalizability studies. *Educational and Psychological Measurement, 54*, 3–7.

Marcoulides, G. A., & Goldstein, Z. (1990). The optimization of generalizability studies with resource constraints. *Educational and Psychological Measurement, 50*, 761–8.

Maxwell, S. E., & Delaney, H. D. (1990). *Designing Experiments and Analyzing Data: A Model Comparison Perspective.* Belmont, CA: Wadsworth.

Messick, S. (1981). Constructs and their vicissitudes in educational and psychological measurement. *Psychological Bulletin, 89*, 575–88.

Messick, S. (1989). Validity. In R. L. Linn (Ed.), *Educational Measurement*, 3rd ed. New York: Macmillan.

Myers, J. L., & Well, A. D. (1991). *Research Design and Statistical Analysis.* New York: Harper-Collins.

Nunnally, J. C., & Bernstein, I. H. (1994). *Psychometric Theory*, 3rd ed. New York: McGraw-Hill.

Nussbaum, A. (1984). Multivariate generalizability theory in educational measurement: An empirical study. *Applied Psychological Measurement, 8*, 219–30.

Pennebaker, J. W. (1982). *The Psychology of Physical Symptoms.* New York: Springer-Verlag.

Pickering, T. G., Harshfield, G. A., Kleinert, H. D., Blank, S., & Laragh, J. H. (1982). Blood pressure during normal daily activities, sleep, and exercise. *Journal of the American Medical Association, 247*, 992–6.

Sarter, M., Berntson, G. G., & Cacioppo, J. T. (1996). Brain imaging and cognitive neuroscience. Toward strong inference in attributing function to structure. *American Psychologist, 51*, 13–21.

Schmidt, F. L., & Hunter, J. E. (1996). Measurement error in psychological research: Lessons from 26 research scenarios. *Psychological Methods, 1*, 199–223.

Shapiro, D., Greenstadt, L., Lane, J. D., & Rubinstein, E. (1981). Tracking-cuff system for beat-to-beat recording of blood pressure. *Psychophysiology, 18*, 129–36.

Shavelson, R. J., & Webb, N. M. (1991). *Generalizability Theory: A Primer.* Newbury Park, CA: Sage.

Shavelson, R. J., Webb, N. M., & Rowley, G. L. (1989). Generalizability theory. *American Psychologist, 44*, 922–32.

Strube, M. J (1989). Assessing subjects' construal of the laboratory situation. In N. Schneiderman, S. M. Weiss, & P. Kaufman (Eds.), *Handbook of Research Methods in Cardiovascular Behavioral Medicine*, pp. 527–42. New York: Plenum Press.

Uebersax, J. S. (1982). A generalized kappa coefficient. *Educational and Psychological Measurement, 42*, 181–3.

Uebersax, J. S. (1987). Diversity of decision-making models and the measurement of interrater agreement. *Psychological Bulletin, 101*, 140–6.

Uebersax, J. S. (1988). Validity inferences from interobserver agreement. *Psychological Bulletin, 104*, 405–16.

Webb, N. M., & Shavelson, R. J. (1981). Multivariate generalizability of general educational development ratings. *Journal of Educational Measurement, 18*, 13–22.

Webb, N. M., Shavelson, R. J., & Maddahian, E. (1983). Multivariate generalizability theory. In L. J. Fyans (Ed.), *New Directions for Testing and Measurement*, no. 18 (Generalizability Theory: Inferences and Practical Application), pp. 67–82. San Francisco: Jossey-Bass.

Whitley, B. E., Jr. (1996). *Principles of Research in Behavioral Science.* Mountain View, CA: Mayfield.

Williams, R. H., & Zimmerman, D. W. (1989). Statistical power analysis and reliability of measurement. *Journal of General Psychology, 116*, 359–69.

Winer, B. J. (1971). *Statistical Principles in Experimental Design.* New York: McGraw-Hill.

Zillmann, D. (1978). Attribution and misattribution of excitatory reactions. In J. H. Harvey, W. Ickes, & R. F. Kidd (Eds.), *New Directions in Attribution Research*, vol. 2, pp. 335–68. Hillsdale, NJ: Erlbaum.

Zimmerman, D. W., & Williams, R. H. (1986). Note on the reliability of experimental measures and the power of significance tests. *Psychological Bulletin, 100*, 123–4.

CHAPTER THIRTY-TWO

SALIENT METHOD, DESIGN, AND ANALYSIS CONCERNS

J. RICHARD JENNINGS & LYNN A. STINE

Science is a method. We observe and then compare observations to find regularities in nature. The method of observation determines what we see and should determine how we interpret our observations. Consider two hypothetical experiments on the same topic. Both ask whether the pupil of the eye dilates during exposure to loud white noise (80 dBA). The first exposes six research participants (referred to as "subjects" in the remainder of the chapter for continuity with the earlier literature) to five minutes of relative quiet (40-dBA white noise) followed by five minutes of loud noise. The second experiment exposes six subjects to five minutes of relative quiet and a different six subjects to five minutes of noise. Both experiments measure pupil size and compare data collected under conditions of relative quiet and relative noise. Yet noise influences pupil size in one experiment but not in the other. Why the discrepancy? We should suspect that the difference in the method of observation caused the discrepancy. This chapter will highlight methodological concerns of particular salience to psychophysiological investigations. Salient issues are those that occur more frequently in psychophysiology than in psychological research in general. General treatments of methodology can be found in Keppel (1991), Kirk (1995), Mitchell and Jolley (1988), and Neale and Liebert (1986). Abelson (1995) offers an enjoyable and wise perspective on statistics and methodology that we recommend highly as well.

A number of earlier considerations in this book of psychophysiological methodology permit us to constrain our coverage in this chapter. Our emphasis will be on experimental design and its relationship to statistical analysis, although we shall also discuss issues of data collection and response representation. The other chapters in Part Five expand the discussion of psychometrics, signal processing, and advanced statistical techniques of particular applicability to psychophysiology. Methodological issues that are specific to particular measures (e.g., event-related poten-

tial, heart rate) will not be covered here. Such coverage is available in measurement-oriented handbooks (Brown 1967; Hugdahl 1995; Martin & Venables 1980; Venables & Martin 1967) and in specific texts – for example, on event-related potential (Rugg & Coles 1995; van Boxtel 1998) or on pupil of the eye (Loewenfeld 1993). A series of publication guidelines on specific measures have also been published in the journal *Psychophysiology*: for skin conductance (Fowles et al. 1981), heart rate (Jennings et al. 1981), electromyography (EMG; Fridlund & Cacioppo 1986), electroencephalography (EEG; Pivik et al. 1993), impedance cardiography (Sherwood et al. 1990), and blood pressure (Shapiro et al. 1996). Basic issues of experimental control are addressed well in a chapter on methodology by Johnson and Lubin (1972). We shall not repeat their review of variables to control in the experimental situation (e.g., environmental temperature) and in the participant; they provide an interesting discussion of controlling the experimental set and activation state in addition to the usual concerns about comparability of age, gender, race, and education. We will attempt to discuss statistical issues salient to psychophysiologists, but we urge the reader also to consult Johnson and Lubin (1972) for a chapter, written by an outstanding practical statistician in collaboration with a psychophysiologist, discussing issues of current relevance (despite its early publication). Stemmler and Fahrenberg (1989) provide a more contemporary chapter on psychophysiological methods that may also prove useful.

Planning the Research

DESIGNING THE OBSERVATIONS

The key principle of methodology is as simple to state as it is difficult to implement: The methods must be chosen to answer the primary question posed by the research. Implementing this principle requires stating the experimental question concretely, assessing the means available for measurement, identifying factors that could confuse the answer to the question, and employing statistics that answer the question precisely.

The psychophysiologist typically starts with a psychological concept of interest, assesses the concept with a physiological measure, and observes the correlation between the measure and the concept across an experimental manipulation or across a relevant dimension of individual differences. We will leave the choice of psychological concept to the reader. The choice of a physiological measure typically poses the first major challenge to the apparent simplicity of fitting the methods to the question. Often the experiment is conducted to see if measure x acts like a measure of a psychological concept. The basis for this expectation must be carefully reviewed. If a good basis exists, then it may also be possible to identify measures which are similar to measure x that either should or should not covary with variation in the psychological process. Drawing a complete picture of the expected mapping between concept and physiological measures should yield optimum convergent and discriminant validity for the measurement methodology. Cacioppo and Tassinary (1990; see also Jennings 1986) have provided a more formal and detailed discussion of how psychological and physiological concepts can be appropriately related to each other. Once this conceptual exercise is completed, a number of practical concerns must then be weighed against the value of obtaining convergent and divergent measures.

An example should clarify the conceptual and pragmatic issues that must be addressed. Consider an investigator interested in impulsive behavior in children. She wishes to show that positive reward induces impulsive behavior in children classified as impulsive (relative to children scoring low on a scale of impulsivity). Positive reinforcement, a nickel, is contrasted with negative reinforcement, the loss of a nickel. Impulsive behavior is operationalized as responding to a tone occurring just prior to the appearance of a signal to respond. A visual, two-choice reaction time (RT) task is presented requiring a left-hand response to the appearance of a left-pointing arrow and a right-hand response to the appearance of a right-pointing arrow. A hundred milliseconds before each arrow stimulus, however, a tone is presented to one of the two ears. Seventy-five percent of the time, the tone is presented on the same side of the body as the side of the correct response to the upcoming arrow.

How is the investigator to use psychophysiological measures? Note first that the investigator seems to have the modest (but hardly simple) goal of validating a scale or dimension of impulsivity. Impulsivity is operationalized as responding prior to the receipt of complete information. Behaviorally, responding is pushing a button. However, physiologically, responding includes preparatory adjustment of posture and competing motor activity, activation of motor cortex of the appropriate laterality, transmission to peripheral motor units, and electrochemical activation of the myofibrils resulting in flexion sufficient to make the button switch closure. The question of what is "responding" now appears more complicated, but the investigator considers only using the button press. A problem arises: button presses can be initiated impulsively in response to the tone or "correctly" in response to the arrow. Correctly initiated responses are likely to average around 300 msec, but correctly initiated fast button presses could be as fast as 120 msec or so. How can fast appropriate responses be separated from impulsive responses? Furthermore, does the investigator define impulsivity by the inappropriate initiation of a response or by completion of a response? For example, consider two children who both initiate a response precisely at tone offset but who differ in nerve conduction speed (or arm length). One child will press the button a few microseconds prior to the other; is this child more impulsive? Perhaps we need concepts of preparatory impulsivity, motor cortex impulsivity, and peripheral nerve impulsivity. Some reading may convince the investigator that early initiation of preparation isn't highly correlated with faster responding, that conduction time differences are not likely to be a major contributor to reaction speed, but that inhibition can stop a response even after activation of the motor cortex. At this point, the investigator may decide that impulsivity may arise both from aberrant central processing as well as from the coupling of this with peripheral response mechanisms. Measures of motor cortex would seem useful, as well as measures of different aspects of the peripheral response.

At this stage, pragmatic measurement factors may be appropriate to consider. Without losing the fit between our measures and our concept of impulsivity, we would like a measure that is simple to use and analyze, inexpensive, not prone to noise, acceptable and ethical to apply to human subjects, and understandable from our own experience (or allows us time to gain that experience in pilot work). Such considerations might push us, for example, toward the use of surface electrodes for electromyography rather than needle electrodes and toward electroencephalography rather than magnetic resonance imaging.

Investigators can weigh pragmatic factors too much or too little in their considerations. The investigator who places too much weight on practicality may choose a measure already operational in the laboratory (e.g. electrocardiography) rather than the conceptually relevant measure that may not yet be operational (e.g. electromyography). The investigator who places too little weight on pragmatic factors will waste time and money and may also incur slightly more subtle costs. Most seasoned investigators believe that it is easier to collect data than to analyze and interpret data. Collecting 64 channels of EEG when the conceptual question requires only four channels

* INCORRECT! Neg reinforcement is the
withdrawal of an aversive stimulus.
Here they have withdrawal of a positive reinforcer stimulus
H. Thorsheim 6/18/01

may mean that each channel will only receive some one sixteenth of the analytic and interpretive time that the investigator would have placed on one of four channels. Although this numerical argument is specious, it seems reasonable to ask the investigator to consider consciously the trade-off between understanding a small number of variables quite well and understanding a large number of variables less well. The trade-off can also occur during data collection if too many technically difficult measures are attempted. Most investigators would not purposefully violate such common-sense considerations, but most have collected data that were not analyzed or have lost data from an entire measure owing to an unforeseen technical failure. Some problems may be avoided if the investigator collects and completely analyzes pilot data from a few subjects, perhaps including himself as a participant.

In the case of our hypothetical experiment on impulsivity, a practical set of response measures might be the lateralized readiness potential, surface electromyography, and measures of response initiation, force, and completion. Briefly, a rationale (not necessarily the best – this is, after all, a hypothetical experiment) can be cited. With surface cortical electrodes over bilateral motor sites and bilateral comparison sites, the degree of motor activation related to a response on one hand can be identified (for reviews see Coles 1989; Coles, Gratton, & Donchin 1988). Surface electromyography over muscles subserving a selected response, in this case each hand, can detect activation that may not result in an overt response (Lippold 1967; van Boxtel, van den Boogaart, & Brunia 1993). Finally, initiation of a response, the force of that response, and time of completion (standard RT) provide converging information on the intensity of any impulsive response (cf. Zahn & Kruesi 1993). Our measurement choices would not be adequate if the investigator had different goals. If, for instance, she wished to explain impulsivity as due to heightened midbrain activation, then convergent measures of cortical and autonomic activation indices might be required.

SIGNAL PROCESSING

Psychophysiological investigations typically use some form of instrumentation to isolate, amplify, and record physiological changes. The typical choice is a combination of electronic amplifiers designed for biological signals and a personal computer with components for analog-to-digital conversion. Such devices are widely used and designed to flexibly meet a variety of needs.

Noninvasively collected physiological signals result in an electrical signal that is then amplified, filtered, and digitized. Amplification poses few problems with current equipment, but students frequently are concerned with the influence of filtering and the rate of sampling. Thorough and elegant treatments of these topics can be found elsewhere (Cook & Miller 1992; Kamen 1987; Stearns & David

1993; Thede 1996), but a few very elementary points may be useful here. Biological signals should be collected without distorting the features of primary interest to the investigator. Any system used to collect biological signals and digitize them for computer processing will have a sampling rate and filter characteristics. Filtering and sampling can, however, distort the signal of interest to the investigator.

Filtering refers to the electronic selection of the signal of interest as typically defined by a frequency range. Frequency is the number of times per second (hertz, Hz) that a signal cycles around its mean value. In the United States the voltage in a typical house cycles around a mean of zero volts 60 times per second or 60 Hz. As delivered to a home, the voltages will contain not only variation at 60 Hz but also very small voltages at other frequencies (e.g., frequencies used by radio transmitters). If we wished only to see the 60-Hz voltage, we might filter a signal to accept voltages varying between 59 Hz and 61 Hz and reject those below 59 Hz or above 61 Hz. In practice the filter will taper off, so that a significant portion of signals between 59 Hz and 50 Hz will be seen, fewer still between 50 Hz and 40 Hz, tapering further to no signal between 40 Hz and 30 Hz. A comparable tapering will likely occur for the frequencies above 60 Hz.

Filtering of biological signals works in the same way, but the changing voltages over time are not as symmetrical or continuous as household voltage (and we almost always want to reject or filter out 60-Hz "noise"). Figure 1 shows an electrocardiogram signal. It varies over time, but much of the time it is flat and then a complex waveform appears. Filter electronics views the waveform as if it were a set of simple, continuously varying waveforms. The figure illustrates this by extracting two portions of the electrocardiogram waveform and then imagining that they continued to vary in the same way over time. When this is done, the sharp (Q-wave) portion of the electrocardiogram might produce a waveform with a frequency of about 45 Hz, while the slowly increasing portion between the S wave and T wave might produce a frequency of about 0.001 Hz.

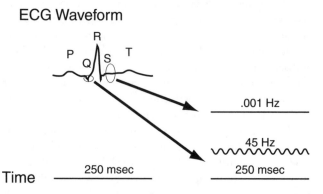

Figure 1. Diagram showing how different segments of a physiological signal can be conceptualized as portions of a sine–cosine wave of a particular frequency.

What will happen to this signal when we apply a low-pass filter[1] that reduces voltages in the signal with frequencies above 35 Hz? The result will be a reduction in amplitude of the Q wave and also of portions of the wave with similar frequencies (e.g., the R wave). Given that the R wave is typically used to determine the time between heart beats, it may well be that we want to shift from a 35-Hz low-pass filter to, say, a 50-Hz low-pass filter. What will happen when we apply a high-pass filter that reduces signals below 1 Hz? The very slow frequencies will be damped, likely eliminating any change in the segment between S and T. This will be fine if we are measuring only interbeat interval but *not* if we are trying to see if heart disease has altered the voltage level of the segment of the signal between the S and T waves. The prudent investigator should estimate the interesting frequency components in the signal and then ensure that filtering via either the amplifier settings (hardware filtering) or computer programming (software filtering) does not influence these signal components. An empirical way of doing this prior to an experiment is to run an artificial signal from a waveform generator similar to your signal of interest through the entire measurement system, noting whether particular frequencies are attenuated by the system.

An analog-to-digital converter transforms a continuous signal into a series of numbers corresponding to the voltages sensed at a particular instant. As the investigator, you will then likely re-represent the signal to yourself as if it were continuous. The converter will make your continuous signal a series of discrete dots of voltage that hopefully will be sufficient to re-create the signal when you "connect the dots." Under ideal conditions, the sampling rate of an analog-to-digital converter will be at least twice the frequency of the highest frequency of interest in your signal; in practice, sampling at four or more times the highest frequency is advisable. The signal is missed or distorted when the sample rate is too low. This is illustrated in the top of Figure 2. An EEG-like signal is shown for two time frames of 300 msec each. The analog-to-digital converter is shown to be sampling at a rate of 10 Hz (less than the cyclic variation of about 12 Hz). The regular waveform on the left is digitized to three points that form a straight line when the dots are connected – the actual signal has been lost. On the right, a signal with slightly higher frequency and lower amplitude is digitized at the same 10-Hz rate. When the dots for this example are connected, an signal is formed that appears to be part of a cycle waveform with a frequency of approximately 1.3 Hz – our original signal has been distorted (aliased).

The bottom of Figure 2 shows a complication arising from oversampling. A slow, respiratory-like signal is

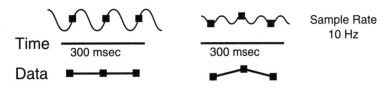

EEG with Sample Points Shown

Sample Rate 10 Hz

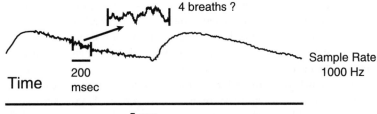

Respiration with Sample Points

4 breaths ?

Sample Rate 1000 Hz

Figure 2. Illustration of how sampling rate will alter the obtained signal. The upper portion illustrates how distortion can occur from sampling a relatively high-frequency signal with too low a sampling rate. The bottom portion of the figure illustrates how a relatively high-frequency sampling rate may emphasize high-frequency noise in a signal, potentially obscuring the low-frequency component of interest.

shown with a good signal-to-noise ratio – that is, the slowly changing component of the signal is very clear visually without much noise. The signal is sampled at a high rate, 1,000 Hz, resulting in about 200 sample points for a 200-msec interval (which also creates very large data files). The sample points are not shown separately because they are so close in time that they are essentially identical to the signal as drawn in the figure. The result of the high sampling rate for the 200-msec segment, shown as amplified, is that the fine structure of peaks and valleys (noise, from our perspective) in the signal is digitized into our data. A computer program designed for respiratory detection may find cyclic high and low points in our data and call them respiratory breaths; it will find four or so "breaths" in this noise. Oversampling problems can be circumvented by creating "smarter" software and by filtering the signal, but simply sampling at a lower frequency (plus filtering) may be easier and will permit the same computer program to do an adequate scoring job (with less data storage required). A frequently practical approach to filtering and sampling is to low-pass filter your signal electronically and then sample the signal at five times the frequency of the filter cut-off frequency (Stearns & David 1993). Additional filtering may be useful for noise that is close in frequency to the signal of interest.

The choice of gain, sampling rate, and filtering rate should be checked throughout the experiment by visually monitoring the output of the hardware–software collection system. Ideally, this is done as the data are collected, displaying the signal at one or more points in processing and also the digitized data as it is stored. A display that shows a relatively "raw" signal and concurrently shows the digitized, processed signal will indicate how sampling and filtering have altered the signal. Filtering can cause time delays as well, so a comparison of when an event occurs relative to your signal in raw and processing displays is also important. Some software programs will also alter the data by excluding points assumed to be invalid. For example, cardiac interbeat intervals shorter than 300 msec or greater than 1,750 msec might be coded as missing data. It is useful to know immediately, or at least after individual participants have completed their session, whether such automatic editing has been done for a large or small amount of the data. The investigator should know when and how data are being transformed and should be able to control such transformations – for example, to adjust the high cut-off for interbeat interval duration to 2,000 msec for an athlete with average interbeat intervals in the range of 1,750 msec. When hardware data displays are not available, software can be written to check on data transformations in a number of ways (Tukey 1977; see also section entitled "Data Collection and Reduction"). Any time spent ensuring that data collection is working as planned is worthwhile. Typically, psychophysiological data requires as much or more processing time as collection time. Collecting good data will make the processing time worthwhile and most often considerably shorter.

RESPONSE DEFINITION AND INTERMEASURE DEPENDENCIES

Many psychophysiological investigations are directed at subjects' responsivity to an environmental event or a psychological process initiated by such events. Responsivity must then be defined objectively. How will the onset of the response be defined? What measures will be used to characterize the response? How will electrical noise influence these definitions? In our previous example, an examination of the lateralized readiness potential of impulsive children will require the definition of a procedure to reveal this response. Electrodes must be placed bilaterally (usually over C3 and C4). Background voltage fluctuations, 60-Hz interference, and other electrical noise are likely to obscure the readiness potential on any single trial. This will force us to use multiple trials so that the results can be ensemble averaged (aligning time samples with the stimuli and then averaging over trials to yield a mean waveform). The obtained potentials must then be assessed in some way. Are potentials examined from stimulus onset to 100 msec after stimulus? From 100 msec before the stimulus to 299 msec after? From the stimulus to when maximum negativity is reached within 500 msec? Answers to these questions define the response for your research and can also guide the design of filters and software scoring systems. An efficient, accurate, and automated response scoring procedure can

save hours of tedious work. As our example implies, response identification and scoring issues are largely specific to the psychophysiological measure studied. Law, Levey, and Martin (1980) provide a relatively general orientation to response scoring. After reading this chapter, more recent measure-specific articles should be consulted.

Psychophysiological responses must typically be defined by exclusion criteria as well as inclusion criteria. Physiological measures respond to many events and not just to the events that are the subject of our research. A cortical negativity just after stimulus onset may meet most criteria for a readiness potential yet still be suspect if it is associated with an eye movement (which could elicit an electrical negativity in the absence of any stimulus). Similarly, by assessing a number of cortical sites with our electrodes, we can determine whether the cortical negativity shows a pattern consistent with a motoric readiness response. If the poststimulus negativity was smaller at central sites than at occipital sites, we may again hesitate in defining our response as a readiness potential. Note that both of these possible exclusion criteria require the investigator to collect additional measures (i.e., an eye movement index and additional scalp sites). Adequate experimental design requires the identification of all factors other than the one we seek to manipulate that may influence our dependent measure.

The application of this dictum is not always clear. Our scientific question determines what is artifact and what is a factor we seek to manipulate. In the case of the impulsive children, we are examining the lateralized readiness potential to find out whether premature responses were organized more frequently in these children than in controls, so our conceptual outcome variable is impulsivity as indexed by the lateralized readiness potential. Impulsivity might also be indexed by eye movements, however. An eye movement toward the source of the irrelevant stimulation may reliably precede an (inappropriate) response to that stimulation. It may even be that the eye movement is such that it produces a frontal negativity that contributes to negativity at central electrodes. The eye movement in this scenario is an index of our conceptual dependent measure and is thus not an artifact. The eye movement creates a negative potential that is assessed at our central scalp sites. This potential will summate with any readiness potential. If the eye movement is toward the direction of the inappropriate response, it might even provide an appropriate amplification of the lateralized readiness potential. In this case we may have a very sensitive index of impulsivity but a contaminated measure of the readiness potential.

More realistic scenarios can be considered for heart rate and respiration. Respiratory movements alter heart rate, and physiological evidence suggests that the central control of heart rate and respiration is integrated to a significant degree (Porges 1995; Richter & Spyer 1990). Preparation for action may well involve an integrated shift in cardiorespiratory regulation toward rapid breathing and heart rate acceleration initiated by a concomitant inspiration and shortening of the time to the next heartbeat. This pattern of response to a stimulus may be centrally organized and thus the most reliable and valid sign of preparation for action. In a resting state, however, respiratory inspiration is reliably associated with cardiac acceleration (sinus arrhythmia). This observation may lead us to correct our experimental data for artifactual influences of respiration by eliminating the heart rate increase associated with respiratory inspiration. Respiratory change is, however, as valid a measurement of preparation for action as heart rate change (see related discussion in Turpin 1986). A critic should argue that respiratory sinus arrhythmia may also be occurring and demand evidence that we have observed a centrally mediated response. Our point here is not to pursue this debate but rather to illustrate how our concepts determine the definition of the appropriate response measure and artifactual influences on that measure.

MEASUREMENT SCALES

The novitiate to psychophysiology is often impressed with the technical equipment and the continuous data flowing from this equipment in objective units such as volts and siemens. This impression can conceal the important measurement issues that psychophysiology shares with the rest of psychology (and most of science). In order to accurately compare groups of people in the same or different conditions, or different conditions in the same people, we must have measures that are the same across people and/or conditions. If we compare the heights of Americans measured by a yardstick with the heights of Dutch people using a "meter stick," we might conclude that the Americans average about 68 inches while the Dutch average about 180 centimeters. No comparison is possible unless a common unit is provided. As scientists we might prefer the metric measure and convert 68 inches into 170 centimeters. We could then say that Dutch and American heights are comparable with, perhaps, a slight height advantage in the Netherlands.

The problems are comparable but more subtle in psychophysiology. Glancing at a polygraph, four signals might be displayed: EEG, ECG (electrocardiograph), blood pressure, and photoplethysmograph. The blood pressure is displayed as signals from a microphone imposed upon a trace reflecting a decreasing pressure within an arm cuff. The other signals are continuous ink tracings. On the chart they all share the same metric, millimeters of deflection assessed from the center line on a polygraph channel. Even so, we realize that we cannot say someone has more ECG than EEG simply because the ECG deflection is larger; the two channels measure different physiological responses. Exploring this further, we could learn that the chart deflections are a direct function of current applied to the pen drivers in the polygraph, which in turn are a function

of the voltages of the amplifier outputs. At the amplifier we might see that an electrical calibration had been performed so that, for example, 50 μV of EEG voltage yielded the same amplifier output as did 25 mV of ECG voltage. The measurements share the same units (volts), but this does not mean they are the same measure. The EEG and ECG are both measurements of biologically generated electricity, so voltage is an appropriate unit of measurement. However, the signals are from different sites, and we know more about the source and exact localization of the ECG signal. The ECG is largely derived from cardiac smooth muscle activity. Some variation in individual heart position does affect voltage levels, but between-subject voltage comparisons can still be made and are clinically useful. For example, a depression in the S-T segment of 1 mV below the level of the T-P segment is taken as a clinical indicant of myocardial ischemia.

The EEG voltage level is dependent on skull thickness and the location of sources of electrical activity. Between-subject comparisons of voltage levels are difficult, given that the exact nature and source of the electrical generator is typically unknown for a specific subject. A similar statement can be made about the photoplethysmography signal (Jennings, Tahmoush, & Redmond 1980). The signal appears to be a complex function of blood pressure and blood flow that is influenced by the precise distance and geometry of the placement of the photoplethysmograph relative to the vascular bed. Voltage measures from such a technique cannot be directly compared between individuals. In short, even though some psychophysiological indices are assessed in units of a common yardstick, those units are not meaningful if we do not know what physiological process is being measured.

Common metrics permitting the direct comparison of individuals can sometimes be based on a feature of a signal that itself is uncalibrated or derived from the outcome of a procedure. The assessment of heart rate and blood pressure are good examples. Although with careful calibration the voltage produced by the cardiac muscle can be compared between individuals, psychophysiologists are rarely interested in this voltage (except for those interested in T-wave amplitude – Contrada et al. 1989; Furedy, Heslegrave, & Scher 1992; Schwartz & Weiss 1983). Typically, interbeat interval is assessed by measuring the time between the R waves of successive beats occurring in the ECG signal. The metric is time, typically assessed in milliseconds. This measure is comparable between individuals as long as the R wave of the ECG can be reliably detected in each individual.

Blood pressure values result from a measurement procedure. Using the cuff technique, calibrated pressures in the cuff are applied to an artery; the pressure within the artery is then inferred from the behavior of the artery when cuff pressure is varied. A common unit of pressure (mmHg) is employed. By convention (Fifth Report

1993), systolic blood pressure is defined as the cuff pressure at the occurrence of the first sound produced by the flow of blood as the cuff is deflated after total occlusion. This measure is comparable between subjects as long as the measurement procedure is conducted appropriately – that is, pressure devices are calibrated, appropriate cuff sizes are used, deflation is well controlled, and detection sensitivity is adequate.

Measures suitable for comparing individuals directly should typically have good scale properties. Physical measures of time and pressure have equally spaced units and ratio properties, so that arithmetic operations performed on the measures are meaningful; for instance, an interbeat interval of 1,200 msec is twice as long as one of 600 msec (see Stevens 1951). Voltage measures have similar properties and are excellent measures if we are interested in voltage. But let's assume we are interested in blood flow and don't know how the voltage output from a photoplethysmograph is related to blood flow. A photoplethysmographic output of 5 mV is half that of 10 mV, but if we don't know its relation to blood flow then the blood flow associated with the higher voltage could be (say) 10 times or 1.1 times as large as that associated with the lower voltage.

Note that physical measures with excellent scale properties do not necessarily support psychological or physiological inferences. If I am interested in impulsivity, and if one person has an interbeat interval of 600 msec and another an IBI of 900 msec, then I can say that the interbeat interval of the former is one third less than that of the latter. However, I cannot say that the former subject has one third more (or less) impulsivity than the latter, because we don't know precisely how impulsivity alters interbeat interval. Similarly, if we wish to use heart rate to infer the presence or absence of sympathetic and parasympathetic activation, we need to know how these activations affect interbeat interval. For example, Quigley and Berntson (1990) noted that the physiological inference that parasympathetic activation is potentiated in the presence of sympathetic activation may depend on whether measures are expressed as heart rate or interbeat interval. A related point, to which we will return later in the chapter, is that the scaling of a variable can determine whether or not an interaction term is significant in a statistical analysis (Loftus 1978).

How can we compare subjects using measures that may not be scaled with equally spaced units? Typically, our research is directed at groups differing in a psychological characteristic (e.g. impulsivity). One might hope that comparing averages computed across the individuals in each group would be accurate. This hope would be somewhat justified if the scaling distortions were randomly distributed between groups, but scaling distortions are not likely to be random. It is more likely, for example, that a distance of one unit of heart rate reflects a greater change in impulsivity for subjects scoring relatively low on an impulsivity scale than for subjects scoring relatively high. Such non-

random distortions would result in inaccurate variability estimates: the low-impulsivity group will have an inaccurately low variability and the high impulsivity inaccurately high; moreover, the mean distance between groups will be inaccurate.

The claim of inaccuracy applies only with respect to an ideal scale of impulsivity. This epistemological issue has ramifications for how we think about the statistics that we would like to apply to our data. Michell (1986) reviewed a long-standing controversy about the relationship between scaling and statistics. *Representational* theory requires that the assignment of numbers to dimensions such as impulsivity (via self-report or heart rate reactions) should reflect empirical relationships among the individuals that establish known number system properties, such as equally spaced intervals between integers in the scale. Our impulsiveness measure, however, might reliably order individuals yet not have this interval scale property (i.e., the measure does not state that the difference in impulsivity between individuals scoring 30 and 20 is the same as that between individuals scoring 20 and 10). Representational theory suggests that we must empirically test the properties of our scale in order to establish, for example, whether it orders individuals but does not assign values with equally spaced intervals. Representational theory further suggests that applying parametric statistics to measures that exhibit only nominal, ordinal, or interval properties is wrong (or, at least, not meaningful), since parametric statistics is designed for numbers that are representative of fundamental measurement systems in which *ratios* can be accurately compared (e.g., $4/2 = 100/50$).

Operational theory, on the other hand, suggests that impulsivity is what impulsivity scales measure. If such measures are appropriately distributed and meet other analytic assumptions, then the application of parametric statistics is fine. Classical theory similarly accepts the use of statistics and the validity of inferences, but only if the measure of impulsivity can be justified as a valid estimate of "true" impulsivity. Our argument implied both that such impulsivity existed (aligning it with operational and classical theory) and that our empirical data would not scale impulsivity with ratio properties (misaligning it with representational theory).

Luce and colleagues (1990, pp. 294–336) commented upon Michell's review and subsequent work. They support the legitimacy of applying parametric statistics in that the sample statistics can appropriately describe the sample. The interval scale properties are seen, however, as limiting the meaningfulness of certain numerical relationships. For example, positive linear transformations will not distort the relationship between a sample mean and its true value for either ratio or equal-interval scales. The relationship between the difference of the two means and the true difference is, however, distorted in the case of equal-interval but not ratio scales. Thus, scientific inferences about the size of a difference between true means are not meaningful for results scaled with only an interval level of measurement. By their arguments, improving measurement from interval to ratio scales extends the number of relationships that can be meaningfully inferred and generalized.

One solution for assessing measures with unknown properties is to abandon statistical procedures based on the assumption of equal-interval measurement and use statistics based on ordinal or categorical scaling (e.g. Siegal 1956). The cost of this solution is a loss of power (less likelihood of detecting differences that are truly present) for specific comparisons. One also rather obviously loses the use of parametric statistical tests, whose current well-developed forms feature such advantages as testing whole designs at once and controlling for covariates. Incurring this cost may be appropriate if scaling is truly ordinal or less, but in the case of psychophysiological measures most might argue that the scaling is more than ordinal even if ratio or equal-interval scaling has not been established. Short of doing the considerable work to prove that appropriate scale properties are present, the best procedure may be to use parametric statistics to identify potentially significant effects and then use nonparametric statistics to confirm the statistical significance of the identified effects. The most important concern, though, is interpretation. For example, statements of magnitude about impulsivity require a conceptual or empirical scaling that accurately places individuals on an equal-interval continuum. In the absence of such scaling, only ordinal conclusions are appropriate – for example, "individuals with higher impulsivity scores are more likely to show earlier EMG response onsets."

A second approach to making group comparisons with measures having unknown scale properties is to use within-subject analyses. Conceptually, the dependent measure then becomes a difference score. Each subject experiences multiple conditions, and the response differences among conditions form the dependent measure (with variance due to the mean level of responding for each subject; between-subject variance is removed). Our current question is whether this improves the comparability of scores between subjects. We will ask only an ordinal question about impulsivity by testing two groups, an impulsive group and a comparison group. We have two dependent measures collected, blood pressure and photoplethysmographic pulse amplitudes.

One question is whether resting, baseline values of these measures differ significantly between groups. If our technique for measuring blood pressure is applied correctly then the values obtained can be compared with parametric statistics. We cannot be as confident of our pulse amplitude measures, however. We should not unthinkingly apply parametric statistics to compare groups, since the group

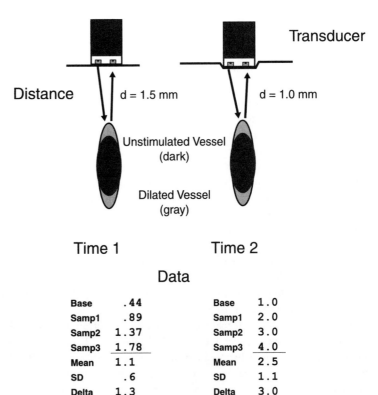

Figure 3. Physiological example of how a nonlinear distortion resulting from variability in placement of a device influences not only the value of measures but also the differences in these measures from baseline measurements (see text).

"main effect" can only compare mean amplitudes of unknown scaling between groups.

A difference score seems helpful if we move to a second question of our experiment. Are the reactions of impulsive subjects greater than those of nonimpulsive subjects? We have administered a mental arithmetic task and measured blood pressure and pulse amplitude. Comparison of blood pressure changes can again be justified. We can now express pulse amplitude as a change from baseline. Have we improved the comparability of our groups? Individual differences in pulse amplitude values are large whereas changes in pulse amplitude are usually more comparable among individuals. The variability of the difference scores may be less than the variability of the amplitudes. Yet this apparent increase in comparability is illusory, because the differencing operation itself cannot change the scale properties of the measure. Figure 3 shows this diagrammatically.

The figure shows a photo transducer placed over a blood vessel, which in the resting state (darkened in the figure) has an identical size for two measurement periods (time 1 and time 2). An experiment is then conducted that induces a vasodilation; for instance, measures are repeated after a 20-min rest between aerobic exercise performed at both time 1 and time 2. The dilation shown is the same for time 1 and time 2, as illustrated with the gray ellipses in the figure. The experiment measures the dilation at three successive time points and scores the maximum change, or delta. The photo device, an optical receiver–emitter, is placed over the vessels: at time 1, it is correctly placed exactly at the skin surface; for time 2, placement is shown as identical but the pressure of attachment has moved the receiver 0.5 mm closer to the vessel measured. The diagram shows the devices working perfectly, but the placement difference has a known effect on the measurement. Reflected light is being measured, and light intensity is known to change as the square of the distance between the light source and receiver. The results shown in the figure incorporate this expected change in light intensity due to the change in distance between emitter and receiver from time 1 to time 2. The consequence of a technical error in device placement is a rescaling of the data between times 1 and 2. The diagram shows how the measurements of the same physiological entity are no longer comparable for mean, standard deviation, or differences.

Our consideration of scaling suggests that caution is warranted with many psychophysiological measures. Parametric statistical procedures can be interpreted with confidence when a measure accurately assesses the range of variability of a physiological parameter of interest with equal units. We cannot safely assume this to be the case when the exact source of a signal is unknown, and thus we cannot calibrate our measure in the equal units appropriate to this signal source. Technical errors or inconsistencies can similarly change measurement scaling between and within individuals on different occasions. Scaling errors can contaminate difference scores as much as absolute measures. Measurement errors may in some cases contribute only to the "random" error of measurement, but consistent biases may also occur.

We have some pragmatic recommendations, which are based on two assumptions: (i) most investigators are primarily concerned with an ordinal hypothesis (e.g., that impulsive subjects show greater reactivity than nonimpulsive subjects); and (ii) the psychophysiological measure is expressed in physical units that can be assumed, relative to the variable of interest, to be monotonic (i.e., larger numbers reliably indicate more of the variable than smaller numbers). In the ideal situation of knowing precisely what the research outcome should be, the preplanned comparison can be set up to test with parametric statistics and checked with a comparable rank-order statistic. More often, though, the investigator has only general expectations and seeks results that may sharpen particular concepts. For example, we may expect impulsive subjects to have more reactive heart rate than nonimpulsive subjects yet be unsure whether this will be expressed primarily in heart rate level, heart rate reactions to the first stimulus, or smaller decreases in heart rate reactions over time. In such a case, parametric statistical analyses could be used to explore the data and identify potential differences that are consistent with the general expectations. The selected comparisons should then be repeated with rank-order statistics to ensure that scaling problems have not created spurious parametric results. Any truly exploratory, post hoc findings could be treated similarly. Interpretations of support for general expectations stated as ordinal differences would seem justified using this strategy, given acceptable levels of significance in the rank-order statistics. Ideally, the current observations would permit us to conceptualize impulsivity and its relation to psychophysiological measures more completely and so provide us with a measurement model for future work.

During the design phase of a research project, scale issues should be considered. A project primarily directed at individual differences must ensure that measures from different individuals are comparable. Thus, the interval versus ratio scale properties of a measure should weigh heavily in measure selection decisions. Projects directed at within-subject investigations of the influence of environmental events on psychophysiological response should also consider scale properties. Difference scores do not solve difficult scale problems, although they are helpful if it is assumed that individual differences and measurement error influence the level of a score and not the scaling of change in level.

SAMPLING: TIME CONSTITUTES SAMPLE IN WITHIN-SUBJECT DESIGNS

Prior to initiation of the research, consideration should be given to data scoring and analysis. Psychophysiologists invariably sample physiological signals that are always present. An experimental psychologist must convince a subject to emit a reaction, but living subjects continually produce brain potentials, heart rate, and skin conductance in the absence of volition. To collect psychophysiological data we must sample an ongoing signal by extracting a time series of data points spanning the course of the time the subject is in our laboratory. Care must be taken to sample these time points without bias and in a fashion that can be replicated by ourselves and other scientists.

As with any sampling, our measures will be more stable and less susceptible to random error if we can collect more time samples from periods sharing the characteristics of interest to us. If we ask a person to do mental arithmetic for five minutes, then blood pressure collected from that period will be estimated better by three samples at 90-sec intervals (close to the maximum number appropriate with a standard cuff technique) than by a single sample. Samples should be spaced at equal intervals unless there are good reasons to sample differently. A psychometric rationale can be offered for this advice. If we assume that our blood pressure measures have a true component and a random error component and that we are sampling the same true component throughout the measurement period, then the true variance in our measure will increase n times as fast as the error variance when we increase the number of measures, where n is defined as the ratio of the increased number of measures taken over the original number (Spearman–Brown prophecy formula; see e.g. Guilford 1954, chap. 13). Kamarck and associates (1992) provided an example of increased measurement stability resulting from applying sampling ideas to the study of cardiovascular reactivity.

An important but simple consideration in sampling is whether the research hypothesis refers to the *tonic level* of a variable (e.g., heart rate levels throughout a 5-min task) or the *phasic response* of a variable (e.g., transient increase in heart rate following a specific stimulus). Counting R-wave spikes for the 5-min task period is an excellent sampling strategy for heart rate level but would not be adequate to resolve heart response in (say) the 5 sec following a stimulus. The heartbeat count uses all the data available in the interval and thus is more reliable than sampling the counts for only a portion of the time period. Sampling must differ for detecting the response to an environmental stimulus. The timing of each individual heartbeat relative to the preceding heartbeat must be saved (ideally, to millisecond accuracy) for heartbeats during the 5 sec preceding and following the stimulus. Tonic and phasic are relative terms, but the point is that, despite differences in sampling time frames, exhaustive sampling within those time frames should yield the most reproducible data.

Some scoring practices are questionable when viewed from the perspective of sampling. Samples of equal length should be compared to ensure that the central tendency and variability of the samples are equally likely to be well estimated between samples. For example, consider the response at the surface of the cortex to a flash of light. The EEG is sampled for 2 sec surrounding the flash, and ensemble averages are computed across multiple flashes. The event-related potential following the flash could be analyzed and graphed solely for the 1 sec following the flash. This would not, however, establish that a cortical response occurred that differed from ongoing EEG activity. The 1 sec prior to the stimulus should also be considered, and the ensemble averaging of this time sample should not yield a waveform comparable to the 1 sec following the light flash. Statistical comparison could verify the existence of a waveform, and graphical presentation of activity before and after stimulus can illustrate the presence of a waveform not present in ongoing EEG.

The scoring of complex waveforms can also be biased from a sampling perspective. A biphasic heart rate response (e.g., deceleration followed by acceleration) can be scored as the difference between the heart rate at stimulus onset and the minimum heart rate following the stimulus within a 10-sec window. It would be tempting to establish that a response occurred by testing whether consistently positive scores were observed for differences formed by subtracting the minimum heart rate from the heart rate at stimulus onset. This scoring scheme, however, is highly biased toward a positive difference, and significant "responses" would likely be found in the majority of random samples of heart rate. A further problem is that the minimum heart rate is a single, extreme sample value that is likely to be an unstable estimate of the size of any response, yet this minimum is compared to a single heart rate at stimulus onset. Stability could be increased by comparing response values to a prestimulus mean of 10 sec of heart rate. Such a measure would remain biased, though, as single points are differenced from a mean value. Adequate scoring requires that the sampling be comparable for pre- and poststimulus periods. This can be done either (i) by including all heart rate values before and after the stimulus for 10 sec in a single analysis (see e.g. Wilson 1967) or (ii) by scoring maximum and minimum values from smoothed data for equivalent samples of pre- and poststimulus heart rate and then using these in analyses.

NUMBER OF SUBJECTS, POWER, AND EFFECT SIZE

In a climate of reduced resources for the support of research, our studies should be large enough to detect the differences we seek (if present) but not significantly larger. Stated differently, it is important to know the power of our studies. Power, then, is the probability of rejecting the null hypothesis when it is false; this complements the more familiar probability of accepting the null hypothesis when it is false (often termed alpha). Power is determined by the ratio of the expected mean differences in behavior and the error variance. Therefore, any parameter affecting the effect size or the error variance plays a role in increasing the power of an experimental design. Such parameters could include the number of subjects in an experiment, the effect size necessary to be meaningful, the variance of the factor of interest, and the error variance. Power analysis has been introduced in some depth to psychology by Cohen (1977, 1992). However, power calculations are influenced by the design of the experiment, and many available tables and programs refer only to between-subject comparisons. A general linear model approach for computing power has been successfully applied to repeated measures by Muller and co-workers (Muller & Barton 1989, 1991; Muller et al. 1992). These authors created software built upon the SAS (1989) package to perform power analyses for repeated measures analyses. General power computation software is now commercially available (e.g. Borenstein, Cohen, & Rothstein 1997).

During the design phase of the experiment, steps should be taken to obtain adequate power. Researchers can increase the treatment variance by selecting groups or conditions that maximize expected differences. Care can be taken to make sure that conditions showing greater differences will be well sampled – for example, ensuring that the high-impulsivity cell of a design is oversampled relative to the prevalence of high impulsivity in the population. In addition, power can be increased by planning comparisons in advance so that precise, one-degree-of-freedom tests can explore the specific expected finding.

Because maximizing the power of your research involves reducing error variance, designing an optimal study and conducting the correct test of the hypotheses becomes critical. Often a step that psychophysiologists take to achieve reduction of error variance is use of a repeated measures design (see next section). Consideration can also be given to measuring covariates that would add variance into the error term if not controlled or to blocking subjects by factors (such as gender or worksite) and then subtracting irrelevant variance due to such blocking factors. Considerations in selecting the appropriate analysis of variance for this design can also optimize power (e.g., a multivariate versus a univariate approach; see discussion in next sections). The most straightforward way to reduce error variance is to increase the number of subjects. This typically increases the time and cost of an experiment, but the impact of the number of subjects on the power of the experiment should not be overlooked. As the number of subjects increases in balanced designs, the use of powerful multivariate statistics becomes appropriate, further increasing power. See Algina and Keselman (1997) for specific guidelines on increasing the power of your design by using a proper sample size and the correct test when, realistically speaking, an estimate of the expected difference between treatment means is not available. O'Brien and Muller (1993) discuss approaches to power for designs that employ repeated measures.

DESIGN: REPEATED MEASURES VERSUS BETWEEN-SUBJECT ASSESSMENT

A final basic design decision is whether to compare the influence of a variable between different groups of subjects or to use a single group and expose them to all levels of the variable. Our initial example of the influence of noise on pupil size compared exposing the same subjects to noise and quiet with exposing different subject groups to noise and to quiet. In the first design, the mean of pupil size under the noise condition is compared to the mean in the quiet condition; in the second design, the mean of one group in noise is compared to the second group in noise. Most psychophysiologists use some form of within-subject design. Why? And what problems does this create? We shall use pupil size as an illustrative example.

As with most psychophysiological measures, the range of differences between individuals in pupil diameter is larger than the range of expected changes due to stimulation. The result is that measures of pupil diameter before and after stimulus will be highly correlated. For example, three subjects could have pupil diameters of 3, 4, and 5 mm. A dilation for each might yield diameters of 3.2, 4.3, and 5.1 mm, respectively. The correlation between pre- and poststimulation values is high, despite the variability among the subjects in the size of change (0.2, 0.3, and 0.1 mm). Consider the statistical result if identical values for pupil size were obtained from one group of subjects for the baseline values and from another for the stimulated values. Such values would be independently collected in the two groups (uncorrelated). A t-test would then be informative if we used a t-test for *dependent* values for the within-subject comparison and an "independent groups" t-test for the other comparison (see e.g. Hays 1994). In both cases, the mean difference between baseline and stimulated pupil is 0.2 mm. This value is divided through by the estimate of the standard error of the mean for the between-subjects design (0.52) or for the within-subjects design (0.01). Hence, the t-value of 0.4 for the between-subjects comparison is dramatically smaller than the value of 20 for the within-subject comparison. Because of the strong correlation between baseline and test values within subject, the within-subject test statistic is markedly more sensitive than the between-subjects test (Hays 1994; Keppel 1991). This difference in sensitivity is the primary argument for using a within-subject design in psychophysiological research.

The main drawback of within-subject designs is dependency (carryover) between conditions. One form of this is dependency within the dependent measure (e.g. pupil size). As discussed later, baseline differences within a dependent measure can be resolved with adjustments conducted during the data analysis. Another form of this within-subject design problem, *serial* dependency, reflects carryover between levels of the independent variable or experimental manipulation (e.g., between a noise condition and a quiet condition). This dependency in the independent variable seriously challenges the interpretation of research results. An example drawn from the extensive discussion of the problem by Poulton (1973; Poulton & Freeman 1966) may be useful. Poulton and Edwards (1979) explicitly compared the results gathered when the influences of a control and three stress conditions were assessed in between-subjects and within-subject groups; they also compared results from both designs to an additional control condition defined by performance during a practice day on the three tasks used as dependent measures. The tasks were a vigilance task, a serial reaction time task, and a dual task with tracking and simple reaction time. Stressors were heat, noise, and heat and noise combined. Each stress condition and a control condition were run on a separate day for the within-subject design, which used a Latin square that assigned different groups of subjects to different orders (see discussion in Winer 1971). The between-subjects design had all subjects trained on the practice day, whereafter the subjects were separated into four groups. Each group received

---

BOX 1. Carryover Diagnostics

Conditions: Noise versus Control

Dependent measure: Heart rate level

Fifty subjects are split into two groups randomly: Noise First group or Control First group

The experiment is then run as follows:

Group	Day 1	Day 2
Noise First ($n = 25$)	Noise	Control
Control First ($n = 25$)	Control	Noise

The standard analysis of this design would have a factor for noise versus control and a factor for order group (between-subjects comparison of Noise First and Control First). The main effect of Noise is the primary outcome of scientific interest. Order has been "controlled," but if a statistically significant (or near-significant) interaction between order group and noise occurs then there is concern that either subject sampling or condition sampling is not independent. Poulton's advice is to run the comparison on the Day-1 data alone, which forms a between-subjects test of the noise effect. If this comparison is not consistent with the main effect from the primary analysis, then again the validity of the results are challenged because now they suggest that Day-2 results were conditioned by the subjects' Day-1 experiences.

---

a single treatment (one of the three stressors or the control) on the next day. All groups were then retested in the control condition on another day. The result of this elaborate and arduous scheme was an opportunity to compare the influence of stressors on performance using the "practice" control, the control from the within-subject Latin square design, and the second-day control results from the between-subjects design. Obviously, if design made no difference then the results should be comparable regardless of the control used in the comparison.

The results indicated significant problems. For example, the influence of heat was significant using the within-subject control condition, but not in practice-day or between-subjects comparisons. More alarmingly, one of the reaction time tasks showed an enhancement in one control comparison and a decrement in another. Similarly, the order of conditions in the within-subject design changed the direction of effect of a stressor on performance. The reader is urged to look at the details of this example in the original publication. The problem of carryover is illustrated well, although the sample sizes of Poulton and Edwards (1979) were minimal and the evident carryover effects not readily explained. One can hope that some of their anomalous results were due to chance and not to reliable serial dependency effects. Nonetheless, the study – as well as Poulton's methodological arguments – clearly warn the investigator using a within-subject design to check its validity. Investigators should first adhere to the general methodological advice to (a) avoid within-subject designs when differential carryover between conditions is likely and (b) isolate conditions experimentally as much as feasible. We also share Poulton's recommendations. Ideally, a study would be run with both within-subject and between-subjects designs. More practically, within-subject designs should vary the order of treatments so that the first treatment received can be analyzed as a between-subjects comparison in order to test whether the direction of influence of any variable is consistent with any within-subject effect obtained. If the direction is inconsistent, then diagnostics should be initiated to understand any carryover effect present in the experiment. The simple example detailed in Box 1 can readily be generalized to more complex designs.

An interesting illustration of carryover effects and their control within an experimental manipulation is provided by Osterhout, Bersick, and McKinnon (1997). These investigators were interested in the influence of word class, frequency, and length upon early negativity in the cortical evoked potential. In experiment 1, words varying in grammatical class, length, and frequency were studied in the context of sentences drawn from paragraphs of meaningful text. Rather clearly, sentence structure induces a dependency between words presented in this fashion. One could expect that some serial predictivity from one word to the next in a sentence would be present and likely vary from word to word (i.e., lower predictivity for the word following "the" than for the word following "grotesque." Put in another way, serial dependency between experimental stimuli is present and variable. Experiment 2 addressed this problem by using similar words but presented without any connecting sentence structure. Their intent was to study the influence on early negativity without the influence of grammar, but methodologically it also varied the nature of the carryover between stimulus items (note, however, that experiment 2 did not eliminate or completely control this carryover). Their key results were robust between experiments, although there were significant differences that were attributed to the influence of grammatical constraints. From a methodological perspective, experiment 2 provided a check on the influence of carryover but also demonstrated that carryover was a confound in experiment 1. In general, this experiment is a good example of both within-manipulation carryover and of checking on this carryover.

Data Collection and Reduction

DATA QUALITY CONTROL

Once the design is set, data collection commences. The experiment should be run exactly as designed. Nonetheless, the results from the first few subjects should be scrutinized carefully to ensure that the assumptions made in designing the study are reasonable – for example, whether a 10-min baseline truly permitted a return of blood pressure to approximately normal values. When data from the design based on the researcher's original assumptions indicate that these assumptions are flawed, redesigning the experiment at this early point is clearly more efficient than completing research with an inappropriate design. The other continuing task during data collection is data quality control.

Psychophysiological data are characteristically fallible, large in quantity, individualistic in quality, and low in intrinsic interest (in their raw form). Studies of the event-related potential, for example, would typically sample data at 100 Hz and might, in a small study, accumulate 100,000 data points per subject. Although averaged electroencephalographic data graphically presented may hold some fascination, the 100,000 numbers constituting the raw data are likely to be low in intrinsic interest. The fallible quality of the data arises from changes in the electrical signal that are large but unrelated to our interest in brain function. For instance, eye and head movements are likely to induce voltage transients that are large and irrelevant to our interests, so editing of these irrelevant values is necessary to maintain the integrity of our data. The massiveness and low interest value of the data pose the first challenge to data editing, one that is likely to overwhelm any attempts at visual editing of the numeric data. How can the data contaminated by such factors as eye movement and head movement be identified efficiently and with appropriate accuracy?

Graphical and statistical techniques combined with human judgment are generally required for appropriate editing. Editing techniques are somewhat specific to different measures and have been discussed by others (Berntson et al. 1990; Cheung 1981; Gratton, Coles, & Donchin 1983). We will provide a brief overview of approaches, in part to emphasize the importance of editing for data integrity.

A number of useful books are available to assist in the graphical presentation of raw data. These will as-sist the investigator in presenting individual data so that outliers can readily be detected. Tukey's classic volume, *Exploratory Data Analysis* (1977), is a useful starting point, as it presents graphical techniques that permit rapid assessment of entire data sets. Techniques of particular relevance are box plots and "stem and leaf" displays, in addition to the usual plotting of the frequency distribution of the data. Box plots, for example, typically display the data as a box centered on the median and extending to the first and third quartiles. Extending beyond the box are lines to the minimum and maximum values present in the data set. The investigator can quickly assess whether the data show the appropriate range of value, central tendency, and balance around the median. Fortunately, many statistical package programs (e.g. Statistica) provide programs to efficiently display raw data in box plot and stem-and-leaf formats.

Once outliers or unusually distributed data are detected, what is to be done? Data can be transformed, outliers can be eliminated, or nothing can be done. Levey (1980) provides a thorough and well-written discussion of the various options. Little absolute advice can be offered beyond that the investigator should first try to understand why a data point is an outlier or why a distribution is distorted. For instance, examining the laboratory notes might reveal that a low–heart rate outlier was from an impulsive child who did not meet study inclusion criteria because medication had been administered just before the study. Such data should be deleted, since it is an error that it was collected and analyzed at all. More typically, heart rate values (e.g., 10 beats per minute) or changes (e.g., 85 beat-per-minute change between heartbeats) will have occurred that are physiologically impossible. Investigation may reveal computer software bugs or data collection errors that might be correctable or may require data deletion. Similarly, distributional characteristics can identify factors such as sampling bias that initially escaped detection by the investigator, who would then have to judge whether interpretation is possible given the bias. If not, then the data set must be discarded; there is no transformation of systematically biased data that will render them interpretable. If no reasons are apparent for the outliers and if neither the sampling nor the manipulations can be faulted, then transformation can be considered.

Transformation is indicated when outliers or the distributional pattern will inappropriately lead to a disproportionate effect on the results owing to a small percentage of the observations. "Appropriate" and "disproportionate" are difficult to define; they remain dependent on the investigator's judgment. For some investigations, outliers may be theoretically expected and indeed the most interesting outcome of the study. The weight given these outliers by the original metric may be appropriate. Given the robustness of common statistics to moderate departures from assumed statistical distributions (see discussion in Levey 1980), transformation may frequently be unnecessary since little disproportionate influence exists. Transformations necessarily make it more difficult to understand how the original measures responded to manipulations or individual differences. This problem is particularly acute when data are scaled on a subject-by-subject basis – for instance, range scores in which a skin conductance response is scored as a proportion of the individual's range of responses (Lykken 1972). A reader interested in the magnitude of skin conductance change in microsiemens will likely be unable to find this number unless the investigators have taken care to provide this information. Transformations can also change the mean results more than most investigators would expect. Levey (1980) and also Cacioppo, Tassinary, and Fridlund (1990) have provided numerical examples in which a typically used transformation changes the mean difference from favoring one condition to favoring another condition. As always, the best approach is to make full use of the graphical and statistical capabilities offered by modern computer programs. The degree of disproportionate influence of outliers or clusters of points can be checked by calculating descriptive statistics with and without these points. Distributions can be examined before and after a transformation to ensure that the rescaling produces conceptually reasonable results. Finally, as with many statistical problems, outliers and distributional problems are frequently solved by increasing the sample size.

When the original scaling does yield outliers and/or distributions in which some observations are having an disproportionate influence, then transformations should be applied. Three topics raised by transformations will be discussed next: transform issues specific to psychophysiology, the use of nonparametric statistics, and dealing with outliers.

The basic unit of measurement for beat-by-beat heart rate and skin conductance has been controversial; thus, we will discuss these two examples although the issues are relevant to most measures. Both the heart rate and skin conductance measures involve a choice between reciprocals. Investigations of beat-by-beat heart rate collect the time of occurrence of the R wave of the electrocardiogram. A *period* or *interval* measure expresses results as the time in milliseconds between R waves, whereas a *rate* measure converts this time to the number of beats to be expected in a minute if the current temporal separation continued – number of milliseconds in a minute (60,000) divided by the number of milliseconds between R waves. An examination of these two metrics (see e.g. Graham 1978a,b; Jennings, Stringfellow, & Graham 1974) revealed different properties of the metrics but no overriding superiority for either; that is, depending on the investigator's scientific question, one or the other may be more suitable. An interesting implication of the metric employed was demonstrated by Quigley and Berntson (1990). These investigators (see also Berntson et al. 1994a) were interested in modeling the influence of joint parasympathetic and sympathetic activation

upon heartbeat timing. Prior work (Levy 1977, Levy & Martin 1984) using electrical stimulation of sympathetic and parasympathetic nerves had suggested that heart rate changes in response to parasympathetic stimulation were greater when sympathetic stimulation was also present, an effect known as accentuated antagonism. The work of Berntson, Uchino, and Cacioppo (1994b) with pharmacological blocking revealed additive sympathetic and parasympathetic influences using interbeat interval as the metric. Quigley and Berntson (1990) reviewed the literature and suggested that no accentuated antagonism was evidenced by the interbeat interval metric; antagonism was evident only with the heart rate metric. Statistically, accentuated antagonism is an interaction term – greater vagal influence at one level of sympathetic activation than at another level of sympathetic activation.

A number of authors have pointed out that the presence of a statistical interaction is particularly sensitive to the measurement scale; Loftus (1978) provided a particularly nice discussion of the issue. In the case of heart rate versus interbeat interval, the effect of the transformation can be intuitively understood from a numerical example. Assume that the interbeat interval increases 60 msec (due to vagal activation) from a baseline during which the heart beats once every 1,000 msec and also 60 msec from another baseline during which the heart beats every 500 msec (the latter baseline is altered by sympathetic stimulation). This example describes an additive, noninteractive relationship. Transforming to the reciprocal, heart rate in beats per minute (bpm), we have a change from 60 bpm to 56.6 bpm and a change from a 120-bpm baseline to 107.1 bpm. A 3.4-bpm change compared to a 12.9-bpm change is consistent with accentuated antagonism. Statistically, an interaction appears to be present: heart rate changes more from the higher level of sympathetic background than from the lower level. But does accentuated antagonism exist? The answer depends on the metric, and the choice of metric depends on the investigator's concept of heartbeat control. Levy and colleagues (e.g. Levy 1977) might argue for the validity of heart rate based on their model of intracellular mechanisms, which yields a nonlinear interaction between sympathetic–adrenergic and parasympathetic–cholinergic activation. Berntson and colleagues (1994a,b; see also Berntson, Cacioppo, & Quigley 1993) might argue for the validity of interbeat interval, given that their mathematical model of additive control is simple and yet provides an excellent fit with their data. Ultimately, the choice of metric will depend upon a preponderance of evidence on control of the heart beat and whether that regulation is best described by interbeat interval or its reciprocal transformation, heart rate. Metric and statistics ultimately cannot be divorced from our interpretations; Loftus (1978) makes the same point for measures of memory in his discussion of how interaction terms are dependent on the unit of measurement.

The development of the electrodermal measure provides an interesting further illustration of this point. The current use of measures of skin conductance to express the change of sweat glands after stimulation is based on a generally accepted model of how sweat glands are anatomically arranged and physiologically activated (Boucsein 1992; Hugdahl 1995). Measures of conductance (in μS) have the added advantage over reciprocal measures of resistance (in $k\Omega$) of reducing the dependency of response magnitude on baseline magnitude (i.e., the conductance measure does not show an interaction between baseline level and response magnitude).

We have already advocated the limited use of a transformation (moving to nonparametric statistics to check parametric results) when the scale properties of our measures are unknown or suspect. Nonparametric statistics convert the original scale to either rank orders or categories. Levey (1980), among many others, pointed out that such a transformation necessarily discards information. When parametric assumptions are correct, parametric statistics will virtually always be more powerful (more sensitive to an existing difference between groups or conditions) than nonparametric tests. Rescaling the data to ordinal or nominal categories does provide the investigator some insight into whether the original scale may give disproportionate weight to certain observations. Significant discrepancies between parametric and nonparametric tests are thus a signal to the investigator to look closely at the scaling and distribution of the data. Another rescaling is frequently done but rarely discussed as such: a continuous measure such as weight is often converted to an analysis of variance factor by splitting values at the mean or median. Scale values have been converted to a nominal scale (i.e., greater weight and lesser weight). The potential loss of information relative to using a statistically equivalent testing procedure such as regression analysis has been argued thoroughly elsewhere (see e.g. Cohen & Cohen 1975).

Bush, Hess, and Wolford (1993) provided an interesting simulation study that addresses the influence of certain transformations as well as outliers on the power of statistical outcomes. These investigators specifically examined within-subject transformations using randomly generated normal and skewed distributions. Varying sample sizes were drawn per subject (i.e., samples within a condition), and the number of subjects and effect sizes were varied also. A thousand or more "experiments" were carried out for each set of parameters tested. All experiments involved a single baseline condition and a single treatment condition, with the baseline-to-treatment manipulation done within each subject. The transformations examined included the arithmetic mean of a subject's data within condition (i.e., averaged over observations within that condition for that subject), log of that mean, a Z-score based on the mean and standard deviations for all observations of that particular subject, a range-corrected score, and a ratio score (expressing score as a fraction of the highest score of that subject). The Z-score measure performed the best overall across variations in sample size, number of observations per subject, skewness, and percentage of data with outliers.

The Z-score continued to do well relative to using medians as well as the other scores across different methods of eliminating outliers. The combination of Z-scores and trimming (eliminating an equal percentage of extreme scores from all subjects) performed the best when outliers were added to the simulation data. Performed "best" was defined as the ability to detect the real difference in conditions that had been added by the experimenters. Very few instances were found in which transformation yielded anomalous results (e.g., baselines higher than treatment) that differed from the original data. Overall, this simulation study suggests that transformations are useful when subjects vary in the degree of variability across observations.

Representation of Results

The results of your research must be presented so their meaning is evident not only to you but also to your peers, students, and ideally to the general public. Toward this end, any tool that is helpful should be used as long as the accuracy of presentation is not sacrificed: graphs, three-dimensional models, or even spatially positioned physical objects. Professor Tryon was known at Berkeley for using helium-filled balloons placed around the office to help him understand the results of cluster analysis. Appropriate representation is important for the evaluation of the quality of your raw data (as noted before), for assessing the meaning of your results, and for the presentation of results to your peers.

A number of books on scientific graphics are available. Most of these rightfully are critical of the modal scientific illustration. Cleveland (1985), for example, found that 30% of the graphs presented in *Science* in 1980 had significant problems: features that were not explained, data points or lines that could not be discriminated, an error in construction, or reproduction so poor that the graph was illegible. Even in the absence of such significant problems, it is common for graphs to obscure rather than highlight the primary feature of the results (e.g., with gridlines that overpower the results, axis numbers or legends that obscure data points) or to be excessively complex.

Different authors provide help in graphical representation in different ways. The history of graphical presentation is used to derive principles for good graphing in the richly illustrated contributions of Tufte (1983, 1990, 1997), which provide an excellent set of examples of how adequate representation leads to appropriate decisions and how disasters can result from inadequate representation (see particularly Tufte 1997). A number of excellent guides focusing more closely on the illustration of typical scientific data are also available (Cleveland 1985; Wainer & Thissen 1981, 1993). We found the Cleveland volume to be a particularly useful "hands-on" guide to graphical representation; like a number of others, it provides ample illustrations of poor graphic representation with correction of the faults identified. A more recent book by Jacoby (1997) offers a pocketbook-sized condensation of graphic advice. Specific information on the plotting and analysis of residuals in regression illustrates the importance of graphing techniques for analyzing as opposed to solely representing results (Cook & Weisberg 1994). Finally, the computer offers a wealth of new approaches to visualizing and modeling results. Collected articles such as those of Earnshaw, Vince, and Jones (1997) may provide ideas for novel ways of using computer representations to understand and communicate results. Representation should help us identify the main outcome of our research, which then must be verified using statistical analysis.

Analysis

The analytic approach should follow directly from the research design and the characteristics of the dependent measures. The basic tool of analysis in most of psychophysiology remains some form of analysis of variance; this approach is complemented by regression techniques, which can be used to calculate analysis of variance terms or as multiple regression analyses. Psychophysiological dependent measures are typically time series (sequential samples over time) of continuous varying quantities that are correlated from one sample to the next. Frequently, these time series are transformed – for example, a mean over a time period or condition is taken – so that the temporal character of the data is changed. An argument can be made for maintaining the time series and using statistical approaches designed specifically for such data. As researchers, rather than statisticians, we will review typical approaches to psychophysiological data and note a few possible improvements recently suggested by statisticians.

THE NULL HYPOTHESIS DEBATE

Most journals publishing psychophysiological work will review statistical results to see if they are "significant." The analysis of variance approach as well as the testing of regression coefficients implies the use of the null hypothesis to test hypotheses by using a fixed probability (e.g., $p < 0.05$) to reject this hypothesis. This approach has been widely criticized (Chow 1996; Cohen 1977, 1994; Harris 1991, 1997; Loftus 1994; Loftus & Masson 1994; see also the special section in vol. 8(1) of *Psychological Science* 1997) for its arbitrariness, its blindness to the size of the effect assessed, and its failure to estimate the likelihood of an empirical claim (Rozeboom 1960). Alternative

approaches to statistical testing have not, however, supplanted null hypothesis testing. Frick (1996) suggested that the continued popularity of null hypothesis testing is due to the appropriate fit between much of our research and the answers provided by this statistical approach. He argued that null hypothesis testing is generally appropriate under the following conditions:

1. when an investigator wishes to test an ordinal hypothesis – for instance, the N400 is or is not sensitive to grammatical errors;
2. when the investigator is *not* attempting to test quantitative predictions or provide guidance for applied situations in which application may require judgments about efficacy of the procedure tested relative to alternatives or countervailing influences;
3. when an investigator requires only sufficient evidence to accept a hypothesis (rather than requiring the probability that a claim is correct); and
4. when power to detect the desired effect is not precisely known.

Many psychophysiological investigations fit these conditions for appropriateness. In addition, establishing even an arbitrary probability value provides a measure that can be used across statistical tests to imply the strength of a relationship (Greenwald et al. 1996).

Nonetheless, critics of the null hypothesis have sound advice, too, which we would also recommend following. For example, Cohen (1994) advised close attention to measurement, careful understanding of data using graphical techniques, attention to effect sizes, reporting of confidence intervals, replicating of experiments, and employing meta-analytic techniques when possible. As the critics point out, null hypothesis testing cannot establish the validity of our hypotheses, null or alternative; null hypothesis testing only estimates the chance that this data would have occurred given that the null hypothesis is true. In reality, our conclusions must be based on thoughtful interpretation in the context of the empirical literature, available concepts, replicability within and across experiments, and available statistical indicants (see Abelson 1995).

COVARIANCE ISSUES AND BASE LEVEL DEPENDENCY

Levey (1980) suggested that base level dependency and data transformation were two issues akin to a bit of sand inside the shell of psychophysiology; by now, a lustrous pearl should have formed or the irritation should have killed the area. He notes that neither has occurred. Instead, these issues, along with arousal and inverted U functions, seem to haunt the area – we don't believe in ghosts but we can't stop thinking about them.

Some of the longevity of the base level dependency issue is based on the plausibility of it as a physiological mechanism. A response system might well be built so that it will respond less when it is operating with a higher output level than with a lower output level. If this were true, then we should certainly take level of function into account when measuring change from that level. This is the so-called law of initial values (Wilder 1958). Does it exist? When a base level–change correlation does appear, what should be done?

The law of initial values is not an empirical law. The preponderance of evidence may well be that baseline and change are unrelated (although we have just pointed out that this may not be true for all transformations of the results). The absence of a relationship in any single study (or even in groups of studies) is typically confounded by differences in the variables measured, the metric employed, the exact statistical approach, and a host of other factors. However, some authors have urged banishing the law – for statistical reasons as well as for empirically based conceptual reasons.

Myrtek and Foerster (1986) analyzed the previously used correlational techniques to see if change was related to base level. They pointed out that the calculations were biased toward finding the negative correlation expected by the law of initial values. They proposed a test eliminating this bias and found that baseline to change showed, if anything, a positive correlation between base level and change. Geenen and van de Vijver (1993) arrived at the same conclusion, but provided a simpler test statistic that was largely equivalent to the Myrtek and Foerster (1986) statistic. Conceptually, the baseline-to-change relationship can be accurately assessed as negative (law of initial values) if baseline variance is substantially larger than response-level variance; conversely, a positive relationship (found to be more likely by Myrtek & Foerster) is present if baseline variance is smaller than response-level variance. Bush and associates (1993) tested the sensitivity of baseline-adjusted scores in the simulation study previously discussed. The Z-score difference scores performed well – and better than not using difference scores – when baselines changed over time within a subject's data. This Z-score difference performed slightly better than the range score, which was designed to address law of initial values issues (covariance-adjusted scores were not tested). The point is, there exist statistical as well as empirical reasons for discarding the law of initial values.

A number of investigators have suggested that a careful assessment of the physiological basis of the response measure is superior to reliance on the dubious law of initial values. The law of initial values is appealing because it seems reasonable; a system may respond more vigorously from a low set point than from one near the maximum of its dynamic range. Different physiological systems may show different response characteristics, however. Furthermore, any corrections for baseline or set point should be based on the specific characteristics of the response in question rather than on a hypothetical relationship.

Berntson and colleagues (1994a,b) developed this point quite well conceptually and empirically for heart rate responses. The latter (1994b) study is an interesting comparison between sitting and standing postures of the influence of individual differences in baseline heart rate on responsivity to a challenge task. The group results showed less response to challenge in the standing relative to the sitting posture; this is in accordance with the "law," since the basal heart rate while standing was higher than the basal heart rate while sitting. The authors suggested that adjusting the baseline via posture yielded consistent correlations between responsivity and baseline because baseline was controlled by autonomic mechanisms. In contrast, individual differences in baseline are not necessarily due to autonomic factors. Individual differences in baseline heart rate were unrelated to response amplitude in both sitting and standing postures. The conclusion was that baseline values arise from a variety of factors. Some of these – for example, constitutional or genetic variation in heart rate – are unlikely to be constrained by the properties of autonomic responsivity. Other factors play upon the sympathetic and parasympathetic regulation of heart rate and thus will be influenced by the properties of these response systems. The researchers advocated further work in understanding the regulation of heart rate level, responsivity, and their relationship.

We summarize our review by suggesting that investigators interested in psychophysiological responses carefully assess how response values might be conceptually and empirically related to basal values for their measures. A statistical or conceptual model of the relation of change and basal state should provide the best response measurement (cf. Stemmler & Fahrenberg 1989). The conceptual assessment should consider the original design decision on choice of baseline and the degree of baseline stability present in the results. Jennings and colleagues (1992) reviewed the importance of baselines and suggested procedures for designing and assessing baselines. As a statistical part of this assessment, the presence of an association between baseline and response could be assessed using the technique of Geenen and van de Vijver (1993). If a significant relationship does not exist, then no correction is necessary. If a relationship does exist, then another attempt should be made to conceptualize the relation. At the very least, covariance adjustments for baseline influences could be made, the results analyzed and then compared to either raw or transformed difference scores. Reporting the noncorrected results is preferable if there are no outcome differences between corrected and noncorrected versions. Presentation of both analyses may be wise if corrected and noncorrected measures yield different results (see similar guidelines in Stemmler & Fahrenberg 1989). Llabre and co-workers (1991) provided a nice overview of the statistical issues involved in using difference scores versus covariance-corrected scores, providing further depth on the issues we have just discussed and extending them to the reliability and generalizability of results.

ANALYSIS OF COVARIANCE

Analysis of covariance can be applied for a multitude of reasons. A frequent use would be to control for factors that are not central to an experiment but might modify the results (e.g., degree of intelligence or anxiety of the participants). Within psychophysiology, however, covariance adjustments are first thought of as a means to "correct" for baseline effects.

As discussed before, such analyses should not be applied automatically. This is a temptation, since using analysis of covariance to assess and/or adjust the influence of basal levels is facilitated by the general availability of package programs performing this analysis. Care must be taken to represent the covariate accurately within the design. Does each subject have a single covariate value? Multiple values? Are the covariate terms pooled across groups? Maxwell, Delaney, and Manheimer (1985) explain, for example, how analysis of covariance results can frequently differ from the results of analysis of variance applied to residuals. The statistical model applied and the resulting differences in pooling across groups and conditions should be understood.

Most programs and statistical discussion of analysis of covariance focus on between- rather than within-subject designs. Adjusting for individual differences in between-subject psychophysiological studies can be important, but studies including at least one within-subject factor are much more common. A paper by Judd, McClelland, and Smith (1996) focused on within-subject designs. The authors addressed the optimal method of obtaining a valid estimate of the influence of the covariate. Standard analyses assume a homogeneity of covariate relationships across treatments; in other words, they assume — across treatments — that all extraneous variables covary in the same way and to the same degree with the dependent variable. Checking this assumption requires testing the interaction between covariate and treatments (by asking the question, "Do the treatments have varying relationships between the covariate and the variate?").

Two covariate situations are assessed for their robustness in the face of failed assumptions and differing analytic approaches. In the first, a single covariate is used for each subject. In psychophysiology this would correspond to the common design in which values from a single baseline period are used as a covariate in the assessment of values obtained from one or more tasks (e.g. mental arithmetic). The covariate in this situation is a between-subjects variable. In the second situation, the covariate is measured multiple times within each subject. For example, a brief baseline period might be used prior to each of a number of tasks. The value for each of these base-

lines could be paired (as a covariate) with the value from the task immediately following the baseline. The covariate in this situation is a within-subject variable. In the former (between-subjects) covariate case, three computational alternatives yield comparable power but vary in the assumptions about error variance that must be made. The simplest approach may be to use a regression technique, which can be implemented readily in SAS (Khatree & Naik 1995). In the latter (within-subject) case, different approaches yield markedly different results. No simple analytic approach can be offered, but Judd et al. (1996) offered guidance for analyzing such designs.

The testing of the homogeneity assumption for the covariances (assumed in most packages) is important but a bit complex. A reasonable compromise may be to plot covariate-treatment scatter diagrams for the cells of a within-subject design to see if any suspicion of inhomogeneity arises. If so, then testing of the assumption should be performed. If analysis of covariance is warranted, the standard programs can be applied once understood. Overall (1994) provided some interesting suggestions on using individual trend scores on repeated measures data to convert within-subject tests to between-subjects tests for certain procedures, including correction for baseline influences.

SEQUENTIAL TIME SAMPLES ARE STATISTICALLY DEPENDENT

Most psychophysiological research involves sequential samples in time from the same subject. Such designs must take the correlation between these samples into account at the time of data analysis (and ideally during design of the research). We have already discussed the enhanced power of repeated measures designs for our type of data and some of the design concerns. A remaining issue is the degree to which available statistical models accurately fit psychophysiological data and thus provide accurate statistical outcomes. The characteristics that make repeated measures a desirable design are precisely those that make analyzing the data a challenge. Psychophysiological measures do not typically meet the requirements of a standard repeated measures analysis: even though correlations between successive measurements of each subject reduce error variance, they violate assumptions of unrelated errors and homogeneity of the variance/covariance matrix (Huynh & Feldt 1970; Jennings & Wood 1976; Keselman et al. 1980; Vasey & Thayer 1987).

When deciding which statistic to use for a repeated measure design, often the choice is assumed to be between univariate or multivariate analysis of variance (ANOVA). One problem encountered in repeated measures is that the assumption of sphericity is usually violated. *Sphericity* requires that the covariance of all pairs of the repeated measures be equal (Huynh & Feldt 1970). Violation of this assumption leads to using a critical test statistic that is too small or to type-I error inflation (Box 1954). In other words, the repeated measures ANOVA assumes that differences between the correlations of any set of pairs of the within-subject treatment are due to chance and that there is an underlying constant correlation (Lavori 1990). Greenhouse and Geisser (1959) and Huynh and Feldt (1976) calculated approximate degrees of freedom (i.e. epsilon-corrected, where epsilon is the degree to which sphericity is violated) to use for repeated measures univariate analysis. These adjusted (reduced) degrees of freedom work well as long as the design employs equal group sizes (Greenhouse & Geisser 1959; Keselman & Keselman 1990; Keselman, Keselman, & Lix 1995). The Greenhouse and Geisser solution suggests reducing the degrees of freedom by a factor of $1/(k-1)$, where k is the number of treatments; in other words, compare the test statistic to the critical value of F with 1 and $n-1$ degrees of freedom. Using these as the entering degrees of freedom to the F distribution table provides the most conservative estimate. A less conservative approximation is available but is suggested as a second step (Greenhouse & Geisser 1959). Greenhouse and Geisser's approach may be too conservative if the number of subjects is small (i.e., if n is less than twice the number of treatments); the Huynh and Feldt epsilon solution is a better adjustment to use for these small-n designs. Both of these procedures are available on major statistical software (e.g., Statistica, BMDP, SAS, SPSS).

Multivariate tests do not require sphericity and thus do not require the epsilon correction factor. There are assumptions of normality and independence across subjects. Certain situations, however, do not favor multivariate analyses. Multivariates seem less robust than corrected univariate analyses for unbalanced designs (Keselman et al. 1995). If the number of variables exceeds the number of subjects, or if the study is designed with a small sample size, then the repeated measures univariate approach with the corrected degrees of freedom may be the more appropriate choice. However, with designs that incorporate large sample sizes, a multivariate analysis is more sensitive than the univariate test (Algina & Keselman 1997; Davidson 1972). Since repeated measures observations are correlated, they can be viewed as an essentially multivariate design (Cole & Grizzle 1966). The multivariate ANOVA estimates all possible correlations of pairs of the within-subject treatment and does not assume they are equal; it therefore allows the influence of the covariation of the pairs to act on the analysis instead of calling it unexplained variability and increasing the error term. The multivariate ANOVA test of differences does not say how the multiple dependent measures may differ, just that they do differ. Additional close examination of planned contrasts is still required (Lavori 1990). As Russell (1990) noted, these subsequent contrasts are not completely protected from "inflated experiment-wise" error. Russell (1990) provided an excellent discussion of the use of multivariate analysis with psychophysiologi-

cal data, noting that multivariate tests are relatively robust and interpretive adjustments can sometimes be made when assumptions are not met.

Other test statistics for repeated measures designs are available in addition to the two salient choices of univariate or multivariate analyses. The Welch–James test for completely randomized designs (James 1951, 1954; Welch 1947, 1951) has been extended to work with unbalanced multivariate designs by Keselman, Carriere, and Lix (1993). This statistic employs nonpooled variance techniques and corrected degrees of freedom; an easy-to-use SAS (1989, 1996) IML program is provided by Lix and Keselman (1995). This should be the statistic of choice for an unbalanced design with unequal group covariances. This procedure does require a relatively large sample size: three to four times the number of within-subject treatments for main effects and five or six times the number of such treatments for interaction effects.

INTERACTIONS

The interpretation and testing of interaction effects often puzzles students. Psychophysiologists cannot afford to be confounded by interactions because our primary interest is often in the interaction term of an analysis of variance. Typically, responses are represented within an analysis of variance by a time factor, with levels corresponding to the time series representing the response – most simply, a mean value for a baseline and one for a response level. We expect this time factor to be statistically significant; that is, we expect a response level to differ from a base level. Our primary interest is the interaction of this time factor with another factor in the experiment (e.g., impulsivity group or item content).

There are many ways to depict interactions, but typically they are interpreted as cell means reflecting a difference between the differences (i.e., a simple effects test; Keppel 1991). Figure 4 illustrates the difference-between-differences interpretation and contrasts the residual interpretation to be discussed shortly. The difference-between-differences technique observes that different means occur for a particular factor but that this difference depends on the concurrent level of an additional factor. When examined using this approach, a meaningful interaction requires that we qualify the meaning of the main effects (Kirk 1995). For example, EMG onset could be earlier for affectively charged items than neutral items, but only among the impulsive group of our example. The difference-between-differences approach would suggest that the item content × impulsivity grouping interaction could be interpreted as EMG onset times being dependent on the affective content of an item but only for impulsive children. Simple effects of task could then be analyzed; that is, we could statistically compare affecting and neutral items only for impulsive children and separately from control children (Meyer 1991).

An alternative approach to interpreting interactions emphasizes removing main effects so that the residuals representing the interaction can be directly examined (Rosnow & Rosenthal 1989a,b, 1991, 1995). This technique is supported by the fact that a cell mean representing an interaction also contains the influence of all lower-level factors (i.e., potential main effects) (Rosenthal & Rosnow 1991; Zuckerman et al. 1993); therefore, interpretation of the cell mean also reflects main effects. To continue with our example, a residual representation of the item content × impulsivity interaction for EMG onset could be interpreted as showing that impulsive and control children react in exactly opposite directions for affectively laden and neutral items. Examining the means for this example, presented in Box 2, should make the removal of main effects clearer to the reader. The data cell means are presented in part A of the table. The marginal means give the magnitude of the mean main effect for item content and group. Part B shows the combination of the main effects (both equal to

---

BOX 2. Extraction of Interactive Effects

A. Cell Means

	Neutral Content	Affective Content	Marginal (Group Main Effect)
Controls	90 msec	90 msec	90 msec
Impulsives	90 msec	10 msec	50 msec
Marginal (Content Main Effect)	90 msec	50 msec	

B. Cell Means Attributable to Additive (Noninteractive) Combination Main Effects

Controls	80 msec	40 msec
Impulsives	40 msec	0 msec

C. Residuals from Main Effect = Interactive Effect

Controls	10 msec	50 msec
Impulsives	50 msec	10 msec

Figure 4. Contrast between the residual and difference-between-differences interpretation of an interaction term. Mean results are shown either with the mean of the individual main effects removed (residual) or without this adjustment (difference between differences).

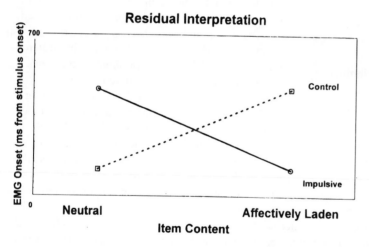

Residual Interpretation

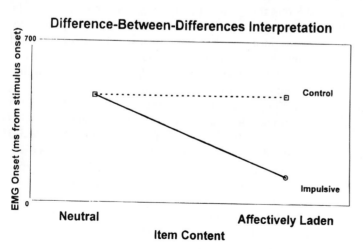

Difference-Between-Differences Interpretation

40 msec in the example). The controls doing neutral items show the addition of both the group and item main effects (i.e., 80 msec), whereas the impulsives performing on affective items show neither main effect (i.e., 0). Subtracting part B from part A yields the residuals. This is the depiction of the interaction with the main effect "controlled." Significant interactions will yield the crossed pattern shown in part C of the table and in the upper panel of Figure 4, because removal of main effect differences will center the data and highlight the differential influences of the variables analyzed.

Both of these approaches (difference-between-differences and residual) result in the same interaction variance (Keppel 1991; Rosnow & Rosenthal 1989b) but lead to different and sometimes conflicting conclusions (Petty et al. 1996). The difference-between-differences approach would say that impulsive children have a different EMG onset that is dependent on the content of the stimuli, whereas the residual approach would say that controls and impulsives have completely opposite reactions to the stimuli content in terms of EMG onset.

Perhaps the guidelines for interpreting interactions should include displaying the main effect residuals that depict the interaction to see if they supply additional, sensible information before a final interpretation is formed. However, many variables that psychophysiologists study do not lend themselves to a residual interpretation. Because interaction residuals always demonstrate a crossover pattern, this pattern should first be indicated by the cell difference approach or by theoretical issues before the residuals are examined.

An example of nonsensical residual information is provided in Petty et al. (1996). An experiment,

Residual Interpretation

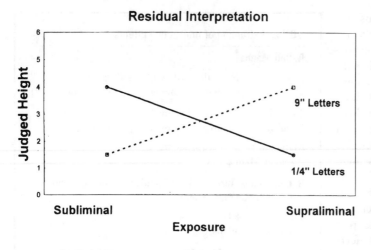

Difference-Between-Differences Interpretation

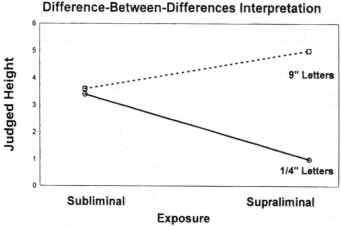

Figure 5. Illustration of the Petty et al. (1996) argument for considering the meaningfulness of the conceptual result when choosing residual versus difference-between-differences interpretations. In the case of subliminal stimuli, the residual interpretation does not appear to be meaningful (see text).

designed to investigate the effects of exposure duration to letters of two different heights (1/4" vs. 9") on a subject's estimation of that height, manipulated duration with a subliminal presentation of 5-msec duration versus a 500-msec supraliminal presentation (see Figure 5). The exposure duration × letter size interaction was significant. The difference-between-differences approach interprets these findings as a greater impact of letter size when the presentation is supraliminal. However, the residual interpretation would deem the traditional interpretation incorrect because it contains the main effect of letter size; instead, the residuals indicate the exposure durations react with letter size in exactly opposite ways. In other words, 9" letters are perceived as larger when supraliminally presented and 1/4" letters appear larger than 9" letters when subliminally presented. Since a subliminal condition indicates that the subject did not even see the letters, this conclusion regarding their reaction to letter size is nonsensical.

PLANNED CONTRASTS AND MULTIPLE REGRESSION: ANALYZING THE INTERACTION

Up to this point, only the interpretation of an interaction has been discussed. Another issue concerns the best statistical test. There do exist alternatives to interaction terms from standard ANOVA packages. *Contrasts* involve comparisons of two or more cell means and thus seem to be an appropriate choice. When constructing contrasts, cell means are orthogonally weighted to correspond to the hypothesized order of their effect. This allows a more focused examination of the data (Rosenthal & Rosnow 1985) than is possible using an interaction term from a standard omnibus *F*-test. Using the Petty et al. (1996) example, we could predict that means would be identical under subliminal conditions but that 9" letters would be judged larger under supraliminal conditions. A contrast could be constructed and tested by assigning equal weights to subliminal conditions (e.g., −2 and −2) and weights of (say) 1 and 3 to the 1/4" and 9" supraliminal conditions, respectively. The weights would directly test your hypothesis rather than depending upon the standard weighting assigned for an interaction in an *F*-test. Indeed, an *F*-test might indicate that the interaction term is significant even if the two letter heights differed under subliminal but not supraliminal conditions – an outcome directly counter to your hypothesis.

Note that, in our contrast test of the "interaction," the variance of the main effect was combined with the interaction variance; the standard ANOVA *F*-statistic would use only the interaction variance and so different results could be obtained. A match between the hypothesis and the statistic is required for appropriate testing. If an interaction is expected then a contrast test may not be appropriate, because the statistic will include the variance of the main effect. If, however, a main effect and an interaction effect are both expected, then a contrast test reflecting this is appropriate because it can incorporate the variance of each. However, if only the main effect contributes meaningful variance then it will not be identified by the contrast test (since an interaction did not occur).

A multiple regression approach can also be used to implement the testing of specific patterns of interaction. First, nonorthogonal contrasts can be tested simultaneously (with the orthogonal contrast) via a multiple regression analysis. Second, several orthogonal contrasts could be specified and simultaneously entered into a regression analysis to determine the partial variance for which the alternative contrasts account (Aiken & West 1991; Rosenthal & Rosnow 1991).[2]

Explaining interactions with an ANOVA model is appropriate when the variables under study are discrete or if the expected relationship between the independent and dependent variable appears as a stepped one (Kenny 1979), but even these instances can be handled with multiple regression techniques (Aiken & West 1991; Cohen & Cohen 1975). Multiple regression is critical when predictor variables are of a continuous nature. As described by a multiple regression equation, an "interaction" means that variable Y regressed on X will have a particular slope for each individual value of Z. This provides a regression line for every point of Z. Each one of this family of regression lines is a simple regression line, and the effect of X on Y is a conditional effect (Darlington 1990).

Appropriate steps for examining the interaction, once named, include plotting the interaction and conducting post hoc tests (Aiken & West 1991). Plotting the interaction involves restructuring the regression equation so that a simple slope of Y on X at Z can be expressed, with several values of Z entered into the equation to provide several solutions. The regression lines of these resolved equations are then plotted so the relationship can be examined. Post hoc questions include asking:

1. whether a specific value of Z generates a regression line significantly different from zero (using a t-test; $t =$ slope divided by standard error with $n - k - 1$ degrees of freedom, where k denotes the number of predictors) (Darlington 1990); and
2. how slopes of any pair of simple regression lines differ from each other (comparing their slope difference score d to zero with a t-test; $t = d/s_d$, where s_d denotes standard error of the differences) (Aiken & West 1991).

Aiken and West (1991) discussed thoroughly the interpretation of multiple regression interaction. An example of this approach to analyzing and presenting interactions within the context of a regression analysis is available in the study-4 analysis of Graziano and associates (1996).

Additional information about the interaction may be gained by estimating its strength as a proportion of the sum of squares of the interaction divided by the total sum of squares. However, this figure technically applies only to the sample under study. An estimated strength of the interaction in the population is:

$$\frac{\text{SS interaction} - (\text{error df} \times \text{MS error})}{\text{SS total} + \text{MS error}}$$

(Hays 1994), where SS denotes sum of squares, df degrees of freedom, and MS mean square.

REGRESSION ALTERNATIVES TO ANOVA FOR REPEATED MEASURES

Analysis of variance can be considered a special case of regression analysis (using dummy variables to express the factor levels). Cohen and Cohen (1975) developed

this technique, which is frequently used in such computational approaches as the general linear model programs within the SAS package. Regression provides considerable flexibility in modeling the data; at a basic level, serial measurements (e.g., a repeated measures time series) can be analyzed as a univariate regression analysis of responses with correlated errors (Ware 1985). This will be further discussed shortly.

At the other end of the spectrum are autoregressive approaches such as ARIMA (autoregressive integrated moving average) that essentially fit periodic components to the data (Box & Jenkins 1970). The strength of the regression approach can also be considered a weakness. A regression model that very closely fits a particular set of sample data may be fitting the variance specific to the quirks of that sample. As such, the population parameters could be inaccurately estimated. This concern makes independent replication of regression models particularly important.

Regression analysis can be a useful tool for psychophysiological studies in that it allows for specific modeling of the inherent correlations of a repeated measures design: it can provide an intraindividual look at data as well as an interindividual perspective provided by a repeated measures ANOVA. Conducting these analyses using several different regression strategies leads to the construction of a more accurate picture of the data. These strategies include individual regression analysis, hierarchical and stepwise regression techniques, and random regression analysis. Appropriately applied, regression techniques can resolve problems of missing data or unbalanced design, serial correlation, and time-varying covariance (Gibbons et al. 1993). A thoroughly argued comparison of different regression and repeated measures approaches to habituation data may be found in Petrinovich and Widaman (1984).

A primary concern with regression analysis techniques is the problem of collinearity. If alternative predictors of the dependent variable are highly correlated, then the one chosen by the analysis as the primary predictor will be dependent on the particular sample in use and so be governed by the quirks of the sample. In this situation especially, the investigator must guard against a literal acceptance of a statistical outcome – for instance, believing that depression but not anxiety predicts school grades solely because of the initial selection of depression by the analysis. For a more complete description of benefits and cautions regarding these techniques, see Cohen and Cohen (1975) and Hays (1994).

Individual regression analysis, also known as growth curve analysis, is a statistical technique that detects a pattern of change in a variable across time within a particular treatment or condition (Sidani & Lynn 1993). The temporal pattern detected by regression analysis provides a qualitative look at relationships that would otherwise be represented as difference scores at different time points by a repeated measures ANOVA. An individual unit of analysis can be a single subject, group, or condition. The linear model, which is employed in the regression technique, assumes that a subject's score on one measure is a function of his or her score on another level, yielding a trend line for each individual (unlike a repeated measures ANOVA, which assumes one common intercept of a trend line for the within-subject variable at each time point; Gibbons et al. 1993). When an individual regression approach is applied to a repeated measures design, the variable of interest is regressed on the time variable. The functional relationship is depicted in the form of a regression line, and the slope of this line provides the magnitude and the direction of change over time. A t-test of the slope compared to a slope of zero tests the difference. This method is useful for describing and evaluating individual differences. Further, comparisons between groups can be examined by finding the regression line for each individual in the sample and testing for group differences with a t-test or ANOVA of the intercept and/or slope. A significant difference between groups on the intercept indicates a baseline difference; a significant difference between groups in slope indicates different patterns of change among the groups.

Individual regression analysis does have some advantages over repeated measures analysis. The former clearly delineates patterns of change across time in terms of magnitude and direction, and it allows for the examination of individual change while still permitting group analysis. In addition, required assumptions are kept to a minimum. Missing data are not as crucial to the identification of the pattern and, when a nonlinear relationship is suspected, polynominal functions can be added to the regression equation to allow an accurate description. However, there are two practical limitations to consider before adopting individual regression analysis. If the variable under study (say, EEG frequency) reacts differently over time (e.g., in different sleep stages), then regression will not be valid because the differences cannot be depicted in a single line. Also, values that change drastically and in different directions require a technique other than linear regression. For a more detailed description of individual regression analysis see Rogosa, Brandt, and Zimowski (1982).

Hierarchical and stepwise regressions may also be of interest to the psychophysiologist. During any multiple regression procedure (anything beyond a bivariate regression), it may be desirable to input predictor variables one at a time to determine the degree of unique variability that each contributes to the model. In hierarchical regression, the entry order of the variables is determined by the experimenter. For example, Jennings and colleagues (1997) were interested in whether age per se or the presence of disease explained the age trends in psychophysiological responses to a battery of challenge tasks. By entering the disease variables first, the additional predictivity of age per se could be examined. Note that all variables are entered into the final model, so

the sequential entry procedure does *not* change the amount of total variance accounted for by a final equation that includes the total set of predictors. Even though the variance explained by each variable individually may depend on the order of their entry into the equation, the influence of any one variable continues to be relative to the influence of other, co-occurring variables. However, hierarchical analysis does provide partial correlations by allowing initial variables to be viewed as "held constant" or "adjusted for."

Stepwise regression differs from hierarchical regression in that the experimenter does not determine the order in which variables are entered into the equation. At each step, the calculation itself determines the variable contributing the most variance to the prediction of a dependent variable. Thus, the first variable to enter the equation is the one that contributes the most variance to the prediction. The next variable to enter is the variable that contributes the most additional variance to the prediction, and so forth. Again, the final results for the total variance explained are the same as when the variables are entered simultaneously, provided that the complete set of predictor variables appear in the equation.

Random regression models (Gibbons et al. 1988), also known as random effects models (Laird & Ware 1982; Ware 1985) or hierarchical general linear models (Bryk & Raudenbush 1987), provide an estimation of random person-specific effects in a manner similar to individual regression analysis. Random regression analysis goes a step beyond individual regression analysis by incorporating information about the population trend across time and providing an estimate of within-subject time trends given the individual's data (Gibbons et al. 1993). In other words, information about other subjects with similar characteristics provides reinforcement for a better estimate of an individual's trend. Similarly, missing data estimation in random regression models is derived from the trends of all other like individuals in the study. These missing data points are not simply interpolated data. They are produced by the model and are consistent with the observed data of the subject yet also differentiate between treatments to the same extent as individuals with complete data do. In addition, measurement at the same time points or for the same number of times is not required of each subject (Gibbons et al. 1993). Examples of missing data estimates produced by random regression are depicted in Gibbons et al. (1993); a more detailed discussion is available in Ware (1985).

In random regression modeling, person-specific estimations are achieved through the use of empirical Bayesian procedures (Casella 1985). These procedures use a weighted average based on the individual's data and data from the entire sample. A subject with the most data receives a weight that is mostly influenced by the individual data. Weights of subjects with less information are more influenced by the group mean. In addition, the variance around a single person's trend is available, resulting in an estimation of the population variance–covariance matrix of person-specific effects. This is not possible with other repeated measures analyses (Bryk & Raudenbush 1987; Gibbons et al. 1993).

Covariates also receive distinctive treatment within a random regression model. Whereas repeated measures models have a problem with time-varying covariates (unlike time-invariant variables, which are adequately handled), such covariates are easily included in a random regression model. The covariance relationships assessed by this model include (a) the overall relationship between the variable of interest and the covariate across time, (b) how this relationship changes over time, and (c) how within-subject change of interest is related to the within-subject change of the covariate (Gibbons et al. 1993).

Related to the issue of covariance is the treatment of unexplained nonrandom errors. Some examples of nonrandom errors (e.g. autocorrelated errors) are allowed in the random regression model – in particular, first-order nonstationary autoregressive errors (Chi & Reinsel 1989). Because these arise when a subject's response at one time point is influenced by the immediately preceding response, this feature is especially important for psychophysiological data. Repeated measures analyses typically employed by psychophysiologists are biased in this case.

Several weaknesses of the random regression modeling technique are evident. The theory from which random regression is derived requires large sample size. This creates an area of caution for psychophysiologists. In addition, a linear trend is assumed, which may not always be the case. Assumption of a linear trend also influences the estimation of missing data points; perhaps missing data would not proceed in a linear fashion. Also, as in most other statistics, a (relatively) normal distribution is expected. Finally, random regression is not appropriate for dichotomous variables, including transformed dummy variables (Stiratelli, Laird, & Ware 1984).

These regression techniques – individual regression analysis, hierarchical or stepwise regressions analysis, and random regression analysis – provide a forward-looking choice for psychophysiologists to optimize their data. However, using a regression technique will lead to different results than those produced by a repeated measures ANOVA and will therefore yield different conclusions. Some of the differences provided by regression are beneficial. The provision of both intraindividual and interindividual information supplies descriptions and evaluations of individual differences. A qualitative look at relationships in terms of their magnitude and direction of change over time offers an alternate view of the data as described by (multivariate) analysis of variance. In addition, regression techniques require a minimum number of assumptions. Missing data is estimated in ways that maximize the influence of individual and group information. Finally, polynomial functions can accurately describe nonlinear relationships when their existence is suspected. A good guide on how to structure

polynomial regression equations is Aiken and West (1991, pp. 62–114).

There are also some limitations when using regression. Most importantly, regression is not appropriate for variables that vary across time or for categorical variables. However, in some cases categorical variables can be transformed into dummy variables to bypass this problem. Also, values that change drastically and in different directions could pose a problem. Lastly, correlated independent variables result in collinearity, which in turn results in large standard error terms and less precise coefficient estimates (Schroeder, Sjoquist, & Stephan 1986) as well as the interpretive problems noted earlier.

As with any decision that researchers must make, the influences of positive and negative factors are present. To decide which is the preferable analysis – regression versus ANOVA – ask two questions. (i) "What aspect of change is of interest?" (That is, are you interested in the existence, magnitude, direction, or rate of change?) (ii) "What is the unit of change that will be analyzed?" (Or is it important to look at individual differences?) For general guides that include understanding and selecting regression as the analysis of choice, please refer to Schroeder et al. (1986) and Hays (1994).

OTHER TIME-SERIES APPROACHES

Spectral variants of time-series analyses have been introduced to psychophysiology largely through the application to heart rate variability by Porges and others (see Porges & Bohrer 1990). The rhythmic (usually sine–cosine) functions present in a sequence of second-by-second heart rate values are identified using frequency (Fourier) or period (ARIMA) analyses. For example, if a 5-min sample of heart rate values is examined, rhythmic fluctuations might be identified at the frequency of respiration (about 0.2 Hz) and around a frequency related to vascular fluctuations (0.1 Hz) along with less well-defined lower frequency fluctuations (Jennings & McKnight 1994; Porges & Bohrer 1990). Porges (1995) related the power (variance at these frequencies) of these components to normal and abnormal early development; later in life, the power in these components is related to vulnerability to heart attack (see the review by van Ravenswaaij-Arts et al. 1993). Other applications of similar or identical techniques have been used to separate the frequency components of the electroencephalogram. For instance, power in the alpha band of the EEG can readily be identified with time-series analyses and related to psychological variables of interest such as affective style (Hoptman & Davidson 1994; Wheeler, Davidson, & Tomarken 1993).

Jones, Crowell, and Kapuniai (1969, 1970), Lobstein, Turpin, and Siddle (1979), and others have proposed that phasic response analyses might benefit from modeling techniques using time-series approaches. The response to an event can be conceptualized as an interruption of the time series. Regression techniques can model the time series over (say) the preceding two minutes and predict the values of the variable for the next few seconds. Any response to an environmental event should produce deviations from that prediction that can then be scored and analyzed. Crowell and co-workers (1979), for example, used a regression technique to predict expected heart rate and EEG and then detected differences from these predictions due to auditory stimulation in hearing-impaired children. We have used a conceptually related technique to look at the sensitivity of heartbeat timing to the phase of the cardiac cycle at which stimuli are presented (Jennings, van der Molen, & Somsen 1998). As psychophysiologists become familiar with regression techniques and time series, such approaches to analysis may become more common.

Closing Comments

We have attempted to highlight methodological concerns relevant at different stages of a psychophysiological research project. The concerns and their discussion drew somewhat on the research literature on methodology and statistics and also upon our own experience. In closing, we ask the reader's forbearance as we draw on that experience again and share our subjective impressions of methodology in psychophysiology.

Our area has a traditional and continuing interest in methodology, most immediately in the technology of non-invasively acquiring physiological signals but also in the general methodology of performing research and drawing appropriate inferences from that research. We have detected no signs of declining interest or flagging of expertise in methodology and statistics. Psychophysiologists remain methodologically sophisticated. Nonetheless, we share methodological problems with other areas of psychology – for example, a relatively unthinking reliance on null hypothesis testing and a rapidly expanding number of statistically significant results that fail to coalesce into conceptual advances.

The major impediments to the use of appropriate scientific methodology may be societal rather than intellectual. An initial stage in working with a conceptual problem is exploring different measures, trying out manipulations, and generally spending some time exploring methods that both follow from the conceptual question and have good measurement properties. Good hypothesis generation should precede the hypothesis testing around which much of our science is structured. Several factors have led to a virtual disappearance of exploratory laboratory time: (a) competition among peers for positions and promotions based on research productivity (often defined numerically); (b) research grants awarded on a similar basis and evaluated in terms of power to confirm existing hypotheses; (c) bureaucratization of human use procedures, making it impractical to vary any

aspect of a research project; and (d) clearly greater rewards for producing research articles than for reading them. In general, the current system seems designed to produce data and reports rather than concepts and explanations. In addition to instilling greater idealism in peers and editors, a solution may be to incorporate exploratory measures and manipulations into larger hypothesis-testing research. This procedure, called leap-frogging by some, permits the authors to get necessary exploration done while continuing to comply with current societal requirements. In the long run, exploratory results should provide the basis of solid research in testing hypotheses.

Having recognized the pressures against good methodology, we would nonetheless urge psychophysiologists to use the best methods. In particular, we urge greater time spent in the conceptualization, initial design, and piloting of projects. Care must be taken to ensure that response definitions, measures, and planned statistical analyses follow directly from the concept of the research. The almost universal dependence of psychophysiological research on within-subject designs implies that we should be particularly wary of carryover effects – the influence of one assessment upon other assessments. Designs should check on and, as necessary, counter such influence.

Once a design is established, care should be taken to use adequate sample sizes. Our success in conceptually replicating our work has not borne out the hope that principles can be uncovered with sample sizes of single digits per cell. Pilot work may help us decide whether we need double or triple digits per cell in our designs. Results should be examined graphically and numerically until the investigator understands the characteristics of the data and how the statistical analyses are expressing those characteristics. Ideally, a graphical presentation and corresponding analysis would be found that convey the same understanding to a reader. Such a presentation should convey the amplitude and conceptual importance of a finding as well as its statistical significance. The process of analyzing the data may reveal that a hypothesis-testing outcome is, in fact, a poor representation of the results. It seems likely that most reports in psychophysiology will show hypothesis-testing outcomes combined with statistically significant but post hoc hypotheses generated in the process of data analysis. Ideally, our priorities would change toward quality over quantity, allowing replications of hypotheses-generating results prior to publication. In practice, the field should be advanced by acknowledging the quasi-hypothesis testing of much of our work and by evaluating this work in terms not of its post-hoc p value but rather of its conceptual importance.

NOTES

1. This wording frequently confuses students. A low-pass filter *passes* frequencies *below* its cutoff point and rejects (or filters out) frequencies above its cut-off point.

2. Contrasts are especially useful when a relationship between more than two factors or levels has to be explained – for example, in a main effect composed of four levels. In addition, they are useful in providing further ways to discuss a linear contrast when the residuals are not significant (significant residuals would imply the linear explanation was not an adequate one). Further contrasts can be performed on the residuals to identify quadratic trends (Abelson 1995; Abelson & Prentice 1997).

REFERENCES

Abelson, R. P. (1995). *Statistics as Principled Argument*. Hillsdale, NJ: Erlbaum.

Abelson, R. P., & Prentice, D. A. (1997). Contrast tests of interaction hypotheses. *Psychological Methods, 2*, 315–28.

Aiken, L. S., & West, S. G. (1991). *Multiple Regression: Testing and Interpreting Interactions*. Newbury Park, CA: Sage.

Algina, J., & Keselman, H. J. (1997). Detecting repeated measures effects with univariate and multivariate statistics. *Psychological Methods, 2*, 208–18.

Berntson, G. G., Cacioppo, J. T., & Quigley, K. S. (1993). Cardiac psychophysiology and autonomic space in humans: Empirical perspectives and conceptual implications. *Psychological Bulletin, 114*, 296–322.

Berntson, G. G., Cacioppo, J. T., Quigley, K. S., & Fabro, V. T. (1994a). Autonomic space and physiological response. *Psychophysiology, 31*, 44–61.

Berntson, G. G., Quigley, K. S., Lang, J. F., & Boysen, S. T. (1990). An approach to artifact identification: Application to heart period data. *Psychophysiology, 27*, 586–98.

Berntson, G. G., Uchino, B. N., & Cacioppo, J. T. (1994b). Origins of baseline variance and the law of initial values. *Psychophysiology, 31*, 204–10.

Borenstein, M., Cohen, J., & Rothstein, H. (1997). *Power and Precision*. Mahwah, NJ: Erlbaum.

Boucsein, W. (1992). *Electrodermal Activity*. New York: Plenum.

Box, G. E. P. (1954). Some theorems on quadratic forms applied in the study of analysis of variance problems: I. Effect of inequality of variance in the one-way classification. *Annals of Mathematical Statistics, 25*, 290–302.

Box, G. E. P., & Jenkins, G. M. (1970). *Time Series Analysis*. San Francisco: Holden-Day.

Brown, C. C. (1967). The techniques of plethysmography. In C. C. Brown (Ed.), *Methods in Psychophysiology*, pp. 54–74. Baltimore: Williams & Wilkins.

Bryk, A. S., & Raudenbush, S. W. (1987). Application of hierarchical linear models to assessing change. *Psychological Bulletin, 101*, 147–58.

Bush, L. K., Hess, U., & Wolford, G. (1993). Transformations for within-subject designs: A Monte Carlo investigation. *Psychological Bulletin, 113*, 566–79.

Cacioppo, J. T., & Tassinary, L. G. (1990). Inferring psychological significance from physiological signals. *American Psychologist, 45*, 16–28.

Cacioppo, J. T., Tassinary, L. G., & Fridlund, A. J. (1990). The skeletomotor system. In J. T. Cacioppo & L. G. Tassinary (Eds.), *Principles of Psychophysiology: Physical, Social, and Inferential Elements*, pp. 325–84. Cambridge University Press.

Casella, G. (1985). An introduction to empirical Bayesian data analysis. *American Statistician, 39*, 83–7.

Cheung, M. N. (1981). Detection of and recovery from errors in cardiac interbeat intervals. *Psychophysiology, 18*, 341–6.

Chi, E. M., & Reinsel, G. C. (1989). Models of longitudinal data with random effects and AR-1 errors. *Journal of the American Statistical Association, 84*, 452–9.

Chow, S. L. (1996). *Statistical Significance: Rationale, Validity and Utility*. Thousand Oaks, CA: Sage.

Cleveland, W. S. (1985). *The Elements of Graphing Data*. Monterey, CA: Wadsworth.

Cohen, J. (1977). *Statistical Power Analysis for the Behavioral Sciences*, rev. ed. Hillsdale, NJ: Erlbaum.

Cohen, J. (1992). A power primer. *Psychological Bulletin, 112*, 155–9.

Cohen, J. (1994). The earth is round ($p < .05$). *American Psychologist, 49*, 997–1003.

Cohen, J., & Cohen, P. (1975). *Applied Multiple Regression/ Correlation for the Behavioral Sciences*, 2nd ed. Hillsdale, NJ: Erlbaum.

Cole, J. W. L., & Grizzle, J. E. (1966). Application of multivariate analysis of variance to repeated measures experiments. *Biometrics, 22*, 810–28.

Coles, M. G. H. (1989). Modern mind–brain reading: Psychophysiology, physiology, and cognition. *Psychophysiology, 26*, 251–69.

Coles, M. G. H., Gratton, G., & Donchin, E. (1988). Detecting early communication: Using measures of movement-related potentials to illuminate human information processing. Special Issue: Event related potential investigations of cognition. *Biological Psychology, 26*, 69–89.

Contrada, R. J., Krantz, D. S., Durel, L. A., & Levy, L. (1989). Effects of beta-adrenergic activity on T-wave amplitude. *Psychophysiology, 26*, 488–92.

Cook, E. W., & Miller, G. A. (1992). Digital filtering: Background and tutorial for psychophysiologists. *Psychophysiology, 29*, 350–67.

Cook, R. D., & Weisberg, S. (1994). *An Introduction to Regression Graphics*. New York: Wiley.

Crowell, D. H., Pang-Ching, G., Kapuniai, L. E., & Bilyk, P. L. (1979). A comparison of clinical behavioral audiometry and autoregression analysis of EEG and heart rate in hearing-impaired children. *Journal of Auditory Research, 19*, 167–72.

Darlington, R. B. (1990). *Regression and Linear Models*. New York: McGraw-Hill.

Davidson, M. L. (1972). Univariate versus multivariate tests in repeated measures experiments. *Psychological Bulletin, 77*, 339–452.

Davidson, R. J. (1995). Cerebral asymmetry, emotion, and affective style. In R. J. Davidson & K. Hugdahl (Eds.), *Brain Asymmetry*, pp. 361–88. Cambridge, MA: MIT Press.

Earnshaw, R. A., Vince, J. A., & Jones, H. (1997). *Visualization and Modeling*. San Diego: Academic Press.

Fifth Report of the Joint National Committee on Detection, Evaluation, and Treatment of High Blood Pressure (1993). *Archives of Internal Medicine, 153*, 154–83.

Fowles, D. C., Christie, M. J., Edelberg, R., Grings, W. W., Lykken, D. T., & Venables, P. H. (1981). Publication recommendations for electrodermal measurements. *Psychophysiology, 18*, 232–9.

Frick, R. W. (1996). The appropriate use of null hypothesis testing. *Psychological Methods, 1,* 379–90.

Fridlund, A. J., & Cacioppo, J. T. (1986). Guidelines for human electromyographic research. *Psychophysiology, 23,* 567–89.

Furedy, J. J., Heslegrave, R. J., & Scher, H. (1992). T-wave amplitude utility revisited: Some physiological and psychophysiological considerations. *Biological Psychology, 33,* 241–8.

Geenen, R., & van de Vijver, F. J. R. (1993). A simple test of the law of initial values. *Psychophysiology, 30,* 525–30.

Gibbons, R. D., Hedeker, D., Elkin, I., Waternaux, C., Kraemer, H. C., Greenhouse, J. B., Shea, M. T., Imber, S. D., Sotsky, S. M., & Watkins, J. T. (1993). Some conceptual and statistical issues in analysis of longitudinal psychiatric data: Application to the NIMH Treatment of Depression Collaborative Research Program Dataset. *Archives of General Psychiatry, 50,* 739–50.

Gibbons, R. D., Hedeker, D., Waternaux, C., & Davis, J. M. (1988). Random regression models: A comprehensive approach to the analysis of longitudinal psychiatric data. *Psychopharmacological Bulletin, 24,* 438–43.

Graham, F. K. (1978a). Normality of distributions and homogeneity of variance of heart rate and heart period samples. *Psychophysiology, 15,* 487–91.

Graham, F. K. (1978b). Constraints on measuring heart rate and period sequentially through real and cardiac time. *Psychophysiology, 15,* 492–5.

Gratton, G., Coles, M. G. H., & Donchin, E. (1983). A new method for off-line removal of ocular artifact. *Electroencephalography and Clinical Neurophysiology, 55,* 468–84.

Graziano, W. G., Smith, S. M., Tassinary, L. G., Sun, C.-R., & Pilkington, C. (1996). Does imitation enhance memory for faces? Four converging studies. *Journal of Personality and Social Psychology, 7,* 874–87.

Greenhouse, S. W., & Geisser, S. (1959). On methods in the analysis of profile data. *Psychometrika, 24,* 95–112.

Greenwald, A. G., Gonzalez, R., Harris, R. H., & Guthrie, D. (1996). Effect sizes and *p*-values: What should be reported and what should be replicated? *Psychophysiology, 33,* 175–83.

Guilford, J. P. (1954). *Psychometric Methods.* New York: McGraw-Hill.

Harris, R. J. (1991). Significance tests are not enough: The role of effect size estimation in theory corroboration. *Theory and Psychology, 1,* 375–82.

Harris, R. J. (1997). Significance tests have their place. *Psychological Science, 8,* 8–11.

Hays, W. L. (1994). *Statistics.* Orlando, FL: Holt, Rinehart & Winston.

Hoptman, M. J., & Davidson, R. J. (1994). How and why do the two cerebral hemispheres interact? *Psychological Bulletin, 116,* 195–219.

Hugdahl, K. (1995). *Psychophysiology: The Mind–Body Perspective.* Cambridge, MA: Harvard University Press.

Huynh, H., & Feldt, L. S. (1970). Conditions under which mean square ratios in repeated measurements designs have exact *F* distributions. *Journal of the American Statistical Association, 65,* 1582–9.

Huynh, H., & Feldt, L. S. (1976). Estimation of the Box correction for degrees of freedom from sample data in randomized block and split-plot designs. *Journal of Educational Statistics, 1,* 69–82.

Jacoby, W. G. (1997). *Statistical Graphics for Univariate and Bivariate Data: Quantitative Applications in Social Science.* Thousand Oaks, CA: Sage.

James, G. S. (1951). The comparison of several groups of observations when the ratios of the population variances are unknown. *Biometrika, 38,* 324–9.

James, G. S. (1954). Tests of linear hypotheses in univariate and multivariate analysis when the ratios of the population variances are unknown. *Biometrika, 41,* 19–43.

Jennings, J. R. (1986). Bodily changes during attending. In M. G. H. Coles, E. Donchin, & S. W. Porges (Eds.), *Psychophysiology: Systems, Processes and Applications,* pp. 268–89. New York: Guilford.

Jennings, J. R., Berg, W. K., Hutcheson, J. S., Obrist, P., Porges, S., & Turpin, G. (1981). Publication guidelines for heart rate studies in man. *Psychophysiology, 18,* 226–31.

Jennings, J. R., Kamarck, T., Manuck, S., Everson, S. A., Kaplan, G., & Salonen, J. T. (1997). Aging or disease? Cardiovascular reactivity in Finnish men over the middle years. *Psychology and Aging, 12,* 225–38.

Jennings, J. R., Kamarck, T., Stewart, C., Eddy, M., & Johnson, P. (1992). Alternate cardiovascular baseline assessment techniques: Vanilla or resting baseline? *Psychophysiology, 29,* 742–50.

Jennings, J. R., & McKnight, J. D. (1994). Inferring vagal tone from heart rate variability. *Psychosomatic Medicine, 56,* 194–6.

Jennings, J. R., Stringfellow, J. C., & Graham, M. (1974). A comparison of the statistical distribution of beat-by-beat heart rate and heart period. *Psychophysiology, 22,* 207–10.

Jennings, J. R., Tahmoush, A. J., & Redmond, D. P. (1980). Noninvasive measurement of peripheral vascular activity. In I. Martin & P. H. Venables (Eds.), *Techniques in Psychophysiology,* pp. 69–137. Chichester, U.K.: Wiley.

Jennings, J. R., van der Molen, M. W., & Somsen, R. J. M. (1998). Changes in heart beat timing, reactivity, resetting, or perturbation? *Biological Psychology, 47,* 227–41.

Jennings, J. R., & Wood, C. C. (1976). The epsilon-adjusted procedure for repeated measures analyses of variance. *Psychophysiology, 13,* 277–8.

Johnson, L. C., & Lubin, A. (1972). On planning psychophysiological experiments: Design, measurement, and analysis. In N. S. Greenfield & R. A. Sternbach (Eds.), *Handbook of Psychophysiology,* pp. 125–58. New York: Holt, Rinehart & Winston.

Jones, R. H., Crowell, D. H., & Kapuniai, L. E. (1969). Change detection model for serially correlated data. *Psychological Bulletin, 71,* 352–8.

Jones, R. H., Crowell, D. H., & Kapuniai, L. E. (1970). Change detection model for serially correlated multivariate data. *Biometrics, 26,* 269–80.

Judd, C. M., McClelland, G. H., & Smith, E. R. (1996). Testing treatment by covariate interactions when treatment varies within subjects. *Psychological Methods, 1,* 366–78.

Kamarck, T. W., Jennings, J. R., Debski, T. W., Glickman-Weiss, E., Eddy, M. J., & Manuck, S. B. (1992). Reliable measures of behaviorally-evoked cardiovascular reactivity from a PC-based test battery: Results from student and community samples. *Psychophysiology, 29,* 17–28.

Kamen, R. (1987). *Introduction to Signals and Systems.* New York: Macmillan.

Kenny, D. A. (1979). *Correlation and Causality.* New York: Wiley.

Keppel, G. (1991). *Design and Analysis: A Researcher's Handbook,* 3rd ed. Englewood Cliffs, NJ: Prentice-Hall.

Keselman, H. J. (in press). Testing treatment effects in repeated measures designs: An update for psychophysiological researchers. *Psychophysiology.*

Keselman, H. J., Carriere, K. C., & Lix, L. M. (1993). Testing repeated measures hypotheses when covariance matrices are heterogeneous. *Journal of Educational Statistics, 18,* 305–19.

Keselman, H. J., Keselman, J. C., & Lix, L. M. (1995). The analysis of repeated measurements: Univariate tests, multivariate tests, or both? *British Journal of Mathematical and Statistical Psychology, 48,* 319–38.

Keselman, H. J., Rogan, J. C., Mendoza, J. L., & Breen, L. J. (1980). Testing the validity conditions of repeated measures F tests. *Psychological Bulletin, 87,* 479–81.

Keselman, J. C., & Keselman, H. J. (1990). Analyzing unbalanced repeated measures designs. *British Journal of Mathematical and Statistical Psychology, 43,* 265–82.

Khatree, R., & Naik, D. N. (1995). *Applied Multivariate Statistics with SAS Software.* Cary, NC: SAS Institute.

Kirk, R. E. (1995). *Experimental Design: Procedures for the Behavioral Sciences,* 3rd ed. Monterey, CA: Brooks/Cole.

Laird, N. M., & Ware, J. H. (1982). Random effects models for longitudinal data. *Biometrics, 38,* 963–74.

Lavori, P. (1990). ANOVA, MANOVA, my black hen: Comments on repeated measures. *Archives of General Psychiatry, 47,* 775–8.

Law, L. N., Levey, A. B., & Martin, I. (1980). Response detection and measurement. In I. Martin & P. H. Venables (Eds.), *Techniques in Psychophysiology.* Chichester, U.K.: Wiley.

Levey, A. B. (1980). Measurement units in psychophysiology. In I. Martin & P. Venables (Eds.), *Techniques in Psychophysiology,* pp. 597–628. Chichester, U.K.: Wiley.

Levy, M. N. (1977). Parasympathetic control of the heart. In W. C. Randall (Ed.), *Neural Regulation of the Heart,* pp. 95–130. New York: Oxford University Press.

Levy, M. N., & Martin, P. (1984). Parasympathetic control of the heart. In W. C. Randall (Ed.), *Nervous Control of Cardiovascular Function.* New York: Oxford University Press.

Lippold, O. C. J. (1967). Electromyography. In P. H. Venables & I. Martin (Eds.), *A Manual of Psychophysiological Methods,* pp. 246–97. New York: Wiley.

Lix, L. M., & Keselman, H. H. (1995). Approximate degrees of freedom tests: A unified perspective on testing for mean equality. *Psychological Bulletin, 117,* 547–60.

Llabre, M. M., Spitzer, S. B., Saab, P. G., Ironson, G. H., & Schneiderman, N. (1991). The replicability and specificity of delta versus residualized change as measures of cardiovascular reactivity to behavioral challenges. *Psychophysiology, 28,* 701–11.

Lobstein, T., Turpin, G., & Siddle, D. A. (1979). Comment on "Correction for sinus arrhythmia in the evoked cardiac response: A timebase problem." *Biological Psychology, 9,* 221–3.

Loewenfeld, I. E. (1993). *The Pupil: Anatomy, Physiology, and Clinical Applications.* Ames: Iowa State University Press.

Loftus, G. R. (1978). On interpretation of interactions. *Memory and Cognition, 6,* 312–19.

Loftus, G. R. (1994). Why psychology will never be a real science until we change the way that we analyze data. Paper presented at the 102nd Annual Convention of the American Psychological Association (August, Los Angeles).

Loftus, G. R., & Masson, M. J. (1994). Using confidence intervals in within-subject designs. *Psychonomic Bulletin and Review, 1,* 476–90.

Luce, R. D., Krantz, D. H., Suppes, P., & Tversky, A. (1990). *Foundations of Measurement,* vol. 3 (Representations, Axiomatizations, and Invariance). San Diego: Academic Press.

Lykken, D. E. (1972). Range correction applied to heart rate and GSR data. *Psychophysiology, 9,* 373–9.

Martin, I., & Venables, P. H. (Eds.) (1980). *Techniques in Psychophysiology.* Chichester, U.K.: Wiley.

Maxwell, S. E., Delaney, H. D., & Manheimer, J. M. (1985). ANOVA of residuals and ANCOVA: Correcting an illusion by using model comparisons and graphs. *Journal of Educational Statistics, 10,* 197–209.

Meyer, D. L. (1991). Misinterpretation of interaction effects: A reply to Rosnow and Rosenthal. *Psychological Bulletin, 110,* 571–3.

Michell, J. (1986). Measurement scales and statistics: A clash of paradigms. *Psychological Bulletin, 100,* 398–407.

Mitchell, M., & Jolley, J. (1988). *Research Design Explained.* New York: Holt, Rinehart & Winston.

Muller, K. E., & Barton, C. N. (1989). Approximate power for repeated measures ANOVA lacking sphericity. *Journal of the American Statistical Association, 84,* 549–55.

Muller, K. E., & Barton, C. N. (1991). Correction to "Approximate power for repeated measures ANOVA lacking sphericity." *Journal of the American Statistical Association, 86,* 255–6.

Muller, K. E., LaVange, L. M., Ramey, S. L., & Ramey, C. T. (1992). Power calculations for general linear multivariate models including repeated measures applications. *Journal of the American Statistical Association, 87,* 1209–26.

Myrtek, M., & Foerster, F. (1986). The law of initial value: A rare exception. *Biological Psychology, 22,* 227–37.

Neale, J. M., & Liebert, R. M. (1986). *Science and Behavior: An Introduction to Methods of Research.* Englewood Cliffs, NJ: Prentice-Hall.

O'Brien, R. G., & Muller, K. E. (1993). Unified power analysis for t-tests through multivariate hypotheses. In L. K. Edwards (Ed.), *Applied Analysis of Variance in the Behavioral Sciences,* pp. 297–344. New York: Marcel Dekker.

Osterhout, L., Bersick, M., & McKinnon, R. (1997). Brain potentials elicited by words: Word length and frequency predict the latency of an early negativity. *Biological Psychology, 46,* 143–68.

Overall, J. E. (1994). Issues in the design and analysis of controlled clinical trials. *Journal of Clinical Psychology, 50,* 95–102.

Petrinovich, L., & Widaman, K. F. (1984). An evaluation of statistical strategies to analyze repeated-measures data. In H. V. S. Peeke & L. Petrinovich (Eds.), *Habituation, Sensitivation, and Behavior,* pp. 155–201. Orlando, FL: Academic Press.

Petty, R. E., Fabrigar, L. R., Wegener, D. T., & Priester, J. R. (1996). Understanding data when interactions are present or hypothesized. *Psychological Science, 7,* 247–52.

Pivik, R. T., Broughton, R. J., Coppola, R., Davidson, R. J., Fox, N., & Nuwer, M. R. (1993). Guidelines for the recording and quantitative analysis of electroencephalographic activity in research contexts. *Psychophysiology, 30,* 547–8.

Porges, S. W. (1995). Orienting in a defensive world. Mammalian modifications of our evolutionary heritage. A polyvagal theory. *Psychophysiology, 32,* 301–18.

Porges, S. W., & Bohrer, R. E. (1990). The analysis of periodic processes in psychophysiological research. In J. T. Cacioppo & L. G. Tassinary (Eds.), *Principles of Psychophysiology,* pp. 708–53. Cambridge University Press.

Poulton, E. C. (1973). Unwanted range effects from using within-subject experimental designs. *Psychological Bulletin, 80,* 113–21.

Poulton, E. C., & Edwards, R. S. (1979). Asymmetric transfer in within-subjects experiments on stress interaction. *Ergonomics, 22,* 945–61.

Poulton, E. C., & Freeman, P. R. (1966). Unwanted asymmetrical transfer effects with balanced experimental designs. *Psychological Bulletin, 66,* 1–8.

Quigley, K. S., & Berntson, G. G. (1990). Autonomic interactions and chronotopic control of the heart: Heart period versus heart rate. *Psychophysiology, 33,* 605–11.

Richter, D. W., & Spyer, K. M. (1990). Cardiorespiratory control. In A. D. Loewy & K. M. Spyer (Eds.), *Central Regulation of Autonomic Function,* pp. 189–207. New York: Oxford.

Rogosa, D., Brandt, D., & Zimowski, M. (1982). A growth curve approach to the measurement of change. *Psychological Bulletin, 92,* 726–48.

Rosenthal, R., & Rosnow, R. L. (1985). *Contrast Analysis: Focused Comparisons in the Analysis of Variance.* New York: Holt, Rinehart & Wilson.

Rosenthal, R., & Rosnow, R. L. (1991). *Essentials of Behavioral Research: Explanation and Prediction,* 2nd ed. New York: McGraw-Hill.

Rosnow, R. L., & Rosenthal, R. (1989a). Definition and interpretation of interaction effects. *Psychological Bulletin, 105,* 143–6.

Rosnow, R. L., & Rosenthal, R. (1989b). Statistical procedures and the justification of knowledge in psychological science. *American Psychologist, 44,* 1276–84.

Rosnow, R. L., & Rosenthal, R. (1991). If you're looking at the cell means, you're not looking at only the interaction (unless all main effects are zero). *Psychological Bulletin, 110,* 574–6.

Rosnow, R. L., & Rosenthal, R. (1995). "Some things you learn aren't so": Cohen's paradox, Asch's paradigm, and the interpretation of interaction. *Psychological Science, 6,* 3–9.

Rozeboom, W. W. (1960). The fallacy of the null hypothesis significance test. *Psychological Bulletin, 57,* 416–28.

Rugg, M. D., & Coles, M. G. H. (1995). *Electrophysiology of Mind.* Oxford University Press.

Russell, D. W. (1990). The analysis of psychophysiological data: Multivariate approaches. In J. T. Cacioppo & L. G. Tassinary (Eds.), *Principles of Psychophysiology,* pp. 775–801. Cambridge University Press.

SAS (1989). *SAS/IML Software: Usage and Reference,* ver. 6. Cary, NC: SAS Institute.

SAS (1996). *SAS/STAT Software: Changes and Enhancements through Release 6.11.* Cary, NC: SAS Institute.

Schroeder, L. D., Sjoquist, D. L., & Stephan, P. E. (1986). *Understanding Regression Analysis: An Introductory Guide.* Newbury Park, CA: Sage.

Schwartz, P. J., & Weiss, T. (1983). T-wave amplitude as an index of cardiac sympathetic activity: A misleading concept. *Psychophysiology, 20,* 696–701.

Shapiro, D., Lane, J. D., Light, K. C., Myrtek, M., Suwada, Y., & Steptoe, A. (1996). Blood pressure publication guidelines. *Psychophysiology, 33,* 1–12.

Sherwood, A., Allen, M. T., Fahrenberg, J., Kelsey, R. M., Lovallo, W. R., & van Doornen, L. J. P. (1990). Methodological guidelines for impedance cardiography. *Psychophysiology, 27,* 1–23.

Sidani, S., & Lynn, M. R. (1993). Examining amount and pattern of change: Comparing repeated measures ANOVA and individual regression analysis. *Nursing Research, 42,* 283–6.

Siegal, S. (1956). *Nonparametric Statistics.* New York: McGraw-Hill.

Stearns, S. D., & David, R. A. (1993). *Signal Processing Algorithms in Fortran and C.* Englewood Cliffs, NJ: Prentice-Hall.

Stemmler, G., & Fahrenberg, J. (1989). Psychophysiological assessment: Conceptual, psychometric, and statistical issues. In G. Turpin (Ed.), *Handbook of Clinical Psychophysiology,* pp. 71–104. Chichester, U.K.: Wiley.

Stevens, S. S. (1951). Mathematics, measurement, and psychophysics. In S. S. Stevens (Ed.), *Handbook of Experimental Psychology,* pp. 1–49. New York: Wiley.

Stiratelli, R., Laird, N. M., & Ware, J. H. (1984). Random-effects models for serial observations with binary response. *Biometrics, 40,* 961–71.

Thede, L. (1996). *Analog and Digital Filter Design using C.* Upper Saddle River, NJ: Prentice-Hall.

Tufte, E. R. (1983). *The Visual Display of Quantitative Information.* Cheshire, CT: Graphics Press.

Tufte, E. R. (1990). *Envisioning Information.* Cheshire, CT: Graphics Press.

Tufte, E. R. (1997). *Visual Explanations: Images and Quantities, Evidence and Narrative.* Cheshire, CT: Graphics Press.

Tukey, J. W. (1977). *Exploratory Data Analysis.* Reading, MA: Addison-Wesley.

Turpin, G. (1986). Cardiac-respiratory integration. In P. Grossman, K. H. L. Janssen, & D. Vaitl (Eds.), *Cardiorespiratory and Cardiosomatic Psychophysiology,* pp. 139–55. New York: Plenum.

van Boxtel, G. J. M. (1998). Computational and statistical methods for analyzing event-related potential data. *Behavior Research Methods, Instruments, and Computers, 30,* 87–102.

van Boxtel, G. J. M., van den Boogaart, B., & Brunia, C. M. H. (1993). The contingent negative variation in a choice reaction time task. *Journal of Psychophysiology, 7,* 11–23.

van Ravenswaaij-Arts, C. M. A., Kolle'e, L. A. A., Hopman, J. C. W., Stoelinga, G. B. A., & van Geijn, H. P. (1993). Heart rate variability. *Annals of Internal Medicine, 118,* 436–47.

Vasey, W. V., & Thayer, J. F. (1987). The continuing problem of false positives in repeated measures ANOVA in psychophysiology: A multivariate solution. *Psychophysiology, 24,* 479–86.

Venables, P. H., & Martin, I. (Eds.) (1967). *A Manual of Psychophysiological Methods.* New York: Wiley.

Wainer, H., & Thissen, D. (1981). Graphical data analysis. *Annual Review of Psychology, 32,* 191–242.

Wainer, H., & Thissen, D. (1993). Graphical data analysis. In G. Keren & C. Lewis (Eds.), *A Handbook for Data Analysis in the Behavioral Sciences,* pp. 391–457. Hillsdale, NJ: Erlbaum.

Ware, J. H. (1985). Linear models for the analysis of longitudinal studies. *American Statistician, 39,* 95–101.

Welch, B. L. (1947). The generalization of Student's problem when several different population variances are unequal. *Biometrika, 29,* 350–62.

Welch, B. L. (1951). On the comparison of several mean values: An alternative approach. *Biometrika, 38,* 330–6.

Wheeler, R. E., Davidson, R. J., & Tomarken, A. J. (1993). Frontal brain asymmetry and emotional reactivity: A biological substrate of affective style. *Psychophysiology, 30,* 82–9.

Wilder, J. (1958). Modern psychophysiology and the law of initial value. *American Journal of Psychotherapy, 12,* 199–221.

Wilson, R. S. (1967). Analysis of autonomic reaction patterns. *Psychophysiology, 4,* 125–42.

Winer, B. J. (1971). *Statistical Principles in Experimental Design.* New York: McGraw-Hill.

Zahn, T. P., & Kruesi, M. J. P. (1993). Autonomic activity in boys with disruptive behavior disorders. *Psychophysiology, 30,* 605–14.

Zuckerman, M., Hodgins, H. S., Zuckerman, A., & Rosenthal, R. (1993). Contemporary issues in the analysis of data. *Psychological Science, 4,* 49–53.

CHAPTER THIRTY-THREE

BIOSIGNAL PROCESSING

GABRIELE GRATTON

Introduction

This chapter reviews issues related to the analysis of psychophysiological data. It will focus on general questions that are relevant to a variety of techniques, rather than on specific issues related to individual methods. The previous chapter of this volume also deals with statistical issues in psychophysiology, focusing on issues of inference and data interpretation.

STAGES OF DATA PROCESSING

In describing the procedures used in analyzing psychophysiological data, it is useful to distinguish among different stages of analysis. The first stage is *signal enhancement* and elimination of observations that are artifactual or that can be considered outliers. This stage, sometimes called "signal conditioning," involves (at least in part) techniques that are specific to each type of physiological measure.

The second stage involves *data reduction* (sometimes called "quantification" or "parameter extraction"). Most psychophysiological experiments involve a large number of observations per subject (i.e. dependent variables). Although this provides data sets that are rich in information content, it also increases the probability of spurious or noisy observations. In general, one of the main objectives of signal processing is maximizing the signal-to-noise ratio. A large number of observations may contain a large number of signals to study but may also contain a large amount of noise. It is therefore advantageous to select information that is relevant and to minimize redundancy between the dependent variables entered in the statistical analysis, since redundant dependent variables will not necessarily increase the signal yet may generate additional opportunities for noise. An important step in signal processing is to reduce the data set to the smallest possible number of dependent variables (each affected by the smallest possible amount of noise) while preserving the information content of the original data set as much as possible. However, a moderate degree of redundancy could be useful in distinguishing random noise from systematic noise and thus in deriving a valid and reliable estimate of the signal.

The third stage of data processing is *statistical analysis,* which may include hypothesis testing, model fitting, parameter estimation, and so forth. As mentioned previously, most psychophysiological experiments are multivariate in nature – that is, they involve repeated observations from the same subjects. The multivariate nature of psychophysiological measures is one of their greatest assets, for it allows the experimenters to view phenomena from different "points of view," thus affording a more complete and detailed picture of bodily phenomena. However, it often introduces special types of problems in the statistical evaluation of multivariate data sets. Two general approaches can be considered: the univariate approach, which considers one dependent variable at a time; and the multivariate approach, which considers all dependent variables (as well as their covariation) together (see Huberty & Morris 1989). Each of these approaches has advantages and disadvantages. In general, when there is a limited number of subjects in the study (relative to the number of dependent variables) and the dependent variables tend to be correlated with each other across conditions (or groups) in the same manner as within conditions (or groups), the univariate approach is more powerful. Conversely, the multivariate approach is preferable when there is a large number of subjects in the study (relative to the number of dependent variables) and when the within- and between-condition (or group) correlations among dependent variables tend to go in opposite directions. (The statistical analysis stage is treated in Chapter 32 and thus will not be considered in detail here.)

John T. Cacioppo, Louis G. Tassinary, and Gary G. Berntson (Eds.), *Handbook of Psychophysiology,* 2nd ed. © Cambridge University Press 2000. Printed in the United States of America. ISBN 62634X. All rights reserved.

In concluding this section, it is important to remind the reader that the output of an analysis is only as good as its input (this is captured by the well-known aphorism "garbage in, garbage out"). Complex and sophisticated data analyses can in no way substitute for clear experimental hypotheses, elegant experimental designs, and accurate data collection procedures. However, they can complement these steps in providing clear and convincing data.

GENERAL ISSUES

Psychophysiological data vary along a number of dimensions, and different types of data propose different types of analytical problems and solutions to the investigator. However, there are a few overarching themes that are valid for most types of measurements. Some general issues are particularly important and worth mentioning at the beginning of this chapter. First, psychophysiological measures are typically *indirect*; in other words, they are measures of events occurring outside the human body that are related to events that occur inside the body. For instance, measures of the electrical activity produced by the body (such as the electrocardiogram and the electroencephalogram, ECG and EEG) are in fact measures of the difference in potential between two electrodes located on the surface of the body; positron emission tomography (PET) measures the arrival of high-energy photons to particular detectors located at some distance around the body, which in turn is related to the concentration of radioactive substances in various areas of the body; and so on. In general, psychophysiological measures are subject to some transformation with respect to the original signal generated within the body (because of physical, physiological, or psychological reasons). This transformation may partially distort the signal (and its statistical properties) and may occasionally generate artifacts that need to be recognized and eliminated from the data before statistical analysis is performed.

Second, most of the data are sampled in a *discrete* fashion – both temporally and spatially. The transformation of analog parameters into discrete measures may distort the signal and require specific solutions to statistical problems. One of the major problems is obtaining a representative sample of the variable of interest over both time and space. In addition, some techniques (such as measures of heart rate acceleration or deceleration) may be based on the observation of internal events (e.g., the occurrence of an R wave in the ECG) whose spacing is variable (and, in the case of heart rate changes, is a function of the variable of interest). This may make it more complicated to compare observations across trials and subjects. Investigators using these measures have developed special approaches to address this problem (see Chapter 9).

Third, most psychophysiological measures are *multiply determined*; that is, they are determined by the interaction of a variety of factors. Some of these factors may be extraneous to and uncorrelated with the experimental manipulations (and thus will contribute to statistical noise), while other factors may be related to the experimental manipulations in ways that differ from those intended by the researcher (and hence will contribute both to statistical noise and to systematic effects). The latter type of confounds are particularly insidious and difficult to eliminate. One of the most important characteristics of good experimental methodology is the use of appropriate control procedures to distinguish between signal and systematic noise.

Fourth, most psychophysiological measures are inherently *noisy*, making it difficult to distinguish between signal and noise in the raw (single-trial) observations. Several techniques have been developed to extract the signal. One of the simplest is signal averaging: the observation is repeated several times and the individual responses are averaged together. Signal averaging is based on the central limit theorem and can therefore be expected to provide reasonable estimates of the expected central tendency of the population in a large number of situations – provided that enough trials are used. Note that, for signal averaging to work appropriately, it is important that the expected value of the noise across trials be equal to zero. Although this is a reasonable assumption in many cases, there are certainly situations in which this is not true. For instance, as we will see later, frequency analysis (such as the Fourier transform) can be used to estimate the "power" or variance associated with a particular frequency. Since this value cannot be less than zero, the average of the power values for a particular frequency obtained in different trials (or in different subjects) will always be greater than zero, even if no systematic activity exists at that frequency.

A problem with signal averaging is that it eliminates potentially relevant information about the variability of the signal from trial to trial (and in some cases from subject to subject): this variability is entirely attributed to stochastic phenomena. In most cases, however, the variability of the signal is not entirely random but rather depends on the influence of intervening variables. For instance, in an experiment evaluating the size of the visual evoked potential as a function of stimulus intensity, the size of the response may also be influenced by subjects' variables (such as allocation of attention, emotional factors, etc.) as well as by contextual conditions (stimulus sequence, noise in the environment, etc.) or still other factors. When signal averaging is used, all of these intervening variables are treated as contributors to stochastic noise and thence ignored. This may lead to loss of information or to systematic errors when contingencies exist between the experimental manipulations of interest and any of the intervening variables. Similar problems have been described with respect to other types of measures (see Estes 1956; Siegler 1987).

Another problem with signal averaging is that the signal may vary along dimensions other than its intensity: in some cases, the latency of the phenomenon or its spatial location

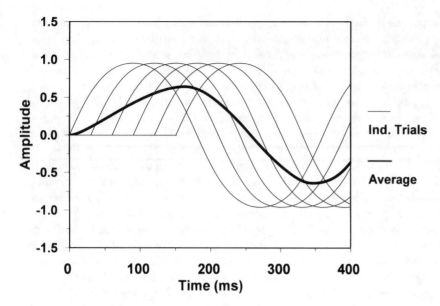

Figure 1. The effect of trial-to-trial variations in latency ("latency jitter") on the amplitude of an averaged psychophysiological activity. In this example, the latency of the first positive peak varies systematically in latency between 90 msec and 270 msec. Although the amplitude of the peak on single trials (indicated by thin lines) is always equal to 1, the amplitude of the peak of the average waveform (indicated by the thick line) is considerably smaller (slightly larger than 0.5). The duration of the activity also appears prolonged.

may vary from trial to trial (partly for the reasons just outlined). In this case signal averaging may produce systematic distortions, the most typical of which is a "smearing" of the response across different data points. The effect of smearing is more intense for signals with a steep gradient. In the case of electrophysiological signals that vary quickly over time, this leads to the phenomenon of "latency jitter": the size of an evoked electrophysiological activity may be underestimated using signal averaging because the activity "peaks" at different latencies on individual trials. A similar problem exists when data from different subjects are pooled together (for a discussion of this problem and some solutions, see Möcks et al. 1988). It is interesting to note that the development of brain imaging methods, which have strong gradients in the spatial domain, has led to the recognition of a similar smearing problem when average spatial maps are computed across subjects (because of intersubject variability in brain anatomy); see Figure 1. This problem is in fact not specific to psychophysiological measures. For instance, investigators in psychology have long recognized that apparently smooth speed–accuracy functions may result from the mixture of distributions of fast responses with a low level of accuracy and slow responses with a high level of accuracy, provided that the two distributions have some degree of partial overlap in response time (Yantis, Meyer, & Smith 1991).

In order to address this problem, several investigators have proposed to measure psychophysiological phenomena on single trials (or subjects). A critical step of this procedure is the development of techniques for identifying target features on single-trial records. These techniques, although quite varied, can be grouped as "pattern recognition" algorithms. Some are based on visual inspection of individual data and are most useful when the target features are much larger than the noise. Others are computer controlled and based on such statistical approaches as cross-correlation, auto-correlation, or other automatic methods. The individual records may then be aligned along the target feature and averaged together. Alternatively, some measure other than the mean can be used to describe the single-record distribution. An example of an alignment methodology in the time domain is the Woody filter (Woody 1967), which is a general-purpose statistical method; an example in the spatial domain is the alignment method proposed by Talairach and Tournoux (1988), a special-purpose approach that has become a standard practice in brain imaging.

General Classifications

Psychophysiological measures are usually defined as non-invasive measures of bodily functions taken with the intent of addressing issues that are relevant to psychologists (i.e., to obtain information that is relevant to the study of the human nature). This broad definition encompasses a large variety of measures that differ along a number of dimensions. Of these dimensions, some are important for the purposes of the present chapter because they result in different types of signal processing problems. I will pay particular attention to three of these dimensions.

FAST VERSUS SLOW MEASURES

As mentioned before, psychophysiological measures reflect bodily changes that are related to psychological phenomena. These changes occur over time. Some of them evolve very quickly (within a few milliseconds) and others quite slowly (over seconds, minutes, or even longer times). Indeed, for each type of psychophysiological measure used, it is possible to consider a parameter that will indicate the speed at which the activity evolves. We may call this parameter the "time constant" of a particular physiological measure. This parameter depends upon three factors: (a) the rate of change of the relevant psychological phenomenon; (b) the time required by the physiological event being measured to track changes in the psychological phenomenon; and (c) the time required for the measurement.

By and large, it is possible to consider individual time-delay functions for each of these steps, although in some cases interaction terms should also be considered. Note that each step may itself comprise several substeps. Each step can be considered as having an input (coming from the previous step) and an output (influencing the next step) – but a delay will usually occur in the operation of translating an input to an output. Here is an example of a function[1] expressing this delay:

$$O_t - O_{t-1} = (I_t - O_{t-1})(1 - e^{-1/tc}). \qquad (1)$$

In this function, the change in the output $(O_t - O_{t-1})$ of a particular step is a delayed function of the difference between its input I_t and its previous level O_{t-1}. The delay is determined by an exponential function whose critical parameter is tc, the *time constant* of this particular step. When several steps are involved, the total time-delay function is determined by a convolution of the individual functions. That is, the total time constant of a measurement is related to the integration of the time constants of each individual step. An example of this cascade, and of its effect on the final output measure, is illustrated in Figure 2. In this example, the initial input is a 3-sec pulse (this may simulate a stimulus of short duration). Four steps were simulated, with time constants of 0.2, 1, 8, and 3 seconds. Note that the final output is substantially delayed with respect to the input and actually peaks well after termination of the pulse (i.e., of the stimulus).

The steps contributing most to the total time constant are called "rate limiting" steps (in the example given, step 3 and, to a smaller extent, step 4). Whereas all factors determining the measurement's time constant – rate of change

Figure 2. Simulated example of a series of individual steps between an input (pulse) and a final output measure. The input is a 3-sec pulse (this may simulate a stimulus of short duration). Each step introduces a delay that is described by a parameter known as the time constant (see text). Four steps were simulated, with time constants of 0.2, 1, 8, and 3 seconds.

of the psychological event, delay of the physiological phenomena, and measurement time – are always present to some extent, there is often only one (or a few) rate limiting factor(s). The nature of the rate limiting factor and the time constant of the measurement vary between different physiological measures. I will label measures with a long time constant "slow" measures and those with a short time constant "fast" measures.

Certain measures of autonomic activity are slow, including measures of electrodermal activity (EDA, in which the psychological and/or the physiological phenomena evolve slowly over time), functional magnetic resonance imaging (fMRI, in which the physiological event under study – a change in blood oxygenation – evolves slowly), and PET (in which the response delay of the hemodynamic or metabolic systems to changes in brain activity is coupled with slow measurement time). Fast measures include those of the event-related brain potential (ERP), magnetoencephalogram (MEG), electromyogram (EMG), and event-related optical signal (EROS). For these measures, all three determining factors are fast. Some other measures, such as heart rate and pupil diameter, are intermediate between these two extremes. Measures with a short time constant have a good temporal resolution (i.e., the effects of two different psychological and/or physiological events occurring in rapid succession can be distinguished), whereas measures with a long time constant have a poor spatial resolution (i.e., events in rapid succession cannot be separated easily). This is illustrated in Figure 3, which compares the time courses of the effect of two stimuli presented in rapid succession on measures with short and long time constants.

Measures with a slow time constant provide few independent observations per unit time. In contrast, measures with a fast time constant provide a large number of independent observations over the same time unit. The processing of psychophysiological data usually requires transformation of the data into a series of numbers sampled over time (i.e., a time series). The issue then arises of the optimal temporal sampling strategy for each measure.

The sampling strategy must preserve as much as possible the information contained in the signal. The minimum sampling frequency at which information is maintained is twice the frequency of the signal (this is called the "Nyquist frequency"). At sampling rates slower than the Nyquist frequency, *aliasing* causes a high-frequency signal to manifest itself as a lower-frequency signal. This phenomenon is illustrated in the top portion of Figure 4. A sampling frequency that is too

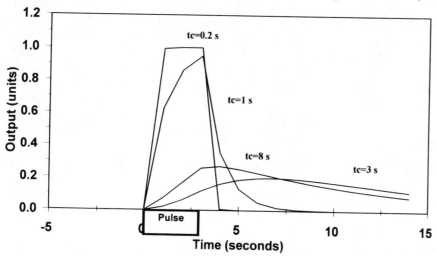

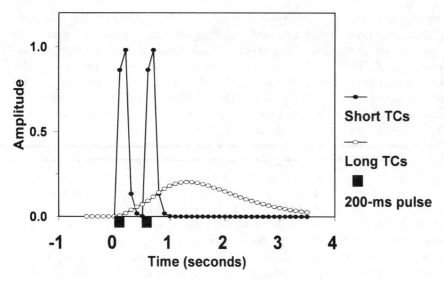

Figure 3. Simulated example of the response of output measures with short and long time constant to two stimulations in rapid succession. Two 200-msec stimulation pulses were presented, separated by an interval of 300 msec (this is intended to simulate two independent psychological events). The closed-circle line is obtained by assuming a cascade of three intervening steps between the stimulation and the measurement system, each introducing a delay characterized by a time constant of 200 msec. The open circle line is obtained by assuming a cascade of three intervening steps with time constants of 5 sec. Note that the short–time constant measure affords easy separation of the two pulses (i.e. psychological events), whereas effects of the two pulses with the long–time constant measure are lumped together.

slow may also completely miss the occurrence of a very fast, transient phenomenon; this is illustrated in the lower portion of Figure 4. This latter consideration may encourage investigators to sample at the highest possible frequency, yet we should also remember that – since each observation will contain both relevant information and noise – it is important to minimize the number of data points (i.e. dependent variables) entered into the statistical analysis. This may be achieved conveniently at the data reduction stage. Finally, some recording systems impose limitations on the maximum sampling rate. However, the issue of aliasing should always be considered when studying a physiological variable. This problem is particularly likely to occur when fast phenomena are studied using a relatively slow sampling rate (e.g., when EEG is measured at less than 20 Hz, ECG at less than 2 Hz, or respiration at less than 0.5 Hz).

DIRECT VERSUS INDIRECT MEASURES

Psychophysiological measures also differ in terms of how many steps intervene between the physiological phenomenon that is the "real" target of the study (e.g., neuronal activity, sympathetic or parasympathetic activation) and the actual physiological measure that is taken (e.g., scalp electrical activity, increased blood flow, in-

creased heart rate or increased EDA). The indirect nature of the measures may have several consequences. First, as mentioned previously, it may introduce a lag between the psychological event of interest and observed changes. Second, each of the intervening steps may introduce distortions in the size and/or shape of the responses with respect to the original signal.

A particularly important issue related to the indirectness of psychophysiological measures is that of linearity of a measure. A measure M is *linear* with respect to its inferential psychophysiological variable ϕ if the following formula is valid:

$$M = k\phi + \text{offset} \quad \text{with} \ k \neq 0. \tag{2}$$

For all practical purposes it may be sufficient that this formula is valid (at least approximately) for only an interval of values of M and ϕ, provided that this interval contains typically observed values of the measure and the expected range of the psychophysiological factor. For the linearity assumption in this formula to be valid, two terms must remain constant across conditions: the factor k and the measurement offset. The proportionality factor k depends on such variables as the relationship between the psychophysiological construct of interest and the physical phenomenon actually measured, the propagation of the physiological measure to the surface, the recording and analysis procedures employed, and so forth. An example of change in the proportionality factor is a change in the way neuronal signals are transformed into a hemodynamic phenomenon. For instance, a similar increase in neuronal activity at occipital and frontal locations may result in a different increase in the scalp electrical signal measured over these two areas. The offset factor may also depend on the effect of variables other than the physiological phenomenon of interest on the observed measure. For instance, an apparent increase in the amplitude of the ERP at frontal electrodes may be the consequence of an increase in the ocular artifact. Similarly, head movements may result in apparent large changes in the MRI signal.

Another interesting example for psychophysiologists is the difference between measures of EDA. Two such measures are possible, of electrical conductivity versus electrical resistance between two locations on the skin; these two measures are inversely related to each other. However, the physiological phenomenon of interest (increase in conductivity associated with the activity of the sweat glands) is directly proportional to conductivity and inversely proportional to resistance. In this case, then, conductivity is a linear measure of the physiological phenomenon whereas resistance is not. Quigley and Berntson (1996) pointed out that a similar case can be made for measures of heart rate versus heart period (which are of course reciprocal to each other): heart period, but not heart rate, appears to vary linearly with basal autonomic activation.

Linearity is useful because it allows for linear transformations of the measure M (such as additions, subtractions, multiplications by a constant, averaging, etc.) to be considered valid also with respect to the physiological variable ϕ. Linear manipulations of the observed measures are commonly performed in the analysis of psychophysiological data. However, if the relationship between M and ϕ is not linear (i.e., if k or the offset are not constant), then such manipulations of the dependent variable may not be valid with respect to the

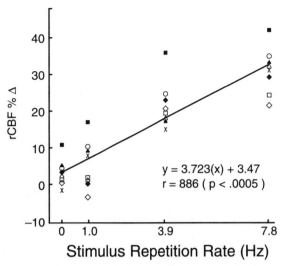

Figure 5. Linearity of the relationship between stimulation frequency and blood flow measures obtained with $^{15}O_2$ PET. Redrawn with permission from Fox & Raichle, "Stimulus rate dependence of regional cerebral blood flow in human striate cortex, demonstrated by positron emission tomography," *Journal of Neurophysiology*, vol. 51, pp. 1109–20. Copyright 1984.

Figure 4. *Top:* The effect of sampling at a frequency lower than the Nyquist frequency (aliasing). The signal (indicated by the thick line) is sampled at 10 Hz (indicated by the open circles), less than the Nyquist frequency of 16 Hz. The result is an apparent 2-Hz signal (indicated by the thin line). *Bottom:* A rapid activity (duration = 62.5 msec) is measured using a 10-Hz sampling rate. In this case, the activity occurs between two sampling points (open circles) and so the peak is not detected by the measurement system.

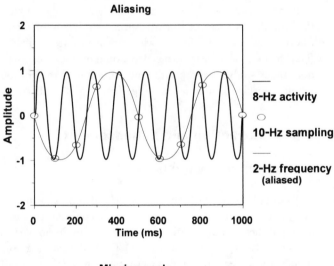

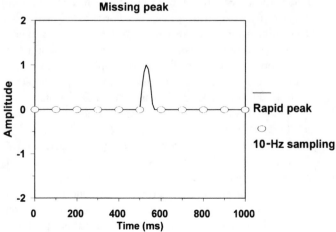

psychophysiological variable, which precludes drawing any inferences (other than potentially misleading ones).

Lack of linearity may occur whenever any of the intervening steps between the observed measure and the psychophysiological construct of interest involve some form of nonlinear transformations. For example, consider the steps occurring between neuronal activity and increased $^{15}O_2$ PET response. The steps include the probable release of some chemical by the active neurons, consequent local vasodilation, increased regional blood flow, and – if radioactive material is introduced into the blood flow – increased radioactivity in a particular volume of the head. In principle, the relationships between causes and effects existing at each step may be nonlinear or even nonmonotonic. In other words, it is not necessarily the case that, for a certain percent increase in neuronal activity, there is an equal percent increase in vasodilation. Therefore, linearity needs to be assessed on a case-by-case basis. For PET responses, Fox and Raichle (1984) observed an almost linear relationship between frequency of visual stimulation (between 0 and 7.8 Hz) and change in blood flow in primary visual cortex as estimated using the $^{15}O_2$ PET method (see Figure 5). The presence of linearity is critical for the application of subtraction methods during the analysis of hemodynamic responses.

Even if the linearity assumption is not met, it is still possible that the relationship between the dependent variable and the physiological phenomenon is monotonic. Whereas a monotonic relationship may limit the use of linear transformations and of parametric statistics, it is still sufficient for the application of nonparametric statistics based on qualitative judgments about effect sizes. Finally, relationships that are nonlinear but follow a more complex function can be handled by transformations that render them linear (as, for instance, the transformation of electrodermal resistance measures into conductance measures).

So far I have discussed the linearity of the relationship between the observed measures and the physiological parameter they intend to measure. To the extent that psychophysiological measures are used to make psychological inferences, it is also important to consider the type of relationship that exists between the physiological parameter and the underlying psychological concept of interest. For example, the purpose of measuring neuronal activity in a certain brain area may be the investigation of memory or attention phenomena, and the purpose of measuring blood pressure may be the investigation of the effect of psychological stressors on the cardiovascular system. Clearly, the issue of linearity (or at least of monotonicity) of the relationship is just as important here as in the case of the relationship between the observed measure and the physiological variable.

CONTINUOUS VERSUS DISCRETE MEASURES

The distinction between continuous and discrete measures refers to the time at which information about the status of the physiological system under study is, in principle, available. Some psychophysiological measures can provide information at any time with no particular restriction. For instance, the diameter of the pupil can be monitored continuously to provide a more or less continuous measure of the level of activation of particular subcomponents of the autonomic system. Likewise, the EMG and the EEG are continuous measures of electric potentials produced by muscles and the brain respectively. However, other physiological measures (e.g., of heart rate, respiration rate) reflect modification of parameters of cyclic events that occur at some intervals within the body. With these measures, information about psychological phenomena may be available only at discrete times. For instance, the state of activation of some subcomponents of the autonomic system can be studied using changes in heart rate, but information is available only when the heart beats (or when a particular electrocardiographic wave, such as the R wave, is produced). Still other measures can only be obtained by using particular maneuvers that elicit special responses in the body. Parameters of the blink reflex, for example, can only be measured by eliciting the blink reflex itself. Therefore, using the blink reflex to monitor changes in status of a particular physiological system (such as one related to emotion) entails that information may be available at specific times only (Bradley, Cuthbert, &

Lang 1991). A similar situation is obtained when the P300 component of the ERP elicited by secondary task probes is used to monitor the level of attention of subjects to primary task stimuli (Wickens et al. 1983).

I will label as "continuous" those measures that can provide information about the state of a physiological system at any time and as "discrete" those measures that provide information only at specific times. An advantage of continuous measures is that information about the time course of psychological phenomena is readily available on single-trial records. Discrete measures can also provide information about the time course of psychological events, but their effective sampling rate is limited by the interval between the successive measurement windows. Finer sampling rates require pooling information obtained across trials and thus are more complicated to obtain. An additional problem with some discrete measures is that the time at which information is available may not be completely under experimental control. For instance, certain measures related to circadian rhythms can only be obtained unobtrusively when the subject is awake. This may result in a "variable" sampling rate that may complicate the analysis. For example solutions to this problem, see Monk and Fookson (1986) and Monk (1987). Measures of heart interbeat interval changes as a function of when (during a cycle) the stimulus is presented create special problems of identification because the time at which measures are available (i.e., the next heartbeat) varies depending on the phenomenon under study. Appropriate representation of the effects requires special techniques (see e.g. Jennings et al. 1991).

Signal Extraction and Enhancement

DOMAINS OF ANALYSIS

Psychophysiological data can be considered as elements of a multidimensional matrix. We can consider the following dimensions that are specific to psychophysiological measures: (a) type of measure; (b) time of sampling (or time with respect to some anchoring event); (c) location in space (itself comprising one, two, or three dimensions). Other dimensions may also be considered, such as experimental condition, subject, group, and so on, but these dimensions are not specific to psychophysiological measures. Since some of the dimensions are grouped together (such as the three spatial dimensions), it is useful to talk about domains of analysis (the temporal domain, the spatial domain, etc.).

For some (or most) experiments, some of these dimensions may have only one cell and are therefore fixed. For instance, we may be recording only one psychophysiological measure or collecting data from only one location. It is important, however, to consider that different values on each of these dimensions all refer to the same individual

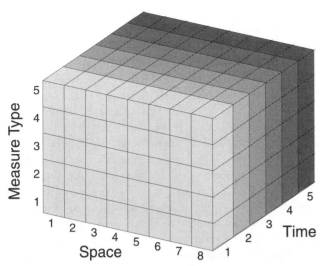

Figure 6. Graphic representation of the multidimensional nature of psychophysiological measures. Only three dimensions (specific to psychophysiological measures) are represented here: space, time, and type of measure. However, space itself may comprise several dimensions, and other dimensions (such as subject, experimental condition, etc.) are not represented. Note that the combination of different dimensions generates a large number of different observations for each subject. Since these are all observations from the same subjects, they may reflect different facets of the same phenomenon. Changes along one dimension may therefore be correlated to changes on another dimension.

case and thus are likely to be correlated. Psychophysiological data can therefore be expressed as elements of a multidimensional measurement matrix:

$$\mathbf{M}_{m,t,x,y,z,c,s}. \tag{3}$$

Note that each element of the measurement matrix $\mathbf{M}$ has several indices corresponding to the type of measure used (m), the time of observation (t), the spatial coordinates of the observation (x, y, z), the conditions of observation (c), and the subject from which the measure is recorded (s). A graphic representation of the multidimensionality of psychophysiological data is presented in Figure 6.

The fundamental multidimensionality of psychophysiological data creates special problems in the statistical analysis. In fact, the probability of spurious observations (i.e., alpha error) increases with the number of observations. It is essential that appropriate steps be taken to reduce the probability of reaching conclusions on the basis of spurious observations (i.e., rejecting the null hypothesis when it is true), and it is equally important to maintain an acceptable probability of reaching some conclusion in the presence of noisy data (i.e., to maintain adequate power).

An additional problem is that the large number of qualifiers (i.e. indices) used for each observation may sometimes render generalization of the results difficult. For example, if an ERP peak is observed at a latency of 400 msec in condition A and at a latency of 600 msec in condition B, should we conclude that the same ERP peak is delayed in

condition B with respect condition A or rather that an altogether different type of ERP activity occurs in the two conditions?

To address these issues it is usually convenient to perform some intermediate analytical (or signal processing) steps between the level of observation of the raw data and the inferential statistical analysis per se, in which the data are used to provide support for or against theoretical arguments. These preliminary steps are known as data reduction or quantification. A consequence of these preliminary analysis steps is that the data should be considered no longer as raw observations but as quantifications of parameters of some intermediate hypothetical construct that has heuristic value and is usually thought to correspond to some anatomical and/or physiological "entity" (activity in a particular brain structure in response to a particular stimulation condition, the blink response, etc.). In all cases, data reduction implies some "interpretation" of the data; that is, an analytical model is applied that (i) makes more or less explicit assumptions about the underlying structure of the phenomenon observed and (ii) involves some mathematical or logical transformation of the original (raw) data in order to reconstruct the value of some parameter of the underlying structure. The quality of the conclusions drawn from an experiment depends critically on the validity of these assumptions.

TEMPORAL DOMAIN

Time Domain and Frequency Domain

The time factor can be analyzed according to either of two basic models. According to the first model, the physiological events in the period under study evolve in a temporally ordered series that exhibits nonstationary properties (i.e., the basic structure of the activity changes over time). An example is the sequence of responses that occur in the brain after presentation of an individual stimulus. Another example is the changes in heart rate before and after the presentation of a critical stimulus. In these cases, it is profitable to use time as the main dimension of analysis (i.e., conduct a time-domain analysis). Usually, particular features of the time series (such as a maximum, a minimum, the integrated amplitude over an interval, a particular wave shape) are considered as target features, and parameters of these features (such as amplitude, latency, or similarity with a particular template) are quantified and entered in the statistical analysis. In addition, time series can be averaged together (with or without alignment with respect to particular features) in order to increase the signal-to-noise ratio. This approach provides for a substantial data reduction, and data can be expressed in terms of properties of the target feature(s).

The second model, in contrast, assumes that the basic structure of the activity does not vary over time and so exhibits stationary properties in which events repeat in a cyclical fashion. Examples include the consistent response of the brain to a regular train of similar stimuli (when habituation is not supposed to play a role) and the oscillation in heart rate associated with respiration (sinus arrhythmia). When this model is appropriate, physiological activity can be analyzed using a set of tools that are able to extract the basic periodic structure of the activity; these methods are called frequency-domain methods. In this case, a new data series is built in which frequency replaces time as the ordering dimension, and data are expressed in terms of how much of the total variability over time is accounted for by fluctuations occurring at particular frequencies. Distinctive features of this new series can then be considered for quantification purposes (e.g., the "dominant" or most represented frequency in the data can be determined) in the same manner as for time-domain analyses. Frequency analysis may also provide information about the relative delay (or phase) at which particular rhythmic oscillations occur with respect to a reference time (such as the time of stimulation).

Fourier Analysis and Autoregressive Methods

Two types of frequency-domain methods are most commonly used: the Fourier transform and autoregressive methods. Both approaches express the original time series in terms of the extent that certain frequencies occur in the data. The Fourier transform is based on a "deterministic" approach; that is, it represents all of the information (variance) contained in the original data in terms of the independent contributions of equally spaced frequencies. In contrast, autoregressive methods (of which there are different varieties) are based on a "modeling" approach: they impose some constraints on the way in which individual frequencies contribute to the original time series. This modeling approach reduces the number of free parameters in the data (i.e., it reduces the dimensionality of the data). This may allow the investigator to separate signal from noise, but it also requires meeting the assumption that the constraints imposed by the procedure are valid.

The Fourier transform is a numerical method commonly used in engineering and other disciplines. A prerequisite for its application is that the sampling rate be constant across a given epoch (for more on frequency analysis techniques with irregular sampling, see Monk 1987). The basic logic of this method is that any given time series (recording epoch) can be expressed in an equivalent manner (i.e., without loss of information and without interpolation or extrapolation) in the time domain and in the frequency domain. In the frequency domain, a time series can be expressed as the sum of several time series, each characterized by the equal-amplitude oscillations of sinusoidal functions with frequencies equal to a multiple of the inverse of the length of the time series (e.g., if the recording epoch is 1 sec long then the frequencies used to describe the time series will be 1 Hz, 2 Hz, 3 Hz, etc.) plus an offset term

related to the mean value across data points (usually called "zero frequency" or DC value). The number of frequencies is equal to the number of elements of the time series divided by 2. Thus, if we are sampling a 1-sec epoch at 128 Hz, the Fourier decomposition will be based on one DC value and 64 basic frequencies (1 Hz, 2 Hz, 3 Hz, ..., 64 Hz). Each basic frequency is associated with an amplitude value (related to how large the oscillation is at that particular frequency) and a "phase" value, which is related to the relative timing of the peak of the first oscillation with respect to the beginning of the time series. Derivation of the Fourier transform is numerically complex and requires a number of exponential operations that is proportional to the square of the number of elements in the time series. Application of the Fourier transform to long time series may therefore be cumbersome. Fortunately, when the number of elements in a time series is a power of 2 (such as 4, 8, 16, 32, 64, 128, ...), the numeric problem simplifies and can be carried out using a procedure called the fast Fourier transform (FFT).

The outcome of the Fourier transform is a complex number associated with each frequency in which the real and imaginary parts both contain information associated with the amplitude and phase of the basic oscillations. The real and imaginary components can be thought of as corresponding to the coordinates of a vector in a complex plane. However, it is most convenient to express the results in terms of the polar coordinates of this vector (length and angle or orientation). This transformation separates the *amplitude* (equivalent to the length of the vector) and *phase* (equivalent to the orientation of the vector) associated with each frequency. Remember that this transformation, although informative, is not linear. Therefore, averaging (or other linear operations) of data is most appropriately conducted prior to this transformation.

The Fourier transform yields a set of phase and amplitude values for each frequency. In most cases, the attention of the investigators focuses on the amplitude data (although there are exceptions, such as in the study of visual evoked potentials; Tomoda, Celesia, & Toleikis 1991). A common way of displaying the results is by plotting amplitude as a function of frequency (this function is also known as the periodogram). In some cases, instead of the amplitude of each oscillation frequency, the data are expressed in terms of the square of this amplitude. This is called the "power" of a particular frequency. *Amplitude and power are equivalent in the frequency domain to standard deviation and variance in the time domain.* Indeed, the sum of the power values for all frequencies is related to the total variance in the data. For this reason, the Fourier transform can also be considered as a method for partitioning the observed variance in a time series into subcomponents with different frequencies. Further, it is possible to apply to power frequency analysis some of the standard tools used for analyzing variance (chi-square test, analysis of variance, etc.).

Finally, it is a common practice to pool together the power for an interval of frequencies within a certain range (i.e., a frequency band). For example, in an EEG study we might be interested in quantifying the total power for frequencies ranging between 8 Hz and 12 Hz (usually called the alpha band) and, in a heart rate study on sinus arrhythmia, the power for frequencies between 0.2 Hz and 0.5 Hz (i.e., the respiration frequency range).

As mentioned before, the Fourier transform is based on the observation that any time series can be decomposed in a number of sinusoidal waves that extend with equal amplitude across the entire time series. Although mathematically valid in all cases, this way of describing the data may produce results that require further interpretation. This may occur for several reasons.

First, there may be cases in which the oscillations in the time series can be best described by functions other than a sinusoid. For instance, the pressure waves that propagate through the arteries after a heartbeat are, at first approximation, triangular in shape (sawtooth; see upper portion of Figure 7). When the shape of the oscillations departs from sinusoidal, the Fourier transform will decompose each wave into subcomponents whose individual frequencies are multiples of the basic frequency at which the wave repeats. These frequencies are labeled "harmonics" and the basic frequency is called the "fundamental." As an example, the periodogram of the sawtooth arterious pressure waves is shown in the lower part of Figure 7. Note that this periodogram indicates activity not only at the basic frequency (around 1.2 Hz) but also at some of its harmonics (such as 2.4 Hz). The pattern of harmonics is related to the particular wave shape of the basic, cyclical pattern. Given that the basic wave shape in most psychophysiological measures is *not* a sinusoid, psychophysiologists are often just as interested in the patterns of harmonics as they are in the fundamental frequency.

Data may also depart from the description underlying the Fourier transform when the type of activity observed in one part of the epoch differs substantially from that in another part. An extreme case is that of "phasic" features, which appear only once in a time series. Phenomena of this type, which are frequently observed in psychophysiological data, may be difficult to study using Fourier transformed data, because the variance associated with them will be distributed in a very complex manner between the DC component and various frequencies (although this variance will still be represented, in some form, in the Fourier transform). In other words, the variance partitioning that is obtained using Fourier transforms is best suited for phenomena that repeat cyclically along the time series (i.e., "stationary" waves).

Figure 7. *Top:* Recording of the peripheral pulse from one subject during a psychological experiment obtained with near-infrared (NIR) optical methods (see Gratton 1997). Note that intensity of the NIR light drops rapidly about every 0.8 sec. These drops correspond to the times at which the arterial blood is pushed into the blood vessels by the beating of the heart. Each drop is followed by a slower increase in the light intensity, reflecting the flow of the arterial blood out of the blood vessels. The quick drop in light intensity followed by the slow increase generate a triangular shaped (sawtooth) wave that repeats about every 0.8 sec. *Bottom:* Amplitude spectrum (periodogram), corresponding to the data reported in the top portion of the figure, obtained using an FFT method (the DC component is omitted). Note that the spectrum is dominated by a 1.2-Hz frequency, which corresponds to the heartbeat frequency. However, activity is also evident at 2.4 Hz and at 3.6 Hz, which are the first and second harmonics of the fundamental 1.2-Hz frequency. The presence of activity at these frequencies indicates that the cyclical pattern is not sinusoidal.

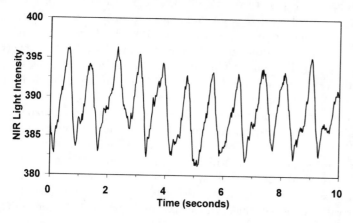

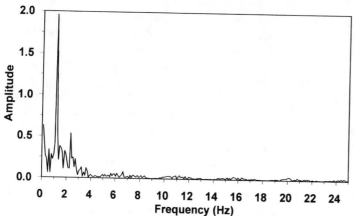

Joint Time–Frequency Domain Analysis

In recent years, combinations of time-domain and frequency-domain approaches have been introduced (see e.g. Stiber & Sato 1997). The major justification for these hybrid techniques is the assumption that the brain processes information via rapid modulation of basic frequencies of activity. A frequency that has been considered as particularly important in brain activity is approximately 40 Hz – the gamma band (see Gray et al. 1989). According to this view, information processing may involve amplitude modulation of 40-Hz activity. When a new stimulus is presented, the oscillations at this frequency increase in size. A converse phenomenon has been observed for the alpha band ("alpha blocking" or "enhancement"; see e.g. Pfurtscheller & Neuper 1992). Another case for hybrid analysis is examining the modulation of sinus arrhythmia over time as a method for studying the time course of vagal activity. Yet another case is given by analysis of the EMG response, which often involves the occurrence of a brief series of high-frequency (typically above 30 Hz) oscillations. In all these cases, the psychological events are transient (and therefore evolve over time) yet their physiological manifestations involve modulation of a cyclical phenomenon. To represent this modulation phenomenon appropriately it is necessary to study the change over time of the amplitude of specific frequencies. This involves segmenting the time series into shorter epochs, determining the amplitude of the frequency of interest in each epoch (this analysis is performed in the frequency domain), and analyzing the time course of modulation of the amplitude of the frequency of interest (this analysis is performed in the time domain). The procedure is known as joint time–frequency analysis or JTFA (e.g. Tallon-Buadry et al. 1996). In the case of EMG, the response is often analyzed entirely in the time domain and involves: (a) recording using a relatively high-frequency bandpass (such as 10–100 Hz), (b) rectification of the wave forms (i.e., transformation of the negative value into positive values), and (c) low-pass filtering (typically below 20 Hz). This process is adequate for determination of latency measures, but it does require recordings with low noise levels.

Amplitude-Domain Measures

All of the temporal-domain data processing steps outlined so far result in descriptions of the observed activity as a function of time, frequency, or a combination of both. However, in some cases, it is preferable to analyze the overall "amount" of activity observed without expressing it as a function of either time or frequency (Cacioppo & Dorfman 1987). This may be appropriate when the time (or frequency) variable is considered irrelevant or when variations of the measurement over time depend on factors that are not related to the physiological (or psychological) variable of interest. For instance, when the stimulation condition cannot be conveniently subdivided into specific time epochs or periodic events, it may be advantageous to consider the overall physiological response observed during an experiment instead of considering the individual responses. An example is the number of electrodermal responses during presentation of a particular videotape, which is not characterized by clearly identifiable time markers. Another case is that of measures that cannot be taken repeatedly, or whose time of acquisition is longer than the time during which the experimental manipulations are conducted. When using the deoxyglucose PET technique, for instance, measures of the amount of radioactive material accumulated in various brain areas are taken at the end of the

experiment (Cherry & Phelps 1996). The temporal dimension in this case is reduced to one data point, and absolute amplitude measures are taken. Finally, in some cases the investigator wants to summarize in a unique number all the variability of observations obtained across an extended epoch (Elui 1969; see also Dorfman & Cacioppo 1990).

SPATIAL DOMAIN
Spatial Dimensions

In recent years there has been a substantial growth of interest in the spatial characteristics of psychophysiological measures insofar as they may correspond to the anatomy of the human body (and particularly of the brain). A particular impulse to this enterprise has been given by the introduction of functional neuroimaging methods (fMRI, EROS, PET, and single-photon emission computerized tomography or SPECT). Because brain anatomy is not conveniently expressed using frequency-domain methods (owing to the fundamental uniqueness of the various structures), other methods of analysis are generally preferred (an exception is the use of Fourier transforms in decoding the spatial information in MRI; see Cohen 1996).

Psychophysiological measures differ in the number of dimensions used and in their relationship with underlying anatomy. Some measures refer to the activity of the brain (such as EEG, ERPs, MEG, fMRI, PET, and EROS), whereas others refer to other body structures (such as ECG and heart rate, EMG, pupillary diameter, measures of the blink response, measures of EDA, blood pressure, respiration). Although both types of measures (of brain activity and of bodily functions) can be taken at different locations, in general the latter are less directly dependent on brain anatomy than the former.[2]

All measures of brain activity produce substantially different results depending on the location at which they are taken. Some of these measures provide data that can be localized to specific brain volumes (e.g., PET and fMRI). For these measures, any recorded value will have three indices, referring to the x, y, z spatial coordinates of the observed value. Other measures (such as ERPs and MEG) provide data that refer to surface observations and thus have only x and y coordinates. For these measures, algorithms have been proposed to allow for the reconstruction of depth information, thus pinpointing brain structures that are responsible for the activity observed at the surface. However, these reconstruction algorithms require a modeling effort that, for both ERPs and MEG, yields multiple solutions that are equally valid from a statistical point of view. Therefore, only limited confidence can be placed in the results.

Maps and tridimensional reconstructions obtained with various techniques can be evaluated on the basis of two major properties: (a) localization power, or the ability to attribute a particular activity to a particular location; and

(b) resolution, the ability to distinguish activity coming from two closely located points. These two properties are different and should not be confused. Some techniques may possess great spatial localization power but limited spatial resolution. This occurs because it is often the case that the larger the activity, the greater is the space over which it can be detected (even outside of the location at which it is generated). Therefore, two closely spaced sources may end up fused into a single blur.

Analysis of Surface Data: Surface Maps and 3D Inference

As previously mentioned, some psychophysiological measures (such as ERPs and MEG) can be used to generate maps of the distribution of a particular physical parameter at the surface of the head (scalp). Usually, these maps are generated using a process of interpolation: a reduced number of surface observations (usually fewer than 50 but in some cases as many as 256) are used to derive representations of the activity over the whole head (or at least a segment of it). The interpolation procedure requires the assumption that the spatial sampling used represents the surface distribution of the underlying phenomenon in a satisfactory way.

As for the time domain, one issue is determining the minimum spatial sampling required to produce representative electrical (and magnetic) maps of brain activity. In general, information theory and common sense indicate that the spatial resolution (but not necessarily the localization) is limited to twice the distance between two adjacent measurement locations (which we can define as the "spatial Nyquist frequency"). At first glance it thus may appear that a greater spatial sampling will result in maps with superior quality. Indeed, some investigators have shown that the information content increases with the number of recording locations (Srinivasan et al. 1996), a result that makes intuitive sense. However, practical and theoretical problems may limit the advantage of increasing spatial sampling of ERP and MEG data. One limiting factor is the cost of devices required to record and analyze data from a large number of channels. Another limiting factor is that measurement errors are also likely to increase with the number of recording channels, resulting in a decreased signal-to-noise ratio.

To illustrate the problem, suppose that an experimenter is interested in running an ERP experiment to determine where a potential reaches its maximum over the scalp. Let us also suppose that, in this experiment, there exists a 0.01 probability that a large, inaccurate value (i.e., an artifact) may influence the measures at any given electrode location and that, if such an artifact occurs, the maps may identify a maximum at an erroneous location. If only a small number of electrodes are used (e.g., fewer than ten), then the probability of a false maximum is relatively small ($p < 0.10$) and some confidence can be put in the results (although the spatial resolution will be very low). However, as the number of recording locations increases, the probability that at least at one location will provide an artifactual value also increases and so likewise the probability of incorrectly localizing the maximum. If enough electrode locations were used (say, over 100), the probability of an incorrect localization would become very high ($p > 0.63$). In this case, little confidence could be placed in the results. This example underscores the need to use the appropriate number of recording locations. It also emphasizes the difference between spatial resolution and localization: procedures that enhance spatial resolution do not necessarily enhance localization, and vice versa.

As mentioned earlier, most maps are constructed using an interpolation process. There exist various algorithms for interpolations. A relatively simple procedure involves using a linear interpolation to derive the values in between the observed locations. One problem with this method is that the maximum of activity in the maps is bound to be at one of the locations at which the recordings were obtained; if two maps are constructed using different locations, they may differ from each other even though the actual physiological situation does not vary. Therefore, more sophisticated techniques are now commonly used. Some of them are based on fitting polynomial surfaces – or other types of surfaces obtained with some form of smoothing function – through the various observed data points (e.g. spline interpolation; Perrin et al. 1987). This interpolation may increase the localization of activity in surface maps, but at the cost of reduced spatial resolution. In addition, assumptions need to be made about the spatial frequencies contained in the data.

Some transformations of the surface maps may be useful for counteracting some limitations of the original observations. For instance, problems with surface maps of electrical potential over the head include: (a) the absolute value at each data point is dependent on the choice of reference; and (b) activity tends to be spread out across extended areas. This may make it difficult to appreciate differences between conditions. Addressing both of these issues is the transformation from maps of voltage difference to those of electric currents ("current source density" or CSD maps). According to Ohm's law, currents flowing between two points are directly related to the differences in potential and inversely related to the resistance between the points. If the resistance is assumed to be constant, then current maps can be easily computed from voltage maps. In the case of the head, the current can be considered to flow almost exclusively along the skin, a path of lower resistance than the skull underneath. The flow of current in two dimensions can then be described as a current density, which is computed using the two-dimensional spatial derivative of the voltage map. This provides a measure of a local gradient, one that is independent of the definition of the reference level (since a local reference system is used) and highlights local details of the maps. However, phenomena that extend across large areas become less visible, and small error variances may be amplified by this method.

Although CSD maps (and other transformed maps) of surface potentials may be useful for highlighting differences between conditions, they should not be interpreted as tridimensional reconstructions of activity inside the head. Such a reconstruction would require a model of (1) how the signal is generated inside the head and (2) how it is transferred from interior sources to the surface. Both problems require different solutions, depending on the type of measure adopted. For electrical activity (EEG and ERPs), understanding propagation of the potential to the scalp requires information about the conductive properties of various media interposed between the sources and the surface electrodes (such as gray and white matter, cerebrospinal fluid, bones, and skin). The transmission of magnetic fields is less influenced by departures from homogeneity in the media. Until recently, all source analysis algorithms were based on abstract constructions (e.g., the "three-sphere model") that modeled the head as a simple geometric shape. In the last few years, more realistic head models have been derived using MRI or computerized axial tomography (CAT) scans, and the propagation of activity to the surface has been computed using finite computation methods. Still, knowledge about the in vivo conductive properties of head tissues is imperfect and may create substantial errors in the computation.

In the last 15 years, substantial developments have been made in the modeling of the sources of electrical and magnetic activity. Three types of approaches can now be used:

1. the regional sources approach, which provides more reliable statements but has low spatial resolution (up to several centimeters);
2. linear source models, in which the influence of various cortical locations is estimated based on the assumption that activity is generated perpendicular to the cortical surface (these models possess intermediate spatial resolution, but their accuracy is difficult to evaluate); and
3. point–dipole models, which usually combine information accrued over time (thus generating a spatiotemporal dipole) – this method has greater spatial resolution and localization power, but it also has a greater level of uncertainty related to the number of sources modeled.

By and large, source modeling of electrical activity (and to some degree of magnetic activity) still requires external validation.

Analysis of Tridimensional Spatial Data

Imaging methods provide three-dimensional descriptions of how the signal is generated inside the body. If the data refer to changes in the strength of the signal as a consequence of the functioning of a particular organ, these methods are called "functional" imaging methods. Examples of such functional techniques include fMRI and PET. Functional imaging methods vary in terms of spatial resolution and localization power, as well as along other dimensions (e.g., how direct the measures are and how much temporal resolution they possess). The great localization power of some of these techniques constitutes their major advantage, but it also creates a number of methodological problems. One of these is that the anatomy of some structures (and of the brain in particular) is quite variable across subjects. Therefore, a signal that appears at one location in one subject may appear at another location in another subject. In order to generalize conclusions across subjects, it is indispensable to "align" the data obtained in different subjects. This process requires rescaling the various anatomical features of each individual to a "standard" anatomy, so that phenomena observed in different subjects can be directly compared. A commonly used procedure to so align different brain anatomies was introduced by Talairach and Tournoux (1988). According to this procedure, structural scans of brains of different individuals (which can be obtained using MRI or CAT scans) are first aligned using a set of basic anatomical features. The brain is then subdivided into areas, and each area is independently rescaled to the dimensions of a standard provided by the Talairach and Tournoux atlas. This allows researchers to compare data across different subjects in assessing the reliability of findings and even to compute "average" brain maps across subjects. Using the standard atlas, it is then possible to associate specific functional data to particular anatomical structures of the brain (such as the Brodmann cytoarchitectonic areas of the cortex). This procedure is likely to introduce small distortions, since the large subdivisions used in the Talairach and Tournoux system may not capture all of the individual differences in anatomy. However, it is a standard method that can provide useful approximations in a number of cases.

An additional problem with three-dimensional spatial data is the huge number of dependent variables used. A three-dimensional scan of the brain based on *voxels* (the small volumes used for sampling a large volume) with a 1.5–3-mm side may generate more than 100,000 data points (each of which should be considered as a dependent variable). The statistical analysis of data sets with such a large number of dependent variables is very complex. Possible solutions to this problem can be found in specialized publications (see Friston 1996).

FILTERING AND ARTIFACT PROBLEMS

One of the major issues in processing any type of data, especially psychophysiological data, is that of distinguishing the signals of interest from noise. Noise can be broadly defined as any phenomena observed in the data other than the signal(s) of interest to the investigator. In general, the ability to distinguish signals from noise can be quantified using a construct called the signal-to-noise ratio (S/N – the amplitude ratio between the signal and the noise). The larger the S/N, the easier it is to identify the signal. As a consequence, more reliance can be made on the observations. One of the major tasks of signal processing is therefore to increase the signal-to-noise ratio. This can be achieved by amplifying the signal, reducing the noise, or both. Procedures or devices that reduce the amount of noise present in the data are generally called *filters*.

Filters are based on the principle that the signal can be distinguished from noise on the basis of some characteristic feature. For instance, the signal may have a particular frequency that is different from that of the noise. Therefore, by amplifying the frequencies carrying the signal and dampening the frequencies carrying the noise, it is possible to increase greatly the S/N. This is common practice in psychophysiological recording, and it can be achieved while the data are recorded (through the use of on-line, usually analog, filters) or at any stage of data analysis (with off-line, usually digital, filters).

Filters are usually described in terms of the frequency at which they attenuate the signal. High-pass filters cut off activity with a frequency lower than a designated frequency, and low-pass filters cut off activity with a frequency higher than a designated frequency; notch filters cut off a selected frequency range and leave unaltered any activity with lower or higher frequencies. Usually, the cut-off point of a filter indicates that, at that frequency, activity is reduced by 3 dB (approximately 70%). However, other parameters are important in describing the performance of a filter. Specifically, the performance operating characteristic (POC) function describes the proportional attenuation of the signal at different frequencies. Ideally, a filter should maintain all of the activity up (for low-pass filters) or down (for the high-pass filters) to the cut-off frequency and eliminate all of the frequency above (or below) the cut-off frequency.

Most psychophysiological recordings involve on-line, analog filters. The advantage of these filters is that they can reduce high frequencies before digitization occurs, which may reduce aliasing of high frequencies. As already mentioned, aliasing occurs when digitization is performed at a rate that is less than twice that of a frequency present in the data. In such cases, activity at a high frequency will be reflected (aliased) as activity at a lower frequency. Aliasing cannot be eliminated once it occurs, so it is very important to prevent it by filtering high frequencies before digitization. Another advantage of on-line filters is that they can be used to cut off large noise oscillations, which usually occur at very low frequencies. These large oscillations may generate signals that are outside the operating range of the analog-to-digital converter, which then will "saturate" (i.e., it will provide an output corresponding to its own maximum or minimum reportable value, not to the actual value).

On-line frequency filters are, however, usually recursive: the filtering is based on activity that has already occurred and not on activity yet to occur. Hence, they introduce a phase distortion in the data. Phenomena may appear to peak at a different time from when they actually do, or their shape may be distorted.[3] On-line low-pass filters (which cut off high frequencies) tend to displace peaks to a later time than when they really occur, and on-line high-pass filters (which cut off low frequencies) tend to displace peaks to an earlier time than when they really occur. In contrast, off-line filters can be nonrecursive and therefore need not produce phase distortion. The extent to which time displacements occur depends on the frequencies that are cut off by the filters. It is therefore preferable that data be recorded on-line using a wide bandpass filter and that filtering used for signal enhancement be mostly carried out off-line using nonrecursive filters.

Various types of off-line digital filters are available. Since they need not be analog, it is relatively simple to produce filters with good performance (i.e., sharp cut-off points). Filters with such characteristics can be built using a frequency-domain transformation of the data, but the operations required are quite complex and may render data processing exceedingly slow. It is possible to construct filters that work in the time domain and approximate the performance of these filters (for reviews see Cook & Miller 1992; Farwell et al. 1993).

Wiener (1964) introduced the concept of "optimal" filter. This is a filter whose POC function is optimized to maximally increase the signal with respect to the noise. For instance, a filter may be built to maximize the between-condition variance with respect to the within-condition variance. To build such a filter it is necessary to define the signal in some manner, so that the frequency carrying the signal can be identified a priori. In addition, an optimal filter can be practically designed only in the frequency domain – and, as just mentioned, filtering in the frequency domain may considerably reduce the speed of signal processing. These problems have limited the use of optimal filters.

In certain cases, the research interest is studying activity characterized by very specific frequencies. For instance, an investigator interested in the response to stimuli presented at regular intervals may assume that the response also should be observed at regular intervals. In this case, the frequency of the signal is well known – either the frequency of stimulation or one of its harmonics. Thus, activity at all other frequencies may be discarded as noise. An inverted notch filter (called a "bandpass" filter) may be used to selectively analyze the response and may greatly enhance the signal-to-noise ratio. Procedures of this type are used to analyze steady-state evoked responses (Tomoda et al. 1991).

So far, our discussion has focused on filters used in the temporal domain to eliminate activity at undesirable frequencies. However, filters can also be built in the spatial domain to amplify selected activity with particular spatial properties; one example is the vector filter procedure proposed by Gratton, Coles, and Donchin (1989a). The vector filter procedure is analogous to a planned contrast executed in the space domain. Gratton et al. (1989b) and Fabiani et al. (1987) showed that this procedure may help identify ERP components.

A special type of noise that is present in most psychophysiological data is known as *artifact*. This term is normally used to indicate large, isolated noise activities that originate outside the system of interest. Examples of artifacts are the potentials associated with blinks and other types of eye movements during the recording of brain electrical activity, susceptibility and other artifacts due to movements during MRI and PET recordings, and missed heart beats in measures of heart rate. Artifacts may be very large – several times larger than the signal – and thus can completely obliterate the signal. Further, they may occur in a systematic fashion; that is, the frequency of artifacts may be consistently greater in one experimental condition than in another. However, artifacts are often easily recognizable because they have specific "signatures" that are readily distinguishable from regular data. For instance, blinks generate electrical potentials that exhibit characteristic spatial distribution over the scalp, and missed heartbeats in heart rate measures produce long intervals that are well outside of the normal variability.

A number of manual and automatic procedures have been developed to detect, eliminate, or compensate for the effects of artifacts. These procedures vary from one physiological measure to another and thus will not be reviewed here. It is important, however, to remember that appropriate procedures for dealing with artifacts are an essential step in the processing of any physiological signal.

Data Reduction and Quantification

QUANTIFICATION

Practically all analyses of physiological measures require a step in which a small number of numerical values are extracted from the large amount of data recorded and are then used for inferential statistics. Usually, this "quantification" itself involves two steps: (1) identifying a particular feature that is considered to represent a particular physiological event; and (2) measuring some parameter of this feature.

Feature Identification

The procedures used to identify the feature of interest are quite variable. In some cases, the feature can be identified by visual inspection of the data. This occurs when the S/N is so large (i.e., greater than 3 : 1) that the feature of interest can easily be distinguished from sources of noise or from other signals. High-S/N examples include blinks in electro-oculographic (EOG) recordings, EMG responses,

and R waves in the ECG. In other cases, the features of interest are buried under variable and sometimes large amounts of noise or under other signals. An example of this is given by various components of the ERP, especially when measured from single trials or from averages of a small number of trials. In this case, identification of the component of interest may be quite complex and require sophisticated pattern recognition algorithms, filtering procedures, or a combination of both. Thus, identifying the P300 component of the ERP on single-trial recordings may require the use of a relatively heavy low-pass filter (band-pass 0–6 Hz or less) and pattern recognition algorithms such as cross-correlation methods etc. (see e.g. Fabiani et al. 1987; Gratton et al. 1989a). A step that is often required for identifying ERP components is the definition of a particular "time window" in which the component is expected to appear. Thus, the P300 may be defined as a positive peak in the ERP appearing in the interval of 300–700 msec; a peak appearing earlier or later may be classified as a different component. Other attributes may also be considered important for classifying data, such as the particular location at which the activity is observed.

Measurement

The second step of the quantification procedure is measuring a particular parameter of the feature of interest. Again, parameters vary along different dimensions. By and large, however, three dimensions are usually considered: (i) temporal dimension, (ii) spatial dimension, and (iii) intensity or frequency of occurrence.

Temporal Dimension. In the case of temporal dimension, activity can be considered as having a particular latency, frequency, or phase. Measures include onset, peak, center-of-gravity, and fitting of particular functions to the data. The two most commonly used measures are onset and peak latency.

Onset measures may be very informative in defining the latency of a particular physiological event (and therefore the maximum latency of the psychological phenomenon it is intended to signal). Onset can be measured as the first data point in the time series exceeding a preset value (this value can be obtained from previous work or from statistical computations of the variability in the measurements; Miller, Patterson, & Ulrich 1998). However, the exact onset time of physiological measures can be difficult to determine when the measures contain even low levels of noise. In the case of noisy measures (such as ERP activity measured on a small number of trials), onset of a particular activity can be estimated by fitting regression lines to different segments of the data (Barrett, Shibasaki, & Neshige 1986) and then determining the point at which the regression line corresponding to the pre- and postonset periods meet. An alternative procedure is to consider the half-amplitude latency, which is the latency required for the signal to reach half of its maximum peak (other proportions of the maximum value can be used; see Smulders, Kenemans, & Kok 1996). This alternative approach is quite reliable (Smulders et al. 1996), but determining what proportion of the maximum value to use is arbitrary and so the measure may not correspond to any particular psychological (or even physiological) phenomenon. In addition, if the maximum value is systematically different across conditions, then any determination of the latency of half-amplitude measures may be misleading. An example is presented in Figure 8.

Peak measures are obtained (in the time or frequency domain) by selecting the time-series data point at which the measure reaches its maximum value. If several peaks are present, the peak point can be defined as the maximum value within a certain interval, or as the "*n*th" peak (the first peak, the second peak, ...). Peak measures tend to be more reliable than onset measures. However, they may be sensitive to high-frequency noise and so it is often advisable to apply a low-pass filter before estimating the peak. The main advantage of peak latency measures is that they are easy to take, even for noisy data. A disadvantage is that, unlike onset measures, they do not necessarily identify a point in time that is of theoretical importance. Whereas we may infer from the onset of a particular activity that a particular psychological process must have been carried out for the activity to occur, the peak of the physiological response may occur some time later and have no specific meaning. An extreme example is given by the time course of the hemodynamic response (measured with fMRI) following the presentation of a train of stimuli. The moment at which the fMRI response reaches its peak may provide little information about the time course of psychological events. On the other hand, onset of fMRI activity in a particular brain area can be considered as a maximum limit for the latency of activation of that area (although, of course, activity in the area may in fact begin some time before it is detected). A similar situation exists for the latency of the peak of the skin conductance response. The peak latency of both fMRI and skin conductance signals may provide little information about the timing of psychophysiological events, yet the onset and the amplitude of either response are useful in understanding the nature of those events.

In general, temporal dimensions are considered as interval measures and hence are most commonly analyzed using parametric statistical approaches. However, temporal measures usually have a limited range. Moreover, in some cases the distribution of the measurement error departs

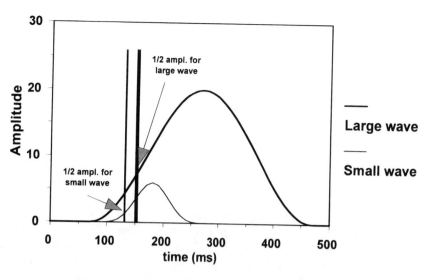

Figure 8. Half-amplitude onset measures for waves of large (thick wave) and small (thin wave) amplitude. The half-amplitude latency of the large wave (thick vertical line) was 170 msec, whereas that of the small wave (thin vertical line) was 147 msec. Using half-amplitude measures to estimate onset latency may lead to the incorrect conclusion that the large-wave onset occurred after the small-wave onset.

substantially from normality, and skewness and platykurtosis may both be present (Fabiani et al. 1987). Both of these problems may lead to reduced power for statistical analysis.

Spatial Dimension. The spatial dimension is most commonly analyzed in terms of the correspondence between the location of a physiological response and a particular anatomical structure (e.g., "the blood oxygenation level–dependent (BOLD) fMRI response was observed in proximity to the calcarine fissure"). With brain imaging techniques, analysis is often carried out in parallel for different data points (known in this field as "voxels"). Then, the voxels showing a response are identified and compared with anatomical maps. There is wide variation in methodology used to determine which voxels (or sets of voxels) show signs of functional activation (i.e., changes in blood flow or BOLD signal). In most cases, some type of statistic is derived for each voxel (or group of voxels). For methods based on hemodynamic or metabolic phenomena, this statistic often involves comparisons across conditions. In this case, the identified voxels are those that show differences between conditions exceeding some criterion, which is often expressed in terms of probability of alpha error.

The response is usually observed over several contiguous voxels. Indeed, given the high probability of false positives in brain imaging studies, responses are often considered meaningful only if they extend over a number of voxels. In this case, the exact location of the activity may be difficult to identify. One procedure is to consider the geometrical center of the region (group of voxels) showing significant effects. An alternative solution is to interpret the data as indicating a response that extends over the whole area where a significant response was observed. There are two possible problems with this latter interpretation.

First, the size of the area where a significant response is observed depends on the criterion used for considering an effect as "significant" and on the power of the measurements. Therefore, the activated area may depend on the number of trials or number of subjects used in the study. Paradoxically, if enough trials were collected (or if the S/N were sufficiently high), then larger areas of the brain could show signs of activation and the response would become *less* localized.

Second, for some measures (e.g. BOLD-fMRI), a large activity in one voxel may actually cause other voxels (both contiguous and noncontiguous) to show activity also. (This response pattern is due to the various procedures used to derive the measure.) For this reason, a strong activity localized in a small volume may produce effects that are difficult to distinguish from those of a weaker response localized to a larger area.

The statistical analysis of spatial information is sometimes undertaken by considering location as a categorical independent variable (a factor). For instance, the analysis of ERP scalp distribution is often carried out using electrode location as a factor in a factorial ANOVA (analysis of variance) design. Effects of experimental variables on scalp distribution would then be visible as interaction between these factors. Although quite popular, this approach has been criticized for two reasons.

First, the ANOVA model is an additive model – so that the contribution of electrode location as a factor to the overall variance is considered as independent from other factors. However, since ERPs always reflect the difference in voltage between locations, if a phenomenon influences the voltage of an ERP activity then it is likely also to influence different electrode locations in a different manner. Therefore an interaction between electrode location and any experimental factor may be due to a change in the overall size of a particular ERP activity, to a change in its spatial distribution (or scalp distribution), or to an interaction between these factors. Some investigators (McCarthy & Wood 1985) have proposed that, before submitting ERP data to an ANOVA, the values obtained at different electrodes should be rescaled by a factor related to the absolute size of the activity (e.g., the range of values or the standard deviation across all electrode locations). This standardization process is intended to eliminate variance across conditions or subjects due to changes

in component amplitude, so that any effects observed as a function of electrode location can be interpreted as being due to a change in the spatial distribution of the ERP activity. This approach appears to be justified when the ERP observed at the scalp (at all scalp locations) is determined by a single component. However, as shown in Figure 9, for overlapping components the standardization procedure does not eliminate the confounding between differences in scalp distribution and differences in component amplitude.

Second, the ERP values measured at different electrode locations are in fact observations of the same phenomenon from different vantage points. For this reason, both the signal and the noise can be correlated. The correlation of the noise observed at different electrode locations (or at different data points) generates a problem in the ANOVA model that is commonly known as "lack of sphericity" (see Jennings & Wood 1976). A solution to this problem is

Figure 9. Effect of standardizing ERP scalp distribution data in conditions with different component amplitude and component overlap. *Top row:* Data from a condition in which there is no component overlap (i.e., all the activity obtained at all electrode locations can be attributed to one component). On the left are plots of the observed and standardized scalp distribution data from a condition in which the component is small (standardization is obtained by dividing the data by the standard deviation across electrode locations). In the middle are similar plots for a condition in which the component has medium size. On the right are plots for a condition in which the component has large size. Note that plots of the standardized scalp distributions are identical for all component sizes. *Bottom row:* Plot from conditions with component overlap. A component with central-maximum scalp distribution and fixed amplitude was added to the observed data presented on the top row. Note that the scalp distribution appears to change from a frontal to a central maximum as a function of component amplitude. Note also that the difference in scalp distribution is not eliminated by standardization.

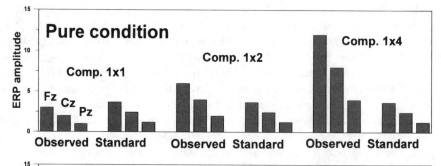

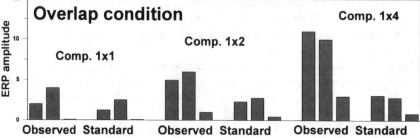

to use a multivariate approach to the analysis of scalp distribution data. Several multivariate approaches have been proposed, including multivariate ANOVA (Vasey & Thayer 1987); multiple regression (e.g. the vector filter; Gratton et al. 1989a); principal component analysis; and single-value decomposition (Lamothe & Stroink 1991).

Other investigators have considered using nonparametric statistics to evaluate location information. A recent example is the use of a "bootstrapping" procedure for studying the location of the peak of a surface distribution of ERPs or optical activity (Fabiani et al. 1998). The purpose of the bootstrap method proposed by Fabiani et al. is to estimate the reliability of maxima of maps of ERP or EROS activity obtained on average data. The bootstrap method involves analysis of a large number of samples of individual trials (bootstrap replications). Each bootstrap replication is obtained by extracting at random (and with re-immission) a number of trials from the original data set equal to the number of trials used to compute the regular average. For each new bootstrap replication, an average map is computed, and the location of maximum is determined. The distribution of the maxima across the different bootstrap replications is then obtained. The location of a maximum is reliable if it is obtained in a large proportion of the bootstrap replications. This bootstrap method does not require that we make assumptions about the distribution of maxima in the population, and it is therefore quite robust. The method can be modified to consider the probability that the maximum is within a certain area. One limitation of the method is that it is ad hoc, although other bootstrap procedures can be used for different applications (see Wasserman & Bockenholt 1989). Some investigators have proposed other "distribution-free" methods for the analysis of spatial distribution data (Karniski, Blair, & Snider 1994).

Intensity

Intensity is usually quantified using one of four approaches: (1) peak amplitude, (2) integrated activity over time (also called area measure), (3) covariance with a template (Fabiani et al. 1987), and (4) frequency of response. These measures are illustrated in Figure 10.

The first two types of measures are heavily dependent on the definition of a "baseline" level (i.e., they are taken by computing the difference between the peak – or the sum of the individual values – and the baseline), whereas the covariance measure requires some hypotheses about the shape of the response to be studied (the response shape can also be obtained with statistical methods – see the next section). Area measures are less sensitive to high-frequency

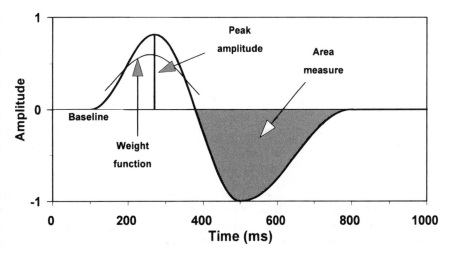

Figure 10. Different measures of the intensity of a psychophysiological response. Three measures are illustrated: peak amplitude, area measure, and weighted amplitude. Note that peak amplitude and area measures require a definition of the baseline value. Weighted amplitude measures can be made independent of the definition of the baseline.

noise than are peak measures. However, empirical studies have shown that if a low-pass filter is applied before the peak measurement, the latter can be at least as reliable as area measures (Fabiani et al. 1987). Covariance measures can be used to separate the contribution of overlapping physiological responses – in this case, a multiple regression approach can be used – and are quite reliable. Examples of covariance measures include estimates of the amplitude of different ERP components obtained with principal component analysis (PCA – Donchin & Heffley 1978) or with stepwise discriminant analysis (SWDA – Donchin 1969; Donchin & Herning 1975; Squires & Donchin 1976). In these cases, the covariance measures are taken with respect to a "weighting" function that has been optimized on the basis of statistical properties of the data (see next section). More recently, multiple regression approaches have been used to analyze hemodynamic data (fMRI, PET, etc.) in the case of complex, factorial designs. An advantage of this approach over the "subtraction" methods traditionally used to analyze such data is that it enables identification of effects associated with interaction terms on the brain image maps. However, the assumptions underlying these methods (i.e., linearity and additivity) remain as critical for these measures as they are for subtraction methods.

All these measures are considered as providing results along interval scales, which can be analyzed using parametric statistics. The error distribution tends to be skewed (since usually the range is limited on the lower end), but platykurtosis is not a problem as it was for latency measures. Amplitude measures may therefore be more reliable than latency measures (Fabiani et al. 1987).

Measures of the frequency of response are used for signals that are quite stereotyped and easily recognizable yet occur only on a certain proportion of the trials or only at irregular intervals. Note that, in many cases (e.g., eye blinks or electrodermal responses), response frequency will not follow a normal distribution; the distributions will have a heavy positive skew, with some subjects exhibiting a large number of responses and others very few or none. In this case, experimental variables will generally produce larger effects for the subjects exhibiting a greater base rate of responses than for those exhibiting a smaller base rate. For instance, all subjects may double their response frequency as a function of experimental manipulations; for those with a low base rate this may generate very little effect, whereas for those with a high base rate the effect may be huge. This results in a large subject × manipulation interaction with consequent reduced statistical power. In cases like this, a logarithmic transformation of the response frequency may help increase the statistical power of the analysis. Alternatively, inferential analysis can be conducted using a log-linear approach (Kennedy 1983). For a discussion of other approaches (standardization, rescaling, etc.), see Ben-Shakhar (1985) and Stemmler (1987).

STATISTICAL APPROACHES TO DATA REDUCTION

As mentioned previously, psychophysiological data are essentially multivariate. One of the major steps in data analysis is the reduction of the sometimes bewildering number of dependent variables to a smaller number that is appropriate for inferential analysis. Statisticians have developed a number of procedures to deal with the problem of data reduction on the basis of the statistical properties of the data. One of the simplest and most popular approaches is PCA (see Donchin & Heffley 1978). Principal component analysis is a statistical procedure for grouping dependent variables in a smaller subset of underlying (or "latent") variables that have the following properties: (a) they explain as much as possible of the variance and covariance of the original set of dependent variables; and (b) they are orthogonal to each other (in other words, they are uncorrelated). The components can be rotated (using procedures such as VARIMAX) to ease interpretability. The PCA components are interpreted in terms of their correlations (or covariances) with the original variables (also called component loadings). Donchin and his collaborators wrote a series of papers outlining the application of PCA to the analysis of ERP data. In this approach, ERP data are viewed as a data matrix in which data points are viewed as variates (i.e., dependent variables in a multivariate approach) while different subjects, conditions, and electrode locations are viewed as individual observations. A standard PCA is then run on the covariance matrix obtained from this data matrix. In most cases, a VARIMAX rotation is run on the results of the PCA. The component loadings are used to describe different components of the ERPs. These loadings

are then used as sets of weights to compute component scores for each subject, condition, and location. The component scores are used as estimates of the amplitude of each component for each of the original waveforms and are submitted to inferential analysis (e.g. ANOVA). This approach has been used in a number of studies (Karis, Fabiani, & Donchin 1984; McCallum & Curry 1984; Ruchkin, Sutton, & Stega 1980; Squires, Squires, & Hillyard 1975), mostly because it provides separate estimates of the amplitude of individual components even when they overlap in time.

This PCA/VARIMAX/ANOVA approach has been criticized (see Möcks 1986; Möcks & Verleger 1985; Wood & McCarthy 1984) on the grounds that variance is misattributed to different components. Indeed, the subdivision of variance into different components as obtained with PCA is entirely arbitrary, since there is an infinite number of ways to subdivide the variance on the basis of the same number of components. Therefore, it is unjustified to consider the components obtained with PCA in terms of physiological entities per se. Further problems with the use of PCA in the analysis of ERPs are the difficulty of incorporating latency shifts within the PCA model (Möcks 1986) and possible correlations between components. However, PCA remains an interesting attempt at a principled way for data reduction, one in which as much as possible of the original variance is retained while the number of independent variables is minimized. As already mentioned, this is one of the major goals of signal processing.

More recently, similar approaches have been proposed to address the issue of data reduction. For instance, Maier and colleagues (1987) used a "spatial" PCA (in which the dependent variables used are spatial locations rather than data points) as a preliminary step for source analysis of ERPs. Spatial PCA has also been used to determine the number of active components at a certain moment in time as a preliminary step for dipole analysis (see the BESA of Scherg & von Cramon 1986). A sequence of spatial and temporal PCAs was employed by Spencer, Dien, and Donchin (1997), whereas Möcks (1988) proposed a multivariate approach that also combines spatial and temporal information. Singular-value decomposition has also been proposed as an alternative model to PCA (see the EMSE of Greenblatt 1996). As with PCA, a problem with most of these approaches is that the result is not unique, since (an infinite number of) alternative descriptions of the data are possible. Further, it is often difficult to interpret the results of the various data reduction procedures used and to compare results obtained in different experiments.

OTHER QUANTIFICATION ISSUES
Absolute versus Relative Effects: The Problem of Baseline and Reference

In a number of cases, psychophysiological measures are intended to reflect a change in a physiological variable from a level that exists prior to the introduction of an experimental manipulation (such as the presentation of a stimulus or the administration of a drug) to a level that exists after the manipulation. The level of the physiological variable before the manipulation begins is called the *resting* or *baseline* level.

For some variables, this level is characterized by the absence of any measurable activity (for instance, there may be little EMG activity in a muscle at rest). Most often, however, the targeted physiological system is already active prior to the experiment and remains active during the experiment (this is clearly true for the heart and the brain). In this case, the baseline level may change as a function of subject, location, and time of measurement. For this reason, most physiological measures are expressed as changes with respect to a baseline level. Determination of an appropriate baseline level is not always simple, because it may not be possible to induce a pure "rest" condition. In most cases, even when the experimental condition does not require a measurable overt response, the subject may be active predicting and evaluating situations from both a cognitive and an emotional point of view. In addition, the subject may be paying attention to internal or external stimuli that are not experimentally controlled.

All of these psychological activities may influence the measurements obtained during the baseline period. If they do so in a manner that is systematically different from that observed at the time of the experimental measurement, or in different ways in different experimental conditions, then there is the possibility the systematic effects may influence the measurement. For instance, in most experiments using ERPs, measurements are taken as differences with respect to a prestimulus baseline level. However, if subjects can anticipate certain properties of the stimulus during the prestimulus period, it is possible that an anticipation component of the ERP (e.g., the contingent negative variation or CNV; Walter et al. 1964) may be elicited during this interval. The differential measures taken at a later time will then be affected by the presence of a CNV during the baseline period. Likewise, if the dependent variable is heart rate then the expectation of an external stimulus may induce heart rate deceleration (Lacey et al. 1963). Note, however, that if the research interest is in comparing conditions in which anticipation is expected to be (on average) the same then this is not necessarily a critical problem, since a similar value is subtracted from both conditions. For this and like reasons, it is generally easier to compare activity observed in different experimental conditions than to draw conclusions from activity observed in a single condition alone. In other words, it is much easier to consider relative than absolute effects.

Whereas the baseline problem is common to most physiological measures, some measures (such as ERPs) also entail the problem of the reference. The term "reference" is used to indicate a comparison value that is valid for all points in space; this contrasts with the term "baseline," which is used to indicate a comparison value that is valid for all points in time. In some cases, physiological measures are obtained by considering the difference in electric potential between two locations. Electric potentials do not possess absolute values and are defined as differences between two energy levels. Therefore, measures of electric potentials should be considered with respect to the locations that are involved. It is, however, possible to compare the difference in potential that exists between point A and point B with that between point C and point B. If the first difference is more positive than the second then we can conclude that point A has a more positive voltage level than point C. In this case, point B will be used as a common reference point. If measures were taken only at a single point in time, which point (A, B, or C) is used as a common reference would make little difference. However, voltage measures are generally taken at different times, and points of maximum difference (or peak values) are identified. The point at which A is most different from B may not be the same point at which A is most different from C. Therefore, the time of the occurrence of the peak on A may differ depending on whether B or C is used as a reference. For this reason, appropriate selection of a reference location is a critical aspect of recording electrical activity.

Historically, there have been three approaches to the problem of reference selection. The first approach is to consider measurements obtained between selected pairs of electrode locations. Such *bipolar* measurements are common practice in the study of EMG, ECG, and EOG. Bipolar derivations can be used to study local phenomena: the two electrodes are placed very close to each other, so that activity generated far away is likely to influence them equally (and therefore to cancel out) whereas activity generated locally is more likely to generate differences. This approach is adequate when the research interest is studying the time course of activity of a relatively simple electric field configuration – such as for EMG, EOG, and (to some extent) ECG. For EEG studies, the bipolar approach fails to account for the complexities of the fields generated by the brain and is therefore used only in certain clinical applications or special cases (e.g., recording auditory brainstem averaged evoked potentials, BAEPs).

A second approach, which uses a *common reference* system, is to consider measurements from a number of locations as differences with respect to the same location (or to a common value). There are a number of choices for the location of the reference value, including the ears, mastoids, nose, forehead, or locations outside the head (extracephalic reference). The latter may pick up electrical activity from the heart (ECG) and therefore require special compensation procedures (Fortgens & de Bruin 1983). Finally, some researchers have advocated the use of an average reference, which is obtained by subtracting or adding a value to all of the observed locations so that the algebraic sum of all of the potential values observed at different locations is equal to zero. Although arguments in favor of one or another of these systems have been proposed (see e.g. Skrandies & Lehmann 1982), there is evidently no clear advantage to using one reference system rather than another: the choice is arbitrary. However, since the selection of the reference may alter the shape of waveforms (including both the amplitude and latency of the peaks), it is very important that the reference selection be made explicit and that the same reference system be used when comparing across different data sets. The common reference system is the one most used in ERP research. Its greatest advantages are ease of computation and the possibility it offers of comparing values obtained at different locations. Its major drawback is the arbitrariness of the choice of the reference.

A third approach is to transform the data so that they are expressed in terms of absolute dimensions (such as current flow) rather than as relative dimensions (such as difference in potential). As we have seen (see the section entitled "Analysis of Surface Data"), this can be achieved by computing the local gradient in potential rather than the difference with a common reference (with the assumption of constant resistance between electrode locations).

Subtraction, Comparisons, and Linearity of the Measures

In most cases, psychophysiologists are interested in comparing physiological responses in two (or more) conditions. The comparison process usually involves a study of the statistical reliability of differences between measures. This, in turn, involves computing several differences across subjects, time points, and locations. Data obtained in different conditions can be interpreted either along ordinal scales (which require using less powerful nonparametric statistics) or along interval scales (which may be analyzed using parametric statistics). The basic assumption of interval scales is that differences between intervals at any level of the scale are directly comparable – for example, the difference between the values 2 and 4 in a given scale has the same significance as the difference between the values 22 and 24. This allows the investigator to subtract common terms and to compare data directly. We previously considered the similar property of linearity (see the section entitled "Direct versus Indirect Measures").

However, most psychophysiological measures depart to some extent from linearity. One of the reasons is that they often have a limited range because physiological systems feature feedback mechanisms that counteract extreme values in order to maintain the body's homeostasis. For example, heart rate is unlikely to drop below 40 beats per minute even under strong vagal activation. There are also other limitations due to the number of units (e.g. neurons) that can respond to particular stimuli. Even so, for most psychophysiological measures there exists an interval of values for which linearity can occur. For practical purposes, it is advantageous for measurements to be taken – if at all possible – in conditions where the psychophysiological measure is within the range in which it exhibits linearity.

Range and scale differences may also vary as a function of subject or of location on the body. For example, certain subjects may exhibit higher variability in a psychophysiological variable than others. Similarly, measures of a psychophysiological variable may have a greater range at one location than another. This will make it more difficult to compare data across subjects or locations. To counteract this problem, standardized measures (in which the data are transformed so as to have equal means and standard deviations) are often used in these types of comparisons.

For a number of psychophysiological variables, it has been found that variability is correlated with the average level of the variable itself for a particular subject or condition. This relationship sometimes takes the form of "ceiling" or "floor" effects, which in psychophysiology often have been considered as examples of the law of initial values (Wilder 1957). Such effects produce departures from linearity, and psychologists have often used special transformations (e.g. logit or probit) to correct such departures. Sometimes the effects are actually proportional to the original value, in which case a logarithmic transformation of the data (or the division by the average value) may equalize variances (and differences) across conditions – and thereby produce a scale that has linear properties. For a discussion of several procedures for comparing conditions with different base rates, see Wainer (1991).

Concluding Remarks

In this chapter we examined several issues related to the analysis of psychophysiological data. In most cases, data analysis procedures can be viewed as an effort to extract meaningful information from data that are often noisy. In these conditions, a major part of the data analyst's work is to increase the signal-to-noise ratio. Although there exist procedures that increase this ratio under all conditions, it is often the case that a priori hypotheses about what type of signal to expect may help in the design of appropriate analysis methodologies. These hypotheses need not be that specific (e.g., suggesting that activity at a particular latency at a particular location is determined by factor A or factor B). Even simple hypotheses – that some activity should be observed somewhere during a latency interval – help in designing appropriate analytical methods. In general, however, the power of the analytical procedure increases with the specificity of the hypotheses that are entertained.

On the other hand, it is often the case that psychophysiological phenomena are quite complex, and unpredicted effects are obtained in a number of studies. In some cases, discovery of these new effects is what affords the greatest scientific advancements. This generates a dilemma for the data analyst: How can maximum power be obtained while maintaining a wide focus in the analysis? In most cases the answer lies in alternating studies conducted with an "exploratory" attitude (enabling investigators to detect unexpected findings) with other, "hypothesis-driven" studies (which provide more rigorous tests of specific hypotheses). This approach emphasizes the need for data analysis to be integrated with experimental design in a bidirectional fashion.

NOTES

I thank Monica Fabiani, John Cacioppo, Lou Tassinary, and Gary Berntson for their comments on previous versions of this manuscript.

1. Note that this formula may not apply to all cases and is only provided as an example of the typical influence of delaying factors on the time course of physiological measures. In fact, not only the time course but also the intensity of the output with respect to the input may vary from case to case.

2. There are, however, notable exceptions to this rule, especially in the study of reflexes. For instance, Hackley and Johnson (1996) used properties of the blink response (a peripheral measure) to determine whether a particular phenomenon (prepulse inhibition) is under the control of cortical or subcortical structures (clearly an issue of function localization within the brain). This indicates that, if appropriate experimental designs are used, peripheral measures can provide some information about the localization of function within the brain.

3. This phenomenon can be minimized by using special types of filters (e.g., elliptical and/or Bessel filters).

REFERENCES

Barrett, G., Shibasaki, H., & Neshige, R. (1986). Cortical potentials preceding voluntary movement: Evidence for three periods of preparation in man. *Electroencephalography and Clinical Neurophysiology, 63*, 327–39.

Ben-Shakhar, G. (1985). Standardization within individuals: A simple method to neutralize individual differences in skin conductance. *Psychophysiology, 22*, 292–9.

Bradley, M. M., Cuthbert, B. N., & Lang, P. J. (1991). Startle and emotion: Lateral acoustic probes and the bilateral blink. *Psychophysiology, 28*, 285–95.

Cacioppo, J. T., & Dorfman, D. D. (1987). Waveform moment analysis in psychophysiological research. *Psychological Bulletin, 102*, 421–38.

Cherry, S. R., & Phelps, M. E. (1996). Imaging brain function with positron emission tomography. In A. W. Toga & J. C. Mazziotta (Eds.), *Brain Mapping: The Methods*, pp. 191–222. San Diego: Academic Press.

Cohen, M. S. (1996). Rapid MRI and functional applications. In A. W. Toga & J. C. Mazziotta (Eds.), *Brain Mapping: The Methods*, pp. 223–58. San Diego: Academic Press.

Cook, E. W., & Miller, G. A. (1992). Digital filtering: Background and tutorial for psychophysiologists. *Psychophysiology, 29*, 350–67.

Donchin, E. (1969). Discriminant analysis in average evoked response studies: The study of single trial data. *Electroencephalography and Clinical Neurophysiology, 27*, 311–14.

Donchin, E., & Heffley, E. (1978). Multivariate analysis of event-related potential data: A tutorial review. In D. Otto (Ed.), *Multidisciplinary Perspectives in Event-Related Brain Potential Research* (EPA-600/9-77-043), pp. 555–72. Washington, DC: U.S. Government Printing Office.

Donchin, E., & Herning, R. I. (1975). A simulation study of the efficacy of stepwise discriminant analysis in the detection and comparison of event related potentials. *Electroencephalography and Clinical Neurophysiology, 38*, 51–68.

Dorfman, D. D., & Cacioppo, J. T. (1990). Waveform moment analysis: Topographical analysis of nonrhythmic waveforms. In L. G. Tassinary & J. T. Cacioppo (Eds.), *Principles of Psychophysiology: Physical, Social, and Inferential Elements*, pp. 661–707. Cambridge University Press.

Elui, R. (1969). Gaussian behavior of the EEG: Changes during performance of mental tasks. *Science, 164*, 328.

Estes, W. K. (1956). The problem of inference from curves based on group data. *Psychological Bulletin, 53*, 133–40.

Fabiani, M., Gratton, G., Corballis, P., Cheng, J., & Friedman, D. (1998). Bootstrap assessment of the reliability of maxima in surface maps of brain activity of individual subjects derived with electrophysiological and optical methods. *Behavior Research Methods, Instruments, and Computers, 30*, 78–86.

Fabiani, M., Gratton, G., Karis, D., & Donchin, E. (1987). Definition, identification, and reliability of measurement of the P300 component of the event-related brain potential. In P. K. Ackles, J. R. Jennings, & M. G. H. Coles (Eds.), *Advances in Psychophysiology*, vol. 2, pp. 1–78. Greenwich, CT: JAI.

Farwell, L. A., Martinerie, J. M., Bashore, T. R., Rapp, P. E., et al. (1993). Optimal digital filters for long-latency components of the event-related brain potential. *Psychophysiology, 30*, 306–15.

Fortgens, C., & de Bruin, M. P. (1983). Removal of eye movement and ECG artifacts from the non-cephalic reference EEG. *Electroencephalography and Clinical Neurophysiology, 56*, 90–6.

Fox, P. T., & Raichle, M. E. (1984). Stimulus rate dependence of regional cerebral blood flow in human striate cortex, demonstrated by positron emission tomography. *Journal of Neurophysiology, 51*, 1109–20.

Friston, K. J. (1996). Statistical parametric mapping and other analyses of functional imaging data. In A. W. Toga & J. C. Mazziotta (Eds.), *Brain Mapping: The Methods*, pp. 363–88. San Diego: Academic Press.

Gratton, G. (1997). Attention and probability effects in the human occipital cortex: An optical imaging study. *NeuroReport, 8*, 1749–53.

Gratton, G., Coles, M. G., & Donchin, E. (1989a). A procedure for using multi-electrode information in the analysis of components of the event-related potential: Vector filter. *Psychophysiology, 26*, 222–32.

Gratton, G., Kramer, A. F., Coles, M. G., & Donchin, E. (1989b). Simulation studies of latency measures of components of the event-related brain potential. *Psychophysiology, 26*, 233–48.

Gray, C. M., Konig, P., Engel, A. K., & Singer, W. (1989). Oscillatory responses in cat visual cortex exhibit inter-columnar synchronization which reflects global stimulus properties. *Nature, 338*, 334–7.

Greenblatt, R. (1996). *Electromagnetic Source Estimation.* San Diego: Source/Signal Imaging.

Hackley, S. A., & Johnson, L. N. (1996). Distinct early and late subcomponents of the photic blink reflex: Response characteristics in patients with retrogeniculate lesions. *Psychophysiology, 33,* 239–51.

Huberty, C. J., & Morris, J. D. (1989). Multivariate analysis versus multiple univariate analyses. *Psychological Bulletin, 105,* 302–8.

Jennings, J. R., van der Molen, M. W., Somsen, R. J., & Ridderinkhof, K. R. (1991). Graphical and statistical techniques for cardiac cycle time (phase) dependent changes in interbeat interval. *Psychophysiology, 28,* 596–606.

Jennings, J. R., & Wood, C. C. (1976). Letter: The epsilon-adjustment procedure for repeated-measures analyses of variance. *Psychophysiology, 13,* 277–8.

Karis, D., Fabiani, M., & Donchin, E. (1984). P300 and memory: Individual differences in the von Restorff effect. *Cognitive Psychology, 16,* 177–216.

Karniski, W., Blair, R. C., & Snider, A. D. (1994). An exact statistical method for comparing topographic maps, with any number of subjects and electrodes. *Brain Topography, 6,* 203–10.

Kennedy, J. J. (1983). *Analyzing Qualitative Data: Introductory Log-Linear Analysis for Behavioral Research.* New York: Praeger.

Lacey, J. I., Kagan, J., Lacey, B. C., & Moss, H. A. (1963). The visceral level: Situational determinants and behavioral correlates of autonomic response patterns. In P. H. Knapp (Ed.), *Expression of the Emotions in Man.* New York: International Universities Press.

Lamothe, R., & Stroink, G. (1991). Orthogonal expansions: Their applicability to signal extraction in electrophysiological mapping data. *Medical and Biological Engineering and Computing, 29,* 522–8.

Maier, J., Dagnelie, G., Spekreijse, H., & van Dijk, B. W. (1987). Principal components analysis for source localization of VEPs in man. *Vision Research, 27,* 165–77.

McCallum, W. C., & Curry, S. H. (1984). A comparison of early event-related potentials in two target detection tasks. Sixth International Conference on Event-Related Slow Potentials of the Brain (EPIC VI): Cognition, information processing, and language (1981, Lake Forest/Chicago). *Annals of the New York Academy of Sciences, 425,* 242–9.

McCarthy, G., & Wood, C. C. (1985). Scalp distributions of event-related potentials: An ambiguity associated with analysis of variance models. *Electroencephalography and Clinical Neurophysiology, 62,* 203–8.

Miller, J., Patterson, T., & Ulrich, R. (1998). Jackknife-based method for measuring LRP onset latency differences. *Psychophysiology, 35,* 99–115.

Möcks, J. (1986). The influence of latency jitter in principal component analysis of event-related potentials. *Psychophysiology, 23,* 480–4.

Möcks, J. (1988). Decomposing event-related potentials: A new topographic components model. *Biological Psychology, 26,* 199–215.

Möcks, J., Kohler, W., Gasser, T., & Pham, D. T. (1988). Novel approaches to the problem of latency jitter. *Psychophysiology, 25,* 217–26.

Möcks, J., & Verleger, R. (1985). Nuisance sources of variance in principal components analysis of event-related potentials. *Psychophysiology, 22,* 674–88.

Monk, T. H. (1987). Parameters of the circadian temperature rhythm using sparse and irregular sampling. *Psychophysiology, 24,* 236–42.

Monk, T. H., & Fookson, J. E. (1986). Circadian temperature rhythm power spectra: Is equal sampling necessary? *Psychophysiology, 23,* 472–9.

Perrin, F., Pernier, J., Bertrand, O., Giard, M. H., & Echallier, J. F. (1987). Mapping of scalp potentials by surface spline interpolation. *Electroencephalography and Clinical Neurophysiology, 66,* 75–81.

Pfurtscheller, G., & Neuper, C. (1992). Simultaneous EEG 10 Hz desynchronization and 40 Hz synchronization during finger movements. *NeuroReport, 3,* 1057–60.

Quigley, K. S., & Berntson, G. G. (1996). Autonomic interactions and chronotropic control of the heart: Heart period versus heart rate. *Psychophysiology, 33,* 605–11.

Ruchkin, D. S., Sutton, S., & Stega, M. (1980). Emitted P300 and slow wave event-related potentials in guessing and detection tasks. *Electroencephalography and Clinical Neurophysiology, 49,* 1–14.

Scherg, M., & von Cramon, D. (1986). Evoked dipole source potentials of the human auditory cortex. *Electroencephalography and Clinical Neurophysiology, 65,* 344–60.

Siegler, R. S. (1987). The perils of averaging data over strategies: An example from children's addition. *Journal of Experimental Psychology: General, 116,* 250–64.

Skrandies, W., & Lehmann, D. (1982). Spatial principal components of multichannel maps evoked by lateral visual half-field stimuli. *Electroencephalography and Clinical Neurophysiology, 54,* 662–7.

Smulders, F. T., Kenemans, J. L., & Kok, A. (1996). Effects of task variables on measures of the mean onset latency of LRP depend on the scoring method. *Psychophysiology, 33,* 194–205.

Spencer, K., Dien, J. & Donchin, E. (1997). Temporal-spatial analysis of the late positive components of the ERP. *Psychophysiology, 34,* S6.

Squires, K. C., & Donchin, E. (1976). Beyond averaging: The use of discriminant functions to recognize event related potentials elicited by single auditory stimuli. *Electroencephalography and Clinical Neurophysiology, 41,* 449–59.

Squires, N. K., Squires, K. C., & Hillyard, S. A. (1975). Two varieties of long-latency positive waves evoked by unpredictable auditory stimuli in man. *Electroencephalography and Clinical Neurophysiology, 38,* 387–401.

Srinivasan, R., Nunez, P. L., Tucker, D. M., Silberstein, R. B., & Cadusch, P. J. (1996). Spatial sampling and filtering of EEG with spline Laplacians to estimate cortical potentials. *Brain Topography, 8,* 355–66.

Stemmler, G. (1987). Standardization within subjects: A critique of Ben-Shakhar's conclusions. *Psychophysiology, 24,* 243–6.

Stiber, B. Z., & Sato, S. (1997). Visualization of EEG using time-frequency distributions. *Methods of Information in Medicine, 36,* 298–301.

Talairach, J., & Tournoux, P. (1988). *Co-planar Stereotactic Atlas of the Human Brain: 3-Dimensional Proportional System: An Approach to Cerebral Imaging.* Stuttgart: Thieme.

Tallon-Buadry, C., Bertrand, O., Delpuech, C., & Pernier, J. (1996). Stimulus specificity of phase-locked and non-phase-locked 40 Hz visual responses in human. *Journal of Neuroscience, 16,* 4240–9.

Tomoda, H., Celesia, G. G., & Toleikis, S. C. (1991). Effect of spatial frequency on simultaneous recorded steady-state pattern electroretinograms and visual evoked potentials. *Electroencephalography and Clinical Neurophysiology: Evoked Potentials, 80,* 81–8.

Vasey, M. W., & Thayer, J. F. (1987). The continuing problem of false positives in repeated measures ANOVA in psychophysiology: A multivariate solution. *Psychophysiology, 24,* 479–86.

Wainer, H. (1991). Adjusting for differential base rates: Lord's paradox again. *Psychological Bulletin, 109,* 147–51.

Walter, W. G., Cooper, R., Aldridge, V. J., McCallum, W. C., & Winter, A. L. (1964). Contingent negative variation: An electrical sign of sensorimotor association and expectancy in the human brain. *Nature, 203,* 380–4.

Wasserman, S., & Bockenholt, U. (1989). Bootstrapping: Applications to psychophysiology. *Psychophysiology, 26,* 208–21.

Wickens, C., Kramer, A., Vanasse, L., & Donchin, E. (1983). Performance of concurrent tasks: A psychophysiological analysis of the reciprocity of information-processing resources. *Science, 221,* 1080–2.

Wiener, N. (1964). *Extrapolation, Interpolation, and Smoothing of Stationary Time Series.* Cambridge, MA: MIT Press.

Wilder, J. (1957). *Stimulus and Response. The Law of Initial Value.* Bristol, U.K.: Wright.

Wood, C. C., & McCarthy, G. (1984). Principal component analysis of event-related potentials: Simulation studies demonstrate misallocation of variance across components. *Electroencephalography and Clinical Neurophysiology, 59,* 249–60.

Woody, C. D. (1967). Characterization of an adaptive filter for the analysis of variable latency neuroelectrical signal. *Medical and Biological Engineering, 5,* 539–53.

Yantis, S., Meyer, D. E., & Smith, J. K. (1991). Analyses of multinomial mixture distributions: New tests for stochastic models of cognition and action. *Psychological Bulletin, 110,* 350–74.

CHAPTER THIRTY-FOUR

DYNAMIC MODELING

ROBERT A. M. GREGSON & JEFFREY L. PRESSING

Introduction

A system is said to be *dynamic* when it evolves through time. If we wish adequately to characterize such a system, and hopefully to predict its future course, it is necessary to study the path of its evolution; in mathematics, this is called its *trajectory*. If the trajectory can be traced in data or expressed succinctly in an equation, then the nature of the dynamics involved is at least partially identified. It follows that dynamical processes are never instantaneous; they occupy real time, and the point at which they terminate – either naturally by attaining some stability or because they are cut short – determines their outcome. The parallels with stimulus–response pairings and their associated response latencies at the psychological level, as well as with the intervening physiological events and internal evolution and feedback, have been long recognized (Gregson 1983).

The last several years have seen a massive expansion in the scope of research into dynamical systems that are not readily treated by traditional sorts of data analysis. In particular, the body of statistical methods that derive from the general linear model – such as analysis of variance, multiple regression, linear time series, and frequency partitioning into energy spectra with an underlying assumption of stability – have been augmented by modeling of systems that change their dynamics over time and can fluctuate aperiodically between states. Models of processes that can float between local stability and periodic or quasiperiodic fluctuations, becoming transiently or permanently chaotic, have been explored both for their intrinsic fascination as mathematics and as analogs of human biological processes in brain and behavior (Basar et al. 1983). The use of these approaches as a replacement for more traditional analyses of data in the frequency domain (e.g., Fourier transforms) is motivated by a belief that the dynamics of the brain are appropriately represented not by a linear model with stochastic noise superimposed but rather by dynamics that have no residual or superimposed random components. By their own evolution in time, these dynamics can create what appears to be noise, even though they are intrinsically deterministic. There are necessarily complications to this view, because systems can be chaotic at one level of organization yet much more simply represented at another, and brain circuitry involves both micro- and mesoscopic dynamics (which mathematical modelers have attempted to link).

It is certainly the case that this area of endeavor is still growing, and for a while the number of publications grew almost exponentially. Difficult intrinsic problems of measurement and system identifiability are slowly being overcome. By its very nature, dynamic analysis is not a methodology that should be approached by looking for standard computer packages and all-purpose theoretical models. The first requirement is a sufficient body of sound data to support the creation of some formal mathematics. Nonlinear equations are intrinsically different from linear equations; they do not satisfy the principle of superposition, which means that effects are not simply additive (as they might be in, say, an analysis of variance model). Nonlinear equations have singularities that may reveal themselves in sharp threshold phenomena, and analytical solutions are rare or nonexistent. When asymptotic solutions do exist, they are often independent of initial conditions. A valuable introductory but rigorous treatment of the area is given by Ingraham (1992).

There are historical reasons why the use of these models did not occur sooner. Partly this is due to the recentness of computing resources adequate for performing calculations of great intrinsic complexity, which were previously impossible to execute in a lifetime. There are many worked examples in the literature of nonlinear dynamics, which appear repeatedly because of their fascination for the

John T. Cacioppo, Louis G. Tassinary, and Gary G. Berntson (Eds.), *Handbook of Psychophysiology,* 2nd ed. © Cambridge University Press 2000. Printed in the United States of America. ISBN 62634X. All rights reserved.

mathematician, but few have been shown to be directly applicable to describing either brain processes or behavioral sequences about which we already know a great deal at the intuitive level. One reason for this can be defined as follows.

There are two approaches to system identification; the distinction is fundamental and should be kept in mind for each section of this chapter. Briefly:

A. starting from the assumed algebra, derive some global properties, and see if they match data; or
B. starting from data, try to work backward to identify the underlying model, which is then taken to be a causal description of the state of affairs.

The latter approach is said to be the *inverse* of the former. Approach **B** is the most important for the psychophysiologist, and it is the more difficult one because we cannot *almost* cheat by assuming the answer in advance. Popular pictorial treatments of chaos – with attractors looking like bundles of wire or with brightly colored fractal boundaries – are examples of approach **A**; they can be an aid to the imagination but are not particularly useful when all we have are long records of brain potentials. In this chapter we will look at examples of both **A** and **B** modeling. It is worth commenting that **A** and **B** can alternate in a series of experiments, and there is also a (rarely used) approach that involves iterative modification of a model **A** converging on-line with data **B** within a single long experiment.

There is perhaps too much enthusiasm about what can be described and predicted, and the apparent insights gained by suspecting that chaos lurks at every turn do require some caution in their acceptance. That much of the new interest in dynamics arose in those sciences where metrics exist to support measurement of rates of change (and of their derivatives) – a situation not universally obtaining in the psychological sciences – should alert us to be cautious about claims of testability. More recently, the emphasis has moved to considering complexity rather than chaos as the core phenomenon (Nicolis & Prigogine 1989).

It is also important to distinguish between nonlinear dynamics and chaotic attractor dynamics. Undoubtedly, many biological processes are intrinsically nonlinear and can "float about" in their structure, exhibiting variable complexity in time, partly as a result of the load that the environment imposes on them in their battle to survive and reproduce. Brain processes can sometimes be described plausibly as exhibiting low-dimensional dynamics, but to show that such activity is chaotic in the strictly mathematical sense is another question. Chaos is an often discussed condition referring to deterministic systems that exhibit apparently random behavior, but there is no universally accepted definition. Mathematically, it can be linked to positive Kolmogorov entropy. In practical terms, many authors would agree that a chaotic data set is nonperiodic, shows sensitive dependence on initial conditions, and has one Lyapunov exponent greater than zero (see details that

follow). However, the status of the Lyapunov exponents in the presence of stochastic noise is uncertain. Demonstrations of chaos based on idealized models, which in their computer realizations are allowed to run for tens of thousands of iterations, are implausible as prototypes for brain activity precisely because the latter does not run in dynamical stability for long periods; it jumps about as in, for example, the switching observed between levels of sleep during dreaming. Chaos is something that a nonlinear system can go into some of the time, but it does not have to be chaotic at all points in time of its observed evolution.

By their nature, psychophysiological data reveal couplings between two or more system levels – for example, (i) microphysiological sequences of physical and chemical events, often changing rapidly over a fine time scale of milli- or microseconds and in distances measured in nanometers, and (ii) behavioral correlates measured much more coarsely in both space and time. Some psychological variables, such as verbal or sensory images, are in time but can hardly be said to be in space in the sense that a neurological response is located. The scientist is naturally concerned with predictability and controllability as fundamental properties of an organism's behavior. Without one (and arguably without both) of these, there is always a feeling that we have not deeply understood behavior. Controllability is, however, an idea originating in engineering applications; it is quite possible to have control without prediction of (say) what a system would do in the long run if the continuous or intermittent intervention via feedback from the controlled subsystem were removed.

We should hope that a choice is available to us of using models either as acausal descriptions or as reflections of what we believe are underlying causalities. In either case, the evidence is in trajectories inferred from the processing of time-series data (or from the predicted time series that models create), and statistically it is some extension of time-series analysis that is used (Tong 1995). When using nonlinear dynamics as a modeling tool, one is employing evolutions that are often no more than locally predictable, matching mathematics to data in a way that is close but can never be shown to be structurally identical. Local predictability is a system variable, not a constant, both in the mathematics and in typical data properties, so exploration to test for predictability in both is necessary. Preceding the possibilities revealed by the use of massively parallel computation, there were repeated suggestions that sensory psychophysiology was so nonlinear that either piecewise linearization was forced upon the investigator – both to describe and to predict conditions for controllability – or that, at best, a descriptive account of all the irregularities that had been observed was a summary of what a system did. Perhaps the fascinating work on tactile sensation and its quirks and surprises, reported by von Békésy (1967) and by Geldard (1975), is one of the most familiar areas we can cite in this regard.

Dynamics strictly refers to mathematical structures, and definitions and proofs of those structures are mathematics, not biology. It is the correspondences between the mathematics (as generators of time series of variables) and the biological strings of data in space and time that make dynamics potentially useful. Properties of dynamical systems that have some a priori plausibility as models of psychophysiological processes can be expected to exhibit some or all of the following characteristics (Gregson 1988).

1. The system is not in static equilibrium; it does not absorb onto a single end state, observed with error contamination, starting from any single input or starting state.
2. The system is locally entropy reducing. However, it is regarded as existing within an organism that eventually dies, and death is a maximization of local entropy.
3. The system as a whole is dissipative; its equations are not reversible in time.
4. The system is quasi-closed; it can be (approximately) treated as closed only locally and with respect to a restricted set of variables.
5. Small changes in input do not necessarily lead to small changes in output.
6. The system is strongly dependent upon its initial conditions.

When we suspect from observations that we are faced with a process involving a physiological substrate to the psychological data in hand, and if qualitatively the situation suggests that some of the properties 1–6 characterize that process, then there is heuristic justification for considering dynamical models. It is fair to warn the investigator that simply taking existing mathematical models from physics "off the shelf" (or via the software package) is a recipe for disaster no matter how popular or well-explored some cases have become. For example, there is a gap between the beautiful, multicolor depictions of Julia sets (and the computer art developed from them) and the actual useful consequences in the experimental sciences of knowing that basins of attraction have fractal edges.

The expansion of results on the capacities of artificial neural networks to learn and to control classes of irregular and partially defined inputs – even when it is not clear exactly what is happening within such networks – has created temptations to see analogies both in neural subsystems and in behaviors that rely on localized brain functions, be they sensory, symbolic or motor. Such inferences require careful empirical support.

Applications within Psychophysiology

There are two main directions from which one can approach the use of dynamics within psychophysiology: as data analysis or as theory construction (which in a restricted sense is modeling).

Historically, data analysis has come first in studies of brain and heart activity, where long data records arise naturally and measures can be collected at millisecond intervals and quantified in physical units. Examples of this way of identifying possible chaotic dyamics in the central nervous system are now diverse (Aertsen & Braitenberg 1992; Babloyantz & Destexhe 1986; Basar et al. 1983; Blinowska & Malinowski 1991; Dunki 1991; Fell, Roschke, & Beckman 1993; Freeman & Skarda 1985; Gallez & Babloyantz 1991; Ganz et al. 1993; Gregson, Campbell, & Gates 1992; Lutzenberger et al. 1992; Mayer-Kress & Layne 1987; Rapp et al. 1993; Stam et al. 1994; Watt & Hameroff 1987; Xu & Xu 1988).

For a psychophysiologically based organism, the environment (which includes other organisms) is one subsystem of the total dynamics that exhibits stimulus–response predictability. Some psychologists in the operant tradition have distinguished between stimulus-bound and response-bound behaviors, and the parallel between this distinction and the difference between open-loop and closed-loop control is not far to seek. In analyzing systems that are controlled, a "slaving" relation within the dynamics arises (Haken 1987) between the driving and the driven, and this extends to multilevel hierarchies of control (Pressing 1999).

In modeling, one is faced with a choice between various algebraic structures. The simplest models are linear and stationary in their parameters. If they fail to fit data, then the linear structure, the degree of parameterization, or the stationarity of the parameters must be abandoned. To accommodate real data that are characteristically unstable over time (outside the highly constrained circumstances of a planned experiment) and simultaneously preserve some economy of theoretical structure, one may move to a nonlinear process whose structure implies jumps in its phase space – so that the model of the process is nonlinear and nonstationary, but still it is stationary in its parameters. This can generally be done with far fewer parameters than would be necessary if progressive complication of a linear model is used as the approach; the metatheoretical problem with nonlinear techniques is simpler in terms of giving each parameter a post hoc psychophysiological interpretation.

One might say that, by the late nineteenth century, there were two forms of description available to a psychophysiologist such as Wundt – deterministic and stochastic – and these dominated all theory construction up until the 1980s. However, most earlier models either were forced to be linear (to make them mathematically tractable) or were essentially linear with superimposed additive Gaussian noise. Nonlinear dynamics added a third type of model, yielding processes that externally could resemble the stochastic yet were intrinsically deterministic – from the traditional perspective, an apparent contradiction. The stochastic models yield predictability in the long run (assuming stationarity), but only in the moments of the distribution of outcomes. They are not predictable in detail, since there is always some uncertainty about the next event in a series. In contrast, the nonlinear deterministic models are highly (locally) predictable in detail under two conditions: (i) if their starting point is known precisely (although this predictability decays exponentially with increasing time); or (ii) in the restricted circumstances of dynamics that are converging onto an attractor. Given noisy data, there is thus always a trade-off among types of explanation with respect to stationarity, linearity, predictability, and complexity (see Kowalik & Elbert 1994).

Marmarelis and Marmarelis (1978) demonstrated that physiological time series, though stationary in their parameters, are not linear and thus require a representation in Volterra or Wiener kernels. This means that even though repeated presentation of the same stimulus does not elicit the same response, the change in response is itself lawful and can be modeled. They remarked:

How do changes in the characteristics of a particular component affect the system function *F*? Paradoxically, a complete solution to this problem may be nearly impossible if the system is linear, while plausible solutions are often obtainable if the system is nonlinear. We explain this apparently perverse viewpoint by noting that in a nonlinear system it is sometimes possible to determine the sequence of underlying events because nonlinear operators do not in general commute, while such a determination is impossible if the system is linear, since linear operators commute. (Marmarelis & Marmarelis 1978, p. 158)

At the same time, nonlinear systems cannot be solved mathematically by linear techniques. Different approaches in analysis are necessary, sometimes drawing on qualitative approaches because analytical solutions do not exist. The choice that seems to arise most often – and to present the greatest difficulties for researchers – is deciding from a given time series of data whether the process is (a) low-dimensional and possibly chaotic or (b) random in the sense of being stochastic and of high dimensionality. Mathematical tests for dimensionality can be unreliable when the apparent dimension is greater than 10, and the finding of an integer dimension does not preclude the dynamics from being fractal in nature (Mayer-Kress 1986). Also, a nonlinear process contaminated by noise can still retain its locally predictable dynamics at low noise levels, albeit with inflated dimensionality.

THE ROLE OF CHAOS IN BRAIN AND BEHAVIOR

What is the significance of chaos for psychophysiology? This is a contentious issue (Doyon 1992). Its role may be quite minor. Glass (1995) argued that convincing evidence of its presence in biological systems is meager. Others have given it a fundamental role to play in cardiac dynamics, although this is disputed. Freeman (see Skarda &

Freeman 1987) presented evidence in favor of the role of chaos in olfactory perception, particularly in the encoding of sensory quality. Gregson (1988, 1992, 1995) suggested that chaotic dynamics can be transitorially involved in a diversity of sensory and perceptual processes that mediate experienced intensity. (See also the section entitled "Nonlinear Psychophysical Dynamics.")

Dynamics Identified without Metric Measures

It is useful to consider as most elementary a case in which there is no precise measurement of the psychological dependent variables and the underlying physiology is complex and not well understood. What we can do depends always on the precision of measurement of response variables and on the rate (in real time) at which observations can be logged. A method that makes minimal assumptions about the metric properties of our response scales (beyond a weak ordering of levels of activation) and that is not critically dependent on having a continuous and differentiable time scale is – from a heuristic perspective – the simplest and most robust tool to use. In terms of our first distinction, this is nearer to the **B** approach. It is still possible to identify some of the dynamical features that persist over a long time span.

Let us suppose that the responses may be categorized as being at any time in one and only one of a set of n mutually exclusive states, $S_1, S_2, \ldots, S_g, \ldots, S_h, \ldots, S_n$, and that the evolution is then a series of transitions between them at times j and $j + k$. If the system is in fact stationary then it converges to a stable set of state probabilities. The data records can be recast in a transition matrix form, where the entries are frequencies of observed jumps between states. The system variables are then the $n \times n$ matrix of transition probabilities $p(S_g \rightarrow S_h)$ and lags k, $1 < k < K$. The maximum lag studied, K, is at the discretion of the investigator. From an incomplete record with a few missing observations, maximum likelihood methods of "filling in" to achieve unbroken runs can be used before modeling is attempted. However, separate sequences cannot be concatenated end-to-end unless strict conditions are met (Gregson 1983). If we define

$$p(S_{g,h,k}) = p(S_g \rightarrow S_h) \quad \text{after } k \text{ steps,}$$

then the transition matrix is

$$\mathbf{T}_{n,k} = \begin{pmatrix} p(S_{1,1,k}) & p(S_{1,2,k}) & \cdots & p(S_{1,n,k}) \\ p(S_{2,1,k}) & p(S_{2,2,k}) & \cdots & p(S_{2,n,k}) \\ \vdots & \vdots & \ddots & \vdots \\ p(S_{n,1,k}) & p(S_{n,2,k}) & \cdots & p(S_{n,n,k}) \end{pmatrix}, \quad (1)$$

where each cell is the transition probability (from a first state at j to a second state k steps later).

If $T_{n,k}$ is fixed in its values in all cells over time, then the process is dynamically stationary, and if $T_{n,k}$ is defined only for $k = 1$ then it is a Markov process. If one of the leading diagonal cells $p(S_{x,x,k})$ is equal to unity, then this x is an absorbing state. If the matrix as a whole is ergodic – which means that, over a finite number of steps, transitions between all states are possible until an absorbing state is entered (if one exists) – then in the limit the process will tend to a steady-state vector whose coordinates are those of an attractor. At time t_0, the initial state probability vector on the system (which is a set of original probabilities $p(S_{x;0})$ at one time point, so two state subscripts are not needed on each S), may be written as

$$S_0 = \{p(S_{1;0}), p(S_{2;0}), \ldots, p(S_{n;0})\}. \qquad (2)$$

This vector affects only the time taken for the process to run to its eventual steady state; it does not affect the terminal values of the system.

The Markov chain is thus a normative model of the system dynamics, and departures from its predictions are themselves informative. If the theoretical final state vector is S_∞, then

$$S_\infty = \{p(S_{1;\infty}), p(S_{2;\infty}), \ldots, p(S_{n;\infty})\} \qquad (3)$$

is reached by repeated postmultiplication by $T_{n,1}$ of the initial vector. In practice this is not necessary to repeat for long; if the system is stationary in its dynamics then it usually converges rapidly to a close approximation of the terminal vector, even if there is no absorbing state in the system.

An example of the use of this approach in studying long series of headaches reported by chronic sufferers is given by Gregson (1987). The raw data were records where each headache was self-rated on experienced intensity (v) from 1 to 5, and its duration (t) in hours from 1 to 24 recorded. The product vt is the severity, and this had a trimodal distribution in most subjects, so that days were marked either by no headache (state N), slight headache (H_1) or severe headache (H_2); these become the three states of the process. If the dynamics of headache generation were stochastic but stationary, then a three-state Markovian process with fixed lag k should be a representation of it. Suppose the lag is $k = 1$, so that the relation

$$T_{n,k} = T_{n,1}^k \qquad (4)$$

holds and predictability decays exponentially with forward time. In fact, headaches do have some periodicities, and their future occurrence is weakly predictable if a long enough data base exists. There are two ways to explore this. The first, for data from a single subject (data may not meaningfully be pooled over subjects), compares the series of empirical $\hat{T}_{n,k}$ ($k = 1, \ldots, N$, $N \gg K$) with the predictions of (4) and then explores the pattern of the leading

TABLE 1. Markovian Representation of Headache Time Series

State (j)	Lag 1			Lag 2		
	H_2	H_1	N	H_2	H_1	N
H_2	0.344	0.125	0.531	**0.194**	0.129	0.677
H_1	0.050	0.500	0.450	0.0	**0.450**	0.550
N	0.097	0.024	0.897	0.126	0.029	**0.845**

Notes: The table shows transition probability matrices for two lags (1-day and 2-day) based on a record of 260 successive days. The states are H_2 = severe headache, H_1 = slight headache, N = no headache. Possible recurrent headache periodicities for this subject were identified: H_2 at 8 and 28 days; H_1 at 8, 16, and 20–24 days.

diagonal terms $p(S_{x,x,k})$ in $\hat{T}_{n,k}$ ($k = 1, \ldots, N$) with the terms in the transition matrix associated with the first severe headache noted. When the transition matrix varies over k but takes the same value for two lags k^* apart, then there is a periodicity of k^*. This is associated with one state, and it may be found that, for example, weak and severe headaches may have different periodicities in the same sufferer. Ljung and Box (1987) provided a statistical test of the fit of a time series to a model.

An example from the data for a single female subject (from Gregson 1987) is shown in Table 1. The transition probabilities in boldface for lag 2 are the values showing persistence beyond that predicted by a three-state, one-lag (j to $j + 1$) chain. Instead of lengths of runs of headaches having a probability distribution that drops off exponentially (as they will in a strictly Markovian process), headaches that occur on one day may then stay for at least some minimum period. We need to know this in order to assess the effects of medication.

A second approach is to use the fact that the series of $p(S_{x,x,k})$ values for increasing $k = 1, 2, \ldots$ is itself a time series, so that it may be cross-correlated with another time series of some biological indicators (e.g. hormonal levels) if the data are sufficiently robust. It is rarely legitimate to pool data across subjects before performing time-series analyses based on Markov chains. One may, however, report the distribution of observed periodicities across subjects as a post hoc description.

When a physically defined measure on responses is available (and the stimuli are physically measured), as in the case of motor skills, then methods involving differential equations can be more traditionally employed.

Attractor Dynamics and Their Indices

In this section we introduce more formally the various descriptive indices used to characterise dynamics; they are equally applicable for describing data (the physicist's phenomenological approach) and for representing complex causality in the abstract.

In order to talk meaningfully about dynamical systems and about the foundations of measures used to identify their stability and predictability, a review of terminology and concepts is needed. In the specific case of electroencephalography (EEG), which is the time series perhaps most often used in psychophysiology, Pritchard and Duke (1995) have provided a tutorial review. The massive work by Nunez (1995) extended the mathematical treatment of the generation of EEG beyond the data analysis approach summarized here.

DIMENSIONALITY

One measure of the degree of complexity of a system's dynamics can be expressed by its dimensionality. There are alternative measures and definitions of this property; the one most often considered in physiological work is the Renyi $D2$. Importantly, we should distinguish between the *degrees of freedom* in a model, which is commonly taken to be the number of independent parameters to be estimated by some statistical criterion, and its *dimensionality*, which is a property of the minimal space in which its attractors can be embedded and is usually fractal (i.e., not an integer) for a well-defined nonlinear process. It is not possible to obtain exact determinations of $D2$ from real biological data, even if the process is stable enough to be characterized by fixed $D2$, but approximate values with relatively small bias are computable and serve to detect systematic shifts in $D2$ from one experimental condition to another. It is the differences in $D2$ induced by stimuli and tasks that are of prime interest to many researchers in psychology and physiology (Lutzenberger et al. 1992).

The estimations of the dimensionality and the Lyapunov coefficients (which we consider in the next section) are interrelated. A review of methods is given by Grassberger, Schreiber, and Schaffrath (1991). So far, the dimensionality of the process has been more readily interpretable in considering processes in the brain or the heart, and their psychological sequelae, than in direct estimation of the Lyapunov coefficients.

Given the trajectory of a hypothetical attractor – which is the path of evolution of dynamics in the *phase space* of system variables – its dimensionality can be defined in a number of ways. The simplest geometrical idea is called *box counting*: the phase space is filled with very small cubes[1] that together just contain the trajectory, and the limit of the necessary number of such cubes as a function of their size is a measure of the dimensionality. If the side of one of these cubes is ε units in length and if $M(\varepsilon)$ is the number of cubes of size ε just sufficient to cover the trajectory, then D_0 is the box-counting dimension (also known as the capacity dimension), which is given by

$$M(\varepsilon) \sim \varepsilon^{-D_0}. \tag{5}$$

This D_0 is crude. It is subject to what are called "saturation" and "depletion" effects (Cutler 1994) that limit its usefulness, so the preference is for calculating $D2$, the *correlation dimension*, which is better behaved. If one of the cubes is C_i and if a measure[2] on the cube is

$$\mu(C_i) \cong 1/M(\varepsilon),$$

then by definition

$$D2 = \lim_{\varepsilon \to 0} \left[\frac{\ln \sum \mu^2(C_i)}{\ln \varepsilon} \right]. \tag{6}$$

EMBEDDING

We now need to introduce a result that derives from a theorem in topology (a more formal treatment is given by Ott, Sauer, & Yorke 1994, chap. 5); here we review the use of this result in dynamical analyses only. If each point on a trajectory in phase space (which is the theoretical basis of an observable data time series) is replaced by a vector X_m made up of the point and $m - 1$ successor points in order, in increments of time τ, then we have replaced one point by some arbitrary number m of points. The theorem shows that points on the trajectory of an attractor with dimension d in the full-system phase space have a one-to-one correspondence with a limited number of variables, and by definition a point in the phase space carries complete information about the current state of the system. (Note that *dimension* here is not like the concept in everyday life as applied to boxes and areas.) By definition, m will be a positive integer, whereas d need not be an integer.

If we pick m carefully and large enough then the attractor can be *embedded* in a subspace of dimension m, so long as $m > 2d$ and $m > 2D_0$. This procedure will tell us about the upper limit on the dimension of the attractor, if it exists, but not necessarily anything about the shape of the attractor. This point illustrates our original distinction between **A** and **B** approaches. If we proceed using **A** then we set up a complete mathematical description of the attractor's shape in advance; but here, using **B**, we can only narrow down some of the attractor's properties: we can say what it is *not* like and how complicated it must at least be. The optimal choice of τ is not a fully resolved problem and in practice calls for some trial and error.

Grassberger and Procaccia (1983) developed an algorithm for estimating $D2$ that (with refinements) has been widely used in applications, partly because of its computational simplicity but also because its statistical properties have since been examined (Ramsey & Yuan 1990) and possible sources of bias identified. This algorithm has been widely influential because it is readily interpreted and calculated; in addition, it has formed a basis for generalization and refinement. The idea behind it is as follows.

Suppose there is a psychophysiological process that we wish to characterize. The process may be due to the effects of a number of different underlying and co-occurring psychophysiological processes. Suppose we could measure all these (interrelated) processes. We could then perform techniques like factor analysis or singular-value decomposition to find the minimum number of factors or dimensions that drive the system being measured. We can call this minimum number of dimensions an estimate of m. In real life, of course, we do not have the luxury of measuring all relevant variables. Often, we may have only a single variable. Can we derive from this the underlying dimensionality of the process? It turns out that, owing to a result known as Takens's theorem, this is possible under certain broad conditions (Takens 1980).

A single time series of N data points, $z_1, z_2, \ldots, z_n, \ldots, z_N$, which corresponds to psychophysiological measurements at regularly spaced intervals of time, is a realization of the trajectory of the dynamics. The interval between successive observations is fixed and very small. From each of these observed data points we can form an m-dimensional vector by embedding as follows:

$$X_m(n) = (z_n, z_{n+\tau}, \ldots, z_{n+(m-1)\tau}). \tag{7}$$

In (7), m is the embedding dimension and τ is a time delay (a certain number of sample times). Takens showed that the true dimensionality of the system can be assessed via this set of $N - m$ vectors, based on univariate measurement. In principle, the same procedure should work for all time delays and all embedding dimensions, provided only that the embedding dimension m is at least one greater than twice the real underlying dimension d. The relative number of pairs of the n points that are separated by less than ε in the embedding space runs to a limit as n increases to infinity. This becomes the *correlation integral* $\hat{C}(\varepsilon)$, where

$$\hat{C}(\varepsilon) = \lim_{N \to \infty} \frac{1}{N^2} \sum_{i,j} U(\varepsilon - r_{ij}). \tag{8}$$

Here U is the unit step function, so that, for all x, $U(x < 0) = 0$ and $U(x > 0) = 1$. The variable r_{ij} is the absolute distance between two vectors X_i and X_j constructed from (7). It can be shown that D2 is then given by

$$D2 = \lim_{\varepsilon \to 0} \frac{\ln \hat{C}(\varepsilon)}{\ln \varepsilon}. \tag{9}$$

To calculate D2, first compute distances between all the vectors $X_m(n)$ in (7). Then compute the correlation integral $\hat{C}(\varepsilon)$, which is just the proportion of these distances smaller than ε. The value of D2 is then given by a plot of $\ln \hat{C}(\varepsilon)$ on $\ln \varepsilon$ over a limited range $\varepsilon_1 < \varepsilon < \varepsilon_2$ that yields a straight line; the slope of this line is an estimate of D2.

Since the limit $\varepsilon \to 0$ can never be experimentally achieved, in practice linearity is sought in this log-log plot of correlation integral versus length for smaller values of length over an appreciable range. The slope of the best straight line yields the correlation dimension; provided the embedding dimension is large enough (i.e., "saturation" has been achieved), the true dimension should emerge and be independent of m. In practice, one looks to calculate D2 for a range of dimensions and assesses the attainment of saturation by some criterion (e.g., by a limitation on their variance over a range of values of m). The fact of saturation can serve to verify that the signal is not white noise. White noise fills whatever dimension in which it is embedded; D2 never saturates but continues to increase with m if the signal is random.

Thus, D2 provides a way to quantify the complexity of the underlying system that is generating the data. In general it will be fractal, and the reliability of estimation decreases with increasing D2. The value of delay chosen is rather arbitrary; in the limit of infinite data sets, its choice is irrelevant. However, in real systems with a limited number of points, a good choice can make a big difference. One common choice is to set τ equal to the value of the first zero crossing of the autocorrelation function. Another approach is to pick τ as one fourth of the dominant frequency found in the power spectrum. Yet another possibility is to choose τ on the basis of the resulting sensitivity of D2 to the experimental manipulations. For further discussion see Rosenstein, Collins, and DeLuca (1993) and Kantz and Schreiber (1997).

Practical issues often intrude in successful D2 estimation with real data, unlike the "data" of experimental mathematics. The number of points required for a stable linear slope can be rather large. Although reliable results for certain time series with low noise values can be obtained for series as short as 500, this is not typical and can depend moreover on the particular distribution of points on the attractor. Under typical conditions of experimental measurement, data sets of minimum size 10^3–10^4 are in order, and some authors recommend data sets as large as 10^6 (Tong 1995), depending on the embedding dimension. Such sizes are unfeasible with psychological data and often impractical with physiological and psychophysiological data.

Furthermore, D2 is not immune to the effects of noise and filtering. Noise added to a completely deterministic time series can change D2 estimates substantially, even if the noise has fairly small amplitude. Filtering of white noise can produce spurious estimates of low dimensionality and assessments of deterministic causation (see examples to follow) if caution is not exercised. Since psychophysical data collection nearly always features filtering to avoid aliasing and other problems, it is essential that filtering *not* remove information relevant to the deterministic attractor geometry if it is to retain its interpretation as underlying system dimensionality. Also, D2 does not cope well with nonstationarity – and biological data often are riddled with it, in the sense that the relevant neural generators are in constant interrelation with the larger and varying physiological system. These often prove to be severe limitations in practice. Hence other indicators have been developed, based on extensions of the Grassberg–Procaccia approach, that are able to minimize these limitations. Farmer, Ott, and Yorke (1983) suggested that the perturbing effects of nonstationarity could be minimized by calculating the dimension relative to particular reference vectors throughout the file. This they called the "pointwise" scaling dimension, $D2_i$.

The serious nonstationarity of psychological data impedes ready implementation of the $D2_i$ algorithm, which thus has been significantly revised by various workers (e.g. Skinner, Molnar, & Tomberg 1994). We deal with an extension particularly useful for biological systems, the $PD2_i$ algorithm, in the section entitled "Point Correlation Dimension Analyses."

The problem with all but very long time series (over 5,000 data points) is that estimates of dimensionality are biased. This need not matter if the interest is only in relative shifts in dimensionality and if the bias is second-order and in the same direction relative to the shifts (criteria met by Gregson et al. 1992). Ramsey and Yuan (1990) identified the expected biases that can arise. Using the Grassberger and Procaccia (1983) algorithm (and others related to it), the authors determined that dimension estimates are always biased upward for pure signals whereas noise can bias them downward. Unsurprisingly, the bias is worse for small samples, and runs of less than 500 data points raise difficulties because estimates are no longer normally distributed over repeated samples. The methods are viable for EEG, ECG (electrocardiogram), or EDR (electrodermal response), but for slow psychophysics they are effectively ruled out.

LYAPUNOV COEFFICIENTS

In this section we will follow the notation of Nicolis and Prigogine (1989); texts vary considerably. Sources up to 1993 are summarized by Ott et al. (1994).

Consider a trajectory that is running onto its attractor in its embedding space, which may grow or shrink in time. The amount that the trajectory changes, projected onto each orthogonal dimension of the embedding space, is expressed in terms of the Lyapunov coefficient of that direction. More precisely, the Lyapunov coefficients (or exponents, as they are sometimes called) are measures of the mean exponential rate of divergence of two initially close trajectories in the designated direction. This is another way of expressing the loss of predictability – or increase of uncertainty and hence of information (in the information theory sense of the word) – as the dynamics evolve in time from any starting point.

Suppose we have two points in the phase space, denoted by

$$\chi_{0,i} \quad \text{and} \quad \chi_{0,i} + \Delta x_{0,i}. \tag{10}$$

Then the separation Δx_i in the immediate neighborhood of $\chi_{0,i}$ is expressed in terms of a linear tangent vector that starts from $\chi_{0,i}$, denoted by Δx_0. Though the process is essentially nonlinear, in this tiny neighborhood we can use a local linear approximation to describe the evolution. This linear part is denoted by L_{ij}, where the j runs over the neighborhood points and the i runs over variables of the dynamic equation. The Lyapunov coefficient for a dimension is then λ_L (dropping the i subscript):

$$\lambda_L(\chi_0, \Delta x_0) = \lim_{\substack{t \to \infty \\ |\Delta x_0| \to 0}} \frac{1}{t} \ln \frac{|\Delta x(\chi_0, t)|}{|\Delta x_0|} \tag{11}$$

(cf. Nicolis & Prigogine 1989, eq. A1.25), and this is the mean exponential rate of divergence of two trajectories that start off close together. The process has an evolution that geometrically is in an embedding space of a priori unknown dimensionality. The actual attractor defining the dynamics has a fractal dimensionality that is noninteger and in general less than that of the space in which it is embedded. If a record of the trajectory of the dynamics is available – of which an EEG trace would be an example – then calculation of all the possible λ_L, one from each independent direction in the phase space, may furnish the sort of information listed in Table 2.

It is the pattern of the coefficients that furnishes a test of whether chaos is present, although brief transient passages into and out of chaos (which are theoretically possible) are not expected to show themselves in such an analysis over long time series of data. The sum of the coefficients will shrink if the process is dissipative over time. It is usually the case that the largest λ_L is easiest to calculate (Rosenstein et al. 1993) and will dominate over large times; the rest add considerably to the computational difficulties.

Calculation of the coefficients is performed by using algorithms based on a time-delay method. There is some possibility of obtaining spurious coefficients, so additional checks are necessary to identify them (see references in Ott et al. 1994, chap. 8; see also Abarbanel 1996).

The problem of short time series of real data arises in all disciplines, and the assumption of stationarity over more than brief interludes is implausible in biological applications. As a result, much effort has been and is being

TABLE 2.

Lyapunov Coefficients	Qualitative Dynamics
all < 0	point attractor, zero dimensionality
one 0, others < 0	one-dimensional attractor
one 0, one < 0	attractor like a folded sheet
at least one > 0	dependent on initial conditions
two > 0	fills a volume in 3-D space

expended on methods for short series. A review issue of the journal *Integrative Physiological and Behavioral Science* gives relevant results (Schiff, Sauer, & Chang 1994). Gençay (1996) developed a statistical test for estimating confidence intervals on Lyapunov coefficients from small data sets, and Marzocchi, Mulargia, and Gonzato (1996) reported some success in estimating dimensionality with data series as short as 50 points (with a 10% noise level present).

Multiple Measure Approaches

The detection of chaos is not a sure thing, and it requires the simultaneous use of a number of measures. These are most often attractor dimension estimation, Lyapunov component estimation, and local prediction. No one of the algorithms invented is universally superior, and studies of the relative performance of algorithms are still few. Heart rate variability has been studied by Vibe and Vesin (1996) using local intrinsic dimension (LID) (Hediger, Passamante, & Farrell 1990; Passamante, Hediger, & Gollub 1989), by Rosenstein et al.'s (1993) MLE method for finding a maximum Lyapunov exponent, and by nonlinear prediction by using the NLP algorithm of Casdagli (1989).

All three methods use the time delay approach, in which the attractor is reconstructed in phase space by associating a vector X with each data point n. If the time delay between successive data points is τ and the embedding dimension is m, then again

$$X_n = (x_n, x_{n+\tau}, \ldots, x_{n+(m-1)\tau}). \qquad (12)$$

Both m and τ must be estimated by recursive computation. The Grassberger–Procaccia algorithm has shown itself unable to distinguish between chaotic attractors and attractors that are fractal in dimension but not chaotic. Thus, it cannot reliably be used for relatively short data runs and so other methods, still vulnerable to ambiguity but more robust, have to be used.

The LID method starts with a guess at a high embedding dimension (say $10 \leq m \leq 40$) and randomly chooses points on the attractor to cover it. Nearest neighbors to each local center X_c are found by assuming a Euclidean space in which the attractor is embedded. A matrix of the local differences from the center is then created and its rank computed, as in principal components analysis. This gives local dimensionality estimates s_i ($i = 1, \ldots, m$), and the probability distribution of these s_i has an expectation that is the d_{LID} sought. Plotting d_{LID} against m gives a characteristic shape for chaotic signals that differs from that obtained for other signals, but the method can fail to recognize high-dimensional chaos.

Computing only the largest Lyapunov coefficient is sufficient for detecting chaos, and Rosenstein et al. (1993) designed a method that will work with shorter time series. It is reasonably robust with respect to noise, and it

will support a classification that is richer than the simple dichotomy of chaos or nonchaos. The drawback is that it presupposes the existence of a positive Lyapunov coefficient. But if the process is indeed chaotic then estimates of $\max(\lambda)$ can be independent of m, which can be set quite low (< 10) for computational exploration.

The NLP method of Casdagli (1989) rests on a theorem proved by Takens (1980). If both the embedding dimension and delay in (12) are chosen suitably, then a smooth map f exists such that

$$x_{n+T} = f(X_n), \qquad (13)$$

where T is a forecasting time ahead from n. Because the map f is smooth, it can be fitted by some piecewise approximation over a local neighborhood of k steps. If the best fit is from a low value of k then, by definition, the signal is deterministic and chaotic. If the best fit is from large k then most probably the signal is linear and stochastic. Intermediate solutions indicate that the process is both stochastic and nonlinear.

Using all methods, Vibe and Vesin (1996) concluded that heart rate is not low-dimensional chaotic. An alternative approach is to detect chaos, if it is present, without using $D2$ or Lyapunov estimates (see e.g. Palus 1995).

Point Correlation Dimension Analyses

The methodology here may be said to be state-of-the-art using a **B** approach. Skinner and associates (Molnar & Skinner 1992; Skinner et al. 1991, 1994) developed the *point correlation dimension*, $PD2_i$. Like $D2_i$ (Farmer et al. 1983), this technique calculates $D2$ by using many reference vectors throughout the data file. This is achieved by calculating the correlation dimension separately for many different points throughout the file, or in the limit for all the points. The value of the correlation integral at point i with embedding dimension m is denoted by $C_i^m(r)$. There are also inbuilt criteria for accepting or rejecting each of the estimates. To be accepted, estimates must: (i) have adequate length for the linear region of the log-log plot of $C_i^m(r)$ versus r, (ii) show sufficient linearity in this region, and (iii) converge to the same estimate over a range of embedding dimensions. The relevant software is available from its developers.

The point correlation dimension appears to have many valuable properties for evaluating nonlinear time series. First, it gives a reference point–based dimensional estimate, so that changes in the state of the system can be localized (if not exactly pinpointed) in time. Second, its average over time is compatible with the full $D2$ estimate, so that system dimensionality still has some interpretable meaning. Third, it can work with relatively short data sets of 500–1,000 points, and it can handle dynamics that are only piecewise stationary (i.e., stationary within these short epochs but not overall). The $PD2_i$ values can change

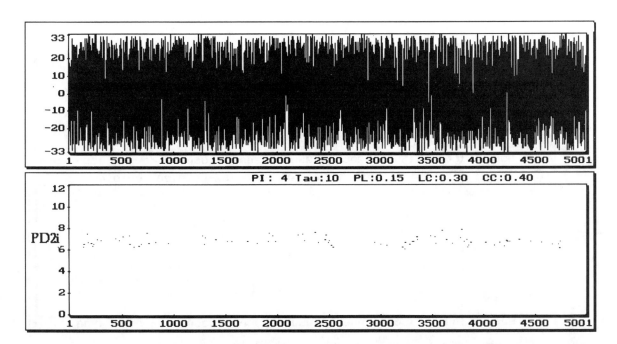

Figure 1. Time series (above) and $PD2_i$ estimates (below) for white noise.

rapidly at boundaries between epochs. Critical jumps between epochs are also potentially detectable by Lyapunov calculations (Kowalik & Elbert 1994). It is the epochs themselves that we would wish to identify with psychological contextual variables.

SAMPLE ANALYSIS WITH EEG DATA

Correlation dimension–based analysis has now been widely applied: to many experimental measurements in physics and chemistry, to financial markets, to nostril ventilation patterns, to electroencephalogram and electrocardiogram data, and to ratings of psychological mood – to mention only a few examples. To show the advantages of the various indicators for the domain of interest here, we will examine a set of EEG data kindly provided by John Trinder of the University of Melbourne Psychophysiology Laboratory. These data were collected under conditions of stage-2 human sleep, with 32 channels of data sampled at 500 Hz. The analysis here is not comprehensive; our goal is simply to illustrate the issues in dimensional analysis.

Dimensional analysis is likely to be most effective when the underlying dimensions are not too great. If the underlying dimension is high, we will need a much higher embedding dimension, and the region of potential linearity will be reduced. For this reason we expect sleep EEG to be more reliably estimable than waking EEG, as has been found experimentally for $D2$. We consider the following series for comparison:

1. white noise;
2. low-pass–filtered white noise;
3. high-pass–filtered white noise;
4. bandpass-filtered white noise;

5. stage-2 sleep EEG before respiratory arousal (electrode FP2);
6. stage-2 sleep EEG after respiratory arousal (electrode FP2);
7. stage-2 sleep EEG with K-complex (electrode Fz);
8. stage-2 sleep EEG with K-complex (electrode Pz).

Low-pass noise was generated from white noise by first-order smoothing; high-pass noise was generated from white noise by first-order differencing; and bandpass noise was generated by first-order smoothing and differencing. The lengths of series 1–4 are 5,000 points, those of series 5–8 are each 5,120 points. Criterion values for $PD2_i$ were those standardly recommended by Skinner: PL = 0.15, LC = 0.30, and CC = 0.40, with $9 \leq m \leq 12$ (Skinner et al. 1994). The optimal discriminative value of τ used was determined by trial and error; variations had minimal effect. Tau was set equal to 50 for the sleep data, 10 for the noise data.

Figure 1 shows the time series and $PD2_i$ plot for white noise. Most of the points are rejected, indicating failure to satisfy at least one of the above criteria. Dimensionality is found to be between 6 and 8 and could not practically be much higher, given the range of embedding dimensions used. The high rejection rate of points suggests that the data do not correspond to a coherent attractor. Similar results are found with low- or high-pass filtering (shown in Figures 2 and 3, respectively), except that the percentage of accepted points is much greater. The additional coherence provided by filtering increases the convergence success of the algorithm.

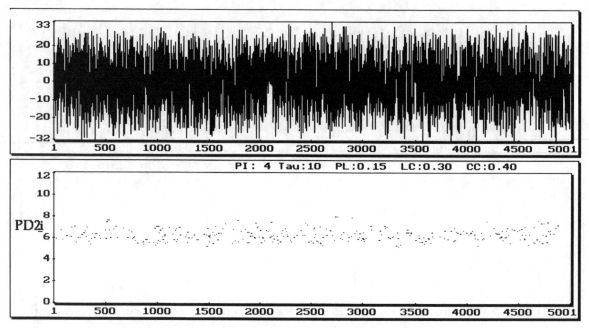

Figure 2. Time series (above) and $PD2_i$ estimates (below) for low-pass–filtered white noise.

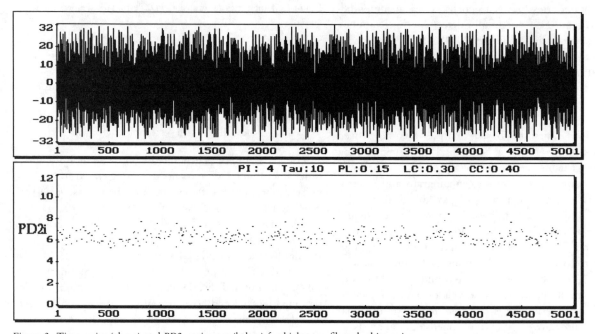

Figure 3. Time series (above) and $PD2_i$ estimates (below) for high-pass–filtered white noise.

The power spectrum of the bandpass noise is shown in Figure 4A; Figure 4B shows the actual series and $PD2_i$. Note that the dimension estimates now center around 4. The additional structure due to bandpass filtering has both reduced the apparent dimension and increased the acceptance rate of reference vectors. In general, colored noise can easily be incorrectly assessed as a deterministic system if one examines only mean values of dimension. Note that all the white-noise–based plots show uniformity of variance across the course of the data.

Figure 5 shows the region preceding a respiration-defined arousal in stage-2 sleep. The electrode site is right prefrontal. The values of $PD2_i$ center around 4 (like the bandpass noise), but there are local fluctuations in variance, $PD2_i$ value, and percentage of reference vectors accepted. We interpret significant drops in acceptance rate to indicate local changes of state, since such nonstationarity will reduce the fraction of points that fulfill the acceptance criteria. Significant increases in variance may indicate critical fluctuations leading possibly to bifurcation. Variations in $PD2_i$ over the course of the data file presumably indicate

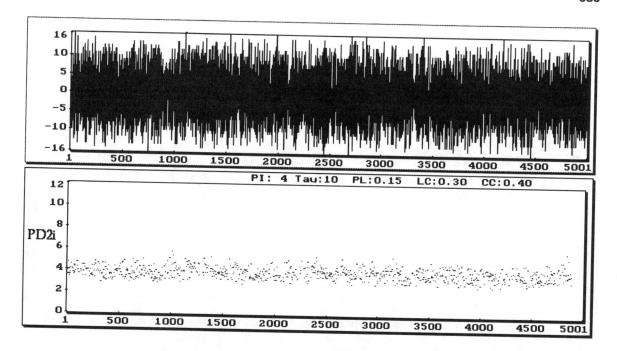

PI: 4 Tau:10 PL:0.15 LC:0.30 CC:0.40

local changes in the involvement of different neural generators of activity.

Figure 6 shows the same electrode site for the same subject, but now *after* the same arousal. The mean $PD2_i$ is significantly lower, there is greater variance, and there are significant stretches of very low acceptance rates, reducing overall acceptance rate. Note that these possible changes of state are not readily apparent in the time series itself, confirming the usefulness of the approach.

Figure 4A. Power spectrum for bandpass-filtered white noise.

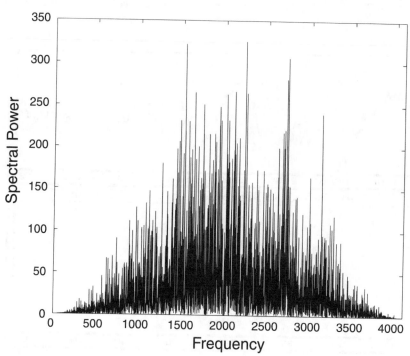

Figure 4B. Time series (above) and $PD2_i$ estimates (below) for bandpass-filtered white noise.

The $PD2_i$ may also yield important insights in modeling specific event classes in the EEG. Its ability to contribute to evoked potential research has been shown by its developers (Molnar & Skinner 1992). Here we illustrate that ability by examining a portion of EEG containing a K-complex, a characteristic transient event in stage-2 sleep known to have a central frontal locus. The K-complex is delineated by a sharp negative wave followed by a positive component (Roschke & Aldenhoff 1991). Figure 7 shows the data and $PD2_i$ plots for the central frontal electrode Fz. The effect of the K-complex occurs on the $PD2_i$ plot before it does on the data plot. The difference here is close to the expected anticipation of $(m-1)\tau$ intrinsic in building the embedded vectors and does not reflect anticipatory cerebral activity. Note that the K-complex reduces dimensionally to a combination of two sources, a single-dimensional source of dim ≈ 1 and (at the end of the plateau) high-dimensional noise. This result is not unique to this K-complex but appears to be quite common (although other types of K-complexes may not show this same signature). Simulations of the K-complex as due to these two factors (a single oscillator burst plus stochastic noise) show the same pattern of results. Hence the $PD2_i$ results suggest a model form for

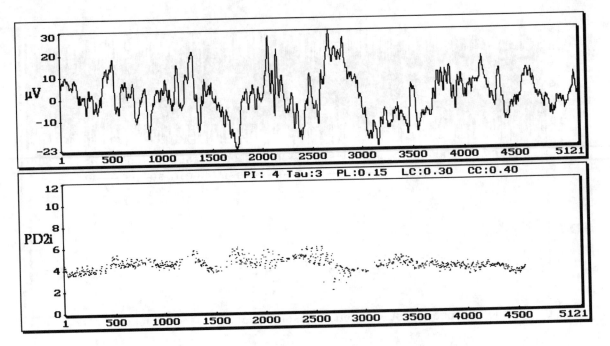

Figure 5. Time series (above) and *PD2$_i$* estimates (below) for stage-2 sleep EEG *before* respiratory arousal (electrode FP2).

at least some types of K-complex, which can be further investigated.

Finally, Figure 8 shows data from the same times, taken at the Pz site, and the corresponding *PD2$_i$* plot. This site does not normally give visual evidence, as judged by EEG experts, of a (frontally centered) K-complex, and indeed that is the case here. Nevertheless, there is a clear increase in dimensionality and gaps in acceptance rate associated with the time of the frontal K-complex, suggesting that related changes of state are also detectable in this site via

PD2$_i$. Local fluctuations in variance are also apparent. The *PD2$_i$* thus appears able to indicate transitions not picked up by conventional expert judgment.

These points are summarized in Table 3, which also includes sample calculations of *D2* for the same time series, based on a single 12-dimensional embedding. The *D2* values are broadly consistent with the *PD2$_i$* averages, with the exception of runs 5 (reason unclear) and 7 (due to data nonstationarity). Note that *D2* does a poor job of distinguishing these particular series from white noise. Our

Figure 6. Time series (above) and *PD2$_i$* estimates (below) for stage-2 sleep EEG *after* respiratory arousal (electrode FP2); same subject as in Figure 5.

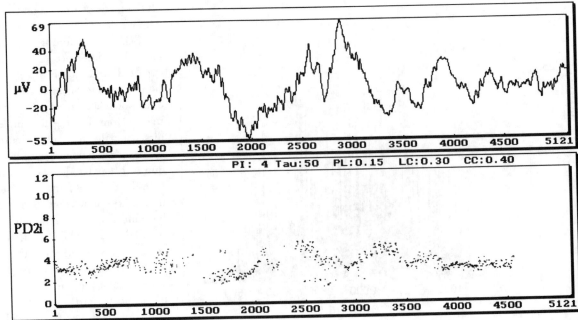

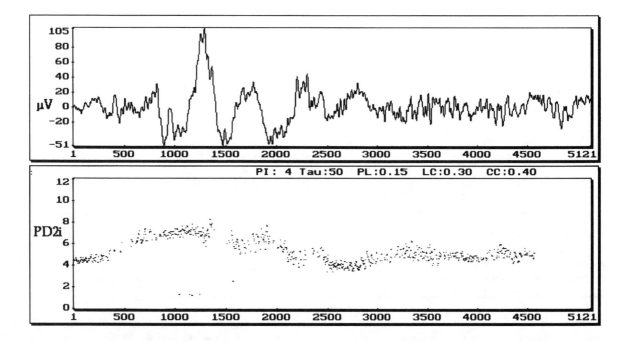

PI: 4 Tau:50 PL:0.15 LC:0.30 CC:0.40

experience is that it must be used with considerable caution. The facile use of $D2$ as a state indicator has received justifiable criticism in recent years (e.g. Rapp 1994). For a more optimistic assessment of the usefulness of $D2$ for sleep analysis, using a time series of 16,384 samples, see Roschke and Aldenhoff (1991). In any case, the mean $PD2_i$ values found here are in good agreement with the range of 4–6 found for stage-2 sleep using $D2$ with much longer data files (Coenen 1996).

Figure 7. Time series (above) and $PD2_i$ estimates (below) for stage-2 sleep EEG with visible K-complex (electrode Fz); same subject as in Figure 5.

Figure 8. Time series (above) and $PD2_i$ estimates (below) for stage-2 sleep EEG corresponding to frontally visible K-complex (electrode Pz); same subject as in Figure 5.

The number of allowed vector points used in $PD2_i$ estimation is 272 for the white-noise case and is in the rough range of 1,500–3,500 for the other series. Hence, standard errors for the mean $PD2_i$ fall in the approximate range 0.01–0.02 (except for the white noise, SE = 0.04), so that all differences of means (except that between the high- and low-pass white noise), which are readily testable by t-test or ANOVA, are highly significant. Note that the separate estimates of $PD2_i$ over the course of the data are essentially

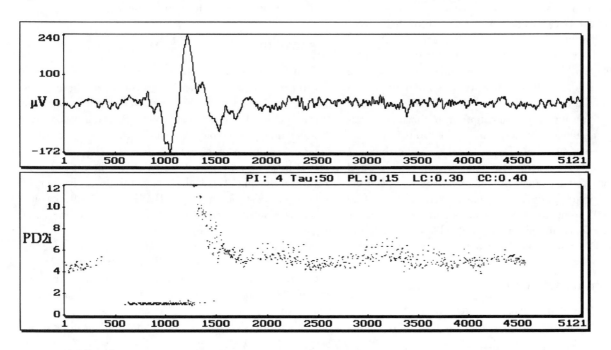

PI: 4 Tau:50 PL:0.15 LC:0.30 CC:0.40

TABLE 3. Comparison of Dimensional Calculations for Various Time Series

Time Series	Source	Mean of $PD2_i$	S.D. of $PD2_i$	Percentage of Vectors Accepted	$D2^a$
1	White noise (WN)	6.78	0.37	5.4	7.43
2	Low-pass WN	6.31	0.64	29.6	5.60
3	High-pass WN	6.35	0.56	28.4	6.65
4	Bandpass WN	3.80	0.54	66.3	3.63
5	Stage-2 sleep before arousal (FP2)[b]	4.27	0.57	70.4	7.98
6	Stage-2 sleep after arousal (FP2)[b]	3.39	0.77	60.6	3.91
7	Stage 2 with K-C(Fz)[c]	4.48	2.10	60.0	8.05
8	Stage 2 with K-C(Pz)[d]	5.29	1.12	57.3	6.10

[a] Noise series: $m = 12$, $\tau = 10$. EEG series: $m = 12$, $\tau = 50$.
[b] Site of EEG recording, 10–20 system.
[c] Stage 2 containing visible K-complex at site (Fz).
[d] Stage 2 corresponding to frontally visible K-complex at site (Pz).

independent (only a very small fraction of the same data may enter into the calculation of more than one point).

It is interesting that the mean dimension is less after arousal than before it, yet the standard deviation increases after arousal. This suggests that postarousal is a simpler state on average than prearousal and that its greater variability may be due to greater fluctuations in (simpler) control mechanisms.

These results are typical of multiple analyses that have been performed. Thus, $PD2_i$ offers a number of advantages in nonlinear analysis of physiological data, and it appears able successfully to distinguish deterministic physiological series from various forms of noise, including autocorrelated colored noise. It can be used to infer changes of state and also, with some caution, to characterize transient events and their generators.

The indicators chosen here were selected for their physiological suitability. They far from exhaust the possibilities. For example, the Hurst exponent (Hurst 1965; see also Feder 1988) has been used in characterizing natural time series with regard to their similarity to white noise and in testing for long-range memory processes (Beran 1994; Mandelbrot 1972); it involves no assumptions of linearity or stationarity. A value of the exponent of close to 0.5 indicates white-noise–like behavior. However, the discriminability of this index was poor here. For example, time series 7 and 8 in Table 1 yielded values of 0.482 and 0.560, respectively (using the original Hurst algorithm), whereas series of 20 runs of 1,000 points each of white noise and high-pass noise (first differencing of white noise) yielded 0.495 ± 0.02 and 0.363 ± 0.034, respectively ($\pm$ figures are standard errors).

Approximate Entropy

In practice, the determination of the Lyapunov exponent is often problematic with actual data. First, even more

data may be required than for the estimation of dimensions (but see Abarbanel 1996 for a contrary opinion). Second, noise can affect the estimation results. It has been shown that positive Lyapunov exponents can occur for noisy systems or, for that matter, in periodic systems with large first derivatives (Glass 1995). Third, what is the actual meaning of the exponent, which is meant to indicate chaotic behavior (i.e. deterministic noise) in the presence of high-dimensional (stochastic) noise? Various solutions to this last issue have been proposed (e.g. Mayer-Kress & Haken 1981; Tong 1995), but the issue remains to be resolved.

Because of these problems, we suggest consideration of an alternative index, developed by Pincus, that computes an approximate entropy (ApEn) and has been shown to produce credible results for short time series.

BACKGROUND

Dimensional calculations have as their foundation the global geometrical structure of an attractor in phase space. Another, independent way to characterize time-series data is via their local sequential structure. For example, we can examine how predictable the series is over short to medium times. A number of techniques for assessing time-series determinism or stationarity are based on the idea of nonlinear forecasting (Casdagli & Eubank 1992; Farmer & Sidorowich 1988; Sugihara & May 1990). A useful evaluation of several such techniques for psychological time series is given by Scheier and Tschacher (1995).

A related concept is that of the *entropy* of a series, which has an analog relation with the thermodynamic and informational uses of this term. Entropy measures the amount of mixing between states and hence the rate-based complexity of the underlying system. Thus, if entropy is high, then disorder is high and predictability will be low.

Many estimators of entropy have been developed in the dynamical literature. Most require large data sets and are designed for mathematically pure systems uncontaminated by noise. The Eckmann–Ruelle entropy is one standard indicator that suffers from such limitations. However, the related family of ApEn index parameters developed by Pincus (1991, 1995) has been shown to have discriminative utility with physiological data (Kaplan et al. 1991; Pincus 1995). Approximate entropy appears to have some desirable properties: it is claimed to be robust to stochastic noise effects and outliers; it can be used with time series as short as 100 points; it is sensitive to typical differences in many biological systems; and it corresponds to the idea of system complexity. The price to be paid for these features is that we no longer have an absolute measure of entropy but only a relative one. Hence, its primary use is in comparing different states and not in providing an absolute characterization.

Mathematically, ApEn is based on the point correlation integral $C_i^m(r)$ defined previously. Let

$$\Phi^m(r) = (N - m + 1)^{-1} \sum_{i=1}^{N-m+1} \ln C_i^m(r). \quad (14)$$

Then the family of approximate entropy statistics is defined as

$$\text{ApEn}(m, r, N) = \Phi^{m+1}(r) - \Phi^m(r). \quad (15)$$

A discussion of the physiological foundation of this algorithm may be found in Pincus and Goldberger (1994). Here we illustrate its use via the series given earlier.

Figure 9. Approximate entropy (ApEn($m, r, 5,000$)) curves for white noise, with $2 \leq m \leq 5$ (series 1, same data as in Figure 1).

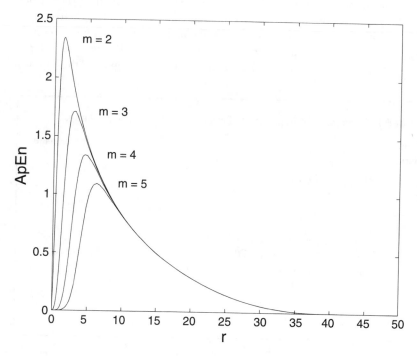

SAMPLE ANALYSIS WITH EEG DATA

Figure 9 shows ApEn(m, r, N) for a range of embedding dimensions from 2 to 5 for white noise (series 1). Figure 10 shows ApEn(m, r, N), for the same dimensional range, for stage-2 sleep EEG with K-complex (electrode Fz, series 7). Note that ApEn is a function of r. The two graph families are readily distinguished by shape, range, and mean. In particular, higher entropy for the white noise over a range of distances is apparent. Pincus suggests that a simple way to document changes of state in entropy is simply to compute point values of ApEn for different states. He suggests choosing ApEn($2, 0.15\sigma; N > 100$) as a basis for comparison of state entropies, where σ is the standard deviation (S.D.) of the embedded series. He has established via Monte Carlo calculations that S.D.s for this indicator are less than 0.055 for a large class of candidate models (Pincus & Goldberger 1994). In Table 4 we show the results of applying this indicator to our eight test series; ApEn provides a ready discrimination of noise sources, including filtered noise sources, from sleep EEG data. As expected, entropy of noise sources is far greater, and white noise shows more disorder than filtered noise.

Because in each case we have a single series, we cannot compute statistical significance. However, this would be simple to do from a set of series in each condition.

In particular, without multiple runs to allow the computation of standard errors, we cannot make any discriminative statements of significance about the different sleep states. However, the results are fully consistent with qualitative expectations. Thus, the ranking of the states a priori in terms of increasing entropy (for the same subject) would be: K-complex (Fz), K-complex (Pz), stage-2 sleep before arousal, stage-2 sleep after arousal. This ranking is based on the frontal origin of the K-complex, its temporal coherence, and disordering (increasing of entropy) effects expected from arousal. The values of Table 4 are in this same order: 0.0049, 0.055, 0.091, 0.112.

SURROGATE DATA

Significance of results with respect to specific null hypotheses can often be refined by the use of surrogate data (Schiff & Chang 1992; Theiler et al. 1992). In this procedure, the original data set is scrambled in some way (e.g., by temporal reordering or by phase randomization of the Fourier transform and then reverse transform) and then the indicator of choice

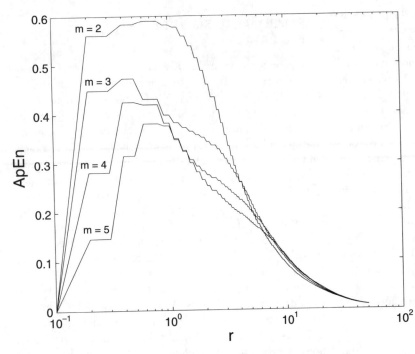

Figure 10. Approximate entropy (ApEn(m, r, 5,000)) curves for stage-2 sleep EEG with K-complex (electrode Fz), with $2 \leq m \leq 5$ (series 7, same data as in Figure 7).

examined to ascertain if a significant difference between the original data and the surrogate data exists. If it does, then support exists for the experimental hypothesis over the null. If not, though, the associated null hypothesis is not disconfirmed; instead, either the data are functionally indistinguishable from the null model or the indicator is insensitive to the differences. Surrogate data techniques are increasingly becoming standard in the refinement of hypothesis testing (see e.g. Kantz & Schreiber 1997).

Nonlinear Psychophysical Dynamics

In this section we begin not with data strings, facing an identification problem whose answers are expressed in Lyapunov or like indices. Rather, we start with a process model so chosen that its algebra will, under some restricted parameter values, generate qualitative phenomena that can match the relatively coarser structure of behavioral data, both sensory and perceptual. We already know a great deal about coarse structure from a century and a half of psychophysical experiments. The strategy may be said to move in reverse, from **B** first and then to the **A** direction, from data to model to more data.

NONLINEAR PSYCHOPHYSICS

Psychophysical studies have always had a very close relationship to psychophysiology. Even when sensory physiology was in its infancy, there was assumed to be a potentially identifiable basis to the stimulus-to-behavioral-response mappings that psychophysics aims to encode. Fechner himself, already in the mid-nineteenth century, called this *psychofysik von unten*. Suppose we have three classes of variables: (i) physical stimuli, (ii) internal physiological responses, and (iii) externally observable behavioral responses. Then psychophysics is (i) $\mapsto$ (iii) with (ii) implicit, or (ii) $\mapsto$ (iii) with (i) implicit; whereas we take psychophysiology in its fullest sense to involve all of (i), (ii), and (iii). The most recent models in nonlinear psychophysics that explicitly rest on dynamics (NPD – nonlinear psychophysical dynamics) do have some parallels with the multiplicity of brain pathways supporting sensation and perception (Gregson 1988, 1992, 1995), and it may be useful here to sketch those parallels briefly. These models have been used in a wide diversity of sensory and perceptual contexts.

MODEL CORE

The basic equation for one sensory channel is the Γ recursion of a complex cubic polynomial. The stimulus level operates on the gain parameter a of the process, but not directly on its internal complex variable Y. After some time – expressed as η, the number of recursions – the process either terminates or is terminated. The value of the real part of Y is then an affine multiple of the output.

TABLE 4. Comparison of Approximate Entropies for the Eight Time Series

Time Series	Source	Approximate Entropy[a]
1	White noise (WN)	2.295
2	Low-pass WN	2.248
3	High-pass WN	2.152
4	Bandpass WN	2.144
5	Stage-2 sleep before arousal (FP2)[b]	0.091
6	Stage-2 sleep after arousal (FP2)[b]	0.112
7	Stage 2 containing visible K-complex (Fz)[b]	0.0049
8	Stage 2 corresponding to frontally visible K-complex (Pz)[b]	0.055

[a] Embedding dimension = 2, $r = 0.15\sigma$; approx. 5,000 data points.
[b] Site of EEG recording, 10–20 system.

Throughout nearly all the analyses (Gregson 1988, 1992, 1995), the recursion has been written and generated as

$$\Gamma: \quad Y_{(j+1)} = -a \cdot (Y_j - 1)(Y_j - ie)(Y_j + ie), \quad (16)$$

where $i = \sqrt{-1}$ and with the recursion given a starting value Y_0 and running $j = 1, \ldots, \eta$. The stimulus input U maps affinely onto a, and e is an internal parameter. Here Y is the state variable in continuous existence before and after the Γ trajectory, which is itself a transient destabilization of the system. This may resemble Freeman's (1994) treatment of the problem. The terminal real value $Y_\eta(\mathrm{Re})$ corresponds to an observable response. The corresponding imaginary part of the trajectory $Y(\mathrm{Im})$ is always second-order. The gain a is the only direct link with the system's environment. There are various forms using (16) within a psychophysical model for repeated trials (Gregson 1988). As used here, e is independent of a in Figure 11 (to follow), the case called $\Gamma V 7$; an alternative, where e is tied to the rate of change of a over successive trials, is called $\Gamma V 1$. Experimental stimulus–response data are thus to be matched to response surfaces $Y(\mathrm{Re}), a \mid e, \eta$.

When writing a general nonlinear psychophysical theory one is not concerned with any particular sensory modality (e.g. taste) or with any specific dimension within a modality (e.g. sweet or salty). The physical units U in which stimulus levels are numerically encoded are arbitrary (meters, feet, cubits even!) but the system gain a is a dimensionless number in a bounded range. Consequently, in the affine mapping $U \mapsto a$, the units of U must themselves be expressed as dimensionless for consistency; hence U is strictly to be taken as U/U_0, a ratio of the input to a base level – or as $(U - U_0)/U_0$ if environmental conditions require such an interpretation. The transformations at output to response units are similarly arbitrary and dimensionless. If responses are expressed as probabilities then the dimensionality problem does not arise, but another response selection mechanism downstream from Γ needs then to be postulated. In previous treatments (Gregson 1992), both the $U \mapsto a$ and $Y(\mathrm{Re}) \mapsto R$ have been written as affine, and the nonlinear dynamics are thus sandwiched between two mappings. It must be emphasized that the Γ recursion has two parts (real and imaginary); also, it is a model not of single-neuron transmission but rather of the function of a pathway that may locally and transiently behave as an almost-closed dual system. When multiple pathways (each carrying different sensory information) are involved then the model is extended: various cases presupposing cross-linkages – which can be facilitatory or inhibitory, mutually or separately on the pathways – can arise simply from the algebra. Of course, the neurophysiology of sensory mappings can involve multiple pathways with variable delays inbuilt as well as pathways that are either specific to a modality or nonspecific and carrying multiple types of information.

When we are concerned with complicated stimuli varying on a diversity of physical dimensions that the receptors can transduce, then the NPD core structure involves (i) the system's state variable $Y(\mathrm{Re}, \mathrm{Im})$ for each channel considered separately, intra- or interdimensionally in sensory inputs, and (ii) the gain a and sensitivity e parameters of the Γ recursion, which carry information on input level and differential responses to inputs. The consequence of inputting a stimulus is to shift Y in a complex manner, and restabilization need not ever bring the system back to an original baseline. The responses are transients at the end of a destabilization and are proportional to $Y(\mathrm{Re})$; the duration η of a destabilization and its interaction λ with parallel channels are predictors of the output.

There are two major options when constructing a representation of fluctuations in outputs:

1. within a single channel, set Γ to generate limit cycling in Y; or
2. store both modes, as mutually exclusive alternatives, in two cross-coupled channels.

With the latter, "$n\Gamma$" option, an interchannel cross-linkage is possible if the e terms in the recursive cubic polynomial Γ for each channel are made to be functions of the maximum of the a terms in the collateral dimensions. Functional coupling between channels has been noted by other workers (Aertsen, Erb, & Palm 1994). For the simplest case of two dimensions (2Γ models) we have

$$e_1 = \lambda_1 \cdot a_2^{-1} \quad \text{and} \quad e_2 = \lambda_2 \cdot a_1^{-1}, \quad (17)$$

where $\lambda_1 > 0$, $\lambda_2 > 0$, and $2.6 < a_{\min} < 4.4$ is a working range for $0.05 < e < 0.40$; approximately $0.20 < \lambda < 1.2$ will avoid the explosive condition (Gregson 1988, chap. 2) of $ae > 1.7$.

The advantage of writing (17) is that the number of parameters in the model is reduced by one, e_1 and e_2 are removed, and λ is introduced with $\lambda_1 = \lambda_2 = \lambda$. But this can be an oversimplification if there is any type of dominance ordering between channels. In the simplest form we have, for dimensions h, k and an unconstrained setting of parameters, that each Γ recursion is of the form

$$Y_{h(j+1)} = -a_h \cdot (Y_{hj}^* - 1)(Y_{hj}^* - i\lambda_h \cdot (a_k)^{-1})$$
$$\times (Y_{hj}^* + i\lambda_h \cdot (a_k)^{-1}) \quad (18)$$

and, correspondingly,

$$Y_{k(j+1)} = -a_k \cdot (Y_{kj}^* - 1)(Y_{kj}^* - i\lambda_k \cdot (a_h)^{-1})$$
$$\times (Y_{kj}^* + i\lambda_k \cdot (a_h)^{-1}) \quad (19)$$

(as before, $i = \sqrt{-1}$). The $n\Gamma$ models extend mathematically to as high a dimensionality n as is required, but saturation is expected to set in for $n \approx 5$ (Gregson 1992).

A graphic way to show what the NPD approach creates as a model is to draw response surfaces. We have found

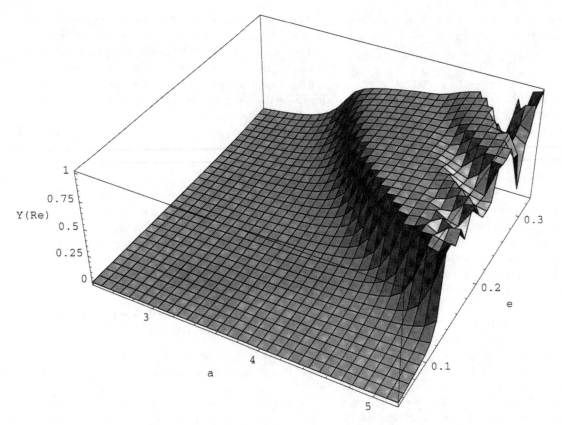

Figure 11. Response surface derived from Γ trajectories: $\eta = 11$, $c = 0.2$.

that useful software for this purpose is Mathematica. The starting point must be the response surface for Γ in its "clean" form, without delay or noise, and corresponding to (16) with

$$2.8 \leq a \leq 5.2, \quad 0.05 \leq e \leq 0.35, \quad \eta = 11.$$

This is shown in Figure 11 in perspective form with axes a and e. There is an escarpment, and sections with fixed e (or fixed a) are the predictions for notional experiments yielding the ubiquitous psychometric almost-ogival functions. The escarpment stabilizes in its shape for low η and is thereafter robust; the chaotic dynamics associated with high ae in the top right corner increase in amplitude and area with increasing η. They are not the focus of prime interest here, where the major concern is rather the preservation or corruption of the escarpment under the influence of contextual variables (such as drug action). We note that the steepness of the escarpment is a function of e for given a or of a for given e; the latter is more usual to consider.

Slower Recurrent Processes

Some recurrent behaviors are not mediated directly by the higher frequencies of brain or heart rhythms yet obviously have a physiological substrate. Examples include music generation and perception as well as some cyclical motor skills. These are of interest because they rest on some internal time-keeping mechanisms, and the search for a biological clock in the brain has been pursued repeatedly (Gregson 1995). We first consider two conceptual problems that have stimulated experimental work: whether an observer can discriminate variations in chaotic dynamics presented in time series of signals (visual or acoustic), and whether a subject can generate or replicate a chaotic series. The same problems of methodology that arose in previous sections are again met here. Gregson and Harvey (1992) showed that some chaotic sequences were discriminable, stochastically, from random noise sequences; typically, the chaotic series have recurrent embedded episodes resembling an arpeggio passage. The evidence that subjects can mimic or locally extrapolate a chaotic series is, however, equivocal; Ward and West (1994) showed that behavior could easily be misidentified in weakly designed experiments.

Another significant source of data for dynamical modeling is found in measurements that focus on a slower time scale than that of electrophysiology: reporting iterative changes in behavioral production, perception, or state assessment. State assessment may, for example, entail self-report of mood or (as earlier) headache intensity as well as clinical assessment of overt behavioral variables such as degree of depression or daily incidence of muscular tics in a patient. Iterated perception includes sequential reports of the orientation of perceptually bistable states (like the Necker cube) or time to report the contents of a 3D binocularly fusable picture of the type commonly appearing in various artistic and popular sources. Iterative production is widely implicated in musical and sports performance and also in many types of temporal and spatial control tasks (e.g., aiming, tracking, tapping, steering) that often have both ecological validity and a track record of use in controlled laboratory experimentation. Such behavioral measures can be coordinated with physiological measurements to establish, for example, correlated neural loci.

Given the orientation of contemporary nonlinear dynamics, it is natural to ask whether such behavioral time series can be successfully modeled as low-dimensional deterministic processes (perhaps with limited amounts of added noise) rather than as processes characterized by high-dimensional noise. Research based on state assessment has suggested that such an approach may bear fruit. Gottschalk, Bauer, and Whybrow (1995) reported evidence – based on observations spanning $1-2\frac{1}{2}$ years – of chaotic mood variation in bipolar disorder. The correlation dimensions of the bipolar group could be clearly distinguished from that of controls, and the power spectrum of the observations showed a $1/f^{\alpha}$ form for both groups with alpha near unity, as has been reported in spectra of other measurements of human cognition such as iterated estimation (Gilden, Thornton, & Mallon 1995; Pressing 1998b). These $1/f^{\alpha}$-type spectra are often considered to point to self-similarity in system trajectories, and they have been modeled by a variety of techniques (Pressing 1998b).

Specific evidence of chaos in depression has been claimed by Heiby (1995) and in schizophrenia by Scheier and Tschacher (1995). The finding that some psychological disorders correspond to low-dimensional organization may have implications for treatment and the understanding of the role of environmental effects. A particular form of dynamical systems theory – synergetics, founded by physicist Hermann Haken – has been influential in attempts to recast clinic practice in a dynamical mold (Haken 1987; Masterpasqua & Perna 1996; Tschacher, Schiepek, & Brunner 1992).

In the area of motor skills, it will be useful to survey experiments involving regular rhythmic motion, such as tapping a repeating temporal pattern or moving the fingers in phased coordination in space (back and forth, say, or in circles). In this domain, it has proved possible to model stable repeating behaviors such as tapping by equations based on linear white noise. In the classic work of Wing and Kristofferson (1973a,b), simple tapping was shown to be based on two types of noise source, central and peripheral. Each is white and independently distributed, but they combine in such a fashion to naturally explain the characteristic experimental finding of a negative value for the autocorrelation function of the interresponse intervals at lag 1. This work was extended to more complex temporal patterns (Jagacinksi et al. 1988; Pressing, Summers, & Magill 1996; Summers & Pressing 1994; Vorberg & Hambuch 1984). Subsequent work involving patients with focal cerebellar or basal gangliar damage (e.g. Parkinson's) has allowed the inference of physiological locations implicated in generation of these different noise sources (Franz, Ivry, & Helmuth 1996; Wing, Keele, & Margolin 1984).

Such linear noise–based models are moving average (MA) models, but the approach has also been extended to conditions of synchronized control (Pressing 1998c, 1999; Pressing & Jolley-Rogers 1997; Vorberg & Wing 1996), which qualify as autoregressive moving average (ARMA) models. In such cases it is not efficacious to postulate a deterministic nonlinear dynamics, because noise effects are experimentally large and the system is stationary and experimentally linear. Estimates of correlation dimension, for example, are typically swamped by white noise.

In contrast, other work emphasizing experimental regions of instability in performance has shown that phase transitions (or bifurcations) can occur between different states of temporal organization in coordination tasks. Such transitions implicate system nonlinearity and determinism. In the classic case of a bimanual finger-wagging or -circling task, there are two natural phase relations between the hands: in-phase or anti-phase (Haken, Kelso, & Bunz 1985). For in-phase movement, the two hands operate with mirror symmetry about the sagittal plane; in the anti-phase condition, the hands operate in parallel relation in space but opposite relative to the sagittal midline plane. (For example, if the left finger circles counterclockwise and the right finger clockwise, we have in-phase circling.)

It is found experimentally that the in-phase motion is stable over the full range of possible movement frequencies whereas the anti-phase relation is stable only for slower speeds, and a sudden transition occurs from anti-phase to in-phase if frequency is incrementally increased (Haken et al. 1985; Kelso 1984). Such transitions show the classic features of the phase transitions of physics, including critical fluctuations, critical slowing, hysteresis, and discontinuity in order parameter (relative phase between the hands) (Kelso 1994; Turvey 1990). These are the hallmarks of nonlinear dynamics, and they allow interpretations of self-organization of the motor system.

The modeling used to describe such systems has exploited simple dynamical maps of the circle map class, differential analogs of them, or differential equations of nonlinearly coupled oscillators (Beek & Beek 1988; Pressing 1998a). These models have been successful in mimicking the phase transition behavior of real motor data. Here the fundamental equations are considered to be deterministic albeit with the presence of high-dimensional noise. This means that, in practice, dimensional and entropic indicators are not efficient discriminators. Instead, the analytical approach has been more geometrical, showing that the qualitative nonlinear and transitional behaviors of the system can be matched by the proposed system equations for a suitable range of parameters. The architects of this method have been Scott Kelso, Michael Turvey, Hermann Haken, and co-workers.

Conclusion

We have chosen and reviewed a range of dynamic models with actual or potential use for describing behavior that simultaneously implicates psychology and physiology. We have illustrated both the **A** and **B** approaches by example, sometimes (but not always) drawing on chaotic dynamics. The mathematical structure of these models necessarily varies as a reflection of the precision and extent of real data that can be represented by them – and also as a reflection of the desire to focus either on the stable end-products of dynamics or on the internal mediating processes between stimulus and response, evolving in real time. There is an infinity of dynamical models that could be created. There is no single counterpart to the ubiquitous general linear model of experimental design statistics, nor should there be.

In choosing between models, the researcher should ideally have high-fidelity records extending through time and identifiably linked to psychological states. The need for metric properties of response measures is greater for nonlinear models, except for the simplest model that we have illustrated. The knowledge of underlying brain processes can be used a priori to eliminate intrinsically implausible theories but *not* to pin down unambiguously which model is most valid. From the formal mathematics of automata theory it is known that this ambiguity is not resolvable (Shannon & McCarthy 1956). Using only externally observable behavior, we cannot sufficiently identify the links between brain and behavior, or between brain and consciousness, which are the proper fundamental concern of the psychologist.

The emergence of real-time data based collectively on MRI (magnetic resonance imaging), PET (positron emission tomography), and EEG recordings of brain activities over wide regions of the cortex, which are synchronous with conscious experience and behavior, will in the long run change the scope of psychophysiology irreversibly. The intrinsic complexity of such recordings, extended in space and time, demands computational dynamics that we can confidently predict will eventually transcend the subtlety and complexity of any examples described in this chapter. Modern literature in the field (e.g. Nunez 1995) shows an increasing focus on making distinctions between levels of cortical action, each with its own dynamics and each level needing its own mathematical representation. We have in the examples chosen here deliberately set out to illustrate such different levels, suggesting representations that can be tractable and interpretable for each.

Glossary of Technical Terms Used in Dynamics

affine   This term describes linear transformations from one set of variables to another. Most simply, an affine transformation from x to x' is of the form $x' = a + bx$.

aliasing   In recording or sampling data, if the sample rate is s then frequencies above $s/2$ cannot be faithfully recorded (Nyquist theorem). Higher frequencies will cause a distortion known as aliasing, which is normally avoided by filtering out higher frequencies from the input before the sampling process.

approximate entropy (ApEn)   An approximate estimation of the entropy of a system based on the *correlation integral*.

ARMA modeling   Autoregressive moving average modeling of time-series data. An ARMA(p, q) model proposes that the current measurement is a linear weighted sum of p previous measurements (autoregression) and white-noise sources with maximum delay q (moving average).

attractor   A locus of points in a *phase space* (e.g., a point, cycle, or surface) that attracts neighboring dynamic trajectories to it. A "chaotic" attractor is one with a positive *Lyapunov exponent* that shows sensitive dependence on initial conditions. A "strange" attractor is one with fractal (noninteger) dimension.

autocorrelation function   The correlation between a time series $x = x_1, x_2, x_3, \ldots, x_N$ and a delayed copy of itself $x^{(k)} = x_{1+k}, x_{2+k}, x_{3+k}, \ldots, x_{N+k}$ as a function of time delay (lag = k). If cov$(\cdot)$ refers to covariance and var$(\cdot)$ to variance, then the lag-k autocorrelation of a time series is given by

$$\rho_x(k) = \text{cov}(x, x^{(k)})/\sqrt{\text{var}(x)\,\text{var}(x^{(k)})}.$$

bistable states   States of a system that can take two different values and may fluctuate in time between them, remaining in either one for an arbitrarily long period.

chaos   Noiselike behavior resulting from a low-dimensional deterministic process. The term is used in a variety of (not quite equivalent) ways, with the most common one referring to a positive *Lyapunov exponent* that indicates sensitive dependence on initial conditions.

correlation dimension   An estimate ($D2$) of the dimension of an attractor based on the *correlation integral*.

correlation integral   A function of r specifying the fraction of pairs of points in a *phase space* or embedding space that are separated by a distance r or less.

dissipative system   A system in which the portion of *phase space* representing the system activity shrinks over time, owing (for example) to energy dissipation processes such as friction.

embedding The process of forming a d-dimensional vector from a single time series by the use of delays. Specifically, if x_n is a time series and τ is a delay that is expressed in units of the sample rate, then the d-dimensional embedding of x_n is $X_n = (x_n, x_{n+\tau}, \ldots, x_{n+(d-1)\tau})$. The embedding space is the d-dimensional space spanned by the variables $x_n, x_{n+\tau}, \ldots, x_{n+(d-1)\tau}$.

entropy A quantitative measure of the degree of disorder of a system.

ergodic system An ergodic system eventually accesses all the potential states of the system, with the possible exception of a set of measure zero.

factor analysis A mathematical technique that looks to model the variation in a set of data on the basis of the effects of a small number of causative factors.

fractal Self-similar at multiple scales (of time or space). The dimension of a fractal structure will be noninteger.

Hurst exponent A parameter H ranging from 0 to 1, developed to characterize persistence and antipersistence in noise sources. Specifically, consider a correlated random walk process with the nth position given by y_n. Then H is defined by

$$\langle \Delta y^2 \rangle = \langle (y_n - y_{n-\tau})^2 \rangle \approx \tau^{2H},$$

where $H = 0.5$ corresponds to white noise and a classical random walk; other values indicate colored noise. $H > 0.5$ indicates persistence (past and future positively correlated), whereas $H < 0.5$ indicates antipersistence (past and future negatively correlated).

Julia set The boundary of the locus of points of the control parameters of a system that leads to stable (bounded) behavior.

Kolmogorov entropy The average rate of the loss of information when proceeding along a trajectory.

LID The local intrinsic dimension of a process estimated from a truncated segment of its evolution as recorded in a time series.

Lyapunov exponent A parameter indicating the rate of divergence of two initially close points in the *phase space* of a deterministic system. Specifically, given two initially close points x_0 and y_0, the trajectories from each point diverge as

$$|x_n - y_n| \approx A \cdot \exp(\lambda \cdot n),$$

where A is some constant and λ is the Lyapunov exponent. In multidimensional phase spaces, there will be a separate Lyapunov exponent in each principal direction; the effect of the largest positive exponent (if there is one) will typically dominate.

Markov process A process whose current state is directly determined by its immediately previous state but not earlier states.

noise The "unwanted" part of a signal. However, (high-dimensional) noise typically arises as a result of the averaging of many small interactions whose processes are deterministic but unknown, producing an apparently random effect. In models of causal processes, noise may occur either additively or multiplicatively.

White noise has a uniform spectral distribution. Colored noise is white noise with a spectral bias in frequency ranges, as may be caused by high- or low-pass filtering. Gaussian noise is noise whose distribution of values forms a Gaussian (normal) distribution.

PD2$_i$ A running indicator of dimensionality of an attractor based on the correlation dimension (*D2*) but with a number of criteria for inclusion and exclusion of points (see text). These criteria, it is claimed, make this indicator particularly robust in handling biological data, which are often difficult to analyze owing to high noise and shortness or nonstationarity of series.

phase randomization A process in which a signal or spectrum is decomposed into its constituent amplitudes and phases; the phases are then randomized. See *surrogate data*.

phase space A normally multidimensional space whose coordinate axes are the system variables, excluding time. A trajectory in this space depicts the time behavior of a particular set of starting conditions.

phase transition A sudden large shift in a system's behavior due to a small change in a control parameter of the system. For example, a liquid changes to a solid under the influence of a very small temperature change at the freezing point. Similar phase transitions have been seen in the nervous system and in overt behavior.

piecewise linearization The fitting of a set of data by (i) partitioning its independent variable range into two or more smaller nonoverlapping intervals and (ii) separately fitting data in each interval to a straight line.

Rényi *D2* Another name for the correlation dimension in this context. A. Rényi (1921–1970) worked extensively on the foundations of conditional probability, entropy, and information theory.

repeller Locus of points in a *phase space* (e.g., a point or a surface) that repels neighboring dynamic trajectories from it.

singular-value decomposition The reduction of a (normally complex) set of data to a small number of principal component dimensions that are primarily responsible for the observed variances in the data. Also known as principal components analysis (PCA).

surrogate data   In assessing the significance of computed nonlinear dynamical indicators like the *correlation dimension* and *Lyapunov exponent,* it is frequently useful to compare the results with those obtained from transformations of the original data, called *surrogate data.* Common types of surrogate data transformations include (i) scrambling the order of the original time series and (ii) taking a Fourier transform of the data, "phase randomizing" all points (retaining amplitude information), and then performing an inverse Fourier transform.

These transformations can help test various null hypotheses. For example, if the correlation dimension of a certain series is not significantly distinguishable from its phase-randomized surrogate, then no evidence exists that the data are in not fact colored noise rather than the results of deterministic processes.

trajectory   A path in *phase space* produced by plotting the progression of system variables in time.

Volterra kernels   A kernel is a function of two variables occurring within an integral equation. For example, in

$$y(t) = \int_{-\infty}^{+\infty} h_1(t, \tau) x(t - \tau) \, d\tau,$$

h_1 is the kernel and the equation is that of a linear time-varying system. The given case is the first Volterra kernel, which corresponds to the first term in an expansion of the function y in terms of the multiple products of x at different times.

Wiener kernels   An extension of the Volterra form, developed for efficiently representing nonlinear systems.

zero crossing   The point at which a function crosses zero.

NOTES

We are pleased to thank David Heleschewitz and Garry Jolley-Rogers for valuable assistance in data analysis and Walter Freeman for valuable discussions.
1. In higher dimensionality these are, strictly speaking, hypercubes.
2. Intuitively, a measure gives us a number indicating the relative size; for a set of formal axioms see Halmos (1950).

REFERENCES

Abarbanel, H. D. (1996). *Analysis of Observed Chaotic Data.* New York: Springer.

Aertsen, A., & Braitenberg, V. (Eds.) (1992). *Information Processing in the Cortex: Experiments and Theory.* Berlin: Springer-Verlag.

Aertsen, A., Erb, M., & Palm, G. (1994). Dynamics of functional coupling in the cerebral cortex: An attempt at a model based interpretation. *Physica D, 75,* 103–28.

Babloyantz, A., & Destexhe, A. (1986). Low-dimensional chaos in an instance of epilepsy. *Proceedings of the National Academy of Sciences U.S.A., 83,* 3513–17.

Basar, E., Flohr, H., Haken, H., & Mandell, A. J. (1983). *Synergetics of the Brain.* Berlin: Springer-Verlag.

Beek, P. J., & Beek, W. J. (1988). Tools for constructing dynamical models of rhythmic movement. *Human Movement Science, 7,* 301–42.

Beran, J. (1994). *Statistics for Long-Term Memory Processes.* New York: Chapman & Hall.

Blinowska, K. J., & Malinowski, M. (1991). Non-linear and linear forecasting of the EEG time series. *Biological Cybernetics, 66,* 159–65.

Casdagli, M. (1989). Nonlinear prediction of chaotic time series. *Physica D, 35,* 335–56.

Casdagli, M., & Eubank, S. (Eds.) (1992). *Nonlinear Modeling and Forecasting.* Redwood City, CA: Addison-Wesley.

Coenen, A. M. L. (1996). Neuronal phenomena associated with sleeping and waking: An integration [Abstract]. *Journal of Sleep Research, 5 (Suppl. 1),* 36.

Cutler, C. D. (1994). A theory of correlation dimension for stationary time series. *Philosophical Transactions of the Royal Society, Ser. A, 348,* 343–55.

Doyon, B. (1992). On the existence and the role of chaotic processes in the nervous system. *Acta Biotheoretica, 40,* 113–19.

Dunki, R. M. (1991). The estimation of the Kolmogorov entropy from a time series and its limitations when performed on EEG. *Bulletin of Mathematical Biology, 53,* 665–78.

Farmer, J. D., Ott, E., & Yorke, J. A. (1983). The dimensions of chaotic attractors. *Physica D, 7,* 153.

Farmer, J. D., & Sidorowich, J. J. (1988). Exploiting chaos to predict the future and reduce noise. In Y. C. Lee (Ed.), *Evolution, Learning, and Cognition,* pp. 277–330. Singapore: World Scientific.

Feder, J. (1988). *Fractals.* New York: Plenum.

Fell, J., Roschke, J., & Beckman, P. (1993). Deterministic chaos and the first positive Lyapunov exponent: A nonlinear analysis of the human electroencephalogram during sleep. *Biological Cybernetics, 69,* 139–46.

Franz, E. A., Ivry, R. B., & Helmuth, L. L. (1996). Reduced timing variability in patients with unilateral lesions during bimanual movements. *Journal of Cognitive Neuroscience, 8,* 107–18.

Freeman, W. J. (1994). Neural mechanisms underlying destabilization of cortex by sensory input. *Physica D, 75,* 151–64.

Freeman, W. J., & Skarda, C. A. (1985). Spatial EEG patterns, nonlinear dynamics and perception: The neo-Sherringtonian view. *Brain Research Reviews, 10,* 147–75.

Gallez, D., & Babloyantz, A. (1991). Predictability of human EEG: A dynamical approach. *Biological Cybernetics, 64,* 381–91.

Ganz, R. E., Weibels, G., Stacker, K.-H., Faustmann, P. M., & Zimmermann, C. W. (1993). The Lyapunov exponent of heart rate dynamics as a sensitive marker of central autonomic organization: An exemplary study of early multiple sclerosis. *International Journal of Neuroscience, 71,* 29–36.

Geldard, F. A. (1975). *Sensory Saltation: Metastability in the Perceptual World.* Hillsdale, NJ: Erlbaum.

Gençay, R. (1996). A statistical framework for testing chaotic dynamics via Lyapunov exponents. *Physica D, 89,* 261–6.

Gilden, D. L., Thornton, T., & Mallon, M. W. (1995). 1/f noise in human cognition? *Science, 267*, 1837–9.

Glass, L. (1995). Chaos in neural systems. In M. Arbib (Ed.), *The Handbook of Brain Theory and Neural Networks*, pp. 186–9. Cambridge, MA: MIT Press.

Gottschalk, A., Bauer, M., & Whybrow, P. C. (1995). Evidence of chaotic mood variation in bipolar disorder. *Archives of General Psychiatry, 52*, 947–59.

Grassberger, P., & Procaccia, I. (1983). Measuring the strangeness of strange attractors. *Physica D, 9*, 189–208.

Grassberger, P., Schreiber, T., & Schaffrath, C. (1991). Nonlinear time sequence analysis. *International Journal of Bifurcation and Chaos, 1*, 512–43.

Gregson, R. A. M. (1983). *Time Series in Psychology*. Hillsdale, NJ: Erlbaum.

Gregson, R. A. M. (1987). The time series analysis of self-reported headache sequences. *Behaviour Change, 4*, 6–13.

Gregson, R. A. M. (1988). *Nonlinear Psychophysical Dynamics*. Hillsdale, NJ: Erlbaum.

Gregson, R. A. M. (1992). *n-Dimensional Nonlinear Psychophysics: Theory and Case Studies*. Hillsdale, NJ: Erlbaum.

Gregson, R. A. M. (1995). *Cascades and Fields in Perceptual Psychophysics*. Singapore: World Scientific.

Gregson, R. A. M., Campbell, E. A., & Gates, G. R. (1992). Cognitive load as a determinant of the dimensionality of the electroencephalogram: A replication study. *Biological Psychology, 35*, 165–78.

Gregson, R. A. M., & Harvey, J. P. (1992). Similarities of low-dimensional chaotic auditory attractor sequences to quasi-random noise. *Perception and Psychophysics, 51*, 267–78.

Haken, H. (1987). *Advanced Synergetics*, 2nd ed. Berlin: Springer-Verlag.

Haken, H., Kelso, J. A. S., & Bunz, H. (1985). A theoretical model of phase transitions in hand movements. *Biological Cybernetics, 51*, 347–56.

Halmos, P. R. (1950). *Measure Theory*. New York: Van Nostrand.

Hediger, T., Passamante, A., & Farrell, M. (1990). Characterizing attractors using local intrinsic dimension calculated by singular-value decomposition and information-theoretic criteria. *Physics Review A, 41*, 5325–32.

Heiby, E. M. (1995). Assessment of behavioral chaos with a focus on transitions in depression. *Psychological Assessment, 7*, 10–16.

Hurst, H. E. (1965). *Long-Term Storage: An Experimental Study*. London: Constable.

Ingraham, R. L. (1992). *A Survey of Nonlinear Dynamics*. Singapore: World Scientific.

Jagacinksi, R. J., Marshburn, E., Klapp, S. T., & Jones, M. R. (1988). Tests of parallel versus integrated structure in polyrhythmic tapping. *Journal of Motor Behavior, 20*, 416–42.

Kantz, H., & Schreiber, T. (1997). *Nonlinear Time Series Analysis*. Cambridge University Press.

Kaplan, D. T., Furman, M., Pincus, S., Ryan, S., Lipsitz, L., & Goldberger, A. (1991). Aging and complexity of cardiovascular dynamics. *Biophysical Journal, 59*, 945–9.

Kelso, J. A. S. (1984). Phase transitions and critical behavior in human bimanual coordination. *American Journal of Physiology: Regulatory, Integrative, and Comparative Physiology, 15*, R1000–R1004.

Kelso, J. A. S. (1994). Elementary coordination dynamics. In S. P. Swinnen, H. Heuer, J. Massion, & P. Casaer (Eds.), *Interlimb Coordination: Neural, Dynamical, and Cognitive Constraints*, pp. 301–18. San Diego: Academic Press.

Kowalik, J. Z., & Elbert, T. (1994). Changes of chaoticness in spontaneous EEG/MEG. *Integrative Physiological and Behavioral Science, 29*, 270–82.

Ljung, G. M., & Box, G. E. P. (1987). On a measure of lack of fit in time series models. *Biometrika, 65*, 297–304.

Lutzenberger, W., Elbert, T., Birbaumer, N., Ray, W. J., & Schupp, H. (1992). The scalp distribution of the fractal dimension of the EEG and its variation with mental tasks. *Brain Topography, 5*, 27–34.

Mandelbrot, B. B. (1972). Statistical methodology for non-periodic cycles: From the covariance to R/S analysis. *Annals of Economic and Social Measurement, 1*, 259–90.

Marmarelis, P. Z., & Marmarelis, V. Z. (1978). *Analysis of Physiological Systems: The White Noise Approach*. New York: Plenum.

Marzocchi, W., Mulargia, F., & Gonzato, G. (1996). Detecting low-dimensional chaos in time series of finite length generated from discrete parameter processes. *Physica D, 90*, 31–9.

Masterpasqua, F., & Perna, P. (1996). *The Psychological Meaning of Chaos: Self-Organization in Human Development and Psychotherapy*. Washington, DC: APA.

Mayer-Kress, G. (1986). *Dimensions and Entropies in Chaotic Systems*. Berlin: Springer-Verlag.

Mayer-Kress, G., & Haken, H. (1981). The influence of noise on the logistic model. *Journal of Statistical Physics, 26*, 149–71.

Mayer-Kress, G., & Layne, S. P. (1987). Dimensionality of the human electroencephalogram. *Annals of the New York Academy of Sciences, 504*, 62–87.

Molnar, M., & Skinner, J. E. (1992). Low-dimensional chaos in event-related brain potentials. *International Journal of Neuroscience, 66*, 263–76.

Nicolis, G., & Prigogine, I. (1989). *Exploring Complexity*. New York: Freeman.

Nunez, P. L. (Ed.) (1995). *Neocortical Dynamics and Human EEG Rhythms*. New York: Oxford University Press.

Ott, E., Sauer, T., & Yorke, J. A. (1994). *Coping with Chaos*. New York: Wiley.

Palus, M. (1995). Testing for nonlinearity using redundancies: Quantitative and qualitative tests. *Physica D, 80*, 186–205.

Passamante, A., Hediger, T., & Gollub, M. (1989). Fractal dimension and local intrinsic dimension. *Physics Review A, 39*, 3640–5.

Pincus, S. (1991). Approximate entropy as a measure of system complexity. *Proceedings of the National Academy of Sciences U.S.A., 88*, 2297–2301.

Pincus, S. (1995). Approximate entropy (ApEn) as a complexity measure. *Chaos, 5*, 110–17.

Pincus, S. M., & Goldberger, A. L. (1994). Physiological time-series analysis: What does regularity quantify? *American Journal of Physiology, 266*, H1643–H1656.

Pressing, J. (1998a). Referential behaviour theory: A framework for multiple perspectives on motor control. In J. P. Piek (Ed.), *Motor Control and Human Skill: A Multidisciplinary Approach*, pp. 357–84. Champaign, IL: Human Kinetics.

Pressing, J. (1998b). Sources for 1/f noise effects in human cognition and performance. *Proceedings of the 4th Conference of the Australian Cognitive Science Society* (Newcastle).

Pressing, J. (1998c). Error correction processes in temporal pattern production. *Journal of Mathematical Psychology, 42,* 63–101.

Pressing, J. (1999). The referential dynamics of cognition and action. *Psychological Review, 106,* 714–47.

Pressing, J., & Jolley-Rogers, G. (1997). Spectral properties of human cognition and skill. *Biological Cybernetics, 76,* 339–47.

Pressing, J., Summers, J., & Magill, J. (1996). Cognitive multiplicity in polyrhythmic performance. *Journal of Experimental Psychology: Human Perception and Performance, 22,* 1127–48.

Pritchard, W. S., & Duke, D. W. (1995). Measuring "chaos" in the brain: A tutorial review of EEG dimension estimation. *Brain and Cognition, 27,* 353–97.

Ramsey, J. B., & Yuan, H.-J. (1990). The statistical properties of dimension calculations using small data sets. *Nonlinearity, 3,* 155–76.

Rapp, P. E. (1994). A guide to dynamical analysis. *Integrative Physiological and Behavioral Science, 29,* 311–27.

Rapp, P. E., Goldberg, G., Albano, A. M., Janicki, M. B., Murphy, D., Niemeyer, E., & Jimenez-Montano, M. A. (1993). Using coarse-grained measures to characterize electromyographic signals. *International Journal of Bifurcation and Chaos, 3,* 525–41.

Roschke, J., & Aldenhoff, J. (1991). The dimensionality of human's electroencephalogram during sleep. *Biological Cybernetics, 64,* 307–13.

Rosenstein, M. T., Collins, J. J., & De Luca, C. J. (1993). A practical method for calculating largest Lyapunov exponents from small data sets. *Physica D, 65,* 117–34.

Scheier, C., & Tschacher, W. (1995). Appropriate algorithms for nonlinear time series analysis in psychology. Technical report no. IFI-AI-95.03, Artificial Intelligence Laboratory, University of Zurich.

Schiff, S. J., & Chang, T. (1992). Differentiation of linearly correlated noise from chaos in a biologic system using surrogate data. *Biological Cybernetics, 67,* 387–93.

Schiff, S. J., Sauer, T., & Chang, T. (1994). Discriminating deterministic versus stochastic dynamics in neuronal activity. *Integrative Physiological and Behavioral Science, 29,* 246–61.

Shannon, C. E., & McCarthy, J. (Eds.) (1956). *Automata Studies.* Princeton, NJ: Princeton University Press.

Skarda, C. A., & Freeman, W. J. (1987). How brains make chaos in order to make sense of the world. *Behavioral and Brain Sciences, 10,* 161–95.

Skinner, J. E., Carpeggiani, C., Landisman, C. E., & Fulton, K. (1991). The correlation dimension of the heartbeat is reduced by myocardial ischemia in conscious pigs. *Circulation Research, 68,* 966–76.

Skinner, J. E., Molnar, M., & Tomberg, C. (1994). The point correlation dimension: Performance with nonstationary surrogate data and noise. *Integrative Physiological and Behavioral Science, 29,* 217–34.

Stam, K. J., Tavy, D. L. J., Jelles, B., Achtereekte, H. A. M., Slaets, J. P. J., & Keunen, R. W. M. (1994). Non-linear dynamical analysis of multichannel EEG: Clinical applications in dementia and Parkinson's disease. *Brain Topography, 2,* 141–50.

Sugihara, G., & May, R. M. (1990). Nonlinear forecasting as a way of distinguishing chaos from measurement error in time series. *Nature, 344,* 734–41.

Summers, J., & Pressing, J. (1994). Coordinating the two hands in polyrhythmic tapping. In S. P. Swinnen, H. Heuer, J. Massion, & P. Casaer (Eds.), *Interlimb Coordination: Neural, Dynamical, and Cognitive Constraints,* pp. 571–93. San Diego: Academic Press.

Takens, F. (1980). Detecting strange attractors in turbulence. In D. Rand & L. Young (Eds.), *Dynamical Systems and Turbulence* (Lecture Notes in Mathematics, no. 898), pp. 366–81. Berlin: Springer-Verlag.

Theiler, J., Galdrikian, B., Longtin, A., Eubank, S., & Farmer, J. (1992). Using surrogate data to detect nonlinearity in time series. In M. Casdagli & S. Eubank (Eds.), *Nonlinear Modeling and Forecasting.* Redwood City, CA: Addison-Wesley.

Tong, H. (1995). A personal overview of non-linear time series analysis from a chaos perspective. *Scandinavian Journal of Statistics, 22,* 399–445.

Tschacher, W., Schiepek, G., & Brunner, E. J. (Eds.) (1992). *Self-Organization and Clinical Psychology: Empirical Approaches to Synergetics in Psychology.* Berlin: Springer-Verlag.

Turvey, M. (1990). Coordination. *American Psychologist, 45,* 938–53.

Vibe, K., & Vesin, J.-M. (1996). On chaos detection methods. *International Journal of Bifurcation and Chaos, 6,* 529–43.

von Békésy, G. (1967). *Sensory Inhibition.* Princeton, NJ: Princeton University Press.

Vorberg, D., & Hambuch, R. (1984). Timing of two-handed rhythmic performance. In J. Gibbon & L. Allan (Eds.), *Timing and Time Perception,* pp. 390–406. New York Academy of Sciences.

Vorberg, D., & Wing, A. (1996). Modeling variability and dependence in timing. In H. Heuer & S. W. Keele (Eds.), *Handbook of Perception and Action,* vol. 3 (Motor Skills). London: Academic Press.

Ward, L. M., & West, R. L. (1994). On chaotic behavior. *Psychological Science, 5,* 232–6.

Watt, R. C., & Hameroff, S. R. (1987). Phase space analysis of human EEG during general anesthesia. In S. H. Koslow, A. J. Mandell, & M. F. Shlesinger (Eds.), *Perspectives in Biological Dynamics and Theoretical Medicine,* pp. 286–8. New York Academy of Sciences.

Wing, A. M., Keele, S., & Margolin, D. I. (1984). Motor disorder and the timing of repetitive movements. In J. Gibbon & L. Allan (Eds.), *Timing and Time Perception,* pp. 183–92. New York Academy of Sciences.

Wing, A. M., & Kristofferson, A. B. (1973a). The timing of interresponse intervals. *Perception and Psychophysics, 13,* 455–60.

Wing, A. M., & Kristofferson, A. B. (1973b). Response delays and the timing of discrete motor responses. *Perception and Psychophysics, 14,* 5–12.

Xu, N., & Xu, J.-H. (1988). The fractal dimension of EEG as a physical measure of conscious human brain activities. *Bulletin of Mathematical Biology, 50,* 559–65.

PART SIX

APPENDICES

CHAPTER THIRTY-FIVE

GENERAL LABORATORY SAFETY

WILLIAM A. GREENE, BRUCE TURETSKY, & CHRISTIAN KOHLER

Several agencies are responsible for the occupational safety and health of the American worker. At the federal level, the primary agency is the Occupational Safety and Health Administration (OSHA). This agency develops guidelines and standards covering millions of workers. In addition, each state can develop regulations for occupational health and safety within its borders. There are currently 25 such state plans: 23 cover both private and public sectors and two cover the public sector only. These state regulations must be at least as effective as the federal program. To learn more about the mission and responsibilities of OSHA consult *All About OSHA* (OSHA 1995a).

Your institutional safety officer should be consulted for guidance when considering specific laboratory safety procedures or designs. This chapter will outline a variety of safety considerations based on OSHA standards as well as other nationally recognized agencies to which federal and state codes look for advice, guidance, and recommendations. These agencies and codes include:

the American National Standards Institute (ANSI);
the American Society for Testing Materials (ASTM);
the National Electrical Code (NEC);
the National Fire Protection Association (NFPA);
the National Institute of Occupational Safety and Health (NIOSH);
the National Safety Council (NSC); and
Underwriters Laboratories, Inc. (UL).

Other sources that advise OSHA can be found by year in the *Federal Register–OSHA*. We will also make specific recommendations to guide principal investigators and laboratory personnel, with specific attention given to the psychophysiological laboratory.

The Development of Safety Concepts

Hammer (1989) argued that the development of effective guidelines, laws, and regulations has been based on two opposing ideas: the cost associated with accident prevention and our moral responsibility for the protection and health of human life. Previously, because of the large loss of human life and great number of accidents, pressure came from a number of sources for effective laws, regulations, and development of agencies to reduce accidents and protect the worker and the public. Slowly, adjustments and compromises yielded current guidelines and recommendations.

Another force that led to contemporary concern for safety was the changing nature of hazards and the public's knowledge and sophistication. Hollister and Trout (1979) commented that hazards in the nineteenth century were more easily recognized and simple in nature; today's hazards are more complex and not as easily recognized. Whereas accidents might previously have been limited to particular individuals or groups of workers, today's accidents may be difficult to control and can affect a large number of individuals. Sobering examples are not hard to find: in the Bhopal (India) disaster of December 1984, at least 3,500 deaths and 200,000 injuries occurred from the leak of methyl isocyanate gas (Andress 1996); the Chernobyl nuclear reactor explosion of 1986 in Northern Central Ukraine killed 31 people (according to Soviet statements) and forced more than 100,000 people to evacuate (Norton et al. 1994). Previously, 1979 witnessed the nuclear power plant accident at Three Mile Island, Pennsylvania: meltdown of the core reactor in unit 2 was 52% complete before emergency measures were able to halt the reaction. This accident resulted in the closing of seven similar plants. Couple these facts with widespread media coverage, insurance claims, and advocacy groups and it is not difficult to understand the concern expressed by federal and state legislatures in improving safety. However, implementing new legislation means new costs to businesses, corporations, and institutions of all sizes, whose resistance to change is understandable.

A perhaps more germane example involved Dartmouth College. A chemistry professor spilled "a couple of drops"

John T. Cacioppo, Louis G. Tassinary, and Gary G. Berntson (Eds.), *Handbook of Psychophysiology*, 2nd ed. © Cambridge University Press 2000. Printed in the United States of America. ISBN 62634X. All rights reserved.

of dimethyl mercury on her latex glove while working in the laboratory in August 1996. Dimethyl mercury penetrates latex gloves immediately and is then absorbed through the skin. The chemist was hospitalized in January 1997 after tests showed 80 times the lethal dosage of mercury in her blood; she died of the exposure in June 1997. OSHA proposed a fine of $13,500 against Dartmouth for not providing proper training regarding the limitations of safety gloves and for having a deficient chemical hygiene plan for the laboratory (*San Diego Union–Tribune* 1997).

The history of compensation and protection to persons and families has come to its present status from early statue law, common law, and the concept of liability. Evolving from this history was the Occupational Safety and Health Act, which became effective in 1971 and whose passage was aimed toward these ends:

To assure safe and healthful working conditions for working men and women: by authorizing enforcement of the standards developed under the act; by assisting and encouraging the State in their efforts to assure safe and healthful working conditions by providing for research, information, education, and training in the field of occupational safety and health; and for other purposes (Public Law 91-596, 1970).

The importance of accident prevention should not be underestimated. According to *Accident Facts* (NSC 1996), the leading causes of death in 1993 for all ages and both sexes were heart disease (743,460 deaths), cancer (529,904 deaths), and stroke (150,108 deaths). However, among persons of all ages, unintentional injuries were the fifth leading cause of death. Motor vehicle accidents claimed 41,893, falls killed 13,141, poison took 7,877, drowning killed 4,390, and fires and burns killed 3,900; all other unintentional injuries resulted in the deaths of 19,322. Of these 19,322 deaths, 548 deaths resulted from electric current (shock). The number of fatalities due to electric current is actually higher, since electrical arcing can ignite fires and explosions and since withdrawal reflexes from shock can result in falls. These electrical dangers are quite pertinent to the psychophysiological laboratory.

Safety Considerations for the Laboratory

OSHA maintains a website, the *Computerized Information System* (http://www.osha-slc.gov/), from which may be obtained current information regarding guidelines, standards, publications, and workplace violence. Here we provide safety checklists based on OSHA publications, information from the Centers for Disease Control, and other sources applicable to the psychophysiological laboratory.

OSHA AND THE ACADEMIC LABORATORY

According to Blanton (1988), the Occupational Safety and Health Act of 1970 did not contain recommendations

for the academic laboratory. It was not until accidents occurred in the 1970s – in which students on several campuses were burned and another student at Columbia University complained that he was being exposed to high levels of radiation in a physics laboratory – did OSHA conduct an investigation. The result was that OSHA began to take a more active interest in academic laboratories.

OSHA's attention was directed at two broad areas: concerns with "substances themselves, such as explosion, fire, and runaway reactions; and those arising from the interaction between substances and lab users, such as poisoning, contamination, and asphyxiation" (Blanton 1988, p. 15). At the time, compliance of colleges and universities to OSHA safety standards was already suspect (Steere 1973). A survey by Blanton (1988) tried to determine the cause of low compliance. Thirty-eight colleges and universities were contacted and questioned regarding problems with compliance. The problems cited most were:

1. safety budgets were too low for compliance;
2. vagueness and sometimes conflicting regulations;
3. excessive paperwork;
4. difficulty in trying to keep current with OSHA's changing standards; and
5. the lack of experience of OSHA inspectors in dealing with the research and teaching workplace.

Departments do not generally have safety budgets, and compliance would require the use of important teaching or research funds. Trying to keep current on OSHA regulations is not considered a priority for many departments, if they are even aware of OSHA standards. One might ask, Who is to do the necessary paperwork – a departmental secretary, a teaching assistant, a senior or junior professor, a special hire for the purpose? Those familiar with academic departments recognize the difficulties for each of these choices. The job may go unfulfilled unless your institution has a safety office or officer. A special assignment within an academic department would probably be resisted.

OSHA standards are often revised. On July 1 of each year, new standards are published; these July 1 standards are the new legal requirements and accordingly should be used. Earlier we referred to the OSHA website, which is continuously updated and can be consulted to obtain the most current information. Still, it is the latest July 1 published standards that are binding. Finally, note that research and teaching institutions have quite low priority within OSHA; the standards have generally been written with industry and business as the primary source of concern.

We have tried to select standards that are applicable to the psychophysiological teaching and research laboratory and that, with some commitment, will make these laboratories a safer place. By reviewing these standards, investigators can become more knowledgeable regarding safety in the laboratory in their own institutions and perhaps become advocates for improved safety.

BUILDING AND LABORATORY

General requirements believed to be applicable to the laboratory and the building housing the laboratory are presented next. The requirements presented in this section are based on OSHA standards and can be utilized as checklists to assess general safety. Many items in the given tables can be evaluated via a walk-through by the appropriate authority. Who has this authority may not be obvious, but possibilities include the institutional safety officer, the departmental chair, and the laboratory supervisor. This walk-through is highly desirable because it shows a commitment to safety by supervisors and administrators to laboratory personnel. It is further suggested that periodic inspections be carried out to determine whether any new safety hazards have developed and to demonstrate a continuing commitment to safety.

Building and Laboratory Safety: General

Table 1 presents safety requirements that can be assessed by a simple walk-through; records should be kept of compliance and discrepancies. Where hazards are noted, every effort should be made to eliminate them.

Items 1, 6, 8, 10, 11, 12, 14, and 15 of Table 1 should be provided in the design of the building. Attempt to make corrections, if this has not been accomplished. For compliance with item 2, it should be noted that there are standard hazard signs for posting. Hammer (1989) discussed some of the properties for warning devices for each of the senses (vision, hearing, etc.). Item 3 addresses emergency evacuation in case of fire, chemical spills, or other emergencies in which rapid egress is necessary. During fires, smoke can restrict vision and exit doors can be confused with nonexit doors. The necessity for clearly marking these exit doors is obvious but not always done. Moreover, some persons do not function well during emergencies and so guidance needs to be obvious and unambiguous for exiting an area. Keeping areas clear (item 9) for freedom of movement protects personnel during emergencies and tends to decrease bruises, abrasions, cuts, and head trauma. Impress on laboratory personnel the necessity for keeping passageways clear and the laboratory neat and orderly. Minor inspections for item 9 can be accomplished each time the supervisor enters the area.

TABLE 1. Building and Laboratory: Safety Checklist

1. Provide exits sufficient for prompt escape in the case of emergency.
2. Post appropriate signs for such items as harmful radiation, biohazards, microwave, room capacities, and exits.
3. Any door that is not an exit but could be mistaken for an exit must be marked NOT AN EXIT.
4. Keep all laboratory areas – including storerooms – in a clean, orderly, and sanitary state.
5. Keep all work surfaces dry. Floors should be slip-resistant.
6. Provide illumination adequate for the laboratory work being done.
7. Keep all aisles and passageways clear and with adequate headroom.
8. Provide elevated surfaces of more than 30 inches (76.20 cm) above the floor or ground with standard guardrails.
9. Stacked supplies, equipment, and materials should be stacked to prevent tipping, falling, rolling, spreading, or collapsing.
10. All exit signs are to be marked and illuminated with a reliable light source.
11. Provide directions to exits with visible signs if point of exit is not apparent.
12. Exit signs must have lettering at least 5 inches (12.7 cm) high, with each letter at least 1/2 inch (1.27 cm) wide.
13. Do not block exits.
14. Doors on cold storage rooms must be provided with an inside release mechanism even when the door is locked from the outside.
15. If a door between two rooms swings in both directions then install a viewing panel.
16. Written standard operating procedures must be available for the use of laboratory equipment.

Item 13 is also important: stacking boxes or other items against the outside of exit doors is easy to do for the unwary. In one case, a rug placed outside an exit door was too thick for the door to open wide enough for exit; the door would open several inches and then bind, completely blocking the passage. To correct this simple oversight required several phone calls, and two weeks elapsed before correction. Item 16 requires the laboratory supervisor to provide written instructions for the use of equipment and suggests that personnel be trained in its use. Particularly in academic settings, many students do not understand the principles of operation of important pieces of equipment. Also, the number of students using the equipment is often large and frequently changing. The necessity of adequate training under these conditions is a constant; printed instructions and training should be of high priority.

Gas Cylinders

The psychophysiology laboratory may have need of pressurized gases for a variety of purposes, including compressed air for cleaning and the use of oxygen and nitrogen with metabolic carts. Hammer (1989) discussed hazards associated with compressed gases and their enclosing cylinders: explosions, the cylinder as a fast-moving projectile, the whipping motion of lines and hoses connected to the cylinder, the cutting and penetrating action on the flesh of gas under pressure, and of course the toxic and explosive

TABLE 2. Compressed Gas Cylinders: Safety Handling

1. Compressed gas cylinders must be regularly inspected for obvious defects, deep rusting, and leakage.
2. Be especially careful of damaging safety valves and relief valves when handling and storing.
3. Keep cylinders away from heat, elevators, stairs, and gangways.
4. Mark empty cylinders and close their valves.
5. In places where cylinders are in use or stored, post signs reading DANGER – NO SMOKING, MATCHES, OR OPEN LIGHTS.
6. When moving cylinders, remove regulators and put on valve protection caps.
7. Use red to identify fuel gas hoses, green for oxygen hoses, and black for inert gas and air hoses.
8. Cylinders with water weight over 30 pounds (13.5 kg) must be equipped with a valve protection device or with a collar or recess for valve protection.
9. Cylinders must be marked to clearly identify their contents.
10. Place valve protectors on cylinders not in use.
11. Close cylinder valves before moving the cylinder, when the cylinder is empty, and when the cylinder is not in use.

effects of some gases on escape. Hammer presents a strong case for securing cylinders:

Spectacular accidents have occurred when such charged cylinders were dropped or struck so the valve breaks off. The cylinder would then take off, in some cases smashing through buildings, rows of vehicles, and creating tremendous havoc that a heavy steel projectile traveling at high speeds can generate. Computations indicate that if a valve is broken off, a cylinder filled to 2,500 psi can reach a velocity of 50 feet per second in 1/10 second. (p. 327)

The use of gas-containing cylinders requires special precautions. In order to be useful, the gas pressure contained in the cylinders must be greater than the surrounding pressure, usually atmospheric (14.7 psi at standard temperature at sea level). Pressure within the cylinder can overcome the containing cylinder or cylinder valves and result in dangerous explosions or hazardous leaks. The pressure within vessels will increase in a nonlinear manner with increasing temperature, which can result from storage in a warm environment produced by the sun, space heaters, or radiators. For example, the vapor pressure of carbon dioxide at 70°F is 835 psi; "doubling" the temperature (to 140°F) more than triples the vapor pressure – to 2,530 psi. Special precautions must always be used in dealing with substances under pressure, and only qualified persons should attempt to repair, remove, or install lines and valves. Table 2 presents OSHA standards for the safe use of pressurized gas cylinders pertinent to the psychophysiology laboratory.

Fire Safety

According to the National Safety Council (1996), there were 6,588 deaths in the workplace in 1994 from all causes. Of these, 105 were due to fire and 97 were caused by explosions; this is 1.6% and 1.4% (respectively) of all deaths

due to accidents. There is always a chance for fire to begin in the laboratory when electrical apparatus is operating or when combustible materials are present. Using data from The National Fire Protection Association Standards (1990), Hoeltge and colleagues (1993) reported that, between 1986 and 1990, there were 101 fires annually in health-care laboratories and 68 in chemical or medical laboratories, resulting in a total of 13 worker injuries and $1,522,000 in property damage. These data do not include many other types of laboratories conducting research in university settings or laboratories not classified as primarily chemical or medical. Hoeltge et al. (1993) also reported that the major ignition source was a short circuit or ground fault (discussed later in the section on electrical safety). Fire safety is very important both for the laboratory worker and for participants in research projects. Table 3 lists safety guidelines and standards consistent with OSHA requirements, and it can be used as a safety checklist. It is also important to consult with local codes and your safety officer regarding compliance, as local codes may be different for your laboratory. An interesting question to pose is whether your safety officer has any idea of the type of equipment and substances you are using, particularly if you are not in a hospital or chemistry laboratory. (See Table 1 for general building and laboratory safety requirements.)

We now comment more extensively on some items listed in Table 3. Item 3 regulates the use of fire extinguishers. Fire extinguishers are not required if the employer has established and implemented a written fire safety policy that requires immediate and total evacuation from the workplace on the activation of an approved fire alarm. Item 4 designates the appropriate type of fire extinguisher for different hazards. OSHA standards require that the distance of travel to a type-A extinguisher for type-A hazards be 75 feet (22.9 m) or less and 50 feet (15.2 m) or less for type-B hazards and extinguishers; type-C extinguishers are to be located in a pattern that is appropriate to the area and to the distribution of class-A and class-B hazards, and type-D extinguishers need to placed within 75 feet (22.9 m) or less from class-D hazards.

Item 5 is particularly important in the academic laboratory because some of the personnel (undergraduate and graduate students) are transitory; thus, a regular training program needs to be maintained whenever new persons join the laboratory team. Items 6 and 7 are especially important in the student environment. A fire extinguisher is a life- and property-saving apparatus, but it may be stolen or utilized for other purposes. The laboratory supervisor must determine that the fire extinguishers are fully charged and that the plastic or wire loop on each trigger is intact.

Item 9 needs to be coordinated with your local safety officer or department, if you have one; if not, then the laboratory supervisor is responsible. Items 10 and 11 are the responsibility of the safety officer, safety department, or building supervisor. However, the laboratory supervisor can assume responsibility for determining whether the evaluations are being carried out. Help on items 12–17 can be obtained from the commercial suppliers who manufacture the hazardous material you may be using. These suppliers can also help choose storage containers for the material.

EMERGENCIES

Planning for emergencies, following safe practices, and designing safe buildings and laboratories is the best preparation for emergencies. Emergencies can occur in the laboratory owing to a number of hazards: fires, explosions, radiation, contact with electrical current, chemical spills, contact or release of pathogens, traumatic injuries to persons, earthquakes, floods, power failure, and one of the latest recognized hazards – workplace violence. In addition, in the psychophysiology laboratory there are cardiovascular risks due to the imposition of stressful psychological or physical conditions. Space limitations restrict treatment of each of the particular hazards, but additional discussion can be found in Hammer (1989) and Keith (1990). In later sections, specific guidelines will be given regarding electrical current, blood-borne pathogens, and cardiovascular risk, since these dangers are more prevalent in the psychophysiology laboratory. In this section we will give general guidelines and standards regarding preparation for – and response to – emergencies. More comprehensive treatments can be found in two manuals produced by OSHA (1992, 1995b) and in Hammer (1989) and Keith (1990). Much of the information presented here is based on these writings.

One of the first questions to be asked and answered by the laboratory director is: What are the hazards for which preparation is necessary? Answering this question will require a "hazards inventory" of the laboratory. Keith (1990) discussed several hazards that are likely to be found in a laboratory: chemical spills, fire, explosions, toxic gas release, and radioactive or biological contamination. We

---

TABLE 3. Fire Safety Checklist and Guidelines

1. Exits must open onto the street or other space that gives safe access to a public way.
2. Two exits are necessary when one of them may be blocked by fire or smoke (see local codes).
3. Determine from your local codes if portable fire extinguishers are necessary for your facility.
4. If fire extinguishers are necessary, then they should be of adequate number and type: type-A, ordinary combustible material files; type-B, flammable liquid, gas, or grease fires; type-C, energized electrical equipment fires; type-D, combustible metals (magnesium, titanium, zirconium, sodium, potassium).
5. If fire extinguishers are present then laboratory personnel must be familiar with the types of extinguishers available and be trained in their use.
6. Fire extinguishers must be serviced, maintained, and tagged at least once per year.
7. Fire extinguishers are to be kept fully charged and in their designated places.
8. Post NO SMOKING signs in areas where flammable or combustible materials are used or stored.
9. If your facility is especially subject to fires or explosions then the local fire department needs to be made aware of your laboratory.
10. Make sure your fire alarm is functional and certified.
11. Responsible parties must test your fire alarms at least once per year.
12. Solvents for cleaning are to have a flash point of 100°F or more.
13. Use approved containers for storage and handling of flammable and combustible liquids.
14. Keep all flammable liquids in closed containers when not in use.
15. Stored flammable and combustible materials must be in rooms with explosion-proof lights.
16. Storage rooms for flammable and/or combustible materials must have mechanical or gravity ventilation.
17. Keep all solvent wastes and flammable liquids in fire-resistant, covered containers.

---

might add the danger of cardiovascular incidents, contact with electrical current, and workplace violence. Hence, the first step in planning for emergencies is to determine what type of emergencies the laboratory is likely to incur.

After the hazards inventory, the next step is developing a written plan of action for each identified type of emergency. This plan should be kept in a central file, and all laboratory personnel should receive a copy. The plan is to include Material Safety Data Sheets for all toxic substances used. These forms are available from the manufacturer and specify precautions regarding handling, storing, and using the material; they also outline emergency and first-aid procedures. It is advisable that the written plan include a rewriting of the data sheets in simple language so that all persons involved can understand them. You should check with your institutional safety officer or safety department, who may have special procedures in place for clean-up of the materials you are using. The written plan must give in detail what is expected of each category of person in the laboratory. Responsibilities range from administering first aid to clean-up or simply sounding the alarm and then leaving the area. For industry, OSHA (1995b) stipulates that, at a minimum, the written plan must contain:

(1) emergency escape procedures and emergency escape assignments, (2) procedures to be followed by employees who remain to perform (or shut down) critical plant [read "laboratory"] operations before the plant is evacuated, (3) procedures to account for all employees after emergency evacuation has been completed, (4) rescue and medical duties for those employees who are to perform them, (5) the preferred means for reporting fires and other emergencies, and (6) names and regular job titles of persons or departments to be contacted for further information or explanation of duties under the plan. (p. 1)

We also view these six items as the minimum; additional features may be required in light of the discussion in this section. The emergency plan needs to be reviewed with laboratory personnel at its inception, when changes to the plan are made, and with all new laboratory workers. It is necessary to assign responsibilities to laboratory personnel. Someone needs to be designated as the in-charge person during all laboratory operations. Specific duties and responsibilities must be spelled out to avoid confusion.

After potential hazards have been identified, Material Safety Data Sheets have been obtained, and a plan has been written and distributed to laboratory personnel, the next step is to train all laboratory personnel regarding (i) every potential hazard to which they might be exposed and (ii) how to protect themselves and laboratory participants. After training, the laboratory director has the responsibility of ensuring the effectiveness of such training. Ideally, this would entail practical examinations and written tests. Review the training and testing for each regular laboratory worker at least twice each year. For all new laboratory personnel, have them undergo the training as soon as they become working members of the laboratory. Different hazards require different plans of action. At the least, personnel should: (a) alert others regarding the emergency; (b) activate the emergency plan relevant to the hazard; (c) contain or neutralize the hazard (or, if this is not possible, call the appropriate emergency numbers); and (d) evacuate the area, if necessary.

The following emergency scenario underscores the importance of designating responsibilities and the need for an emergency action plan. Two students are conducting a stress study, and the participant reports feeling faint and nauseated. The ECG (electrocardiogram) is being monitored and shows significant S-T segment depression (discussed later in the section on monitoring participant safety). Suddenly, the participant slumps forward and strikes her head on the edge of an amplifier; bleeding ensues, and she appears to be unconscious. What is to be done? Assume that both students have been trained in CPR (as they should have been) or even are first-aid certified. If one student has been designated as the in-charge

person by the laboratory supervisor, then responsibilities can be carried out according to the emergency plan. The emergency plan can direct: (a) one person to begin CPR, if necessary; (b) the second person to stop the blood flow (first aid) following universal precautions (discussed in the section on preventing infection); and (c) one of the pair to call the emergency telephone number as soon as possible. Confusion will remain at a minimum if personnel have been trained and the line of authority is clear. Of course, the person using the telephone must know the laboratory room number and must be able to inform emergency personnel how to locate the room. The person telephoning – if not needed for CPR or blood flow control – can then move to a strategic location and direct the emergency team when it arrives. Other types of emergencies will likewise result in efficient action *provided* a plan has been developed, the lines of authority are clear, and each person knows what action to take according to the plan.

Table 4 lists other items to facilitate the emergency plan. Note the necessity of posting telephone and room numbers. Laboratory personnel need to be familiar with the location of the nearest telephone. The suggested posting must be clearly visible at the telephone and other locations in the laboratory, and it should display the following.

1. Telephone number of the laboratory or the nearest telephone.
2. Room number(s) of laboratory.
3. Directions to the laboratory from the nearest main street and the name of that street.
4. A listing of laboratory personnel with their telephone numbers and titles:
   a. laboratory supervisor;
   b. laboratory assistant supervisor;
   c. laboratory personnel.
5. Emergency telephone numbers:
   a. 911, if this service is available;
   b. institutional safety officer or department;
   c. security;
   d. local police department;
   e. local fire department;
   f. nearest medical aid.
6. Location of laboratory first-aid kit (or nearest first-aid kit).
7. Person certified to administer first aid for the laboratory and telephone number.
8. Places of exits from laboratory and building.
9. Place where "spill kit" packages are stored (if available), or name and telephone number of the individuals responsible for spill clean-up.
10. Location of fire alarms (if any).
11. Warning that elevators are not to be used during emergencies.

Basic Safety Training for Laboratory Personnel

We have covered the necessity of developing a safety plan for the laboratory. It was also noted that laboratory personnel should receive training on the plan and should practice emergency responses as specified in the plan. In this section we describe the specific skills and information that are required for safe laboratory operation.

Cardiopulmonary Resuscitation (CPR). All personnel should receive CPR training and have in their possession a valid card. The training can be obtained from either the local fire department or Red Cross chapter. Hospital employees can usually become certified at their place of employment. The CPR card is valid for one year and must then be renewed. The laboratory supervisor should keep a photocopy of this card on file.

First Aid and Safety. First-aid training is advisable and is available from your Red Cross chapter. All laboratory personnel are advised to obtain such training. The first-aid card is valid for three years and then must be renewed. Photocopies of these cards should also be kept on record.

Basic Electricity and Electronics. We recommend that a basic understanding of electricity be obtained. Training gives laboratory personnel a better understanding of the dangers involved in working with electrically powered apparatus and forewarns against making errors. In later sections, we discuss working more safely with electricity and point out errors likely to be made (but we do not cover electricity basics). For basic theory we recommend Marshall-Goodell, Tassinary, and Cacioppo (1990) or Simpson (1995).

Laboratory Apparatus. Each laboratory will have a unique configuration of apparatus for its research needs. Each member of the laboratory should have an understanding of the operation of the equipment, the physiological response that it measures, and basic trouble shooting for malfunction. Such information will result in more reliable and valid data recording, help the operator to detect improper apparatus function, and guide the researcher in determining the difference between equipment malfunction and anomalous responses from participants.

Fire Extinguishers. If your laboratory is responsible for initial containment of fires, then training in the proper use of fire extinguishers is necessary. In addition, laboratory personnel need to be knowledgeable regarding the appropriate type of fire extinguisher for each of the different classes of combustible materials. Relevant information is printed on the fire extinguisher and should be in the emergency action plan. Consult with your fire department for information and advice as needed.

TABLE 4. Emergency Preparation Checklist

1. Post emergency telephone numbers where they can be seen easily.
2. Post the room number(s) of the laboratory and have a written description of how emergency personnel can locate the laboratory.
3. Know the location of the nearest hospital, clinic, or infirmary for medical care. Know what arrangements have been determined for transport to that facility or develop such arrangements.
4. All laboratory personnel who are expected to respond to medical emergencies should: (a) be first-aid certified; (b) have had hepatitis-B vaccination; (c) have had appropriate training to protect themselves from blood-borne pathogens, including universal precautions; and (d) have available and be able to use appropriate protective gear (e.g., gloves and masks) for protection against blood-borne pathogens. OSHA has determined that individuals who give first aid as only an ancillary part of their laboratory work need not have pre-exposure hepatitis-B vaccination. However, following exposure to blood or other potentially infectious materials, the incident must be reported and the exposed individual must be offered the opportunity for hepatitis-B vaccination within 24 hours of the incident.
5. Following exposure, an immediate medical evaluation and then a medical follow-up is necessary.
6. Medically approved first-aid kits should be made available in the laboratory. The kits must be inspected periodically and supplies replenished when necessary.
7. In laboratories working with toxic or corrosive materials, a quick flush system must be available for the eyes and body.
8. Develop a comprehensive emergency plan.

Cardiovascular Risk. Many laboratories intentionally stress participants for research purposes. These stressors are usually benign for the healthy person; with participants who are at risk for cardiovascular or health problems, emergencies are more likely to occur. These concepts are covered at length in a later section, which also lists agencies offering advanced training. However, if at-risk participants are to be processed, then special training and certification should be obtained or a certified person should be present in the laboratory with the necessary emergency equipment.

Universal Precautions. If laboratory personnel must handle blood or other potentially infectious materials, then familiarity with universal precautions is necessary (see the section on preventing infection).

Auditory Stimuli

Auditory stimuli are utilized in the psychophysiological laboratory for several purposes: conditioned stimuli, unconditioned stimuli, masking, startle, discrimination learning, and signal detection. Our concern is the intensity with which these stimuli are presented. Intensity of auditory stimuli is measured with a sound pressure level (SPL) meter, which is designed to measure sound intensity in decibels (dB). An intensity of 10^{-12} W/cm² corresponds to the threshold of hearing for a 1,000-Hz sine wave tone. Decibels are defined as follows:

$$\text{number of decibels} = 10 \log_{10}(I_W/I_{WT}),$$

where I_W denotes intensity (in watts) of the stimulus and I_{WT} is the hearing threshold as just defined. Evaluating this equation shows that the threshold for hearing at 1,000 Hz is 0 dB. Normal speech is about 60 dB, heavy traffic is about 100 dB, and a large jet engine at 22 m is about 120 dB. An SPL meter has three basic scales (A, B, and C) as well as fast and slow response times. The human ear is less sensitive to low-frequency sounds. The A scale approximates the response of the human ear by attenuating low frequencies in measuring dB level; most measurements of auditory stimuli for humans utilize the A scale. The slow scale responds more slowly to peak intensities. Because we are concerned with these peak intensities for sudden onset (startle) tones, it is necessary to use the fast scale when measuring very short-duration stimuli with rapid rise times.

NOISE EXPOSURE LIMITS

In order to avoid damage to hearing, limits on noise exposure have been established by OSHA. In the psychophysiology laboratory the use of noise for experimental purposes and the gathering of data in noisy environments require that investigators be aware of limits of exposure and follow OSHA standards and guidelines. Assessment of noise exposure requires evaluating both the intensity of the noise and its duration. Table 5 presents the exposure limits beyond which a person must wear protective hearing devices. The left column presents the time of exposure in hours for a given intensity of noise; the right column shows the intensity. All measurements are taken with an SPL on scale A with slow response time. For example, a person exposed to 90 dBA for 8 hr or more in a working day must wear hearing protectors that reduce the noise to 85 dBA (as specified by OSHA, which also reviews acceptable

attenuators). However, most exposures to noise are not of constant intensity. Thus, assessing noise exposure requires a "daily dose" (DD) measure of noise, which is calculated as follows:

$$DD = (C_1/T_1 + C_2/T_2 + \cdots + C_n/T_n) \times 100,$$

where C_n denotes the total exposure at a specified noise level and T_n is the total time of exposure at that noise level. If DD exceeds 100 then noise attenuators must be worn. OSHA also stipulates that any worker exposed to noise at 85 dBA for an 8-hr period must have a baseline audiogram completed within six months of the first exposure. If a specified hearing loss is detected at the twelve-month follow-up, then attenuators are required. A hearing loss (standard threshold shift) is defined by OSHA as an average drop of 10 dBA or more at 2 kHz, 3 kHz, and 4 kHz in either ear. Annual audiograms are then required for comparison against the original baseline. Recent OSHA recommendations may change the requirements from 85 dBA to 82 dBA both for required testing and for noise attenuators. If your laboratory may be subject to these standards then the latest OSHA requirements should be consulted. A general discussion of noise exposure can be found in NIOSH (1972).

IMPACT NOISES

No sound should ever be presented to a participant with an intensity of 140 dB or more. Such intense noises can permanently damage the hearing mechanism. Although the ear has a built-in protective reflex to dampen loud sounds, this reflex requires 80 msec to operate (Guyton & Hall 1996) and cannot protect against such intense noises. Because of experimental data (Henderson et al. 1991) and the earlier recommendations of NIOSH (1972), OSHA will probably recommend that unprotected noise exposure at or above 115 dBA not be allowed. We have reviewed recent literature on the utilization of sound stimuli in the journal *Psychophysiology* and found that the proscribed level has not been used. During 1997, the loudest sound used was 110 dBA of 1-sec duration (Gautier & Cook 1997); in 1996, the most intense was 106 dB in 50-msec bursts of white noise (Bradley, Cuthbert, & Lang 1996). These short durations at the intensities used are within the OSHA guidelines. All things considered, it is reasonable to limit exposure to intensities no greater than 115 dBA.

Electrical Safety

The National Safety Council (1996) estimates that the total number of deaths due to "contact with electrical current" was 346 out of a total of 6,588 workplace deaths in 1994, making up 5.3% of fatalities. As the titles of the various chapters in this *Handbook* suggest, it is not

TABLE 5. Comparison Table of Daily Duration to Allowable Sound Level

Daily Duration (hours)	Allowable Sound Level
8.0	90
6.0	92
4.0	95
2.0	100
1.0	105
0.5	110
0.25	115

Note: Sound-level units are dBA, slow-response SPL.
Source: Code of Federal Regulations (1996), Table G-16.

possible to work in the area of psychophysiology without using equipment powered by electrical energy. The hazard of contacting electrical current is always present. This section will present several concepts requisite to understanding electrical hazards and the prevention of electrical accidents.

The damage caused by contact with electrical current can result in involuntary reflexes, burns, cardiac fibrillation, ventricular standstill (asystole), tissue and organ destruction, and death. Reflexes may lead to falls or forceful contact with other hazardous materials or with containers of those materials, leading to spills or fires. Burns result from the heat generated by short circuits, contact with overheated electrical elements, and the passage of high current levels through the skin or deeper tissue. Low levels of current passing through the heart can result in cardiac fibrillation, and higher levels can result in complete cardiac arrest. Current passing through the respiratory muscles can stop the ability to breathe, and higher currents passing through the brainstem can damage the respiratory center and lead to asphyxiation even after the current is withdrawn. The sources of these currents reside in electrically powered apparatus, power lines serving that apparatus, static electricity, and (infrequently) lighting strikes entering equipment or laboratory when buildings or apparatus are improperly grounded.

PROTECTION AGAINST SHOCK: INTRODUCTION

Several strategies may be used to reduce the hazard of contact with injurious electrical current. As mentioned earlier, the possibility of contact always exists when working with electrically powered equipment. In this section we will present means to increase safety by several routes: use of battery-powered equipment, optic fiber connections, electrical isolation, grounds and grounding, ground fault interrupter circuits, double insulation, and minimizing the possibility of injury by lightning strikes.

Use of Battery-Powered Equipment

The battery voltages used to power electrophysiological monitoring equipment are generally quite low, usually 9 V DC or less; current flow through the skin is therefore minimal. Cleaned, abraded, intact skin may have as few as 5,000 ohms between recording electrodes. All 9-V battery voltage applied to the recording electrodes would only produce a current flow ($I = E/R$) of 1.8 mA. Batteries are completely isolated from ground, so no current can flow from battery to ground. Battery-operated equipment is very safe, but there are disadvantages and some dangers. Remember that pacemakers and implantable defibrillators for the heart can apply a brief voltage to keep the heart operating and can reverse a fibrillating heart; the circuits powered by the battery step up the voltage, thereby

dropping the current. However, once the protective skin layer is broken, impedance drops precipitously and even a 9-V battery supplying current across the heart is unsafe. Furthermore, battery-powered devices may be connected to recording devices that are usually line powered, so the safety features of the battery can be defeated unless isolating or current-limiting circuits are used. Batteries need recharging or replacement, which can prove inconvenient and incur extra costs. Finally, some batteries will explode if improperly connected to the charger or if overheating occurs. For example, in 1979 the Federal Aviation Administration disallowed the use of all lithium sulfur dioxide batteries in U.S. registered aircraft because of several explosions (Hammer 1989).

Optic Fiber Connections

Another safety option is to connect the participant with sensors that are coupled to amplifiers by optical cables. Using this method, no shock is possible. The fiber optical cables are nonconductive – light is used to carry the information from the subject to the amplifiers. This method gives protection from shock due to accidental ground contact and avoids ground loops (shock from contact with ground and ground loops is discussed two sections hence). However, special circuits are required for optical amplifiers. Also, because no ground contact is used, the signals can be quite noisy in an electrically active environment.

Electrical Isolation

Electrical hazards may be reduced by isolating the participant from ground. In the psychophysiology laboratory this technique is made more difficult when the participant is connected directly to the monitoring apparatus. Isolation transformers separate energized equipment from the grounded primary circuits of the transformer. Therefore, the inadvertent touching of a "hot" source and any earth ground by the experimenter or the participant does not result in a shock, since there is no pathway back to earth ground. Isolation transformers may be purchased for just this purpose. Some commercial equipment is designed with isolation circuits already installed. The popular Minnesota Impedance Cardiograph™ uses such circuitry. When purchasing equipment, determine if the apparatus is designed with isolating circuitry.

When using an isolated circuit, shock hazards are still present. If a person contacts both the hot wire and the neutral wire of an isolation transformer, a shock will be delivered. Unqualified personnel should not attempt repairs. Apparatus should be de-energized when being repaired, connected to, or disconnected from other energized equipment. A second danger occurs if a conductor from the secondary system accidentally contacts ground. Because there is no return path to the grounded neutral of the line power in an isolated system, usual protective devices like fuses or circuit breakers do not operate. Hence, if the second conductor contacts ground, "a short circuit will occur with possible disastrous consequences, such as ignition of ether vapors by arc or a lethal shock to personnel" (McPartland & McPartland 1996, p. 1121). Therefore, an ungrounded isolation system must give visual and auditory warning if such a contact to ground occurs. Suppliers can give the necessary specifications of transformers for a particular laboratory use. You should determine whether the isolation transformer is constructed with the necessary warning alerts should a ground contact occur.

Grounds and Grounding

Electrical service systems for most laboratory apparatus appear at the electrical receptacle into which cords are plugged for powering apparatus. The voltage is about 120 V AC in the United States and Canada. The plug is generally three-pronged and of a standard configuration. The small short blade contacts the ungrounded or "power" source and the wider blade contacts the grounded side of the power source in the receptacle. The plug inserted into the wall receptacle carries current to the resistance loads in the apparatus. The third pin on the plug makes contact with a conductor in the receptacle that leads back to the grounded side of the receptacle and to physical grounds: this pin is the grounding pin. This grounding pin is longer than the other two pins and is U-shaped. Because of this configuration, the plug can be inserted only one way, and the grounding U-shaped pin is the first to make contact when inserted and the last to make contact when the plug is removed. The grounding pin detects ground faults and protects participants, operators, and equipment. The use of a grounding pin should never be circumvented by using a "cheater" adapter that permits use of a three-pronged plug with a two-slot receptacle.

A *ground fault* is said to occur when an unwanted connection is made between a power-carrying conductor and ground. When such a contact is made the object of the contact rises to the voltage level of the power source. For example, if the ungrounded current-carrying conductor in a piece of apparatus were frayed and contacted the equipment housing, the housing would rise to the voltage of the power conductor. Such contact can also be made from insulation breakdown or a broken power wire. Figure 1 shows two different conditions and the danger involved to a person contacting a faulted system. The sink is connected to earth ground through cold-water pipes with a very low-resistance path to earth. Part A of the figure shows

apparatus with a power line directly touching the metal part of the chassis. Note that the chassis is connected to earth ground by way of the grounding conductor of the third pin and also is connected with the grounded conductor (not shown). When the fault occurred, the current-carrying capacity of the circuit breaker or fuse (usually 20 or 30 amps in the laboratory) was exceeded and opened, thereby removing the fault: the chassis fell to ground potential. A person touching the apparatus and a ground, such as the sink, would not be shocked. The opening of the circuit protection device can easily be shown by Ohm's law: $I = E/R$. Assume that the voltage E at the receptacle is 120 V and that the resistance R of the chassis to ground is very low, about 1 ohm. The resulting current flow is 120 A, enough to open the circuit protection device immediately.

Now examine Part B of Figure 1, where the ground wire to earth is broken or nonexistent. What happens to the person touching the faulted chassis that has risen to 120 V? First, the equipment will continue to operate, since no large currents are detected by the circuit protector. The theoretical minimum resistance between the two hands is

Figure 1. Part A: A fault has occurred between the hot wire and the chassis; the grounding wire is intact and the circuit breaker or fuse is opened, and the person is not shocked. Part B: The grounding wire is broken, no fault is detected, and the person receives a dangerous shock.

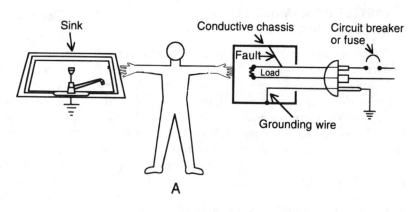

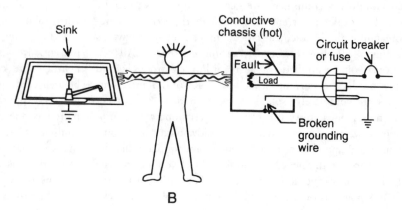

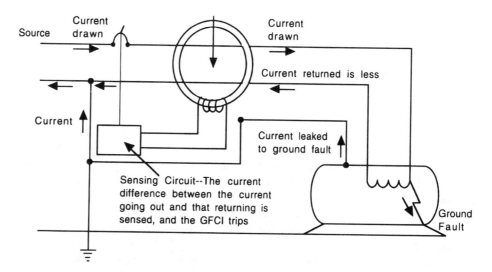

Figure 2. The ground fault circuit interrupter senses the difference between current flowing out of the power source and current returning. If a difference of 5 mA or greater is detected, power is shut off within 5 msec. Redrawn from OSHA (1983), *An Illustrated Guide to Electrical Safety,* p. 109.

500 ohms; the actual resistance is usually higher. If we use a more reasonable value of 1,500 ohms, then what is the amount of current flowing between the two hands and across the heart? Again using Ohm's law, we see that $I = 80$ mA. This 80 mA is a very dangerous shock and is within the range for initiating ventricular fibrillation. The 80 mA is much too small to activate the circuit protector, which requires 20 or 30 amps to open. If the person cannot let go of either the sink or the chassis then the person's resistance will drop even further, and current through the body and across the heart will rise.

To increase safety in the laboratory, all equipment grounding, terminals, insulation, and plugs should be checked at least twice each year (Moak 1994). We present a checklist for electrical safety in a later section. On a daily basis, it only takes a moment to determine whether grounding is intact before operating equipment.

Ground Fault Circuit Interrupter

The ground fault circuit interrupter (GFCI) should be utilized in all laboratories where the possibility exists for either the experimenter or subject to contact both the power side of electrical lines and ground – in Figure 1, this was indeed the case. The GFCIs should be installed to serve as the interface between the receptacle and the power cords supplying the equipment. In fact, GFCIs are required by electrical codes if receptacles are near cold-water pipes or water that contacts drains. It is preferable to have the GFCIs installed during laboratory construction. Figure 2 shows the mechanism of action for a GFCI. The current drawn from the power source is compared with the current returning. If a discrepancy as small as 5 mA is detected by the sensing circuit in the GFCI, the power output of the GFCI is interrupted in as little as 25 msec. Figure 2 depicts a ground fault between power and a grounded tank. If we replace the tank with a person, it can be seen that the GFCI will stop current flow through the person and prevent a severe shock.

Double Insulation

Double insulation is built into some tools and appliances (e.g., heaters, toasters, hand drills). Devices with double insulation do not have a grounding conductor to any of the conducting but non–current-carrying surfaces, so only a two-pronged plug is used to access wall receptacles. Double insulation means that, in addition to functional insulation (like the winding on a coil), there is also installed a second insulation designed to protect the user if the functional insulation should fail. If you intend to use a device that has only a two-pronged plug, first determine that the device has been approved by a recognized safety agency like Underwriters Laboratories (UL 1983).

OTHER CONCEPTS AND CONSIDERATIONS

Several miscellaneous considerations regarding electrical safety are presented next: ground loops and leakage current; the physiological effects of current; electrical polarity; lighting strikes; and current limits.

Ground Loops and Leakage Currents

Electrical charge differentials always seek to neutralize by current flow from a higher voltage to a lower one; paths to ground are one such neutralizing process. Unwanted paths can occur through: (a) frayed wiring; (b) insulation breakdown due to aging, heat, contact with corrosive chemicals, or mechanical abuse; and (c) damp or wet environments. Capacitive coupling will also induce current flow in normally non–current-carrying parts of apparatus. Any contact made between the higher voltage source and ground through any of these means will result in current flow. If the person becomes the path, shock can occur.

Another, more subtle path for current flow occurs when two or more pieces of apparatus are connected to ground at different resistances. In this case a ground loop can occur, and current will flow between the pieces of apparatus to ground if contact is made between the different devices. This contact can be made by the laboratory worker when two or more devices are touched simultaneously. Furthermore, if a laboratory participant is connected to the ground of different electronic devices with different resistances to ground, then current can flow through that individual. In addition, leakage current will flow through a subject if one piece of apparatus has a faulty ground connection.

One protection against such occurrences is to connect all pieces of apparatus to a common ground at one point in the laboratory. This can be accomplished easily by plugging equipment into a small strip outlet (but do not use multiple outlets that plug directly into the wall receptacle). The strip outlet must have a place for the ground on its plugs, and only the strip is plugged into the wall receptacle; of course, all receptacles on the strip must have a place for ground from the apparatus plug. One can measure the individual resistance of each (U-shaped) ground socket on the receptacle. Differences might be detected if a connection is loose or broken within the body of the strip. For safety, always make these measurements with the power strip unplugged from the power receptacle. To determine whether the apparatus has good ground connection, check the resistance between the U-shaped prong on the plug of the apparatus and the conductive surfaces of the apparatus (metal housing, screws, metal operating knobs, etc.). In both cases – power strip and apparatus surfaces to U-shaped prong – the ohmmeter should read a dead short: 0 ohms.

Finally, to establish whether the participant will be grounded on connection to the apparatus, determine the resistance between the ground lead (which will be attached to the subject) and the U-shaped prong on the power cord running from the device as follows. Unplug the power cord from the wall receptacle, and place one end of an ohmmeter on the ground probe of the plug and the other on the ground lead; if the measured resistance is 0 ohms then the participant will be grounded when attached. The subject will usually be grounded unless your apparatus is electrically isolated or battery-powered. Again, the importance of proper intact grounding of apparatus should be apparent.

Staewen (1994) indicated that the maximum leakage for hospital conditions – when a patient is connected to equipment – is 10 μA for source current and sink current. Source current is current that flows from connected apparatus through the person to ground; sink current (patient isolation risk current) is "current flowing from the patient to ground through a part applied to the patient due to the unintended introduction of a voltage from an external source on the patient" (p. 132). Leakage current maxima for enclosures of cord-connected apparatus remain at 100 μA under normal operating conditions and 300 μA under single-fault conditions, which include "open ground conductors; short circuit of either barrier or double insulation; failure of a single component; the application of line voltage on an isolated patient-applied part; the application of line voltage to an input or output part (or to accessible conductive hardware of the enclosure) of equipment that is not intended to be grounded" (p. 131). However, under single-fault conditions, only 50 μA are allowed for isolated patient connections and 100 μA for nonisolated connections.

If surface electrodes are to be used, then the psychophysiology participant should be treated as if in a hospital. Standard practice in the psychophysiological laboratory is to reduce skin resistance through cleaning and sometimes abrading. The protective skin resistance is purposely circumvented under some conditions, among which are: puncturing the skin for single-cell muscle fiber recording, using needle electrodes for electroencephalographic recording, and inserting indwelling catheters for automatic blood withdrawal and heparin injections. Finally, recording devices inserted into body cavities will reduce the electrical resistance between apparatus and participants. In all of these cases, adherence to appropriate low levels of leakage current (as prescribed by electrical codes) is necessary. Determine from specifications whether your laboratory equipment meets these standards.

The Physiological Effects of Electrical Current

Electrical current magnitudes that contact the body can range from the small microampere levels found in leakage currents to above 200 kA in lightning strikes. Small currents are quite likely to occur, whereas the larger currents of lightning require improbable circumstances (which do, however, occur each year). The following paragraphs enumerate the physiological effects of 60-Hz current when contact is made through intact skin (Bernstein 1994).

1. About 0.5 mA is the threshold of detection for electrical current. At this level, a small tingle is perceived.

2. At 5 mA, a definite shock is felt. This level may lead to involuntary muscle contractions and a vigorous withdrawal reflex from the electrical source. Some persons cannot let go at this intensity. The "let-go threshold" is the point at which involuntary contractions are so strong that the individual can no longer release the electrically charged object. If the person is not removed from the current then the skin impedance will continue to drop, with a simultaneous current increase.

3. At 6–25 mA (women) and 9–30 mA (men), the shock becomes quite painful and the let-go threshold is exceeded.

4. At 50–150 mA there is extreme pain. If the current is across the chest, then respiratory arrest will occur (owing

to involuntary tonic spasms of the respiratory muscles). Currents of 50 mA for 2 sec or longer can result in ventricular fibrillation. If current is not removed, death will follow. However, once fibrillation occurs, the heart seldom reverts unaided to its normal rhythm. Cardiac fibrillation is an uncoordinated twitching of cardiac fibers that generates no pumping action; CPR must be administered immediately and qualified help summoned.

5. At 500 mA, ventricular fibrillation can occur in only 0.2 sec.

6. At 1,000 mA, nerve and muscle damage occur, as well as cardiac arrest; death is highly likely. At this level, the heart will sometimes resume normal pumping action when current is removed – provided that excessive destruction of heart tissue has not occurred. Note that the lower current levels induce fibrillation whereas the higher levels induce cardiac arrest.

7. Above 10,000 mA, severe internal and external burns occur and death is most probable.

Maintaining Proper Polarity in Plugs and Receptacles

The use of receptacles, plugs, and connectors requires maintaining correct polarity between the ungrounded (hot) conductor, the grounded (neutral) conductor, and the grounding conductor. The insulation of the ungrounded conductor can be of any color except white or green. It is usually black and should be connected to the brass or black terminal on the plug (remember, "black to brass" or "black to black"). The grounded conductor must be connected to the light or nickel-colored terminal ("white or gray to light"). Finally, the grounding conductor (used to ground equipment and connected to the U-shaped probe) is to be green, green with stripes, or bare; it should be connected to the green hexagonal-head terminal screw. (Remember, "green to green" or "green to ground.") Reversal of polarities puts the operator at risk for shock.

The most dangerous reversal occurs when the ungrounded (hot) conductor is inadvertently connected to the green hexagonal terminal on the plug, the grounding conductor is connected to the brass terminal, and the grounded conductor is properly connected to the light (nickel-colored) terminal. This reversal would result in the hot conductor energizing the housing of the equipment or tool. The circuit protector would not operate, and severe shock would occur if the operator touched the housing and any ground. A less serious but still hazardous situation occurs when the ungrounded and neutral conductors are reversed. In this case, the neutral wire would be placed across the On–Off switch of the apparatus. When the switch is Off, the hot wire would still be connected to the internal parts of the device. Probing inside the tool or apparatus could result in shock. Follow these guidelines when you find it necessary to replace a plug or to check on the polarities of plugs already rewired. Clearly

understandable polarities are described and illustrated in *An Illustrated Guide to Electrical Safety* (OSHA 1983).

The laboratory worker assumes that the receptacles were wired correctly during building construction. Whether the receptacle has correct polarity is best left to a qualified electrician. However, safe plug-in testing devices (outlet circuit testers) are available in hardware stores. Skuggevig (1992) reported the results of a survey in the homes of Underwriters Laboratories employee volunteers in the 1950s to determine the percentage of receptacles wired incorrectly. The results of the survey showed that 83% of the polarized receptacles were wired correctly; 6% were incorrectly wired polarized receptacles, and 11% were non-polarized.

Comparison of the Physiological Effects of Different Frequencies

Direct current is less hazardous (at the same amperage) than 60-Hz (alternating) current; the value needed to produce a startle reflex or ventricular fibrillation is about three times higher for direct current. Moreover, there is no let-go phenomenon for DC; instead of increases in muscular contraction with increases in amperage, as occurs in AC, the experience is increasing heat. However, the act of letting go of a DC line is extremely painful: as the body part is removed, the contact area decreases and amperage per unit area rises rapidly. Reilly (1992) combined data from several sources regarding the let-go current for DC. Whereas 99.5% of volunteers refused to let go of a DC wire at 99 mA, 99.5% of volunteers could *not* let go at only 22 mA AC. This relationship also holds for the startle reflex and ventricular fibrillation; that is, the amount of current for an effect is always higher for DC than AC.

The commonly used 60 Hz is most dangerous for mammals. In the range of 10–100 Hz, let-go current is approximately the same. However, below 10 Hz and above 500 Hz, the amount of current required for a given effect increases rapidly. For example, at 5,000 Hz the let-go current is about 65 mA, whereas at 5 Hz the let-go current is approximately 50 mA (Dalziel 1943, 1972). Considerably higher currents are required for physiological damage (and for the let-go threshold) as frequencies increase or decrease from 60 Hz.

Lightning

Grounding of systems and circuit conductors is required by the *National Electrical Code* (1996). That is, the electrical system and circuits supplying a building must be grounded and have a grounding system. The purposes of such grounding are (a) to limit voltages in the supply circuits and laboratory due to lightning, power surges from the supply, and unintentional contact with lines of greater voltage, and (b) to provide stability of power to ground during use. In addition, the grounding of conductors provides a path for activation of circuit protectors if a ground fault occurs.

Lightning strikes kill and injure persons around the world, and about 400 are struck each year (Bernstein 1991a). According to *Accident Facts* (NSC 1996), lightning in the United States was the cause of 75 deaths in 1991, 53 deaths in 1992, 57 deaths in 1993 and 72 deaths in 1994. The states with the highest casualty rates were Florida, North Carolina, and Texas. The nature of a lightning strike is one of high voltage and high amperage discharge. Lightning discharges occur from cloud to cloud, cloud to atmosphere, and cloud to earth or water. The strike may reach earth by a path through trees, ships, high points on the earth, buildings, towers, and animals. If you are conducting research outdoors during lightning discharges, all personnel must immediately seek low ground (such as ravines or gullies) or take shelter within buildings. As lightning strikes traverse an area, high points become a target for discharge. Seeking shelter under a tree can be disastrous; a lightning strike will move down the tree to ground. From the ground around the tree, current flows through the earth and will flow through objects on the earth. In addition, side flashes will occur to a person or other object in proximity to the tree or object receiving the strike. Amperage values for these strikes range between 5 kA to 200 kA, with voltages in the millions. The strike lasts about 100 μsec. The damage to a person receiving a lightning strike may include: burns at the point of entry, internal lesions, skeletal fractures from falls or muscle contractions, neurologic damage, paralysis, muscle pain, photophobia of intense light, internal abdominal bleeding, cerebral cortical splitting, and subarachnoid hemorrhage (Critchley 1934; Silversides 1964).

When lightning strikes a building, the current flow moves to ground over lines of smallest resistance. The grounding of power circuits within the building results in this current shunting to ground, provided the building is grounded according to code specifications. Without proper grounding of the electrical circuits, the current flow will be essentially random, with side flashes to conductive elements within the structure. Because devices are connected to the electrical circuits, some of this current or even side flashes can appear in or on the electrical apparatus. One of the authors (W.A.G.) of this chapter experienced a lightning strike event. During his service in the Army, he was housed in an old wooden barracks. A thunderstorm occurred and moved directly over the barracks. Lightning struck the building (or nearby) and appeared in the latrine. Side flashes were observed between water pipes in the latrine, accompanied by loud crackling sounds. These strikes and side flashes occurred approximately three times before the storm moved on. This building was not properly grounded! Protection against lightning for buildings, equipment, and personnel was discussed at some length by Bernstein (1991b), to which the interested reader is referred for a comprehensive examination of details and further references. You should shut down and disconnect partic-ipants from any apparatus if you are in a building that does not have adequate lightning protection when a storm occurs. Temporary and older buildings may be vulnerable.

Current Limits

The 50–60-Hz frequency has cost advantages for the transmission of power. Unfortunately, this range of frequencies generates the maximal physiological response. Underwriters Laboratories (1990), in advising the Consumer Product Safety Commission, recommended current limits for electrical apparatus. The values were taken from the work of several investigators and are set so as to be applicable to persons with the lowest thresholds. Because of large individual differences, the threshold current values are higher in many persons for a given effect. In general, children have the lowest values, women have intermediate values and men have the highest values. Sweeney (1992) developed a physiological model to explain these age and gender differences. The limits for the startle reaction and let-go are based largely on the work of Dalziel and Mansfield (1950) and Dalziel and Massoglia (1956). The limit for ventricular fibrillation is based on work reported by Ferris and associates (1936), Kourvenhoven (1949), and Geddes and Baker (1971).

ELECTRICAL CHECKLIST

It is helpful to have a checklist for evaluating the electrical safety of the laboratory. We have compiled the list below from our own experience and several other sources. Sources are identified unless it is our personal recommendation.

1. Metal ladders must be legibly marked "CAUTION – Do Not Use Around Electrical Equipment – Severe Shock Danger" or an equivalent warning (OSHA 1996).

2. All cord-connected portable electrically operated tools must be effectively grounded or have approved double insulation (OSHA 1996).

3. All non–current-carrying metal parts of electrically operated tools and equipment must be effectively grounded (OSHA 1996).

4. Every six months, routine maintenance should be performed on all electrical devices in the laboratory. Checks should be carried out on grounding connections, current leakages, and electrical cords. Current leakages are best detected by qualified biomedical personnel. A local hospital or your engineering department should be contacted for advice (Moak 1994).

5. Have laboratory personnel report any hazards associated with electrical equipment or power-carrying cords (OSHA 1996).

6. Each time an electrical apparatus is used, inspect the grounding and the GFCI.

7. When service to electrical apparatus is necessary, switches must be opened, locked out, and tagged – if

permanently installed (OSHA 1996). Otherwise, open switches and unplug the apparatus.

8. Extension cords must have a grounding conductor (OSHA 1996). Inspect the grounding conductor before each use.

9. Exposed wiring and cords that are frayed or have deteriorated insulation are to be replaced immediately (OSHA 1996).

10. Flexible cords should be free of splices (OSHA 1996).

11. Provide the means for securing flexible cords at plugs, receptacles, tools, and electrical equipment (OSHA 1996).

12. Do not use metal measuring tapes (or measuring tapes with metallic thread woven into them) if there is any possibility of contact with energized equipment (OSHA 1996).

13. Before drilling through floors or walls, determine the location of electrical power lines (OSHA 1996).

14. Disconnect power before replacing fuses (OSHA 1996).

15. Ground all interior metal electrical raceways and enclosures (OSHA 1996).

16. All energized parts of electrical circuits and equipment must be guarded against accidental contact by approved cabinets and enclosures (OSHA 1996).

17. Mask unused openings of electrical enclosures with appropriate covers, plugs, or plates (OSHA 1996).

18. Remove all metal jewelry before working on or around energized equipment (OSHA 1996).

19. Observe proper voltages and polarities when installing or charging batteries (OSHA 1996).

20. Turn equipment off before unplugging.

21. Have operating manuals of all equipment available. Laboratory personnel should be familiar with the manual and the apparatus (Moak 1994).

22. Label each piece of equipment with its current requirements so as not to overheat the circuit supplying the equipment (Moak 1994).

23. Do not use "cheater" plugs to bypass the grounding probe on the apparatus or extension cord (Moak 1994).

24. Avoid using extension cords for equipment because of the possibility of overheating and increased leakage current (Moak 1994).

25. Special care should be taken so that leads attached to a participant do not contact potentially grounded areas: floors, equipment chassis, or other metal (Moak 1994).

26. Leakage current must be 10 μA or less for any equipment in direct contact with the participant (*National Electrical Code* 1996).

Prevention of Infection

The acquired immunodeficiency syndrome (AIDS) pandemic has brought to the forefront issues of protection against accidental transmission of infectious diseases. The risk of transmission of body-fluid–borne or blood-borne

infection during routine EEG recording, for example, is believed to be extremely low and not documented in the literature – except for transmission under special conditions, such as depth electrode placement in patients with Creutzfeldt–Jakob disease (CJD) (Bernoulli et al. 1977). Although the vast majority of psychophysiological evaluations are performed in people who do not suffer from major medical illnesses, infectious diseases most prone to blood-borne transmission (AIDS, CJD, hepatitis) can present with symptoms that frequently go undiagnosed or unrecognized in the early phases of illness.

Since 1988, the Centers for Disease Control (CDC) has published recommendations for prevention of HIV (human immunodeficiency virus, which causes AIDS), hepatitis B, and other blood-borne pathogens in health-care settings. These recommendations urge the adoption of universal blood and body fluid precautions – that is, all probands are considered to be infected with HIV. We have amended and incorporated parts of the CDC guidelines (1987, 1988, 1989) in the following recommendations for prevention of communicable diseases.

DISEASES

Infectious diseases can be transmitted by any of the following routes: air, contact, vehicle (water, food), and vector (e.g., mosquito, flea, tick). The following section deals with the two routes – air and contact transmission – that are factors to consider in the set-up and maintenance of the psychophysiology laboratory.

Airborne Diseases

Airborne diseases may be caused by inadequate cleaning of the laboratory, a defective ventilation system (legionella), and infected technicians or probands (common respiratory viruses, varicella, tuberculosis). Maintenance of the psychophysiology laboratory and the ventilation system falls under general maintenance guidelines for health facilities and will not be discussed here. Likewise, technicians need to follow health screening and procedures as outlined by their employee health guidelines. Additionally, appropriate care must be exercised so that seemingly trivial – but, for immunocompromised patients, life-threatening – infections such as chicken pox, shingles, measles, and influenza are not transmitted to these patients.

Blood-Borne Diseases

Blood-borne diseases are transmitted in the health-care or laboratory setting by transmission of blood-borne organisms from one person to another, typically entering the bloodstream through an open wound or via penetration injury from sharp objects.

AIDS. The AIDS that is caused by the human T-cell lymphotropic virus type III is characterized by severe and eventually lethal suppression of the immune system. This virus makes patients susceptible to a variety of opportunistic infections and neoplasms involving the central nervous system. The main route of transmission is sexual contact, which is followed in frequency by blood-borne transmission in intravenous drug abusers and patient groups (e.g., hemophiliacs and recipients of blood transfusions or blood products).

Previous studies have shown that health-care workers in frequent contact with AIDS patients and their blood have remained seronegative (Hirsch, Wormser, & Schooley 1985). The risk of transmission of AIDS is very low unless there is direct blood contact – such as occurs with an accidental stick from a needle used in an infected person immediately prior (Wormser, Rabkin, & Joline 1988). Once exposed to air, the AIDS virus is quickly destroyed and can be inactivated by disinfectants such as sodium hypochlorite (household bleach), hydrogen peroxide, and alcohol at concentrations below those recommended for use as disinfectants (Martin, McDougal, & Loskoski 1985; Rutala 1990) or by way of gas, heat, and chemical sterilants (CDC 1987).

Viral Hepatitis. There are several types of viral hepatitis, including the three types most likely to be encountered in the psychophysiology laboratory: A (infectious), B (serum), and C (serum). Hepatitis A is transmitted enterically by way of fecal contamination, whereas hepatitis B and C are typically transmitted by infected blood (e.g., via transfusions, needle sticks, tattooing, or ear piercing) but also by much less apparent means: toothbrushes, razors, baby bottles, and toys. Infection with hepatitis A causes a circumscribed clinical syndrome consisting of general malaise followed by clinical jaundice and subsequent complete recovery, altogether lasting 2–12 weeks. Hepatitis B and C present with a similar syndrome of longer duration in about 75% of cases. The remaining 25% may experience a prolonged phase of illness with eventual complete recovery; however, about 15% of all cases experience either chronic persistent or chronic active hepatitis.

Unlike HIV, viruses that cause viral hepatitis and CJD are resistant to many conventional disinfectants or sterilants and require adherence to strict sterilizing procedures. The hepatitis A virus is inactivated by boiling for 1 min or ultraviolet irradiation. The hepatitis B virus is inactivated by boiling for 1 min, heating at 60°C for 1 hr, steam autoclaving, or a 5% sodium hypochlorite solution (*Journal of Clinical Neurophysiology* 1994); the hepatitis C virus can probably be inactivated by these same procedures. Scientists are strongly advised to apprise themselves of current state laws and OSHA standards regarding prevention.

Creutzfeldt–Jakob Disease (CJD). This disease is a rare infectious disorder associated with a proteinaceous particle (prion); it occurs in a familial pattern in 10%–15% of cases. It produces a progressive and terminal spongiform encephalopathy. Mode of transmission is not adequately known. However, the virus resists many common techniques of sterilization and disinfection, including boiling, ultraviolet irradiation, and 70% alcohol. The recommended method of sterilization is steam autoclaving at 121°C at 15 psi for at least 1 hr (Brown et al. 1990).

PREVENTION OF BLOOD-BORNE DISEASES

This section discusses guidelines for preventing the transmission of blood-borne diseases that are uniformly (CJD, AIDS) or potentially (hepatitis B and C) lethal.

The major risk of body-fluid disease transmission in psychophysiological research is related to the routine preparation of the subject's skin or scalp by abrasion with chemical cleansing agents. This practice carries the potential to produce breaks in the skin with resultant leakage of blood or plasma, which can carry the infectious viral agents just described. According to the classification scheme for infection control, objects and instruments are listed as noncritical, semicritical, or critical with respect to their potential for disease transmission (Garner & Rutala 1986; Rutala 1990).

Noncritical Items

Noncritical items are those that contact intact skin and carry the lowest risk of disease transmission. Such items are surface electrodes, stethoscopes, ultrasonic surface probes, tabletops, and floors. Clean such equipment with a low-level disinfectant before use. Common low-level disinfectants include isopropyl alcohol (70%–90%), sodium hypochlorite (100 ppm available chlorine), and phenolic-, iodophor-, or quaternary ammonium germicidal detergent solution (follow the product label for dilution). Because fluid precautions are to be universally applied, as if all probands were potentially infected with HIV (CDC 1987), technicians should wear nonsterile gloves for procedures involving noncritical items. Because electrodes are commonly placed on abraded skin in the psychophysiological laboratory, the electrodes are considered semicritical rather than noncritical items.

Semicritical Items

Semicritical items are those that contact either mucous membranes or skin that has lost its integrity – as frequently occurs with the process of disinfection and placement of EEG, EMG, ECG, and EDR surface electrodes – or when the skin has sustained cuts, scratches, chapping, or any disease. Surface electrodes should be considered semicritical items, which means they must be free of micro-organisms and so require high-level disinfection. In addition, materials such as gauze pads and cotton swabs used to abrade skin are considered semicritical items and need to be sterilized before use. Semicritical items need to undergo disinfection by wet pasteurization or chemical germicides aimed at "eliminating many or all pathogenic microorganisms in inanimate objects, with the exception of bacterial spores" (Rutala 1990, p. 100).

To reduce the risk of disease transmission between tester and proband, technicians should wash their hands before and after the procedure in addition to wearing disposable sterile gloves. Once surface electrodes are removed, they should be discarded or cleaned with soap and water; if so cleaned for re-use then the electrodes should be rinsed thoroughly and disinfected according to standard hospital sterilization procedures (CDC 1987). Disinfection procedures may involve the same agents used for sterilization at much shorter exposure time (typically 10–20 min). Agents for disinfection include steam, gas, dry heat sterilization, and immersion in chemical germicides registered as "sterilants" with the U.S. Environmental Protection Agency. Commonly used disinfectants are solutions of sodium hypochlorite (AAEE 1986) or 2% glutaraldehyde for disinfecting electrodes otherwise corroded by bleach (Putnam, Johnson, & Roth 1992). Up-to-date information about the use of registered sterilants and the prevention of hazardous exposure can be obtained from the National Pesticide Communications Network (1-800-858-7378) and the electrode manufacturer. After disinfection, semicritical items require storage that will prevent microbial contamination.

Critical Items

Critical items are those that enter sterile tissue or the vascular system (Rutala 1990). In the psychophysiology laboratory, critical items include subdermal electrodes, needles, and the lancets used for skin preparation. Critical items must be sterile at the time of use – free of all forms of microbial life (Rutala 1990) – and must be handled with extreme caution. Their use in the psychophysiology laboratory should be avoided unless absolutely necessary. The risk of disease transmission from an accidental stick from a needle just used on an infected patient has been estimated to be between 6% and 30% for hepatitis (CDC 1989) and 0.35% for HIV (Wormser et al. 1988). After use, subdermal electrodes, needles, and lancets should be discarded immediately in a puncture-resistant container. Subdermal electrodes that are not discarded must be sterilized immediately after use; follow the specific instructions of the electrode manufacturer, then store to ensure continued sterility. Sterilization is accomplished by physical or chemical means. Sterilization procedures typically involve one of five methods (Rutala 1990): steam under pressure; ethylene oxide gas; liquid chemicals such as 2% glutaraldehyde–based formulas (at manufacturer's recommendations); demand release chlorine dioxide (6 hr); and 6% hydrogen peroxide (6 hr).

CONCLUSIONS ON PREVENTION OF INFECTION

Existing disease prevention guidelines demand that universal precautions be used during evaluations and management of all participants. However, considerable latitude exists in interpretation of what constitutes precautions that are necessary to limit the transmission of blood-borne diseases. Medical situations may range from those with low potential for disease transmission (office visits and physical examinations) to those with high potential for disease transmission – for example, vascular or orthopedic surgeries, which can result in large-volume blood loss with the attendant risk for exposure to a blood-borne pathogen. The laboratory researcher needs to keep in mind the degree of potential disease transmission from these medical considerations. Constitutional symptoms of malnourishment, malaise, discoloration of skin, and chronic cough may herald a chronic and potentially infectious disease process.

The risk of body-fluid or blood-borne disease transmission during standard procedures in the psychophysiology laboratory is extremely low. Routine cleaning of the electrophysiology laboratory and apparatus, use of gloves, and reprocessing of electrodes according to recommended disinfection or sterilization procedures will minimize the risk. Standard sterilization and disinfection procedures are adequate for reprocessing equipment contaminated with HIV or the more resistant hepatitis B virus. More stringent procedures are necessary if the proband is known or suspected to suffer from Creutzfeldt–Jakob disease. These recommendations are formulated on the basis of the best information currently available. Specific recommendations will be revised as public health policies undergo reassessment and new electrodes and sterilants become available.

Health and Risk Assessment

Although testing procedures in the psychophysiological laboratory are generally benign, it is incumbent upon investigators to understand the medical history of participants if anything more than minimal stress is involved or if physical or psychological problems would be relevant to the safety of the participant. In ACSM (1995) may be found the components of a medical history, which can serve as a guide in considering assessment. The American College of Sports Medicine may be consulted for further discussion, with the understanding that ACSM is mainly concerned with exercise testing and prescription. We have used some of these components as a guide for compiling a medical history but have altered the content for relevance to psychophysiology.

Physician Diagnosis. If a diagnosis is relevant to the procedures then it should be obtained. The screening questionnaire will alert the investigator to problem areas that may require follow-up. Relevance, of course, depends on the level of stress imposed on the participant and the purpose of the experiment. Conditions such as diabetes, hypertension, cancer, pregnancy, history of heart disease, and many others may be relevant.

Results of a Physical Examination. If necessary, the results of previous physical examinations can be acquired with permission of the participant. Relevant findings might include strokes, fainting, abnormal blood findings, or cardiac abnormalities.

Current and Previous Symptoms. The *Health Problems Checklist* (Schinka 1989) is a fairly comprehensive self-administered questionnaire that can be followed by an interview to determine the significance of the symptoms reported. For stress-related research, cardiovascular symptoms could be noteworthy – including pain in jaw, chest, neck, or arms – especially if precipitated by stress.

Recent Problems. Again, each of these must be assessed with regard to its relevance and risk in the experiment. Problem areas here may include recent accidents, illnesses, surgeries, or hospitalizations.

Muscle, Joint, Tendon, or Ligament Problems. If the experiment requires ambulation, manipulation, heavy lifting, or rapid movements (as in tracking), then such problems may preclude participation or require some modification of procedures.

Determine Which Medications Are Being Used and Their Effects. Some medications may suppress heart rate or ventricular function (beta blockers). If, for example, the investigator is trying to stress or exercise a participant to a particular heart rate or blood pressure and the medications are limiting the response, then this must be known.

Use of Other Psychoactive or Performance-Altering Substances. Determine the use of tobacco, alcohol, steroids, caffeine, or other nonprescription substances and whether these substances will affect the participant's safety in the study.

Level of Physical Conditioning. If you are requiring the participant to exercise, you should know the fitness level of your participant to prevent excessive stress.

Genetic Influences. Assess the family history of your participant to help evaluate risk. Such factors in the family as hypertension, cardiac and pulmonary disease, and sudden death should be known.

Table 6 presents the Physical Activity Readiness Questionnaire (PAR-Q; Reading & Shepard 1992), whose original version was used as a screening device for beginning a low to moderate exercise program. The revised version (presented in Table 6) is less likely to produce false positives, especially in older people. It is designed for people between the ages of 15 and 69. A subject who answers Yes to any of the questions should be advised to consult a physician before beginning an exercise program or having a fitness appraisal. A participant who answers No to all questions can become more

physically active or undergo a fitness appraisal. This questionnaire can also be found in ACSM (1995), which includes forms that may be copied for use and contain more information for the participant, including informed consent. The PAR-Q may be useful in screening for the psychophysiology laboratory if exercise is involved; it can also serve as an alerting mechanism for potential problems.

We have discussed two screening tests. We now present a list of all screening devices we examined.

1. The revised PAR-Q just discussed (Reading & Shepard 1992).
2. The *Health Problems Checklist,* discussed previously (Schinka 1989).
3. The Cardiovascular Rehabilitation History Questionnaire (Wilson, Fardy, & Froelicher 1981). Although slanted toward cardiac rehabilitation programs, this questionnaire contains sections on social history, medical history, and cardiovascular risk factors.
4. The Medical History Questionnaire, which is reprinted in Pollock and Wilmore (1990). This questionnaire was designed by the Institute for Aerobics Research in Dallas, Texas. Sections include general information, present history, past history, family medical history, cardiovascular risk factors, a 24-hour history, and special questions for women. Enough information is requested to enable informed decisions regarding health and cardiovascular risk.

STRESSORS AND RISK FACTORS

Psychophysiologists can use numerous stressors in investigations: noise, electric shock, cold, heat, social challenges,

---

TABLE 6. The Physical Activity Readiness Questionnaire (PAR-Q)

Yes	No	
○	○	1. Has a doctor ever said that you have a heart condition and recommended only medically supervised activity?
○	○	2. Do you have chest pain brought on by physical activity?
○	○	3. Have you developed chest pain in the past month?
○	○	4. Do you tend to lose consciousness or fall over as a result of dizziness?
○	○	5. Do you have a bone or joint problem that could be aggravated by the proposed physical activity?
○	○	6. Has a doctor ever recommended medication for your blood pressure or a heart condition?
○	○	7. Are you aware, through your own experience or a doctor's advice, of any other physical reason against your exercising without medical supervision?

Note: If you have a temporary illness, such as a common cold, or are not feeling well at this time, then postpone the activity.

Source: Shepard, Thomas, & Weller, "The Canadian Home Fitness Test: 1991 Update," *Sports Medicine,* vol. 11, p. 359. Copyright 1991 by Adis International Inc. Adapted with permission of the authors and publisher.

intellectual (mental arithmetic, the Stroop test, problem solving), exercise, and public speaking, to name several. Although the stressors have not been ranked regarding their physiological import, at this time an absolute ranking is probably not possible because reactions vary as a function of a participant's history, age, gender, health, and genetic makeup. Nevertheless, the investigator should take into account risk factors and health status before subjecting a participant to high levels of stress, especially exercise. Further guidance to the investigator is available by obtaining information regarding factors that predict cardiovascular (CV) disease. We emphasize CV risk because high levels of stress may precipitate CV incidents. If they choose to process an at-risk subject, laboratory personnel must be capable of recognizing a CV incident or an impending incident and be prepared for correct action. Laboratory personnel must also know when not to include a particular participant in a study, and so a careful evaluation of the medical history is necessary.

Common risk factors for CV disease (and hence for the increased possibility of a CV incident) can be assessed by interview, blood pressure, and serum cholesterol. There are currently no specific guidelines for imposing stressors in the psychophysiology laboratory. In our opinion, data need to be obtained and interpreted to help the psychophysiologist assess the medical implications of stress for laboratory work. Here, at least, we can present the common risk factors that are predictive of CV disease; these factors are especially important for evaluating a participant who is to undergo exercise testing or who is to begin an exercise program. Common risk factors for CV disease that should be assessed include:

1. age – men older than 45 and women older than 55;
2. cigarette smoking;
3. systolic blood pressure measured at rest (greater than 140 mmHg systolic or greater than 90 mmHg diastolic or both);
4. total serum cholesterol greater than 200 mg/dl (note: high-density lipoprotein cholesterol greater than 60 mg/dl is considered a *positive* risk factor; i.e., it lessens the CV risk);
5. insulin-dependent diabetes mellitus; and
6. a sedentary life style.

A fuller discussion of these risk factors can be found in ACSM (1995) and Gordon and Mitchell (1993).

SPECIAL CASES AT RISK

There is a peculiar lack of studies from the psychophysiological laboratory regarding electrocardiographic (ECG) analysis – other than the usual measurement of R-R wave intervals for calculating heart rate and the work of Furedy and his associates (Furedy, Heslegrave, & Scher 1992) on T-wave amplitude changes during stressful tasks. One method the cardiologist uses to help diagnose heart disease entails analysis of the waveforms and intervals of the ECG. Perhaps this paucity of psychophysiological data reflects the lack of interest in these changes as they might reflect psychological processes or, perhaps, the lack of training of investigators in recognizing and evaluating such changes. Electrocardiographic research could provide data for normal subjects and for participants with different degrees of risk (or with disease) at baseline and during various stressful situations.

Studies have reported on diagnosed CV participants who were subjected to psychological stress in order to assess CV function during stress, as indexed (at least partially) by ECG and blood pressure. Our purpose here is not to review that literature but to present a few paradigmatic reports – which will indicate the diagnoses and the CV changes found – to alert the psychophysiological investigator regarding such diagnoses and the CV risk.

Rasmussen and co-workers (1984) used cold pressor (CP) and hyperventilation as stressors on male and female patients admitted for coronary angiography due to attacks of chest pain. An S-T segment elevation or depression (see later section on terminating a session) greater than 0.1 mV or significant T-waves were seen in 25 of 105 patients (23.9%). Coronary angiography indicated that the abnormal ECG changes were due to reduced diameters in the ischemic related vessels. Specchia and colleagues (1984) had 122 patients perform mental arithmetic during coronary anteriography and found significant S-T segment abnormalities in 22 of them. Of these 22 patients, the 20 who were given an exercise stress test all showed S-T segment abnormalities.

In a study using radionuclide ventriculography, Rozanski and associates (1988) used several stressors: mental arithmetic, the Stroop task, simulated public speaking, and reading. The responses were then compared with those induced by exercise for 39 patients with coronary artery disease and 12 control subjects. In the patient group, 23 (59%) had ventricular wall abnormalities while undergoing the mental stressors and 14 (36%) had a statistically significant fall in ejection fraction (the percentage of blood ejected from the heart on a given beat). It is interesting to note that the magnitude of the cardiac abnormality during the personally relevant speaking task was similar to the abnormality caused by exercise and proved to be the most potent mental stressor. Finally, in 19 of the 23 patients (83%) showing abnormal wall motion, no symptoms were experienced (silent ischemia). Regarding safety of the participant, this study shows that processing at-risk subjects who have significant physiological symptoms may not report such symptoms; thus, it seems obvious that ECG monitoring is necessary for persons at high risk or with known disease.

More recently, Legault and colleagues (1995) worked with 46 patients with stable coronary artery disease. They found that 23 of the patients (50%) showed an ischemic response to mental stress (giving a 3–5-min speech about their own faults or bad habits) as assessed by a decrease of $\geq 5\%$ in left ventricular ejection fraction. When the patients wore Holter monitors during 48 hours of ambulation, the investigators found that mental stress–induced ischemia in the laboratory was significantly associated with ambulatory ischemia, as indicated by S-T segment depression. In other words, ambulatory ischemia was predicted by mental stress–induced ischemia. Again, for participants at risk – in this case, diagnosed coronary artery disease – mental stress produced a potentially dangerous circumstance; without monitoring the S-T segment, depression would have not been detected.

WHO IS AT RISK?

It is recommended (ACSM 1995) that laboratory personnel be trained and certified in CPR in all situations where exercise testing is undertaken. We apply this recommendation to the psychophysiological laboratory when any stress testing (psychological or physical) is performed or when any electronic devices are attached to a participant. This recommendation, along with the protocols discussed previously, will make the processing of subjects much safer.

However, the question of risk still remains. Can we safely process any participant? If not, then who is to be excluded? Do we need physician screening for some participants? With regard to exercise, the investigator should consult ACSM (1995); further guidelines may be found in Fletcher et al. (1990). However, if a person has known disease then the principal investigator is responsible for taking acceptable precautions. Should a medical examination be recommended, then discussion with the examining physician is prudent in order to obtain an informed medical opinion regarding whether to proceed with exercise testing. For psychological stress testing, the criterion established for minimal risk by the National Institutes of Health (1993) may be followed:

A risk is minimal where the probability and magnitude of harm or discomfort anticipated in the proposed research are not greater, in and of themselves, than those ordinarily encountered in daily life or during the performance of routine physical or psychological examinations or tests.... For example, the risk of drawing a small amount of blood from a healthy individual for research proposes is no greater than the risk of doing so as part of routine physical examination. (p. G-8)

Using this minimal risk criterion, the investigator can proceed with testing for most participants without physician consultation; additional safety can be added using a medical screen. Stressors are certainly encountered in daily life that are of greater intensity than those usually employed in the psychophysiology laboratory. Even so, if

an investigator accepts a participant into a study then responsibility for the well-being of that participant shifts to the investigator. Simple screens and interviews will help to avoid the criticism, "You should have known." Finally, the research reviewed in the previous section provides further data on reactions to stress for persons with known cardiovascular disease.

Safety Monitoring of Participants

We have just discussed risk assessment prior to accepting a participant in a study that involves physical or psychological stress. We now go on to monitoring participants via ECG and blood pressure (BP). If screening has determined that a person has cardiovascular disease or is at high risk, then medical clearance should be obtained and the ECG and BP should be monitored to detect ECG and BP changes which signal that, without medical supervision, a test should be stopped. The full set of criteria for stopping an exercise test can be found in ACSM's (1995) Table 4-6 for apparently healthy adults and Table 5-4 for clinical testing. We recommend that the full ACSM (1995) guidelines be obtained for laboratory use if exercise is part of your protocol. The monitoring of the ECG requires training and experience. Several references can be consulted to begin learning about ECG monitoring (ACSM 1995; Durstine et al. 1993; Froelicher 1987; Goldberger & Goldberger 1994; Scheidt 1986). The American College of Sports Medicine provides training, certification programs, and testing for different levels of skill and knowledge for those interested (ACSM 1995). In the next sections we will give some common-sense and technical criteria for terminating a session.

TERMINATING A SESSION

If the investigator – after screening the participant – has decided to proceed, then special criteria can be used that will help determine when a session should be ended. These criteria include real-time observation of the subject as well as the subject's ECG and BP. The criteria given here are not exhaustive (see ACSM 1995) but are listed so that investigators and laboratory personnel may, without extensive training, make informed decisions (see also Figures 3–6). The following events constitute criteria for termination of an exercise session (see the next section for details):

1. the S-T segment shows a downsloping, horizontal, or upsloping depression > 2.0 mm from a baseline determination;
2. the S-T segment is upsloping from the baseline > 2.0 mm;
3. ventricular tachycardia is suspected;
4. three or more premature ventricular contractions in 1 min or less;

5. atrial fibrillation or atrial flutter;
6. elevation of systolic BP > 260 mmHg or diastolic BP > 115 mmHg;
7. moderate to severe angina;
8. cold, clammy skin or cyanosis;
9. mental confusion or dizziness;
10. verbalizations of distress or discomfort; or
11. participant requests termination.

Although these criteria are taken from guidelines on exercise, they can also provide guidance for other types of stress testing.

THE ELECTROCARDIOGRAM

The electrocardiogram is measured by affixing electrodes near the heart. There are agreed-on configurations used in clinical work that enable interpretation of the resultant waveforms. Full monitoring is accomplished using a 12-lead system, which electrically views the heart from different perspectives; with the 12-lead system it is more likely that an abnormality can be detected. Determining heart rate and interbeat intervals requires only one lead, so long as some particular aspect of the ECG is reliably obtained. Clinical work requires that the stream of ECG signals be traced on an oscilloscope, computer screen, or other recording media at 25 mm/sec with the amplification set to 1 mV/cm. (Other criteria for recording the ECG can be found in Chapter 9 of this volume.) This section augments the previous section, where test termination criteria were set forth.

Many laboratories do not have the necessary apparatus to record a 12-lead ECG; nor is this necessary for most psychophysiological research purposes. It is possible to use a single-lead system, which can detect S-T segment changes and arrhythmias but is not as sensitive as the 12-lead system. Pollock and Wilmore (1990) discussed the most sensitive of the single, bipolar leads: the manubrium-to-V_5 lead, termed the CM_5. Using the CM_5 with the bipolar attachment (left arm negative and V_5 placement positive) and the V_1 configuration yields a three-lead system that is quite sensitive to abnormal ECGs; this configuration was made popular by Ellestad (1986). However, if only one lead is to be used then the CM_5 is recommended. To obtain the CM_5 configuration, place the negative electrode on the manubrium and the positive electrode on V_5. To find the V_5, place a mark in the fifth intercostal space at the midclavicular line; then place the electrode at the same level as the mark but at the anterior axillary line.

Figure 3 shows three types of S-T segment depressions: upsloping, downsloping, and horizontal. The S-T segment depression can be caused by an ischemic condition in the heart, although other causes are possible (e.g., drug effects, hyperventilation, electrolyte abnormalities). To be significant, the depression must occur 0.08 sec after the end of the QRS waves and be ≥ 1 mm. Downsloping S-T

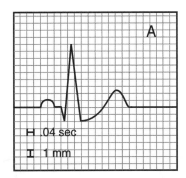

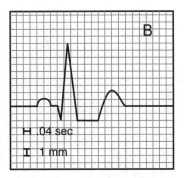

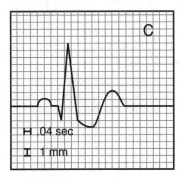

Figure 3. ECG patterns showing upsloping (part A), horizontal (part B), and downsloping (part C) S-T segment depressions; these depressions many times indicate myocardial ischemia. Adapted with permission from Scheidt, *Basic Electrocardiography,* illustrated by Frank H. Netter, M.D. Copyright 1986 by Novartis. All rights reserved.

segment depression is considered to be the most specific for ischemia, followed in significance by horizontal and then upsloping forms (Scheidt 1986). The ECG in Figure 3 shows the P wave, the Q wave, the R wave and the S wave. The S wave begins where the downswing of the R wave crosses the "isoelectric" line, which is the level of a line extending from the end of the T wave to the beginning of the next P wave. It can be seen that each of the three insets have greater than 1 mm depression at the 0.08-sec point. The S-T segment change may be accompanied by chest pain or other signs of angina: jaw pain, arm pain (especially left arm), or throat pain. Ischemia is not always accompanied by pain; there can be silent myocardial ischemia. The S-T segment depression does not always accompany ischemia, and the actual depression may be

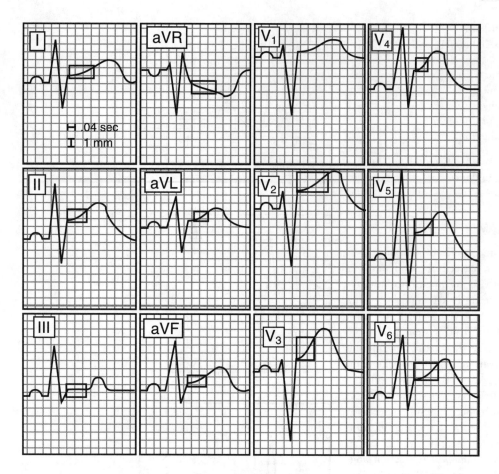

Figure 4. A 12-lead ECG recording showing S-T segment elevations. Such elevations may be due to myocardial ischemia, vasospasm, as a normal variant of early repolarization, pericarditis, myocardial infarction, or aneurysm. Adapted with permission from Scheidt, *Basic Electrocardiography,* illustrated by Frank H. Netter, M.D. Copyright 1986 by Novartis. All rights reserved.

very subtle. Other ECG abnormalities (e.g., T-wave flattening or inversions) may accompany myocardial ischemia even when S-T segment depression is absent (Goldberger & Goldberger 1994).

Another possibility is S-T segment elevation. Figure 4 shows a 12-lead ECG recording with elevations occurring in all leads except V_1. The generalized elevations shown in so many leads are probably diagnostic of pericarditis (Scheidt 1986). However, elevations can result also from cardiac inflammation, strong myocardial ischemia caused by cardiac arterial occlusion or vasospasm (Prinzmetal's angina), ventricular aneurysm, myocardial infarction, and early repolarization (i.e., the T wave begins during the S-T segment).

Figure 5 shows premature ventricular contractions (PVCs), which can be recognized by three characteristics: (i) they occur before the next normal beat is usually expected; (ii) the QRS complex is abnormally wide (i.e., ≥ 0.12 sec); and (iii) the QRS and the T wave are (usually) of opposite polarity. Several conditions can initiate PVCs, including cardiac stimulating drugs (e.g. caffeine),

anxiety, underlying cardiac disease, acute myocardial infarctions, electrolyte disturbances, hypoxemia, and irritable foci in the ventricle itself. Although PVCs are fairly common, even in young healthy people, frequent PVCs can be serious. Ventricular tachycardia is, by definition, a run of three or more successive PVCs. A longer series can lead to hypotension, syncope, or even ventricular fibrillation and death. Should PVCs begin to occur, it is necessary to stop the experiment, relax the participant, monitor the ECG, and prepare for an emergency. Part A of Figure 5 shows three PVCs occurring successively; part B illustrates full ventricular tachycardia. The ECG record shown in part B is life-threatening and so immediate emergency measures would be needed. The sequel can be ventricular fibrillation during which no blood is pumped from the heart; death is imminent without immediate intervention.

The last of the cardiac arrhythmias discussed here are atrial flutter and atrial fibrillation; these two conditions are presented in parts A and B (respectively) of Figure 6. Atrial flutter and fibrillation are the result of a focus or many foci in the atria that stimulate the atria to contract – the stimulus is no longer the standard pacemaker of the heart. Atrial flutter produces a characteristic sawtooth wave call the F wave. Atrial flutter rarely occurs in the normal heart but is found in patients with valvular heart disease, chronic ischemic heart disease, hypertensive heart disease, and other cardiac myopathies. Paroxysmal atrial flutter may also occur in the healthy heart because of psychological stress or excessive alcohol consumption (Goldberger & Goldberger 1994). The rate of depolarization is quite rapid, about 250–350 beats per minute (bpm). The ventricular rate is usually some fraction of the flutter rate: 1/2, 1/4, or 1/8.

In atrial fibrillation, the heart rate is in the range of 400–600 bpm. The waveform is irregular and wavy instead of the usual P wave. The fibrillatory waves are called f waves. The ventricular rate is quite rapid, but the interbeat interval is very irregular because only some of the f waves are able to stimulate the atrioventricular node. Because the pumping action of the atria is not coordinated, the amount of blood reaching the ventricles is less than normal and so cardiac output is lowered, which can result in hypotension and myocardial ischemia. Obviously, if these conditions develop then testing should be stopped and emergency measures taken.

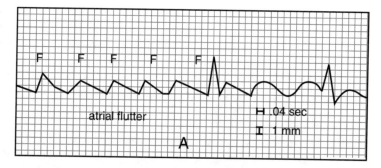

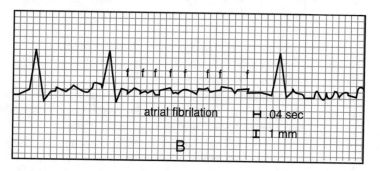

Figure 6. Part A: Atrial flutter with characteristic F waves. Part B: Atrial fibrillation with characteristic f waves. Redrawn with permission from Goldberger & Goldberger, *Clinical Electrocardiography: A Simplified Approach*, 5th ed. Copyright 1994 C. V. Mosby Company.

This brief discussion of the abnormal ECG is very incomplete. However, the conditions presented should allow the investigator to recognize some abnormalities and stop a session. Usually, however, some diagnosis will have been made; again, the importance of health and risk screening is evident, and the laboratory supervisor needs to obtain medical advice before proceeding in some cases. If any of the conditions develop unexpectedly, the session can be stopped. A great deal has been written covering the ECG and how to read and interpret the various waveforms. The interested reader can certainly pursue this area but should receive special training and certification to achieve competency.

BLOOD PRESSURE MONITORING

To ensure that blood pressure does not rise to dangerous levels during a procedure, it is necessary to monitor correctly. A procedure described by the American Society of Hypertension (1992) is reprinted as an appendix of the ACSM (1995) *Resource Manual*.

One aspect of monitoring that is not always covered in descriptions of methods is the auscultatory gap. When a cuff is inflated into the range of pressures below the systolic and above the diastolic, one expects to hear Korotkoff sounds. If these sounds are not heard, then the operator assumes that the artery has been occluded and cuff pressure is above systolic pressure. However, this may not

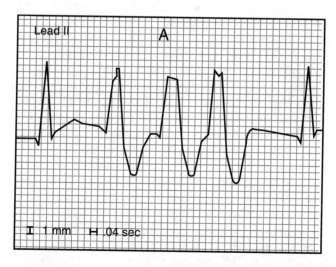

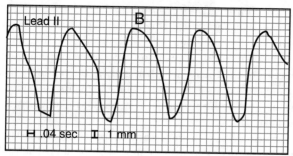

Figure 5. Part A: A normal QRS waveform followed by three successive premature ventricular contractions (PVCs); three or more successive PVCs define ventricular tachycardia. Part B: Full development of ventricular tachycardia – a very dangerous condition (see text). Redrawn with permission from Goldberger & Goldberger, *Clinical Electrocardiography: A Simplified Approach*, 5th ed. Copyright 1994 C. V. Mosby Company.

always be the case, since some individuals have a range of pressures between systolic and diastolic where *no* sounds are heard; this range is called the auscultatory gap. To verify that cuff pressure is above systolic, the radial pulse must be palpated until the inflating cuff pressure stops the pulse. At that point, one can be certain that systolic pressure has been exceeded by the cuff. Then merely continue rapidly inflating the cuff to 30 mmHg above the disappearance of the radial pulse before beginning deflation. Care must be taken when deflating the cuff that, upon entering the auscultatory gap, the operator does not assume that diastolic pressure has been obtained; continue deflating the cuff and the Korotkoff sounds will re-appear.

We have recommended terminating procedures when systolic pressure exceeds 260 mmHg or diastolic pressure exceeds 115 mmHg. Although these values are recommended by ACSM during exercise testing, there are no recommended values for terminating psychological tests; moreover, psychophysiologists use exercise as a stressor and for other purposes (Delistraty et al. 1992). Because regulatory mechanisms of blood pressure for psychological stress are different from that of exercise, we can only present the ACSM guidelines and suggest that the investigator consider these as stop-points in stress testing.

However, it is unlikely that stress testing of a psychological nature will drive blood pressures to exercise levels. We searched the journal *Psychophysiology* (1992 through May 1997) to determine the magnitude of blood pressure values reported. The highest values were reported by Sundin et al. (1995). Average systolic BP values of 153 mmHg and diastolic BP values of 106 mmHg were reported for postmyocardial patients on an arithmetic task, and similar values for the cold pressor task were also found. Healthy controls produced an average diastolic BP of 104 mmHg for the cold pressor test and 98 mmHg for mental arithmetic. Although standard deviations and ranges were not reported, we can assume that diastolic BP of 115 mmHg was approached or exceeded in one or both groups by some participants.

Summary and Recommendations

Four general nonmandatory principles were established by OSHA (1996) to guide the development and maintenance of an effective safety and health program. When dealing with laboratory safety, these principles can be used as general guidelines:

1. commitment of management and involvement of employees;
2. analysis of the worksite;
3. prevention and control of hazards; and
4. proper training of personnel.

The following discussion is based on these principles.

Principle 1 effectively requires the principal investigator or department head to provide resources and control activities in the laboratory with an effective commitment toward the safety of laboratory personnel and participants. Involvement of members of the department and of laboratory personnel in setting up guidelines is essential and promotes their commitment. The means by which this goal may be accomplished should include at least: (a) a stated policy, so that all involved clearly comprehend the importance of the safety and health policy; (b) establishment of clear safety goals; (c) a means of showing that supervisors and the department head are clearly involved; (d) active involvement of laboratory personnel and department members in the development of policies and procedures; (e) designation of specific responsibilities to all those actively involved in the laboratory and department; (f) allocation of adequate authority and resources to those in positions of responsibility; (g) a means of assessing the accountability of those responsible; and (h) a review of the program, at least annually.

Principle 2 requires an examination of the laboratory to identify hazardous or potentially hazardous conditions. The following are recommendations for achieving that goal: (a) conduct a comprehensive survey of the laboratory; (b) analyze any new laboratories, additions to the laboratories, changes in systems, and new equipment; (c) routinely re-evaluate the laboratory; (d) provide a way for laboratory personnel to notify supervisors and department heads regarding hazardous conditions; (e) carefully investigate accidents or "near-misses" for effective prevention in the future; and (f) analyze any illnesses or accidents over time to identify patterns for future prevention.

Principle 3 is intended to prevent hazards or, at least, to control hazardous conditions if they cannot be eliminated – as in the presence of blood-borne pathogens. Means towards the realization of this principle include: (a) engineering techniques – for example, use of soundproofing materials to reduce noise; (b) safe laboratory procedures and effective enforcement of such procedures; (c) reducing length of exposure to hazardous conditions; (d) supplying protective equipment; (e) requiring regular maintenance of equipment to prevent malfunction; (f) developing an effective plan for emergencies and periodic practice of the emergency plan; and (g) developing a medical plan that includes CPR, immediate first aid, and a means of mobilizing the nearest physician or emergency medical care.

Principle 4 is concerned with the training of supervisors and laboratory personnel. Laboratory personnel must be made aware of the potential hazards in the laboratory and of effective means of avoiding such hazards. Laboratory supervisors need training to identify and anticipate hazards, and they should reinforce the training of employees regarding hazardous conditions and the need for protective measures.

Blanton (1988) discussed the relationship between safety, OSHA, and the academic laboratory. He found safety considerations to be severely lacking, in part because OSHA has not generally been concerned with academic laboratories but rather with small businesses and industry. However, hazardous conditions do exist in the academic laboratory, as this chapter readily attests. Academic laboratories need special consideration because: (a) students who work in the laboratory are transitory and not well-trained in safety principles; (b) the need for training of new laboratory personnel is generally not a high priority; and (c) the allocation of funds and resources for safety compete with funds used for supplies, equipment, and salaries. The protection of all persons involved in laboratory research needs to move to a much higher position in the hierarchy of concerns.

Blanton asked academic institutions how safety could be improved. A number of suggestions were given. First, make OSHA requirements more clear and relevant to the academic environment. (Interestingly, more contact with OSHA was seen as desirable.) Second, periodic inspections by OSHA were seen as welcome. Third, respondents wanted more training of personnel and a stronger commitment by the administration to safety matters. Fourth, Environmental Protection Agency (EPA) qualified personnel were seen as needed to supervise disposal of materials. Fifth, consultants were needed to help with allocation of institutional funds for compliance. Finally, the respondents suggested that – because education is the purpose of academic institutions and since laboratory training is a necessary part of that mission – the community should share more in the financing of safety.

NOTE

The authors wish to thank Ginette Blackhart for bibliographic and figure preparation and Cherie Jackman for bibliographic preparation.

REFERENCES

AAEE [American Association of Electromyography and Electrodiagnosis] (1986). Suggested infection control guidelines for performing electrodiagnostic studies in HTLV-III positive patients. *Muscle Nerve, 9,* 762–3.

ACSM [American College of Sports Medicine] (1995). *ACSM's Guidelines for Exercise Testing and Prescription,* 5th ed. Baltimore: Williams & Wilkins.

American Society of Hypertension (1992). Recommendations for routine blood pressure measurement by indirect cuff sphygmomanometry. *American Journal of Hypertension, 5,* 207–9.

Andress, J. M. (1996). Bhopal. In *The Encyclopedia Americana: International Edition,* vol. 3, p. 642. Danbury, CT: Grolier.

Bernoulli, C., Siegfried, J., Baumgartner, G., Regli, F., Rabinowicz, T., Gajdusek, D. C., & Gibbs, C. J., Jr. (1977). Danger of accidental person-to-person transmission of Creutzfeldt–Jakob disease by surgery. *Lancet, 1,* 478–9.

Bernstein, T. (1991a). Electrical systems, terminology, and components-relationship to electrical and lightning accidents and fires. In E. K. Greenwald (Ed.), *Electrical Hazards and Accidents: Their Cause and Prevention,* pp. 1–27. New York: Van Nostrand.

Bernstein, T. (1991b). Lightning protection for buildings, equipment, and personnel. In E. K. Greenwald (Ed.), *Electrical Hazards and Accidents: Their Cause and Prevention,* pp. 135–55. New York: Van Nostrand.

Bernstein, T. (1994). Electrical injury: Electrical engineer's perspective and an historical review. In R. C. Lee, M. Capelli-Schellpfeffer, & K. M. Kelley (Eds.), *Electrical Injury: A Multidisciplinary Approach to Therapy, Prevention, and Rehabilitation,* vol. 720, pp. 1–11. New York: Annals of the New York Academy of Sciences.

Blanton, C. (1988). OSHA and the academic laboratory. *Professional Safety, 13,* 14–16.

Bradley, M. M., Cuthbert, B. N., & Lang, P. J. (1996). Lateralized startle probes in the study of emotion. *Psychophysiology, 33,* 156–61.

Brown, P., Liberski, P., Wolff, A., & Gajdusek, D. (1990). Resistance of scrapie infectivity to steam autoclaving after formaldehyde fixation and limited survival after ashing at 360°C: Practical and theoretical implications. *Journal of Infectious Diseases, 161,* 467–72.

CDC [Centers for Disease Control] (1987). Recommendation for prevention of HIV transmission in health-care settings. *Morbidity and Mortality Weekly Report, 36 (Suppl. 2S),* 1s–18s.

CDC (1988). Update: Universal precautions for prevention of transmission of human immunodeficiency virus, hepatitis B virus and other blood borne pathogens in health-care settings. *Morbidity and Mortality Weekly Report, 37,* 377–82, 387–8.

CDC (1989). Guidelines for prevention of transmission of human immunodeficiency virus and hepatitis B virus to health-care and public-safety workers. *Morbidity and Mortality Weekly Report, 38 (Suppl. S-6),* 1–37.

Code of Federal Regulations (1996). *Title 29, OSHA Standards 1910.* Washington, DC: U.S. Government Printing Office.

Critchley, M. (1934). Neurological effects of lightning and of electricity. *Lancet, 1,* 68–72.

Dalziel, C. F. (1943). Effect of waveform on let-go currents. *AIEE Transactions, 62,* 739–44.

Dalziel, C. F. (1972). Electric shock hazard. *IEEE Spectrum, 9,* 41–50.

Dalziel, C. F., & Mansfield, T. H. (1950). Effects of frequency on perception currents. *AIEE Transactions, 69,* 1162–8.

Dalziel, C. F., & Massoglia, F. P. (1956). Let-go currents and voltages. *AIEE Transactions Part II, 75,* 49–56.

Delistraty, D. A., Greene, W. A., Carlberg, K. A., & Raver, K. K. (1992). Cardiovascular reactivity in Type A and B males to mental arithmetic and aerobic exercise at an equivalent oxygen uptake. *Psychophysiology, 29,* 264–71.

Durstine, J. L., King, A. C., Painter, P. L., Roitman, J. L., Zwiren, L. D., & Kenny, W. L. (Eds.) (1993). *ACSM's Resource Manual for Guidelines for Exercise Testing and Prescription.* Media, PA: Williams & Wilkins.

Ellestad, M. S. (1986). *Stress Testing Principles and Practices,* 3rd ed. Philadelphia: Davis.

Ferris, L. P., King, B. G., Spence, P. W., & Williams, H. B. (1936). Effects of electric shock on the heart. *AIEE Transactions, 55,* 498–515.

Fletcher, G. F., Froelicher, V. F., Hartley, L. H., Haskell, W. L., & Pollock, M. L. (1990). Exercise standards. A statement for health professionals from the American Heart Association. *Circulation, 82*, 2286–2322.

Froelicher, V. F. (1987). *Exercise and the Heart: Clinical Concepts*, 2nd ed. Chicago: Year Book Medical Publishers.

Furedy, J. J., Heslegrave, R. J., & Scher, H. (1992). T-wave amplitude utility revisited: Some physiological and psychophysiological considerations. *Biological Psychology, 33*, 241–8.

Garner, J. S., & Rutala, M. S. (1986). Guideline for handwashing and hospital environmental control. *American Journal of Infection Control, 14*, 110–26.

Gautier, C. H., & Cook, E. W. III (1997). Relationship between startle and cardiovascular reactivity. *Psychophysiology, 34*, 87–96.

Geddes, L. A., & Baker, L. E. (1971). Response to passage of electric current through the body. *Journal of the Association for the Advancement of Medical Instrumentation, 5*, 13–18.

Goldberger, A. L., & Goldberger, E. (1994). *Clinical Electrocardiography*, 5th ed. St. Louis, MO: Mosby.

Gordon, N. F., & Mitchell, B. S. (1993). Health appraisal in the nonmedical setting. In J. L. Durstine, A. C. King, P. L. Painter, J. L. Roitman, & L. D. Zwiren (Eds.), *Resource Manual for Guidelines for Exercise Testing and Prescription*, 2nd ed. Philadelphia: Lea & Febiger.

Guyton, A. C., & Hall, J. E. (1996). *Textbook of Medical Physiology*, 9th ed. Philadelphia: Saunders.

Hammer, W. (1989). *Occupational Safety Management and Engineering*, 4th ed. Englewood Cliffs, NJ: Prentice-Hall.

Henderson, D., Subramaniam, M., Gratton, M. S., & Saunders, S. S. (1991). Impact noise: The importance of level, duration and repetition. *Journal of the Acoustical Society of America, 89*, 1350–7.

Hirsch, M. S., Wormser, G. P., & Schooley, R. T. (1985). Risk of nosocomial infections with human T-cell lymphotrophic virus III (HTLV-III). *New England Journal of Medicine, 312*, 1–4.

Hoeltge, G. A., Miller, A., Klein, B. R., & Hamlin, W. B. (1993). Accidental fires in clinical laboratories. *Archives of Pathology and Laboratory Medicine, 117*, 1200–4.

Hollister, H., & Trout, C. A., Jr. (1979). On the role of system safety in maintaining "affordable" safety in the 1980s. Paper (no. SAND 79-1671C) presented at the Fourth International System Safety Conference (San Francisco).

Journal of Clinical Neurophysiology (1994). Report of the committee on infectious diseases. *Journal of Clinical Neurophysiology, 11*, 128–32.

Keith, F. R. (1990). *Handbook of Laboratory Safety*, 3rd ed. Boca Raton, FL: CRC Press.

Kourvenhoven, W. B. (1949). Effects of electricity on the human body. *Electrical Engineering, 68*, 199–203.

Legault, S. E., Langer, A., Armstrong, P. W., & Freeman, M. R. (1995). Usefulness of ischemic response to mental stress in predicting silent myocardial ischemia during ambulatory monitoring. *American Journal of Cardiology, 75*, 1007–11.

Marshall-Goodell, B. S., Tassinary, L. G., & Cacioppo, J. T. (1990). Principles of bioelectric measurement. In J. T. Cacioppo & L. G. Tassinary (Eds.), *Principles of Psychophysiology*, pp. 113–48. Cambridge University Press.

Martin, L. S., McDougal, J. S., & Loskoski, S. L. (1985). Disinfection and inactivation of the human T lymphotropic virus type III/lymphadenopathy-associated virus. *Journal of Infectious Diseases, 152*, 400-3.

McPartland, J. F., & McPartland, B. J. (1996). *McGraw-Hill's National Electrical Code Handbook: Based on the Current 1996 National Electrical Code*, 22nd ed. New York: McGraw-Hill.

Moak, E. (1994). AANA journal course: Update for nurse anesthetists – An overview of electrical safety. *Journal of the American Nursing Association, 62*, 69–75.

National Electrical Code (1996). Quincy, MA: National Fire Protection Association.

National Fire Protection Association Standards (1990). *National Electrical Code*. Quincy, MA: National Fire Protection Association.

National Institutes of Health (1993). *Protecting Human Research Subjects: Institutional Review Board Guidebook*. Washington, DC: U.S. Government Printing Office.

NIOSH [National Institute of Occupational Safety and Health] (1972). *Criteria for a Recommended Standard: Occupational Exposure to Noise* (NIOSH Publication no. HSM 73-11001). Washington, DC: U.S. Government Printing Office.

Norton, P. B., et al. (Eds.) (1994). *The New Encyclopædia Brittanica: Micropaedia*, 15th ed., vols. 1–29. Chicago: Encyclopedia Britannica.

NSC [National Safety Council] (1996). *Accident Facts*, rev. ed. Itasca, IL: NSC.

OSHA [Occupational Safety and Health Administration] (1983). *An Illustrated Guide to Electrical Safety* (Publication no. 3073). Washington, DC: U.S. Government Printing Office.

OSHA (1992). *Principle Emergency Response and Preparedness Requirements in OSHA Standards and Guidelines for Safety and Health Programs* (Publication no. 3122). Washington, DC: U.S. Government Printing Office.

OSHA (1995a). *All About OSHA* (Publication no. 2056). Washington, DC: U.S. Government Printing Office.

OSHA (1995b). *How to Prepare for Workplace Emergencies* (Publication no. 3088). Washington, DC: U.S. Government Printing Office.

OSHA (1996). *OSHA Handbook for Small Business* (Publication no. 2209). Washington, DC: U.S. Government Printing Office.

Pollock, M. L., & Wilmore, J. H. (1990). *Exercise in Health and Disease*. Philadelphia: Saunders.

Public Law 91-596, 91st Congress, S.2193, 29 December 1970, as amended by Public Law 101-552, section 3101, 5 November 1990.

Putnam, L. E., Johnson, R., Jr., & Roth, W. T. (1992). Guidelines for reducing the risk of disease transmission in the psychophysiology laboratory. *Psychophysiology, 29*, 127–49.

Rasmussen, K., Bagger, J. P., Bittzauw, J., & Henningsen, P. (1984). Prevalence of vasospastic ischaemia induced by cold pressor test or hyperventilation in patients with severe angina. *European Heart Journal, 5*, 354–61.

Reading, T. S., & Shepard, R. J. (1992). Revision of the Physical Activity Readiness Questionnaire (PAR-Q). *Canadian Journal of Sport Science, 17*, 338–45. [Based on the British Columbia Department of Health, PAR-Q Validation Report, 1975.]

Reilly, J. P. (1992). *Electrical Stimulation and Electropathology*. Cambridge University Press.

Rozanski, A., Bairey, C. N., Krantz, D. S., Friedman, J., Resser, K. J., Morell, M., Hilton-Chalfen, S., Hestrin, L., Bietendorf, J., & Berman, D. S. (1988). Mental stress and the induction of silent myocardial ischemia in patients with coronary artery disease. *New England Journal of Medicine, 318*, 1005–12.

Rutala, W. A. (1990). APIC guideline for selection and use of disinfectants. *American Journal of Infection Control, 18*, 99–117.

San Diego Union–Tribune (1997). Dartmouth accused in research death. 19 August, p. A-5.

Scheidt, S. (1986). *Basic Electrocardiology*. West Caldwell, NJ: Ciba-Geigy.

Schinka, J. A. (1989). *Health Problems Checklist*. Odessa, FL: Psychological Assessment Resources.

Shepard, R. J., Thomas, S., & Weller, I. (1991). The Canadian home fitness test: 1991 update. *Sports Medicine, 11*, 358–66.

Silversides, J. (1964). The neurological sequelae of electrical injury. *California Medical Association Journal, 91*, 195–204.

Simpson, C. D. (1995). *Principles of Electronics*. Upper Saddle River, NJ: Prentice-Hall.

Skuggevig, W. (1992). Standards and protective measures. In J. P. Reilly (Ed.), *Electrical Stimulation and Electrical Pathology*, pp. 429–65. Cambridge University Press.

Specchia, G., de Servi, S., Falcone, C., Gavazzi, A., Angoli, L., Bramucci, E., Ardission, D., & Mussini, A. (1984). Mental arithmetic stress testing in patients with coronary artery disease. *American Heart Journal, 108*, 56–63.

Staewen, W. S. (1994). Electrical safety reconsidered – The new AAMI electrical safety standard. *Biomedical Instrumentation Technology, 28*, 131–2.

Steere, N. V. (1973). Research needed for laboratory safety standards – Part I. *Journal of Chemistry Education, 50*, A539–A543.

Sundin, O., Öhman, A., Palm, T., & Strom, G. (1995). Cardiovascular reactivity, Type A behavior, and coronary heart disease: Comparisons between myocardial infarction patients and controls during laboratory-induced stress. *Psychophysiology, 32*, 28–35.

Sweeney, J. D. (1992). Muscle response to electrical stimulation. In J. P. Reilly (Ed.), *Electrical Stimulation and Electrical Pathology*, pp. 285–327. Cambridge University Press.

UL [Underwriters Laboratories] (1983). *Double Insulation Systems for Use in Electrical Equipment* (UL 1097). Santa Clara, CA: Underwriters Laboratories.

UL (1990). *Standards for Safety: Laboratory Equipment* (UL 1262). Santa Clara, CA: Underwriters Laboratories.

Wilson, P. D., Fardy, P. S., & Froelicher, V. F. (1981). *Cardiac Rehabilitation, Adult Fitness and Exercise Testing*. Philadelphia: Lea & Febiger.

Wormser, G. P., Rabkin, C. S., & Joline, C. (1988). Frequency of nosocomial transmission of HIV infection among health care workers. *New England Journal of Medicine, 319*, 307–8.

CHAPTER THIRTY-SIX

FUNCTIONAL MRI

Background, Methodology, Limits, and Implementation

PETER A. BANDETTINI, RASMUS M. BIRN, & KATHLEEN M. DONAHUE

Introduction

Over the past decade, magnetic resonance imaging (MRI) has developed into a powerful diagnostic technique, advancing rapidly from the creation of the first images in 1973 [1] to the current state of providing detailed information about both anatomy and function. This explosive growth is partially due to the fact that many tissue parameters can affect the MR signal. Signal acquisition can be manipulated in a variety of ways, enabling the user to control image contrast. More recently, advances in scanner hardware have enabled the collection of an entire image in 50 msec or less. Consequently, MRI has evolved from a technique able to provide images with superb soft tissue contrast to one that is also capable of imaging fast physiological processes.

The goal of this chapter is to provide the conceptual background for understanding MRI, with a particular emphasis on functional MRI (fMRI) contrast mechanisms, methods, and pertinent issues. The next section introduces the basic principles of MR imaging – that is, the creation of spatial information using magnetic field gradients. This includes a brief overview of conventional, fast, and echo planar imaging sequences, followed by a discussion of the use of these sequences to evaluate function. We then devote an entire section to explaining the use of MRI to observe human brain function.

Basic Principles of Magnetic Resonance Imaging

MAGNETIC RESONANCE PHENOMENON
Nuclei in a Magnetic Field

The first step in creating a magnetic resonance image is placing the subject in a strong magnetic field. The magnet set-up is shown in Figure 1. This field is typically in the range of 0.5 to 3 Tesla, which is ten to sixty thousand times the strength of the earth's magnetic field. The presence of such a strong magnetic field causes the nuclear spins of certain atoms within the body – namely, those with a nuclear spin dipole moment – to orient themselves either parallel or antiparallel to the main magnetic field (B_0). The nuclei precess about B_0 with a frequency, called the resonance or Larmor frequency (ν_0), which is directly proportional to B_0:

$$\nu_0 = \gamma B_0, \tag{1}$$

where γ is the gyromagnetic ratio, a fundamental physical constant for each nuclear species. Since the proton nucleus (^1H) has a high sensitivity for its MR signal (a result of its high gyromagnetic ratio, 42.58 MHz/Tesla) and a high natural abundance, it is currently the nucleus of choice for magnetic resonance imaging. Because the parallel state is the state of lower energy, slightly more spins reside in the parallel configuration. This creates a net magnetization, which is represented by the vector M_0.

Radiofrequency Field

Magnetic *resonance* occurs when a radiofrequency (RF) pulse, applied at the Larmor frequency, excites the nuclear spins and so raises them from their lower to higher energy states. Classically, this can be represented by a rotation of the net magnetization M_0 away from its rest or equilibrium state. The amount of this rotation is given in terms of the *flip angle,* which depends on the strength and duration of the RF pulse. Common flip angles are $90°$, where the magnetization is rotated into a plane perpendicular to B_0 to create transverse magnetization (M_T), and $180°$, where the magnetization is inverted or aligned antiparallel to B_0. A vector diagram of magnetization during a $90°$ pulse is schematically shown in Figure 2. Once the magnetization is deflected, the RF field is switched off

John T. Cacioppo, Louis G. Tassinary, and Gary G. Berntson (Eds.), *Handbook of Psychophysiology,* 2nd ed. © Cambridge University Press 2000. Printed in the United States of America. ISBN 62634X. All rights reserved.

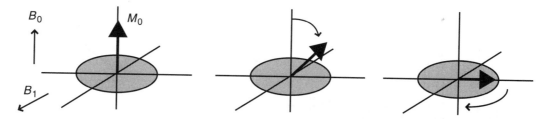

and the magnetization once again freely precesses about the direction of B_0. According to Faraday's law of induction, this time-dependent precession will induce a current in a receiver coil, the RF coil. The resultant exponentially decaying voltage, referred to as the free induction decay (FID), constitutes the MR signal. The FID is shown in Figure 3. Since precession occurs at the Larmor frequency, the resulting MR signal also oscillates at a frequency equal to the Larmor frequency.

During the period of free precession the magnetization returns to its original equilibrium state by a process known as *relaxation,* which is characterized by two time constants, T1 and T2. These constants depend on certain physical and chemical characteristics unique to tissue type, therefore contributing substantially to the capability of MRI to produce detailed images of the human body with unprecedented soft tissue contrast.

Relaxation Phenomenon

Spin–Lattice Relaxation (T1). Radiofrequency stimulation causes nuclei to absorb energy, lifting them to an excited state. The nuclei in their excited state can return to the ground state by dissipating their excess energy to the lattice. This return to equilibrium is termed spin–lattice relaxation and is characterized by the time constant T1, the spin–lattice relaxation time. The term "lattice" de-

Figure 2. A series of vector diagrams illustrating the excitation of a collection of spins by applying an alternating magnetic field, in this case a 90° radiofrequency (RF) pulse (represented here as B_1); B_0 indicates the direction of the main magnetic field. The first two vector diagrams are in a frame of reference rotating with the radiofrequency pulse. As a result, the alternating magnetic field can be represented by a vector in a fixed direction. Application of the RF pulse flips the magnetization into the transverse plane, after which the magnetization continues to precess about the main magnetic field.

scribes the magnetic environment of the nuclei. To better understand T1 relaxation, consider the following example. Suppose that, in the equilibrium state, M_0 is oriented along the z-axis. A 90° RF pulse rotates M_0 completely into the transverse plane so that M_z (the z component of M_0) is now equal to zero. After one T1 interval, $M_z = 0.63M_0$. After two T1 intervals, $M_z = 0.86M_0$, and so on. Thus, the T1 relaxation time characterizes the exponential return of the M_z magnetization to M_0 from its value following excitation.

The inversion recovery sequence that is most sensitive to T1 effects consists of a 180° RF pulse followed by a delay (TI, the inversion time), which in turn is followed by a 90° RF pulse and signal acquisition (AQ). Hence, this sequence is denoted by

$$180° -- TI -- 90° -- AQ. \qquad (2)$$

At time $t = 0$, M_0 is inverted by a 180° pulse, after which M_z ($= M_0$) lies along the negative z-axis. Because of spin–lattice relaxation, M_z will increase in value from $-M_0$ through zero and back to its full equilibrium value of $+M_0$. A 90° pulse is applied at a time TI after the initial 180° pulse. The 90° pulse rotates the partially recovered magnetization, M_z, into the transverse plane, resulting in a detectable MR signal or FID. The FID reflects the magnitude of M_z after a time TI. By varying the TI, the rate of return of M_z to its equilibrium position can be monitored, as shown in Figure 4. If we assume that M_z is initially equal to $-M_0$ after the 180° pulse and recovers with an exponential decay rate 1/T1, then the equation describing the recovery of M_z is given by

$$M_z(t) = M_0[1 - 2e^{-t/T1}]. \qquad (3)$$

Figure 1. A schematic of a typical MR imaging system. The essential components include the magnet producing the main magnetic field, shim coils, a set of gradient coils, an RF coil, and amplifiers and computer systems (not shown) for control of the scanner and data acquisition.

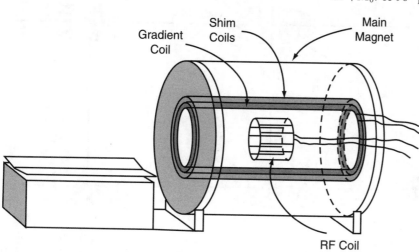

Gradient Coil

Shim Coils

Main Magnet

RF Coil

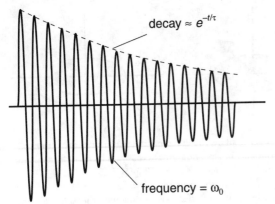

Figure 3. The signal acquired after excitation in the absence of applied magnetic field gradients is a decaying sinusoid, called the free induction decay (FID). This signal is characterized by two parameters – the amplitude and the frequency, which depend on the number and type of spins being studied and the magnetic environment that the spins are in.

Spin–Spin Relaxation (T2, T2*). Immediately after an RF pulse, the magnetic moments (or spins) are in phase. Because of natural processes that cause nuclei to exchange energy with each other, the spins lose their phase coherence. As a result, the net transverse magnetization (M_T) decays to zero exponentially with time, yielding spin–spin relaxation. This decay is characterized by the time constant T2. However, processes other than inherent spin–spin interactions also cause the spins to dephase. The main magnetic field is not perfectly homogeneous, so nuclei in different portions of the sample experience different values of $\mathbf{B_0}$ and precess at slightly different frequencies. This is described in more detail later. When both natural processes and magnetic imperfections contribute to M_T decay, the decay is characterized by the time constant T2*, which

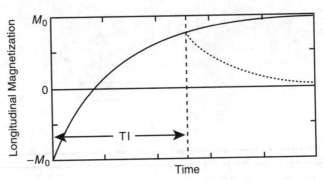

Figure 4. In an inversion recovery sequence, an initial 180° RF pulse flips the magnetization along the $-z$-axis. The magnetization then relaxes back to its equilibrium state with a time constant T1. At a time TI after the 180° pulse, a 90° pulse is applied, flipping the partially recovered magnetization into the transverse plane. This acquired signal (dotted line) is modulated by the T1 relaxation of the tissue.

is less than T2. Typically, both T2* and T2 are much less than T1.

The spin–echo pulse sequence was designed to correct for the transverse decay due to field inhomogeneities. It consists of a 90° RF pulse followed by a 180° RF pulse and signal acquisition:

$$90° \text{ -- } \tau \text{ -- } 180° \text{ -- } \tau \text{ -- AQ.} \qquad (4)$$

Figure 5. A series of vector diagrams illustrating the formation of a spin echo. The diagrams are shown in a frame of reference rotating with the resonance frequency of water. The magnetization is excited by an RF pulse, flipping it into the transverse plane (a). Because of magnetic field inhomogeneities, the spins dephase – shown here as a "fanning out" of the vector (b). At a time t (c), a 180° RF pulse is applied that flips the spins to the other side of the transverse plane (d). The spins then continue to precess as before, but now the slower precessing spins are ahead of the faster ones (e). The spins refocus, forming an echo of the original transverse magnetization at time $2t$ (f).

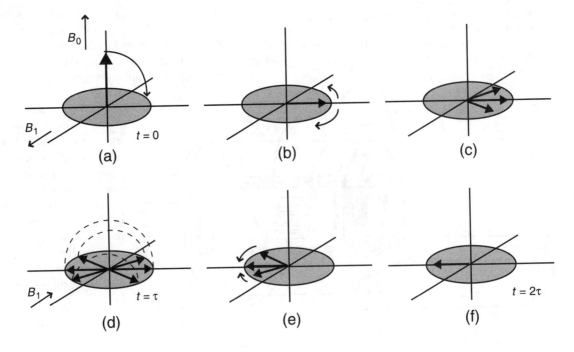

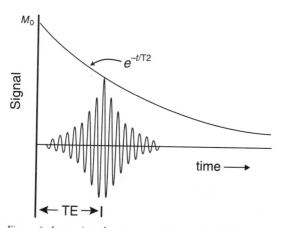

Figure 6. In a spin–echo sequence, the amplitude of the acquired signal (shown here as a spin echo) is modulated by the T2 relaxation of the spins. Signals acquired at a longer TE will be smaller.

As illustrated in Figure 5, following the 90° RF pulse, spins experiencing the slightly higher fields precess faster than those experiencing the lower fields. Consequently, the spins "fan out" or lose coherence. Then, at some time τ after application of the 90° pulse, a 180° pulse is applied and the spins will be flipped into mirror image positions; that is, the fast spins will now trail the slow spins. Hence, at a time τ later, the fast spins will have caught up with the slow spins, so that all are back in phase and a *spin echo* is created. The total period between the initial 90° pulse and the echo is denoted the echo time (TE $= 2\tau$). Thus, the spin echo reflects the magnitude M_T after time TE.

Spins lose phase coherence not only because of field inhomogeneities but also because of the natural processes responsible for spin–spin relaxation. These natural processes are irreversible and cannot be refocused. Therefore, the spin–echo signal amplitude at time TE reflects T2 decay. Consequently, as the value of TE is increased, the echo amplitudes will decrease. This is shown in Figure 6 and can be simply described as follows:

$$M_T(t) = M_0 e^{-t/T2}. \tag{5}$$

IMAGING CONCEPTS

The basic goal of MR imaging is to measure the distribution of magnetization within the body, which depends on both the variation in the concentration of water and the magnetic environment between different tissues. In a completely uniform field, all of the hydrogen protons of water resonate at the same frequency. The RF coil used to detect the signal, as shown in Figure 1, is sensitive only to the frequency, amplitude, and phase of the precessing magnetization and not to the spatial location. It cannot distinguish two spins at different locations that are precessing at the same frequency; it can only distinguish spins precessing at different frequencies. To make an image it is necessary to make the spin's precessional frequency depend on the location of the spin. This is accomplished

by superimposing linear magnetic field gradients on the main magnetic field. The term "gradient" indicates that the magnetic field is altered along a selected direction. Referring to the Larmor equation (1), we note that if the field is varied linearly along a certain direction then the resonance frequency also varies with location, thus providing the information necessary for spatial localization.

We will first review the conventional method by which gradients are applied to acquire a two-dimensional image. Understanding these principles will aid in the understanding of more advanced techniques (e.g., fast gradient echo and echo planar imaging) that are described in subsequent sections.

Obtaining a two-dimensional image requires three steps. The first step is to excite only the spins in the slice of interest; this is called *slice selection*. The next steps are to localize the spins within that slice using the techniques of *frequency encoding* and *phase encoding*. For convenience, let z denote the direction for slice selection, x the direction for frequency encoding, and y the direction for phase encoding. These designations are arbitrary and unrelated to the actual physical orientation of the x, y, and z gradient coils. These concepts are introduced by building up a conventional spin–echo imaging sequence, which consists of a combination of RF and gradient pulses.

Slice Selection

The first step is the selection of a slice, which is achieved by applying a magnetic field gradient along the z-axis (G_z) during a 90° RF pulse of a specific frequency bandwidth (period 1 of Figure 7). When the slice selection gradient G_z is applied along the z-axis, the resonance frequencies of the protons become linearly related to positions along the z-axis. Individual resonance frequencies correspond to individual planes of nuclei. In this example, these planes are oriented perpendicular to the z-axis. When the frequency-selective 90° pulse is applied while G_z is energized, only nuclei in the plane with corresponding frequencies will be excited; thus, a slice will be selected. This is indicated as the dark gray area in Figure 8. The frequency bandwidth of the excitation pulse, together with the gradient, confines the excitation to the nuclei in the slice. No signals are excited or detected from areas outside the defined slice.

The RF pulse that is transmitted to the patient contains not just one frequency but rather a narrow range, or *bandwidth,* of frequencies. Quantitatively, the thickness of the excited slice (Δz) in centimeters is related to the gradient amplitude G_z and RF bandwidth Δf as follows:

$$\Delta z = \Delta f / \gamma G_z. \tag{6}$$

If Δf is increased so that more frequencies are present in the RF pulse, then a larger slice will be excited. Alternatively, if the strength of the gradient is decreased then

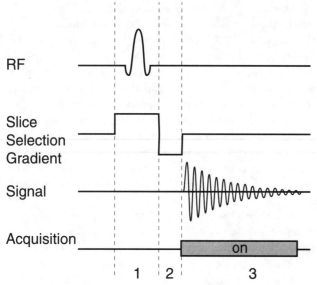

Figure 7. The sequence of RF power and gradient strength used for slice selection. To excite only one slice, a magnetic field gradient is applied during the excitation RF pulse.

more spins are resonating in a given range of frequencies, and again a larger slice is excited. Therefore the thickness of the slice excited can be varied in two ways: by changing the strength of the gradient, as indicated in Figure 9, or by varying the bandwidth of the transmitted RF pulse, as shown in Figure 10.

The slice-selection gradient G_z has two effects on the MR signal, the desired one of aiding in spatial localization and the unwanted one of dephasing the signal (since the phase of the spins is also proportional to field strength).

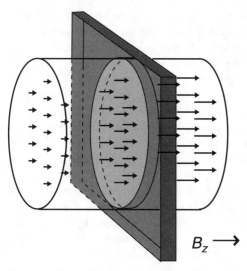

Figure 8. The application of a magnetic field gradient in slice selection creates a stronger magnetic field at one end of the sample than at the other end, shown here as arrows of varying length. When the RF pulse is transmitted into the sample, only those spins whose precessional frequency matches the frequencies in the RF pulse are excited, shown here as a dark gray slab.

Therefore, after the slice selection gradient (period 1), a negative z gradient follows (period 2 of Figure 7) to compensate for the dephasing effects of the slice selection gradient. Ideally, this gradient will result in an accumulated phase that is equal and opposite to the phase accumulated from the initial slice selection gradient, thereby canceling its dephasing effects. This type of gradient is often referred to as a "time-reversal" or "rephasing" gradient.

Frequency Encoding

After slice selection, the next task is to distinguish signals from different spatial locations within the slice. This is accomplished in the x direction by applying a gradient G_x, the *frequency encoding* gradient, during the acquisition of the signal (time period 3 in Figure 11). Because the MR signal is sampled during the time that G_x is on, this period is also commonly referred to as the "readout" period and G_x as the "read" gradient. This signal can come from either the FID or a spin–echo sequence, the latter formed by applying a 180° pulse at a time TE/2 after the 90° excitation pulse, as shown in Figure 11(b). Sequences that collect the signal from the FID are known as gradient–echo (GRE) sequences; those that collect the signal from the spin echo are known as spin–echo (SE) sequences. The two differ in the contrast that they provide. For example, because of the refocusing pulse, spin–echo sequences are less susceptible to magnetic field inhomogeneities and thus reflect differences in T2 rather than T2* relaxation times between the tissues. These differences will be discussed in detail later. The next few sections will deal mainly with the spin–echo sequence.

The way in which the linear gradient encodes the spatial information can be more easily seen by considering a sample consisting of two vials of water, aligned with the y-axis and placed some distance apart in the x direction (see Figure 12). All of the signal comes from these two sources of water. If signal from this sample is collected without the application of any gradients, both areas are

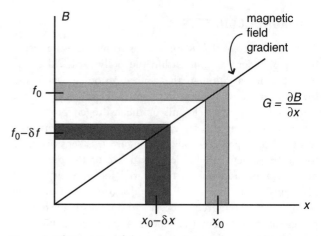

Figure 9. The position of the excited slice can be varied by changing the frequency of the transmitted RF pulse.

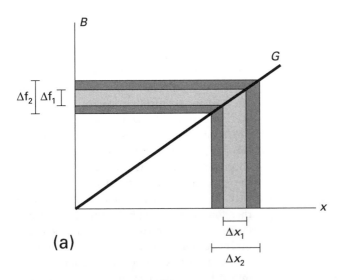

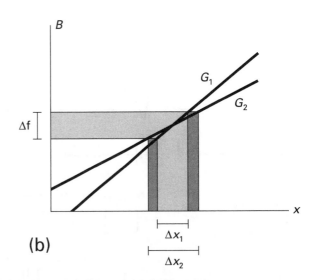

Figure 10. The thickness of the excited slice can be varied either by (a) changing the bandwidth of the transmitted RF pulse or by (b) changing the amplitude of the slice selection gradient. Here Δf_1 = frequency 1, corresponding to slice thickness Δx_1; Δf_2 = frequency 2, corresponding to slice thickness Δx_2; and G = magnetic field gradient.

precessing at the same frequency. Consequently, the signal will appear as a pure sinusoid, and applying a mathematical process called the Fourier transform will show that it contains only one frequency. (Whereas the FID represents the time evolution of M_{xy}, the Fourier transform of the signal represents its frequency distribution.) The amplitude of this frequency peak corresponds to the total amount of water from both vials.

However, if a gradient is applied during the acquisition of the signal, then the spins in one vial are in a slightly higher magnetic field than those in the other vial. According to the Larmor relation, one group of spins will precess faster than the other group, and the signal will be an interference pattern composed of both of these frequencies. A Fourier transform applied to this signal will reveal two distinct frequencies. Since a spatially linear gradient was applied, the frequencies of these peaks exactly correspond to the position of the vials. Also, the amount of signal at a given frequency is determined by the number of spins precessing at that frequency, so it is directly related to the amount of magnetization at a given location. In other words, the Fourier transform of the signal is simply a projection of the distribution of magnetization onto the frequency encoding axis.

Figure 13 shows the phases of the magnetization vectors in one slice at three time points during frequency encoding. The presence of the gradient induces the spins at one end to precess faster than those at the other end, causing an increasing amount of phase shift along this direction. As time progresses (when the gradient has been applied for a longer duration), the amount of "phase twisting" is increased. One effect of this is that the peak of the signal (when it is least dephased) will be at the beginning of the acquisition. In order to move the peak signal to the center of the acquisition window, a negative gradient lobe (time reversal gradient) with exactly half the area of the frequency encoding gradient is applied just *before* the frequency encoding gradient. This initially dephases

the spins, which are then brought back in phase by the applied frequency encoding gradient (see Figure 14). In the spin–echo sequence, the gradient lobe is positive and occurs before the 180° inversion pulse.

The details of the frequency encoding procedure dictate the image size (in centimeters) or *field of view* along the x-axis:

$$\text{FOV}_x = \frac{\text{BW}}{\gamma G_x}, \tag{7}$$

where BW is the receiver bandwidth. Note that the receiver bandwidth should not be confused with the excitation RF bandwidth, which dictates the slice thickness (see equation (6)). Here, the bandwidth is the effective range of frequencies that can be properly detected, as determined by the Nyquist criterion [2]. The BW is controlled by the digital sampling rate, which in turn is determined by the number of points N_x on the signal to be digitized and the length of time the receiver is on (the acquisition time, AQ):

$$\text{BW} = \frac{N_x}{\text{AQ}}. \tag{8}$$

Accordingly, from these two equations, the pixel size along the frequency encoding axis can be derived as follows:

$$\text{pixel size} = \frac{\text{FOV}_x}{N_x} = \frac{1}{\gamma G_x(\text{AQ})}. \tag{9}$$

Phase Encoding

The final spatial dimension can be encoded into the signal by applying a programmable phase encoding gradient G_y, simultaneous with the rephasing gradient in period 2, in the time between the excitation and the acquisition (see

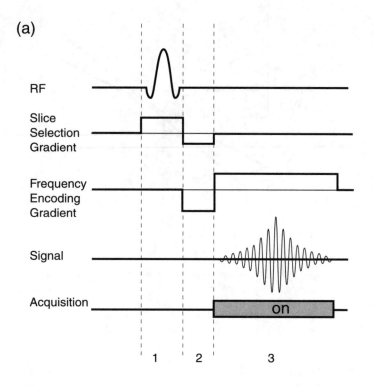

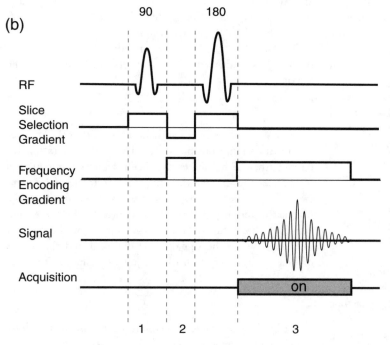

Figure 11. The sequence of RF power and gradient ampitudes used to excite one slice and encode the positions of the spins within that slice into the signal. In this *frequency encoding*, the positions of the spins are encoded by applying a magnetic field gradient in one of the directions in the excited slice during the acquisition. Note that the signal can come either from (a) the FID or (b) a spin echo (an echo of the FID). Sequences using signals from the FID are called gradient–echo sequences; sequences using signals from the spin echo are called spin–echo sequences.

Figure 15). During the phase encoding period, nuclei in each column of voxels along the y direction experience different magnetic fields. Nuclei subjected to the highest magnetic field precess fastest. This is no different from the effect of the frequency encoding pulse. However, the state of magnetization during the phase encoding pulse is less important than the phase shift accumulated after the phase encoding gradient has been turned off. When the gradient is on, the nuclei that experience the highest field advance the farthest and therefore acquire a phase angle, ϕ_y, that is larger than that in voxels experiencing smaller magnetic fields. After G_y is turned off, the nuclei revert to the resonance frequency determined by the main magnetic field. However, they "remember" the previous event by retaining their characteristic y-dependent phase angles. The field of view in the y direction (FOV_y) is quantitatively defined in a manner similar to (7):

$$FOV_y = \frac{1}{\gamma T_y G_{y\,max}}, \qquad (10)$$

where T_y is the duration and $G_{y\,max}$ is the maximum amplitude of the phase encoding gradient.

Although the signal obtained from one acquisition (slice selection, phase encoding, and frequency encoding) contains information from all voxels in the imaging slice, the information gathered from a single iteration of this sequence is not sufficient to reconstruct an image. Consequently, the sequence must be repeated with different settings of the phase encoding gradient G_y.

When a phase encoding gradient of a particular value has been applied, the effect of that gradient is to shift the phases of the spins by an amount depending on their position (in this case, in the y direction) and the amplitude of the phase encoding gradient. For example, spins near the isocenter experience no phase shift, whereas spins at positions off center are shifted by a certain amount depending on their distance from the center. The net result of this spin dephasing is simply a decrease in the signal. It is only through varying the amount of this dephasing (thus varying the amount of signal decrease) – by stepping through the phase encoding gradient's range of amplitudes – that the location of structures along the phase encoding gradient can be identified.

If the data at each cycle of the G_y setting were plotted, it would show sinusoidal curves with a frequency

Sample

Gradients

B

Signal

↓ FT

Frequency content of signal

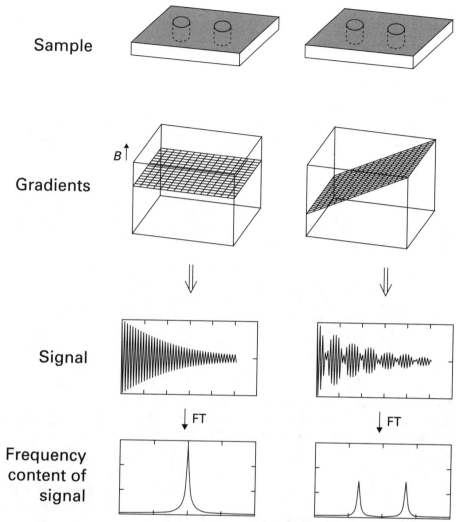

dictated by the rate of phase change (between each iteration of the pulse sequence), which, in turn, depends on location. A similar curve is derived during frequency encoding, but with a difference: each sample along this curve originates from a different MR signal. Each of these MR signals follows a phase encoding gradient pulse of different amplitude. However, as with frequency encoding, the frequency components of the curve are identified by the Fourier transform and the magnetization is ascribed to a given location.

In summary, for a matrix of size $N_y \times N_x$, the required number of iterations is N_y. The N_y signals, each corresponding to a different value of G_y, are sampled N_x times during the read period. Subsequent two-dimensional Fourier transformation yields the intensity values of each of the $N_y \times N_x$ pixels.

Image Formation Mathematics: *k*-Space

The key to image formation is encoding the location of the magnetization in the phase of the MR signal. It is worthwhile to look at this encoding process in more detail. Consider the encoding of spatial information along

Figure 12. A series of steps illustrating the concept of frequency encoding to distinguish the signal coming from two point sources of magnetization (e.g., small vials of water) in an object. *Left*. When no gradient is applied, both sources of magnetization resonate at the same frequency, and the signal is a simple decaying sinusoid. When this signal is Fourier transformed, the signal is shown to contain only one frequency. *Right*. When a gradient is applied, one of the sources of magnetization precesses at a higher frequency than the other. The resulting signal is an interference pattern of the two frequencies, which is shown (by Fourier transformation) to contain two distinct frequencies. Notice that the Fourier transformed signal is the projection of the amount of magnetization along the axis along which the gradient was applied. That is, in this one-dimensional case, the frequency content of the signal *is* the image.

one dimension within the plane after the slice has been excited. A collection of spins along one dimension can be thought of as a column of vectors, as shown in Figure 16. After the slice has been excited, all of the spins within the slice are in phase. Once a magnetic field gradient is applied, the spins will precess at different frequencies depending on their location. At any given moment, certain spins will have accumulated more phase than others. These gradients can thus be thought of as "twisting" the

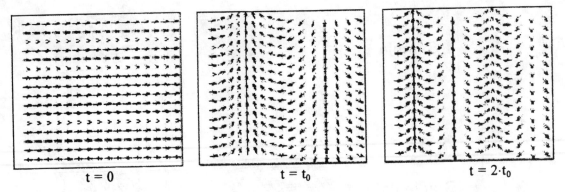

$$t = 0 \qquad\qquad t = t_0 \qquad\qquad t = 2 \cdot t_0$$

Figure 13. At each time increment when the signal is acquired in frequency encoding, the gradient has been applied for a longer period of time. This causes an increasingly greater variation in the phase in the direction in which the gradient was applied.

initially aligned column of spins. This twisting of the magnetization vectors by the gradients can be expressed as a rotation of the magnetization by an angle ϕ, which depends on the strength of the magnetic field experienced by that particular location:

$$M = M_T(x, y)e^{-i\phi} = M_T(x, y) \exp\left\{-i \int_0^t \gamma B \, dt'\right\}. \quad (11)$$

(For notational convenience, we observe the convention $e^x \equiv \exp\{x\}$.) At each point in time, the RF coil integrates this magnetization over the entire volume; thus, the signal at a given point in time can be expressed as

$$S(t) = \int M_T(x, y) \exp\left\{-i \int_0^t \gamma B \, dt'\right\} dx \, dy. \quad (12)$$

For imaging, linear gradient fields are applied and so the magnetic field $\mathbf{B}$ experienced by the spins can be rewritten as

$$\mathbf{B} = \int G_x \, dx + \int G_y \, dy = G_x x + G_y y. \quad (13)$$

If it is assumed that the position of the magnetization with respect to the coils does not change with time (i.e., the patient does not move), then the signal can be written as

$$S(t) = \int M_T(x, y) \exp\left\{-i\left(x\gamma \int_0^t G_x \, dt' + y\gamma \int_0^t G_y \, dt'\right)\right\}. \quad (14)$$

If we make the substitutions

$$k_x = \gamma \int_0^t G_x \, dt' \quad \text{and} \quad k_y = \gamma \int_0^t G_y \, dt', \quad (15)$$

then (14) becomes

$$S(k_x, k_y) = \int M_T(x, y) \exp\{-i(k_x x + k_y y)\} \, dx \, dy. \quad (16)$$

This signal is a Fourier transform of the magnetization, by virtue of the gradients applied. A measure of the magnetization, $M(x, y)$, can be obtained by taking a two-dimensional Fourier transform of the signal.

Figure 14. Diagrams showing the gradient amplitude, the phase of two spins subjected to these gradients, and the profile of the resulting signal. When an initial negative gradient is applied (right), the spins are in phase in the center of the acquisition window. This leads to a greater net signal.

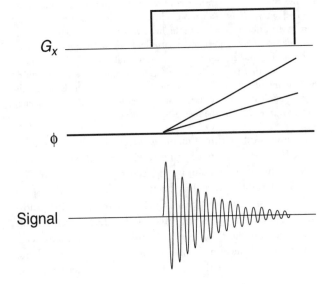

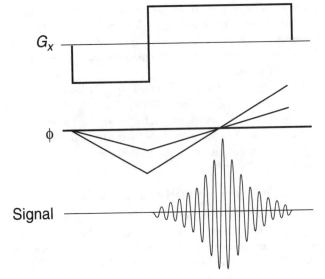

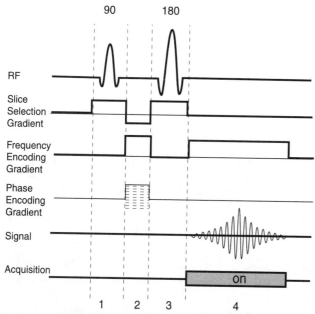

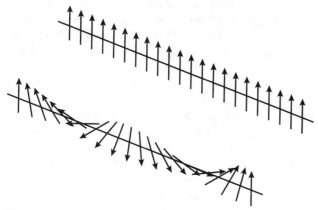

Figure 15. A complete pulse sequence diagram for the spin–echo sequence. Spatial locations of the spins are encoded into the signal by applying three orthogonal gradients, techniques known as slice selection, frequency encoding, and phase encoding. In period 1, a 90° pulse and a slice selection gradient excite one slice. In period 2, the initial frequency encoding gradient and the phase encoding gradient are applied. In period 3, a 180° pulse is applied, along with a slice selection pulse (such that only the spins in the same excited slice are "flipped"); in period 4, the frequency encoding gradient is applied and the signal is acquired. The sequence shown here is repeated numerous times (128, 256, 512, etc., depending on the desired resolution), each time with a different strength of the phase encoding gradient.

Because of the way the gradients are applied during the imaging scan, it is natural to think of the MR signal as being collected in spatial frequency space, or "k-space" [3–5], as implied by the terms in equation (15). This representation is often much more convenient in discussing the details of pulse sequences. In this space, usually plotted in two dimensions, each point describes the amount of a particular spatial frequency present in the imaged object.

Figure 16. The application of a magnetic field gradient can be thought of as twisting the initially aligned column of spins. These spins are then summed at every point in time using the RF coil.

The strongest signal of imaged objects is typically in the center of k-space, where all gradient values are equal to zero. The regions farther out in k-space correspond to higher spatial frequencies, which are especially important in discerning sharp differences in signal (e.g. at edges). Therefore, the highest spatial frequency sampled (or the furthest sample from the center of k-space) determines the resolution of the final image. The further out, the higher the resolution. In contrast, the interval between the samples in k-space, or the resolution in k-space, determines the field of view of the image – in other words, the largest spatial extent that can be acquired. The smallest sample interval corresponds to a large field of view. Care must therefore be taken to acquire samples that are both (i) fine enough to image the entire region of interest and (ii) far enough out in k-space to obtain the desired resolution.

Sampling different points in k-space is accomplished by applying magnetic field gradients, as demonstrated in equation (15). The center of k-space corresponds to the time immediately after excitation and immediately prior to the application of magnetic field gradients. Application of a magnetic field gradient causes the phases of the spins to twist by an increasing amount that corresponds to the amplitude and duration of the gradients, as implied by equation (15). Collecting the signal at this time will cause increasingly higher spatial frequencies to be sampled. In other words, the gradients allow movement in k-space, as shown in Figures 17 and 18.

The figures offer a brief example of how pulse sequences are commonly described in the context of k-space.

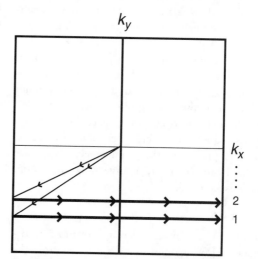

Figure 17. A k-space diagram showing the path through k-space taken to acquire the signal for the gradient–echo (GRE) sequence. For each excitation, the phase encoding gradient moves us a fixed distance in the negative k_y direction and the initial negative frequency encoding gradient moves us in the negative k_x direction. The signal is then sampled moving in the positive k_x direction as the frequency encoding gradient is applied. The signal is then allowed to relax, and the sequence is repeated with a different value for the phase encoding gradient. In this manner, a sufficient range of k-space can be scanned.

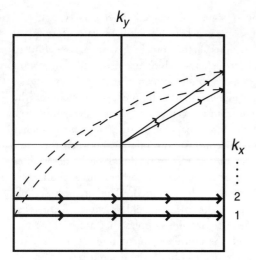

Figure 18. A k-space diagram for the spin–echo (SE) sequence. After the spins are excited, gradients in the positive x and y directions are applied, moving us in the positive k_x and positive k_y direction. The 180° pulse flips us through the center of k-space to the negative k_x, negative k_y direction, after which the positive frequency encoding gradient moves us in the positive k_x direction, allowing us to sample the frequencies as before. This sequence of steps is repeated with different values for the phase encoding gradient.

In the gradient–echo sequence described earlier, we started at the origin of k-space after the excitation. The initial negative x-gradient lobe moves us to the left (negative x frequency) and the phase encoding gradient moves us a specific amount in the y direction of k-space. The final application of an x gradient moves us in the positive x direction, during which time we acquire the signal. The signal is then allowed to relax, and with the next excitation, the value of the phase encoding gradient is changed, allowing us to scan a different line in k-space (Figure 17). For the spin–echo sequence, the initial positive x-gradient lobe moves us in the positive x direction, and the initial phase encoding gradient moves us a specified amount in the positive y direction. The application of a 180° RF pulse flips us through the origin of k-space to the negative x, negative y direction, after which point the signal acquisition occurs just as in the gradient–echo sequence (see Figure 18). In this manner, a large range of spatial frequency space is sampled.

Image Contrast

Although T1, T2, and proton density are intrinsic tissue parameters over which the user has no control, the operator can alter tissue contrast and the signal-to-noise ratio (S/N) by the choice of the pulse sequence parameters. Specifically, images can be obtained in which tissue contrast is primarily determined by (i.e. weighted toward) T1, T2, or proton density characteristics. With the spin–echo imaging sequence, for example, the type of image weighting is determined by the repetition time (TR) and the echo time (TE). The effects of TR and TE on im-

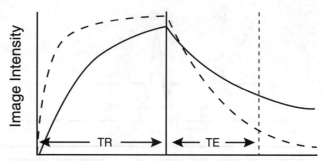

Figure 19. Schematic depicting the effects of TR and TE on the weighting of image intensity. The solid and dashed curves represent two tissues with different T1 and T2 values. The choice of TR (position of solid vertical line) dictates the degree of T1 weighting, while the choice of TE (position of dashed vertical line) determines the amount of T2 weighting.

age weighting are depicted schematically in Figure 19 for the case of two tissues with different T1 and T2 relaxation times. The repetition time TR determines the extent of T1 relaxation. The initial 90° RF pulse completely tips the existing longitudinal magnetization into the transverse plane, leaving zero longitudinal magnetization. If the spins were again excited at this time, no signal would be produced. Therefore, a time interval (TR) is allowed to elapse between excitations so that the spins can undergo T1 relaxation and recover at least part of their longitudinal magnetization.

It is apparent from Figure 19 that the maximum T1 contrast between tissues occurs when TR is greater than zero and less than some time when both tissues have completely recovered their longitudinal magnetization. A long TR (i.e., $\gg$ 5T1) allows enough time to elapse so that almost complete T1 relaxation occurs, rendering signal intensity not a function of T1. The maximum magnetization to which the signal returns is determined by proton density. Likewise, the amount of T2 contrast is dictated by the choice of TE. The longer the time interval TE, the greater the extent of T2 relaxation. Therefore, spin–echo images acquired with short TR (TR $\approx$ T1) and short TE (TE < T2) are T1-weighted. With shorter TR values, tissues such as fat (which have short T1 values) appear bright; tissues that have longer T1 values, such as tumors and edema, take more time to relax toward equilibrium and therefore appear dark. The short TE value diminishes the importance of tissue T2 differences. Similarly, images acquired with long TR (to diminish T1 differences) and long TE (TE $\approx$ T2) are T2-weighted. Therefore, tissues with long T2 (tumors, edema, and cysts) appear bright, whereas tissues that have short T2 (e.g., muscle and liver) appear dark. Images acquired with long TR (TR $\gg$ 5T1) and short TE (TE < T2) are called "proton density–weighted" images. Tissues with increased proton density appear moderately bright. It should be noted that both T1- and T2-weighted images are always partly weighted toward proton density as well.

Sequence Timing

Conventional spin–echo and gradient–echo sequences are repeated at time intervals equal to TR, the repetition time. The number of times the sequence is repeated (for one average) is determined by the desired spatial resolution (proportional to the number of voxels) along the phase encoding direction and is equal to the number of phase encoding steps (N_y). For NEX (number of excitations) averages, the total time required to obtain an image slice is

$$TR \times N_y \times NEX. \qquad (17)$$

Typical parameters for conventional spin–echo sequence are a TR of 2 sec, 128 phase encoding steps, and two averages, giving a total acquisition time of 8.5 min.

To decrease imaging time, one or more of these parameters can be decreased. Decreasing the number of averages by two will halve the imaging time, but with the additional effect of decreasing the S/N by $\sqrt{2}$ or 41%; this will increase the graininess of the image. Motion artifacts (which are also decreased by averaging) could become significant if imaging time were reduced by decreasing the number of averages. Reducing the image matrix size or the number of phase encoding steps decreases imaging time at the expense of spatial resolution. Moreover, the larger pixels result in an increased S/N. The simplest way to speed up an ordinary SE scan would be to drastically reduce TR. However, the signal produced depends on the amount of T1 relaxation that occurs during the interval TR and thus on the available signal for the next excitation. A short TR relative to T1 would result in significant signal losses. Consequently, the T1 relaxation times of tissue protons limit the degree to which the pulse repetition times (TR) can be shortened. Two techniques that overcome TR limitations include gradient–echo (GRE) and echo planar imaging (EPI) techniques. These fast imaging sequences are discussed in the following sections.

An alternate procedure to speed up acquisition of spin–echo images has been developed in which several 180° pulses follow each 90° RF excitation pulse, creating several spin echoes with each echo differently phase encoded. Consequently, if four spin echoes follow each 90° excitation pulse, then the total acquisition time would be one fourth of that with the conventional approach of acquiring one phase encoding step per excitation pulse. This principle underlies the RARE (rapid acquisition with relaxation enhancement) imaging technique [6]. Obviously, acquisition of signals at different effective echo times lends strong T2 weighting to RARE images.

PULSE SEQUENCE AND CONTRAST TOPICS
Fast Gradient–Echo Imaging

In its most basic form, the GRE pulse sequence, as shown in Figure 11(a), consists of one RF pulse with a flip angle α, followed at some time later by the acquisition of the gradient echo. The time between the excitation and the acquisition of the gradient echo is defined as the echo time, TE:

$$\alpha \text{ degrees } -- TE -- \text{gradient echo.} \qquad (18)$$

Because GRE sequences lack a 180° refocusing pulse, images generated with these sequences are sensitive to artifacts from magnetic field inhomogeneities (i.e., T2* effects).

Gradient echo sequences are typically used as fast sequences because data are acquired before the dephasing of spins from previous application of the pulse sequences is complete; that is, T2* decay is not complete. In most cases, the TR is less than the time for more than 90% of the spins to dephase (three times the T2 time). Consequently, GRE sequences may be further divided into two categories according to how they handle the residual magnetization after data acquisition: those that attempt to maintain it in a steady-state condition and those that simply eliminate it. Those techniques that maintain it – refocused FLASH (fast low-angle shot), FISP (fast imaging with steady-state precession), and GRASS (gradient-recalled acquisition steady state) – rephase the spins along one or more axes prior to reapplication of the next RF pulse.

Gradient echo sequences that eliminate the residual transverse magnetization (e.g., spoiled FLASH or spoiled GRASS sequences) typically use a "spoiler" pulse to accelerate the dephasing (see Figure 20). Specifically, a high-amplitude, long-duration gradient ruins (spoils) the residual transverse magnetization by disturbing the local magnetic field homogeneity. The best results occur when the spoiler gradient is applied across the slice selection direction. Other spoiling schemes include the use of random RF pulse phases (RF spoiling) and variable TR. See [7] for a more thorough review of these and other fast gradient echo sequences.

Gradient–Echo Image Contrast

In SE imaging, tissue contrast may be manipulated by changes in the TR and TE, as described previously. With GRE sequences, the image contrast is varied by changing TR, TE, and the flip angle α, depending on the pulse sequence [8]. The amount of T2 weighting is dictated by the TE, TR, and type of sequence. A short TE, long TR, and transverse-spoiled sequence all serve to decrease the degree of T2 weighting. For a given TE, low flip angles increase proton density weighting whereas high flip angles increase T1 weighting. At very short TRs, however, the images become weighted toward T2/T1 – that is, structures with larger T2/T1 ratios (e.g. liquids) appear bright. Yet, with very fast GRE sequences (TR $\approx$ 3 msec) and $\alpha < 5°$, soft tissue contrast almost disappears [9]. The signal becomes dominated by spin density. However, if conventional MR experiments are placed before the whole GRE imaging

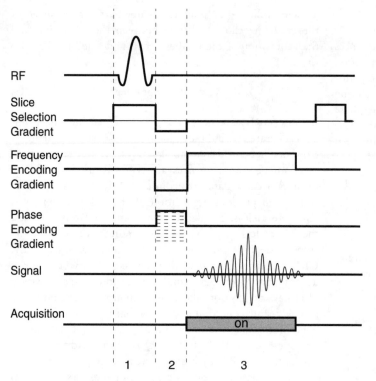

Figure 20. A complete pulse sequence diagram for a gradient–echo sequence. Spatial locations of the spins are encoded into the signal by applying three orthogonal gradients. The sequence shown here is repeated numerous times (128, 256, 512, etc., depending on the desired resolution), each time with a different strength of the phase encoding gradient. The gradient–echo sequence has an advantage over the spin–echo sequence for fast imaging in that it does not use a 180° pulse and does not rely on a 90° excitation pulse.

sequence, images of any desired contrast can be achieved without changing the measuring time. The turbo-FLASH imaging technique is one technique that implements this idea.

The turbo-FLASH method employs an initial 180° RF pulse to invert the spins. Next, an inversion delay (TI) is allowed to elapse, during which differences in longitudinal magnetization (T1 contrast) evolve depending on the T1 relaxation times of various tissues. Finally a very rapid gradient-echo acquisition using an ultrashort TR (e.g., 4 msec) and an ultrashort TE (e.g., 2 msec) is performed. The total time for data acquisition (32 phase encoding steps) is on the order of 100 msec. When using a contrast agent, an appropriate TI value can be selected so that signal from the tissue that does not receive contrast agent is eliminated; this enables wash-in of a contrast agent to be easily visualized [10].

Gradient–Echo Timing

Like the spin–echo sequence, the GRE sequence is repeated at time intervals equal to TR; the total time required to obtain an image slice is TR × N_y × NEX. However, because the TRs used in GRE imaging are typ-

ically very much shorter ($\approx$ 10 msec) than those used in SE imaging ($\approx$ 1 sec), GRE images can be acquired in seconds rather than minutes. For example, using an image matrix of 128 × 128, a TR of 10 msec, and two averages, our total image acquisition time is 2.56 sec. Because the short TRs preclude an interleaved multislice acquisition (as discussed for SE imaging), there simply is not enough time within TR for excitation and detection in other slices. Therefore, the total acquisition time for multislice imaging is

$$(\text{number of slices}) \times (\text{number of views per slice}) \times \text{NEX} \times \text{TR.} \qquad (19)$$

Echo Planar Imaging Sequences

Echo planar imaging (EPI) is significantly different from standard two-dimensional Fourier transform (2DFT) imaging methods. With 2DFT methods, only one projection (or line in k-space) is acquired with each TR interval, so image acquisition time is relatively lengthy. In contrast, the EPI method acquires k-space lines needed to create an image after a single RF excitation (hence, one "plane" is acquired with one RF excitation and subsequent "echo"). First, as in a 2DFT SE sequence, a spin echo is produced by application of a 90° and a 180° RF pulse, with the echo peaking at the echo time (TE). However, rather than apply a single phase encoding gradient and a constant frequency encoding gradient, we rapidly oscillate the frequency encoding gradient during the build-up and decay of the spin echo. A series of gradient echoes is thereby produced, each one of which is separately phase encoded by application of a brief phase encoding gradient pulse. Because all of the data are acquired after a single RF pulse, the images are free from T1 weighting and can be strongly T2 weighted, with the degree of T2 weighting dependent on the value of TE.

In addition to spin–echo EPI images, it is possible to obtain gradient–echo EPI images. The acquisition method is similar to that for spin–echo EPI, except that the series of separately phase encoded gradient echos is acquired under the envelope of a gradient–echo signal produced by a single RF pulse. The measuring time of EPI methods lies in the range of 32–128 msec. Echo planar imaging requires special hardware to allow for rapid gradient switching, whereas gradient–echo techniques can be readily implemented on standard imaging systems.

Functional MRI

The use of fMRI has grown explosively since its inception [11–15]. Among the reasons for this explosive growth are the noninvasiveness of fMRI, the wide availability of

MR scanners capable of fMRI, and the relative robustness and reproducibility of fMRI results. With these reasons for using fMRI came a proportional need for caution. The technology can be easily misused and results can be over-interpreted. A solid understanding of the basics of fMRI is necessary. In this section, we clarify these basic concepts, discuss several practical issues related to fMRI's use, and suggest potential innovations.

MAGNETIC SUSCEPTIBILITY CONTRAST

Magnetic resonance imaging emerged in the 1970s and 1980s as a method by which high-resolution anatomical images of the human brain and other organs could be obtained noninvasively [1; 16–19]. The first types of image contrast used in MRI were proton density spin–lattice relaxation (T1) and spin–spin relaxation (T2) contrast [20–24]. The many degrees of freedom in MR parameter space has allowed MR contrast types to expand from physical to physiological [25]. The types of intrinsic MRI physiological contrast that have been discovered and developed include blood flow [25–28], diffusion [25; 29–33], perfusion [25; 31–40], and magnetization transfer [25; 41; 42]. Chemical shift imaging has been able to provide information about relative concentrations and distributions of several chemical species [25; 43; 44].

The effects of endogenous and exogenous paramagnetic materials and, more generally, of materials having different susceptibilities have also been characterized. An understanding of susceptibility contrast is an essential prerequisite to the exploration of fMRI contrast mechanisms.

Magnetic susceptibility, χ, is the proportionality constant between the strength of the applied magnetic field and the resultant magnetization established within the material [45]. In most biological materials, the paired electron spins interact weakly with the externally applied magnetic field, resulting in a small induced magnetization – oriented opposite to the applied magnetic field – that causes a reduction of field strength inside the material. These materials are *diamagnetic* and have a negative magnetic susceptibility.

In materials with unpaired spins, the electron magnetic dipoles tend to align parallel to the applied field. If the unpaired spins are in sufficient concentration, this effect will dominate, causing the induced magnetization to be aligned parallel with the applied field and thus an increase in magnetic field strength inside the material. These materials are *paramagnetic*. Figure 21 illustrates magnetic field flux through diamagnetic and paramagnetic materials.

As mentioned earlier in this chapter, the Larmor relationship entails that spins will precess at a faster frequency when experiencing a higher magnetic field. In the presence of a magnetic field perturber with susceptibility that differs from surrounding tissue, spins will precess at different frequencies depending on their location relative to

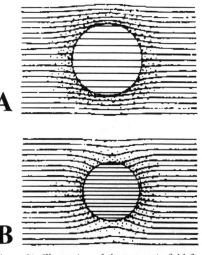

Figure 21. Illustration of the magnetic field flux through (A) diamagnetic and (B) paramagnetic materials. Within diamagnetic materials, the net flux is less; within paramagnetic materials, the net flux is greater. Magnetic field distortions created around the material are proportional to the object geometry and the difference in susceptibility between the object and its surroundings.

the perturber. In this case, the spins will rapidly become out of phase and the MRI signal will therefore be decreased. When the susceptibility differences between the perturber and its surroundings are large, the field distortions are large. Conversely, field distortions decrease when the susceptibility of the perturber becomes more similar to its surroundings; this causes more protons to have similar precession frequencies, allowing them to stay in phase longer. Increased phase coherence increases the MRI signal by decreasing the T2* and T2 decay rate. As an example, Figure 22 shows two plots of MRI signal intensity based on the simplified gradient–echo signal intensity relationship $S(\mathrm{TE}) = S_0 e^{-\mathrm{TE}/\mathrm{T2}^*}$, where $S(\mathrm{TE})$ is the signal as a function of echo time. The signal is usually described as decaying in an exponential manner; T2* is the signal decay rate. In Figure 22, the T2* values used are 48 msec and 50 msec, and R2* = 1/T2* (the relaxation rate).

If the signal decay over time is described as an exponential, then the natural log (Ln) of that signal will produce a straight line when plotted against time. This makes the slope more readily measurable. The slope of such a curve is simply the value 1/T2* (i.e., the relaxation rate R2*). Given

$$\mathrm{Ln}(S) = \mathrm{TE}/\mathrm{T2}^*, \qquad (20)$$

$$\mathrm{Ln}(S)/\mathrm{TE} = 1/\mathrm{T2}^* = \mathrm{R2}^*, \qquad (21)$$

it follows that R2* may be obtained from the slope of $\mathrm{Ln}(S)$ versus TE, as shown in Figure 23.

If we assume that signal changes are affected by changes *only* in R2*, then the change in relaxation rate ($\Delta \mathrm{R2}^*$) may be estimated by measuring S_r (signal during rest) and S_a (signal during activation), using only one TE value and the expression

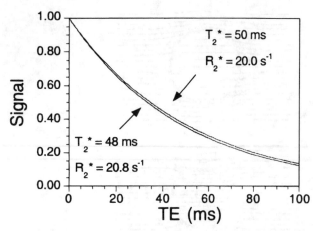

Figure 22. Plot of signal versus TE. The two curves represent typical values of R2* in the brain. The difference in relaxation rates represent typical differences between resting (20.8 sec^{-1}) and activated (20.0 sec^{-1}) R2* in the brain (-0.8 sec^{-1}). These signals are referred to as S_r (resting signal) and S_a (active signal) in the text (in general, the MR signal is denoted S).

$$\frac{-\mathrm{Ln}(S_a/S_r)}{\mathrm{TE}} = \Delta \mathrm{R2}^*. \qquad (22)$$

The expression relating percent change to $\Delta \mathrm{R2}^*$ is

$$\text{percent signal change} = 100(e^{-\Delta \mathrm{R2}^*(\mathrm{TE})} - 1). \qquad (23)$$

Figure 24 is a plot of the percent signal change versus TE between the synthesized resting and activated curves. An approximately linear fractional signal increase with TE is apparent. As TE is increased, the fractional signal change increases. However, as we will show, the contrast (what really matters in an fMRI experiment) has a peak at one specific TE value.

If $\Delta \mathrm{R2}^*$ is small relative to R2*, then the signal difference between the two curves will be maximized at TE $\approx$ T2* (typically shorter and measured by gradient–echo pulse

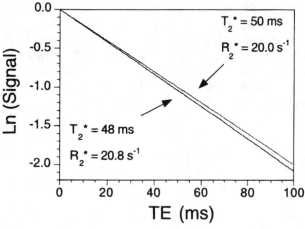

Figure 23. Ln(S) versus TE. Transverse relaxation rates (R2 and R2*) are measured by applying a linear fit to curves such as these. Here, activation-induced changes in S_0 are considered zero and single exponential decays are assumed.

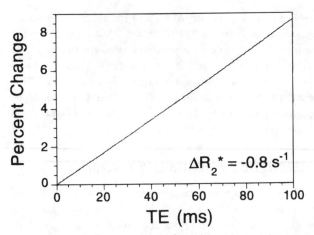

Figure 24. Percent change versus TE from the synthesized data set (see text). Given a $\Delta \mathrm{R2}^*$ value typically obtained, a linear dependence of percent change on TE is observed in the TE range typically used.

sequences) or T2 (typically longer and measured by spin–echo pulse sequences), as demonstrated in what follows. The contrast between the two signal intensities (S_a and S_r) with a difference in relaxation rate of $\Delta \mathrm{R2}^*$ can be approximated by

$$S_a - S_r = \exp\{-\mathrm{TE}(\Delta \mathrm{R2}^* + \mathrm{R2}_r^*)\} - \exp\{-\mathrm{TE}(\mathrm{R2}_r^*)\}, \qquad (24)$$

where $\mathrm{R2}_r^*$ is the relaxation rate associated with a measured S_r at a given TE value. The TE value at which equation (24) is maximized is given by

$$\mathrm{TE} = \frac{\mathrm{Ln}((\Delta \mathrm{R2}^* + \mathrm{R2}_r^*)/\mathrm{R2}_r^*)}{\Delta \mathrm{R2}^*}. \qquad (25)$$

In the limit as $\Delta \mathrm{R2}^*$ approaches 0, the TE value at which contrast is maximized approaches $1/\mathrm{R2}_r^*$ or $\mathrm{T2}_r^*$. A graphical demonstration of this contrast maximization is shown in Figure 25. Even though the percent change increases, as shown in Figure 24, the contrast or signal *difference* does not increase monotonically with TE.

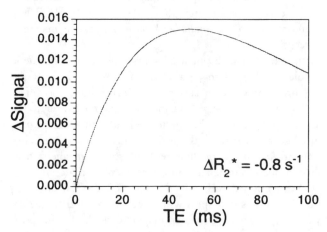

Figure 25. Plot of ΔS versus TE from the same synthesized data sets shown in the previous figures. A maximum is reached at TE $\approx$ T_r^* (approximately 48 msec).

Bulk susceptibility changes (either endogenous or exogenous) lead to MRI signal changes primarily in the manner just described. A more detailed description of the precise effects of susceptibility perturbers will be provided later.

Endogenous Susceptibility Contrast

One of the three fMRI contrast mechanisms described in this section (blood oxygenation level–dependent contrast, BOLD) is based on the understanding that blood has oxygenation-sensitive paramagnetic characteristics [45–48]. Hemoglobin is the primary carrier of oxygen in the blood. Hemoglobin that is not bound to oxygen, called deoxyhemoglobin (deoxy-Hb), contains paramagnetic iron; hemoglobin that is carrying oxygen, called oxyhemoglobin (oxy-Hb), contains diamagnetic oxygen-bound iron [45–48]. The modulation in the magnetic susceptibility of blood by changes in oxygenation is the basis of BOLD contrast. Using MR susceptometry [49], the susceptibility of completely oxygenated red blood cells was measured to be $-0.26 \pm 0.07 \times 10^{-6}$ (cgs units). With this technique, blood susceptibility was also shown to be linearly proportional to blood oxygenation (it decreases linearly as oxygenation increases). The susceptibility of completely deoxygenated red blood cells is $0.157 \pm 0.07 \times 10^{-6}$, so the susceptibility difference between completely oxygenated and completely deoxygenated red blood cells is therefore 0.18×10^{-6}. The profound effects of blood oxygenation changes on MR signal intensity have been demonstrated since 1979 [47–58].

Exogenous Susceptibility Contrast

Exogenous paramagnetic substances, which include both Gd(DTPA) and Dy(DTPA), can give useful information regarding several aspects of organ function [59]. When injected into the brain, these intravascular agents can give information on blood volume and vascular patency [49; 58–65]. The effects of these agents on tissue T1, T2*, and T2 are highly dependent on chemical environment and compartmentalization, as has been observed [49; 58–65] and modeled [59; 61–64; 66–79].

One mechanism of action for these compounds is dipolar interaction, which has an effect on intrinsic T1 and T2 relaxation times [59; 61]. This effect relies on the direct interaction of water with unpaired spins. Homogeneous distributions of solutions containing paramagnetic ions display relaxivity changes that can be predicted by the classical Solomon–Bloembergen equations [61], but in the healthy brain these injected agents remain compartmentalized within the intravascular space, which contains only about 5% of total brain water. The extent of agent–proton interaction is reduced by the limited rate at which diffusing or exchanging protons in the other 95% of brain water pass through the intravascular space, which is also less accessible owing to the blood–brain barrier. These combined effects greatly limit the agent-induced T1 effects,

which rely on direct interaction of protons with the paramagnetic agents. In this case, T2* and T2 shortening effects – caused by contrast agent–induced bulk susceptibility differences between intravascular and extravascular space [61–64; 66–75] – dominate over classical dipolar relaxation effects.

HEMODYNAMIC CONTRAST

Many types of physiological information can be mapped using fMRI, including baseline cerebral blood volume [25; 62], changes in blood volume [11], baseline and changes in cerebral perfusion [35; 38; 80–84], and changes in blood oxygenation [12; 13; 15; 85–88]. Recently, quantitative measures of CMR (cerebral metabolic rate) O_2 changes with activation have been derived from fMRI data [89–91].

Blood Volume

A technique developed by Belliveau and Rosen et al. [62; 64; 92] utilizes the susceptibility contrast produced by intravascular paramagnetic contrast agents and the high-speed capabilities of echo planar imaging (EPI) to create maps of human cerebral blood volume (CBV). A bolus of paramagnetic contrast agent is injected (the technique is slightly invasive), and T2- or T2*-weighted images are obtained at the rate of about one image per second using echo planar imaging [39; 93–95]. As the contrast agent passes through the microvasculature, magnetic field distortions are produced. These gradients (which last the amount of time that it takes for the bolus to pass through the cerebral vasculature) cause intravoxel dephasing, resulting in a signal attenuation that is linearly proportional to the concentration of contrast agent [62; 64; 76], which, in turn, is a function of blood volume.

Changes in blood volume that occur during hemodynamic stress or during brain activation can then be visualized by "subtracting" the maps imaged during a resting state from one imaged during hemodynamic stress or neuronal activation [11]. The use of this method marked the first time that hemodynamic changes accompanying human brain activation were mapped with MRI.

Blood Perfusion

An array of techniques now exist for mapping cerebral blood perfusion in humans. The MRI techniques are similar to those applied in other modalities such as positron emission tomography (PET) and single photon emission computed tomography (SPECT) in that they all involve arterial spin labeling. The MRI-based techniques hold considerable promise of high spatial resolution without the requirement of contrast agent injections. They use the fundamental idea of magnetically tagging arterial blood outside the imaging plane and then allowing flow of the tagged blood into the imaging plane. The RF tagging pulse is usually a 180° pulse that "inverts" the magnetization.

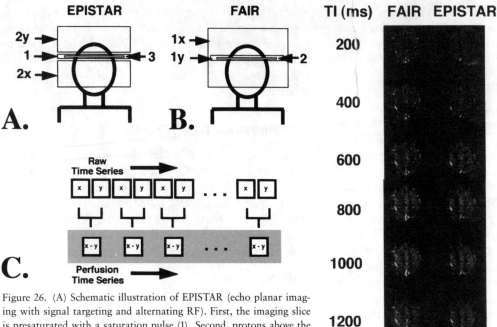

Figure 26. (A) Schematic illustration of EPISTAR (echo planar imaging with signal targeting and alternating RF). First, the imaging slice is presaturated with a saturation pulse (1). Second, protons above the imaging plane and below the imaging plane are alternately inverted or tagged (2x and 2y). Third, the image is collected after a delay time, TI, to allow the tagged protons to perfuse into the imaging plane (3). Alternate images collected in the sequential time series correspond to either the tag below (2x) or above (2y) the plane. (B) Schematic illustration of FAIR (flow-sensitive alternating inversion recovery). First, protons either within the plane or everywhere are alternately inverted or tagged (1x and 1y). Second, the image is collected after a delay time, TI, to allow the tagged protons (1x) to perfuse into the imaging plane. Alternate images collected in the sequential time series correspond to either the tag everywhere (1x) or only within (1y) the imaging plane. (C) Method by which the time series of perfusion images is created from the pulse sequences shown in (A) and (B). The alternate images, x and y, are collected in time. These images, with different tags applied, are different only in the degree to which flowing spins contribute to the signal. Therefore, a perfusion signal–only time series of images is created by pairwise subtraction of the images.

Generally, these techniques can be subdivided into (i) those that use continuous arterial spin labeling, which involves continuously inverting blood flowing into the slice [80] and (ii) those that use pulsed arterial spin labeling, periodically inverting a block of arterial blood and measuring the arrival of that blood into the imaging slice. Examples of these techniques include:

1. echo planar imaging with signal targeting and alternating RF (EPISTAR), schematically illustrated in Figure 26(A), which involves alternately inverting slabs of magnetization above and below the imaging slice [38; 39]; and

2. flow-sensitive alternating inversion recovery (FAIR), schematically illustrated in Figure 26(B), which involves the alternation between slice-selective and non–slice-selective inversion.

The latter was introduced by Kwong et al. [81; 96; 97] and referred to as FAIR by Kim et al. [84]. More recently, a

Figure 27. Comparison of EPISTAR and FAIR at corresponding TI values. As TI is lengthened, tagged blood distributes from large arteries into smaller vessels and capillary beds. In the capillaries, the tagged blood water exchanges almost completely with tissue water. Short TIs highlight rapidly flowing blood; long TIs highlight capillary bed perfusion.

pulsed arterial spin labeling technique known as QUIPSS (quantitative imaging of perfusion using a single subtraction) was introduced [83; 98]. In the case of the pulsed techniques, pairwise subtraction of sequential images – illustrated in Figure 26(C) with and without application of the RF tag outside the plane – gives a perfusion-related signal.

Varying the delay time between the inversion or tag outside the imaging plane and the acquisition of the image yields perfusion maps that highlight blood at different stages of its delivery into the imaging slice. Because there is necessarily a gap between the proximal tagging region and the imaging slice, there is a delay in the time for tagged blood to reach the arterial tree. This delay time can be highly variable, ranging from about 200 msec to about 1 sec for a gap of 1 cm. At 400 msec, typically only blood in larger arteries has reached the slice and so the pulsed arterial spin labeling signal is dominated by focal signals in these vessels; whereas at 1,000 msec, tagged blood has typically begun to distribute into the capillary beds of the tissue in the slice. Images acquired at late inversion times can be considered qualitative maps of perfusion. Figure 27 shows perfusion maps created at different TI times using both the FAIR and the EPISTAR technique. As TI is lengthened, tagged blood distributes from large arteries into smaller vessels and capillary beds. In the capillaries, the tagged blood water exchanges almost completely with tissue water. To quantify perfusion using these techniques, it is necessary to more carefully model the phenomena and relevant variables [84; 97; 99; 100]. For quantification, a minimum of two subtractions at different TIs is required in order to calculate the rate of entry (perfusion) of tagged blood into the slice [100].

For the mapping of human brain activation (i.e., to observe only activation-induced *changes* in blood perfusion), a more commonly used flow-sensitive method is performed by applying the inversion pulse always in the same plane. In this case, the intensity of all images obtained will be weighted by modulation of longitudinal magnetization by flowing blood and also by other MR parameters that normally contribute to image intensity and contrast (proton density, T1, T2). Therefore, this technique allows only for observation of changes in flow that occur over time with brain activation. This technique was first implemented by Kwong et al. [13] to observe activation-induced flow changes in the human brain. In this seminal paper, activation-induced signal changes associated with local changes in blood oxygenation were also observed.

Blood Oxygenation

In 1990, work of Ogawa et al. [85; 101; 102] and Turner et al. [86] demonstrated that MR signals in the vicinity of vessels and in perfused brain tissue decreased with a decrease in blood oxygenation. This type of physiological contrast was coined "blood oxygenation level dependent" (BOLD) contrast by Ogawa et al. [85].

The use of BOLD contrast for the observation of brain activation was first demonstrated in August 1991 at the 10th Annual Society of Magnetic Resonance in Medicine meeting [103]. The first papers demonstrating the technique, published in July 1992, reported human brain activation in the primary visual cortex [13; 14] and motor cortex [12; 13]. Two [12; 13] of the first three reports of this technique involved the use of single-shot EPI at 1.5 Tesla. The other [14] involved multishot FLASH imaging at 4 Tesla. Generally, a small local signal increase in activated cortical regions was observed using gradient–echo pulse sequences – which are maximally sensitive to changes in the homogeneity of the main magnetic field.

The working model constructed to explain these observations with susceptibility contrast imaging is that an increase in neuronal activity causes local vasodilation, which in turn causes an increase in blood flow. This results in an excess of oxygenated hemoglobin beyond the metabolic need, thus *reducing* the proportion of paramagnetic deoxyhemoglobin in the vasculature. This hemodynamic phenomenon was previously suggested by non-MRI techniques [104–106]. A reduction in deoxyhemoglobin in the vasculature causes a reduction in magnetic susceptibility differences in the vicinity of veinuoles, veins, and red blood cells within veins, thereby causing an increase in spin coherence (increase in T2 and T2*) and thus an increase in signal for T2*- and T2-weighted sequences.

Presently, the most widely used fMRI technique for the noninvasive mapping of human brain activity is gradient–echo imaging using BOLD contrast. There are several reasons for this. (a) Gradient–echo T2*-sensitive techniques have demonstrated higher activation-induced signal change contrast (by a factor of 2 to 4) than T2-weighted, flow-sensitive, or blood volume–sensitive techniques. (b) The BOLD contrast can be obtained using more widely available high-speed multishot non-EPI techniques. (c) The T2*-weighted techniques are sensitive to blood oxygenation changes in vascular structures, including large vessels that may be spatially removed from the focus of activation. For most applications, techniques that are more sensitive to microvascular structures entail a too severely compromised ratio of functional contrast to noise. This last issue will be further discussed shortly.

Figure 28 gives a summary of the cascade of hemodynamic events that occur on brain activation and of their effects on the appropriately weighted MRI signal.

ISSUES IN fMRI

Although rapid progress continues, many issues in fMRI remain incompletely understood. Here we provide a description of the current state of understanding regarding some general fMRI issues, grouped under headings of interpretability, temporal resolution, spatial resolution, dynamic range, and sensitivity.

Interpretability

The question of interpretability regards the concern of exactly what the relationship is between the fMRI signal and underlying neuronal activation. Two "filters" separate direct observation of neuronal processes using fMRI. The first is the relationship between neuronal activation and hemodynamic changes, and the second is the relationship between hemodynamic changes and MR signal changes.

In the past five years, considerable progress has been made in the characterization of the second relationship: that between activation-induced hemodynamic changes and the fMRI signal changes. Here we discuss the issue of MRI-achievable hemodynamic specificity, as well as the dynamic range and the upper limits of temporal and spatial resolution of fMRI.

A high priority in fMRI is to correlate accurately the activation-induced MR signal changes with underlying neuronal processes. It is generally accepted that perfusion and oxygenation changes in capillaries are closer in both space and time to neuronal activation than changes arising in arteries or veins. As mentioned, different pulse sequences can be made sensitive to specific populations of vessel sizes, blood flow velocities, and contrast mechanisms.

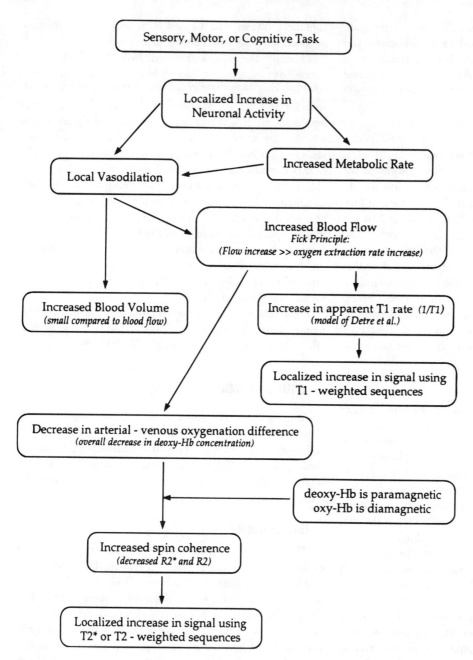

Figure 28. Flow chart summarizing the cascade of hemodynamic events that occur with brain activation and their corresponding effects on the appropriately sensitized MRI signal.

The fMRI pulse sequence that gives the highest functional contrast-to-noise ratio is a T2*-weighted gradient–echo sequence, which is likely to have contrast weighting that includes large draining vein effects and, in the case of short-TR–high flip-angle sequences (short TR values are required for non-EPI fMRI sequences), large vessel arterial inflow effects. Sequences that may be able to more selectively observe capillary oxygenation (spin–echo with velocity nulling) or perfusion (arterial spin labeling with velocity nulling) effects are less robust. They have a lower functional contrast-to-noise ratio, are generally less time-efficient, and may not allow extensive multislice imaging. The tremendous need for high fMRI contrast-to-noise ratio, high image acquisition speed, and flexibility (e.g., multislice imaging) has to date outweighed the need, in most cases, for selective observation of capillary effects. Enhancements in fMRI sensitivity may allow these hemodynamically selective pulse sequences to be more commonly used. The strategies for achieving hemodynamic specificity include not only pulse sequence modifications but also simple vein and artery identification strategies or even activation strategies that remove draining vein effects. For a review of these sequences, see [107].

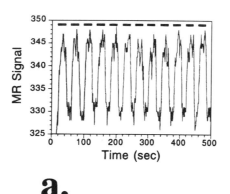
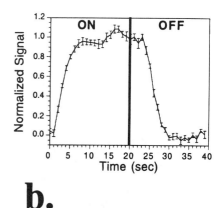

a.

b.

Temporal Resolution

The temporal resolution of fMRI has been variably defined in the literature. These definitions include the image acquisition rate, the time it takes for the activation-induced response to rise or fall a given amount (otherwise known as the time constant of the measured changes), the maximum rate at which activation can be turned on and off and still generate a detectable response, the smallest detectable activation duration, the smallest detectable difference in latency (between two identical activations that have different onset times) in an individual voxel or region of interest (ROI), and the smallest detectable difference in latency across separate voxels or ROIs. These aspects of fMRI temporal resolution will be discussed next.

Image Acquisition Rate. The rate at which images are acquired is determined by the pulse sequence used. Multishot functional imaging techniques do not generally require specialized gradient hardware, but they usually require at least 3 sec for image acquisition [14; 108–111]. A faster technique, single-shot echo planar imaging [94; 95; 112], generally requires specialized gradients or gradient switching hardware. The readout window width of an echo planar image is about 20–40 msec. Hybrid techniques, such as multishot EPI [113; 114], provide a good compromise in spatial resolution and time but suffer from the shot-to-shot instability characteristic of all multishot techniques. These instabilities, caused primarily by respiration and cardiac cycle effects, are reduced by spiral scanning strategies [110; 111], retrospective *k*-space realignment techniques [115], and navigator pulses [116].

In the context of fMRI, a TE in the range of 30–60 msec is optimal (≈ T2* of gray matter from 4 Tesla to 1.5 Tesla, respectively); the minimum time between successive image acquisitions (TR) is typically about 100 msec. With the use of partial *k*-space acquisition techniques and a shorter (and hence nonoptimal) TE, image acquisition rates as high as 60 images per second have been reported [117]. Issues regarding the trade-offs between image acquisition rate and functional contrast have not yet been fully resolved. From a practical standpoint, collection of a mul-

Figure 29. (a) Typical BOLD response from an ROI in motor cortex during repeated cycles (20 sec on, 20 sec off) of finger tapping. The time series of echo planar images of the motor cortex were obtained using EPI at 1.5 Tesla (TR = 2 sec, TE = 40 msec). (b) Average of the twelve on–off cycles shown in (a).

tislice whole-brain volumetric EPI data set requires a TR of about 2 sec. The limitations of a long TR can be overcome in the context of cyclic on–off activation time series. Finer temporal sampling of the cyclic on–off activation cycle is achievable using a TR that is not an even multiple of the cycle time [118].

Basic Dynamic Characteristics of the BOLD Signal. Figure 29 shows a typical BOLD contrast response from an ROI in motor cortex during repeated cycles of finger tapping (20 seconds on, 20 seconds off). Figure 29(b) is the average of the twelve on–off cycles shown in Figure 29(a). Several aspects of the BOLD contrast are illustrated here. First, the signal is generally stable over time, although Frahm and colleagues observed a small downward drift of the baseline and the activation-induced signal change magnitude within the first minutes of either continuous or cyclic on–off visual stimulation [119; 120].

With activation, the time for the BOLD response to first significant increase from baseline is approximately 2 sec [13; 120; 121]. The time to plateau in the "on" state is approximately 6–9 sec [121]. With cessation of activation, the time to return to baseline is longer than the rise time by about one or two seconds [122]. As mentioned, several groups have reported a "pre-undershoot" or initial dip during the first 500 msec [123] to 2 sec of the signal [124; 125]. More commonly observed is a post-undershoot, which is observed more in the visual than motor cortex and has an amplitude that is dependent on stimulus duration [126]. On cessation of activation, the post-undershoot signal can take up to a minute to return to baseline [120; 127].

The hemodynamic response can be thought of as a low-pass filter [128]. A straightforward method of determining the filter characteristics is to modulate the input and observe the output. Figure 30 demonstrates the effect of modulating the on–off motor cortex activation rate

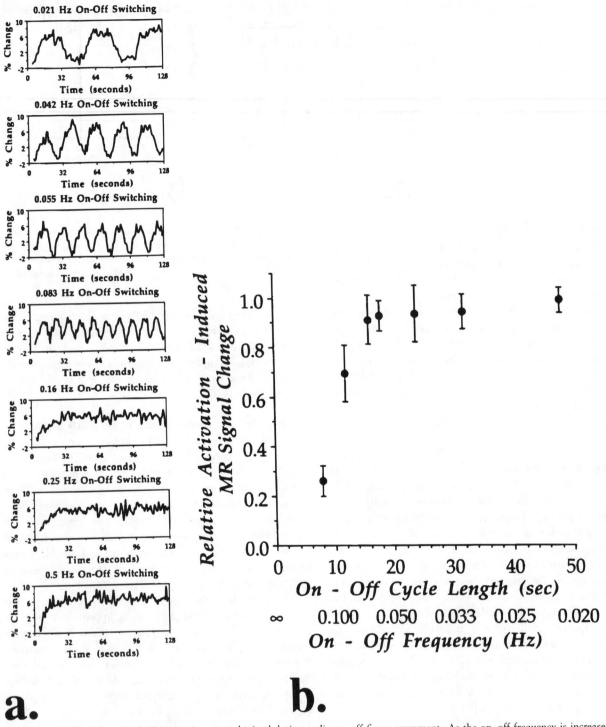

Figure 30. (a) Signal from an ROI in motor cortex obtained during cyclic on–off finger movement. As the on–off frequency is increased from 0.021 Hz to 0.5 Hz, the activation-induced amplitude becomes decreased and the signal becomes saturated in the "on" state. (b) Summary of the dependence of the relative amplitudes of the activation-induced signal on switching frequency shown in (a). The relative signal change amplitude is reduced at on–off rates above 0.06 Hz.

from 24 sec on and 24 sec off to 1 sec on and 1 sec off. Because the time to reach a baseline after cessation of activity is slightly longer than the time to plateau in an "on" state, the signal becomes saturated in that state with the faster on–off frequencies. The relative activation-induced signal

amplitude in the motor cortex does not show a significant decrease until the switching frequency is higher than 0.06 Hz (8 sec on and 8 sec off), and it does not follow the activation timing above 0.13 Hz. Other work has shown that, with sufficient averaging, a constant on–off rate of 2 sec on and 2 sec off can induce a measurable hemodynamic response [129; 130]. Also, the time to reach the saturated "on" state decreases as the on–off rate increases.

The Hemodynamic Response to Transient Activation. Linear deconvolution of a neuronal input function from the measured hemodynamic response gives a hemodynamic "impulse response" that resembles the type of response that is induced by a brief stimulus – modeled as a Poisson function [128] and a Gamma function [131], among others. The implicit assumption in this analysis is that the hemodynamic response is linear and that the neuronal input is a binary "boxcar" function. Issues related to the linearity of the hemodynamic response become important when considering experimental design and signal interpretability issues (discussed later in this chapter). Regardless, a brief "impulse" of activation elicits a response that quite closely resembles the shape of a deconvolved neuronal "impulse response." The first event-related fMRI experiments were performed using primary visual and motor activation [122; 132–135], demonstrating the critical fact that a single transient activation (2 sec or less) can induce a measurable hemodynamic response. The general response was shown to peak at about 4–6 sec following activation and then return to baseline at about 10 sec after activation. Details of this transient activation-induced hemodynamic response are discussed next.

The Minimum Detectable Stimulus Duration. One of the first questions asked after fMRI was discovered was, "How brief of a stimulus can one give and still elicit a measurable response?" First, Blamire et al. [132] reduced a visual stimulus duration to 2 sec, successfully showing a response. Then, Bandettini et al. [122; 133] demonstrated a response to 500-msec–duration finger tapping. Figure 31 shows these early results obtained from a region in motor cortex. The time series consist of two finger-tapping durations of 5 sec, 3 sec, 2 sec, 1 sec, and 500 msec.

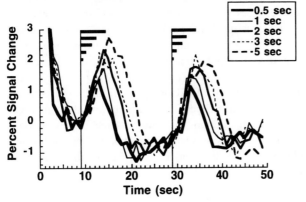

Figure 31. Signal from an ROI in motor cortex across five separate runs during which the subject was cued to perform finger tapping for 0.5, 1, 2, 3, and 5 sec twice during the time series. The time between the two finger tapping periods was 20 sec (TR = 1 sec).

The responses are clearly delineated from each other based on the finger-tapping duration. The amplitude and time to peak systematically shift with stimulus duration. Also, even after waiting 20 sec between stimuli, the baseline has shifted to a lower level owing to the time it takes for the post-undershoot to dissipate.

Savoy et al. [134; 135] reduced the stimulus duration further, performing a study in which the fMRI response to stimulus durations of 1,000 msec, 100 msec, and 34 msec were compared. A measurable response was obtained using all stimulus durations. The responses to the 100-msec and 34-msec stimuli were considerably smaller than the response to the 1,000-msec stimulus, and the former were similar in shape and amplitude to each other. These results suggest that the minimum stimulus duration has not yet been determined but that, below a specific stimulus duration, the hemodynamic response remains constant.

A Paradigm Shift in Experimental Design: Event-Related fMRI. A critical question in event-related fMRI was whether a transient cognitive activation could elicit a significant and usable fMRI signal change. In 1996, Buckner and colleagues [136] demonstrated that, in fact, event-related fMRI lent itself quite well to cognitive activation questions. In their study, a word-stem completion task was performed using a "block design" strategy and an event-related strategy. Robust activation in the regions involved with word generation were observed in both cases.

Given the substantial amount of recent publications that describe event-related fMRI [123; 129; 130; 137–154], it can probably be said that this is one of the more exciting developments in fMRI since its discovery. Several papers describing event-related signal change characteristics and analysis techniques have recently been published [95; 141; 142; 150; 151; 155; 156].

The advantages of event-related activation strategies are many [152]. These include the ability to more completely randomize task types in a time series, the ability to selectively analyze fMRI response data based on measured behavioral responses to individual trials, and the option of incorporating overt responses into a time series. Separation of motion artifact from BOLD changes is possible by the use of the temporal response differences between motion effects and the BOLD contrast-based changes [137; 157].

Experimental Design Issues in Event-Related fMRI. Experimental design and interpretation issues depend on whether the activation-induced hemodynamic response behaves like a linear system. The evidence is somewhat conflicting. Boynton et al. [150] demonstrated that, under most circumstances, the hemodynamic response behaves in a linear manner. Nevertheless, they also observed that the amplitude of the response to brief stimuli is larger than a linear system would predict. This observation was supported by Bandettini et al. [129; 130].

Reasons for nonlinearities in the event-related response can be neuronal, hemodynamic, or metabolic in nature. The neuronal input may not be a simple boxcar function. Instead, an increased neuronal firing rate at the onset of stimulation (neuronal "bursting") may cause a slightly larger amount of vasodilation that later plateaus at a lower steady-state level. The amount of neuronal bursting necessary to significantly change the hemodynamic response, assuming a linear neuronal–hemodynamic coupling, is quite large. For example, to account for the almost double functional contrast for the experimental relative to the linear convolution-derived single-event responses, the integrated neuronal response over 2 sec must double. Assuming that neuronal firing is at a higher rate for only about the first 50 msec of brain activation, the neuronal firing rate must be 40 times greater than steady state for this duration.

As is well known, BOLD contrast is highly sensitive to the interplay of blood flow, blood volume, and oxidative metabolic rate. If, with activation, any one of these variables changes with a different time constant, then the fMRI signal can show fluctuations until a steady state is reached [119; 158; 159]. For instance, an activation-induced increase in blood volume would slightly reduce the fMRI signal, since more deoxyhemoglobin would be present in the voxel. If the time constant for blood volume changes were slightly longer than that of flow changes, then the activation-induced fMRI signal would first increase and then be reduced as blood volume later increased. The same could apply if the time constant of oxidative metabolic rate were slightly slower than that of flow and volume changes. Evidence for increased oxidative metabolic rate after 2 min of activation is given by Frahm et al. [119], but no evidence suggests that the time constant of the increase in oxidative metabolic rate is only seconds longer than the flow increase time constant – as would be required for it to be applicable only to relatively high-amplitude single-event responses. These hemodynamics, which may also differ on a voxelwise basis, have yet to be characterized fully.

From this information it is clear that, when using a constant interstimulus interval (ISI), the optimal ISI is about 10–12 sec and the response is somewhat nonlinear. Nonlinearities have also been demonstrated by other studies [140; 156]. Dale and Buckner [151] have nevertheless shown that responses to visual stimuli, presented as rapidly as once every 1 sec, can be adequately separated using overlap correction or deconvolution methods. These methods are possible if the ISI is varied during the time series. Burock et al. [139] demonstrated that remarkably clean activation maps can be created using an average ISI of 500 msec and deconvolution methods to extract overlapping responses. Assuming that the hemodynamic response is essentially a linear system, there is no obvious minimum ISI; rather, there exists an optimal ISI *distribution*. An exponential

distribution of ISIs (with a mean as short as psychophysically possible) is optimal from a statistical standpoint. Of course, the rapidity with which stimuli can be presented ultimately depends on the study being performed. Many cognitive tasks may require a lower presentation rate. Several cognitive studies have been successfully performed using intermixed, rapidly presented trials [138; 149].

Although excellent activation maps can be created using rapidly presented stimuli and deconvolution methods, interpretation of details of the deconvolved responses depends on the linearity of the system. Future work in event-related experimental optimization rests in what further information can be derived from these responses. Between-region, between-voxel, between-subject, and stimulus-dependent variations in amplitude, latency, shape, and responsivity of the event-related fMRI responses are still relatively uncharacterized. Reasons for these differences are also still unclear.

Single-Event fMRI: Single-Thought Measurement. Individual responses to individual events are easily detectable even at relatively low field strengths, but it should be noted that the studies described in previous sections involved relatively long time series and considerable averaging or "binning" of the individual responses into specific categories. These approaches are extremely powerful, but repeatability of individual activation patterns is likely to be somewhat imperfect, especially across trials spaced several minutes apart.

Several studies have demonstrated the ability to create functional maps and to derive useful information using only a single response to a single input. Richter and colleagues were able to derive the relative onset of activation of supplementary motor cortex relative to primary motor cortex using a delayed motor task following a readiness cue [160; 161]. Also, Richter et al. [162] demonstrated the ability to correlate individual response widths to the duration of a mental rotation task. The larger the angle that an object was mentally rotated, the longer the task took and the wider was the event-related parietal region response.

These types of studies represent yet another exciting new direction in fMRI paradigm design. It is imagined that measurement of complex responses from large arrays of cognitive manipulations are achievable in a single time series using this approach, which may represent a large jump in one aspect of fMRI temporal resolution: usable information per unit time. The combination of single-event fMRI paradigm design with analysis techniques that involve linear regression of multiple expected responses in a single time series [163] may expand even further the utility of fMRI.

Latency Discernibility within a Voxel or Region of Interest. If a task onset or duration is modulated, such as in the aforementioned motor cortex tasks or mental rotation studies [160–162], the accuracy with which one can temporally correlate the modulated input parameters to the measured output signal depends on the variability of the signal within a voxel or region of interest.

Savoy and colleagues [135] have addressed this issue of latency estimation accuracy. Variability of several temporal components of an activation-induced response function were determined. Six subjects were studied, and ten activation-induced response curves were analyzed for each subject. The relative onsets were determined by finding the latency with which each of the temporal "components" was maximized with each of three reference functions, representing three "components" of the response curve: the entire curve, the rising section, and the falling section. The standard deviations of the entire curve, rising phase, and falling phase were found to be 650 msec, 450 msec, and 1,250 msec, respectively. The reason for the difference between the rising phase and falling phase variability remains an open question.

Latency Discernibility across Voxels or Regions of Interest.
Researchers have reported observing across-region differences in the onset and return to baseline of the BOLD signal during cognitive tasks [136; 164]. For example, during a visually presented event-related word-stem completion task, Buckner et al. [136] reported that the signal in the visual cortex increased about 1 sec before the signal in the left anterior prefrontal cortex. One might argue that this is expected, since the subject first observes the word stem and then, after about a second, generates a word to complete this task. Others would argue that the neuronal onset latencies should not be more than about 200 msec. Can inferences regarding the spatial–temporal cascade characteristics of networked brain activation be made on this time scale from fMRI data? Without controlling for the intrinsic temporal variability of the BOLD signal over space, such inferences cannot be easily made for temporal latency differences below about 4 sec. If appropriate controls are performed, then the variability approaches that of a single response in an individual voxel.

Lee et al. [165] were the first to observe that the fMRI signal change onset within the visual cortex during simple visual stimulation varied from 6 sec to 12 sec. These latencies were also shown to correlate somewhat with the underlying vascular structure. The earliest onset of the signal change appeared to be in gray matter; the latest onset appeared to occur in the largest draining veins. This basic observation was also made in the motor cortex [107; 166]. In one study, latency differences did not show a clear correlation with draining veins [167].

Figure 32 demonstrates three sources of temporal variability. Figure 32(a) shows us a plot of the average time course from the motor cortex resulting from 2-sec finger tapping. As mentioned, the first source of variability is the intrinsic noise in the time-series signal (the standard deviation of the signal is on the order of 1%). The second source of variability is that of the hemodynamic response, which ranges from 450 msec to 1,250 msec, depending on whether one is observing the rising or the falling phase of the signal. The third source of variability is the latency spread over space.

The plot in Figure 32(a) was used as a reference function for correlation analysis and allowed to shift ±2 sec. Figure 32(b) is a histogram of the number of voxels in an activated region that demonstrated a maximum correlation with the reference function at each latency (relative to the average latency) to which the reference function was shifted. As can be seen, the spread in latencies is over 4 sec. Figure 32(c) includes a map of the dot product (measure of signal change magnitude) and latency, demonstrating that the regions showing the longest latency roughly correspond to the regions that show the largest signal changes. These largest signal changes are likely to be downstream draining veins.

To obtain information about relative onsets of cascaded neuronal activity from latency maps, it is important to characterize the underlying vasculature-related latency distribution at which one is looking. Savoy et al. [134; 135] demonstrated that activation onset latencies of 500 msec were discernible using a visual stimulation timing described as follows. First, the subject viewed a fixation point for 10 sec. Then, the subject's left visual hemifield was activated 500 msec before the right; both hemifields were activated for 9 sec, and then the left hemifield stimulus was turned off 500 msec before the right.

With careful choice of ROI from which the time-course plot is made, these onset differences can be shown. However, maps of latency cannot reveal the onset differences because, as mentioned, the variability over space (about 4 sec) dominates the inserted 500-msec variability from left to right hemifield. In addition, the onset latency – as derived from a time course obtained from a region of interest – is extremely sensitive to the choice of ROI, since the spatial variability is so extreme.

Modulation of the stimulation timing has allowed *relative* latency differences to be mapped. In the study shown, the left–right onset order was switched so that, in the first run, the left hemifield was activated and turned off 500 msec and 250 msec prior to the right; in the second run, the right hemifield was activated and turned off 500 msec and 250 msec prior to the left. Latency maps were made for each onset order and subtracted from each other to reveal clear delineation between right and left hemifield that was not apparent in each of the individual maps. This operation is shown in Figure 33. It should be noted that maps are of the change in onset of one area relative to another and not of absolute latency. Maps such as these may be extremely useful in determining which regions of activation are modulated relative to other areas, given a specific and measurable task timing or response variation.

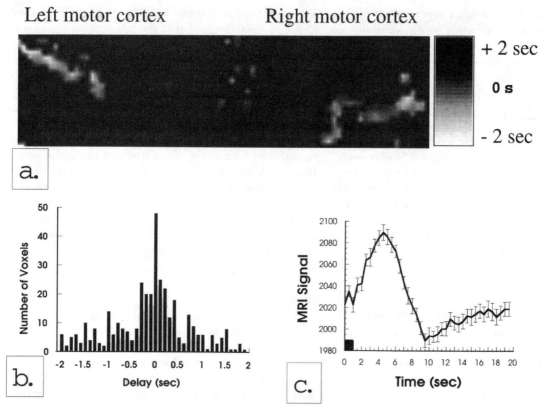

Figure 32. Demonstration of several of the limits of fMRI temporal resolution. Echo planar imaging was performed at 3 Tesla using a Bruker Biospec 3T/60 equipped with a local head gradient coil. A time-course series of axial images (matrix size = 96 × 96, FOV = 20 cm, TE = 40 msec, TR = 500 msec, flip angle = 80°) through the motor cortex was obtained. Bilateral finger tapping was performed for 2 sec, alternating with 18 sec of rest. These figures demonstrate that the upper temporal resolution is determined by the variability of the signal change in time and space. (a) Time course of the signal elicited by tapping fingers for 2 sec. The standard deviation at each point was in the range of 1%–2%. The standard deviation of the hemodynamic change, in time, is in the range of 450–650 msec. (b) Map of the dot product (a measure of the activation-induced signal change magnitude) and the relative latencies or delays of the reference function (the plot in (a) was used as the reference function) at which the correlation coefficient was maximized. The spatial distribution of hemodynamic delays has a standard deviation of about 900 msec. The longest delays approximately match the regions that show the highest dot product and the area where veins are shown as dark lines in the T2*-weighted anatomical image. (c) Histogram of relative hemodynamic latencies; this was created from the latency map in (b).

A similar study by Luknowski et al. [168] showed that the mean accuracy of latency measures from multivoxel ROIs is ±27 msec, which is comparable to that of electrophysiological experiments.

Spatial Resolution

As with temporal resolution, the upper limit on functional spatial resolution is likely determined not by MRI limits but by the hemodynamics through which neuronal activation is transduced. Evidence from in vivo high-resolution optical imaging of the activation of ocular dominance columns [104; 105; 169] suggests that neuronal control of blood oxygenation occurs on a spatial scale of less than 0.5 mm. Magnetic resonance evidence suggests that the blood oxygenation increases occurring with brain activation are more extensive than the actual activated regions [165; 170–173]. In other words: it is possible that, whereas the local oxygenation may be regulated on a sub-millimeter scale, the subsequent changes in oxygenation

may occur on a larger scale owing to a spillover effect. An example of this difference in activated region is given in Figures 34 and 35.

Figure 34 shows a comparison of a spin-tagging technique (FAIR) with BOLD contrast functional imaging. Low-resolution (64 × 64) and high-resolution (128 × 128) anatomical and functional (correlation maps) BOLD contrast images (gradient–echo, TE = 40 msec) were obtained of an axial slice through the motor cortex. Single-shot EPI was performed using a local gradient coil [174] and a 3T/60 Bruker Biospec scanner. The images were 5 mm thick and the FOV was 20 cm. The task was bilateral finger tapping. Resting and active state perfusion maps, created using FAIR (TI = 1,400 msec, TR = 2 sec, spin–echo TE = 42 msec), are also shown. Functional correlation maps using BOLD contrast at the two different resolutions are compared with a functional correlation map using the FAIR perfusion time-course series. The magnified images, shown in Figure 35, illustrate that the areas of activation obtained

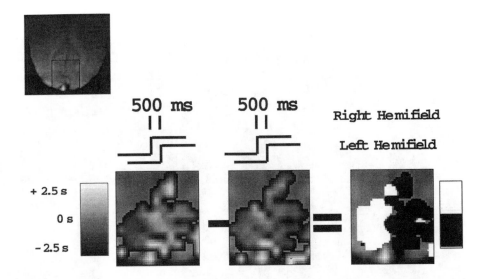

Figure 33. Activation within a region of visual cortex is shown for two separate conditions. In one condition (left), the right visual hemifield stimulation precedes the left by 500 msec (top) and 250 msec (bottom). In the other condition (middle), the left precedes the right by 500 msec and 250 msec. Latency maps from both of these conditions show an intrinsic spread of ±2.5 sec, which is too large to clearly identify the relative latencies across hemifields. However, once the data are normalized for this intrinsic variance (by directly comparing the hemodynamic response from the two different lags within individual voxels), the offset between left and right hemifield can be observed (right). This demonstrates that normalization of the hemodynamic lag can allow small *relative* temporal offsets to be identified. These normalized offsets can then be compared across regions to make inferences about neuronal delay. For this experiment, the TR was 400 msec.

using FAIR and BOLD contrast generally overlap but also have some significant differences. These spatial shifts in activation are likely to be due to the differences in hemodynamic sensitizations of the two sequences. The FAIR technique using a TI of 1,400 msec is optimally sensitized to imaging capillary perfusion, as shown in the resting and active state flow maps. The BOLD contrast functional images are strongly weighted by the effects of large draining veins.

In general, achieving the goal of high–spatial resolution fMRI requires a high functional contrast to noise and reduced signal contribution from draining veins. Greater hemodynamic specificity – accomplished by proper choice of pulse sequence (selective to capillary effects), innovative activation protocol design (phase tagging), and/or proper interpretation of signal change latency (latency mapping) – may allow for greater functional spatial resolution. If the contribution to activation-induced signal changes from larger collecting veins and arteries can be easily identified and eliminated, then (i) our confidence in localization of brain activation will increase and (ii) the upper limits of spatial resolution will be determined by scanner resolution and functional contrast to noise rather than by variations in vessel architecture.

Currently, voxel volumes as low as 1.2 μl have been obtained by functional FLASH techniques at 4 Tesla [175], and experiments specifically devoted to probing the upper limits of functional spatial resolution (using spiral scan techniques) have shown that fMRI can reveal activity localized to patches of cortex having a size of about 1.35 mm [176]. These studies and others using similar methods [121; 176–179] have observed a close tracking of MR signal change along the calcarine fissure as the location of visual stimuli was varied.

The voxel dimensions typically used in single-shot EPI studies are in the range of 3–4 mm in plane, with 4–10-mm slice thicknesses. These dimensions are determined by practical limitations such as readout window length, sampling bandwidth, S/N, limits of dB/dt, and data storage capacity. Other ways to bypass the practical scanner limits in spatial resolution include partial k-space acquisition [95] and multishot mosaic or interleaved EPI [95; 113; 114]. In many fMRI situations, multishot EPI may be the optimum compromise between spatial resolution, S/N, and temporal resolution for fMRI.

Dynamic Range

It is important not to interpret spatial differences in fMRI signal change magnitude as indications of differences in the degree of neuronal activation, because the signal is highly weighted by hemodynamic factors such as the distribution of blood volume across voxels. Nonetheless, it is possible to observe differences in fMRI signal change in the same regions but across incrementally modulated tasks. This may be a useful method for extracting more direct neuronal information from the fMRI time-course series.

The first demonstration that fMRI response is not simply binary was made by Kwong et al. [13]. Both flow- and oxygenation-sensitized MR signal in V1 were measured as flicker rate was modulated. The signal behavior corresponded closely with that obtained with a previous

(a)   (b)   (c)   (d)

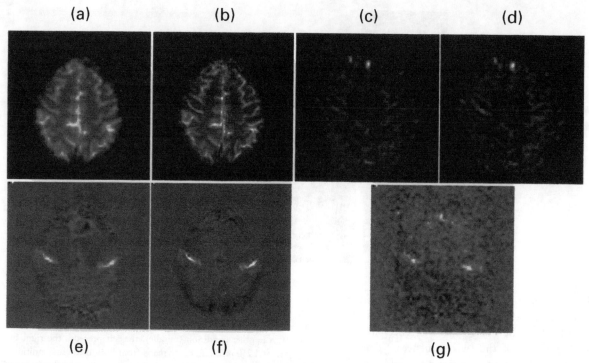

(e)   (f)   (g)

Figure 34. Comparison of perfusion-weighted and BOLD-weighted functional echo planar images at 3 Tesla. Echo planar imaging was performed using a Bruker 3T/60 scanner and a local head gradient coil. All images were created of the same plane in the same experimental session. The slice thickness was 5 mm and the FOV was 20 cm. An axial plane was chosen which contained the motor cortex. (a) 64×64 gradient–echo anatomical image (TE = 50 msec, TR = ∞). (b) 96×96 gradient–echo anatomical image (TE = 50 msec, TR = ∞). (c) Perfusion image created during the resting state using a FAIR time course series (TI = 1,400 msec, spin–echo TE = 60 msec, TR = 2 sec). (d) Perfusion image created from the same time course series as (c) during bilateral finger tapping. (e) 64×64 BOLD contrast functional correlation image created from the time series of images in which image (a) was the first of the series. Bilateral finger tapping was performed. (f) 96×96 BOLD contrast functional correlation image created from the time series of images in which image (b) was the first of the series. Bilateral finger tapping was performed. (g) 64×64 perfusion-only functional correlation image created from the same time series of perfusion images from which the resting state (c) and active state (d) images were created. Note the difference in spatial location of the area of activation between the flow-weighted and perfusion-weighted functional images. The "hot spot" in the BOLD contrast images is likely to be a draining vein, which does not appear in the perfusion-weighted functional image created using FAIR.

PET study [180]. Other studies have revealed a responsivity in higher visual areas to contrast and flicker rate [181; 182]. In the primary motor cortex, a linear signal dependence on finger tapping rate has been demonstrated [183]. In the primary auditory cortex, a sublinear dependence on syllable presentation rate has been demonstrated [184].

Sensitivity

Extraction of a 1% signal change (which is typical of fMRI) against a backdrop of motion, pulsation, and noise requires careful consideration of the variables influencing the signal detectability. These variables span factors that increase signal, increase fMRI contrast, reduce physiologic noise, and reduce artifactual signal changes. Next we present a list of some salient variables that are important to consider in relation to optimizing fMRI sensitivity.

Averaging. Averaging of sequentially obtained images increases the S/N by the square root of the number of images collected. One difficulty is that, if averaging is performed over too long a period (exceeding $\approx$ 5 min), then systematic artifacts (i.e., slow movement or drift) tend to outweigh the benefits obtained from averaging for that duration.

Field Strength. As previously discussed, S/N and functional contrast increase with field strength. However, such difficulties as increased shimming problems, increased physiologic fluctuations, and limitations on the possible RF coils used also increase with field strength. It has yet to be determined if gains in sensitivity and contrast obtained by increasing field strength cannot be achieved by other methods at lower fields, or if the gains in sensitivity and contrast outweigh the disadvantages of imaging at high field strengths.

Filtering. In most fMRI studies using EPI, the noise over time is dominated not by system noise but by physiologic fluctuations. These fluctuations correspond to specific frequencies (i.e., heart and respiration rates). Filtering out of these frequencies can increase the functional contrast-to-noise ratio, or at least make the noise closer to Gaussian so that parametric statistical tests can be applied.

Gating. Gating is a technique whose one serious drawback has at least a potential solution. Gating involves triggering of the scanner to the heart beat so that an image is always collected at a specific phase of the cardiac cycle. This is advantageous because a primary source of noise is collection of images at different phases of the cardiac cycle, which causes head misregistration (the brain moves with every heartbeat) and pulsatile flow artifacts. Image collection at a single phase would eliminate this misregistration, thereby reducing the noise and potentially increasing the spatial resolution of fMRI (i.e., the brain would be imaged at a single position all of the time). The drawback to gating is that if the heart rate changes during the collection of images then the MR signal intensity also changes, depending on the tissue T1 and the average TR used. This generally causes very large fluctuations in the data – which makes gating relatively worthless in the context of fMRI. However, a technique has been developed to correct for the global fluctuations that occur with heart rate changes [185], which would make gating a feasible option in fMRI. Gating would be especially useful for identifying activation in structures at the base of the brain, since that is where pulsatile motion is greatest, where activation is most subtle, and where activated regions are the smallest – requiring the most consistent image-to-image registration.

Paradigm Timing. The choice in fMRI timing is usually determined by the sluggishness of the hemodynamic response (it is seldom useful to go much faster than an on–off cycle of 8 sec on, 8 sec off), the particular brain system that is being activated (cognitive tasks may have a more delayed response), and the predominant frequency power of the noise. As a rule of thumb, the goal is to maximize both the number of on–off cycles and the amplitude of the cycle in order to maximize the power of postprocessing techniques such as correlation analysis [186] to extract functional information. Generally, contrast-to-noise ratio is maximized and artifact is minimized by cycling the activation at the highest rate that the hemodynamics can keep up with and by having a time-course series of no longer than about 3–4 min.

Postprocessing. Many approaches have been used to extract from fMRI data estimates of the significance, amplitude, and phase of the functional response, yet there is still surprisingly little agreement on the appropriate techniques. A review has recently been published on statistical software packages for fMRI [187]. Generally speaking, if one knows the exact shape and phase of the expected signal response then a matched filter (i.e. correlation) approach may be optimal. If the shape is unknown, then use of a single expected response function (boxcar function or a sine wave) may miss unique activation patterns. The challenge of accurately determining regions of sig-

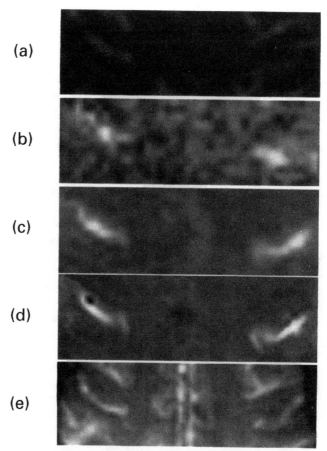

Figure 35. Magnification of selected images displayed in Figure 34 to emphasize the differences in the activation locations that appear with different hemodynamic sensitizations. (a) Baseline 64 × 64 perfusion image – magnification of Figure 34(c). (b) 64 × 64 perfusion-only–sensitive functional correlation image – magnification of 34(g). (c) 64 × 64 BOLD contrast functional correlation image – magnification of 34(e). (d) 96 × 96 BOLD contrast functional correlation image – magnification of 34(f). (e) 96 × 96 gradient–echo anatomical image – magnification of 34(b). Dark lines in the image are likely due to deoxygenated veins (lower T2* and phase difference from other tissue in voxel, thereby causing dephasing).

nificant activation from fMRI data is nontrivial and has yet to be solved. Some of the techniques for addressing this issue include: (a) development of accurate and robust motion correction/suppression methods; (b) determination of the noise distribution [121; 188; 189]; (c) determination of the temporal [128] and spatial [190] correlation of activation-induced MR signal changes and of baseline MR signal; (d) characterization or assessment of the temporal behavior or shape of activation-induced signal changes [121; 164; 184; 191; 192]; and (e) characterization of how the aforementioned factors vary in time and space [165; 193], across tasks [121; 191; 192], and with different pulse sequence parameters [13].

It is important always to inspect the data for motion and not to assume too much about the expected response and yet, at the same time, to use all of the current a priori information about hemodynamic responses and neuronal activation to extract meaningful information.

Pulse Sequence. Pulse sequences that can be used for fMRI have a wide range of sensitivities; gradient–echo sequences are the most sensitive and time-efficient. Standard clinical multishot techniques (i.e., FLASH or GRASS) suffer from significantly more motion-related noise than EPI techniques or spiral multishot techniques [110; 111; 194]. Also, application of navigator echoes [110; 116] or other types of image reconstruction–related postprocessing of multishot data can significantly reduce artifactual fluctuations.

Choice of RF Coil. The trade-off here regards spatial coverage versus sensitivity. The smaller the coil used, the less brain tissue it couples to. This gives a higher S/N but much less brain coverage; larger RF coils yield more brain coverage but lower S/N. Where sensitivity is critical, a surface coil in a specific region may be desirable. Where whole-brain imaging is desirable, a whole-brain quadrature RF coil is optimal [195]. This coil is generally as close to the head as possible and couples only to the brain region. It should noted that typical whole *head and neck* coils used clinically are suboptimal for whole-brain fMRI, since they couple also to the face and neck regions (only adding noise) and since they are generally not as close as possible to the head.

Voxel Size. The signal-to-noise ratio is directly proportional to voxel volume. Functional contrast to noise is optimized by matching the volume of the active region to the voxel volume. Because functional region sizes are not well characterized and are likely to vary widely, the optimal voxel size is difficult to predict. Many have generally matched the voxel slice to the cortical thickness. Other groups have used a slightly thicker slice to increase brain coverage given a limitation in the number of slices obtainable. As described before, spatial resolution may actually be *reduced* with the use of smaller voxels if the contrast-to-noise ratio is not high enough to detect more subtle capillary effects. In such a case of low contrast to noise, primarily downstream draining veins would be detected. This phenomenon may explain the exclusive detection of large vessels by Lai and Haacke et al. [172; 173] using small voxels. Overall, small voxels are desirable as long as the sensitivity remains high enough to detect a 1% signal change.

COMMON fMRI PLATFORMS

In an attempt to bring together much of what has been discussed so far, in this section we describe some of the most commonly used platforms for fMRI. The three types of fMRI pulse sequences examined here are EPI, conventional multishot imaging, and spiral scanning.

Echo Planar Imaging

Echo planar imaging is an ultrafast MRI technique [39; 93–95] that has been (and continues to be) ubiquitous in the ongoing development and application of fMRI. In most of the growing number of centers with EPI capability, it is the fMRI method of choice for most applications.

The EPI technique has several drawbacks (low spatial resolution, high sensitivity to off-resonance effects, need for specialized hardware, potential for peripheral nerve stimulation, and need for specialized image reconstruction algorithms). The advantages of EPI (high temporal resolution, high flexibility for imaging several types of physiological processes, high stability, low imaging duty cycle, low sensitivity to motion) still greatly outweigh the disadvantages for most purposes related to fMRI. Following is a brief description of some of these EPI characteristics.

Spatial resolution in single-shot EPI is limited either by the area of k-space that can be sampled in approximately one T2* period or by the system bandwidth [196]. The area of k-space that can be covered is limited by either the velocity in k-space (gradient amplitude) or the acceleration in k-space (gradient slew rate) – and typically by both.

The requirement with EPI for strong and rapidly switching gradients is satisfied by (1) increasing the gradient amplifier power or using a speed-up circuit; (2) implementing resonant gradient technology; (3) reducing the inductance of the gradient coils so that they can be driven by conventional gradient amplifiers; or (4) increasing the field of view and/or lowering the resolution to match the speed at which standard gradient amplifiers can keep up.

The first strategy is probably the least commonly used, whereas the second strategy is likely the most common EPI technique. Strategies (1) and (2) both use whole-body gradient coils, which allow performance of EPI for functional and/or kinematic studies on the heart, lungs, digestive system, kidneys, throat, joints, and muscles. In the context of fMRI, whole-body gradients allow more accessibility for patients with mobility problems and for easy delivery of brain activation stimuli.

The third strategy is used primarily by several centers that have home-built gradient coils. This strategy is implemented by using a gradient coil that is localized only to the head. The gradient fields are optimized for a region that usually covers the brain and/or the region of RF sensitivity. Finally, single-shot EPI can be carried out on a conventional imaging system without the use of local gradient coils (i.e., using the whole-body gradient coil) by simply using a large FOV and/or a small image matrix size [197]. Functional MRI using EPI with voxel sizes of about 10 mm × 10 mm × 10 mm (the approximate resolution of a PET scanner) have been performed on a standard GRE 1.5-Tesla Signa system with excellent results [198]. This type of echo planar imaging capability exists on practically every clinical scanner in the world.

The requirements for successful implementation of EPI for fMRI are not limited to hardware. In most cases, phase correction algorithms (applied during image reconstruction) are necessary to compensate for timing errors related to imperfections in the gradients, gradient-induced eddy currents, or static field inhomogeneities. A major non–hardware-related limitation on gradient slew rate is the biological threshold for neuronal stimulation due to time-varying magnetic fields. At present, high-performance gradient systems (either local gradient coils or high-powered whole-body systems) are capable of exceeding the FDA guidelines on gradient field slew rate (dB/dt). This is a large determinant of the upper limit on the resolution possible using single-shot EPI to image humans.

Because of the long sampling time and artifactual phase modulation, EPI is sensitive to two types of off-resonance artifacts: signal dropout and image distortion. Signal dropout is primarily due to intravoxel phase dispersion resulting from through-plane variation of magnetic field. The problem of signal dropout in gradient–echo sequences can be reduced by reduction of the TE, reduction of the voxel volume, and/or localized shimming. Also, this effect is greatly reduced in spin–echo EPI because the macroscopic off-resonance effects are refocused at the echo time.

Image distortion is caused by an off-resonance phase modulation that occurs during data acquisition. In EPI, this linear phase modulation creates a primarily linear distortion of the image in the phase encoding direction. Several postprocessing methods have been put forward for correcting image distortion in EPI [198; 199].

With the use of EPI, approximately ten images may be obtained per second – allowing the option to image the entire brain in under 2 sec or to sample a smaller number of imaging planes and so allow a more dense sampling of the time course. Another possibility in EPI is to sample less densely in space but to cover a large volume in a single shot; this technique is known as echo volume imaging (EVI) [93; 200].

A practical but significant factor to be considered when performing fMRI with EPI is the rapidity with which large amounts of data are collected. This data may then go through several additional transformations (adding to the total required data storage capacity) before a functional image is created. If 10 slices of 64×64 resolution are acquired every 2 sec. (typical for multislice fMRI), then the data acquisition rate is approximately 2 MB per minute.

Conventional Multishot Imaging

High-resolution fMRI techniques developed for use with conventional gradients include multishot FLASH [14; 108; 173; 201–204], turbo-FLASH [205], low-resolution EPI [132; 206], multishot or interleaved EPI [113; 114], echo-shifted flash [207; 208], keyhole imaging [209], and fast spin–echo [210].

Several centers have been able to successfully implement conventional multishot techniques in a routine and robust manner for fMRI [108; 172; 175; 201]. The advantages to multishot techniques are relatively high in-plane spatial resolution, less sensitivity to off-resonance effects, and availability on most clinical scanners. The disadvantages are: lower temporal resolution; increased noise due to non-repeated shot-to-shot misregistration of k-space lines [110; 111; 194] owing to variable sampling of low-frequency lines at different phases of the cardiac cycle; lower signal due to the need for short TR and low flip angles; reduced capability to perform multislice fMRI as rapidly as with EPI; and less flexibility or "dead time" (which comes with the long TR typically used for EPI) for other types of pulse sequence manipulations. More time-efficient and stable multishot techniques include fast spin–echo [210] and spiral scan imaging [110; 111; 194].

Spiral Scanning

Of non-EPI techniques, the most temporal stability has been exhibited by multishot spiral scan sequences, which involve traveling outward from the center of k-space in a spiral manner and are used in conjunction with a single-point phase correction scheme [194; 211]. Spiral scanning also involves oversampling at the center of k-space – where the acquisitions are intrinsically gradient-moment nulled – providing less sensitivity to phase errors caused by brain, blood, or cerebral spinal fluid pulsations with the cardiac cycle.

Spiral scanning has been used for many fMRI applications [176; 177; 190; 212] and has demonstrated, when used in conjunction with a phase-tagging activation scheme, the highest functional resolution (1.35 mm) to date [176]. In studies where high spatial resolution is important or where EPI is unavailable, spiral scan appears to be the method of choice.

Several review articles and chapters on fMRI techniques and applications are available [107; 122; 166; 190; 213–221].

Epilogue

Since its inception in 1991, fMRI has evolved rapidly into a highly robust and widely used technique. It is fraught with technical difficulties, most of which are fully solvable. The technique is also full of surprises and likely to have at least several uses and new directions not yet uncovered. Our hope is that the reader of this chapter will come away with a clear sense of the sophistication necessary to conduct fMRI well and with a solid understanding of successful fMRI implementation.

NOTE

This work was supported in part by grant MH51358 from the National Institutes of Health.

REFERENCES

[1] Lauterbur, P. C. (1973). Image formation by induced local interactions: Examples employing nuclear magnetic resonance. *Nature, 242,* 190–1.

[2] Bracewell, R. N. (1965). *The Fourier Transform and Its Applications.* New York: McGraw-Hill.

[3] Twieg, D. B. (1983). The k-trajectory formulation of the NMR imaging process with applications in analysis and synthesis of imaging methods. *Medical Physics, 10,* 610–21.

[4] Mezrich, R. (1995). A perspective on k-space. *Radiology, 195,* 297–315.

[5] Ljunggren, S. (1983). A simple graphical representation of Fourier-based imaging methods. *J. Magn. Reson., 54,* 338–43.

[6] Hennig, J., Nauerth, A., & Friedburg, H. (1986). A fast imaging method for clinical MR. *Magn. Reson. Med., 3,* 823–33.

[7] Chien, D., & Edelman, R. R. (1991). Ultrafast imaging using gradient echoes. *Magn. Reson. Quart., 7,* 31–56.

[8] Buxton, R. B., Fisel, C. R., Chien, D., & Brady, T. J. (1989). Signal intensity in fast imaging. *J. Magn. Reson., 83,* 576–85.

[9] Haase, A., Frahm, J., Matthaei, D., Hanicke, W., & Merboldt, K.-D. (1986). FLASH imaging. Rapid NMR imaging using low flip-angle pulses. *J. Magn. Reson., 67,* 258–66.

[10] Atkinson, D. J., Burstein, D., & Edelman, R. R. (1990). First pass cardiac perfusion: Evaluation with ultrafast MR imaging. *Radiology, 174,* 757–62.

[11] Belliveau, J. W., Kennedy, D. N., McKinstry, R. C., Buchbinder, B. R., Weisskoff, R. M., Cohen, M. S., Vevea, J. M., Brady, T. J., & Rosen, B. R. (1991). Functional mapping of the human visual cortex by magnetic resonance imaging. *Science, 254,* 716–19.

[12] Bandettini, P. A., Wong, E. C., Hinks, R. S., Tikofsky, R. S., & Hyde, J. S. (1992). Time course EPI of human brain function during task activation. *Magn. Reson. Med., 25,* 390–7.

[13] Kwong, K. K., Belliveau, J. W., Chesler, D. A., Goldberg, I. E., Weisskoff, R. M., Poncelet, B. P., Kennedy, D. N., Hoppel, B. E., Cohen, M. S., Turner, R., Cheng, H. M., Brady, T. J., & Rosen, B. R. (1992). Dynamic magnetic resonance imaging of human brain activity during primary sensory stimulation. *Proc. Nat. Acad. Sci. USA, 89,* 5675–9.

[14] Ogawa, S., Tank, D. W., Menon, R., Ellermann, J. M., Kim, S.-G., Merkle, H., & Ugurbil, K. (1992). Intrinsic signal changes accompanying sensory stimulation: Functional brain mapping with magnetic resonance imaging. *Proc. Nat. Acad. Sci. USA, 89,* 5951–5.

[15] Frahm, J., Bruhn, H., Merboldt, K. D., Hanicke, W., & Math, D. (1992). Dynamic MR imaging of human brain oxygenation during rest and photic stimulation. *JMRI, 2,* 501–5.

[16] Mansfield, P., & Grannell, P. K. (1973). NMR diffraction in solids? *J. Phys. C., Solid State Phys.,* L422–L426.

[17] Mansfield, P., & Grannell, P. K. (1975). "Diffraction" and microscopy in solids and liquids by NMR. *Phys. Rev. B, 12,* 3618–34.

[18] Mansfield, P., & Morris, P. G. (1982). *NMR Imaging in Biomedicine.* New York: Academic Press.

[19] Morris, P. G. (1986). *Nuclear Magnetic Resonance Imaging in Medicine and Biology.* Oxford University Press.

[20] Edelstein, W. A., Bottomly, P. A., Hart, H. R., & Smith, L. S. (1983). Signal, noise, and contrast in nuclear magnetic resonance (NMR) imaging. *J. Comput. Assist. Tomogr., 7,* 391–401.

[21] Young, I. R., Burl, M., & Bydder, B. M. (1986). Comparative efficiency of different pulse sequences in MR imaging. *J. Comput. Assist. Tomogr., 10,* 271–86.

[22] Fox, R. A., & Henson, P. W. (1986). A general method for optimizing tissue discrimination in magnetic resonance imaging. *Med. Phys., 13,* 635–43.

[23] Buxton, R. B., Edelman, R. R., Rosen, B. R., Wismer, G. L., & Brady, T. J. (1987). Contrast in rapid MR imaging: T1- and T2-weighted imaging. *J. Comput. Assist. Tomogr., 11,* 7–16.

[24] Wehrli, F. W., MacFall, J. R., Glover, G. H., Grigsby, N., Haughton, V., & Johanson, J. (1984). The dependence of nuclear magnetic resonance (NMR) image contrast on intrinsic and pulse sequence timing parameters. *J. Magn. Reson. Imag., 2,* 3–16.

[25] Moonen, C. T. W., vanZijl, P. C. M., Frank, J. A., LeBihan, D., & Becker, E. D. (1990). Functional magnetic resonance imaging in medicine and physiology. *Science, 250,* 53–61.

[26] Wedeen, V. J., Meuli, R. A., Edelman, R. R., Geller, S. C., Frank, L. A., Brady, T. J., & Rosen, B. R. (1988). Projective imaging of pulsatile flow with magnetic resonance. *Science, 230,* 946–8.

[27] Edelman, R. R., Mattle, H. P., Atkinson, D. J., & Hoogewood, H. M. (1990). MR angiography. *AJR, 154,* 937–46.

[28] Listerud, J. (1991). First principles of magnetic resonance angiography. *Magn. Reson. Quart., 7,* 136–70.

[29] Carr, H. Y., & Purcell, E. M. (1954). Effects of diffusion on free procession in nuclear magnetic resonance experiments. *Phys. Rev., 94,* 630–5.

[30] Stejskal, E. O., & Tanner, J. E. (1965). Spin-diffusion measurements: Spin echoes in the presence of a time-dependent field gradient. *J. Chem. Phys., 42,* 288–92.

[31] LeBihan, D., Turner, R., Moonen, C. T., & Pekar, J. (1991). Imaging of diffusion and microcirculation with gradient sensitization: Design, strategy, and significance. *JMRI, 1,* 7–28.

[32] LeBihan, D., Breton, E., Lallemand, D., Aubin, M.-L., Vignaud, J., & Laval-Jeantet, M. (1988). Separation of diffusion and perfusion in intravoxel incoherent motion MR imaging. *Radiology, 168,* 497–505.

[33] SMRM Workshop (1991). Future directions in MRI of diffusion and perfusion. *Magn. Reson. Med., 19,* 209–333.

[34] LeBihan, D. (1990). Magnetic resonance imaging of perfusion. *Magn. Reson. Med., 14,* 283–92.

[35] Detre, J. A., Leigh, J. S., Williams, D. S., & Koretsky, A. P. (1992). Perfusion imaging. *Magn. Reson. Med., 23,* 37–45.

[36] LeBihan, D. (1992). Theoretical principles of perfusion imaging: Applications to magnetic resonance imaging. *Invest. Radiol., 27,* S6–S11.

[37] Detre, J. A., Zhang, W., Roberts, D. A., Silva, A. C., Williams, D. S., Grandis, D. J., Koretsky, A. P., & Leigh, J. S. (1994). Tissue-specific perfusion imaging using arterial spin labeling. *NMR in Biomedicine, 7,* 75–82.

[38] Edelman, R. R., Sievert, B., Wielopolski, P., Pearlman, J., & Warach, S. (1994). Noninvasive mapping of cerebral perfusion by using EPISTAR MR angiography [Abstract]. *JMRI, 4(P),* 68.

[39] Edelman, R., Wielopolski, P., & Schmitt, F. (1994). Echoplanar MR imaging. *Radiology, 192,* 600–12.

[40] Edelman, R. R., Siewert, B., Adamis, M., Gaa, J., Laub, G., & Wielopolski, P. (1994). Signal targeting with alternating radiofrequency (STAR) sequences: Application to MR angiography. *Magn. Reson. Med., 31,* 233–8.

[41] Wolff, S. D., & Balaban, R. S. (1989). Magnetization transfer contrast (MTC) and tissue water proton relaxation in vivo. *Magn. Reson. Med., 10,* 135–44.

[42] Balaban, R. S., & Ceckler, T. L. (1992). Magnetization transfer contrast in magnetic resonance imaging. *Magn. Reson. Quart., 8,* 116–37.

[43] Brown, T. R., Kincaid, B. M., & Ugurbil, K. (1982). NMR chemical shift imaging in three dimensions. *Proc. Nat. Acad. Sci. USA, 79,* 3523–6.

[44] Maudsley, A. A., Hilal, S. K., Perman, W. H., & Simon, H. E. (1983). Spatially resolved high resolution spectroscopy by "four dimensional" NMR. *J. Magn. Reson. Med., 52,* 147–51.

[45] Schenck, J. F. (1992). Health and physiological effects of human exposure to whole-body four-tesla magnetic fields during MRI. *Annals of the New York Academy of Sciences, 649,* 285–301.

[46] Pauling, L., & Coryell, C. D. (1936). The magnetic properties and structure of hemoglobin, oxyhemoglobin, and carbonmonoxyhemoglobin. *Proc. Nat. Acad. Sci. USA, 22,* 210–16.

[47] Thulborn, K. R., Waterton, J. C., Matthews, P. M., & Radda, G. K. (1982). Oxygenation dependence of the transverse relaxation time of water protons in whole blood at high field. *Biochim. Biophys. Acta, 714,* 265–70.

[48] Brindle, K. M., Brown, F. F., Campbell, I. D., Grathwohl, C., & Kuchell, P. W. (1979). Application of spin-echo nuclear magnetic resonance to whole-cell systems. *Biochem. J., 180,* 37–44.

[49] Weisskoff, R. M., & Kiihne, S. (1992). MRI susceptometry: Image-based measurement of absolute susceptibility of MR contrast agents and human blood. *Magn. Reson. Med., 24,* 375–83.

[50] Brooks, R. A., & Chiro, G. D. (1987). Magnetic resonance imaging of stationary blood: A review. *Med. Phys., 14,* 903–13.

[51] Gomori, J. M., Grossman, R. J., Yu-Ip, C., & Asakura, T. (1987). NMR relaxation times of blood: Dependence on field strength, oxidation state, and cell integrity. *J. Comput. Assist. Tomogr., 11,* 684–90.

[52] Matwiyoff, N. A., Gasparovic, C., Mazurchuk, R., & Matwiyoff, G. (1990). The line shapes of the water proton resonances of red blood cells containing carbonyl hemoglobin, deoxyhemoglobin, and methemoglobin: Implications for the interpretation of proton MRI at 1.5 T and below. *Magn. Reson. Imag., 8,* 295–301.

[53] Hayman, L. A., Ford, J. J., Taber, K. H., Saleem, A., Round, M. E., & Bryan, R. N. (1988). T2 effects of hemoglobin concentration: Assessment with in vitro MR spectroscopy. *Radiology, 168,* 489–91.

[54] Janick, P. A., Hackney, D. B., Grossman, R. I., & Asakura, T. (1991). MR imaging of various oxidation states of intracellular and extracellular hemoglobin. *AJNR, 12,* 891–7.

[55] Wright, G. A., Nishimura, D. G., & Macovski, A. (1991). Flow-independent magnetic resonance projection angiography. *Magn. Reson. Med., 17,* 126–40.

[56] Wright, G. A., Hu, B. S., & Macovski, A. (1991). Estimating oxygen saturation of blood in vivo with MR imaging at 1.5 T. *JMRI, 1,* 275–83.

[57] Thulborn, K. R., & Brady, T. J. (1989). Iron in magnetic resonance imaging of cerebral hemorrhage. *Magn. Reson. Quart., 5,* 23–38.

[58] Hoppel, B. E., Weisskoff, R. M., Thulborn, K. R., Moore, J. B., Kwong, K. K., & Rosen, B. R. (1993). Measurement of regional blood oxygenation and cerebral hemodynamics. *Magn. Reson. Med., 30,* 715–23.

[59] Lauffer, R. B. (1990). Magnetic resonance contrast media: Principles and progress. *Magn. Reson. Quart., 6,* 65–84.

[60] SMRM Workshop (1991). Contrast enhanced magnetic resonance. *Magn. Reson. Med., 22,* 177–378.

[61] Bloembergen, N., Purcell, E. M., & Pound, R. V. (1948). Relaxation effects in nuclear magnetic resonance absorption. *Phys. Rev., 73,* 679.

[62] Rosen, B. R., Belliveau, J. W., & Chien, D. (1989). Perfusion imaging by nuclear magnetic resonance. *Magn. Reson. Quart., 5,* 263–81.

[63] Villringer, A., Rosen, B. R., Belliveau, J. W., Ackerman, J. L., Lauffer, R. B., Buxton, R. B., Chao, Y.-S., Wedeen, V. J., & Brady, T. J. (1988). Dynamic imaging with lanthanide chelates in normal brain: Contrast due to magnetic susceptibility effects. *Magn. Reson. Med., 6,* 164–74.

[64] Rosen, B. R., Belliveau, J. W., Vevea, J. M., & Brady, T. J. (1990). Perfusion imaging with NMR contrast agents. *Magn. Reson. Med., 14,* 249–65.

[65] Donahue, K. M., Burstein, D., Manning, W. J., & Gray, M. L. (1994). Studies of Gd-DTPA relaxivity and proton exchange rates in tissue. *Magn. Reson. Med., 32,* 66–76.

[66] Kennan, R. P., Zhong, J., & Gore, J. C. (1994). Intravascular susceptibility contrast mechanisms in tissues. *Magn. Reson. Med., 31,* 9–21.

[67] Fisel, C. R., Ackerman, J. L., Buxton, R. B., Garrido, L., Belliveau, J. W., Rosen, B. R., & Brady, T. J. (1991). MR contrast due to microscopically heterogeneous magnetic susceptibility: Numerical simulations and applications to cerebral physiology. *Magn. Reson. Med., 17,* 336–47.

[68] Yablonsky, D. A., & Haacke, E. M. (1994). Theory of NMR signal behavior in magnetically inhomogeneous tissues: The static dephasing regime. *Magn. Reson. Med., 32,* 749–63.

[69] Gillis, P., & Koenig, S. H. (1987). Transverse relaxation of solvent protons induced by magnetized spheres: Applications to ferritin, erythrocytes, and magnetite. *Magn. Reson. Med., 5,* 323–45.

[70] Hardy, P. A., & Henkleman, R. M. (1991). On the transverse relaxation rate enhancement induced by diffusion of spins through inhomogeneous fields. *Magn. Reson. Med., 17,* 348–56.

[71] Hardy, P. A., & Henkleman, R. M. (1989). Transverse relaxation rate enhancement caused by magnetic particulates. *Magn. Reson. Imag., 7,* 265–75.

[72] Chu, S. C.-K., Xu, Y., Balschi, J. A., & Springer, C. S., Jr. (1990). Bulk magnetic susceptibility shifts in NMR studies

of compartmentalized samples: Use of paramagnetic reagents. *Magn. Reson. Med., 13,* 239–62.

[73] Weisskoff, R. M., Hoppel, B. J., & Rosen, B. R. (1992). Signal changes in dynamic contrast studies: Theory and experiment in vivo [Abstract]. *JMRI, 2(P),* 77.

[74] Boxerman, J. L., Weisskoff, R. M., Hoppel, B. E., & Rosen, B. R. (1993). MR contrast due to microscopically heterogeneous magnetic susceptibility: Cylindrical geometry. In *Proceedings of the 12th Annual Meeting of the SMRM* (New York), p. 389.

[75] Edmister, W. B., & Weisskoff, R. M. (1993). Diffusion effects on T2 relaxation in microscopically inhomogeneous magnetic fields. In *Proceedings of the 12th Annual Meeting of the SMRM* (New York), p. 799.

[76] Weisskoff, R. M., Zuo, C. S., Boxerman, J. L., & Rosen, B. R. (1994). Microscopic susceptibility variation and transverse relaxation: Theory and experiment. *Magn. Reson. Med., 31,* 601–10.

[77] Ogawa, S., Menon, R. S., Tank, D. W., Kim, S.-G., Merkle, H., Ellerman, J. M., & Ugurbil, K. (1993). Functional brain mapping by blood oxygenation level–dependent contrast magnetic resonance imaging: A comparison of signal characteristics with a biophysical model. *Biophysical J., 64,* 803–12.

[78] Wong, E. C., & Bandettini, P. A. (1993). A deterministic method for computer modelling of diffusion effects in MRI with application to BOLD contrast imaging. In *Proceedings of the 12th Annual Meeting of the SMRM* (New York), p. 10.

[79] Li, C. S., Frisk, T. A., & Smith, M. B. (1993). Computer simulations of susceptibility effects: Implications for lineshapes and frequency shifts in localized spectroscopy of the human head. In *Proceedings of the 12th Annual Meeting of the SMRM* (New York), p. 912.

[80] Williams, D. S., Detre, J. A., Leigh, J. S., & Koretsky, A. S. (1992). Magnetic resonance imaging of perfusion using spin-inversion of arterial water. *Proc. Nat. Acad. Sci. USA, 89,* 212–16.

[81] Kwong, K. K., Chesler, D. A., Weisskoff, R. M., & Rosen, B. R. (1994). Perfusion MR imaging. In *Proceedings of the 2nd Annual Meeting of the SMR* (San Francisco), p. 1005.

[82] Wong, E. C., Buxton, R. B., & Frank, L. R. (1997). Implementation of quantitative perfusion imaging techniques for functional brain mapping using pulsed arterial spin labeling. *NMR in Biomedicine, 10,* 237–49.

[83] Wong, E. C., Buxton, R. B., & Frank, L. R. (1998). Quantitative imaging of perfusion using a single subtraction (QUIPSS and QUIPSSII). *Magn. Reson. Med., 39,* 702–8.

[84] Kim, S.-G. (1995). Quantification of relative cerebral blood flow change by flow-sensitive alternating inversion recovery (FAIR) technique: Application to functional mapping. *Magn. Reson. Med., 34,* 293–301.

[85] Ogawa, S., Lee, T. M., Kay, A. R., & Tank, D. W. (1990). Brain magnetic resonance imaging with contrast dependent on blood oxygenation. *Proc. Nat. Acad. Sci. USA, 87,* 9868–72.

[86] Turner, R., LeBihan, D., Moonen, C. T. W., Despres, D., & Frank, J. (1991). Echo-planar time course MRI of cat brain oxygenation changes. *Magn. Reson. Med., 22,* 159-66.

[87] Ogawa, S., & Lee, T. M. (1992). Functional brain imaging with physiologically sensitive image signals [Abstract]. *JMRI, 2(P) (WIP Suppl.),* S22.

[88] Haacke, E. M., Lai, S., Reichenbach, J. R., Kuppusamy, K., Hoogenraad, F. G. C., Takeichi, H., & Lin, W. (1997). In vivo measurement of blood oxygen saturation using magnetic resonance imaging: A direct validation of the blood oxygen level–dependent concept in functional brain imaging. *Human Brain Mapping, 5,* 341–6.

[89] Davis, T. L., Kwong, K. K., Weisskoff, R. M., & Rosen, B. R. (1998). Calibrated functional MRI: Mapping the dynamics of oxidative metabolism. *Proc. Nat. Acad. Sci. USA, 95,* 1834–9.

[90] Kim, S.-G., & Ugurbil, K. (1997). Comparison of blood oxygenation and cerebral blood flow effects in fMRI: Estimation of relative oxygen consumption change. *Magn. Reson. Med., 38,* 59–65.

[91] vanZijl, P. C. M., Eleff, S. M., Ulatowski, J. A., Oja, J. M. E., Ulug, A. M., Traystman, R. J., & Kauppinen, R. A. (1998). Quantitative assessment of blood flow, blood volume, and blood oxygenation effects in functional magnetic resonance imaging. *Nature Medicine, 4,* 159–67.

[92] Belliveau, J. W., Rosen, B. R., Kantor, H. L., Rzedzian, R. R., Kennedy, D. N., McKinstry, R. C., Vevea, J. M., Cohen, M. S., Pykett, I. L., & Brady, T. J. (1990). Functional cerebral imaging by susceptibility-contrast NMR. *Magn. Reson. Med., 14,* 538–46.

[93] Mansfield, P. (1977). Multi-planar image formation using NMR spin echoes. *J. Phys., C10,* L55–L58.

[94] Stehling, M. K., Turner, R., & Mansfield, P. (1991). Echo-planar imaging: Magnetic resonance imaging in a fraction of a second. *Science, 254,* 43–50.

[95] Cohen, M. S., & Weisskoff, R. M. (1991). Ultra-fast imaging. *Magn. Reson. Imag., 9,* 1–37.

[96] Kwong, K. K. (1995). Functional magnetic resonance imaging with echo planar imaging. *Magn. Reson. Quart., 11,* 1–20.

[97] Kwong, K. K., Chesler, D. A., Weisskoff, R. M., Donahue, K. M., Davis, T. L., Ostergaard, L., Campbell, T. A., & Rosen, B. R. (1995). MR perfusion studies with T1-weighted echo planar imaging. *Magn. Reson. Med., 34,* 878–87.

[98] Wong, E. C., Buxton, R. B., & Frank, L. R. (1996). Quantitative imaging of perfusion using a single subtraction (QUIPSS). In *Proceedings of the 2nd International Conference on Functional Mapping of the Human Brain* (Boston), p. 5.

[99] Chesler, D. A., & Kwong, K. K. (1995). An intuitive guide to the T1 based perfusion model. *Int. J. Imag. Syst. & Tech., 6,* 171–4.

[100] Buxton, R. B., Wong, E. C., & Frank, L. R. (1995). A quantitative model for EPISTAR perfusion imaging. In *Proceedings of the 3rd Annual Meeting of the SMR* (Nice), p. 132.

[101] Ogawa, S., Lee, T.-M., Nayak, A. S., & Glynn, P. (1990). Oxygenation-sensitive contrast in magnetic resonance image of rodent brain at high magnetic fields. *Magn. Reson. Med., 14,* 68–78.

[102] Ogawa, S., & Lee, T.-M. (1990). Magnetic resonance imaging of blood vessels at high fields: In vivo and in vitro

measurements and image simulation. *Magn. Reson. Med.,* 16, 9–18.

[103] Brady, T. J. (1991). Future prospects for MR imaging. In *Proceedings of the 10th Annual Meeting of the SMRM* (San Francisco), p. 2.

[104] Grinvald, A., Frostig, R. D., Siegel, R. M., & Bratfeld, E. (1991). High-resolution optical imaging of functional brain architecture in the awake monkey. *Proc. Nat. Acad. Sci. USA,* 88, 11559–63.

[105] Frostig, R. D., Lieke, E. E., Ts'o, D. Y., & Grinvald, A. (1990). Cortical functional architecture and local coupling between neuronal activity and the microcirculation revealed by in vivo high-resolution optical imaging of intrinsic signals. *Proc. Nat. Acad. Sci. USA,* 87, 6082–6.

[106] Fox, P. T., & Raichle, M. E. (1986). Focal physiological uncoupling of cerebral blood flow and oxidative metabolism during somatosensory stimulation in human subjects. *Proc. Nat. Acad. Sci. USA,* 83, 1140–4.

[107] Bandettini, P. A., & Wong, E. C. (1997). Magnetic resonance imaging of human brain function: Principles, practicalities, and possibilities. *Neurosurgery Clinics of North America,* 8, 345–71.

[108] Frahm, J., Merboldt, K.-D., & Hanicke, W. (1993). Functional MRI of human brain activation at high spatial resolution. *Magn. Reson. Med.,* 29, 139–44.

[109] Kim, S.-G., Ashe, J., Georgopoulos, A. P., Merkle, H., Ellermann, J. M., Menon, R. S., Ogawa, S., & Ugurbil, K. (1993). Functional imaging of human motor cortex at high magnetic field. *J. Neurophysiol.,* 69, 297–302.

[110] Noll, D. C. (1995). Methodologic considerations for spiral *k*-space functional MRI. *Int. J. Imag. Syst. & Tech.,* 6, 175–83.

[111] Glover, G. H., & Lee, A. T. (1995). Motion artifacts in fMRI: Comparison of 2DFT with PR and spiral scan methods. *Magn. Reson. Med.,* 33, 624–35.

[112] Schmitt, F., Stehling, M., & Turner, R. (1998). *Echo-Planar Imaging: Theory, Technique, and Application.* Berlin: Springer-Verlag.

[113] Butts, K., Riederer, S. J., Ehman, R. L., Thompson, R. M., & Jack, C. R. (1994). Interleaved echo planar imaging on a standard MRI system. *Magn. Reson. Med.,* 31, 67–72.

[114] McKinnon, G. C. (1993). Ultrafast interleaved gradient-echo-planar imaging on a standard scanner. *Magn. Reson. Med.,* 30, 609–16.

[115] Le, T. H., & Hu, X. (1996). Retrospective estimation and correction of physiological artifacts in fMRI by direct extraction of physiological activity from MR data. *Magn. Reson. Med.,* 35, 290–8.

[116] Hu, X., & Kim, S.-G. (1994). Reduction of signal fluctuations in functional MRI using navigator echoes. *Magn. Reson. Med.,* 31, 495–503.

[117] Biswal, B., Jesmanowicz, A., & Hyde, J. S. (1997). High temporal resolution fMRI. In *Proceedings of the 5th Annual Meeting of the ISMRM* (Vancouver), p. 1629.

[118] Buxton, R. B., Luh, W. M., Wong, E. C., Frank, L. R., & Bandettini, P. A. (1998). Diffusion-weighting attenuates the BOLD signal change but not the post-stimulus undershoot. In *Proceedings of the 6th Annual Meeting of the ISMRM* (Sydney), p. 7.

[119] Frahm, J., Krüger, G., Merboldt, K.-D., & Kleinschmidt, A. (1996). Dynamic uncoupling and recoupling of perfusion and oxidative metabolism during focal activation in man. *Magn. Reson. Med.,* 35, 143–8.

[120] Fransson, P., Kruger, G., Merboldt, K.-D., & Frahm, J. (1998). Temporal characteristics of oxygenation-sensitive responses to visual activation in humans. *Magn. Reson. Med.,* 39, 912–19.

[121] DeYoe, E. A., Bandettini, P., Neitz, J., Miller, D., & Winans, P. (1994). Functional magnetic resonance imaging (fMRI) of the human brain. *J. Neuroscience Methods,* 54, 171–87.

[122] Bandettini, P. A., Wong, E. C., Binder, J. R., Rao, S. M., Jesmanowicz, A., Aaron, E. A., Lowry, T. F., Forster, H. V., Hinks, R. S., & Hyde, J. S. (1995). Functional MRI using the BOLD approach: Dynamic characteristics and data analysis methods. In D. LeBihan (Ed.), *Diffusion and Perfusion: Magnetic Resonance Imaging,* pp. 335–49. New York: Raven.

[123] Hennig, J., Janz, C., Speck, O., & Ernst, T. (1995). Functional spectroscopy of brain activation following a single light pulse: Examinations of the mechanism of the fast initial response. *Int. J. Imag. Syst. & Tech.,* 6, 203–8.

[124] Menon, R. S., Ogawa, S., Strupp, J. P., Anderson, P., & Ugurbil, K. (1995). BOLD based functional MRI at 4 Tesla includes a capillary bed contribution: Echo-planar imaging correlates with previous optical imaging using intrinsic signals. *Magn. Reson. Med.,* 33, 453–9.

[125] Hu, X., Le, T. H., & Ugurbil, K. (1997). Evaluation of the early response in fMRI in individual subjects using short stimulus duration. *Magn. Reson. Med.,* 37, 877–84.

[126] Davis, T. L., Weisskoff, R. M., Kwong, K. K., Savoy, R., & Rosen, B. R. (1994). Susceptibility contrast undershoot is not matched by inflow contrast undershoot. In *Proceedings of the 2nd Annual Meeting of the SMR* (San Francisco), p. 435.

[127] Bandettini, P. A., Kwong, K. K., Davis, T. L., Tootell, R. B. H., Wong, E. C., Fox, P. T., Belliveau, J. W., & Weisskoff, R. M. (1997). Characterization of cerebral blood oxygenation and flow changes during prolonged brain activation. *Human Brain Mapping,* 5, 93–109.

[128] Friston, K. J., Jezzard, P., & Turner, R. (1994). Analysis of functional MRI time-series. *Human Brain Mapping,* 2, 69–78.

[129] Bandettini, P. A., & Cox, R. W. (1998). Contrast in single-trial fMRI: Interstimulus interval dependency and comparison with blocked strategies. In *Proceedings of the 6th Annual Meeting of the ISMRM* (Sydney), p. 161.

[130] Bandettini, P. A., & Cox, R. W. (submitted). Functional contrast in event-related fMRI: Theory and experiment. *Human Brain Mapping.*

[131] Cohen, M. S. (1997). Parametric analysis of fMRI data using linear systems methods. *NeuroImage,* 6, 93–103.

[132] Blamire, A. M., Ogawa, S., Ugurbil, K., Rothman, D., McCarthy, G., Ellermann, J. M., Hyder, F., Rattner, Z., & Shulman, R. G. (1992). Dynamic mapping of the human visual cortex by high-speed magnetic resonance imaging. *Proc. Nat. Acad. Sci. USA,* 89, 11069–73.

[133] Bandettini, P. A., Wong, E. C., DeYoe, E. A., Binder, J. R., Rao, S. M., Birzer, D., Estkowski, L. D., Jesmaniowicz,

A., Hinks, R. S., & Hyde, J. S. (1993). The functional dynamics of blood oxygen level dependent contrast in the motor cortex. In *Proceedings of the 12th Annual Meeting of the SMRM* (New York), p. 1382.

[134] Savoy, R. L., O'Craven, K. M., Weisskoff, R. M., Davis, T. L., Baker, J., & Rosen, B. (1994). Exploring the temporal boundaries of fMRI: Measuring responses to very brief visual stimuli. In *Book of Abstracts of the 24th Annual Meeting of the Society for Neuroscience* (Miami), p. 1264.

[135] Savoy, R. L., Bandettini, P. A., Weisskoff, R. M., Kwong, K. K., Davis, T. L., Baker, J. R., Weisskoff, R. M., & Rosen, B. R. (1995). Pushing the temporal resolution of fMRI: Studies of very brief visual stimuli, onset variability and asynchrony, and stimulus-correlated changes in noise. In *Proceedings of the 3rd Annual Meeting of the SMR* (Nice), p. 450.

[136] Buckner, R. L., Bandettini, P. A., O'Craven, K. M., Savoy, R. L., Peterson, S. E., Raichle, M. E., & Rosen, B. R. (1996). Detection of cortical activation during averaged single trials of a cognitive task using functional magnetic resonance imaging. *Proc. Nat. Acad. Sci. USA, 93*, 14878–83.

[137] Birn, R. M., Bandettini, P. A., Cox, R. W., & Shaker, R. (1999). Event-related fMRI of tasks involving brief motion. *Human Brain Mapping, 7*, 106–14.

[138] Buckner, R. L., Goodman, J., Burock, M., Rotte, M., Koutstaal, W., Schacter, D., Rosen, B., & Dale, A. M. (1998). Functional-anatomic correlates of object priming in humans revealed by rapid presentation event-related fMRI. *Neuron, 20*, 285–96.

[139] Burock, M. A., Buckner, R. L., & Dale, A. M. (1998). Understanding differential responses in event related fMRI through linear simulation. In *Proceedings of the 6th Annual Meeting of the ISMRM* (Sydney), p. 245.

[140] Friston, K. J., Josephs, O., Rees, G., & Turner, R. (1998). Nonlinear event-related responses in fMRI. *Magn. Reson. Med., 39*, 41–52.

[141] Friston, K. J., Fletcher, P., Josephs, O., Holmes, A., Rugg, M. D., & Turner, R. (1998). Event-related fMRI: Characterizing differential responses. *NeuroImage, 7*, 30–40.

[142] Josephs, O., Turner, R., & Friston, K. (1997). Event-related fMRI. *Human Brain Mapping, 5*, 243–8.

[143] McCarthy, G., Luby, M., Gore, J., & Goldman-Rakic, P. (1997). Infrequent events transiently activate human prefrontal and parietal cortex as measured by functional MRI. *J. Neurophysiology, 77*, 1630–4.

[144] Rosen, B. R., Buckner, R. L., & Dale, A. M. (1998). Event-related functional MRI: Past, present, future. *Proc. Nat. Acad. Sci. USA, 95*, 773–80.

[145] Schacter, D. L., Buckner, R. L., Koutstaal, W., Dale, A. M., & Rosen, B. R. (1997). Late onset of anterior prefrontal activity during true and false recognition: An event related fMRI study. *NeuroImage, 6*, 259–69.

[146] Hickok, G., Love, T., Swinney, D., Wong, E. C., & Buxton, R. B. (1997). Functional MR imaging during auditory word perception: A single-trial presentation paradigm. *Brain and Language, 58*, 197–201.

[147] Luknowsky, D. C., Gati, J. S., & Menon, R. S. (1998). Mental chronometry using single trials and EPI at 4T. In *Proceedings of the 6th Annual Meeting of the ISMRM* (Sydney), p. 167.

[148] Konishi, S., Yoneyama, R., Itagaki, H., Uchida, I., Nakajima, K., Kato, H., Okajima, K., Koizumi, H., & Miyashita, Y. (1996). Transient brain activity used in magnetic resonance imaging to detect functional areas. *NeuroReport, 8*, 19–23.

[149] Clark, V. P., Maisog, J. M., & Haxby, J. V. (in press). An fMRI study of face perception and memory using random stimulus sequences. *J. Neurophys.*

[150] Boynton, G. M., Engel, S. A., Glover, G. H., & Heeger, D. J. (1996). Linear systems analysis of functional magnetic resonance imaging in human V1. *J. Neuroscience, 16*, 4207–21.

[151] Dale, A. M., & Buckner, R. L. (1997). Selective averaging of rapidly presented individual trials using fMRI. *Human Brain Mapping, 5*, 329–40.

[152] Zarahn, E., Aguirre, G., & D'Esposito, M. (1997). A trial-based experimental design for fMRI. *NeuroImage, 6*, 122–38.

[153] Buckner, R. L., & Koutstaal, W. (1998). Functional neuroimaging studies of encoding, priming, and explicit memory retrieval. *Proc. Nat. Acad. Sci. USA, 95*, 891–8.

[154] Buckner, R. L., Koutstaal, W., Schacter, D. L., Wagner, A. D., & Rosen, B. R. (1998). Functional-anatomic study of episodic retrieval using fMRI. *NeuroImage, 7*, 151–62.

[155] Friston, K. J., Frith, C. D., Turner, R., & Frackowiak, R. S. J. (1995). Characterizing evoked hemodynamics with fMRI. *NeuroImage, 2*, 157–65.

[156] Vasquez, A., & Noll, D. (1998). Nonlinear aspects of the BOLD response in functional MRI. *NeuroImage, 7*, 108–18.

[157] Birn, R. M., Bandettini, P. A., Cox, R. W., & Shaker, R. (1998). fMRI during stimulus correlated motion and overt subject responses using a single trial paradigm. In *Proceedings of the 6th Annual Meeting of the ISMRM* (Sydney), p. 159.

[158] Buxton, R. B., Wong, E. C., & Frank, L. R. (1998). Dynamics of blood flow and oxygenation changes during brain activation: The balloon model. *Magn. Reson. Med., 39*, 855–64.

[159] Menon, R. S., Ogawa, S., & Ugurbil, K. (1995). High-temporal-resolution studies of the human primary visual cortex at 4T: Teasing out the oxygenation contribution in fMRI. *Int. J. Imag. Syst. & Tech., 6*, 209–15.

[160] Richter, W., Andersen, P. M., Georgopolous, A. P., & Kim, S.-G. (1997). Sequential activity in human motor areas during a delayed cued finger movement task studied by time-resolved fMRI. *NeuroReport, 8*, 1257–61.

[161] Kim, S.-G., Richter, W., & Ugurbil, K. (1997). Limitations of temporal resolution in functional MRI. *Magn. Reson. Med., 37*, 631–6.

[162] Richter, W., Ugurbil, K., Georgopoulous, A., & Kim, S.-G. (1997). Time-resolved fMRI of mental rotation. *NeuroReport, 8*, 3697–3702.

[163] Courtney, S. M., Ungerleider, L. G., Keil, K., & Haxby, J. V. (1997). Transient and sustained activity in a distributed neural system for human working memory. *Nature, 386*, 608–11.

[164] Binder, J. R., Jesmanowicz, A., Rao, S. M., Bandettini, P. A., Hammeke, T. A., & Hyde, J. S. (1993). Analysis of phase differences in periodic functional MRI activation

data. In *Proceedings of the 12th Annual Meeting of the SMRM* (New York), p. 1383.

[165] Lee, A. T., Glover, G. H., & Meyer, C. H. (1995). Discrimination of large venous vessels in time-course spiral blood-oxygen-level-dependent magnetic-resonance functional neuroimaging. *Magn. Reson. Med., 33*, 745–54.

[166] Bandettini, P. A. (1995). Magnetic resonance imaging of human brain activation using endogenous susceptibility contrast. Doctoral dissertation, Medical College of Wisconsin.

[167] Saad, Z. S., Ropella, K. M., Carman, G. J., & DeYoe, E. A. (1996). Temporal phase variation of FMR signals in vasculature versus parenchyma. In *Proceedings of the 4th Annual Meeting of the ISMRM* (New York), p. 1834.

[168] Luknowsky, D. C., Gati, J. S., & Menon, R. S. (1998). Mental chronometry using single trials and EPI at 4T. In *Proceedings of the 6th Annual Meeting of the ISMRM* (Sydney), p. 167.

[169] Frostig, R. D. (1994). What does in vivo optical imaging tell us about the primary visual cortex in primates? In A. Peters & K. S. Rockland (Eds.), *Cerebral Cortex*, vol. 10, p. 331. New York: Plenum.

[170] Turner, R., Jezzard, P., Bihan, D. L., & Prinster, A. (1993). Contrast mechanisms and vessel size effects in BOLD contrast functional neuroimaging. In *Proceedings of the 12th Annual Meeting of the SMRM* (New York), p. 173.

[171] Frahm, J., Merboldt, K.-D., Hanicke, W., Kleinschmidt, A., & Boecker, H. (1994). Brain or vein-oxygenation or flow? On signal physiology in functional MRI of human brain activation. *NMR in Biomedicine, 7*, 45–53.

[172] Haacke, E. M., Hopkins, A., Lai, S., Buckley, P., Friedman, L., Meltzer, H., Hedera, P., Friedland, R., Thompson, L., Detterman, D., Tkach, J., & Lewin, J. S. (1994). 2D and 3D high resolution gradient-echo functional imaging of the brain: Venous contributions to signal in motor cortex studies. *NMR in Biomedicine, 7*, 54–62.

[173] Lai, S., Hopkins, A. L., Haacke, E. M., Li, D., Wasserman, B. A., Buckley, P., Friedman, L., Meltzer, H., Hedera, P., & Friedland, R. (1993). Identification of vascular structures as a major source of signal contrast in high resolution 2D and 3D functional activation imaging of the motor cortex at 1.5T: Preliminary results. *Magn. Reson. Med., 30*, 387–92.

[174] Wong, E. C., Bandettini, P. A., & Hyde, J. S. (1992). Echo-planar imaging of the human brain using a three axis local gradient coil. In *Proceedings of the 11th Annual Meeting of the SMRM* (Berlin), p. 105.

[175] Ugurbil, K., Garwood, M., Ellermann, J., Hendrich, K., Hinke, R., Hu, X., Kim, S.-G., Menon, R., Merkle, H., Ogawa, S., & Salmi, R. (1993). Imaging at high magnetic fields: Initial experiences at 4 T. *Magn. Reson. Quart., 9*, 259–77.

[176] Engel, S. A., Rumelhart, D. E., Wandell, B. A., Lee, A. T., Glover, G. H., Chichilnisky, E. J., & Shadlen, M. N. (1994). fMRI of human visual cortex. *Nature, 369*, 525. [Erratum, vol. 370, p. 106.]

[177] Schneider, W., Noll, D. C., & Cohen, J. D. (1993). Functional topographic mapping of the cortical ribbon in human vision with conventional MRI scanners. *Nature, 365*, 150–3.

[178] Sereno, M. I., Dale, A. M., Reppas, J. R., Kwong, K. K., Belliveau, J. W., Brady, T. J., Rosen, B. R., & Tootell, R. B. H. (1995). Functional MRI reveals borders of multiple visual areas in humans. *Science, 268*, 889–93.

[179] DeYoe, E. A., Carman, G., Bandettini, P., Glickman, S., Weiser, J., Cox, R., Miller, D., & Neitz, J. (1996). Mapping striate and extrastriate areas in human cerebral cortex. *Proc. Nat. Acad. Sci. USA, 93*, 2382–6.

[180] Fox, P. T., & Raichle, M. E. (1985). Stimulus rate determines regional brain blood flow in striate cortex. *Ann. Neurol., 17*, 303–5.

[181] Tootell, R. B. H., Reppas, J. B., Kwong, K. K., Malach, R., Born, R. T., Brady, T. J., Rosen, B. R., & Belliveau, J. W. (1995). Functional analysis of human MT and related visual cortical areas using magnetic resonance imaging. *J. Neuroscience, 15*, 3215–30.

[182] DeYoe, E. A., Schmit, P. W., & Neitz, J. (1995). Distinguishing cortical areas that are sensitive to task and stimulus variables with fMRI. In *Book of Abstracts of the 25th Annual Meeting of the Society for Neuroscience* (San Diego), p. 1750.

[183] Rao, S. M., Bandettini, P. A., Binder, J. R., Bobholz, J., Hammeke, T. A., Stein, E. A., & Hyde, J. S. (1996). Relationship between finger movement rate and functional magnetic resonance signal change in human primary motor cortex. *J. Cereb. Blood Flow & Metab., 16*, 1250–4.

[184] Binder, J. R., Rao, S. M., Hammeke, T. A., Frost, J. A., Bandettini, P. A., & Hyde, J. S. (1994). Effects of stimulus rate on signal response during functional magnetic resonance imaging of auditory cortex. *Cognitive Brain Research, 2*, 31–8.

[185] Guimaraes, A. R., Baker, J. R., & Weisskoff, R. M. (1995). Cardiac-gated functional MRI with T1 correction. In *Proceedings of the 3rd Annual Meeting of the SMR* (Nice), p. 798.

[186] Bandettini, P. A., Jesmanowicz, A., Wong, E. C., & Hyde, J. S. (1993). Processing strategies for time-course data sets in functional MRI of the human brain. *Magn. Reson. Med., 30*, 161–73.

[187] Gold, S., Shristian, B., Arndt, S., Zeien, G., Cizadlo, T., Johnson, D. L., Flaum, M., & Andreasen, N. C. (1998). Functional MRI statistical software packages: A comparative analysis. *Human Brain Mapping, 6*, 73–84.

[188] Jezzard, P., LeBihan, D., Cuenod, C., Pannier, L., Prinster, A., & Turner, R. (1993). An investigation of the contributions of physiological noise in human functional MRI studies at 1.5 Tesla and 4 Tesla. In *Proceedings of the 12th Annual Meeting of the SMRM* (New York), p. 1392.

[189] Weisskoff, R. M., Baker, J., Belliveau, J., Davis, T. L., Kwong, K. K., Cohen, M. S., & Rosen, B. R. (1993). Power spectrum analysis of functionally-weighted MR data: What's in the noise? In *Proceedings of the 12th Annual Meeting of the SMRM* (New York), p. 7.

[190] Cohen, J. D., Noll, D. C., & Schneider, W. (1993). Functional magnetic resonance imaging: Overview and methods for psychological research. *Behavior Research Methods, Instruments, and Computers, 25*, 101–13.

[191] Binder, J. R., Rao, S. M., Hammeke, T. A., Bandettini, P. A., Jesmanowicz, A., Frost, J. A., Wong, E. C., Haughton, V. M., & Hyde, J. S. (1993). Temporal characteristics of

functional magnetic resonance signal changes in lateral frontal and auditory cortex. In *Proceedings of the 12th Annual Meeting of the SMRM* (New York), p. 5.

[192] DeYoe, E. A., Neitz, J., Bandettini, P. A., Wong, E. C., & Hyde, J. S. (1992). Time course of event-related MR signal enhancement in visual and motor cortex. In *Proceedings of the 11th Annual Meeting of the SMRM* (Berlin), p. 1824.

[193] Lee, A. T., Meyer, C. H., & Glover, G. H. (1993). Discrimination of large veins in time-course functional neuroimaging with spiral *k*-space trajectories [Abstract]. *JMRI, 3(P),* 59–60.

[194] Noll, D. C., Cohen, J. D., Meyer, C. H., & Schneider, W. (1995). Spiral *k*-space MR imaging of cortical activation. *JMRI, 5,* 49–56.

[195] Wong, E. C., Boskamp, E., & Hyde, J. S. (1992). A volume optimized quadrature elliptical endcap birdcage brain coil. In *Proceedings of the 11th Annual Meeting of the SMRM* (Berlin), p. 4015.

[196] Farzaneh, F., Riederer, S. J., & Pelc, N. J. (1990). Analysis of T2 limitations and off-resonance effects in spatial resolution and artifacts in echo-planar imaging. *Magn. Reson. Med., 14,* 123–39.

[197] Blamire, A. M., & Shulman, R. G. (1994). Implementation of echo-planar imaging on an unmodified spectrometer at 2.1 Tesla for functional imaging. *Magn. Reson. Imag., 12,* 669–71.

[198] Jezzard, P., & Balaban, R. S. (1995). Correction for geometric distortion in echo planar images from B_0 field distortions. *Magn. Reson. Med., 34,* 65–73.

[199] Weisskoff, R. M., & Davis, T. L. (1992). Correcting gross distortion on echo planar images. In *Proceedings of the 11th Annual Meeting of the SMRM* (Berlin), p. 4515.

[200] Song, A. W., Wong, E. C., & Hyde, J. S. (1994). Echo-volume imaging. *Magn. Reson. Med., 32,* 668–71.

[201] Duyn, J. H., Moonen, C. T. W., vanYperen, G. H., de Boer, R. W., & Luyten, P. R. (1994). Inflow versus deoxyhemoglobin effects in BOLD functional MRI using gradient-echoes at 1.5 T. *NMR in Biomedicine, 7,* 83–8.

[202] Connelly, A., Jackson, G. D., Frackowiak, R. S. J., Belliveau, J. W., Vargha-Khadem, F., & Gadian, D. S. (1993). Functional mapping of activated human primary cortex with a clinical MR imaging system. *Radiology, 188,* 125–30.

[203] Cao, Y., Towle, V. L., Levin, D. N., & Balter, J. M. (1993). Functional mapping of human motor cortical activation with conventional MR imaging at 1.5 T. *JMRI, 3,* 869–75.

[204] Constable, R. T., McCarthy, G., Allison, T., Allison, A. W., Anderson, A. W., & Gore, J. C. (1994). Functional brain imaging at 1.5 T using conventional gradient echo MR imaging techniques. *Magn. Reson. Imag., 11,* 451–9.

[205] Hu, X., & Kim, S.-G. (1993). A new T2*-weighting technique for magnetic resonance imaging. *Magn. Reson. Med., 30,* 512–17.

[206] Wong, E. C., & Tan, S. G. (1994). A comparison of signal to noise ratio and BOLD contrast between single voxel spectroscopy and echo-planar imaging. In *Proceedings of the 2nd Annual Meeting of the SMR* (San Francisco), p. 663.

[207] Liu, G., Sobering, G., Olson, A. W., von Gelderen, P., & Moonen, C. T. (1993). Fast echo-shifted gradient-recalled MRI: Combining a short repetition time with variable T2* weighting. *Magn. Reson. Med., 30,* 68–75.

[208] Moonen, C. T., Liu, G., von Gelderen, P., & Sobering, G. (1992). A fast gradient-recalled MRI technique with increased sensitivity to dynamic susceptibility effects. *Magn. Reson. Med., 26,* 184–9.

[209] Shaw, D. W., Weinberger, E., Hayes, C. E., Yuan, C., Stark, J. E., White, K. S., Radvilas, M., Young, G., & Foo, T. (1993). Reduced K-space (keyhole) functional imaging without contrast on a conventional clinical scanner. In *Proceedings of the 12th Annual Meeting of the SMRM* (New York), p. 1430.

[210] Constable, R. T., Kennan, R. P., Puce, A., McCarthy, G., & Gore, J. C. (1994). Functional NMR imaging using fast spin echo at 1.5 T. *Magn. Reson. Med., 31,* 686–90.

[211] Glover, G. H., Lee, A. T., & Meyers, C. H. (1993). Motion artifacts in fMRI: Comparison of 2DFT with PR and spiral scan methods. In *Proceedings of the 12th Annual Meeting of the SMRM* (New York), p. 197.

[212] Cohen, J. D., Forman, S. D., Casey, B. J., & Noll, D. C. (1993). Spiral-scan imaging of dorsolateral prefrontal cortex during a working memory task. In *Proceedings of the 12th Annual Meeting of the SMRM* (New York), p. 1405.

[213] Turner, R., & Jezzard, P. (1994). Magnetic resonance studies of brain functional activation using echo-planar imaging. In R. W. Thatcher, M. Hallett, T. Zeffiro, E. R. John, & M. Huerta (Eds.), *Functional Neuroimaging: Technical Foundations,* pp. 69–78. San Diego: Academic Press.

[214] Schulman, R. G., Blamire, A. M., Rothman, D. L., & McCarthy, G. (1993). Nuclear magnetic resonance imaging and spectroscopy of human brain function. *Proc. Nat. Acad. Sci. USA, 90,* 3127–33.

[215] Binder, J. R., & Rao, S. M. (1994). Human brain mapping with functional magnetic resonance imaging. In A. Kertesz (Ed.), *Localization and Neuroimaging in Neuropsychology,* p. 185. San Diego: Academic Press.

[216] Prichard, J. W., & Rosen, B. R. (1994). Functional study of the brain by NMR. *Journal of Cerebral Blood Flow and Metabolism, 14,* 365–72.

[217] Cohen, M. E., & Bookheimer, S. Y. (1994). Localization of brain function using magnetic resonance imaging. *TINS, 17,* 1994.

[218] Orrison, W. W., Lewine, J. D., Sanders, J. A., & Hartshorne, M. F. (1995). *Functional Brain Imaging.* St. Louis, MO: Mosby.

[219] Bandettini, P. A., Binder, J. R., DeYoe, E. A., & Hyde, J. S. (1996). Sensory activation-induced hemodynamic changes observed in the human brain with echo planar MRI. In D. M. Grant & R. K. Harris (Eds.), *Encyclopedia of Nuclear Magnetic Resonance,* pp. 1051–6. Chichester, U.K.: Wiley.

[220] Bandettini, P. A., Binder, J. R., DeYoe, E. A., Rao, S. M., Jesmanowicz, A., Hammeke, T. A., Haughton, V. M., Wong, E. C., & Hyde, J. S. (1995). Functional MRI using the BOLD approach: Applications. In D. LeBihan (Ed.), *Diffusion and Perfusion: Magnetic Resonance Imaging,* pp. 351–62. New York: Raven.

[221] Schneider, W., Casey, B. J., & Noll, D. (1994). Functional MRI mapping of stimulus rate effects across visual processing stages. *Human Brain Mapping, 1,* 117–33.

INDEX